Clinical Electroencephalography

Oriano Mecarelli
Editor

Clinical Electroencephalography

Springer

Editor
Oriano Mecarelli
Department of Human Neurosciences
Sapienza University of Rome
Rome
Italy

Clinical Electroencephalography is partially based on the Italian volume "Manuale Teorico Pratico di Elettroencefalografia" by Oriano Mecarelly published in 2009 by Wolters Kluwer Health.

ISBN 978-3-030-04572-2 ISBN 978-3-030-04573-9 (eBook)
https://doi.org/10.1007/978-3-030-04573-9

This Springer imprint is published by the registered company Springer Nature Switzerland AG
The registered company address is: Gewerbestrasse 11, 6330 Cham, Switzerland

This book is dedicated to my daughters Valeria and Giulia, to my nephew Diego and to those in my family who supported me throughout the long period in which I was busy in its preparation.

Preface

Thirty years have elapsed since the first Italian edition of my EEG Handbook in 1988 [1], followed by a second one in 1995 [2] and the last totally rewritten in 2009 [3]. It is now a great honour for me to publish the present textbook on "Clinical Electroencephalography" in English.

This textbook is based largely on my personal experiences of learning, practising, and teaching Clinical Electroencephalography at the Sapienza University of Rome. Therefore, it reflects the influence of the Roman School of EEG which I attended, where I was trained, and to the development of which I have contributed over the last 30 years. Moreover, in this book, I have benefited from the precious collaboration of the most important Italian and European specialists of this field. This is the first EEG manual published in English and written almost entirely by Italian authors, reflecting the importance of electroencephalographic culture in our country.

This textbook has an educational purpose, and it is recommended for neurologists and neurophysiologists, for residents in neurology and related branches, and also for EEG technicians and aims to providing them with an in-depth knowledge applicable in the clinical field.

All the EEG features are debated, from the most basic technical notions to the description of normal and pathological EEG patterns and their correlation with neurological and systemic diseases.

During the last 30 years, electroencephalography has undergone a thorough revolution, not only for the discovery and description of new patterns or for its application in different fields but also for its technological development, which has led to the complete digitization of the equipment, the acquisition, the recording, and the storage of the cerebral bioelectric signals.

When in the late 1970s I started dealing with EEG reporting, tracings were recorded on paper. The physician had to analyse voluminous packages of paper looking for possible alterations, basing on EEG tracings with fixed montages and notes directly marked with a pencil by the technician. Presenting EEG tracings for didactic purposes was possible only by using photography or by copying the page of interest superimposing a sheet of transparent paper and patiently copying the underlying EEG traces. Strange as it may seem, the whole iconography of my first handbook was prepared in this way!

Nowadays, EEGs are acquired exclusively in digital form and are displayed on monitors for reporting. EEG traces can be transferred to different computers and reviewed in any hospital department or even outside the hospital walls; the physician can also modify the displayed parameters of EEG after the acquisition to facilitate the report. The traces of interest can also be easily captured using simple computer softwares for graphics. Therefore, in the last few years, the optimization of techniques for recording and reviewing has greatly enhanced the clinical and educational use of EEG, increasing its fields of application.

Compared to other neuroimaging techniques, EEG still remains a useful, non-expensive, easily accessible, therefore—irreplaceable diagnostic tool to assess cerebral functions. However, sometimes EEG reporting is made by neurologists without specific expertise in the field of electroencephalography. In Italy, for instance, no specific certification attesting an in-depth knowledge of neurophysiology is required to interpret the EEG findings. Currently, Italian universities train excellent neurophysiology technicians (who graduate in 3 years in a first-level degree course, which can be followed by a specialization course of 2 years), but the Specialization in Clinical Neurophysiology has been abolished.

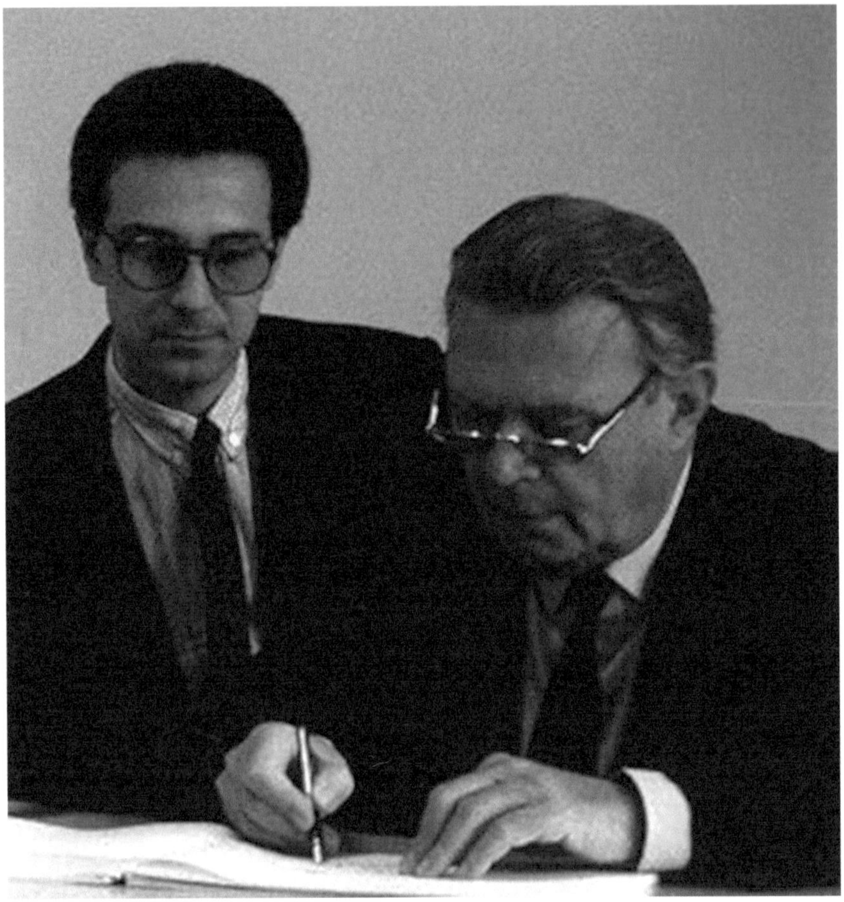

Me and Professor Gianfranco Ricci in 1992, reporting an EEG on paper

Therefore, the aim of this text is to provide the reader with theoretical and practical information on clinical electroencephalography, in a comprehensive but synthetic way, without aiming to replace the most traditional and irreplaceable textbooks published overseas.

Just as in the 2009 Italian edition, I dedicate this work to my dearest mentor, Professor Gianfranco Ricci (Palermo 1925–Roma 2000), who introduced me to the field of electroencephalography and with whom I worked until his retirement, in 1997. Professor Gianfranco Ricci was also the master of those who dedicated themselves to the knowledge of EEG in Italy from the 1960s. I will never forget his absolute human and intellectual honesty and his availability to anyone. It is impossible not to recognize how he was able to make people passionate on their daily work, teaching us to draw inspiration for research projects, always to be carried out with a rigorous scientific method. Professor Gianfranco Ricci was a great "maestro" and a physician appreciated by everyone, particularly by his patients, but he was also a pioneer of clinical neurophysiology in Italy. In 1972, he founded, at the Sapienza University of Rome, the Special School for Technicians of Neuropathophysiology, which in the same year—thanks to Professor Elio Lugaresi—was also inaugurated at the University of Bologna. Subsequently, his entire academic career was dedicated to the training of neurophysiology technicians and physicians involved in EEG and epilepsy.

I would also like to thank my co-workers (fellows, residents, and students) who supported me during the planning and preparation of this textbook and who helped me in the choice of figures, mostly taken from our laboratories.

I am proud that EEG technicians have contributed to some sections of the manual. Technicians are often relegated to the role of mere executors of diagnostic investigation. I strongly believe, instead, that they should be always involved in neurophysiological matters, both from an educational and scientific perspective, providing their active contribution.

The last and most sincere thanks go to those who have believed in this editorial project and have given me the necessary support to be able to complete it.

Rome, Italy
2018

Oriano Mecarelli

References

1. de Feo MR, Mecarelli O. Testo-Atlante di Elettroencefalografia clinica. Editore Marrapese. I Edizione. 1988. pp. 1–231.
2. de Feo MR, Mecarelli O. Testo-Atlante di Elettroencefalografia clinica. Editore Marrapese. II Edizione. 1995. pp. 1–552.
3. Mecarelli O. Manuale Teorico Pratico di Elettroencefalografia. Wolters Kluwer Health – Springer Healthcare Communications. 2009. pp. 1–649.

Acknowledgements

I am grateful to all my colleagues and friends who have contributed in various ways to this book. In particular I would like to thank:

- Patrizia Pulitano (MD, PhD), my colleague and main collaborator
- The EEG technicians of my institution (Liliana Barbagallo, Leonardo Davì, Daniela De Santis, Giuseppe Iannuzzi, Maurizio La Riccia, Nicoletta Panella, and Marco Tiribelli)
- The neurology residents and the students in Neuropathophysiologic Techniques of the Department of Human Neurosciences at Sapienza University

Contents

Contributors

Lara Alvisi IRCCS Istituto delle Scienze Neurologiche di Bologna, Bologna, Italy

Department of Biomedical and Neuromotor Sciences, University of Bologna, Bologna, Italy

Aldo Amantini SODc Neurofisiopatologia, Dipartimento Neuromuscolo-Scheletrico e degli Organi di Senso, AOU Careggi, Florence, Italy

Unità di Riabilitazione Neurologica, Fondazione Don Carlo Gnocchi, IRCCS, Florence, Italy

Nicoletta Azzi Department of Medicine and Surgery, Sleep Medicine Center, University of Parma, Parma, Italy

Sándor Beniczky Department of Clinical Neurophysiology, Aarhus and Danish Epilepsy Centre, Dianalund, Denmark

Department of Clinical Neurophysiology, Aarhus University Hospital, Aarhus, Denmark

Francesca Bisulli IRCCS Istituto delle Scienze Neurologiche di Bologna, Bologna, Italy

Department of Biomedical and Neuromotor Sciences, University of Bologna, Bologna, Italy

Marianna Brienza Department of Human Neurosciences, Sapienza University of Rome, Rome, Italy

Azienda Ospedaliero-Universitaria Policlinico Umberto I, Rome, Italy

Francesco Brigo Department of Neurosciences, Biomedicine and Movement Sciences, University of Verona, Verona, Italy

Department of Neurology, Hospital Franz Tappeiner, Merano, Italy

Mario Brinciotti Department of Human Neurosciences, Neurophysiopathology - Epilepsy Centre (C.I.M.S.), Sapienza University of Rome, Rome, Italy

Maria Paola Canevini Department of Health Sciences, Epilepsy Center—Child and Adolescent Neurology and Psychiatry, University of Milan, Milan, Italy

Gaetano Cantalupo Child Neuropsychiatry, University of Verona, Verona, Italy

Chiara Davassi Department of Human Neurosciences, Sapienza University of Rome, Rome, Italy

Lidia Di Vito IRCCS Istituto delle Scienze Neurologiche di Bologna, Bologna, Italy

Maurizio Elia Unit of Neurology and Clinical Neurophysiopathology, Oasi Research Institute, IRCCS, Troina, Italy

Giovanna Fanelli Department of Neurology, Ospedale San Raffaele, Milan, Italy

Elena Gardella Danish Epilepsy Center, University of Southern Denmark, Dianalund, Denmark

Department of Clinical Neurophysiology, Danish Epilepsy Centre, Danish Epilepsy Hospital—Filadelfia, Dianalund, Denmark

University of Southern Denmark, Odense, Denmark

Antonello Grippo SODc Neurofisiopatologia, Dipartimento Neuromuscolo-Scheletrico e degli Organi di Senso, AOU Careggi, Florence, Italy

Unità di Riabilitazione Neurologica, Fondazione Don Carlo Gnocchi, IRCCS, Florence, Italy

Matteo Impellizzeri Department of Neurology, Ospedale San Raffaele, Milan, Italy

Dorothee Kasteleijn-Nolst Trenite Department of Neurosurgery and Epilepsy, University Medical Center Utrecht, Utrecht, The Netherlands

Faculty of Medicine and Psychology, Nesmos Department, Sapienza University, Rome, Italy

Laura Licchetta IRCCS Istituto delle Scienze Neurologiche di Bologna, Bologna, Italy

Department of Biomedical and Neuromotor Sciences, University of Bologna, Bologna, Italy

Roberto Mai "Claudio Munari" Epilepsy Surgery Centre, Niguarda Hospital, Milan, Italy

Valeria Mariani "Claudio Munari" Epilepsy Surgery Centre, Niguarda Hospital, Milan, Italy

Massimo Mastrangelo Pediatrics Department, V.Buzzi Children Hospital, ASST Fatebenefratelli Sacco, Milan, Italy

Maria Matricardi Department of Human Neurosciences, Epilepsy Centre (C.I.M.S.), Sapienza University of Rome, Rome, Italy

Oriano Mecarelli Department of Human Neurosciences, Sapienza University of Rome, Rome, Italy

Stefano Meletti Department of Biomedical, Metabolic, and Neural Science, OCSAE Hospital, University of Modena and Reggio Emilia, Modena, Italy

Andrea Melpignano Department of Medicine and Surgery, Sleep Medicine Center, University of Parma, Parma, Italy

Elena Merli IRCCS Istituto delle Scienze Neurologiche di Bologna, Bologna, Italy

Department of Biomedical and Neuromotor Sciences, University of Bologna, Bologna, Italy

Giulia Milioli Department of Medicine and Surgery, Sleep Medicine Center, University of Parma, Parma, Italy

Fabio Minicucci Department of Neurology, Chief of Epilepsy Center, Ospedale San Raffaele, Milan, Italy

Barbara Mostacci IRCCS Istituto delle Scienze Neurologiche di Bologna, Bologna, Italy

Ferruccio Panzica Clinical and Biomedical Engineering Unit, Department of Neurophysiology, Fondazione IRCCS Istituto Neurologico "C. Besta", Milan, Italy

Liborio Parrino Department of Medicine and Surgery, Sleep Medicine Center, University of Parma, Parma, Italy

Giusy Carfi' Pavia Rare and Complex Epilepsy Unit, Department of Neuroscience and Neurorehabilitation, Bambino Gesù Children's Hospital, Rome, Italy

Veronica Pelliccia "Claudio Munari" Epilepsy Surgery Centre, Niguarda Hospital, Milan, Italy

Nicola Pietrafusa Department of Neuroscience, Bambino Gesu' Children's Hospital, IRCCS, Rome, Italy

Francesco Pisani Medicine and Surgery Department, Parma University, Parma, Italy

Patrizia Pulitano Azienda Ospedaliero-Universitaria Policlinico Umberto I, Rome, Italy

Department of Human Neurosciences, Sapienza University of Rome, Rome, Italy

Claudia Rinaldi IRCCS Istituto delle Scienze Neurologiche di Bologna, Bologna, Italy

Department of Biomedical and Neuromotor Sciences, University of Bologna, Bologna, Italy

Cristiano Rizzo Micromed S.p.A., Mogliano Veneto, Italy

Guido Rubboli Danish Epilepsy Center, Filadelfia/University of Copenhagen, Dianalund, Denmark

Barbara Scelsa Pediatrics Department, V.Buzzi Children Hospital, ASST Fatebenefratelli Sacco, Milan, Italy

Praveen Sharma Department of Neurology, King George's Medical University, Lucknow, India

Nicola Specchio Rare and Complex Epilepsy Unit, Department of Neuroscience and Neurorehabilitation, Bambino Gesù Children's Hospital, Rome, Italy

Andrea Stabile Division of Clinical and Experimental Epileptology, Foundation IRCCS Neurological Institute "Carlo Besta", Milan, Italy

Department of Neurology, San Gerardo Hospital ASST Monza, University of Milano Bicocca, Monza, Italy

Pasquale Striano Pediatric Neurology and Muscular Diseases Unit, Department of Neurosciences, Rehabilitation, Ophthalmology, Genetics, Maternal and Child Health, "G. Gaslini" Institute, University of Genoa, Genoa, Italy

Salvatore Striano Department of Neurological Sciences, Epilepsy Centre, Federico II University, Naples, Italy

Laura Tassi "Claudio Munari" Epilepsy Surgery Centre, Niguarda Hospital, Milan, Italy

Carlo Alberto Tassinari University of Bologna, Bologna, Italy

Paolo Tinuper IRCCS Istituto delle Scienze Neurologiche di Bologna, Bologna, Italy

Department of Biomedical and Neuromotor Sciences, University of Bologna, Bologna, Italy

Irene Trippi Department of Medicine and Surgery, Sleep Medicine Center, University of Parma, Parma, Italy

Marina Trivisano Rare and Complex Epilepsy Unit, Department of Neuroscience and Neurorehabilitation, Bambino Gesù Children's Hospital, Rome, Italy

Anna Elisabetta Vaudano Department of Medicine and Surgery, Sleep Medicine Center, University of Parma, Parma, Italy

Edoardo Vicenzini Azienda Ospedaliero-Universitaria Policlinico Umberto I, Rome, Italy

Department of Human Neurosciences, Sapienza University, Rome, Italy

Aglaia Vignoli Department of Health Sciences, Epilepsy Center—Child and Adolescent Neurology and Psychiatry, University of Milan, Milan, Italy

Flavio Villani Epilepsy Monitoring Unit "Paolo Zorzi", Division of Clinical and Experimental Epileptology, Foundation IRCCS Neurological Institute "Carlo Besta", Milan, Italy

Part I

Technical Aspects and Normal EEG Patterns

Past, Present and Future of the EEG

1

Oriano Mecarelli

The historical bases for the possibility to record bioelectric signals date back to the experiments of Italian scientists (Luigi Galvani, 1737–1798, and Alessandro Volta, 1755–1832), as well as of the British scientists (Georg Ohm, 1787–1854, and Michael Faraday, 1791–1867), who proved that biological tissues, especially muscle tissue, have considerable electrical properties. Another Italian physic and neurophysiologist, Carlo Matteucci (1811–1868), started in 1830 experiments using the astatic galvanometer of Leopoldo Nobili (1784–1835) and proved that biological tissues were excitable and generated direct electrical currents [1–3]. The first attempts to record an electroencephalographic signal from the cerebral cortex of experimental animals (rabbits and monkeys) were carried out at the Liverpool Royal Infirmary from 1870, by the British physiologist Richard Caton (1842–1926) [4] and, in the following years, other European scientists (Adolf Beck and Napoleon Cybulski in Poland, Vasili Danilevsky in Russia, etc.) kept pursuing these experimental studies.

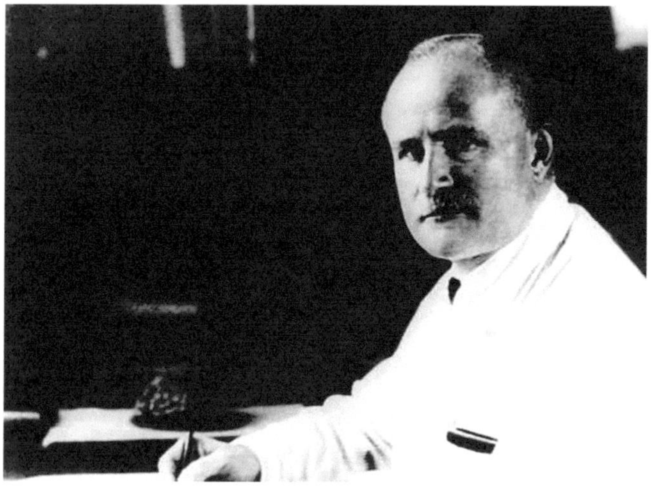

Fig. 1.1 Hans Berger (1873–1941), the father of electroencephalography and rector of Friedrich Schiller University of Jena (1927–1937)

However, it was a German neuropsychiatrist from Jena, Hans Berger (born in 1873 and died by suicide in 1941), who discovered human Electro Encephalo Gram (EEG) (Fig. 1.1) [5, 6]. From 1902 to 1910, Berger studied the electrocortical activity of dogs and, successively, recorded the human EEG tracings; Berger made the first human EEG on July 6, 1924 during a neurosurgical operation on a 17-year-old boy. Berger worked very closely with neurosurgeons and started his studies with recording attempts achieved by positioning the electrodes directly on the cerebral cortex, in patients with large bone windows caused by war head injuries. Afterwards, he addressed the EEG recordings from the scalp, with the application of two electrodes, one frontal and one occipital, using his own son as a volunteer. It must be taken into consideration that, at the time, Berger only had a rudimentary device at his disposal, built by the engineer Mr. Siemens with a double-coil galvanometer that guaranteed a sensitivity of 130 μV/cm (Fig. 1.2). The first EEGs recorded by Berger on photographic paper lasted for 1–3 min and they consisted of one EEG channel, with frontal-occipital bipolar derivation, one channel for simultaneous recording of the electrocardiogram and one channel for time marking (Fig. 1.3). In his first scientific report in 1929, [7] Hans Berger described the characteristics of the alpha rhythm and also defined the beta activity. In fact, it was Berger who identified with the Greek letter "alpha" the normal occipital background rhythm (reported in awake state, with the eyes closed and with responsiveness to eye opening) and, with the letter "beta", the more rapid frequency activity [6, 7].

A year later, Berger had accumulated 1133 recordings from 76 subjects; these essential experiences allowed Berger to publish, from 1929 to 1937, 14 scientific reports which were not given, however, much credit or diffusion and mainly because they were written in German.

O. Mecarelli (✉)
Department of Human Neurosciences,
Sapienza University of Rome, Rome, Italy
e-mail: oriano.mecarelli@uniroma1.it

O. Mecarelli (ed.), *Clinical Electroencephalography*, https://doi.org/10.1007/978-3-030-04573-9_1

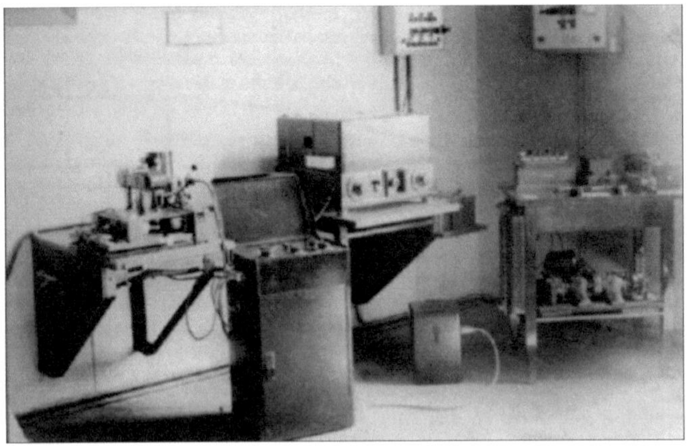

Fig. 1.2 The recording apparatus used by Berger and built by Siemens

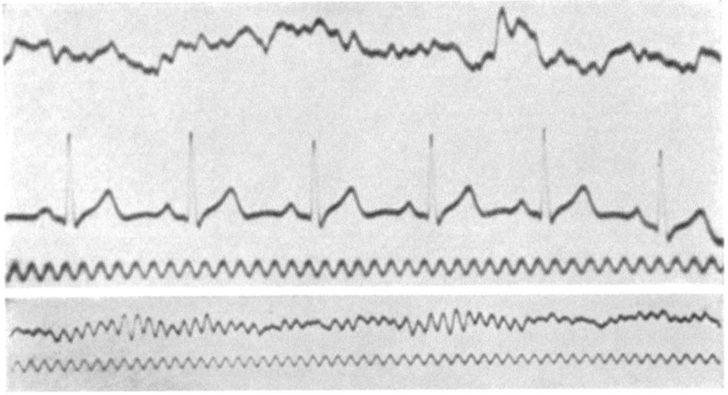

Fig. 1.3 The first human EEG recorded by Berger

In 1934 Lord Edgar Adrian (1889–1977) and Brian Matthews (1906–1986), of the Cambridge Physiological Laboratory, confirmed Berger's research using copper gauze electrodes and introducing differential amplifiers with valves into the systems. They published their results in English in the journal *Brain*, making them more easily accessible from the Anglophone scientific community [8]. They corroborated unequivocally that the "Berger rhythm" was real and that it had a cortical origin (not related to muscular activity or artifacts). Always in England, from 1936, William Grey Walter (1910–1977) became the pioneer of clinical EEG. Grey Walter built an oscilloscope able to record three EEG channels and this method began to be used for the diagnosis of cerebral tumours and as a rudimentary monitoring system, both during surgery and to confirm the effects of anaesthesia. It was Grey Walter who, following Berger's example, identified with the Greek letter "delta" and "theta" the slow EEG activity and who, as early as 1943–1944, introduced the first methods for automatic analysis of the cerebral bioelectric signal [9, 10].

In America, from 1935 onwards, EEG science developed rapidly, also because many European scientists moved to work across the Atlantic in North America, escaping from dictatorship and the imminent war. The most eminent EEG scientists were Hallowell Davis (1896–1992) and Frederick Gibbs (1903–1992), at Harvard Medical School in Boston, Herbert H. Jasper (1906–1999), at Brown University in Providence and Lee E. Travis (1896–1987), at University of Iowa. In those years, the most important clinical EEG studies on epileptic patients were carried out, conducted mainly by F. Gibbs and William G. Lennox (1884–1960). Erna Gibbs (1904–1987), the wife of Frederick Gibbs, was one of the first self-trained EEG technician in the world, and she immediately collaborated with these studies and the "Gibbs-Gibbs-Lennox era" proved to be one of the most productive periods in the history of clinical electroencephalography. The *Atlas of Electroencephalography* by Gibbs and Gibbs has allowed the dissemination of knowledge about the EEG all over the world, becoming the "bible" of electroencephalographers for many decades [11, 12]. WG Lennox was the president of the International League Against Epilepsy (ILAE) from 1935 to 1946 and the editor of *Epilepsia* from 1945 to 1950. He founded the Seizure Unit in Boston and led in clinical and electroencephalographic research.

Furthermore, at that time, at the still-prestigious Montreal Institute of Neurology (McGill University) in Canada, the neurosurgeon Wilder Penfield (1891–1976) (Fig. 1.4) and

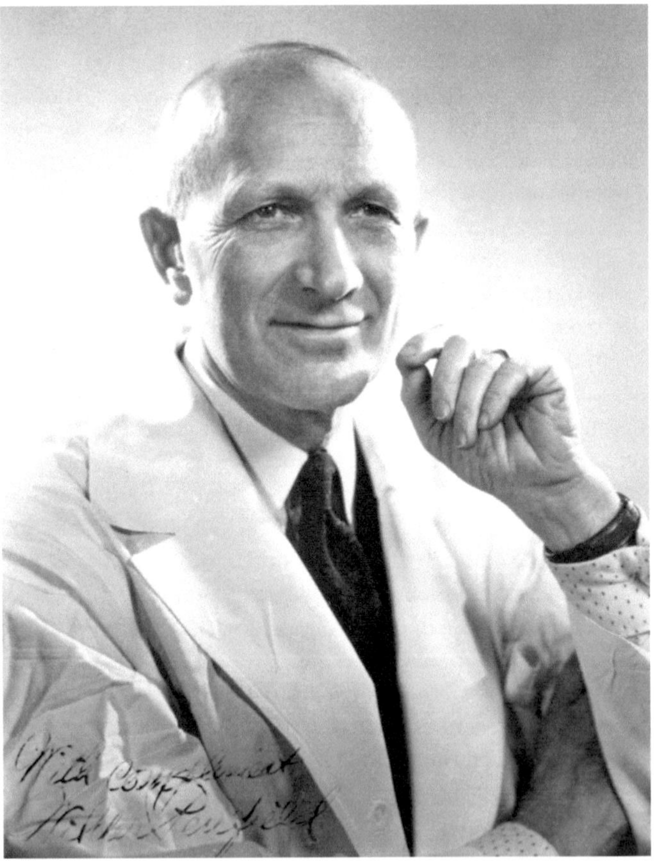

Fig. 1.4 Wilder G. Penfield (1891–1976) (photograph of Author's personal property)

the neurophysiologist Herbert Jasper (who came from Brown University and who had previously studied the EEG in children with behavioural disorders) used superficial and deep intraoperative recordings to determine brain function and to study the various types of epilepsy. Jasper founded the EEG laboratory in Montreal in January 1939 and, during the subsequent months, he carried out 1000 recordings in 500 epileptic patients, more than half of whom were considered suitable candidates for neurosurgical treatment of epilepsy. In a few years, thanks to the works of Penfield and Jasper, Montreal became the most important centre of reference for neurosurgical treatment of focal epilepsies and the publication, in 1954, of the book *Epilepsy and the Functional Anatomy of the Human Brain* crowned this intense and fruitful collaboration between Jasper and Penfield [13].

In Italy, the first human EEG studies started with scientists Mario Gozzano in Rome (from 1935) and Agostino Gemelli in Milan (from 1937). Agostino Gemelli (1878–1959) was a psychologist and philosopher, and he was interested in the influence of the psyche on EEG. Mario Gozzano (1898–1986) was professor of clinical neurology in Bologna and later, from 1951 to his retirement, in Rome at Sapienza University (Fig. 1.5). Gozzano produced his major experimental EEG work at the Berlin-Buch Brain Institute, under the guidance of Oskar Vogt (1870–1959) and Alois E. Kornmüller (1905–1968). The results of the studies carried out by Gozzano in Berlin were published in 1935 but, unfortunately, only in Italian; these study did not have therefore the international relevance, but opened the way for the EEG culture among the Italian neurologists [14, 15]. Besides, Mario Gozzano himself was the founder of the Italian EEG and Clinical Neurophysiology Society and he organized the 5th Congress of International Federation of Societies for EEG and Clinical Neurophysiology (IFSECN) in Rome, in 1960.

After the Second World War, electroencephalography developed even further, both in Europe and in America. In 1947, the first International Congress of EEG was held in London (and just during this scientific event the IFSECN society was founded, with H. Jasper as its first president), followed by the second Congress in Paris in 1949. These two pivotal congresses helped to define the first international parameters to be used in EEG recordings, parameters that were later published on the journal *Electroencephalography and Clinical Neurophysiology* (better known as the EEG Journal, now *Clinical Neurophysiology*). The journal is still the official organ of International Federation of Clinical Neurophysiology (IFCN). In Europe, during the post-war period, the most prestigious epileptological and electroencephalographic school was that of Henri Gastaut (1915–1995), at the Centre Saint-Paul in Marseille (France). In 1946, Gastaut went to the laboratory of Grey Walter in Bristol to learn the basic of EEG and in 1949 for a sabbatical year at the Montreal Neurological Institute with Jasper and Penfield. On his return to Marseille, he founded the Centre Saint-Paul for epileptic children. Gastaut, together with his collaborators (in particular Robert Naquet, Joseph Roger, Annette Beaumanoir, Michelle Bureau, Charlotte Dravet, etc.), represented for many years the point of reference for neurologists and child neuropsychiatrists in Europe and beyond, organizing - from 1950 to 1980 - the famous series of "Colloquia" at Marseille. Gastaut's school also formed the most known and experienced Italian epileptologists (Fig. 1.6).

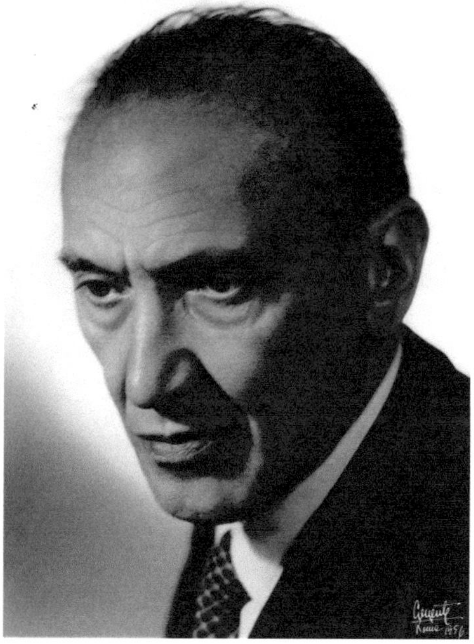

Fig. 1.5 Mario Gozzano (1898–1986), neurologist at Sapienza University of Rome, in 1956. Mario Gozzano was one of the founders and the first president of the Italian League Against Epilepsy (Lega Italiana Contro l'Epilessia, LICE) in 1955 (photograph of Author's personal property)

From 1960 onwards, EEG was clinically used not only as a means to study and diagnose epilepsy and space-occupying lesions, but also as a useful diagnostic and prognostic test in many other fields. At the same time, EEG also helped to define and to standardize the various sleep stages, and it provided useful information on the study of sleep disorders. In 1968, Rechtschaffen and Kales published the first manual, with the definition of the scoring system for the sleep stages in human subjects, still used for the characterization of sleep macrostructure [16].

The history of EEG is simultaneous with the evolution of the equipment required for its recording [17]. The first commercial EEG machine was built up and marketed by Albert Grass in 1935–1936. It was the Grass Model I, with three differential amplifiers, three channels and an ink-writer that recorded on rolls of paper. At the time of its introduction, the Model I was the only commercial system available with a bandwidth of 1.0–10,000 Hz. Successively, in 1939, the Grass Model II appeared, with four-channel and six-channel capability. The "console" Grass Model III was marketed in

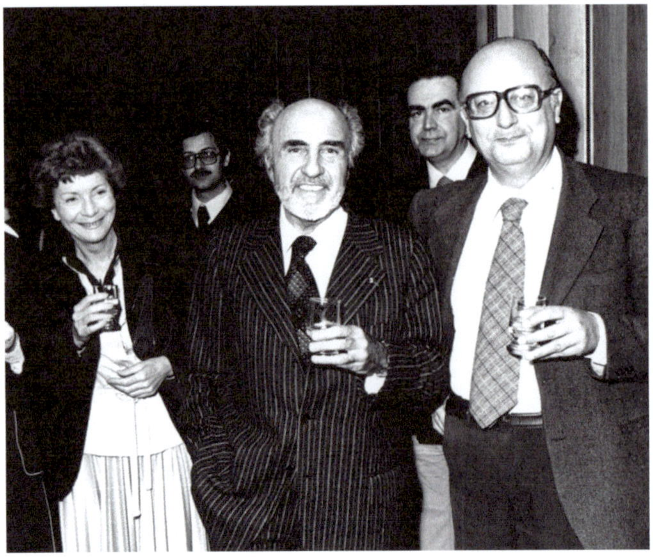

Fig. 1.6 Henri Gastaut (1915–1995) in the centre, between Anne Beaumanoir (1923)—one of his excellent collaborators in Marseille—and Professor Raffaello Vizioli (1926–2006), a famous Italian neurologist who taught at the University of Naples and then at the Sapienza University of Rome (photograph of Author's personal property)

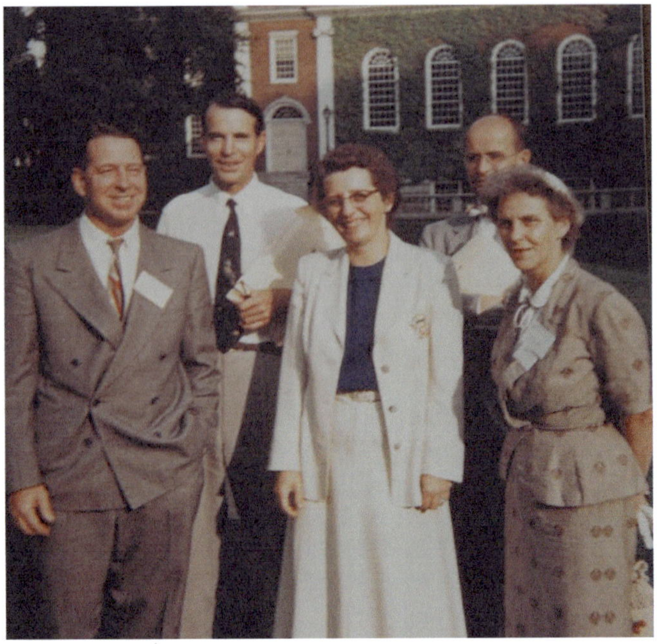

Fig. 1.7 From left to right: Albert Grass, Frederic Gibbs, Ellen Grass, Robert Morison and Erna Gibbs at the third International Congress of Electroencephalography and Clinical Neurophysiology, held in Boston in 1953 (from SJ Zottoli, The Origin of the Grass Foundation, Biol Bull. 2001;201:218–226; with permission by SJ Zottoli and the Grass Foundation)

1946 and included the first 8-channel and 16-channel EEGs ever made. About 5000 systems of this model were shipped worldwide after the war. The collaboration between Frederic Gibbs and Albert Grass at Harvard was very interesting. In May 1935 Gibbs asked Grass to build a three-channel electroencephalograph. This EEG device was built in a few months and this allowed Grass to become a research instrument engineer at the Harvard Medical School, where he remained in this position from 1935 until 1943. At Harvard, Grass met Ellen Robinson, a biologist who devoted herself to the study of evoked responses of the brainstem. Albert Grass and Ellen Robinson married in 1936 and continued to work at Harvard, in close collaboration with Frederic and Erna Gibbs, and this was a good example of the fruitful collaboration between neuroscientists and bioengineers that made major and rapid progress to EEG studies (Fig. 1.7).

In 1950, Franklin Offner produced a portable EEG system (Offner Type T), using the first transistorized amplifiers invented in 1947 at Bell Laboratories. This technology developed rapidly and, in few years, it became indispensable for all high-quality EEG systems. Besides Grass Instruments and Offner Electronics, in the post-war period, many other companies started the production of electroencephalographs in the USA, in Japan and in Europe: to name just a few, this list included Alvar in France, Marconi in England, Schwarzer in Germany, Van Gogh in the Netherlands, etc. By mid-1950s, nearly every teaching hospital was equipped with EEGs.

From 1960s thereafter, EEG laboratories kept growing considerably in number and many other companies appeared on the market, producing more and more compact and less bulky systems; international market leadership was taken over by Nihon Kohden, Nicolet and Telefactor.

From 1960 to 1980, there were great developments in methods for computerized analysis of the various EEG parameters, made possible by the introduction in the market of the first digital EEG systems and by their incredible gradual improvement. At the same time, technology allowed to have access to increasingly smaller devices, also useful for neuromonitoring techniques, like ambulatory EEG and video EEG. As a matter of fact, the development of the television-related technologies stimulated their use for clinical monitoring. In 1954, Gastaut and Bert stressed the importance of EEG recording in conditions "as close as possible to those of life itself" [18]. At Montreal Institute, as early as the 1950s, a complex system was used and, through a camera and mirrors, enabled the recording of EEG combined with video for seizure monitoring. However, this was a system that did not allow the synchronization between video and EEG recording; this was perfomed only in 1962 by E.S Goldensohn and R. Koehle, at Neurological Institute of New York, where the first split-screen closed-circuit video/EEG TV system for epilepsy monitoring was constructed [17].

Starting from the 1970s, the image storing systems on videotapes and the methods of computerized telemetry progressively improved. The improvements in technology created the opportunity to use on a large scale videotapes for the storage of synchronized video and EEG information, ensuring a reliable and low-cost system. Since 1980, the advent of digital technology has allowed the marketing of multifunctional, expandable and more and more sophisticated computerized systems that have completely revolutionized the electromedical devices. At the beginning, digital electroencephalographs were received with scepticism by clinical neurophysiologists, because of the insufficient screen resolution of the monitors and because of an initial difficulty of working without the EEG layout on paper. For few years, the discussion took place on the fact that digital EEG recordings were not entirely reliable and, in any case, not equivalent to those made with analog systems.

Today, all the electroencephalographs consist of a computer, fixed or portable, equipped with specific software which can execute standard EEG, video EEG, long-term monitoring, etc. Once the initial reluctance had been overcome, it was acknowledged that digital EEG has doubtless more advantages compared to traditional electroencephalography, especially concerning storage, review and offline reformatting of the acquired data. Moreover, digital traces can be transmitted over the network and they allow remote reporting and easier exchange of opinions between different neurophysiologists.

Almost 90 years after the publication of the first report on human EEG by Hans Berger, it can be affirmed that electroencephalography maintains its interest and usefulness, both in the diagnostic branch as well as a neurophysiological technique to be used in the experimental fields. If it's true that the fundamental physiologic and pathologic EEG patterns had already been described in the period between 1940 and 1960, thanks to technological development, much progress was then made in the following years, both on the acquisition and the processing of the recorded bioelectric signal.

It is undeniable that the EEG, after the advent of neuroimaging, has lost much of its importance in the diagnostic field. Today's neuroimaging systems allow us to study the morphology of brain areas with high precision, and the EEG can no longer be used - as it was decades ago - for purely localizing purposes, except but in the epileptological field. Nonetheless, it cannot also be denied that EEG still maintains its important role as a test to explore brain functions. Moreover, the co-registration of EEG with functional radiologic imaging of MRI, PET and SPECT provides more information to identify the functional cerebral networks and to better estimate the epileptogenic zone, optimizing surgical results.

In the third millennium, the role of EEG (now digitally acquired and stored) needs to be reconsidered and its fields of application better defined. Clinical epileptology is still based on the EEG execution, with various modalities and registration systems (standard EEG, video EEG, ambulatory EEG, long-term monitoring, etc.). The role of EEG is important for the diagnostic classification of epilepsy and for differential diagnosis; furthermore, EEG has a significant role also during the management of chronic diseases (objective evaluation of the epileptiform abnormalities and the neurotoxic effects of drugs, monitoring during the withdrawal of pharmacological treatment, presurgical evaluation, etc.). In emergency, EEG is fundamental for the diagnosis of status epilepticus (especially non-convulsive) and for the control of the efficacy of its treatment.

Beyond epilepsy, EEG is still important in a high number of neurological diseases, always bearing in mind that this neurophysiological method of evaluation allows the exploration of the dynamic functionality of the whole brain structures over time, also highlighting alterations of the complex cerebral networks.

In the last two decades, EEG has increasingly acquired an important role in the monitoring of critically ill patients, since EEG is a useful tool in evaluating coma. Changes in EEG patterns may indicate coma level, and EEG patterns may be suggestive of either favourable or poor prognosis. During coma, EEG is also essential to detect electrical seizures and to document their duration and response to therapy. It is useful to monitor pharmacological-induced coma and, in several countries, it is mandatory for the diagnosis of brain death. With the actual digital technology, it is also possible to carry out continuous or seriated recordings of both EEG and evoked potentials in intensive care units (ICUs) and, in comatose patients, this multimodal neuromonitoring can further provide useful information for patients' prognosis.

Neurophysiological Intra Operative Monitoring (NIOM) is another important field of EEG application in the current era and it is generally based on the recordings of several types of evoked potentials and the EEG. In the surgery room, EEG is used to evaluate the level of anaesthesia, to monitor the cerebral perfusion and oxygenation and to identify any focal neurological impairment or epileptic seizures.

To conclude, EEG remains an indispensable method for the study of brain functional status from a clinical point of view and it still maintains the characteristics of a laboratory test of relatively simple execution, non-invasive, reproducible and not expensive. Beyond its well-established fields of clinical use, EEG is also of interest in various experimental areas. The infraslow and ultrafast EEG activity are nowadays studied to better understand the neurocognitive processes. The MagnetoEncephaloGraphy (MEG) allows the recording of brain signals without distortion by the skull and the scalp and, therefore, combined with EEG techniques, better clarifies the source of the signals themselves. Quantitative EEG analysis also provides relevant information on functional and effective connectivity between brain areas. Finally, the combined registration of EEG with functional and metabolic neuroimaging techniques allows the identification of the brain networks involved in various pathophysiological processes.

References

1. Brazier MAB. A history of the electrical activity of the brain. The first half-century. London: Pitman Medical; 1961.
2. Goldensohn ES. Animal electricity from Bologna to Boston. Electroenceph Clin Neurophysiol. 1998;106:94–100.
3. Sutter R, Kaplan PW, Schomer DL. Historical aspects of electroencephalography. In: Schomer DL, Lopes da Silva FH, editors. Niedermeyer's electroencephalography. Basic principles, clinical applications, and related fields. 7th ed. New York: Oxford University Press; 2018. p. 3–19.
4. Caton R. Interim report on investigation of the electric currents of the brain. Br Med J. 1877;1(Suppl):62.
5. Gloor P. Hans Berger and the discovery of the electroencephalogram. Electroenceph Clin Neurophysiol. 1969; Suppl 28: 21–36.
6. Gloor P. Hans Berger on the electroencephalogram of man. The fourteen original reports on the human electroencephalogram. Amsterdam: Elsevier; 1969. p. 1–350.
7. Berger H. Uber das Elektrenkephalogramm des Menschen. Arch Psychiatr Nervenkr. 1929;87:527–70.
8. Adrian ED, Matthews BHC. The Berger rhythm: potential changes from the occipital lobes in man. Brain. 1934;57:355–85.
9. Walter WG. The location of cerebral tumours by electroencephalography. Lancet. 1936;II:305–8.
10. Walter WG, Dovey VJ. Electroencephalography in cases of subcortical tumours. J Neurol Neurosurg Psychiatr. 1944;7:57–65.
11. Gibbs FA, Gibbs EL. Atlas of electroencephalography, Methodology and controls, vol. 1. 2nd ed. Cambridge: Addison-Wesley; 1951.
12. Gibbs FA, Gibbs EL. Atlas of electroencephalography, Epilepsy, vol. 2. Cambridge: Addison-Wesley; 1952.
13. Penfield WG, Jasper HH. Epilepsy and the functional anatomy of the human brain. Boston: Little, Brown; 1954. p. 1–896.
14. Gozzano M. Ricerche sui fenomeni elettrici della corteccia cerebrale. Riv Neurol. 1935;8:212–61.
15. Mazza S, Pavone A, Niedermeyer E. Mario Gozzano: the work of an EEG pioneer. Clin Electroenceph. 2002;33:155–9.
16. Rechtschaffen A, Kales A. A manual of standardized terminology, techniques and scoring system for sleep stages of human subjects. Washington, DC: Washington Public Health Service, US Government Printing Office; 1968.
17. Collura TF. History and evolution of electroencephalographic instruments and techniques. J Clin Neurophysiol. 1993;10:476–504.
18. Gastaut H, Bert J. EEG changes during cinematographic presentation. Electroenceph Clin Neurophysiol. 1954;6:433–44.

Neurophysiological Basis of EEG

2

Marianna Brienza and Oriano Mecarelli

2.1 Central Nervous System: Anatomo-physiological Considerations

Nervous tissue is composed of nerve cells, the neurons, together with a supporting tissue called neuroglia, which is found only in the brain and medulla spinalis [1]. Neurons are highly differentiated and specialized cells, and they are distinguished from the other cells because of their complex and polarized structure. They are constituted of: 1) a cell body called "soma" whose morphology characterizes the cell type, qualifying it as stellate, pyramidal, etc. ; 2) two types of cytoplasmic prolongations: the dendrites and the axon, anatomically and functionally different: while dendrites converge on the soma, the axon conveys activity to distant locations.

Dendritic arbors receive synaptic inputs. The various dendritic morphologies have been used for classifying neuronal types by Cajal. Type-specific dendritic morphology is directly linked to the neuronal function. The location and density of the dendritic arbors determine the type and the number of inputs that a neuron can sample. The size and shape of dendritic trees govern their passive electrotonic properties, while the dendritic distribution of ion channels endows active membrane conductance [2–4].

In the mature nervous system, the primary purpose of the axon is to propagate and regenerate action potentials at a consistent speed and, secondarily, to provide support for the energetic and signalling needs of its distal processes [5].

Morphologically, each neuron consists of two distinct domains: the somatodendritic domain contains the cell body (soma), multiple dendrites and a short region of the proximal axon adjacent to the soma (axon hillock); the axonal domain projects a long axon away from the axon hillock toward the next neuron, in the neural circuitry or toward a target tissue where it branches into multiple axon terminals that form the synapses. Functionally, information flow starts from the somatodendritic domain, which receives synaptic input from neighbouring or distant neurons, and it is subsequently transmitted to the axonal domain which s sends signals to the next neuron in the neural circuitry or to a target tissue (Fig. 2.1) [6].

Glial cells are more numerous than neurons. The generic term "glial cells" includes various cell types (astrocytes, oligodendrocytes, microglia, ependymal cells, etc.) with a trophic and supportive function: they are essential for providing metabolic support to neurons and for myelination of axon fibers [7].

Macroscopically, human Central Nervous System (CNS) is composed of different structures that, in the cranio-caudal sense, are the spinal cord, the brainstem (oblongata, pons, midbrain), the cerebellum, the diencephalon and the telencephalon (basal ganglia, white matter and cortex). The telencephalon is divided into two hemispheres by the interhemispheric fissure. Each hemisphere is divided in lobes and each lobe is crossed by the sulci that delimit the circumvolutions.

On the basis of the cytoarchitectural characteristics, the cerebral cortex is organized in six layers with different functions, depending on the type of cortex (visual, somatosensory, motor, etc.), but with a similar columnar organization. In rostro-caudal sense, they are numerated from I to VI and they are composed of different cellular types, reflecting their differentiation in function and connectivity. Although apparently separated, cortical layers are structurally inter-connected: for example, layer IV contains spiny apical dendrites of layer V pyramids and spiny basal dendrites of layer III pyramids. As a matter of fact, we can distinguish an ascending and a descending pathway. The first pathway has layer IV as a primary target, also called the "granular layer" that receives inputs from the thalamus and relays signals to layers III, II and IIIb [8]. The descending pathway does not instead involve the middle layers. Inputs from layers II-III reach the layers V (of the giant pyramidal cells) and VI which are interconnected. Layer V proj-

M. Brienza · O. Mecarelli (✉)
Department of Human Neurosciences, Sapienza University of Rome, Rome, Italy
e-mail: oriano.mecarelli@uniroma1.it

O. Mecarelli (ed.), *Clinical Electroencephalography*, https://doi.org/10.1007/978-3-030-04573-9_2

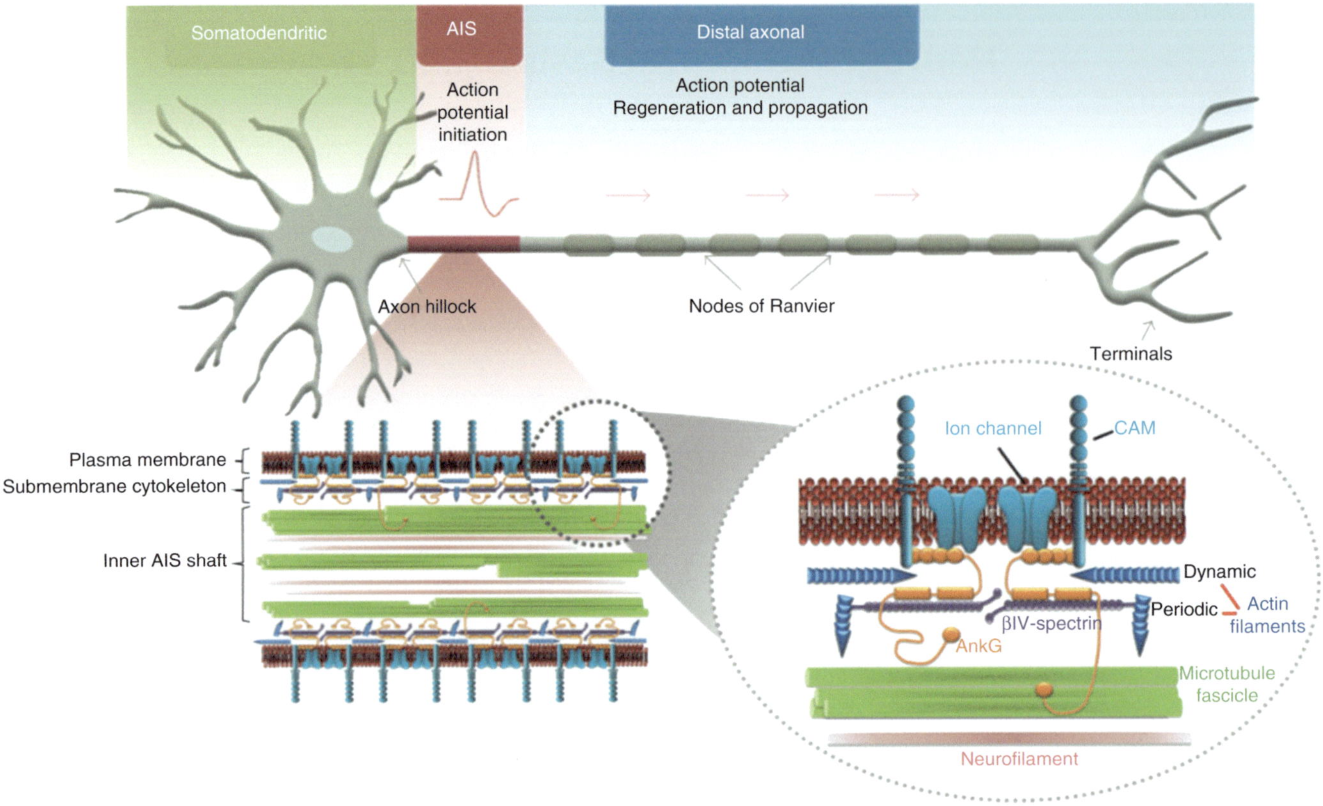

Fig. 2.1 Architecture of the Axon Initial Segment (AIS) and its key protein components. Polarized neurons receive synaptic inputs in the somatodendritic domain (green), which transmits the signals through the axon hillock to the axon initial segment (red). The AIS integrates synaptic inputs and initiates an action potential that propagates along the distal axon (blue) and is amplified at nodes of Ranvier. Molecular organization of the AIS (bottom part of the figure). The AIS can be divided into three layers, the plasma membrane, submembrane cytoskeleton and inner AIS shaft (left), each having AIS-specific features (zoomed view at bottom right). The scaffolding protein Ankyrin G (AnkG) recruits many other proteins to the AIS and can interact with components in the different AIS regions. In the plasma membrane, AnkG - through its N-terminal membrane-binding domain - binds voltage-gated ion channels, important for action potential initiation and regulation, and Cell Adhesion Molecules (CAMs). The submembrane cytoskeleton contains AnkG, βIV-spectrin and actin filaments. These proteins form a periodic network along the entire length of the AIS. Periodic actin is spaced ~190 by at least two βIV-spectrin subunits, which attach to the membrane through interactions with AnkG. In addition to periodic actin, relatively long, randomly oriented, dynamic actin filaments also exist in the submembrane cytoskeleton, and these filaments may have functions distinct from periodic actin. The inner AIS shaft contains microtubule bundles (fascicles), neurofilaments and potentially also actin filaments (not shown). AnkG can extend its C-terminal tail into the inner AIS shaft where it is predicted to interact with microtubule fascicles (modified from Jones SL and Svitkina TM. Axon Initial Segment Cytoskeleton: Architecture, Development, and Role in Neuron Polarity. Neural Plast. 2016;2016:6808293,with permission)

ects to the subcortical structures through the axon that originates from the cell body or from one of the basal dendrites and, after being covered by the myelin sheath, constitutes the projection and association fibres. Layer VI contains multiple distinct classes of pyramidal neurons defined by their apical dendritic arborization patterns, a broad category of oddly shaped excitatory neurons and a variety of inhibitory neurons; however, the typical neurons are short and tall pyramidal neurons, which constitute the majority of excitatory cells in layer VI (Fig. 2.2) [9].

It is important to underline that the ascending and descending pathways represent only a schematization of the cerebral circuits, organized with much more complexity: in addition to the "vertical" information flow, many signals run also "horizontally" and/or reverberate among the various layers, to optimize and integrate the final output (associative fibres).

The functionality of the neuron is guaranteed by the cell membrane. The cell membrane is a selective filter, extremely thin (0.005 μm) and consists of a phospholipids double layer. Specific receptors for chemicals (exogenous and endogenous) and specific ion channels are located on the cell membrane. The voltage-dependent channels on the presynaptic cell membrane perform a double function: to depolarize the presynaptic membrane then triggering the action potential and to produce a current of such intensity to generate a variation of action potential also in the postsynaptic cell. All the neurons, pyramidal and nonpyramidal, establish interneuro-

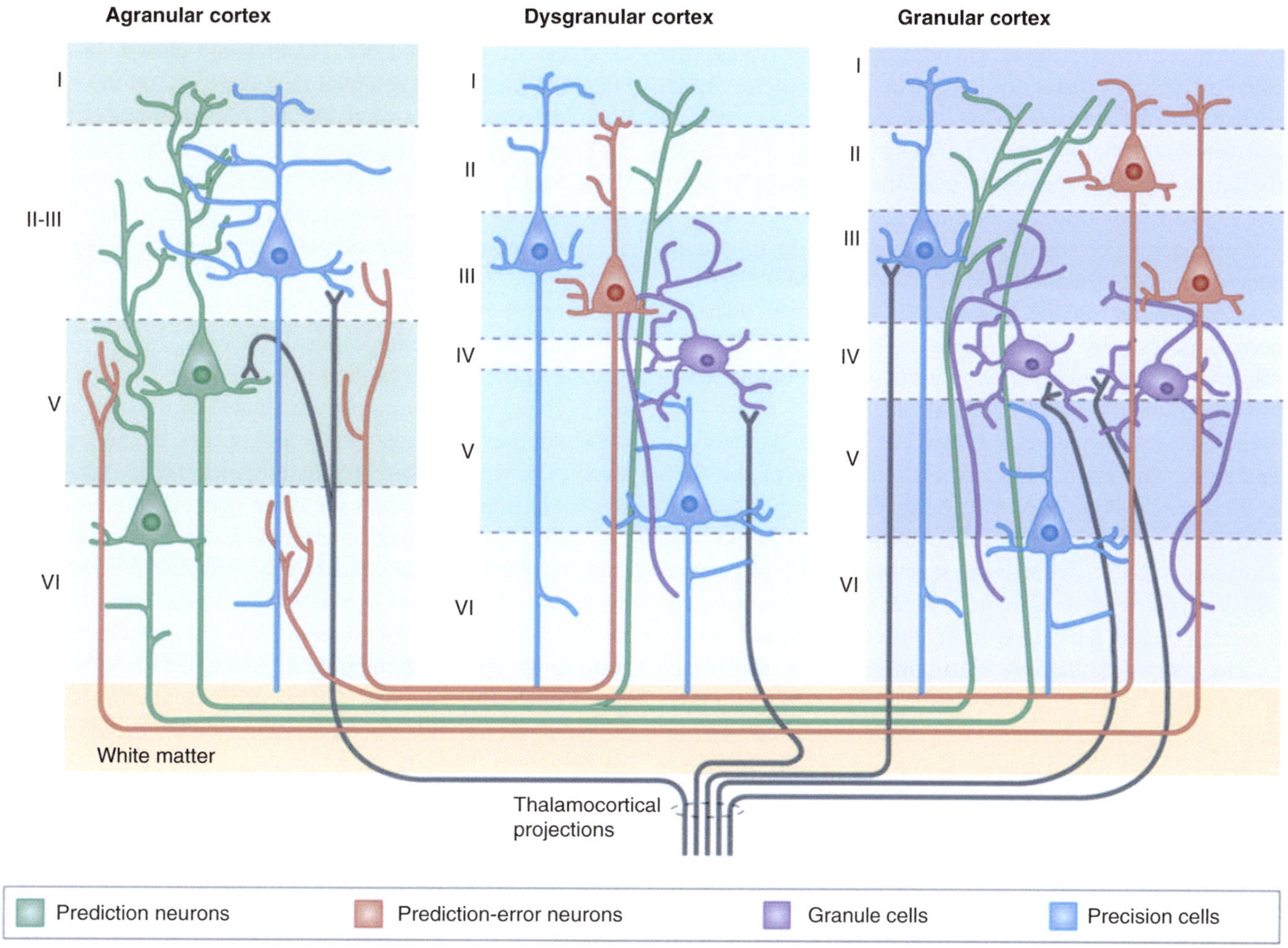

Fig. 2.2 Organization and cellular architecture of cortical layers. Cortical columns are defined by different numbers of layers (also called laminae), with each layer having characteristic cell types and pathways of intracortical and intercortical connectivity. Granular cortex (right) is characterized by six differentiated laminae (layers I-VI), with layer IV containing granule cells, which are excitatory spiny stellate neurons (purple) that amplify and distribute thalamocortical inputs throughout the column. Granular cortex also contains many spiny pyramidal neurons throughout its infragranular and supragranular layers. Pyramidal neurons have a triangular soma, from which basal dendrites project; an ascending apical dendrite, often with large dendritic tufts in layer I; and a single axon that descends and projects out of the cortical column (sometimes with multiple collaterals). Conversely, agranular cortex (left) does not have a fully expressed layer IV and has a poorly differentiated boundary between layer II and layer III. These upper laminae contain relatively fewer pyramidal neurons than does granular cortex. However, agranular cortex contains relatively greater numbers of large pyramidal neurons in layer V and layer VI than in its upper layers. Despite not having a defined layer IV with granule cells, agranular cortex still receives thalamic projections; however, the sensory information that enters agranular cortex is less amplified and less well redistributed throughout the column than in granular cortex. Dysgranular cortex is found in transition zones between granular and agranular regions and contains a small but defined layer IV and a distinctive (although rudimentary) layer II and layer III (modified from Barrett LF, Simmons WK. Interoceptive predictions in the brain. Nat Rev Neurosci. 2015;16:419–429, with permission)

nal connections through the synapses that can be achieved at the level of the cell body, of the dendrites and of the axon.

Synaptic transmission can be electrical or chemical. In the case of electrical synapses, there is a cytoplasmic continuity between the pre- and postsynaptic terminal (gap junction). Nerve transmission through the electrical synapses is very rapid, because it is the result of the direct passage of the current generated by the voltage-dependent channels of the pre-synaptic cells, with a virtually absent delay. Electric synapses often interconnect entire populations of neurons and, in these cases, the function is to synchronize their responses. When many cells are interconnected by electric synapses, the threshold necessary to evoke an action potential becomes high and, if this threshold is exceeded, the whole group of electrically coupled neurons will tend to discharge synchronously and maximally as the action potential is "all-or-nothing". These synapses are typical of the pyramidal cells. Most of the electrical synapses are able to transmit both depolarizing and hyperpolarizing currents [10]. In the chemical synapses the presynaptic and postsynaptic terminals are divided by the synaptic cleft, an intersynaptic space of 30–50 nm. The electrical potential generated in the axonal terminal induces release of a chemical neuromediator by the presynaptic vesicles which spreads in the synaptic cleft binding specific receptors and determining the opening of ionic channels which then modify the postsynaptic membrane potential. The synaptic delay ranges in this case from 0.3 to several ms.

Postsynaptic potentials may be excitatory or inhibitory, depending on the neuromediator released. The action of a neurotransmitter on the postsynaptic membrane does not depend necessarily on the chemical structure of the neurotransmitter, but rather on the properties of the binding receptors: acetylcholine is almost always an excitatory transmitter; noradrenaline, dopamine and serotonin can be excitatory or inhibitory. The main inhibitory neuromediator of the CNS is the Gamma-Amino Butyric Acid (GABA); postsynaptic GABA receptors form permeable channels to Cl^- ions. The activation of these channels determines the entry of Cl^- ions which hyperpolarize the membrane of the neurons and increases their conductance during the resting state.

The main excitatory neurotransmitter is Glutamate (Glu). Many types of postsynaptic receptors for Glu have been identified, basically represented by α-Amino-3-hydroxy-5-Methyl-4-isoxazol-Propionic Acid receptors (AMPA), quisqualate and kainate, and *N*-Methyl-D-Aspartate) (NMDA) receptors. AMPA receptors form permeable channels to both Na^+ and K^+ ions. Ionic currents that pass through these channels are responsible for the early stage of a fast excitatory postsynaptic potential. The NMDA receptors form a channel that is permeable to Ca^{++}, Na^+ and K^+ ions; this receptor-channel complex is also voltage-sensitive. In resting conditions, the channel is blocked by extracellular Mg^{++} ions. To open the NMDA channel, the neurotransmitter Glu and a depolarizing current are necessary. Given the delay with which this channel opens, the ionic currents crossing the channel cause the appearance of a late component of the postsynaptic excitatory potential.

Excitatory synapses are usually located on dendrites, while inhibitory synapses are mainly found on neurons cell body where they are able to effectively counteract the effects of excitatory afferents from the axon and the dendrites. The final integration of synaptic inputs is made at the axon hillock, which is the area of the cell body closest to the initial segment of the axon. It has the highest density of Na^+ channels of the whole cell and, therefore, it will also have the lowest threshold for triggering an action potential.

Nerve cells communicate through direct or mediated synaptic contacts, and the electrical impulse is generated and transmitted through the input and output of ions with positive or negative electrical charges. In resting conditions, the concentration of K^+ ions inside the cell is about 30–50 times higher than outside, and Na^+ ions are 10 times more concentrated outside than inside. The ion concentrations are kept stable by an active ion pump and, in resting conditions, K^+ channels are open and Na^+ channels are closed. In resting state, the membrane potential then depends: on the electrochemical gradient created by the transmembrane Na^+/K^+ ATPase, located at the plasma membrane of all mammalian cells, which utilizes energy from ATP hydrolysis to extrude three Na^+ cations and import two K^+ cations into the cell [11]; on the high membrane permeability to the K^+ ions and, on the other hand, by the low permeability to the Na^+ ions. This corresponds to a potential difference of about −70 mV, with more negative charges inside the cell.

Due to the high basal K^+ permeability, the resting potential of living cells is normally dominated by the high and low concentration of K^+ ions inside and outside the cell, respectively. The action potential that underlies the propagation of the nerve impulse reflects the rapid opening and closing of Na^+- and K^+-selective channels in response to changes in the transmembrane potential. After a stimulus, the very fast opening of voltage-activated Na^+ (Nav) channels causes a depolarization of the membrane. While the Nav channels are transiently open, the membrane potential is briefly dominated by the different Na^+ ions concentrarion, low inside and high outside the cell. The transient membrane depolarization subsequently triggers the slower opening of the voltage-activated K^+ (Kv) channels, which then repolarize the membrane toward the resting potential [12].

One of the most critical functional aspects of Kv channels is their high selectivity for K^+ over Na^+ ions. In comparison, Nav channels, which serve as a trigger to initiate the action potential with their fast-gating kinetics, do not need to be as highly selective as Kv channels. Thus, the difference in selectivity is consistent with the respective functional contribution of these channels to the generation of the action potential. The large conductance and high selectivity of K^+ channels, in particular, are absolutely critical to ensure rapid return to the resting potential after membrane depolarization [13]. The action potential is generated in 1 ms; repolarization occurs in 2–3 ms. Immediately after the genesis of an action potential, the membrane is refractory to other stimulations, initially in an absolute and then in a relative way (raising the threshold of excitability). Changes of the electrical charges between inside and outside the cell, less important than those that determine the action potential, can generate other electric potential differences. Excitatory neurotransmitters can make the neuronal membrane highly sensitive to Na^+ ions for 1–2 ms (Fig. 2.3).

During this short time, Na^+ ions enter the cell reducing the negativity of the resting potential of 1–5 mV and realizing an Excitatory PostSynaptic Potential (EPSP), that takes about 15 ms to completely disappear. On the other hand, inhibitory neuromediators can determine an increase in resting potential (−70 mV) up to values of about −75 mV, allowing entry of the Cl^- ion into the cell and the exit of K^+ ions: the Inhibitory PostSynaptic Potential (IPSP) will be achieved, and it will also persist for about 15 ms (Fig. 2.4).

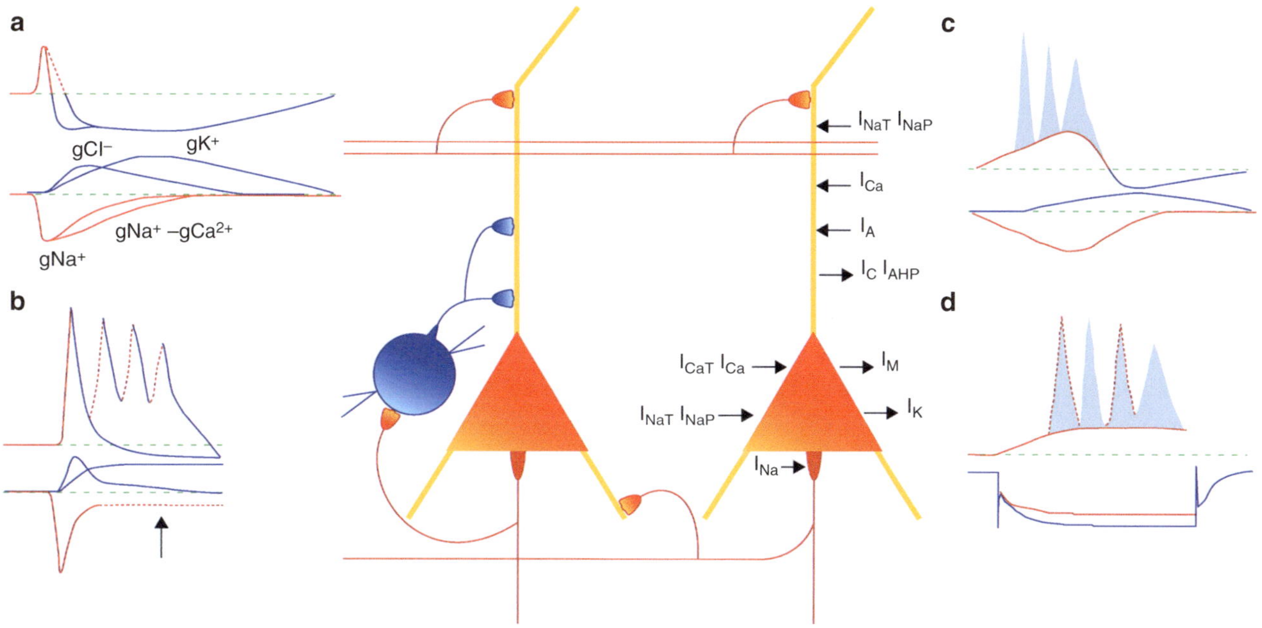

Fig. 2.3 Ionic currents that cause the excitability of cortical neurons. In (**a**–**d**), the upper graph represents voltage recorded with the current clamp technique and the lower graph shows the current signals related to ionic conductance (g) through the open channel. NMDA receptors mediate a long Excitatory PostSynaptic Potential (EPSP; broken red line in **a**). The pyramidal neurons (red) receive inhibitory synaptic input via feedback circuits from local GABAergic interneurons (blue). The action of GABA on postsynaptic receptors generates Inhibitory PostSynaptic Potentials (IPSPs; blue trace in **a**). Membrane depolarizations activate voltage-gated sodium channels producing the rising phase of the action potential (**b**, red traces). Subsequently, various voltage-gated potassium channels, which are involved in the repolarizing phase (**b**, blue traces), are activated. The few channels that fail to inactivate carry the persistent fraction of the sodium current (I_{NaP}; broken red trace in **b**, arrow). The calcium ion-dependent currents (unbroken red lines in **c**) shape the depolarization after an action potential and ultimately sustain hyperpolarizing afterpotentials, which mainly depend on the various potassium currents activated by entry of calcium ions into the cell (Ic, I_{AHP}; blue traces). Under inhibition by muscarine, the membrane may undergo more intense depolarization (**d**, red traces), which favours recurrent, closely spaced action potentials and burst activity (from Avanzini G and Franceschetti S. Cellular biology of epileptogenesis. Lancet Neurol. 2003;2:33–42, with permission)

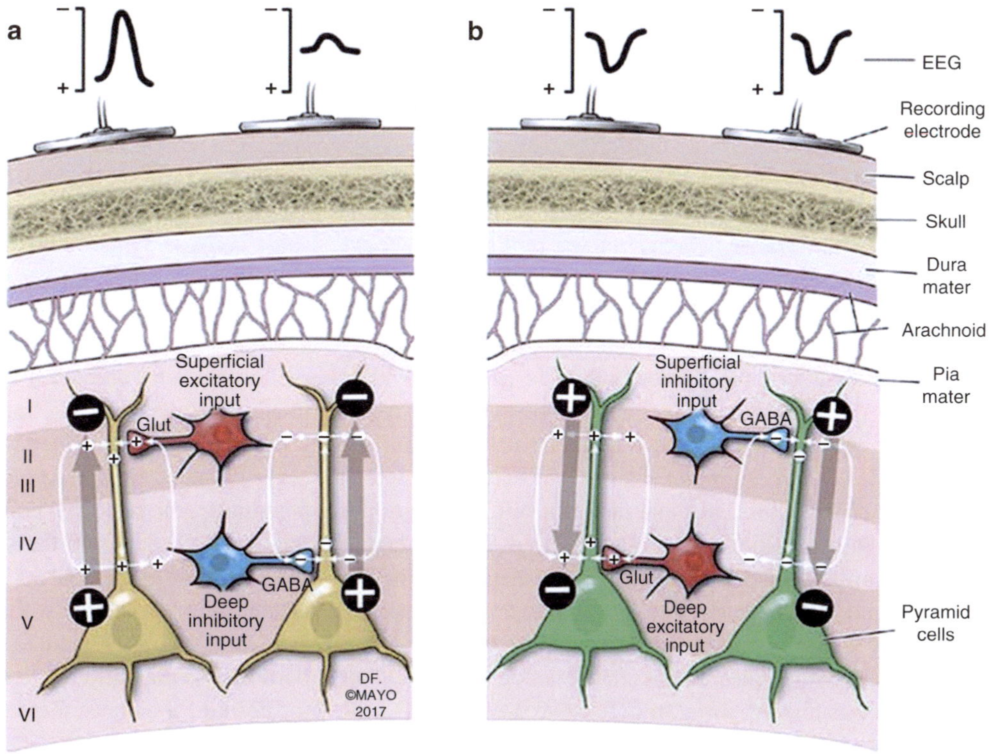

Fig. 2.4 Schematic drawing of the scalp EEG registering negative (**a**) and positive (**b**) deflections elicited from summated EPSPs and IPSPs derived from pooled pyramidal cells. Cells releasing glutamate and GABA provide excitatory and inhibitory superficial and deep synaptic connections resulting in an electrophysiological sink or source. *EEG* electroencephalography, *EPSP* Excitatory PostSynaptic Potentials, *GABA* Gamma-AminoButyric Acid, *IPSPs* Inhibitory PostSynaptic Potentials (Figure courtesy of Anteneh Feyissa M.D. and Mayo Clinic. From Tatum WO, Rubboli G, Kaplan PW, et al. Clinical utility of EEG in diagnosing and monitoring epilepsy in adults. Clin Neurophysiol. 2018;129:1056–1082, with permission)

2.2 Origin of the Electrical Activity of the Brain

Electroencephalography is a graphic representation of the difference in voltage between two different cerebral locations plotted over time [14]. Therefore, the Electro Encephalo Gram (EEG) consists of the recording of the bioelectric activity of the brain from the scalp. The synchronized activity of large cell aggregates can be detected by extracellular recordings; in this case, the signals that are recorded are called field potentials. Surface EEG can be considered the result of field potentials that are produced by fluctuations in the electrical activity of large populations of cortical neurons; these extracellular current flows are generated by the spatial summation of the postsynaptic potentials of the activated cells (Fig. 2.5).

EEG is the graphical representation of the potential difference between an "active" electrode, placed above the seat where the neuronal activity takes place, and an "indifferent electrode", located at a certain distance from the first. It is a dynamic measure, as the potential difference is represented as a function of time. Therefore, the surface EEG measures the electric potential difference between different areas of the scalp and reflects the current flowing in the cerebral cortex during synaptic activation of the dendrites of many pyramidal neurons, which lie just below the surface of the skull.

Although the action potentials - as the larger electrical potentials generated by the neurons - may appear to be the most obvious source of the electrical potentials recorded by the scalp, they contribute minimally to the genesis of EEG graphoelements.

Action potentials cannot be the main cause of the EEG genesis for two main reasons: the amplitude of the electric field produced by the propagation of an action potential decreases much more rapidly than the amplitude of the fields produced by the postsynaptic potentials; the duration of action potentials is very short, 1 ms, and this time is insufficient to obtain an adequate synchronization of large cortical neuronal populations (even a minimal asynchrony of a few milliseconds would make the summation of action potentials impossible). Conversely, the flows of synaptic currents in the extracellular space last for about 10–40 ms, so the postsynaptic potentials can add up together more efficiently than the action potentials and create electric fields large enough to be able to be registered from outside, even without a perfect synchronization.

Moreover, the excitatory or inhibitory postsynaptic potential show other peculiarities that makes it different from the action potential: it does not have a threshold; it is graduated (i.e. its amplitude is proportional to the magnitude of the stimulus and, therefore, does not respond to the "all or none" law, as the action potential); it is a local; it has no tendency to propagate without decrement (as the action potential), but it decreases as moving away from its source.

We have already stated that the genesis of EEG is based on the flow of ionic currents generated by the neurons in the extracellular space. To understand the origin of postsynaptic extracellular potentials, we can imagine an ionic current that flows inward towards the cell through the synaptic membrane and outward through the large surface of the extrasynaptic membrane. The net ionic current is then recorded as the voltage existing through the resistance of the extracellular space. Since the extracellular resistance is very low, compared to the high resistance of the membrane, transmembrane voltage is equal to the product of the current for the resistance of the membrane. Furthermore, the ionic current flowing through the high resistance of the membrane determines a potential difference higher than that caused by the current when it flows through the extracellular resistance. This is one of the reasons why the intracellular potentials are much larger (mV) than the extracellular ones (μV).

The electrical conductivity of biological tissues depends on the distance between generator and recording electrode, on the spatial diffusion and on the orientation of the generator: if the neurons of a population are oriented in parallel and activated synchronously, the amplitude of the signal recorded remotely is greater.

To further understand the importance of the synchronization of cortical cells for EEG genesis, it is also necessary to consider that the electrical contribution of each cortical neuron is very poor and that the signal must cross several layers of non-neural tissues, including the meninges, the cephalorachidian liquid, the bones of the skull and the skin. Each layer has different conduction properties that attenuate the electric signal before it reaches the electrodes on the scalp. As a result, thousands of simultaneously activated neurons are necessary to generate an EEG signal strong enough to be detected from the electrodes on the scalp surface.

Synchronous activation of over 100 cortical neurons in an area of at least 6 cm^2 is required to determine a visible EEG signal from the scalp. Therefore, the amplitude of the EEG signal depends, above all, on the synchronization of the activated cells. If synchronous activation of this group of cells repeats many times, the resulting EEG will be characterized by broad and rhythmic waves. When a layer of pyramidal neurons is not activating coherently, the excitatory current will not be zero, and our baseline EEG signal will consist of fluctuations in the baseline excitatory current. The zero potential surface is located halfway between the positive and negative poles of the dipole. To understand how electrical potentials generated by populations of the pyramidal neurons are recordable on the scalp, it is important to consider the solid angle concept of the volume conduction theory. According to this therory, the potential generated by a dipole layer in a volume conductor (brain and its environs) is proportional to the solid angle subtended by the dipole layer at the point of the measurement.

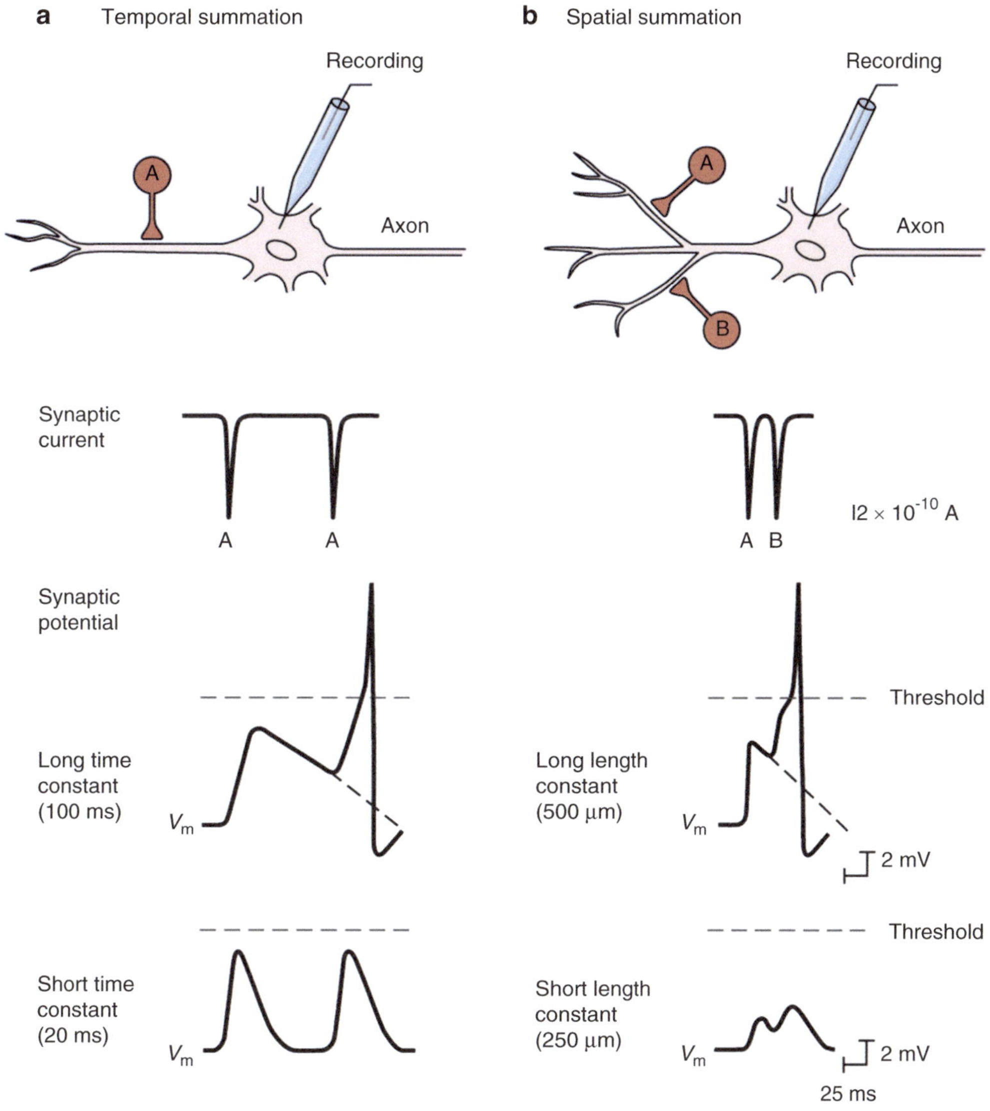

Fig. 2.5 Central neurons are able to integrate a variety of synaptic inputs through temporal and spatial summation of synaptic potentials. (**a**) The time constant of a postsynaptic cell affects the amplitude of the depolarization caused by consecutive Excitatory PostSynaptic Potentials (EPSPs) produced by a single presynaptic neuron (*A*). Here the synaptic current generated by the presynaptic neuron is nearly the same for both EPSPs. In a cell with a long time constant, the first EPSP does not fully decay by the time the second EPSP is triggered. Therefore, the depolarizing effects of both potentials are additive, bringing the membrane potential above the threshold and triggering an action potential. In a cell with a short time constant, the first EPSP decays to the resting potential before the second EPSP is triggered. The second EPSP alone does not cause enough depolarization to trigger an action potential. (**b**) The length constant of a postsynaptic cell affects the amplitudes of two EPSPs produced by two presynaptic neurons (*A, B*). For illustrative purposes, both synapses are the same (500 μm) distance from the postsynaptic cell's trigger zone at the axon initial segment and the current produced by each synaptic contact is the same. If the distance between the site of synaptic input and the trigger zone in the postsynaptic cell is only one length constant (i.e. the postsynaptic cell has a length constant of 500 μm), the synaptic potentials produced by each of the two presynaptic neurons will decrease to 37% of their original amplitude by the time they reach the trigger zone. Summation of the two potentials results in enough depolarization to exceed threshold, triggering an action potential. If the distance between the synapse and the trigger zone is equal to two length constants (i.e. the postsynaptic cell has a length constant of 250 μm), each synaptic potential will be less than 15% of its initial amplitude, and summation will not be sufficient to trigger an action potential (from Kandel ER, Schwartz JH, Jessell TM. Principles of neural sciences. 5th ed. New York: McGraw-Hill; 2012; with permission)

What we observe in EEG is a baseline signal of about 30 μV, which suggests that the fluctuations in the excitatory current during periods of minimal activity are about 2% of the maximum excitatory current during fully coherent excitation. The polarity of the potential recorded from the scalp depends on the site and depth of the synaptic activity onset. To explain this concept, it is important to make a distinction between the site from which the current starts

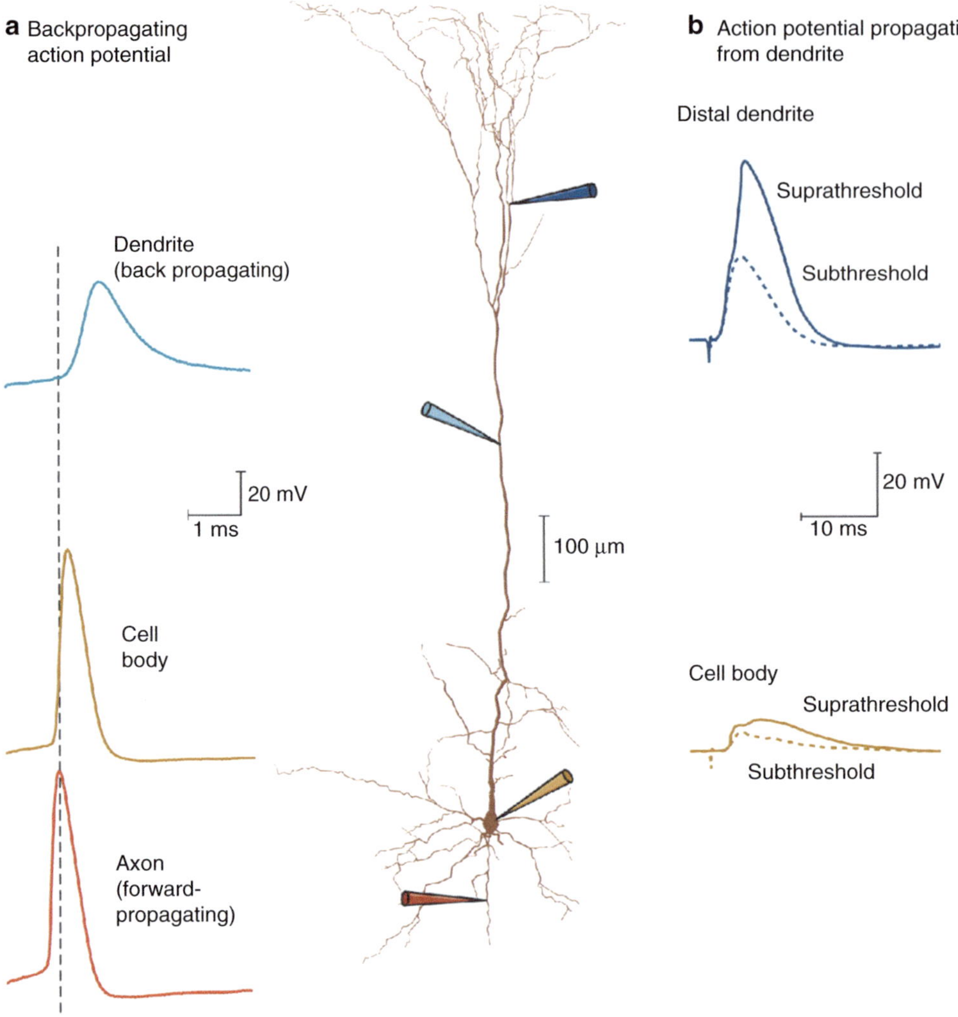

Fig. 2.6 Dendrites support propagation of action potentials to and from the axon initial segment. The figure illustrates an experiment in which several electrodes are used to record membrane voltage and pass stimulating currents in the axon, the soma and at several locations along the dendritic tree. The recording electrode and corresponding voltage trace are matched according to colour. (Adapted, with permission, from Stuart et al. 2000.) (**a**) An action potential can be propagated from the axon initial segment to the dendrites. Such backpropagation depends on activation of voltage-gated Na^+ channels in the dendrites. Unlike the action potential that is continually regenerated along an axon, the amplitude of a backpropagating action potential decreases as it travels along a dendrite due to the relatively low density of voltage-gated Na^+ channels in dendrites. (**b**) A strong depolarizing excitatory postsynaptic potential at a dendrite can generate an action potential that travels to the cell body. Such forward-propagating action potentials are often generated by dendritic voltage-gated Ca^{2+} channels and have a high threshold. They propagate relatively slowly and decrement with distance, often failing to reach the cell body. The solid line shows a suprathreshold response generated in the dendrite and the dotted line shows a subthreshold response (from Kandel ER, Schwartz JH, Jessell TM. Principles of Neural sciences. 5th ed. New York: McGraw-Hill; 2012; with permission)

and moves away (source) and the site to which the current approaches (sink). The activity recorded by EEG is that of the most superficial layers of the cortical grey matter. The potential changes in the cortical EEG are due to the current flow in the fluctuating dipoles formed by the dendrites of the cortical cells and the cell bodies; namely, the current to flow through the volume conductor between "source" at the soma and basal dendrites and the "sink" at the apical dendrites, sustaining the EPSP. At the incoming current (sink), an upward deflection of the potential will be obtained, indicating a negative potential of depolarization (EPSP); at the outgoing current (source), a downward deflection, which indicates a positive hyperpolarization potential (IPSP), will be obtained (Fig. 2.6).

The flows of ionic charges caused by the EPSP-IPSP generate the extracellular field potentials, whose recording from the scalp constitutes the EEG activity. The synapses located on the cell body, near the axon hillock, are generally inhibitory, while those on the dendritic spines are mainly excitatory. The recorded EEG signals are generated mainly by neurons located near the recording electrode and only in small parts by more distant neurons: the broader the population of neurons under the recording electrode, the greater the EEG signal will result.

Moreover, the more the electrode (REF) is placed near the site where the recorded bioelectric activity originates (REC), the more the signal amplitude decreases as a function of the square root of the distance. The small amplitude of the extracellular recorded potentials is due, in addition, to the low value of the extracellular resistance and to their rapid decrease as a function of distance. The amplitude of these potentials becomes a critical factor when the tip of the electrode is far from the activated neurons, as occurring when we record from the scalp with a macro electrode. In such cases, it is not possible to record the activity of individual neurons, because the amplitude of the potentials is too small and the macroelectrodes are not sufficiently selective to discriminate the activity of these neurons from that of neighbouring cells. The EEG recorded from the scalp is, instead, the summary of the activity of a large number of neurons.

Thalamic afferences synchronously activate thousands of cortical neurons. The first response of the cortex to a signal originating from the thalamus is a sink in the deep layers (where excitatory synapses are located) and a source in the superficial layers. A recording electrode placed on the scalp is closer to the source than to the sink. The polarity of the electrical signals will be different depending on the site of the excitatory synapses (in the superficial or deep layers).

In extracellular recordings, an upward deflection indicates a negative potential when the recording electrode is near the synapse in which current is entering. When the recording electrode is located at level of the deeper cortical layers, far from the synapse, the same excitatory postsynaptic potential is recorded as a downward deflection. At rest, there is no potential difference between the soma and the dendrites of pyramidal cells, as both exhibit uniformly positive charges on the membrane surface and negative charges inside the membrane. This changes when, for example, due to the effect of afferent messages, there is a depolarization of the dendrites and an EPSP occurs. Therefore, there is a flow of current from the cell body (source) to the dendrites (sink), generating an electric field whose intensity can be measured as a potential difference between two points on the same line of force generated by two electric charges of opposite sign; this constitutes a dipole, its entity depending on the resistance of extracellular fluids. In practice, neurological generators do not correspond precisely to simple one-dimensional dipoles. Any source of activity large enough to be recorded in EEG will comprise at least a small area of cortex whose neurones are synchronously active. This source may be regarded as a three-dimensional sheet, polarized across its thickness. If it is small enough, it may still be conveniently represented as an "equivalent dipole." A larger area of cortex may be curved or even convoluted, and the equivalent dipole then becomes a complex sum of all the vectors. Furthermore, when many widely scattered generators are active, an infinite number of combinations may give rise to the same pattern of surface potential [15].

While the vector's magnitude is a function of the distance from the recording electrode (regarding the brain bioelectrical signals, the signal strength is inversely proportional to the square of the distance), the vector's direction always remains the same. If two or more vectors are oriented simultaneously towards the same electrode, they can be added together: the result of this sum will correspond to the arithmetic sum of their magnitudes. Depending on the orientation of the dipole compared to the cortical surface, we can distinguish a *vertical* (or radial) dipole oriented vertically to the cortical surface, a *horizontal* (or tangential) dipole located in a groove or in the interhemispheric fissure and an *oblique* dipole, if the positive and negative extremities are not aligned. Therefore, scalp electrodes can record different kinds of signal depending on dipole orientations (Fig. 2.7). The amplitude of signal

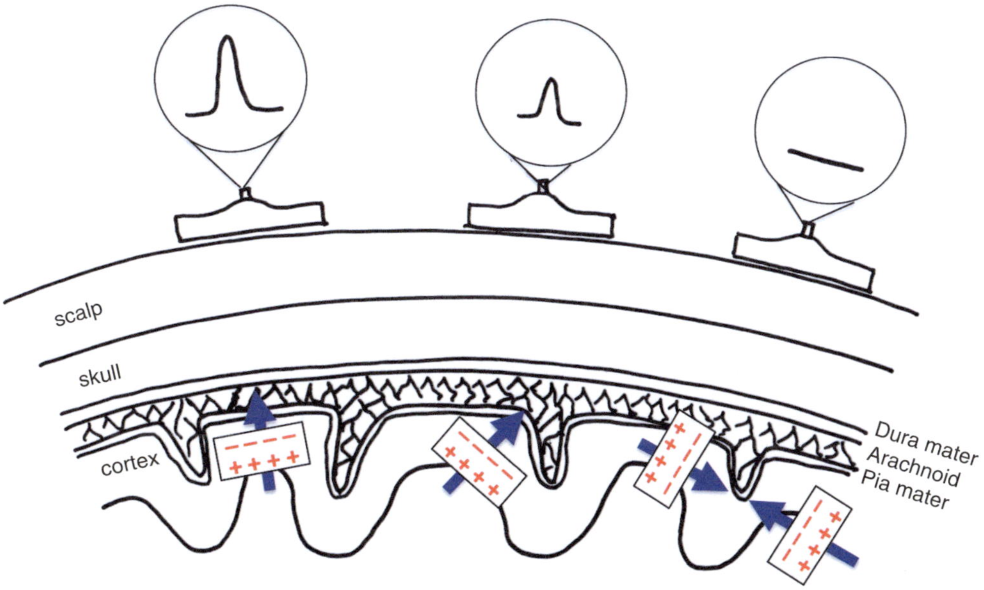

Fig. 2.7 Example of bioelectric signals recordable from the scalp, depending on the orientation and the underlying dipole: vertical, oblique, horizontal

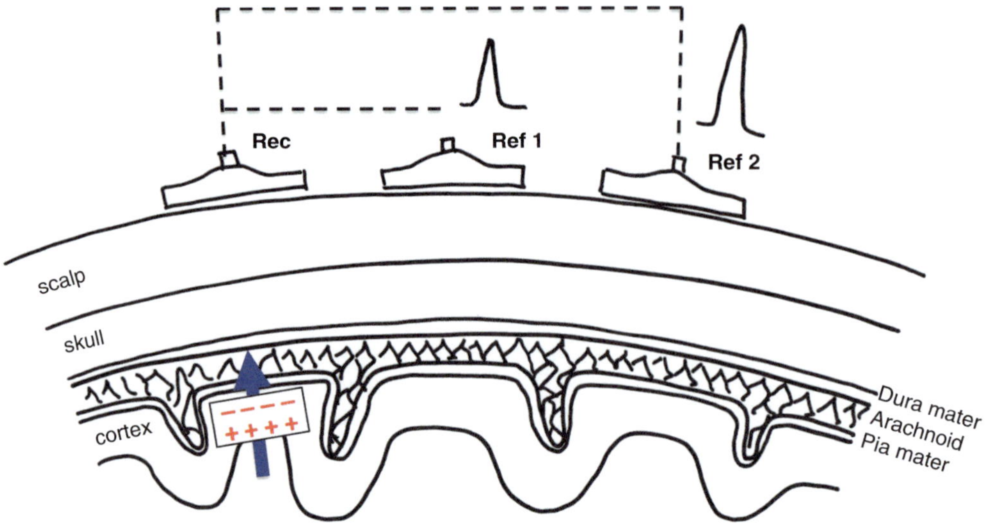

Fig. 2.8 Schematic representation of a population of cortical pyramidal cells. The amplitude of the recorded signals depends on the interelectrode distance: it grows as the distance increases

depends on the distance between the two electrodes and it grows as the distance between the electrodes increases (Fig. 2.8).

Furthermore, the position of the two electrodes compared to the dendrites is very important: for example, the best condition to record a potential gradient is when an electrode is placed on the surface at the main axis of the apical dendrites and the other is located more laterally. If the two electrodes are placed symmetrically and in a lateral position compared to the arborization of the dendrites, it is not possible to record any electrical gradient, as the two recording points are equipotential.

An electrical gradient between cell body and apical dendrites can also occur when the soma is hyperpolarized, due to an IPSP, while dendrites are in rest conditions; in this case the current flow goes from the cell body to the dendritic terminations.

A question that has always been asked over the years and which has found, to date, only partial answers is about the origin of the EEG rhythms. The dorsal thalamus is considered to be the chief subcortical EEG rhythm generator, synchronizing populations of neocortical neurons as voltage generators. In normal conditions, both thalamic nuclei and cortical regions interact to produce the synchrony of cortical PostSynaptic Potentials (PSPs) during wakefulness and sleep. The facultative pacemaker theory assumes that thalamocortical relay neurons send fibres to the cortex as well as give off branches that turn back and end on thalamic inhibitory interneurons (biofeedback servomechanism). Nucleus reticularis hypothesis attributes the pacemaker properties to the nucleus reticularis thalami, whose cells release the inhibitory neurotransmitter GABA in rhythmic bursts of depolarizations directed to the neurons of the dorsal thalamus and rostral brainstem [14]. The thalamus is the major gateway for the flow of information toward the cerebral cortex and is the first station at which incoming signals can be blocked by synaptic inhibition during sleep. This mechanism contributes to the shift that the brain undergoes as it changes from an aroused state, open to signals from the outside world, to the closed state of sleep [16].

2.3 Focus on Alpha Rhythm

Many studies on the normal EEG alpha rhythm have been performed, and they have demonstrated that the Posterior Dominant Rhythm (PDR) changes continuously during life and continues to mature throughout adolescence into early adulthood. It is difficult, therefore, to infer what the age-related increases in PDR frequency observed in human developmental studies actually mean in terms of maturation of the underlying brain functions [17, 18]. In addition to the genesis of the alpha rhythm, the thalamus seems to have a fundamental role. Although the exact contribution of thalamic activity as a generator of alpha rhythm is still not fully clarified, the pulvinar - among the posterior nuclei - is more likely associated with the spontaneous modulation of posterior alpha rhythm and its extensive connections with the entire cortex make it well-suited to finally modulate the alpha rhythm. More generally, the thalamic nuclei, in particular the dorsal ones, can be considered anatomo-functional stations of the ascending reticular activating system; this could explain how the alpha rhythm is closely related to them as it depends on the arousal levels [19]. In this context, alpha waves, defined as the oscillatory activity of the EEG recorded primarily on occipital regions with a frequency range between 8 and 12 Hz [20], behave like sleep spindles, inhibiting incoming information from sensory systems at the thalamic and early cortical level. Recordings from single thalamocortical relay cells (which are responsible of spindle generation) have demonstrated that hyperpolarization of the membrane potential when these cells are less receptive may

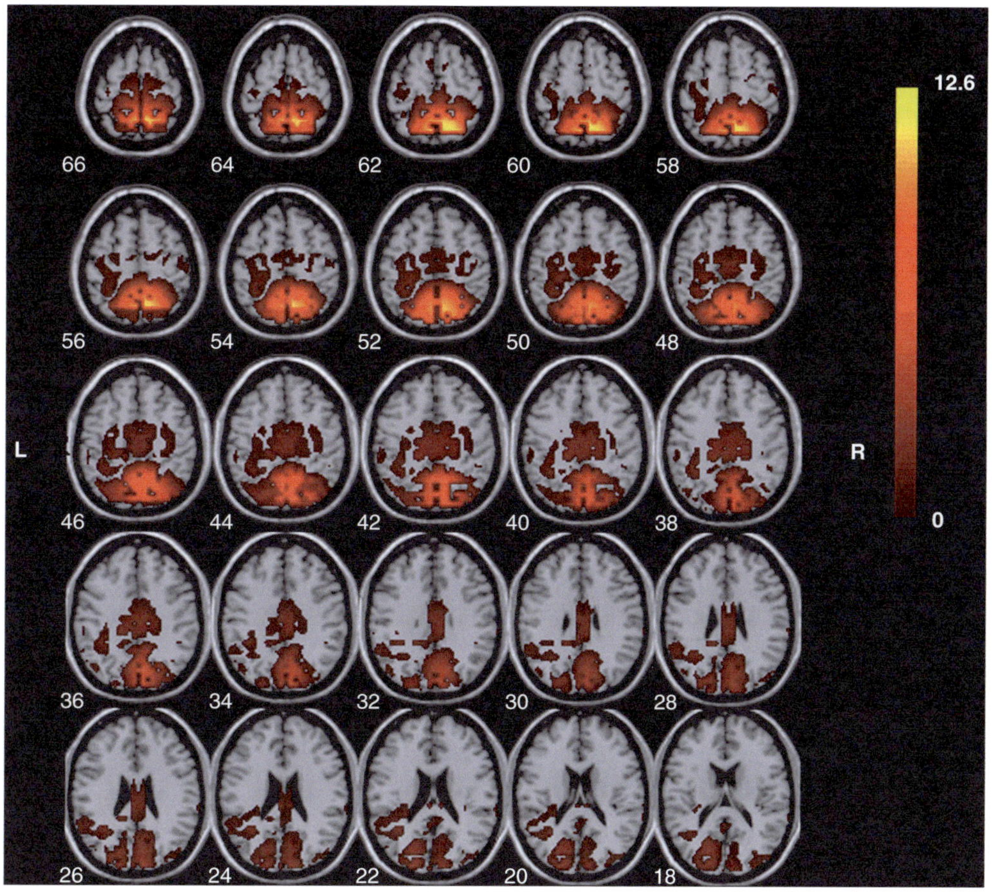

Fig. 2.9 Spatial pattern of the alpha band Default Mode Network (DMN) component that was identified in rest with the eyes closed condition and showed the highest correlation with self-referential-thought-scale (From Knyazev GG, Slobodskoj-Plusnin JY, Bocharov AV, Pylkova LV. The Default Mode Network and EEG alpha oscillations: an independent component analysis. Brain Res. 2011.21;1402:67-79, with permission)

give rise to an oscillation in the alpha range [21]. These kinds of oscillations in the primary visual area may represent a mechanism to stop incoming information and they are at the basis of the "gating function theory", along with the classical alpha desynchronization predicting higher alpha activity in inhibited cortical areas and lower activity in areas engaged in information processing [22]. Great attention has been focused, in recent years, on the study of the correlation between alpha rhythm and Default Mode Network (DMN). DMN is a resting state network, typically defined to include regions of the Medial PreFrontal Cortex (MPFC), Anterior Cingulate Cortex and Posterior Cingulate Cortex (PCC), cuneus/precuneus and temporoparietal junction/angular gyrus. These brain areas appear to be particularly active in resting state, while their activity decreases during the execution of specific tasks: increased activations within this network are related to the processes of memorization and creating associations, being related to the learning and integration processes [23]. Therefore, the relationship between DMN and alpha rhythm is not surprising, if we consider that the alpha rhythm is typically recorded during the quiet awakening and is selectively suppressed during the performance of specific tasks [24]. Correlation studies between EEG and Magnetic Resonance Imaging (MRI) have shown the relationship between alpha rhythm and DMN with conflicting opinions. Some areas of the DMN, such as orbital and medial PFC and PCC, seem to be active during quiet awakening in concomitance with the registration of the alpha activity, while some areas, such as posterior cingulate and parietal cortex, superior frontal cortex and medial frontal and bilateral temporal cortex, seem to have been suppressed [25]. However, given the great overlap and integration between these and other cortical areas, further studies are necessary to confirm and corroborate these results (Fig. 2.9).

2.4 Origin of Slow Brain Rhythms

There are at least two cellular sources of delta activities, originating in the thalamus and in the cortex. The combination of the intrinsic electrophysiological properties of the thalamic and cortical neurons, together with their synaptic connections and glial cells, are responsible for the generation of these oscillations. Thalamocortical neurons are able to display a clocklike delta rhythm, either induced by imposed hyperpolarizing current pulses or spontaneously. It has been described that thalamocortical neurons, recorded in vitro, display rhythmic bursts of high-frequency spikes with an interburst frequency of 1–2 Hz. This oscillation results from the interplay between two membrane currents: [26] the transient calcium current and a hyperpolarization-activated cation current. Thalamic neurons can be found in two different physiological states: a transmission mode and a burst mode. When the membrane potential of a thalamic neuron is close to the threshold of the action potential, the neuron is in the transmission mode: the synaptic excitatory potentials generated by the afferent signals generate a discharge whose characteristics depend on the sensory stimulus. These thalamic discharges produce low-amplitude signals in a desynchronized EEG pattern. On the other hand, when the thalamic neuron is hyperpolarized by inhibitory afferent signals, it is in the burst mode, because they react to brief depolarization with a burst of action potentials. Each burst produces a volley of EPSPs in cortical dendrites that generates a slow, synchronized and rhythmic EEG activity (delta activity). This pattern is observed in deep sleep and it is also recorded when the blocking of thalamocortical transmission occurs, such as in coma or in some epileptic seizures [27].

However, the presence of a delta rhythm after thalamectomy also suggests its further cortical genesis. Cortical neurons throughout layers II-VI displayed a spontaneous oscillation recurring with periods of 1–1.54–5 s, consisting of prolonged depolarizing and hyperpolarizing components. The long-lasting depolarizations of the slow oscillations consisted of EPSPs, fast IPSPs and fast pre-potentials, reflecting the action of synaptically coupled GABAergic local-circuit cortical cells [28]. A contribution of both NMDA-mediated synaptic excitatory events and a voltage-dependent persistent sodium current to the depolarizing component of the slow oscillation was also demonstrated [29].

A recent comparative study during simultaneous EEG and functional MRI recording in 14 patients after sleep deprivation evaluated positive and negative Blood Oxygenation Level Dependent signal (BOLD) correlations with delta and theta rhythms for left and right temporal electrodes. The two rhythms were almost entirely distinct in either anatomic distribution or correlation. Essentially, the delta rhythm had negative correlations within the frontal and temporal lobes, deep grey nuclei and cerebellum and positive correlations within the occipital and parietal lobes the theta rhythm had negative correlations within the occipital and parietal lobes and positive correlations within the frontal and temporal lobes, cerebral nuclei and cerebellum [30]. Another study by Hofle et al. assessed the EEG delta power with positron emission tomography on subjects progressing from wakefulness to slow wave sleep. They found that delta slow activity had negative correlation with thalamus, brainstem reticular formation, cerebellum, anterior cingulate cortex and orbitofrontal cortex. Positive correlation was indeed present in visual and auditory cortices [31]. However, the high variability of the results of correlation studies is mainly due to the different recording and processing methods and, therefore, needs further investigation.

References

1. Standring S. Gray's anatomy: The anatomical basis of clinical practice. 40th ed. London: Churchill-Livingstone/Elsevier; 2008.
2. London M, Hausser M. Dendritic computation. Annu Rev Neurosci. 2005;28:503–32.
3. Li L, Gervasi N, Girault JA. Dendritic geometry shapes neuronal cAMP signalling to the nucleus. Nat Commun. 2015;6:6319.
4. Luo J, McQueen PG, Shi B, Lee CH, Ting CY. Wiring dendrites in layers and columns. J Neurogenet. 2016;30:69–79.
5. Kirkcaldie MT, Collins JM. The axon as a physical structure in health and acute trauma. J Chem Neuroanat. 2016;76:9–18.
6. Jones SL, Svitkina TM. Axon initial segment cytoskeleton: architecture, development, and role in neuron polarity. Neural Plast. 2016;2016:6808293.
7. Philips T, Rothstein JD. Oligodendroglia: metabolic supporters of neurons. J Clin Invest. 2017;127:3271–80.
8. Shipp S. Structure and function of the cerebral cortex. Curr Biol. 2007;17:R443–9.
9. Briggs F. Organizing principles of cortical layer 6. Front Neural Circuits. 2010;4:3.
10. Kandel ER, Siegelbaum SA. Overview of synaptic transmission. In: Kandel ER, Schwartz JH, Jessell TM, editors. Principles of neural sciences. 5th ed. New York: McGraw-Hill; 2012.
11. Holm TH, Lykke-Hartmann K. Insights into the pathology of the α3 Na^+/K^+-ATPase ion pump in neurological disorders; lessons from animal models. Front Physiol. 2016;7:209.
12. Lacroix JJ, Campos FV, Frezza L, Bezanilla F. Molecular bases for the asynchronous activation of sodium and potassium channels required for nerve impulse generation. Neuron. 2013;79:651–7.
13. Roux B. Ion channels and ion selectivity. Essays Biochem. 2017;61:201–9.
14. Olejniczak P. Neurophysiologic basis of EEG. J Clin Neurophysiol. 2006;23:186–9.
15. Henderson CJ, Butler SR, Glass A. The localization of equivalent dipoles of EEG sources by the application of electrical field theory. Electroencephalogr Clin Neurophysiol. 1975;39:117–30.
16. Steriade M. Alertness, quiet sleep, dreaming. In: Peters A, Jones EG, editors. Cerebral cortex. New York: Plenum; 1991.
17. Marcuse LV, Schneider M, Mortati KA, Donnelly KM, Arnedo V, Grant AC. Quantitative analysis of the EEG posterior-dominant rhythm in healthy adolescents. Clin Neurophysiol. 2008;119:1778–81.
18. van der Stelt O. Development of human EEG posterior alpha rhythms. Comment on quantitative analysis of the EEG posterior-dominant rhythm in healthy adolescents. Clin Neurophysiol. 2008;119:1701–2.
19. Vaudano AE, Ruggieri A, Avanzini P, et al. Photosensitive epilepsy is associated with reduced inhibition of alpha rhythm generating networks. Brain. 2017;140:981–97.
20. Horne JA. Why we sleep: the functions of sleep in humans and other animals. Oxford: Oxford University Press; 1988.
21. Lopes da Silva F. Neural mechanisms underlying brain waves: from neural membranes to networks. Electroencephalogr Clin Neurophysiol. 1991;79:81–93.
22. Toscani M, Marzi T, Righi S, Viggiano MP, Baldassi S. Alpha waves: a neural signature of visual suppression. Exp Brain Res. 2010;207:213–9.
23. Buckner RL, Andrews-Hanna JR, Schacter DL. The brain's default network: anatomy, function, and relevance to disease. Ann N Y Acad Sci. 2008;1124:1–38.
24. Knyazev GG, Slobodskoj-Plusnin JY, Bocharov AV, Pylkova LV. The default mode network and EEG alpha oscillations: an independent component analysis. Brain Res. 2011;1402:67–79.
25. Bowman AD, Griffis JC, Visscher KM, et al. Relationship between alpha rhythm and the default mode network: an EEG-fMRI study. J Clin Neurophysiol. 2017;34:527–33.

26. Amzica F, Lopes Da Silva FH. Cellular substrates of brain rhythms. In: Shomer DL, Lopes da Silva FH, editors. Niedermeyer's electroencephalography: basic principles, clinical applications and related fields. 7th ed. Philadelphia, PA: Lippincott Williams & Wilkins; 2017.
27. Kandel ER, Schwartz JH, Jessell TM. Principles of neural sciences. 5th ed. New York: McGraw-Hill; 2012.
28. Steriade M, Nunez A, Amzica F. A novel slow (<1 Hz) oscillation of neocortical neurons in vivo: depolarizing and hyperpolarizing components. J Neurosci. 1993;13:3252–65.
29. Contreras D, Timofeev I, Steriade M. Mechanisms of long-lasting hyperpolarizations underlying slow sleep oscillations in cat corticothalamic networks. J Physiol. 1996;494:251–64.
30. Marawar RA, Yeh HJ, Carnabatu CJ, Stern JM. Functional MRI correlates of resting-state temporal theta and delta EEG rhythm. J Clin Neurophysiol. 2017;34:69–76.
31. Hofle N, Paus T, Reutens D, et al. Regional cerebral blood flow changes as a function of delta and spindle activity during slow wave sleep in humans. J Neurosci. 1997;17:4800–8.

3 Scalp and Special Electrodes

Oriano Mecarelli and Ferruccio Panzica

3.1 General Characteristics of Electrodes

Electrodes are the connecting system between the tissues where bioelectric activity is generated, or through which it is conducted, and the amplifier inputs. The electrical current in the human body is the result of ion flow, while the current in electronic circuits and instrumentation is due to electron flow. In order to record bioelectric signals, such as EEG and EMG, the ionic currents must be converted. This function is carried out by electrodes, transducers that sense the ion flow on the surface of the tissue, and convert it into an electron current.

Electrodes can be of different types and shapes, but they are still an interface between the patient and the recording device. The ideal electrode should not distort the signal nor generate significant artifacts. However, in reality, this is very difficult to accomplish. As the first component of the EEG signal acquisition chain, the characteristics of electrodes, namely, electrode–tissue interface, polarisation and impedance, are factors influencing the overall system performance and patient comfort.

The flow of electric current from body to electrode can be understood by examining the electrode–electrolyte interface [1]. When a metal is placed in an electrolyte, such as in the saline environment of tissue or skin, at the electrode–electrolyte interface, reduction/oxidation (redox) reactions occur. Assuming that the metal of the electrode and the cations (positive ions) in the solution are the same, the following reactions occur:

$$\mathrm{C} \rightleftarrows \mathrm{C}^{n^+} + ne^- \tag{3.1}$$

$$\mathrm{A}^{m^-} \rightleftarrows \mathrm{A} + me^- \tag{3.2}$$

In (Eq. 3.1) an atom C gives up electrons (oxidation) and discharges it into a solution as a positively charged ion, while the electrons remain as a charge carrier in the electrode. In (Eq. 3.2) the reaction involves an anion which can become a neutral atom giving off one or more free electrons to the electrode.

When a metal is brought into contact with a solution, the above reactions occur immediately; therefore, the local concentration of cations and anions in the solution at the electrode–electrolyte interface changes, and neutrality of charges is not maintained between the electrode and electrolyte where two layers of oppositely charged ions are produced, called the electrical double layer, similarly to that existing along electrically active biological cell membranes. This charge distribution establishes a potential difference known as the half-cell potential. It mainly depends on the metal involved, the concentration of its ions in the solution and the temperature.

Therefore, when a metal such as silver (of which traditional electrodes are made of) comes into contact with a solution containing ions, a stable electric potential between the metal and the solution can be measured (electrode potential). This property is used, for example, in batteries and accumulators to create a potential difference between the two poles. The stable electrode potential does not distort the bioelectric activity recorded by the electrode, but it adds a fixed value that can be even larger than 1 V; in the case of silver/silver chloride (Ag/AgCl), the half-cell potential is 222 mV. This value of half-cell potential is much larger than the EEG amplitude. Ideally, this would not be problem, because if the electrode potentials of two electrodes - both connected to a differential amplifier - are of the same amplitude, they will simply cancel each other because their difference will be equal to zero, thus permitting a correct recording of potentials. If, however, the electrode potentials are unequal and/or variable, this could generate unreliable signals that

O. Mecarelli (✉)
Department of Human Neurosciences, Sapienza University of Rome, Rome, Italy
e-mail: oriano.mecarelli@uniroma1.it

F. Panzica
Clinical and Biomedical Engineering Unit, Department of Neurophysiology, Fondazione IRCCS Istituto Neurologico "C. Besta", Milan, Italy
e-mail: ferruccio.panzica@istituto-besta.it

O. Mecarelli (ed.), *Clinical Electroencephalography*, https://doi.org/10.1007/978-3-030-04573-9_3

would add to the bioelectrical activity and could be present at the output of the differential amplifier.

Theoretically, if two electrodes are of the same shape and made of the same metal, their electrode potential should be exactly the same (and the potential difference should be equal to zero), but light impurities and contaminations of the surface can cause imbalances of potentials, in the amount of several mV, for a pair of similar electrodes. Moreover, neurophysiological signal distortion can also happen on the electrode surface because of the metal with which it is built. Silver electrodes, coated with silver chloride, are stable and particularly suitable for surface EEG recordings.

The half-cell potential described above refers to the equilibrium when no electric current exists between the electrode and the electrolyte. In many metal electrodes, the electrochemical interface does not allow electric charge to cross with equal ease in both directions, resulting in a higher electrode resistance to current flow in one direction than the other. Therefore, if there is a current flow, the electrode half-cell potential value could vary from its reference value depending on the direction and magnitude of electrode current flow [2]. In electrochemistry, this process is known as *electrode polarisation*. Electrode polarisation generally refers to the change of electric potential difference at the electrode–electrolyte interface due to the electric current passing through it, so that the equilibrium initially existing is disturbed and altered leading to an overpotential.

Theoretically, two types of electrodes are possible, those that are perfectly polarisable and those that are perfectly nonpolarisable. Ideally, polarisable electrodes are those in which no actual charge (faradic current) crosses the electrode–electrolyte interface (the electrical double layer) when a current is applied between the electrode and the electrolyte. This kind of electrodes are, therefore, characterised by an absence of net faradic current between the electrode surface and the electrolyte. The electrode–electrolyte interface behaves like a capacitor and the current across it is a displacement current. No Direct Current (DC) can flow between it and, therefore, the electrode–electrolyte interface acts as a high-pass filter reducing the transduction and transmission of low-frequency components. Moreover, it shows a very large change in potential upon the passage of small currents.

Perfectly nonpolarisable electrodes are those in which charges can move freely across the electrode–electrolyte interface. Its half-cell potential does not change from its equilibrium value upon application of the current and, therefore, there is no overpotential.

Electrodes made of noble metals such as platinum, iridium and gold behave similarly to perfectly polarisable electrodes. These materials are indeed electrochemically inert and, therefore, they are difficult to be oxidised and dissolved. An electric current changes the concentration of ions at the electrode–electrolyte interface, so the overpotential seen in this type of electrodes is mainly due the concentration of change.

Electrode polarisation could be associated with electric instability and could give rise to high impedance and high noise levels.

The best electrode–electrolyte interfaces for biopotential recordings are those made of a combination of metal and one of its metallic salts, usually chloride. Metallic salt is used as a coating on the metal and acts as an intermediary in the electrode–electrolyte process. A chloride electrode consists of a metallic electrode, placed in contact with one of its insoluble salts and immersed in a solution of soluble salt of the same anion (e.g. silver, in contact with silver chloride, immersed in sodium chloride).

The AgCl outer layer is highly reversible with chloride ions in physiologic electrolytes and the silver is highly reversible with its salt. Thus, current can reversibly flow across the electrode by the following two-stage chemical reaction:

$$Ag \leftrightarrow Ag^{+} + e^{-}$$

$$Ag^{+} + Cl^{-} \leftrightarrow AgCl$$

With the flowing of an external current, so that the silver electrode becomes positive, silver atoms lose an electron and discharges as ions (Ag^{+}) into the solution and immediately combine with the chloride ions (Cl^{-}) of the solution to produce neutral insoluble silver molecules that attach themselves on the electrode. Chloride ions are thus removed from the solution.

$$NaCl \rightarrow Na^{+} + Cl^{-}; Ag^{+} + Cl^{-} \rightarrow AgCl.$$

If the current passes through the double electric layer in the opposite direction, silver ions in the solution regain electrons and settle as metallic silver on the surface of the electrode; the solution becomes unsaturated and silver chloride splits into silver and chloride ions:

$$Ag^{+} + \text{electron} \rightarrow Ag; AgCl \rightarrow Ag^{+} + Cl^{-}.$$

In this way, chloride ions pass through the solution. The passage of small amounts of charges through the electrode, in both directions, makes the chloride layer thinner or thicker, but it does not change its properties. Unless a substantial amount of charges passes through in the same direction (as what can happen, for example, when executing an imprudent electrode impedance test through a DC source), the electrochemical state of the electrode surface remains stable and the electrode potential unvaried.

This process of electric charge transfers greatly lowers electrode resistance to solution, reduces electrode polarisation to near zero, improves electrode potential stability and reduces electrochemical noise. Therefore, the Ag/AgCl electrodes have characteristics similar to those of an ideal nonpolarisable electrode.

When a pair of electrodes is connected to a differential amplifier input, the difference between the two electrode potentials, if stable, can be removed by capacitors, called coupling capacitors, acting as low-cut filters (or high-pass filters) and so the potential difference will not be displayed in the recorded signal.

The situation worsens when potentials slowly change in time because of the changes in the conditions of the skin-electrode interface.

The ability to record low frequencies is also strictly connected to the electrode surface: the lower the surface of the electrode, the lower its electric capacity, the bigger the cut to lower frequencies as a result of polarisation. Paradoxically, smaller electrodes are often built with non-chloridisable materials and, therefore, susceptible to polarisation, but there are practical reasons for this:

- Needle electrodes, used for electromyography but also for EEG recordings of the scalp, must be made of stiff metal, like stainless steel, which can also be sharpened.
- Intracerebral electrodes can't be manufactured with non-polarisable materials, like silver chloride, because they are toxic if introduced into the brain. Stainless steel intracerebral electrode also contains a layer of chromic oxide on its surface, acting as another serial capacitor, lowering the resulting capacity value.

Finally, another artifact source not mentioned earlier is the connection between the electrode to a metallic wire of a different material (electrode-copper wire bimetallic junction), used for the connection to the amplifier. Should this junction (weld joint) not be correctly insulated and come into contact with the electrolyte (gel, etc.), it could function as a battery and produce fluctuating potentials of high amplitude, which generate artifacts.

In conclusion, electrodes are of vital importance in the chain of instruments used to record bioelectric signals; therefore, in order to record reliable data, it is necessary that they be prepared and treated with great care.

3.2 Electrode Chloridation

To make traditional silver electrodes nonpolarisable, an electrolytic method is used. Before re-chloriding previously used electrodes, it is necessary to carefully remove the existing layer of silver chloride; this can be achieved electrolytically by immersing the above-mentioned electrodes in a saline solution and making them electronegative (at more or less 9 V) compared with another silver electrode for a few minutes, until the surface is clear of any coloured chloride residue. Electrodes are then placed in a glass container with a saline solution, each of them attached to the positive pole of a 1.5 V battery. The negative pole of the battery is connected to another silver electrode, also immersed in the saline solution. With this method, after approximately 30 s, the electrodes connected to the positive pole will be covered with a layer of silver chloride and they will gain a dark brown or violet colour. The current passes at about 2.5 mA per cm^2 of electrode surface and it must flow for about a minute. The chemical reactions taking place when silver electrodes are immersed in saline solution are described by the following equations: $NaCl \rightarrow Na^+ + Cl^-$; $Cl^- + Ag^+ \rightarrow AgCl$. Na^+ ions react to the cathodic surface, producing hydrogen ions: $2Na^+ + 2H_2O + 2$ electrons $\rightarrow 2NaOH + H_2$.

Electrode chloridation is not necessary - of course - when using newly developed electrodes (gold-plated silver, gold or sintered metal electrodes).

3.3 Standard Recording Electrodes

Electrodes for scalp EEG recordings are: bridge electrodes, cup electrodes and needle electrodes. A bridge or pad electrode is an Ag/AgCl electrode, composed of a distal enlarged plate covered with a cotton pad, and a proximal segment, extended and usually threaded, to which wire connectors are fastened. The electrode is mounted on a plastic bridge (or a tripod) and various kinds of connectors can be attached (alligator clip, spring plug or touch proof) (Fig. 3.1a).

The main benefit of these electrodes is that they guarantee reliable recordings, with flexible and easily adjustable positioning. However, the tampon (impregnated with saline solution) tends to dry over time and this causes an increase in impedance. Moreover, the pressure on the patient's head (caused by the rubber bands of the cap) creates a certain physical annoyance over time and the montage becomes unstable in the event of a seizure or lack of cooperation; lastly, the junction between the electrode and the connector can generate artifacts (Fig. 3.1b).

Cup electrodes (or disc electrodes) are usually composed of an Ag/AgCl disc plate, partially concave in its inner part, with a small hole in the middle. In this case, the cup is integrated with the wire connecting it to the amplifier and this cable can be directly welded to the plate or detachable (bayonet connector). Gold-plated silver or sintered metal cup electrodes are currently available on the market (Fig. 3.2).

Cup electrodes can be secured on the patient's skin by applying them directly or with the help of a small gauze pad soaked in collodion or with a specific adhesive paste (see Chap. 7). To secure the electrodes to the skin with collodion, after having separated the hair and scrubbed the skin, small gauze pads soaked in liquid collodion can be used. Alternatively, liquid collodion can be poured slowly on the

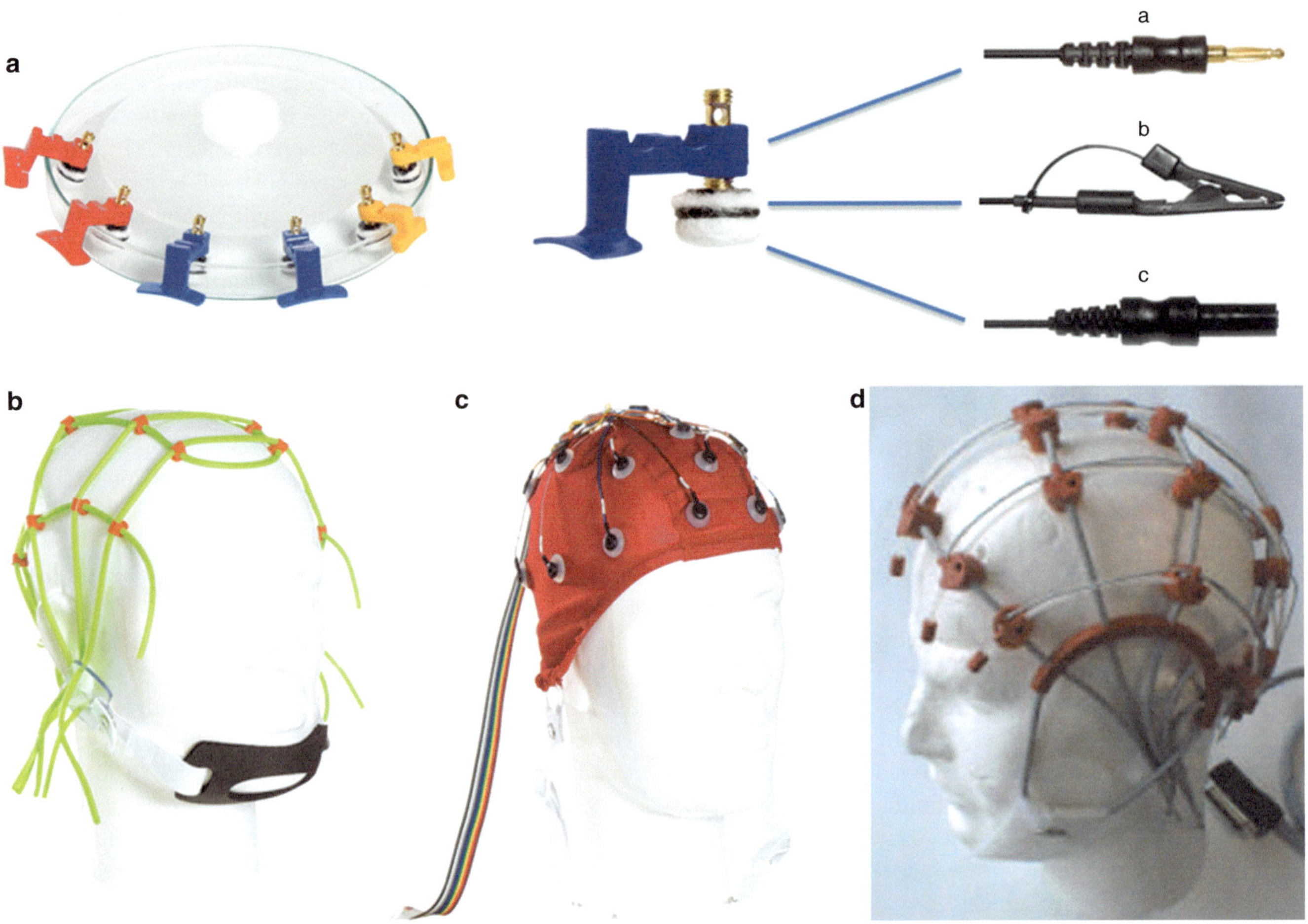

Fig. 3.1 (**a**) Bridge electrodes and their connectors: (*a*) spring plug; (*b*) alligator clip; (*c*) touch proof. (**b**) Cap with rubber bands for positioning bridge electrodes. (**c**) Prewired cap for standard EEG recording. (**d**) Elastic cap with electrodes pre-inserted in junctures

cup electrode with a syringe without a needle. A stream of cold air, discharged by a compressor or a simple hair-drier, can be used to dry the collodion. Once all the electrodes are placed, a conductive gel must be inserted into the hole at the centre of the cup and an impedance check must be carried out. The conductive gel can also be inserted into the concave side of the disc, before it is applied on the skin. This method is consistent over time and is more resistant to wire movements and traction; therefore, it is more suitable for long-term EEG monitoring. Disadvantages include longer preparation times, non-flexibility of the electrode montage and the use of collodion. Collodion is an unpleasant-smelling, flammable and toxic adhesive solution. Since its vapours are heavier than air, they tend to spread along the ground, and thus the room needs to be ventilated and equipped with a vapour extractor. Moreover, when applying collodion, particular care has to be be taken to cover the eyes and other mucous membranes which could accidentally come into contact with it. Removal of the collodion-placed electrodes can be carried out with an acetone-soaked cotton ball. Acetone inhalation can produce nasal and conjunctival irritation, respiratory effects, nausea and vomiting.

Traditional adhesive pastes (such as bentonite paste) can be used instead of collodion, but they don't guarantee the same adhesion to the skin and they also require special storage procedures. In addition, they can cause undesired skin reactions.

New types of adhesive pastes can now be found on the market (e.g. EC2, whose main ingredient is propyl paraben); they don't release vapours, they are non-toxic and they don't require special preservation methods. In addition, their removal can be accomplished with a simple aqueous solution. Electrode positioning with this method has shown stability for a long time and is therefore also appropriate for long-term video-EEG monitoring [3, 4].

Contact electrodes can also be placed on the scalp using prewired caps (Figs. 3.1c and 3.3). They are elastic caps of a textile material (skullcap) in which the electrodes are permanently embedded. These electrodes usually consist in silver discs, contained in a plastic shell with a hole in the middle.

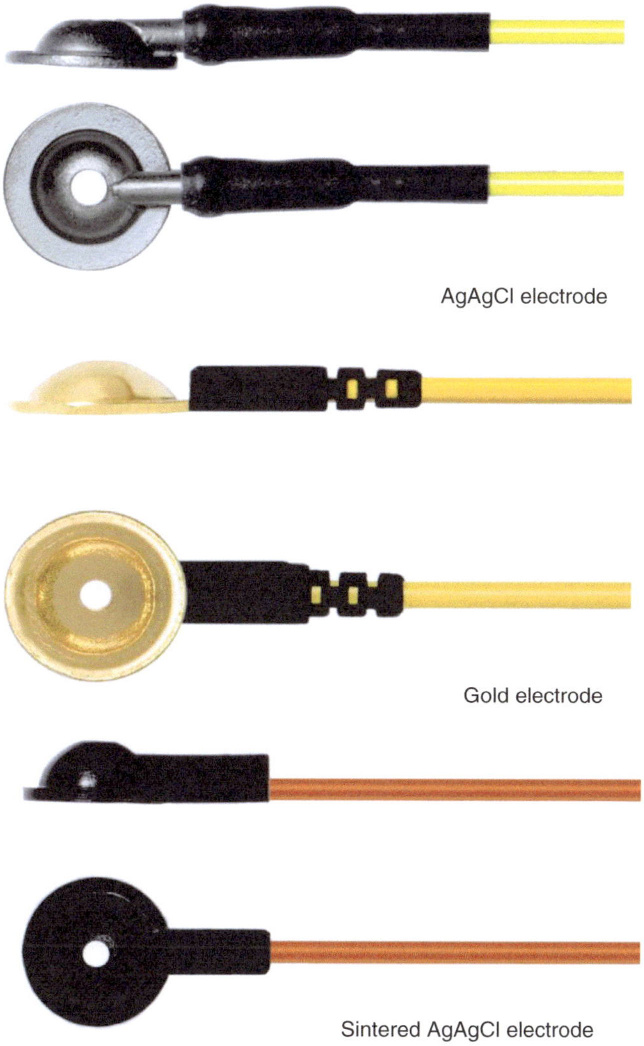

Fig. 3.2 Examples of casted silver Ag/AgCl, stamped gold (Au) and sintered Ag/AgCl cup electrode with central hole

Once the cap is positioned on the patient's head, it is possible to insert a conductive gel through the hole on the electrodes, to facilitate their contact with the skin. All electrodes inserted into the cap are firmly connected to the wires, which in turn are connected to a single cable, inserted into the amplifier through its connector. This method of preparation is usually more comfortable for the patient and it guarantees montages with multiple electrodes achieved in a relatively short time, with good recording reliability, especially in the case of long-term monitoring or motor seizures (electrodes are flat and are not easily moved). Using these caps, however, it is not possible to reduce easily skin-electrode impedances and the electrode placement cannot be modified in case of any particular cranial conformations, skin wounds or pulse artifacts. Slow and large "sliding" artifacts can also occur easily, when an excessive amount of gel is inserted between the skin and the electrode.

Caps having the advantages of both traditional and prewired caps are the rubber band caps in which the contact electrodes are already inserted into the junctures between the rubber bands themselves and they are permanently connected to the wires, which in turn are covered by a single shielded cable; by using this type of cap, the patient preparation time can be reduced and the position of the electrodes can be changed according to individual needs (Fig. 3.1d).

Needle electrodes are made of stainless steel or platinum–iridium needles, about 1.5–2 cm long and about 0.3–0.4 mm in diameter, directly connected to a wire, which ends up in a connector to be then inserted into the amplifier. It must be positioned subcutaneously and obliquely to the surface (30°), after proper disinfection of the affected skin area. To avoid asymmetry in magnitude of the recorded signal, it is essential that the needles be aligned in parallel, in the anteroposterior direction.

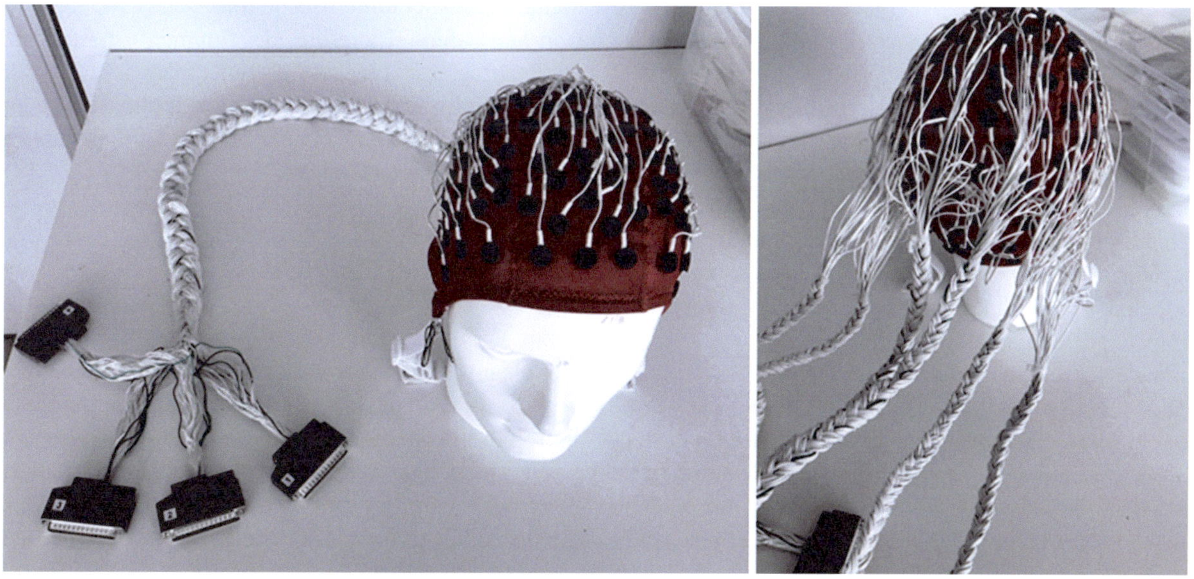

Fig. 3.3 Examples of prewired elastic cap for high density EEG

The American Clinical Neurophysiology Society (ACNS) guidelines do not recommend these electrodes for routine clinical use, because of their higher impedances, patient discomfort, risk of injuries to personnel and infection risks [5, 6]. Sterilisation of welded cable electrodes is possible with ethylene oxide (not in autoclave though), but this problem is currently solved with the use of presterilised disposable needles. Actually, this type of electrode is very easy to use for recordings in the intensive care unit or, more generally, in patients with low levels of consciousness, including operating room recordings or for brain death ascertainment. In any case, needle electrodes, by their intrinsic properties, attenuate EEG frequencies lower than 1 Hz and this must be taken into account.

3.4 Recent Developments: Dry and Active Electrodes

Ag/AgCl electrodes with wet conductive gel are still almost universally used for biopotential recordings in clinical and research applications. With proper preparation, they are characterised by a low skin-electrode impedance that reduces artefacts or interference induced by cable movement; they show an excellent signal quality and good Signal-to-Noise Ratio (SNR). However, wet electrodes require skin preparation and professional personnel in order to place them properly. In addition, their impedance could deteriorate in a few hours after gel application and the gel itself can dry out. These drawbacks limit the use of Ag/AgCl electrodes for long-term EEG monitoring, especially when a large number of electrodes should be placed on the scalp.

In order to overcome these drawbacks, in recent years, dry (gel-free) electrodes have been developed. The main advantages are that they do not require the use of conductive gel or paste nor any skin/scalp preparation, thus reducing the setup time and improving subject comfort. However, dry electrodes present a higher impedance comparing with Ag/AgCl electrodes leading to high susceptibility to movement artifacts and to a significant increase in the noise and interference picked up from the environment; moreover, they are much more sensitive to the condition of the skin. Typical dry-electrode impedance ranges from a few hundreds of kΩ to a few tens of MΩ [7]. Therefore, dry electrodes should be used coupled with differential amplifiers with a very high input impedance and shielding in order to come near to the performance of wet electrodes [8].

State-of-the-art superficial dry electrodes for EEG can be grouped in two categories: contact electrodes and non-contact - or capacitive-coupling - electrodes. Dry non-contact sensors isolate the electrode from the skin, but this leads to even higher electrode impedance and makes EEG recordings more susceptible to movement and muscular artifacts. Regarding to subject comfort, dry electrodes implemented with conductive rigid metal pins can provide long-term EEG recordings but at the cost of pain and discomfort. Recently, dry electrodes with soft contact to the skin and an electrode impedance ranging from 20 to 500 kΩ have been developed [9–13].

Recent advances in integrated circuits and sensor techniques have allowed the development of dry Active Electrode (AEs) [12]. These are electrodes with integrated amplifiers that locally buffer and amplify EEG signals. The closeness of electrode to amplifier reduces interference and noise pickup. Furthermore, the low output impedance of the integrated amplifier allows the use of high-impedance dry electrodes, reducing cable motion artefacts, noise and interference from the environment. On the other hand, an AE-based EEG system require more wires (e.g. for power supply) compared to a conventional EEG, especially when additional functions (e.g. impedance measurement) are integrated in AEs.

Early AEs included simple analog buffers, i.e. voltage followers. This is at present the most popular architecture, because of its balanced performances. Moreover, it makes the use of the active shielding technique simpler to reduce the interferences [8, 14].

The main limitation of this classic AE architecture is that an analog buffer only performs impedance conversion without providing any voltage gain. Therefore, follow-on readout circuits are needed, leading to additional power consumption. Other configurations involve the use of inverting or non-inverting amplifiers, each with proper advantages and disadvantages.

Clearly, AE-based EEG systems should be designed to meet the requirements compliant with medical standards, which impose constraints on the electrical performance in terms of input impedance, noise, electrode offset tolerance, signal quality, common-mode rejection ratio, power dissipation and safety. Therefore, development of AEs remains a challenging task [15]. At present, there is an increase for EEG recording systems for research application and mobile, wearable applications, mainly because of their robustness to environmental interference.

3.5 Special Electrodes

From early on in the history of electroencephalography, it was clear that some cerebral regions were difficult to analyse with conventional surface electrodes. In order to obtain more thorough information, adjunctive electrodes, also known as basal electrodes, began to be used. In particular, these electrodes can be useful when identifying epileptiform abnormalities in the mesial and basal surfaces of the temporal and frontal lobes. They are generally invasive or semi-invasive and they can only be used in specific cases and in adequately specialised laboratories.

3.5.1 Sphenoidal Electrodes

Sphenoidal electrodes were introduced into EEG practice in 1951 [16] to analyse areas of the temporal lobe not recordable from the scalp. They are composed of a stainless steel or platinum wire, insulated along its entire length, except for the 3–5 mm at the extremity (Fig. 3.4). Sphenoidal electrodes are positioned under local anaesthesia, in a sterile environment, using as a guide, a lumbar puncture needle, inserted 3 cm anterior to the external auditory canal, below the zygomatic arch, and through the mandibular notch, targeting the lateral border of foramen ovale (Fig. 3.5). Sphenoidal electrodes denomination is Sp1 and Sp2. These electrodes are generally reliable regarding the quality of the recording, and they can be left in place for up to 3 weeks. As an alternative, shorter sphenoidal electrodes (mini-sphenoidal) can be used; their insertion is associated with less discomfort, but the results of few studies do not demonstrate particular advantages. Sphenoidal electrodes are mostly well tolerated by patients and they cause little artifactual activity. Infrequently, they can cause bleeding, penetration of the salivary duct or lesions of the trigeminal branches with consequent facial pain.

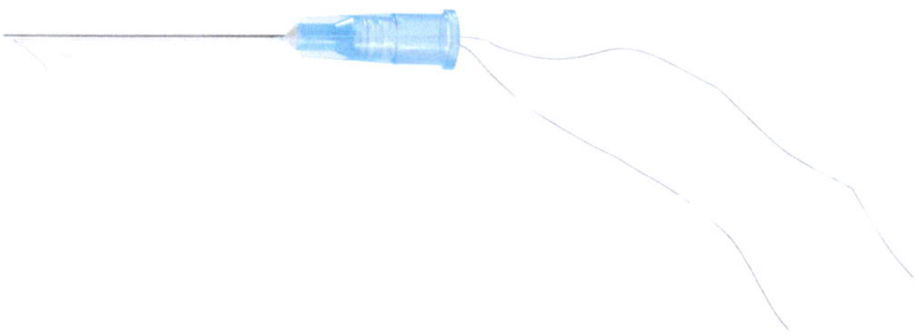

Fig. 3.4 Hook wire electrode, usable also as sphenoidal electrode

3.5.2 Naso-Ethmoidal Electrodes

These curved-end electrodes are applied under local anaesthesia. They are inserted in an upward direction, between the nasal septum and the nasal concha, coming close to the lamina cribrosa of the ethmoid bone. They can be useful for recordings of the basal surface of the frontal lobe. Once in place, this type of electrode is well tolerated, even though at times it can cause irritation of the conjunctiva.

3.5.3 Nasopharyngeal Electrodes

The nasopharyngeal electrodes consist of a solid or semi-solid insulated silver rod, with a small silver ball at the tip. After their lubrication, the electrodes are inserted bilaterally through the nares until they reach the nasopharynx posterior wall. They don't require local anaesthesia nor a sterile environment and are placed in the nasopharynx for the recording time only. This method is not considered invasive and, therefore, these electrodes can be positioned by an adequately trained technician and removed at the end of the recording session.

The nasopharyngeal electrodes may record the bioelectric activity generated in the inferior-mesial surface of the temporal and frontal lobes and so their indications are similar to those of sphenoidal electrodes, although with greater disadvantages. In fact, relevant artifacts can be generated by breathing and pharyngeal muscle contraction and, in relation to motor seizures, electrodes can cause injury to the pharynx itself. For these reasons, nasopharyngeal electrodes are currently rarely used.

3.5.4 Zygomatic Electrodes

The zygomatic electrodes are considered a non-invasive replacement for sphenoidal electrodes, suitable for routine recordings in the study of focal epileptic seizures (Fig. 3.6).

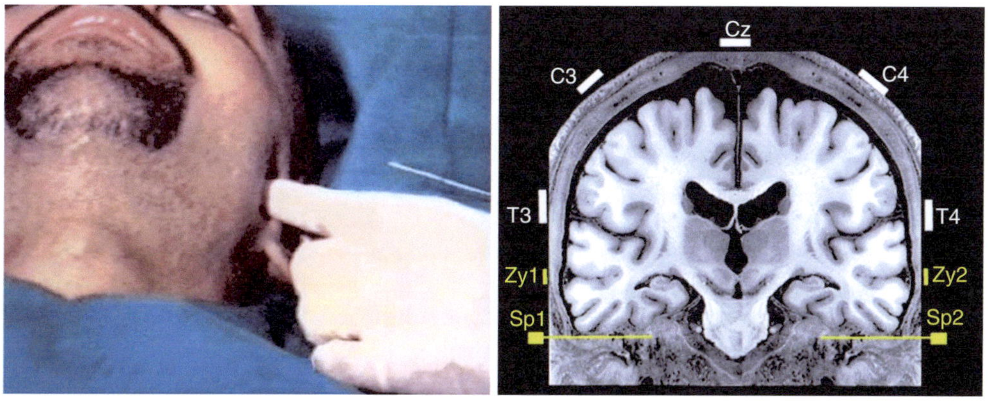

Fig. 3.5 Positioning of bilateral sphenoidal electrodes (courtesy of Francesca Bisulli and Paolo Tinuper, IRCCS Institute of Neurological Sciences, and Department of Biomedical and Neuromotor Sciences, University of Bologna, Italy)

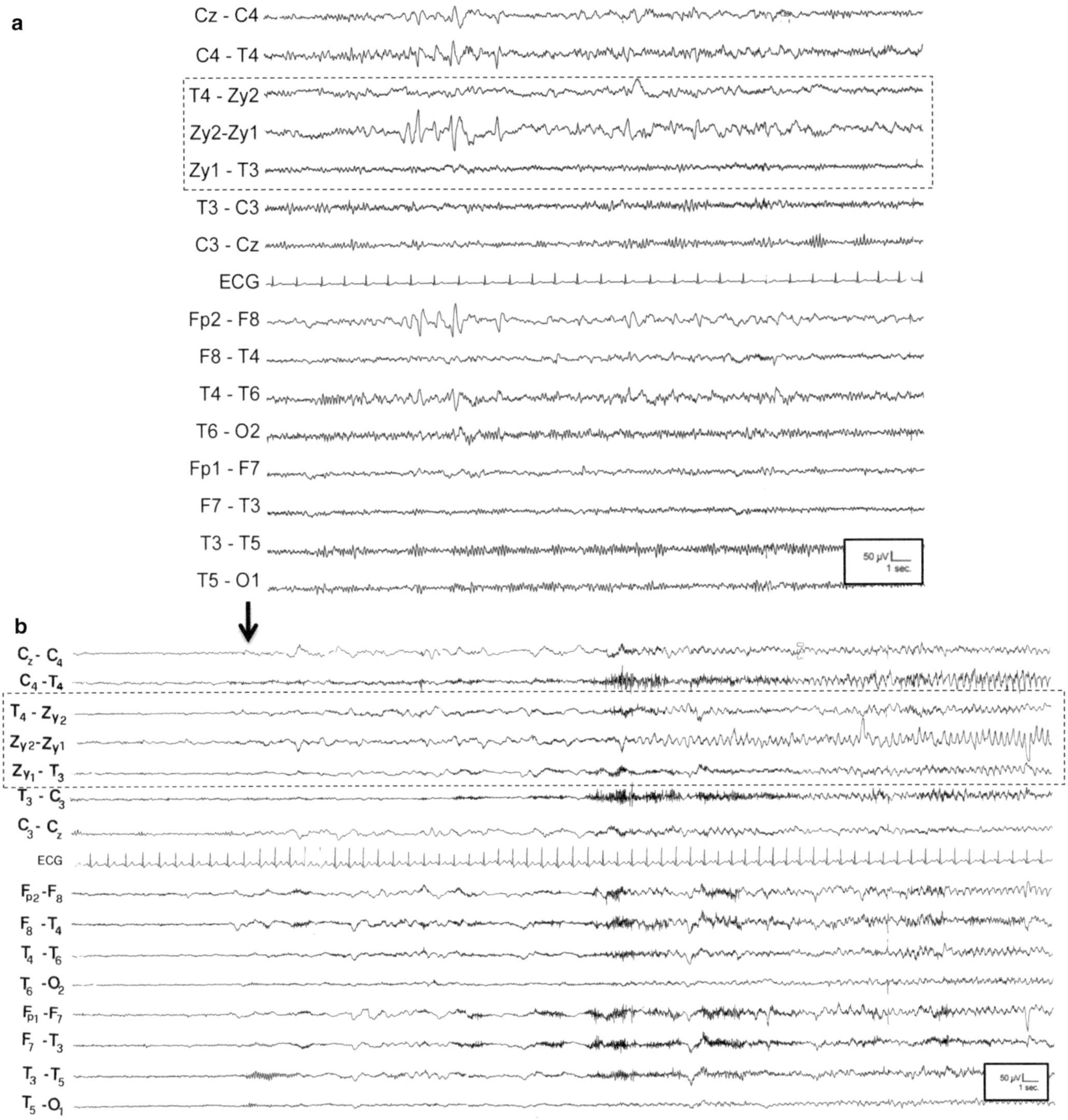

Fig. 3.6 An example of EEG recording with additional zygomatic electrodes in a 35-year-old woman with temporal epilepsy: interictal (**a**) and ictal (**b**, onset of discharge at arrow) epileptic pattern (courtesy of Francesca Bisulli and Paolo Tinuper, IRCCS Institute of Neurological Sciences, and Department of Biomedical and Neuromotor Sciences, University of Bologna, Italy)

Zygomatic electrodes are simple cup electrodes, applied in front of the tragus, on the zygomatic arch, along the line connecting the tragus and the nasion. However, their ability to highlight epileptiform abnormalities that arise from basal and mesial frontotemporal regions is lower than sphenoidal electrodes.

3.5.5 Supraorbital Electrodes

Supraorbital electrodes are cup electrodes which can be applied, with collodion or adhesive paste, below and into the third medialis of the superciliary arch. They can be used when the aim is a more thorough study of the frontal pole activity. Given their positioning, these electrodes are particularly sensitive to eye movement-generated artefacts and the activity recorded with them must always be compared to the purely electrooculographic one. These electrodes are named as So2 and So1 and they are referred in bipolar derivation to Fp2 and Fp1.

3.5.6 Tympanic Electrodes

Tympanic electrodes are an additional mean of recording brain areas that cannot be explored from the scalp and traditionally they are composed of a small S-shaped, insulated tube, about 6 cm long, terminating in a soft little sphere, of 7 mm in diameter, soaked in physiologic solution. These electrodes are inserted through the ear canal until their soft extremity touches the tympanic membrane (this requires experience and manual sensitivity). They can be used to study epileptic abnormalities that originate from the lower part of the temporal lobe, but they can be useful, rather than for EEG, to better visualise the first component of acoustic evoked potentials. Nowadays, for the evoked potential recording, a miniaturised version can be used, wet EEG electrodes positioned at discreet scalp and ear locations, useful for recording EEG on an everyday basis, and this will increase user acceptance and open up new avenues for the monitoring of the human brain function during daily life situations and actions.

3.6 Infection Control

The problem of transmissibility of certain pathogens, especially in a hospital environment, has always existed, but the attention in this regard has increased after the advent of HIV infection. Many diseases, from viral hepatitis to Creutzfeldt-Jakob disease (CJD), are at risk of being transmitted from patient to staff or other patients, through the use and reuse of contaminated electrodes. The problem is also relevant with regard to forensics.

Detailed recommendations regarding sterilisation of electrodes (or other instruments) were issued by the American Electroencephalographic Society [17] and recently reviewed [18]. For a continuous update on the procedure, you can also consult the Neurodiagnostic Society site at http://www.aset.org.

The highest risk of infection occurs when using needle electrodes. The technician can get infected either by needle pricks or through contact between blood and broken skin. Risks of transmission from patient to patient obviously exists with the reuse of the same electrodes. The preparation of the patient's skin before the electrodes are positioned can also cause bleeding or serous exudates, which can contaminate both the electrodes and the technician's hands. It is, therefore, advisable to avoid abrasions of the scalp, caused by excessive rubbing or by sharp objects, even blunt ones, used - for example - to clear out the hair. Blunt needles used to apply the conductive gel under the electrodes on prewired caps are particularly susceptible to contamination risk.

Disposable gloves can be worn by technical staff during the placement, removal and washing of the electrodes. Particular attention must be paid in trying not to touch other instruments when wearing potentially infected gloves. Application of the electrodes on patients who are known (or suspected) to be suffering from highly transmissible diseases must be carried out using all adequate physical protections: surgical masks, disposable overalls and latex gloves. EEG needle electrodes should be sterile and disposable; otherwise, they must be accurately cleaned and autoclaved (e.g. at 121 °C for 15 min). Needles used to inject conductive gel require similar measures. Bridge electrodes or cup electrodes must be cleaned with an adequate detergent after each use and they should be brushed in order to remove fragments of gel or adhesive paste; subsequently, they must be immersed in a sodium hypochlorite solution for at least 10 min, after each application. In cases of a highly infectious patient (e.g. with CJD), the preferred solution is to use disposable electrodes, to be later destroyed in an incinerator. Intracranial electrodes are at the highest risk of the transmission of diseases like CJD and so they should also be destroyed after use.

The recording system should be cleaned as well, with sodium hypochlorite, if contaminated with fluids at high biological risk. Two percent glutaraldehyde is a very powerful disinfectant for almost any infective disease (except for CJD), but it is not suitable for ordinary cleaning, as it can sensitise the staff. All contaminated linen should be treated according to locally recommended procedures. It is clear, however, that the precautions to be adopted to prevent the risk of infections (especially if not excessively high) should never affect the patient's dignity.

Appendix: Electro-Physical Characteristics of Electrodes

M. Mistretta

Silver (Ag): it is a transition, pliable, biocompatible metal for non-invasive use only. It is characterised by a higher electrical conductivity than the other metals and by a medium/low level of electrode potential. It is subjected to a fast oxidation in contact with ozone and therefore the air. It is often used as a basic material in the production of surface electrodes, and in order to reduce to the minimum the inherent noise, it is essential to use the 999% pure one. The pure silver is a non-magnetic metal.

Silver/silver chloride (Ag/AgCl): it is a mixed material with pure silver base and an external layer of silver chloride. The external match between silver metal and silver chloride salt guarantees unique features for the electrode. This mixed material is characterised by a fixed and specific electrode potential and by a low electrode/skin contact impedance. Therefore, it is perfect for recordings of low levels of AC and DC potentials and shows lower noises in low frequency in comparison with gold and pure silver. The layer of chloride silver that covers silver can be achieved through a chemical or electrolytic process. Both treatments make the electrode to get a characteristic dark grey colouring. Being of a least thickness, this external coat can deteriorate in the long term if high-saline content pastes and gel are used and if they are not removed at the end of use conveniently. Moreover, it is necessary to pay a particular attention to external mechanical abrasions that could take the treatment away. In case of a continuous employment, a treatment of re-chlorinating is needed when you notice the surface of the electrode has lost its original colour.

Sintered silver/silver chloride (Sint Ag/AgCl): it has the same electrical features of Ag/AgCl as it is formed by a mixture of Ag and AgCl very thin powders that are compacted through the sintering process. Therefore, you get an electrode of uniform thickness characterised by a greater stability of electrical features in the long term compared to an average Ag/AgCl. With regard to maintenance, this type of electrode does not need to be re-chlorinated but only to remove the remains of gel and conductive paste carefully.

Gold (Au): it is a transition, pliable, biocompatible metal used also for invasive employment. It is characterised by an excellent electrical conductivity, by a medium/low electrode potential and by the fact it is resistant to most chemical compounds. These features make it perfect for an employment with strong saline-based electrolytes and adhesives or diluents of a various nature. It is often employed as an external coat in the production of cup electrodes to be used in long terms monitoring or for sleep studies, as adhesives and diluents strong like collodion and acetone are applied with the electrode. Owing to a high biocompatibility, it is often used for invasive electrodes for recording of both potentials and electric stimulation.

Tin (Sn): it is a post-transition, pliable and resistant to metal corrosion. It is characterised by a good electrical conductivity, low level of electrode potential and a low level of innate noise. It is the material with the best value/quality relationship in the production of electrodes, and historically it is used in the production of head caps with prewired electrodes.

Carbon/graphite (C): it is a non-metal material with a good electrical conductivity; it has a very low level of electrode potential and shows a low level of noise similar to Ag/AgCL. Moreover, it has the quality to be radium-opaque and non-magnetic. Often, the graphite powder is inserted into plastics and paints to be employed in the production of electrodes. This solution makes the electrical features of this material worse but makes it easily usable in manufacturing systems.

Steel (alloys AISI 304,316): biocompatible, of high hardness and elastic alloy, characterised by a remarkable resistance to corrosion in water and in the air. It gives a medium electrical conductivity. Owing to mechanical and ductile features, it is used in the production of medical needles. Given its wide employment in the medical field, it guarantees the best quality/price relationship.

Platinum (Pt): it is a transition, pliable metal; it has a strong resistance to corrosion and is biocompatible. Usually it is used in alloy with iridium to improve its mechanical resistance. It is recognised for its good electrical conductivity and is employed for cortical electrodes and needles. It is a non-magnetic material.

Titanium (Gr. 5): it is a light and resistant metal, both mechanically and chemically. It is a biocompatible material and customarily is employed in prostheses. As far as the electrical characteristics, they are similar to tins. It is a non-magnetic material and for this feature it is used for MRI compatible products, especially needle electrodes, owing to its physical characteristics like steel. Given its high level of biocompatibility and resistance, it is also used for long-duration applied electrodes and implantable electrodes.

References

1. Neuman MR. Biopotential electrodes. In: Webster JG, editor. Medical instrumentation: application and design. 4th ed. Hoboken, NJ: John Wiley & Sons Inc.; 2010. p. 189–240.
2. Rowe BC. Bioelectricity and its measurement. In: Kutz M, editor. Standard handbook of biomedical engineering and design. New York: McGraw-Hill; 2003. p. 1–50.
3. Falco C, Sebastiano F, Cacciola L, et al. Scalp electrode placement by EC2 adhesive paste in long-term video-EEG monitoring. Clin Neurophysiol. 2005;116:1771–3.
4. Dash D, Dash C, Primrose S, et al. Update on minimal standards for electroencephalography in Canada: a review by the Canadian Society of Clinical Neurophysiologists. Can J Neurol Sci. 2017;44:631–42.
5. Epstein CM, et al. Guidelines Review Committee. American Clinical Neurophysiology Society. Guideline 1: minimum techni-

cal requirements for performing clinical electroencephalography. J Clin Neurophysiol. 2006;23:86–91.
6. Sinha SR, Sullivan S, Sabau D, et al. American Clinical Neurophysiology Society Guideline 1: minimum technical requirements for performing clinical electroencephalography. J Clin Neurophysiol. 2016;33:303–7.
7. Searle A, Kirkup L. A direct comparison of wet, dry and insulating bioelectric recording electrodes. Physiol Meas. 2000;21:271–83.
8. Metting van Rijn AC, Peper A, Grimbergen CA. High-quality recording of bioelectric events. Part 2. Low-noise, low-power multichannel amplifier design. Med Biol Eng Comput. 1991;29:433–40.
9. Lin CT, Liao LD, Liu YH, Wang IJ, Lin BS, Chang JY. Novel dry polymer foam electrodes for long-term EEG measurement. IEEE Trans Biomed Eng. 2011;58:1200–7.
10. Grozea C, Voinescu CD, Fazli S. Bristle-sensors-low-cost flexible passive dry EEG electrodes for neurofeedback and BCI applications. J Neural Eng. 2011;8:1–14.
11. Lee SM, Kim JH, Byeon HJ, Choi YY, Park KS, Lee SH. A capacitive biocompatible and adhesive electrode for long-term and cap-free monitoring of EEG signals. J Neural Eng. 2013;10:036006.
12. Chen YH, Op de Beeck M, Vanderheyden L, Mihajlovic V, Grundlehner B, Van Hoof C. Comb-shaped polymer-based dry electrodes for EEG/ECG measurements with high user comfort. Conf Proc IEEE Eng Med Biol Soc. 2013;2013:551–4.
13. Fiedler P, Pedrosa P, Griebel S, Fonseca C, Vaz F, Supriyanto E, Zanow F, Haueisen J. Novel multipin electrode cap system for dry electroencephalography. Brain Topogr. 2015;28:647–56.
14. Metting van Rijn AC, Peper A, Grimbergen CA. High-quality recording of bioelectric events. Part 1. Interference reduction, theory and practice. Med Biol Eng Comput. 1990;28:389–97.
15. Xu J, Mitra S, Van Hoof C, Yazicioglu RF, Makinwa KAA. Active electrodes for wearable EEG acquisition: review and electronics design methodology. IEEE Rev Biomed Eng. 2017;10:187–98.
16. Jones D. Recording of the basal electroencephalogram with sphenoidal electrodes. Electroencephalogr Clin Neurophysiol. 1951;3:100.
17. American EEG Society. Report of the committee on infectious diseases. J Clin Neurophysiol. 1994;11:128–32.
18. Scott NK. Infection prevention: 2013 review sand update for neurodiagnostic technologists. Neurodiagn J. 2013;53:271–88.

4 Electrode Placement Systems and Montages

Oriano Mecarelli

4.1 Traditional International 10-20 System

When Hans Berger recorded the first human EEG, he only had two electrodes available, positioned them in the anterior and posterior regions of the head. Berger kept using this method for many years, considering it an efficient system to measure the global cortical activity. Later on, other researchers highlighted how, in reality, EEG activity varied significantly depending on the area of the scalp from which it was recorded. Observation of different regional cerebral rhythms encouraged the use of multiple electrodes and of more recording channels, but standardization of the recording methods soon became necessary, so that the resulting data could be comparable with one another. A committee of International Federation of Societies for EEG and Clinical Neurophysiology (IFSECN), led by H. Jasper, started then working on a specific electrode positioning system to be used in all laboratories. The first standardized system was presented at the 2nd International Congress of IFSECN in Paris in 1949 and published by Jasper in 1958; it is still universally used and known as the International 10-20 System (IS 10-20) [1].

In the development of IS 10-20, the following concerns were addressed:

- Definition of a measuring system for electrode positioning, taking into account clearly defined anatomical landmarks, so that the measurements were as proportional as possible to the shape of the skull
- Electrode distribution in order to guarantee that they cover every part of the skull and electrode identification according to standard positions, regardless whether all, or only some, are used in a specific recording
- Identification of the various electrode positions depending on the underlying brain area (frontal, central, temporal, parietal and occipital), rather than just using numbers, so that communication is more immediate and intuitive
- Execution of appropriate anatomical studies to safely localize brain area projections which, presumably, match the electrode standard positions.

Correct positioning of the electrodes on the scalp according to IS 10-20 is achieved by tracing imaginary lines, starting from specified anatomical landmarks. These circumferential lines are mutually perpendicular and they are represented by:

– Anteroposterior sagittal midline, connecting nasion to inion, through the vertex. Nasion is the depression between the eyes, just above the nasal bridge, at the insertion of the frontal bone and the nasal bones. Inion is the highest point in the midline of the protuberance of the occipital bone.
– Along this sagittal midline, there are five standard positions called frontopolar (Fpz), frontal (Fz), central (Cz), parietal (Pz) and occipital (Oz). The letters F, C, P, and O indicate the underlying cerebral area and the letter z stands for zero. Considering the total distance between nasion and inion in centimeters, Fpz and Oz points are located at 10% of the total distance, respectively, from the nasion and the inion. All other positions are calculated at 20% of the distance between Fpz and Oz (the 10-20 denomination originated precisely from this percentage calculation). The ideal placing along the skull would set the central electrode (Cz) exactly in the middle of the line between nasion and inion; anatomical studies showed that C electrodes are located 1 cm within the central sulcus [2] (Fig. 4.1a).

O. Mecarelli (✉)
Department of Human Neurosciences, Sapienza University of Rome, Rome, Italy
e-mail: oriano.mecarelli@uniroma1.it

O. Mecarelli (ed.), *Clinical Electroencephalography*, https://doi.org/10.1007/978-3-030-04573-9_4

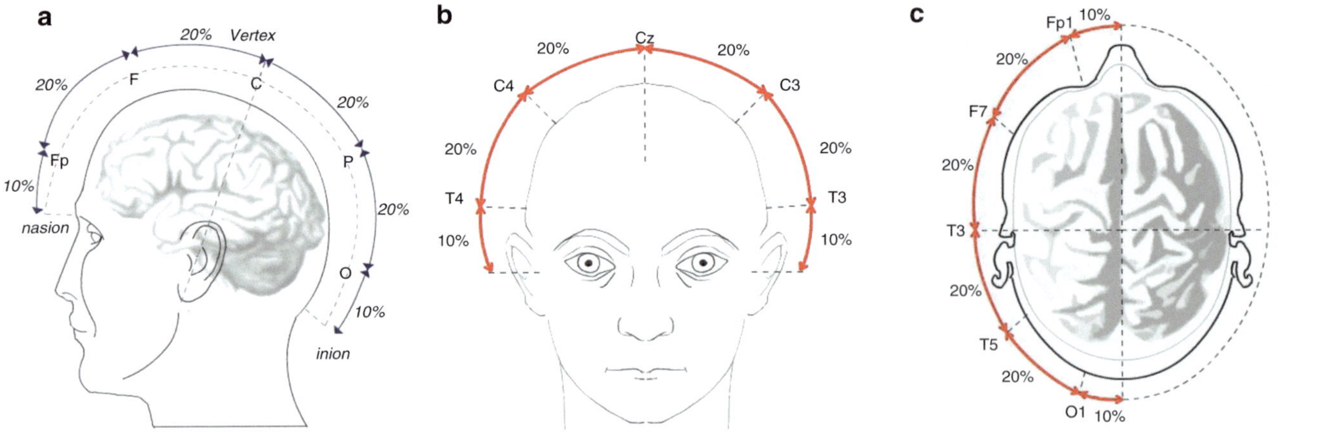

Fig. 4.1 Traditional 10-20 system. (**a**) Anteroposterior mesial line, connecting nasion and inion; (**b**) latero-lateral coronal line, connecting the two preauricular points, through the vertex; (**c**) sagittal lateral longitudinal line, connecting nasion and inion

– Latero-lateral coronal line, from the right to the left preauricular point, through the vertex. The preauricular points are identified as depressions at the root of the zygoma, just anterior to the auditory canal. Along this line, temporal electrodes (T4 to the right and T3 to the left) must be placed at 10% of the total distance, starting from the preauricular point while lateral central electrodes (C4 to the right and C3 to the left) must be placed at 20% from the temporal points (T4 and T3) and from the vertex (Cz) (Fig. 4.1b).

Starting from these two lines(i.e. the antero-posterior sagittal and the latero-lateral coronal) it is then possible to trace another two pairs of circumferential longitudinal lines in the anterior-posterior direction: lateral longitudinal line, from Fp2 to O2, through F8, T4 and T6 on the right; from Fp1 to O1, through F7, T3 and T5 on the left (Fig. 4.1c); longitudinal parasagittal line, from Fp2 to O2, through F4, C4 and P4 on the right; from Fp1 to O1, through F3, C3 and P3 on the left. Frontopolar electrodes (called Fp2 in the right and Fp1 in the left) are placed along the longitudinal line, at 10% of the distance to the side of Fpz, while for occipital electrodes (called O2 and O1) the 10% is measured with reference to Oz. Positions of the inferior frontal electrodes (F8 and F7) and posterior temporal electrodes (T6 and T5) are calculated at 20% of this line starting, respectively, from Fp2/Fp1 and O2/O1. The remaining frontal electrodes (F4 and F3) and parietal electrodes (P4 and P3) are placed along the frontal and parietal coronal lines, equally distant between the mesial and temporal lines on each side.

Standard numbering of the traditional 10-20 system establishes the disposition of even-numbered electrodes on the right side of the skull and of odd-numbered electrodes on the left side, identifying with letters the brain area above which they are positioned: Fp2, F4, F8, C4, P4, T4, T6 and O2 for the right hemisphere and Fp1, F3, F7, C3, P3, T3, T5 and O1 for the left hemisphere.

This measuring system identifies 21 standard electrode positions, including electrodes on the medial line (Fz, Cz, and Pz) and two reference auricular electrodes (A2 and A1) (Fig. 4.2a).

The International 10-20 system defined, in a short period of time, a standard scalp electrode positioning, allowing reliable comparisons of the acquired data from the various laboratories around the world. Nevertheless, the system is not exempt from criticisms. First of all, this system does not take into account that most human heads are asymmetrical. The posterior part of the skull is larger than the anterior one. Moreover, when dividing the skull in four quadrants (starting from nasion, inion and preauricular points), it can be noted that right-handed patients' heads temd to have a larger posterior quadrant on the left side and a larger anterior quadrant on the right side. For this reason, it would be necessary to arrange the electrodes proportionally not to the whole skull, but dividing it into four quadrants, meaning that the montage should be individualized.

For this reason, it is impossible that the interelectrode distances are the same along the longitudinal and transverse lines and, since interelectrode distance has a significant effect on the amplitude of the recorded signal, this problem should be carefully considered.

Furthermore, the relationship between the superficial positioning of the electrodes and the underlying anatomical structure was not correctly identified and, for this purpose, modern neuroimaging techniques should be better utilized. The 21 standard electrodes montage is not necessarily extensive enough to overlay all brain areas. For a correct detection of basal frontotemporal and mesial temporal areas, for example, specific additional electrodes are required.

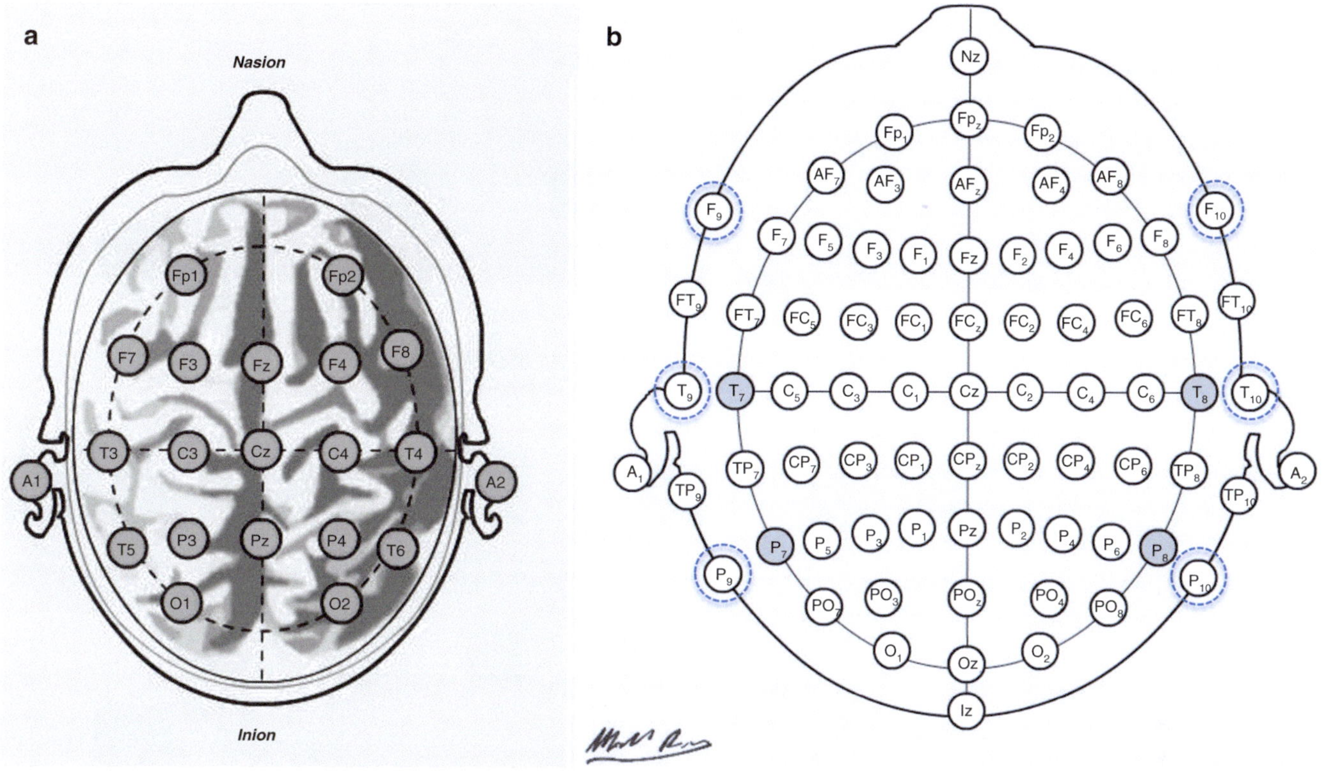

Fig. 4.2 (**a**) Standard positions of the 19 scalp electrodes and of the 2 ear reference electrodes, according to traditional 10-20 system; (**b**) modified 10-10 system, with 73 electrode positions on the scalp and 2 ear reference electrodes (note that the electrodes T8, P8, T7 and P7 replace the electrodes formerly named T4, T6, T3 and T5); the electrodes of the inferior temporal chain F10, T10, P10, F9, T9 and P9 (dotted circles) are actually recommended as new standard montage with 25 electrodes

4.2 Modification of 10-20 System (10-10 System)

Digital-EEG development and the introduction of high-density EEG and source localization methods made it necessary to increase the electrode arrays. Therefore, a modification of 10-20 nomenclature with the definition of 10-10 combinatorial nomenclature has been proposed and accepted by the American Clinical Neurophysiology Society (ACNS) and by the International Federation of Clinical Neurophysiology (IFCN) [3–7].

The modified combinatorial nomenclature is an extension of the 10-20 system and it entails the positioning on the scalp of more than 70 electrodes, placed along 11 sagittal chains and 9 coronal chains. The modified 10-10 terminology replaces the inconsistent T4/T3 and T6/T5 terms with the consistent T8/T7 and P8/P7 (Fig. 4.2b). The advantage of this new labelling is that all electrodes designated by the same letter are placed in the same coronal line and that all electrodes positioned along the same sagittal line have the same post-scripted number (except for Fp2/Fp1 and O2/O1); however, the disadvantage of the new nomenclature is represented by the fact that the letter "P" might suggest a *parietal* location, whereas P8/P7 are electrodes placed over the posterior temporal lobe. According to ACNS guidelines in the clinical context, it is still an acceptable alternative to continue to use T4/T5 and T6/T7 [6]. Electrodes between the frontal and central rows are named "FC", between the frontal and temporal rows "FT", between the central and parietal rows "CP" and between the parietal and occipital rows "PO". The electrodes between the frontopolar and frontal rows are named "AF", indicating "Anterior Frontal" placement [7].

The 10-10 system added also 10% contacts that are inferior to the standard frontotemporal and temporal-occipital chain. These electrodes are named F10/F9, FT10/FT9, T10/T9, TP10/TP9 and P10/P9. This inferior temporal chain may be completed with electrodes Fp10/Fp9, AF10/AF9, PO10/PO9 and O10/O9.

During the routine recordings with the traditional 10-20 system, the placement of the 19 standard scalp electrodes does not always detect the activity originating or propagating from mesial temporal structures. For this reason, the IFCN recommends a new standard array for clinical practice that includes the six electrodes of inferior temporal chain (F10/F9, 10% inferior to F8/F7; T10/T9, 10% inferior to T8/T7; P10/P9, 10% inferior to P8/P7): this results in a total of 25 electrodes placed on the scalp (Figs. 4.2b, 4.3 and 4.4) [7].

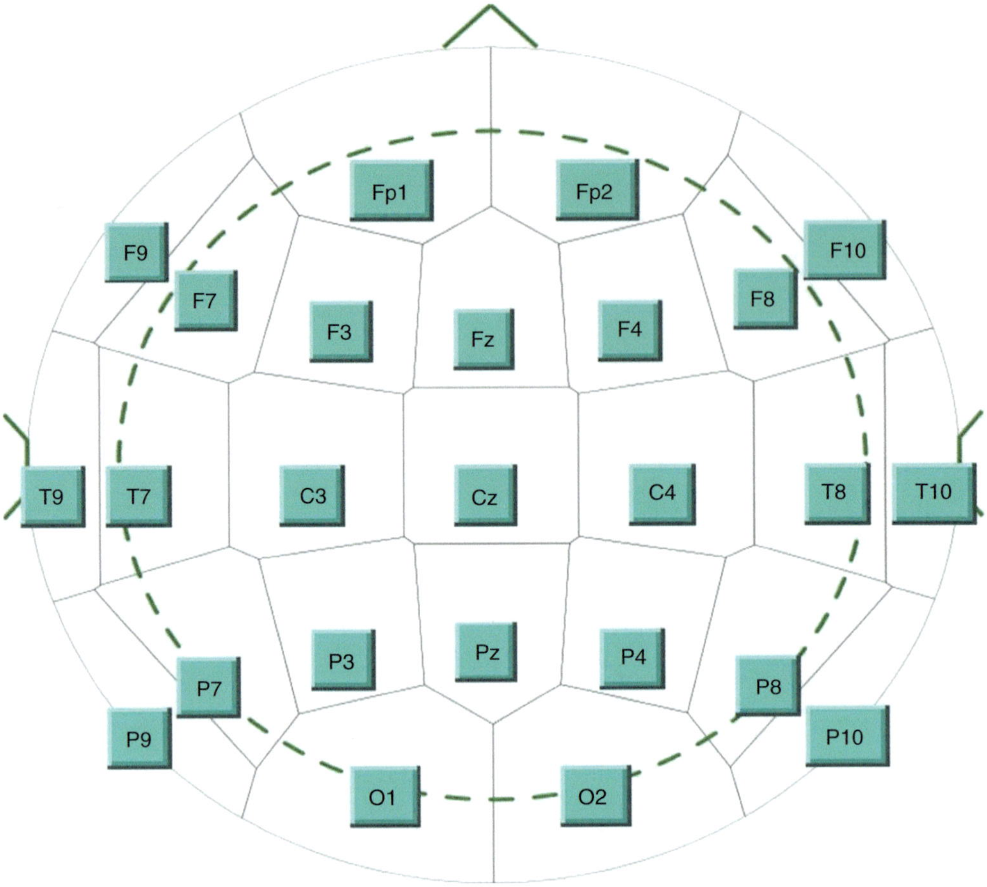

Fig. 4.3 New standard montage with additional coverage of the inferior and anterior brain regions, according to the recent recommendations of International Federation of Clinical Neurophysiology (from ref. [7], with permission)

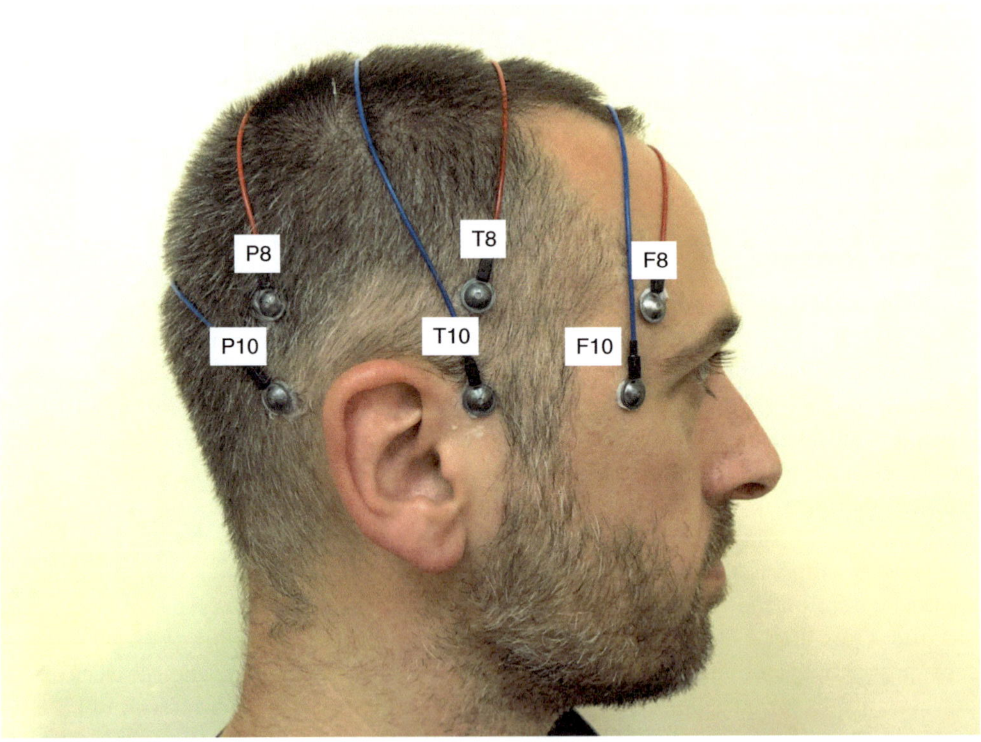

Fig. 4.4 Electrodes of the right inferior temporal chain according to new recommendations of IFCN (T8 = ex T4; P8 = ex T6)

Recently, it has been demonstrated that adding six electrodes in the inferior temporal chain to the traditional 10-20 system improves the identification of EEG abnormalities originating from the basal part of the temporal lobes [8].

4.3 Proposed 10-5 System for High-Resolution EEG

A further extension of 10-10 system, named 10-5 system, was proposed in 2001, but it has not yet been accepted by ACNS and IFCN [9]. The 10-5 proposed extension defines the position and nomenclature of 345 locations on the head and it can accommodate a homogeneous distribution of a subset containing, for example, 128 or 256 electrodes (Fig. 4.5a, b). The nomenclature of this system uses the combination of two letters to indicate the contours lying halfway between the original 10-20 system contours (the electrodes between the F and C contour were labelled FC and so on for others) [9]. In this way, the locations for the coronal contours from anterior to posterior were named: AF, AFF, F, FFC, FC, FCC, C, CCP, CP, P, PPO and PO. Electrodes for high-density EEG are applied by using expandable nets or caps with embedded electrodes and their localization is determined by digitization in three-dimensional space (Figs. 4.6 and 4.7).

4.4 Final Recommendations

Although in clinical practice the electrode placement method should be individualized on the basis of the clinical needs of the individual patient, the following recommendations should be considered, according to the guidelines of ACNS and IFCN: [6, 7].

- The 10-20 traditional system (21 electrodes) may be adequate for most of the patients, even for ambulatory or video-EEG long-term monitoring.
- In the suspicion of epilepsy or in epileptic patients without a clear visualization of the epileptic focus, supplementing the 10-20 EEG array with six electrodes for the inferior temporal chain (25 electrodes in total) is recommended.
- In children, except for special cases, the same number of electrodes as in adults is usually recommended.
- The 10-10 system should be used in epileptic patients undergoing pre-surgical evaluation and for source localization purpose.
- For the transition from the traditional system to the new larger arrays, the modification of EEG machine headboxes and a gradual process of educating operators on the new terminology are necessary.

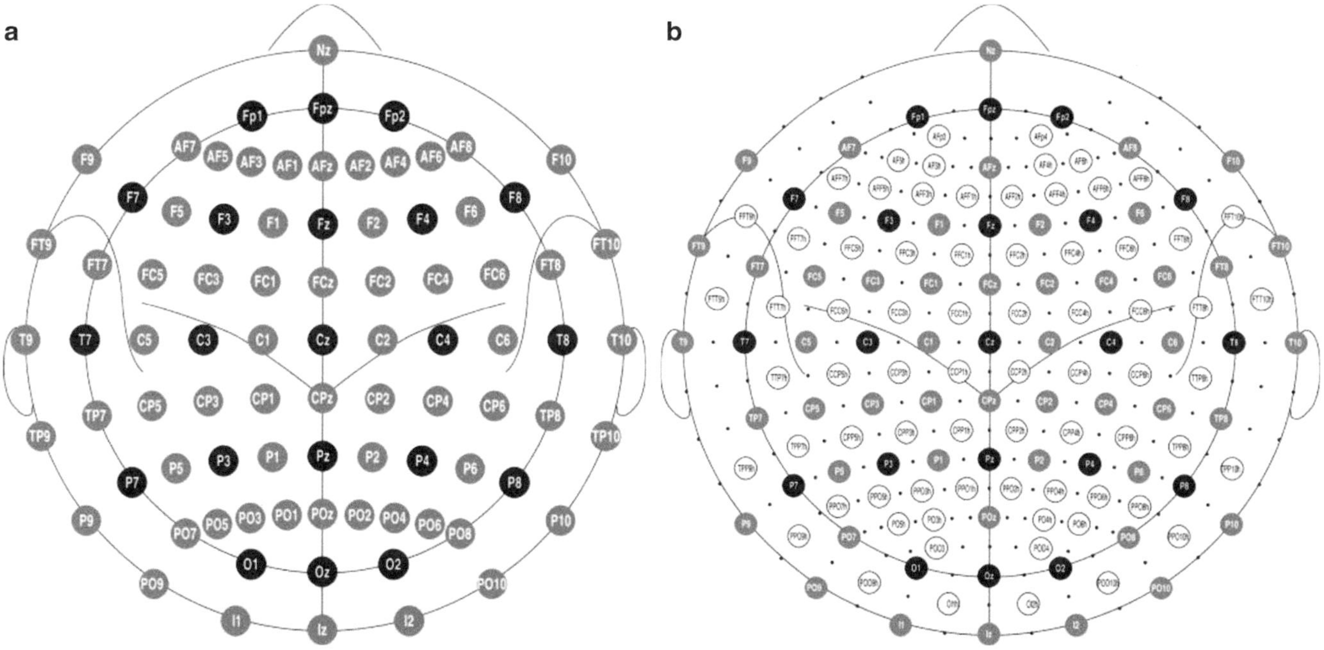

Fig. 4.5 The 10-10 and 10-5 extension of traditional 10-20 system. In (**a**) black circles indicate positions of the original 10-20 system and grey circles indicate additional positions introduced in the 10-10 extension. In (**b**) electrode positions in the proposed 10-5 system: additional positions to the 10-10 system are indicated with dots; a selection of additional positions useful for a 128 channel EEG system is indicated with open circles (from ref. [9], with permission)

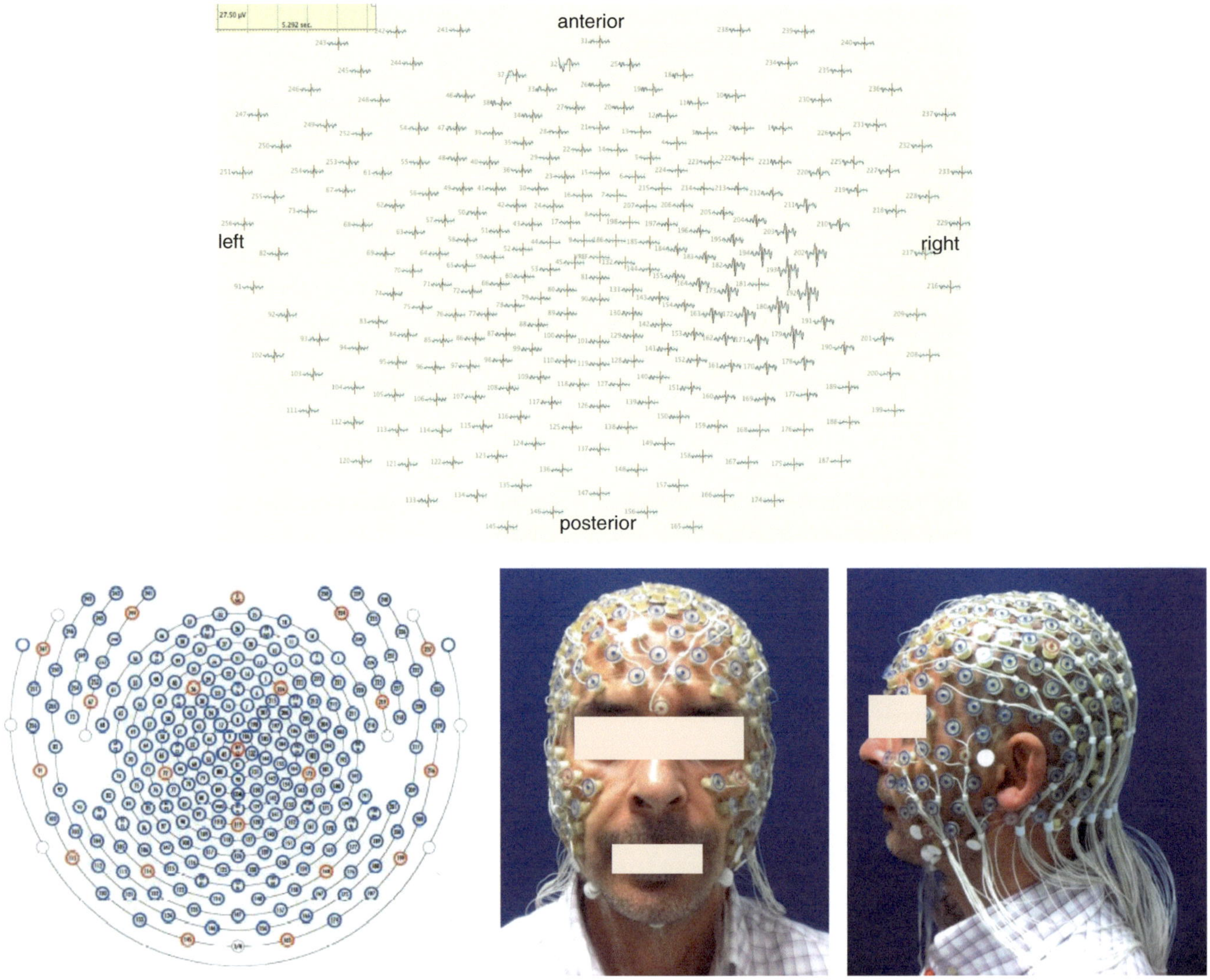

Fig. 4.6 An example of 256-channel high-density EEG, with projected locations of the electrodes on the scalp (courtesy from: Paolo Manganotti, Clinical Neurology Unit, University of Trieste—Italy)

4.5 Electrode Derivations and Montages

Brain electrical signals are displayed on the monitor depending on how the electrodes are connected to the amplifiers. Each amplifier has two electrode inputs (1 and 2) and the *potential measurement* represents the *potential difference* between these two points. From the electrical point of view, one of these points is called "common" or "ground" and its potential is deemed to be *zero*: unfortunately, ground points generate potentials and do not correspond to a real zero. This can be overcome by connecting two amplifiers together at the ground point and comparing the potential difference between their active inputs. Then, if two amplifier inputs (1 and 2) have the same polarity and voltage, the output will be zero (*in-phase rejection*) while, when these potentials are different, the recorded output value will be proportional to the difference between the two input values. Using differential amplifiers, only the difference between two inputs is known and not the absolute value of the potentials of electrodes attached to either inputs 1 or 2. Comparing a large number of electrode positions, EEG allows—with a good approximation—the localization of an abnormal activity on the scalp. In summary, on the monitor or recording paper, the signal is displayed with two fundamental characteristics: voltage and polarity. With regard to polarity, by convention, if the relative voltage difference is negative, the signal deflects upward and, if the voltage difference is positive, it goes downward. Therefore, if input 1 is more negative than input 2, the output signal will deflect upward, whereas if input 1 is more positive than input 2, the output signal will deflect downward. Finally, when inputs 1 and 2 have the same polarity and voltage, the output signal will be a flat line (Fig. 4.8).

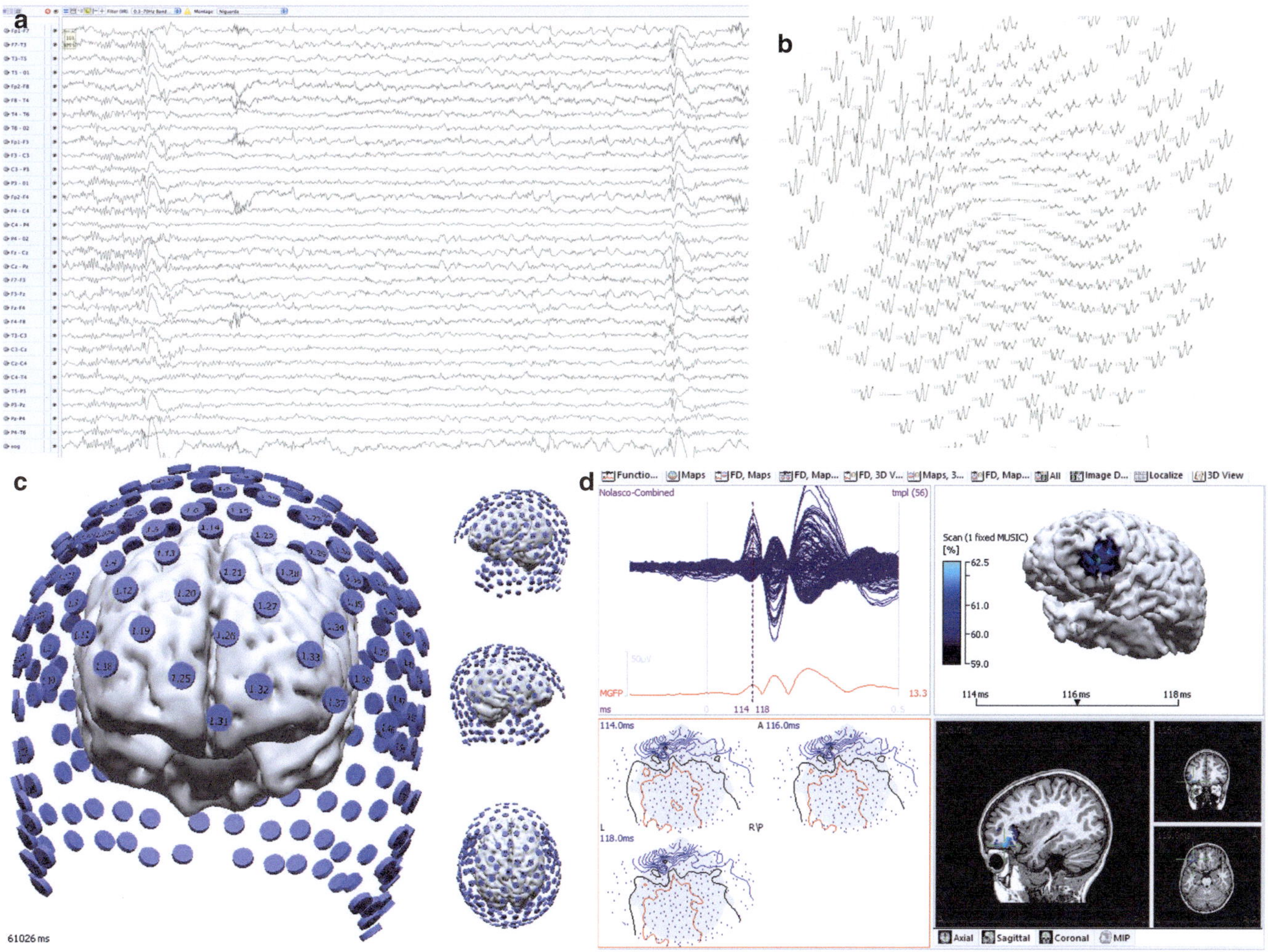

Fig. 4.7 Comparison of standard and high-density EEG in a patient with epileptic left temporal focus; (**a**) standard EEG recording with placement of electrodes according to 10-20 system; (**b**) recording of a single spike by 256 electrodes placed on the scalp; (**c**) the 256 placed electrodes projected onto a 3D image of the patient's brain, obtained by MRI; (**d**) source analysis of epileptic focus (56 spikes average) (courtesy from: Annalisa Rubino, Lino Nobili, Epilepsy Surgery Centre—Niguarda Hospital, Milan, and Child Neuropsychiatry, Department of Neurosciences, University of Genoa)

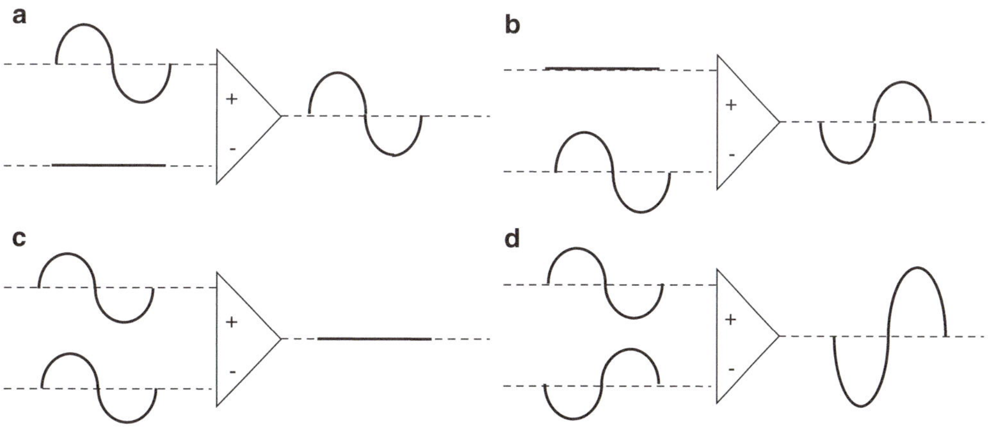

Fig. 4.8 Morphology and amplitude of different input signals of differential amplifiers and the respective output signals. The figure shows obviously ideal circumstances. If the signal is confined to a single channel (**a**, **b**), the output signal will have a different polarity, depending on the characteristics of input signal. If, instead, the two input signals are identical (with the same polarity), the output will be zero (**c**). Finally, if the two input signals have different polarity, the output signal will be the result of their summation (**d**)

Since there are endless input combinations that can generate the same output value, it is impossible to know the value of two inputs only knowing the output value of a differential amplifier. Back to EEG, if we imagine the electric fields on the surface of the scalp as the surface of the sea, rippled by waves of different sizes intersecting with each other, an EEG is rarely like a pond with almost imperceptible waves (when this happens, it means we are close to cortical activity suppression, characteristic of severe clinical conditions as brain death). Continuing with this analogy, electrodes are like corks, floating on the water, and the only thing we can do is to measure the height differences among them. This analogy would be perfect if the corks were correctly positioned, with regular distances, and if they were arranged in an orthogonal grid. A fixed point is then needed, as the shore to which all corks should refer.

In electroencephalography, aside from electrode positioning on the scalp (according to IS 10-20), a fundamental role is played by electrode combination (montage) and their type of connection to the amplifier (derivation). For historical and practical reasons, EEG is usually displayed as a set of traces showing how potential differences change over time. In a traditional EEG tracing (analog EEG), each trace is the result of the connection of two electrodes to the amplifiers and filters, with the signal sent to the galvanometer and to the writing device. With the introduction of digital EEG, the whole system has been replaced by computer software and hardware, but every trace continues to be called *channel*.

4.5.1 Reference Derivations

4.5.1.1 Common Reference

With this recording method, each electrode placed on the scalp is referred to as a common electrode, placed at a point x, on the scalp or elsewhere. The principle is similar to a geographical map, where the altitude of every location is measured in relation to the sea level. The common reference electrode should be as neutral as possible from the electrical point of view (not contaminated by cerebral electric potential nor by other biological electrical signals), which is a really rare occurrence. Fig. 4.9 shows the fundamental principles of the so-called *"inactive" common reference.* A potential with a negative voltage peak at the F3 electrode generates a surrounding electric field with gradient marked by the circular lines. The bilateral occipital and right parietotemporal areas are considered to have a uniform potential, which we can arbitrarily establish as zero. Therefore, the scalp electrodes T4, T6, P4, O2 and O1 and the A2 ear reference electrode have zero potential and they are consequently positive when compared to the other cerebral electrodes; they are also very different from F3 (which has the maximum negative peak). Starting from this situation, any point of the head can be chosen as a reference but, to better demonstrate the distribution of the potential generated under F3, the best option would be to choose an electrode not "contaminated" by this activity, like the A2 contralateral ear electrode or non-

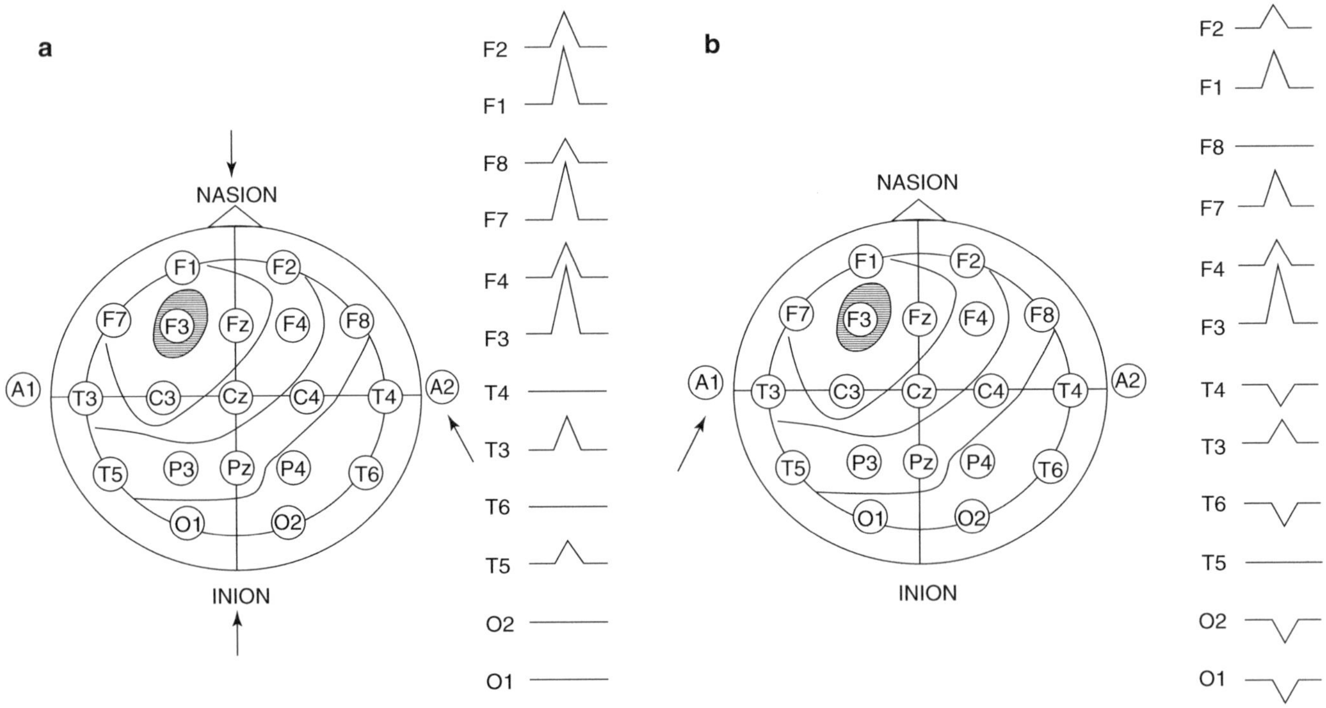

Fig. 4.9 Common reference recording (see text for explanation; F2 and F1 = Fp2 and Fp1). (**a**) reference electrode A2; (**b**) reference electrode A1

cephalic reference. Using A2 as a reference, the signals in this virtual situation would be displayed like in Fig. 4.9a.

Choosing the A1 left ear electrode as a reference, which is located inside the F3 electrical field and which has a low-amplitude negative potential when compared to the arbitrary zero (a common occurrence in normal practice), a very different pattern will be drawn: the channels showing lack of activity will be the ones with the same potential as the reference and, therefore, will be evened out; a downward deflection, caused by the relative negativity of the common reference, will be found instead on the electrodes placed in the area of zero potential (Fig. 4.9b).

An active scalp electrode can also be chosen as the *active common reference*. Figure 4.10 shows a virtual situation in which the electrode placed at F3 is chosen as the common reference. F3 is over the maximum electrical field on the scalp and it records the highest negative signal. Since, in this case, the reference is negative in comparison to other electrodes, all amplifiers will produce downward deflections. Moreover, since the electrodes surrounding the activity peak (F1, Fz, F7, C3) differ only slightly in potential from the reference, their corresponding channels will show smaller deflections than the ones farther away (the longer the distance from the reference, the higher the deflection).

The major drawback produced by active common reference is the *reference contamination*: when the reference electrode is placed close to a maximal peak potential, all the corresponding electrodes will be subjected to a change in voltage; all electrodes equipotential to the reference will be evened out, while the one least affected by the reference will show a pseudo-positivity. So, theoretically, given a known electric field (see Fig. 4.9), it would not be hard to estimate the shape of the wave that will appear on the EEG channel, depending on the reference. In practice, the concept must be reversed as we need to understand the distribution of the potentials on the scalp without knowing *a priori* - in a better way - the precise localization and the origin of the signal nor its positive or negative polarity.

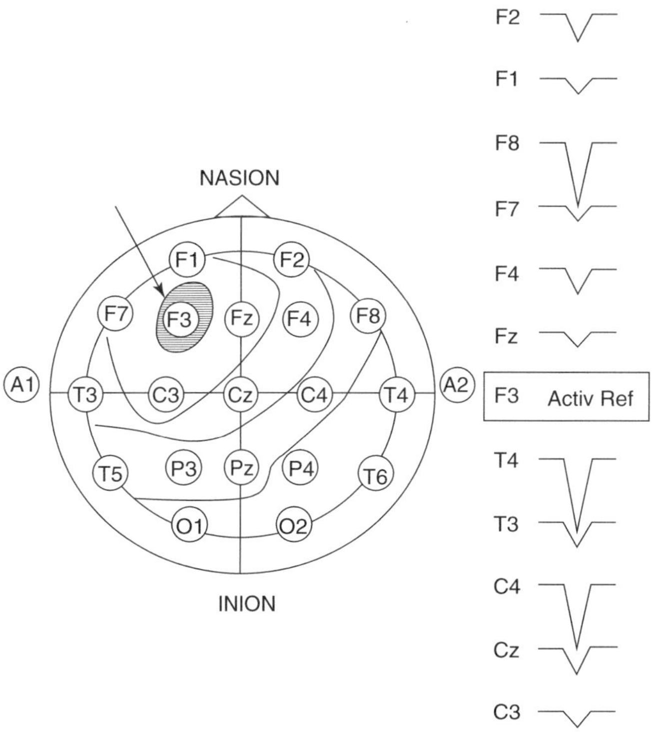

Fig. 4.10 Active common reference recording (see text for explanation; F2 and F1 = Fp2 and Fp1)

There are, however, more complex conditions than those mentioned above. For example, when it is necessary to analyse multiple events, localized to various electrodes, both synchronous and asynchronous, it could be difficult to interpret the resulting patterns.

All the problems analysed so far could be overcome by choosing an acceptable inactive reference electrode, placed in non-cephalic areas, named *physical* reference (neck-chest reference). Auricular or nuchal electrodes can be also chosen as the reference, but they cannot be considered completely "inactive". For example, electrical events generated from the temporal lobes can be recorded with auricular or mastoid electrodes; also nasal or mental electrodes can record activities originating from the orbital surfaces of the frontal lobes. On the other hand, when using a non-cranial reference, there is the risk of recording many artifacts: when they are in-phase in all channels, there is no problem for the interpretation, but when this does not occur, the EEG tracings can be completely obscured. Vertical eye movements produce high potential differences between scalp electrodes and the nasal or mental reference. Equally important are interferences produced by muscles and the ECG.

In conclusion, common reference tends to "contaminate" differential amplifiers, reducing in-phase rejection and increasing interferences; for this reason, depending on the particular situation, a specific reference should be chosen: auricular lobe or mastoid, omolateral or contralateral to the analysed activity (not recommended in the case of bilateral activity); electrodes placed along the mesial line in frontal region or at the vertex (not recommended in case of drowsiness or sleep because arousal phenomena mostly affect the reference electrode); nasal or mental electrodes (not recommended for alert patients because they produce larger artifacts).

Current digital EEG systems always refer the cerebral bioelectric signal to a common reference electrode, which typically has an input in patient headbox named G2 and which can be positioned on the scalp or elsewhere (usually, it is placed medially on the scalp, anterior to Fz or between Fz and Cz). The G2 common electrode is the common point referring to which all potentials of the single electrodes are measured (Fig. 4.11).

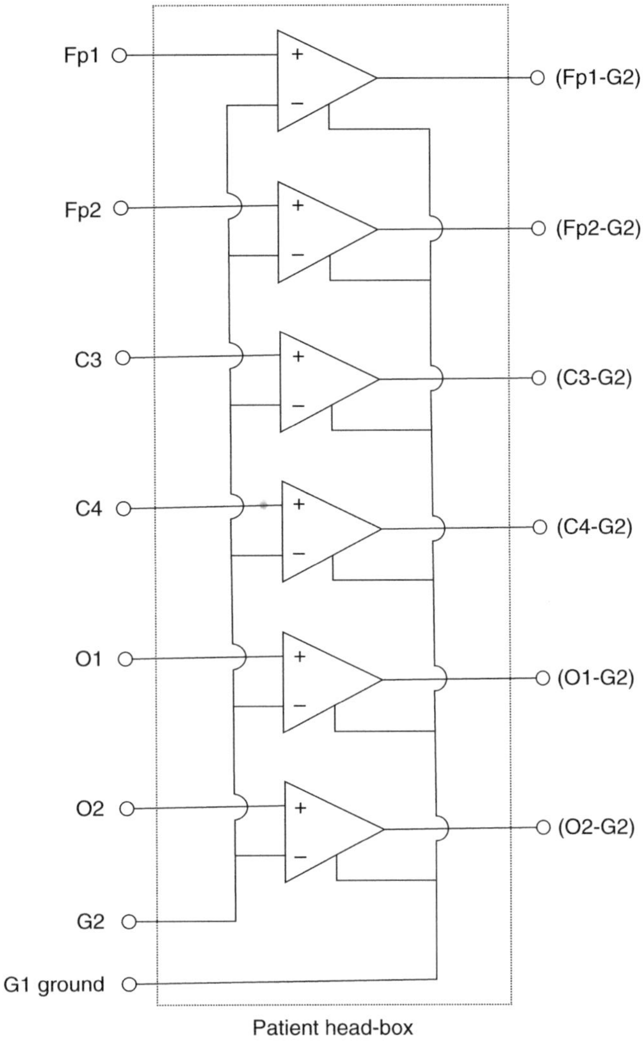

Fig. 4.11 G2—common reference recording. G2 electrode is connected to the inverting input (negative) of all amplifiers, while the electrode to be measured is connected to the non-inverting input. What the machine physically measures is the potential difference between each electrode and G2 (Fp1–G2, etc.)

4.5.1.2 Common Average Reference

Many of the problems encountered with the use of common reference can be overcome by average reference (AVG), a mathematical reference, introduced in electroencephalography by Goldman and Offner in 1950 [10, 11]. In this case, the potentials of single electrodes are referred to an instant average value obtained by adding together the potentials of all applied electrodes. The higher the number of electrodes, the closer to zero the reference average potential will be. In fact, one of the properties of the mathematical average of a series of numerical values is that the sum of the average differences equals zero. Regarding the results on the EEG tracings, this means that we will always have positive or negative deflections, with respect to the zero value of the reference.

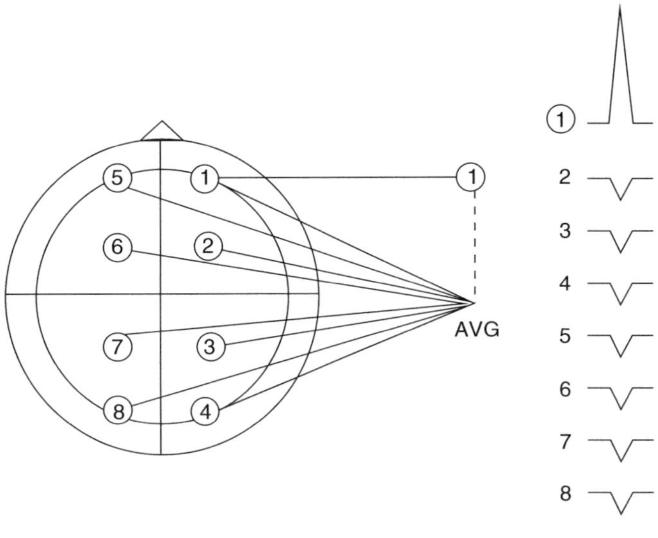

Fig. 4.12 Average reference (AVG) recording (see text for explanation)

In analog systems, this derivation method is achieved by joining all electrodes to a high resistor placed in a common place inside the device. Modern digital systems calculate the mathematical average of the potential differences of all the electrodes used at the same time, and moment by moment. Figure 4.12 exemplifies how AVG reference works. In this case, an ideal situation is presented with only eight electrodes applied to the scalp; electrode 1 has a more significant potential difference than the others (−80 μV), while the other electrodes remain at arbitral values of *zero*. The average of all electrodes will be:

$$\frac{-80+0+0+0+0+0+0+0}{8}=-10\mu V$$

As a result, electrode 1 will have a negative potential equal to:

$$-70\mu V\rightarrow\left[-80-(-10)=-70\mu V\right],$$

other electrodes will have a small positive potential equal to:

$$10\mu V\rightarrow\left[0-(-10)=10\mu V\right]$$

Therefore, the first electrode will have an upward deflection equal to −70 μV, while other electrodes will have a downward deflection equal to 10 μV.

More generally, when an electrode has a potential of value P, the AVG reference of that electrode will record a potential difference P_1 equal to:

$$\frac{P(n-1)}{n}$$

The higher the value of n, the closer P_1 will get to the value of P and the lower the deflections on the other channels will be. This means that the number of electrodes which contribute to average calculation should be as high as possible.

In digital electroencephalography, calculation of the average reference is achieved as follows (in this case, with application of 19 standard electrodes):

$$\frac{\left[(\text{Fp1}-\text{G2})+\text{Fp2}-\text{G2})+\ldots+(\text{O1}-\text{G2}\right)}{19}$$
$$=\frac{\left[\text{Fp1}+\text{Fp2}+\ldots+\text{O1}+\text{O2}\right]}{19}-\frac{19\times\text{G2}}{19}=\frac{[0]}{19}-\text{G2}=-\text{G2}$$

All above described is valid assuming that the average value of the 19 electrodes is 0. In this case, AVG value constitutes the absolute value of point G2. The AVG reference trace tells us that:

$$(\text{Fp1}-\text{AVG})=(\text{Fp1}-\text{G2})-(-\text{G2})=\text{Fp1}-\text{G2}+\text{G2}=\text{Fp1}$$

The recorded potential should then be the absolute potential of the Fp1 electrode.

Some systems are equipped to eliminate some of the electrodes from the total summation, but this can cause reviewing errors. Every average common derivation, whose deflections summation is other than zero, should be carefully and cautiously evaluated.

When we use an AVG reference, a localized event affects multiple channels, though the electrodes directly above the focal fields can usually be identified as the ones with higher amplitude deflections and of opposite polarity, compared to the majority of the other electrodes.

An accurate localization of a specific event is not easy in the case of multifocal and not in-phase potentials recorded by various electrodes, which will lead to activity resets.

Furthermore, the problem of contamination exists also in this case and it is accentuated in the case of high-amplitude localized activities on the scalp, including artifactual activity. To avoid this, the *correct average reference* can be calculated by excluding, from the average, the electrodes in which an excessively high-voltage or artifactual activity is recorded.

4.5.1.3 Source Derivation

Finally, a particular type of average reference is source derivation, introduced for the first time by Hjorth in 1975 [12] to improve the localization of focal activity on the scalp.

In this case, each electrode potential is referred to a reference making the weighted average of the electrodes around it. Its basic principle is that each cerebral generator causes a wave, which is much wider than the starting focal point. Source derivation tries to view focal generators as radial currents, travelling along the scalp, starting from the generator itself. This method is based on the application of Laplace's equation, according to which the radial current of a given point can be calculated by the second derivative of the electric field potential of that point. Basically, the radial current is calculated by the summation of the potential differences of the dipole created by the electrode in question and by the four surrounding electrodes. The resulting currents are called Laplacian. In the ideal situation where the focal point is located underneath the electrodes that are being observed, the Laplacian current will be the only visible one, while the value of the currents underneath the neighbouring electrodes will be zero. Source derivation, then, is nothing more than the visualization of a single electrode potential, compared to the weighted average of its neighbouring electrodes and the average weightings are inversely proportional to the distance between the electrode in question and its neighbours, from which the reference is calculated.

However, this technique has considerable limitations, including alteration of the real width of a potential and the generation of false opposition of polarity.

Figure 4.13a shows the differences that can be encountered using source derivation, starting from an "ideal" situation in which a high potential, placed under the F3 electrode and transmitted to the neighbouring electrodes in a variable manner, is recorded on the scalp with common reference (the F3 absolute potential is of 100 μV). With the source derivation method, considering the potential of F3 with respect to the weighted average of the four surrounding electrodes (Fp1, F7, C3, Fz), the resulting potential will be of 20 μV, significantly lower than the one we started from.

$$\text{F3}=100-\frac{80+80+80+80}{4}=20\mu V$$

Conversely, if the electrode F8 has an absolute potential of 0 (as in Fig. 4.13b), with source derivation method an opposite polarity (−40 μV) will be obtained, in comparison to the weighted average of the surrounding electrodes Fp2, F4, C4 and T4.

$$\text{F8}=0-\frac{40+80+40+0}{4}=-40\mu V$$

4.5.1.4 Bipolar Derivations

In bipolar derivations, the potential difference is calculated between electrode pairs, placed along chains (longitudinal or transversal) in which an electrode is shared with two following channels.

In this way, an event localized underneath a specific electrode will generate a deflection with the same voltage, but opposite polarity, in the two adjacent points in the chain of the electrode.

Figure 4.14a shows how the previously described theoretical example of common reference (maximum negative potential at F3 electrode) appears using bipolar derivation. The phenomenon known as *phase-reversal*, typical of bipo-

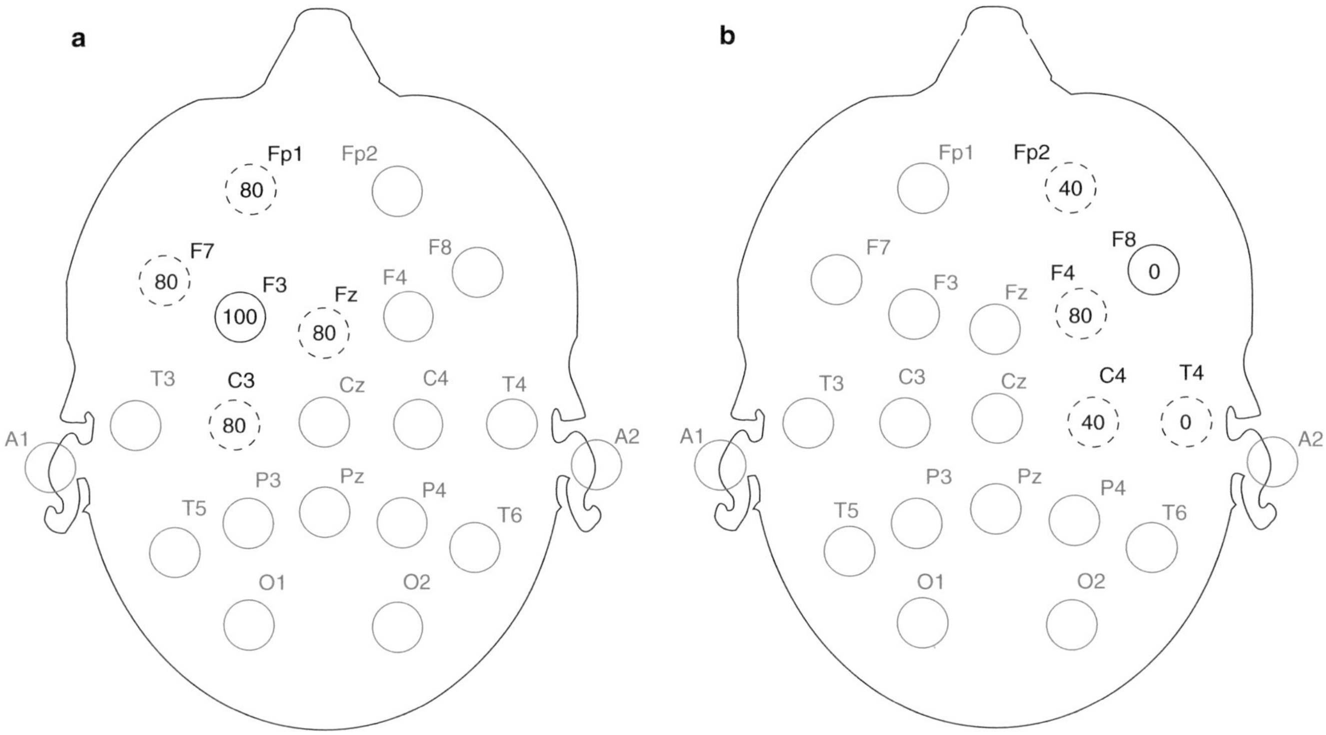

Fig. 4.13 Comparison between the absolute potential of F3 and F8 obtained with "inactive" common reference (CR) and that deriving from source derivation (SD) method. The dotted circles indicate the electrodes used for the source derivation. In (**a**) the absolute potential of F3. In (**a**) the absolute potential of F3 with CR is 100 μV and with SD 20 μV. In (**b**) the absolute potential of F8 is 0 μV with CR and—40 μV with SD

lar montages and caused by the fact that an electric event affects the electrode in the middle of the chain, occurs between channels 1 and 2. In this case, F3 localizes the maximum field and the reverse phase is due to the fact that it is a common electrode to the first and second channel. This is an *instrumental phase reversal,* because it is the instrument that causes the phase reversal; it must be distinguished from a *true phase reversal*, due to two different polarities simultaneously present in adjacent cortical areas.

When the maximum potential field is equally distant from the F3 and C3 electrodes (Fig. 4.14b), the second channel will not record any potential difference (zone of isopotentiality), while the phase reversal will be observed between the first and the third channel. Finally, if the maximum potential field takes place at the end of the chain (Fig. 4.14c), the only positive deflection will be detected in the channel connecting C3 with P3, possibly causing a wrong interpretation of the phenomenon. The phenomenon of phase reversal is shown also in Fig. 4.15.

Using bipolar derivations for a correct focal localization of the bioelectrical events, it is necessary to simultaneously display two electrode chains, placed perpendicular to each other: an accurate and exact localization is possible only when the phase reversal occurs at the point where the two lines intersect. In Fig. 4.16, the maximum focal field is localized in the quadrangle enclosed between the Fz, F4, C4 and Cz electrodes, with its relating isoelectric line on the channels connecting orthogonally the F4–C4 and C4–Cz electrodes. In conclusion, bipolar derivations have a remarkable localization ability but, in order to achieve this, it is essential that the various interelectrode chains are displayed simultaneously (anteroposterior and transversal).

With the bipolar montage, it is harder to compare the asynchrony between two homologous regions and it is difficult to map the voltage of a specifically localized event. It is also important to remember that in-phase activities affecting both inputs of the differential amplifier are evened out: therefore, spikes generating a fairly extensive area can be completely obscured or only partially shown. The opposite can also happen though: if a spike is positive in F4 and negative in C4, by pairing F4–C4 we will see a "false" spike of higher amplitude (addition-out-of-phase).

As already pointed out, recent digital EEG systems always use a reference derivation in signal acquisition, measuring the potential of each electrode with reference to a common electrode (G2).

With these systems it is possible, both online and offline, to reformat any type of montage and, thus, to display the tracing both in reference (common or AVG) and in bipolar derivation. To reformat a bipolar derivation starting from the one using G2 as a common electrode, the computer executes the following process:

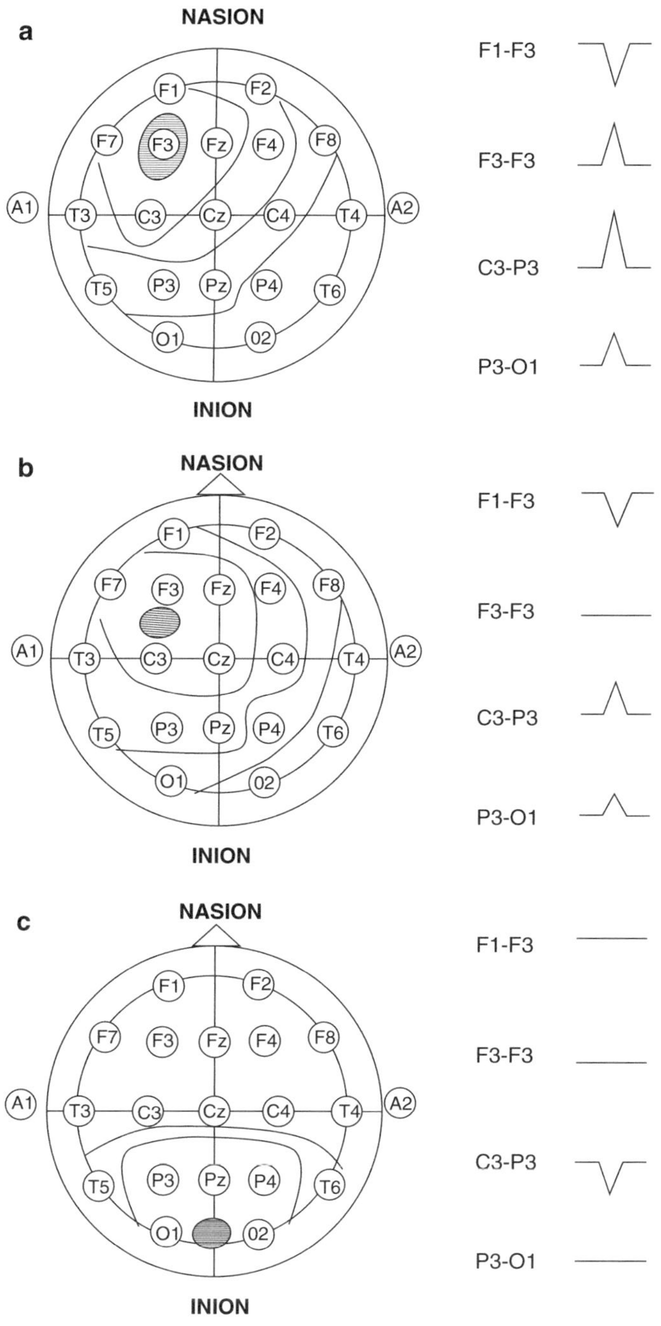

Fig. 4.14 Bipolar derivation recording (see text for explanation). (**a**) maximum negative potential at F3 electrode, phase reversal phenomenon; (**b**) zone of isoipotentiality when maximum potential field is equally distant from F3 and C3; (**c**) maximum potential field at the end of the chain: only positive deflection will be detected in the channel connecting C3 with P3

$$(\mathrm{Fp2} - \mathrm{G2}) = \mathrm{A}$$

$$(\mathrm{F4} - \mathrm{G2}) = \mathrm{B}$$

$$\mathrm{A} - \mathrm{B} = (\mathrm{Fp2} - \mathrm{G2}) - (\mathrm{F4} - \mathrm{G2}) = \mathrm{Fp2} - \mathrm{G2} - \mathrm{F4} + \mathrm{G2} = \mathrm{F2} - \mathrm{F4}$$

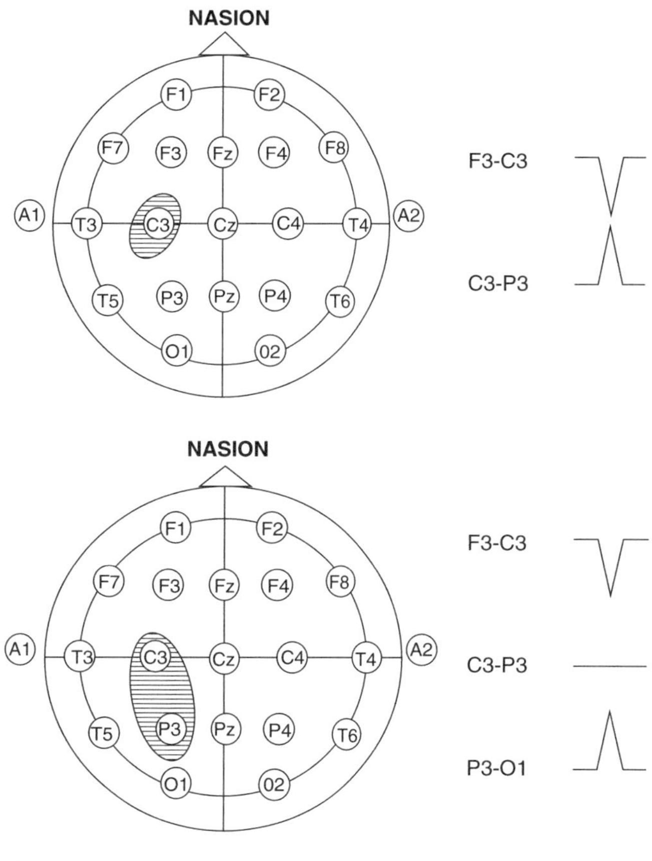

Fig. 4.15 Schematic representation of an instrumental phase reversal phenomenon between F3–C3 and C3–P3 channels. A maximum field potential underneath C3 will be observed in phase reversal on the two channels having C3 in common (*above*) while, if the event equally affects the two adjacent electrodes C3 and P3, the potential will be cancelled on the channel connecting these two electrodes (*below*)

Through this simplified mathematical calculation, the computer is able to reformat the montage and show it as bipolar, subtracting the value of G2 electrode, used as reference.

4.5.1.5 Choice of Derivation in Clinical Practice

Since EEG patterns are variable (focal or diffuse, transient or persistent), there is not one single ideal derivation to highlight all cerebral activities. A first important factor to take into account in the choice of derivation is the *interelectrode distance*, and this is particularly valid for active common references and bipolar derivations. In bipolar derivations, distances between the paired electrodes are small and equal, favouring the detection of the fast EEG activities; in active common reference, distances are bigger and unequal, facilitating the amplification of the signal, thus better showing the slower activities.

Focal epileptic activity is a phenomenon that provokes a change in the potential, limited to a small part of the scalp. In order to accurately localize a strictly isolated focal potential with bipolar derivations, it is necessary to demonstrate the simultaneous phase reversal at the point of intersection between two electrode chains placed perpendicular to each

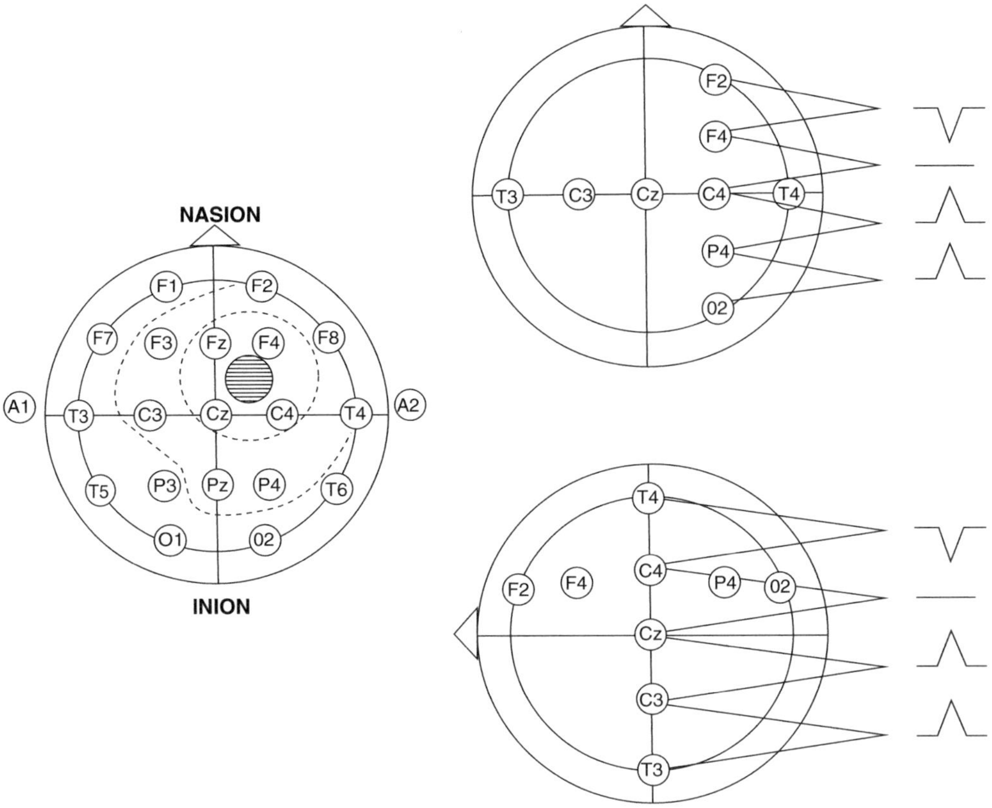

Fig. 4.16 In bipolar derivations the correlation between longitudinal and transversal interelectrodic chains allows a more accurate localization of focal event with the identification of phase reversal and isopotentiality phenomena (see text for further explanation)

other: therefore, it is necessary to use a suitable montage and, sometimes, to also apply additional electrodes.

Common reference does not present such limitations and it has some advantages, especially for the detection of an epileptic activity with a not very good localized focus; it is important, though, to be sure that the chosen reference is not contaminated by the activity of the phenomenon itself (e.g., in case of a focus with centrotemporal spikes, the ideal common reference is placed on the contralateral auricular lobe).

Average reference seems to be the preferable technique, even if the problem of contamination still exists for all channels (it is thus advisable to calculate the correct average reference, obtained by excluding the most active electrodes from the average calculation). When the focus is recorded by multiple electrodes, the phenomenon is better showed using common reference (preferably inactive), which provides a better definition of the potential distribution and of the shape of the wave.

In order to correctly identify and localize any focal activity, it should always be best to use more than one derivation. Generally, it is important to bear in mind some important considerations:

- Common reference allows to locate focal activity with higher voltage and with the same polarity.
- Average reference shows a wider signal underneath one or more electrodes, but of opposite polarity than the majority of other electrodes.
- Bipolar derivation localizes focal activity highlighting the phase reversal or cancellation of the signal (zone of isopotentiality).

Figure 4.17 shows how visualization of a real right temporal epileptic focus, recorded with a digital system, which varies depending on the displayed derivations.

Most of EEG diffuse activities are correctly evidenced by bipolar derivations, while average reference (AVG) can be misleading, possibly showing a localized phenomenon as a diffuse one. However, with bipolar derivation, the potential differences between adjacent electrodes are recorded and there are no indications regarding the activity of each electrode with respect to a distant reference point; in addition, bipolar derivation can show a reduction in signal amplitude or, within a widespread pattern, it can underestimate focal amplitude reductions, which has the same localization value as spikes. Generally, EEG diffuse activities are better evidenced by a common reference derivation, but the reference electrode should not be affected by the studied activity and so, when this is not possible, it should be placed in a way that allows equal recording of both hemispheres. An extracranial medial reference, for example, can be used. Fig. 4.18 shows a widespread spike-wave discharge, predominant anteriorly, with the three recording methods.

To summarize, the main advantages and disadvantages of the derivation systems are the following:

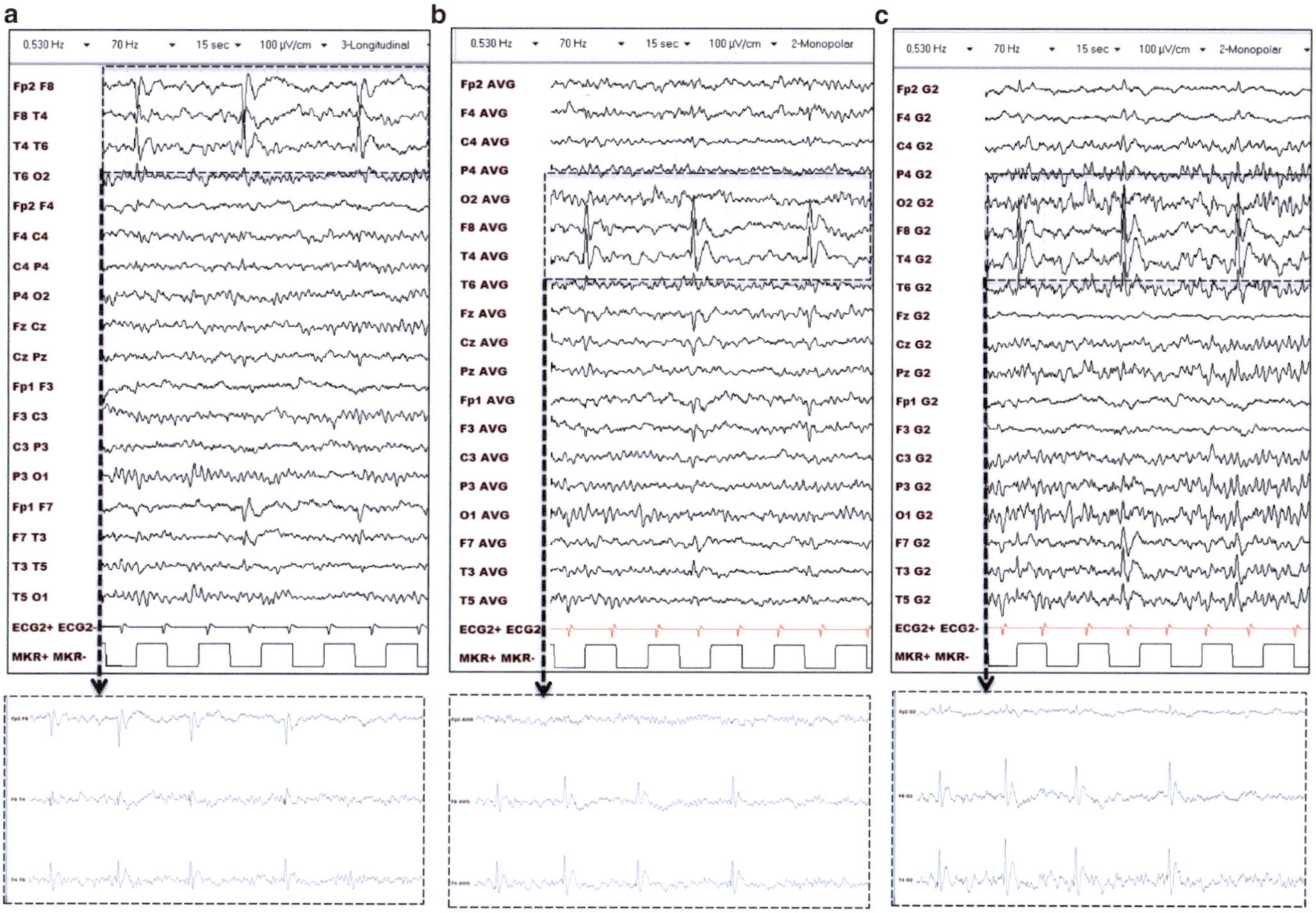

Fig. 4.17 The same EEG epoch of 5 s shows a right temporal epileptic focus in bipolar, AVG reference and common active reference derivations. In (**a**) (bipolar derivation) the phase reversal phenomenon in the first and third channel is evident, with almost total cancellation of the spikes in the intervening channel F8–T4 (these electrodes are placed over the focus and their potentials presumably have the same polarity and voltage as input to the differential amplifiers); note the poor spread of spikes to the homologous contralateral areas. The AVG reference derivation (**b**) confirms the higher negative signals at F8 and T4 electrodes; note, however, that positive signals are present also in Fz, Cz, Fp1 and F3, and negative in F7 and T3. When a common active electrode of reference is used (**c**) (G2, placed on midline in Fpz), the signal shows the same negative higher voltage in F8 and T4, with the evidence of synchronous lower negative signals contralaterally in F7, T3 and T5. However, in this practical example, all three derivations allow to localize the epileptogenic focus with good reliability (T4, T6, T3, T5 = T8, P8, T7, P7 according to the new nomenclature)

1. Common reference derivation.
   (a) Good localization of any kind of focal activity (including low-voltage or flat activity).
   (b) Good wave-shape definition.
   (c) Acceptable localization of the most common artefacts.
   (d) Good mapping of diffuse activity.
   (e) Acceptable evaluation of bilateral synchrony of homologous areas.
   (f) If the reference is not inactive, its activity will “contaminate” the related electrodes, compromising the above-listed advantages.
2. Average reference derivation.
   (a) Acceptable localization of transient focal graphoelements
   (b) Poor wave-shape definition (except for sharp focal potentials on a low-voltage background activity)
   (c) Unsatisfactory highlighting of areas with low-voltage activity
   (d) Poor artifact localization
   (e) Unreliable in cases with high-voltage asynchronous diffuse activity
   (f) Unreliable when one or several electrodes record high-amplitude activity, influencing the calculation of the average too much
3. Bipolar derivation
   (a) Good localization of transient focal activity
   (b) Good definition of bilateral synchrony-symmetry of homologous areas
   (c) Good localization of the most common artefacts

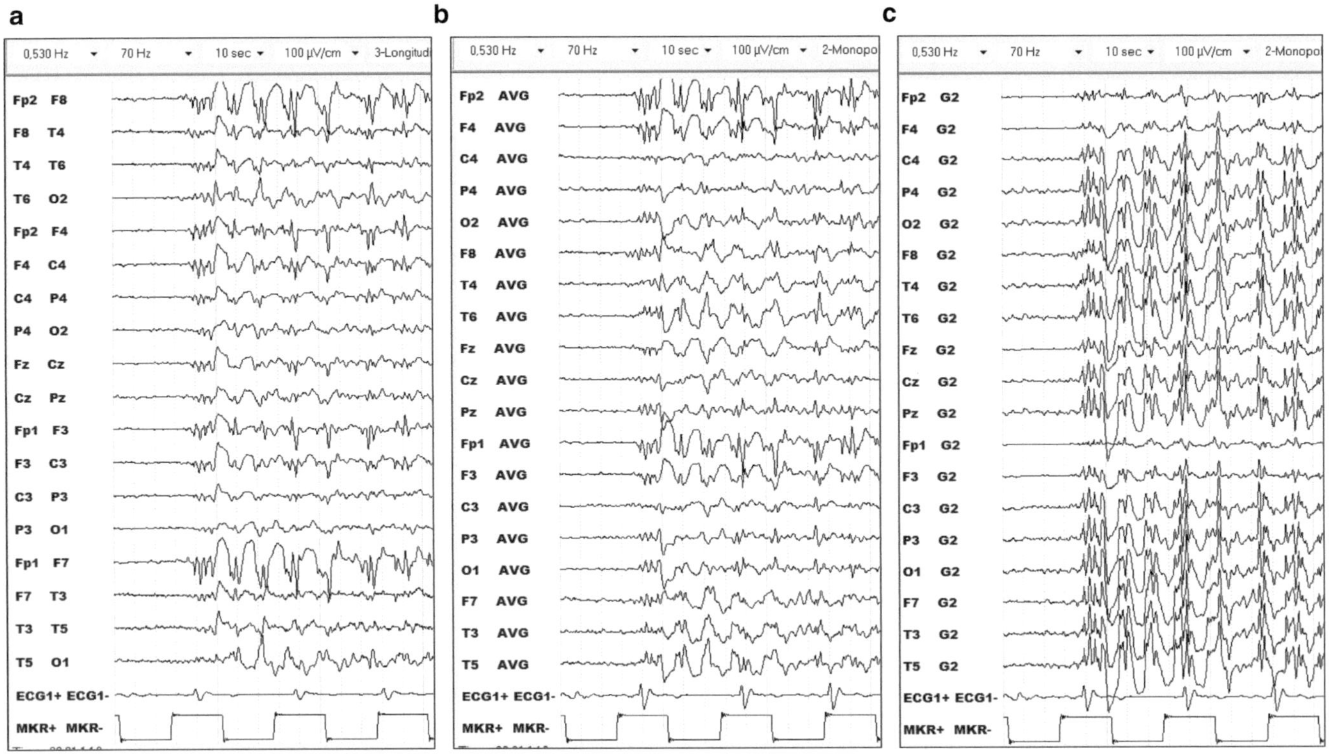

Fig. 4.18 Diffuse discharge of polyspikes and spike-and-wave complexes, predominantly in anterior areas. The bipolar (**a**) and AVG reference derivation (**b**) show the real characteristic of discharge, while the common active reference derivation (with G2-reference electrode placed in Fpz) is misleading (**c**). In (**c**) the contamination reference is very evident and the electrodes with larger signals are precisely those closest to the reference electrode; in them, therefore, the recorded activity is significantly reduced in voltage (T4, T6, T3, T5 = T8, P8, T7, P7 according to the new nomenclature)

(d) Poor mapping of diffuse activity
(e) Poor or non-existent emphasizing of areas with absence or reduction in signal voltage
(f) Suppression or reduction in amplitude of in-phase activity on a pair of electrodes (isopotentiality areas)
(g) Not always good wave-shape definition

4.5.2 Montages

A montage is the specific method of electrode connection to the recording channel of the electroencephalograph. With 21 electrode positions in the 10-20 system and 16 channels on display, the number of possible montages is 21. The 10-10 system, with more than 70 electrode positions, allows the creation of an even higher number of montages and the modern digital EEG machines allow the display of up to 256 channels.

A wide range of montages, many of which are complex and inadequate, is used in EEG laboratories for routine recordings. This dissimilarity prevents the correct exchange of information between experts in the field. To counteract this, both the International Federation of Clinical Neurophysiology (IFCN) and the American Clinical Neurophysiology Society (ACNS) have published some guidelines which include ad hoc recommendations [7, 13].

The montages for routine EEG recording are designated as Longitudinal Bipolar (LB), Transverse Bipolar (TB), or Referential (R). Montages are designed for 18, 20, 26 and more channels. Here we report a list of the main recommendations drawn from the above-mentioned guidelines:

- Not less than 16 channels of simultaneous recording should be used (a larger number of channels would be encouraged).
- At least 21 electrodes should be placed following the 10-20 system (the IFCN recommend at least 25 electrodes, including the inferior temporal chain) [7].
- Both bipolar and referential montages should be used for clinical interpretation.
- The electrode derivations of each channel should be clearly identified at the beginning of each montage, so that the pattern of electrode connection is made as simple as possible and easily comprehensible.
- In bipolar derivations, electrode pairs should run in straight lines and their interelectrode distance should be kept equal.
- Channel progression must be anterior-posterior.

Guidelines also recommend that a single channel Electro Cardio Gram (ECG) should be included on one EEG channel.

According to IFCN and ACNS, channels obtained by connecting the left-side electrodes should be above the right-sided ones. This recommendation coincides with the prevailing practice of the vast majority of EEG laboratories in North America and in other areas, but it is not followed in Italy and in many other European countries. In this book, according to the tradition of the Italian and European neurophysiological academic school and the totality of clinical practice in our country, the right-sided leads are placed above the left-sided leads for either blocks of derivations.

Regarding referential montages, the choice of reference is critically important. For the ACNS, a midline electrode (as Cz) would be a better choice of reference than A1 or A2. However, the referential suggested montages by ACNS establish the right auricular electrode (A2) as reference for the electrodes on the right side and the left auricular electrode (A1) for the ones on the left side.

Currently, in digital electroencephalography, the G2 reference electrode can be used as an "active" reference, placing it on the midline, anteriorly to Fz.

Figures 4.19 and 4.20 show suggested bipolar longitudinal and transverse montages with the extended standard array. Table 4.1 shows bipolar (old and new) and referential suggested montages. According to 10-10 position nomenclature, T4, T6, T3 and T5 should be changed to T8, P8, T7 and P7.

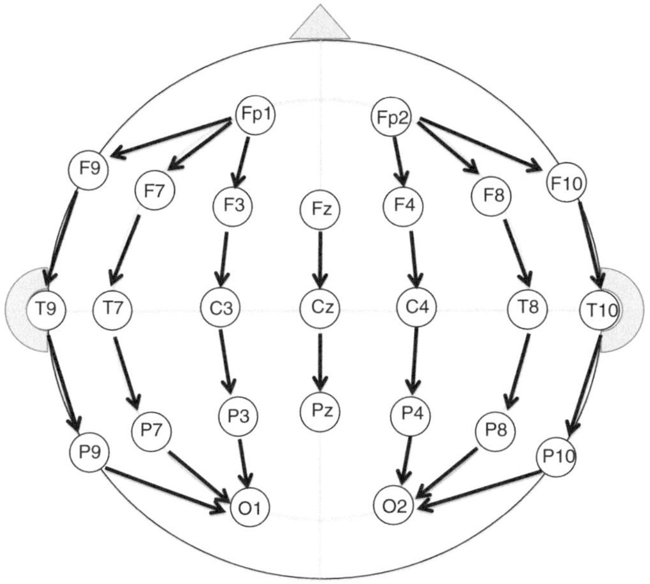

Fig. 4.19 New longitudinal bipolar montage proposed by International Federation of Clinical Neurophysiology (IFCN) [7]

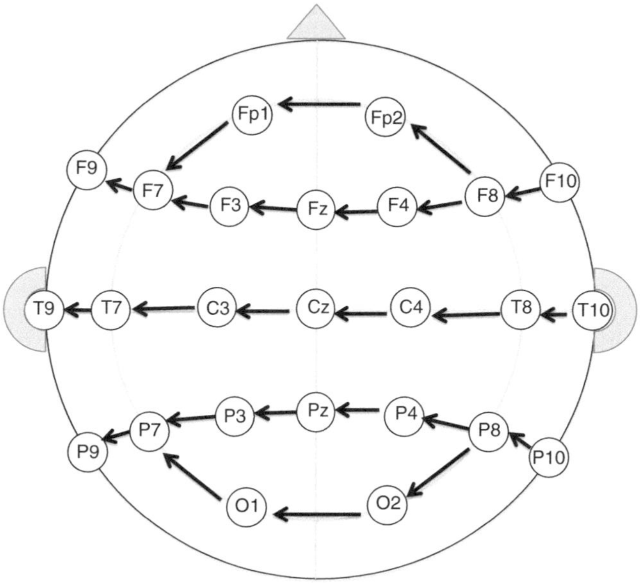

Fig. 4.20 New transverse bipolar montage proposed by International Federation of Clinical Neurophysiology (IFCN) [7]. Note that the interelectrode distance between the inferior and superior temporal electrodes is shorter (10%) compared to the other interelectrode distances (20%)

Table 4.1 Suggested old/new Longitudinal Bipolar (LB) and Transverse Bipolar (TB) and referential montages with the extended standard array [7]

No. channel	LB montage (old)	No. channel	LB montage (new)	No. channel	TB montage (old)	No. channel	TB montage (new)
1	Fp2—F8	1	Fp2—F10	1	F8—Fp2	1	F8—Fp2
2	F8—T8 (F8–T4)	2	F10—T10	2	Fp2—Fp1	2	Fp2—Fp1
3	T8—P8 (T4–T6)	3	T10—P10	3	Fp1—F7	3	Fp1—F7
4	P8—O2(T6–O2)	4	P10—O2	4	F8—F4	4	F10—F8
5	Fp2—F4	5	Fp2—F8	5	F4—Fz	5	F8—F4
6	F4—C4	6	F8—T8	6	Fz—F3	6	F4—Fz
7	C4—P4	7	T8—P8	7	F3—F7	7	Fz—F3
8	P4—O2	8	P8—O2	8	T8—C4 (T4–C4)	8	F3—F7
9	Fz—Cz	9	Fp2—F4	9	C4—Cz	9	F7—F9
10	Cz—Pz	10	F4—C4	10	Cz—C3	10	T10—T8
11	Fp1—F3	11	C4—P4	11	C3—T7 (C3–T3)	11	T8—C4
12	F3—C3	12	P4—O2	12	P8—P4 (T6–P4)	12	C4—Cz
13	C3—P3	13	Fz—Cz	13	P4—Pz	13	Cz—C3
14	P3—O1	14	Cz—Pz	14	Pz—P3	14	C3—T7
15	Fp1—F7	15	Fp1—F3	15	P3—P7 (P3–T5)	15	T7—T9
16	F7—T7 (F7–T3)	26	F3—C3	16	P8—O2 (T6–O2)	16	P10—P8
17	T7—P7 (T3–T5)	27	C3—P3	17	O2—O1	17	P8—P4
18	P7—O1 (T5–O1)	18	P3—O1	18	O1—P7 (O1–T5)	18	P4—Pz
19	ECG	19	Fp1—F7	19	ECG	19	Pz—P3
		20	F7—T7			20	P3—P7
		21	T7—P7			21	P7—P9
		22	P7—O1			22	P8—O2
		23	Fp1—F9			23	O2—O1
		24	F9—T9			24	O1—P7
		25	T9—P9			25	ECG
		26	P9—O1				
		27	ECG				

References

1. Jasper HH. The ten-twenty electrode system of the International Federation. Electroencephalogr Clin Neurophysiol. 1958;10:371–5.
2. Klem GH, Luders HO, Jasper HH, Elger C. The ten-twenty electrode system of the International Federation of Clinical Neurophysiology. Electroencephalogr Clin Neurophysiol Suppl. 1999;52:3–6.
3. American Electroencephalographic Society. Guideline thirteen: guidelines for standard electrode position nomenclature. J Clin Neurophysiol. 1994;11:111–3.
4. Nuwer MR, Comi G, Emerson R, et al. IFCN standards for digital recordings of clinical EEG. Electroencephalogr Clin Neurophysiol. 1998;106:259–61.
5. American Clinical Neurophysiology Society. Guideline 5: guidelines for standard electrode position nomenclature. J Clin Neurophysiol. 2006;23:107–10.
6. Acharya JN, Hani A, Cheek J, Thirumala P, Tsuchida TN. American clinical neurophysiology society guideline 2: guidelines for standard electrode position nomenclature. J Clin Neurophysiol. 2016;33:308–11.
7. Seeck M, Koessler L, Bast T, et al. The standardized EEG electrode array of the IFCN. Clin Neurophysiol. 2017;128:2070–7.
8. Justesen AB, Johansen ABE, Martinussen NI, et al. Added clinical value of the inferior temporal EEG electrode chain. Clin Neurophysiol. 2018;129:291–5.
9. Oostenveld R, Praamstra P. The five percent electrode system for high resolution EEG and EPR measurements. Clin Neurophysiol. 2001;112:713–9.
10. Goldman D. The clinical use of the "average" reference electrode in monopolar recording. Electroencephalogr Clin Neurophysiol. 1950;2:209–12.
11. Offner FF. The EEG as potential mapping: the value of the average monopolar reference. Electroencephalogr Clin Neurophysiol. 1950;2:213–4.
12. Hjorth B. An on-line transformation of EEG scalp potentials into orthogonal source derivation. Electroencephalogr Clin Neurophysiol. 1975;39:526–30.
13. Acharya JN, Hani AJ, Thirumala PD, Tsuchida TN. American clinical neurophysiology society guideline 3: a proposal for standard montages to be used in clinical EEG. J Clin Neurophysiol. 2016;33:312–6.

5 EEG Signal Acquisition

Cristiano Rizzo

5.1 Introduction

Electroencephalography (EEG) signal acquisition originated in the 1930s, but not until the development of digital systems in the 1980s was there a significant impact on the technology, particularly with respect to EEG signal analysis.

Before digital technology, EEG systems were analogues, recording signals using pens directly onto paper that didn't allow any further modifications or processing. It was only possible to inspect or "read" the ink tracing and add some handwritten comments or observations.

The adoption of digital technologies allowed the data to be stored into a computer and subsequently processed and displayed. This has opened new opportunities for the user to analyse and display the data which has changed the way EEG data is "read". Not only is the EEG now read on a high-resolution PC screen and manipulated, but the screen can display additional information that is of added value to the reporting process.

In order to appreciate the significance of digital electroencephalograph, this chapter will explore the structure of a modern data collection system to identify the different components and understand their function. The next chapter describes some of the ways data can be processed and/or analysed.

This chapter presents information that is essential for the overall understanding of a digital electroencephalograph system. Other information that is not essential will be found as notes or in the appendix and can be read only if deemed necessary. This is to simplify the text for those who want an overview of the topic but also provides more detailed information for those who wish to understand more.

5.1.1 Digital EEG System Structure

A digital electroencephalograph (Fig. 5.1) is a system composed of the following main elements:

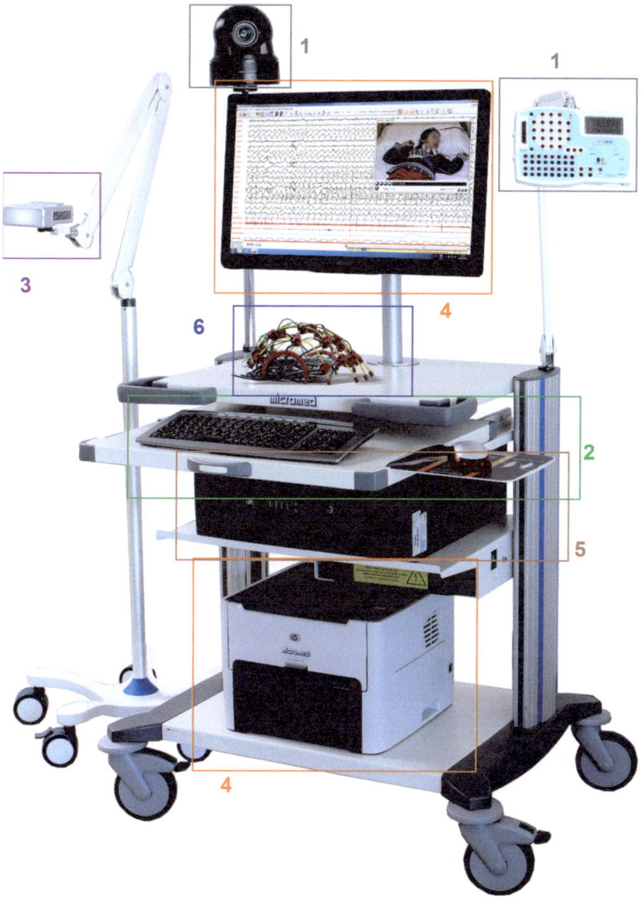

Fig. 5.1 Digital electroencephalograph

C. Rizzo (✉)
Micromed S.p.A., Mogliano Veneto, Italy
e-mail: cristiano.rizzo@micromed.eu

O. Mecarelli (ed.), *Clinical Electroencephalography*, https://doi.org/10.1007/978-3-030-04573-9_5

1. Data acquisition devices
   (a) EEG "headbox" - Amplifier
   (b) Video camera
2. Manual input devices
   (a) Keyboard
   (b) Mouse
3. Stimulation devices
   (a) Photic stimulator
4. Output devices
   (a) Monitor
   (b) Printer
5. Processing devices
   (a) Computer
6. Recording accessories
   (a) Electrodes
   (b) Caps
   (c) Conductive gel
7. Supports
   (a) Carts
   (b) Arms/stands

The *data acquisition devices* are the core of the system and convert the analogue signals and visual images collected from the patient to a digital representation that can be stored in a computer. The main component of the entire EEG system is the *headbox* and collects the EEG data from the patient and will be the subject of most of this chapter. The *video camera* is the device that records the continuous image (video) of the patient and is closely synchronized with the electrical (EEG) information. Section 5.5 describes the Video in more detail.

The *input devices*, usually a *keyboard* and *mouse*, allow the user to enter additional information into the system and to control the system functionality.

The *stimulation devices* are used to deliver controlled stimuli to the patient with the objective of stimulating a controlled response, for example, to induce an epileptic seizure. The most common example of a *stimulation device* is the *photic stimulator* that emits a powerful flash (up to 2 J/stimuli) at a given frequency and intensity and for a selectable duration. The first photic stimulators used a xenon lamp to generate the light. These lamps had the ability to deliver very powerful bursts of light for very short durations. However, they have now been replaced with high-power LED (light-emitting diode) systems which have similar, or even better, characteristics. For additional information on the use of the photic stimulator, see Chap. 13.

The *output devices* provide the user with feedback and output from the system. This includes the *monitor*, where the EEG and additional information is displayed (see Sect. 5.4.3), and the *printer*, where information and results can be printed for a permanent record (see also Sect. 5.4.4).

The *processing devices* include the *computer*, which always hosts a *processor*, that performs all the basic analysis, an internal *RAM—random access memory*—to temporarily store the data (typical values are 4–8 Gb) and programmes necessary to run the analysis, at least one *hard disk* to permanently store the data (typical values are 500 Gb to 1 Tb) and usually a *CD/DVD reader/writer* to read and/or write data onto external media that can be read on any PC. The computer will have several interfaces or *communication ports* (i.e. network,[1] serial port,[2] USB port[3]), allowing the computer to communicate with the various peripherals including the *input and output devices*. One particular type of interface are the *synchronization devices* commonly referred to as *trigger IN* and *trigger OUT*; these are communication ports that allow the user to send and receive very simple signals (typically TTL[4]) used to synchronize devices. The trigger IN port of an EEG system receives synchronization signals from external devices (e.g. a photic stimulator), while the trigger OUT port of an EEG system can send synchronization signals to peripheral devices that need to be driven or controlled. In general, the role of the computer is to process all the data coming from input devices and data acquisition devices and provide the user with feedback and control through the output devices.

The *recording accessories* are the *electrodes*, *caps*, *conductive gel* and other transducers that interface or connect the patient to the headbox. Information about these accessories can be found in Chap. 3 of this book.

The *supports* consolidate the system into a single unit for ease of use and functionality. They are typically the *cart* and the various arms and support frames that hold the amplifiers, computer and other devices.

5.2 Analogue Components

5.2.1 EEG Signal Detection: The Electrodes

The electrodes, which include all the signal detection devices like the caps, wire electrodes, belts and other transducers, connect directly to the patient and play a fundamental role in

[1]The *network* interface supports very fast communication between PCs. The kind of interface depends on the communication standard, but currently all PCs use the Ethernet standard 10/100 or Gigabit Ethernet. Wireless networks are also common, often called WiFi (technical name of IEEE 802.11) which support speeds from 11 to 54 Mbps or even higher with the new standards.

[2]The *serial port* is a standard serial communication that transmits data at low speeds between different devices. This has been replaced with the USB Port (see next note).

[3]The *USB port* (*Universal Serial Bus*) is a standard serial communication protocol for high speed communication between different devices. It is now the most common standard and is available on almost any PC or device with multiple different connector types.

[4]The *standard TTL* (transistor-transistor logic) is a binary standard, using just 0 and 1, where "0" is associated with a voltage between 0 and 0.8 V and "1" is associated with a voltage between 2 and 5 V. This is why it is often referred to as the 0–5 V standard.

Fig. 5.2 Differential amplifier

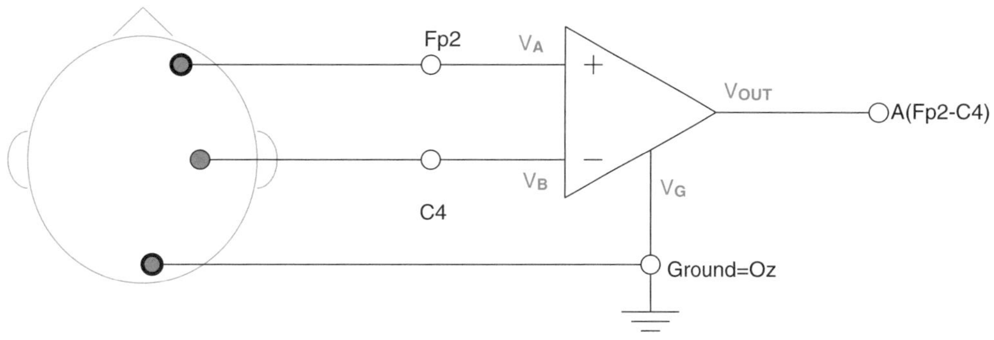

the EEG signal acquisition. They represent the connection between the location where the signal is measured and the amplifier. Given their fundamental importance and the number of different electrodes available on the market, this book has a dedicated chapter on this topic (Chap. 3).

5.2.2 EEG Acquisition System: The Differential Amplifier

EEG signals are normally acquired using a differential amplifier. This is a component that measures small electrical potential difference between two points and then amplifies several times that potential for recording.The general design of a differential amplifier, connected to two points on the scalp, can be represented by Fig. 5.2.

The amplifier has two inputs, normally referred to as inverting input and non-inverting input. The amplifier then measures and amplifies the difference of potential between these two inputs, that is[5]:

$$V_{\mathrm{OUT}} = A\left(V_{\mathrm{A}} - V_{\mathrm{B}}\right)$$

where V_{OUT} is the measured voltage, V_{A} the voltage at the inverting input, V_{B} the voltage at the non-inverting input and A is the amplification factor. In the case of an EEG signal, the amplification factor is in the range of 10,000 and increases the measured voltage, normally in the range of 500 μV, to become compatible with the voltage normally used in electronic circuits that are in the range of a few volts. The exact value of this amplification factor is not relevant for the user because it is made redundant by the signal processing, and for the sake of simplicity, it will be omitted, and a simplified version of the formula will be used:

$$V_{\mathrm{OUT}} = \left(V_{\mathrm{A}} - V_{\mathrm{B}}\right)$$

The measured voltage V_{OUT} is theoretically referenced to a potential normally called "ground"[6] and highlighted in Fig. 5.2 as V_{G}, so that:

$$V_{\mathrm{OUT}}=(V_{\mathrm{A}}-V_{\mathrm{G}})-(V_{\mathrm{B}}-V_{\mathrm{G}})=V_{\mathrm{A}}\cancel{-V_{\mathrm{G}}}-V_{\mathrm{B}}\cancel{+V_{\mathrm{G}}}=V_{\mathrm{A}}-V_{\mathrm{B}}$$

The formula shows that the value of the measured voltage is independent of the ground potential. However, this is only true if the amplifier can effectively measure the voltages $(V_{\mathrm{A}} - V_{\mathrm{G}})$ and $(V_{\mathrm{B}} - V_{\mathrm{G}})$; if not, the amplifier could "saturate" and measure V_{OUT} incorrectly. As a result, although the electrode that detects the ground potential could, theoretically, be placed in any location on the patient, its position must actually consider the possible saturation effect and should always be positioned close to all the other electrodes to minimize the difference of potential between them.

In reality, signal amplification is not perfect and cannot be simplified to the extent shown in the formula. As a result, several parameters have been defined to evaluate the ability of an amplifier to amplify the signal. The most common parameters for this evaluation are the CMRR (Common Mode Rejection Ratio), the *internal noise* of the amplifier, its *input impedance* and its *bandwidth.*

CMRR is an index of the rejection of common noise between two inputs of the amplifier (inverting and non-inverting). If the same noise is present at the two inputs (very common in practice), this noise should be completely cancelled by the amplifier because of its "differential" nature. In other words, because the amplifier is only detecting the difference of potentials between the two inputs, any common

[5]Note that, according to the electronic naming convention, the non-inverting input should be highlighted with the symbol "+" that, in the above example, corresponds to Fp2, and the inverting input should be highlighted with the symbol "−" that, in the above example, corresponds to C4. Consequently, the signal Fp2-C4 should have positive signals going up and negative signals going down. However, in the EEG naming convention, for historical reasons, all signals are drawn in reverse, and the notation Fp2-C4 implies that a positive Fp2 signal will go down (i.e. an eye blink). This inversion is commonly done by the display system together with inverting the amplifier input. For the sake of simplicity, the electronic naming convention is used in this text, assuming that the inversion is performed by the display system.

[6]The name "ground" for the reference potential is misleading because it is not in contact with the real ground or earth of the power supply but is in fact just a "common" potential for the measurement. Despite "common" being a more appropriate term, "ground" is used in this text following the common terminology used in the EEG field.

noise should be eliminated. In practice, the common noise is not perfectly cancelled but is significantly attenuated. For example, a common noise of 1 V will not be cancelled entirely but will result in a component of noise typically about 1 μV. The value of the CMRR is measured in dB to highlight the attenuation factor and is calculated as follows[7]:

$$\mathrm{CMRR} = 20\log_{10}\left(V_{\mathbf{IN}} / V_{\mathbf{OUT}}\right)$$

Using the values of the example this becomes:

$$\mathrm{CMRR} = 20\log_{10}\left(1\,\mathrm{V} / 1\,\mu V\right) = 20\log_{10}\left(1{,}000{,}000\right) = 20\times 6 = 120\,\mathrm{dB}$$

The value recommended by [1] is 110 dB, and amplifiers currently on the market have values around 100 dB or higher.

The *internal noise* of the amplifier is the value of the output when all inputs are set to zero. Theoretically according to the formula, the output should be zero, but, in practice, the circuits that compose the amplifier produce some noise that by design should be minimized. Normal values for this noise[8] are a few μV, if measured peak to peak (indicated as μV_{PP}), or below 1 μV, if measured as effective value (indicated as μV_{RMS}).[9]

The *input impedance* of the amplifier is a parameter that indicates the resistance to current flow through the amplifier as a function of the applied voltage. Its value should be as high as possible and is typically in the range of hundreds of MΩ or higher.

The *bandwidth* of the amplifier defines the operating frequency range of the amplifier. If the lower limit of the bandwidth is 0 Hz, the amplifier is called a DC-amplifier (direct current) and can record very slow potentials.[10] In all other cases, the amplifier is called an AC-amplifier (alternating current) and will have a cut-off frequency below which all potentials will be significantly attenuated.[11] The lower limit of the amplifier bandwidth should be selected based on the signal to be recorded, typically in the range of a tenth of a Hertz (i.e. 0.1 Hz). Values for this limit are shown in Table 5.1 and in Sect. 5.3.4 where the upper limit of the bandwidth is shown and which is always correlated to the anti-aliasing filter that is necessary for sampling.

5.2.3 EEG Acquisition Technique: Common Reference and Bipolar Electrodes

One of the biggest advantages offered by digital EEG is that the signals are no longer recorded in an unmodifiable way on paper but acquired and stored in a format capable of post-processing and display. This big advantage is used by digital systems to record not the potential differences between only two electrodes, as on paper EEG, but to record the potential difference between each electrode and, through a common electrode, any other electrode. For this reason the common electrode is called a common reference. A common reference amplifier design is shown in Fig. 5.3.

Figure 5.3 only shows four electrodes with common references, but this can be extended to any number of channels in a recording system. The common reference electrode is connected internally to the inverting input of each differential amplifier, and the ground electrode is connected internally to each differential amplifier. Consequently in order to record, for example, a 19-channel EEG, it is necessary to apply 21 electrodes to the patient, 19 so-called active electrodes plus the common reference and the ground. Generally speaking, to record N channels, N + 2 electrodes have to be applied.

Once all the active electrode potentials are recorded with respect to a common reference, any specific signal between any two electrodes can be calculated using simple subtraction[12] for example:

$$(\mathrm{Fp2\text{-}Ref})\text{-}(\mathrm{C4\text{-}Ref}) = \mathrm{Fp2}\text{-}\cancel{\mathrm{R}}\mathrm{ef}\text{-}\mathrm{C4}+\cancel{\mathrm{R}}\mathrm{ef}=\mathrm{Fp2}\text{-}\mathrm{C4}$$

The formula illustrates that the result does not depend on the position of the common reference electrode, at the condi-

[7] Note that the CMRR value can vary as a function of the frequency of the signal. As a result, when a CMRR value is specified, it should always be accompanied by the frequency, or the bandwidth, of the signals.

[8] Note that the internal noise of the amplifier can vary as a function of the bandwidth of the signal so that when an internal noise value is specified, it should always be accompanied by the frequency, or the bandwidth, of the signals used for the measurement.

[9] The approximate value of the internal noise, measured as peak to peak, can be obtained from the internal noise measured as the effective value (or RMS—Root Mean Squared) using the following formula:

$$V_{\mathrm{PP}} = 2\times\sqrt{2}\times V_{\mathrm{RMS}}$$

The approximation is that this formula is valid only for sinusoidal signals.

[10] With respect to DC amplifiers, see Chap. 3 where the problems generated by the coupling with the recording electrodes are discussed.

[11] Note that below the *cut-off frequency* of a *high-pass filter*, the signal is not completely cancelled but only attenuated, and its attenuation becomes higher and the signal approaches zero the further the signal is away from the cut-off frequency. The same applies for the low-pass *filter*: above the cut-off frequency, the signal is not completely attenuated, and its attenuation becomes higher the further the signal is away from the cut-off frequency. Note that, by definition, at the cut-off frequency, the signal has an attenuation of 70% meaning that a signal of 100 μV is attenuated to 70.7 μV.

[12] This assumption depends on the fact that the EEG fields have been demonstrated to be *conservative fields*, which means that given three points A, B and C and measuring $V_A - V_C$ and $V_B - V_C$, the potential $V_A - V_B$ can be obtained as the difference of the first two.

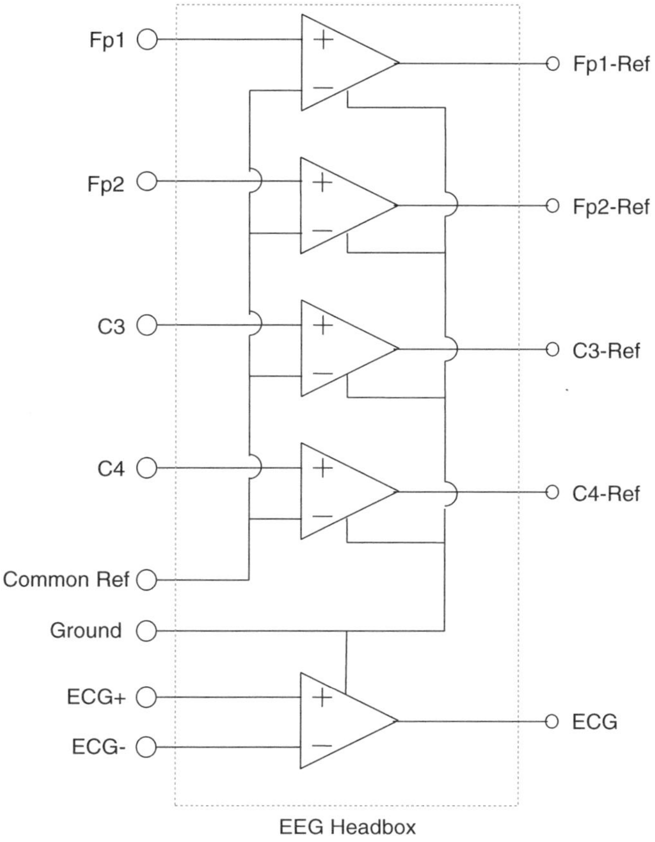

Fig. 5.3 Common reference acquisition

tion to avoid any saturation of the recorded signal. Saturation can occur in two different ways:

1. Both recorded potentials (Fp2-Ref) and (C4-Ref) saturate: in this case, the display of Fp2-C4 will be a flat line because the difference between two saturated signals (which implies they are both at the maximum value) is zero. This situation is typical in cases where the potential of the common reference electrode increases due to artefact. In a unipolar montage, this artefact will be seen easily, while in any bipolar montage, only a short flat line will be seen.
2. Only one of the two recorded potentials (Fp2-Ref) or (C4-Ref) saturates: in this case, the display of Fp2-C4 will be the signal from the electrode that does not saturate; thus, this problem is very difficult to detect.

Note that in Fig. 5.3, there are a couple of bipolar electrodes (ECG), to show examples of polygraphy electrodes (ECG, respiration and others) that are recorded in bipolar mode and only share the ground electrodes with the EEG channels.[13]

Note that the physical bi-auricular reference is a common reference where two earlobe electrodes are shorted and used as a common reference as shown in Fig. 5.4:

5.2.4 EEG Acquisition System: Noise

What has been described for the differential amplifier is valid under ideal circumstances; however, we must consider the "true" characteristics of the amplifier operating under nonideal circumstances. The main problem is that the contact between the electrodes and the scalp is never perfect. This imperfect contact is defined as the *contact impedances* and is measured on all the electrodes, including the common reference and ground electrodes, and leads to the susceptibility of unwanted noise detected through the electrodes and the connecting cables. The complete analysis of this interference is very complex and depends on a large number of variables; however, a simplified analysis can be made using the following diagram (Fig. 5.5):

In the diagram, I_P indicates the micro-current that can flow through the patient due to electromagnetic induction (the patient acts as an antenna for the electromagnetic noise) and that reaches the ground. I_C indicates the micro-current that can flow through the cables again caused by electromagnetic induction (the cables form a loop, and an electromagnetic force is induced in the cables following Faraday's Law). Z_A, Z_B and Z_G represent the contact impedances at input A, B and ground respectively, while Z_{IN} represents the input impedance of the differential amplifier. By applying the law of electronic circuits,[14] the output voltage, V_{OUT}, can be calculated as:

$$V_{OUT} = [V_A - V_B] + [I_P \times Z_G (Z_B - Z_A)/Z_{IN}] + [I_C (Z_A - Z_B)] = \text{Signal} + \text{Noise}$$

It is clear that the output is two components: the desired signal $V_A - V_B$[15] plus an undesired noise component. To understand the origin of this noise component, representative values can be used for the variables: if it is assumed that the induced micro-current caused by the patient and cable is, respectively, I_P = 0.2 μA and I_C = 10 nA and the contact impedances are Z_A = 10 kΩ, Z_B = 5 kΩ and Z_G = 20 kΩ (which are representative of values seen in practice) and the input impedance of the differential amplifier Z_{IN} = 100 MΩ. The result is:

$$V_{OUT} = [V_A - V_B] + [0.2\,\mu A \times Z_G (Z_B - Z_A)/Z_{IN}] + [10\,\text{nA}(Z_A - Z_B)]$$

[13]Note that to record polygraphy channels, it is necessary to always have a ground electrode applied to the patient; otherwise the differential amplifier of these bipolar channels will not have a reference potential and may not work correctly.

[14]Consider the current I_P flows through Z_A and Z_B and then Z_G. Then consider the current I_C in the loop $Z_A - Z_B$, and apply Ohm's Law.

[15]Note that for simplicity, the amplification factor has been omitted.

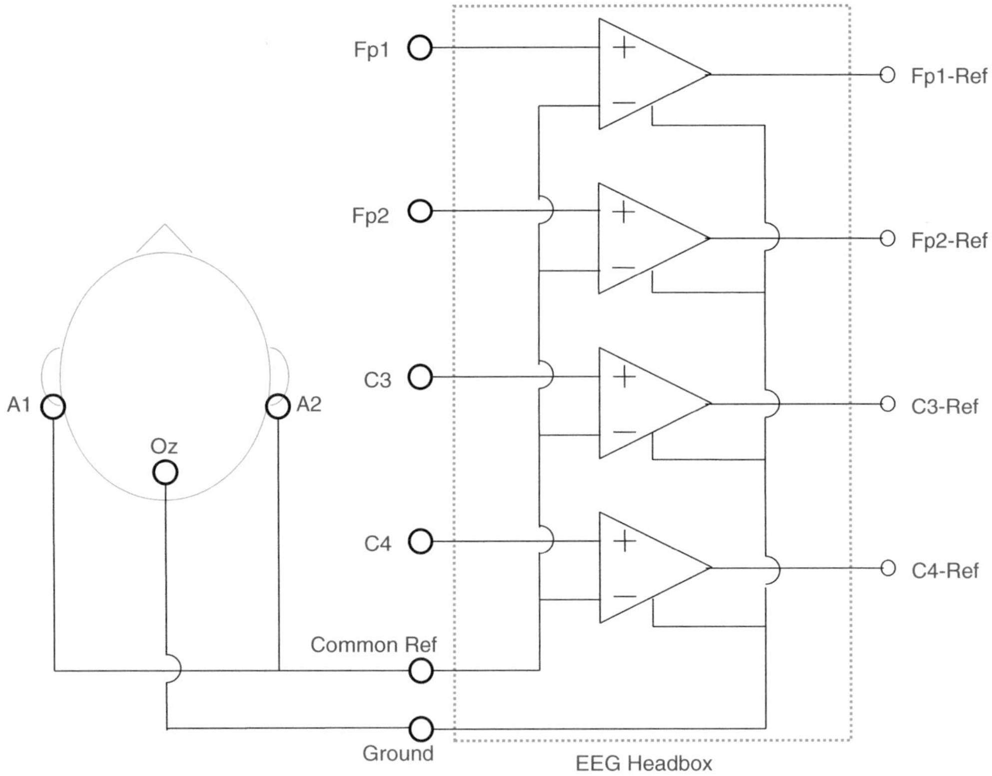

Fig. 5.4 Physical bi-auricular common reference acquisition

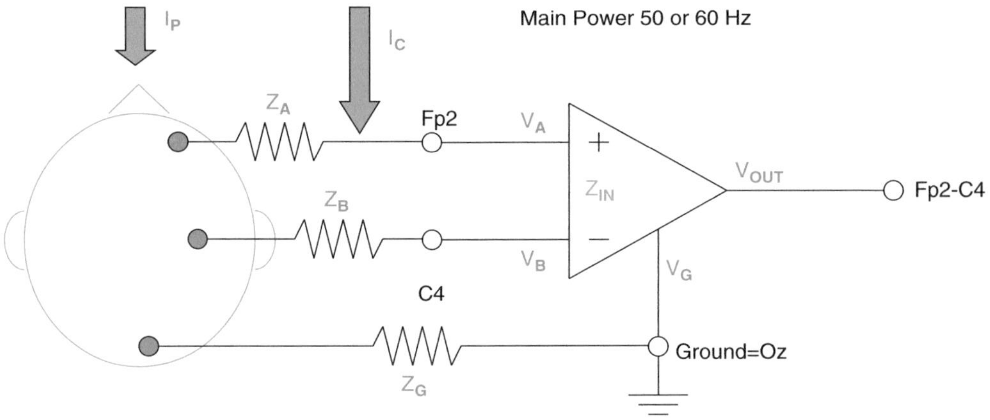

Fig. 5.5 Diagram of noise detected by a differential amplifier

$$V_{\text{OUT}} = [V_A - V_B] + [0.2\,\mu V] + [50\,\mu V]$$

Clearly, the majority of the noise is generated by the induction through the cables and can have significant values that are in the same range, or even greater, than the signal. Typical EEG signals are normally in the range of hundreds of μV, so it is clear that a component in the range of 50 μV can significantly impact the recording. The most common noise detected by the electrode cables is induced by the mains power (in Europe 220 V at 50 Hz, in the US 110 V at 60 Hz) and is generated by almost every electronic device. Typically, the induced noise has a frequency of 50 Hz (or 60 Hz in the US).[16] This is the reason why all EEG systems feature a stop-band filter, centred at 50 Hz. This filter, commonly called a *notch filter*,[17] is designed to eliminate the undesired component (i.e. 50 Hz) and is often called *50 Hz Filter.*[18] The transfer function of the filter is shown in Fig. 5.6.

Unfortunately, given the growing number of electronic devices that are present in a hospital environment, plus old or poorly installed main lines, the noise is not only a sinusoidal component at 50 Hz but 50 Hz signal contaminated by other components which quite often create harmonics of the mains

[16] Note that several other countries than the USA have a mains frequency of 60 Hz, so the notch filter needs to be centred appropriately depending on the country.

[17] The notch filter (or multi-notch) is usually a digital filter that is run during the signal display process so that it can be activated or deactivated as the signal is displayed to the user.

[18] Note that the term *50 Hz* should only be used to indicate just the 50 Hz noise component and not all the other noise components discussed. Often, *50 Hz* is used improperly to refer to any kind of noise visible on the EEG.

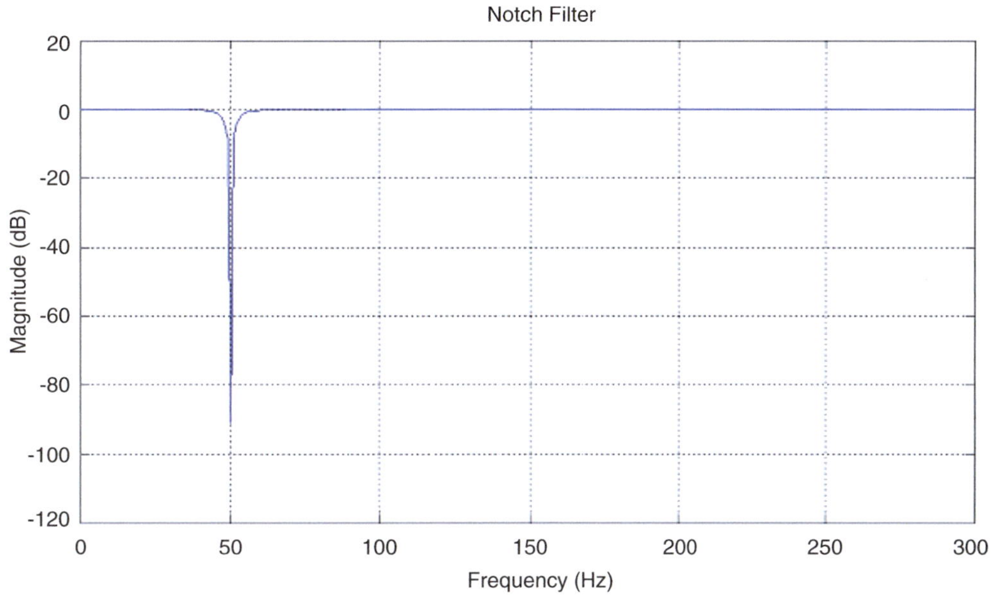

Fig. 5.6 Notch filter transfer function

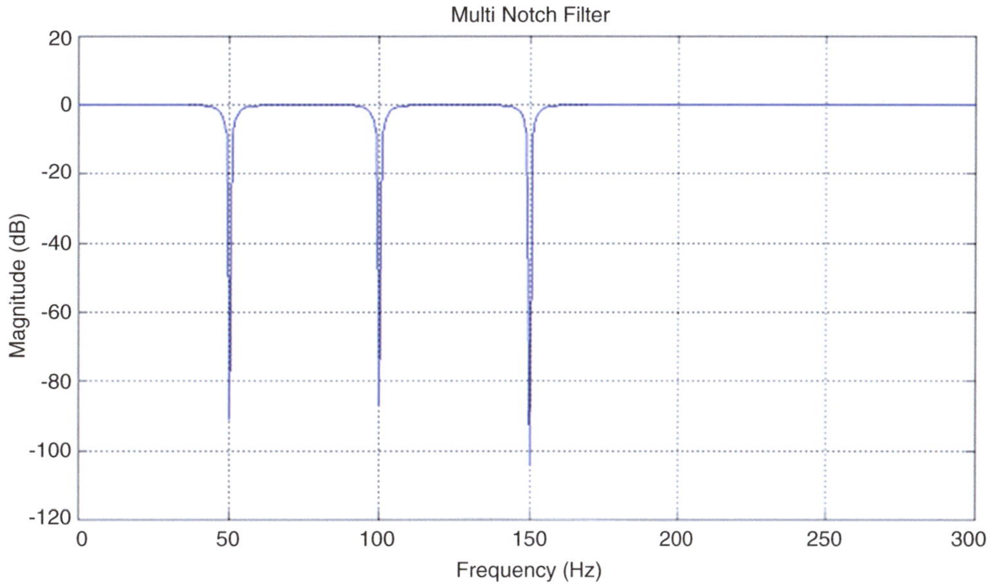

Fig. 5.7 Multi-notch filter transfer function

frequencies, or multiple frequencies, each a multiple of the original mains frequency. The most typical example of this is the 50 Hz sinusoidal signal with multiple peaks associated with its cycles that are caused by switching systems. The notch filter eliminates the 50 Hz component, but all the peaks remain, contaminating the signal. These problems have resulted in the design of *multi-notch filters* that can be set to eliminate several frequency components of the original signal, starting from 50 Hz and moving forward with each main harmonic, for example, 100 Hz, 150 Hz, 200 Hz and further if necessary. The transfer function of such a filter is shown in Fig. 5.7:

Another important reason to consider the formula for the noise with respect to the output voltage is that both additional noise terms are functions of $(Z_A - Z_B)$. This means that noise does not depend on the "value" of the impedance of a single electrode but on the "difference" between the values of two electrodes. As a result, to minimize the noise, it is necessary to make the two impedances equal to each other. Clearly, this is not possible so the only available strategy to minimise noise is to *reduce all the contact impedances as much as possible*, including those of the common reference and the ground electrodes, so that their difference will be minimal.

5.3 Analogue-To-Digital Conversion

The analogue-to-digital conversion of a signal is a process that converts an analogue signal waveform to a sequence of numbers that can be processed and stored in a PC. The analogue-to-digital conversion is very common in our daily

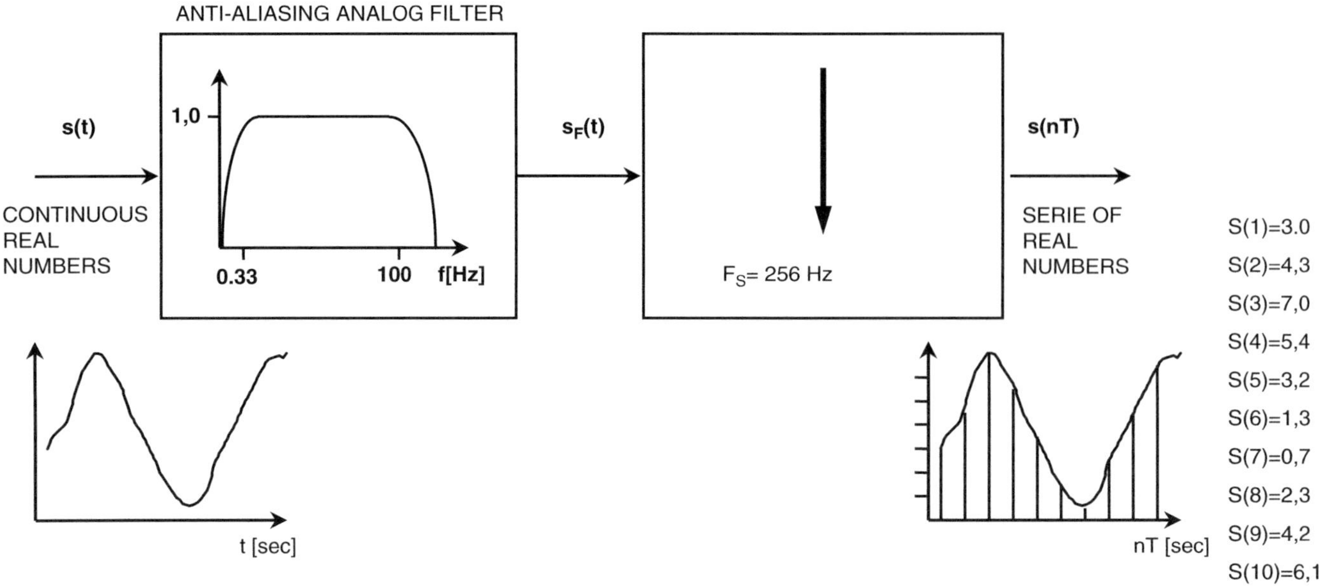

Fig. 5.8 Sampling process equivalent scheme

life, used for music, telephones, televisions and many other applications. This is discussed in Sect. 5.3.5.

5.3.1 Sampling

Sampling is a very simple process that, given an analogue signal properly amplified, consists of "measuring" the signal a given number of time per second and then storing the measured values instead of the entire analogue signal. An example of an analogue-to-digital conversion is shown in Fig. 5.8.

As shown in the diagram, the analogue signal is measured at regular periodic intervals. The frequency of this measurement is defined as the *sampling frequency*, indicated as F_S. Sampling is a no-loss process, which means that no information is lost, if and only if the sampling frequency is at least twice F_{MAX}, the maximum frequency that occurs in the signal.

This is known as the sampling theorem[19] and can be written as a formula:

$$F_S > 2 \times F_{MAX}$$

If the sampling theorem is not followed, the resulting digital signal can be corrupted, so all sampling systems filter the analogue signal at least at half the sampling frequency before sampling. This is usually called an anti-aliasing filter, where the name aliasing is taken from the typical error that can appear if the sampling is not performed correctly.[20] For example, if we assume that the bandwidth of the EEG does not exceed 100 Hz, an adequate sampling rate, in agreement with [1], is 256 Hz,[21] which means that the low-pass anti-aliasing filter should have a cut-off frequency of approximately 100 Hz as shown in the diagram. Note that the cut-off frequency of the anti-aliasing filter is never exactly half the sampling frequency. This is because at the cut-off frequency, the signal is not completely cancelled but only attenuated to about 70% of its value. Normal cut-off frequencies are in the range of 1/3 or even 1/4 of the sampling frequency to ensure that frequencies above half of the sampling frequency are properly cancelled.

Note that with the sampling process, we represent a set of continuous real numbers (the signal to measure) with a set of real numbers (the sampled signal).

5.3.2 Quantization

The objective of the quantization process is to complete the analogue-to-digital conversion process by reducing the measured samples to a set of finite numbers. It is important to note that the values measured by the sampling process are

[19]The mathematician and electric engineer Claude Elwood Shannon, known as "the father of information theory," formulated the sampling theorem in 1948. It was the first step toward the "digitization" of communications and started the revolution in digital technology.

[20]Aliasing is the phenomenon that represents signals associated with frequencies that exceed half of the sampling frequency appearing in the reconstructed signal as "duplicates" of the original signal. This means they will appear at frequencies that are specular to the original pivoting on the sampling frequency. For a better understanding, see Appendix 1—The Aliasing

[21]Note that for the sampling rates, most of the time a power of 2 value is selected (i.e. 256, 512, 1024 and so on) as this makes data processing by a PC more time efficient.

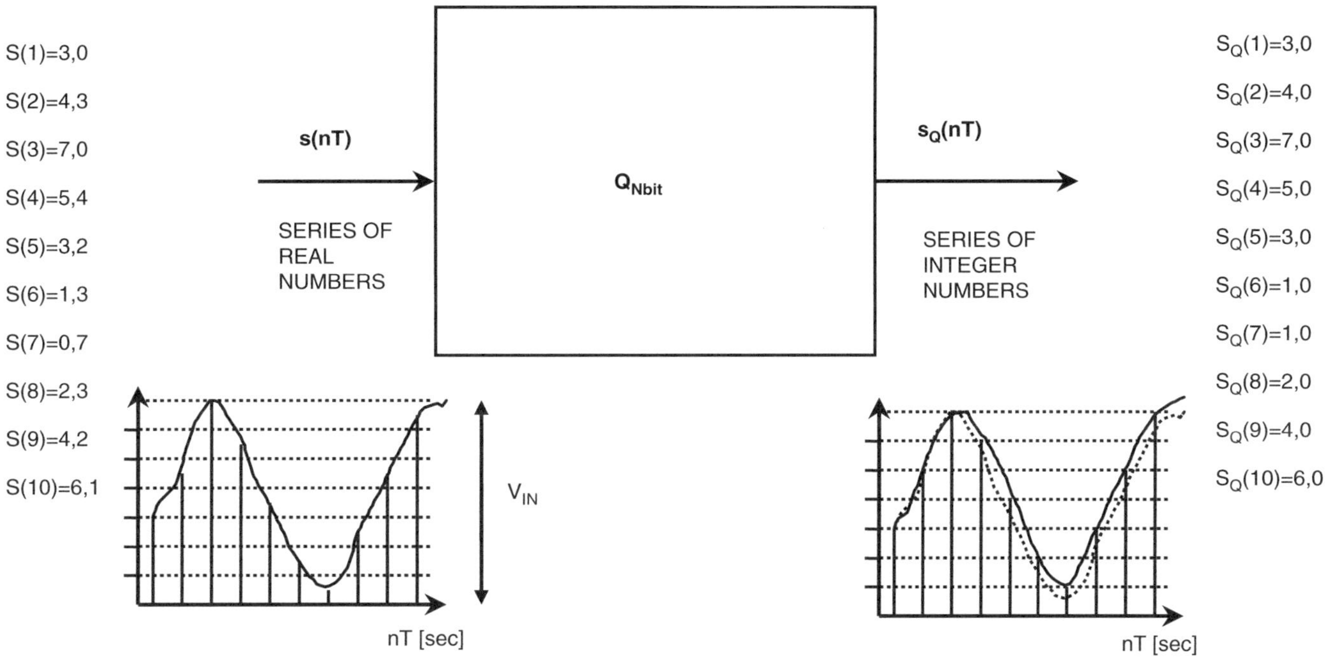

Fig. 5.9 Quantization process equivalent diagram

real numbers, so they have practically infinite resolution. This makes it impossible to store them in a simple form like a byte. Quantization approximates the real measured value to a close integer value.

A diagram of such a process could be that of Fig. 5.9

As the diagram highlights, quantization happens in a finite range of amplitudes, often referred to as the *maximum signal input* (indicated in Fig. 5.9 as V_{IN}), which defines an upper and lower limit for the signal to be converted. This parameter plays a very important role in the EEG signal acquisition process, because it needs to encompass the signal to be converted to avoid the *saturation* phenomenon. This happens when the measured signal exceeds the maximum signal input with the result that the value above the maximum signal input appears as the maximum signal input instead of the real signal, "cutting" the signal at the upper or lower value.[22] This saturation phenomenon should not be confused with the saturation of the amplifier, even though the result is very similar (as described in Sect. 5.2.3).[23] An example of saturation is shown in Fig. 5.10.

Another very important parameter for the quantization process is the precision of the measurement. In a digital system, this is determined by the *number of bits* used for the quantization of the signal (indicated in Fig. 5.9 as Nbit). The number of bits used is directly proportional to the *number of intervals* (or more correctly *number of digits*) in which the maximum input signal is split. The relation is the following:

Nbit = 8 → 2^8 digit = 256 digit
Nbit = 12 → 2^{12} digit = 4,096 digit
Nbit = 16 → 2^{16} digit = 65,536 digit
Nbit = 22 → 2^{22} digit = 4,194,304 digit
Nbit = 24 → 2^{24} digit = 16,777,216 digit

We can define the *precision of the measurement* or *resolution* as the ratio between the maximum input signal and the number of intervals in which such a range is split:

$$\text{Resolution} = \frac{\text{Maximum input signal}}{\text{Number of intervals}}$$

This value identifies the precision of the measurement of the quantization process and is expressed in [V/digit]. Note that the precision of the process is not uniquely identified by the number of bits, as often specified, but by a well-defined ratio between two values where only the denominator is proportional to the number of bits.[24]

[22]This phenomenon is similar to what happened with paper EEG systems when the pens reached their maximum excursion. In those systems, the limit was set by the physical limit of the excursion of the pens; in the digital systems, the limit is defined by the maximum signal that can be quantified.

[23]The main difference is that the saturation of the amplifier has a minimum recovery time before it functions correctly (the ability to amplify properly), while the saturation of the maximum signal input is a reversible problem, and the correct signal is shown as soon as the signal returns to within limits.

[24]The number of bits is quite often used as an indicator of the precision in those systems that can use several different values of maximum input signals, having multiple precision values (one for each different maximum signal input value).

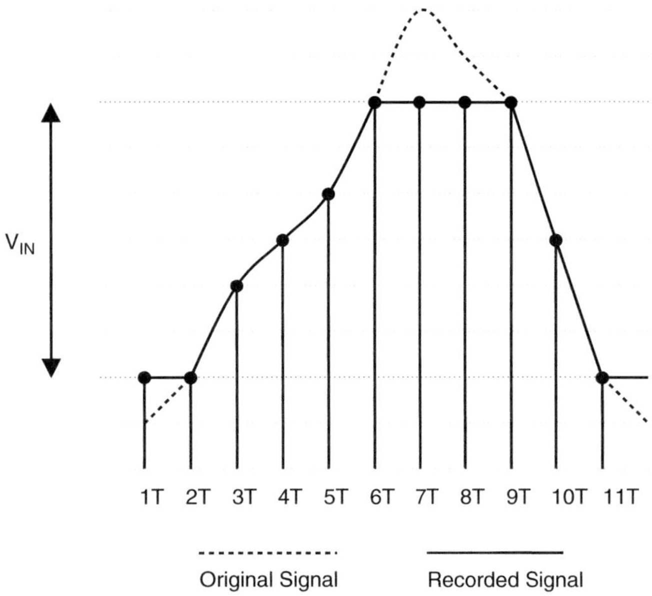

Fig. 5.10 Example of saturation of the input signal

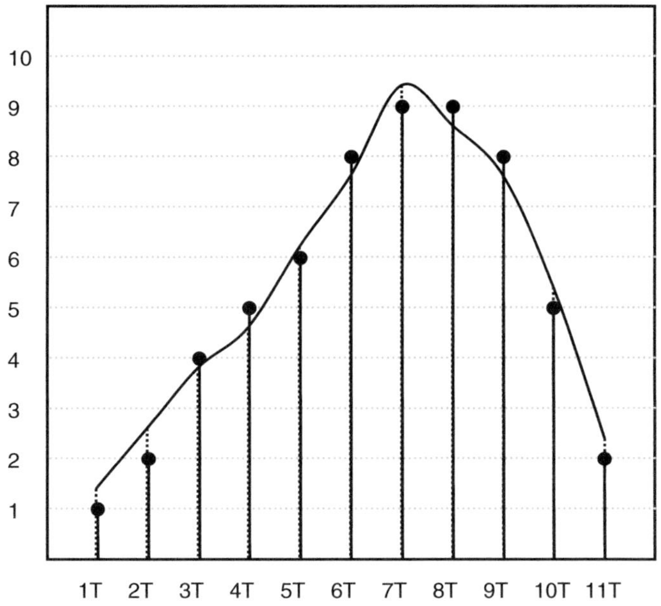

Fig. 5.11 Example of approximation of the signal due to quantization

As the quantization process induces an error in the measurement, it is necessary to quantify the magnitude of such an error to evaluate its importance. Considering how the process is performed, by "measuring" the signal using the closest interval, it is evident that the average quantization error is half the interval into which the maximum input signal is divided, as shown in Fig. 5.11.

As shown in Fig. 5.11, a signal is represented by the closest quantization level either above it (samples 3 T, 4 T, 6 T, 8 T, 9 T of Fig. 5.11) or below it (samples 1 T, 2 T, 5 T, 7 T, 10 T, 11 T of Fig. 5.11).

More precisely this can be written as:

$$\text{Average measurement error} = \frac{\text{Quantization interval amplitude}}{2}$$

In systems on the market, the number of bits normally used for quantization is typically 16 (with a minimum value recommended by [1] of 12) combined with a maximum input signal of at least 1 mV for EEG (±500 μV), which leads to the following values:

$$\text{Resolution} = \frac{1000[\mu V]}{65536[\text{digit}]} = 0.015[\mu V / \text{digit}] = 15[\text{nV} / \text{digit}]$$

Because this resolution is more than sufficient for most applications, quite often systems use maximum input signals higher than 1 mV to handle intracranial signals and various polygraphic signals (i.e. ElectroCardioGram, ElectroOculoGram and others).

5.3.3 Decimation

Decimation is an advanced technique that is not essential for the comprehension of the EEG signal acquisition process. This paragraph describes some of the more sophisticated aspects of the process. *Decimation* is basically a digital process which reduces the number of samples collected. For example, sampling a signal at 512 Hz and then keeping one sample for every two (which means one sample is kept and one sample discarded) results in a signal sampled at half the original sampling rate or 256 Hz. This operation is often referred to as *downsampling*, as it leads to a reduction of the original sampling rate.

In order to obtain the correct result from decimation, the sampling theorem (seen in Sect. 5.3.1) must be honoured. This means that the signal to be decimated must not contain any frequencies higher than half of the new sampling frequency resulting from the decimation. As a result an additional anti-aliasing filter should be applied to the signal before decimation. The advantage is that this filter operates on a sampled signal and is therefore a *digital filter*. This is the main reason over-sampling techniques are used. The original signal is sampled at very high frequencies (i.e. 8 kHz) and then decimated to obtain the desired sampling rate with a digital anti-aliasing filter, which has a much better performance than a similar analogue filter. A second advantage, which is more complicated and will not be addressed in this book, is the reduction of background noise (minimal) that results using this technique.

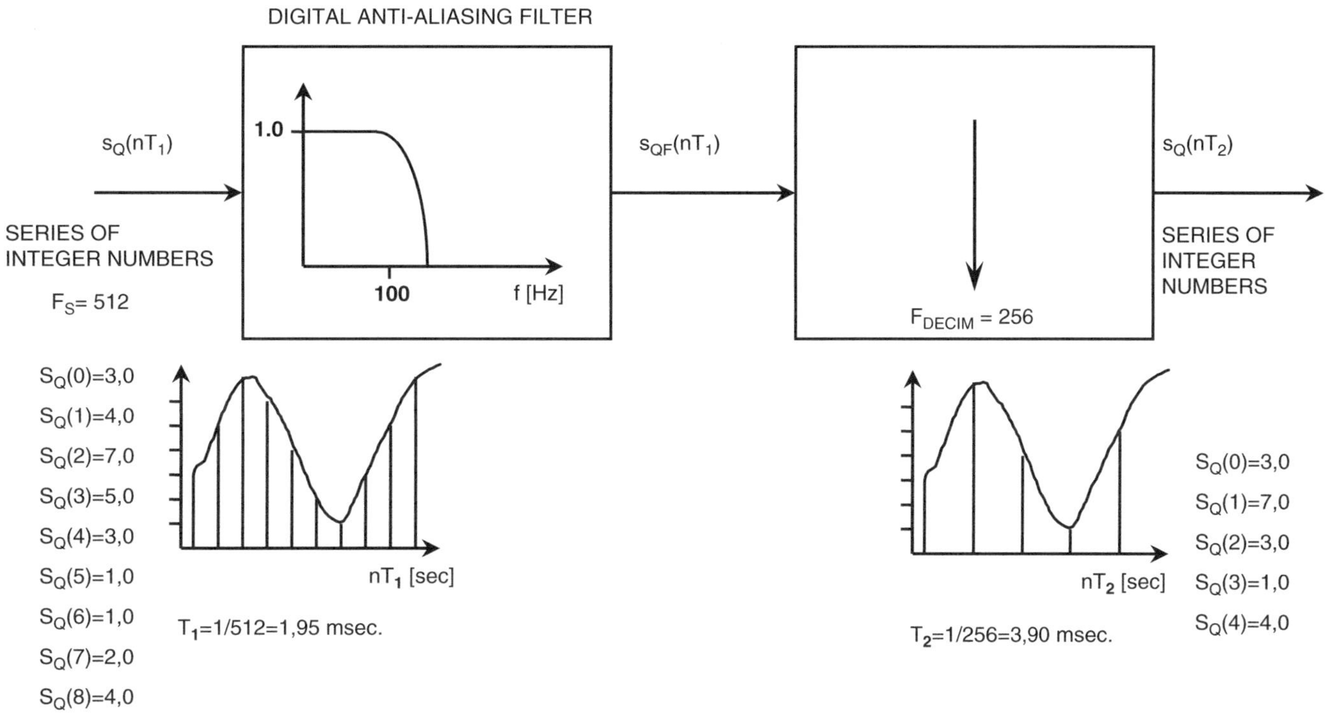

Fig. 5.12 Decimation equivalent scheme

A possible scheme for the decimation process is shown in Fig. 5.12:

As shown in Fig. 5.12, assuming an input signal $S_Q(nT_1)$ sampled at 512 Hz, to perform a decimation of 2 to 1 (which means moving from a sampling rate of 512 Hz–256 Hz), the first process is to apply an anti-aliasing filter with a cut-off frequency that is at least half of the resulting sampling rate (i.e. lower than 256/2 = 128 Hz). In the example this frequency has been chosen to be 100 Hz. The decimation process of keeping just one sample for every two can only be completed after the filtering, obtaining the desired output signal $S_Q(nT_2)$.

In reality the decimation process is often used to convert a signal from very high sampling rates (e.g. 8192 Hz) to much smaller values (e.g. 256 Hz) to take advantage of having a single analogue anti-aliasing filter in the circuits and the rest of the process performed by the software (or firmware) with digital filters to allow the selection of the desired sampling rate.

5.3.4 Summary of the Parameters of EEG Signal Acquisition

As discussed in the previous paragraphs, the parameters that must be known to sample EEG signals correctly are:

B = *signal bandwidth*[25]
A_{MAX} = *maximum signal amplitude*

Consequently, the following parameters must be set in the recording system:

F_S = *sampling frequency*, which must be at least twice the maximum frequency composing the signal (i.e. the upper limit of the bandwidth)
V_{IN} = *maximum signal input*, which must be larger than the maximum signal amplitude to guarantee correct signal recording

The most common parameters for typical EEG signals are shown in Table 5.1, derived from recommended standards [1], and calculated with a 16 bit quantization:

[25]For the sampling process, the upper limit of the bandwidth is the important parameter, while the lower limit of the bandwidth is more important for the selection of the high-pass filter.

Table 5.1 Recording parameters for EEG and polygraphic signals

Signal type	A_{MAX}	V_{IN} (μV)	Resolution (nV/digit)	Bandwidth (Hz)	F_S (Hz)
EEG—adult	50–400 μV	800	12.2	0.3–70	256
EEG—children	100–1000 μV	1600	24.4	0.3–70	256
EEG—intracranial	1–2 mV	3200	48.8	0.3–150	512
ElectroCardioGram	0.5–3 mV	3200	48.8	1.6–70	256
Muscle	10 μV to −10 mV	12,800	0.19	50–500	1024
ElectroOculoGram	50–400 μV	800	12.2	0.3–70	256

Table 5.2 Example parameters for analogue-to-digital conversion of common signals

	Signal type	Band	FC	N_{BIT}	Channels	Data throughput (kbytes/s)
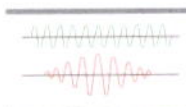	EEG	120 Hz	256 Hz/channel	16	20	10
	Acoustic EP	8 kHz	16 kHz/channel	16	2	32
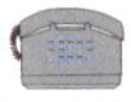	Telephone	4 kHz	8 kHz	8	1	8
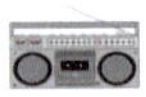	Audio	20 kHz	44.1 kHz/channel	16	2	172

5.3.5 Examples of Other Analogue-To-Digital Conversion Processes

The analogue-to-digital conversion process described for EEG signals is common to many other applications of daily life such as telephones, music and others. For example, voice transmitted by our mobile phones is sampled at 8 KHz with a quantization at 8 bit, with a resulting bandwidth of less than 4 KHz, which works correctly for a normal conversation. However, when we consider high-fidelity audio, because the audible signal that can be heard by humans is in the range of 20 KHz, the music must be sampled at 44.1 KHz and 16 bit to sound correct. Examples of analogue-to-digital conversion of signals are shown in Table 5.2:

5.4 The Digital Component

Once the analogue EEG signal is converted to digital, the signal goes through additional processes such as *storing*, *display*, *printing* and other manipulations for further analysis. The following paragraphs describe these processes.

5.4.1 EEG Signal Storage

Once the EEG signal is converted to a digital format, most EEG systems immediately store it. The first destination for data is the *hard disk* of the recording PC or another disk over the network. Subsequently the data is normally transferred to a disk over the network which provides reading station access for viewing, analysis and reporting. Once the signal has been displayed, analysed and reported, the signal (or just a part of it[26]) is transferred to a permanent storage media, which could be another disk or a non-rewritable media like *CD-R*[27] or *DVD-R*,[28] through an application that is normally part on the reporting system. These media allow the data to be permanently stored (or at least for several years) in an unmodifiable way, as required by some national laws. It's important to remember that in modern systems, the EEG is normally stored as "raw" data, that is, exactly as the signal was acquired by the amplifier. This means that all EEG channels are stored with a common reference, with only the filters performed by the hardware system and without any additional filter (including the notch filter), and these processes are performed when displaying the signal on the screen, as described in the next paragraphs.

[26] It's a common practice to select only parts of the EEG and video to be permanently stored. This is necessary to reduce the amount of data stored while keeping all the relevant information (e.g. seizures) for subsequent review and/or analysis.

[27] CD-R is a non-rewritable optical media (not the same as rewritable CD, which should not be used for this purpose) with a capacity of 650 or 700 Mb.

[28] DVD-R is a non-rewritable optical media (once again, not to be confused with rewritable DVD which should not be used for this purpose) with a capacity of 4700 Mb, often referred as 4.7 Gb even if in the informatics standard 4.7 Gb should be 4.7 × 1024 Mb = 4812 Mb.

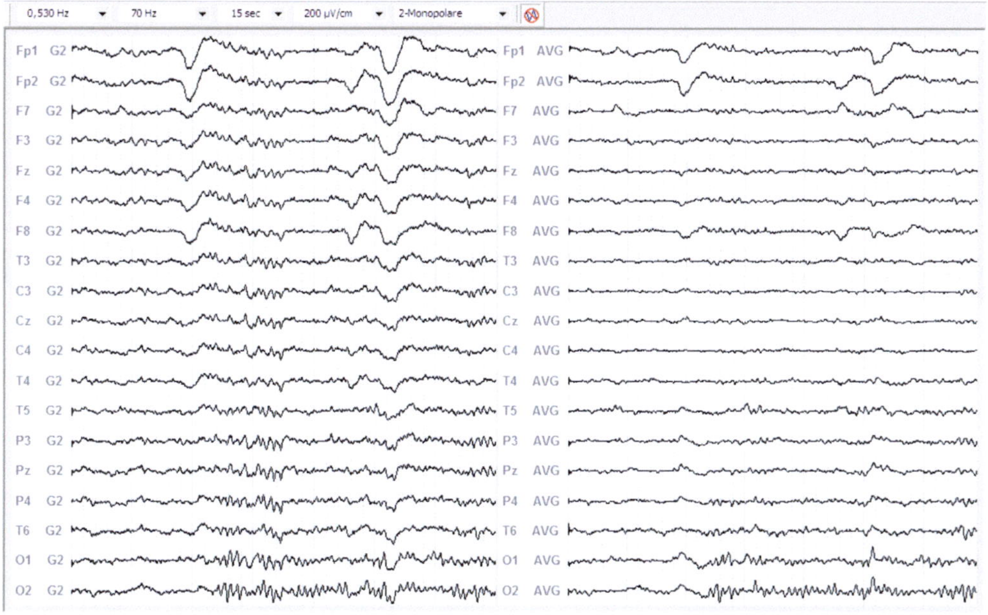

Fig. 5.13 Example of EEG signal with a common reference and average reference

5.4.2 EEG Signal Digital Processing

Before being displayed, the EEG signal goes through various processes, which include some or all of the following:

1. The original signal, where all channels are recorded in Common Reference, can be re-referenced, that is, calculating for each signal the *Average Reference* or the *Source Reference.*
   - *Average Reference* yields the absolute potential of each recorded electrode, as discussed in Sect. 5.2.3. For example, for the electrode C3 recorded as (C3-Ref), the average reference yields $C3_{ABS}$. This is obtained by calculating the average of all the common reference electrodes (which should ideally be the absolute potential of the common reference electrode—named AVG) and subtracting this value from the signal of each channel. Written as a formula, this is:

$$AVG = \frac{(Fp1\text{-}Ref)+(Fp2\text{-}Ref)+..+(O2\text{-}Ref)}{19} = \frac{(Fp1+Fp2+\ldots+O2)-19\cdot Ref}{19}$$

$$= \cancelto{0}{\frac{(Fp1+Fp2+\ldots+O2)}{19}} - \frac{\cancel{19}\cdot Ref}{\cancel{19}} = -Ref_{ABS}$$

The first term of the formula should tend to zero as the arithmetic average of a large number of uncorrelated signals, so the result will be the real "absolute" potential of the common reference electrode Ref_{ABS}. By simply re-montaging the signals with this newly calculated reference, the result is:

$$C3_{ABS} = (C3\text{-}Ref)\text{-}AVG = C3\text{-}\cancel{Ref}+\cancel{Ref} = C3_{ABS}$$

The disadvantage of this process is that the number of averaged signals is normally not as large as required (should be infinite), so the AVG potential obtained is not the "real" potential of the common reference electrode but is contaminated by all the high-amplitude signals that are present in the various electrodes (e.g. eye blink artefact). When this signal is subtracted from each electrode, the contaminated signal spreads to all the electrodes.[29] This phenomenon, known as *average reference contamination*, can be avoided by increasing the number of electrodes to be recorded (which in most cases is not possible) or by excluding those electrodes where artefacts are most often present (e.g. Fp1, Fp2 for Eye Blinks) from the calculation of the AVG potential.

Figure 5.13 shows two set of signals displayed in unipolar montage. The signals on the left are shown in common reference and the signals on the right in average reference, including the fronto-polar electrodes in the average calculation.

As the figure shows, the artefact due to eye blinks that is present in the common reference display, mainly in the frontal area (i.e. Fp1 and Fp2), contaminates other electrodes (i.e. O1, O2 with reverse polarity) with the average reference display.

The average reference is rarely used for the visual interpretation of EEG, but it is often necessary for processing that requires an absolute value for the potentials, such as mapping.

Also, note that the average reference does not affect the display with a bipolar montage because the same potential is

[29] The signal is spread into any other channel attenuated by a factor that is the number of channels used for the calculation, with reverse polarity (inverted) due to the subtraction performed by the re-montaging.

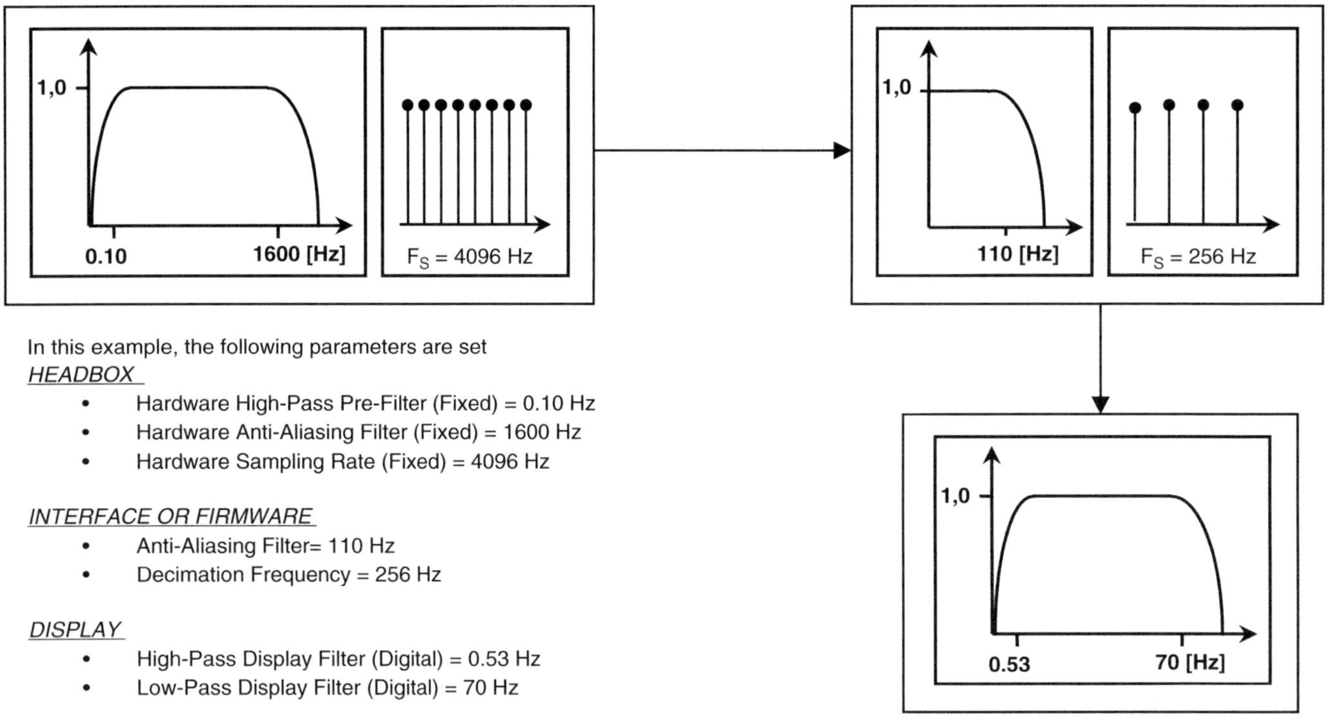

Fig. 5.14 Example of a complete filtering chain for an EEG signal

subtracted from all the electrodes so that the difference of potentials between two electrodes remains the same.

- *Source Reference* is a signal processing technique that aims to highlight the "source" of the potentials. In other words, the potential will be higher in the electrode that is closest to the source of the potentials. A complete analysis of this technique is complicated and described in Appendix 2—Source Reference.

2. The *Montage* defines how signals are recombined and selected for display. This could be *unipolar* (each signal with the reference selected at the previous point) or *bipolar* (the difference between two channels recorded with the same reference). Refer to Sect. 5.2.3: Common Reference and Bipolar Electrodes—for further details.
3. Signals are *filtered* (using correctly designed digital filter) to reduce the recorded bandwidth for the display and to cut noise (e.g. a digital notch filter). These filters represent additional processing over and above the filters already applied by the hardware as seen in the previous paragraphs. For example, Fig. 5.14 shows a diagram of the complete filtering chain for a typical acquisition and display process.

As Fig. 5.14 shows, the system works to progressively narrow the bandwidth of the signal until it is compatible with the display.

These three processes are all digital and allow any of their parameters to be modified to prepare the signal for display on the screen and/or for printing.

5.4.3 EEG Signal Display

Signal display is a very important process, often under evaluated, because it defines the quality of the final "presentation" of the recorded EEG to the user and can therefore influence correct data interpretation.

Data are drawn on a matrix of points, called *pixels*, that compose the LCD[30] screen. The size of the pixel matrix is a characteristic of the graphic card of the PC and the screen that is connected to the graphic card. In fact, to display an image on the screen, the matrix must exist in the memory of the graphic card, and the screen has to be capable of displaying the matrix of pixels, or interpolations have to occur. Typical matrix is 1440 × 900, 1680 × 1050 (mainly used on laptops) and 1920 × 1080 (Full HD). It is worth noting that the size of the pixel depends on the resolution and the size of

[30] *LCD* is the acronyms of liquid crystal display and is the most common display type. Depending on the brand and model, its size ranges typically from a minimum of 15″ up to 24″, 27″ or even 30″. The screen proportions are always 16:9 or 16:10, or in other words, the horizontal size is 16/9 of the vertical size. The resolution again depends on the brand and model but is often 1920 × 1080 as this is a common TV standard (full HD resolution), but there are also even higher resolutions.

Table 5.3 Typical pixel sizes

Monitor	Proportion	Resolution	Monitor size	Pixel size
17″	16:9	1440 × 900	37.6 × 21.2 cm	0.29 × 0.29 mm
19″	16:9	1600 × 900	42.1 × 23.7 cm	0.26 × 0.26 mm
21″	16:9	1920 × 1080	46.5 × 26.2 cm	0.24 × 0.24 mm

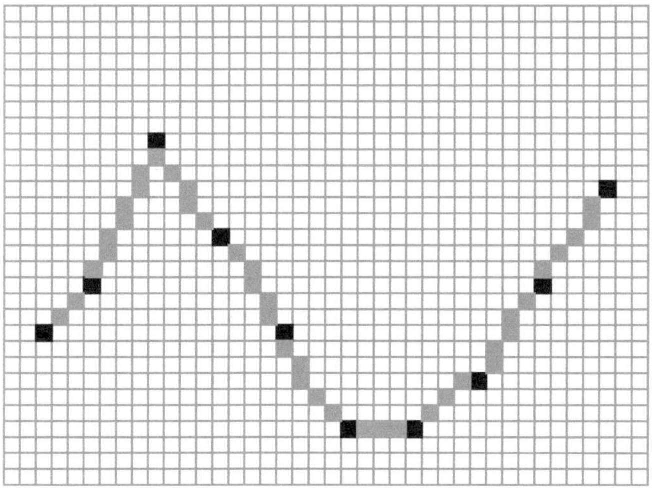

Fig. 5.15 EEG signal drawn on a pixel matrix 40 × 30

the screen. Typical values for pixel size are shown in Table 5.3.

The display of the EEG signal is presented by drawing on the pixel matrix of the graphic card the sequence of signal samples connecting each point, in the simpler hypothesis, with a line identified by "on" pixels. The result, on a different scale, is shown in Fig. 5.15, where the digital signal $S_Q(i)$ = [3.0; 4.0; 7.0; 5.0; 3.0; 1.0; 1.0; 2.0; 4.0; 6.0] is drawn.

As Fig. 5.15 shows, the value of a signal sample is associated with a specific pixel (drawn in black in Fig. 5.15). The vertical coordinate is proportional to the value of the sample, while the horizontal coordinate is time (in Fig. 5.15 the proportion factor is 4 pixel/digit). These pixels are then linked by additional pixels (drawn in grey in Fig. 5.15).

The vertical scaling factor determines the *video gain*, often improperly called its *sensitivity*, that is calibrated by the EEG system manufacturer with proportions that are, for example, 100 μV/cm, 200 μV/cm, 400 μV/cm, 800 μV/cm for the EEG and other values for other signal types.[31] It is worth noting that typically a signal that is quantized at 16 bit, that is 65,536 digits, is then drawn in about 200 vertical pixels[32]; this means that all the efforts made to increase the precision of the quantization vanish when the signal is displayed.

The horizontal scaling factor determines the so-called *base time*, that is, the number of seconds of EEG drawn on the screen. This factor is also calibrated by the EEG system manufacturer to display an integer number of seconds on the screen (typically 10, 15 or 20 s) or to represent a proportion, for example, 1.5 cm/s or 3.0 cm/s. It is worth noting again that a signal, for example, sampled at 256 Hz is then drawn in about 96 horizontal pixels.[33] This quite often contaminates the signal (most of the time unperceivably) due to the number of samples that are drawn on the same horizontal position.

It is clear that for an optimal display of EEG signals, both the horizontal and vertical resolution of the screen must be chosen as high as possible. For the screen of an EEG reporting station, a minimum resolution of 1920 × 1080 pixel is recommended.

5.4.4 EEG Signal Printout

Signal printout is also a very important process but is less and less common as the display interpretation is now preferred. Printouts still occur, for example, to give patients a few pages of EEG together with the report and/or for medical-legal reasons. Printouts are normally done in two ways:

Single sheet printout, typically on A4 paper format (or "Letter" in the US) and with laser technology on standard paper. The process is very much the same as the display described in the previous paragraph: the paper is divided into a matrix of points that can be switched "on" or "off." In the case of a printer, the number of points is determined by the resolution of the printer that is often at least 600 dpi,[34] which is four times larger than the video, minimizing the resolution issue described for the screen. This is also the reason why EEG signals printed on paper look "thinner" than the same signals on the screen: they are plotted on a matrix of much smaller points and consequently the lines are thinner.

Continuous module printout is rarely used. This was done on thermal paper that, by heating, became darker. The reso-

[31] Values range from 1, 2, 5, 10 μV/cm plus all their multiples 20, 50, 100 μV/cm up to 1, 2, 5 mV/cm for polygraphic signals which have typically higher amplitudes.

[32] The calculation is done assuming a vertical resolution of 1080 pixel with 10 EEG signals on the screen. Every signal will occupy at maximum the space between the signal above and the signal below. So, considering a space between lines of 1080/10 = approx. 100 pixel, the space occupied by a signal will be 2 × 100 = 200 pixel.

[33] The calculation is done with a horizontal resolution of 1920 and 20 s of EEG signals drawn on the screen, that is, 1920/20 = 96 pixels per second of signal.

[34] DPI is the acronym for "dots per inch" and is the number of dots per inch of the matrix. One inch corresponds to 2.54 cm, so 600 dpi corresponds to 600/2.54 = 236 points/cm. As an A4 sheet size is 29.7 × 21 cm, assuming a border of 1 cm, the matrix of points on an A4 sheet is (29.7–2) × 236 = 6537 and (21–2) × 236 = 4484 or 6537 × 4484 points.

Fig. 5.16 Block diagram of a digital video EEG acquisition system

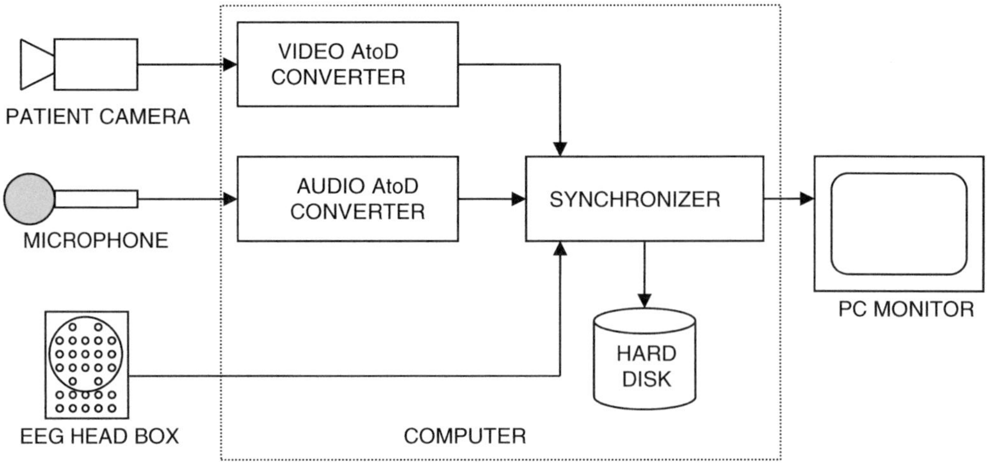

lution of these printers, typically 16 points/mm, was not as high as the laser printers but still better than the screen resolution.

In both printout cases, vertical and horizontal scaling factors are properly calibrated by the EEG system manufacturer to reach the desired *gain on paper* and *base time*.

5.5 Synchronized Digital Video

Recording the patient video synchronously with the EEG is a technique used for many years and has evolved to its current form of synchronized digital video.

The first systems were composed of a camera filming the pens writing the EEG data onto the scrolling paper, while a second camera filmed the patient; the two signals were then mixed together and the video EEG was obtained.

With the first digital EEG, recording of the video started on videotape and the synchronization signal was encoded into the video tape. This kind of system is often referred to as the *analogue video* option for digital EEG.

In the middle 1990s, the first *digital video* systems were developed, which involved recording the video into a file, together with the EEG; the recording PC and its software performed the synchronization. It is worth noting that in many of these systems, analogue or digital, audio was always recorded.

Main advantages of digital video over analogue are:

- Digital video is easier to store and transfer as both EEG and video can be written on the same media (hard disk, CD or DVD or any other).
- Digital video offers direct access to any time instant of the video, without the need to rewind or fast forward the tape as with the analogue video.

However, it is worth noting that digital video has introduced new variables such as the resolution of the image, the codec used for the compression and the codec used to play the video on a PC. The following paragraphs describe these parameters in detail and how the digital video is recorded and stored.

5.5.1 Digital Video EEG Acquisition

A digital video EEG acquisition system is basically a PC that performs three digitizing processes simultaneously: analogue-to-digital conversion of the EEG, the video and the audio. Figure 5.16 shows a diagram for such a video EEG acquisition system:

Analogue-to-digital conversion of the EEG has already been reviewed in Sect. 5.3. The analogue to digital conversion of the audio, as discussed in Sect. 5.3.5, is the same as EEG, just with different parameters; the next paragraph will analyse the digitizing process for the video.

5.5.2 Video Signal Digitalization

The video signal normally acquired by a standard camera is composed of 25 images per second,[35] captured by the camera itself.[36] The complete analogue to digital conversion consist of digitizing every image and storing the entire sequence of

[35]The 25 images/s. Comes from the PAL video standard adopted in Europe for all TV signals. In the USA the TV standard is NTSC which uses 30 images/s (originally 29.97 fps but now adapted to digital cameras using 30 fps).

[36]Note that the video signal has already been sampled in the time domain by acquiring 25 images per second. This means that, according to the sampling theorem discussed previously, there should not be any movement in the signal faster than 12.5 movements/s. In reality there's no way to apply an anti-aliasing filter to this signal, so if a movement is faster than 12.5 times/s, it will be displayed incorrectly. A typical example is the wheels shown in older western movie that appear to turn backward.

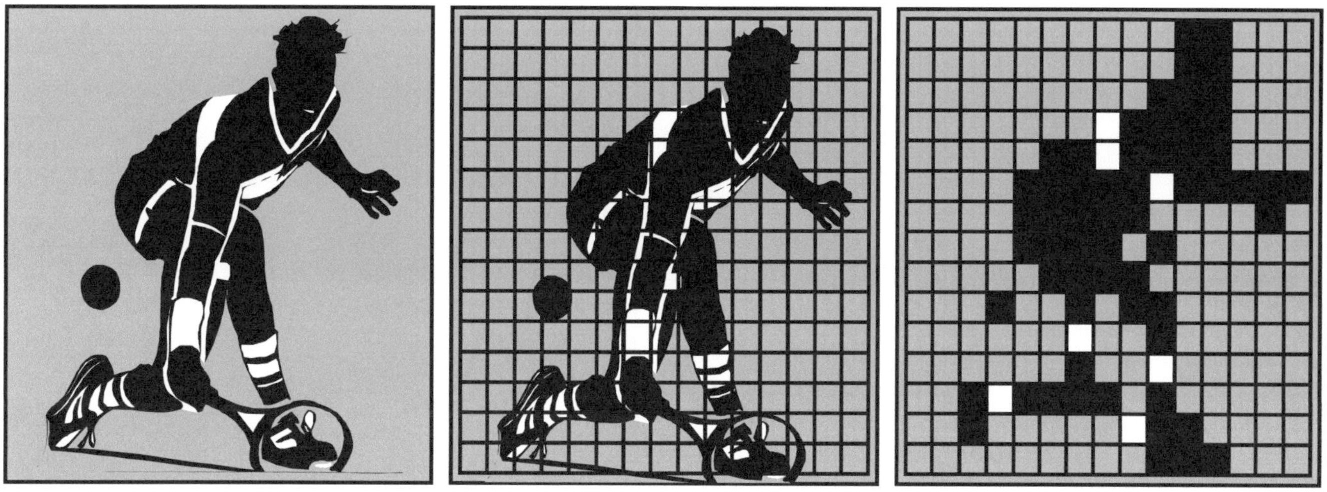

Fig. 5.17 Digitalization of an image

Table 5.4 Video resolution

Name	Image resolution
Full HD—1080i/p	1920 × 1080
HD—720p	1280 × 720
CIF[a]	384 × 288

[a]CIF is the acronym of Common Interchange Format that was a common format representing a good compromise between quality and size

25 images per second, or less if necessary,[37] into a file. The *number of images* or *frames per second (fps)* is the number of images per second that is recorded into the file. The *resolution* of the video is the number of pixels used for the digitization of each image, which defines the quality of the images and of the video, as shown in Fig. 5.17.

As shown in Fig. 5.17—if the resolution of the image is too small, there is the "pixelisation" effect where the border of the original image is no longer visible in the digitized image. In practice resolution is much better than this, and typical values are shown in Table 5.4:

Once the video signal has been digitized, it is never stored in its original form because its size would be too large and not practical to manage. To solve this problem, a process of *compression of the video signal* is performed to obtain more acceptable file sizes. Compression is a very complex process that is reviewed in the next paragraph.

5.5.3 Digital Video Compression

Digital video compression is a widely used process that is performed on all digital video signals currently used.

The first compression used in digital video was called *MJPEG* (Motion JPEG[38]), in which every single image was compressed into a JPEG format and the sequence of images stored. This technique, despite being intuitive, didn't exploit the fact that the difference between one image and the next could be minimal, so that new techniques have been developed, all of them named *MPEG* (Motion Picture Experts Group), that exploit this concept of only storing the difference between sequential images.

It is simple to understand that several different algorithms can be developed for this type of compression, so the MPEG standard has evolved enormously over time taking advantage of the increasing computational power of digital systems and optimizing the results. As a result, from the initial *MPEG-1* standard, the *MPEG-2* was developed (used by DVDs) up to the most recent *MPEG-4*. All these standards have their own peculiar characteristics but, as far as video EEG is concerned, their differences stand out in the fact that a similar quality result can be obtained with smaller file sizes, as shown in the following table:

The calculation in Table 5.5 was performed on a CIF resolution video and using a similar image quality factor. By changing these parameters, it is possible to get very different results that make any comparison looking at the file size, very difficult to identify the compression.

[37]In some applications, like sleep, it is not always necessary to record at 25 frames/s. As most of the time there's no need to monitor detailed movement and a lower number of frames/second is sufficient, typically 12.5 or 5 or 1, reducing the file size proportionally.

[38]JPEG is the acronym of Joint Photographic Experts Group and is the most used standard for the picture compression, allowing high-compression factor that can be selected according to the desired image quality.

Table 5.5 Video file sizes

Codec	File size	
MJPEG	28.1 Mb/min	1.65 Gb/h
MPEG-1	8.2 Mb/min	495 Mb/h
MPEG-2	5.2 Mb/min	315 Mb/h
MPEG-4	4.3 Mb/min	260 Mb/h

5.5.4 Digital Video File Display

As discussed in the previous paragraph, digital video files are always compressed, and there are several different compression standards. As each compression standard corresponds to a different compression algorithm, to display the video on a PC, it is necessary to have the complementary decompressor algorithm. The union of the two words (COmpressor–DECompressor) has created the word *codec* that identifies the software and algorithm that a computer should use for the compression of a video and which to use to display a compressed video. According to the compression type and the operating system used, it is possible to have different problems displaying a video, so it's strongly recommended to always have the codec software available when moving a video to a different PC (i.e. for a presentation at a conference or simply on another PC).

It is worth noting that the file extension does not automatically identify the compression. Files with the same extension (typically .AVI) can have very different codecs.

Acknowledgments Thanks to Raffaele Orsato MEng, PhD for Figs. 5.6 and 5.7, Marco Cursi MEng for Fig. 5.17, Arianna, Laura and Piergiorgio for revising this chapter and most of all to David and Kristen for revising the entire English text.

Appendix 1: The Aliasing

Aliasing is the phenomenon that "replicates" signal components that exceed half of the sampling rate into the part of the spectrum below half the sampling rate. The replication happens specular to the sampling rate. For a better comprehension of this phenomenon, one can think of taking the spectrum of the analogue signal and replicating it specular starting from the selected sampling rate. The resulting spectrum after the sampling will be the sum of the two spectrums: the original one and the replicated one. It is evident that if the two spectrums don't overlap, there's no error in the sampling. Vice versa, if the two spectrums overlap, some "unwanted" component will be generated on the signal and called "aliasing."

As an example, consider the EEG signal spectrum of Fig. 5.18 that is an EEG contaminated by 50 Hz. The signal has a main Theta component, a good Alpha peak and another

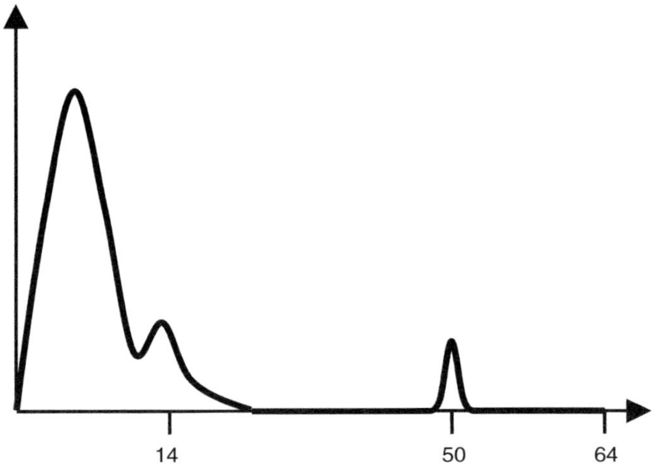

Fig. 5.18 Original spectrum of the analog signal

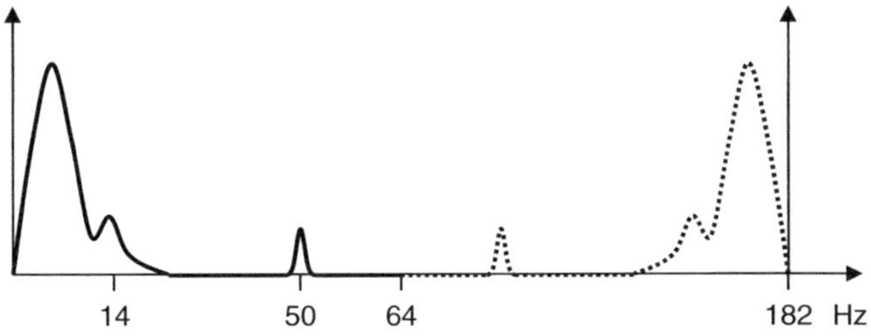

Fig. 5.19 Overlapped spectrum F_S = 128 Hz

peak at 50 Hz created by the noise. If the signal is sampled at 128 Hz, the original spectrum is replicated (symmetrically) starting from 128 Hz.

In this case the "replicated" spectrum does not overlap with the original thus there's no aliasing effect, as shown in Fig. 5.19. The maximum frequency that composes the original signal is around 50 Hz, which is lower than half the sampling rate used.

However, if the signal is sampled at 64 Hz without a proper anti-aliasing filter, the replicate of the spectrum (symmetrically) starts at 64 Hz as shown in Fig. 5.20 with the dashed line and in this case, the overlap is clear and their sum would lead to the spectrum of Fig. 5.21 which does not represent the original signal.

As shown in Fig. 5.21, the 14 Hz peak is increased by the replication of the 50 Hz component (that replicates exactly at 64–50 = 14 Hz) and the result on the signal would be a "pseudo" alpha over all the EEG.

Appendix 2: Source Reference

Source reference is a signal processing technique that aims to identify where (in terms of which electrode) the signal originates or finding the "source" of the signal. In practice, the

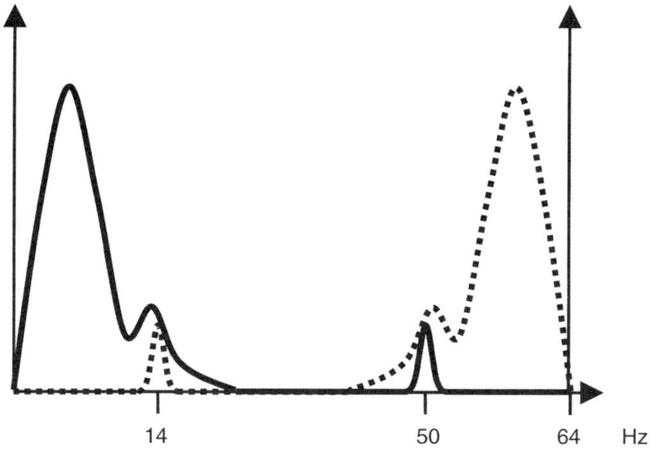

Fig. 5.20 Overlapped spectrum $F_S = 64$ Hz

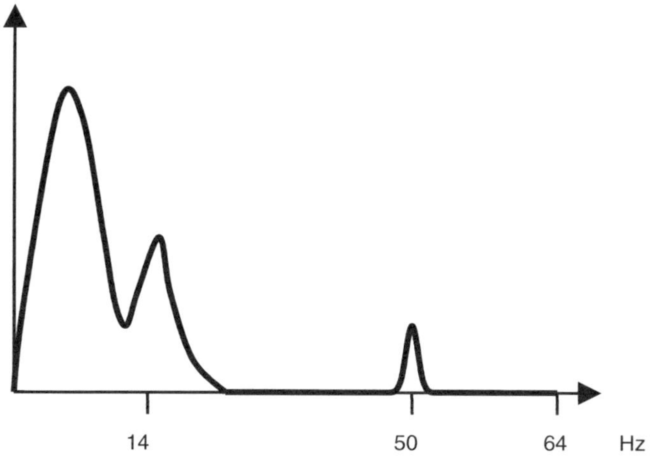

Fig. 5.21 Resulting spectrum $F_S = 64$ Hz

potential of an electrode will be higher if the source of the potential is located close to the electrode.

The fundamental concept of this principle is that the surface electrical fields are the expression of currents originating in points of the scalp that correspond to perpendicular field lines and there exists an equation that links the *source current* to the measured potentials, known as *Laplace's equation* (an alternative name for this technique is *Laplacian*). Such a current multiplied by a constant resistance becomes a potential, known as the *source potential* that can be calculated for every electrode. Using this technique the spatial dependent information is embedded into a new potential, i.e. $C3_{SRC}$, that highlights the topographic origin of the observed potentials. This results in the higher source potentials being located where the difference between the nearest potential is highest, thus localizing the source.

From a purely mathematical standpoint, the analysis is far too complex for this text, but the result is simple: The source potential of an electrode is the average of the difference of potentials between the electrode and its neighbouring electrodes. Consider, for example, the Cz electrode, recorded as (Cz-Ref), the source potential of Cz, will be indicated as Cz_{SRC} and can be calculated, under the hypothesis of using only four neighbouring electrodes, by the following formula:

$$Cz_{SRC} = \frac{(Cz - Fz) + (Cz - Pz) + (Cz - C3) + (Cz - C4)}{4}$$

Visually, the impact of calculating the source potentials for all the electrodes on the scalp is shown in Fig. 5.22:

As can be seen from Fig. 5.22, the potential of the Cz electrode, that is, the source of the signal, is the only location that the source potential calculation has increased, which highlights the source of the signal itself.

It is worth noting that the source reference can be seen as an average reference where the term to subtract *SRC* varies from electrode to electrode instead of being the same for each electrode. If we write this in formulas, we get

$$Cz_{SRC} = \frac{(Cz - Fz) + (Cz - Pz) + (Cz - C3) + (Cz - C4)}{4} = \frac{4(Cz - Ref) - [(Fz - Ref) + (Pz - Ref) + (C3 - Ref) + (C4 - Ref)]}{4}$$
$$= (Cz - Ref) - [0.25(Fz - Ref) + 0.25(Pz - Ref + 0.25)(C3 - Ref + 0.25))(C4 - Ref] = (Cz - Ref) - SRC$$

It becomes then a problem of calculating the weights that every neighbouring channel should have for the calculation of the SRC potential and to define how many neighbouring electrodes one wants to consider, typically 4 or 8. On a real EEG signal, the effect of the calculation of the source reference is shown in Fig. 5.23:

The figure shows clearly that the eye movement becomes visible only on the Fp1 and Fp2 electrodes (that are close to where they generate) and does not contaminate other electrodes as was the case with the average reference. Similarly the alpha-rhythm is only seen on the occipital electrodes O1 and O2.

Note that, unlike the average reference, the potential of the electrodes varies in a non-uniform way so that the source reference changes the display of the signals in all bipolar montages, not only in the unipolar montages.

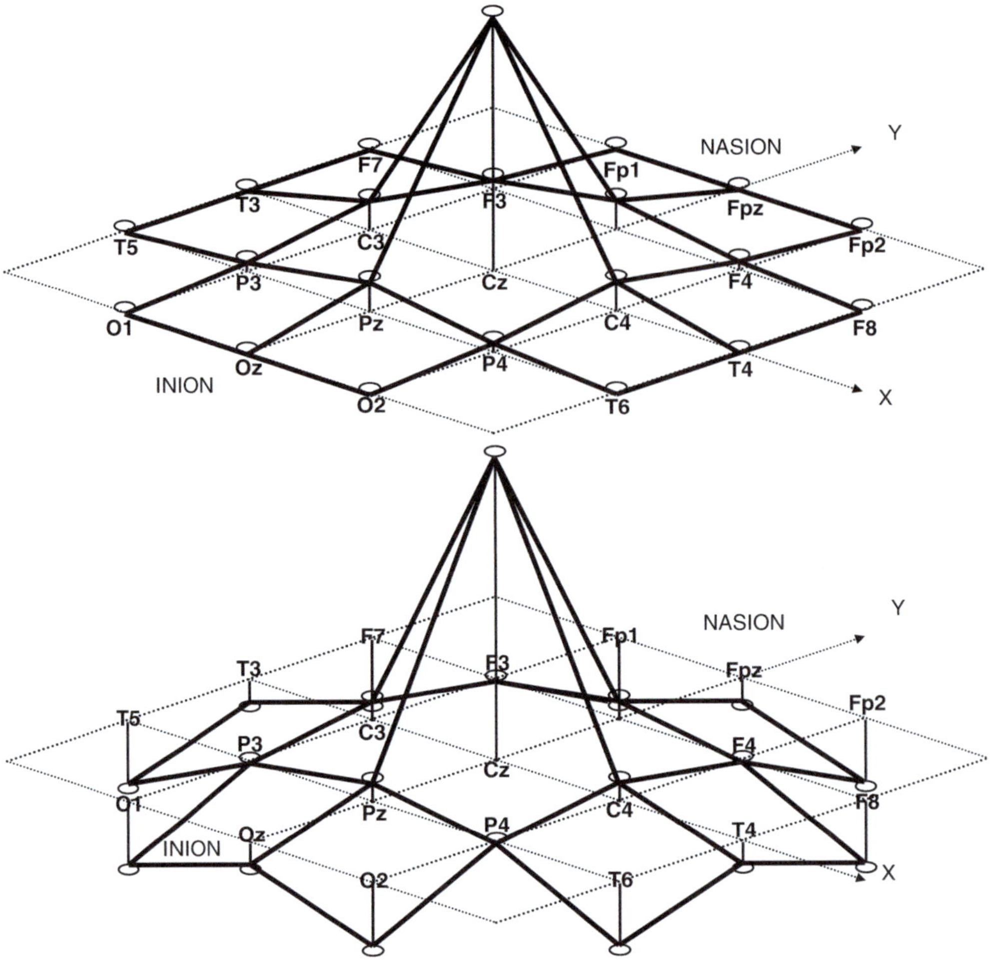

Fig. 5.22 Example of calculation of source potentials

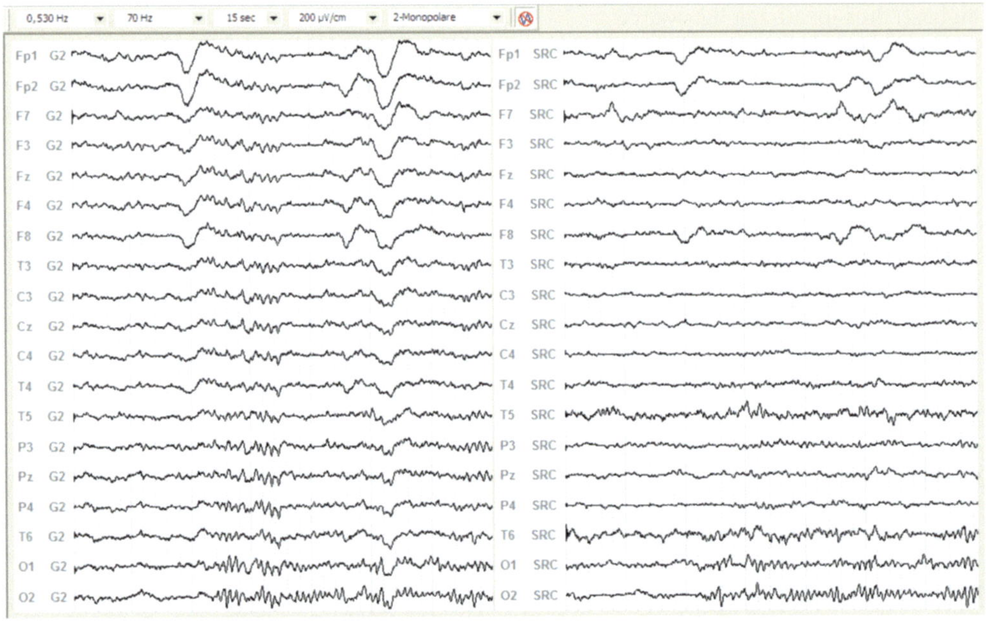

Fig. 5.23 Effect of the source reference on an EEG signal

Reference

1. Recommendation for the practice of clinical neurophysiology: guidelines of the International Federation of Clinical Neurophysiology. Electroencephalogr Clin Neurophysiol Suppl. 1999;52:1–304.

EEG Signal Analysis

6

Cristiano Rizzo

6.1 Introduction

The analysis process of the EEG signal is to obtain values that can highlight a particular property of the signal itself, thus characterizing it. Any value obtained also needs to be displayed correctly through an accurate drawing technique in order to make the value useful and clearly legible to the user.

Given the definition, it is clear that there are many different EEG signal analyses and display techniques, so to list them would not be useful.

As such, given the objective of this section, we have chosen to list only some of the most diffused techniques of signal analysis and possible display techniques. We have selected the classic *spectral analysis*, the calculation of *parameters in the time domain* and their main display techniques as *cerebral mapping*, *trending over time* and *time-frequency graphics.*

6.2 EEG Signal Analysis in the Frequency Domain

Signal analysis in the frequency domain, or *spectral analysis*, is a technique widely used in several scientific fields and is the basis of many common processes such as MRI. By definition, spectral analysis is a statistical analysis of data, and its complete technical description is far too complicated for the purposes of this section, so it will not be included here. We will instead try to highlight its importance without getting too much into theory. The terminology used will not be the most precise from an engineering point of view, but hopefully this would allow a better understanding of the point.

We can start by stating that spectral analysis is based on the transformation of the EEG signal from the time domain (a series of samples in time) into the frequency domain (a series of samples for each frequency). The greatest advantage of this operation is the condensation into a few values of the information contained in some seconds to some hours. As this is by definition a statistical analysis, the result will be an average information on the structure of the EEG signal and will not highlight any very short signal patterns or any signal that has a weak power.

The basic principle is that any signal can be obtained as sum of pure sinusoidal components, with different amplitudes and phases as shown in Fig. 6.1.

In this example the 2 seconds of EEG signal are obtained as the sum of just four components at 4, 10, 11 and 20 Hz, each of them with different amplitudes (10 μV the 4 Hz component, 50 μV the 10 Hz component, 30 μV the 11 Hz component, 14 μV the 20 Hz component). The signal in the frequency domain in Fig. 6.1 shows, for each frequency, the amplitude of the component (to be exact, half of the peak to peak amplitude).

The display of the signal as a *spectrum*, as in Fig. 6.2, is a graphic that shows, for each pure component in the frequency domain, the power of the signal at that frequency and is called power spectral density (PSD). This graphic should be represented as a bar graphic, but, in reality, it is always drawn as a continuous graphic where the *X*-axis is the frequency (measured in Hz or cycle/s) and the *Y*-axis is the power density of each frequency quantum (measured in μV^2/Hz). The calculation of this decomposition is obtained by means of the Discrete Fourier Transform (DFT) that in the version that allows a very fast calculation, introduced in 1970 [1], takes the name of Fast Fourier transform (FFT).

Please note that Fourier analysis is just one of the possible spectral estimation techniques; other techniques like autoregressive modelling can be found in the literature [2].

Spectral analysis consists of cutting the EEG signal into epochs of 2 s or more and then transforming, according to the Fourier technique, every epoch to obtain the PSD. Finally, an average of all the spectrum is performed and the result is displayed as a graphic.

C. Rizzo (✉)
Micromed S.p.A., Mogliano Veneto, Italy
e-mail: cristiano.rizzo@micromed.eu

O. Mecarelli (ed.), *Clinical Electroencephalography*, https://doi.org/10.1007/978-3-030-04573-9_6

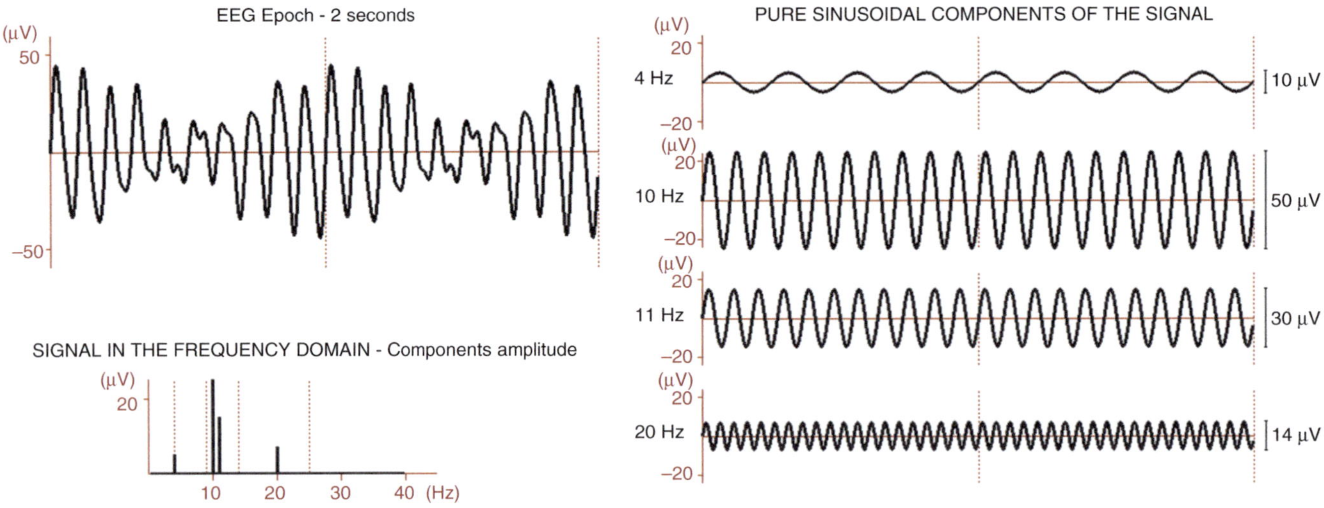

Fig. 6.1 Decomposition of an EEG signal into pure sinusoidal components

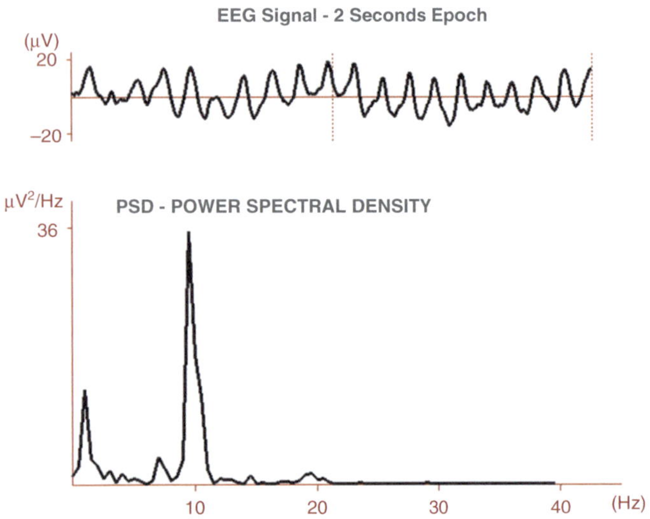

Fig. 6.2 Spectrum, or PSD, of an EEG signal characterized by alpha rhythm

As already discussed, spectral analysis is not a precise method but an average method as it highlights the harmonic content of the signal in predefined epochs; adding to the fact that several spectrums are averaged, it is clear that this technique cannot highlight short signal transient or very low-power signals.

In order to improve the performance of the spectral analysis, several techniques are often used, such as *overlapping*, *detrending* and *tapering*.

Overlapping consists of running the analysis on epochs that are overlapped, that is, analysing fixed epochs of 2 s, starting every second as shown in Fig. 6.3. This allows the analysis of every element of the signal in a way that in one epoch, or in the next one, the element is centred.

Detrending consists of removing continuous components or slopes from each epoch. Technically this means removing from the EEG signal the "line" that best approximates the evolution of the signal in the given epoch, as shown in Fig. 6.4:

Figure 6.4 shows the line that best interpolates the EEG signal and the signal resulting after the subtraction of this line. The resulting spectrum highlights a modification of the power in a way that best represents what an EEG expert could see in the signal itself. The "slow" components of the signal that are removed are rarely of interest for the analysis, while the faster components are highlighted, and they are quite often most important for the analysis.

Tapering, or windowing of the signal, aims to reduce the spectral leakage phenomenon that, spreading the power of a signal among the spectrum, tends to hide important components of the signal that might have a weaker power. The improvement obtained with this technique is important especially in those cases where a dominant signal of high power (i.e. slow EEG waves) could "mask" other significant components (i.e. alpha rhythm). Technically speaking, this operation consists of multiplying any signal epoch by a given function that usually is equal to 0 at the extremes of the epoch.

6.2.1 EEG Parameters in the Frequency Domain

Once standard spectral analysis has been performed on an EEG signal, properly split into epochs and conditioned with the techniques described in the previous paragraph, the average spectrum of the analysed EEG signal is obtained. This spectrum is then split into parts that are normally used for the description of the EEG rhythm, which are delta, theta, alpha and beta, as shown in Fig. 6.5.

Splitting the spectrum this way allows the calculation of several other data that could summarize interesting charac-

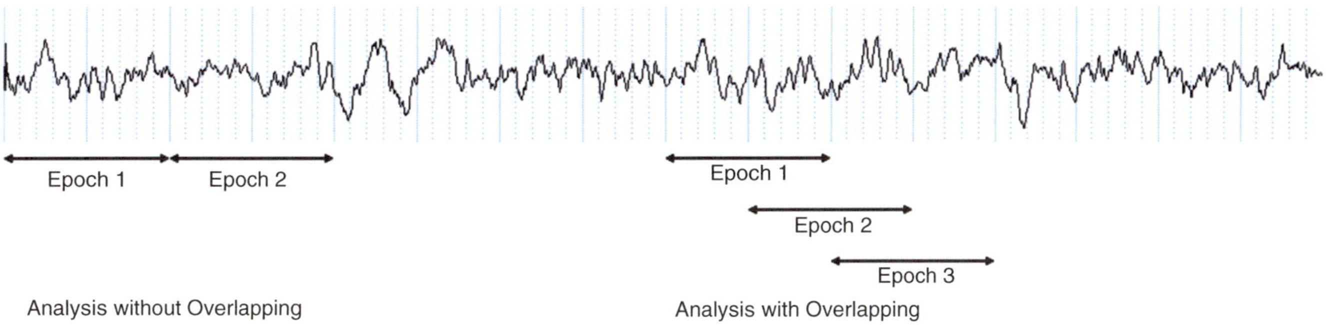

Fig. 6.3 Epoch selection with and without overlapping

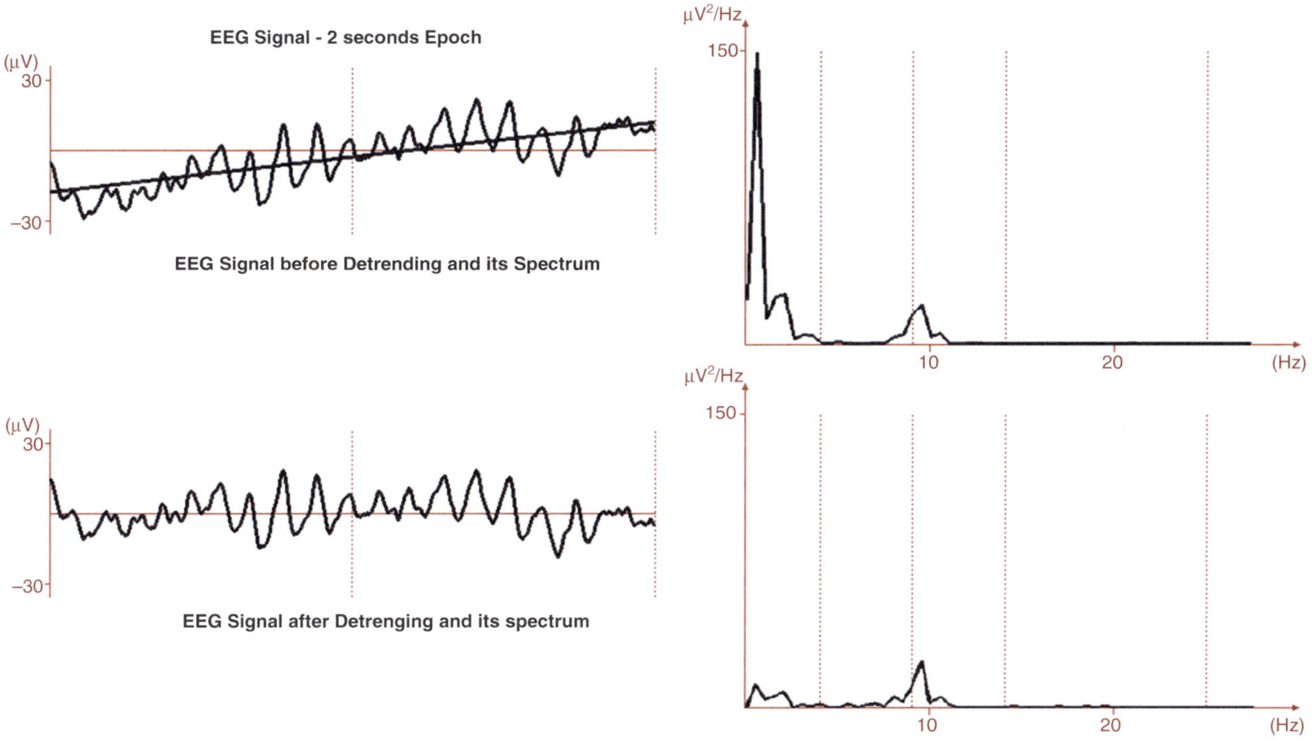

Fig. 6.4 Example of detrending of an EEG signal epoch

teristics of the EEG signal that quantify something that is normally determined with the visual inspection, like the following:

- *Absolute Power* in the different bands. These values are calculated as the area underlying the spectrum of the signal in the interval of frequency that defines each band,[1] as shown in (Fig. 6.6). Their measurement unit is μV^2.
- *Relative Power* in the different bands. These values are calculated as the ratio between absolute power in a band and the total power (i.e. the sum of the power in all the bands). Under the assumption to use the four standard bands, one could obtain:

$$P_{REL}(\text{alfa}) = \frac{P_{ABS}(\text{alfa})}{P_{ABS}(\text{delta}) + P_{ABS}(\text{theta}) + P_{ABS}(\text{alfa}) + P_{ABS}(\text{beta}) +}$$

- As a ratio between two homologous values, the result is a-dimensional and is normally expressed as a percentage.
- *PPF—Peak Power Frequency*. This refers to the frequency where the spectrum has its peak, as shown in Fig. 6.7. This calculation could be restricted to the frequency interval defined by each band. The measurement unit is that of frequency, that is, Hz or cycle/s.

[1] Mathematically it is the integral, in the frequency domain, of the PSD.

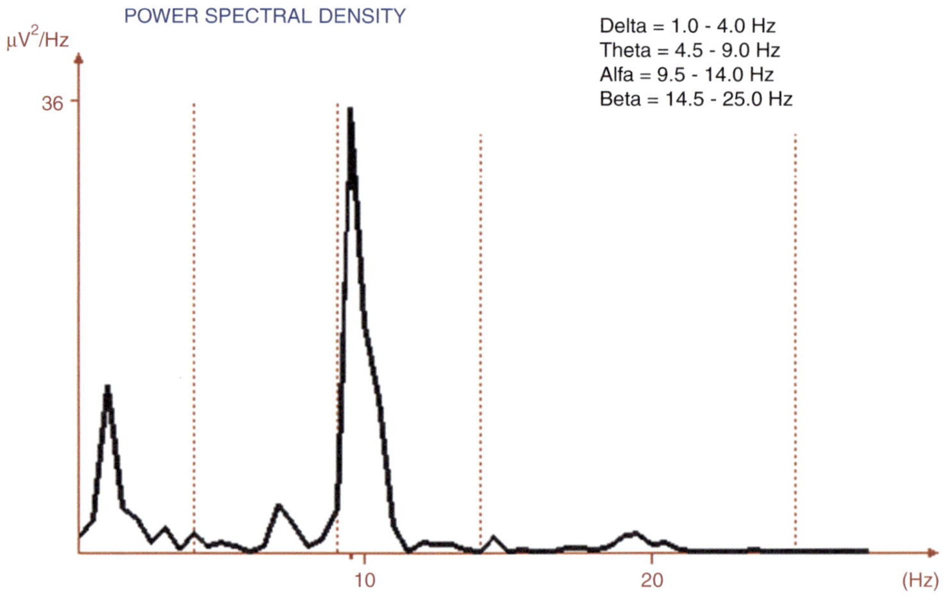

Fig. 6.5 PSD of an EEG signal split into standard bands

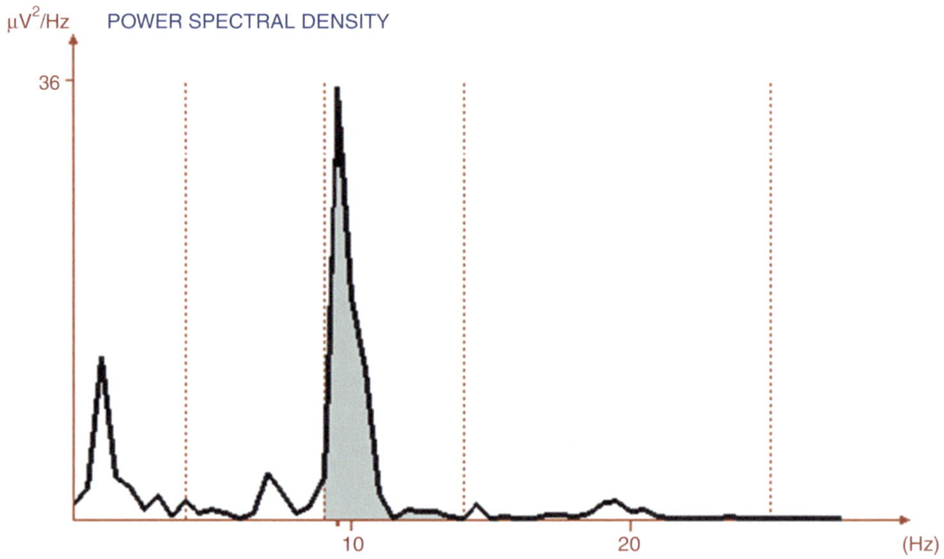

Fig. 6.6 Absolute power of the alpha band shown as area underlying the spectrum

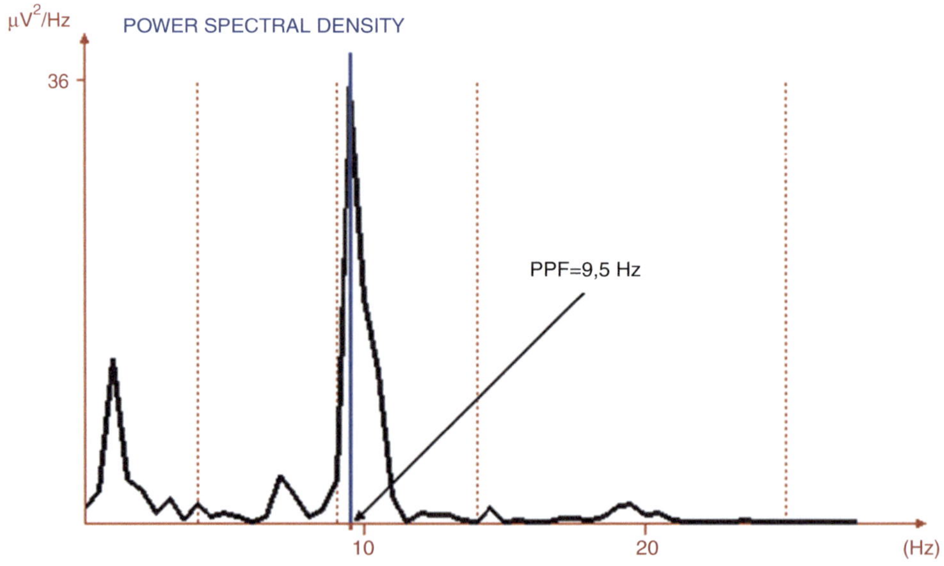

Fig. 6.7 Example of calculation of PPF on the spectrum of an EEG signal

- *MF—Median Frequency*. This is the frequency that splits the spectrum into two regions, each underlying 50% of the total power, as shown in Fig. 6.8. The measurement unit is that of frequency, that is Hz or cycle/s.
- *SEF—Spectral Edge Frequency*. This is defined as "size" of the spectrum. It can be obtained with different techniques, and quite often, it is defined as the interval of the spectrum that underlines 95% of the total power, as shown in Fig. 6.9. The measurement unit is that of frequency, that is, Hz or cycle/s.
- *MDF—Main Dominant Frequency*. This is the dominant frequency of the spectrum, defined as an average of the frequencies weighted by the power at each frequency. The calculation formula is:

$$\mathrm{MDF} = \frac{\sum_{f=0}^{f_{\mathrm{MAX}}} f \cdot \mathrm{PSD}[f]}{\sum_{f=0}^{f_{\mathrm{MAX}}} \mathrm{PSD}[f]}$$

- The measurement unit is that of frequency, that is, Hz or cycle/s.

All of these parameters can be used by themselves or in combination with each other to define new variables, often called *indexes*. A common example in the literature is the theta/alpha quotient that is calculated as the ratio between the absolute power in the theta band and the absolute power in the alpha band of the same signal. It is easy to understand that several other indexes could be defined as a function of

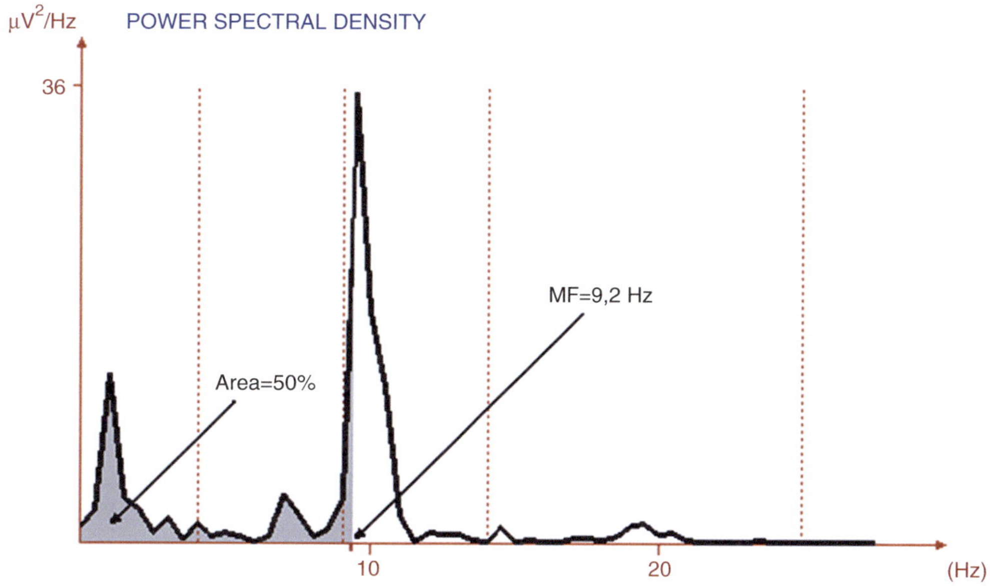

Fig. 6.8 Example of calculation of MF on the spectrum of an EEG signal

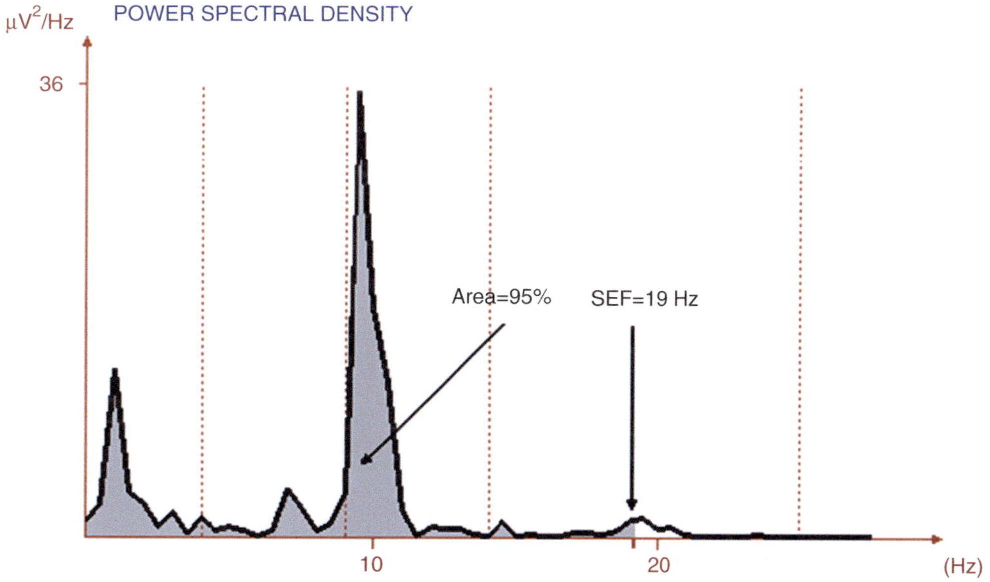

Fig. 6.9 Example of calculation of SEF on the spectrum of an EEG signal

parameters of the same signal, as well as function of parameters of different signals. An example of the latter could be the ratio between the same parameter of two electrodes on different sides of the brain, defining then a sort of asymmetry index.

Those indexes, being often the ratio between homologous entities, have some advantages:

- They can represent very complex characteristics of the signal in a very concise way.
- They are in general less sensitive to artefact, at least to those contaminating the electrodes in a similar way.
- They are generally less sensitive to big differences in the absolute power of the signal of different subjects, characteristics that they share with the relative power.

6.2.2 Data Calculation

A "historic" problem of the spectral analysis is the complexity of the calculation—the enormous amount of effort necessary to obtain and display data. For example, the fast Fourier transform (FFT) of a single epoch of one EEG channel sampled at 256 Hz requires 2048 multiplications plus the operations necessary to acquire data, its memorization and its display. This means that 1 min of 20 channels of EEG data requires over two million multiplications. This is to understand that, before the recent evolution of digital technology, such a calculation was very difficult thus limiting the diffusion of the technique. Today, the modern computer can easily perform such calculations, allowing for the deployment of the technique more widely.

6.3 EEG Signal Analysis in the Time Domain

EEG parameters calculated in the time domain are all measurements and/or calculations performed directly on the original signal, without any transformation as in the case of the spectral analysis.

6.3.1 EEG Parameters in the Time Domain

There exist several EEG parameters in the time domain, and, given the scope of this book, we will consider only those parameters that are often used and cited in the literature:

- *Zero Crossing*: defined as the number of times the EEG signal crosses the baseline, as shown in Fig. 6.10. Unfortunately, this parameter does not always represent what is referred to in EEG as the rhythm of the signal. Quite often the rhythm of interest is embedded into slow waves that make the calculation false. An example of this is in Fig. 6.10.
- Note that in the mentioned example, there are 32 crossings in 2 s, that is, 16 per second, which should lead to a rhythm of the signal of 8 Hz, but, in reality, it is about 10 Hz. The problem is in the crossings lost due to the drift the signal has in a certain interval that avoid it crossing the baseline.
- *Burst Suppression Ratio*: this is a parameter that quantifies the degree of suppression of an EEG signal [3]. It is calculated, on an epoch of fixed duration, as the ratio between the time the signal remains stable below a given threshold, i.e. ±5 μV, and the duration of the epoch itself as shown in Fig. 6.11. In order to consider an EEG signal suppressed, the signal doesn't have to exceed the threshold for at least 400–500 ms. If within an epoch there are multiple intervals of suppression, they should be added. This parameter sets, practically speaking, which percentage of the epoch is occupied by a suppressed signal.
- In this example there is a suppression interval of 0.810 s on an epoch of 2 s, giving then a BSR of 0.810/2.000 = 0.405, that is, 40.5%.

6.4 Data Display Technique

Data display is fundamental in any kind of analysis. This is why some paragraphs are dedicated to this point, dealing with the most commonly used display techniques.

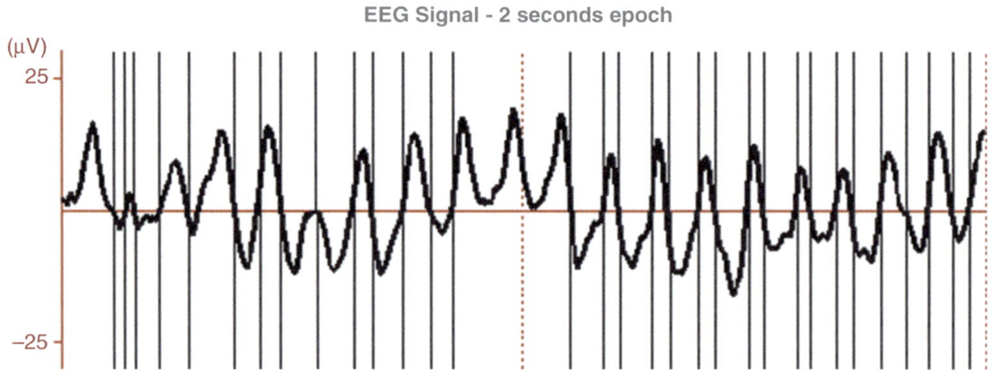

Fig. 6.10 Example of calculation of "Zero Crossing" of an EEG signal

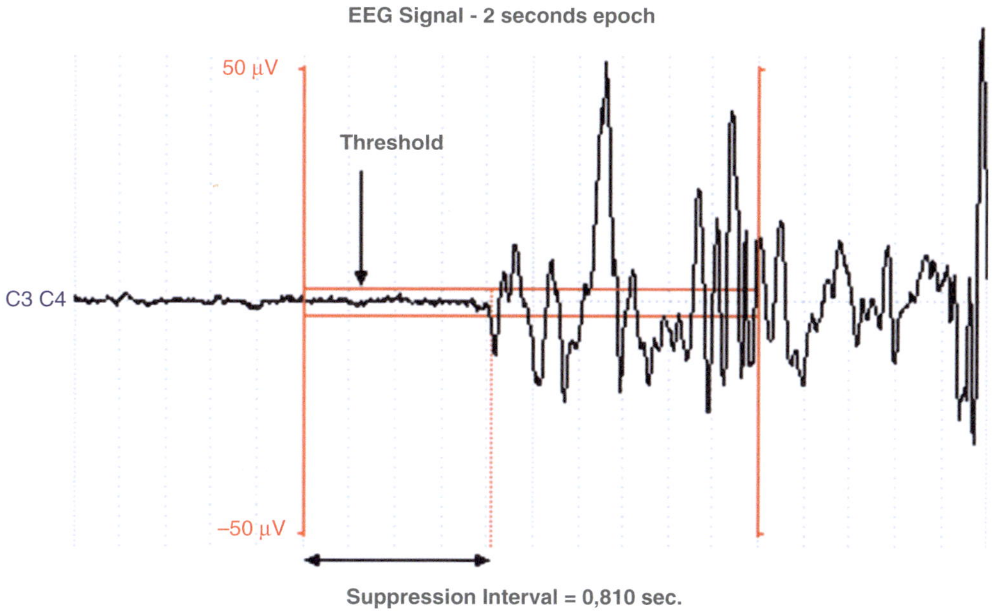

Fig. 6.11 Calculation of "Burst Suppression Ratio (BSR)" on an EEG signal

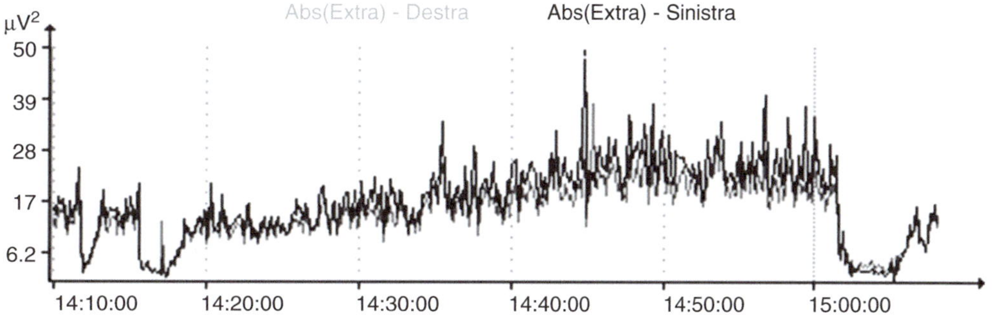

Fig. 6.12 Trend of absolute power on the right and left hemisphere

When choosing the display technique, one should focus on which characteristics should be highlighted:

- Evolution of the data over time
- Spatial distribution of the data

We will now analyse the most diffused display technique according to these two choices.

6.4.1 Display of Data Evolution over Time

All display techniques of data evolution over time share the same characteristic: a time axis along which all information are drawn. In order of complexity, some of the possible techniques are:

- *Histograms and Trends*. These are the simpler techniques, often the most efficient, to display time evolution of a parameter, with the down side of not allowing the display of a lot of variables on the same graphic in order to avoid compromised legibility. The display consists in a Cartesian graphic with the time in an axis (often the horizontal one), more or less compressed, on the other axis the parameter to display. This graphic can display any kind of parameter, calculated both in time and frequency domains. The example in Fig. 6.12 shows a trend with two absolute power calculated on all derivation of the right (light grey) and left (dark grey) hemisphere of an EEG recorded during carotid endarterectomy.
- *Compressed Spectral Array (CSA)*. This is a type of display often used in the past to display the spectral analysis. It was used for the first time in 1971 for the advantages it offers for the display of power spectrum over time. It consists in a vertical successive display of power spectrum obtained over time as shown in Fig. 6.13, obtaining then a graphic with a prospect effect.
- The *X*-axis shows frequency, the *Y*-axis shows the power and the step between each spectrum is the time between each interval so that *Z*-axis shows time. This kind of display is helpful and can easily show the variation over time of background rhythm. It still needs to be interpreted by an expert and is problematic in that big artefacts can easily hide all the graphic behind the last drawn spectrum. This is the reason this technique has been supplanted by the DSA.

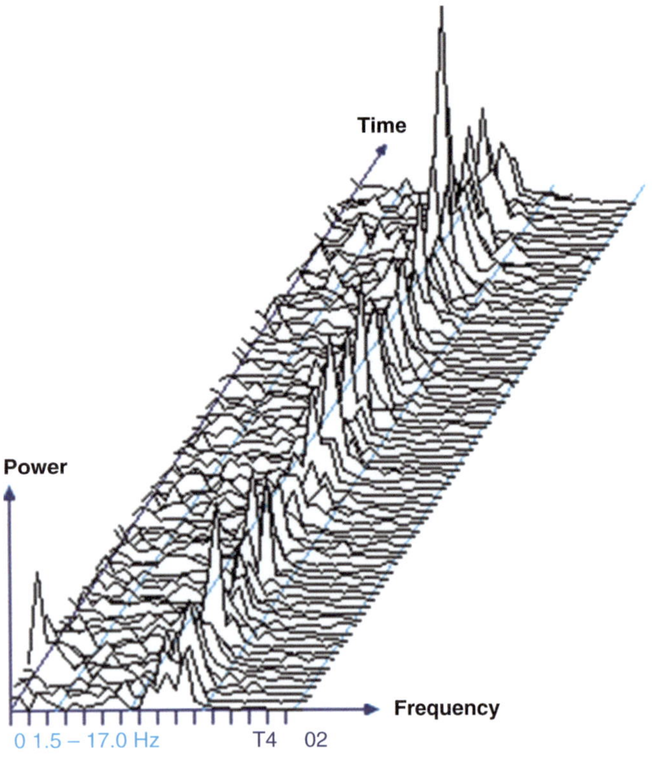

Fig. 6.13 CSA of an EEG characterized by an alpha rhythm

- *Density Spectral Array (DSA)*. This is another technique to display time evolution of the spectral analysis that uses a chromatic scale to display the power of each frequency quantum of the spectrum. This means that every power spectrum is represented by a coloured stripe (or greyscale stripe) where the *Y*-axis represents the frequency of the point; the colour of the point represents the power of the frequency spectrum at that frequency. The succession of such stripes represents the time evolution of the spectrums, that is, the DSA, as shown in Fig. 6.14.
- This type of display does not mask the previous components, as is the case with CSA, and can easily display very long sequences; however, the presence of very weak modification of power is not always as easy to localize as it was with the CSA.
- *Wavelet*. This is a technique very similar to DSA, which is a time-frequency graphic that uses a chromatic scale to display the power of each frequency component at a given time. The difference with the DSA stands in the spectral analysis technique used, not a simple Fourier transform but a more complex wavelet transform, which allows a better indication of the power of the frequency components for even the shortest intervals, in the order of milliseconds. This allows a more detailed data analysis, unfortunately losing the global overview characteristics, which is one of the bigger advantages of DSA. Wavelet transform is therefore used to analyse short time interval like evoked potentials or particular EEG pattern (i.e. spike) as shown in Fig. 6.15 but can in principle be used for longer EEG interval.
- *aEEG — Amplitude Integrated EEG*. This is a technique to display EEG in time domain that performs special data processing that can be summarized as follows:
  - Selective band-pass filter between 2 and 15 Hz
  - Transformation of the signal in semilogarithmic scale[2]
  - Rectification of the signal[3]
  - Smoothing to identify only maximum and minimum peaks of the resulting signal
  - Graphic of the result
- The graphic obtained with this technique shows condensed information about the amplitude of the signal, mainly showing the amplitude of the biggest peaks and that of the smallest peaks, as shown in Fig. 6.16.

  This technique, introduced decades ago [4] but still often used especially in neonatal intensive care units, is normally identified as CFM (cerebral function monitor), which is the name of the first device that used this technique.

6.4.2 Display of Spatial Distribution of Data

Brain Mapping is a technique that aims to display the spatial distribution on the scalp of an activity that is measured only on a few points of the scalp itself. Once such a distribution is calculated from the values at these points, it can be displayed obtaining the so-called maps.

The calculation performed to obtain such a mapping is an interpolation of the activity that is effectively measured on the scalp, and, depending on the kind of activity, the following results can be obtained:

- *Amplitude Maps*: this is a display of the distribution on the scalp of the amplitude of the EEG signal measured at a given time, that is, for a digital signal, at a given sample.
- *Frequency Maps*: this is a display of the distribution on the scalp of the average power in a given frequency band

[2] Semilogarithmic scale means that all values up to 10 μV remains linear and all values above 10 μV are transformed in a logarithmic scale.

[3] Rectification means turning to positive all negative signals. Mathematically this is the module of the value.

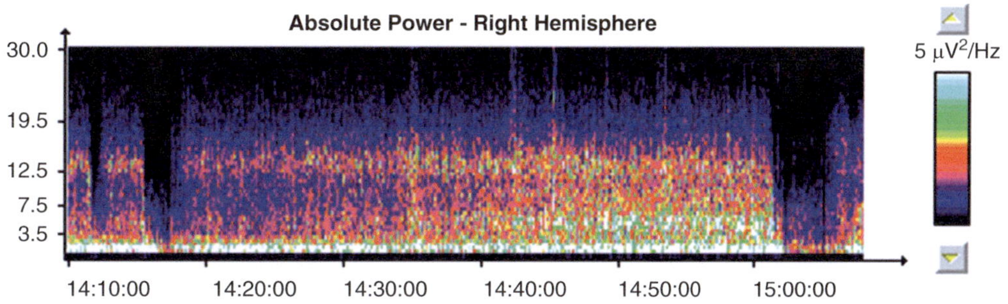

Fig. 6.14 DSA of an EEG trace

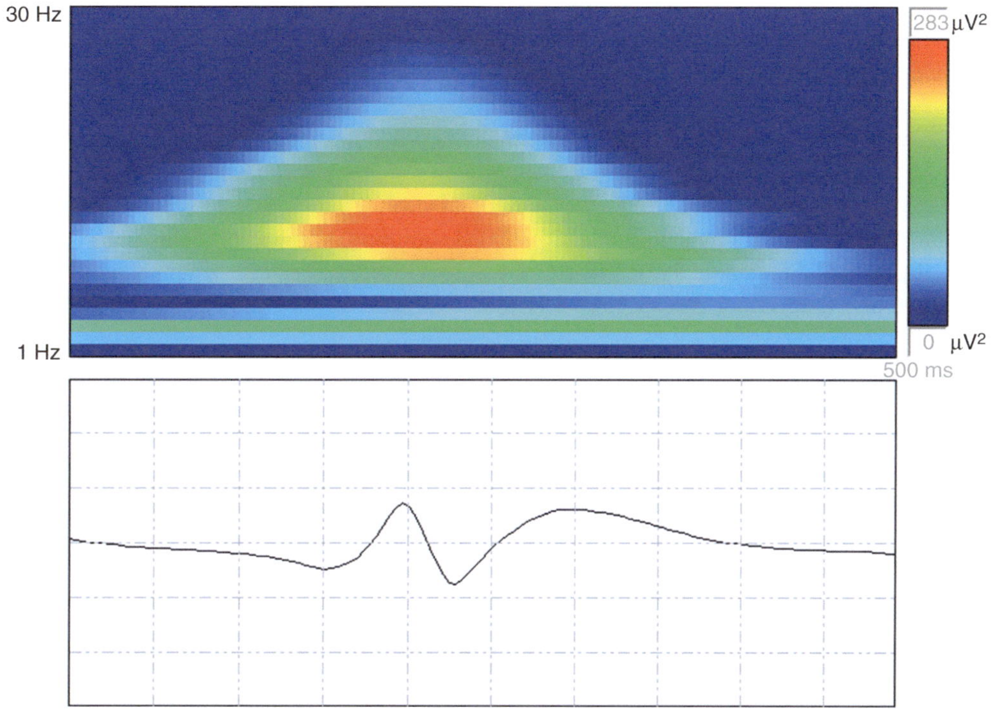

Fig. 6.15 Wavelet transform of a spike and wave signal

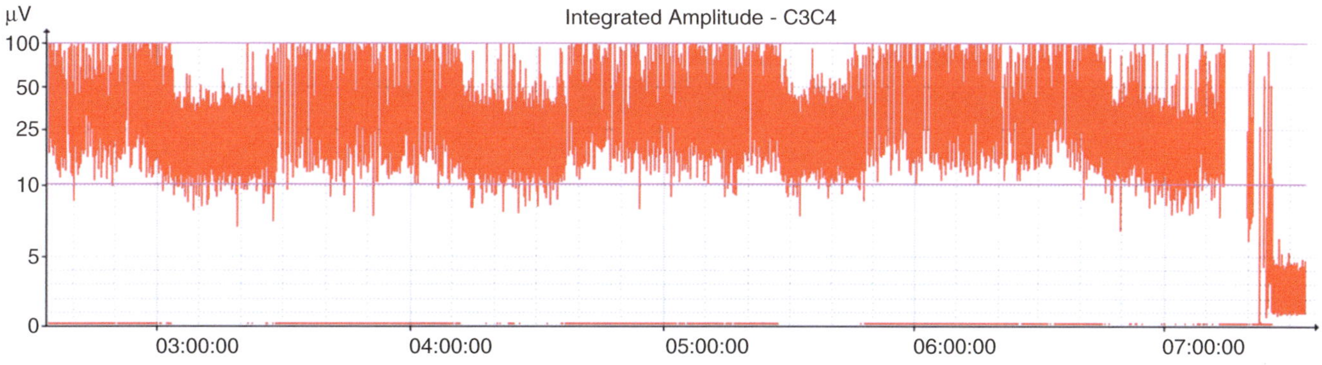

Fig. 6.16 EEG trace displayed as aEEG

of the EEG signal calculated in one or more selected time interval on which spectral analysis is performed.

- *Coherence Maps*: this is a display of the distribution on the scalp of the average coherence in a given frequency band of the EEG signal calculated in one or more selected time interval on which spectral analysis is performed.

This technique has evolved in recent time thanks to the integration of functional data (EEG, EP) with the structural data supplied by the MRI. In fact, if we were to display the activity all over the scalp, we have a few choices to create a model of the scalp, like using a simple mathematical model of the scalp, which is normally a circle (planar) or a sphere, or generating a realistic model of the scalp from the MRI.

In the following paragraphs, we will provide an overview of the basic elements of a correct brain mapping, always referring to a general entity to be mapped (amplitude, power or others).

6.4.2.1 Spatial Sampling

Brain mapping is based on the principle of spatial sampling. The theoretical fundamentals of this are the equivalent of the sampling theorem of EEG signals analysed on Chap. 5 but extended to two dimensions. A deep analysis of the spatial sampling is probably too complex in this context; it is only important to point out the principle that, in the different spatial directions, the signal should not have a too high modification compared to the number of measures (point of measure being the electrodes). If, as in the example in Fig. 6.17, in a space of 10 cm we apply 10 electrodes, getting then 10 measures (F_{SAMP} = 100 sample/m), the signal cannot exceed 50 "waves" per metre (50 = Max spatial frequency, that is, $F_{SAMP}/2$), which means a maximum of 5 "waves" in 10 cm under test. This, assuming a uniform spatial sampling, should be verified in all possible directions of the space.

Given that it is not possible to restrict the signal from having a certain spatial modification, one can simply adapt the number of point of measurement on the scalp in a way to properly cover all possible spatial modification of the signal to be examined.

Several experiments have been performed in order to properly identify the amount of spatial variation of the EEG signals, which is how the activity is different from one point to another, and the results led to the following:

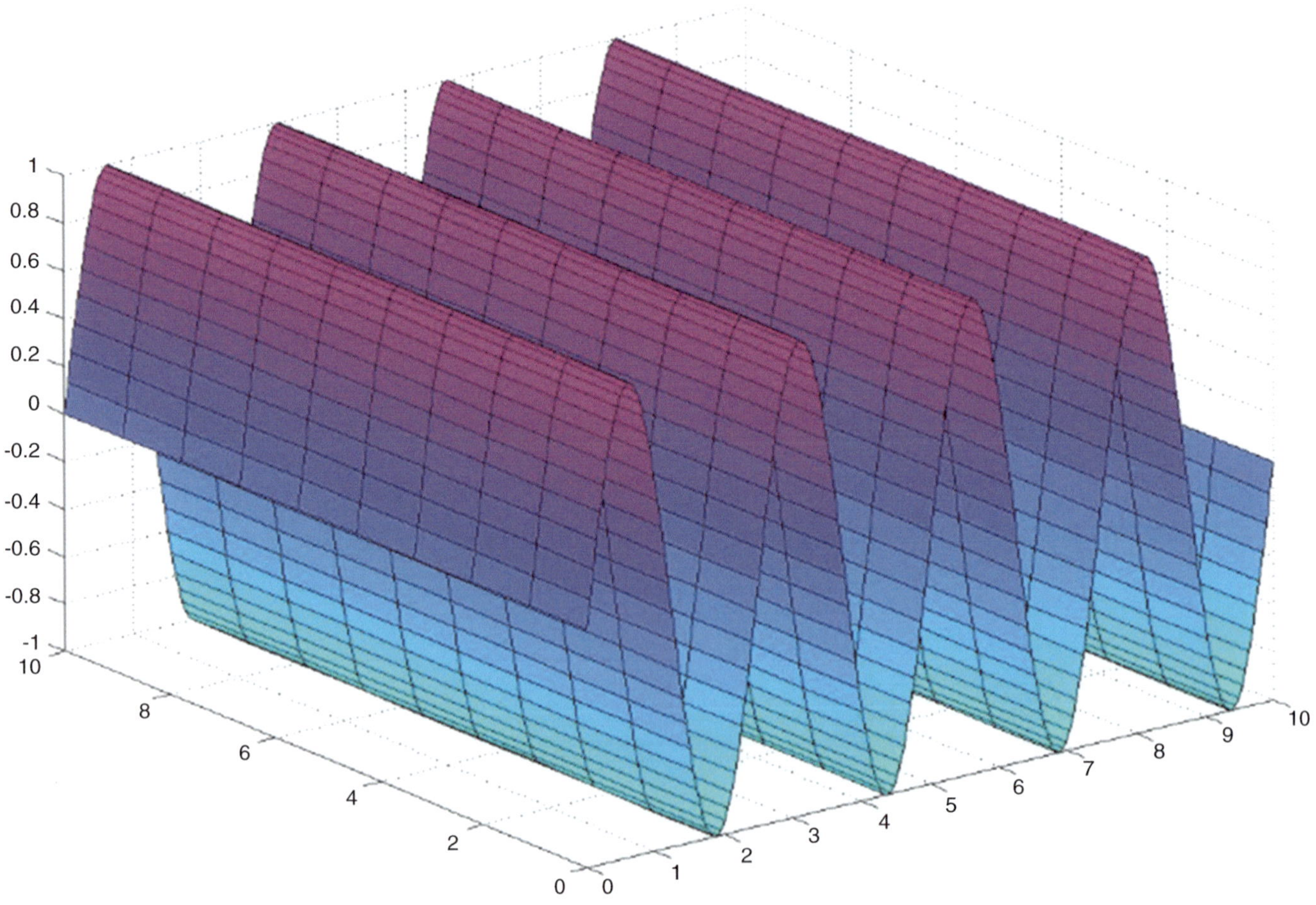

Fig. 6.17 Signal with four "waves" along the *X*-axis

- For a correct mapping of the cerebral EEG activity in *standard clinical application*, the minimum number of electrodes to be used is *25*, with positions based on the 20% and 10% of standardized measurements from anatomical landmarks on the skull [5]. These 25 electrodes, which used to be 19 [6], are Fp1, Fp2, F9, F7, F3, Fz, F4, F8, F10, T9, T7 (ex T3), C3, Cz, C4, T8 (ex T4), T10, P9, P7 (ex T5), P3, Pz, P4, P8 (ex T6), P10, O1 and O2, positioned according to the scheme in Fig. 6.18.
- For a correct mapping of the cerebral EEG activity requiring a *precise spatial localization* like source localization, a minimum number of *64* electrodes is required, positioned according to the scheme in Fig. 6.18. This kind of recording, using 64 up to 256 electrodes, is often referred as high-density EEG (HD-EEG) [5] and is nowadays widely used in clinical practice.

6.4.2.2 Scalp Models

As seen in the previous paragraphs, in order to achieve proper brain mapping, a correct scalp model needs to be defined. Once the scalp model is defined, the electrode positions need to be measured (or defined) using the same coordinate system of the model. Scalp models can be basically divided into three categories:

- *Planar Models*: these are models defined on a planar surface, where contours can be a circumference or a contour similar to that of a head or a brain (in this last case quite often, the brain circumvolution is drawn on the plane as well). These models, given their simplicity, have been and still are widely used. The coordinate system is Cartesian, which means that the position of each electrode is specified by a pair of numbers (x, y). The value of such coordinates is obtained as projection on the axial plane of the measured (or supposed) electrode positions.
- *Three-Dimensional Spherical Models*: these are more refined models as they approximate the scalp with a hemisphere on which electrodes are placed. These models have often been used in research, and their efficacy has proven to be better than the planar models. The coordinate system, in this case, could be specified by three coordinates (x, y, z), but very often, for the sake of simplicity, one assumes the sphere with unitary radium so that for each electrode one specifies just two coordinates, called

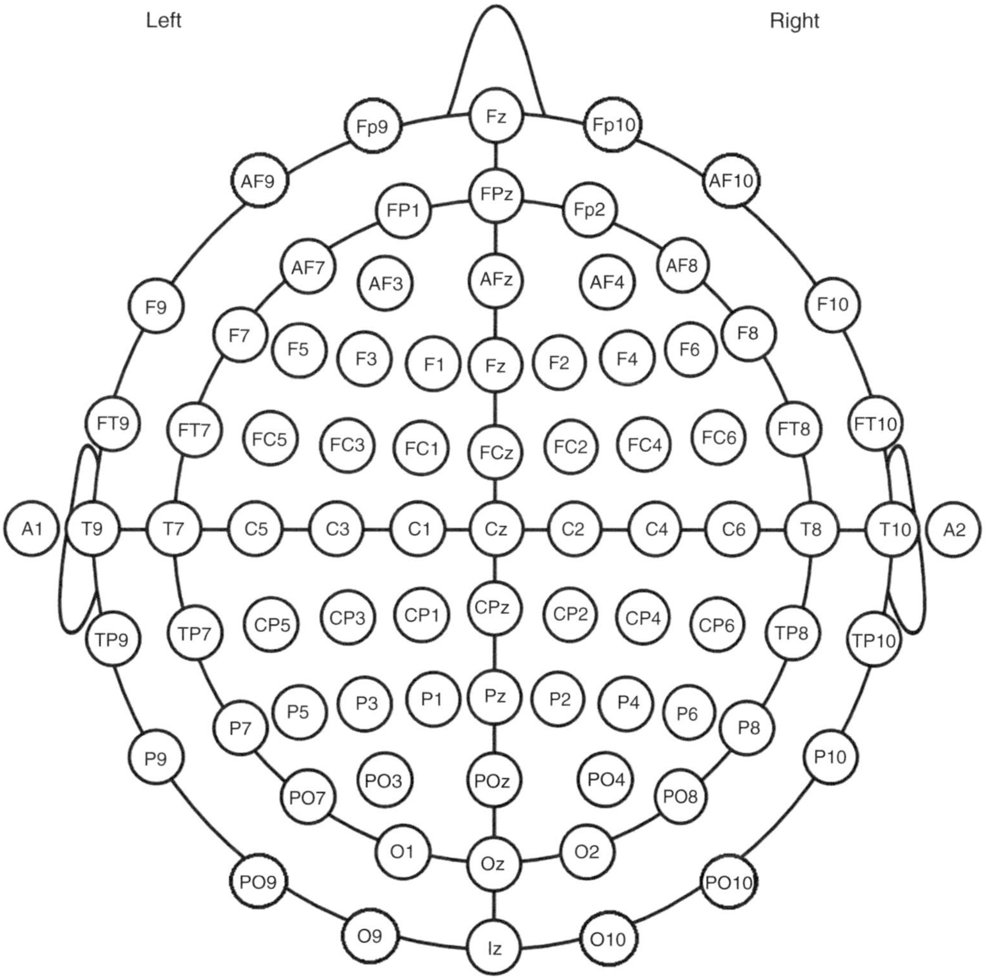

Fig. 6.18 Name and standard position of the IFCN standard 10/10 electrode system

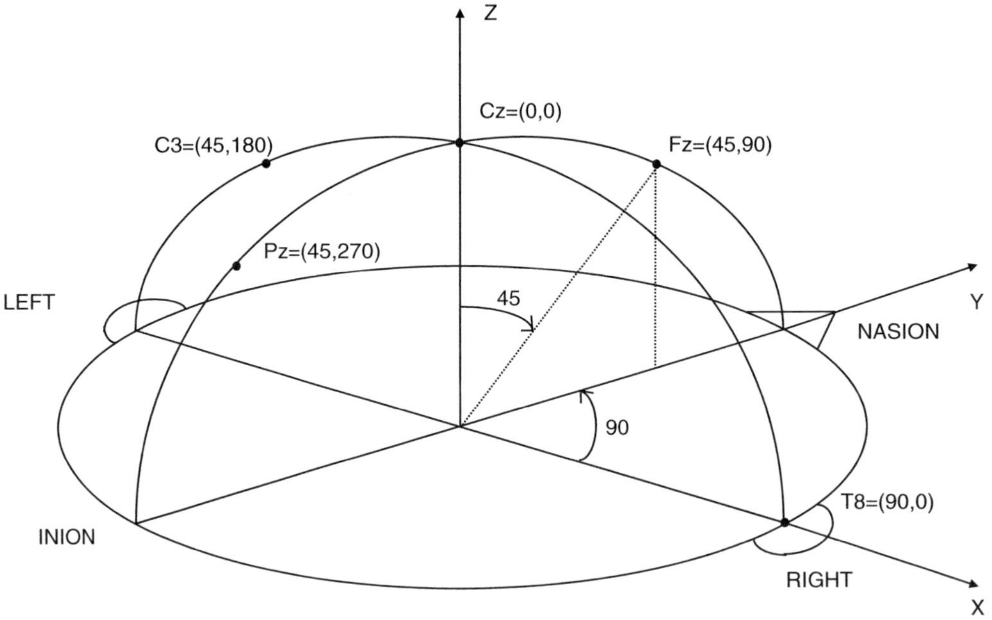

Fig. 6.19 Coordinate system for three-dimensional spherical models

latitude and longitude. Normally latitude is calculated with 0 in Cz, longitude with 0 in T8 (ex T4) as shown in the following picture (Fig. 6.19).

- An example of coordinates for the 10/10 system electrodes in Fig. 6.18 (excluding the lower ones), as latitude and longitude, could be those in Table 6.1.
- *Realistic Three-Dimensional Models*: these are models that try to minimize approximation by processing the MRI of the patient to obtain a model of the scalp surface. In order to do this, one needs dedicated software that reads MRI data, which is then processed to get a three-dimensional model of the head made of voxels and then create the model by, for example, drawing triangles that perfectly match the scalp surface. An example of such three-dimensional model and the related approximation of the scalp is shown in Fig. 6.20.

  The coordinate system, in case of realistic models, has to be Cartesian, defined by three coordinates (*x*, *y*, *z*). Such coordinates have to be precisely measured with dedicated tools that measure the exact position of a point in space, in all three dimensions, and use easy markers as a reference for the axis (i.e. nasion, inion, earlobes — easily identified in the MRI).[4]

6.4.2.3 Interpolation Techniques

As already discussed, brain mapping is the display of values of a certain signal on the scalp when the signal has been measured only on certain points. The fundamental operation is then the interpolation of the missing data, which can be obtained by means of several different algorithms; three of those algorithms, often used in practice, are analysed below:

1. *K-NN interpolation*: the K-NN method, which stands for K-Nearest Neighbours, is used to interpolate the value of the signal in a given point, by means of the values measured on the K nearest electrodes to the point itself. In general the value of the point can be calculated as a weighted average of the values of the K nearest electrodes, where the weight is proportional to the distance of the point from the electrodes. This is a very simple and fast technique that involves the placement of electrodes on the scalp and was the most used technique for brain mapping in the past, before technology provided automated calculation. It is a so-called "local" method, meaning that for the estimation of the value of the signal at a point, one uses a limited number of known measures, within the proximity of the point. This method shows another evident problem: the maximum and minimum values of the signal will always be located in one of the electrode positions, and this, clearly, is not likely to be accurate. This interpolation technique can be used with any of the scalp models discussed in the previous paragraphs.
2. *Interpolation based on planar SPLine*: this technique, which is applied in several other scientific domains [7], is a "global" technique versus "local", as all values of the measured electrodes are used to calculate the interpolated signal in a given point of the scalp model. Mathematically it is a very complex process, where the result is obtained by minimizing the curves of a plane that is forced to pass by all known points that can be placed at any position on the scalp. The continuous surface that is obtained is regular, and its maximum and minimum are not necessarily

[4]The devices that perform such measures are often called "3D tracker" and allow to measure with very good precision the position of the electrodes on the scalp.

Table 6.1 Coordinates of the standard electrodes as latitude and longitude

Electrode	Latitude	Longitude
Fp1	90	108
Fp2	90	72
F7	90	144
F3	61.8	130.7
Fz	45	90
F4	61.8	49.3
F8	90	36
T7 (ex T3)	90	180
C3	45	180
Cz	0	0
C4	45	0
T8 (ex T4)	90	0
P7 (ex T5)	90	216
P3	61.8	229.3
Pz	45	270
P4	61.8	310.7
P8 (ex T6)	90	324
O1	90	252
O2	90	288
Oz	90	270
Fpz	90	90
FC2	30	45
FC1	30	135
CP1	30	225
CP2	30	315
AF4	72.5	68
AF3	72.5	112
PO3	72.5	248
PO4	72.5	292
FC6	69.5	20
FC5	69.5	160
CP5	69.5	200
CP6	69.5	340
FT8	90	18
AF8	90	54
FPz	90	90
AF7	90	126
FT7	90	162
TP7	90	198
PO7	90	234
Oz	90	270
PO8	90	306
TP8	90	342
AFz	67.5	90
F5	75.5	139
F1	50	113
F2	50	67
F6	75.5	41
FC3	48	152.5
FCz	21	90
FC4	48	27.5
C5	67.5	180
C1	22.5	180
C2	22.5	0
C6	67.5	0
CP3	48	207.5
CPz	21	270
CP4	48	332.5
P5	75.5	221
P1	50	247
P2	50	293
P6	75.5	319
POz	67.5	270

located at the position of the electrodes. This interpolation technique can be applied to all scalp models discussed in previous paragraphs with minor adaptation.

3. *Interpolation based on spherical SPLine*: this technique is fairly similar to the previous one in terms of characteristics and properties and obtains the value of the interpolated signal by minimizing the curves of a sphere that is forced to pass by all known points. This is again a "global" interpolation technique that results in a continuous and regular surface that allows placing the electrodes at any position on the scalp but can be used only in conjunction with a three-dimensional model.

6.4.2.4 Choice of the Reference in Cerebral Mapping

As brain mapping aims to display the values of a signal in all points of the scalp, this signal should be measured in an absolute sense. In our case, such a signal is an electric potential that, as seen in the previous chapter, instruments measure only as difference of potential between two points. The measured values are then all referred to a "common electrode" that could have two fundamental characteristics:

- *Common electrode located in a neutral point:* in such hypothesis (which can be approximated by connecting both earlobes to the recording system common reference), the potentials could be used as they are recorded, without prior processing, as they should already identify an absolute value for each electrode.
- *Common electrode located in an active point:* in such hypothesis (which is usually the case as the common reference of the amplifier is connected to an electrode located in an active point of the scalp), the potentials need to be processed in order to subtract from them the activity of the common electrode. *Average Reference* and *Source Reference* are often used in this case, and they are described in the previous chapter.

6.5 Examples

This paragraph aims simply to show examples of application of the analysis and display techniques seen in this chapter. The first example is a spectral analysis with "frequency mapping". Figure 6.21 shows the 20-s segment of a 19-channel EEG (old standard 10/20) to be analysed. The data is displayed with average reference, expressly selected for mapping. Spectral analysis is performed with overlapping, detrending and tapering.

Figure 6.22 shows the results of the spectral analysis of each of the 19 channels that is the PSD. Figure 6.23 shows, instead, the frequency maps in the four main EEG bands (delta, theta, alpha, beta) for the very same EEG segment. The scalp model is three-dimensional and spherical with electrode coordinates expressed as latitude to longitude; the interpolation used is SPLine spherical. Please note that the chromatic scale has very different boundaries for the four different maps. One can notice the distribution of the alpha rhythm in the occipital region (but asymmetric as clearly evident in the EEG) with a power that is much higher than the other bands (see the boundary of the chromatic scale to better understand the real value).

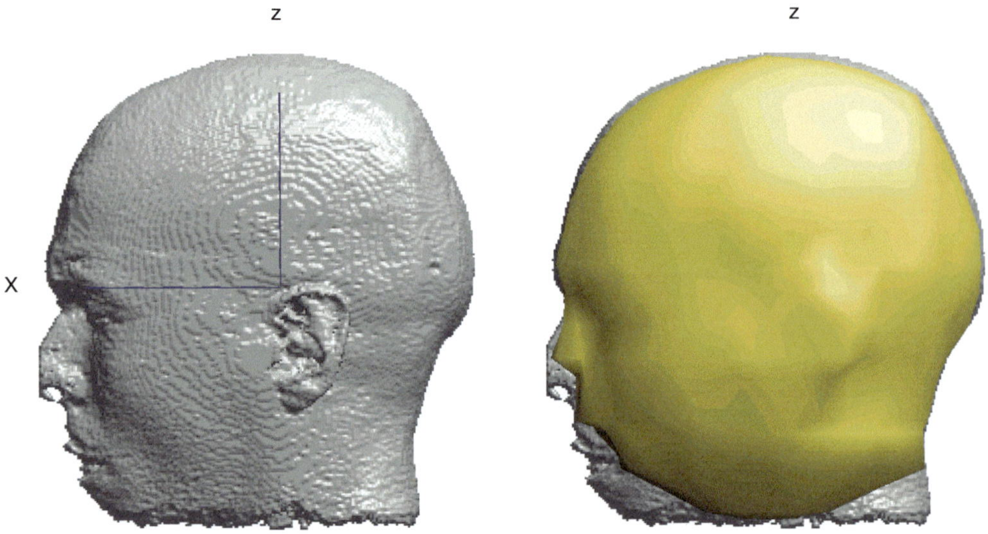

Fig. 6.20 3D head model obtained by MRI (left) and scalp model (right in yellow)

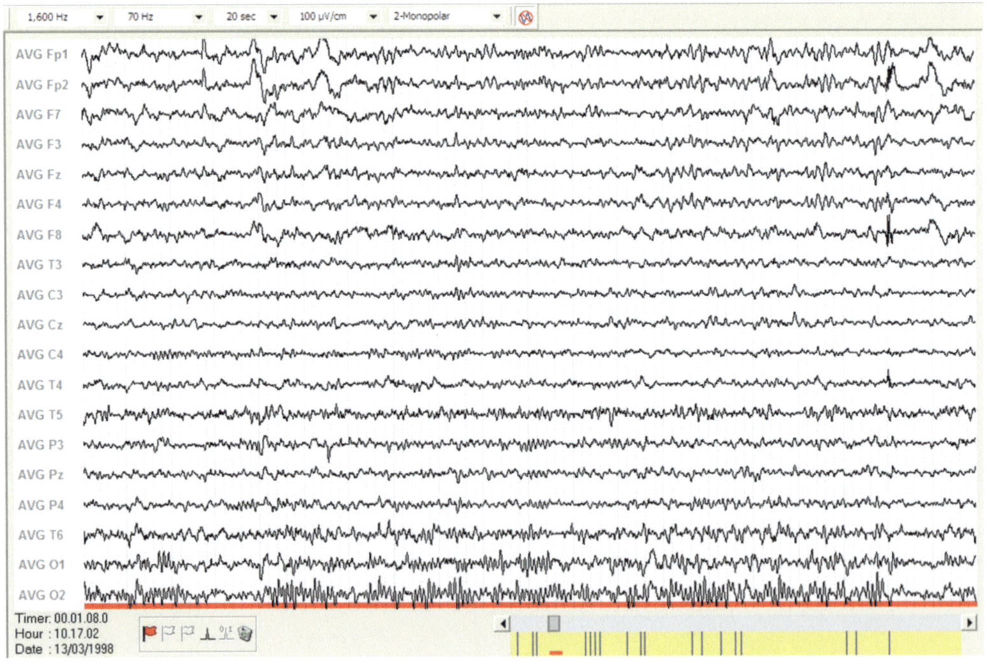

Fig. 6.21 EEG segment selected for spectral analysis

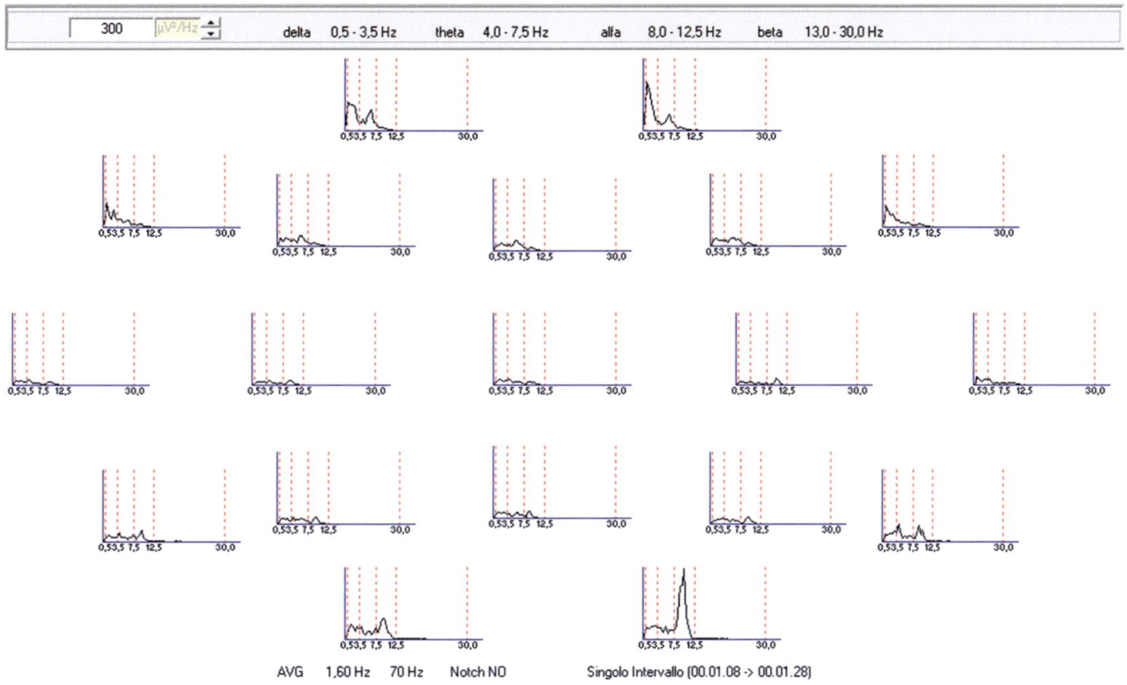

Fig. 6.22 PSD of the EEG segment in Fig. 6.21

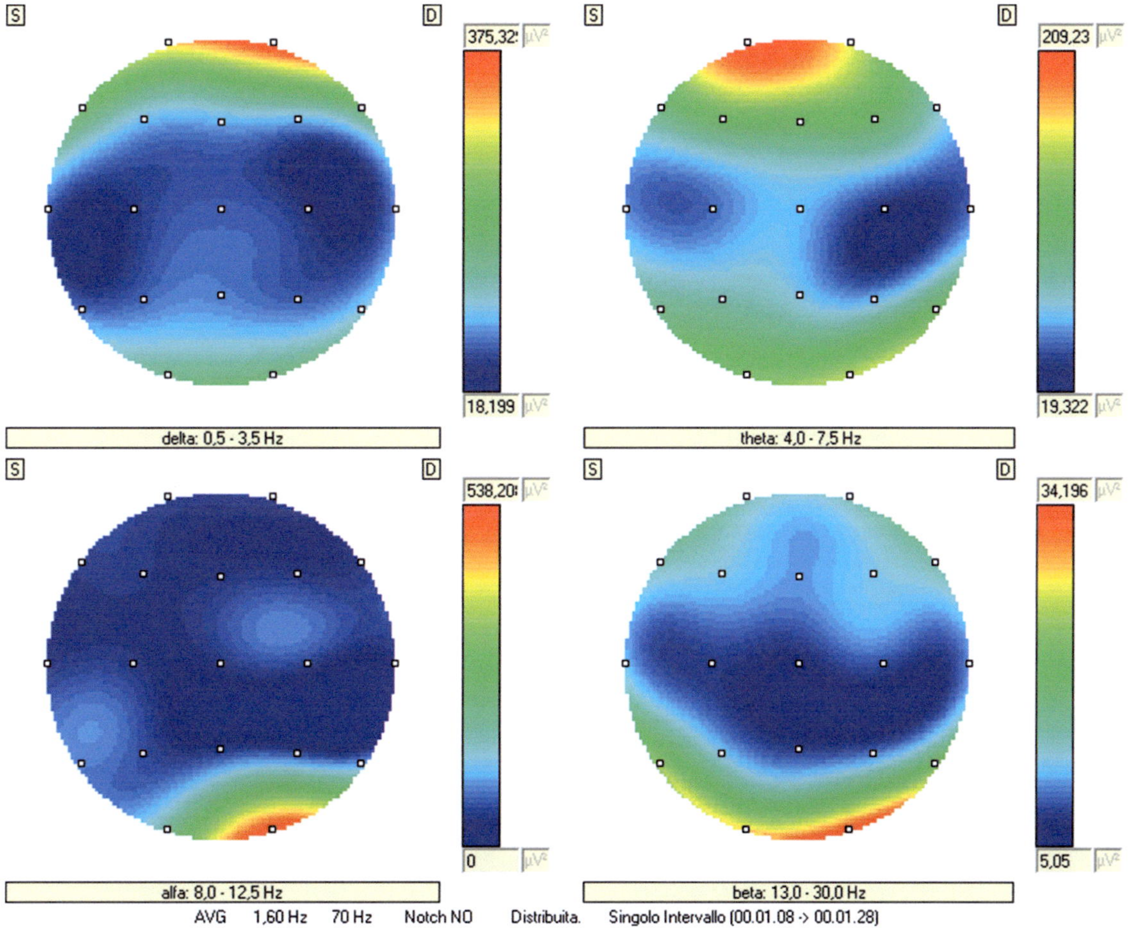

Fig. 6.23 Frequency maps of the EEG segment in Fig. 6.21

Acknowledgement Thanks to Arianna, Laura and Piergiorgio for revising this chapter and most of all to David and Kristen for revising the entire English text.

References

1. Cooley JW, Tukey JW. An algorithm for the machine calculation of complex Fourier series. Math Comput. 1965;19:297–301.
2. Kay SM, Marple SL. Spectrum analysis—a modern perspective. Proc IEEE. 1981;69(11):1380–419.
3. Rampil IJ. Electroencephalography. New York: Raven Press; 1994.
4. Maynard DE, Prior PF, Scott DF. Device for continuous monitoring of cerebral activity in resuscitated patients. Br Med J. 1969;4:545–6.
5. Seeck M, et al. The standardized EEG electrode array of the IFCN. Clin Neurophysiol. 2017;128:2080–77.
6. Nuwer MR, Comi G, Emerson R, Fuglsang-Frederiksen A, Guérit JM, Hinrichs H, Ikeda A, Luccas FJ, Rappelsburger P. IFCN standards for digital recording of clinical EEG. International Federation of Clinical Neurophysiology. Electroencephalogr Clin Neurophysiol. 1998;106:259–61.
7. Wahba SG. Spline interpolation and smoothing on the sphere. SIAM J Sci Stat Comput. 1981;2:5–16.

EEG Laboratory: Patient Care and the Role of the EEG Technician

7

Oriano Mecarelli

7.1 Environment, Patient Care, and Recording Preparation

Before each recording session, the EEG technician must check that all the necessary equipment is available and fully functional. The laboratory room must be tidy and cozy, and it should also be equipped with toys to amuse children or anything that can help to recreate the conditions triggering a seizure (television, food, etc.). If it is necessary to administer medications or to analyze the online tracings, the neurologist must be alerted.

To ensure an accurate and reliable recording, the technician should read the examination request form from the referring physician before admitting the patient, and he should also view eventual previous EEG exams. This will support the examination and planning the monitoring of specific polygraphic parameters that can supply useful additional information. The technician also has the task to collect all the information regarding the patient: complete personal data (first and last name, gender, date of birth, address, handedness); the reasons for the referral and relevant medical and neurological history, particularly concerning epileptic seizure details (type of seizure, time elapsed since the last seizure, triggers, etc.); current medications (particularly CNS drugs); information on other diseases that can require the exam limitation; the presence and location of any skull defects; previous EEG results (if available); neuroimaging results (computed tomography and/or magnetic resonance imaging).

Digital EEG systems allow the recording and storing of all of these informations as a separate text file or in the same file as the EEG data, and the technician must be sure that the information about the patient are correctly related to the recording. The neurophysiologist can then review all the patient's clinical data, which will help him to interpret the results of the EEG recording.

An accurate preliminary explanation of the procedure to the patient is essential: what for us is a simple routine procedure may instead be cause of concern for the patient. Many people still falsely believe that electricity flows between the system and the patient's head during the exam. In the collective imaginary, EEG is still sometimes associated with a kind of electroshock or, at any rate, to an examination that is capable of revealing mental processes. Explanation of the procedure must be of course adjusted to the patient's comprehension ability, but it is usually useful to point out that EEG is a harmless, diagnostic and not a therapeutic exam, through which the spontaneous electric activity of the brain is recorded and during which no electricity is absolutely administered. This approach is helpful because it facilitates the patient's relaxation, and it ensures better cooperation. Moreover, excessive anxiety can cause muscle and movement artifacts that disturb the recording, and an anxious subject will unlikely reach the necessary state of relaxation or even drowsiness, during which significant diagnostic abnormalities are more likely to arise.

After the complete and accurate explanation from the technician, the patient (or the person accompanying them) should sign an informed consent form, in particular when specific procedures carry the risk of triggering a seizure.

The same technician should carry out the entire recording; a production-line approach that involves application of electrodes and recording by different technicians is not good practice. During the EEG recording, the technical staff must not express opinions on the exam nor on other matters, and it is important to avoid unnecessary entry or exit in and out the recording room.

Recordings on young children or non-cooperating adults may present additional difficulties. The presence of a parent, a nurse, or a therapist who knows the patient well is often useful or even indispensable. On the other hand, experienced technicians can usually recognize those parents who are excessively anxious and who, instead of helping, can be

O. Mecarelli (✉)
Department of Human Neurosciences, Sapienza University of Rome, Rome, Italy
e-mail: oriano.mecarelli@uniroma1.it

O. Mecarelli (ed.), *Clinical Electroencephalography*, https://doi.org/10.1007/978-3-030-04573-9_7

counterproductive. In this case, it's better to respectfully and gently ask them to leave the room. Examinations on very young children are preferably carried out while a parent is holding them. In these circumstances, especially after a meal, it is easier for them to fall asleep. When carrying out a recording on a non-cooperating subject, the technician must be able to cope with the situation. In these cases, it's pointless to immediately position the head cap and electrodes, since it is necessary to first establish a physical connection with these patients, trying to get them to feel comfortable with us and with the surrounding environment. For that purpose, books, toys or other objects of interest can be used, in order to distract them from the technical procedure.

The electrodes placement on the scalp should be managed with the patient in a sitting position, accessible from all the sides. Children may be reassured by showing them a simulation of electrode positioning it on the head of a doll or on the back of the technician's hand. Sometimes, children can be scared by the noise of the air compressors used, in certain laboratories, to attach the electrodes with collodion. In these cases, the use of a hair dryer, an object well-known to children, or of adhesive paste, is recommended.

The time necessary for the electrodes placement is very important, because it gives the technician a chance to obtain the trust of the patient, to verify the contents of the request and to obtain more details on the medical history. During a relaxed conversation with the technician, who is usually less intimidating than a physician, the patient will often spontaneously give important information, not mentioned during the formal interview with the neurologist. Thus, new information obtained should be added to the request form. Moreover, the technician must indicate:

- conformational cranial abnormalities (which can determine inevitable asymmetries in the electrodes positioning, causing an incorrect interpretation of the EEG);
- scalp and/or skull defects (burr holes, post-craniotomy scars, etc.) that can preclude the standard positioning of the electrodes or be a cause of peculiar EEG patterns like breach rhythm;
- patient's mental state and level of awareness at the beginning of and during the recording;
- hand preference (which could also explain possible asymmetries).

During a standard EEG execution, the patient should be as relaxed as possible and this can be achieved by letting them lay on a bed in the supine position or sitting on a slightly reclined couch. The room must be dimly lit and as soundproof as possible. During the recording, the technician must be able to always monitor the patient's behavior. If they're particularly restless or experiencing a seizure, the use of a mattress on the floor or a hospital bed with cot sides can be required. In this case, continuous surveillance by a nurse or another technician is needed, to avoid dangerous falls. If a patient has physical deficits and arrives on a wheelchair, it would be more appropriate to leave him sitting in the chair during the execution of the exam.

Before the recording starts, the patient must be given the opportunity to use the toilet, so that it is not further needed during the exam. The patient can be asked to take off too tight or heavy items of clothing, to feel more comfortable and to avoid them sweating. In case of a hearing impairment or in foreign patients with language barriers, it may be useful to agree upon a system of signals to request the subject to open and close the eyes and to perform other procedures.

7.2 Electrode Placement and Control

The impedance of the electrodes must be checked after their placement on the scalp and it should be checked again after the patient is settled on the bed or couch. Modern electroencephalographs always measure impedance values, but this operation can also be carried out with portable instruments (impedance meter). The impedance check system is based on the use of a sinusoidal signal at about 10 Hz, generated by the instrument and transmitted to the electrodes connected to it, with reference to a common electrode. To determine which electrodes have suitable impedance, headboxes are equipped with a LED display, and the same display can be shown on the computer monitor.

Surface electrodes should have an impedance lower than 5 kΩ; with modern digital EEG recording equipments, impedances up to 10 kΩ are acceptable, but it is important that the impedances are balanced. Impedances should also not be below 100 Ω: this value indicates a shunt or short circuit, due to a salt bridge on the scalp [1]. Impedance of small, non-polarizable electrodes (i.e., needle electrodes) is higher than that of cup electrodes, but they are stable and may be used in special situations and for prolonged EEG recordings in comatose patients. In any case, perseverance in the attempt of lowering the impedance to try improve the recording is always beneficial, although this is not always possible, especially with young children and non-cooperating patients.

Electrodes are an essential element of electroencephalography and the technician must check that they are placed correctly and have low impedance. However, in order to lower the impedance, it is not necessary to produce abrasion on the skin. With modern high input impedance amplifiers and accurate digital filters for power line noise (60 or 50 Hz), high-quality EEG can indeed be recorded without skin abrasion [2]. Skin breakdown during placement of electrodes is quite frequent especially in children, and it must be avoided also because it can cause infections [2–4]. Electrodes used for EEG recordings must be disinfected with the appropriate procedures, especially when used in patients with contagious diseases. In these cases, however, disposable electrodes are recommended [1, 5].

The electrodes are of various types and they can be applied on the scalp by different methods (see Chap. 3 and 4). The use of collodion is one of the best techniques for securing EEG electrodes to the scalp, especially for long-term monitoring. However, the use of collodion, because of its inflammability and toxicity, requires accurate safety procedures for storage and utilization. Furthermore, the collodion can be removed only with acetone and its inhalation can produce nasal and conjunctival irritation, respiratory effects, nausea and vomiting, etc. When using collodion in the EEG laboratory, a simple vapor extraction system must be operative; nevertheless, collodion is not recommended for short routine recordings. The electrolyte adhesive paste, such as EC2, may substitute collodion in the electrodes placement, also for long-term monitoring, with an optimal cost-benefit ratio (Fig. 7.1) [6].

The 10-20 system is the only one officially recommended by the International Federation of Clinical Neurophysiology (IFCN) for the placement of all 21 electrodes [7]. The development of high-density EEG system and source localization methods (which refers to the use of 64–256 electrodes) has subsequently made necessary modifications of this system, and the 10-10 system has been accepted by the American Clinical Neurophysiology Society (ACNS) and IFCN for almost two decades (see Chap. 4) (Fig. 7.2) [8–11].

In the 10-10 system some electrodes from the 10-20 system were renamed: T3 and T4 were renamed to T7 and T8, and T5 and T6 were renamed to P7 and P8. In 2001, the 10-5 system was introduced [12], but the nomenclature was not yet formally accepted by the ACNS and IFCN. Very recently, the IFCN strongly recommends an array of 25 electrodes for standard EEGs including 6 electrodes of the inferior temporal

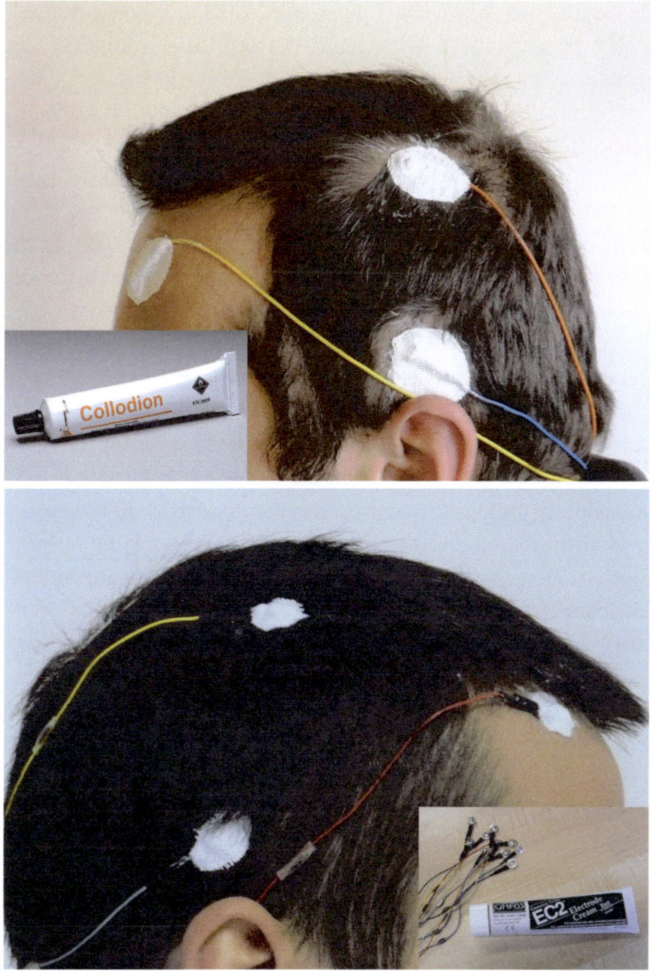

Fig. 7.1 Placement of electrodes on the scalp with collodion and EC2 adhesive paste

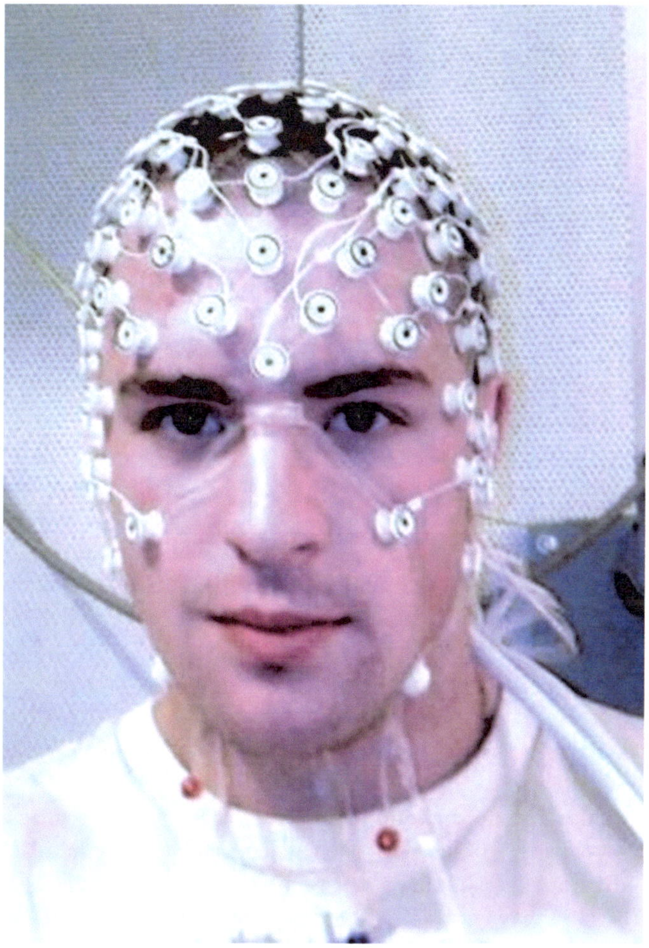

Fig. 7.2 An example of a head cap for the EEG high-density recording (photograph of public domain on web)

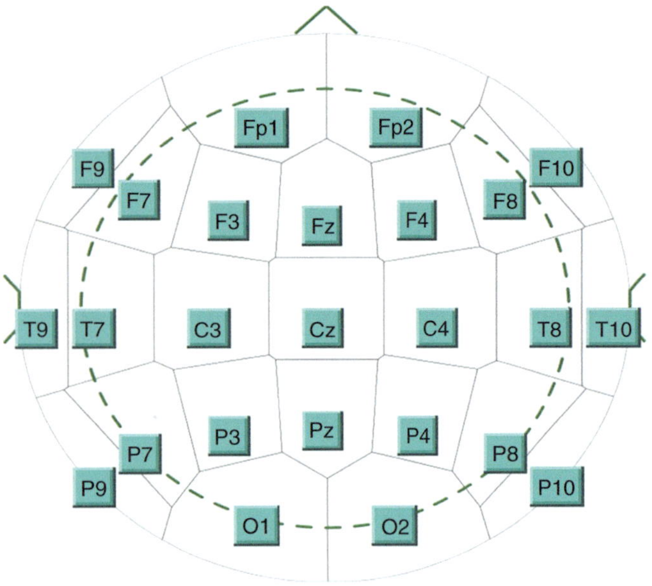

Fig. 7.3 New standard montage, with the coverage of the inferior-basal and anterior part of the temporal lobe. From ref. [11], with permission

chain (Fig. 7.3). The standard 10-20 system did not indeed include electrodes to record the activity of the inferior-basal and anterior part of temporal lobe. These electrodes are named, according to 10-10 system, F9-T9-P9 and F10-T10-P10 [11].

In conclusion, the 10-20 system is clinically adequate and efficient for routine standard EEG; the 10-10 system should be used in patients undergoing presurgical evaluation in Long-Term Epilepsy Monitoring Unit (LTEMU) or for additional digital analysis (i.e., electrical source imaging). Additional electrodes from the 10-10 system may also be used, sometimes, during standard EEG, especially to make a better localization of an epileptic focus.

For both clinical and educational purposes, it would be desirable to switch to T7/T8 and P7/P8 instead of T3/T4 and T5/T6, but the new terminology must be gradually accepted by the electroencephalographers and the EEG machine headboxes modified. At present, it would be an acceptable alternative to continue using the old terms or both [10]. In children, all 21/25 electrodes recommended for adults should be used [11, 13] even if, in the case of poor compliance or in critically ill children or for prolonged monitoring, the application of a smaller number of electrodes is also acceptable (Fig. 7.4).

Furthermore, in addition to scalp electrodes, it is necessary to apply other electrodes and devices to the record of polygraphic parameters, particularly ElectroCardioGram (ECG, always considered indispensable, in all recordings), ElectroOculoGram (EOG) and ElectroMyoGram (EMG) (see Chap. 15–16).

7.3 EEG Recording

With older analog systems, the technician had only one opportunity to acquire a satisfactory tracing to be presented to the electroencephalographer compiling the EEG report; all efforts then had to be concentrated toward achieving a sufficiently long and reliable tracing, with a modest quantity of artifacts and with a correct acquisition parameters set up. With digital technology, a wrong choice of online visualization parameters is not a real problem, since EEG can be reformatted and read offline with modified filters, sensitivity and baseline periods. However, if the tracing is not visualized correctly during the acquisition, the risk for the technician is to underestimate important elements and not act accordingly, thus impairing the correct interpretation of the exam.

In many laboratories, technical-methodological aspects are strictly standardized: a sequence of montages, not excluding any applied electrodes, is visualized; opening and closing of the eyes must follow a specific sequence; acoustic and tactile stimuli are regularly administered; photostimulation is carried out following a planned sequence, often automatically programmed, with fixed periods of stimulation and pause.

Sometimes, however, a more flexible approach is necessary. If the EEG duration itself gives an indication of the quality of the work carried out, a better quality indicator is actually represented by the variability of the average duration of the tracing, because it reflects the flexibility of the recording procedure. Although following standard procedures is fundamental, the technician must always consider that each patient is different and that even EEG recordings must have a physiological degree of variability. If the goal is, for example, to verify how the background EEG activity is altered in a disoriented subject, a few minutes of recording can be enough. On the contrary, if a patient with suspected epileptic seizures shows a normal EEG during wakefulness, extending the recording period can be helpful, both to increase the possibility to detect interictal abnormalities and to record under lower alertness conditions. With very young children, the tracings could initially be unreadable, but if the technician is patient, the child will probably fall asleep, allowing a sleep recording without artifacts.

A standard EEG is initially acquired and displayed according to predefined parameters. The sensitivity of EEG equipment is usually set in the range of 50–100 μV/cm of trace deflection [1].

A sensitivity >100 μV/cm does not allow the detection of a significant low amplitude activity, while a sensitivity <50 μV/cm increases excessively the EEG activity and limits the identification of peculiar waveforms or frequencies (Fig. 7.5).

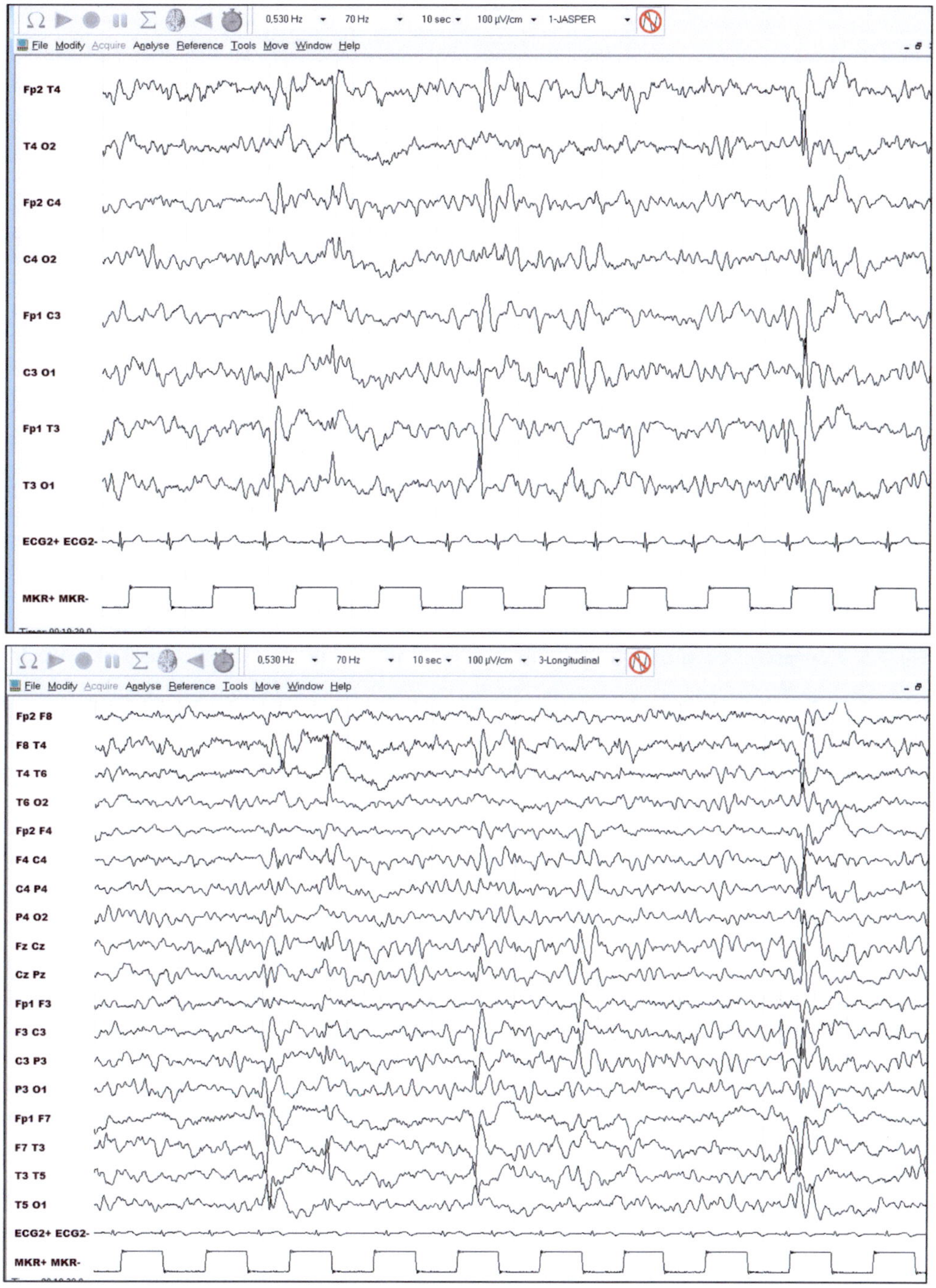

Fig. 7.4 An 8-year-old child with multifocal epileptic abnormalities. Visualization of 8 (upper) and 18 (bottom) channels of the same 10 s EEG epoch

Using digital equipments, the signals are filtered at two levels: the first analog filter is applied at the actual amplifier before digitation and cannot be changed by user; the second digital filter processes only the data for display, and its improper use does not allow the technician to evaluate correctly the recording, without however permanently altering the recorded data. The low-pass filter (High-Frequency Filter, HFF) during standard EEG recording should normally be set at 70 Hz, while the high-pass filter (Low-Frequency Filter, LFF) should be no higher than 1 Hz (corresponding to a time constant with at least 0.1 s for analog systems) (Fig. 7.6).

The increase of LFF should not be used routinely to attenuate slow artifacts, because this can also result in the disappearance of delta pathological activity. On the other hand, the reduction of HFF, to reduce excessive muscular artifacts,

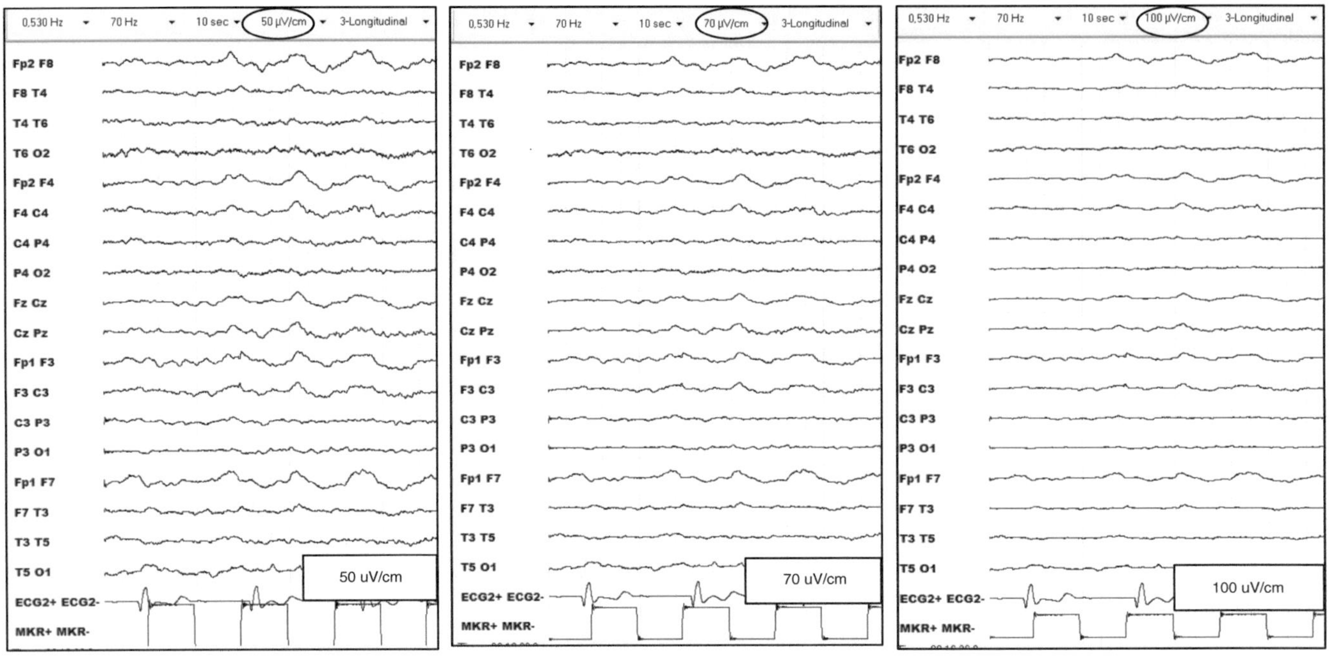

Fig. 7.5 Examples of the same EEG epoch, displayed with different sensitivities (50, 70, and 100 μV/cm)

can distort and attenuate the sharp abnormalities. Rather than working with filters, the technician should try to prevent eye movements as much as possible and to reduce muscle activity by relaxing the patient and asking him not to contract his facial muscles. LFF can be increased to attenuate the excessive slow activities, clearly artifactual in nature (perspiration, arterial pulse, etc.).

To eliminate fast activities due to electrical interference, a 60 Hz (in North America) or 50 Hz (in Europe) *notch filter* should be used (Fig. 7.7); a noise source can remain however active, and it must be removed before resorting to the filter, because the presence of a disturbance can denote other technical problems like, for example, disconnection of one electrode. The notch filter should not be routinely used, but its use should be restricted to special environments (i.e., ICU recordings).

The abovementioned settings may need to be modified according to what is being displayed.

Sensitivity must be reduced if the underlying activity is so large that it saturates the channel; on the other hand, it must be increased if the tracing is less evident. However, a judicious use of low- and high-frequency filters, in the end, is advisable to emphasize or clarify specific types of EEG patterns.

Acquisition of EEG data onto a digital storage should occur at the minimum sampling rate of 256 Hz and at the resolution of at least 16 bits [14].

For the storage of various EEG recordings (standard EEG, video-EEG, A-EEG, etc.), it is preferable to use newer storage technologies, in particular digital server systems, which can facilitate review in remote locations and whose data protection with backups is on charge of hospital engineer staff. The EEG data can be reviewed on the computer screen with sufficient temporal and spatial resolution. A standard horizontal scaling should be available, with a minimum resolution of 128 data points/s on the screen for a 10-s page, but more expanded horizontal scales should also be available. A standard vertical scaling with a minimum spacing of 10 mm per channel should be used for a display of up to 21 channels [14].

With analog instruments, the most widely used paper speed was 30 mm/s, but some laboratories also used a paper speed of 15 mm/s or intermediate (20 or 25 mm/s) (Fig. 7.8).

Nowadays, with the use of digital systems and visualization of the EEG tracings on the monitor, it's easy to change the baseline periods according to the specific needs. Users accustomed to reading the tracing on paper at 30 mm/s will continue to use this setting on the monitor and vice versa. A display of 10–20 s/page (depending on its size) corresponds roughly to a paper speed of 30 mm/s, and it should be used for routine exams. In reality, a flexible method is advised. Sometimes, it will be necessary to compress the recorded EEG tracing, in order to follow an event in its evolution or to evaluate its fluctuations (display of >20 s/page). In other cases, it may be necessary to display a short period of the recording on the monitor; this is useful, for example, to study the morphology of a graphoelement or for its correlation to polygraphic parameters. In any case, the use of nonstandard parameters can be confusing when the tracings, digitally

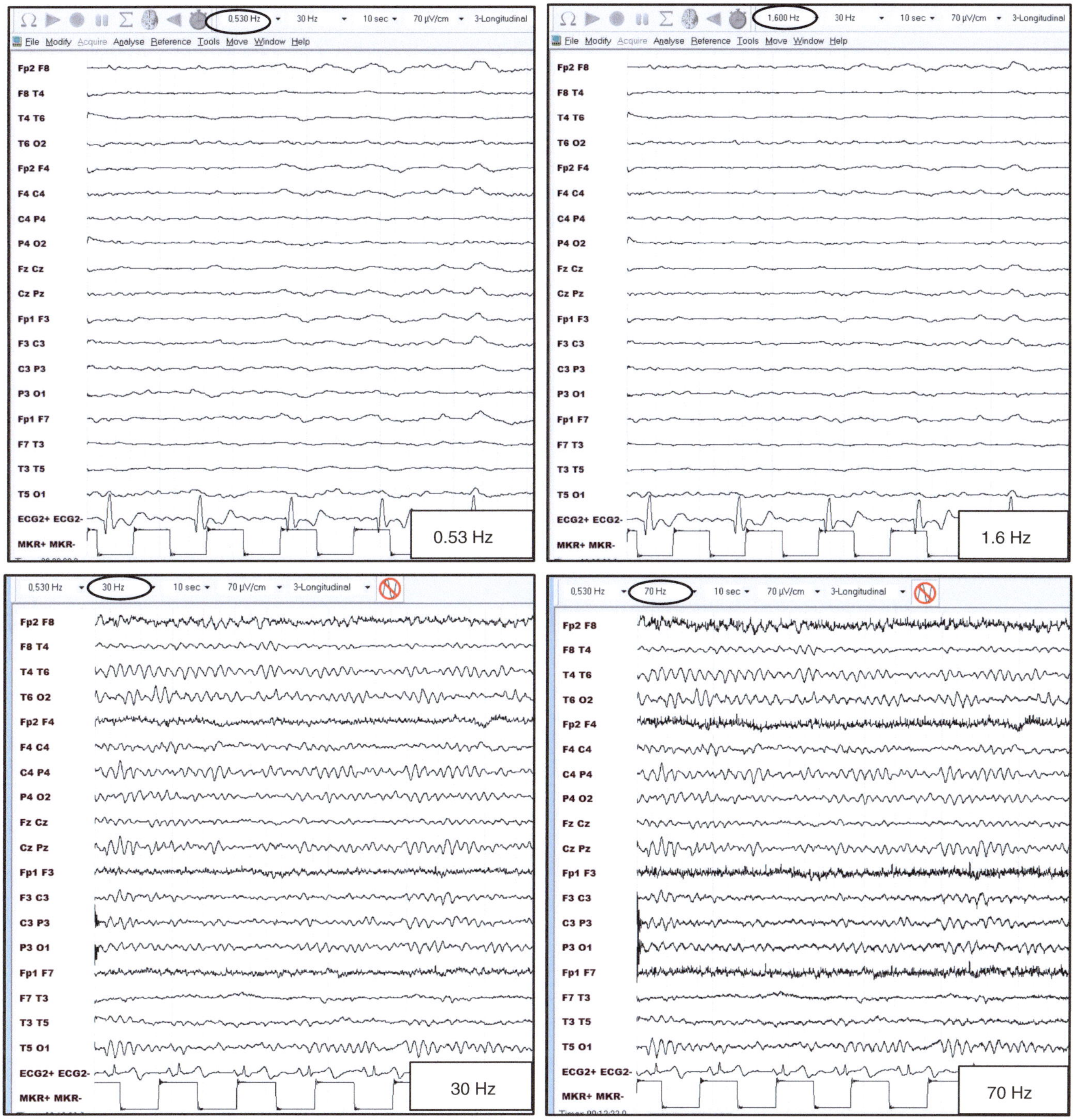

Fig. 7.6 Top: same EEG epoch displayed with high-pass filter at 0.53 Hz and 1.6 Hz. Bottom: same EEG epoch displayed with low-pass filter at 30 and 70 Hz

recorded and then printed on paper, are read by physicians with different habits and preparation; for this reason, it is important that each EEG tracing clearly shows the time marker and the acquisition parameters.

Up to 16–18 and more channels can be displayed on the monitor at the same time, both in bipolar (longitudinal and transverse) and in referential derivations. With 21 electrode positions (10-20 system) and 16 channels, the number of possible montages is 21. The 10-10 system, with more than 70 electrode positions, allows the creation of a much larger number of montages [10, 15].

Additional channels must be dedicated to visualizing the polygraphic parameters, basically represented by ECG, EOG, EMG as already stated above.

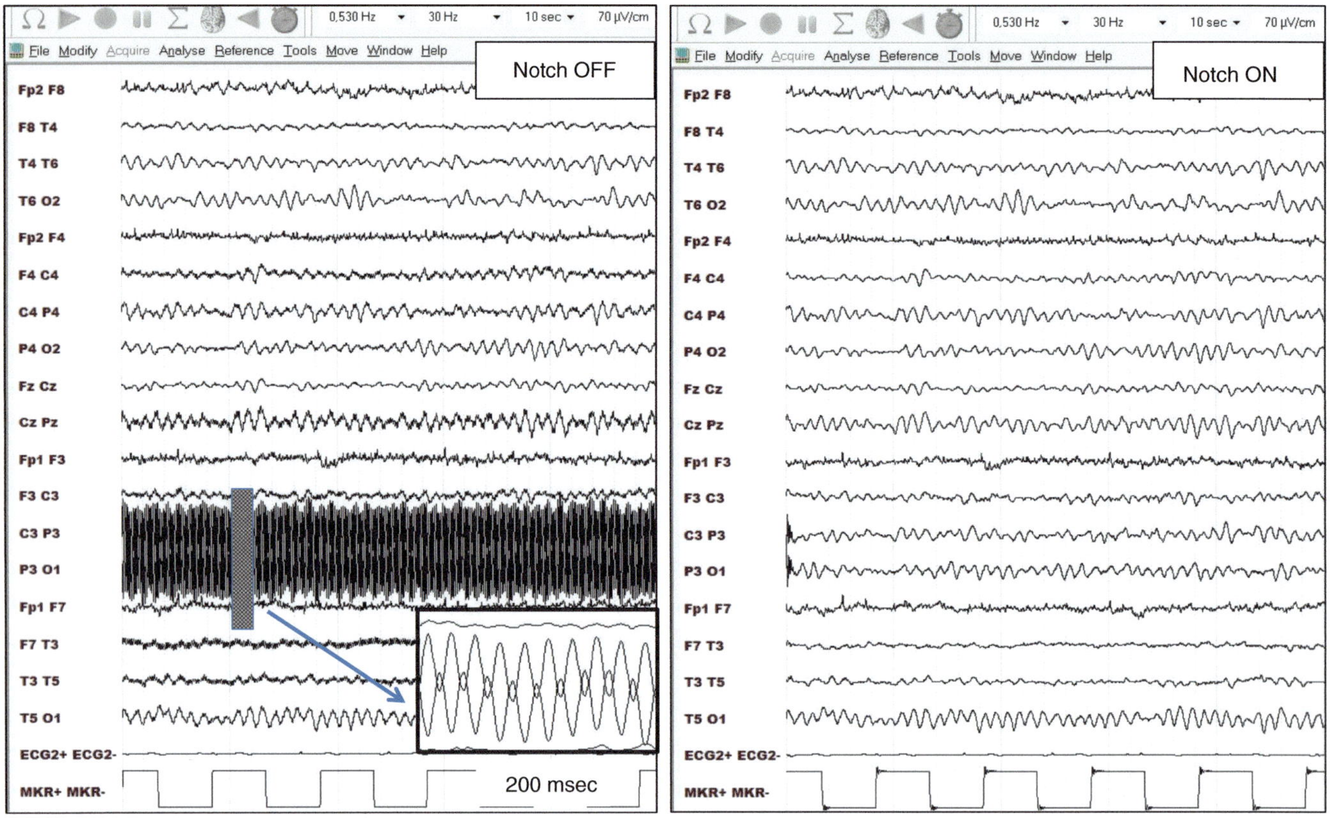

Fig. 7.7 Alternating current artifact at 50 Hz (left), removed by notch filter (right)

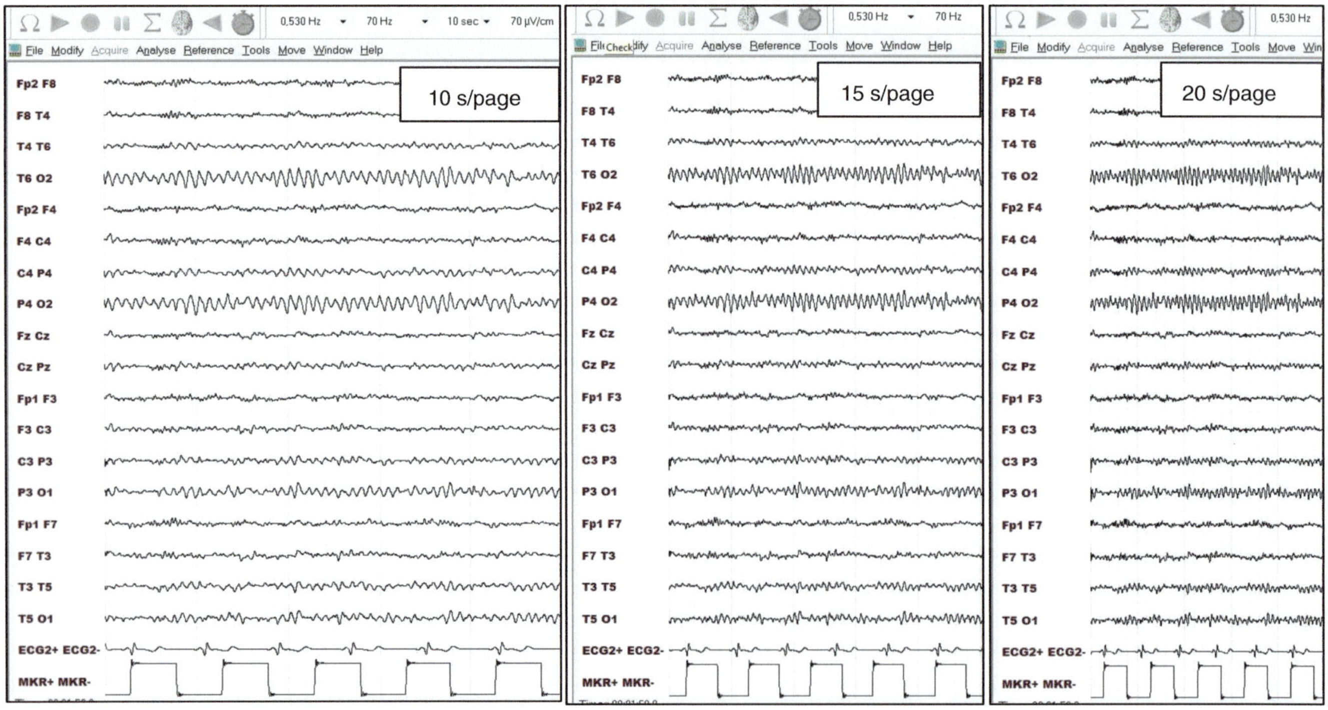

Fig. 7.8 The same EEG epoch displayed on the screen with different modalities (at 10, 15 and 20 s per page)

The duration of standard EEG recordings varies widely among laboratories. European guidelines recommend EEG recordings of at lest 30 min [16]. Results from studies conducted on epileptic patients suggest that in epilepsy-related indications, the shortest duration of standard EEG should be 20 min [17]. Also ACNS has recently established that standard EEG recordings under baseline conditions should consist at least of 20 min of reliable and without artifacts recording, to which activation procedures (intermittent photic stimulation and hyperventilation) must follow [1].

The possibility offered by digital EEG to display many more channels simultaneously and to modify acquisition parameters and montages during review must absolutely not entail a reduction in the recording time. The EEG technician should view the EEG in bipolar (longitudinal and transverse) and referential montages during the recording, both to identify the good connection in all electrodes and to appreciate subtle abnormalities requiring, for example, additional electrode placements.

During EEG recording in basal condition, it is necessary to assess EEG changes corresponding to eye-closed and eye-open conditions, both voluntary and on request. The closing and opening of the eyes induce, respectively, the appearance and block the background alpha rhythm. In the periods immediately after eye closure, short sequences of faster alpha rhythms can appear (squeak phenomenon). Some physiological rhythms or graphoelements (i.e., mu rhythms, lambda waves) are visible only when the opening of eyes has blocked the alpha activity. The spontaneous movements of the eyes may induce artifacts that simulate frontotemporal slow activity and the eyes opening and closing helps to differentiate between pathological and artifactual activity. In addition, epileptic discharges in photosensitive subjects often manifest only in coincidence with eye closure. For all these reasons, during a standard EEG recording, unless we want the patient to fall asleep, eye opening and closing must be tested several times (every 2–3 min); if the subject is not cooperating, the technician must manually perform the opening-closing of the eyes. Finally, the patient's response to the closing-opening eye command also allows the technician to evaluate the drowsiness and mental status of the subject.

During the EEG recording, the technician must report on the tracing all the significant events that occur, particularly the events disturbing the recording or the maneuvers and stimuli applied to the patient.

After recording under baseline conditions, activation procedures must be carried out, especially hyperventilation and photic stimulation (see Chap. 14) [1]. Execution methods for these tests must always be carefully explained to the patient and caregivers, in order to get them to cooperate and to avoid artifacts. During Hyper Ventilation (HV), the patient must carry out deep breathing, consisting of short but intense inhalations followed by prolonged exhalations, at a higher frequency than normal (normal, 10–12 breaths/min; HV, 18–20 breaths/min), for a period of 3–5 min. During hyperventilation, the patient must try to keep his head as still as possible and the eyes closed; the technician should encourage the patient to perform the test correctly, noting the quality of its effort during HV on EEG recording.

Intermittent Photic Stimulation (IPS) must be carried out before hyperventilation or at least 3 min after its conclusion. Biochemical variations and eventual EEG modifications induced by hyperventilation can indeed be prolonged for a few minutes after its interruption; consequently, performing this test before IPS can be confusing. However, as some patients can only relax after hyperventilation, in these patients it can be done before IPS, waiting a few minutes before testing the photic stimulation. Some children, however, can find photic stimulation amusing and, in these cases, it can be useful to carry it out at the beginning of the recording, to obtain a better cooperation. The correct standard procedure for performing IPS and HV is extensively described in Chap. 14. During the recording, the decision to follow a different procedure can be developed; each patient is an individual and the modality of EEG recording must sometimes be "tailored," based on questions that the technician can deduce from the request form, previous exams or decision taken together with the doctor. IPS and HV are activation procedures that may show epileptiform interictal abnormalities that potentially may induce epileptic seizure in susceptible patients and both the patient and the caregivers must be informed of this possibility.

In our laboratory, when a clear PhotoParoxysmal Response (PPR) was recorded, the IPS is retested with the use of Z1 blue lenses of an ultraviolet material with an 80% luminance cut. The Z1 lens are indeed highly effective in controlling PPR in a large number of photosensitive patients (Fig. 7.9) [18].

Sleep recording is useful to highlight otherwise non-detectable epileptiform EEG abnormalities, in patients with a clinical history that suggests epileptic seizures. Furthermore, in very young children, sleep recordings can be essential to obtain a tracing without artifacts, as much as possible. In these cases, the recording can be carried out in the laboratory in the early afternoon, possibly shortly after lunch (*nap* EEG), with one of the parents holding the child who is put to sleep after electrodes application. When the child is asleep and after having verified that the EEG changes distinctive of the first NREM stages are being recorded, acoustic stimuli will have to be administered to elicit physiological graphoelements like K-complexes. Sleep EEG recordings in laboratory on adults can be achieved by putting special care into making the patient as comfortable as possible (have them take off their shoes or any tight items of clothing; supply

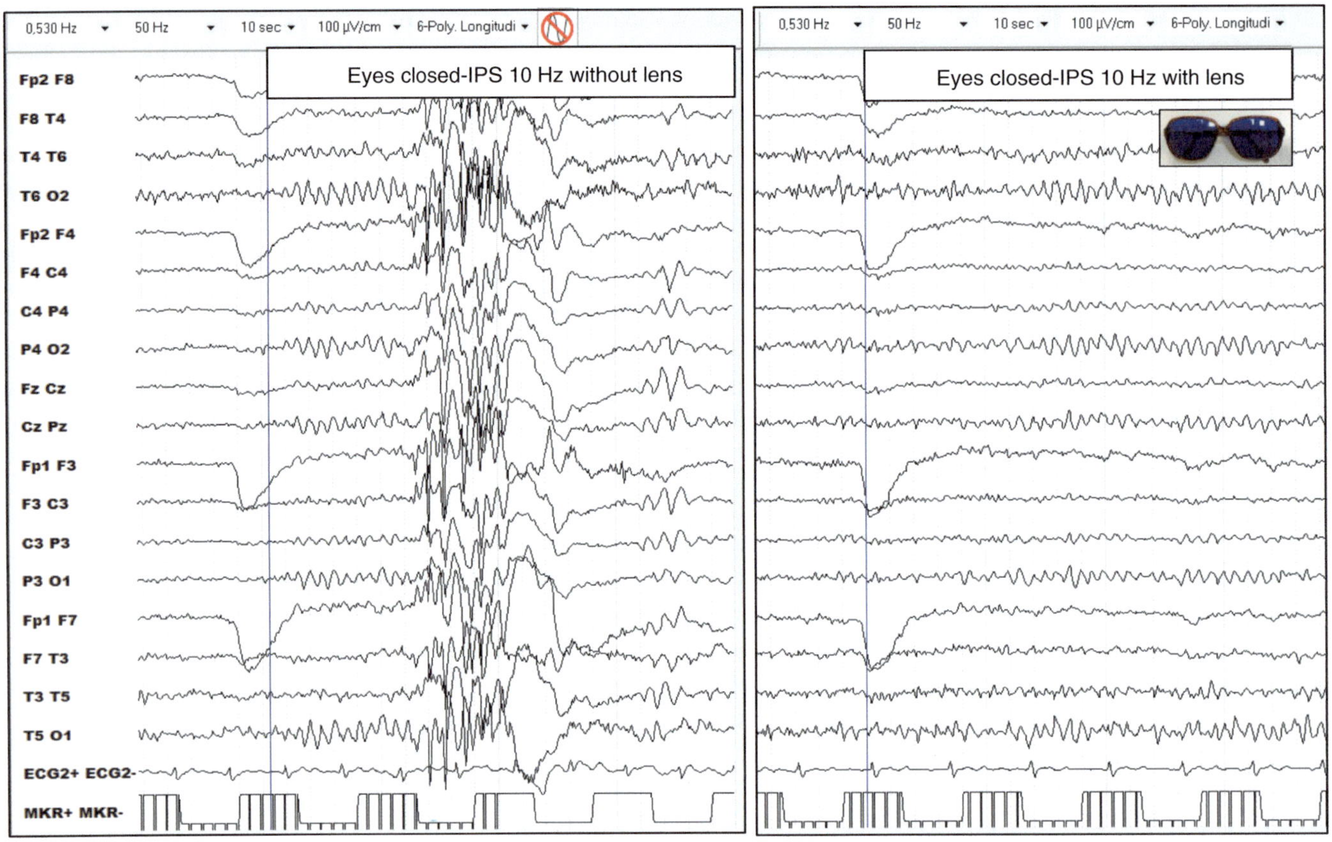

Fig. 7.9 Photoparoxysmal response with photostimulation at 10 Hz, suppressed by Zeiss-Claret 1.5 KF 133 lens

them with a blanket; allow them to use the toilet before beginning of the acquisition; use cup electrodes or pre-cabled caps; carry out the recording in a dimly lit and soundproof room).

In some patients, EEG is required precisely to assess their state of alertness or the atypical tendency for excessive daytime sleepiness, in a state of psychosensory relaxation.

When a patient who tends to fall asleep needs to be kept awake, acoustic stimuli must be periodically administered, as well as the request to open their eyes. If the awake EEG is needed for quantitative analysis (e.g., to assess the effects of drugs), the patient can be asked to open and close their eyes alternatively every 20–30 s. Tracing epochs of 8–10 s are thus obtained, selected 5 s after each eye opening or closure, discretely stable and reliable for the computer analysis. The patient can also be engaged in mental tasks that favor concentration and retention of alertness, or they can be asked to maintain continuous pressure on a button.

Specific tests to assess alertness and/or the tendency for excessive daytime sleepiness are the *Maintenance of Wakefulness Test* (*MWT*) and the *Multiple Sleep Latency Test (MSLT)*.

The *MWT* measures a patient's ability to stay awake: the patient should not smoke for at least 30 min before the test and should not have caffeinated beverages after the awakening. Then, after applying the electrodes, he will be placed in a comfortable sitting position in a quiet dimly lit room and he will be instructed to remain awake as long as possible. Four or five polygraphic recordings, each lasting for 40 min (with a 2-h interval between each recording), must be executed, starting 1.5–3 h after waking up. A PolySomnoGraphy (PSG) before MWT is not required. Each recording ends after 40 min if no sleep occurs or after the onset of sleep onset; the sleep onset during MWT is defined as three consecutive epochs of N1 or one epoch of any other sleep stages. Even if there are no universally accepted normative data for the MWT, a mean sleep latency of <8 min is considered abnormal, whereas values of >8 min and <40 min of sleep latency are of uncertain significance.

The MSLT is a better-standardized method for the study of excessive daytime sleepiness. This test must be preceded by a nocturnal PSG and starts 2–3 h after its conclusion. The patient is asked to relax and fall asleep while sitting comfortably on a recliner or lying down on a bed, in a dimly lit quiet room. No sedative or exciting drugs should be taken before the recording. The MSLT consists of four to five nap recordings at 2-h intervals, each recording must last a maximum of 20 min. The patient preparation must include the necessary polygraphic parameters to assess the various sleep stages (EMG, EOG). The evaluated parameters are the mean sleep-onset latency and the occurrence of sleep-onset REMs within the first 15 min of sleep onset. If no sleep occurs, the recording stops after 20 min whereas, if the patient falls asleep, the test is ended 15 min after the first period of 30 s epoch in any stage of sleep. A mean sleep latency <8 min is considered pathological; values between 8 and 10 min are consistent with mild sleepiness and a mean sleep latency of 10–15 min is normal [19].

7.4 Ictal Event Recordings and EEG report

Clinical ictal events are more often observed by EEG technicians than physicians or any other medical staff. Although the first concern must be the patient's safety if a sezure would arise during the examination (therefore the first thing to do is ensure that they don't hurt themselves falling or aptly intervene in the case of suffocation or dangerous behavior), the technician should not interrupt the EEG recording. In fact, the possibility to observe seizures (like those reported on the medical history) and simultaneously record the EEG correlates constitutes a unique opportunity for the diagnostic purposes. Technicians should therefore be prepared for the phenomenology and semeiology of the various epileptic seizures, to better detect and test manifestations that need to be documented. The technician should indeed be able to carry out other actions, such as to test whether the patient is able to respond when questioned (asking him to name objects or to answer simple quesions), to test mucle tone, pupils responsiveness and to examine some reflexes. A European task force from the ILAE has recently developed a standardized ictal testing battery for patient's testing during seizures [20]. Most of EEG laboratories are now equipped with a video-EEG system and the technician should always be ready to film the patient's behavior in sync with the EEG recording. Obviously, the video recording does not relieve the technician from carefully observing and testing the patient during a seizure. The Video-EEG recordings can be performed if the patient or the caregivers signed the informed consent according to the institutional policies.

To obtain a reliable and useful ictal EEG recording, the electrodes must be securely placed and resistant to any sudden movements or automatisms. Should the patient have a seizure when the montage is still incomplete, the technician must start the recording as soon as possible, to try collecting as much data as possible, even with an incomplete montage. During a seizure, the technician's task are: to give assistance to the patient to ensure they do not hurt themselves; to keep the EEG recording going and to prevent detachment of the electrodes (e.g., placing the headbox closer to the patient's head, thus avoiding that the cables are distracted to any pulling loads); to observe the seizure and to test the patient's interaction with the environment; to take note, as soon as the circumstances will allow it, of the observed details so that they will not be forgotten or inaccurately reported. EEG technicians should also be able to use (under the doctor's supervision) suggestion provoking techniques, to induce non-epileptic seizures, to be differentiated from epileptic ones. Video-EEG is, in these cases, also fundamental. The suggestion provoking techniques, in addition to intermittent photic stimulation and hyperventilation, include the compression of body parts, the placing of moistened patches on the skin, verbal stimulation, etc. (Fig. 7.10).

At the end of the recording, the technician should immediately send the EEG recordings to the neurophysiologist with the electrographic or clinical seizures, as well as with other significant clinical events that occurred in the laboratory. In some patients, there may be indeed the need for other diagnostic examinations or acute medications. Some special procedures that may be riskful for the patient should be carried out only in the presence of a qualified physician, with the informed consent, in an environment with adequate resuscitation equipment.

The technician's abilities to interpret the recorded tracing vary from case to case and from country to country, but they have certainly improved in the last few years. In the USA, several levels of specialization of the neurodiagnostic technologists are identified (please note web site https://www.aset.org). The Canadian Society of Clinical Neurophysiologists recently published a review of the laboratory standards and recommendations for EEG technologists. [21] In Italy, various universities currently operate a 3-year Bachelor Degree Course in Neurophysiopathology Techniques, which can be followed by a Master Degree Course in Diagnostic Techniques, lasting 2 more years. The Italian degree is valid and approved in the European Union; nevertheless, to provide general or specific information regarding the exam report is to-date not considered a technician's task. The technician must explain the patient that the medical report needs a qualified physician's expertise and that the results must be assessed and completed with the other clinical data. In many cases, active cooperation between the technician who carried out the EEG and the physician compiling the offline medical report is needed; the correct interpretation of the EEG patterns is often possible with the information provided by the technician.

To conclude, the technician's responsibility toward the patient does not end until the patient has left the laboratory. In the case of hospitalized patients, it may be necessary to take them back to their ward or ensure that the auxiliary staff or the ambulance takes care for their transportation. In the case of outpatients, it is possible to verify whether an appoint-

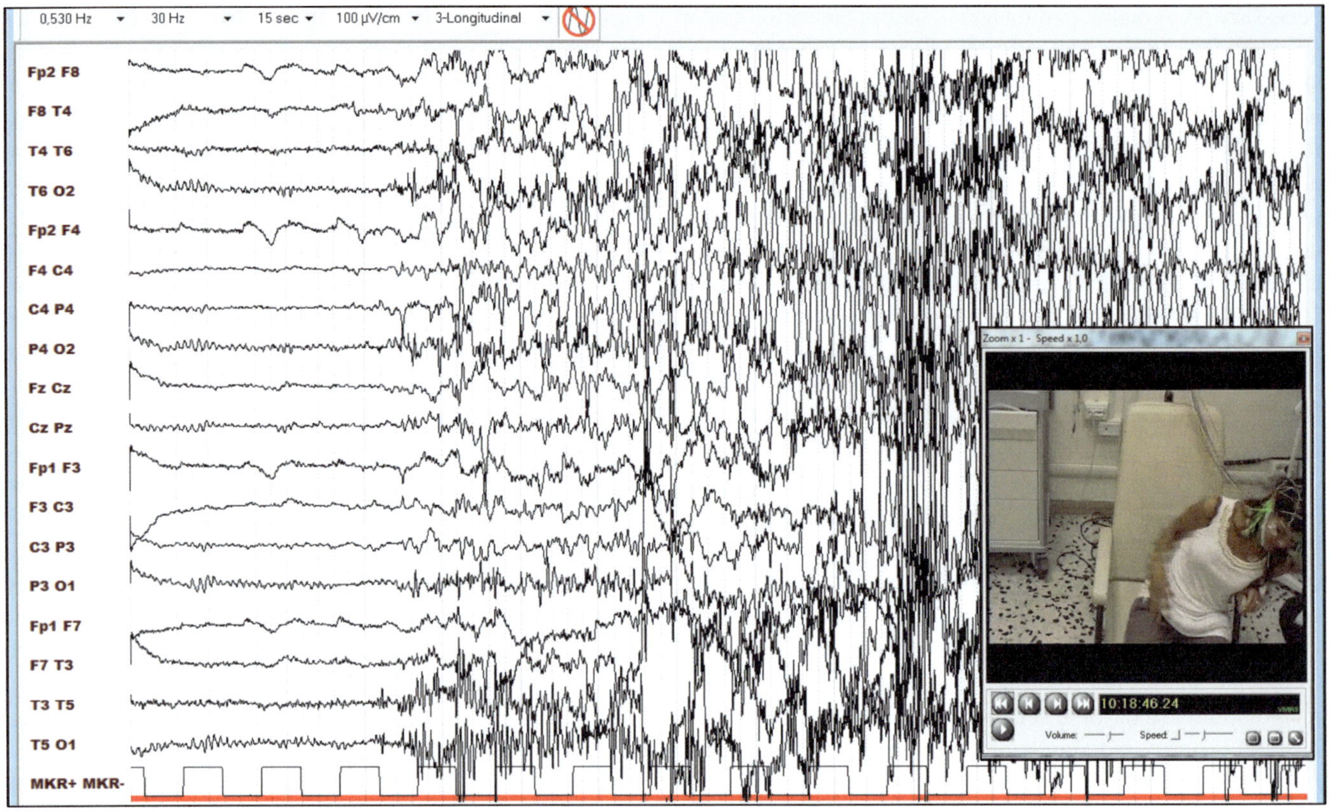

Fig. 7.10 A video-EEG recording of psychogenic non-epileptic seizure induced by a suggestion provoking technique

ment has been fixed with the referring physician. It would be also desirable to organize a neurophysiopathology unit so that the patient can be visited, if necessary, immediately after the EEG execution.

7.5 Networked EEG Laboratory.

A computer network is a system that allows information to be shared between computers located in different places, even at distance from each other. Networking has revolutionized the computer system, making it possible to move from large powerful but very expensive data processors to a series of independent but interacting computers.

A network topology describes the arrangement of systems on a computer network. It defines how the computers, or nodes, within the network are arranged and connected to each other: the *bus* or *line topo*logy is a network setup in which each computer is connected to the others in a linear way; in the *star topology* all nodes are individually connected to a central connection point, which functions as a control of the network itself; a *ring topology* is a network configuration in which device connections create a circular data path, therefore the nodes of the network are joined by point-to-point links in a closed way; in the *mesh topology* each computer is interconnected with one another, allowing for most transmissions to be distributed, even if one of the connections goes down.

A computer network basically allows:

1. The sharing of resources: if multiple computers are connected to each other, each of them can reach the others' private resources. The most functional model for communication and use of information is represented by the client/server structure. Various users (clients) can connect to a superior machine (server), which shares programs into the network and can manage the database.
2. Communication between different users: examples of real-time communication possibilities between remote users are represented by chat lines, audio conference and/or teleconference, etc. Thanks to the existence of networks, files can be transferred or copied from one computer to another, databases created and used by many operators; working on a remote computer (virtual terminal) is also possible. The worldwide network connection (*Internet*) allowed a real revolution in the communications field: e-mails made it possible to exchange correspondence between different users, even when very far away from each other, connected to the same network.

Information on the network can be transmitted mainly through the use of electric cables, optical fibers and radio waves.

Coaxial cables allow little interference and great transmission speed, but they are now disused. Information travels above all through already installed telephone lines. When the transmission passes through the telephone network, the digital signal must be transformed into analog and then digital. This happens inside the modem, a device that allows the circulation of information via the Internet. In reality, the modem modulates and demodulates: inside it there are A/D converters, which convert the data from analog to digital and vice versa. The Integrated Services Digital Network (ISDN) and Asymmetrical Digital Subscriber Line (ADSL) networks, on the other hand, allow the direct transmission of digital data (without the need for conversion) and, therefore, they enable very high transmission speeds. Transmission through optic fiber cables allows currently a much faster transmission speed and is immune to electromagnetic disturbances, and for these reasons its use will be increasingly implemented.

At local level, wireless transmission is spreading increasingly through radio waves or infrared rays (wireless local area network, Bluetooth, or Wi-Fi technology) which offer though a limited coverage. For long-distance transmission, the most widely used system nowadays is the satellite Internet with a transmitter that sends signals to a satellite sending them back with minimal delay to a receiver.

Precisely based on their geographic coverage, networks must therefore be distinguished into *local* (*Intranet*) or *global* (*Internet*) networks. Local networks can extend for a few meters (e.g., connecting several rooms in the same building: PAN, personal area network) or even for a few kilometers (connecting several floors of the same building or neighboring areas: LAN, local area network). Local networks also include the internal network of a university campus (CAN: campus area network) or the metropolitan network, which extends within a city (MAN: metropolitan area network). To protect local networks from external connections, router firewalls are used.

Networks that extend beyond the aforementioned limits and which use the *Internet* to communicate (the Internet is the real *network of networks*, capable of interconnecting billions of computers anywhere in the world) are defined as *geographical* or *global networks* (WAN: wide area network). Both in the MAN and WAN networks, public transmission channels are used and, therefore, to access the network, it will be necessary to contact a network provider. The provider will manage data received from the user and transfer it to the recipient according to the best possible route, through a device called a router.

There are official rules for the interaction between the various network components, validated and issued by the ISO (International Standards Organization). These rules are quite complex, so much so that hardware device manufacturers have to comply with the more practical standards of the Internet protocol suite (TCP/IP).

The digital technological evolution that has been briefly described above has substantially changed communication possibilities in every type of sector and also in the hospital environment. As a matter of fact, in most public hospitals there is a complex hospital information system (HIS). This system handles the administrative part, the collection of all clinical laboratory and instrumental data relating to both inpatients and outpatients; with the appropriate security measures, this database will allow to access clinical laboratory documentation by healthcare professionals. Figure 7.11 shows schematically the various network connection possibilities.

With modern digital systems, an EEG tracing can be adequately recorded anywhere and, therefore, the concept of an EEG laboratory must also be reviewed, in a broader and more dynamic perspective. Portable EEG systems can indeed reach the patients in any hospital ward and also record EEGs in emergency conditions. Permanent EEG acquisition devices can be installed in neurophysiological laboratories as well as many other departments. Therefore, nowadays, the role of EEG technicians must be reviewed: they no longer have to wait for the patient at the laboratory, but they also move to where the intervention is needed.

The recorded data can be stored inside the same recording system and then transmitted to other units (both for final storage and reporting) in various ways. Once technicians have returned to the lab, they can simply connect their laptop with a cable to the central unit (which also serves as a data storage) and then transfer all the tracings performed bedside. As an alternative, tracings can be transferred on a mobile device (like a pen drive) and then sent to the central unit. Finally, there is the more interesting possibility of remotely transferring the recorded material, using the hospital's internal network (Intranet) or the external public network (Internet). In this modern perspective, the networked EEG laboratory can be organized in different ways, which are of increasingly complexity, but also easy to implement. Following, some examples:

1. The networking of the various existing systems within a Neurophysiology Operative Unit.

   The various digital systems available, placed either on the same floor or on different floors of a hospital building, can be attached to a "direct" network (via cable connection), with the possibility of communicating between them and above all with the possibility of channeling all

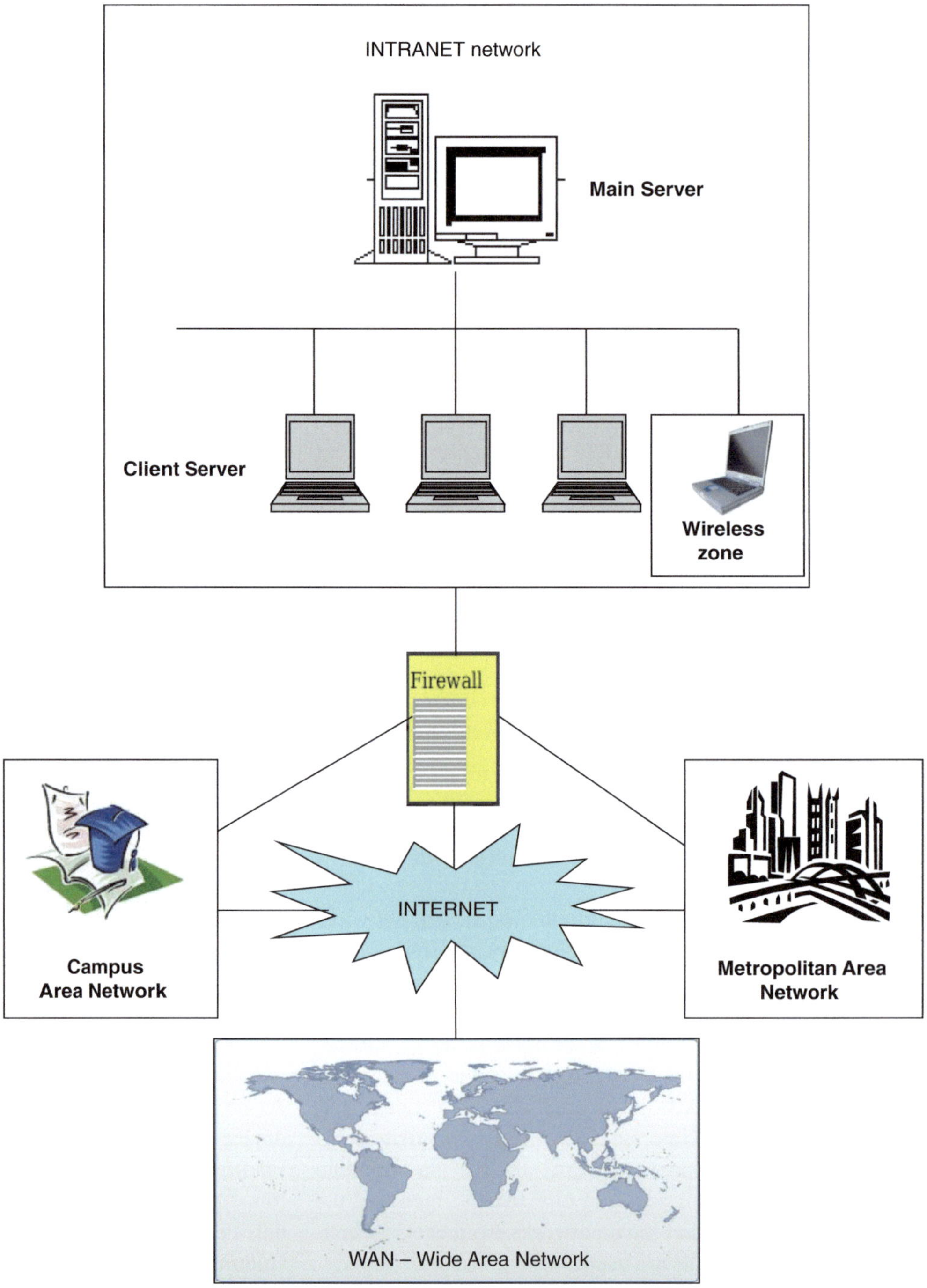

Fig. 7.11 Schematic description of the various network connection possibilities for computers located in very different and distant geographic locations

the acquired data to a central unit, which will also act as the main storage unit.

A simple network model of this type can include:

(a) Two or more EEG recording machines (e.g., named EEG1, EEG2, etc.)
(b) One or more review station
(c) One central unit for review and storage (file server)

With this type of organization, all EEGs recorded in the various rooms can be viewed remotely or even online, by referring physicians and then stored, both for medical and legal purposes and for their subsequent use (teaching, research, follow-up, etc.). The report can either be printed directly by the physician or sent to the computerized reception desk (Fig. 7.12).

2. Local network connection of recording units located on different floors or buildings, within the same hospital or associated hospitals.

As already mentioned, one of the most important advantages of digital technology has been that it made available small, portable, or easily movable EEG devices,

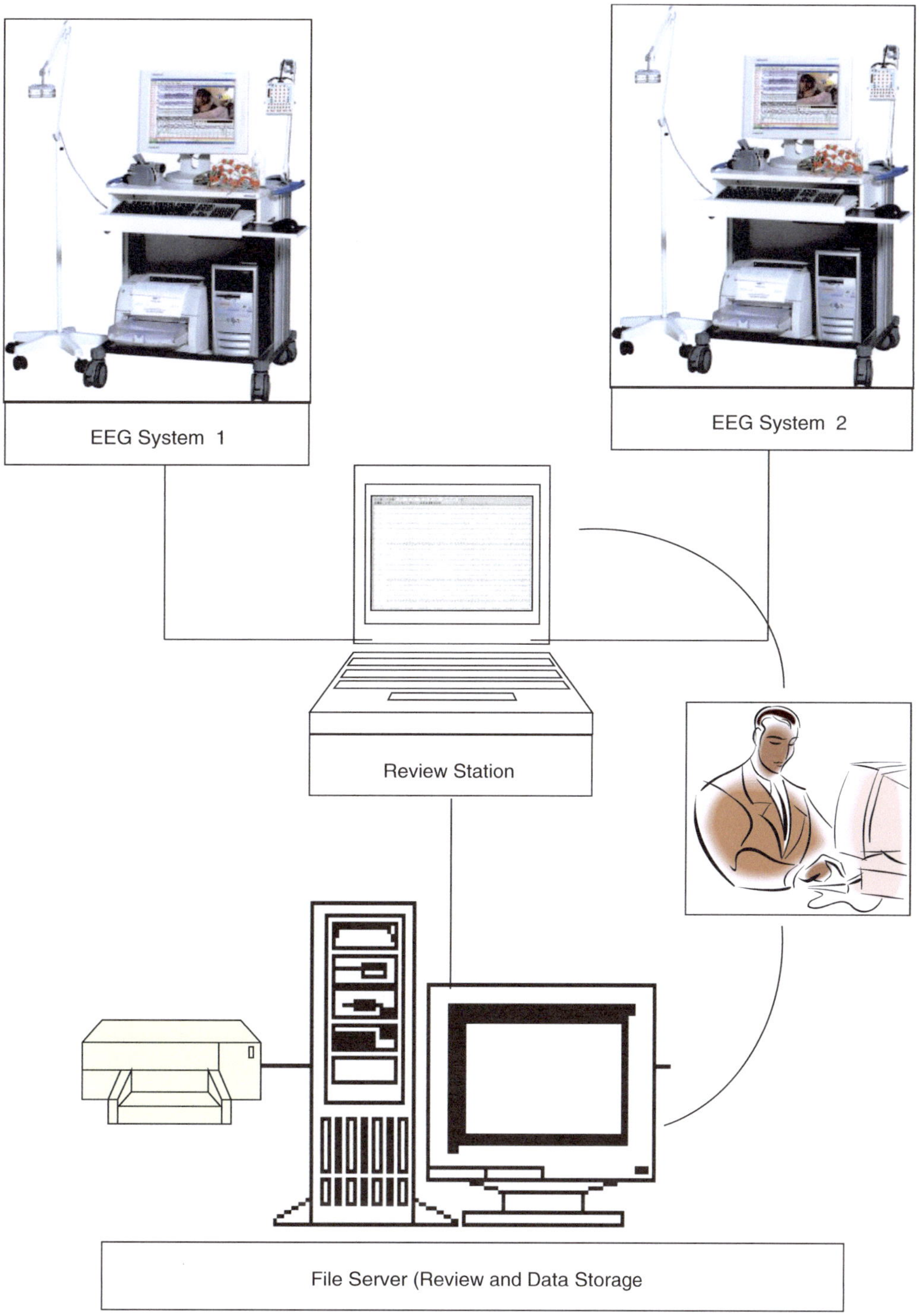

Fig. 7.12 A simple network in which two EEG recording systems are connected to a review station and a file server (for review and data storage)

suitable for recordings in particular environments (even when disconnected from the power grid). At present, it is therefore possible, within the same hospital, to record tracings anywhere (emergency department, intensive care unit, surgery room, etc.) and then to transmit what is recorded via the Internal hospital network (Intranet) to the central unit for reporting and storage. From the same central unit, the reports can then be sent to the requesting department (Fig. 7.13).

3. Remote sharing of EEG tracings

The most innovative possibility, however, is to be able to transmit the recorded EEG traces using the Internet, and this is achievable through the creation of a web server or a restricted virtual private network (VPN).

The connection via a web server is accessible from any Internet workstation and may not necessarily require the installation of specific software for review. The procedures in this case are the following: the tracings can be

Fig. 7.13 Example of a complex EEG network that allows the connection of various digital EEG systems, positioned in different departments of the same hospital or associated hospitals

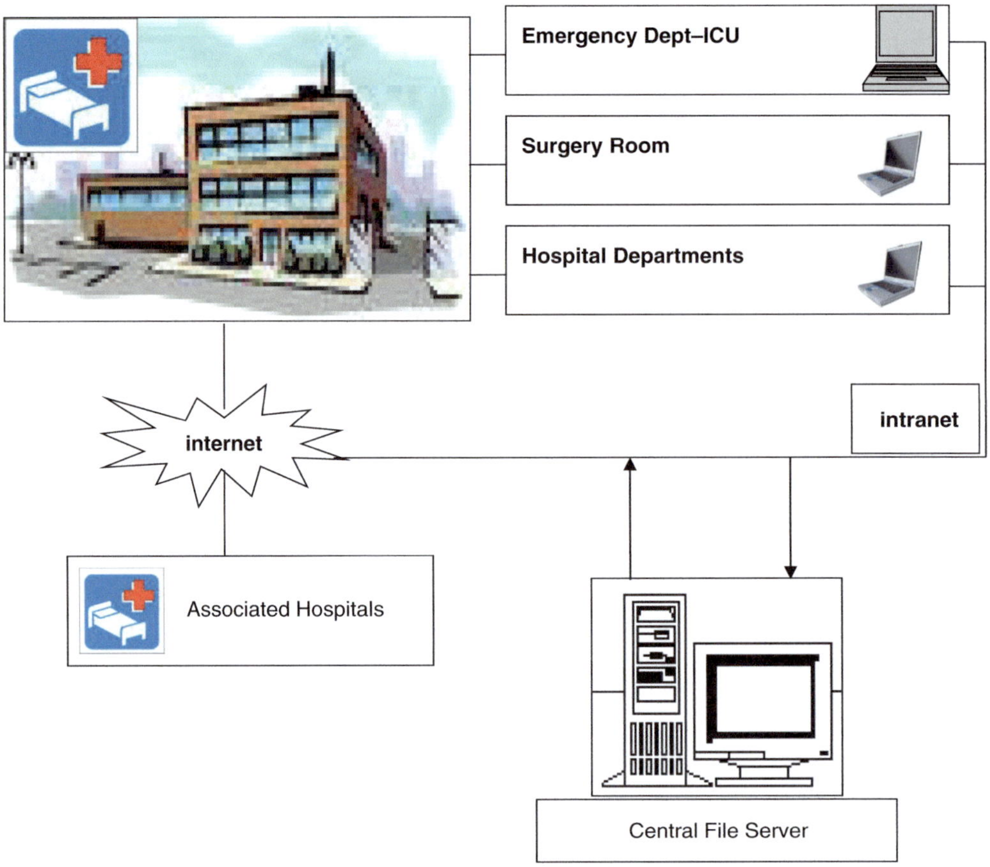

recorded from any workstation inside the hospital and then transferred to the web server in an accredited area; the physician gains access to the protected area with a username and password from any other workstations, both inside and outside of the hospital; once the tracing has been evaluated, the physician can generate the report in various ways, for example, by e-mail.

With the VPN, the EEG tracing is always transferred to the hospital's internal server, which the doctor can only access with his own computer, but not necessarily while being inside the hospital. Therefore, he will be able to view the trace even at home and generate a report according to standard methods.

Thinking of a more complete organization, connected to the HIS (hospital information system), the following networked structure can be easily and inexpensively devised:

(a) The HIS sends the list of the ongoing exams to the Acquisition Units (according to internal and external requests)
(b) The EEG tracing is recorded anywhere inside the hospital
(c) The EEG is transferred to the internal review station (which is nothing more than a slot on the specific hospital or associated hospital server)
(d) The electroencephalographer connects to the VPN with their computer, regardless of where they are (at the hospital, at home, traveling, etc.), views the EEG and sends the report immediately to the HIS, which then makes it available online to the applicant.

All the procedures for the acquisition, transmission, review and storage of digital EEG data must be performed respecting the patient's privacy to protect the abuse of patient's information. Adequate security measures must protect against unauthorized users, computer viruses and accidental destruction of files.

References

1. Sinha SR, Sullivan S, Sabau D, et al. American clinical neurophysiology society guideline 1: minimum technical requirements for performing clinical electroencephalography. J Clin Neurophysiol. 2016;33:303–7.
2. Ferree TC, Luu P, Russel GS, Tucker DM. Scalp electrodes impedance, infection risk, and EEG quality. Clin Neurophysiol. 2001;112:536–44.
3. Jarrar R, Buchhalter J, Williams K, McKay M, Luketich C. Technical tips: electrode safety in pediatric prolonged EEG recordings. Am J Electroneurodiagnostic Technol. 2011;51:114–7.

4. Berlin F, Carlile JA, de Burgo MI, et al. Technical tips: electrode application and preventing skin breakdown techniques. Am J Electroneurodiagnostic Technol. 2011;51:206–19.
5. Scott NK. Infection prevention: 2013 review and update for neurodiagnostic technologists. Neurodiagn J. 2013;53:271–88.
6. Falco C, Sebastiano F, Cacciola L, et al. Scalp electrode placement by EC2 adhesive paste in long-term video-EEG monitoring. Clin Neurophysiol. 2005;116:1771–3.
7. Jasper HH. The 10–20 electrodes system of the International Federation. Electroencephalogr Clin Neurophysiol. 1958;10:367–80.
8. American Electroencephalographic Society. Guideline thirteen: guidelines for standard electrode position nomenclature. J Clin Neurophysiol. 1994;11:111–3.
9. Nuwer MR, Comi G, Emerson R, et al. IFCN standards for digital recording of clinical EEG. Electroencephalogr Clin Neurophysiol. 1998;106:259–61.
10. Achaya JN, Hani A, Cheek J, Thirumala P, Tsuchida TN. American clinical neurophysiology society guideline 2: guidelines for standard electrode position nomenclature. J Clin Neurophysiol. 2016;33:308–11.
11. Seeck M, Koessler L, Bast T, et al. The standardized EEG electrode array of the IFCN. Clin Neurophysiol. 2017;128:2070–7.
12. Oostenveld R, Praamstra P. The five percent electrode system from high-resolution EEG and ERP measurements. Clin Neurophysiol. 2001;112:713–9.
13. Kuratani J, Pearl PL, Sullivan L, et al. American clinical neurophysiology society guideline 5: minimum technical standards for pediatric electroencephalography. J Clin Neurophysiol. 2016;33:320–3.
14. Halford JJ, Sabau D, Drislane FW, Tsuchida TN, Sinha SR. American clinical neurophysiology society guideline 4: recording clinical EEG on digital media. J Clin Neurophysiol. 2016;33:317–9.
15. Acharya JN, Hani AJ, Thirumala PD, Tsuchida TN. American clinical neurophysiology society guideline 3: a proposal for standard montages to be used in clinical EEG. J Clin Neurophysiol. 2016;33:312–6.
16. Flink R, Pedersen B, Guekht AB, et al. Guidelines for the use of EEG methodology in the diagnosis of epilepsy. International league against epilepsy: commission report commission on European affairs: subcommission on European guidelines. Acta Neurol Scand. 2002;106:1–7.
17. Craciun L, Gardella E, Alving J, et al. How long shall we record electroencephalography? Acta Neurol Scand. 2014;129:9–11.
18. Capovilla G, Gambardella A, Rubboli G, et al. Suppressive efficacy by a commercial available blue lens on PPR in 610 photosensitive epilepsy patients. Epilepsia. 2006;47:529–33.
19. Chokroverty S, Vetrugno R. Polysomnography: technical and clinical aspects. In: Schomer DL, Lopes da Silva FH, editors. Niedermeyer's electroencephalography. Basic principles, clinical applications, and related fields. 7th ed. Oxford: Oxford University Press; 2018. p. 897–967.
20. Beniczky S, Neufeld M, Diehl B, et al. Testing patients during seizures: a European consensus procedure developed by a joint taskforce of the ILAE—commission on European Affairs and the European Epilepsy Monitoring Unit Association. Epilepsia. 2016;57:1363–8.
21. Dash D, Dash C, Primrose S, et al. Update on minimal standards for electroencephalography in Canada: a review by the Canadian Society of Clinical Neurophysiologists. Can J Neurol Sci. 2017;44:631–42.

8 Artifacts

Marianna Brienza, Chiara Davassi, and Oriano Mecarelli

8.1 Artifact Classification

In this chapter, artifacts are classified into three groups:

- Physiological artifacts
- Artifacts caused by the acquisition system
- Artifacts caused by electrical interference and external equipment

8.1.1 Physiological Artifacts

Physiological artifacts are generated from the patient, arising from sources other than the brain [1], and they are mostly represented by eye movements, muscular, electrocardiographic and respiratory activities.

8.1.1.1 Eye Movement Artifacts

Eye movements are primarily recorded from the frontal electrodes, although they can also be extended to other regions. The strength of the interference depends upon the proximity of the electrodes to the eyes and upon the direction the eye is moving to. Eye movements can be lateral, vertical, oblique, or rotational. They can also be conjugated or disconjugated.

The main vertical movements are eye-blinking and eye-opening, while the principal lateral ones that can show also oblique and rotational characteristics are:

- *Saccadic eye movements*—fast eye movements that are required to bring the objects of interest on the fovea (they can be voluntary or reflex).
- *Smooth pursuit eye movements*— allowing the eyes to closely follow a moving object.

M. Brienza · C. Davassi · O. Mecarelli (✉)
Department of Human Neurosciences, Sapienza University of Rome, Rome, Italy
e-mail: oriano.mecarelli@uniroma1.it

Finally, *nystagmus* is a rapid, rhythmic, repetitive and involuntary eye movements which can be horizontal, vertical, or rotational.

The EEG signal is produced by the eyeball acting as a dipole, with the positive pole oriented anteriorly (cornea) and the negative pole oriented posteriorly (retina), that generates a large-amplitude alternate current field, detectable by any of the electrodes near the eyes. If there are no ocular movements, the corneo-retinal resting potential, being stable, cannot be recorded on EEG derivations with normal amplifiers. During ocular and/or palpebral movements, the dipole rapidly changes direction and, therefore, the related electric field is recordable on the frontotemporal derivations in the form of high-voltage potentials (up to 100–200 μV).

Eye-blinking is the most typical vertical movement observed on the EEG, useful to identify the normal waking state, especially during ambulatory-EEG and polysomnography. When individuals close their eyes, ocular globes deviate upward (Bell's phenomenon) and the positive charge of the cornea is recorded by the scalp electrodes. In a typical bipolar montage, eye-blinks induce characteristics sharp positive deflections in the anterior electrodes, Fp1 and Fp2, and - to a lesser degree- in the F3 and F4 (Fig. 8.1). It is also believed that the eye-blinking artifacts originate from the eyelids, functioning as a conductor between the corneal surface and the frontopolar region of the scalp rather than from the eyeball movement itself, creating a positive potential in the frontal electrodes during the blink. Blinks typically occur about 20 times a minute. Repeated blinking, of lower width and higher frequency, is called *flutter* (Fig. 8.2). When opening the eyes, the eyeball rotates downward; the electronegative retina draws nearer to the frontal electrodes increasing their negative charge and therefore creating a wide negative signal. The eyeball downward movement thus generates an artifact which is similar to the eye-opening one.

Lateral eye movements mostly involve the anterior temporal electrodes, F7 and F8, that are the best placed to perceive the positivity of the cornea, as the eye globe moves

O. Mecarelli (ed.), *Clinical Electroencephalography*, https://doi.org/10.1007/978-3-030-04573-9_8

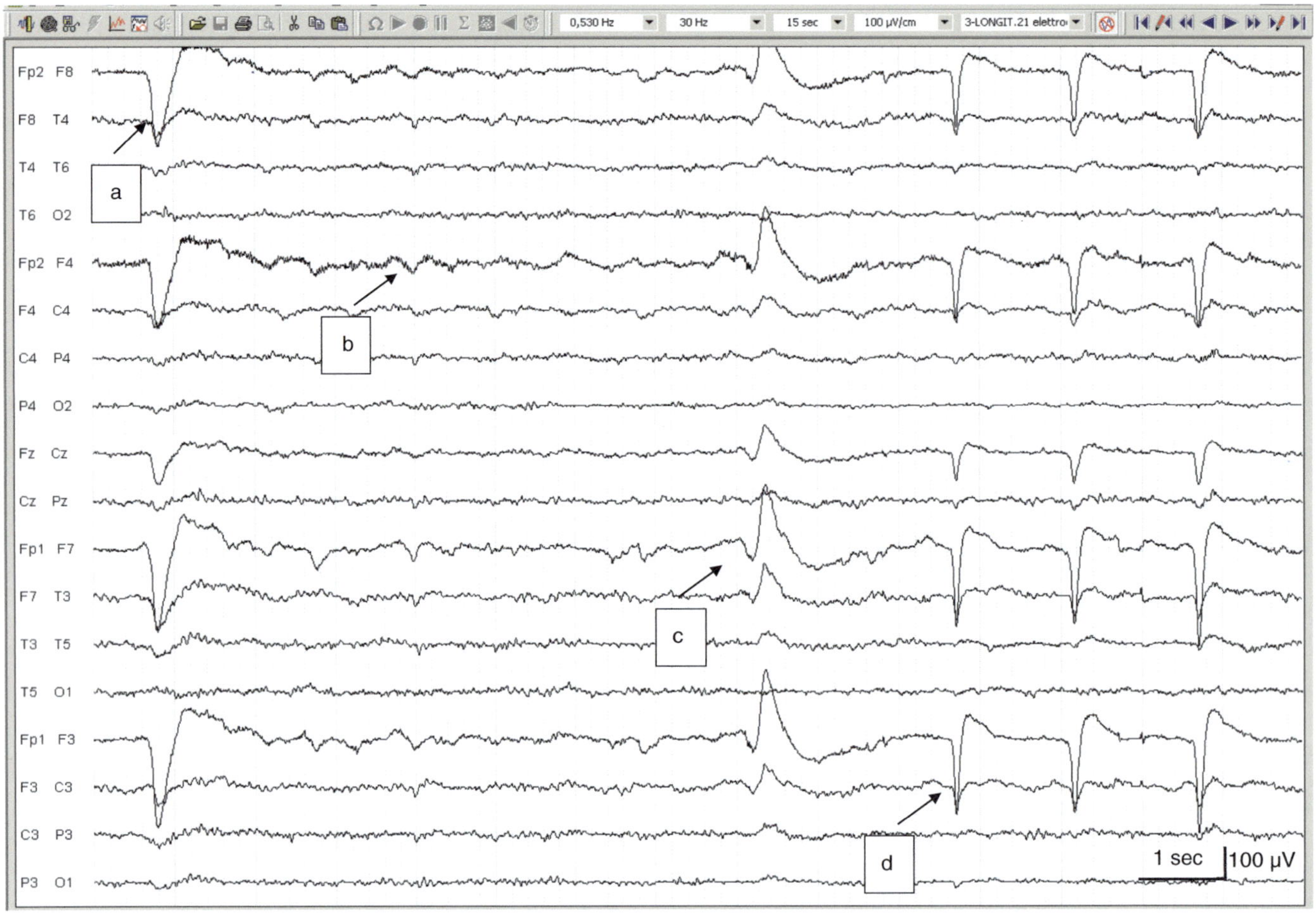

Fig. 8.1 Standard EEG: eye-closing (a), slow eye movements with eyelids closed (b), eye-opening (c), blinking artifacts on the anterior derivations (d)

from side to side on the horizontal plan. When moving the eyes to the right, the electropositive cornea draws closer to the F8 electrode, positively charging it, while the electronegative retina draws closer to the F7 electrode, negatively charging it. When moving the eye to the left, the electropositive cornea draws closer to the F7 electrode, positively charging it, while the electronegative retina draws closer to the F8 electrode, negatively charging it. This artifact is also due to the activation of the lateral rectus muscles that produces motor unit potential artifact during rapid eye movements in the F7 and F8 electrode derivations. An important example of lateral eye movement artifact is represented by *slow roving eye movements* of drowsiness. Like the lateral eye movements, they present a positive phase reversal in the anterior temporal electrodes - on the side where the eyes are moving - and a negative phase reversal in the contralateral anterior temporal electrodes. These movements are characterized by a rounded, more prolonged shape when compared with those occurring during wakefulness or REM sleep and with tendency to be quicker and have a more squared-off onset [2, 3].

Nystagmus consists of eyes repetitive and involuntary oscillations, with a slow deviation of the eyeballs toward one side and with a rapid movement in the opposite direction. In most cases, nystagmus, if not very wide, does not cause a variation in the corneo-retinal dipole interfering with the EEG signal. However, it is possible that it generates an artifactual activity easily mistaken for theta band potentials or for artifacts caused by a high interelectrode impedance. The side of the positive phase reversal indicates the direction of the fast component of the nystagmus [4].

Eye movements monitoring, through the placement of electrodes above and below the eyes, helps to distinguish the polarity and, consequently, the source of the signal: when the signals are *in phase* with one another, they arise from the brain; when they are *out of phase*, they indicate an eye origin [4]. There are various possibilities for the electrodes positioning to record ocular movements (Electro Oculo Gram, EOG). *Lateral horizontal electrodes* should be placed 1 cm laterally to the right and left epicanthus or 1 cm laterally and medially to the epicanthus of each eye; they can be referred to one another or to A1–A2 (Fig. 8.3a, c) and they

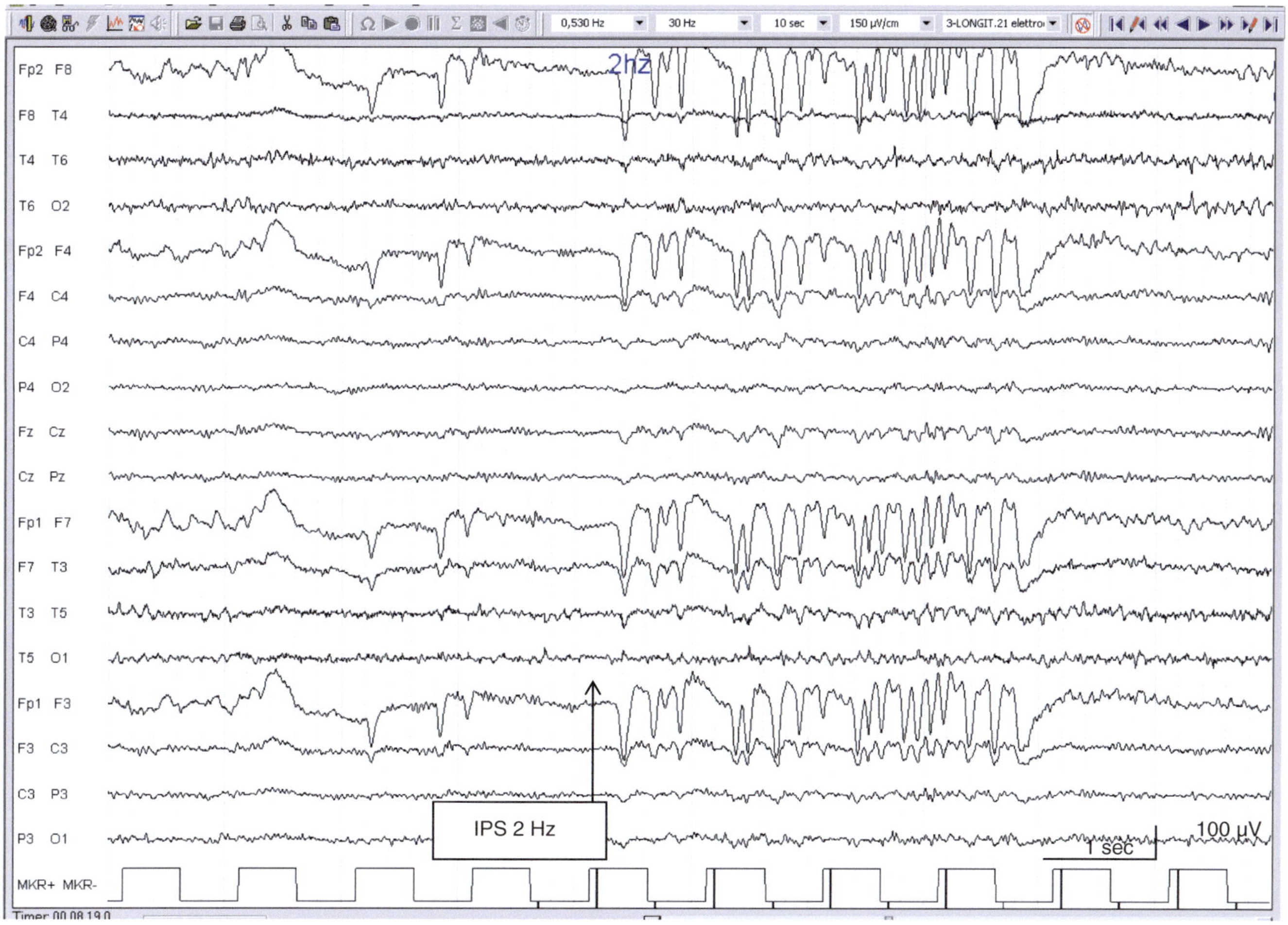

Fig. 8.2 Blinking artifacts with high frequency during Intermittent Photic Stimulation (IPS) at 2 Hz

Fig. 8.3 Placement of ocular electrodes for ElectroOculoGram (EOG): (**a**) bilateral electrodes for horizontal movements, (**b**) supra- and suborbital electrodes for vertical movements, (**c**) placement of electrodes for vertical movements of the right eye and horizontal movements of the left eye, (**d**) bilateral diagonal electrodes for both horizontal and vertical movements. All these electrodes can be referred to each other (bipolar) or to auricular references A1–A2 (referential). RE: Right Eye, LE: Left Eye

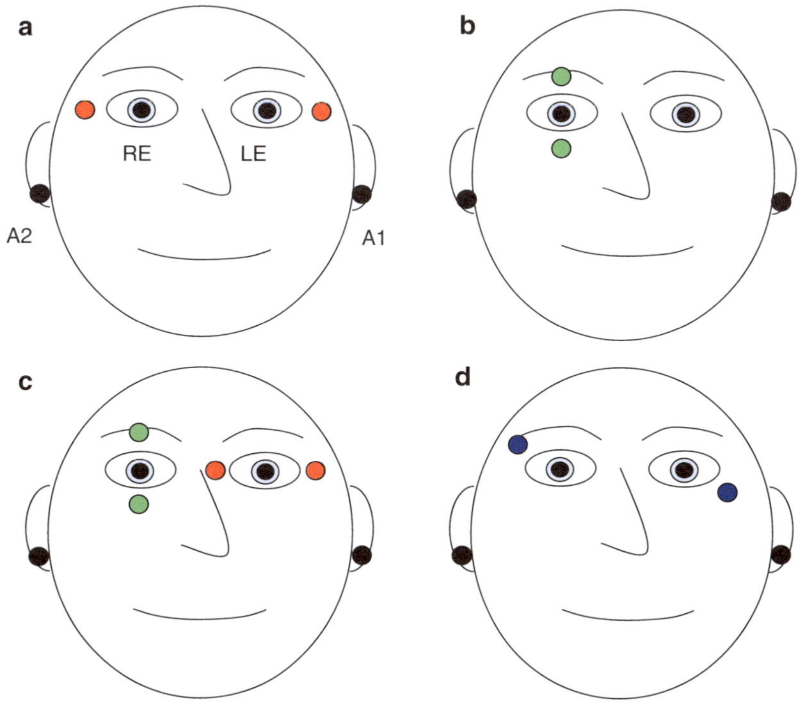

are useful for horizontal ocular movement recordings. *Infraorbital and supraorbital electrodes* should be placed 1 cm below and above the medial orbital axis; they can be referred to one another or to the auricular electrodes (A1–A2) (Fig. 8.3b, c). These electrodes are very useful for vertical ocular movement recordings, the most frequent in EEG recordings. Finally, *diagonal lateral electrodes* should be placed laterally on the epicanthus, the right 1 cm above and the left 1 cm below it; they can be referred to one another or to the omo- or contralateral auricular electrode (Fig. 8.3d). With this type of montage, it is possible to record both horizontal and vertical ocular movements, but it is not possible to distinguish them from one another. Figure 8.4 summarizes ocular movement artifacts that can be visualized at the same time both on the EEG and the EOG, depending on the type and direction of the eye in space.

EOG is important when the nature of a bioelectric activity in the medial-anterior areas is equivocal and it is necessary to differentiate the EEG from the electric activity generated by the eye movements. This is particularly true in scarce cooperating patients who continuously keep moving their eyes. The type of ocular movement monitoring to perform is up to the technician's decision and it should be based on patient's characteristics and the specific clinical issue. At the beginning of each recording, it is always useful to ask the patient to carry out simple eye movements (like opening and closing the eyes, lateral and vertical movements) to better identify the artifactual graphoelements, in order to be able to recognize them afterward. If the patient is keeping the eyes closed and have slow ocular movement artifacts, which could remind a slow pathologic activity, these are observed on the frontal derivations, and the technician should then ask the patient to keep eyelids closed with two fingers, applying a slight downward pressure. Sometimes, it is necessary for the technician to carry out this task, to feel the subpalpebral ocular movements.

8.1.1.2 Muscle Artifacts

The appearance of high-frequency muscle bioelectrical activity, superimposed onto the EEG tracings, is very common, especially in frontotemporal areas (due to the contraction of temporal muscles), in frontal areas (due to the contraction of facial muscles) and in temporo-occipital areas (contraction of the muscles of the neck) (Fig. 8.5). Muscle artifacts usually show with bursts of potentials at high frequency, may have different morphologies without a repetitive or stereotyped shape, and don't present sustained trends with incremental/decremental frequency as in epileptic seizures. Single motor units may represent an exception because of their repetitive firing, but as they do not produce an electric field, they are not observed in adjacent electrodes [2]. To avoid muscle activity, the patient should be relaxed, with his/her mouth slightly open to decontract the jaw and the temporal muscles; a suitable position of the patient's head allows them to relax their neck muscles.

In specific cases, for example, during recordings in patients under mechanical ventilation, curariform drugs can be used to suppress muscle activity. Botulinum toxin, injected into the scalp, have been also tested to record seizures during video-EEG monitoring.

8.1.1.3 Glossokinetic Artifact

The tongue, as the eyeball, has a net dipole and its movements generate the glossokinetic artifact. The shape of this artifact may show both slow waves and spiky components and its field can extend over the whole scalp [2].

8.1.1.4 Electrocardiogram Artifact

The electric field generated by cardiac activity can be detected through volume conduction from the heart to the scalp electrodes. Since the cardiac electric field is equipotential at the scalp, it is often not detectable with bipolar derivations, while it is clearly recognizable as a spike with low-medium amplitude, synchronous with the QRS complex, using inactive common reference derivations.

As extrasystolic beats or prolonged cardiac arrhythmias can also appear on the EEG and as ECG artifacts are difficult to be avoided, it is preferable, even during routine EEG recordings, to monitor cardiac activity (Fig. 8.6). The ECG artifact is difficult to be eliminated; the patient could be asked to change his position or the technician try to slightly move the most contaminated electrodes, but the best option is, however, to document the artifact by adding an ECG channel (Fig. 8.7).

The ECG artifact is well evident in comatose patients, in whom the residual brain activity is poor or absent: in these patients, EEGs are displayed with high amplification and the ECG artifact appears clearly and diffuse (Fig. 8.8).

It is important to distinguish the ECG artifact from *the ballistocardiogram*, a particular artifact caused by the rhythmic movements of the head and related to the cardiac pulsatility, which cause oscillations in the electrode wires.

8.1.1.5 Pulse Artifact

This artifact is observed when one electrode is placed directly on - or near - an artery on the scalp (often the superficial temporal artery), creating an artifactual waveform related to the pulsation [2]. It appears as a rhythmic activity at the same frequency as the heartbeat (Fig. 8.9). Pulse artifacts are more pronounced with bridge electrodes, held in place by elastic caps, and they are due to the rhythmic increase-decrease of impedance and to the variation of pressure on the electrode-skin interface. Pulse artifacts appear to be slightly delayed, compared to the QRS complex recorded by the ECG, because of the time lapse between the electrical contraction of the

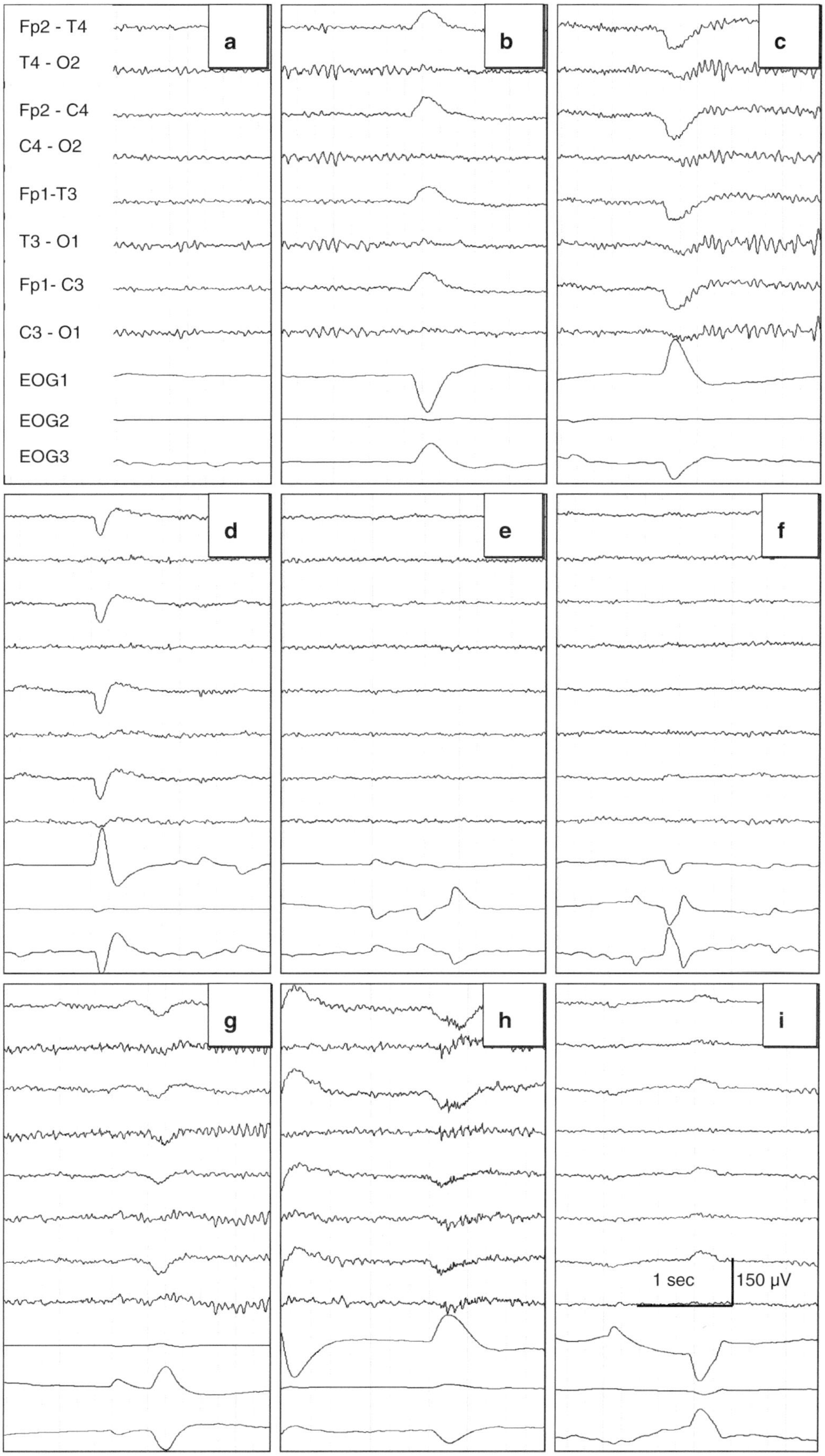

Fig. 8.4 Ocular movement artifacts visible on EEG and EOG derivations. (**a**) Recording with eyes closed and without ocular movements; (**b**) eyes opening; (**c**) eyes closing; (**d**) blinking; (**e**) saccades; (**f–i**) ocular movements toward right, left, up and down, respectively. EOG1 ocular electrodes for vertical movements of the right eye; EOG2 ocular electrodes for horizontal movements of the right eye; EOG3 ocular diagonal electrodes for movements of right and left eye. Bipolar derivations. Filters: 0.53–30 Hz

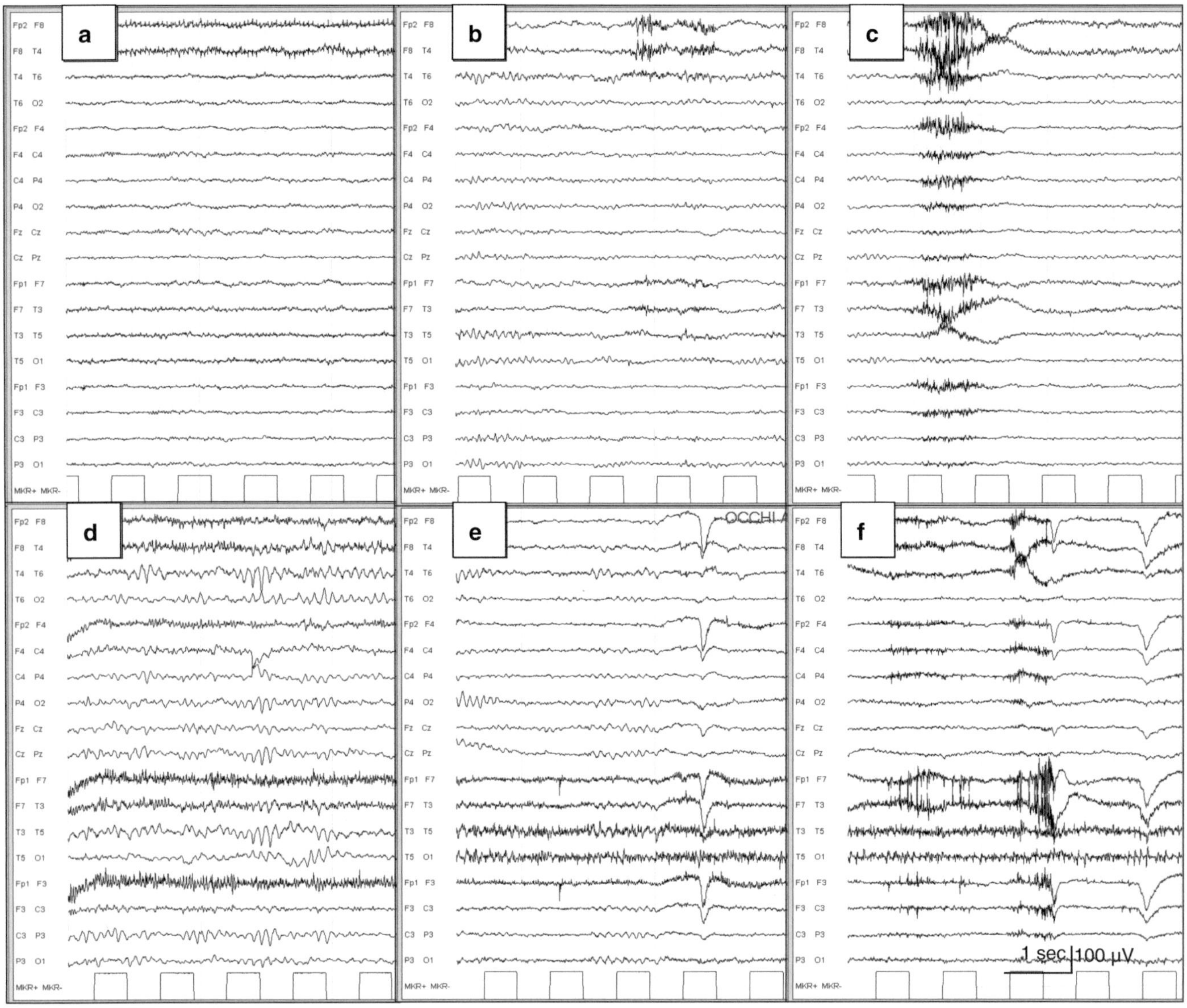

Fig. 8.5 Different muscular artifacts (**a**–**f**) visible on EEG traces. Filters: 0.53–70 Hz

heart muscle and the arrival of the blood flow in the vessel under the electrode. To remove this artifact, it is necessary to move the electrode about 1 cm from the artery and/or slightly loosen the headcap.

8.1.1.6 Cardiac Pacing Artifact

This artifact is difficult to be classified; it should be included among the artifacts of non-biological origin but, since the cardiac pacemaker is implanted under the skin, we can also consider it a particular kind of biological artifact. The pacemaker generates rhythmic spikes, if it is continuously active, or random spikes, if it is active only during cardiac arrhythmias. It is impossible to be eliminated, so that ECG monitoring is mandatory in these cases.

8.1.1.7 Electrodermogram Artifacts

They occur as slow oscillations (0.5–0.2 Hz), caused by the difference of impedance between the skin and the electrodes, due to the sweating of the skin on which the electrode is placed or to the excess of saline solution or gel. It is particularly accentuated by the use of badly chloridated electrodes and it is generally recordable by several electrodes simultaneously (Fig. 8.10). This artifact often reflects the non-triggered sympathetic skin response and, therefore, it depends on the level of the patient's anxiety. To avoid this, electrodes and their wires must be fixed; the EEG should be performed in a cool, dry environment; the skin should be cleaned of excessive gel and sweat; the patient should be relaxed as much as possible.

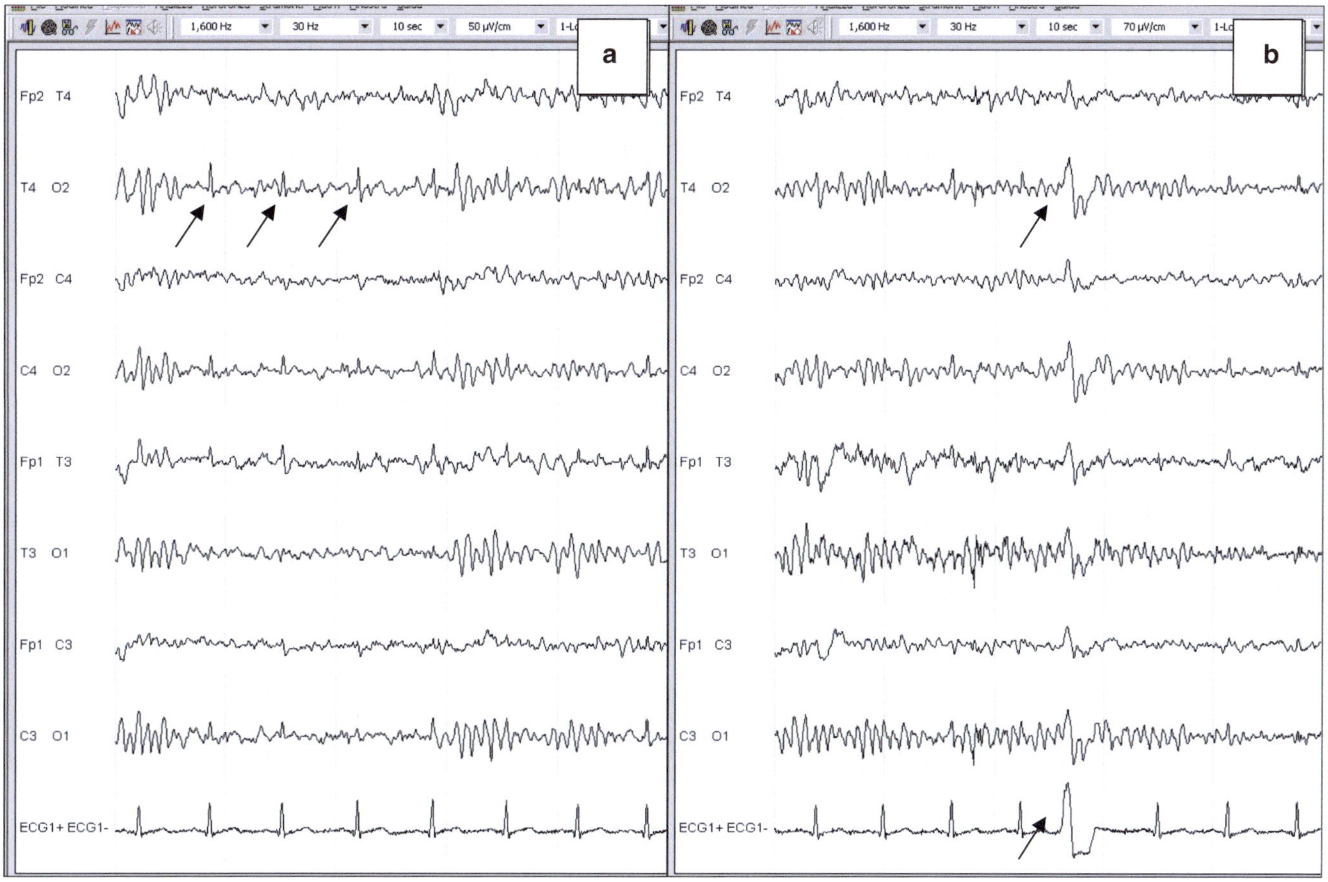

Fig. 8.6 (**a**) ECG artifacts, better evident on T4-O_2. (**b**) Sharp wave of cardiac origin (ventricular extrasystole)

8.1.1.8 Respiratory Artifacts

Respiratory artifact occurs when breathing causes a gentle movement of the head along with each breath. Slow oscillations are usually more evident in the posterior areas, they are synchronous with breathing and they can be observed during hyperventilation. They are frequently observed in patients whose head rests on a pillow or on the headrest of an armchair, because of the rhythmic variations of the pressure between the electrodes and the scalp during breathing. To eliminate this artifact, it is therefore sufficient to avoid the contact of the electrodes with the pillow or the armchair.

8.1.1.9 Tremor Artifact

A continuous or sub-continuous tremor, affecting the head and/or limbs, often determines the appearance of diffuse or localized theta rhythmic oscillations (Fig. 8.11). This artifact is caused by the oscillations of the electrode wires. To eliminate it, it is necessary to position the wires as firmly as possible and to ask the patient to assume positions in order to limit the tremor. Avoid blocking the body segment affected by the tremor, since blocking a limb does not stop muscle contraction that generates the tremor and the artifact will increase.

8.1.1.10 Other Movement Artifacts

Other movement artifacts, often rhythmic, involuntary and impossible to eliminate, are caused by suction, hiccups, mastication, deglutition and swinging of the head or trunk (Fig. 8.12). In these cases, it is essential that the EEG technician indicates the type of movement responsible for the artifact on the tracing, and it would also be useful to video-monitor the movements themselves.

8.1.2 Artifacts due to the Acquisition System

8.1.2.1 Interelectrode "Salt Bridge" Artifact

This artifact appears as a flattening of the trace in bipolar derivations, in which some channels have one or more common electrodes. The large increase in conduction on the skin area between two electrodes referred to each other, caused by the presence of excessive conductive material (gel, water,

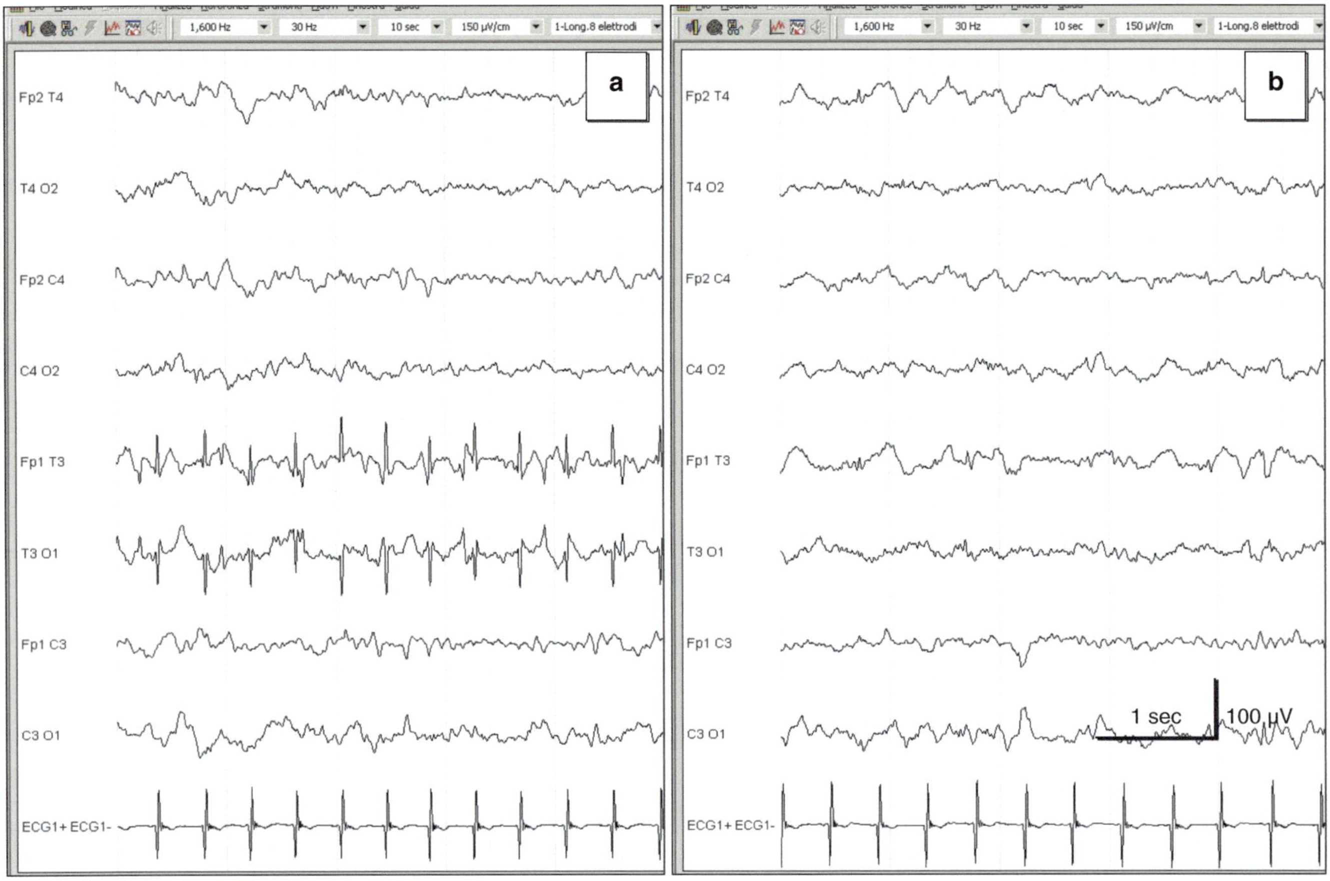

Fig. 8.7 ECG artifacts in the left temporal area, recorded in a 2-year-old child during sleep (**a**); the artifact disappears when the patient changes head position (**b**)

etc.), reduces to zero - or to values very close to zero- the difference in electric potential between the electrodes themselves (Fig. 8.13a). To eliminate this artifact, it is necessary to clean and dry the skin under the electrodes. The same phenomenon (abnormal flattening of the trace) can occur when two electrodes, coupled in bipolar derivation, are placed too close to one another; in this case, similarly, the potential difference tends to decrease proportionally to the interelectrode distance.

8.1.2.2 Bad Skin-Electrode Contact Artifact

When an excessively high impedance is present between the skin and the electrode - due to sebaceous excess (more frequent in hairless subjects), interposition of hair, excess of conductive substances, etc. - various types of artifacts may occur, varying from the appearance of alternating current to slow and/or sharp high-amplitude graphoelements (Fig. 8.13b). Electrode "pop" is the characteristic artifact that occurs as a consequence of an abrupt impedance change, deriving from subtle electrode movement due to drying of electrode gel or paste, a poor connection of the electrode to the wire, a broken lead wire, or a faulty connection between the electrode pin and the jackbox [4]. Strictly confined to a single electrode, this artifact tends to maintain a characteristic morphology, with a fast increase and a slow decrease. Nevertheless, the electrode popping may assume other shapes as well. Usually in an isolated phenomenon, when repetitive, it may resemble a seizure discharge [2]. Sometimes, the impedance change is not so abrupt, and the artifact may mimic a low-voltage arrhythmic delta wave pattern.

To eliminate this artifact, it is necessary to thoroughly clean the skin, to use a good conductive solution, to wet the electrode pads and to make sure the electrode is not too dry or non-chlorinated. The electrodes responsible for the artifact should be replaced and repositioned by checking the skin-electrode impedance again.

8.1.2.3 Electrode Pressure Artifacts

When one or more electrodes press against any surface or object, artifacts appear on the respective EEG channels. They can be characterized by large slow and/or sharply

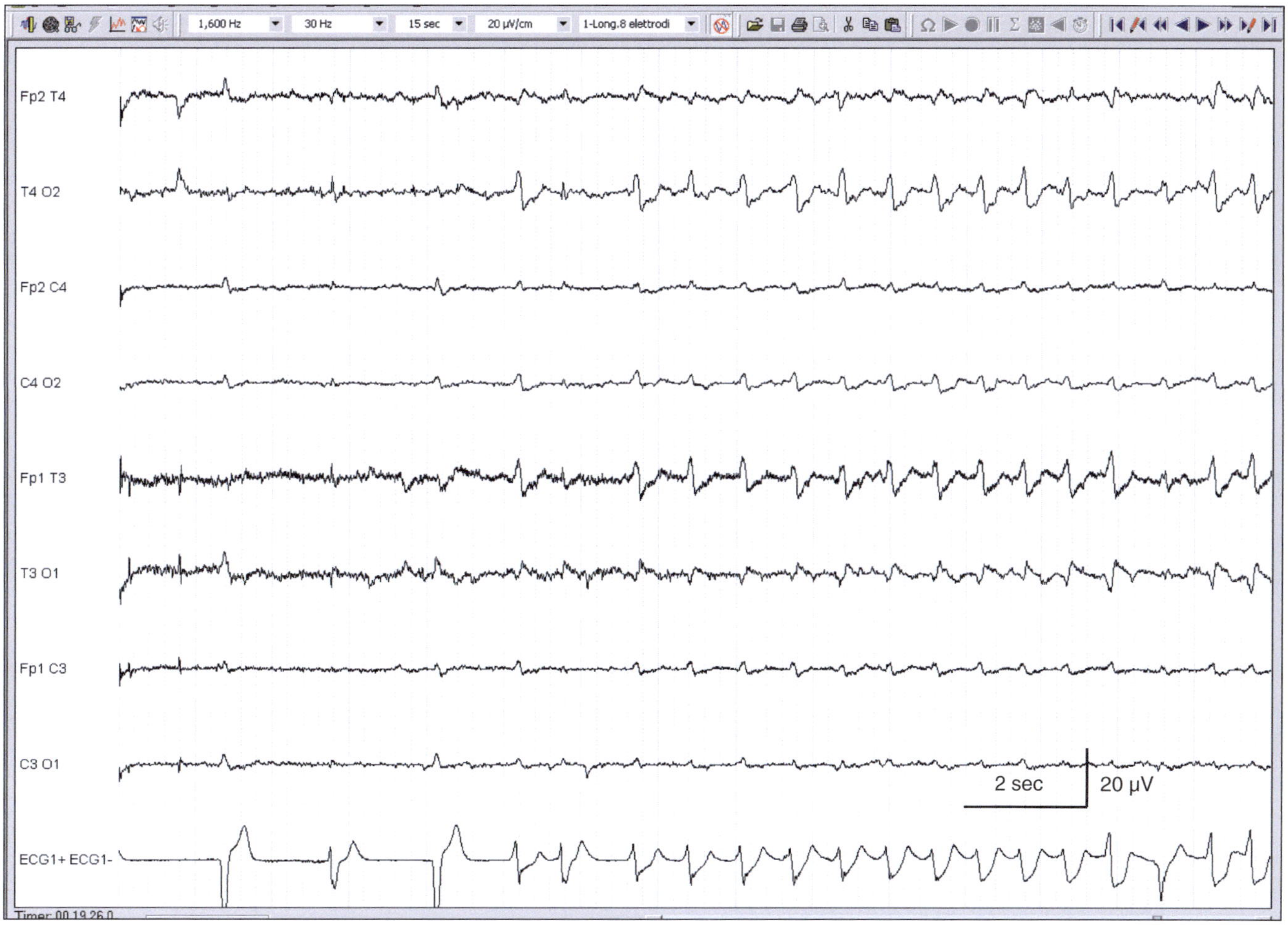

Fig. 8.8 Seventy-nine-year-old patient with severe cardiac arrhythmia and brain anoxia. On the EEG trace, the bioelectrical cerebral activity is absent, even at high amplification of the signal (20 µV/cm), while a widespread cardiac artifact is clearly evident (atrial fibrillation), more evident in T4-O_2 and Fp1-T3 derivations

countered deflections, alternating current, etc. At the beginning of each recording, the technician should produce pressure artifacts on the electrodes, to verify their correct positioning and connection (Fig. 8.14). To avoid pressure artifacts, the patient's head should not lay directly on the headrest or on the bed.

8.1.2.4 Bad Electrode-Clamp and Connector-Headbox Contact Artifacts

These artifacts can present with different characteristics in distribution and shape, although they are generally characterized by sharp or slow, isolated, or in rhythmic sequences, high-voltage graphoelements (Fig. 8.15). Sometimes, these artifacts can simulate fast, low-amplitude epileptic spikes. They are mostly caused by oxidation or deterioration of the cable connector on the electrode or headbox side. To eliminate them, it is necessary to replace the electrode and/or the electrode headbox connecting cable or to work on the headbox connector input.

8.1.2.5 Artifacts Generated from Rhythmic Oscillations of the Cables

Rhythmic oscillations of the cables induce the appearance of artifactual activities which are very similar to those caused by tremor. In an EEG laboratory, there are many causes of cable oscillations, from the flow of ventilated air to the vibrations impressed on the floor and/or the armchair where the patient is sitting (Fig. 8.16). These artifacts are then particularly abundant in special environments such as intensive care units. In these cases, the wires often lay on the bed, on the tubes of the ventilator, or on other electric cables and vibrations are very easily transmitted to the wires, generating rhythmic artifacts. The technician should, therefore, ensure the absence of contacts between the wires and the sources of

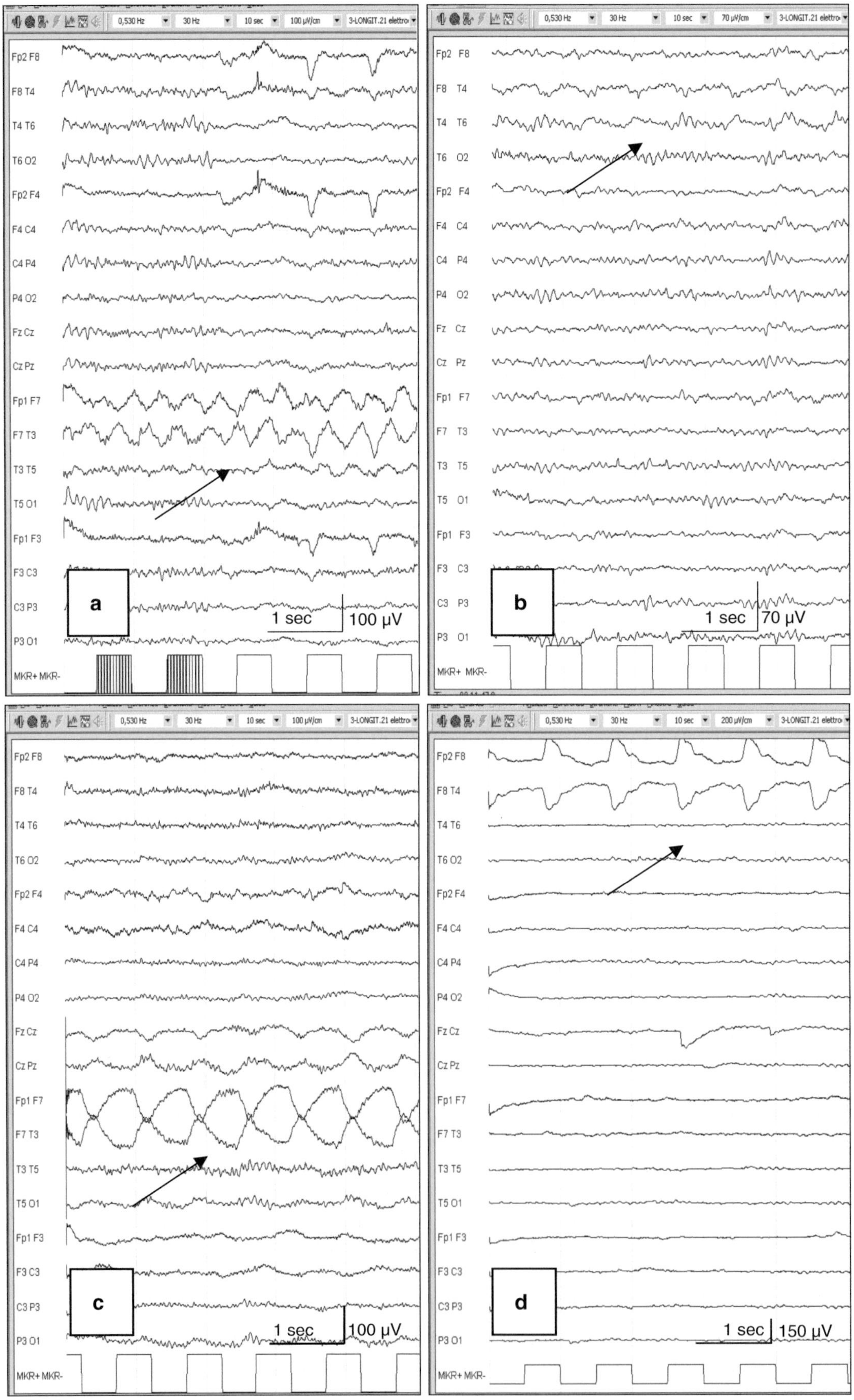

Fig. 8.9 Different kinds of pulse artifacts (**a**–**d**)

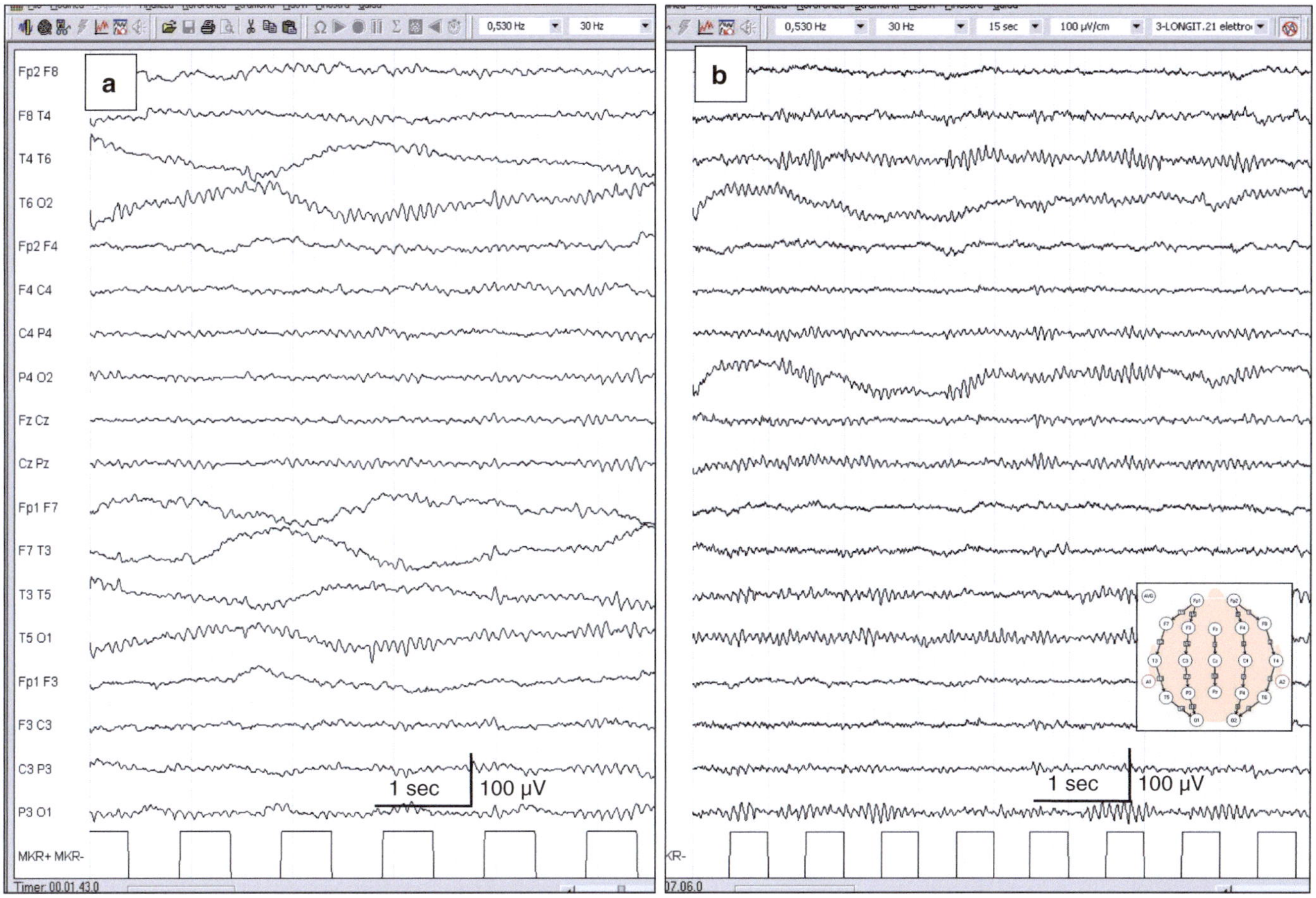

Fig. 8.10 ElectroDermoGram (EDG) artifacts: two examples (**a**, **b**) in different scalp regions

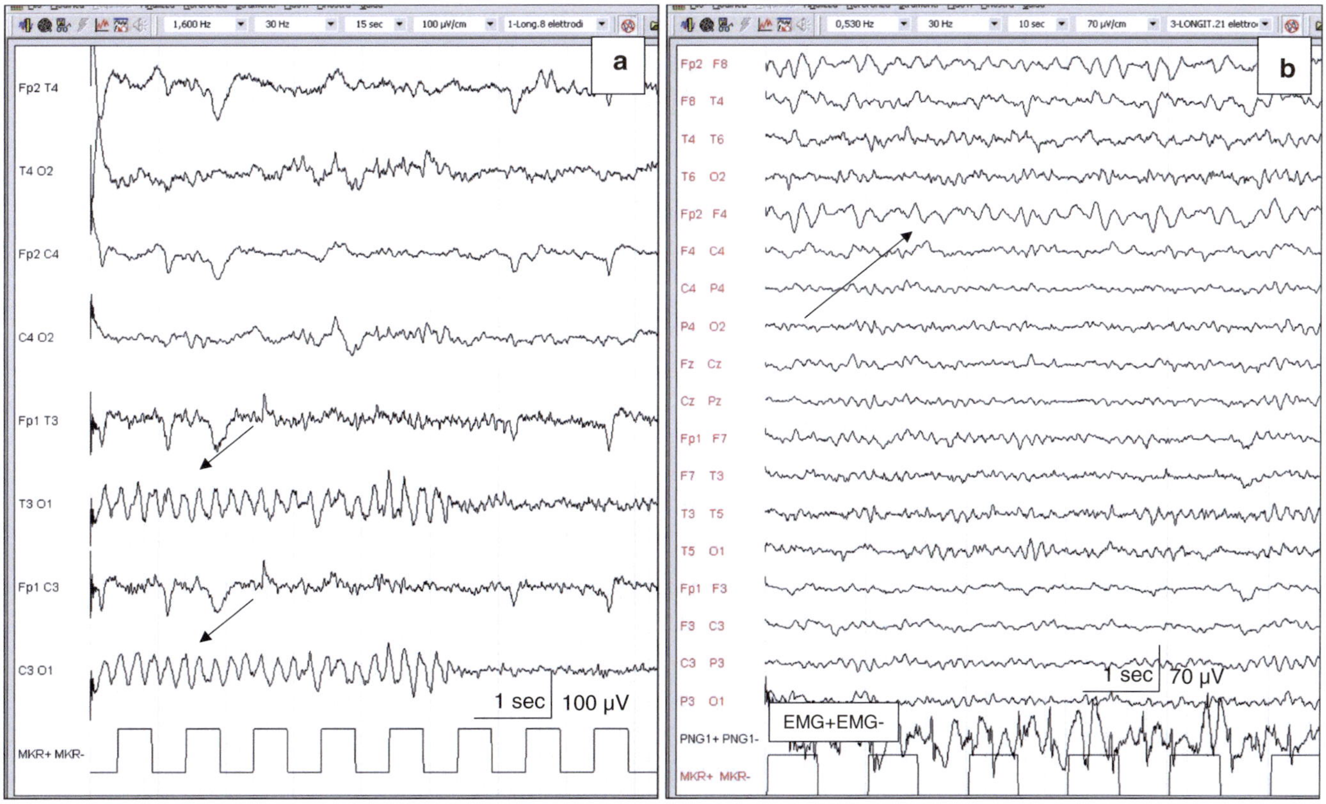

Fig. 8.11 Tremor artifacts in left posterior (**a**) and right anterior (**b**) areas

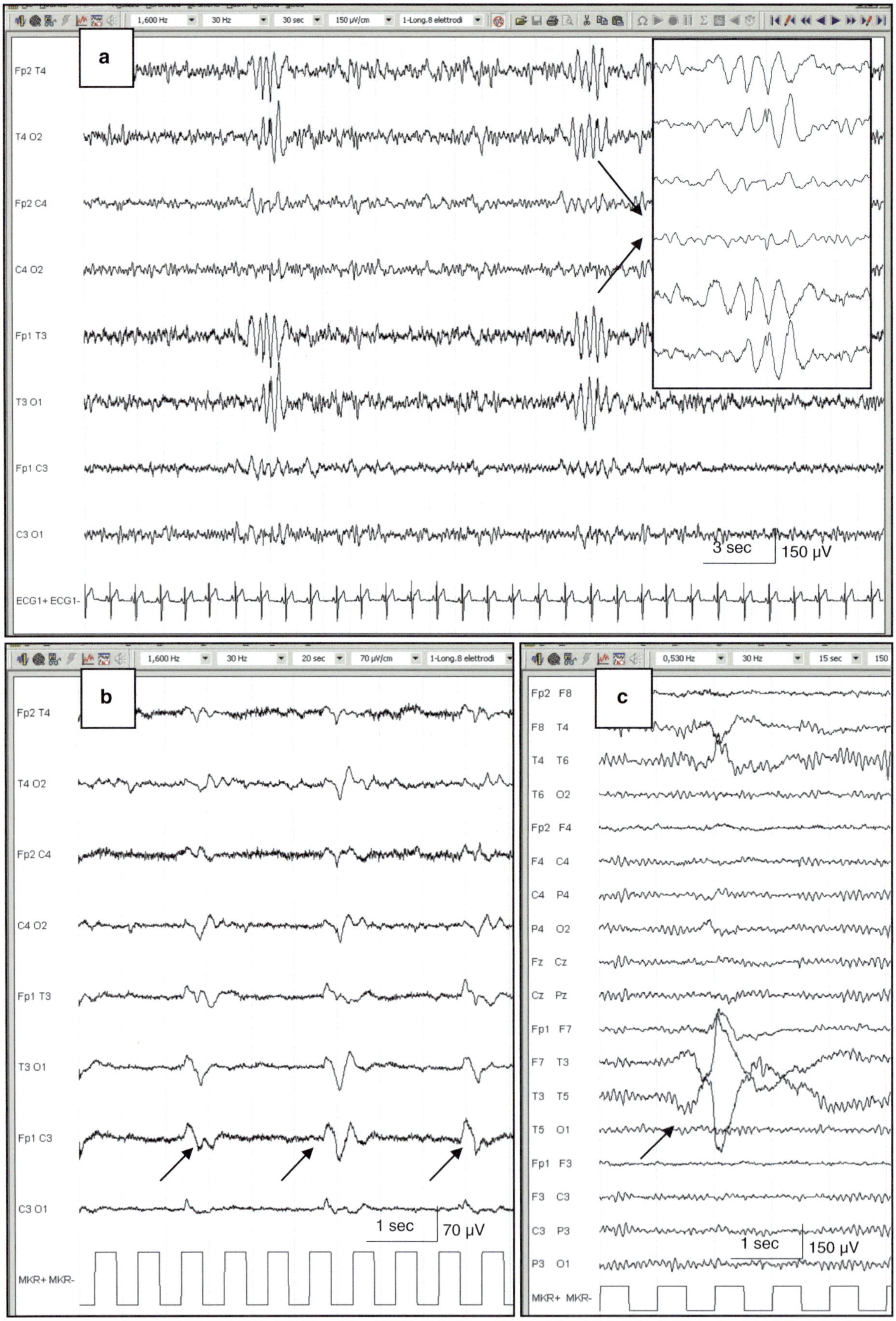

Fig. 8.12 (**a**) Rhythmic suction artifact in a vegetative state patient; (**b**) hiccup artifact in a patient with hepatic encephalopathy; (**c**) swallowing artifact

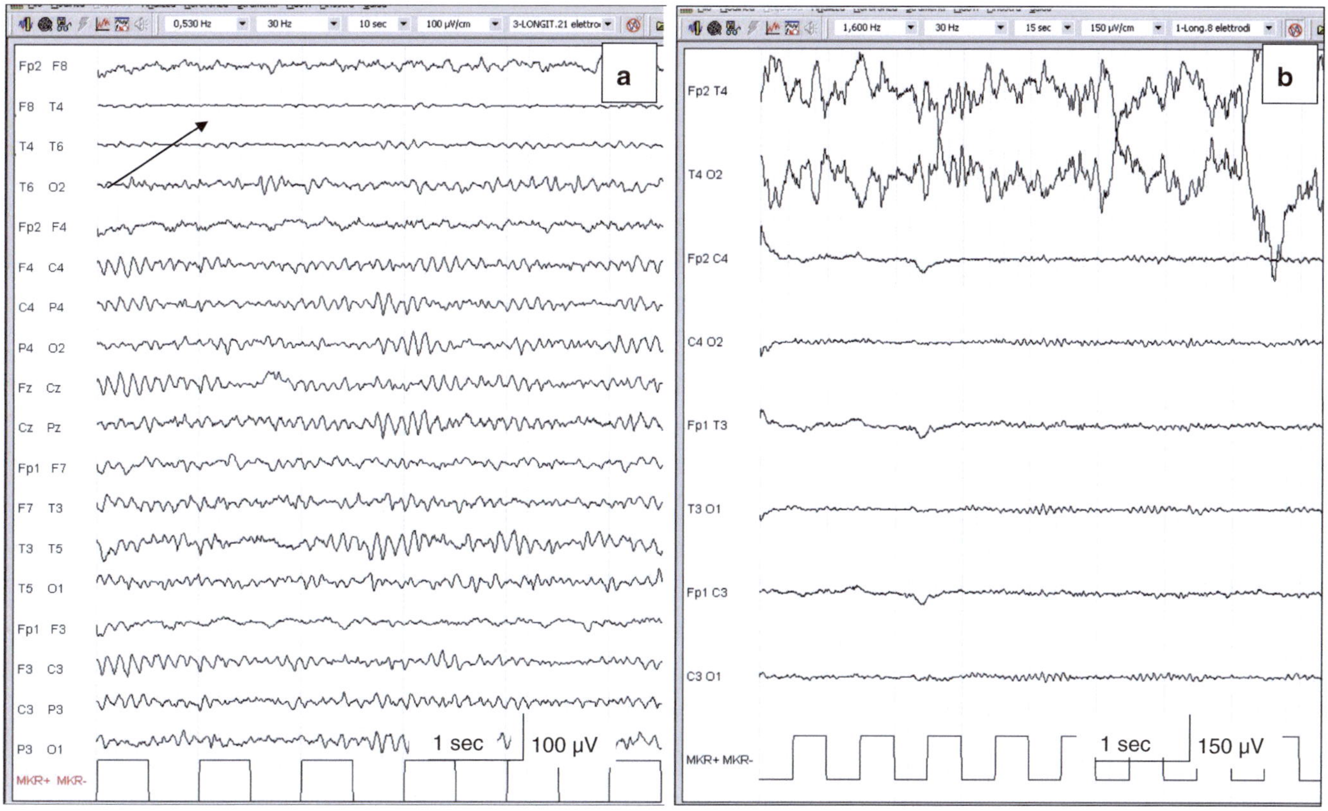

Fig. 8.13 (**a**) Interelectrode bridge artifact; (**b**) bad skin-electrode contact artifact on T4

oscillations, possibly binding them into a single cable. Any monomorphic and rhythmical activity, localized or diffuse, in the theta frequency range must everytime be carefully evaluated to differentiate it from cerebral or extra-cerebral origin.

8.1.3 Electrical Interference and External Equipment Artifacts

8.1.3.1 Alternating Current Artifact

Alternating electrical interference from main power supply is definitely the most common instrumental source of artifact. This artifact is represented by a continuous rapid activity (at 50 Hz in Europe and at 60 Hz in the United States and some other countries) of variable amplitude. It consists of an electromagnetic signal generated by electric cables or equipment connected to the electrical network (even if not in operation), which overlaps the recorded cerebral signal, often making it not evaluable. Solutions to eliminate these artifacts are: lowering the skin-electrode impedance as much as possible, to balance the differential amplifier input impedances; switching off and disconnecting from the power supply all nonessential equipment; removing headbox, cables and the patient from the artifact source (this artifact is also sensitive to the variation in distance of the artifact source from the recording system); positioning the electrode cables all close to each other (this operation facilitates the entry of the alternating current in all the channels in the same quantity, facilitating the differential amplifier subtraction task). In EEG laboratories, it is difficult to record alternating current artifacts, since all electrical systems are built according to specific criteria to avoid interferences and according to the current regulatory provisions. Conversely, it is easier to record alternating current in particular environments such as in intensive care units or in surgery operating rooms, because of the interference from other systems. In these cases, portable digital devices are very useful, since they can be disconnected from the network and powered by batteries.

Finally, it should be reminded that all EEG devices have a special filter (notch filter) that specifically removes the 50 Hz frequencies (Fig. 8.17).

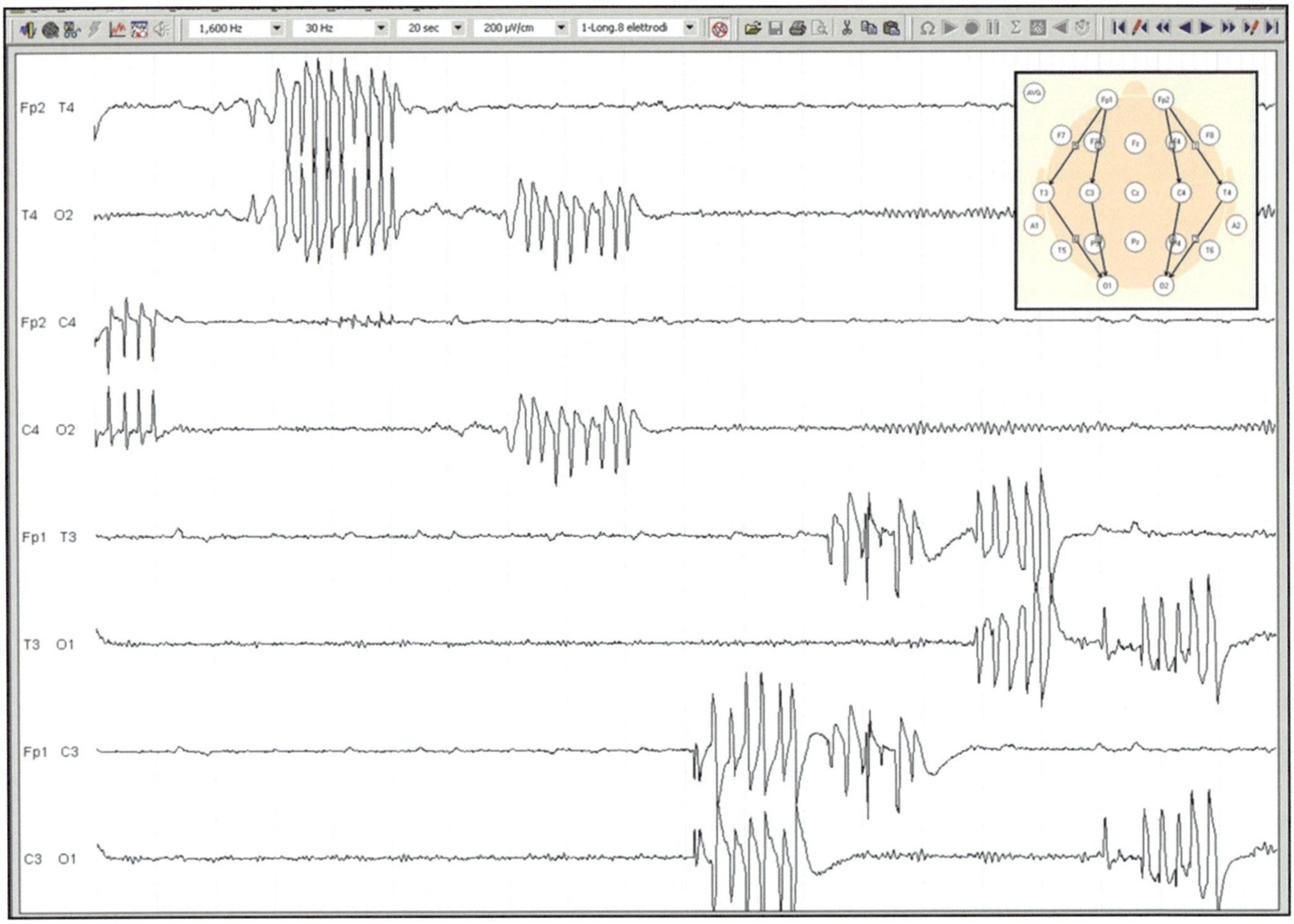

Fig. 8.14 Artifact due to the percussion on cup electrodes by technician, in order to check their correct positioning and connection

8.1.3.2 Telephone Artifact

When the artifact is due to the ringing of a landline telephone, positioned in the room where the EEG is recorded, it appears on the trace as sequences of rapid rhythms, present on one or more channels (Fig. 8.18a). In this case, the electromagnetic signal generated by the device and by the oscillating circuit that underlies the telephone ring is captured. The artifact will therefore be particularly evident in the presence of old telephones with electromechanical bells. To avoid this, it is necessary to disconnect the telephone from the power socket or lift the handset (reducing the volume of the ring does not eliminate the artifact). Even mobile phones may cause artifacts, which usually occur in the form of widespread discharges of sharply countered graphoelements (Fig. 8.18b, c). This artifact is always electromagnetic, but it appears before the phone rings, when the device is connecting to the net to send or to receive a call. To avoid this, it is advisable to turn off any mobile phone during the recording.

8.1.3.3 Switch Artifacts

The switching on/off of electrically powered equipments determines the appearance of rapid spikes or of sharply countered and slow high-voltage graphoelements on one or more EEG channels (Fig. 8.19). To avoid these artifacts, it is first necessary to ensure that the electrical system of the environment in which the recording takes place is in accordance with the law. It is then necessary to identify the artifact source and, in special cases, to disable the responsible devices.

8.1.3.4 Mechanical and Device-Related Artifacts

Mechanical Ventilation

In ICUs, it is very frequent to record a slow and/or sharp-countered artifact, synchronous with ventilation. This artifact is due to the thoracic expansion, which determines the movement of both the trunk and the head of the patient,

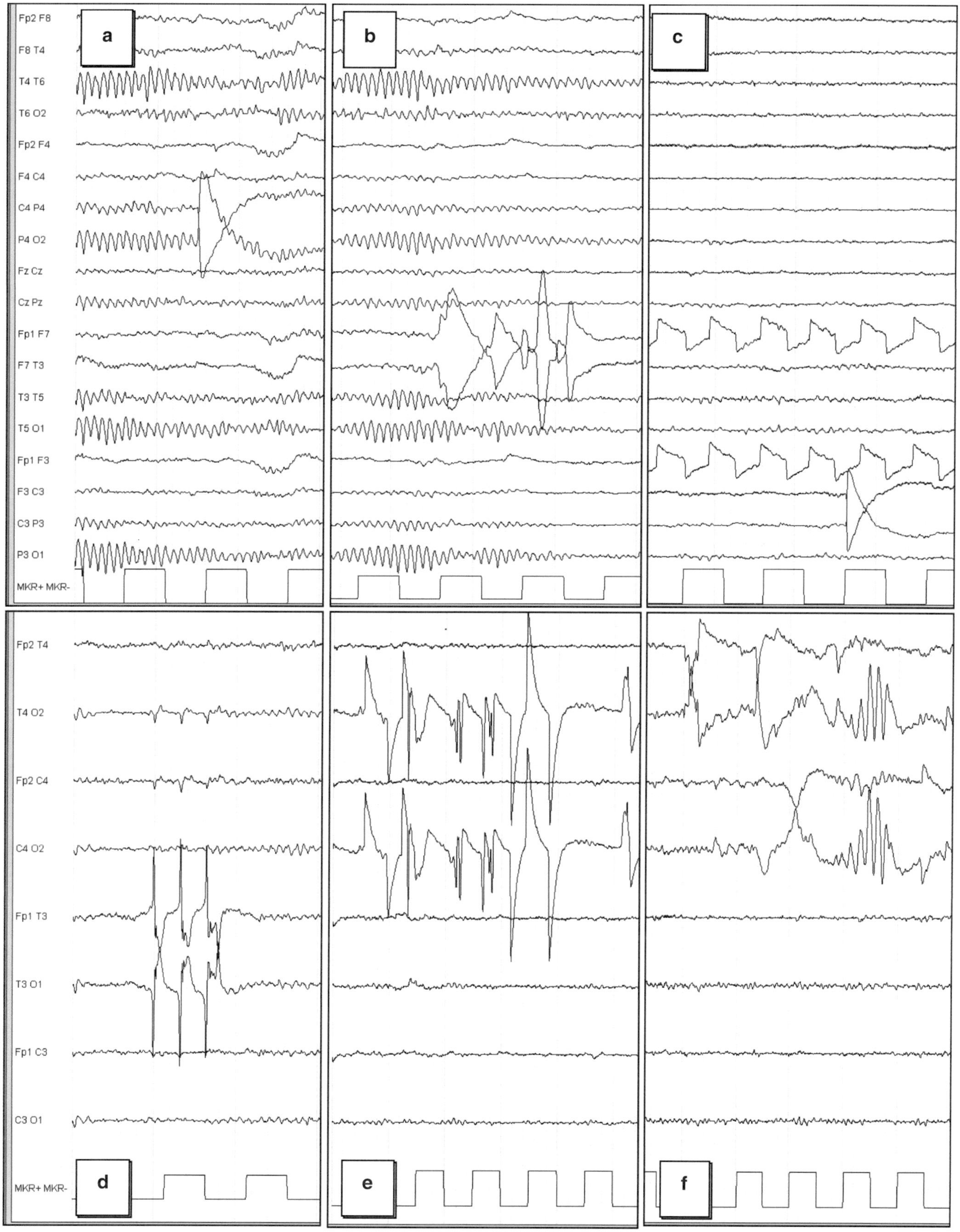

Fig. 8.15 Bad electrode-clamp-headbox contact artifacts. (**a**) Pop artifact on P4; (**b**) clamp artifact on F7; (**c**) clamp artifact on Fp1; (**d–f**) clamp and headbox contact artifact on T3, O_2, T4-O_2

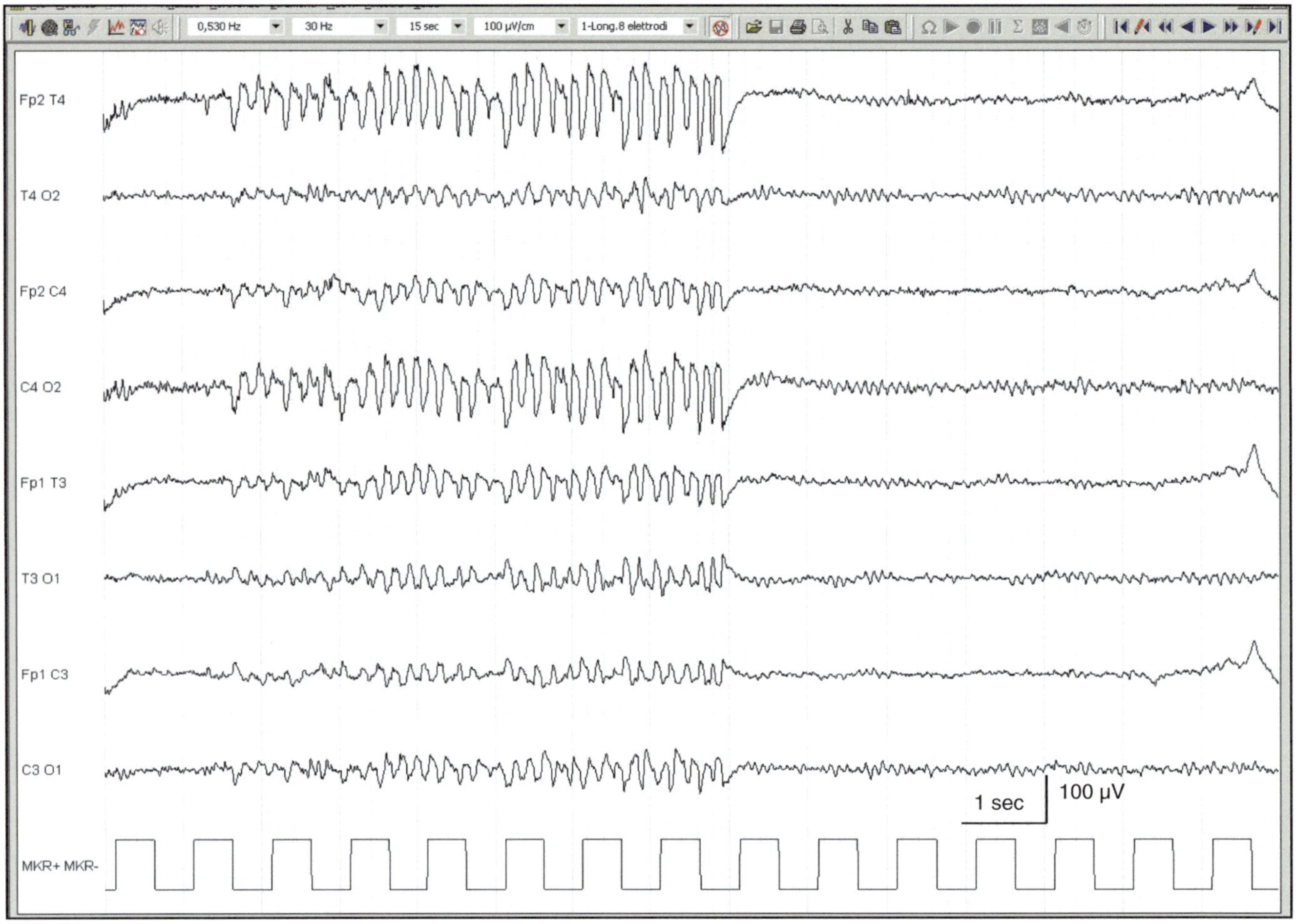

Fig. 8.16 Rhythmic wire oscillation artifact

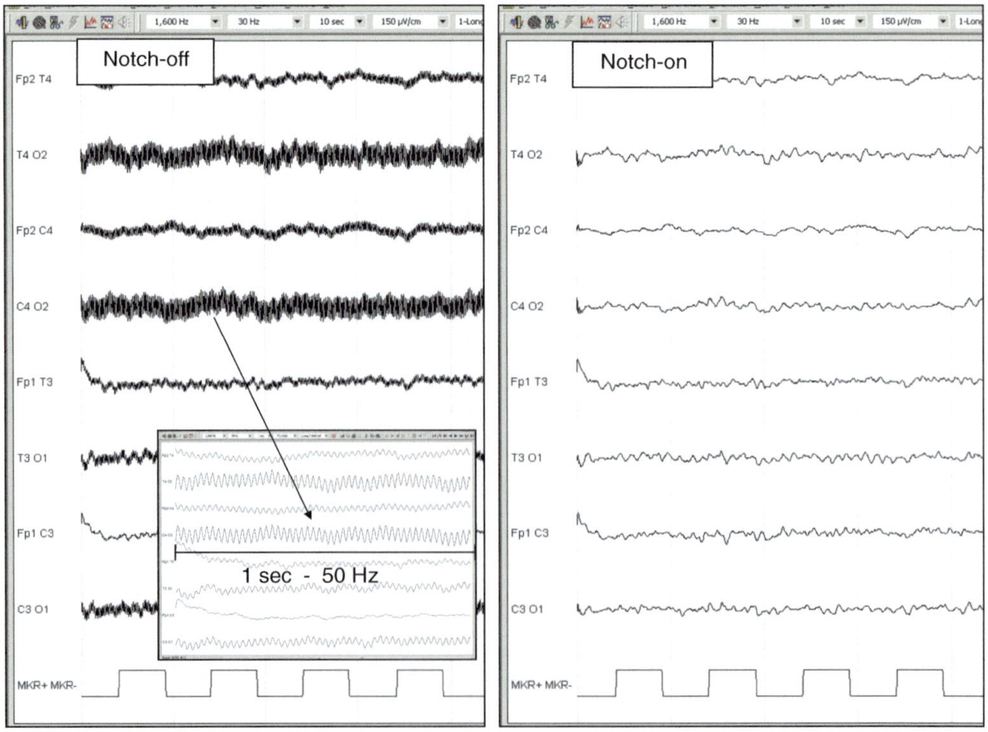

Fig. 8.17 EEG recording in ICU: without the notch filter, alternating current artifact (50 Hz) makes bioectrical brain activity not evaluable (on the left). Notch filter removing the 50 Hz frequencies allows the correct EEG visualization (on the right)

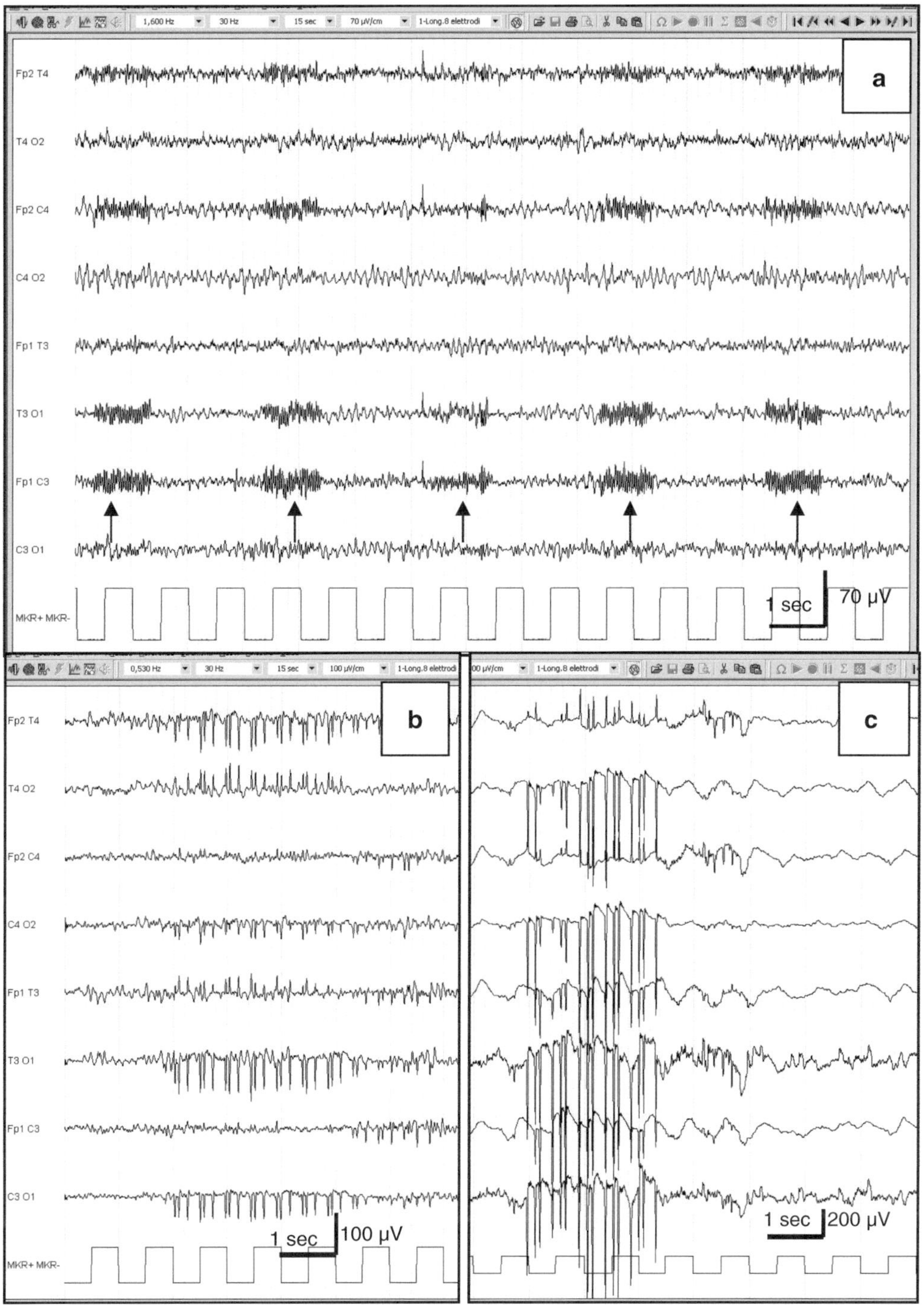

Fig. 8.18 (**a**) Landline phone ring artifact. (**b**, **c**) Two examples of mobile phone artifacts

transmitting to the cables, usually laying right in contact with the ventilator tube. To be sure of the artifact source, it is sufficient to compare its rhythm with the frequency of the breathing acts. To remove this artifact, it is necessary to limit the movements of the body and the oscillations of the cables (trying to group them as much as possible and to avoid contact with the tubes) and to eventually request the interruption of the assisted ventilation for a few seconds.

Hemodialysis and Hemofiltration Devices

The activation of the "step-by-step" electric motors of peristaltic pumps present in the hemodialysis machine, connected to the patient under examination or to neighboring patients, determines an artifact characterized by continuous sequences of rhythmic spikes or sharply countered sinusoidal waves (generally at 5–7 Hz), on various channels (Fig. 8.20). This artifact often completely prevents the EEG recording and

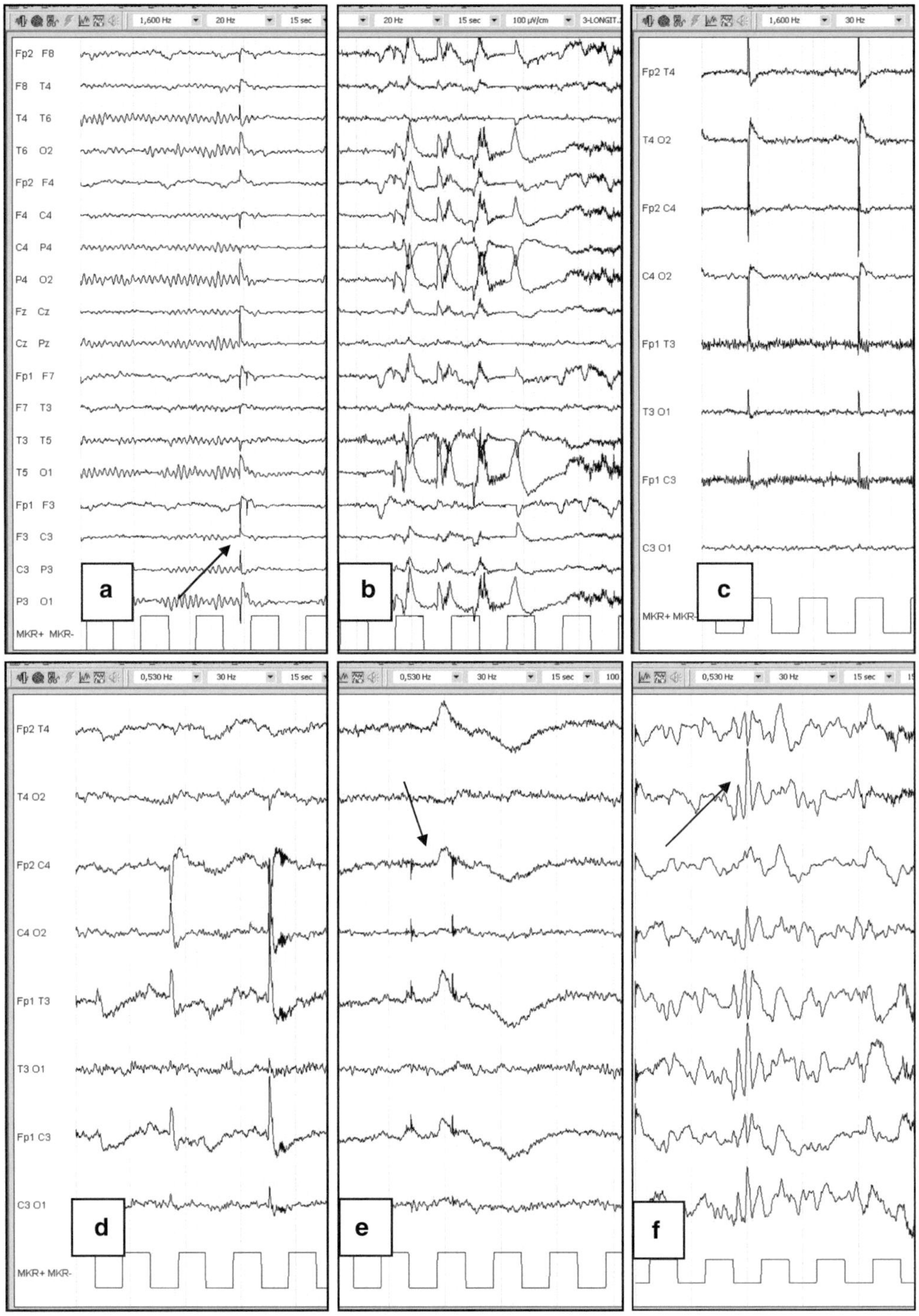

Fig. 8.19 Electrical interferences artifact: (**a**) turning on the light switch in the room; (**b**, **c**) neon lamp artifact; (**d**–**f**) different types of peristaltic pump artifact, recorded in ICU

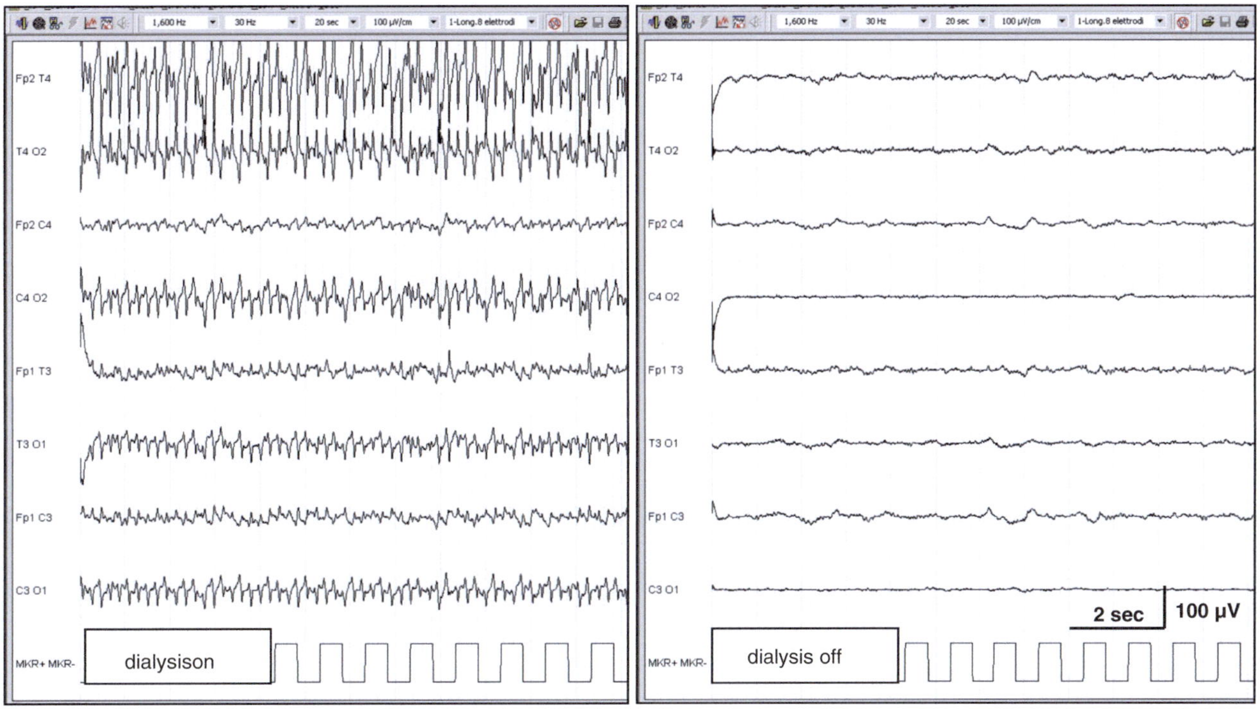

Fig. 8.20 Hemodialysis equipment artifact, disappearing after its deactivation

cannot be eliminated unless the hemodialysis machine is switched off. Extracorporeal oxygenation devices can also generate an irregular square-wave artifact that can be reduced moving the device away from the patient's head.

Electrosurgical Devices

During EEG monitoring in the operating room, widespread discharges of wide and rapid spikes induced by the use of electrosurgical devices are frequent. These artifacts interrupt the EEG visualization on all channels and often determine the flattening of the traces, for a short block in saturation of the amplifiers (Fig. 8.21). This type of artifact cannot be eliminated and, to avoid it, the recording should be interrupted before each electric scalpel is switched on. It is also necessary to make sure, from the manufacturer of the electroencephalograph, that the system is able to deal with such electric shocks without being damaged.

Swan-Ganz Catheter

The Swan-Ganz catheter, or pulmonary arterial catheter, is a device used for invasive monitoring of hemodynamic parameters, such as central venous pressure and pulmonary artery pressure. Its functioning is based on the use of a resistance, which heats the surrounding blood, and of sensors that evaluate the timing and the way of moving the heated blood. The catheter acts cyclically and intermittently, but not rhythmically. This type of artifact, recorded in the intensive care unit and in the surgery room, is presented in the form of a rapid, wide-ranging, apparently nonrhythmic artifact (Fig. 8.22a). If the trace is not displayed compactly (30–60 s/page), the repetitiveness of the artifactual cycle is often missed, due to the activation of the heater and, therefore, the cause of the artifact cannot be pinpointed. To eliminate the artifact, it is necessary to ask the anesthesiologist-resuscitator to deactivate the catheter for the time necessary to record the EEG.

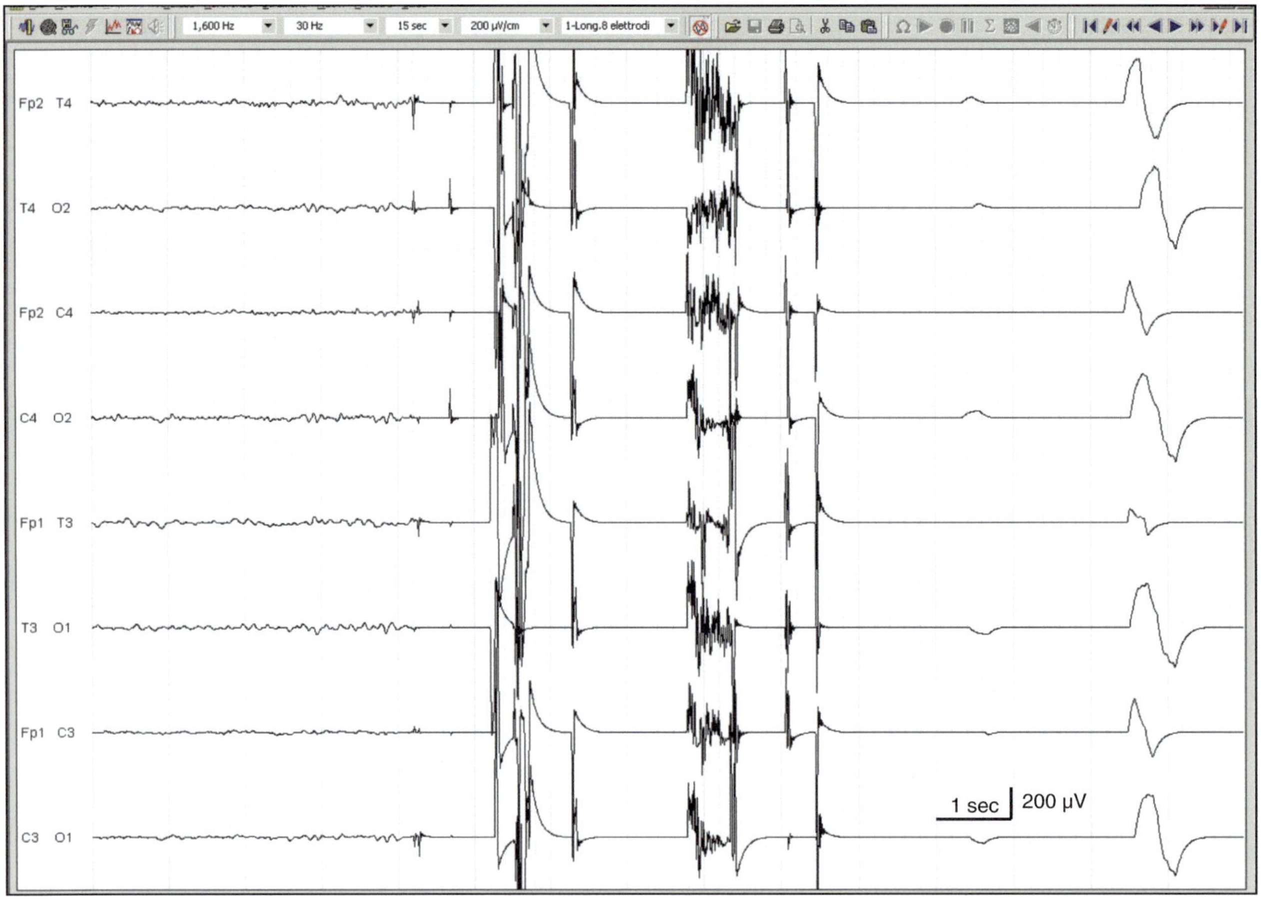

Fig. 8.21 Artifact by electric scalpel

External Cardiac Pacemaker Artifact

Sometimes, in the intensive care units it is possible to record an artifact from an external cardiac pacemaker, a type of pacemaker that is applied externally to the patient's chest through adhesive electrode pads (Fig. 8.22b). It is generally not possible to remove it, but the anesthesiologist can be asked to interrupt the stimulation for few seconds, monitoring the patient's vital functions.

Acknowledgment We wish to thank all our technicians (Liliana Barbagallo, Leonardo Davì, Daniela De Santis, Giuseppe Iannuzzi, Nicoletta Panella, Marco Tiribelli) and the neurophysiologist Patrizia Pulitano for their help in acquiring EEG artifacts samples.

Fig. 8.22 (**a**) Swan-Ganz catheter artifact; (**b**) external pacing artifact that disappears when it turns off

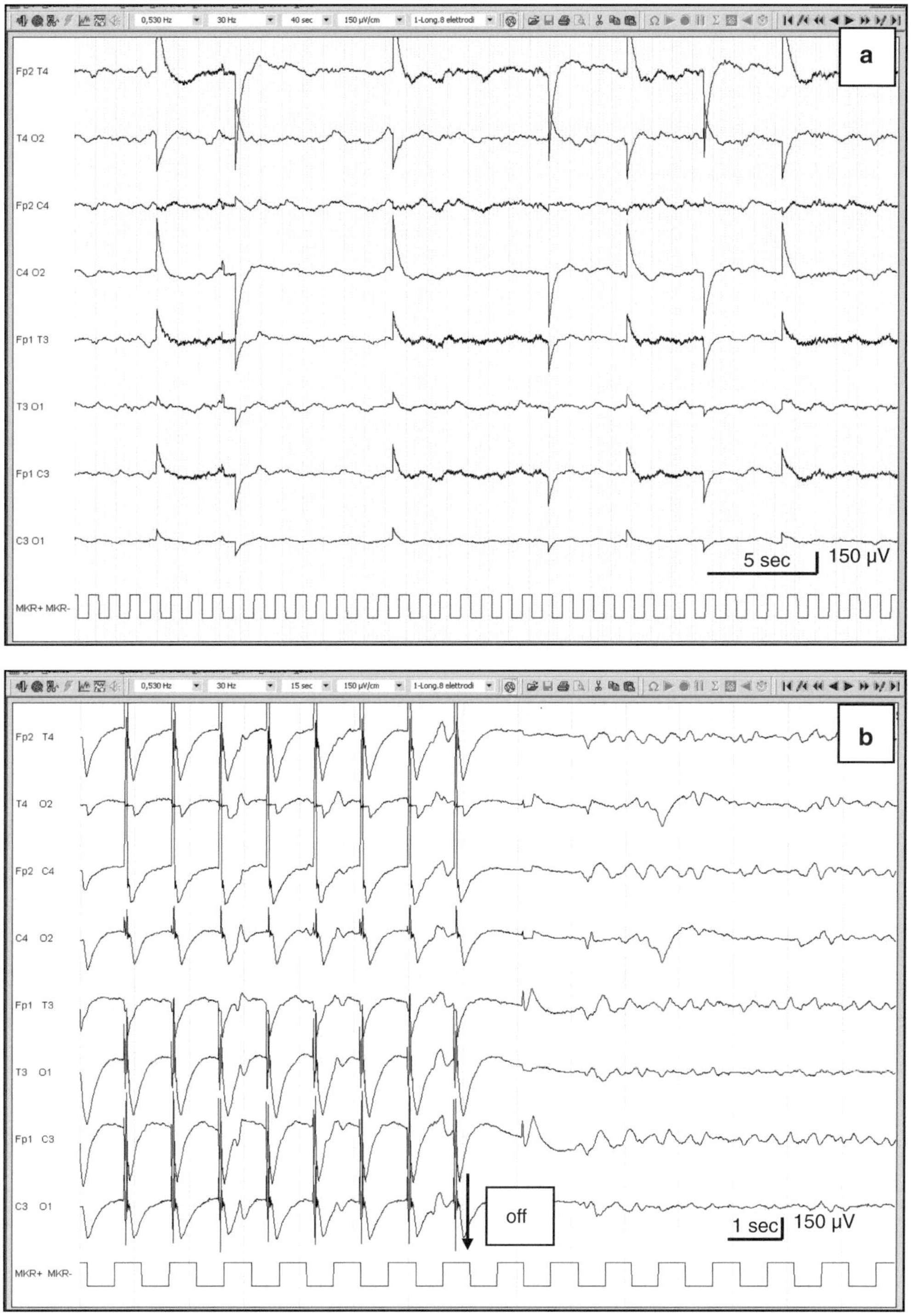

References

1. Urigüen JA, Garcia-Zapirain B. EEG artifact removal-state-of-the-art and guidelines. J Neural Eng. 2015;12:031001.
2. Libenson MH. Electroencephalographic artifacts. In: Libenson MHPractical approach to electroencephalography. 1st; Philadelphia, Saunders Elsevier, pp 124–145, 2010.
3. Iwasaki M, Kellinghaus C, Alexopoulos AV, et al. Effects of eyelid closure, blinks, and eye movements on the electroencephalogram. Clin Neurophysiol. 2005;116:878–85.
4. Tatum WO, Reinsberger C, Dworetzky BA. Artifacts of recording and common errors in interpretation. In: Shomer DL, Lopes da Silva FH, editors. Niedermeyers electroencephalography: basic principles, clinical applications and related fields. 7th ed. New York: Oxford University Press; 2018. p. 266–316.

Normal Awake Adult EEG

9

Oriano Mecarelli

9.1 General Characteristics of the EEG Signals

In order to properly describe the various components of an EEG recording and to subsequently determine whether it can be classified as normal or abnormal, the first step is the detailed recognition of the isolated or repeated EEG waveforms. The main features used to describe EEG signals are principally the wave shape (morphology), the voltage (amplitude), the frequency of repetition, the spatial distribution (localization), and the modality of appearance (rhythmicity, continuity, synchrony, symmetry). These EEG features vary with age, mental state, consciousness level and individual characteristics also in physiological conditions and, therefore, these factors have to be taken into account to define an EEG as normal or abnormal.

EEG waveforms can be defined as "slow" or "sharp/spiky" on the basis of their shape or morphology (Fig. 9.1a). Slow signals are represented by rounded waveforms with a long duration in milliseconds (ms). The duration of a signal is considered as the time between the beginning of the signal and the end of a single wave or a complex of waves.

If the shape of the slow signals is particularly regular, these are defined as "monomorphic"; on the other hand, if irregularities are observed on the rounded shape, these are called "polymorphic."

The "sharp" or "spiky" signals have a shorter duration in time. The spiky transients have various characteristics and they are pathological in relation to epileptic syndromes. However, certain sharp graphoelements can be observed also in healthy subjects, particularly in drowsiness and in sleep.

The morphology of an EEG signal is then described by the phase, which is defined from the point at which the signal leaves the isoelectric line to the point where it returns to the baseline. Depending on how many phases a signal presents, it will be classified as monophasic, biphasic, triphasic and polyphasic (Fig. 9.1b).

Transient or repeated EEG signals may occur apparently simultaneously in two or more locations of the one or both hemispheres: this EEG feature is described as *synchronous*. When there is a time difference between the appearance of signals in various channels, the EEG feature is - on the contrary - described as *asynchronous*. Sometimes, there is a short time difference between two or more deflections. However, since subtle asynchronies may also be of clinical relevance, asynchrony can be clearly demonstrated either by

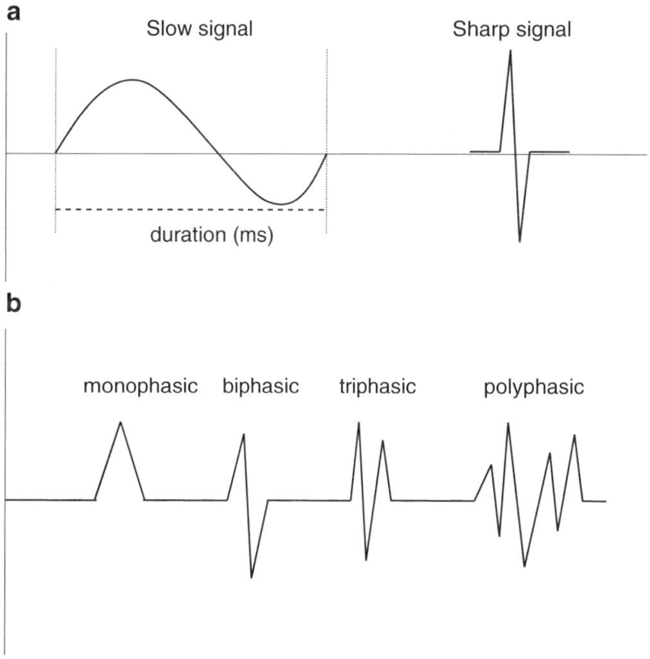

Fig. 9.1 Morphologic characteristics of EEG signals (**a**) Signal with slow or sharp shape. (**b**) Various types of signals, differentiating by their phases

O. Mecarelli (✉)
Department of Human Neurosciences, Sapienza University of Rome, Rome, Italy
e-mail: oriano.mecarelli@uniroma1.it

O. Mecarelli (ed.), *Clinical Electroencephalography*, https://doi.org/10.1007/978-3-030-04573-9_9

expanding the time scale or by using special measurement techniques.

The *amplitude* of an EEG signal (expressed in microvolts, μV) is also important for its characterization, from a morphological point of view. The amplitude of a wave is measured by evaluating the height of the wave, assessed in mm measured peak-to-peak, and multiplying it by the sensitivity of the amplifier, thus obtaining a value in μV/mm. The amplitude depends on various factors (i.e., location and derivation of electrodes) and the visual assessment of amplitude of EEG phenomenon in mm/μV can be very arbitrary. The exact measurement of the amplitude of an EEG signal should be performed using a special cursor at various epochs of the tracing, where the EEG phenomenon is clearly present.

When comparing the signals amplitude obtained in two or more channels of an hemisphere with those recorded from the same regions of the contralateral hemisphere, we must also describe the *symmetry/asymmetry* of the signals. An EEG transient - or rhythm - is symmetric when it has more or less the same amplitude in the two or more channels compared. On the contrary, an EEG phenomenon is asymmetric when its peak-to-peak amplitude is significantly lower - or higher - than that of the contralateral side.

Finally, an EEG phenomenon must be described according to the number of times that waveforms repeat themselves over a 1-s period. This characteristic is defined the *frequency* of the EEG signals and it is usually measured in Hertz (Hz). The frequency is the most important parameter for characterizing the ongoing EEG activities and the physiological rhythms.

Figure 9.2 schematically describes the amplitude and the frequency characteristics of different EEG signals repeating in form of rhythms.

A fundamental parameter for characterizing an EEG pattern is the recognition of its spatial representation in the scalp. For the spatial localization of EEG transients, it is fundamental to know the electrode positions and the derivations. An EEG signal is defined as *focal* when it is present on a single area of a cerebral hemisphere and as *multifocal* if it is present on different areas of a hemisphere or of both hemispheres, but asynchronously. The waveforms can be instead defined as *diffuse* or *generalized* when synchronous in all brain areas of both the hemispheres (Fig. 9.3).

Some rhythmic activities are characteristically located in specific regions of the scalp (alpha rhythm, mu rhythm, sleep spindles, etc.) and for the description it is important to define their localization, in addition to their frequency and symmetry.

A sporadic single EEG signal, clearly distinguished from the background activity, is defined as a *"transient"*. A stereotyped succession of two or more EEG signals represents instead a *"complex"*, that may be isolated or - more frequently - organized in sequences (ongoing activity). The EEG transient event and/or complexes are apparently spontaneous, or evoked by intrinsic or extrinsic stimuli. Both the

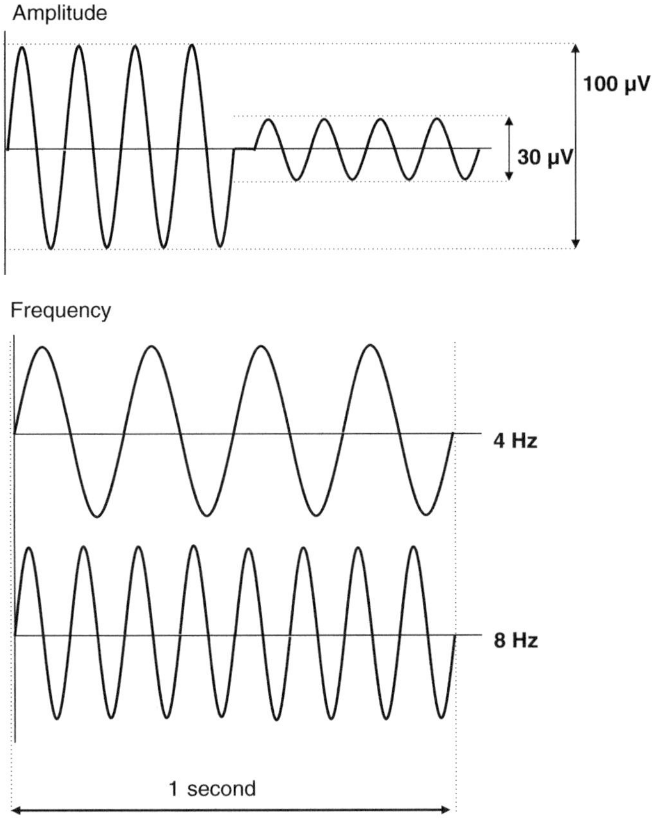

Fig. 9.2 Different amplitude and frequency of EEG rhythm

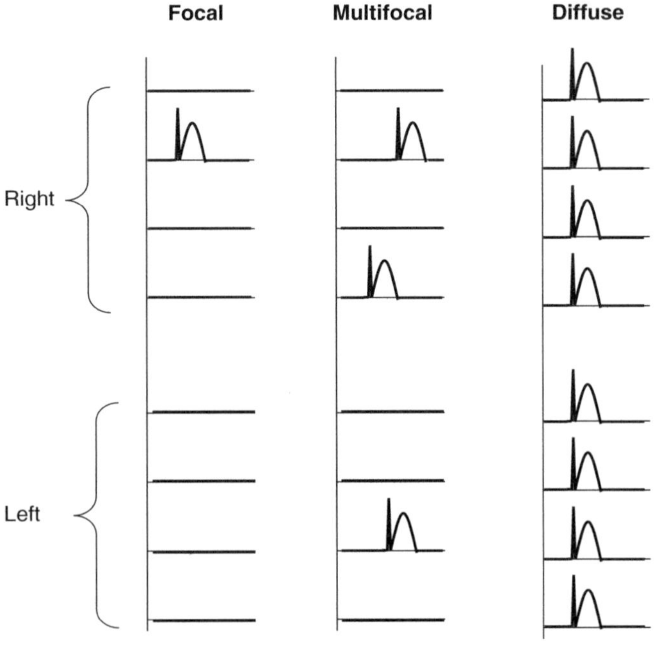

Fig. 9.3 Different localization of EEG signals on two cerebral hemispheres

transient signals and the complexes may have recurred over time at periodic or quasi-periodic intervals (*continuity*). These features are typical of many pathological EEG patterns and will then be described later.

9.2 EEG Frequencies

The wide spectrum of EEG frequencies are grouped in bands and historically named using the Greek letters. EEG activity recorded at the scalp with routine EEG instruments usually exclude the frequencies below 0.5–0.3 Hz and normally do not exceed 30 Hz. The classical frequency bands of EEG are defined as follows (Fig. 9.4):

- Delta (δ): 0.1 to <4 Hz
- Theta (θ): 4 to <8 Hz
- Alpha (α): 8 to <13 Hz
- Beta (β): > 13–30 Hz

The *delta band* was first described by Walter in 1936 [1] as an EEG marker for cerebral tumors and it includes the slowest EEG frequencies (<4 Hz); these can often be confused on visual inspection with artifactual oscillations and then improperly "cutted" by technicians with high-pass filters. The visual analysis of the physiological awake adult EEG is not always able to highlight the effective amount of the delta component which is masked by the other frequencies, or represents electrical artifacts. The quantitative frequency analysis of EEG tracings usually shows, also in adults, the presence of an appreciable amount of delta power. Currently, however, there is great interest in ultraslow components (0–0.3 Hz) which are termed Direct Current (DC) potentials and represent shifts of the baseline. The identification and characterization of ultraslow activity play no significant role in the clinical EEG, but they have a great interest in various experimental fields (e.g., for the study of immature cortical activity, the identification of epileptogenic zone, the

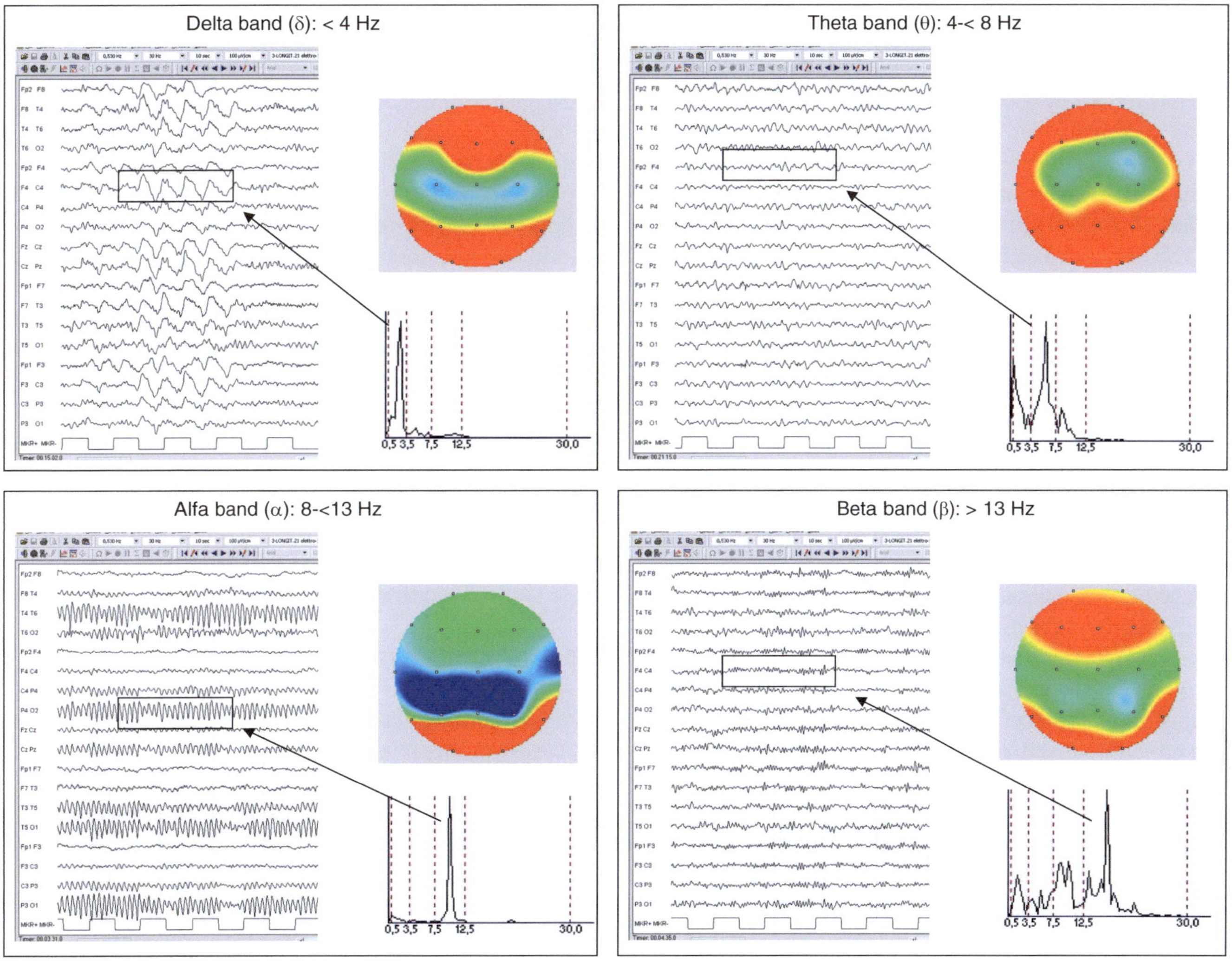

Fig. 9.4 Qualitative and spectral representation of the main EEG frequency bands

relation with cortical spreading depression in migraine attacks, etc.) [2].

The *theta band* (4.0 to <8.0 Hz) should be divided into theta 1 (theta slower: 4.0 to <6.0 Hz) and theta 2 (theta faster: >6.0 to <8.0 Hz). Even the term "theta band" was first introduced by Walter, in 1944 [3], associated with the presence of thalamic tumors (he had chosen *theta* to stand for *thalamus* because he presumed these waves had a thalamic origin). In normal adult subjects, the theta band is poorly represented but its incidence is variable, dependent on age, individual characteristics, level of vigilance, etc. The appearance of anterior theta activity in adults can be facilitated by a particular emotional states or mental processes of problem-solving. Furthermore, when a gradual disappearance of the alpha rhythm substituted by theta activity is observed in an EEG tracing of an awake adult, this means that the subject is sleepy. Sometimes, it is difficult to attribute a physiological or pathological significance to theta activity registered in an awake adult and the decision can only be facilitated by careful assessment of the specific situation.

The *alpha band* (8.0 to <13 Hz) is proper for an EEG tracing registered in adults during quiet wakefulness with eyes closed. The term *alpha* was introduced by Berger in 1929 [4] and this frequency band is characteristic of the physiological alpha rhythm that will be described subsequently in detail.

Even within this frequency band, we can distinguish slow alpha (8.0–9.0 Hz), intermediate alpha (9.0–11 Hz) and fast alpha (11 to <13 Hz).

The *beta band* includes the frequencies between 13 and 30 Hz; it was first named by Berger [4]. In the experimental psychophysiologic literature, this frequency band is divided into beta 1 (13 to <20 Hz) and beta 2 (>20 to 30 Hz). A beta activity of low amplitude (<30 μV) is normally recorded over the fronto-centro-temporal regions in awake EEG of normal adults. It is sometimes more appreciable with open eyes or mental activity because, with closed eyes, it is masked by the much higher amplitude and synchronization of the alpha rhythm. The beta activity is related to mental and cognitive processes of various types, anxiety and state of alert; it is also induced or increased by drowsiness and light sleep. Furthermore, numerous drugs (barbiturates, benzodiazepines, neuroleptics, antihistamines, amphetamines, cocaine, etc.) are potent beta-activators. During the recording of a routine EEG, the anterior beta activity arising from the brain can be confused with electrical activity generate by the muscles ("muscle artifact") and, therefore, suppressed by the technician with specific filters.

Currently, there is a great scientific interest in more rapid EEG frequency bands that are not detectable during the recording of a traditional EEG, but can be recorded with modern digital equipments. The frequencies above the beta band are traditionally defined *gamma band* (γ, 30–80 Hz). Successively, Curio [5] has been proposed by the following designations for the ultrafast activity: omega band (ω, 80–120 Hz), rho band (ρ, 120–500 Hz), and sigma band (σ, 500–1000 Hz). In epilepsy, experimental studies over the past decade have focused particularly on interictal High-Frequency Oscillations (HFOs) >80 Hz that seems to be promising new biomarkers in epilesy. HFOs are defined as spontaneous EEG events consisting of at least four oscillations (*ripples*) that clearly stand out from the background activity. HFOs are subdivided into *ripples* (80 to 250 Hz), *fast ripples* (250–500 Hz), and *ultrafast ripples* (>500 Hz). The ripples can be recorded by MagnetoElectroencephaloGraphy (MEG) and EEG with automatic detection methods, whereas fast and ultrafast ripples can be recorded only with intracranial EEG methods. The principal clinical application of HFOs was in the context of epilepsy surgery, followed by the assessment of epilepsy severity and monitoring of drugs response [6, 7]. Several artifacts, due to muscle contractions, movements or bad electrode contacts, should be distinguished from epileptic HFOs. The HFOs appear also to be correlated with both cognitive and perceptual-motor processes.

Including the ultraslow and ultrafast frequencies, recordable EEG frequencies with the current technology can be classified as shown in Table 9.1.

Table 9.1 Frequency EEG bands

Hz	EEG bands
0–0.3	Ultraslow
0.3 to <4	Delta—δ
4 to <8	Theta—θ
8 to <13	Alpha—α
13 to <30	Beta—β
30 to <80	Gamma—γ
	HFOs
80–250 Hz	Ripples
250–500 Hz	Fast ripples
>500–1000 Hz	Ultrafast ripples

9.3 The Physiological Rhythms and Normal Graphoelements

9.3.1 Alpha Rhythm

First described by Berger in 1929 [4, 8], the *alpha rhythm* (or *posterior dominant rhythm*) is the hallmark of the awake EEG in older children and adults, with eyes closed or visually inattentive and during the psychosensorial relaxed condition [9]. The alpha rhythm has a typical location in the posterior head regions; in some subjects, the alpha rhythm is strictly confined to the occipital areas, but in others it also spreads forward to all the posterior quadrants (posterior temporal, parietal, and occipital regions). Sometimes, the posterior rhythm may even spread to the central and frontal

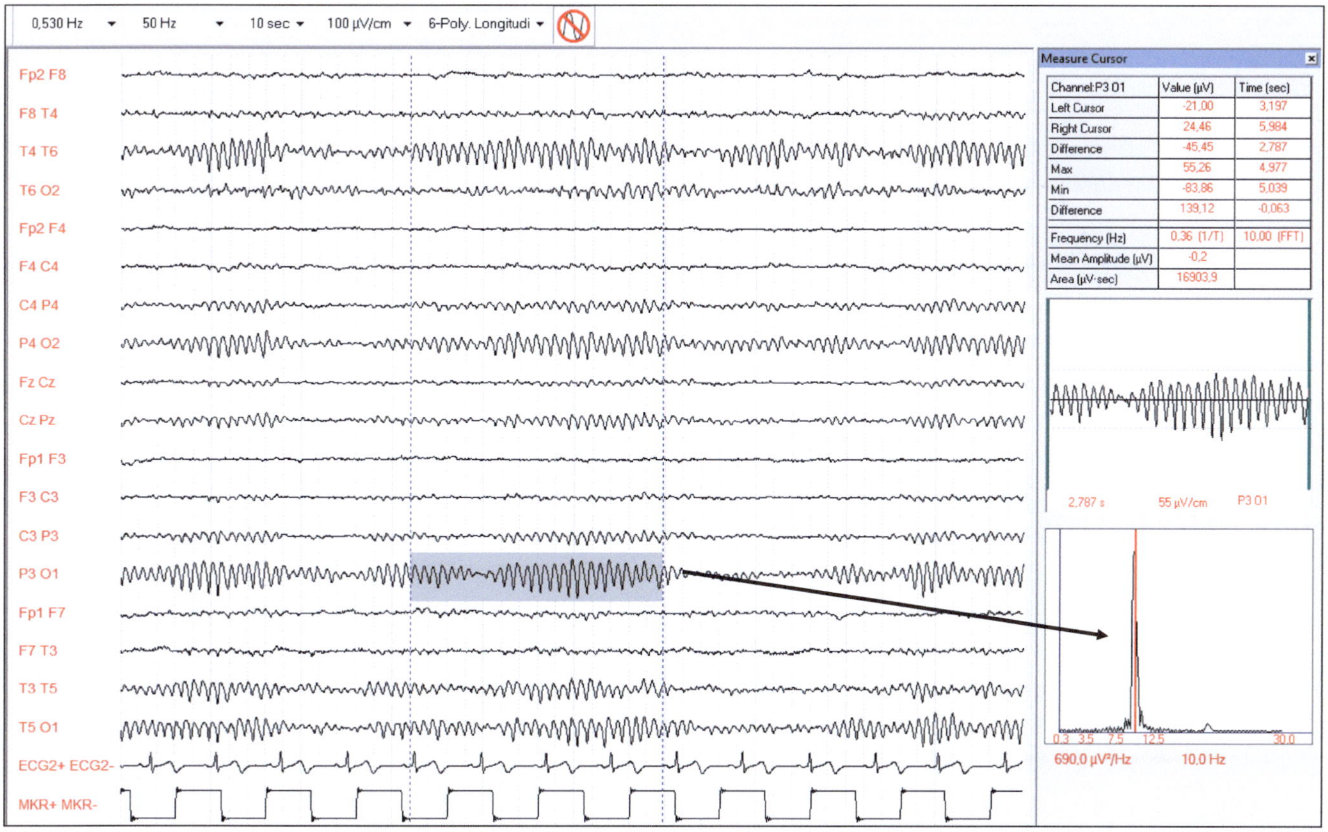

Fig. 9.5 An example of alpha rhythm in an awake adult subject with eyes closed. The tract delimited by the dotted lines shows a background alpha rhythm with a frequency of 10 Hz and with a peak of amplitude of 55 µV/cm. Alpha rhythm is typically visible on the posterior regions with a regular and sinusoidal morphology

areas (F4 and F3 electrodes), mainly in aged subjects or during drowsiness (Figs. 9.5 and 9.6).

Even the subjects blind from birth have an alpha rhythm localized in parieto-occipital areas, but the rhythm has a significant reduction of power in the blind when compared to the normally-sighted controls [10]. The morphology of alpha rhythm is mostly regular (monomorphic rhythm) with sinusoidal or fusiform shape (increase and gradual decrease in amplitude, "waxing and waning"; peaks and troughs of the waveform rounded and regular). Rarely, the alpha rhythm has a sharpened morphology ("spiky alpha," with the negative sharp component of wave and the positive rounded component) and it is considered a normal variant, especially in older children and in young adults.

The alpha rhythm has a frequency within the range of alpha band (8 to <13 Hz), generally ranging from 9 to 11 Hz in adults. The frequency is usually the same in both hemispheres but, in the same individual, it may vary in terms of 1 or even 2 Hz. Some frequency variations of the alpha rhythm may be dependent on menstrual cycle (acceleration of alpha frequency in the premenstrual phase with reduction of its amount) [11] or be related to body temperature (higher frequencies during temperature increase) [12, 13].

Recently, it has been demonstrated that the posterior alpha rhythm is significantly slower in adult patients in the wake periods of sleep recordings (before and after sleep), compared to standard wake recordings [14].

Brief faster than baseline alpha rhythm sequences can also be recorded immediately after eyes closing (squeak phenomenon) (Fig. 9.7) [15].

Sometimes, the normal sequences of alpha rhythm are substituted by slower or faster frequencies (slow or fast alpha variants) [9, 16]. The term "slow alpha variant" is referred to the appearance of a subharmonic of the fundamental rhythm (with a ratio of 1:2 or 1:3; if, e.g., the alpha rhythm has a frequency of 12 Hz, its slow variants will have a frequency of 6 or 4 Hz, respectively) (Fig. 9.8) [17].

The alpha slow variants have the same topography and reactivity as the fundamental rhythm, but they can also be unilateral or asymmetric. More rarely, the appearance of fast variants of alpha can also be observed (16–20 Hz), for the most part endowed with alpha activity and with the same topography and reactivity. The fast variants can be activated by Intermittent Photic Stimulation (IPS) and induced by benzodiazepines.

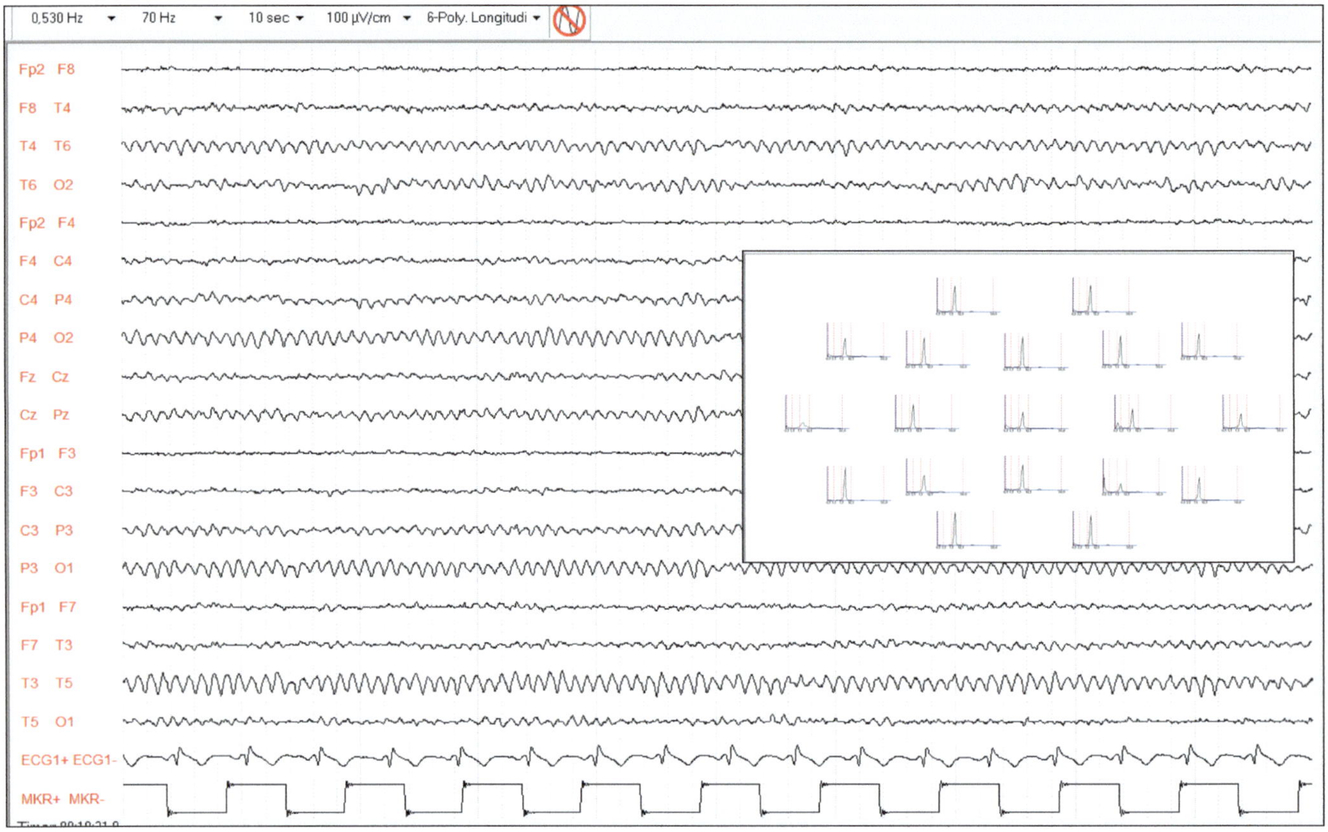

Fig. 9.6 An example of alpha rhythm recorded in a normal 57-year-old subject with eyes closed, during drowsiness. Alpha activity spreads from the posterior regions to the central and frontal areas, as demonstrated by the spectrograms

The amplitude of posterior alpha rhythm in most adults is less than 50 µV. In order to be able to measure the amplitude in an objective manner, a digital measurement cursor must be used, checking the amplitude values randomly at various points in the tracing and then calculating a mean value. This procedure is difficult to implement during a routine EEG inspection and, therefore, visual assessment of the alpha activity amplitude can be very arbitrary; it is then preferable to make subjective quantification of the amplitude in terms of low, medium, and high. Usually, the amplitude of posterior alpha rhythm is asymmetrical on the two hemispheres, with a lower voltage in the dominant hemisphere (the left in right-handed individuals and the right in the left-handed) [18]. However, the difference in the posterior alpha rhythm amplitude between the two hemispheres usually does not exceed 20%. An asymmetry of posterior alpha rhythm is considered to be abnormal when, in the non-dominant hemisphere, its amplitude is more than threefold greater than that of the dominant hemisphere. On the other hand, when the voltage of the alpha rhythm is higher in the dominant hemisphere, the difference is considered abnormal if the amplitude is twofold higher, compared to contralateral side. Differences of amplitude less than 50% are not, however, considered to be pathological (Fig. 9.9).

The reason why the amplitude of the alpha rhythm is higher in the posterior regions of the non-dominant hemisphere is not actually well known. To explain this phenomenon, we still refer to the theory that the cortical EEG signals are always of higher amplitude in brain areas that are not too much involved in mental processes [18]. However, it is probable that the mild interhemispheric asymmetry of the alpha rhythm does not depend on hemispheric dominance, but is to be related to differences in skull thickness [19].

There are also normal EEG tracings in which the alpha activity is poorly appreciable (low amplitude or desynchronized tracings). In these cases, the desynchronization of background activity is often correlated to the state of anxiety for the examination or due to the characteristic of the subject, or it is dependent on the non-relaxing registration environment (Fig. 9.10) [16].

In addition to the frequency, the localization and the amplitude, the other fundamental characteristic of the posterior alpha rhythm is its peculiar reactivity. This physiological posterior rhythm, very well synchronized with closed eyes and in a relaxed state of wakefulness, suppresses dramatically when the eyes are opened and/or during heightened mental activity (such as arithmetic calculation), somatosensory stimuli, etc. This phenomenon is called the "blocking

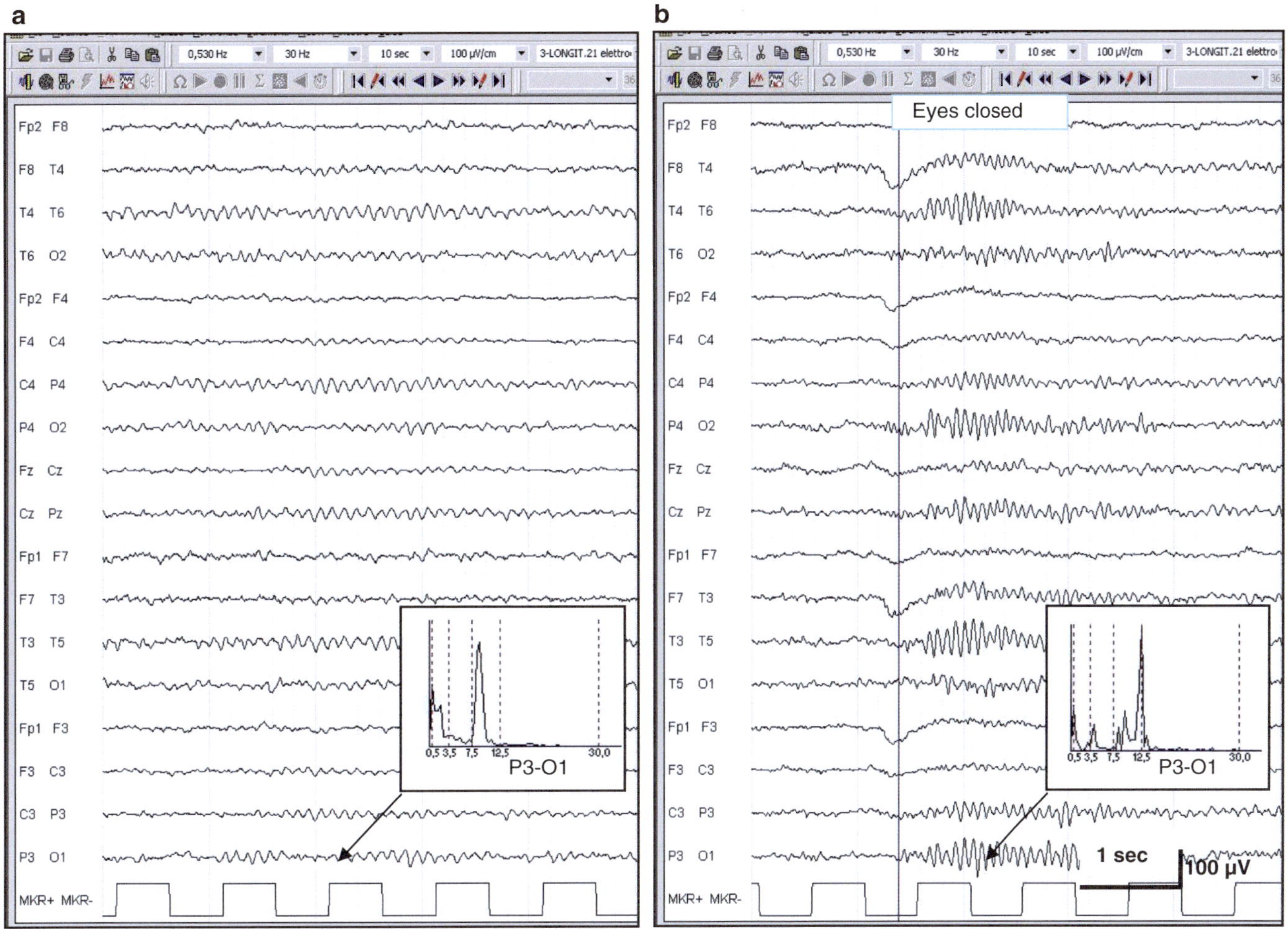

Fig. 9.7 (**a**) Sequences of alpha rhythm at 8–9 Hz, recorded during baseline with eyes closed; (**b**) in the same subject, a brief faster sequence of alpha rhythm at 10.5–11 Hz, immediately after eyes closure (squeak phenomenon)

arrest of alpha," discovered in his first report by Berger [4]: during EEG recording with eyes closed it is usually observed in the synchronized alpha rhythm that disappears immediately as the technician asks the subject to open his eyes or to perform specific mental tasks. However, it must be emphasized that sensory stimulation and mental activity block the alpha rhythm in less pronouncedly than the opening of the eyes [20]. Sometimes, blocking reactivity is only partial and with open eyes an alpha rhythm, poorly modulated, persists (Fig. 9.11).

On the other hand, the blocking reactivity of alpha rhythm is defined as "paradoxical" when, in subjects with eyes closed, a background activity of theta frequency, often related to drowsiness, prevails; the command to open eyes determines, as awakening reaction, the reappearance of alpha rhythm absent before.

9.3.1.1 Genesis of the Alpha Rhythm

The majority of authors who have studied the genesis of the alpha rhythm have established that it is a rhythm of cortical origin, but with an important thalamic influence. Bishop, in 1936, first proposed the concept of corticothalamic reverberating circuits, a concept that was later reaffirmed by many others [21]. Andersen and Andersson, in 1968, [22] proposed the theory of the *thalamic pacemaker*, based on similarities between human alpha activity and experimental spindle activity induced in animals by barbiturates. According to this theory, the alpha rhythm is generated on the basis of rhythmic inputs that originate from the thalamic centers. These inputs, through specific thalamocortical fibers, activate the upper cortical centers, inducing their synchronization. This type of thalamocortical excitation would also involve the activation of inhibitory interneurons, acting only at the level of the thalamic circuits. Therefore, according to this theory, an alternation of excitation/inhibition is then determined in the thalamus, which would be at the basis of the synchronization and the rhythmicity of the cortical activity.

In recent decades, the genesis of the alpha rhythm has not been further clarified and demonstrated. From both clinical and experimental data, it can be assumed that cortical alpha rhythm is the result of cortico-cortical and thala-

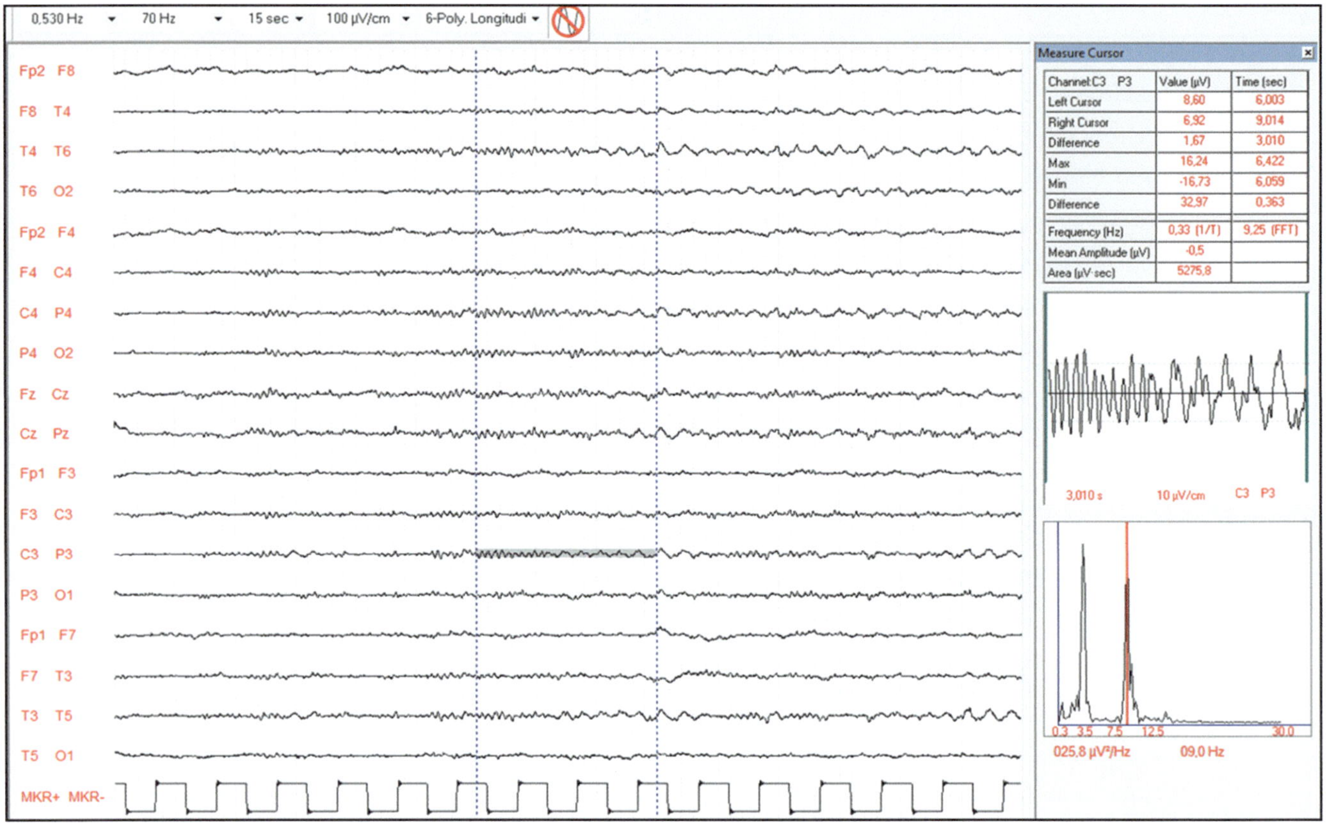

Fig. 9.8 A combination of posterior alpha rhythm at 9 Hz and its subharmonic at 3 Hz (slow alpha variant)

mocortical systems, interacting with each other in very complex way [23].

The neurophysiological mechanisms underlying the reactivity of the alpha rhythm (i.e., the blocking of alpha with eyes open or during mental activities) are also not well elucidated, but it is supposed that, in the desynchronization of the tracing, a fundamental role of the ponto-mesencephalic reticular formation, through its activating action toward the cerebral cortex, is involved.

9.3.2 Mu Rhythm (μ)

Described for the first time by Gastaut in 1952 [24], the mu rhythm (also known by discouraged terms such as rhythm en arceau, comb rhythm, rolandic rhythm, wicket rhythm and somatosensory alpha rhythm) [9, 18] is characterized by brief and/or prolonged rhythmic sequences of waves with the frequency similar to that of an alpha posterior rhythm, but with a different location and reactivity. The most typical frequency of the mu rhythm fluctuates from 7 to 11 Hz and it is often mixed with beta activity. This rhythm is typically observed in wakefulness, but it can also be observed in stages N1, N2, and R of sleep. The amplitude of the mu rhythm is generally less than 50 μV (usually lower than the amplitude of the alpha rhythm) and its maximum spatial representation is in the central regions of scalp (below the C4, C3, and Cz electrodes). The waves which constitute the mu rhythm are arciform (with sharpened negative phase and rounded positive phase) and they appear either at eyes opened or closed, in subjects with motor inactivity (Fig. 9.12) [12].

The prevalence of the mu rhythm reported in the literature during the registration of EEGs in healthy subjects or patients is very variable with values of 10–20% in young adults and with a lower incidence in children and the elderly. Probably, the prevalence of mu rhythm is higher; as a matter of fact, during closed-eye recordings, the mu rhythm can be confused with the alpha rhythm transmitted into the central regions. In addition, during routine EEG recordings, the traits of tracings performed at eyes open are very short and, therefore, the mu rhythm may not be highlighted. With more sophisticated quantitative EEG analysis, the mu rhythm in almost all healthy adult subjects may be highlighted [12, 18, 19].

The mu rhythm may be unilateral or bilateral, asynchronous and/or asymmetrical in the two hemispheres, with no particular correlation with the hemispheric dominance. Isolated reports have suggested that a unilateral mu rhythm can be associated with a structural ipsilateral cortical lesion, even in the absence of additional EEG abnormalities [25].

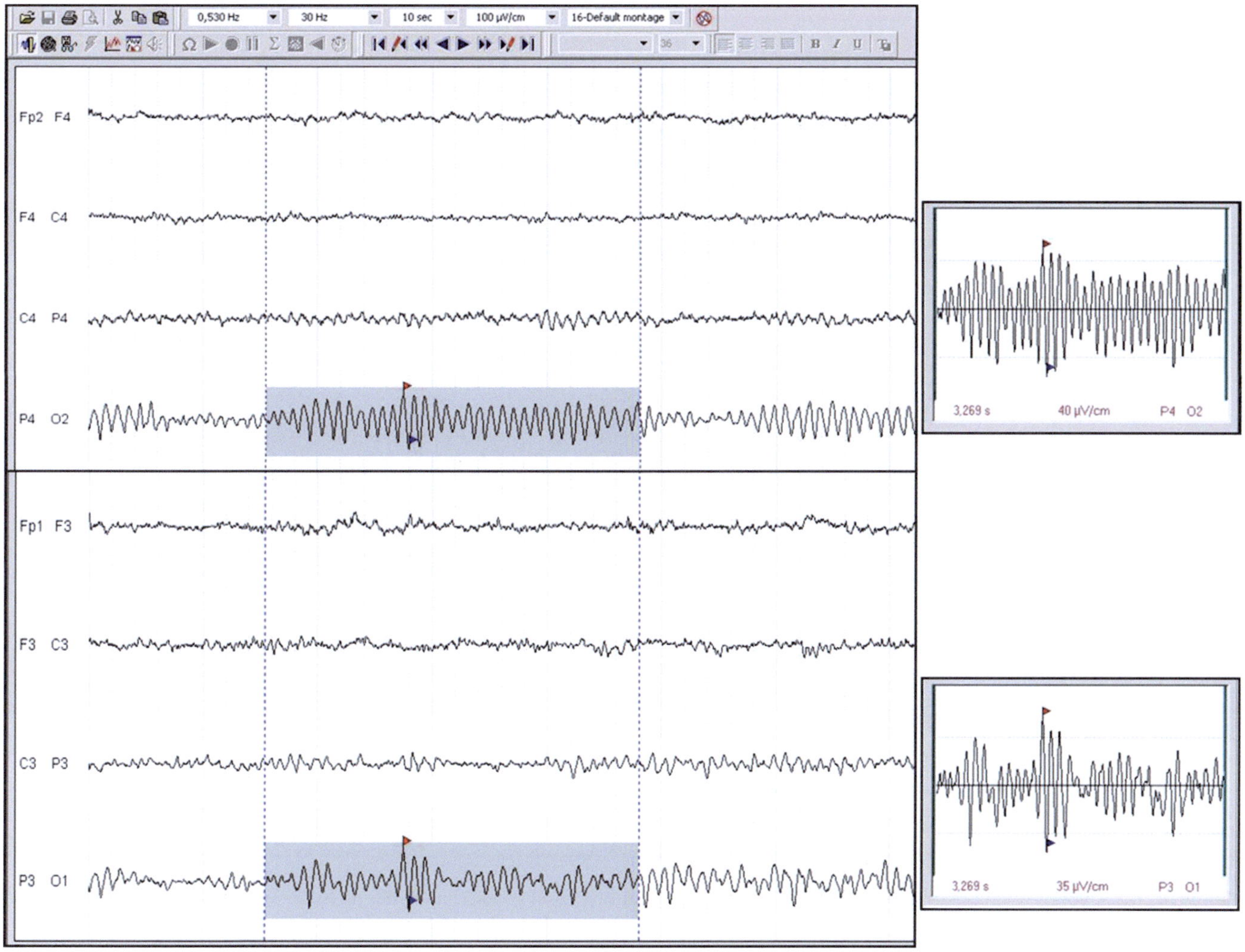

Fig. 9.9 Normal asymmetry (left < right) of the posterior alpha rhythm in a right handed subject.

The most important peculiarity of the mu rhythm is its reactivity. The mu rhythm is indeed blocked by movements (active, passive, or reflex), by the tactile stimulation of body areas, or even by mental movement planning. If the mu rhythm is well evident only from one side, the best manoeuver to visualize its reactivity is to ask the subject to tighten the contralateral hand or think about performing this action (Fig. 9.13).

The proof that thinking to perform a movement is sufficient to block the mu rhythm is shown by the fact that the rhythm stops a few millisecond before the beginning of the voluntary movement itself [26]. In addition, even subjects with an amputated limb show this reactivity of the contralateral mu rhythm after thinking about the execution of the movement in the phantom limb [27].

Finally, it was noted that the mu rhythm is enhanced or sometimes facilitated by Intermittent Photic Stimulation (IPS) and pattern vision, validating the idea that, for this rhythm, the integration of sensory and visual function is relevant [12].

The mu rhythm in the scalp central areas was correlated with the beta activity (around 20 Hz) described in the motor cortex in patients during electrocorticographic recording. Also this activity could be blocked by contralateral movement or with thinking about the execution of movement [28].

Although the mu rhythm is present in a high percentage of healthy subjects and it represents a physiological normal EEG pattern, in the past it has often been attributed to a pathological significance, or interpreted as a "borderline pattern."

One of the historical theories on the genesis of the mu rhythm was in fact that it was an expression of hyperexcitability of the rolandic cortex.

More recent studies have instead proposed to interpret the mu rhythm as an important information processing function that connects the perception with the action; specifically, it would be the expression of the processes involved in the transformation of "seeing" and "hearing" into "doing." [29]

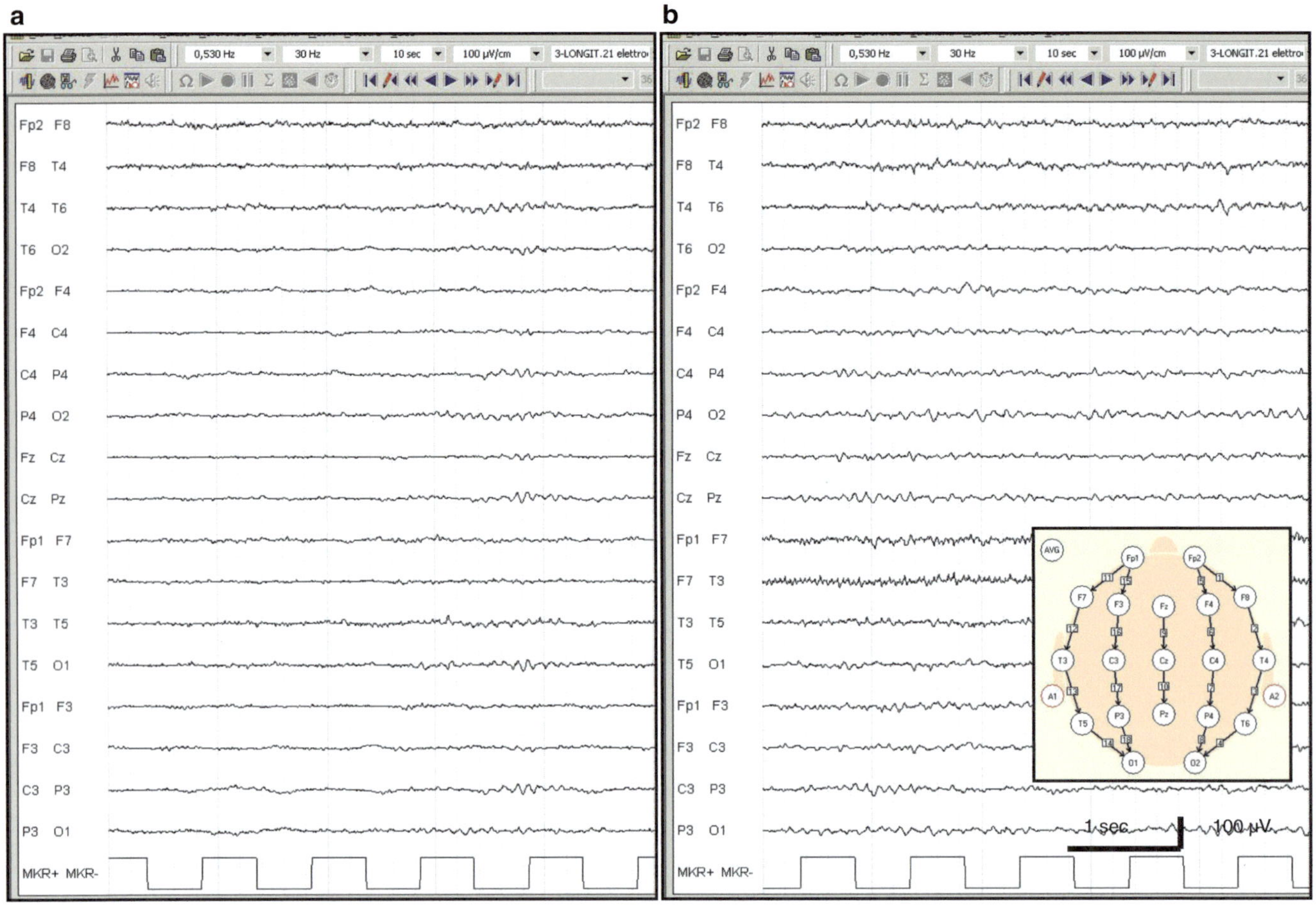

Fig. 9.10 (**a**) A poorly appreciable alpha rhythm in an adult subject during basal condition; (**b**) during hyperventilation alpha activity appears better synchronized

Table 9.2 and Fig. 9.14 summarize and compare the fundamental characteristics of the alpha rhythm and the mu rhythm.

9.3.3 Breach Rhythm

Breach Rhythm (BR) consists of focal sequences of rhythmic or pseudorhythmic mixed activity (theta, alpha and beta), sometimes associated with focal slowing or sharp activity, or isolated spikes. The breach rhythm develops over - or near - the area of bone skull defects, such as after craniotomy for neurosurgery or traumatic lesions, and it is not indicative of brain dysfunctions [9, 30, 31]. The breach rhythm may be considered as a consequence of the skull defect and not as an epileptiform abnormality (Figs. 9.15 and 9.16).

The genesis of BR is not fully understood, but the bone defects cause a reduced filtering effect and reduced electrical impedances. Sharpening and irregular morphology of BR may be misinterpreted, leading to a misdiagnosis of epilepsy. Therefore, a correct differential diagnosis is important for the relevant clinical consequences [32]. BR occurs in wakefulness, but it may persist also during sleep. If located in the central regions, it may be blocked by contralateral movements, because of the coexistence of an underlying mu rhythm, but this reactivity is not observed in the temporal region.

9.3.4 Lambda Waves

Lambda (λ) waves are physiological sharp waves occurring during visual scanning in awake subjects [9]. Their prevalence has been reported to vary between 2% and 88%, with the highest occurrence in children and in young adults [33]. They appear in occipital regions, with minimal spread to parietal and posterior temporal areas. The lambda waves morphology is biphasic or triphasic and the most prominent phase is positive. Their amplitude is usually low (20–40 µV), their duration between 200 and 300 ms, and their frequency of repetition is at intervals from 200 to 500 ms. They are mostly bilateral, synchronous and symmetrical, but they may also be unilateral or otherwise asymmetrical (Fig. 9.17).

Lambda waves are best elicited when the subject visually scans a textured or a complex picture, in a well-lit labora-

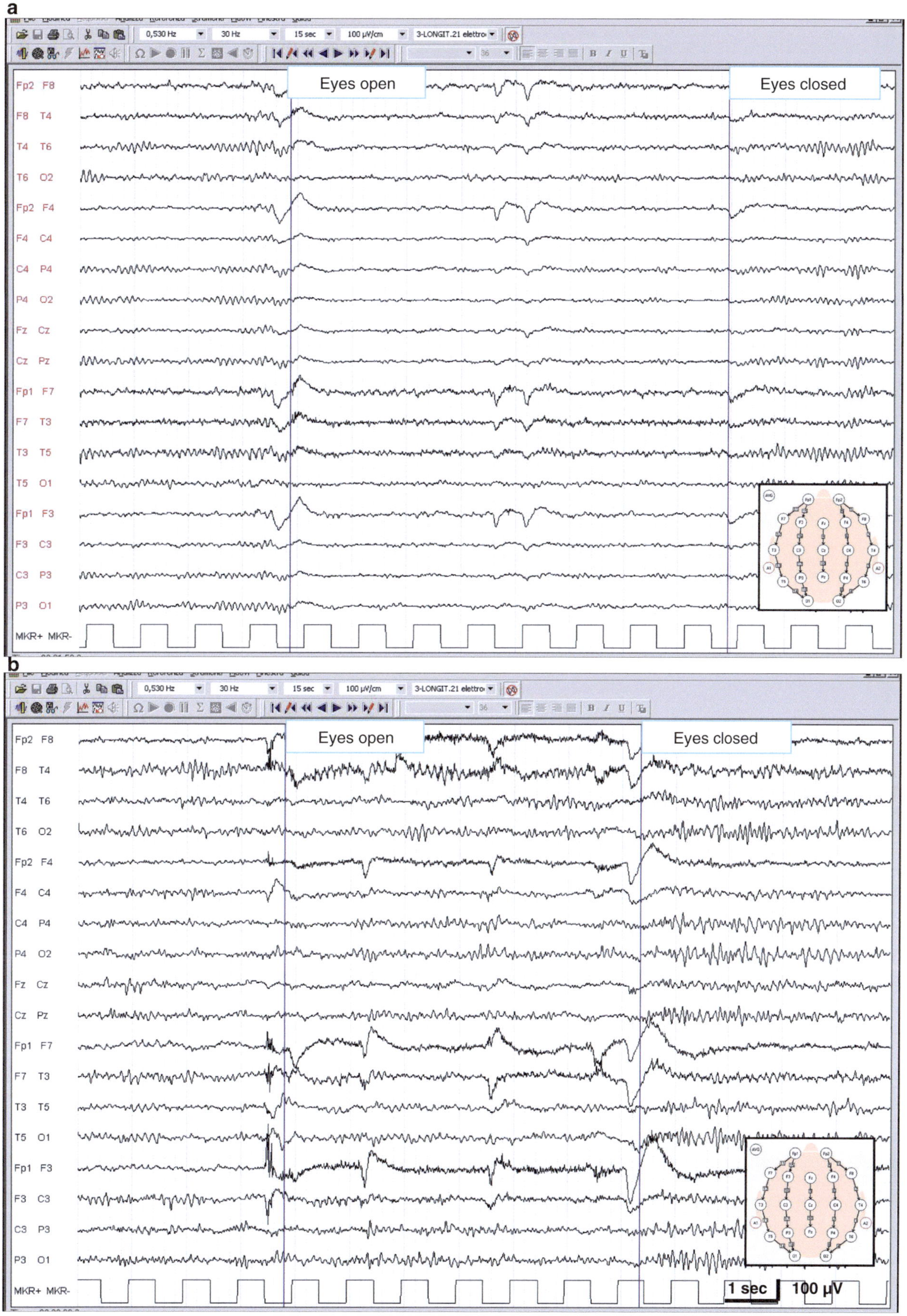

Fig. 9.11 (**a**) Normal reactivity of alpha rhythm with eyes opening; (**b**) incomplete reactivity of alpha rhythm that partially persists at eyes open

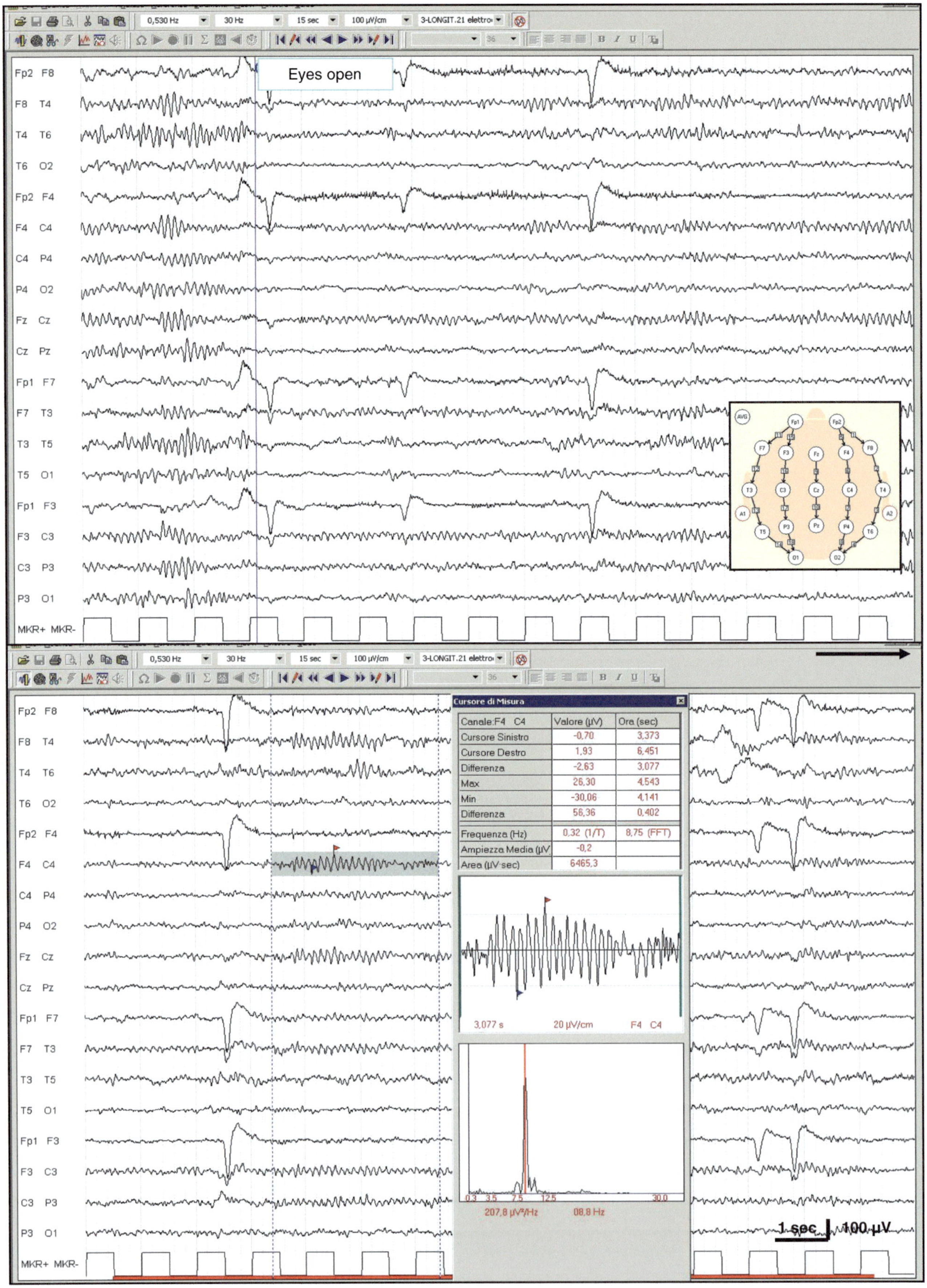

Fig. 9.12 Mu rhythm, better evident with eyes open; the peak of frequency is at 8.8 Hz and maximum spatial representation is on the central areas, bilaterally

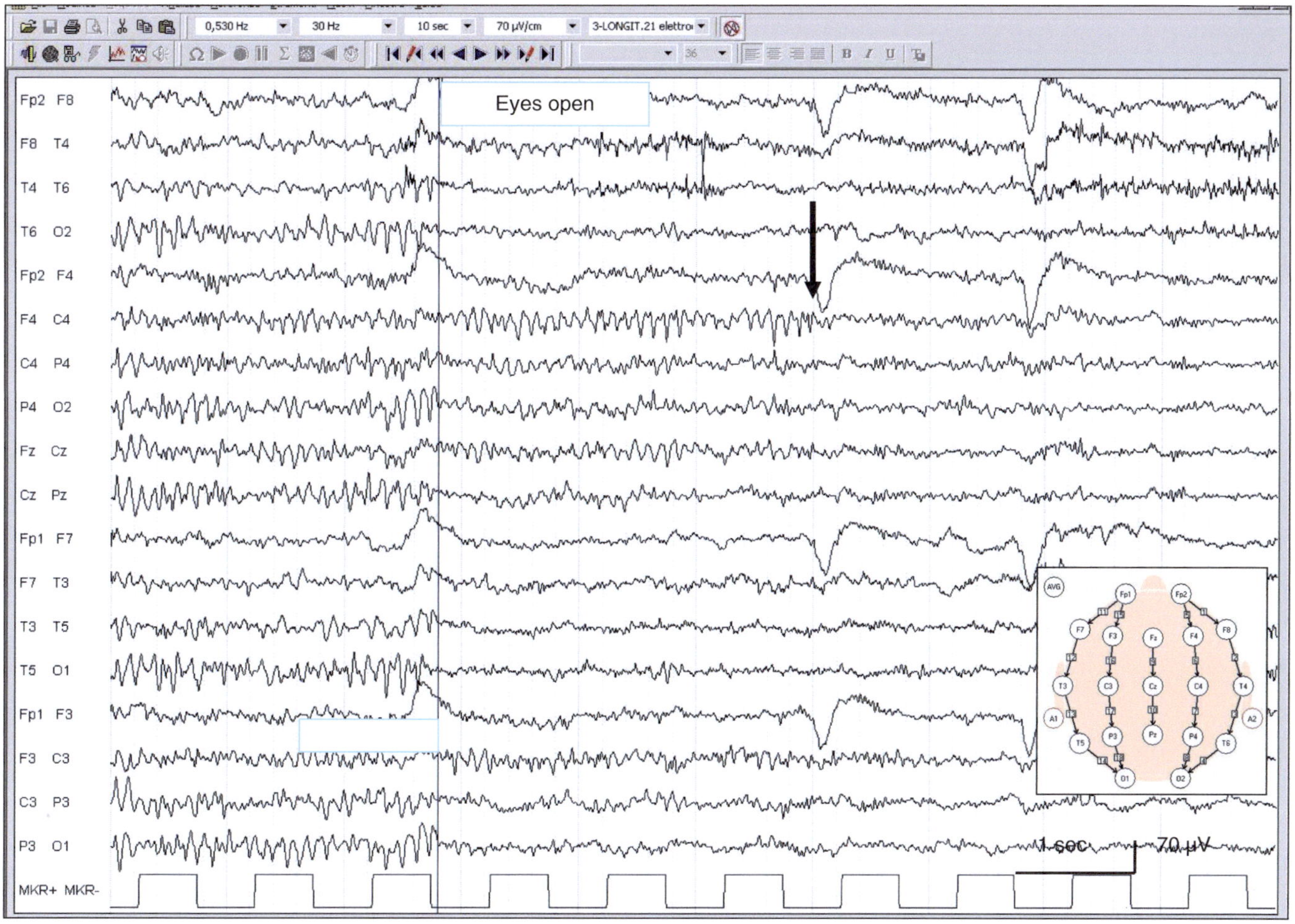

Fig. 9.13 Sequences of mu rhythm, more evident on right central region, blocked by asking the subject to tighten the contralateral hand (at arrow)

Table 9.2 Characteristics of the alpha rhythm and the mu rhythm

	Alpha rhythm	Mu rhythm
Frequency (Hz)	8 to <13	>7–11
Variants	Slow to fast	Absent or rare
Amplitude (µV)	<50	<50
Localization	Posterior areas	Central areas
Conditions of occurrence	Closed eyes	Either closed and open eyes
Reactivity	Opening of the eyes	Movement, tactile stimulus, mental movement planning

tory; they are closely correlated with fast saccadic eye movements (*saccadic movement* means the eye movement in space exploration, rapid and unconscious, followed by a fixation pause). Lambda waves appear after a saccadic movement with a latency of 70–80 ms. The disappearance of lambda waves is obtained with closing the eyes, the decrease of the ambient lighting level, or by placing a completely white sheet of paper in front of the eyes of the subject (*fixation off*). Therefore, from a neurophysiological point of view, lambda waves represent a sort of visual evoked responses and they are the expression of oculomotor and visual integration.

According to Billings [34] there are two different types of lambda waves. The first type would be generated by the faster conducting fibers of the optic nerve (Y-type fibers), immediately after the primary saccadic movement. The second type would be instead related to the visual impulses coming through the slower optical fibers (X-type fibers), with return to central vision during or slightly before the locking phase of the secondary corrective saccadic movement.

Recently, Alvarez et al. [35] studied the occurrence of lambda waves in adult outpatients, during prolonged EEG monitoring for unclear diagnosis of epilepsy. Lambda waves were found in 32% of prolonged recordings, mainly during watching TV, in relation to normal EEGs. Furthermore, all recordings with lambda waves also had Positive Occipital Sharp Transients of Sleep (POSTS) (Fig. 9.18). This study showed that watching TV likely represents a powerful stimulus for lambda waves appearance and confirms the physiological

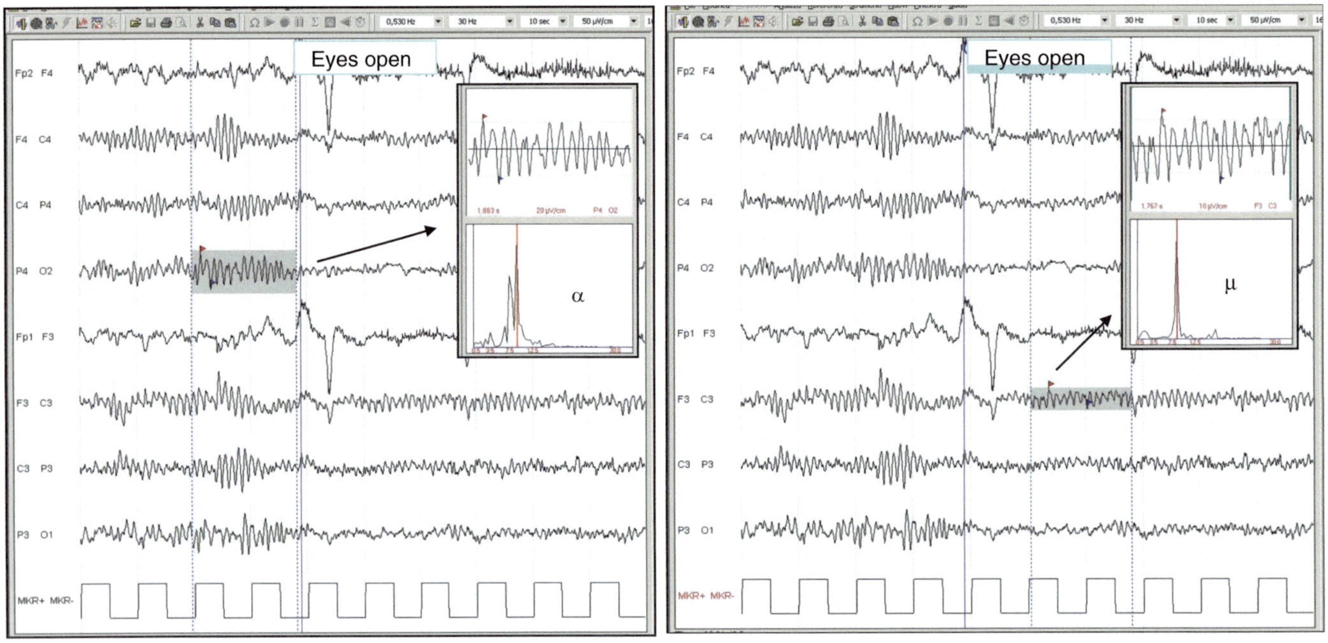

Fig. 9.14 Comparison between alpha and mu rhythm in a healthy 36-year-old man

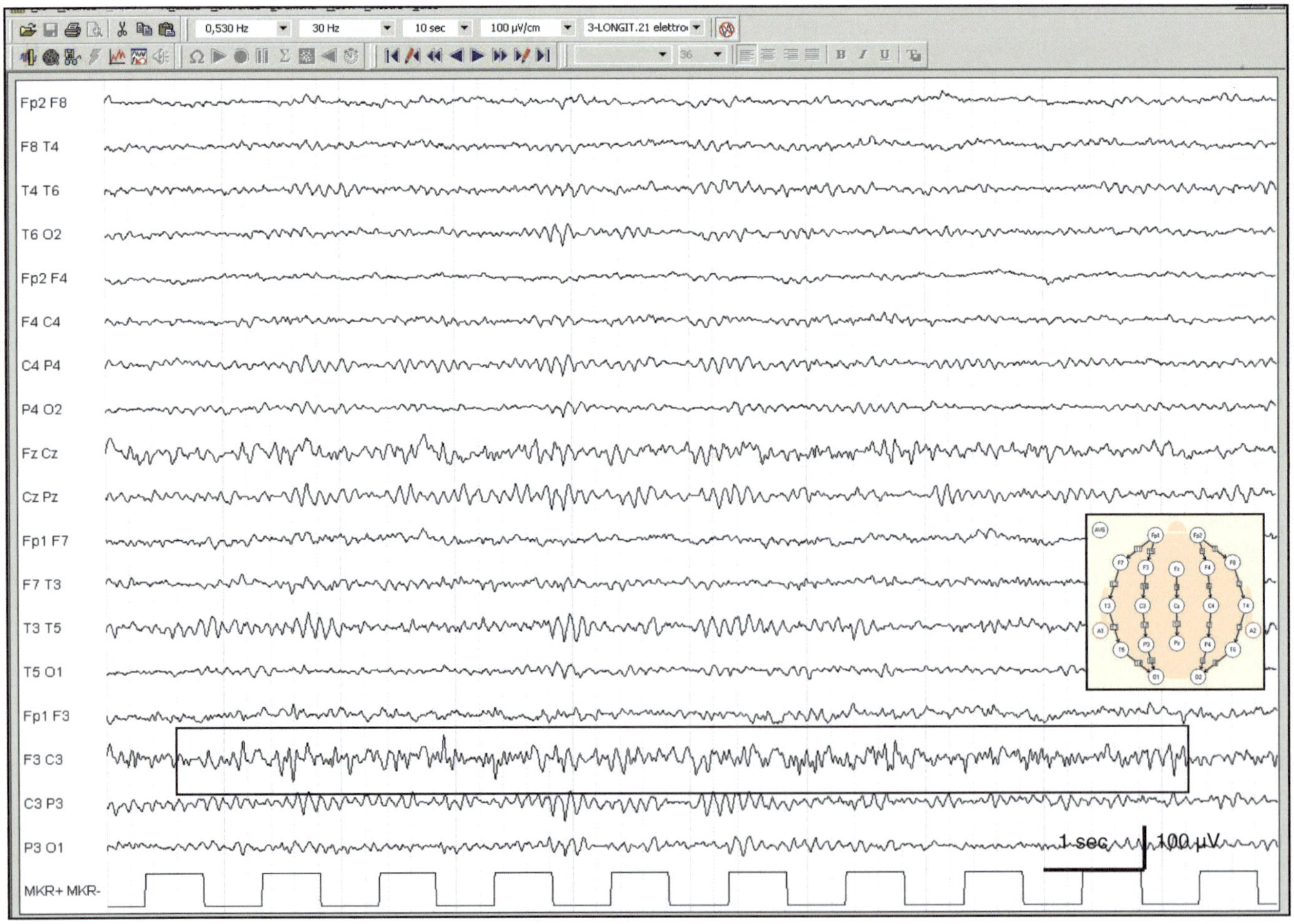

Fig. 9.15 Breach rhythm recorded on left fronto-central region in a man who underwent craniotomy in the same site

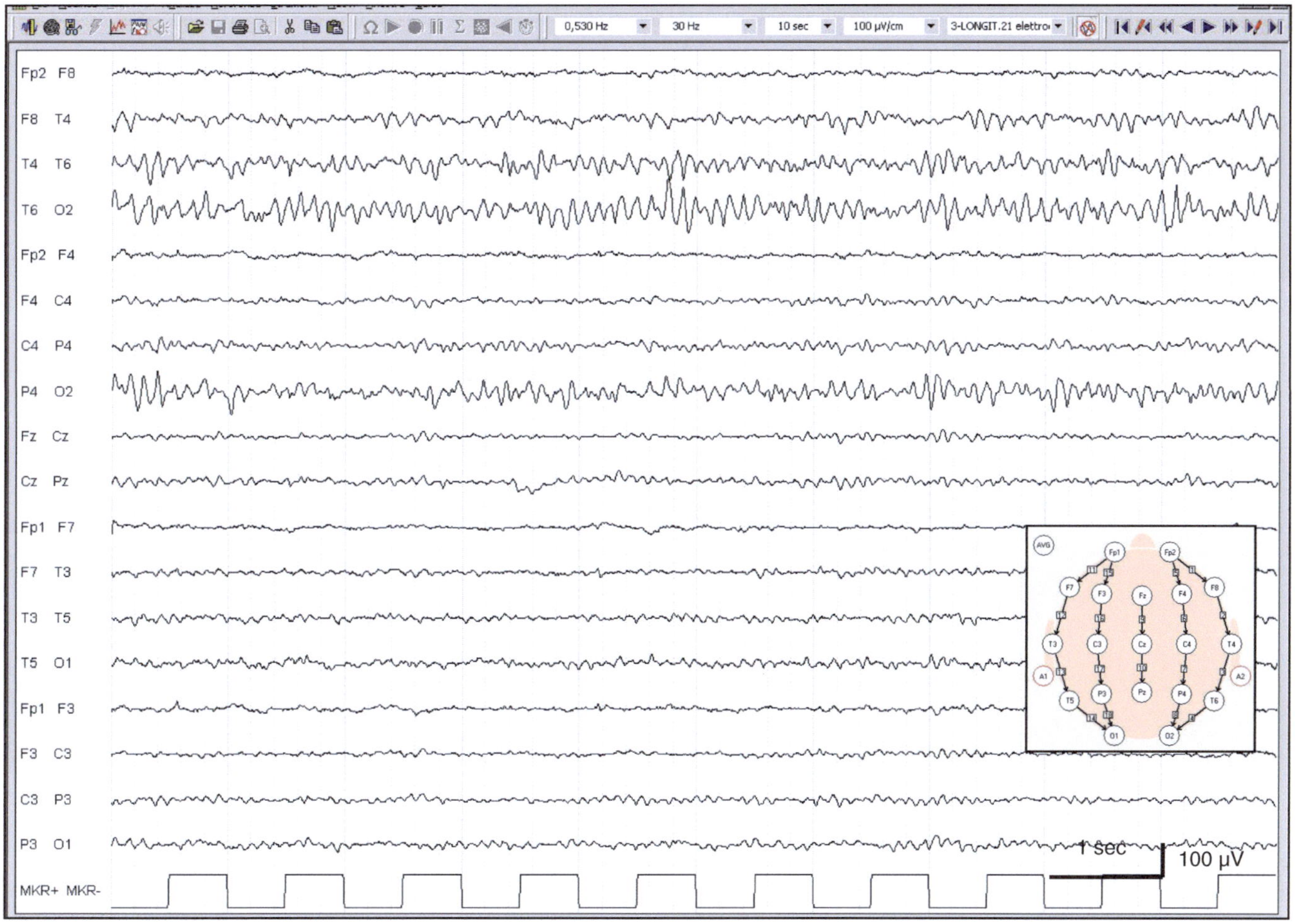

Fig. 9.16 Breach rhythm on right posterior parietotemporal region in a 48-year-old patient who underwent craniotomy to remove a ganglioglioma

benign nature of this EEG pattern. Finally, the lambda waves are of principal interest for the study of the visual system and should not be misinterpreted as epileptiform abnormalities.

9.4 Intraindividual and Interindividual Variability of the Normal Awake Adult EEG

The EEG of a single subject may present variations both during a specific recording session, as well as in separate recordings over time. This intraindividual variability is due to several factors, endogenous (arousal or drowsiness, anxiety, mental activity, blood sugar level, body temperature, etc.) or exogenous (laboratory lighting level and temperature, noise, etc.).

However, the changes in background activity observed in the same individual during a recording session depend mainly on the modifications in the alert level. As a matter of fact, if you can maintain in the same subject the same level of alertness and the same environmental conditions, there is a good correlation between seriated EEG tracings performed at different times (intraindividual stability of EEG).

EEG intraindividual differences have been reported also in women in relation to the various ovulatory and menstrual phases. Summarizing, in preovulatory and premenstrual phases substantially, it has been observed an increase in alpha frequency and beta power; in postovulatory and menstrual phase, instead, the alpha rhythm decreases in frequency, and the absolute power of theta and alpha activity increases, while the beta power decreases [11, 12].

The interindividual EEG variations, usually in the alpha rhythm, seem to be correlated with individual characteristics (personality, intellectual level, gender, genetic factors, etc.) [36].

As regard to the gender, some very old studies reported a more symmetric distribution of alpha frequency and also a higher beta amplitudes in females. However, other authors have successively found that the alpha rhythm is better represented in males than in females [37] or that there is no correlation between the EEG and sex of the subjects [38]. These discordant reports probably depend on dissimilar - and not comparable - experimental methods in EEG studies.

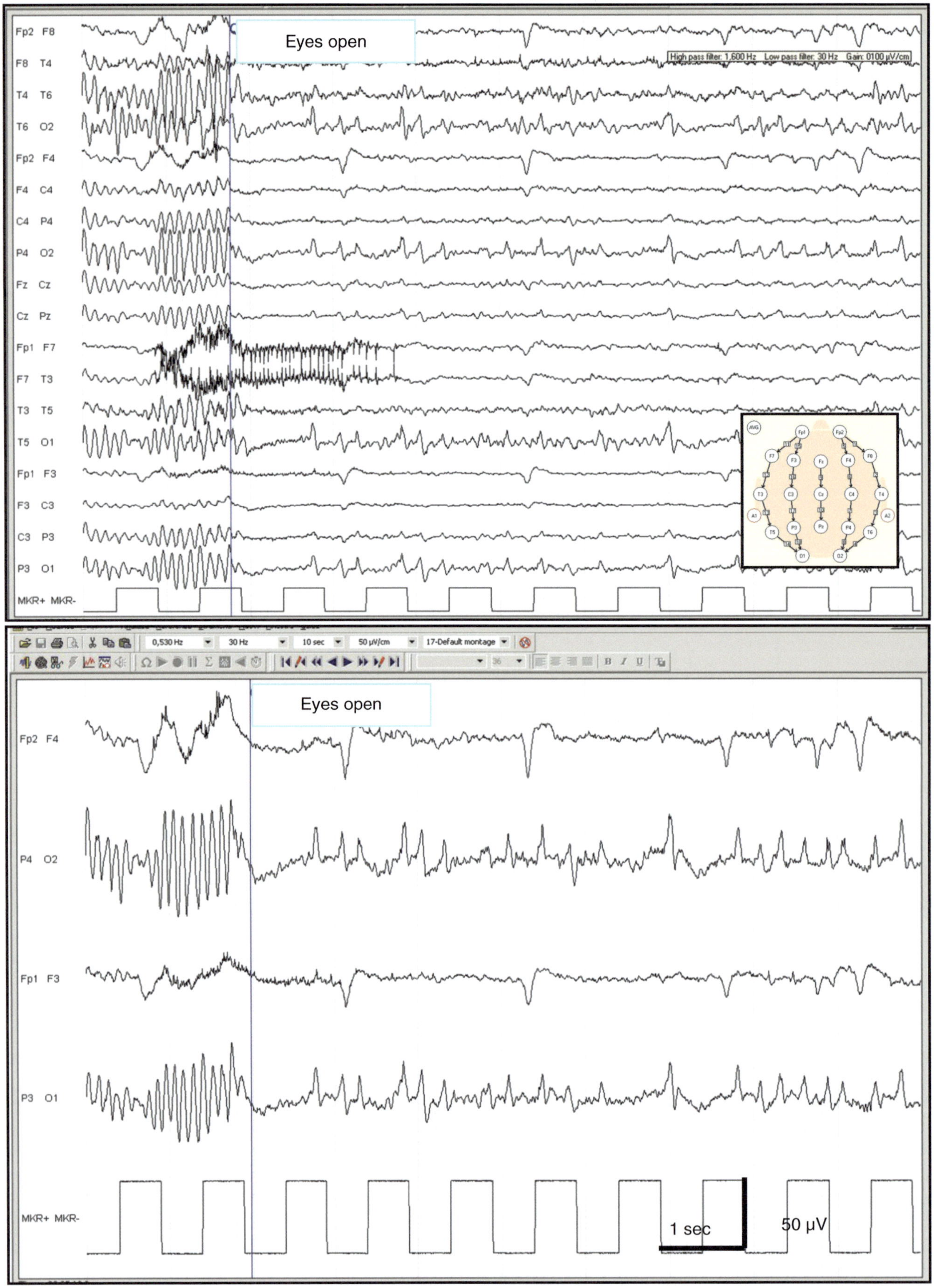

Fig. 9.17 Bilateral, synchronous, and symmetric lambda waves, with eyes open

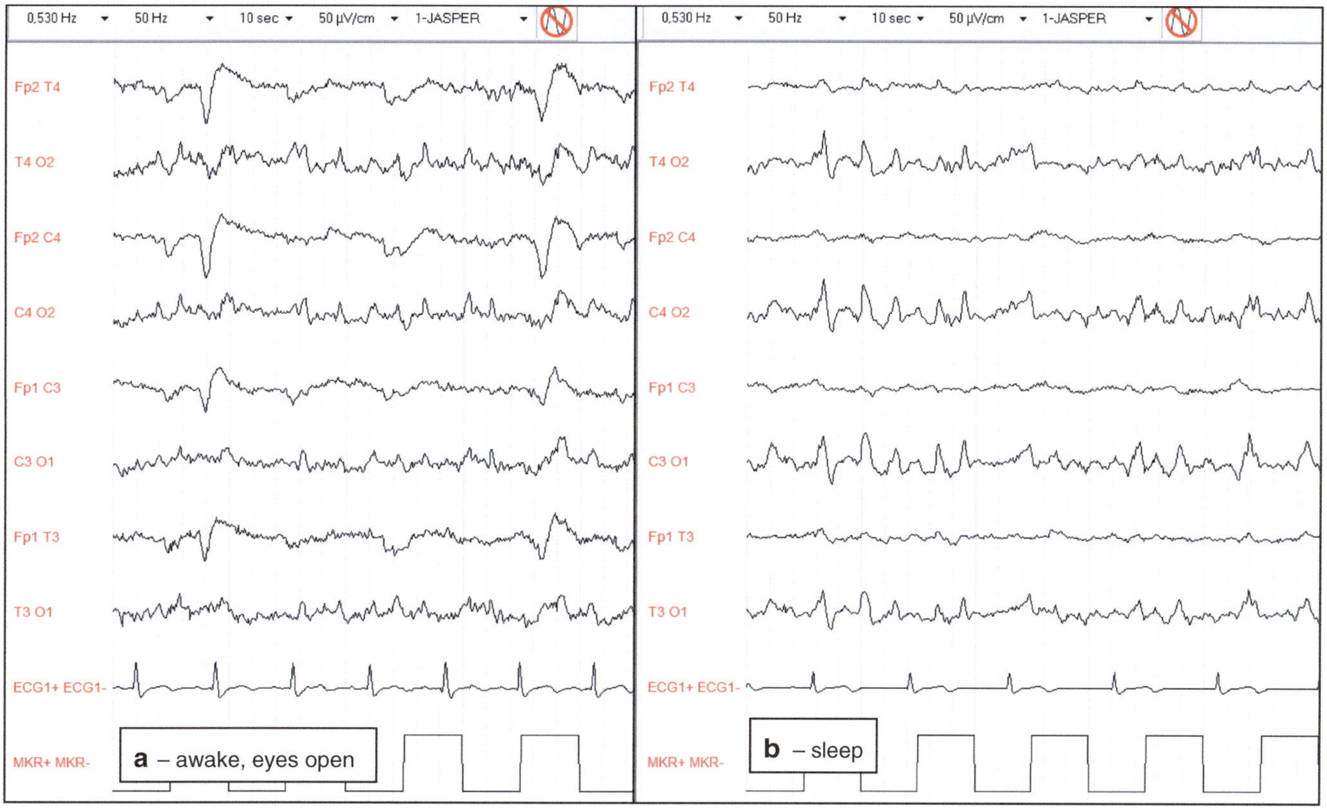

Fig. 9.18 In the same adult subject, lambda waves during awake, with eyes open (**a**), and POSTS during N1 stage of sleep (**b**)

9.5 Age Effect on the EEG of Wakefulness

The characteristics of neonatal EEG are treated in detail in Chap. 11.

In the first few years of life (1–3), the awake EEG is dominated by diffuse slow delta-theta activity, with high amplitude. This slow activity gradually tends to become rhythmic and with a prevalence in the central and parietal regions. In particular, from 3 to 12 months of life, the posterior background activity - considered a precursor of the subsequent alpha rhythm - has a frequency of about 4 Hz, is quite rhythmic, and is partially reactive to the opening-closing of the eyes. In the 2nd year of life, this activity reaches the frequency of about 6–7 Hz and in the third year of age it is around 7–8 Hz, with a more evident reactivity. From the 3rd year of age, therefore, an *immature* alpha rhythm, with low frequency and partial posterior localization, is already recognizable. The mid-posterior background activity at this age is of high amplitude and mixed with slower rhythms at 2–5 Hz.

From 3 to 5 years of age, the posterior rhythm is maintained at a frequency around 8 Hz, interrupted at intervals by 1.5–4 Hz sequences, and the tracing shows abundant theta activity in anterior regions and/or diffuse, at 5–7 Hz. Hyper Ventilation (HV, activation procedure that can be tested in laboratory with a good cooperation already from 3 to 4 years) shows mostly a widespread, hypersynchronous, wide-voltage slow activity; a photic driving response, particularly at low frequencies, is observed during the Intermittent Photic Stimulation (IPS).

From 6 to 12–15 years, the alpha rhythm progressively reaches the frequency of about 10 Hz, although it is always of high amplitude and mixed with slower theta activity ("*posterior slow waves of youth*"); sometimes, this theta activity, confined in temporal posterior regions, is rhythmic and at subharmonic alpha frequency (slow alpha variant) (Figs. 9.19 and 9.20).

From 12 to 15 years onward, EEG acquires progressively all the characteristics of the adult, both in basal and during activation tests, with final mature pattern at around 18–20 years. In the EEG maturative process, however, the interindividual variability must always be taken into great consideration, since it has a decisive influence on when a mature waking EEG pattern can be achieved [39–43].

From about 20 years, the physiological awake EEG maintains stable characteristics. From the age of 50 onward, a slight increase in theta activity and/or a slight decline in alpha frequency may begin to appear, although consistent with a normal EEG for age. According to some authors, the alpha rhythm slows down by 0.08 Hz per year from the age of 60, but this fact has not been confirmed by others [44–46].

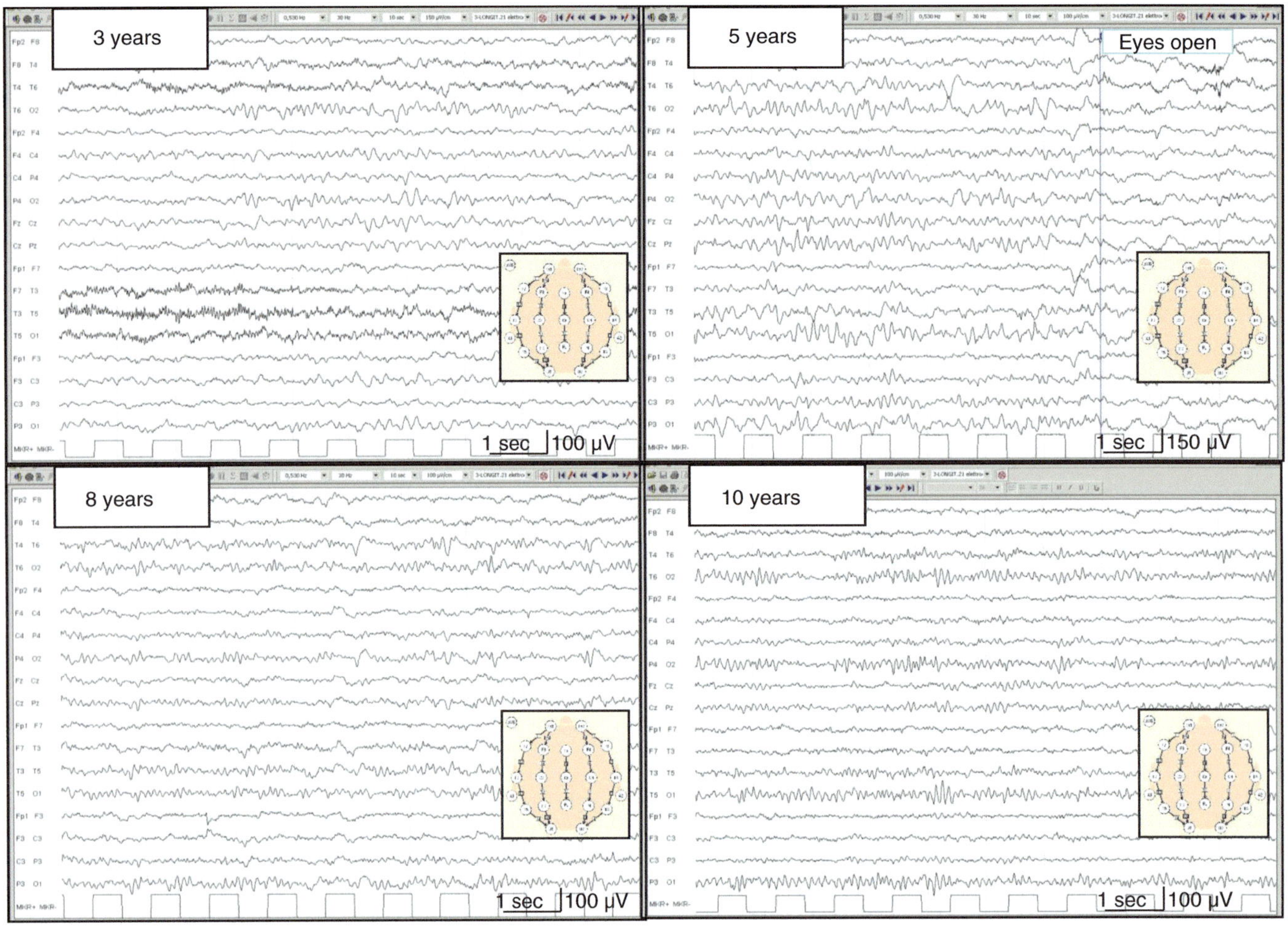

Fig. 9.19 Maturation of EEG. Examples of background activity with eyes closed in subjects of various age: 3 years old, 5 years old, 8 years old, and 10 years old

A more recent review by Rossini et al. [47] describe resting EEG changes across physiological aging, with gradual amplitude decrease of alpha rhythm and a global slowing of the background activity. However, an alpha rhythm at a frequency of 7.5–8 Hz in subjects over 80 years can be considered completely normal. Furthermore, in the elderly, the posterior physiological rhythm is of lower amplitude and tends to spread to the anterior regions (Figs. 9.21 and 9.22). Frequently, the slow alpha variants are also observed in the posterior regions.

In subjects over the age of 60, theta activity is frequently observed in temporal regions, mainly in the left side; this slow activity is considered physiological if it does not exceed 10–15% of the total registration period. HV increases slow activity and IPS less frequently induces posterior photic driving responses. In conclusion, however, even during aging, the interindividual variability of EEG must be taken into account; in fact, 90-year-olds or even centenarians can still present an alpha rhythm at a frequency of 9–10 Hz.

9.6 The Concept of Normality of EEG

First of all, it must be premised that the interpretation of an EEG is always subjective and that it can be influenced by multiple factors, mainly dependent on the experience of the technologists and of the clinical neurophysiologists. If the technician has not been able to recognize and eliminate from the recording an artefactual activity that can be easily mistaken for pathological changes, this can obviously lead to misinterpretations. It is also very important that the technician assesses the level of awareness of the patient during the recording session: focal and/or diffuse slowings may depend on variations in the subject's state of arousal or attention, which could also lead to incorrect interpretation of the tracing. In a routine EEG laboratory, the tracings should always be accompanied by an anamnestic data sheet containing complete information on the patient, from the personal data to the more specific clinical ones. Even if it is a laboratory test, the EEG must be interpreted in light of the patient's age, their clinical history, the reasons for the request, any pharma-

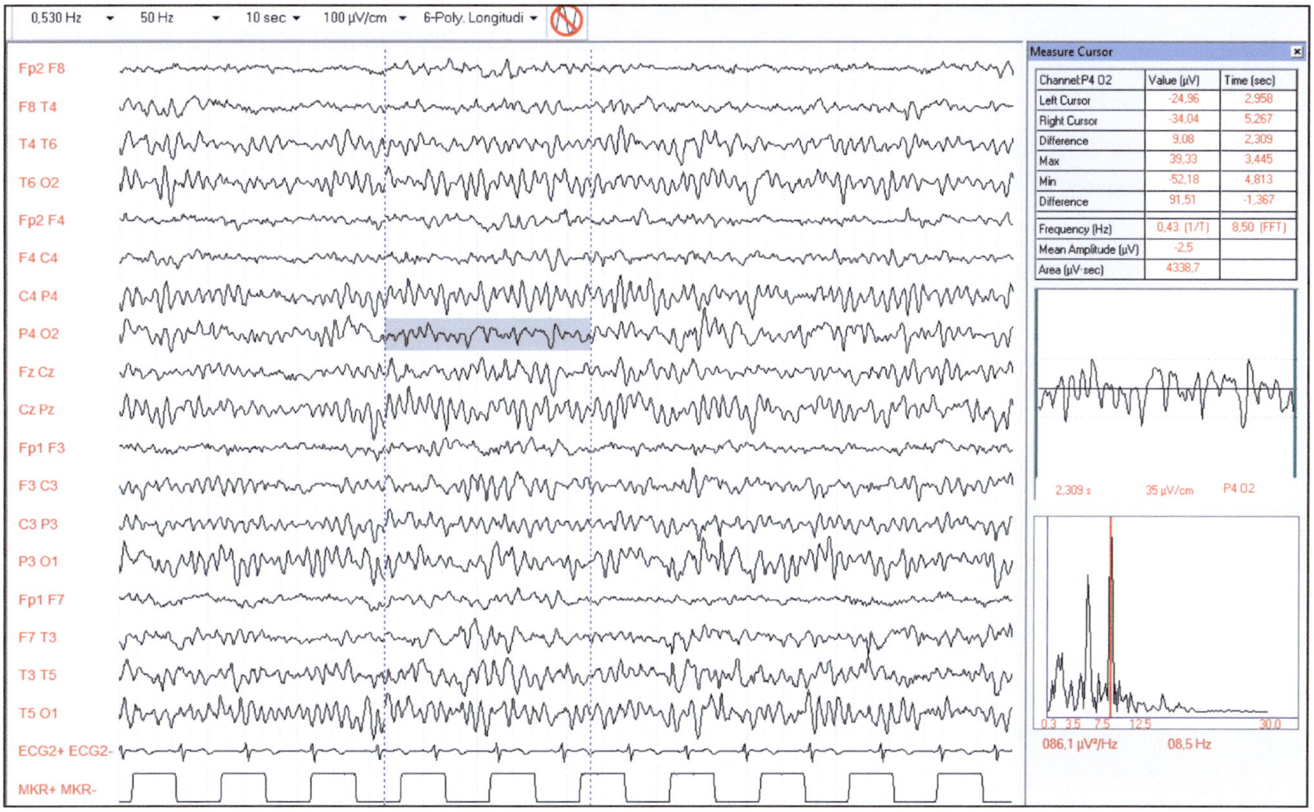

Fig. 9.20 Posterior slow waves of youth in a normal subject 12 years old

cological therapies, etc. Given that the tracing has been acquired correctly by technicians and that it is accompanied by all the necessary information, the interpretation of the EEG recording as normal or abnormal depends on the clinical neurophysiologist, who will prepare a report based on his theoretical preparation and on his practical experience. The theoretical knowledge of clinical EEG is obviously indispensable and it would be preferable that those who dedicate themselves to the reporting of EEG examinations are specialized in Clinical Neurophysiology or have attended at least specific residential courses. The theoretical preparation, however, has very little value if not accompanied by extensive experience in EEG, which should be certified only after a large number of tracings actually evaluated under supervision. It is well known that routine EEGs are frequently misinterpreted by neurologists without neurophysiology fellowship training (as the majority of neurologists interpreting EEG are). Misinterpretation of routine EEGs leads to the misdiagnosis of epilepsy and the inappropriate use of antiepileptic drugs, as well as to an inadequate diagnosis and treatment of non-epileptic seizures [32, 48]. Only with appropriate practical experience will neurologists be able to correctly differentiate a normal EEG recording from an abnormal one, taking into account that there are unusual and/or borderline patterns and that what can be considered "normal" for an individual is not necessarily for another. In general, however, for a correct interpretation of EEGs, it is essential that there is a continuous exchange of information between the technician and neurophysiologist and that the technician participates directly, where possible, in the reporting phase. Equally important is that the neurophysiologist does not get stuck in his position and that he is also able to acquire an EEG independently. In the initial training periods, all medical doctors interested in electroencephalography should spend a period in a laboratory, in close contact with the patient, the technician and the equipment. We must never forget that a normal EEG in basal conditions could become pathological during activation tests and that they must be performed according to correct and universally accepted criteria. However, activation tests can sometimes highlight EEG modifications with respect to the baseline tracing which, although they are completely physiological for that subject or that situation, can be instead interpreted as abnormal and, therefore, as pathological. Equally, it is sometimes necessary to repeat the EEG recording because, in some pathologies, seriated tracings have a higher probability of highlighting pathological changes: so it is not universal that a first EEG considered normal may not be followed by successive registrations with clear abnormalities. When you are not sure that a certain pattern is normal or pathological, it is always advisable to repeat the EEG recording, with the perspective that the repetition of a diagnostic exam is always

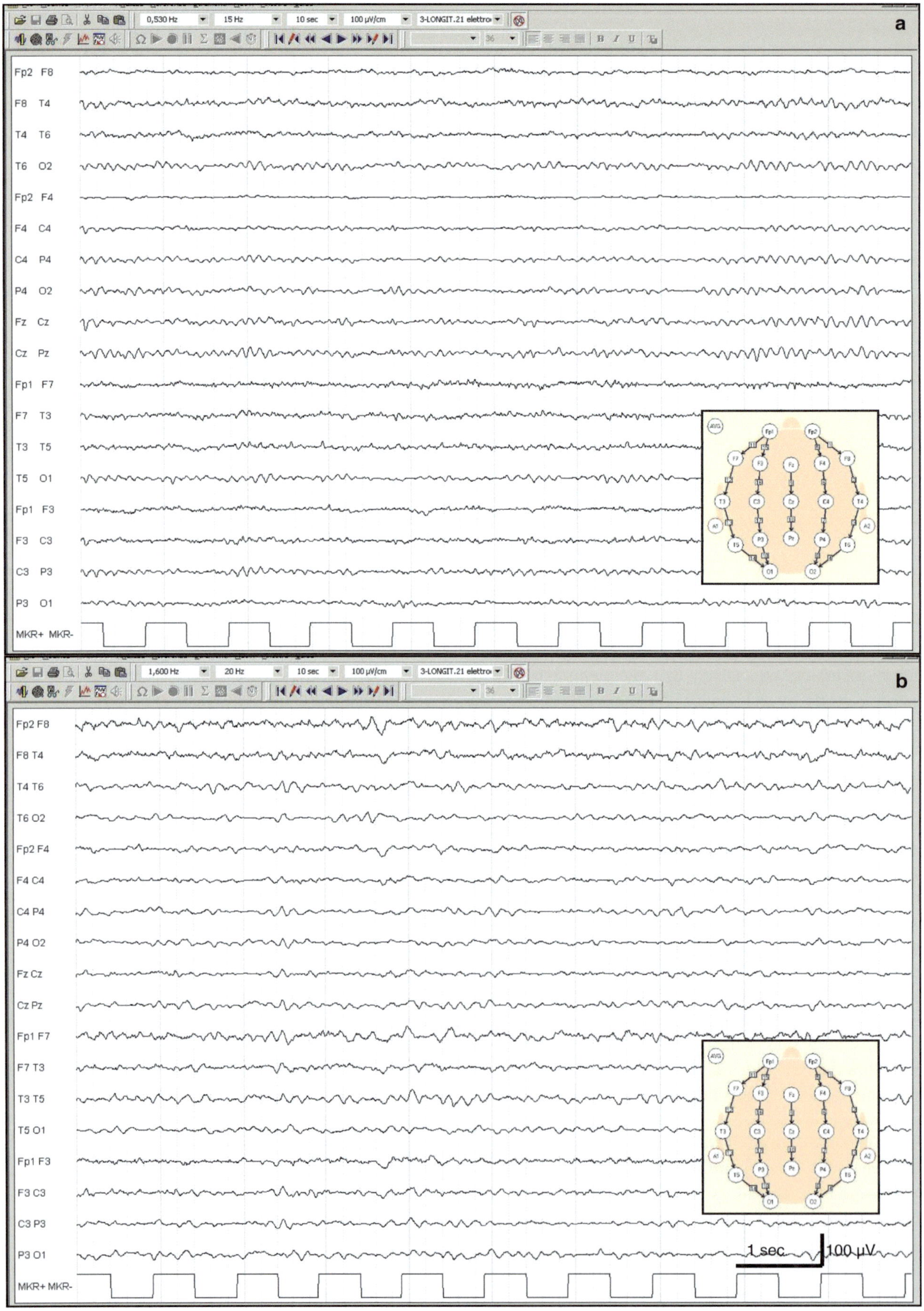

Fig. 9.21 Examples of background activity with eyes closed in two old subjects (**a**, 83 years old, and **b**, 95 years old)

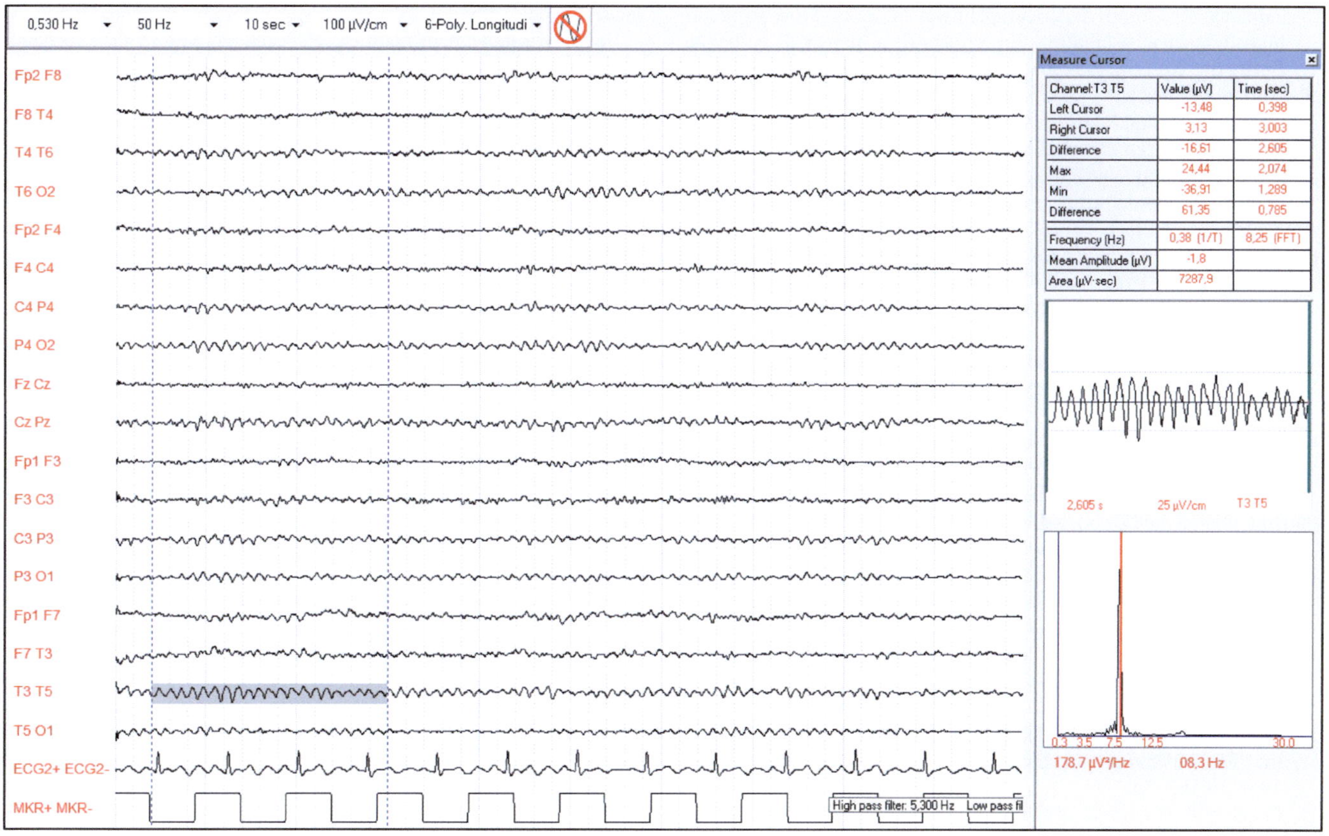

Fig. 9.22 Poorly localized alpha activity with low amplitude and peak of frequency of 8.3 Hz in an 85-year-old subject

better than an incorrect report. It can also happen that the neurophysiologist is so uncertain in the assessment of an EEG that they request the opinion of a second expert; in this case it is better that the second evaluation is carried out blindly, without knowing the clinical data. Subsequently, the two experts can cooperate together an electro-clinical correlation and reach a shared EEG report.

However, the variability of interindividual assessment is notable [49]. A recent study of Halford et al. [50] has shown that interrater agreement among academic neurophysiologists in epileptiform transients identification varies considerably and that the American Board of Clinical Neurophysiology certification is associated with improved performance.

To overcome the problem of interindividual evaluation variability of EEG features, there is a need to find a computerized tools to improve the quality of EEG assessment and reporting in clinical practice and to improve education in EEG [51].

Finally, there is the possibility of referring to specific automated software for objective EEG evaluations (computerized signal analysis, brain mapping, automatic detection of epileptiform transients, etc.). How these methods are useful in clinical practice to a better discern, compared to the visual inspection, between normal and abnormal EEGs, is questionable. With these devices, it will be easier to characterize and quantify some EEG parameters, but current abnormality detection softwares have an insufficient sensitivity requiring, however, a neurophysiologist to examine each EEG.

Acknowledgment I am grateful to neurophysiologist Dr Patrizia Pulitano for her help in selecting and editing the EEG figures and to neurologist Dr Edoardo Vicenzini in editing the manuscript.

References

1. Walter WG. The location of cerebral tumours by electroencephalography. Lancet. 1936;II:305–8.
2. Vanhatalo S, Voipio J, Kaila K. Infraslow EEG activity. In: Schomer DL, Lopes da Silva FH, editors. Electroencephalography. Basic principles, clinical applications, and related fields. 6th ed. Philadelphia: Lippincott Williams & Wilkins; 2011. p. 741–8.
3. Walter WG, Dovey VJ. Electroencephalography in cases of subcortical tumours. J Neurol Neurosurg Psychiatry. 1944;7:57–65.
4. Berger H. Uber das Elektrenkephalogramm des Menschen. Arch Psychiatr Nervenkr. 1929;87:527–70.
5. Curio G. Ultrafast EEG activities. In: Niedermeyer E, Lopes Da Silva F, editors. Electroencephalography. Basic principles, clinical applications, and related fields. 5th ed. Philadelphia: Lippincott Williams & Wilkins; 2005. p. 495–504.
6. Frauscher B, Bartolomei F, Kobayashi K, et al. High frequency oscillations: the state of clinical research. Epilepsia. 2017;58:1316–29.

7. Zijmans M, Worrell GA, Dumpelmann M, et al. How to record high-frequency oscillations in epilepsy: a practical guideline. Epilepsia. 2017;58:495–504.
8. Adrian ED, Mathews BHC. The Berger rhythm: potential changes from the occipital lobes in man. Brain. 1934;57:355–85.
9. Kane N, Acharya J, Benickzy S, et al. A revised glossary of terms most commonly used by clinical electroencephalographers and updated proposal for the report format of the EEG findings. Clin Neurophysiol Pract. 2017;2:170–85.
10. Kriegseis A, Henninhausen E, Rosler F, Roder B. Reduced EEG alpha activity over parieto-occipital brain areas in congenitally blind adults. Clin Neurophysiol. 2006;117:1560–73.
11. Harding GFA. Thompson CRS. EEG rhythms and the internal milieu. In: Remond A, editor. Handbook of electroencephalography and clinical neurophysiology, vol. 6A. Amsterdam: Elsevier; 1976. p. 176–94.
12. Chang BS, Schomer DL, Niedermeyer E. Normal EEG and sleep: adults and elderly. In: Schomer DL, Lopes da Silva FH, editors. Electroencephalography. Basic principles, clinical applications, and related fields. 6th ed. Philadelphia: Lippincott Williams & Wilkins; 2011. p. 183–214.
13. Tatum WO IV. Normal adult EEG. In: Ebersole JS, editor. Current practice of clinical electroencephalography. 4th ed. Philadelphia: Wolters Kluwer Health; 2014. p. 90–124.
14. Meritam P, Gardella E, Alving J, et al. Diagnostic yield of standard-wake and sleep EEG recordings. Clin Neurophysiol. 2018;129:713–6.
15. Stom van Leeuwen W, Bekkering DH. Some results obtained with the EEG-spectrograph. Electroencephalogr Clin Neurophysiol. 1958;10:563–70.
16. Cooper R, Binnie C, Billings R. Techniques in clinical neurophysiology. EEG phenomenology. Amsterdam: Elsevier; 2003. p. 169–221.
17. Kuhlo W. Slow posterior activities. In: Chatrian GE, Lairy GC, editors. The EEG of waking adult. Handbook of electroencephalography and clinical neurophysiology, vol. 6A. Amsterdam: Elsevier; 1976. p. 89–104.
18. Libenson MH. Visual analysis of the EEG: wakefulness, drowsiness and sleep. In: Libenson MH, editor. Practical approach to electroencephalography. Philadelphia: Saunders Elsevier; 2010. p. 5–30.
19. Krishnan V, Chang BS, Schomer DL. Normal EEG in wakefulness and sleep: adults. and elderly. In: Schomer DL, Lopes da Silva FH, editors. Neidermeyer's electroencephalography. Basic principles, clinical applications, and related fields. Oxford: Oxford University Press; 2018. p. 202–28.
20. Niedermeyer E, Krauss GL, Peyser CE. The electroencephalogram and mental activation. Clin Electroencephalogr. 1989;20:215–26.
21. Bishop GH. The interpretation of cortical potentials. Cold Spring Harb Symp Quant Biol. 1936;4:305–19.
22. Andersen P, Andersson SA. Physiological basis of the alpha rhythm, Neuroscience series, vol. 1. New York: Appleton Century Crofts; 1968: 235p.
23. Steriade M, Gloor P, Llinas RR, et al. Basic mechanisms of cerebral rhythmic activities. Electroencephalogr Clin Neurophysiol. 1990;76:481–508.
24. Gastaut H. Etude électrocorticographique de la réactivité des rythmes rolandiques. Rev Neurol. 1952;87:176–82.
25. Yamak R, Beydoun AA, Dirani MM, et al. Unilateral mu rhythm and associated cortical lesions on brain MRI. J Clin Neurophysiol. 2017;34:144–50.
26. Chatrian GE. The mu rhythm. In: Remond A, editor. Handbook of electroencephalography and clinical neurophysiology, vol. 6. Amsterdam: Elsevier; 1976. p. 46–69.
27. Gastaut H, Naquet R, Gastaut Y. A study of the mu rhythm in subjects lacking one or more limbs. Electroencephalogr Clin Neurophysiol. 1965;18:720–1.
28. Jasper HH, Penfield W. Electrocorticograms in man: effects of voluntary movement upon the electrical activity of the precentral gyrus. Arch Psychiatr Nervenkr. 1949;183:163–74.
29. Pineda JA. The functional significance of mu rhythms: translating "seing" and "hearing" into "doing". Brain Res Rev. 2005;50:57–68.
30. Cobb WA, Guiloff RJ, Cast J. Breach rhythm: the EEG related to skull defects. Electroencephalogr Clin Neurophysiol. 1979;47:251–71.
31. Brigo F, Cicero R, Fiaschi A, Bongiovanni LG. The breach rhythm. Clin Neurophysiol. 2011;122:2116–20.
32. Benbadis SR, Tatum WO. Overinterpretation of EEGs and misdiagnosis of epilepsy. J Clin Neurophysiol. 2003;20:42–4.
33. Chatrian GE. The lambda waves. In: Remond A, editor. Handbook of electroencephalography and clinical neurophysiology, vol. 6A. Amsterdam: Elsevier; 1976. p. 123–49.
34. Billings RJ. The origin of the occipital lambda wave in man. Electroencephalogr Clin Neurophysiol. 1989;72:95–113.
35. Alvarez V, Maeder-Ingvar M, Rossetti A. Watching television: a previously unrecognized powerful trigger of lambda waves. J Clin Neurophysiol. 2011;28:400–3.
36. Shaw JC. The Brain's alpha rhythms and the mind. Amsterdam: Elsevier; 2003.
37. Matsuura M, Yamamoto K, Fukuzawa H, et al. Age development and sex differences of various EEG elements in healthy children and adults. Electroencephalogr Clin Neurophysiol. 1985;60:394–406.
38. Ehlers CL, Kupfer DJ, Buysse DJ, et al. The Pittsburgh study of normal EEG sleep in young adults: focus on the relationship between waking and sleeping EEG spectral patterns. Electroencephalogr Clin Neurophysiol. 1998;106:199–205.
39. Petersen I, Eeg-Olofsson O. The development of the electroencephalogram in normal children from the age of 1 through 15 years. Neuropediatrie. 1971;2:247–304.
40. Eeg-Olofsson O, Petersen I, Selden U. The development of the electroencephalogram in normal children from the age of 1 through 15 years. Paroxysmal activity. Neuropaediatrie. 1971;2:375–404.
41. Eeg-Olofson. The development of the electroencephalogram in normal adolescents from the age of 16 through 21 years. Neuropaediatrie. 1971;3:11–45.
42. Duffy FH, Albert MS, McAnuty G, Garvey AJ. Age-related differences in brain electrical activity of healthy subjects. Ann Neurol. 1984;16:430–8.
43. Marcuse LV, Schneider M, Mortati KA, et al. Quantitative analysis of the posterior-dominant rhythm in healthy adolescents. Clin Neurophysiol. 2008;119:1778–81.
44. Wang HS, Busse EW. EEG of healthy old persons. A longitudinal study. I. Dominant background activity and occipital rhythm. J Gerontol. 1969;24:419–26.
45. Giaquinto S, Nolfe G. The EEG in the normal elderly: a contribution to the interpretation of aging and dementia. Electroencephalogr Clin Neurophysiol. 1986;63:540–6.
46. Klass DW, Brenner RP. Electroencephalography of the elderly. J Clin Neurophysiol. 1995;12:116–31.
47. Rossini PM, Rossi S, Babiloni C, et al. Clinical neurophysiology of aging brain: from normal aging to neurodegeneration. Prog Neurobiol. 2007;83:375–400.
48. Benbadis SR. Errors in EEGs and the misdiagnosis of epilepsy: importance, causes, consequences, and proposed remedies. Epilepsy Behav. 2007;11:257–62.
49. Williams GW, Luders HO, Brickner A, et al. Interobserver variability in EEG interpretation. Neurology. 1985;35:1714–9.
50. Halford JJ, Arain A, Kalamangalam GP, et al. Characteristics of EEG interpreters associated with higher interrater agreement. J Clin Neurophysiol. 2017;34:168–73.
51. Beniczky S, Aurlien H, Brogger JC, et al. Standardized computer-based organized reporting of EEG: SCORE—second version. Clin Neurophysiol. 2017;128:2334–46.

10 Normal Sleep EEG

Anna Elisabetta Vaudano, Nicoletta Azzi, and Irene Trippi

10.1 Sleep EEG Recordings, Why and When

It is well known that many epileptic discharges may be absent during the waking state and occur only (or at least more easily) in sleep. For this reason, brief sleep recordings during spontaneous sleep or after sleep deprivation are generally performed in regular EEG laboratories to disclose such paroxysms. These recordings are often not longer than 30 min, representing de facto a nap. A nap shows normally the process of falling asleep from the waking state to drowsiness and from drowsiness to light NREM sleep. These stages are usually the most informative stages for the epileptologist who is searching for clinically relevant abnormalities and especially for epileptic discharges not demonstrable in the waking state. However, additional information can be obtained only during deeper and REM sleep.

Nocturnal sleep and daytime nap, besides the difference in circadian phase, differ in multiple important aspects, such as total sleep time, the amount of sleep spindle-rich stage 2 sleep, slow-wave sleep (SWS), and REM sleep [1]. A more complete sleep study can be performed in sleep laboratories, with the aim of recording a whole night sleep or a 24 h time span and analyzing not only EEG but also other physiologic parameters with a complete polysomnography (or video-polysomnography, representing the gold standard for sleep investigation-PSG), in order to get a more complex perspective about the dynamics of patient's sleep, the trend of cardiovascular parameters, and the presence of abnormal movements during sleep.

The principal indications to perform all night PSG study are the following:

1. To differentiate between epileptic and non-epileptic nocturnal events (e.g., parasomnias, syncope due to nocturnal arrhythmias, sleep-related movement disorders)
2. To diagnose electrical status epilepticus during slow-wave sleep (ESES)
3. To demonstrate the absence of REM atonia in patients with REM behavior disorder (RDB)
4. To investigate sleep-related breathing disorders (especially in suspected obstructive sleep apnea syndrome (OSAS) with clinical signs of comorbid sleep disorders and/or significant pulmonary, cardiovascular, neuromuscular diseases)
5. To investigate sleep-related movements disorders (i.e., periodic limb movement (PLM))
6. To investigate, together with other diagnostic tests (multiple sleep latency test-MSLT) daytime sleepiness of unknown origin (e.g., suspected narcolepsy)

10.2 General Rules of Sleep Stages Scoring

Normal human sleep comprises two states—rapid eye movement (REM) and non-REM (NREM) sleep—that alternate cyclically across a sleep cycle. State characteristics are well defined: NREM sleep includes synchronous cortical EEG phenomena (sleep spindles, K-complexes, and slow waves) together with low muscle tonus; during the REM sleep, EEG is desynchronized, muscles are atonic, and dreaming occurs. A nightly pattern of sleep in mature humans sleeping on a regular schedule includes reliable features. Sleep begins in NREM and progresses through deeper NREM stages (stages N2 and N3) before the first episode of REM sleep occurs, approximately 80–100 min later. Thereafter, NREM sleep and REM sleep cycle with a period of approximately 90 min. NREM stage N3 concentrate in the early NREM cycles, and REM sleep episodes lengthen across the night (Fig.10.1). In the usual 6.5–8.0 h of sleep of young adults, stage N1 makes up about 5% of total sleep time (TST), stage N2 50–55%, stage N3 20%, and REM sleep 20–25%. Age affects the pattern of sleep stages across the night. In the newborn the sleep cycle is much shorter, approximately 40–45 min, slow-wave sleep (stage N3) more abundant, and REM sleep also much

A. E. Vaudano (✉) · N. Azzi · I. Trippi
Department of Medicine and Surgery, Sleep Medicine Center, University of Parma, Parma, Italy

O. Mecarelli (ed.), *Clinical Electroencephalography*, https://doi.org/10.1007/978-3-030-04573-9_10

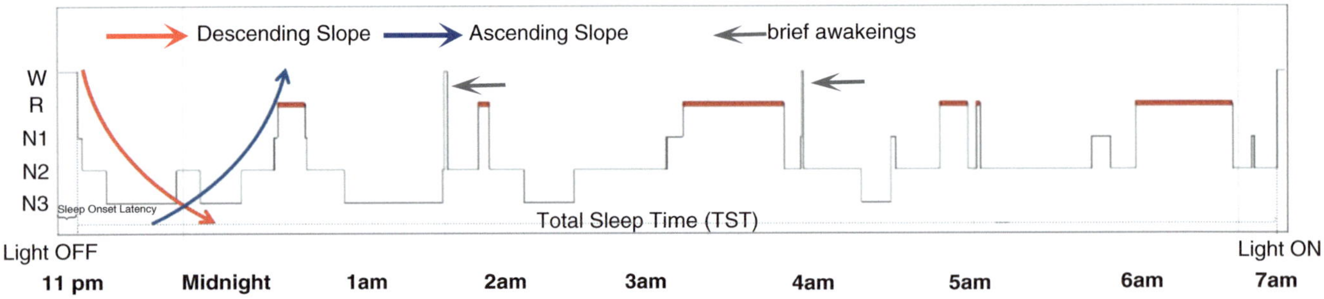

Fig. 10.1 Sleep pattern from a healthy human. An exemplary hypnogram depicting the different sleep stages over 8 h of nocturnal sleep. *W* wake, *R* REM, *N1* N1 sleep stage, *N2* N2 sleep stage, *N3* N3 sleep stage. The ascending-descending of the sleep cycle are represented by the red and blue arrow, respectively. Note that this pattern is less evident in the second part of the night particularly toward the last cycle

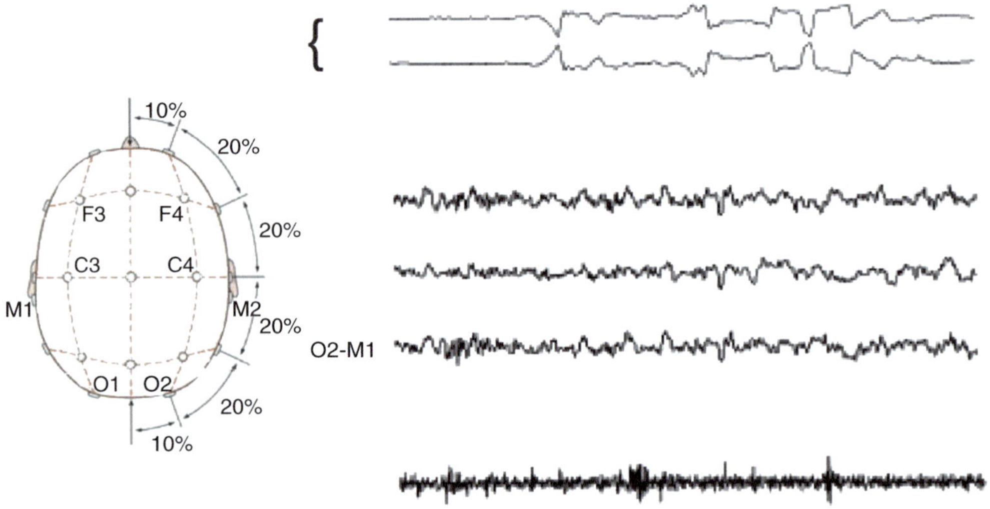

Fig. 10.2 Minimal recommended derivations for PSG recordings according to the AASM manual: two EOG derivations (E1, left EOG; E2, right EOG); three EEG channels (F4, C4, O2) referred to the contralateral mastoid (M1); one EMG derivation placed over the chin muscle. *F* frontal, *C* central, *O* occipital

higher, about 50% of TST. Moreover, sleep onset directly into the REM state may happen, and sleep is dispersed throughout the 24-h period. In late infancy and childhood, sleep becomes nocturnal with an afternoon nap. NREM sleep always occurs first, the sleep cycle lengthens progressively toward the 85 min of the adult, and slow sleep and REM sleep decrease. In old age there is a marked diminution of stages N3, slight reduction of REM sleep, a decrease of total sleep time, and increasing episodes of wakefulness.

The official rules for sleep stage classification in sleep laboratories were first established during an international expert consensus in 1968, described by Rechtschaffen and Kales [2], and then updated and modified in 2007 by the American Academy of Sleep Medicine (AASM) [3] and subsequent versions.

The AASM manual, despite some intrinsic limitations and weakness, represents the international approved standard for sleep and associated events (arousal, cardiac, respiratory, and movement events) scoring rules. Actually the latest AASM version regarding rules for scoring of sleep dated 2018 [3].

At least three EEG channels, one EOG (electrooculogram) and one chin EMG (electromyography) are necessary to score sleep stages (Fig. 10.2 and Table 10.1). Sleep staging is based on visual analysis of 30-s subsequent epochs, recognizing the main features of each single epoch in order to classify the latter as one of five distinct stages: one stage of wake (W) and four different sleep stages (N1, N2, N3, R) (Fig. 10.3).

The general rules for sleep stage scoring, according to AASM manual [3], are reassumed in the Table 10.2.

10.3 Bases of Sleep Regulation

The neurobiological bases of sleep and wake and the regulation of the cyclic alternation of these two states are extremely complexes, and their detailed description goes beyond the objectives of this chapter. This paragraph aims to delineate the principal elementary mechanisms of sleep, but it not constitutes an exhaustive review of this fascinating but complicated topic.

Table 10.1 Technical specifications for EEG, EOG, and EMG according to AASM manual [3]

EEG*:* at minimum 3 EEG channels (frontal, central, and occipital derivations)	Recommended derivations are: (a) F4-M1 (b) C4-M1 (c) O2-M1 (d) Backup electrodes should be placed at F3, C3, O1, and M2 to allow display of F3-M2, C3-M2, and O1-M2 if electrodes malfunction during the study *Note*: M1 and M2 refer to the left and right mastoid processes. M1 is the standard reference electrode for recording EEG	Acceptable EEG derivations are: (a) Fz-Cz (b) Cz-Oz (c) C4-M1 (d) Backup electrodes should be placed at Fpz, C3, O1, and M2 to allow substitution of Fpz for Fz, C3 for Cz or C4, O1 for Oz, and M2 for M1 if electrodes malfunction during the study
EOG	The recommended EOG derivations and electrode positions are: (a) Derivations: E1-M2 (left) and E2-M2 (right) (b) Electrode positions: E1 is placed 1 cm below the left outer canthus and E2 is placed 1 cm above the right outer canthus	Acceptable EOG derivations and electrode positions are: (a) Derivations: E1-Fpz and E2-Fpz (b) Electrode positions: E1 is placed 1 cm below and 1 cm lateral to the outer canthus of the left eye, and E2 is placed 1 cm below and 1 cm lateral to the outer canthus of the right eye
CHIN EMG	Three electrodes should be placed to record chin EMG: (a) One in the midline 1 cm above the inferior edge of the mandible (b) One 2 cm below the inferior edge of the mandible and 2 cm to the right of the midline (c) One 2 cm below the inferior edge of the mandible and 2 cm to the left of the midline	The standard chin EMG derivation consists of both the electrodes below the mandible referred to the electrode above the mandible. The other inferior electrode is a backup electrode to allow for continued display of EMG activity if one of the primary electrodes malfunctions

EEG electroencephalogram, *EMG* electromyography, *EOG* electrooculography, *C* central, *F* frontal, *P* parietal, *O* occipital, *M* mastoid

The balance of sleep (S) and wake (W) states is related to reciprocal interactions between sleep-promoting systems (located in the medial part of brainstem, dorsal reticular substance of the medulla, ventrolateral preoptic nucleus (VLPO), and basal forebrain) and wake-promoting systems (ascending reticular activating system (ARAS) that includes the pontine and midbrain tegmental region, the posterior hypothalamus, and the basal forebrain cholinergic neurons).

Regulation of wakefulness is principally delegated to the neurons of the reticular activating system that modulates the cortical activation throughout two pathways [4]:

- A dorsal path from cholinergic neurons of latero-dorsal and pedunculo-pontine tegmental nuclei that activate glutamatergic thalamocortical projections.
- A ventral path that involves the aminergic arousal system from the brainstem compounded of serotoninergic (dorsal raphe nuclei), noradrenergic (locus coeruleus), histaminergic (tuberomammillary nucleus), and dopaminergic (ventral periaqueductal grey) neurons. This route receives also contributions from orexinergic neurons and melanin-concentrating hormone neurons of lateral hypothalamus and cholinergic neurons from the basal forebrain.

Sleep occurs when the VLPO, anterior hypothalamus, and basal forebrain are activated and inhibit the ARAS principally throughout GABAergic and galaninergic projections.

Transition between W and S represents hence the result of reciprocal inhibition between arousal- and sleep-promoting systems. This relationship can be modelled as a "flip-flop switch" circuit [5] in which the two competing sides inhibit each other generating a bistable feedback loop with two alternative states (W and S) without intermediate patterns. Mathematical models based on physiological data proposed a dynamic sleep-wake cycle regulation that assumes the existence of transitional states depending on the strength of the external (sensory) inputs [6–8] and the intracycle sleep dynamic regulation [9]. Simplifying, the effect of a stimulus during sleep is influenced by the state dominance of sleep- or wake-promoting forces on the descending or ascending slopes of the cycles. [10]. A sleep cycle begins with a descending slope, where the sleep stages follow a deepening tendency (from stage N1 to N3), followed by an ascending slope, characterized by an "ascending" sequence of stages—going from deep to more superficial (from N3 toward stage N1 and then REM sleep) (Fig.10.1). This pattern is less clearly observed in the second half of night sleep. Descending slope carries sleep-promoting tendencies, whereas the ascending one results from wake/rapid eye movement (REM)-promoting force. The dynamic interplay between ascending and descending slope in each sleep cycle is strictly related to the sleep homeostatic regulation, i.e., the accumulation of sleep pressure (propensity) during waking and its dissipation during sleep [11, 12]. When the homeostatic

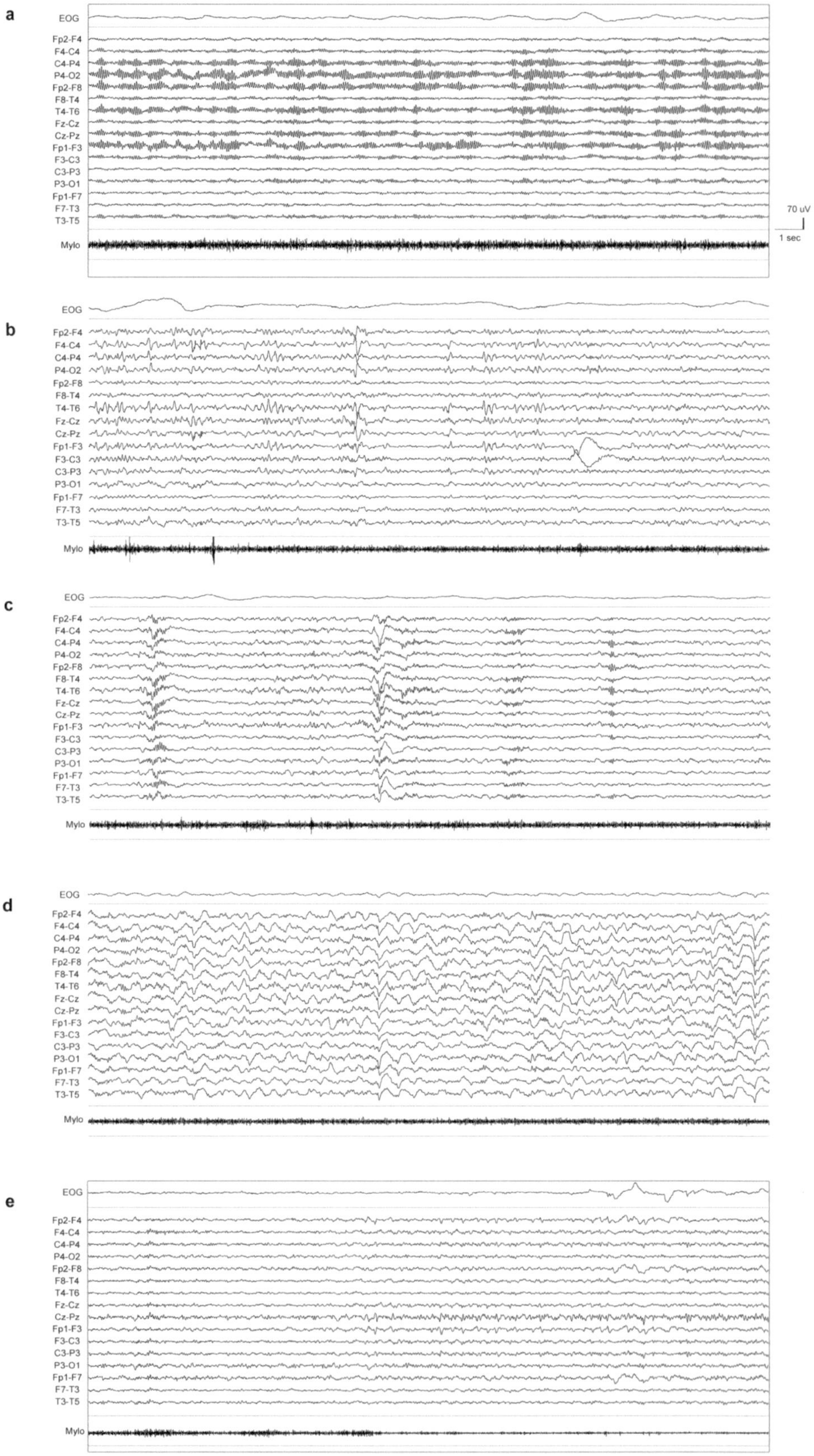

Fig. 10.3 Sleep stages. (**a**) stage W; (**b**) stage N1; (**c**) stage N2; (**d**) stage N3; (**e**) stage R. The representative EEG pages correspond to a time window of 30 s. EEG traces are displayed in bipolar montage. *EOG* electrooculogram. EMG derivation is represented by the activity of the mylohyoid muscle (mylo)

Table 10.2 General rules for sleep stages scoring

The following terminology should be used for the stages of sleep in adults	(a)	Stage W (wakefulness)
	(b)	Stage N1 (NREM1)
	(c)	Stage N2 (NREM2)
	(d)	Stage N3 (NREM3)
	(e)	Stage R (REM)
Score epochs using the following parameters	(a)	Score sleep stages in 30-s, subsequential epochs commencing at the start of the study
	(b)	Assign a stage to each epoch
	(c)	If two or more stages coexist during a single epoch, assign the stage comprising the greatest portion of the epoch
Score in accordance with the following definitions for EEG frequencies	(a)	Slow-wave activity: frequency of 0.5–2.0 Hz and minimum amplitude of 75 μV peak to peak in frontal derivations
	(b)	Delta waves are 0–3.99 Hz
	(c)	Theta waves are 4–7.99 Hz
	(d)	Alpha waves are 8–13 Hz
	(e)	Beta waves are greater than 13 Hz

pressure is high (that is during the descending slope of cycles), it drives the hypothalamic sleep-promoting neurons to high level of firing, which keeps the wake-promoting arousal system inhibited. This allows the thalamic burst-firing system to produce spindling and slow-wave oscillations that protect the continuity of sleep against arousals. When the homeostatic pressure decreases, the firing of the VLPO nucleus declines gradually, accompanying the sleeper to progressively higher levels of arousal along the ascending slopes of the sleep cycle preparing the next REM period [13]. Depending on the level of the homeostatic pressure, the same sensory input can elicit "traditional" arousal-like or sleep-like responses. A sleep-like response may be K-complexes, a series of K-complexes with spindles, or a sudden increase in slow-wave synchronization in deeper sleep [10]. From a functional point of view, the two slopes are essentially different, and apparently identical sleep stages are in fact not the same in descending and ascending slopes. Stage N2 during the descending slope differs from stage N2 sleep during the ascending one, reflecting the balance between sleep- and wake-promoting force at any point of the sleep cycle [10].

10.4 EEG Changes During Sleep, General Concepts

EEG changes during sleep might be of long duration (termed "tonic events") or transient (termed "phasic events"). The classical macrostructural dimension of sleep dynamics based on the 30-s epochs analysis mainly relates to the "tonic" events, i.e., the relatively long-lasting backgrounds patterns. Long periods of EEG desynchronization characterized REM sleep as well as wakefulness, while prolonged synchronization pattern occur during deep sleep, like stage N3. The microstructure of sleep refers to transient phenomena that occurs spontaneously or evoked. These events occur during specific parts of wakefulness or REM sleep (such as rapid eye movements) or during various stages of NREM sleep, being the classical hallmarks of sleep stages (as the occurrence of spindles and K-complex (KC) during N2). In addition, the cycling alternating pattern (CAP) framework provides a microcyclicity measure of NREM sleep representing an indicator of physiological and pathological sleep instability and playing a role in gating pathological and physiological sleep events. The CAP phases are built by variously combined EEG phasic events (KC, slow-wave activity). The distribution of transient sleep events across sleep, including CAP, seems to clearly follow the interplay of sleep- and wake/REM-promoting forces both within the individual cycles and through the whole night course, in association with the interactions of reciprocal antagonistic brain stem networks determining cortical responsiveness [14]. The following paragraphs describe in details the macrostructural and microstructural EEG elements of sleep, emphasizing their reciprocal relationships as a continuous evolving process that insures good sleep quality and contributes to a maintain individual brain resilience [13].

10.5 Sleep Onset

The onset of sleep under normal circumstances in healthy adults is through NREM sleep. This fundamental principle of normal human sleep reflects a highly reliable finding and is important in considering normal versus pathologic sleep. For example, the abnormal entry into sleep through REM sleep can be a diagnostic sign in adult patients with narcolepsy. According to the AASM manual, sleep onset is defined by the first epoch scored as any stage other than stage W (generally corresponding to the first epoch of stage N1) (Table 10.3). This approach, while is helpful to characterize the macrostructure of a 7–8 h of nocturnal EEG activity, is unsatisfactory for determining the microstructure of the sleep onset process. A common example is the waxing and waning of alpha activity just before and during stage N1. By just checking whether the percentage of alpha activity is over or under 50% (as required to distinguish stage W from N1), the scorer ignores potentially interesting micro-oscillations along the arousal continuum. The available tests that measure sleepiness or vigilance (as MSLT or maintenance of wakefulness test-MWT) are based on calculating the time to sleep onset, that is, according to official guidelines, as the first epoch of any sleep stage. However, this criterion could be too rigid or too permissive, making the test poorly

Table 10.3 AASM rules for sleep stages [3]

W	*Onset*: more del 50% of the epoch contains either one or both: 1. Alpha rhythm (posterior dominant rhythm) over the occipital region 2. Other findings consistent with stage W (all individuals) (i) Eye blinks (0.5–2 Hz) (ii) Rapid eye movements associated with normal or high chin muscle tone (iii) Reading eye movements *End:* transition to stage N1, N2. The earliest sign of drowsiness is the absence of eye blinks
N1	*Onset:* more del 50% of the epoch contains low-amplitude mixed-frequency EEG (LAMF) and/or the appearance of any of the following phenomena: (a) EEG activity in range of 4–7 Hz with slowing of background frequencies by ≥1 Hz from those of stage W (b) Vertex sharp waves (c) Slow eye movements *End*: transition to stage W, N2, and R
N2	*Onset*: co-occurrence of: (a) delta waves must not exceed the 20% of the epoch (b) either or both the following occur during the first half of that epoch or the last half of the previous epoch: 1. One or more K-complexes unassociated with arousals 2. One or more sleep spindles *End*: transition to stage W, N3, R, an arousal followed LAMF (stage N1), or a major body movement followed by LAMF and slow eye movement (SEM)
N3	*Onset*: ≥20% of an epoch consists of SWA irrespective of age *End*: transition to stage W, N2, N1, R
R	*Onset*: co-occurrence of: (a) low-amplitude LAMF activity without K-complexes or spindles; (b) low chin EMG tone (no higher than in any other sleep stage and usually at the lowest level of the entire recording) for the majority of the epoch; (c) rapid eye movements (REMs) at any position within the epoch *End*: one of the following: (a) transition to stage W or N3; (b) increase in chin EMG tone above the level of stage R for the majority of the epoch and criteria for stage N1 are met; (c) occurrence of an arousal or a major body movement followed by LAMF and SEM (score the epoch as stage N1); (d) one or more non-arousal-associated K-complexes or sleep spindles in the first half of the epoch in the absence of REMs, even if chin EMG tone remains low (score the epoch as stage N2)
Arousal	Arousal during sleep stages N1, N2, N3, or R if there is an abrupt shift of EEG frequency, including alpha, theta, and/or frequencies greater than 16 Hz (but not spindles) that lasts at least 3 s, with at least 10 s of stable sleep preceding the change. Scoring of arousal during REM requires a concurrent increase in submental EMG lasting at least 1 s

sensitive or specific. It can be argued that a brief "micro-sleep" intruding into wake state cannot be considered as unequivocal sleep; by counterpart, it has been demonstrated that performances, as driving reaction time, may be altered in drowsiness state, before definite sleep onset [15]. Light drowsiness represents a specific brain state. Neurophysiological studies have demonstrated event-related potentials peculiarities during light drowsiness [16], and both altered inter- and intrahemispheric EEG coherence when compared with wakefulness, suggesting that cerebral functional organization changes during light drowsiness [17, 18]. While physiological and behavioral features show large intersubjective variability and ambiguity, analysis of EEG seems to be the most reliable method with respect to detection of sleep onset. In adults, the earliest indication of transition from wakefulness to stage N1 usually consists of a combination of dropout of alpha activity and slow rolling eye movements (Fig. 10.4). The alpha waves are replaced by low-voltage slow activity, mainly in the range of 2–7 Hz. In late infancy and early childhood, drowsiness is characterized by typical diffuse 4–6 Hz rhythmic theta activity (hypnagogic hypersynchrony), while later in childhood and, in many cases, in the declining years of life, the onset of drowsiness is characterized by greater amounts of slow activity mingling with the posterior alpha rhythm. An electroencephalographically defined drowsy state does not exist in the neonate, and, in elderly, abrupt transitions from wakefulness to light sleep are quite common. Deepening of drowsiness is associated with enhancement of slow activity. At this stage, arousing stimuli lead to immediate return of the posterior alpha rhythm, called "paradoxical alpha response" [19]. When alpha rhythm is reactivated in deep drowsiness or in NREM sleep, the maximum is usually frontal rather than occipital named "short microarousals."

10.6 Deep Drowsiness (Stage N1 Sleep)

Following the AASM scoring rules (Table 10.3), stage N1 (Fig. 10.3, panel b) is defined by the attenuation of the alpha rhythm and the occurrence of low-amplitude, mixed-frequency activity (defined as low-amplitude, predominantly 4–7 Hz activity) for more than 50% of the epoch. Burst of relatively high-voltage very synchronous theta activity is

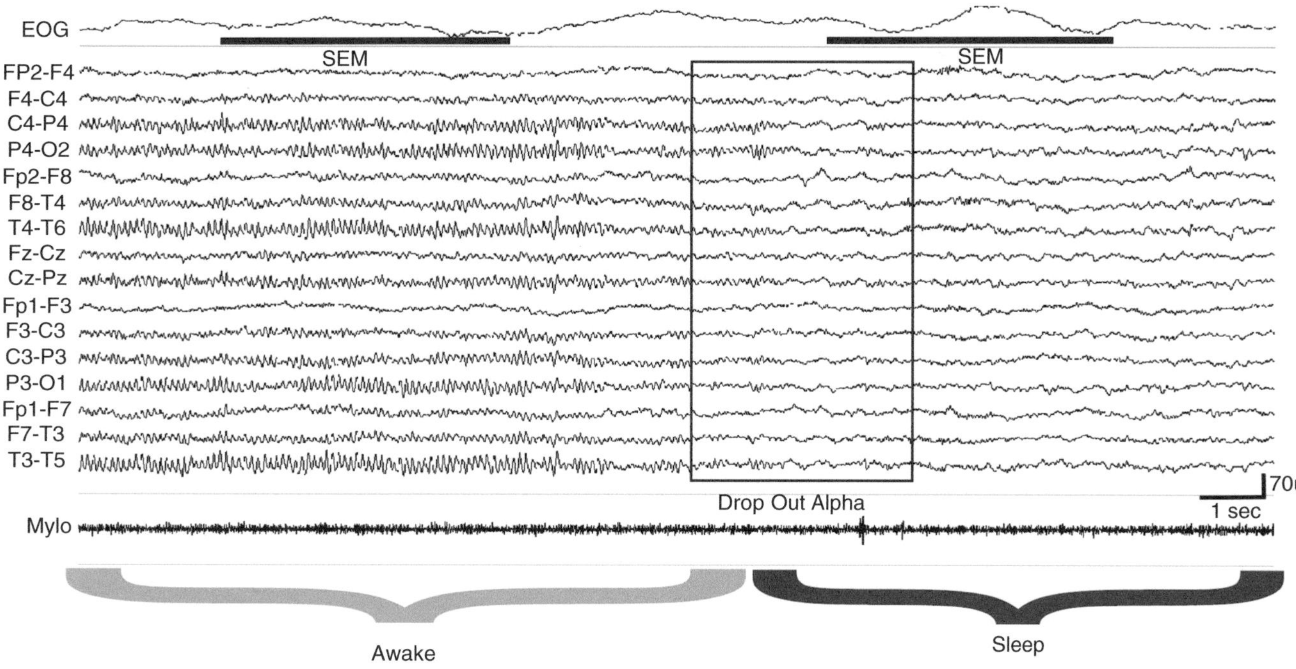

Fig. 10.4 The sleep onset. Representative EEG showing the combination of the alpha rhythm dropout and SEM, thus indicating the sleep onset. EEG traces are displayed in bipolar montage. *EOG* electrooculogram. EMG derivation is represented by the activity of the mylohyoid muscle (mylo)

common during the onset of N1 in children and young adolescent. Slow eye movements (SEM) commonly precede the EEG transition from W to N1. Although the onset of SEM usually leads the EEG transition by only 1 or 2 min, the lead time may occasionally—particularly during daytime sleep—be as long as 15 min. SEM are very useful to distinguish stage N1 transition occurring during stage N2 or R sleep.

The characteristic neurophysiologic elements of this stage, but not mandatory to N1 scoring, are vertex sharp waves and positive occipital sharp transients of sleep.

10.6.1 Vertex Sharp Waves (V Wave)

V wave (VWs): Vertex Sharply contoured waves with duration <0.5 s maximal over the central region and distinguishable from the background activity [3].

Vertex sharp waves (also named "vertex waves," "V waves," "vertex sharp transients," or "vertex spikes") are sharply contoured compounded electroencephalographic potentials characterized by a main negative component, preceded and followed by brief and low-voltage positive components. VWs are 50–200 ms long, with a variable voltage (until 250 μV) and a maximal topographic expression over the central region, often with a phase opposition on median derivations (Fig. 10.5, panel a). They are typically bilateral and symmetric, but they may show also asymmetries, especially in children or in pathological conditions [20, 21]. VWs may appear as isolated events, clearly standing out over the background activity, or they can occur in repetitive salvos firing at a range of about 1/s or faster. VWs usually appear in deep drowsiness/stage N1 and may persist during stage N2.

It is generally accepted that VWs are comparable to different sensory modalities evoked potentials, presenting analogies to evoked acoustic responses in wake state, which have maximum expression on vertex areas. The most common neurophysiological interpretation is that VWs are either a direct response to an external stimulus or a mechanism to maintain sleep (indirect response) after a stimulus [22]. This is similar to the common understanding of the K-complex and is based on the evidence that both VWs and K-complexes may be elicited by sudden stimulation irrespective of the sensory modality. In neurophysiologic studies, VWs have been associated with the N300 and N350 evoked potential responses [22, 23]. MEG and fMRI studies have attempted to determine the sources of these distinct waveforms and have found that the maximum amplitude of vertex waves localized over midline areas of the cortex [24–26]. In particular, VWs represent the activity of integrated functional system mainly involving the sensory-motor cortices

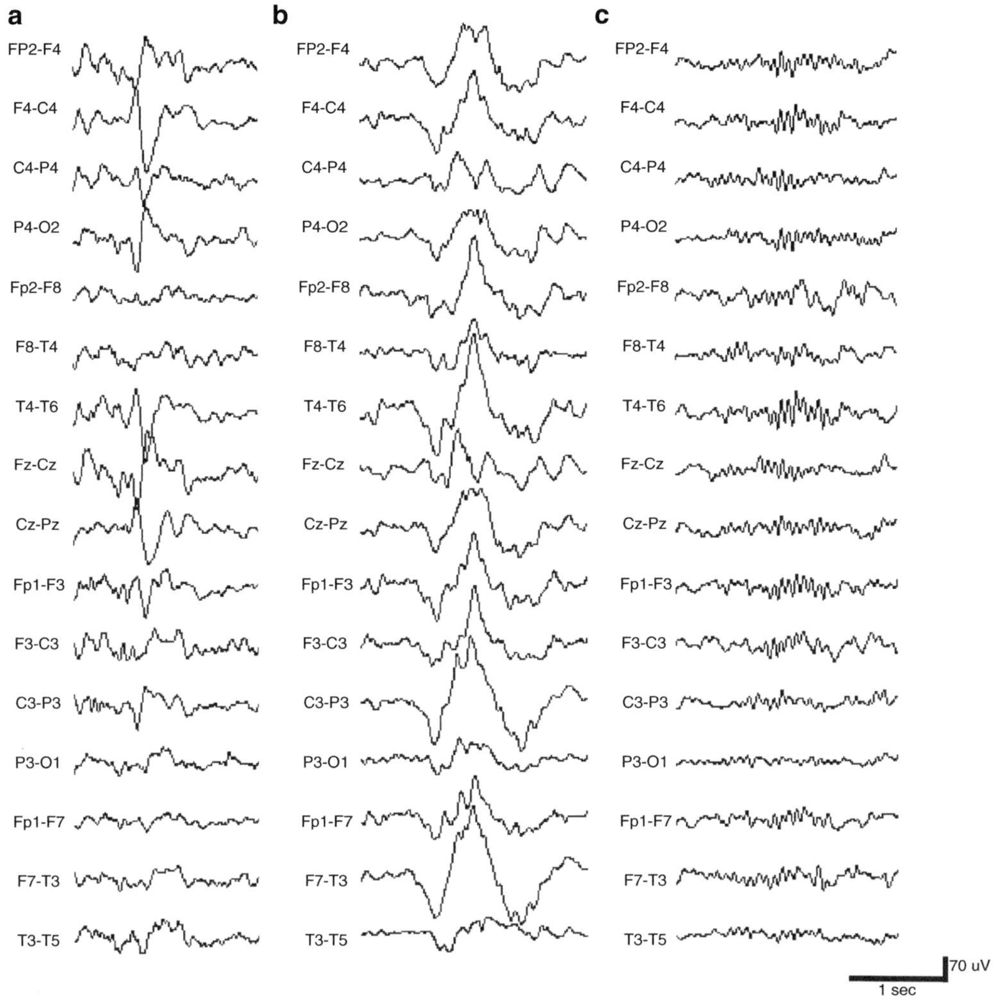

Fig. 10.5 Representative examples of vertex waves (panel **a**), K-complex (panel **b**), sleep spindles (panel **c**) recorded during sleep. EEG traces are displayed in bipolar montage

(probably the generator) and the posterior medial regions (medial occipital cortices). Interestingly, no thalamic involvement was documented with fMRI [26].

10.6.1.1 Vertex Sharp Waves Across the Life Span

VWs may occur as infrequent broad components by 6 months of age but are seen as prominent elements around 16 months, becoming sharper with a shorter duration by 24 months and repetitive by 30 months [27, 28] (Fig.10.6). VWs expression is maximal between 2 and 12 years, when they show a greater amplitude, longer duration, and a more frontal expression. In school-age children, vertex waves may show moderate amplitude asymmetries with asymmetrical spread into the vicinity. Under these circumstances, the physiologic vertex activity may be confused with cerebral rolandic spikes. Rolandic spikes, usually picked up by electrodes C3 or C4 over central areas, may occasionally arise from the vertex itself. When such a coexistence of vertex potentials exists, the physiologic vertex waves are usually of longer duration and of somewhat higher voltage than the abnormal spikes [21]. Vertex waves may become small and inconspicuous in aged individuals and are often poorly demonstrable in such persons.

10.6.2 POSTs (Positive Occipital Sharp Transients of Sleep)

POSTs are an EEG activity of deep drowsiness and sleep, characterized by positive spike-like waves localized on occipital areas, mainly in theta range. POSTs are often bilateral and synchronous but may be also asymmetrical [29] (Fig. 10.7).

POSTs are not strictly connected to a specific sleep stage. These elements appear mostly during superficial sleep and may persist during deep sleep, but they are practically absent in REM.

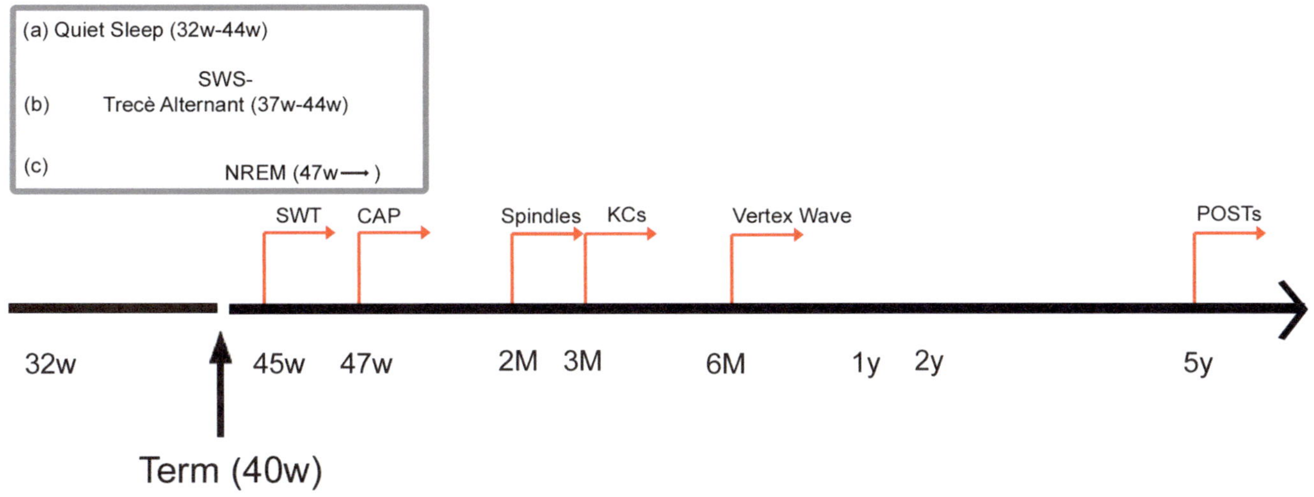

Fig. 10.6 Schematic diagram of temporal evolution of main neurophysiological features of sleep in infancy. The grey box indicates periods of appearance of main behavioral stages: (**a**) Quiet sleep (QS) is commonly described from 32nd postconceptional weeks until the 44th and is characterized by long-lasting bursts of large amplitude delta activity; (**b**) *Tracé alternant* pattern alternated with high amplitude delta activity starts after the 37th postconceptional age. The *Tracé alternant* is defined as bursts of slow waves, sometimes mixed with sharp waves, alternating with periods of relative quiescence; from the 44th to the 47th postconceptional week, the QS shows important changes that foreshadows to the sleep stages appearance: *tracé alternant* disappears as the proportion of slow waves increases, and the term "slow-wave sleep" (SWS) can be used. Further categorization of sleep states into the stages of sleep becomes possible. (**c**) From the 47th postconceptional age, NREM sleep, similar to the one structured in adults, occurs. The red arrows indicate the age of appearance of the main sleep phasic features. *POSTs* positive occipital sharp transients of sleep, *CAP* cycling alternating pattern, *KCs* K-complexes, *SWS* slow-wave sleep, *w* weeks, *y* year

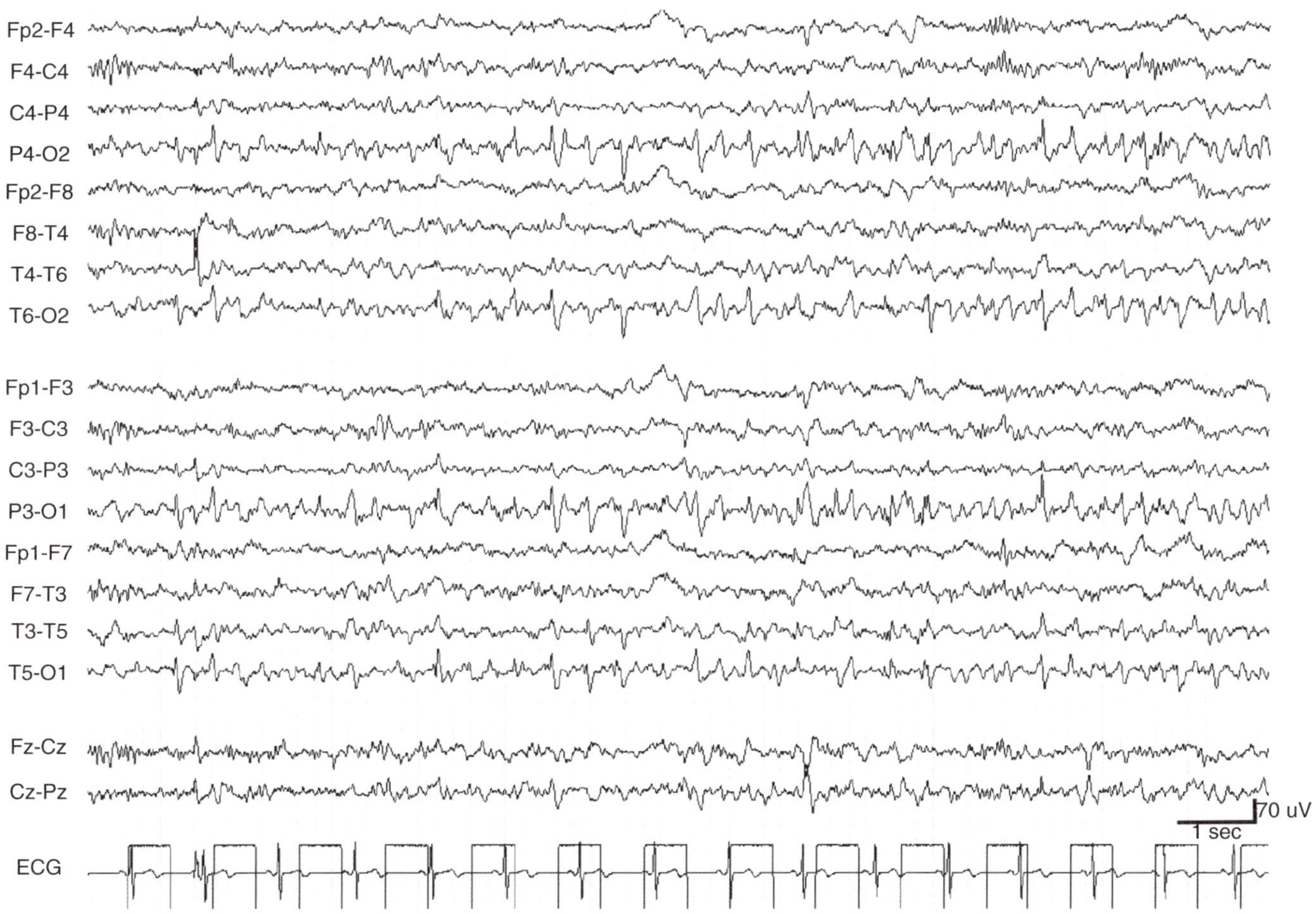

Fig. 10.7 POSTs. Representative EEG page showing bilateral POSTs in N2. Note the presence of frequent sub-continuous positive spike-like waves and theta activity localized on the parieto-occipital and temporo-occipital areas. EEG is displayed in bipolar montage

POSTs are not consistently established before 5 years of age (Fig. 10.6), although they may be prominent in some children from about 3 years. This pattern is most commonly found in adolescents and young adults, whereas their prevalence declines in elderly, with a slight female prevalence [30].

Although POSTs have anecdotally been correlated to various abnormal conditions [31, 32], they are generally considered as a normal variant of physiological sleep EEG activity, and their real significance remain uncertain. It has been hypnotized that POSTs may be related to visual function, representing a "playback" of visual information collected during the day [33].

The connection to visual activity is also supported by their absence in blind or severely amblyopic people [34] and by the similarities of these potentials to lambda waves, a posterior EEG activity during wakefulness elicited by visual exploration or by looking geometric patterns.

10.7 Light Sleep (Stage N2 Sleep)

Stage N2 is characterized by the appearance of peculiar EEG figures (K-complex and spindles) standing over a background activity mainly constituted by medium voltage theta and delta activity (Fig. 10.3, panel c). Beside slow-frequency background activities, fast frequencies are often observed in N2 in the range of 15–30 Hz even in unsedated patients with no history of chronic intake of sedatives. AASM rules for scoring N2 sleep are summarized in the Table 10.3.

10.7.1 K-Complexes

> *K-complex*: A well-delineated, negative, sharp wave immediately followed by a positive component standing out from the background EEG, with total duration ≥0.5 seconds, usually maximal in amplitude when recorded using frontal derivations. For an arousal to be associated with a K-complex, the arousal must either be concurrent with the K-complex or commence no more than 1 second after termination of the K-complex [3].

K-complexes (KCs) were discovered in the early 1930s by Loomis and colleagues [35], as electric potentials both evoked by auditory stimuli (knocking on the door of the experimental chamber, thus the letter "K" in the name of these elements) and spontaneous. KCs are characterized by an initial biphasic (and not seldom multiphasic) sharp positive component followed by a slow negative wave, often mixed with superimposed final fast components (12–14 Hz sleep spindles) (Fig. 10.5, panel b). The slow component may exceed 1000 ms in duration, and its length and degree of prominence depend on filter setting. KCs are >0.5 s in duration and >75 μV in amplitude and show a frontal prominence, just like the rest of sleep slow-wave activity [36]; they can occur isolated or grouped in series. When KCs are averaged, the peaks of positive and negative waveforms are seen as P200, N550, and P900 components in the averaged event-related potential (ERP), with the N550 and P900 components typically largest over frontal electrode sites. Because the N550 amplitude can be in excess of 100 μV, it is thought to reflect the synchronized activity of a large number of cortical neurons [37] and has been hypothesized to reflect cortical integrity [38].

10.7.1.1 KC Across the Life Span

KCs appear during the same age span of spindles (3–6 months) (Fig. 10.6), becoming larger in older children and in early adolescence and showing a progressive reduction in amplitude and frequency in elderly. The frequency of KCs decreases from cycle to cycle, parallel with the decrease in the depth of sleep [39].

The underlying cellular mechanism of K-complexes is based on a slow (<1 Hz) oscillation of cortical neurons associated with fluctuations of the membrane potential between a depolarized and hyperpolarized level [40] very similar to the up- and downstates of below 1 Hz sleep slow oscillations [10].

The physiological significance of KCs has been the subject of significant debate. On the one side, KCs are arousal-related phenomena being supported by accompanying activation patterns such as an increase of heart rate and phasic increases in muscle tone. However, the fact that KCs activity mirrors other slow waves in NREM sleep supports the idea that KC is a promoter of sleep [10, 13, 41].

10.7.1.2 KC as Arousal Phenomena

KCs can be elicited by sensory stimuli [42], are associated with signs of autonomic activation [43], and are sometimes followed by an EEG arousal. These evidences suggest that they may be functionally related to arousal systems. Several studies have shown that KCs can be elicited by any sensory modality but with different cortical activation patterns, depending on the type of stimulation [37, 42, 44–46]. In 2014, Laurino and colleagues [47] identified the topological/dynamic features of evoked KCs depending on stimulus modality or local cortical properties. The earliest wave (the initial positive element of the K-complex, also called P200) was topographically located on the stimulation-related primary sensory areas; this potential acts as traveling cortical excitation that elicits a bistable cortical response, appearing on the EEG as a biphasic slow wave over fronto-central regions (the giant negative deflection (N550) and the subsequent positive one (P900), respectively, reflecting downstate and upstate of <1 Hz oscillations), depending on the reactivity of cortex in different NREM sleep levels. In their conclusion the authors confirm the KC's Janus-faced dual properties: on the one hand, they are evoked by an input-related cortical excitation, and on the other hand, they represent an induced, cortical slow wave in the fronto-central region.

10.7.1.3 KC as Slow Wave

Some features of KCs are common with slow waves, the hallmark of sleep homeostasis. As slow-wave sleep (SWS), frequencies of KCs tend to decrease in stage N2 from evening to morning and from cycle to cycle [39] and show a rebound effect elicited by sleep deprivation [48]. The amplitude of KCs is proportional to the depth of the sleep cycle in which it is measured [49]. Furthermore, the decreasing trend of number, amplitude, and density during aging is similar in KCs and in SWS and reflects the progressive reduction of cortical thickness [38, 50, 51].

10.7.2 Sleep Spindles

> *Sleep spindle*: A train of distinct waves with frequency 11–16 Hz (most commonly 12–14 Hz) with a duration ≥0.5 s, usually maximal in amplitude in the central derivations [3].

Spindles are defined as waxing-and-waning EEG waves oscillating at a frequency of 11–16 Hz and predominant over central EEG derivations; spindles characterize NREM N2 but can also be found during NREM N3 (Fig. 10.5, panel c). Spindles are discrete events, a feature that distinguishes them from spindling activity (i.e., the continuous EEG activity between 11 and 16 Hz, often reported as the EEG power in this frequency band). Minimum spindle's duration is set to 0.5 s, while no maximal duration value has been proposed. The spindle frequency range is typically between 11 and 16 Hz, although some authors report much slower (9–10 Hz [52, 53]) and faster (18 Hz [54]) spindles. Furthermore, (at least) two types of spindles are reported in humans: late slow frontal (9–12 Hz) and early fast centro-parietal (13–15 Hz) spindles (reviewed in [55]). This dichotomy was reported in various EEG and MEG studies [53, 56, 57] but also with functional magnetic resonance imaging (fMRI) [58] and after pharmacological manipulation [59]. This distinction, based on the spindle time onset, frequency, and topography, also corresponds to different relationships with sleep cycling. The first spindle trains show a frequency around 14 Hz, while the 12 Hz spindles appears a little later with deepening sleep although the patient is still in N2. With deepening sleep (at the transition between N2 and N3), an even slower spindle occurs (around 10 Hz) with maximum topography over the frontal leads. This activity is likely to be a forerunner of rhythmic discharges in the 6–10 Hz range, which is commonly observed in N3.

Fast centro-parietal and slow frontal spindles reflect the involvement of different neocortical regions [53]. Fast centro-parietal spindles reflect a more local synchronization mainly constrained to the thalamus, precentral/premotor cortices, and hippocampus, while late slow frontal spindles are the results of a more global brain synchronization [58]. These findings suggest the presence of multiple generator areas for spindles in humans and support the notion that sleep arises from activities of local circuits [53]. On average fast centro-parietal spindles precede slow frontal spindles by 200–500 ms; timing differences among cortical spindles reflect propagation along the thalamic reticural nucleus (RE).

The neurophysiological mechanisms of spindle generation reflect the intrinsic properties and interactions between inhibitory cells in the RE and bursting thalamocortical (TC) relay neurons. According to the model of Steriade [40], sleep spindles rhythm is initiated in GABAergic thalamic reticular neurons, which impose onto thalamocortical neurons rhythmic inhibitory postsynaptic potentials, thus de-inactivating a low-threshold Ca2+ current, which promotes burst firing. These bursts are transferred to the cortex that is responsible of generating rhythmic excitatory postsynaptic potentials at spindles' frequency. Spindle generation involves inhibition of thalamocortical afferents, hence suggesting that they constitute the stones of loss of responsiveness to external stimuli observed during NREM sleep. The "sensory gate" notion assigned to the thalamus and mediated by the spindles confers a useful role of spindling bursts to preserve sleep continuity by inhibiting sensory inputs [13].

10.7.2.1 Sleep Spindles Across the Life Span

Mature sleep spindles usually appear during the second month of life (for review, see [60] [Fig. 10.6]). Before that time, the dominant EEG pattern spindle-like activity is termed "delta brushes" seen in premature infants and in utero. They consist of spindle-like oscillations of 8–20 Hz, riding on top of delta (0.3–1.5 Hz) waves. These oscillations can occur during any stage (sleep or waking); however, as the brain matures, they become restricted to sleep. Spindles are initially seen over central areas of the brain and gradually develop over frontotemporal areas during the first year of life [61]. During adolescence, density reaches a relative maximum with equal distribution across frontal, central, and parietal leads. In aging, there is a return to the same pattern seen earlier in development, with highest density at central leads. Spindles are most impressive in childhood and adolescence; their voltage tends to become smaller throughout adulthood. In old age, spindles of low voltage are very common; this is probably not due to old age alone but to cerebrovascular disease. Sleep spindles share this decline of voltage with vertex and K-complexes as age advances. Spindles have been reported to be more frequent in women than in men [62].

10.7.2.2 Spindles and Slow-Wave Activity (SWA)

With respect to slow waves, spindles tend to occur preferentially at upstates [40, 63]. Given that slow waves propagate from prefrontal cortex toward posterior regions [64, 65], and spindles occur sooner in posterior regions (see above), the result is that frontal spindles occur later during slow-wave upstates.

In stage N3 when SWA is maximal, spindle density is reduced. In early NREM sleep, when SWA is highest, spindle density and spindle frequency are significantly lower. Moreover, spindle density and frequency are lower in the middle of NREM cycles when SWA is maximal and higher toward the transition to REM sleep when SWA tapers off.

10.8 Deep Sleep (Stage N3 Sleep)

Stage N3 (slow-wave sleep or deep sleep) represents the sum of previous stage S3 and stage S4 of Rechtschaffen and Kales (R&K) nomenclature. The hallmark of this stage is the so-called slow-wave activity (SWA), formed by high-voltage slow waves of delta frequency, between 0.5 and 2 Hz measured over the frontal regions (Fig.10.3, panel d). The frequency range of SWA is not universally defined as for different authors it is considered between 0.5 and 4.5 Hz [21, 64, 66]. AASM rules for scoring N3 stage are summarized in the Table 10.3. In previous R&Ks scoring rules, deep sleep was divided in two different stages, depending on the percentage of the epoch dominated by SWA (20–50%, stage S3; ≥50%, stage S4) (Fig.10.8). Sleep spindles may persist during stage N3, but they become less relevant; also KC may be present, whereas eye movements are not usual. Chin EMG is often lower than in light sleep. Small sharp transients may be superimposed on the slope of a slow wave, forming a pattern recalling a mitten, with a "thumb section," represented by the sharp component and a "hand section" formed by the subsequent slow wave. The "Mitten pattern" can only be recorded with a monopolar referential montage during relatively deep sleep stages. This activity is usually prevalent over the frontal and central regions and is considered a normal variant [21]. Another physiological EEG pattern is called "alpha sleep pattern," and it typically reaches its maximum in stage N3. It is characterized by rhythmical 7–11 Hz activity, often combined with slow delta activity, prevalent over the frontal leads. The alpha sleep pattern must be differentiated from alpha-delta sleep, a pattern associated with delta sleep deficit and often noted in patients with fibromyalgia [67], chronic fatigue syndrome [68], and depressive disorders [69]. By contrast, the alpha sleep pattern has been found to be associated with a stable sleep organization [70].

10.8.1 Slow-Wave Activity (SWA)

> *Slow-wave activity*: Waves of frequency 0.5–2 Hz and peak-topeak amplitude >75 μV, measured over the frontal regions referenced to the contralateral ear or mastoid (F4-M1, F3-M2) [3].

Slow waves are the surface-EEG visible epiphenomenon of slow (<1 Hz) oscillations in membrane potential of cortical neurons, alternating between a hyperpolarization phase (*downstate*), when virtually all cortical neurons remain silent for a few hundred milliseconds, and a subsequent depolarization phase (*upstate*) when neurons fire at high rate, more than in quiet wakefulness [71, 72]. This phenomenon is due to intrinsic currents and intracortical network interactions [73–76] depending on the function of the cerebral cortex alone [71, 73, 77, 78].

The slow oscillations occur during any stage of NREM sleep with an increasing rate as sleep deepens [64]; the sporadic oscillations occurring during light sleep (stages N1–N2) seem to correspond to K-complexes, whereas during deep sleep, they are related to slow waves in the frequency <1 Hz. The spatiotemporal dynamics of these oscillations are the same regardless the sleep stage, supporting the theory about a continuum of reactive sleep EEG elements (i.e., transient phenomena which may occur both spontaneously and evoked by sensory stimuli) like vertex waves, KC, and SWA [10]. During the first phases of light sleep (stages N1 and N2), an acoustic stimulus may evoke vertex waves (comparable to an amplified acoustic evoked potential—N350). From stage N2 the stimulus may elicit a KC, characterized by a first element comparable to a residue of evoked potential (P200) followed by a SW (N550 and P900). In deepening of sleep, the response becomes more complex and nonspecific (as SW activity configuring CAP A1 phases—see below). This theory is consistent with recent EEG-fMRI findings [26, 79, 80] and HdEEG studies [47, 81].

Slow-wave oscillation during sleep thus represents the fundamental stone by which the sleep process builds its proper rhythms. Using high-density electroencephalogram recordings in humans, Massimini and colleagues [64] have shown that each wave originates at a definite site and travels over the scalp at an estimated speed of 1.2–7.0 m/s. Waves originate more frequently in prefrontal- orbitofrontal regions and propagate in an anteroposterior direction. Each slow

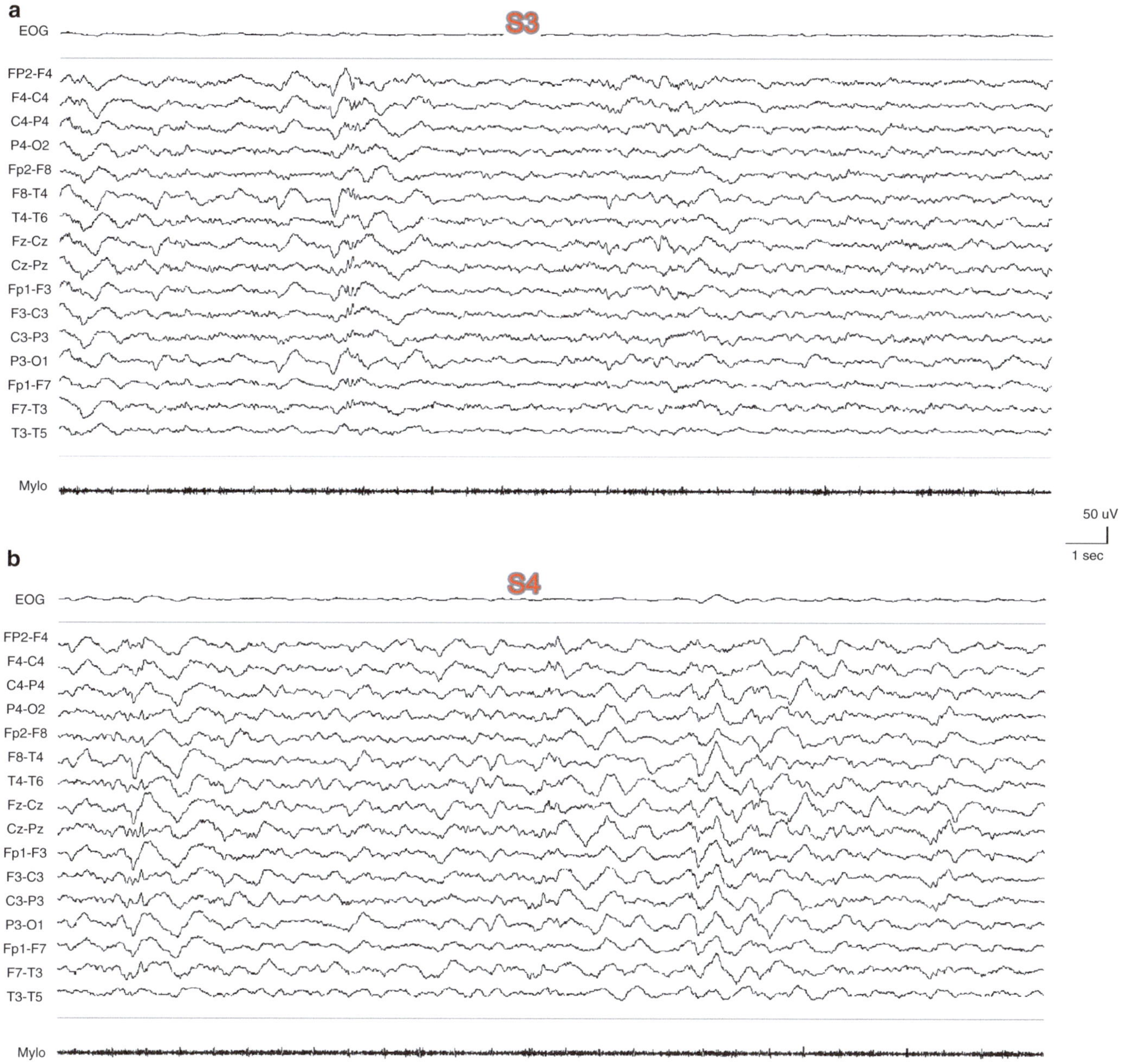

Fig. 10.8 Representative EEG pages of deep human sleep. According to the Rechtschaffen and Kales scoring rules, deep sleep was divided in two different stages (actually founded in a single stage N3), depending on the percentage of the epoch dominated by SWA (20–50%: stage S3, panel **a**; ≥50%: stage S4, panel **b**). EEGs are displayed in bipolar montage. *EOG* electrooculogram. EMG derivation is represented by the activity of the mylohyoid muscle (mylo)

oscillation starts small and becomes progressively larger and finally dissolves, suggesting that an initial small depolarizing event involves a progressively wider population of neurons through cortico-cortical connections, as it extends through the cortex.

The amount of SWA is related to sleep pressure and homeostatic regulation of sleep, increasing in function of previous wake and returning to baseline during sleep. It has been proposed that, in adults, the homeostatic decline of SWA along consecutive sleep cycles is related to a progressive reduction in synaptic strength, which is thought to increase during wakefulness due to learning processes and decrease during sleep through a sleep-dependent process of synaptic downscaling, leading to restoration of energy and space resources [11, 12, 82]. Computered models [83], studies of LFP rats recordings [84] and of human EEG [81], have been demonstrated that these well-established sleep pressure-related modifications in SWA during the course of sleep are not limited to a decrease of the total number of SW but they are associated with changes in specific electrophysiologic parameters of the individual slow waves. In particular, compared to a relative small reduction of the density of slow waves (i.e., the total number of SW/hour of sleep), there is a more relevant decrease of high-amplitude SW and of the slope of SW, as well as an increase in waves with multiple peaks [81, 85].

10.8.1.1 SWA Across the Life Span

SWA undergoes remarkable changes during development that parallel the time course of cortical maturation. In studies including children and adolescents, the topographical distribution of SWA was analyzed with scalp and high-density electroencephalography [86, 87]. The results showed age-dependent differences in SWA topography: SWA was highest over posterior regions during early childhood and then shifted over central derivations to the frontal cortex in late adolescence [88]. This trajectory of SWA topography matches the course of cortical gray maturation [86].

The SW delta activity (total SW counts, amplitude, and slope) decreases with aging starting from adolescence [89]. Homeostatic sleep regulation seems however unaffected in adolescence [88]. In adults, significant reduction of SWA prosecutes, and this SWA impairment becomes especially prominent in older adults (for review, see [66]). The maximal age-related decrements in absolute SWA are observed over the prefrontal cortex (PFC) derivations and in the first NREM sleep cycles, with reductions of 75–80% on average relative to young adults.

10.9 REM Sleep

REM sleep is the third major physiological state of vigilance, beside wakefulness and NREM sleep. REM sleep is characterized by rapid eye movements associated with a decreased amplitude of EEG activity, similar to that seen during wakefulness and a loss of muscle tone. The co-occurrence of an EEG signal similar to that of the waking state and a behavior of unresponsiveness leaded to the term of "paradoxical sleep." In the course of the decades, REM sleep has also been called "activated sleep" or, for the evidence that subjects awakened from REM sleep reported usually vivid dreams, "dream sleep." REM sleep is defined by the co-occurrence of electroencephalographic, electrooculographic, and electromyographic characteristics. Therefore, REM sleep should be assessed certainly only with polygraphic methods. Whenever the electroencephalographer must search specifically for REM periods, attention must be laid on the use of two channels for electrooculography (two additional canthus electrodes, connected to the ears), one channel for cutaneous electromyography (submental region) and a thermocouple or strain gauge for pneumographic documentation [21]. Nevertheless, even in routinely EEG recordings (without oculographic leads), electroencephalographs can recognize the REM sleep occurrence being the ocular potentials mostly quite impressive and almost always leading to marked eye movement artifacts in frontopolar and anterior temporal leads [90].

Background activity during REM is low-amplitude, polyrhythmic, and mixed-frequency characterized by fast activity and a small amount of 3–7 Hz theta rhythms, usually similar to that seen in stage N1, with trains of "Sawtooth waves" (SWTs) as superimposed rhythm (Table 10.3; Fig. 10.3, panel e). Sequences of alpha activity, 1–2 Hz slower than during wakefulness, are common. The first REM phase of the night is often shorter than those seen in the last part of the sleep time, and it can be characterized by a mixture of REM and sleep spindles and/or K-complexes. The typical hallmarks of REM stage are the occurrence of rapid eye movements (REMs), low chin EMG tone, and sawtooth waves (SWTs) (Fig.10.9).

REMs: Conjugate, irregular, sharply peaked eye movements with an initial deflection usually lasting <500 ms.
Low chin EMG tone: Baseline EMG activity in the chin derivation no higher than in any other sleep stage and usually at the lowest level of the entire recording.
SWTs: Trains of sharply contoured or triangular, often serrated, 2–6 Hz waves maximal in amplitude over the central head regions and often, but not always, preceding a burst of rapid eye movements [3].

10.9.1 SWTs (Sawtooth Waves)

STWs were first described by Jouvet et al. [91] and Berger et al. [92] decades ago, but their source and neurophysiologic meaning have not been defined yet. STWs are bursts of sharply contoured or triangular, often serrated, surface positive waves, in the frequency range of 2–6 Hz, with an amplitude comprised between 20 and 100 μV. These waves are bilateral and symmetrical, and widely distributed over the scalp, but maximal in amplitude over the central or frontal areas [93, 94] appearing at about 5 weeks of age [95] (Fig. 10.6). STWs' mean density seem to be lower during the first REM period compared to subsequently sleep cycles [96]. STWs' trains are correlated with other phasic events of REM sleep, usually following transient muscle activities and preceding/occurring in conjunction with bursts of rapid ocular movements [97–99]. Despite the prevalence of STWs over the vertex, animal models sug-

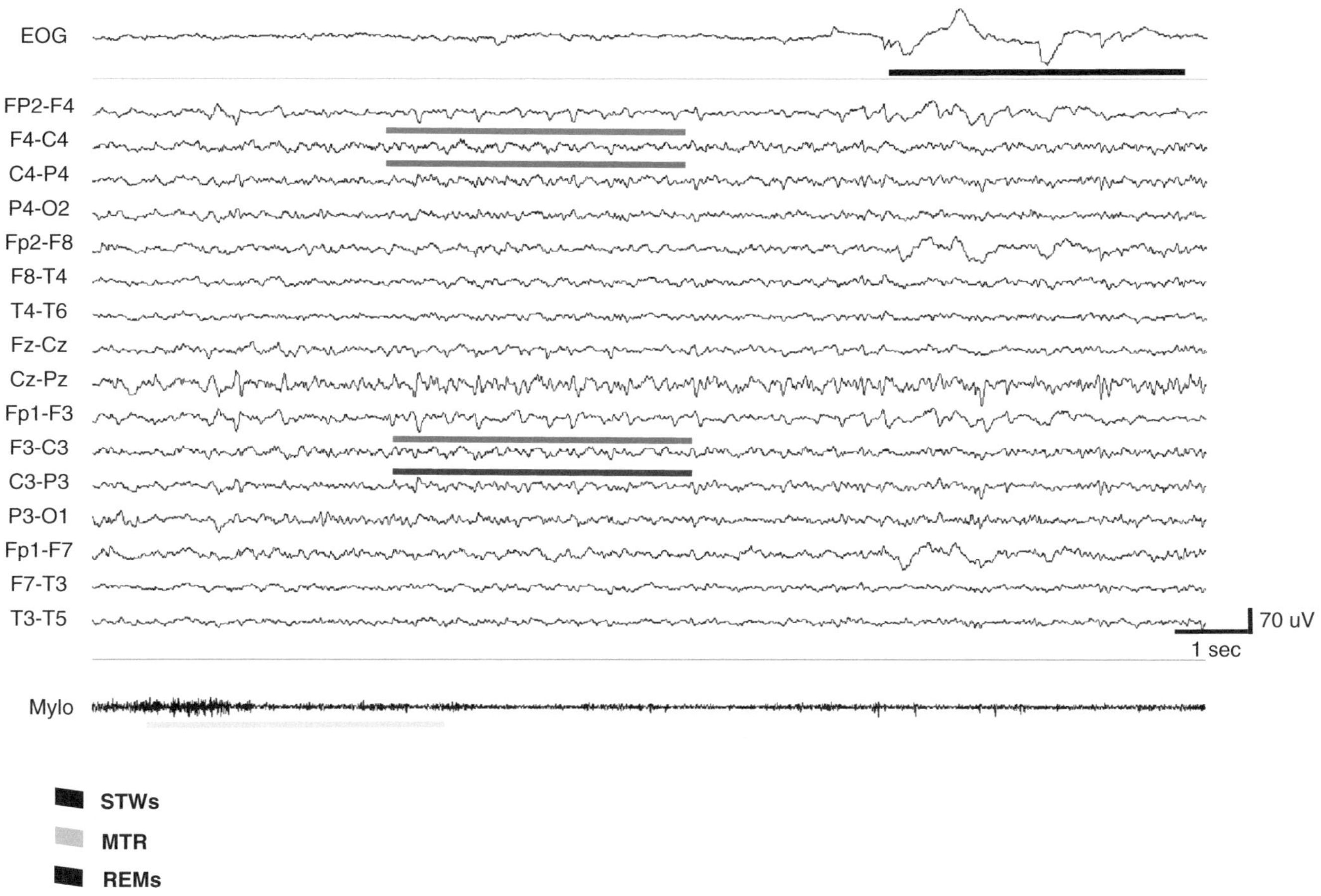

Fig. 10.9 REM sleep. Note the 2.5 Hz notched waves, prominent in F3-C3, F4-C4, Fp1-F3, Fp2-F4 occurring before REMs. The characteristic sequence of MTR, SWT, and REMs at the onset of stage REM is demonstrated. *MTR* muscle tone reduction, *SWT* sawtooth waves, *REMs* rapid eye movements. EEG is displayed in bipolar montage. *EOG* electrooculogram. EMG derivation is represented by the activity of the mylohyoid muscle (mylo)

gested that STWs are possibly related to ponto-geniculo-occipital spikes, a potential related to REM sleep and documented only in animals, originating in the pons, involving the lateral geniculate nucleus, and terming over the occipital regions [100]. This relationship is consistent with the evidence that in patients affected by brainstem pathologies as post-polio syndrome [101] or vegetative states [102], abnormalities in STWs have been documented. Surprisingly, however, anomalies in STW have been demonstrated also in supratentorial disorders as hemispheric stroke [103] and temporal lobe epilepsy [104].

10.10 Microstructure of Sleep and the Cyclic Alternating Pattern (CAP)

The 30 s epoch scoring confers a stepwise outline to the sleep histogram characterized by periods of static configuration (sleep stages) interrupted by rapid shifts (stage changes). This method of scoring neglects short-duration events lasting less than the scoring epoch, although such events also carry important information. Transient EEG phenomena have been described within the sleep recordings allowing identification of what is known as the microstructure of sleep [105, 106]. These brief phenomena are related to the sleep instability and arousals.

According to the AASM definition (Table 10.3), arousal is defined as an abrupt shift of EEG frequency including alpha, theta, and/or frequencies greater than 16 Hz (but not spindles). It can be accompanied by an increase of electromyographic activity and of cardiac frequency or by body movements. An arousal must be preceded by at least 10 s of continuous sleep. Nevertheless, this definition may be not complete, as other EEG elements, characterized by slow activity, as K-complexes or delta bursts, are considered arousal-related phenomena but are not scored as arousals unless they are associated with an EEG frequency shift toward theta, alpha, or beta rhythms (Fig. 10.10, panel a). Furthermore, the AASM criteria of arousal does not include the concept of periodicity.

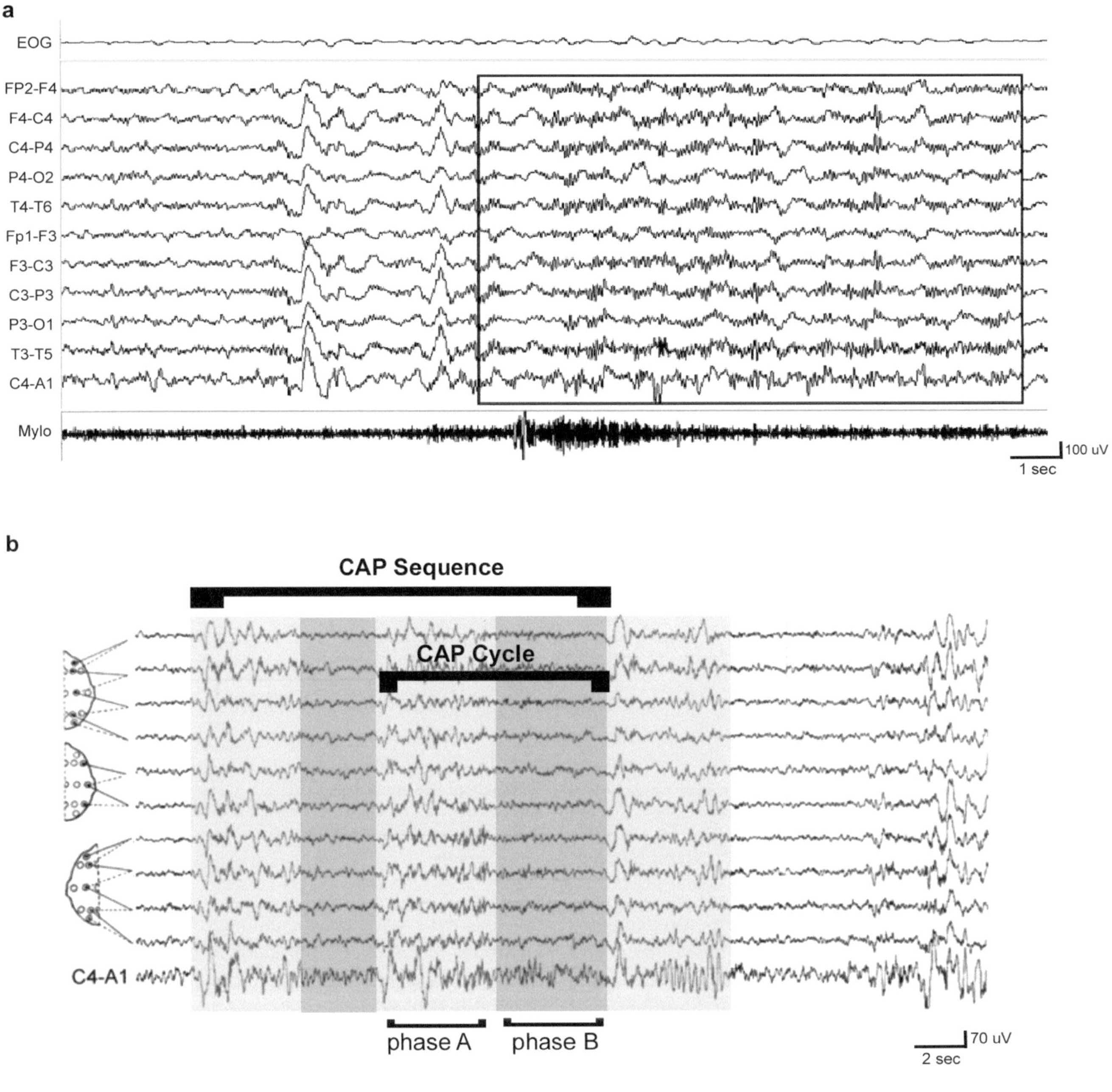

Fig. 10.10 Panel (**a**) Arousal according to AASM criteria (arousal is described by the black box). Only rapid rhythms are considered. Slow waves preceding the shift toward rapid frequencies are excluded. EEG is displayed in bipolar montage. *EOG* electrooculogram. EMG derivation is represented by the activity of the mylohyoid muscle (mylo). Panel (**b**) A CAP cycle is defined as a sequence of two alternating stereotyped EEG patterns, each lasting more than 2 and less than 60 s, called phase A and phase B, which are the expression of a sustained fluctuation between "greater arousal" level (phase A: usually 8–12 s) and "lesser arousal" level (phase B: usually 16–25 s). At least two full CAP cycles in succession are needed to define a CAP sequence; all CAP sequences begin with a phase A and end with a phase B. The phase A that terminates a CAP sequence is counted as non-CAP

In the middle of the 1980s, Terzano and co-workers [107] recognized a microstructural cyclicity in NREM sleep, named cyclic alternating pattern (CAP). The introduction of the CAP framework provides a substantial departure from the general consensus about arousals during sleep either conceptually and as EEG criteria. The conceptual basis of arousals as proposed by the American Sleep Disorders Association and reported in the AASM manual is that arousals, being a transient cortical activation, are markers of sleep disruption representing a detrimental and harmful feature for sleep [108] and thus excluded from the conventional staging procedures. According to the CAP theory, arousal is an integral part of sleep texture taking part in the sleep regulation processes [41] and represents a complex phenomenon involving not only cortical areas but also other brain centers and peripheral neural components [13, 41]. The activating pattern occurring within the somato-vegetative systems do not always correspond to a cortical activation, as the arousal definition seems to suggest. The outcome of stimulation can also be a mild cortical activation expressed as a mixed slow-rapid EEG pattern (as for subtypes A2 of CAP) or can evoke a protective reaction of the sleeping brain (as for subtypes A1 of CAP) as described below.

10.10.1 Definitions of CAP and Non-CAP

The cyclic alternating pattern (CAP) is a specific type of periodic activity of NREM sleep characterized by phases of EEG activation (**A** phase) and subsequent phases of return to background activity (**B** phase), both ranging between 2 and 60 s, evolving in a cycling pattern.

A phase **A** and the following phase **B** compose a CAP cycle, and a succession of cycles defines a CAP sequence. All CAP sequences begin with a phase **A** and end with a phase **B** (Fig. 10.10, panel b).

The absence of CAP for >60 s is scored as non-CAP, considered as a phase of sustained physiologic stability. An isolated phase **A** and the phase **A** that terminates a CAP sequence is considered as non-CAP (Fig. 10.11). CAP sequences have no upper limits for duration and number of CAP cycles. Each CAP sequence is usually formed by five to six CAP cycles.

CAP sequences usually precede the transition from non-REM to REM sleep. REM sleep is characterized by the lack of EEG synchronization; thus phase **A** in REM sleep consists mainly of desynchronized activities (fast low-amplitude rhythms), which are separated by a mean interval of 3–4 min. Consequently, under physiologic circumstances, CAP is not present in REM sleep. However, pathologic conditions characterized by repetitive **A** phases recurring at intervals <60 s, as periodic REM-related sleep apnea events, can produce CAP sequences in REM sleep. Within non-REM sleep, a CAP sequence is not interrupted by a sleep stage shift if CAP scoring requirements are satisfied. Consequently, because CAP sequences can extend across adjacent sleep stages, a CAP sequence can contain a variety of different phase **A** and phase **B** activities.

10.10.1.1 CAP Phase A Boundaries

Amplitude Limits

Phasic activities initiating a phase **A** must be 1/3 higher than the background voltage, calculated during the 2 s before onset and 2 s after offset of a phase **A** itself. However, in some cases, a phase **A** can present ambiguous limits due to inconsistent voltage changes. Onset and termination of a phase **A** are established on the basis of an amplitude/frequency concordance in the majority of EEG leads.

Temporal Limits

Each phase **A** or **B** is 2–60 s in duration. If two consecutive phase **A** are separated by an interval <2 s, they are combined as a single phase **A**. If they are separated by a >2 s interval, they are scored as independent events.

10.10.1.2 Phase A EEG Events and Subtypes

Compared to background activity, phase **A** can be composed of slower, higher-voltage rhythms, faster lower-voltage rhythms, or by mixed patterns including both. They may include delta bursts, sequences of vertex sharp transients, K-complex sequences, polyphasic bursts, K-alpha, intermittent alpha, and EEG arousals (Table 10.4).

Based on the reciprocal proportion of EEG synchrony (high-voltage slow waves) and EEG desynchrony (low amplitude rapid activities), phase **A** can be classified into three subtypes (Fig. 10.12):

- *Subtype A1:* EEG synchrony is the predominant activity. If present, EEG desynchrony occupies <20% of the entire phase **A** duration. Examples of **A1** include delta bursts, K-complex or vertex sharp transient sequences, and polyphasic bursts with <20% of EEG desynchrony.
- *Subtype A2:* The EEG activity is a mixture of slow and fast rhythms with 20–50% of phase **A** characterized by EEG desynchrony. Examples of **A2** include polyphasic bursts with more than 20% but less than 50% of EEG desynchrony.
- *Subtype A3:* The EEG activity is predominantly low-voltage fast rhythms with >50% of phase **A** occupied by EEG desynchrony. Examples of **A3** include K-alpha, EEG arousals, and polyphasic bursts with >50% of EEG desynchrony. A movement artefact within a CAP sequence is also classified as subtype **A3**.

Different **A** phases show distinct topographic distribution. **A1** can be considered as frontal lobe arousals, as they prevail in anterior regions, whereas **A3** are localized principally over the posterior areas. **A2** share both spectral and topographic characteristics of A1 and A3. They origin over the anterior regions with an initial slow component, and then they spread toward parieto-occipital areas acquiring the characteristics of **A3** subtypes (fast low-voltage activity) [109]. Subtype **A1** is most common as sleep EEG synchrony increases (from light to deep non-REM sleep) and when synchrony predominates (stage N3). **A1** phases are concentrated during the descending branch of the sleep cycle and follow the homeostatic decay of slow-wave oscillation both within one cycle

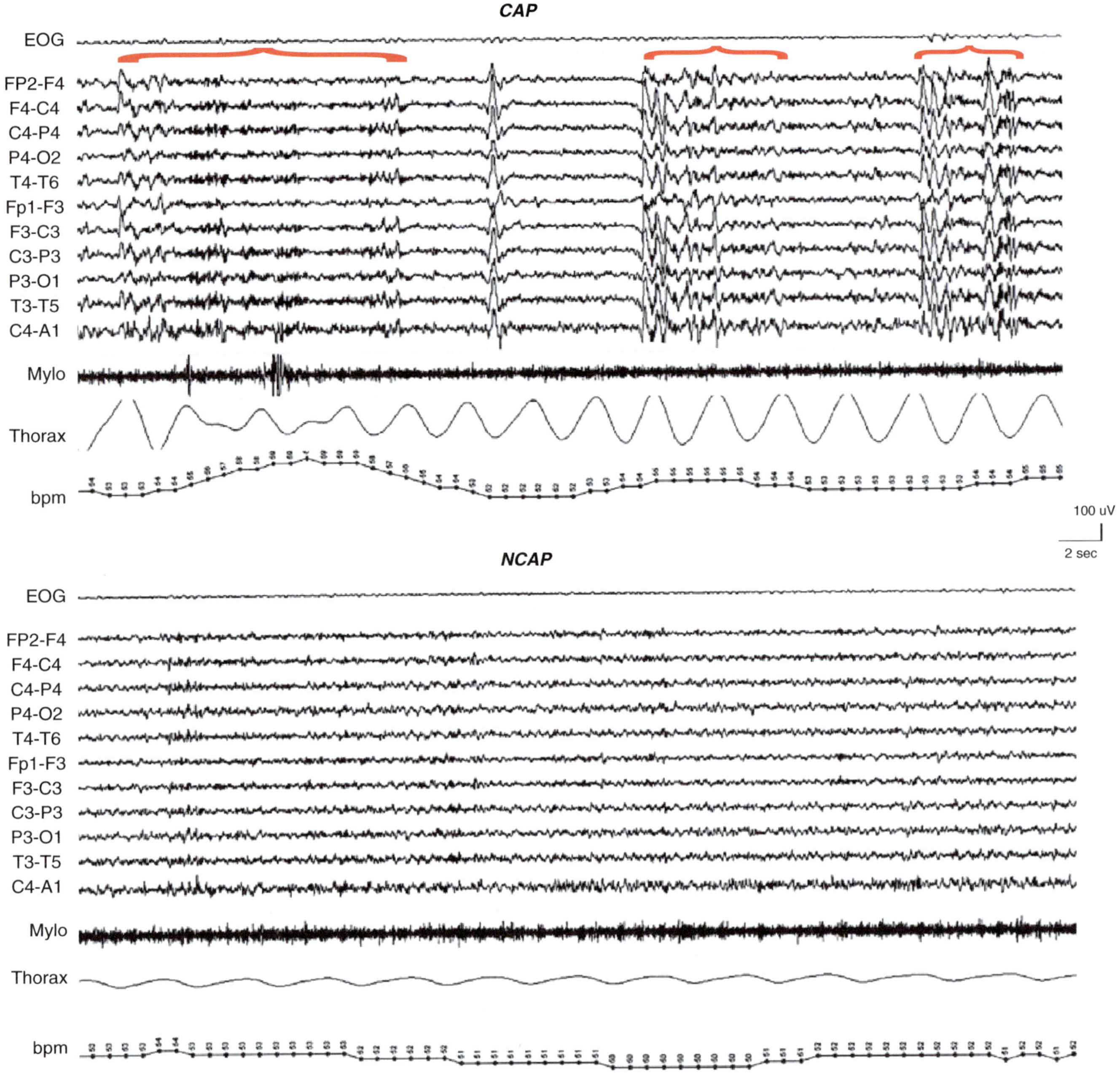

Fig. 10.11 Examples of CAP and NCAP during N2. *Top image*: CAP during N2. Three A phases are highlighted by red brace brackets. Note the correspondent increase in heart frequency (bpm) during CAP A phases. *Bottom image*: NCAP during N2. Note the absence of EEG, heart frequency, and respiratory fluctuations. EEG is displayed in bipolar montage. *EOG* electrooculogram. EMG derivation is represented by the activity of the mylohyoid muscle (mylo). Thorax: respiratory effort. Bpm: heart rate

Table 10.4 Example of A phases

Delta bursts	Sequence of at least two waves in delta frequency and with an amplitude at least 1/3 higher than the background activity
Polyphasic bursts	Clusters of high-voltage delta waves, intermixed with faster rhythms (in the theta, alpha, or beta frequency bandwidth)
K-alpha	A K-complex followed immediately by an alpha burst with an overall duration of ≥2 s
Intermittent alpha	Intermittent sequences of alpha activity, usually localized more anteriorly and often increased in amplitude and decreased in frequency than during wakefulness. It is normally seen during the first phases of sleep, when stage N1 remerges in the ascendant branch of sleep cycle, or during REM sleep
EEG arousals	Abrupt shift of EEG frequency including alpha, theta and/or frequencies greater than 16 Hz (but not spindles) that shortly interrupt the sleep continuity, lasting at least 3 s, with at least 10 s of stable sleep preceding the change and, if scored during REM, with a concurrent increase in submental EMG lasting at least 1 s

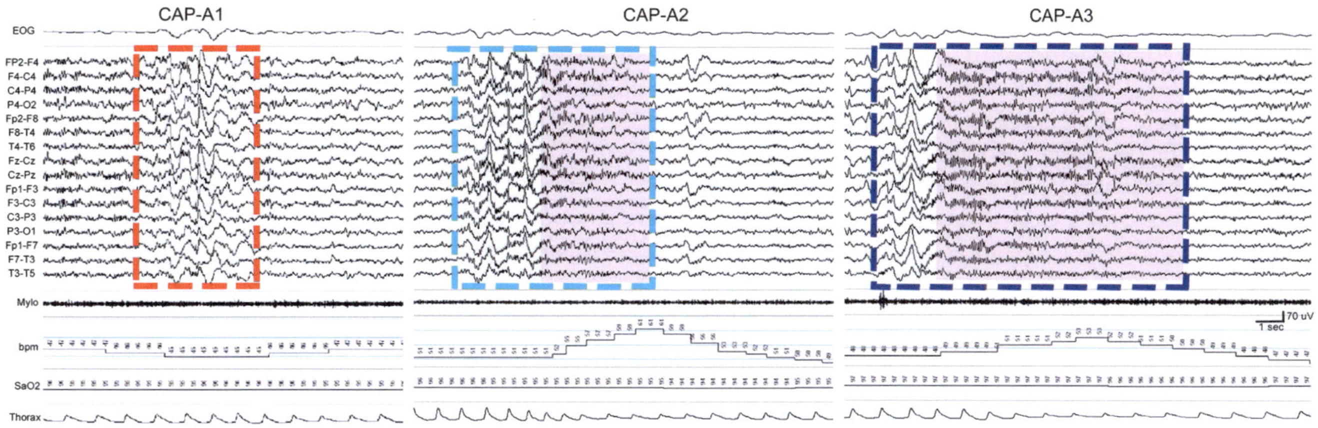

Fig. 10.12 Examples of CAP-A subtypes. The red box identifies the limits of A1 phase, the light blue one the A2 phase, and the blue box the A3 phase. The pink box shows the amount of EEG desynchronized activity in each A phase: less than 20% in A1 (note that in this example A1 is constituted only by SWA), between 20 and 50% in A2 and >50% in A3. Notably during A2 and A3 subtypes, EEG activity is accompanied by changes in heart rate and respiratory effort. EEG is displayed in bipolar montage. *EOG* electrooculogram. EMG derivation is represented by the activity of the mylohyoid muscle (mylo). Thorax: respiratory effort. Bpm: heart rate. SaO_2: oxyhemoglobin saturation

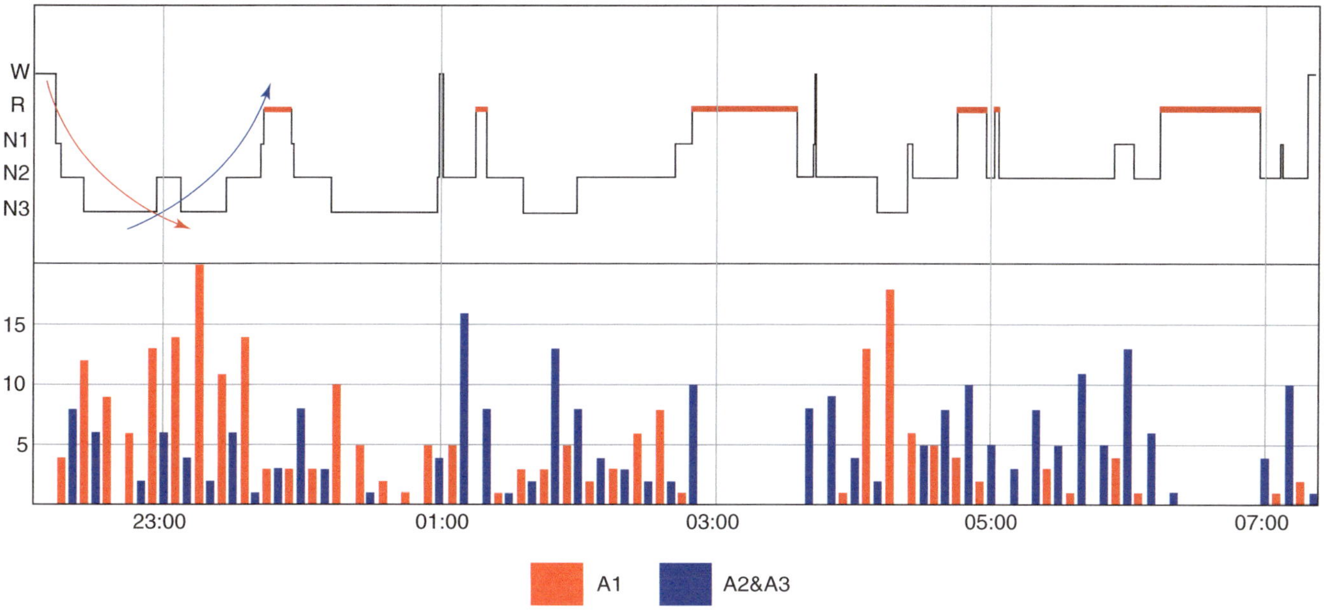

Fig. 10.13 Distribution of A phases matched with hypnogram. Red bars: number of synchronization phases (A1) each 10 min. Blue bars: number of desynchronization phases (A2 + A3) each 10 min. A1 phases prevail during the descendent branch (identified by the red arrow on the hypnogram) and the plateau of deep sleep, whereas A2 and A3 phases are localized primary during the ascending branch (identified by the blue arrow on the hypnogram), preceding the appearance of REM sleep. The progressive decline of A1 along the night reflect the homeostatic sleep process

and from cycle to cycle. Subtypes **A2** and **A3** are mostly concentrated as sleep-related brain activity progresses from synchrony to greater desynchrony (e.g., in stage N2 preceding the onset of REM sleep), and they prevail during the ascending branch of the sleep cycle [10] (Fig.10.13). The same perturbation can evoke a **A1** or **A2/A3** response depending on the sleep propensity and intracycle dynamic regulation. The elicitation of the CAP **A1** pattern by acoustic stimuli during CAP B phases has proven that a certain amount of (reactive) sleep slow waves are evoked by sensory stimulation [47, 110]. Based on these observations, the CAP system can be viewed as a short range homeostatic process in which the amount of slow-wave activity is buffered instantly (fast homeostatic reaction), therefore preserving sleep continuity: a natural "slow-wave injection," protecting sleep against perturbations.

10.10.2 Measures of CAP and CAP trend During Age Span

CAP is a marker of sleep instability, as well as other EEG features, and it highly depends on brain development. Among the various CAP parameters, CAP rate is the most extensively used for clinical purposes. Calculated as the percentage ratio of total CAP time to non-REM sleep time, CAP rate is the measure of arousal instability; it can be enhanced when sleep is disturbed by internal or external factors and its variations correlate with the subjective appreciation of sleep quality with higher values of CAP rate associated with poorer sleep quality.

CAP rate in normal sleepers shows a low intraindividual variability from night-to-night [111]; CAP rate has a complex evolution during development.

In newborns, as soon as the NREM sleep emerges, CAP begins to develop, and the oscillating pattern of the different phasic EEG activities becomes evident. The gradual appearance of an oscillating pattern of slow EEG activities representing the first prototype of CAP appears at 46–55 weeks of conceptional age (Fig.10.6). During infancy, CAP rate shows a gradual increase with a peak in adolescence and then a gradual decrease in adulthood followed by an increase in the elderly [112–116] (Fig.10.14).

These age-related changes of CAP rate reflect the biological growth processes that lead to adolescence, the development maturational consolidation, and finally the process of senescence that is accompanied by the increasing of sleep instability.

The peripubertal peak of CAP rate is associated with the maximum of the A1 subtypes percentage, which shows a bell-shaped course during the life (Fig. 10.15). In contrast, subtypes **A2** and **A3** undergo a linear increase from infants, preschool children to the old age, similar to the arousal evolution across the life span [110, 112, 117]. The ratio between A1 and A2/A3 is higher in school-age children, supporting the notion that sleep in this age range (6–10 years) may be considered as the "gold standard" for sleep quality [118] because of its length, continuity, and restorative features. On the other hand, the increase of the percentage of A2 in preschoolers might represent the higher sleep instability of this age period. In school-aged children, the increased values of CAP rate during N3 and the greater percentage of **A1** subtypes indicate that in this age group, the homeostatic process requires a higher number of oscillations in order to maintain the restorative function of sleep [113, 115, 119].

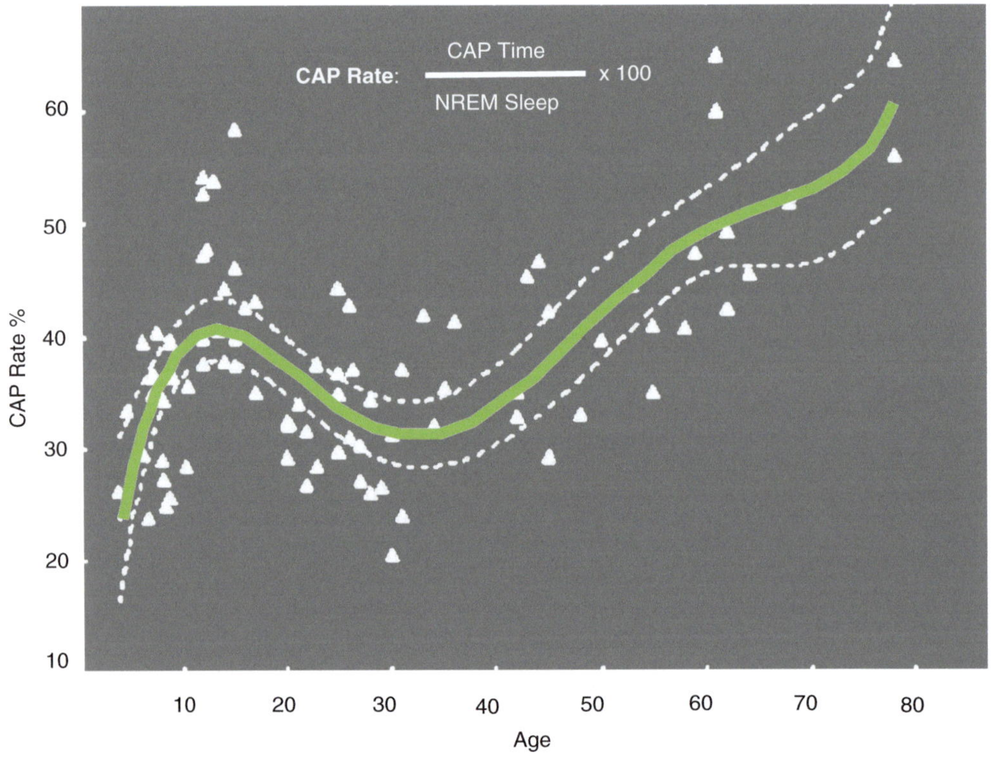

Fig. 10.14 Age-related modifications of CAP rate along the normal life span. Note a bimodal distribution with a first peak around the puberty followed by a decrease during adult life and a subsequent new increase in senescence. The green line identifies the average physiological distribution of CAP rate across ages, while dotted white lines show the related standard deviations. White triangles refer to the CAP rate of single subjects included in the analysis. The present figure has been extrapolated from the data presented in [110]. Age is expressed in years

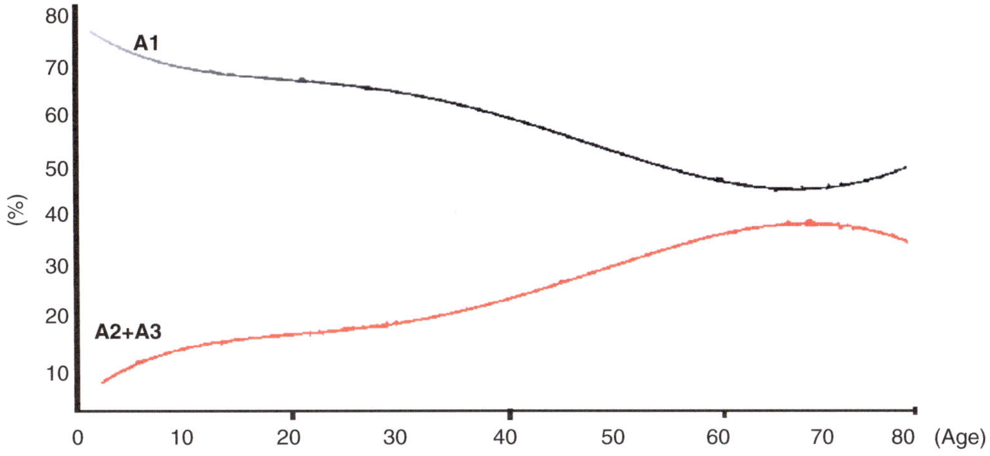

Fig. 10.15 Normative age-related changes of phase A subtypes. The percentages of subtypes A1 (black line) tend to decrease along the lifespan mirrored by the reciprocal increase of subtypes A2 and A3 (red line). The opposite trends converge approximately at the age of 60–70 years. The present figure has been extrapolated from the data presented in [110]. Age is expressed in years

References

1. Lo JC, Dijk D-J, Groeger JA. Comparing the effects of nocturnal sleep and daytime napping on declarative memory consolidation. PLoS One. 2014;9:e108100.
2. Rechtschaffen A, Kales A. A manual of standardized terminology, techniques and scoring system for sleep stages of human subjects. Oakland, CA: University of California; 1968.
3. AASM Manual. For the scoring of sleep and associate events. Rules, terminology and technical specifications. Westchester, IL: American Academy of Sleep Medicine; 2007.
4. Saper CB, Scammell TE, Lu J. Hypothalamic regulation of sleep and circadian rhythms. Nature. 2005;437:1257–63.
5. Saper CB, Chou TC, Scammell TE. The sleep switch: hypothalamic control of sleep and wakefulness. Trends Neurosci. 2001;24:726–31.
6. Lo C-C, Chou T, Penzel T, Scammell TE, Strecker RE, Stanley HE, et al. Common scale-invariant patterns of sleep-wake transitions across mammalian species. Proc Natl Acad Sci U S A. 2004;101:17545–8.
7. Behn CGD, Brown EN, Scammell TE, Kopell NJ. Mathematical model of network dynamics governing mouse sleep-wake behavior. J Neurophysiol. 2007;97:3828–40.
8. Halász P, Bódizs R. Dynamic NREM sleep regulation models. In: Dynamic structure of NREM sleep. London: Springer; 2013. p. 7–11.
9. Halász P. The role of micro-arousals in the regulation of sleep. Ideggyogyaszati Szle. 2006;59:252–60.
10. Halász P. The K-complex as a special reactive sleep slow wave—a theoretical update. Sleep Med Rev. 2016;29:34–40.
11. Tononi G, Cirelli C. Sleep and synaptic homeostasis: a hypothesis. Brain Res Bull. 2003;62:143–50.
12. Tononi G, Cirelli C. Sleep and the price of plasticity: from synaptic and cellular homeostasis to memory consolidation and integration. Neuron. 2014;81:12–34.
13. Parrino L, Vaudano AE. The resilient brain and the guardians of sleep: new perspectives on old assumptions. Sleep Med Rev. 2018;39:98–107.
14. Takahashi K, Kayama Y, Lin JS, Sakai K. Locus coeruleus neuronal activity during the sleep-waking cycle in mice. Neuroscience. 2010;169:1115–26.
15. Ruyi Foong, Kai Keng Ang, Chai Quek, Cuntai Guan, Aung Aung Phyo Wai. An analysis on driver drowsiness based on reaction time and EEG band power. 37th Annual International Conference of the IEEE Engineering in Medicine and Biology Society (EMBC). IEEE, Milan; 2015 [cited 2018 May 15]. p. 7982–5.
16. Sekine A, Niiyama Y, Kutsuzawa O, Shimizu T. A negative component superimposed on event-related potentials during light drowsiness. Psychiatry Clin Neurosci. 2001;55:473–8.
17. Wada Y, Nanbu Y, Koshino Y, Shimada Y, Hashimoto T. Inter- and intrahemispheric EEG coherence during light drowsiness. Clin EEG Electroencephalogr. 1996;27:84–8.
18. Vecchio F, Miraglia F, Gorgoni M, Ferrara M, Iberite F, Bramanti P, et al. Cortical connectivity modulation during sleep onset: a study via graph theory on EEG data. Hum Brain Mapp. 2017;38:5456–64.
19. Goldie L, Green JM. Paradoxical blocking and arousal in the drowsy state. Nature. 1960;187:952–3.
20. Niedermeyer E, Pribram HF. Unilateral suppression of vertex sharp waves in the sleep electroencephalogram (case report). Electroencephalogr Clin Neurophysiol. 1966;20:401–4.
21. Chang BS, Schomer DL, Niedermayer E. Normal EEG and sleep; adults and elderly. In: Schomer DL, Lopes de Silva FH, editors. Niedermeyer's electroencephalography: basic principles, clinical applications and related fields. Philadelphia, PA: Lippincott Williams & Wilkins; 2010. p. 183–214.
22. Colrain IM, Campbell KB. The use of evoked potentials in sleep research. Sleep Med Rev. 2007;11:277–93.
23. Bastien CH, Crowley KE, Colrain IM. Evoked potential components unique to non-REM sleep: relationship to evoked K-complexes and vertex sharp waves. Int J Psychophysiol. 2002;46:257–74.
24. Gora J, Colrain IM, Trinder J. The investigation of K-complex and vertex sharp wave activity in response to mid-inspiratory occlusions and complete obstructions to breathing during NREM sleep. Sleep. 2001;24:81–9.
25. Lu ST, Kajola M, Joutsiniemi SL, Knuutila J, Hari R. Generator sites of spontaneous MEG activity during sleep. Electroencephalogr Clin Neurophysiol. 1992;82:182–96.
26. Stern JM, Caporro M, Haneef Z, Yeh HJ, Buttinelli C, Lenartowicz A, et al. Functional imaging of sleep vertex sharp transients. Clin Neurophysiol. 2011;122:1382–6.
27. Grigg-Damberger M, Gozal D, Marcus CL, Quan SF, Rosen CL, Chervin RD, et al. The visual scoring of sleep and arousal in infants and children. J Clin Sleep Med. 2007;3:201–40.
28. Hughes JR. The development of the vertex sharp transient. Clin EEG Electroencephalogr. 1998;29:183–7.
29. Rey V, Aybek S, Maeder-Ingvar M, Rossetti AO. Positive occipital sharp transients of sleep (POSTS): a reappraisal. Clin Neurophysiol. 2009;120:472–5.
30. Pristasová E, Procházka M, Cigánek L. Theta rhythms and positive bioccipital waves in the EEG during sleep. Psychiatr Neurol Med Psychol (Leipz). 1983;35:656–60.

31. Hughes JR, Means ED, Stell BS. A controlled study on the behavior disorders associated with the positive spike phenomenon. Electroencephalogr Clin Neurophysiol. 1965;18:349–53.
32. Saito M, Ishida T, Nakamura M, Ihara M, Murase I. Factors affecting the occurrence of high-frequency positive occipital sharp transients of sleep. Keio J Med. 2003;52:25–9.
33. Vignaendra V, Matthews RL, Chatrian GE. Positive occipital sharp transients of sleep: relationships to nocturnal sleep cycle in man. Electroencephalogr Clin Neurophysiol. 1974;37:239–46.
34. Brenner RP, Zauel DW, Carlow TJ. Positive occipital sharp transients of sleep in the blind. Neurology. 1978;28:609–12.
35. Loomis AL, Harvey EN, Hobart GA. Distribution of disturbance-patterns in the human electroencephalogram, with special reference to sleep. J Neurophysiol. 1938;1:413–30.
36. Cote KA, de Lugt DR, Langley SD, Campbell KB. Scalp topography of the auditory evoked K-complex in stage 2 and slow wave sleep. J Sleep Res. 1999;8:263–72.
37. Colrain IM. The K-complex: a 7-decade history. Sleep. 2005;28:255–73.
38. Colrain IM, Sullivan EV, Rohlfing T, Baker FC, Nicholas CL, Padilla ML, et al. Independent contributions of cortical gray matter, aging, sex and alcoholism to K-complex amplitude evoked during sleep. Sleep. 2011;34:787–95.
39. Curcio G, Ferrara M, Pellicciari MC, Cristiani R, De Gennaro L. Effect of total sleep deprivation on the landmarks of stage 2 sleep. Clin Neurophysiol. 2003;114:2279–85.
40. Steriade M. Neuronal substrates of sleep and epilepsy. Cambridge; New York: Cambridge University Press; 2003.
41. Halász P, Terzano M, Parrino L, Bódizs R. The nature of arousal in sleep. J Sleep Res. 2004;13:1–23.
42. Riedner BA, Hulse BK, Murphy MJ, Ferrarelli F, Tononi G. Temporal dynamics of cortical sources underlying spontaneous and peripherally evoked slow waves. Prog Brain Res. 2011;193:201–18.
43. Tank J, Diedrich A, Hale N, Niaz FE, Furlan R, Robertson RM, et al. Relationship between blood pressure, sleep K-complexes, and muscle sympathetic nerve activity in humans. Am J Physiol Regul Integr Comp Physiol. 2003;285:R208–14.
44. Niiyama Y, Satoh N, Kutsuzawa O, Hishikawa Y. Electrophysiological evidence suggesting that sensory stimuli of unknown origin induce spontaneous K-complexes. Electroencephalogr Clin Neurophysiol. 1996;98:394–400.
45. Roth M, Shaw J, Green J. The form voltage distribution and physiological significance of the K-complex. Electroencephalogr Clin Neurophysiol. 1956;8:385–402.
46. Sallinen M, Kaartinen J, Lyytinen H. Precursors of the evoked K-complex in event-related brain potentials in stage 2 sleep. Electroencephalogr Clin Neurophysiol. 1997;102:363–73.
47. Laurino M, Menicucci D, Piarulli A, Mastorci F, Bedini R, Allegrini P, et al. Disentangling different functional roles of evoked K-complex components: mapping the sleeping brain while quenching sensory processing. NeuroImage. 2014;86:433–45.
48. Nicholas CL, Trinder J, Colrain IM. Increased production of evoked and spontaneous K-complexes following a night of fragmented sleep. Sleep. 2002;25:882–7.
49. Halász P. Hierarchy of micro-arousals and the microstructure of sleep. Neurophysiol Clin. 1998;28:461–75.
50. Crowley K, Trinder J, Kim Y, Carrington M, Colrain IM. The effects of normal aging on sleep spindle and K-complex production. Clin Neurophysiol. 2002;113:1615–22.
51. Colrain IM, Crowley KE, Nicholas CL, Afifi L, Baker FC, Padilla M, et al. Sleep evoked delta frequency responses show a linear decline in amplitude across the adult lifespan. Neurobiol Aging. 2010;31:874–83.
52. Mölle M, Bergmann TO, Marshall L, Born J. Fast and slow spindles during the sleep slow oscillation: disparate coalescence and engagement in memory processing. Sleep. 2011;34:1411–21.
53. Andrillon T, Nir Y, Staba RJ, Ferrarelli F, Cirelli C, Tononi G, et al. Sleep spindles in humans: insights from intracranial EEG and unit recordings. J Neurosci. 2011;31:17821–34.
54. Nader RS, Smith CT. Correlations between adolescent processing speed and specific spindle frequencies. Front Hum Neurosci. 2015;9:30.
55. De Gennaro L, Ferrara M. Sleep spindles: an overview. Sleep Med Rev. 2003;7:423–40.
56. Lüthi A. Sleep spindles: where they come from, what they do. Neurosci Rev J Bring Neurobiol Neurol Psychiatry. 2014;20:243–56.
57. Astori S, Wimmer RD, Lüthi A. Manipulating sleep spindles—expanding views on sleep, memory, and disease. Trends Neurosci. 2013;36:738–48.
58. Schabus M, Dang-Vu TT, Albouy G, Balteau E, Boly M, Carrier J, et al. Hemodynamic cerebral correlates of sleep spindles during human non-rapid eye movement sleep. Proc Natl Acad Sci U S A. 2007;104:13164–9.
59. Ayoub A, Aumann D, Hörschelmann A, Kouchekmanesch A, Paul P, Born J, et al. Differential effects on fast and slow spindle activity, and the sleep slow oscillation in humans with carbamazepine and flunarizine to antagonize voltage-dependent Na+ and Ca2+ channel activity. Sleep. 2013;36:905–11.
60. Clawson BC, Durkin J, Aton SJ. Form and function of sleep spindles across the lifespan. Neural Plast. 2016;2016:6936381.
61. Hagne I. Development of the EEG in normal infants during the first year of life. A longitudinal study. Acta Paediatr Scand Suppl. 1972;232:1–53.
62. Gaillard J-M, Baudat J, Blois R. The effect of sex depressive state and minor tranquilizers on K potentials and spindles during sleep. Clin Neurol Neurosurg. 1987;89:172–3.
63. Mölle M, Marshall L, Gais S, Born J. Learning increases human electroencephalographic coherence during subsequent slow sleep oscillations. Proc Natl Acad Sci U S A. 2004;101:13963–8.
64. Massimini M, Huber R, Ferrarelli F, Hill S, Tononi G. The sleep slow oscillation as a traveling wave. J Neurosci. 2004;24:6862–70.
65. Nir Y, Mukamel R, Dinstein I, Privman E, Harel M, Fisch L, et al. Interhemispheric correlations of slow spontaneous neuronal fluctuations revealed in human sensory cortex. Nat Neurosci. 2008;11:1100–8.
66. Mander BA, Winer JR, Walker MP. Sleep and Human Aging. Neuron. 2017;94:19–36.
67. Vijayan S, Klerman EB, Adler GK, Kopell NJ. Thalamic mechanisms underlying alpha-delta sleep with implications for fibromyalgia. J Neurophysiol. 2015;114:1923–30.
68. Van Hoof E, De Becker P, Lapp C, Cluydts R, De Meirleir K. Defining the occurrence and influence of alpha-delta sleep in chronic fatigue syndrome. Am J Med Sci. 2007;333:78–84.
69. Jaimchariyatam N, Rodriguez CL, Budur K. Prevalence and correlates of alpha-delta sleep in major depressive disorders. Innov Clin Neurosci. 2011;8:35–49.
70. Scheuler W, Kubicki S, Marquardt J, Scholz G, Weiβ KH, Henkes H, et al. The alpha-sleep pattern—quantitative analysis and functional aspects. In: Koella WP, Obal F, Schulz H, Visser P, editors. Sleep, vol. 1988. Stuttgart: Fischer; 1986.
71. Steriade M, Contreras D, Curró Dossi R, Nuñez A. The slow (<1 Hz) oscillation in reticular thalamic and thalamocortical neurons: scenario of sleep rhythm generation in interacting thalamic and neocortical networks. J Neurosci. 1993;13:3284–99.
72. Steriade M, Timofeev I, Grenier F. Natural waking and sleep states: a view from inside neocortical neurons. J Neurophysiol. 2001;85:1969–85.
73. Timofeev I, Grenier F, Bazhenov M, Sejnowski TJ, Steriade M. Origin of slow cortical oscillations in deafferented cortical slabs. Cereb Cortex. 2000;10:1185–99.
74. Sanchez-Vives MV, McCormick DA. Cellular and network mechanisms of rhythmic recurrent activity in neocortex. Nat Neurosci. 2000;3:1027–34.
75. Bazhenov M, Timofeev I, Steriade M, Sejnowski TJ. Model of thalamocortical slow-wave sleep oscillations and transitions to activated states. J Neurosci. 2002;22:8691–704.

76. Compte A, Sanchez-Vives MV, McCormick DA, Wang X-J. Cellular and network mechanisms of slow oscillatory activity (<1 Hz) and wave propagations in a cortical network model. J Neurophysiol. 2003;89:2707–25.
77. Timofeev I, Steriade M. Low-frequency rhythms in the thalamus of intact-cortex and decorticated cats. J Neurophysiol. 1996;76:4152–68.
78. Shu Y, Hasenstaub A, McCormick DA. Turning on and off recurrent balanced cortical activity. Nature. 2003;423:288–93.
79. Caporro M, Haneef Z, Yeh HJ, Lenartowicz A, Buttinelli C, Parvizi J, et al. Functional MRI of sleep spindles and K-complexes. Clin Neurophysiol. 2012;123:303–9.
80. Jahnke K, von Wegner F, Morzelewski A, Borisov S, Maischein M, Steinmetz H, et al. To wake or not to wake? The two-sided nature of the human K-complex. NeuroImage. 2012;59:1631–8.
81. Riedner BA, Vyazovskiy VV, Huber R, Massimini M, Esser S, Murphy M, et al. Sleep homeostasis and cortical synchronization: III. A high-density EEG study of sleep slow waves in humans. Sleep. 2007;30:1643–57.
82. Tononi G, Cirelli C. Sleep function and synaptic homeostasis. Sleep Med Rev. 2006;10:49–62.
83. Esser SK, Hill SL, Tononi G. Sleep homeostasis and cortical synchronization: I. Modeling the effects of synaptic strength on sleep slow waves. Sleep. 2007;30:1617–30.
84. Vyazovskiy VV, Riedner BA, Cirelli C, Tononi G. Sleep homeostasis and cortical synchronization: II. A local field potential study of sleep slow waves in the rat. Sleep. 2007;30:1631–42.
85. Vyazovskiy VV, Olcese U, Lazimy YM, Faraguna U, Esser SK, Williams JC, et al. Cortical firing and sleep homeostasis. Neuron. 2009;63:865–78.
86. Colrain IM, Baker FC. Changes in sleep as a function of adolescent development. Neuropsychol Rev. 2011;21:5–21.
87. Ringli M, Huber R. Developmental aspects of sleep slow waves: linking sleep, brain maturation and behavior. Prog Brain Res. 2011;193:63–82.
88. Kurth S, Ringli M, Geiger A, LeBourgeois M, Jenni OG, Huber R. Mapping of cortical activity in the first two decades of life: a high-density sleep electroencephalogram study. J Neurosci. 2010;30:13211–9.
89. Feinberg I, Campbell IG. Sleep EEG changes during adolescence: an index of a fundamental brain reorganization. Brain Cogn. 2010;72:56–65.
90. Matsuo F. Recognition of REM sleep in standard EEG. Electroencephalogr Clin Neurophysiol. 1981;52:490–3.
91. Jouvet M, Michel F, Mounier D. Analyse électroencépholographique comparée du sommeil physiologique chez le chat et chez l'homme. Revue Neurologique. 1960;103:189D–205D.
92. Berger RJ, Olley P, Oswald I. The EEC, eye-movements and dreams of the blind. Q J Exp Psychol. 1962;14:183–6.
93. Yasoshima A, Hayashi H, Iijima S, Sugita Y, Teshima Y, Shimizu T, et al. Potential distribution of vertex sharp wave and saw-toothed wave on the scalp. Electroencephalogr Clin Neurophysiol. 1984;58:73–6.
94. Broughton R, Hasan J. Quantitative topographic electroencephalographic mapping during drowsiness and sleep onset. J Clin Neurophysiol. 1995;12:372–86.
95. Curzi-Dascalova L. Waking and sleeping E.E.G. in normal babies before 6 months of age (author's transl). Rev Electroencephalogr Neurophysiol Clin. 1977;7:316–26.
96. Pearl PL, LaFleur BJ, Reigle SC, Rich AS, Freeman AAH, McCutchen C, et al. Sawtooth wave density analysis during REM sleep in normal volunteers. Sleep Med. 2002;3:255–8.
97. Sato S, McCutchen C, Graham B, Freeman A, von Albertini-Carletti I, Alling DW. Relationship between muscle tone changes, sawtooth waves and rapid eye movements during sleep. Electroencephalogr Clin Neurophysiol. 1997;103:627–32.
98. Takahara M, Kanayama S, Hori T. Co-occurrence of sawtooth waves and rapideye movements during REM sleep. Int J Bioelectromagn. 2009;11:144–8.
99. Kober SE, Wood G, Kampl C, Neuper C, Ischebeck A. Electrophysiological correlates of mental navigation in blind and sighted people. Behav Brain Res. 2014;273:106–15.
100. Balzamo E. States of wakefulness and ponto-geniculo-cortical activities (PGC) in Papio anubis (author's transl). Electroencephalogr Clin Neurophysiol. 1980;48:694–705.
101. Siegel H, McCutchen C, Dalakas MC, Freeman A, Graham B, Alling D, et al. Physiologic events initiating REM sleep in patients with the postpolio syndrome. Neurology. 1999;52:516–22.
102. Oksenberg A, Gordon C, Arons E, Sazbon L. Phasic activities of rapid eye movement sleep in vegetative state patients. Sleep. 2001;24:703–6.
103. Bassetti CL, Aldrich MS. Sleep electroencephalogram changes in acute hemispheric stroke. Sleep Med. 2001;2:185–94.
104. Vega-Bermudez F, Szczepanski S, Malow B, Sato S. Sawtooth wave density analysis during REM sleep in temporal lobe epilepsy patients. Sleep Med. 2005;6:367–70.
105. Terzano MG, Parrino L, Mennuni GF. Associazione Italiana di Medicina del Sonno, editors. Eventi fasici e microstruttura del sonno = phasic events and microstructure of sleep. Martano: Lecce; 1997.
106. Terzano MG, Parrino L. Origin and significance of the cyclic alternating pattern (CAP). Sleep Med Rev. 2000;4:101–23.
107. Terzano MG, Mancia D, Salati MR, Costani G, Decembrino A, Parrino L. The cyclic alternating pattern as a physiologic component of normal NREM sleep. Sleep. 1985;8:137–45.
108. Bonnet MH, Carley DW, Carskadon MA, Easton PA, Guilleminault C, Harper RM, et al. EEG arousals: scoring rules and examples: a preliminary report from the Sleep Disorders Atlas Task Force of the American Sleep Disorders Association. Sleep. 1992;15:173–84.
109. Ferri R, Bruni O, Miano S, Terzano MG. Topographic mapping of the spectral components of the cyclic alternating pattern (CAP). Sleep Med. 2005;6:29–36.
110. Parrino L, Ferri R, Bruni O, Terzano MG. Cyclic alternating pattern (CAP): the marker of sleep instability. Sleep Med Rev. 2012;16:27–45.
111. Terzano MG, Parrino L, Fioriti G, Spaggiari MC, Piroli A. Morphologic and functional features of cyclic alternating pattern (CAP) sequences in normal NREM sleep. Funct Neurol. 1986;1:29–41.
112. Parrino L, Boselli M, Spaggiari MC, Smerieri A, Terzano MG. Cyclic alternating pattern (CAP) in normal sleep: polysomnographic parameters in different age groups. Electroencephalogr Clin Neurophysiol. 1998;107:439–50.
113. Bruni O, Ferri R, Miano S, Verrillo E, Vittori E, Della Marca G, et al. Sleep cyclic alternating pattern in normal school-age children. Clin Neurophysiol. 2002;113:1806–14.
114. Bruni O, Ferri R, Miano S, Verrillo E, Vittori E, Farina B, et al. Sleep cyclic alternating pattern in normal preschool-aged children. Sleep. 2005;28:220–30.
115. Lopes MC, Rosa A, Roizenblatt S, Guilleminault C, Passarelli C, Tufik S, et al. Cyclic alternating pattern in peripubertal children. Sleep. 2005;28:215–9.
116. Miano S, PiaVilla M, Blanco D, Zamora E, Rodriguez R, Ferri R, et al. Development of NREM sleep instability-continuity (cyclic alternating pattern) in healthy term infants aged 1 to 4 months. Sleep. 2009;32:83–90.
117. Boselli M, Parrino L, Smerieri A, Terzano MG. Effect of age on EEG arousals in normal sleep. Sleep. 1998;21:351–7.
118. Carskadon M, Keenan S, Dement WC. Nighttime sleep and daytime sleep tendency in preadolescents. In: Guilleminault C, editor. Sleep and its disorders in children. New York: Raven Press; 1987.
119. Bruni O, Ferri R, Vittori E, Novelli L, Vignati M, Porfirio MC, et al. Sleep architecture and NREM alterations in children and adolescents with Asperger syndrome. Sleep. 2007;30:1577–85.

Normal Neonatal EEG

11

Massimo Mastrangelo, Barbara Scelsa,
and Francesco Pisani

In this chapter, the peculiar aspects of neonatal EEG are discussed, alongside with the recording modalities and the characteristic and age-specific electroencephalographic physiological patterns of the newborn, from preterm birth to the end of the neonatal period. In the Appendix, the terms utilized to describe the neonatal EEG will be defined.

The iconographic material is taken from electroencephalographic exams performed during daily clinic practice at V. Buzzi Children Hospital, in Milan (Pediatric Neurology Unit and Neonatal Intensive Care Unit). The children to whom the iconography refers have been evaluated by at least one of the authors and are not affected by any neurological condition.

11.1 Neonatal EEG Features

The EEG is a relatively easy, reproducible, non-traumatic method of functional exploration of the cortical and subcortical cerebral activity. It can be performed also at the patient's bed and with ventilatory assistance. Together with clinical signs and neuroimaging investigation, the EEG allows a global and dynamic evaluation of the brain functioning, and it has also an early prognostic value since the neonatal period [1]. It is important to underline the French author's statement in which a methodological fundamental message is contained: especially in the neonatal period, compared to all the other periods of life, the EEG interpretation cannot be made regardless of the clinical and neuroradiologic data. The integration of EEG characteristics, anamnestic data with gestational age (GA) and conceptional age (CA), clinical features (neurological examination and behavioral state during the EEG recording), and morphological elements (cerebral ultrasound and magnetic resonance image (MRI) is an essential condition for an accurate definition of the functional state of the brain of the newborn. In addition, the fetal and neonatal brain maturation from the 24th week of GA up to the term age is responsible for significant modifications of neonatal behavioral and EEG patterns. Therefore, the reference parameters vary, from prematurity to the at term age, depending on the CA.

11.2 Historical References

The first EEG recordings were performed by Hans Berger in 1929, becoming more and more frequent and technically satisfactory during the following decades. Only at the end of the 1950s, thanks to the contribution of French authors in particular, the electric patterns of preterm and full-term newborns were relatively defined. The peculiarities of cerebral electrical activity were emphasized, such as the presence of "inactive" periods, i.e. without electrical activity, of longer duration, the greater the prematurity; moreover the different patterns and graphic elements were also defined depending on the different CA. In parallel, since the second half of the 1950s and in the following decade, German authors focused their interest on the behavioral patterns of the newborn: wake, sleep, and different types of sleep states, defining their characteristics and relative percentages, in the development of the brain from prematurity to the end of gestation.

From the second half of the 1960s, but especially from the second half of the 1970s, thanks to the contribution of Parmelee et al. [2], Dreyfus-Brisac and Monod [3], Monod and Tharp [4], Watanabe et al. [5, 6], Tharp et al. [7], and Lombroso [8], a relatively standardized and adopted "normative" is in fact available, regarding the technical characteristics of recording and the normal and pathological EEG patterns in the premature and term infant, to which we sub-

M. Mastrangelo (✉) · B. Scelsa
Pediatrics Department, V.Buzzi Children Hospital, ASST Fatebenefratelli Sacco, Milan, Italy
e-mail: massimo.mastrangelo@asst-fbf-sacco.it

F. Pisani
Medicine and Surgery Department, Parma University, Parma, Italy

O. Mecarelli (ed.), *Clinical Electroencephalography*, https://doi.org/10.1007/978-3-030-04573-9_11

stantially refer today. Within the aforementioned papers, the interested reader can find the historical bibliographic references relating to the EEG in the neonatal period.

11.3 Qualitative Analysis of the Signal

The qualitative analysis and interpretation is based on the visual examination of the EEG [9, 10]. It involves the observation and definition of the EEG background activity and of the typical developmental EEG features specific to each CA. Therefore, the knowledge (of the examiner) and the possibility to define the parameters of "normality" must take into account the individual variability and influence that extra-neurological factors may have on the EEG patterns. This becomes the conditio sine qua nonotherwise it is impossible to correctly address and define what is pathological.

Related to the anatomic-functional brain maturation, it is known that from the 24th week of GA up to the period corresponding to the term age, there are changes in both the clinical behavior and the electro-cerebral activity, which vary specifically for epochs of 2 weeks. Literature is consistent in defining the normal findings of a recording at different conceptional ages, the severity grade of the brain impairment, the prognostic value of serial recordings at standardized times, the diagnostic meaning of some specific EEG patterns, the definition of the EEG findings of the epileptic seizures (which may be both electroclinical and electrographic only seizures), the ability to evaluate the effects of anticonvulsant therapy taking into account the phenomenon of the "electroclinical dissociation," and the possibility of obtaining information on the cerebral functioning of patients which are difficult to examine (newborns in coma or curarized). Moreover, extreme caution is necessary in formulating a judgment of abnormal recording, particularly in the context of extreme prematurity where there could be a modest disproportion between the observed electrical pattern and the CA of reference.

Since we discuss the normal criteria of the neonatal EEG in this chapter, it is necessary to point out the concept of "normality" at different gestational ages. Given that a physiological pregnancy has a duration of 38–42 weeks, it seems paradoxical to speak of "normality" in case of a baby born at 24 or 25 weeks of GA. On the other hand, the scientific progress in the perinatal medicine has led to a significant increase in the number of extremely preterm newborns; therefore, it is essential to investigate features of normal brain functioning even in the preterm newborns less than 27 weeks of GA.

These are obviously "extreme" clinical conditions often associated with a "low or very low birth weight." However, extreme prematurity could also be due to a maternal cause, and it is not uncommon to observe apparently healthy extremely premature infants (not affected by major neurological pathologies). In these cases, the knowledge and definition of "normality" features, while taking into account the individual variability and the extra-neurological conditions, is the essential prerequisite for tackling the problem of "pathology."

In summary, a methodological approach to interpreting the neonatal EEG that can be agreed upon is the one proposed by Janet E. Stockard-Pope [11], to which we add, however, the two points related to the clinical condition of the patient. The EEG is in fact a technique whose diagnostic potential is strongly enriched when it is strongly integrated into the general (clinical-neurologic-neuroradiological) context of the newborn:

- To know the GA and CA.
- To define the clinical condition.
- To define the cerebral ultrasound picture.
- To define the behavioral state.
- To define the polygraphic EEG findings according to the conceptional age and the behavioral state, with particular reference to the spatial and temporal organization of the background EEG activity, to the synchrony, to the presence of specific age patterns, to the reactivity, and to the EEG-behavioral state.

With some simplification, the gestalt approach to the neonatal EEG, from the extreme prematurity to the term age, involves the definition of the findings during the inactive EEG epochs and of the findings during the epochs with electrical activity and their evolution and modification over the weeks.

Only after the acquisition of such a methodological approach, it will be possible to take into consideration the characteristics of the pathological EEGs [12–14].

Before concluding this first introductory part, it is necessary to point out the research carried out by the group of Mizrahi, Kellaway, and Hrachovy of the University of Houston, Texas [15], from the end of the 1990s on the attempt to develop automatic and semiautomatic signal analysis systems in this particular field of application: prolonged monitoring in infants at risk of seizures. This approach is outside the scope of this manual, but the reader might find further information in Karayannis et al. [16]. Finally, Stevenson and Boylan [17] have reviewed and deepened the topic of automated seizure detection concluding that despite recent progress, it is not yet possible to apply these technologies into routine clinical practice.

11.4 Registration Techniques

The EEG recording in the neonatal period represents some peculiar difficulties related to the type of patient and the environment in which it is registered (incubator, thermal cradle).

The reader can refer to the guidelines of the American Clinical Neurophysiology Society (ACNS) [18, 19], to the ones of the International Federation of Clinical Neurophysiology [20], and to the work of Chang and Tsuchida on continuous EEG monitoring [21].

Here, we only want to highlight some significant aspects.

11.5 Preparation of the Newborn

The behavioral state of the newborn is a very important variable to consider in order to perform a recording that includes an entire cycle of spontaneous sleep and quiet wake phases, if age and general clinical conditions allow it. Therefore, it is suggested to breastfeed the newborn before the recording, provide a diaper change, and start recording even when awake but prolong it until the required behavioral states are achieved.

11.6 Positioning of the Electrodes

Chlorinated silver cup electrodes are used, with electroconductive paste, applied with ring-shaped patches, better if then fixed with a net that covers the scalp collecting the wires toward the electroencephalograph head. A cotton ball is placed above each electrode, under the patch, to improve grip. In the newborn, especially in a thermal cradle, the use of collodion (toxic) is prohibited.

A rapid application variant, used in our laboratory, consists of "preborn" button electrodes, inserted into perforated rubber bands. Needle electrodes are not recommended; being traumatic, they can be a source of infection.

The electrodes are positioned according to the International System 10–20 [22], modified for the newborn, taking into account both the size of the skull, especially in the extreme premature babies, and the immaturity of the frontal lobes of the newborn that do not extend so anterior to the skull.

Although it is obvious that the higher the number of electrodes on the scalp, the finer the signal can be, in our experience, nine head positions can be considered sufficient to acquire a properly differentiated signal in relation to the spatial organization.

No more than 8–10 electrodes are used: generally F3-4, C3-4, O1-2, T3-4, Cz., connected according to a double longitudinal montage (F4-C4, C4-O2, F4-T4, T4-O2, F3-C3, C3-O1, F3-T3, T3-O1) and a transverse montage that includes the vertex (T4-C4, C4-Cz, Cz-C3, C3-T3). Furthermore, an additional extracephalic reference lead is applied.

Before applying the electrodes, the baby's scalp is prepared with a slight abrasion in each electrode seat with a medium abrasive gel using the cotton end of an applicator stick; this can cause a slight erythema but it is only temporary and transitory.

For prolonged EEGs, it is necessary to apply a new dose of conductive paste to the cup electrodes—once or twice a day.

The optimal recording time of an examination is not less than 90 minutes, and therefore usually it takes at least 2 hours, considering the preparation time of the newborn and the adjustment of the child to the optimal recording. Even for the premature baby, the recording should not take less than 40 min and must allow to obtain relatively stable periods with a continuous and discontinuous electric EEG pattern.

Generally the reactivity of the child, and of the EEG traces, must be systematically studied at the end of the recording with auditory stimuli (hand clapping) or tactile stimuli; the technician must be constantly present during the recording to make the necessary adjustments in the surrounding environment (artifacts) and for the newborn care.

The EEG parameters used in our laboratory are high-pass filter of 0.53 Hz; low-pass filter of 30 Hz; notch filter for network noise, active; signal sensitivity of 100 mcV for 10 mm; and scrolling speed of 15–30 mm/s.

11.7 Polygraphic Parameters

In clinical practice, with the exception of specific medical indications, the polygraphic parameters are not recorded in critically ill neonates and in extreme preterm neonates (especially if intubated) that must be handled with extreme caution. In the others, the acquisition of polygraphic parameters is necessary to document and characterize the different behavioral states. Until the third month of post-conceptional age (PCA), cup electrodes are used with electroconductive paste, fixed with a plaster.

- Electrooculogram (EOG). The electrodes are positioned laterally to the external chant, on the two sides, respectively, above and below the median, to acquire both the lateral and the vertical eye movements.
- Recording parameters used are high-pass filter of 0.53–1.6 Hz, low-pass filter of 30 Hz, and signal sensitivity, to be adapted according to the deflection caused by the movement of the ocular globe—generally 100–200 mcV for 10 mm.
- Electromyogram (EMG). Muscle activity can be documented by placing a pair of skin electrodes under the chin on the chin muscle.
- The recording parameters used are high-pass filter of 5.0 Hz, low-pass filter of 70 Hz, and sensitivity, to be adapted according to the deflection caused by the suction movement—generally 100–150 mcV for 10 mm.
- Electrocardiogram (ECG). An electrode is located above the midline of the thorax and refers to other one in the left side of the thorax for recording a single channel that allows to identify the heart rhythm and especially a waveform certainly due to the electrical deflection of cardiac origin (see artifacts and constantly low-voltage EEG trace).
- The recording parameters used are high-pass filter of 5.0 Hz, 15 Hz of low-pass filter, and sensitivity, to be

modified according to the amplitude and the acquired waveform that varies with respect to the positioning of the electrodes (since the ECG is a wide signal, a sensitivity of 700–800 mcV is used).

- Respiratory activity. The respiratory rate is recorded at the thoracic and abdominal level using band transducers able to appreciate chest wall movements; in addition, the measurement of the airflow from the nostrils and the mouth is associated allying thermocouple devices placed under the nostrils and the registration of the saturation of O_2 and CO_2 by means of a distal oximeter.
- The recording parameters used are high-pass filter of 0.016 Hz, low-pass filter of 15 Hz, and sensitivity, to be adapted according to signal characteristics (150–200 mcV).
- Other nonstandard parameters can be recorded in particular clinical conditions: measurement of systemic blood pressure, global body movements, and contact EMG on different muscle groups.

11.8 Digital Video EEG

In recent years, with particular reference to the study of the semiology of neonatal seizures, considerable interest has been placed on this type of method that allows to obtain a video recording synchronized to the EEG recording. In order to obtain a good recording, it is essential to have a proper preparation of the surrounding environment: in particular, it is important to check temperature and lighting and avoid interference between the recording instruments and those used for the newborn care. During paroxysmal events and in any case where unusual events occur, nursing staff should not interfere with video recording, and the newborn should be kept uncovered to allow observation of the face and limbs.

The EEG technician, adequately trained in the management of the newborn, has the task of recording important events for the interpretation of the EEG. It is up to him, in any case, to prepare and properly follow the EEG registration. The video-EEG does not replace the human eye but provides the possibility of an off-line review of what happened during the recording phase [14, 23].

11.9 Maturation of Behavioral and EEG Patterns: From Prematurity to the End of the Neonatal Period

11.9.1 Behavioral Patterns

In the term infant, it is possible to recognize "behavioral states" with cyclic and predictable trends, defined on the basis of the presence of specific motor, neurovegetative, and affective-relational behaviors.

These states defined by Prechtl and Beintema [24], on the basis of changes in breathing, eye movements, body movements, and crying, are clearly identifiable from the 37th week of GA. Each specific behavioral state corresponds to a specific cerebral electrical activity.

State I: Regular breathing, eyes closed, and no movement of the body (quiet sleep)
State II: Irregular breathing, closed eyes, and small movements of the body (active sleep)
State III: Open eyes and rare and slow movements of the body (quiet alert)
State IV: Open eyes and movements of great amplitude (active alert)
State V: Open or closed eyes, intense motor activity, and crying

In the preterm newborns, the behavioral states are less clearly defined. In infants aged under 28 weeks of GA, sleep and wakefulness are not always discernible (indeterminate state). Historically, it has originated the statement that a newborn of GA under 27 weeks is never awake and never sleeps [4]. Actually, a clear difference between wakefulness and sleep is only possible from 32 weeks of GA. Before this age, it seems more appropriate to define rest phases and phases of activity (rest-activity cycles). On the other hand, some authors hypothesize the emergence of a rudimentary sleep differentiation even in earlier ages; however, the definition of states is constantly based on the use of the EEG. Vecchierini et al. [25] analyzed the characteristics of EEG and ocular motility in a preterm sample at a conception age of between 24 and 26 weeks and documented the presence of two sleep patterns: the first one characterized by the presence of eye movements and a more continuous cerebral electrical activity of greater amplitude and the second one from the absence of ocular movements and from a more discontinuous and lower-amplitude electrical activity. At 28–31 weeks of GA, from the EEG and polygraphic point of view, we begin to recognize epochs of activity in part similar to the active sleep and alert states recognized in the full newborn, alternating with epochs of "quiet sleep." From 31 to 34 weeks' GA, these epochs of active sleep-wakefulness are more easily identifiable with behavioral and polygraphic parameters and prevail over the phases in which the newborn appears inert and the polygraphic-behavioral parameters suggest a phase of quiet sleep. Only from 35 weeks of GA, a clear differentiation between wakefulness, active sleep, and quiet sleep is recognizable. From 38 to 42 weeks of GA, the behavioral states are stable and well differentiated with progressive reduction of the active sleep phases and parallel increase in the phases of quiet sleep.

Active sleep (REM sleep) corresponds to Prechtl's state II, and it is ontogenetically the most ancient sleep because it originates from subcortical structures (it originates in the rostral part of the brainstem with projections to the hypothalamus). The newborn shows small-body movements, sometimes smiles or makes facial grimaces, and presents rapid lateral movements of the eyeballs; breathing is irregular and the muscle tone is decreased (especially bulbar muscles). Up to 34 weeks' GA, this is the predominant type of sleep. The full-term newborn falls asleep directly into REM sleep. Two EEG patterns are distinguished within the active sleep cycle. The first is recognizable at the beginning of the cycle: high-voltage continuous (HVC) or mixed activity. The second is called low-voltage irregular (LVI), and it is observed after a non-REM sleep cycle. In some cases, the active sleep that follows a calm sleep appears completely indistinguishable from the wake EEG pattern (activité moyenne).

Quiet sleep (non-REM/NREM sleep) corresponds to a more developed status (Prechtl's state I). It is a more evolved status than the previous one because it originates from the caudal structures of the brainstem with projections to the hypothalamus, to the thalamus, and subsequently into the cortex. It appears well differentiated from the 35th week of GA and is recognizable by the presence of regular breathing (short respiratory irregularities are still possible, especially in infants with respiratory disorders), absence (or rare) of eye movements, and constant tonic muscle activity. Body movements are rare and similar to sursauts. In this behavioural state, two patterns are discernible: the first is called alternating pattern (tracé alternant), and the second is continuous slow-wave pattern [continuous slow waves (CSW) or high-voltage slow (HVS)]. For practical purposes, even at lower GA, the discontinuous patterns are more often associated with states in which the newborn lies motionless with closed eyes, and most of the authors believe that this electroclinical condition can be assimilated to a quiet sleep phase.

Indeterminate (or transitional) is defined as a sleep period that does not meet the criteria described above for active sleep or quiet sleep. It is generally observed just before REM sleep and between REM sleep and quiet sleep.

11.9.2 Physiological EEG Patterns

In general, the EEG recording of the premature infant is characterized by the discontinuity of the brain electrical activity. The recording of the full-term infant, and in any case with a CA over 35–36 weeks, is characterized by the continuity of the electrical activity in all the states [15, 25, 26].

The visual analysis of the neonatal EEG, from prematurity to the term CA, involves in the first instance the definition of the features during either the inactive trace or the traces with electrical activity, with their respective spatial and temporal characteristics. In the context of the so-called developmental process, there is a gradual change from a discontinuous pattern to a continuous one, which simultaneously loses the typical electrical features of the previous CA to be enriched with graphic elements typical of later CA. At the same time, the EEG patterns associated with the different behavioral states of wakefulness and sleep, which are organized proportionally to the CA, must be identified. The comparison of certain shapes and electrical EEG patterns characteristic of the appropriate CA is an indication of behavioral electrical concordance and ultimately of probable physiological functionality of the CNS. On the contrary, the absence of concordance and the alteration of EEG patterns must be at least a suspicion sign of pathology. However, it should be kept in mind that for each CA, typical figures and EEG patterns can coexist with figures and patterns of earlier ages and that the EEG patterns are very sensitive to extracerebral variables. It follows that the conclusion on the EEG recording, especially in preterm babies, should be expressed with caution and based on repeated recordings at appropriate times. Dealing with a full-term infant, in the ideal recording conditions, a complete sleep wake cycle can be obtained during a 60–90 min-EEG recording; wakefulness → active sleep → quiet sleep → wakefulness (sometimes after a quiet sleep cycle it is also possible to observe a second phase of the active sleep with an activité moyenne-like pattern).

A summary of the peculiar EEG features and patterns in the different CA is reported below (see also Table 11.1):

Before 27 weeks GA: EEG recording is characterized by discontinuous electrical activity as follows: short bursts of a duration varying from 1 to 46 s (or more) and with amplitude around 50 μV are interspersed with inactive epochs lasting generally less than 60 s. The presence of slow waves at 0.5–1 Hz of variable amplitude up to over 300 μV, with variable localization, sometimes widespread, often temporal or occipital, mono-/biphasic, often in short sequences, rarely associated with rapid activity at 5–9 Hz that is superimposed on the slow waves when located in the central regions. The presence of isolated high-amplitude and variable morphology frontal sharp waves (200–300 μV). Short burst, diffuse, or temporal and occipital localization of sharp theta activity of high amplitude up to 300 μV might also be observed.

The greater the prematurity, the longer the duration of the epochs in which no electrical activity is recognized on the EEG recording; reciprocally, the greater the prematurity, the lower the duration of the epochs with continuous electrical activity.

Significant interhemispheric synchrony of the bursts. Monomorphic occipital delta, in short runs of a few seconds, bilaterally synchronous and symmetric. Poor or no reactivity of the background EEG activity to stimulations (Figs. 11.1, 11.2, 11.3, and 11.4).

By 27 to 29 weeks GA: EEG recording with an overall discontinuous electric activity, more continuous in active

Table 11.1 Developmental EEG patterns and behavioral states

Conceptional age (week)	Specific waveforms[a]	Continuity of electrical activity and specific patterns[a]	Behavioral state
24–27	Hypersynchronous bursts Occipital delta of 0.5–1 Hz Infrequent central (occipital) delta brushes	Discontinuous tracing No reactivity to stimulation	Undetermined state
28–31	Occipital delta Central delta brushes Rhythmic temporal theta activity Sharp temporal theta bursts	Discontinuous tracing Electrical activity becomes continuous during active sleep No reactivity to stimulation	Active sleep (Wake±/Quiet sleep±)
32–34	Frequent occipital-temporal delta brushes Synchronous occipital delta Rhythmic temporal and alpha bursts Both positive and negative, temporal and Rolandic sharp waves	Discontinuous tracing (in quiet sleep) Continuous tracing in active sleep Inconstant reactivity to stimulation	Active sleep (Wake±) (Quiet sleep±)
35–37	Encoches frontales ASD[b] (infrequent) Infrequent occipital delta brushes Multifocal slow sharp waves	Activité moyenne LVI[c] Tracé alternant Reactive to stimulation	Wake Active sleep Quiet sleep Undetermined/ transitional sleep
38–44	Encoches frontales ASD[b] Isolate Rolandic and temporal sharp waves	Activité moyenne Mixed activity LVI[c] Tracé alternant HVS[d] Reactive to stimulation	Wake Active sleep Quiet sleep Transitional sleep

Adapted from Lombroso [12], Tharp [27], Anders et al. [28], Kellaway [29], Ferrari et al., [30] Mastrangelo et al., [31], André et al. [32]
[a]Both for the specific waveforms and patterns, refer to the following iconography (Figs. 11.1, 11.2, 11.3, 11.4, 11.5, 11.6, 11.7, 11.8, 11.9, 11.10, 11.11, 11.12, 11.13, 11.14, 11.15, 11.16, 11.17, 11.18, 11.19, 11.20, 11.21, 11.22, 11.23, 11.24, 11.25, 11.26, 11.27, 11.28, 11.29, 11.30, 11.31, 11.32, 11.33, and 11.34)
[b]*ASD* anterior slow dysrhythmia
[c]*LVI* low-voltage irregular
[d]*HVS* high-voltage slow

sleep state. Rolandic and occipital delta brushes, in active sleep state. Initial representation of theta rhythmic temporal activity (temporal sawtooth) in sequences (runs) up to 2 s—bilateral symmetric and synchronous occipital delta waves in sequences of variable duration (less than 60″). Less interhemispheric synchrony of the bursts compared to the aforementioned age. Poor or no reactivity of the background EEG activity to stimulations (Figs. 11.5, 11.6, 11.7, 11.8, 11.9, 11.10, 11.11, and 11.12).

By 30 to 34 weeks GA: EEG recording with an overall discontinuous electrical activity during calm sleep, greater representation of continuous epochs during active sleep state.

Frequent occipital and temporal delta brushes in active sleep state (from 33 weeks of CA in quiet sleep)—reduction of temporal theta temporal activity (from 32 weeks of CA) replaced by temporal rhythmic alpha activity that disappears before 35 weeks of CA.

Significant interhemispheric asynchrony (especially in quiet sleep state). Initial reactivity of the background EEG activity to stimulation (Figs. 11.13 and 11.14).

By 35 to 37 weeks GA: continuous electric activity in all the states (mixed activity) in wakefulness/active sleep state, although transient and short periods of low-voltage background EEG activity may occur in quiet sleep state. Reduction of delta brushes with occipital and temporal localization, more evident in quiet sleep state. Frontal sharp waves in sleep state (more often bilaterally synchronous). Initial appearance of anterior slow dysrhythmia (ASD). Isolated multifocal sharp waves. Resumption of the interhemispheric synchrony. Background activity reactive to stimulation (Figs. 11.15, 11.16, 11.17, 11.18, 11.19, 11.20, and 11.21).

More than 38 weeks GA: continuous electrical activity in all states. Frontal sharp waves and ASD more frequent in the transition from active sleep state to quiet sleep state. Isolated Rolandic or temporal spikes. Significant interhemispheric synchrony from 40 weeks of CA. Five EEG states can be distinguished: wakefulness, active sleep (two patterns) and quiet sleep (two patterns) states (see Appendix):

Wakefulness: Activité moyenne

Active sleep (REM sleep):

- Mixed activity: at the beginning of the sleep cycle
- Low-voltage irregular (LVI): low-voltage irregular pattern after a quiet sleep state

Quite sleep state (NREM sleep):

- Tracé alternant (TA)—alternating tracing, intermittent pattern
- High-voltage slow (HVS)—high-voltage slow pattern:

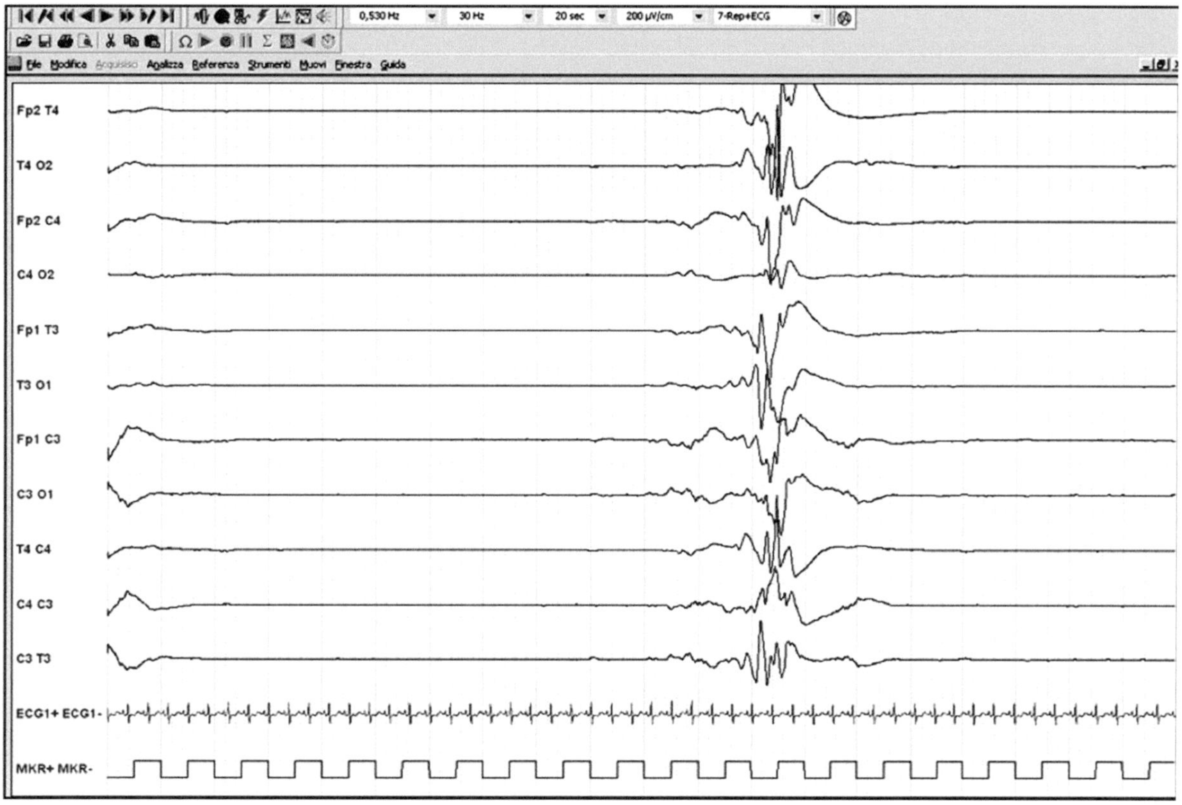

Fig. 11.1 24 weeks GA, 24.4 weeks CA. Discontinuous tracing with electrical quiescence. Bilateral synchronous 3–4 s burst with sharp theta activity (4–5 Hz, 50–350 µV), predominant over temporal regions. An isolated diffuse delta wave (up to 350 µV) is intermingled or follows immediately the burst. This newborn (the same in Figs. 11.1, 11.2, 11.3, and 11.4) was mechanically ventilated for non-neurological reasons. Spontaneous motility and cerebral ultrasound were normal. The inter-bursts interval is CA dependent and has its longest duration at this age

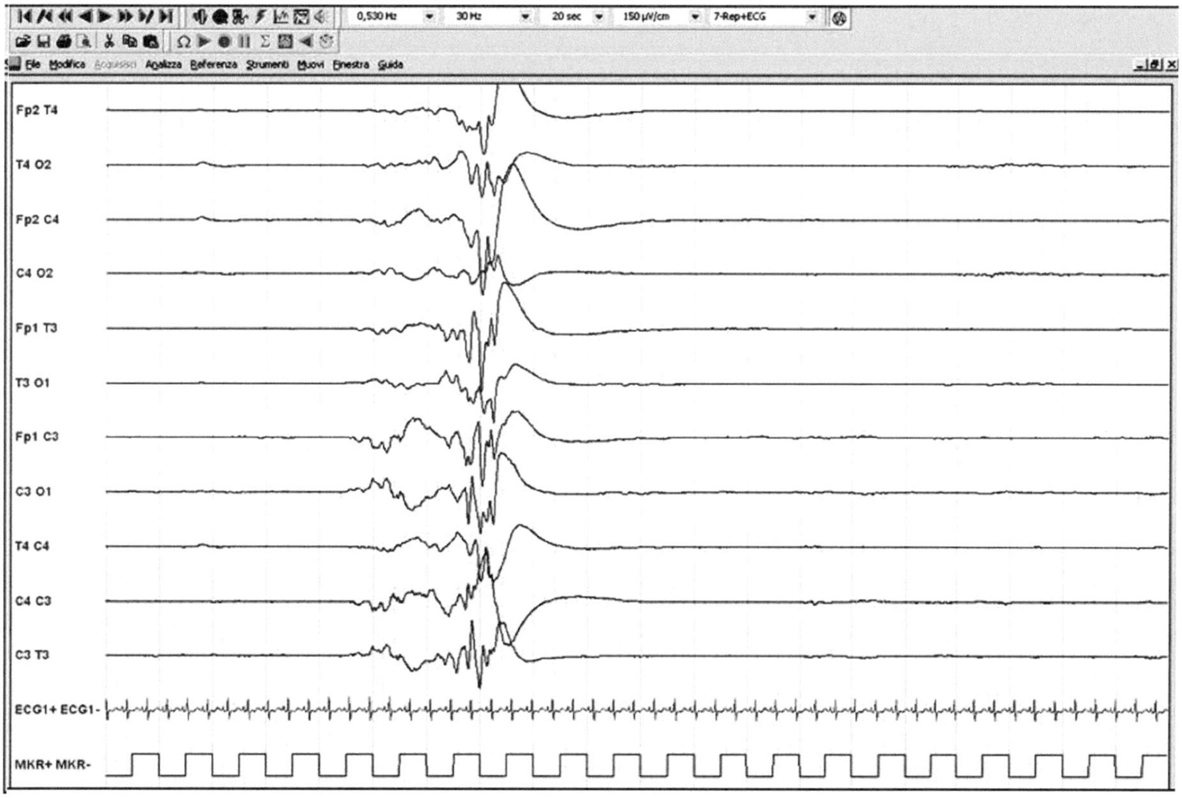

Fig. 11.2 24 weeks GA, 24.4 weeks CA. Discontinuous tracing with electrical quiescence. Synchronous bilateral burst in a discontinuous tracing. Notice that the activity in the burst is not symmetrical

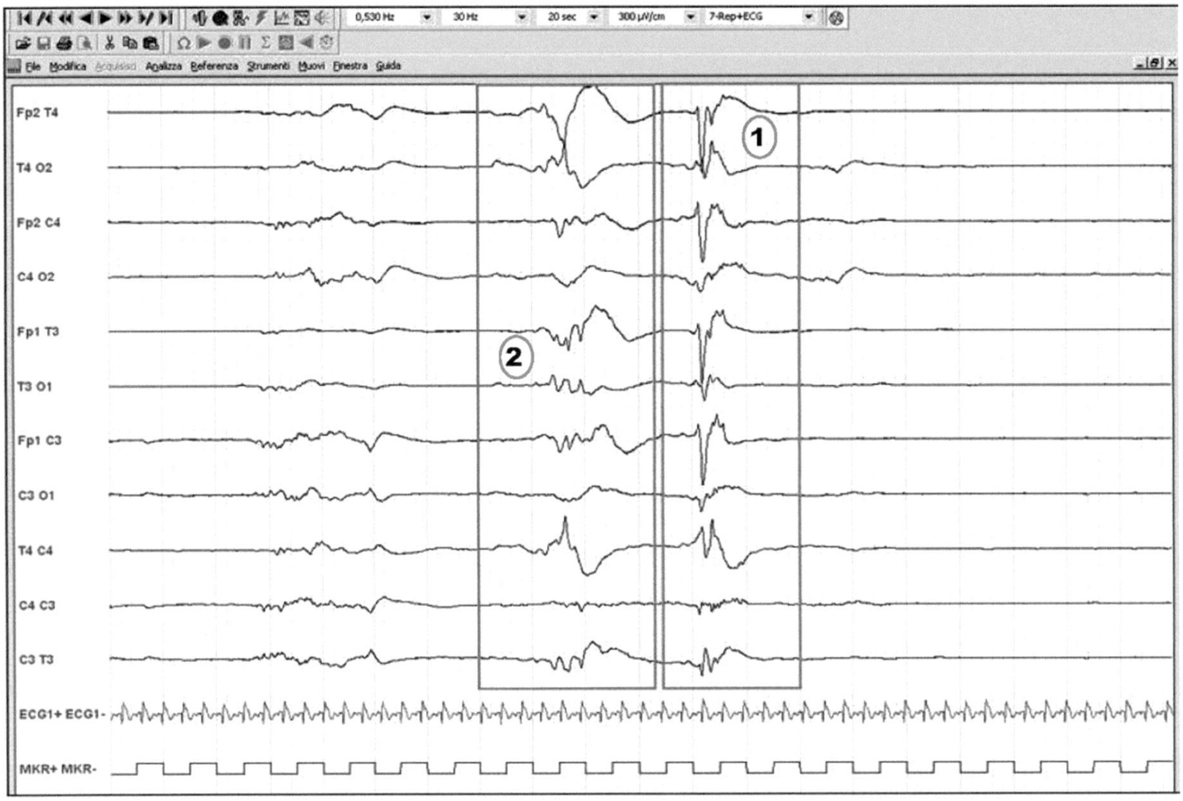

Fig. 11.3 24 weeks GA, 25.2 weeks CA. Discontinuous tracing with electrical quiescence. Notice in the burst (*1*) sharp and dysphasic frontal slow waves (negative-positive course up to 400 µV), (*2*) temporal theta activity (up to 120 µV), associated with a diffuse delta wave of high amplitude (up to 350 µV), predominately over temporal regions. The electrical quiescence periods decrease progressively

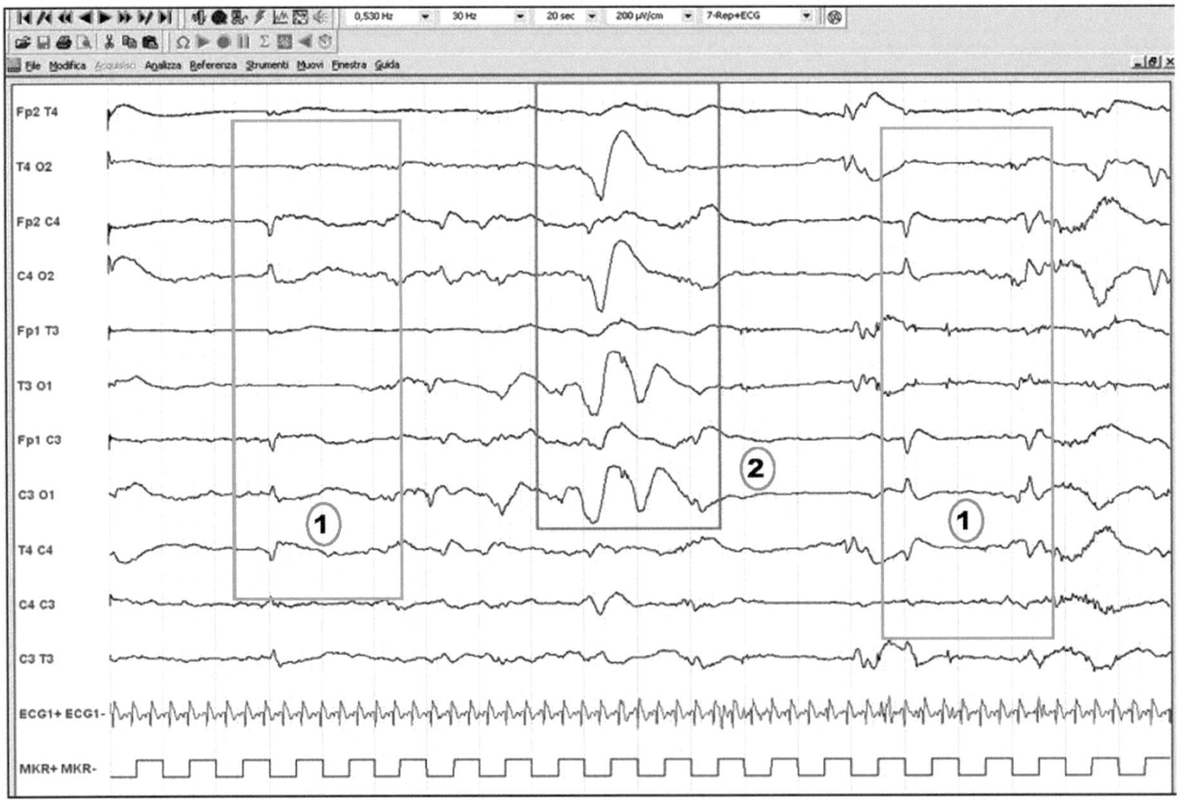

Fig. 11.4 24 weeks GA, 25.2 weeks CA. Discontinuous tracing: (*1*) period of more continuous and diffuse low-voltage activity (less than 150 µV). (*2*) Bilateral delta activity over occipital regions up to 400 µV, isolated or in short sequences

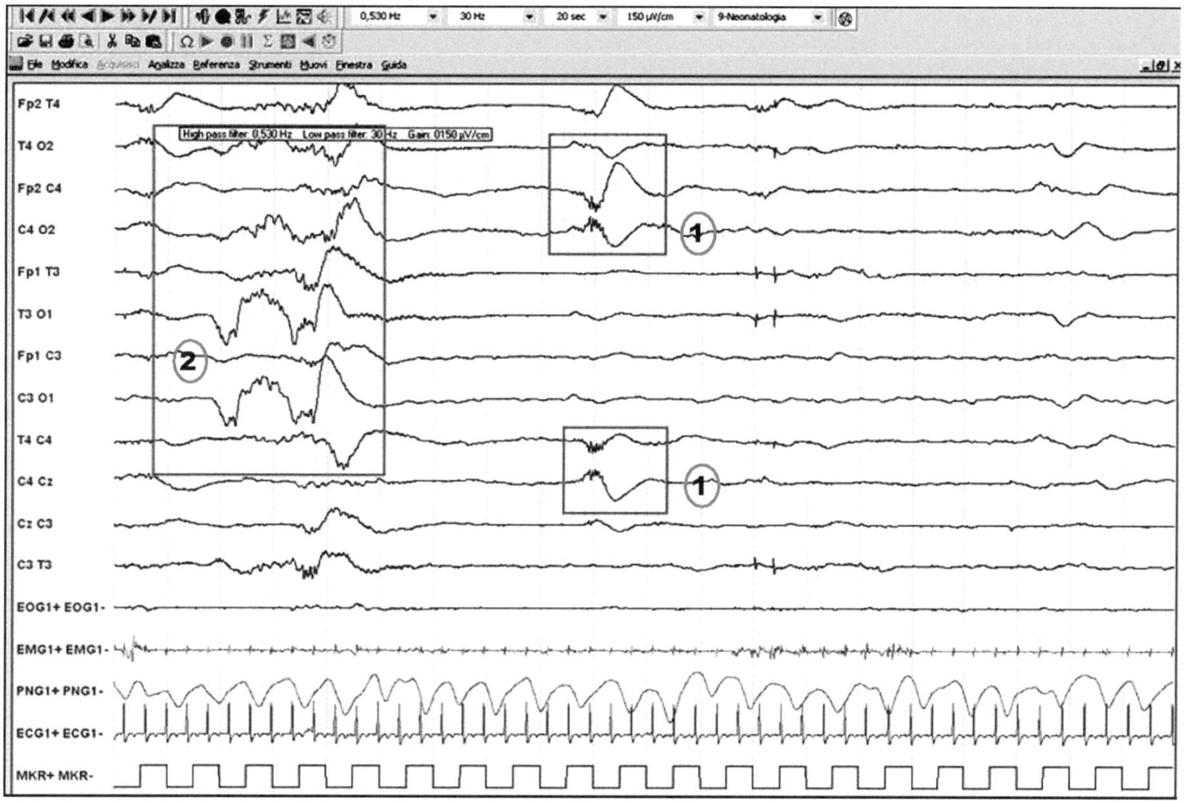

Fig. 11.5 27 weeks GA, 29–30 weeks CA. Discontinuous tracing: (*1*) Rolandic and (*2*) occipital delta brushes (delta wave with superimposed beta complexes): the amplitude of the slow wave is between 150 and 300 μV, while beta activity is generally less than 40 μV

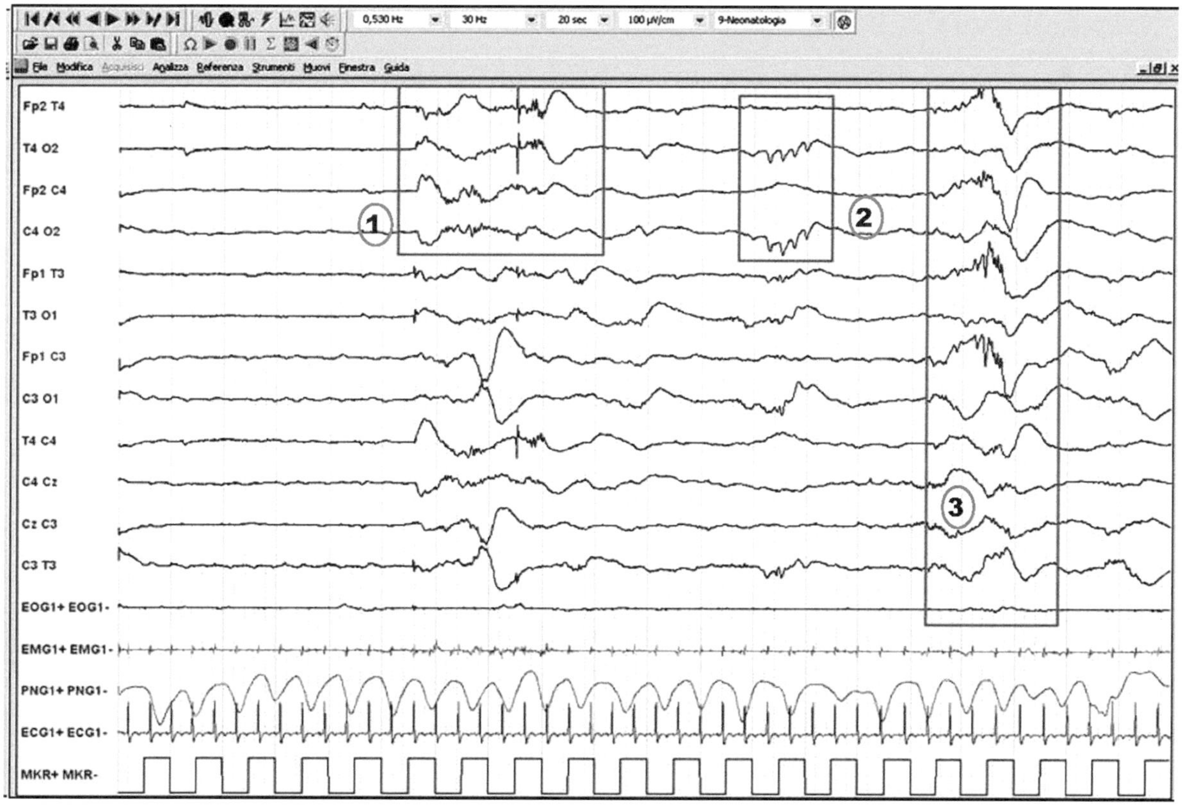

Fig. 11.6 27 weeks GA, 29–30 weeks CA. Discontinuous tracing: (*1*) Rolandic and occipital delta brushes (delta wave amplitude is less than 100 μV); (*2*) occipital rhythmic theta activity (less than 70 μV) in the right side; (*3*) notice in the bursts a diffuse delta activity

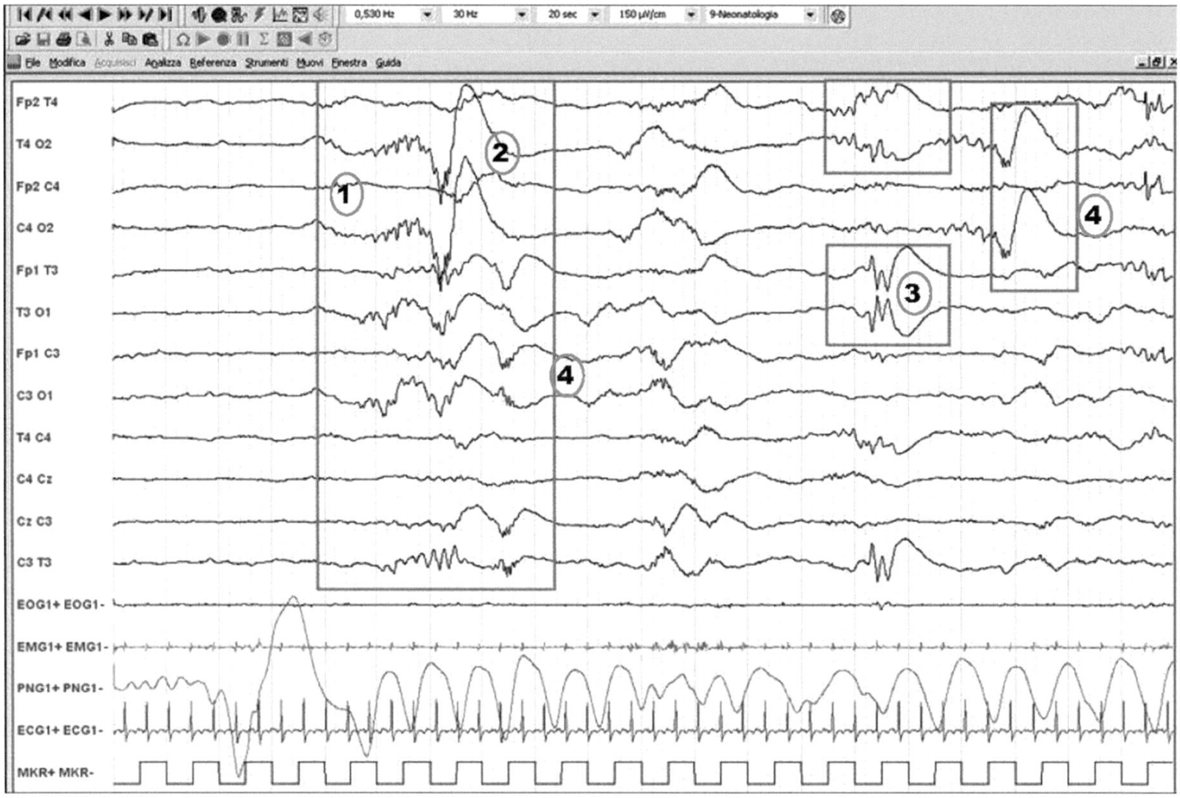

Fig. 11.7 27 weeks GA, 29–30 weeks CA. Discontinuous tracing: notice a 20 s epoch with continuous activity related to active sleep. (*1*) rhythmic theta occipital activity; (*2*) bilateral occipital delta activity (up to 400 μV); (*3*) sharp and bilateral temporal theta (up to 150 μV); (*4*) Rolandic and occipital delta brushes (delta wave amplitude between 150 and 300 μV)

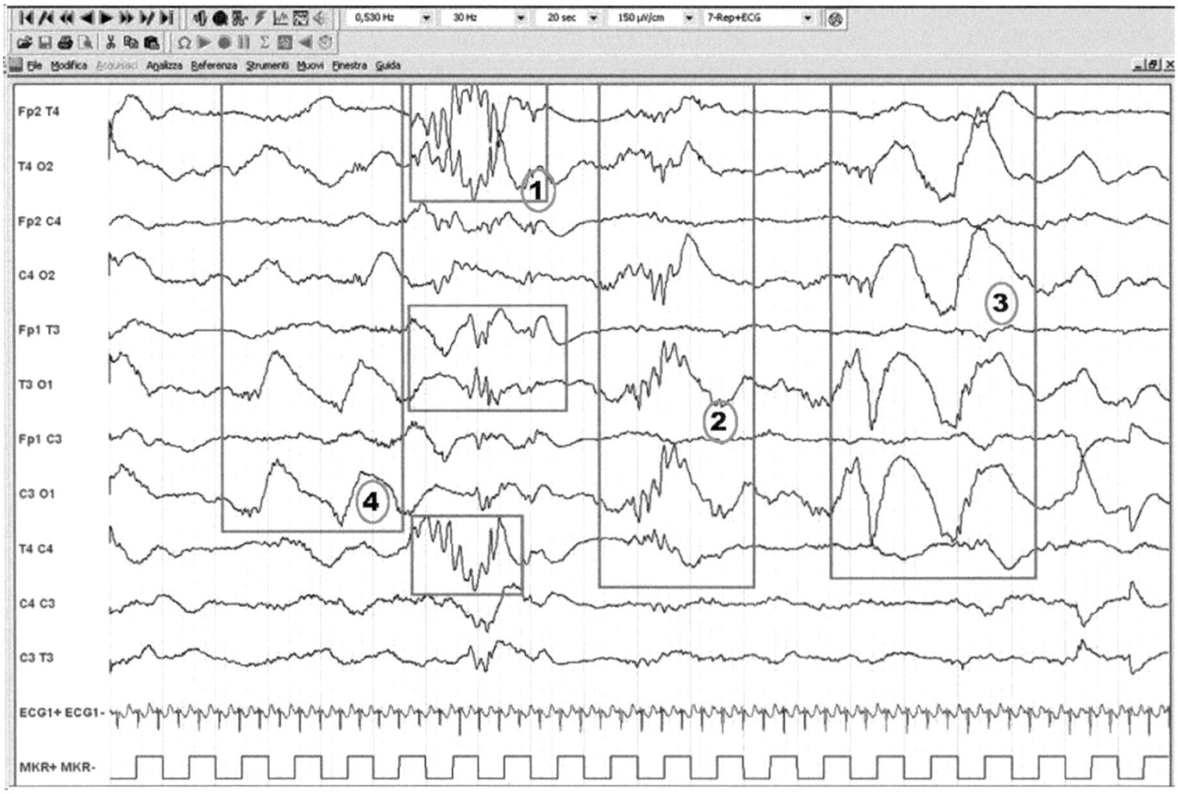

Fig. 11.8 24 weeks GA, 29–30 weeks CA. In a discontinuous tracing epochs lasting 20 s with continuous electrical activity consistent with active sleep. Electrical pattern overlapping the description in Fig. 11.7 (same CA, different GA in the two newborns): (*1*) bilateral sharp theta temporal activity for 2 s; (*2*) bilateral occipital theta rhythmic activity; (*3*) occipital rhythmic delta wave, bilateral and synchronous; (*4*) occipital delta brushes

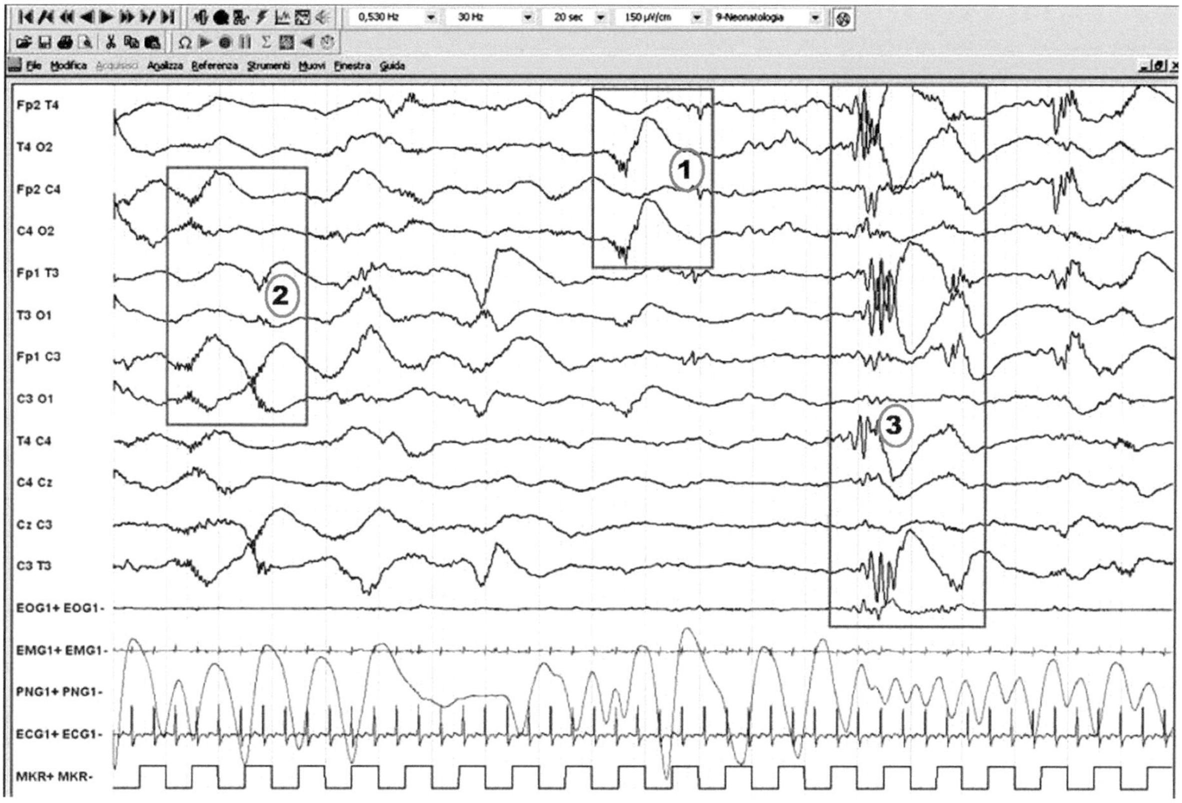

Fig. 11.9 27 weeks GA, 29–30 weeks CA. In a discontinuous tracing epochs lasting 20 s with continuous electrical activity consistent with active sleep: delta brushes (*1*) occipital and (*2*) Rolandic; (*3*) sharp and rhythmic bilateral temporal theta activity

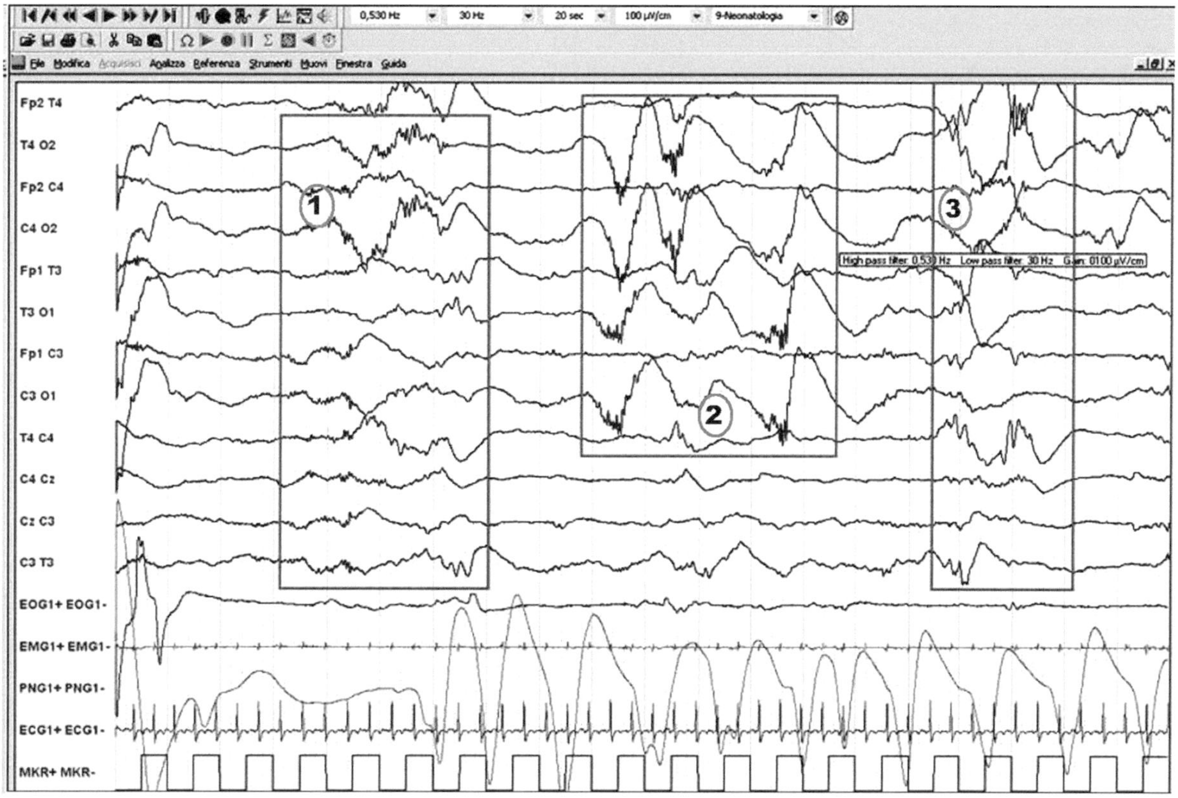

Fig. 11.10 27 weeks GA, 29–30 weeks CA. Discontinuous tracing: (*1*) Low-voltage alpha activity over right occipital and left central regions; (*2*) bilateral and synchronous delta brushes over occipital regions; (*3*) sharp rhythmic theta activity over right temporal region. Between the three patterns described there are brief (1–2 s-long) with quiescent activity. This condition is related to active sleep

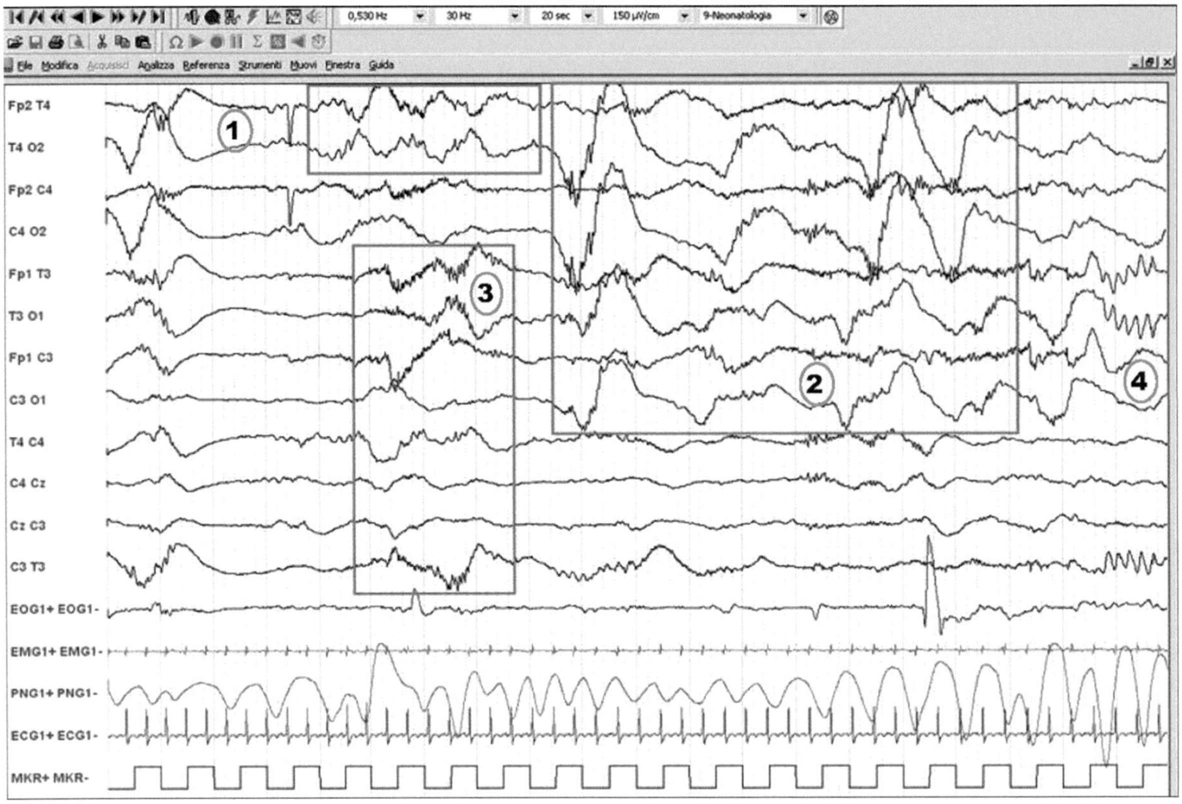

Fig. 11.11 27 weeks GA, 29–30 weeks CA. Transition from active to quiet sleep: (*1*) temporal alpha activity; (*2*) bilateral occipital delta activity (up to 300 μV); (*3*) occipital and Rolandic delta brushes; (*4*) 2 s theta rhythmic activity over left temporal region

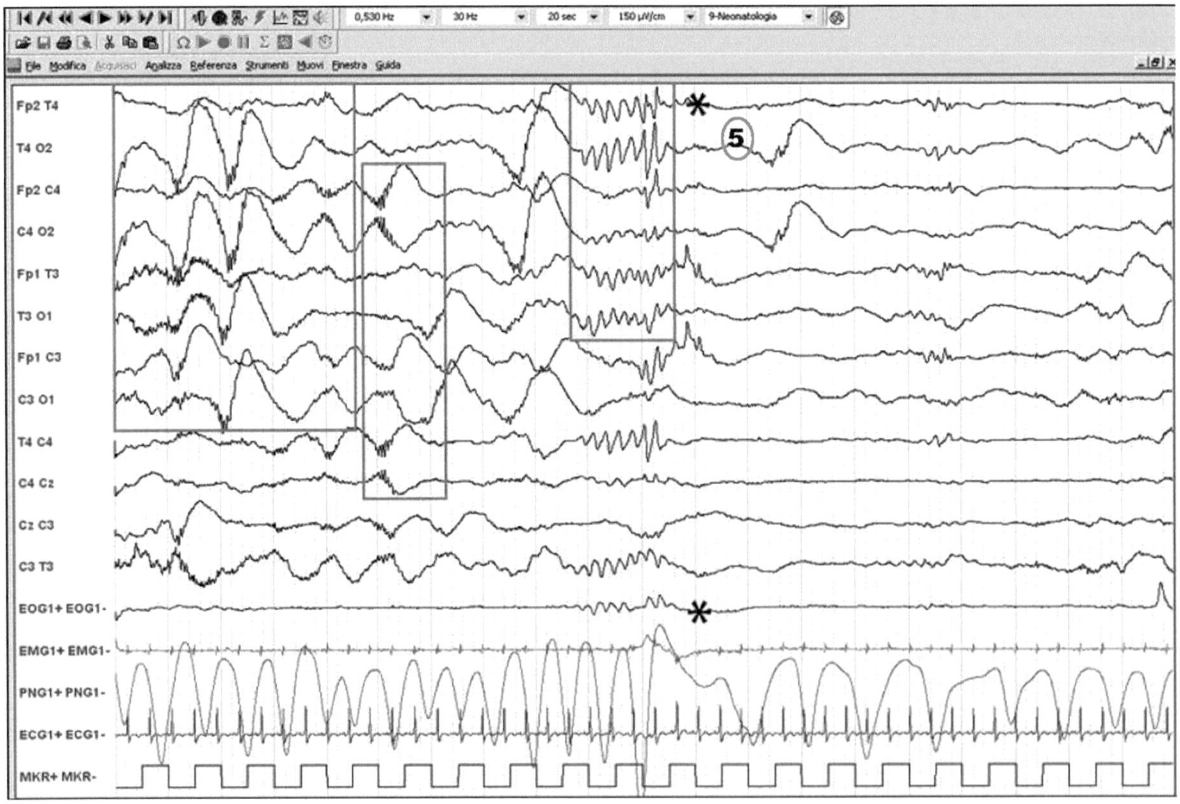

Fig. 11.12 27 weeks GA, 29–30 weeks CA. Same patient of Fig. 11.11 with overlapping features. Moreover (*5*) transition pattern to discontinuous tracing

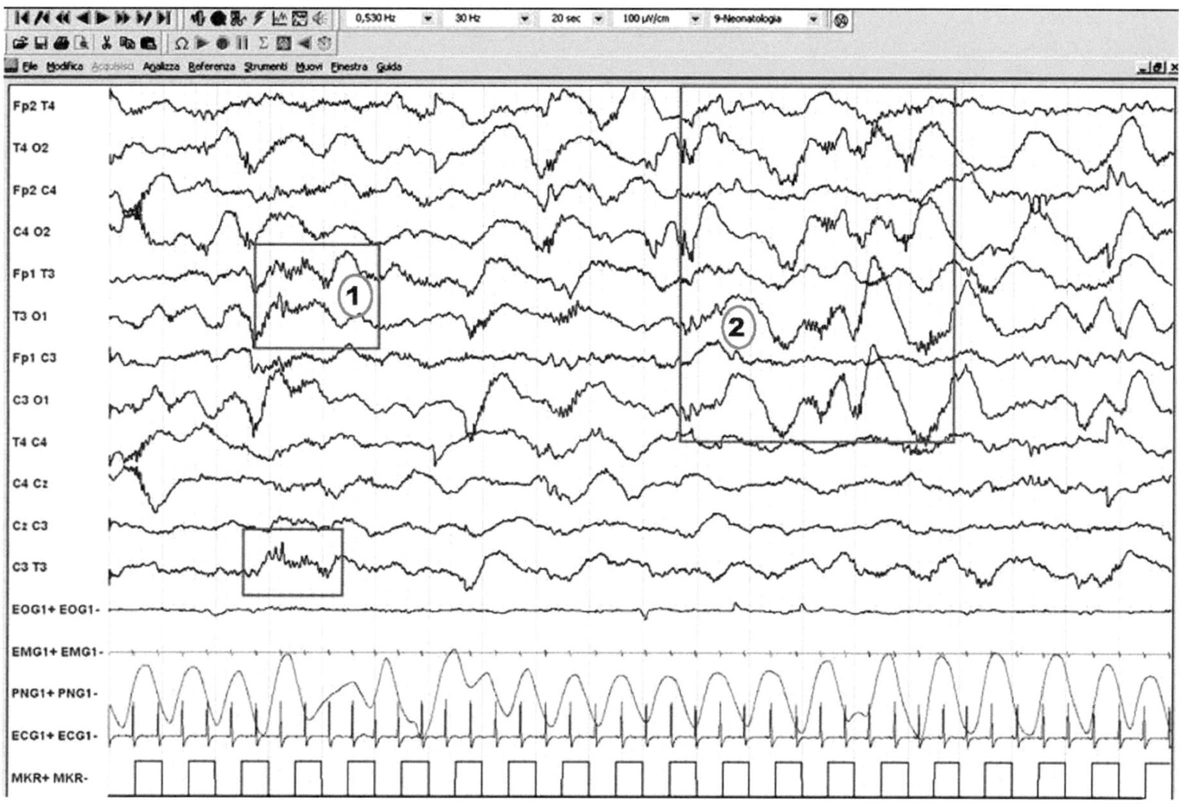

Fig. 11.13 27 weeks GA, 33–34 weeks CA. Continuous electrical activity in REM/active sleep: (*1*) slow amplitude temporal rhythmic alpha activity; (*2*) sequence of delta brushes over bilateral occipital regions

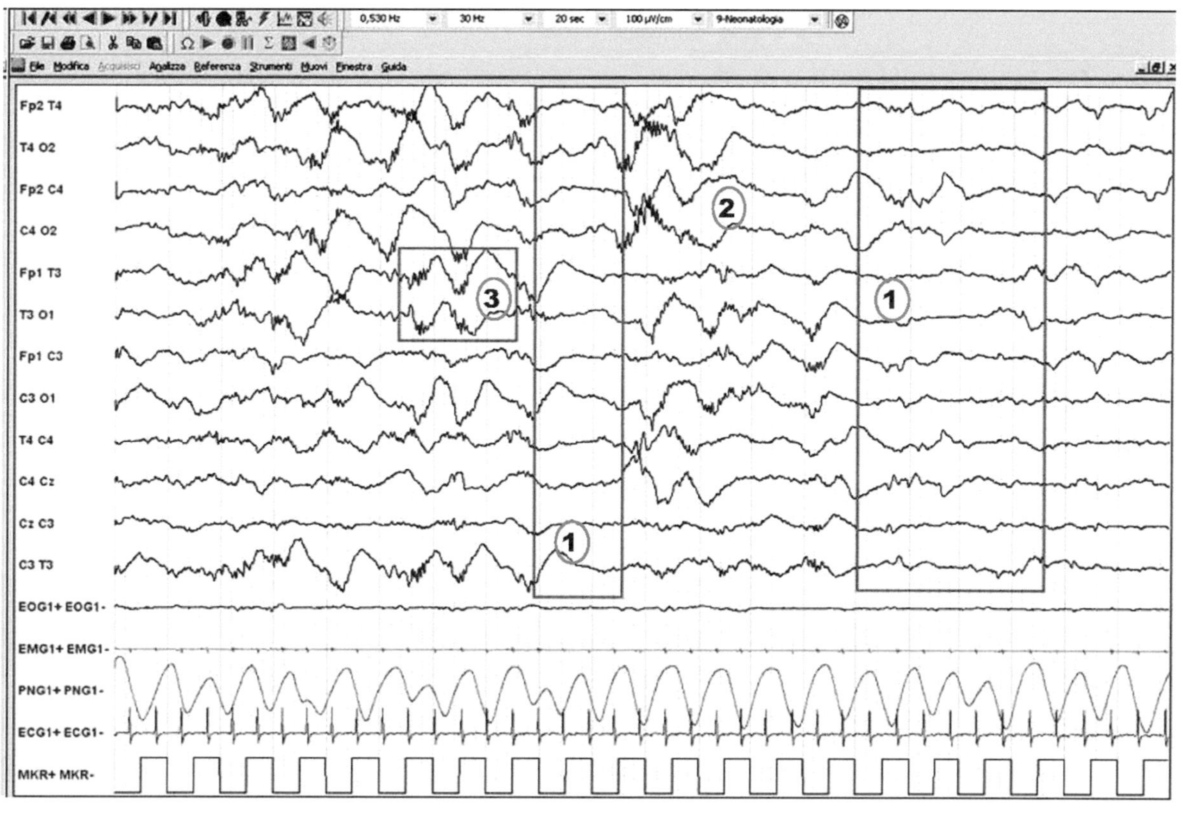

Fig. 11.14 27 weeks GA, 33–34 weeks CA. NREM/Quiet sleep. The pattern is still discontinuous, but (*1*) interbursts of inactivity are progressively reduced in duration comparing to previous CA; (*2*) bilateral delta activity over occipital regions; (3) temporal and occipital delta brushes

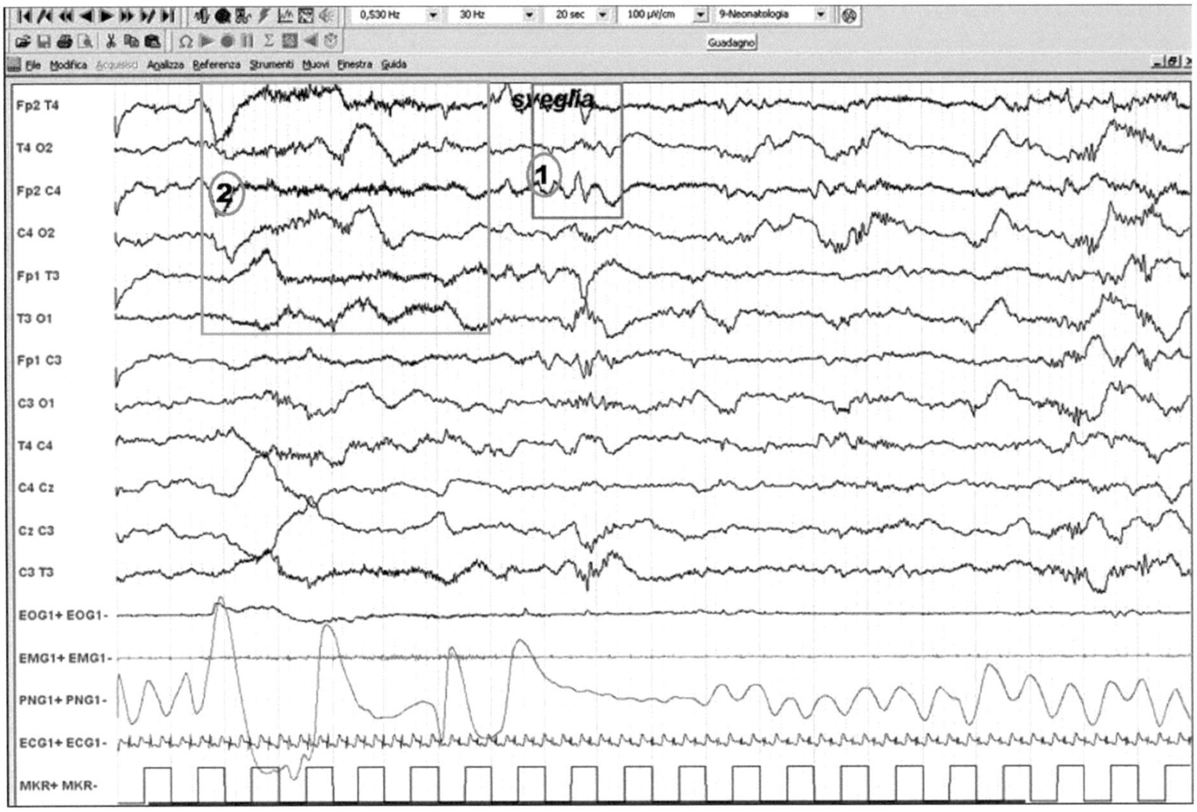

Fig. 11.15 32 weeks GA, 35–36 weeks CA. Quiet alert: diffuse continuous electrical activity, mostly theta (less than 60 μV), several delta and alpha waves (sveglia = awake). (*1*) Anterior sleep frontal transients over the right side; (*2*) artifactual fast activity (muscles) in the frontal right leads and temporal left region related to a global movement documented by the artifact of pneumogram polygraphic channel

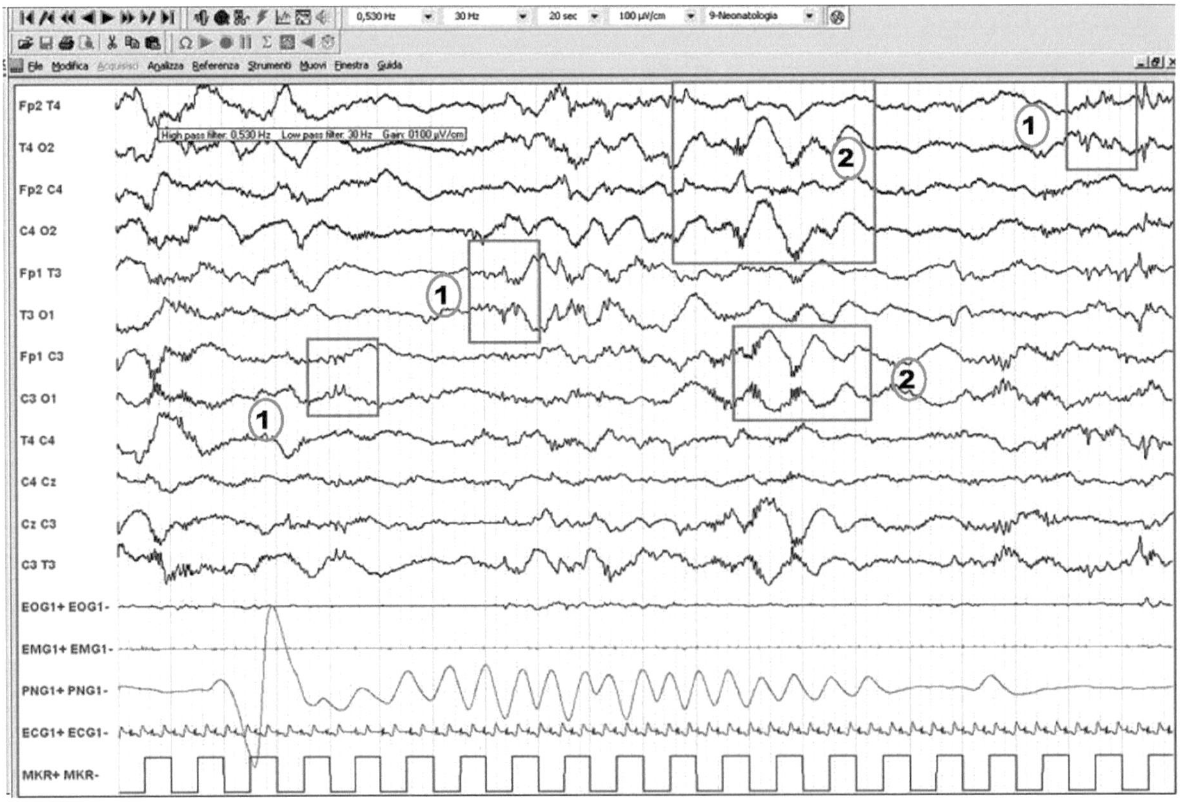

Fig. 11.16 32 weeks GA, 35–36 weeks CA. Continuous electrical activity in transitional sleep pattern. (*1*) Multifocal and isolated slow spikes over central and temporal left regions; (*2*) delta brushes over right occipital and left central regions

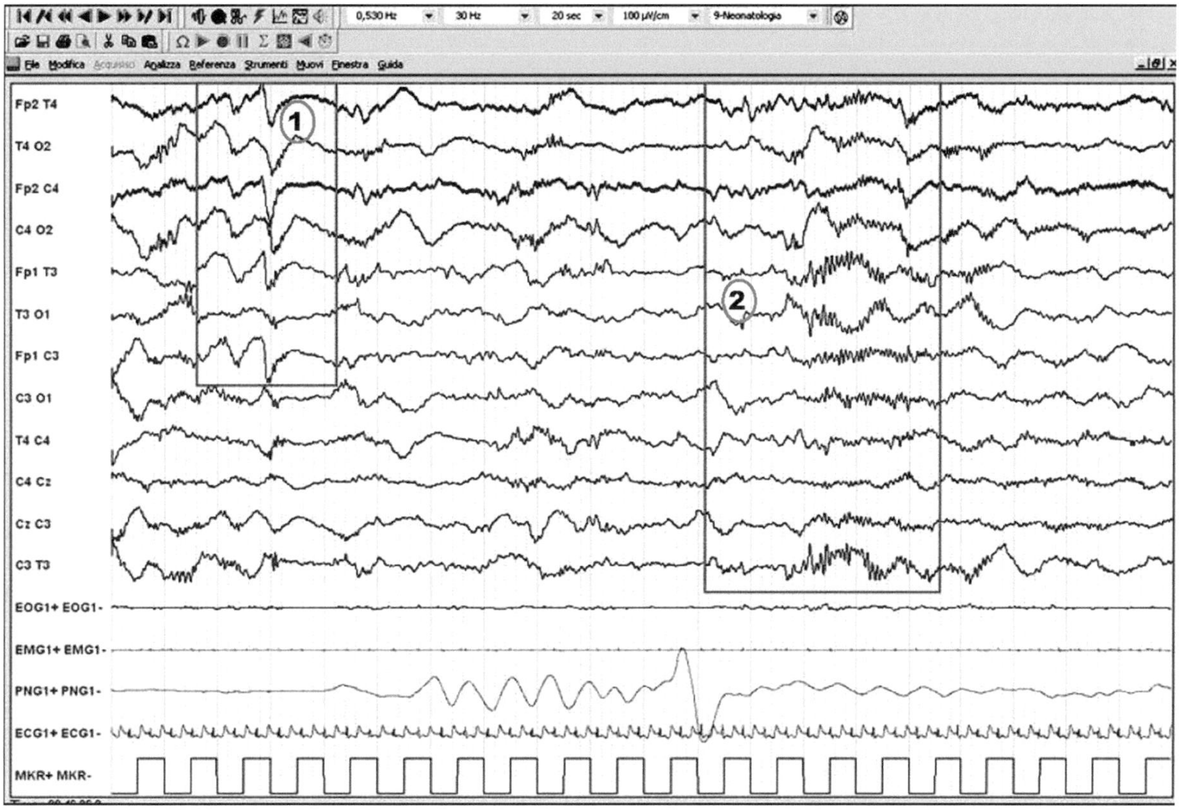

Fig. 11.17 32 weeks GA, 35–36 weeks CA. Active sleep: continuous diffuse theta-delta activity. (*1*) Bilateral frontal sharp transients (*encoche frontale, Dreyfus-Brisac, 1962)*; (*2*) bilateral central and temporal alpha-beta activity. Irregular activity in the PNG polygraphic channel

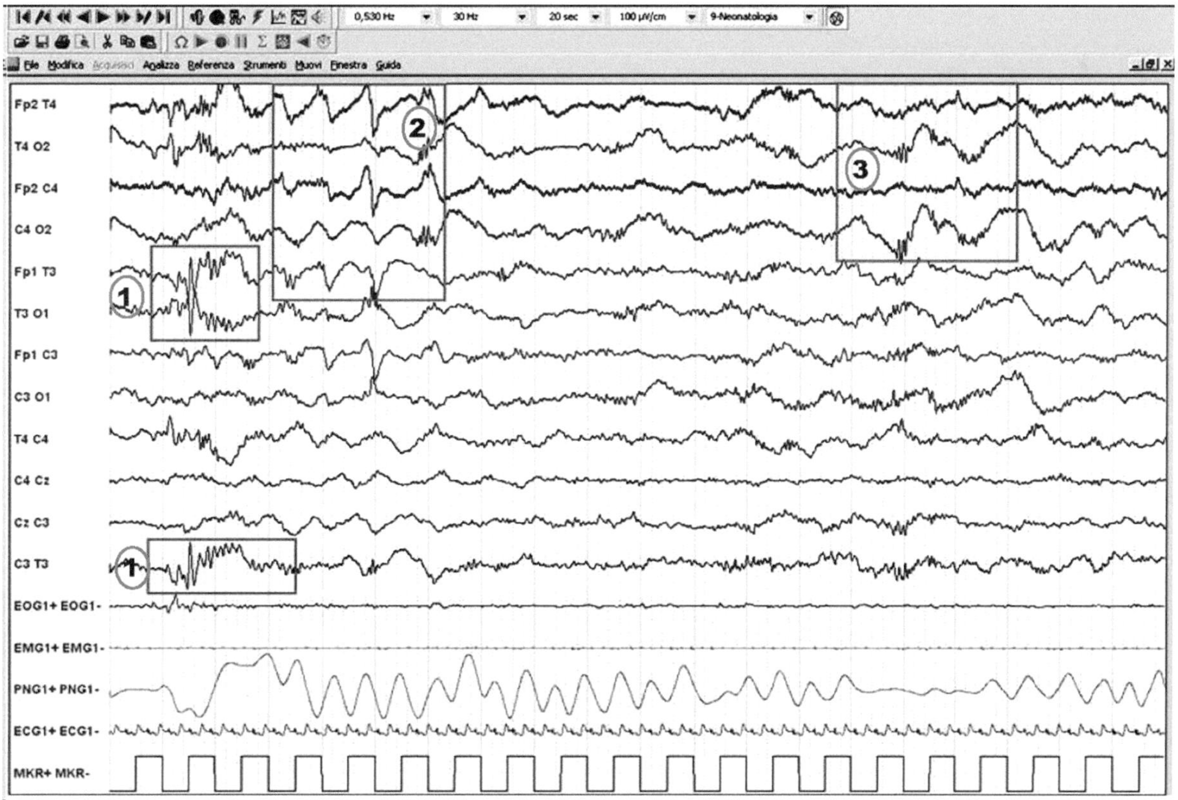

Fig. 11.18 32 weeks GA, 35–36 weeks CA. Active sleep: continuous background activity with (*1*) left theta-alpha activity associated with temporal medium voltage isolated sharp wave; (*2*) rhythmic bifrontal delta activity associated with frontal sharp transients; (*3*) occipital delta brushes over the right side

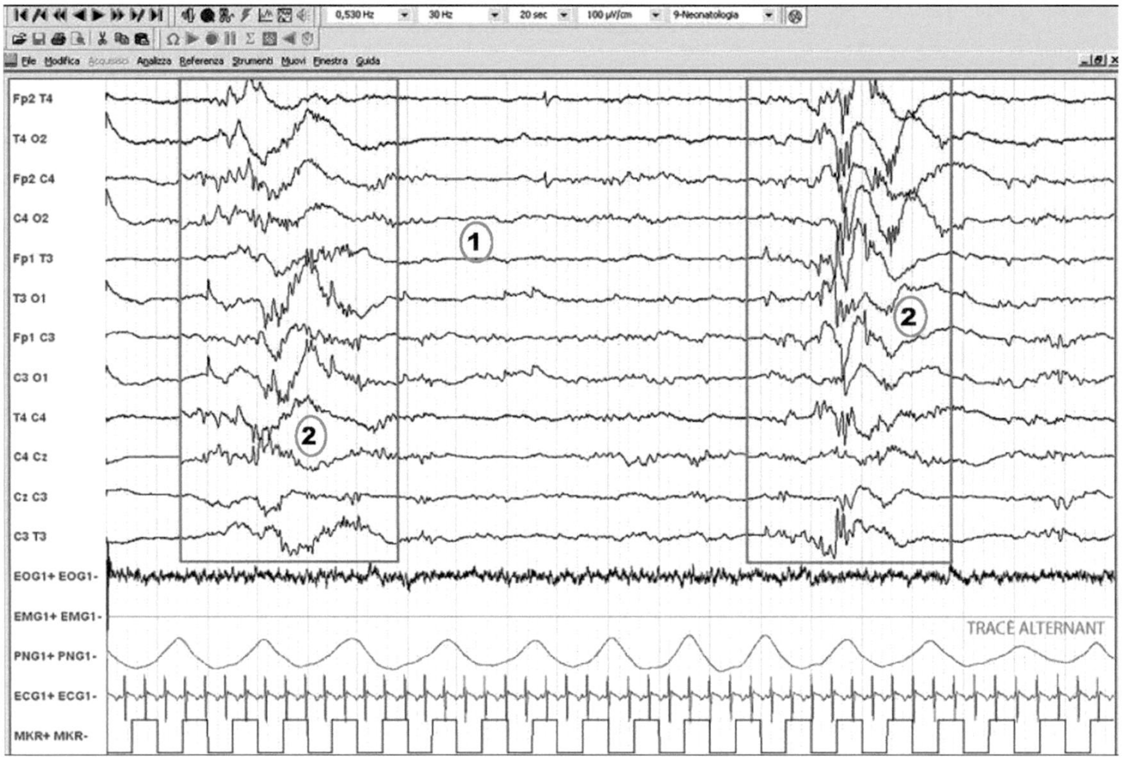

Fig. 11.19 33 weeks GA, 37–38 weeks CA. *Tracé alternant* pattern in deep non-rapid eye movement (NREM/quiet) sleep: (*1*) periods (8–10 s) of discontinuity with low-voltage (less than 50 µV) theta activity; (*2*) bilateral bursts (3–5 s) with theta (50–100 µV) and delta (up to 300 µV) activity with intermingled low-voltage beta activity. Concordance of polygraphic parameters: absent ocular movements; regular breathing and heart rate frequency

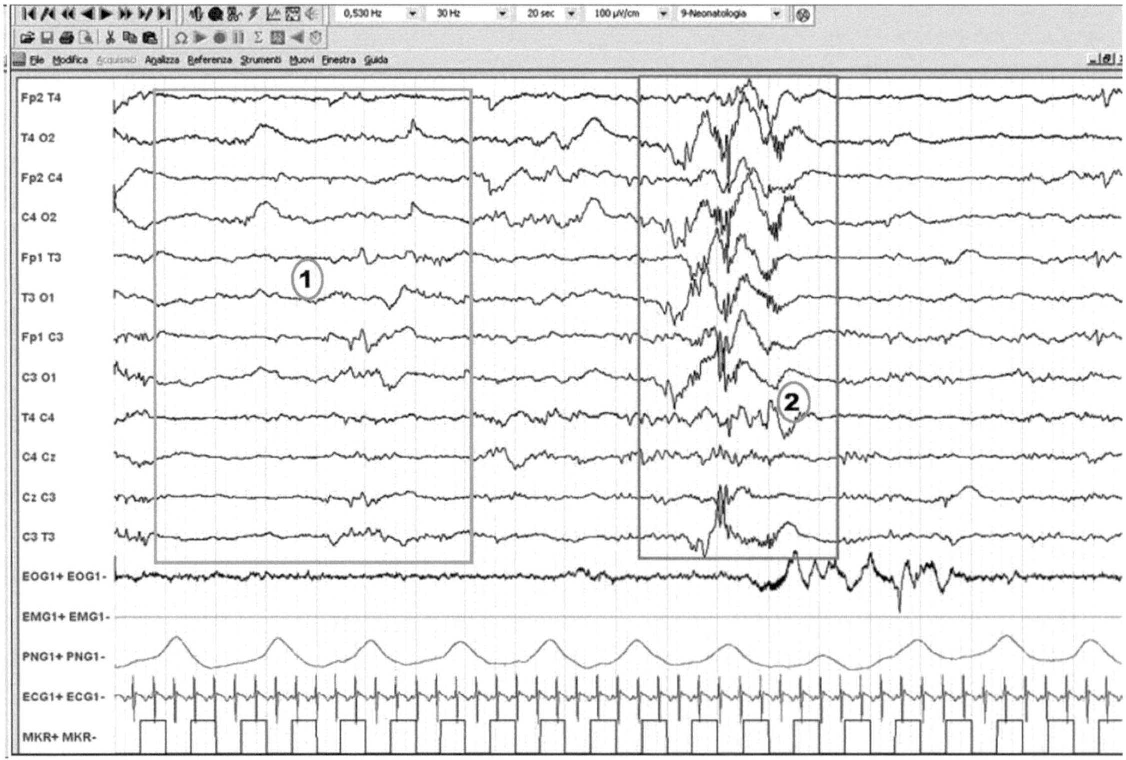

Fig. 11.20 33 weeks GA, 37–38 weeks CA. *Tracé alternant* pattern in deep non-rapid eye movement (NREM/quiet) sleep: (*1*) periods (8–10 s) of discontinuity with low-voltage (less than 50 µV) theta activity; (*2*) bilateral bursts (3–5 s) with theta (50–100 µV) and delta (up to 300 µV) activity with intermingled low-voltage beta activity. Concordance of polygraphic parameters: in the EOG channel artifacts related to abnormal electrode contact; regular breathing and heart rate frequency

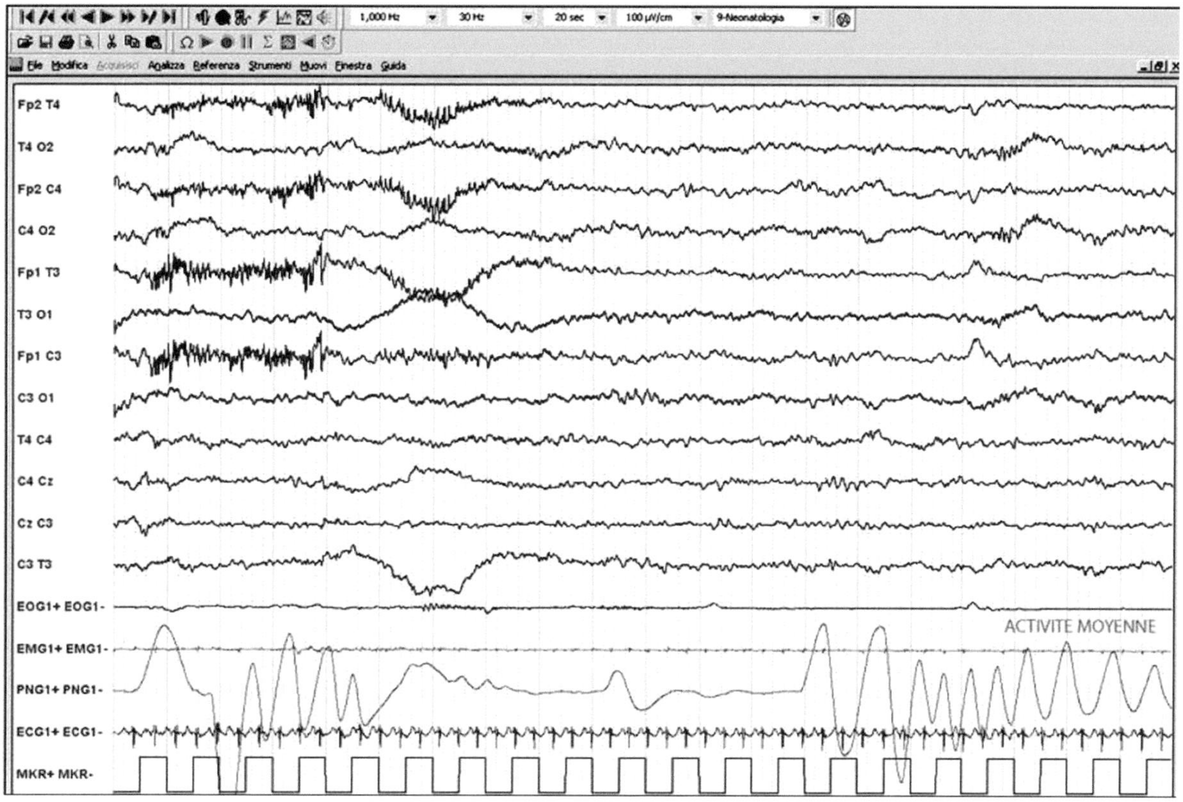

Fig. 11.21 29 weeks GA, 37–38 weeks CA. A*ctivité moyenne* pattern: in quiet awake state with open eyes, continuous diffuse theta (4–6 Hz, 40–60 µV) activity. Medium voltage EMG activity in anterior leads. Polygraphic parameters: in the EOG rapid eyes movements; irregular breathing and increasing heart rate frequency

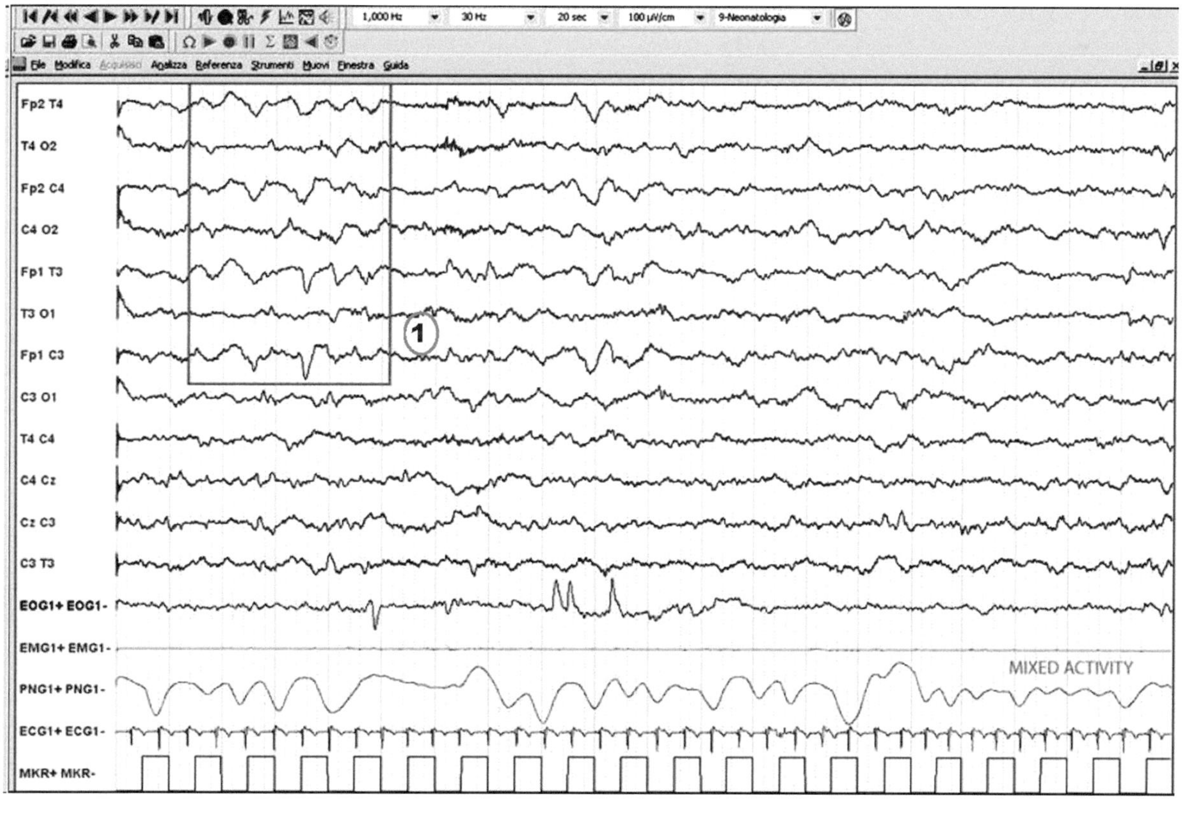

Fig. 11.22 38 weeks GA, 39 weeks CA. Active sleep before quiet sleep: continuous diffuse theta (4–6 Hz, 40–60 µV) activity with superimposed diffuse slow delta activity; (*1*) rhythmic bifrontal delta activity and frontal sharp transients on the left side

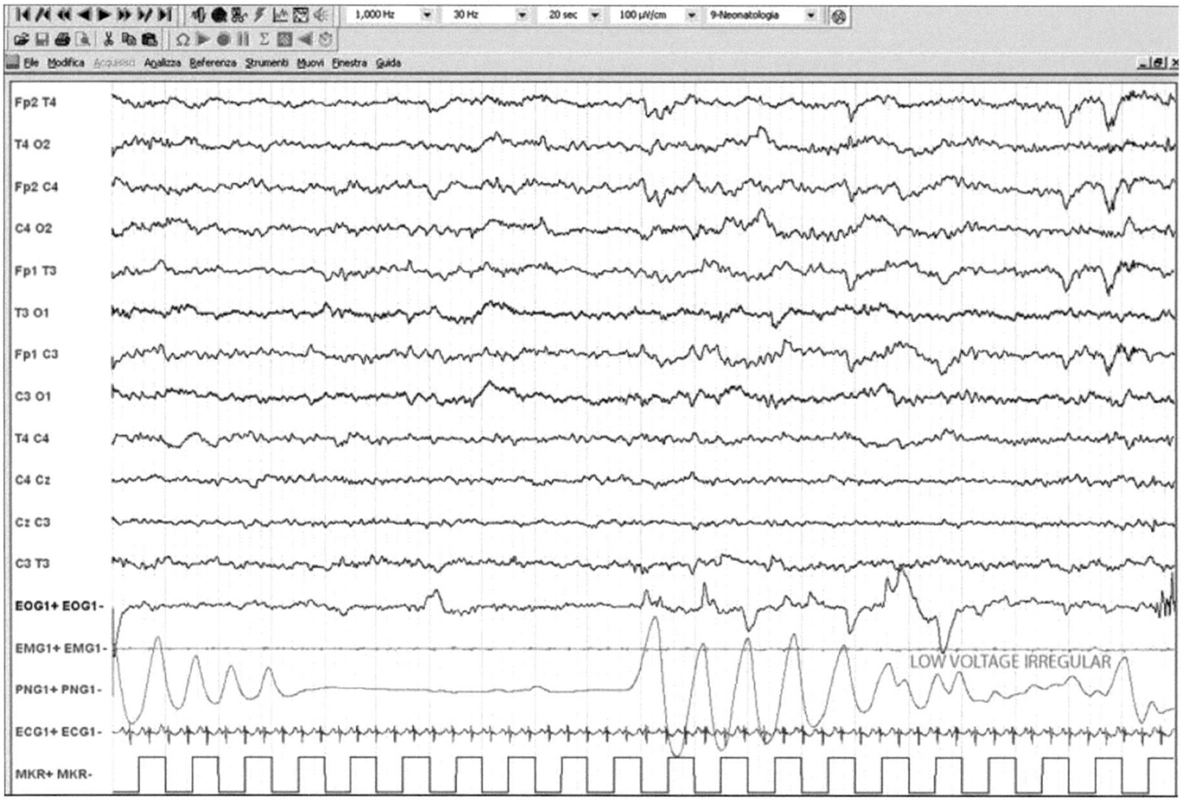

Fig 11.23 29 weeks GA, 38 weeks CA. Low-voltage irregular pattern: REM/active sleep after NREM/quiet sleep: mixed diffuse theta (4–6 Hz, 40–60 µV) activity. Polygraphic parameters: in the electrooculogram channel rapid eyes movements, irregular breathing with a 6 s breathing pause

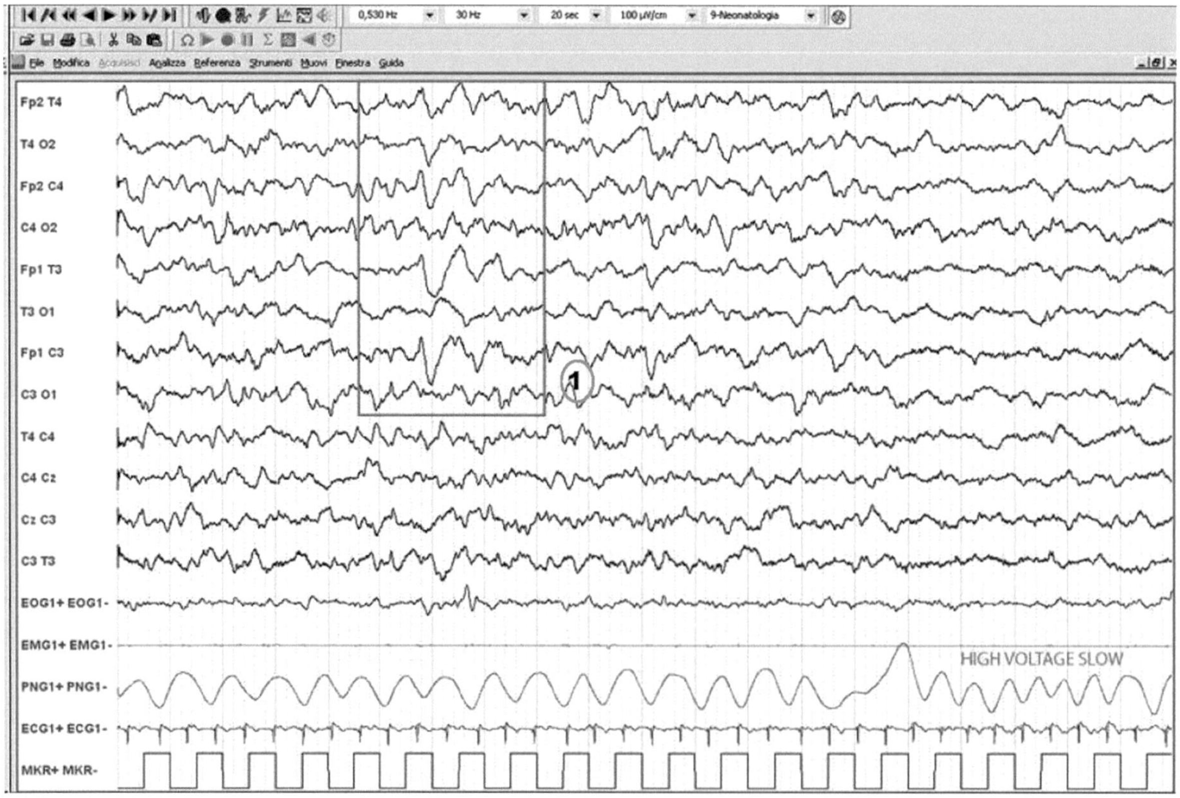

Fig. 11.24 38 weeks GA, 39 weeks CA. High-voltage slow (HVS) pattern: quiet sleep with diffuse and bilateral slow (delta-theta, 0.5–4 Hz, up to 150 µV) activity. (*1*) Rhythmic bifrontal delta activity and frontal sharp transients on the left side

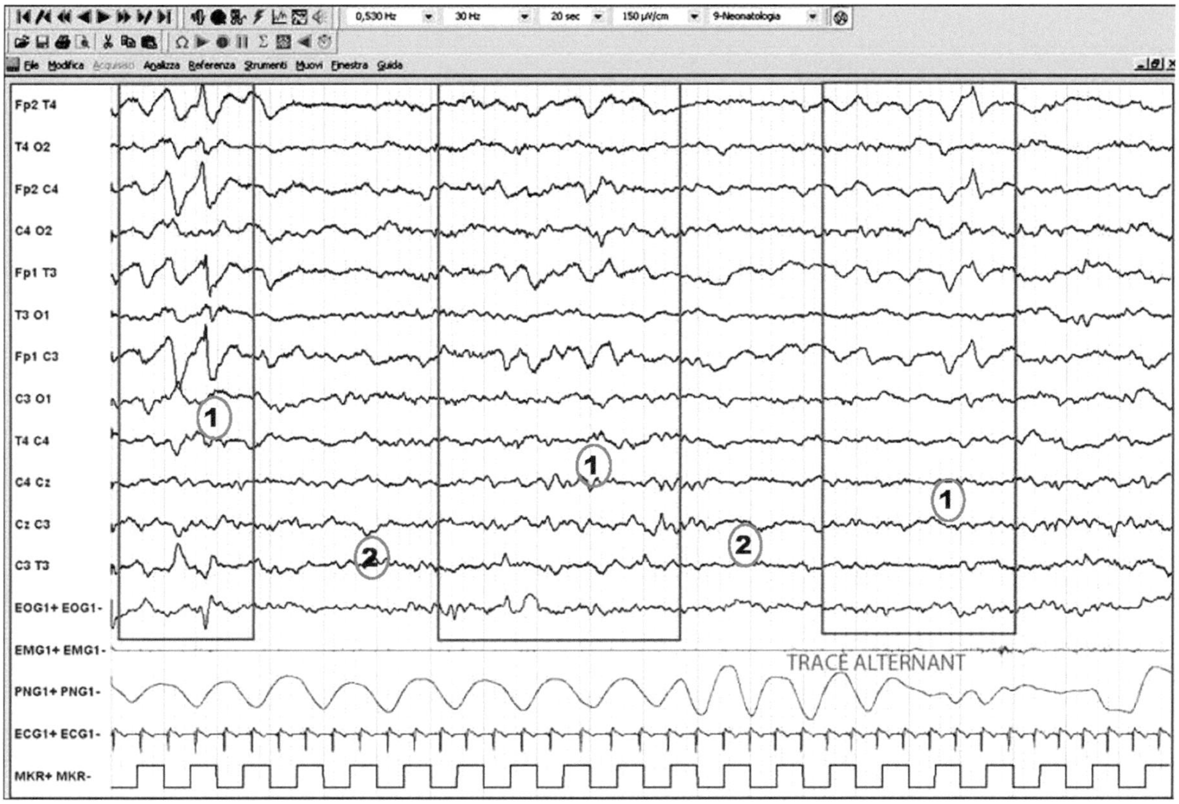

Fig. 11.25 38 weeks GA, 39 weeks CA. *Tracé alternant* pattern during NREM/quiet sleep: (*1*) 2–4 s periods with diffuse delta (up to 100–200 µV) activity intermingled with (*2*) 4–10 s periods with diffuse theta (4–6 Hz, 25–50 µV) activity. Notice within the first burst (*1*): bifrontal rhythmic delta activity with frontal sharp transients

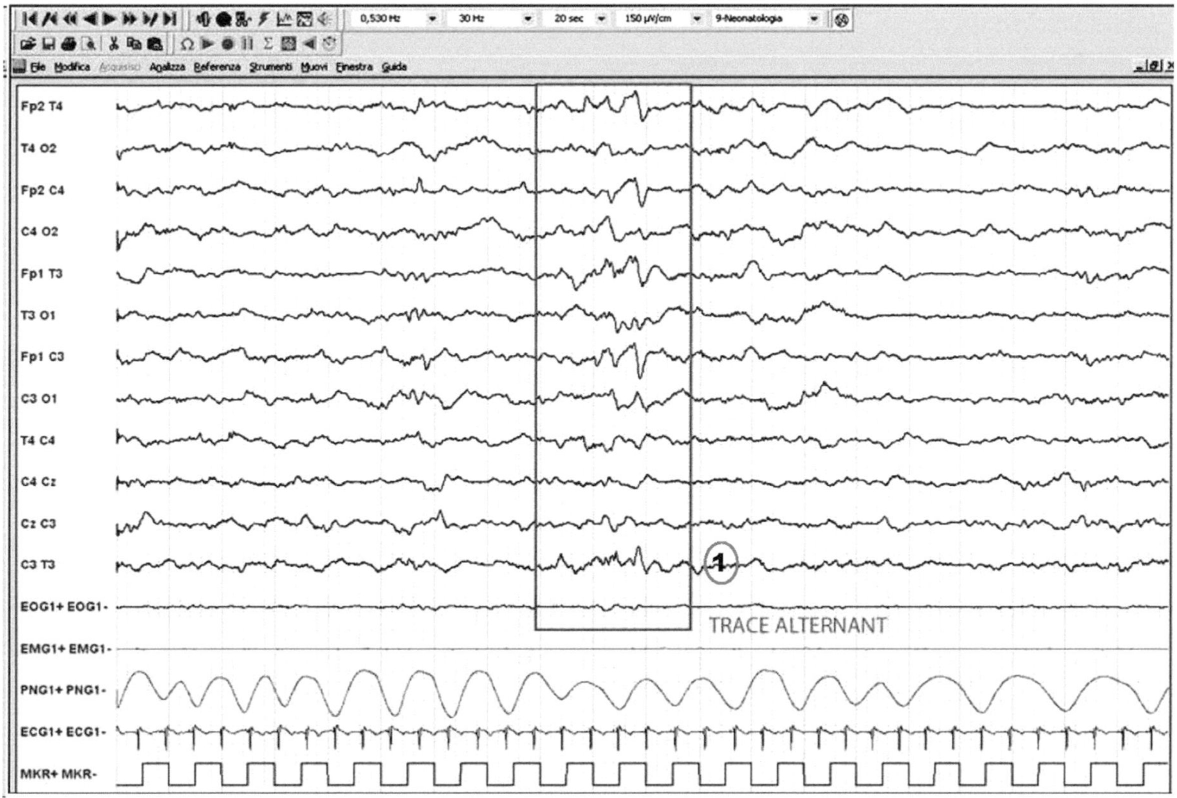

Fig. 11.26 38 weeks GA, 39 weeks CA. *Tracé alternant* pattern evolving to transitional sleep pattern: within 8–10 s periods with diffuse theta (4–6 Hz, 25–60 µV) activity, arise (*1*) a 3–4 s burst with bilateral delta (100–250 µV) activity and frontal sharp transients

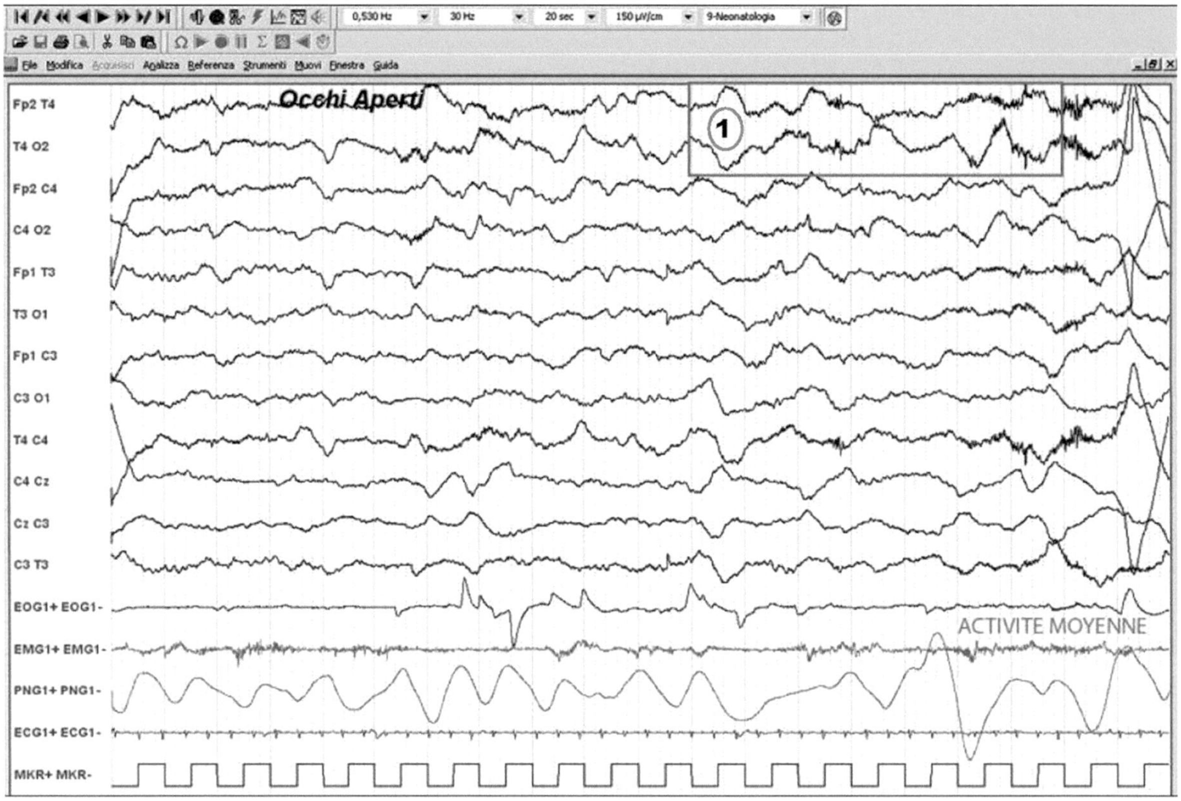

Fig. 11.27 40 weeks GA, 41 weeks CA. A*ctivité moyenne* pattern during awake: within continuous diffuse theta (4–6 Hz, 40–60 μV) activity 1) EMG activity due to sucking bilateral but more evident in the temporal right regions. Polygraphic parameters: according to the awake condition: eyes movements, muscular activity and irregular breathing. (Occhi Aperti = eyes open)

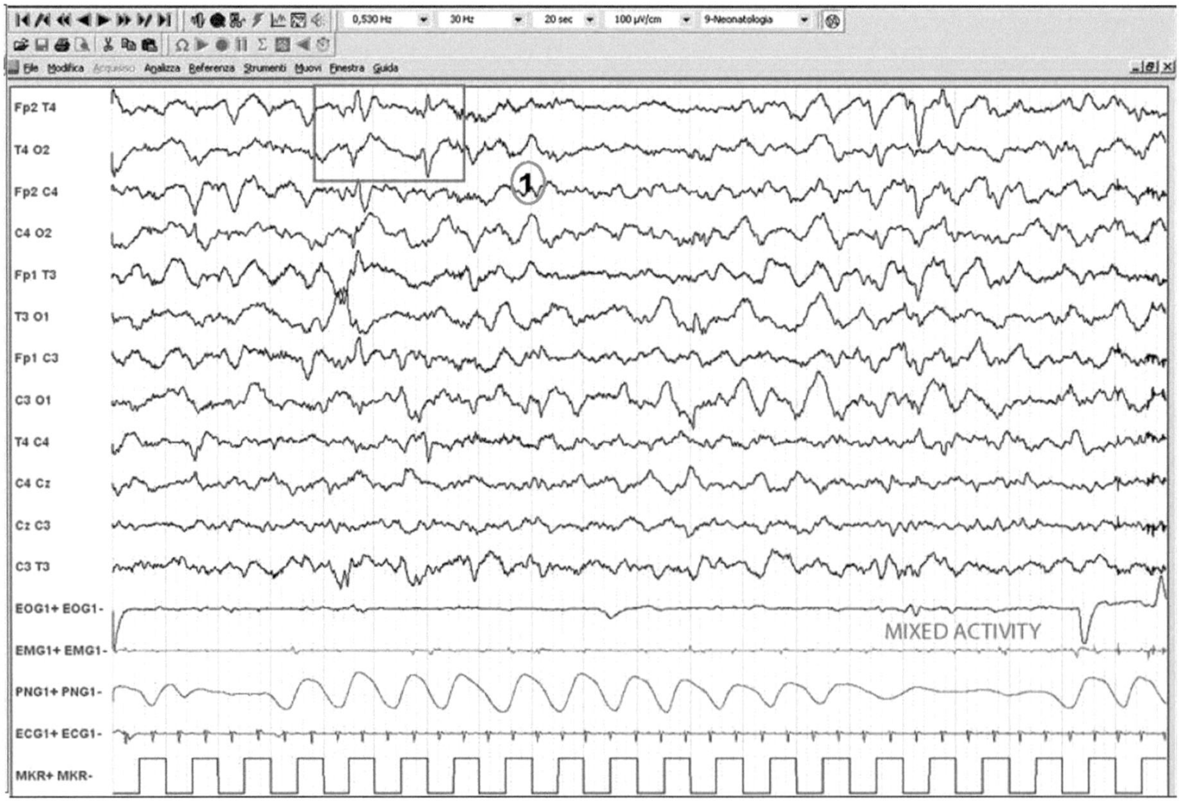

Fig. 11.28 40 weeks GA, 41 weeks CA. Mixed activity pattern before NREM/quiet sleep: prevalence of delta activity compared to theta activity with (*1*) isolated sharp waves in the right temporal region

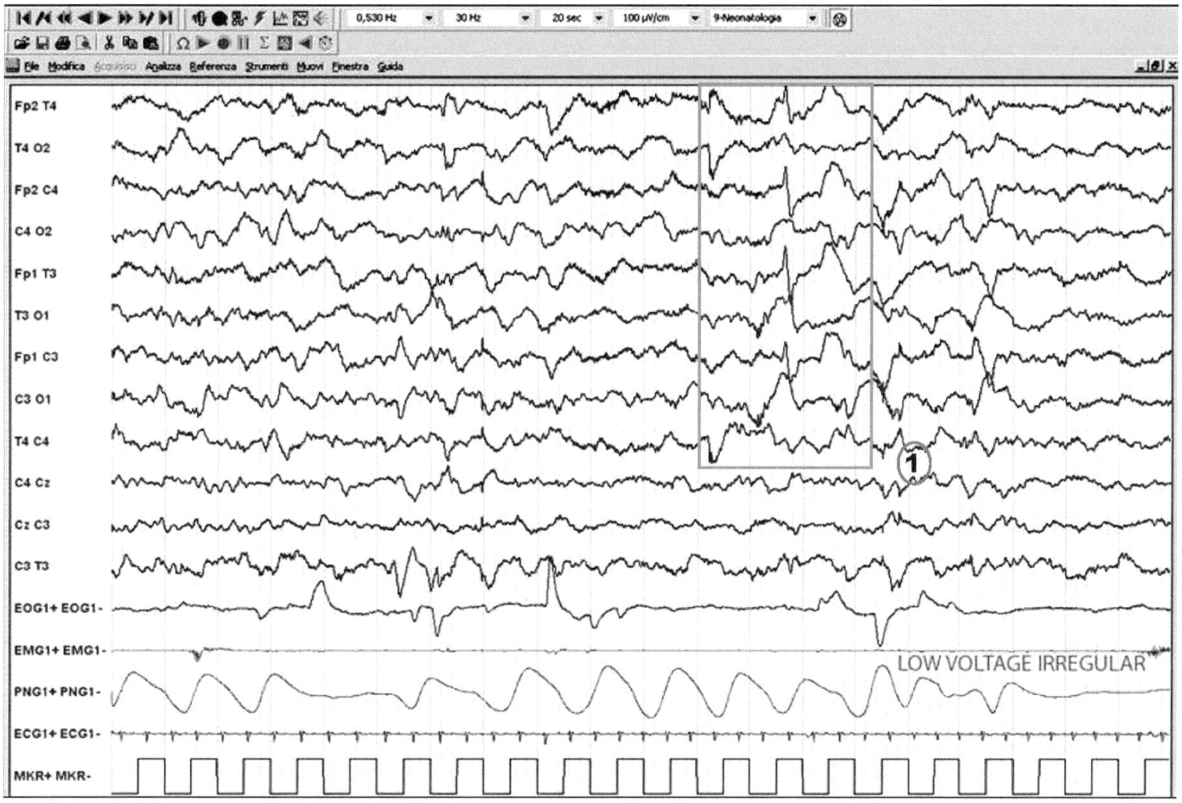

Fig. 11.29 40 weeks GA, 41 weeks CA. Low-voltage irregular pattern: REM/active sleep after NREM/quiet sleep: mixed diffuse theta (4–6 Hz, 40–60 µV) activity with few delta activity intermingled; (*1*) frontal sharp transients. Polygraphic parameters: EOG with rapid eyes movements; in EMG channel infrequent mylohyoid muscle brief contractions; in PNG irregular breathing

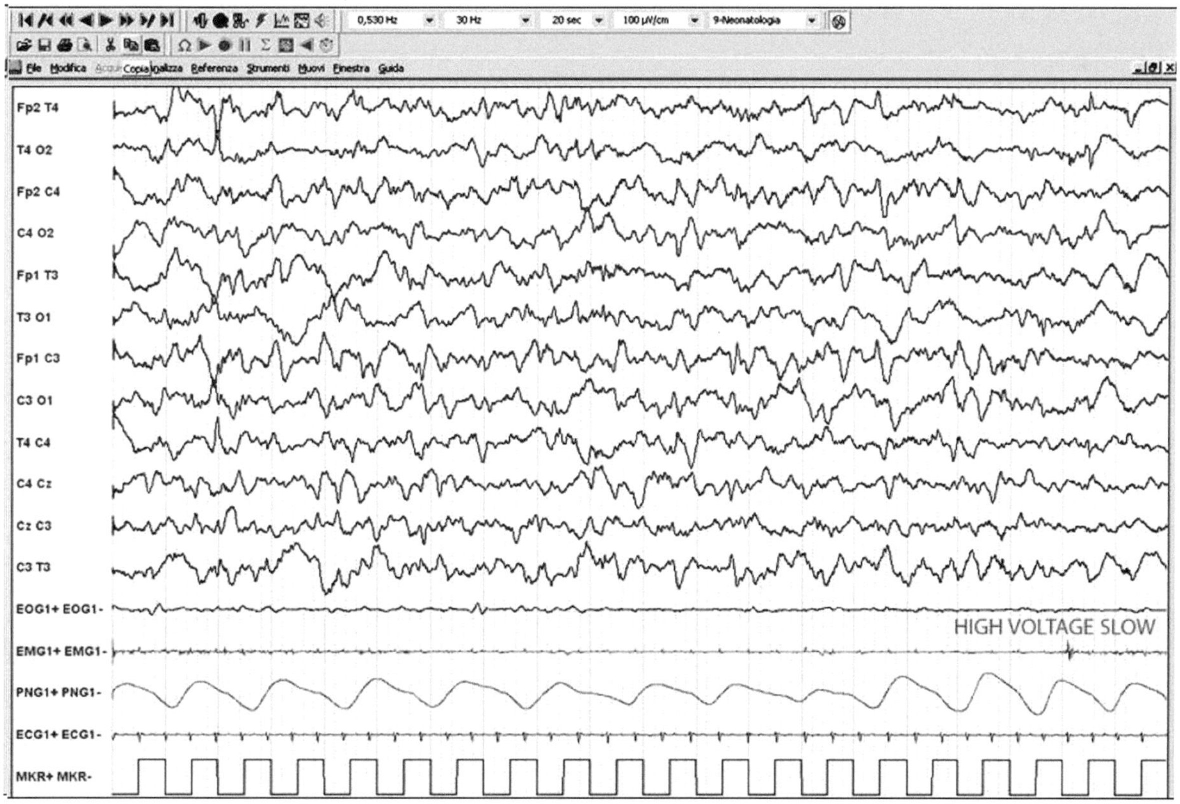

Fig. 11.30 40 weeks GA, 41 weeks CA. High-voltage slow (HVS) pattern: quiet sleep with diffuse and bilateral slow (delta-theta, 0.5–4 Hz, up to 200 µV) activity. Notice the most abundance of delta activity compared to Fig. 11.24. Polygraphic parameters in accordance with EEG pattern

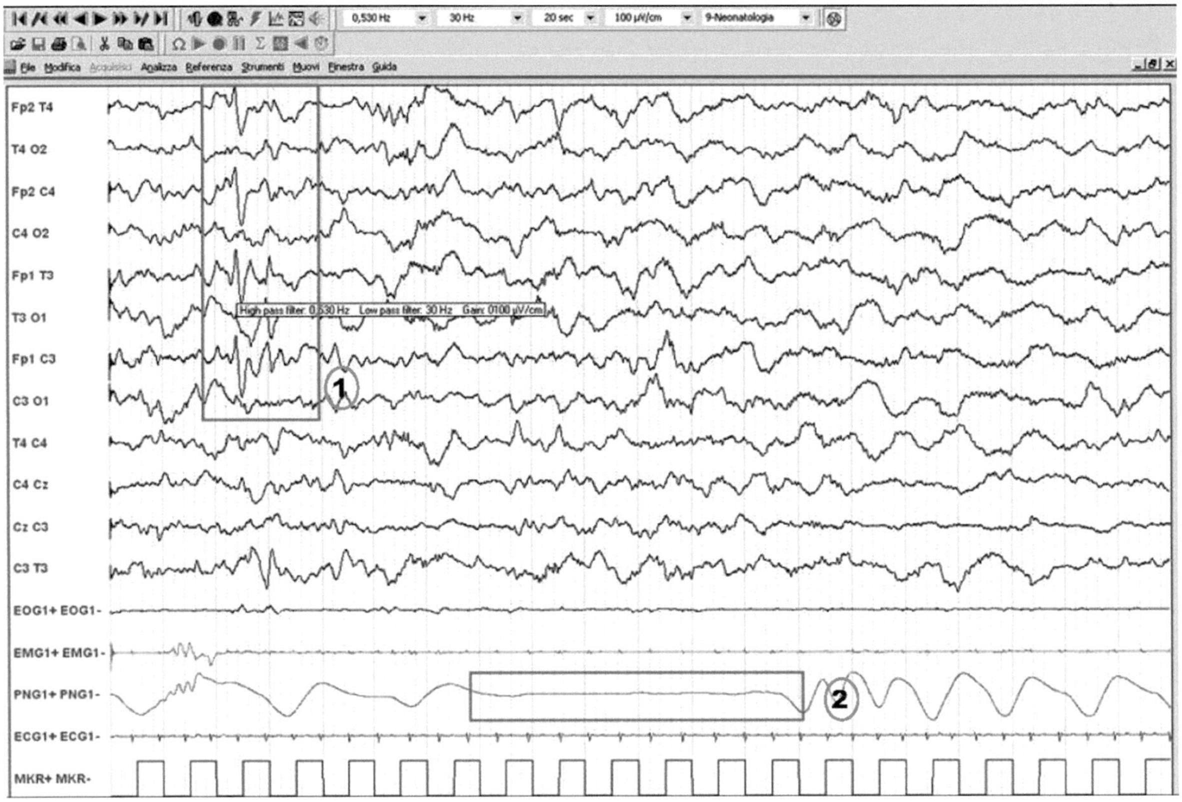

Fig. 11.31 40 weeks GA, 41 weeks CA. Transitional sleep from REM/active sleep to NREM/quiet sleep. (*1*) Bilateral frontal sharp transients; (*2*) 6 s breathing pause at the beginning of quiet sleep

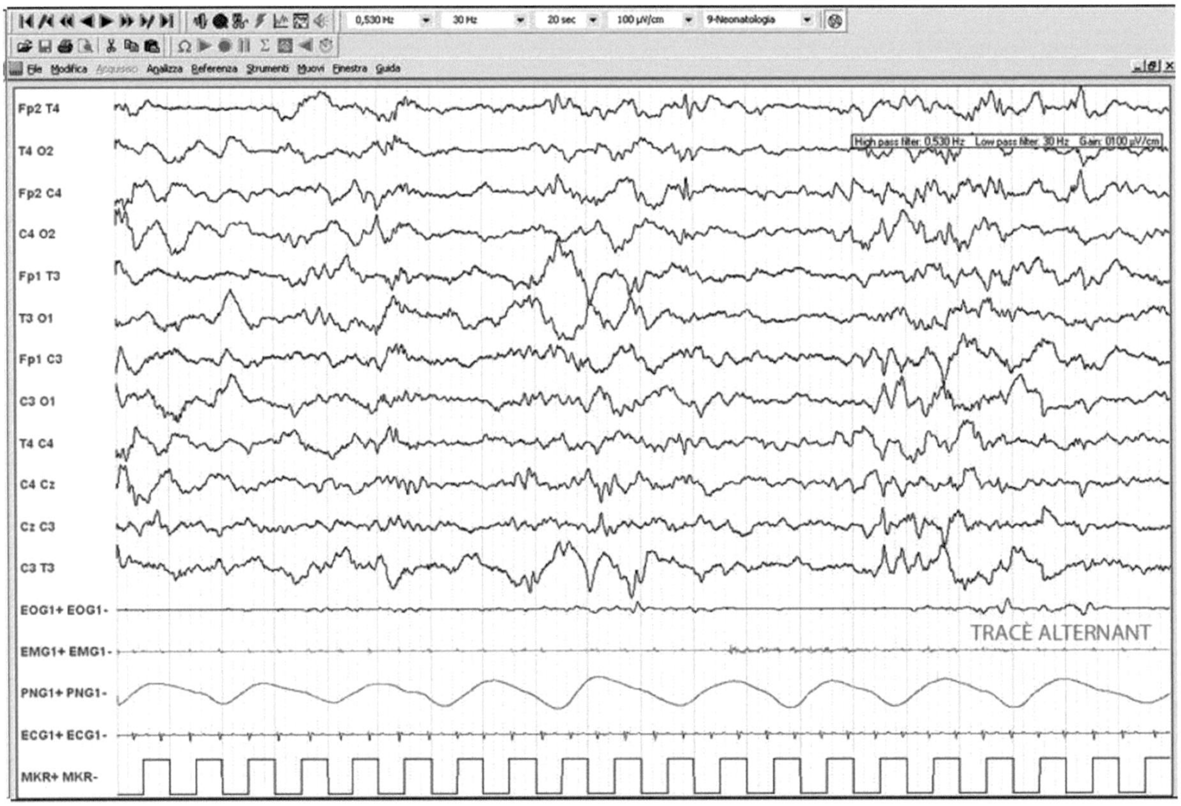

Fig. 11.32 40 weeks GA, 41 weeks CA. *Tracé alternant* pattern: within the bursts the most rapid and sharp activities disappeared compared to what is observed in previous CA (see Figs. 11.19 and 11.20). Burst amplitude is less than 200 µV. The interbursts activity has an amplitude up to 40–50 µV. Polygraphic parameters in accordance with EEG pattern

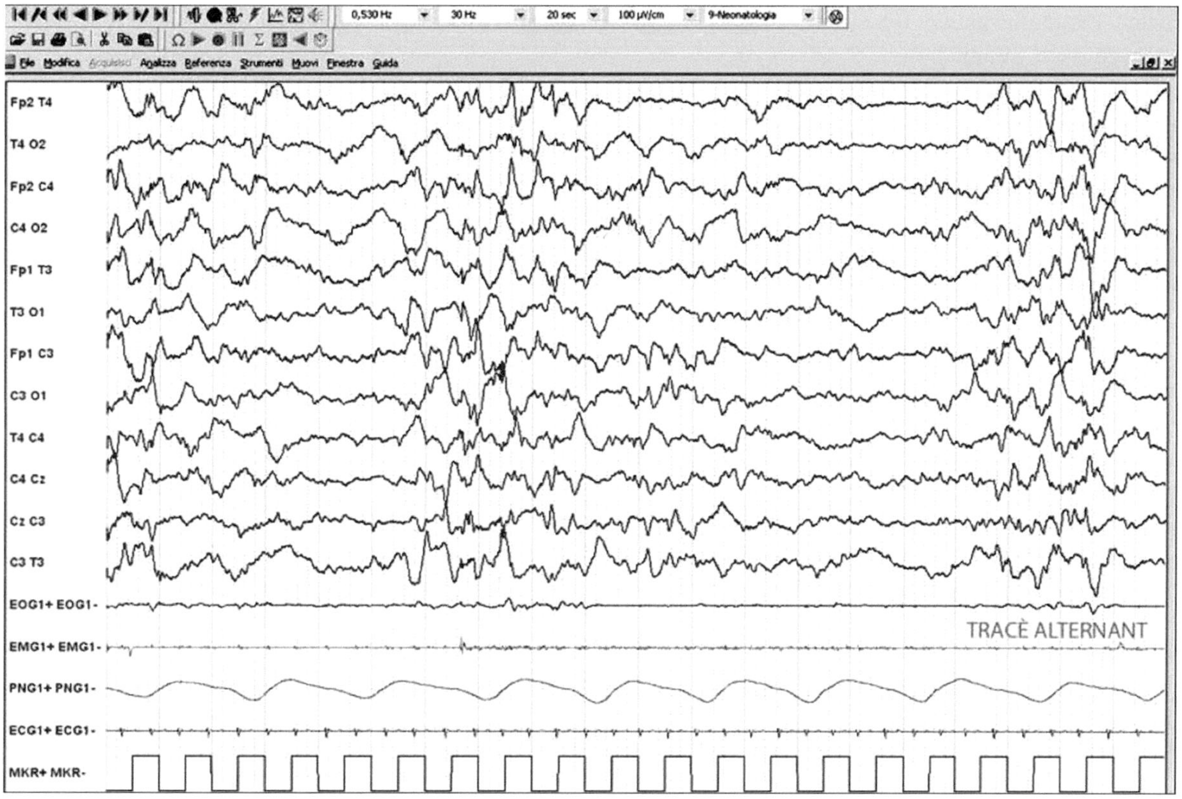

Fig. 11.33 40 weeks GA, 41 weeks CA. *Tracé alternant* pattern: the same characteristics of Fig. 11.32

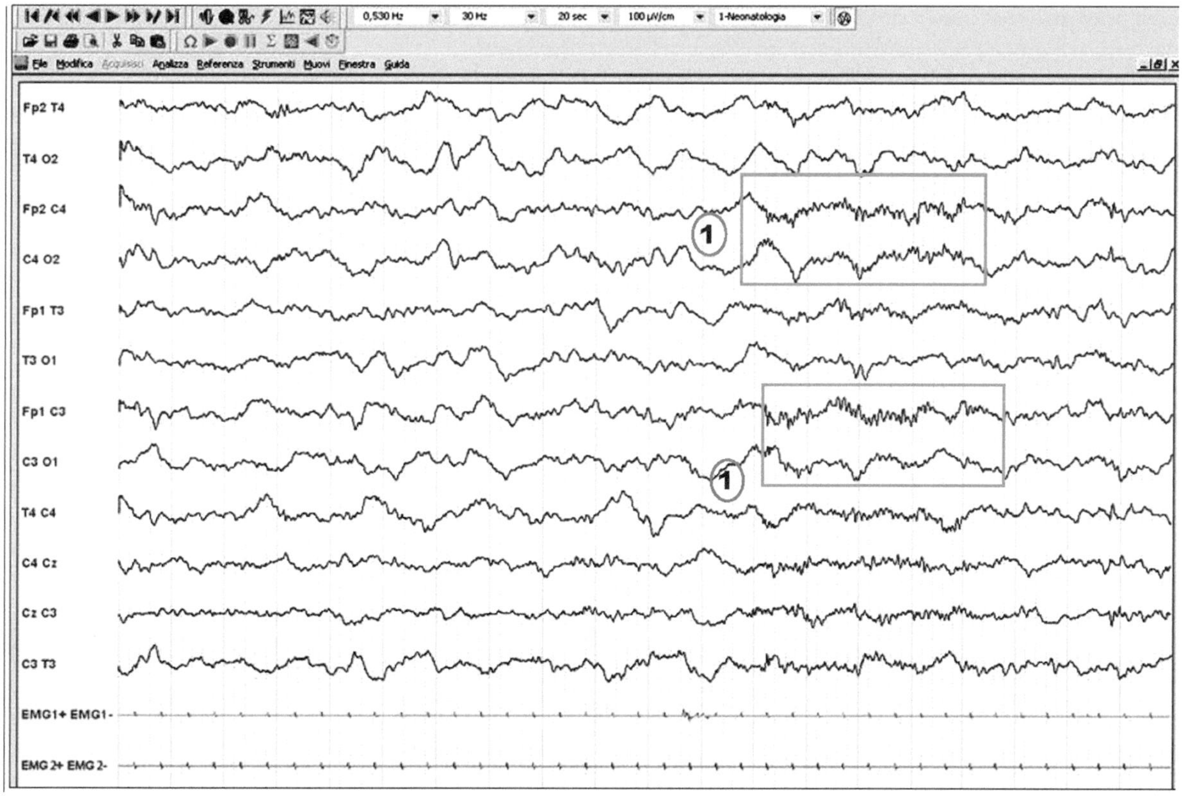

Fig. 11.34 39 weeks GA, 44 weeks CA. NREM/quiet sleep pattern with prevalence of diffuse and continuous theta-delta activity up to 200 μV; (*1*) rudimentary sleep spindles in the midline central region

Persistent interhemispheric synchrony. The background activity is reactive to stimulation.

Forty-four weeks: (by convention, it is considered the end of the neonatal period). In quiet sleep, the intermittent pattern progressively evolves toward a continuous slow pattern with the initial appearance of the sleep spindles (Fig. 11.34).

The table summarizes the main development graphoelements in the EEG of the newborn, in parallel with the differentiation of behavioral states.

11.10 Amplitude-Integrated EEG (aEEG)

With the widespread use of the therapeutic hypothermia, there has been a significant impulse into the spreading of amplitude-integrated EEG (aEEG) use in neonatal intensive care units (NICU). It has some strengths such as the easiness of use [33], the immediate availability even for prolonged recordings, the compressed time scale, and the reduced montage, which shortens the technical time required for the execution and interpretation of recordings. aEEG is a reliable tool to monitor background brain activity in infants [34, 35], particularly if used with two channels and with the raw EEG data and if compared to the 1-h multichannel EEG recording [36, 37]. aEEG should be considered as a screening tool [38, 39] for seizure detection because there is general agreement regarding the fact that aEEG can miss infrequent, focal, low-amplitude, brief seizures with a duration <30 s [40–42]. For these reasons, reference to conventional or "raw" EEG should be made in order to increase its sensitivity and specificity whenever suspicious neonatal seizures are detected [43, 44]. Furthermore, the environment in NICU is not favorable for the neurophysiological monitoring of newborns because of the presence of several NICU equipment that can potentially lead to important artifacts. These can easily mimic a neonatal ictal discharge on aEEG, and sometimes raw EEG traces of the aEEG are not enough to clarify the real nature of these doubtful episodes [39, 45, 46].

Acknowledgments

- To the EEG technicians of the Pediatric Neurology Unit: Francesca Tabarelli, Deborah Meroni, and Gaetano Turi for their competence and sensitivity, constantly expressed in the management of newborns and in the acquisition of EEG recordings.
- To the colleagues of the Pediatric Neurology Unit and Neonatology and Neonatal Intensive Therapy Unit of the Buzzi Children's Hospital, for the daily fruitful collaboration.
- To Dr. Alfredo Radaelli and Davide Radaelli, for their essential advices in preparing the figures and the manuscript.

Appendix

Glossary

Activité moyenne: EEG pattern of the full-term newborn corresponding to wakefulness or to active sleep after quiet sleep state. Continuous electric activity with prevalent frequencies between 4 and 7 Hz (1–10 Hz), with an amplitude between 25 and 50 μV, with intermixed low-voltage delta activity.

- **Activity at 0–3 Hz**: slow waves at 0.3–3 Hz, of amplitude up to 300 μV, in the preterm newborn of less than 26 weeks GA.
- **Activity at 3–7 Hz activity**: occipital and isolated or in short runs of 1–2 s, of amplitude between 50 and 200 μV, in the preterm newborn of less than 27 weeks GA.
- **Activity at 8–13 Hz**: in short runs of 1–2 s, of amplitude between 25 and 30 μV, prevalent on Rolandic and occipital regions, in the preterm newborn of less than 28 weeks GA.

Anterior slow dysrhythmia (ASD): physiological pattern of the term newborn. In the neonatal period, the word dysrhythmia is still accepted—the ASD is characterized by a short sequence of 1–2 s of anterior slow waves at 2–3 Hz and of amplitude between 50 and 150 μV, synchronous (and asynchronous), sometimes associated with the frontal sharp transients.

Background activity: it includes the predominant frequencies and amplitudes with their variability, in relation to the spatial and temporal parameters, during the EEG recording. The background activity can be continuous or discontinuous depending on the presence, or not, in a given recording period, significant changes in the frequency, and/or amplitude of the electrical activity. However, the term "discontinuous" is used to define the recordings in which there are sections of significant voltage attenuation up to the absence of electrical activity. In relation to the clinical meanings of the "discontinuous tracing," the reader might refer to the iconography of this chapter and of the following chapter concerning the pathologic neonatal EEG recordings.

Conceptional age (CA): GA plus the weeks since birth; gestational age, measured from the time of the last menstrual period + chronological age.

Concordance and discordance: the presence or absence of regularly structured electrical and behavioral parameters, in relation to the specific state in the different GA.

Delta brush: physiological transient of the preterm and healthy newborn, with variable localization depending on the GA. It is a complex transient in which fast activity at 8–22 Hz, generally of low voltage (10–70 μV), immediately precedes; it is superimposed or immediately follows a high-amplitude slow wave at 0.3–1.5 Hz, between 75 and 250 μV of amplitude. The characteristics of both fast activity and slow wave vary according to the degree of prematurity.

Dysmaturity: EEG characteristic due to the presence of an electric pattern corresponding to a lower GA than expected for that specific GA.

Encoches frontales (frontal sharp transients): typical physiological features since 35 weeks' GA, characterized by a biphasic wave (negative-positive) of amplitude variable between 50 and 200 μV, anteriorly localized, bilaterally synchronous and asynchronous; observable until the end of the neonatal period in quiet sleep state.

Gestational age (GA): the number of weeks since the beginning of the last menstrual.

High-voltage slow (HVS): slow pattern of high voltage—electric pattern of the full-term newborn during the quiet sleep state: frequencies between 0.5 and 4 Hz, of amplitude between 50 and 150 μV, irregularly rhythmic.

Liability: poorly definable or unstable behavioral state.

Low-voltage irregular (LVI): low-voltage irregular pattern—electric pattern of the full-term newborn, corresponding to the active sleep that appears after a quiet sleep phase: frequencies between 1 and 8 Hz with amplitude lower than 40–60 μV.

Mixed activity: electric pattern of the full-term infant corresponding to the active sleep that generally appears at the beginning of a sleep cycle. It is constituted by the moyenne activité pattern over which theta-delta activity at 2–4 Hz is superimposed, with an amplitude of less than 100 μV.

Neonatal period: the first 4 weeks of life for the full-term newborn (40 weeks' GA) and in any case up to the 44 weeks of GA for the preterm newborn:

- **Preterm newborn**: born before 37 weeks of GA.
- **Term newborn**: born between 38 and 42 weeks of GA.
- **Post-term newborn**: born over 42 weeks of GA.

Paroxysmal: mode of appearance of an electrical event that begins and ends abruptly, clearly distinguishing itself from the background activity, generally of higher but sometimes of lower amplitude.

Positive and negative (temporal/Rolandic sharp waves): phase reversal in a bipolar derivation with variable localization, generally isolated and with voltage lower than 100 μV. Otherwise, they have a connotation of focal pathological transients and/or white matter involvement (positive Rolandic sharp waves).

Reactivity: modification of the background activity after external stimulation.

Sharp transients: spike or sharp wave transients that maintain the same morphological definition usually used in electroencephalography at any age but in the neonatal period are frequently typical physiological features of specific GA.

State: well-defined behavioral modality characterized by physiological events that occur in specific epochs of postnatal life both in the full-term and in the preterm newborn, with a predictable and cyclical trend.

Temporal spike and sharp waves: physiological elements, of variable amplitude, peculiar to an age between 29 and 32 weeks' and at 37 weeks' GA (multifocal interburst sharp waves).

Temporal theta burst or temporal sawtooth: peculiar physiological elements of the preterm newborn <33 weeks' GA—short sequences of 3–5 s of diffuse rhythmic activity at 4–7 Hz, of amplitude between 50 and 250 μV, synchronous on the same hemisphere or more evident in the temporal region, bilaterally synchronous and asynchronous.

Tracé alternant (TA, alternating tracing): electric pattern of the full-term newborn observable in the quiet sleep—epochs of 3–8 s with delta activity at 0.5–3 Hz of amplitude between 50 and 200 μV, with superimposed fast activity of lower voltage, interspersed with sections of 3–8 s with theta activity at 4–6 Hz of amplitude between 25 and 40 μV.

References

1. Lamblin MD, Andre M, Auzoux M, et al. Indications of electroencephalogram in the newborn. Arch Pediatr. 2004;11(7):829–33.
2. Parmelee AH Jr, Schulte FJ, Akiyama Y, et al. Maturation of EEG activity during sleep in premature infants. Electroencephalogr Clin Neurophysiol. 1968;24:319–29.
3. Dreyfus-Brisac C, Monod N. The electroencephalogram of full term newborn and premature infants. In: Remond A, editor. Handbook of electroencephalography and clinical neurophysiology, vol. 6B. Amsterdam: Elsevier; 1975. p. 6–23.
4. Monod N, Tharp B. Activité electroencéphalographique normale du nouveau-né et du prématuré au cours des états de veille et de sommeil. Rev Electroenceph Neurophysiol Clin. 1977;7:302–15.
5. Watanabe K, Iwase K. Spindle-like fast rhythms in the EEGs of low birthweight infants. Dev Med Child Neurol. 1972;14:373–81.
6. Watanabe K, Iwase K, Hara K. Developmental of slow-wave sleep in low birth weight infants. Dev Med Child Neurol. 1974;16:23–32.
7. Tharp BR, Cukier F, Monod N. Valeur prognostique de l'EEG du prématuré. Neurophysiology. 1977;7:386–91.
8. Lombroso CT. Quantified electrographic scales on 10 pre-term healthy newborns followed up to 40–43 weeks of conceptional age by serial polygraphic recordings. Electroencephalogr Clin Neurophysiol. 1979;46:460–74.
9. Lombroso CT. Neonatal electroencephalography. In: Niedermeyer E, Lopes da Silva F, editors. Electroencephalography: basic principles, clinical applications and related field. Munich: Urban & Schwartzenberg; 1982. p. 725–62.
10. Tharp BR. Electrophysiological brain maturation in premature infants: an historical perspective. J Clin Neurophysiol. 1990;7(3):302–14.
11. Stockard-Pope JE, Wener SS, Bickford R. Atlas of neonatal electroencephalography. 2nd ed. New York: Raven; 1992.
12. Lombroso CT. Neonatal polygraphy in full-term and premature infants: a review of normal and abnormal findings. J Clin Neurophysiol. 1985;2:105–55.
13. Hrachovy RA, Mizrahi EM, Kellaway P. Electroencephalography of the newborn. In: Daly DD, Pedley TA, editors. Current prac-

tice of clinical electroencephalography. 2nd ed. New York: Raven; 1990. p. 201–42.
14. Mizrahi EM, Kellaway P. Neonatal electroencephalography. In: Diagnosis and management of neonatal seizures. Philadelphia, PA: Lippincott-Raven; 1998. p. 99–143.
15. Mizrhai EM, Hrachovy RA, Kellaway P. Atlas of neonatal electroencephalography. 3rd ed. Philadelphia, PA: Lippincott Williams & Wilkins; 2004.
16. Karayiannis NB, Xiong Y, Tao G, et al. Automated detection of videotaped neonatal seizures of epileptic origin. Epilepsia. 2006;47(6):966–80.
17. Stevenson NJ, Boylan GB. Advances in neurophysiology and neonatal seizures: automated seizures detection. In: Nagarajan L, editor. Neonatal seizures. Current management and future challenges. London: Mac Keith Press; 2016. p. 56–75.
18. Kuratani J, Pearl PL, Sullivan L, et al. American Clinical Neurophysiology Society Guideline 5: minimum technical standards for pediatric electroencephalography. J Clin Neurophysiol. 2016;33(4):320–3.
19. Shellhaas RA, Chang T, Tsuchida T, et al. The American Clinical Neurophysiology Society's Guideline on continuous electroencephalography monitoring in neonates. J Clin Neurophysiol. 2011;28(6):611–7.
20. De Weerd AW, Despland PA, Plouin P. Neonatal EEG. The international federation of clinical neurophysiology. Electroencephalogr Clin Neurophysiol Suppl. 1999;52:149–57.
21. Chang T, Tsuchida TN. Conventional (continuous) EEG monitoring in the NICU. Curr Pediatr Rev. 2014;10(1):2–10.
22. Jasper HH. The ten-twenty electrodes system of the International Federation. In: International Federation of Societies for Electroencephalography and clinical neurophysiology: recommendations for the practice of clinical neurophysiology. Amsterdam: Elsevier; 1983. p. 3–10.
23. Nagarajan L, Gosh S. The role of the video EEG in neonates with seizures. In: Nagarajan L, editor. Neonatal seizures. Current management and future challenges. London: Mac Keith Press; 2016. p. 12–29.
24. Prechtl HFR, Beintema D. The neurological examination of the full term newborn infant. Clinics in Dev Med 12. London: Spastics Society and Heinemann; 1964.
25. Vecchierini MF, d'Allest AM, Verpillat P. EEG pattern in 10 extreme premature neonates with normal neurological outcome: qualitative and quantitative data. Brain and Development. 2003;25:330–7.
26. Biagioni E, Frisone MF, Laroche S, et al. Occipital sawtooth: a physiological EEG pattern in very premature infants. Clin Neurophysiol. 2000;111:2145–9.
27. Tharp B. Neonatal and pediatric electroencephalography. In: Aminoff M, editor. Electrodiagnosis in clinical neurology. New York: Churchill Livingston; 1986. p. 77–124.
28. Anders T, Emde R, Parmelee AH Jr. A manual of standardized terminology, techniques and criteria for scoring of states of sleep and wakefulness in newborn infants. Los Angeles: UCLA Brain Information Service, NIDS Neurological Information Network; 1971.
29. Kellaway P. Introduction to plasticity and sensitive periods. In: Kellaway P, Noebels JL, editors. Problems and concept in developmental neurophysiology. Baltimore: The Johns Hopkins University Press; 1989. p. 3–28.
30. Ferrari F, Biagioni E, Cioni G. Neonatal electroencephalography. In: Levene MI, Chervenak FA, Whittle M, editors. Fetal and neonatal neurology and neurosurgery. 3rd ed. London: Churchill Livingston; 2001. p. 155–80.
31. Mastrangelo M, Scelsa B, Fiocchi I, et al. EEG neonatale. In: Mecarelli O, editor. Manuale Teorico Pratico di Elettroencefalografia. 1st ed. Philadelphia, PA: Wolters Kluwer Health; 2009. p. 166–93.
32. André M, Lamblin MD, d'Allest AM, et al. Electroencephalography in premature and full-term infants. Developmental features and glossary. Neurophysiol Clin. 2010;40(2):59–124.
33. Boylan G, Burgoyne L, Moore C, et al. An international survey of EEG use in the neonatal intensive care unit. Acta Paediatr. 2010;99:1150–5.
34. Toet MC, Van Der Meij W, De Vries LS, et al. Comparison between simultaneously recorded amplitude integrated electroencephalogram (cerebral function monitor) and standard electroencephalogram in neonates. Pediatrics. 2002;109(5):772–9.
35. Hellström-Westas L. Comparison between tape-recorded and amplitude-integrated EEG monitoring in sick newborn infants. Acta Paediatr. 1992;81(10):812–9.
36. Lavery S, Shah DK, Hunt RW, et al. Single versus bihemispheric amplitude-integrated electroencephalography in relation to cerebral injury and outcome in the term encephalopathic infant. J Paediatr Child Health. 2008;44(5):285–90.
37. Mathur AM, Morris LD, Teteh F, et al. Utility of prolonged bedside amplitude-integrated encephalogram in encephalopathic infants. Am J Perinatol. 2008;25(10):611–5.
38. Shelhaas RA, Chang T, Tsuchida T, et al. The American clinical neurophysiology society's guideline on continuous electroencephalography monitoring in neonates. J Clin Neurophysiol. 2011;28:611–7.
39. Abend NS, Wusthoff CJ. Neonatal seizures and status epilepticus. J Clin Neurophysiol. 2012;29:441–8.
40. Mastrangelo M, Fiocchi I, Fontana P, et al. Acute neonatal encephalopathy and seizures recurrence: a combined aEEG/EEG study. Seizure. 2013;22(9):703–7.
41. Rennie JM, Chorley G, Boylan GB, et al. Non-expert use of the cerebral function monitor for neonatal seizure detection. Arch Dis Child Fetal Neonatal Ed. 2004;89:F37–40.
42. Shellhaas RA, Soaita AI, Clancy RR. Sensitivity of amplitude-integrated electroencephalography for neonatal seizure detection. Pediatrics. 2007;120:770–7.
43. Shah DK, Mackay MT, Lavery S, et al. Accuracy of bedside electroencephalographic monitoring in comparison with simultaneous continuous conventional electroencephalography for seizure detection in term infants. Pediatrics. 2008;121:1146–54.
44. Zimbric MR, Sharpe CM, Albright KC, et al. Three-channel electroencephalogram montage in neonatal seizure detection and quantification. Pediatr Neurol. 2011;44:31–4.
45. McCoy B, Hahn CD. Continuous EEG monitoring in the neonatal intensive care unit. J Clin Neurophysiol. 2013;30:106–14.
46. Shah DK, Boylan GB, Rennie JM. Monitoring of seizures in the newborn. Arch Dis Child Fetal Neonatal Ed. 2012;97:F65–9.

12 Normal Variants and Unusual EEG Patterns

Francesca Bisulli, Claudia Rinaldi, Elena Merli, and Paolo Tinuper

12.1 Normal Variants

Normal variants consist of non-pathological variants of the background rhythm usually seen in the occipital (slow physiological posterior activities) or centroparietal areas (mu rhythm). Like background activity, these rhythms react to certain physiological changes or provocations like eye opening or repetitive movements of the extremities [1].

12.1.1 Slow Physiological Posterior Activities

Slow physiological posterior activities can be rhythmic or arrhythmic. Rhythmic activities account for 1–2% of the posterior activities, and they include the slow alpha variant and posterior theta rhythm. Arrhythmic activities consist of slow posterior waves and lambda waves [2].

12.1.1.1 Slow Alpha Variant

First described by Goodwin in 1947 [3], the slow alpha variant pattern appears as a rhythm in which a subharmonic frequency of the posterior rhythm is either superimposed on or replaces the posterior rhythm itself [2]. Usually the alpha variant fires at half the frequency of the patient's more typical background rhythm.

Like the normal background rhythm, the slow alpha variant has a sinusoidal appearance. It is mostly seen in posterior head regions when the subject's eyes are closed or when visual attention is lacking. The slow alpha variant is promptly suppressed by eye opening [1] (Fig. 12.1a, b).

F. Bisulli (✉) · C. Rinaldi · E. Merli · P. Tinuper
IRCCS Istituto delle Scienze Neurologiche di Bologna, Bologna, Italy

Department of Biomedical and Neuromotor Sciences, University of Bologna, Bologna, Italy
e-mail: francesca.bisulli@unibo.it

The slow alpha variant is considered a normal EEG variation, and it seems unrelated to the diagnosis of epilepsy. Sometimes it occurs in short bursts and could have a notched appearance mimicking interictal epileptiform abnormalities. Caution is needed to avoid overinterpretation. On a subject's tracing, the alpha variant usually alternates with periods of normal-appearing alpha discharges. Recognition of the variant could be aided by the transition to regular alpha rhythm [1].

12.1.1.2 Posterior Theta Rhythm

Les rhythmes postereurs a 4 cycles/seconde was first described by Pitot and Gastaut in 1956 [4] and later renamed "posterior theta rhythm" in 1964 [5]. It has a repetition rate of 4 Hz with a range of 3–5 Hz and is characterized by a high voltage (50–100 μV) and a regular (usually sinusoidal) shape [2]. Its slow waves intermix either with the subharmonic or harmonic posterior theta rhythm itself, or with the alpha posterior rhythm. The posterior theta rhythm usually occurs bilaterally in long bursts lasting 10–60 s, it is confined to the occipital areas [2] (Fig. 12.2). The posterior theta rhythm can be suppressed by eye opening and is most commonly of higher voltage in the right hemisphere [2]. The activity is most frequently in children and has been considered a genetic trait in childhood epilepsy [6].

12.1.1.3 Posterior Slow Waves

Gastaut first described posterior slow waves in infants in 1955 [7]. In 1959, Gastaut and Aird studied these waves in young adults [8].

Posterior slow waves are theta and delta waves that intermix with the posterior rhythm. They are mainly seen in early adolescence, become less common over the years, and disappear in adulthood. They are slow waves typically lasting 350–500 milliseconds with a voltage range of 50–200 μV and can be considered a slow variant of the alpha rhythm with which they are always associated [2] (Fig. 12.3).

Like the alpha rhythm, posterior slow waves are bilateral and confined to the posterior temporal, parietal, and occipital

O. Mecarelli (ed.), *Clinical Electroencephalography*, https://doi.org/10.1007/978-3-030-04573-9_12

areas. The amplitude of the posterior slow waves usually differs between the two hemispheres and is often of lower voltage on the left. These waveforms behave just like normal waking background rhythms: they disappear completely with eye opening and during drowsiness, whereas they increase with hyperventilation [2].

Posterior slow waves can bear some resemblance to spike or spike-and-wave discharges. They must be recognized as normal variants to avoid misleading interpretations [2]. The presence of incisures of the background alpha posterior rhythm on top of the slow wave proves the physiological nature of these waves and hence aids the differential diagnosis (Fig. 12.3) (see magnification).

12.1.1.4 Lambda Waves

Lambda waves were first described by Gastaut in 1951 [9] and then by Evans in the following year [10]. Evans described their electrographic morphology as "monophasic triangular waves," calling these potentials "lambda waves" as their shape resembles the Greek letter lambda (λ). They are low-

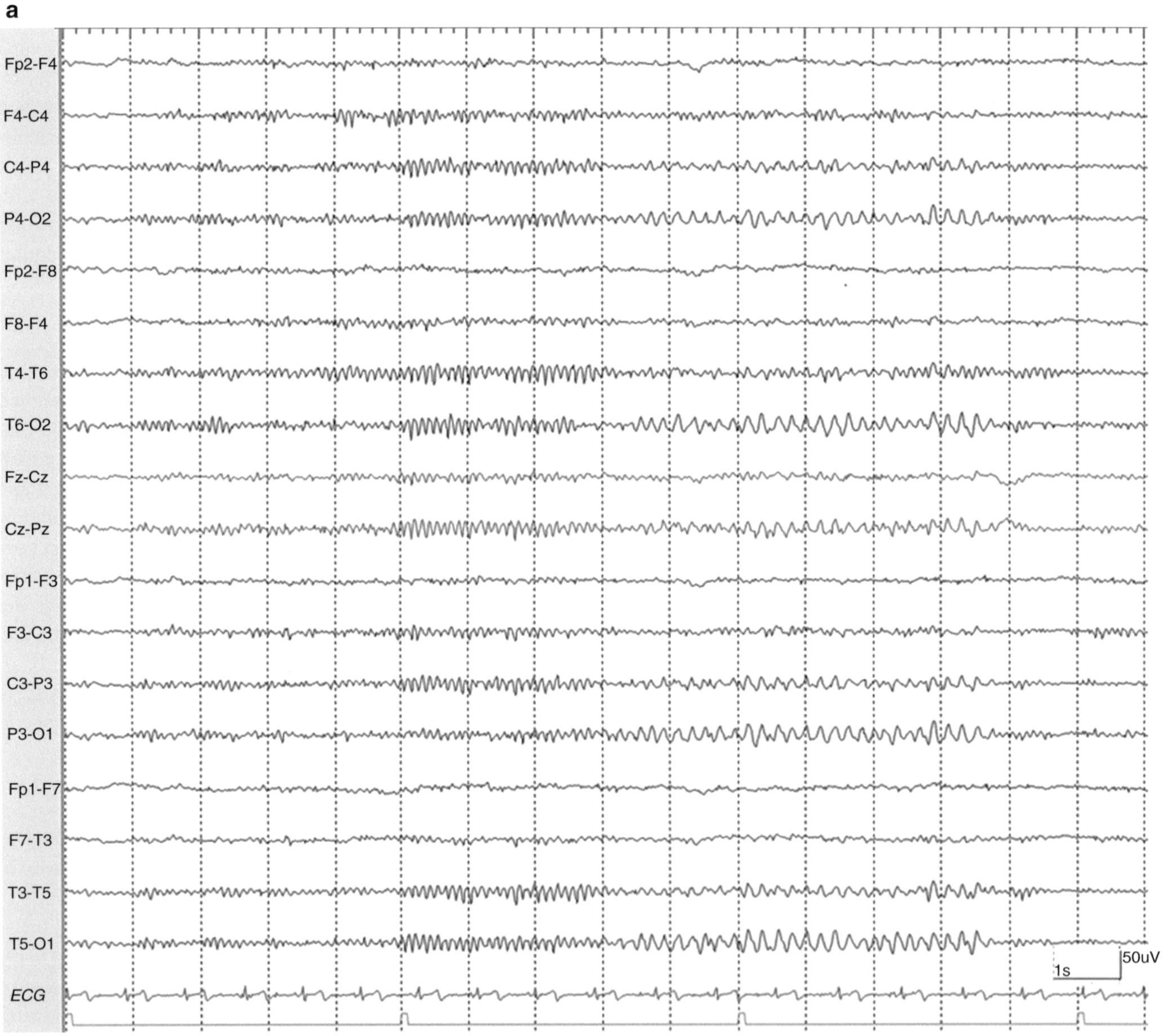

Fig. 12.1 (**a**) (F, 36 years) The transition between an occipital alpha sinusoidal background activity to a subharmonic half-frequency posterior rhythm. This activity clearly replaces the posterior rhythm itself and maintains its characteristics, such as the sinusoidal appearance and occipital localization. (**b**) (M, 67 years) Magnification of the slow alpha variant. A convenient technique to recognize normal variants is to look for their relation with the background activity. If the pattern is physiological, it normally contains the incisures of the background rhythm. As an example, in this case you can see posterior alpha rhythm's incisures over the slow alpha variant rhythm

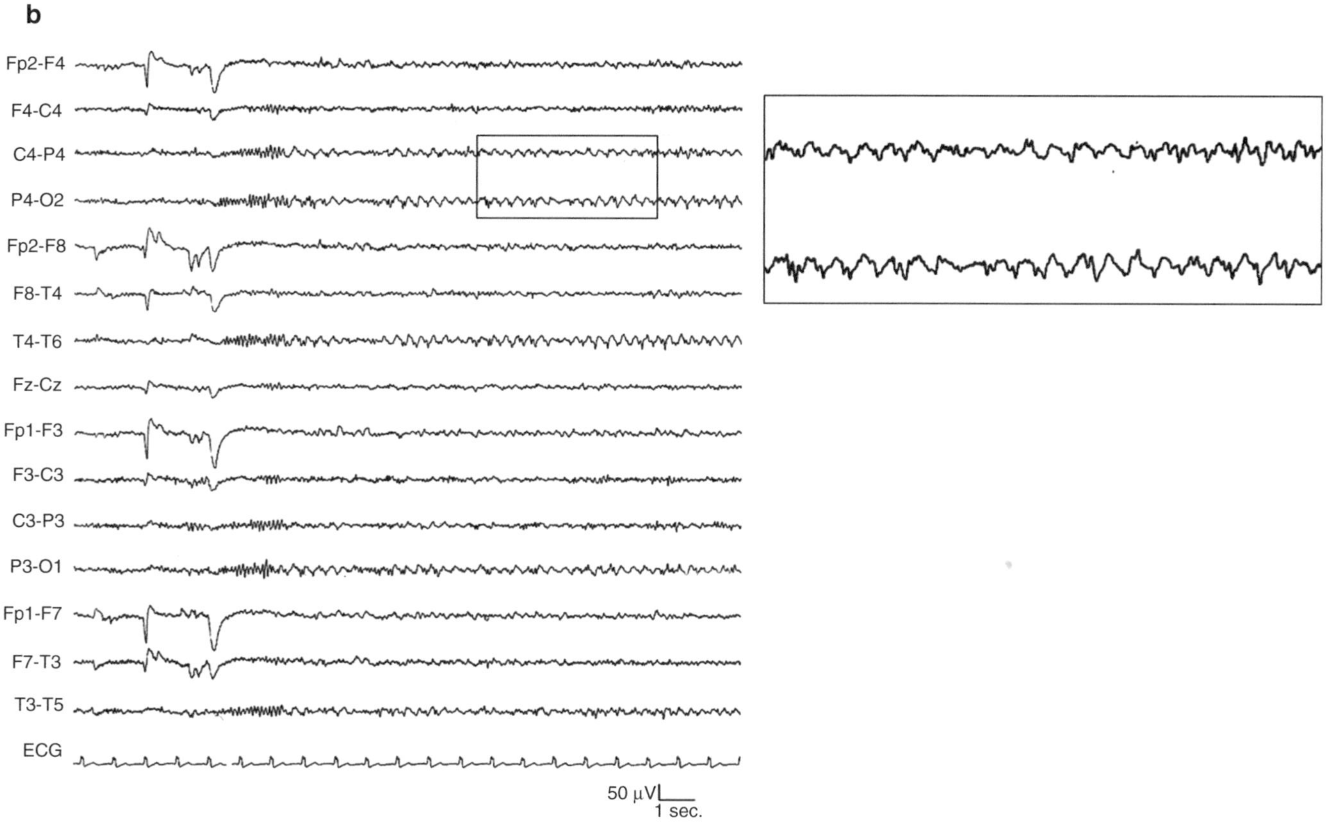

Fig. 12.1 (continued)

voltage sharp transient waves that appear over visual areas exclusively with eyes opened [10] (Fig. 12.4).

Lambda waves occur exclusively as random bi- or triphasic waveforms lasting 20–30 ms [9]. They generally fire at a rate of 1–3 Hz but can be totally arrhythmic. Lambda waves are usually bilateral and synchronous, although they may occasionally be unilateral. Voltage asymmetry is not considered abnormal [2]. These waveforms are more frequently seen in children aged 2–15 years than in adults [12].

There is no consensus in the literature on the incidence of lambda waves in normal individuals. They may be present one day and undetectable the next, and their degree of expression may also vary from time to time. Their presence also depends on the recording's setting. All these factors have made it difficult to establish the true incidence of the lambda rhythm in the normal population [2].

Lambda waves appear during wakefulness when the patient's eyes are open in a well-lit room and are associated with horizontal searching eye movements. They are inhibited during visual fixation (they disappear when vision is fixed on a point and reappear on the cessation of fixation) and enhanced during viewing a patterned field of high contrast (they disappear when the field being viewed is uniform). Evans suggested that the mechanism necessary for their production is an abrupt change in the retinal afferent impulses due to fast eye movements [10]. All cases presenting lambda waves show a strong response to photic stimulation, suggesting a possible common generator [10].

12.1.2 Mu Rhythm

First described as *rythme rolandique en arceau* by Gastaut and colleagues in 1952 [11], the mu rhythm is an arch-shaped rhythm most often seen from late childhood to adulthood. Walter designated this rhythm with the Greek letter mu (μ) owing to its morphology [12]. It is present as a visually detectable rhythm in 10% of normal adults [2].

Mu waveforms occur at a frequency similar to that of the patient's posterior rhythm and vary with age. They typically fire at a rate of 7–11 Hz with a voltage range of 30–100 μV [2]. They can be unilateral or bilateral; when bilateral they are usually asymmetric and asynchronous.

Mu rhythms are synchronized waveforms generated by electrical activity involving large numbers of neurons in the brain area responsible for voluntary movement. This is why

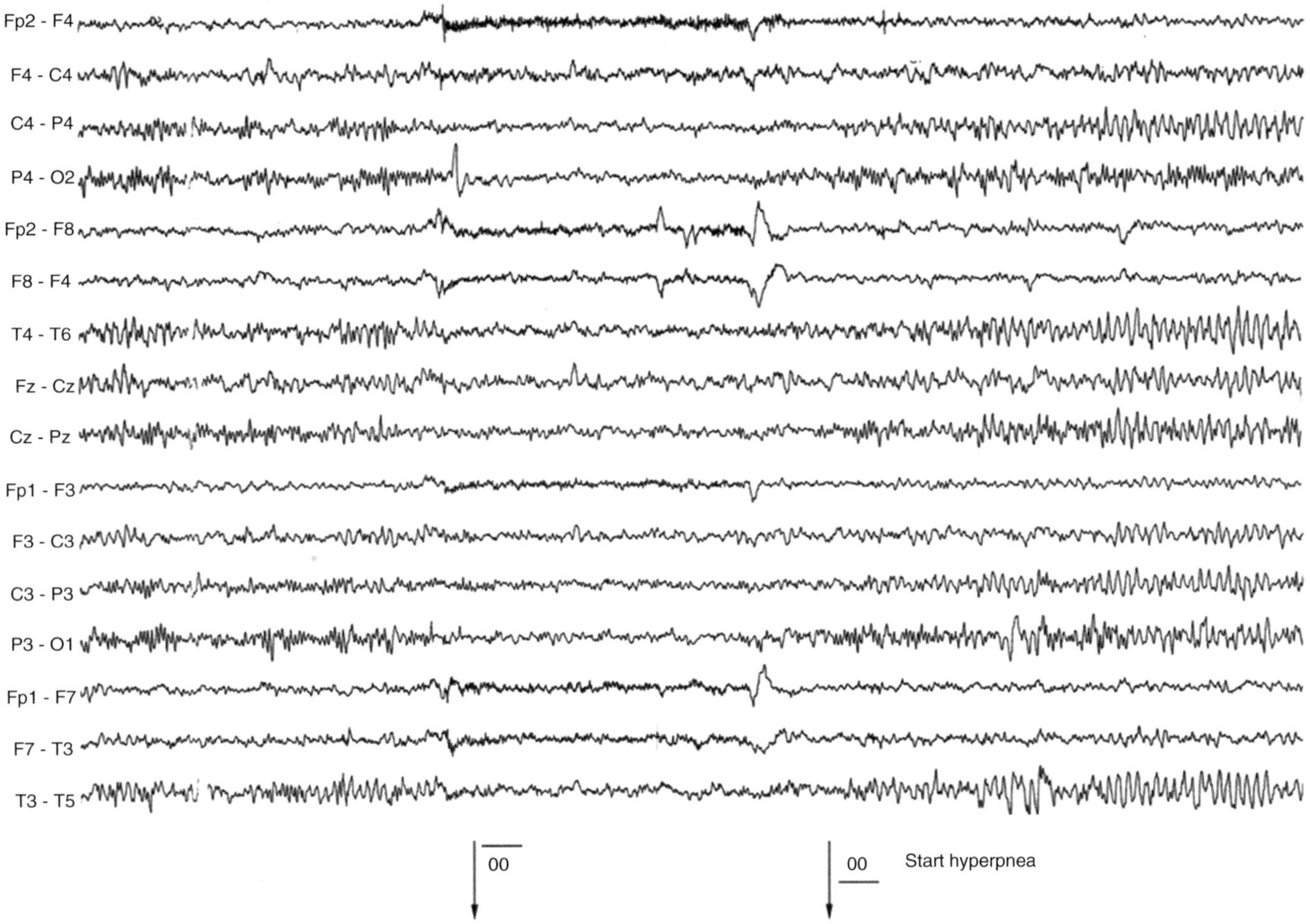

Fig. 12.2 (M, 8 years) The posterior theta rhythm consists of long bursts of a high-voltage, regular, sinusoidal, theta activity that occurs bilaterally and remains confined to the occipital areas. It presents intermixed with other background activities. In this case, it appears mixed with subharmonic or harmonic frequencies of the posterior theta rhythm itself or with the alpha posterior rhythm. The posterior theta rhythm can be suppressed by eye opening and is elicited by hyperpnea

these rhythms are best seen in the centroparietal area during relaxed wakefulness and best recorded by C3 and C4 electrodes.

The mu rhythm is particularly labile and exhibits physiological reactivity. It is in fact the rhythm of the sensorimotor cortex at rest [13]: it attenuates or completely disappears with movement, imagining a movement or somatosensory stimulation of the contralateral limb [12] (Fig. 12.5a, b).

Sometimes the mu rhythm is sharpened on one side and rounded on the other and therefore can be commonly confused with epileptiform activity. In order to distinguish between a sharp central rhythm and a mu rhythm, reactivity should be tested by asking patients to open their eyes (to make alpha rhythm disappear) and then move their contralateral hand, noting that the mu discharges disappear and the posterior alpha rhythm is enhanced [12].

A high-voltage mu activity may be recorded unilaterally in the central region over a focal skull breach. It has been called the *volet* rhythm (the French term *volet* means breach) and was described by Fischgold et al. in 1952 [14]. Mu rhythm pathogenesis has been under debate: some authors considered it the result of an overexpression of natural rhythms through the skull defects [14], whereas others, like Naquet, considered it the result of a discharge originating from the corticomeningeal scar [15].

In the setting of a focal skull breach, the mu rhythm usually has a sharp configuration mixed with slower frequency activities: it may falsely mimic an epileptogenic focus. For this reason, it is important to test the physiological reactivity of the mu rhythm: a reactive breach rhythm will rule out an abnormal pattern. However, a lack of reactivity does not exclude the possibility of a normal variant [16].

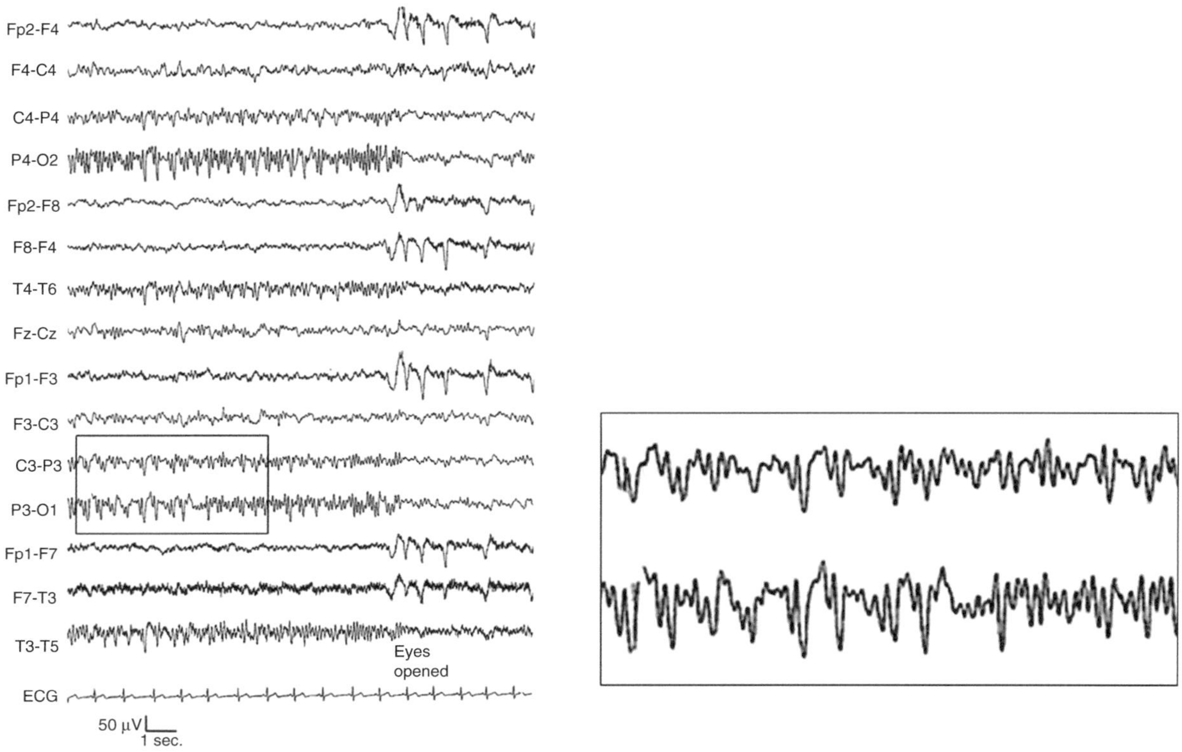

Fig. 12.3 (M, 12 years) Posterior slow waves are theta and delta waves. Even though they occasionally present with a spiky component, they can be recognized as normal variants because of their association with the background posterior rhythm. They appear over the posterior regions, are intermixed with posterior alpha activity, and react to eye opening. The magnification shows the incisures of the background alpha posterior rhythm as proof of the physiological nature of these waves

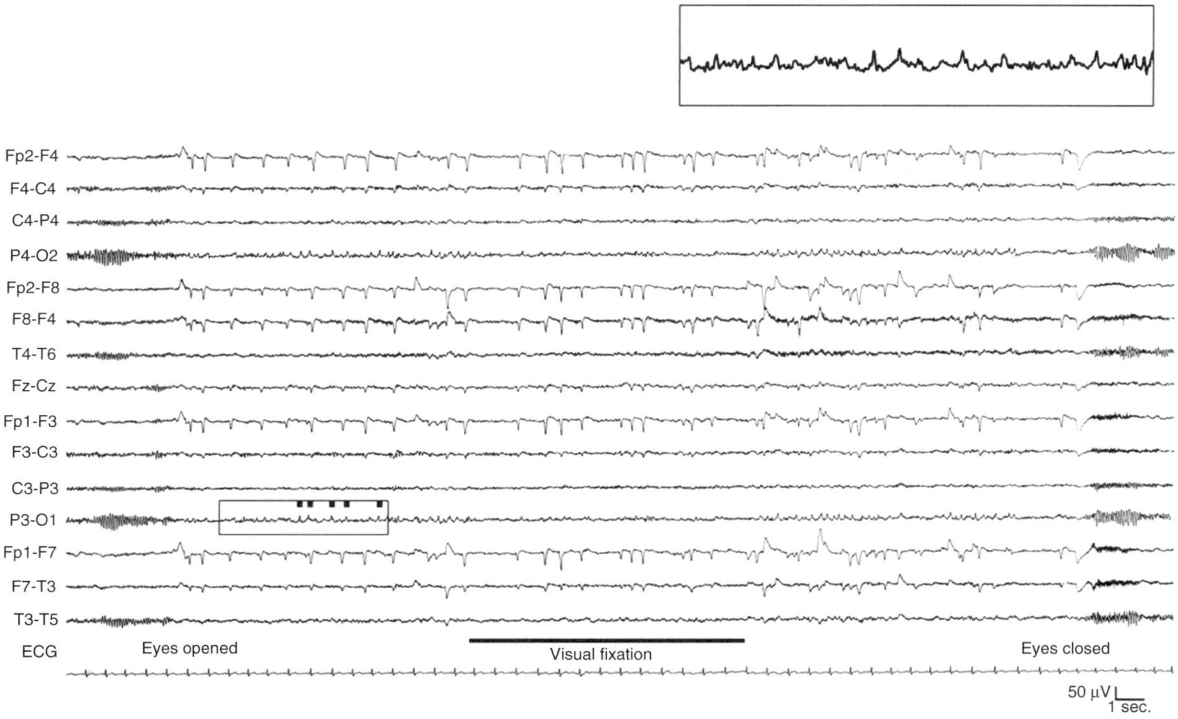

Fig. 12.4 (F, 31 years) Lambda waves (filled square) have a characteristic shape resembling the Greek letter lambda (λ). Their typical aspect can be seen in the magnification. Lambda waves are usually bilateral and synchronous (as in this figure), although occasionally they may be unilateral, over the occipital derivations. As they are the electroencephalographic representation of the patient's horizontal searching eye movements, they appear with the patient remaining eyes opened in a well-lit room and are inhibited during visual fixation. Artifacts derived from eye movements can be seen over the anterior derivations

Differential diagnosis with the breach rhythm. The breach rhythm is a focal high-voltage physiological activity developing over or near a skull defect (mostly a surgical craniotomy site) [16, 17] (Fig. 12.6). It occurs in wakefulness and sometimes disappears during sleep. The breach rhythm generally fires at a rate of 6–11 Hz and has an arch-shaped morphology. Sometimes it may be spiky and irregular due to a mix of beta, alpha, mu, and theta activity [18]. This makes a clear-cut diagnosis between epileptiform discharges in the same area of the breach rhythms particularly challenging [18]. Breach rhythms sometimes bear a resemblance to mu rhythms or wicket rhythms: if they are located over the central area, it is important to test mu reactivity asking patients to move their contralateral limb [18]. In itself, the breach rhythm is not indicative of a brain dysfunction [16]. The mechanism underlying the genesis of breach rhythms remains unsettled. They may be the final consequence of a change in the transmission of EEG waves: the waveforms appear enhanced as they are unfiltered due to the absence of bone, which represents the major resistive element between the cortex and the scalp electrode [16]. However, some data suggest a more complex underlying mechanism than simply the reduced filtering effect of the EEG signal [16, 17]. Sometimes the breach rhythm is better seen over an EEG electrode that is not only placed over the skull defect. Moreover, bone replacement does not always reduce the breach rhythm. Finally, the breach rhythm develops a few weeks or months after surgery in many patients.

12.2 Unusual Benign Epileptiform Patterns

Benign epileptiform variants (BEVs) are various distinctive unusual waveforms that have no established relationship with clinical seizures despite bearing some

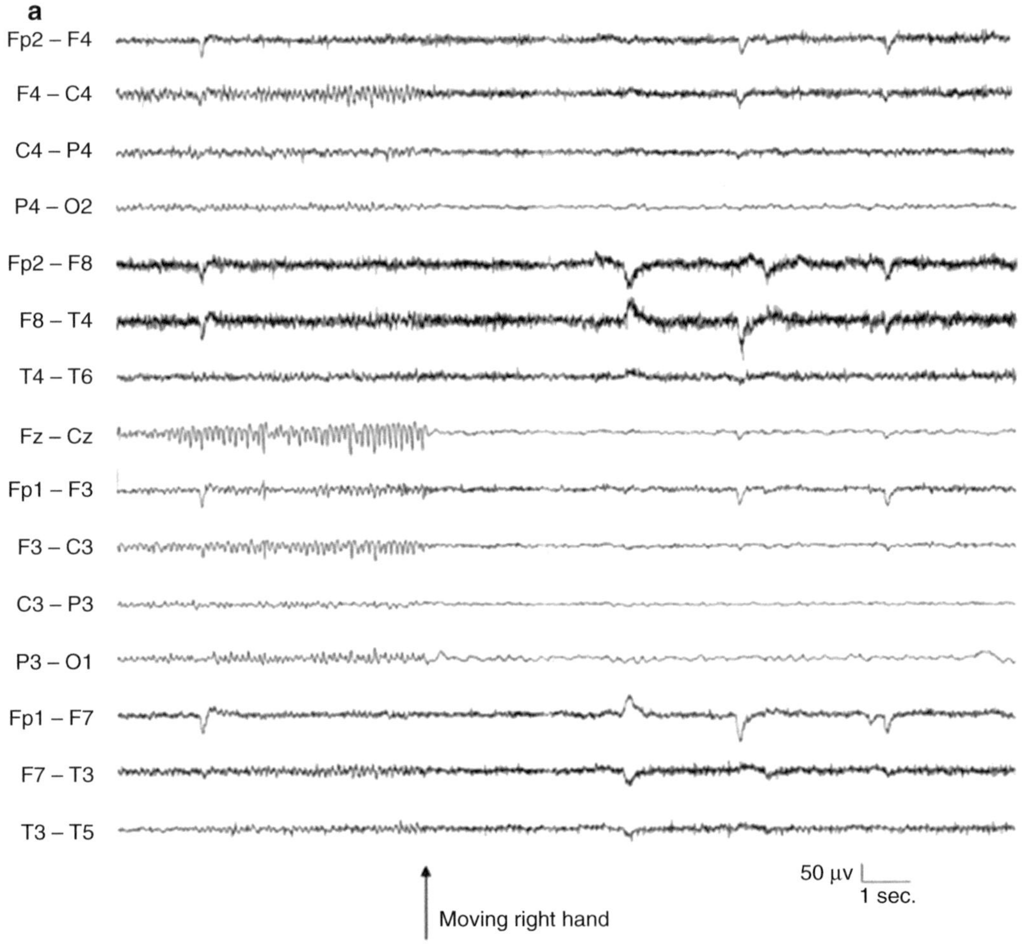

Fig. 12.5 (**a**) (F, 40 years) and (**b**) (F, 45 years). The mu rhythm is an arch-shaped rhythm whose morphology resembles the Greek letter mu (μ). It usually occurs with a frequency similar to that of the patient's posterior rhythm. The mu rhythm can be unilateral or bilateral (asymmetric and asynchronous) and is generated by the synchronous discharge of neurons in the brain area responsible for voluntary movements, so that it is seen in the centroparietal areas (C3 or C4 (Fig. 12.5a) or CZ (Fig. 12.5b) electrodes). It attenuates or disappears with movement, imagining a movement or somatosensory stimulation of the contralateral limb (Fig 12.5a), frequently with a strict anatomical correspondence. Reactivity is major evidence distinguishing a sharp or mu central rhythm from epileptiform activity

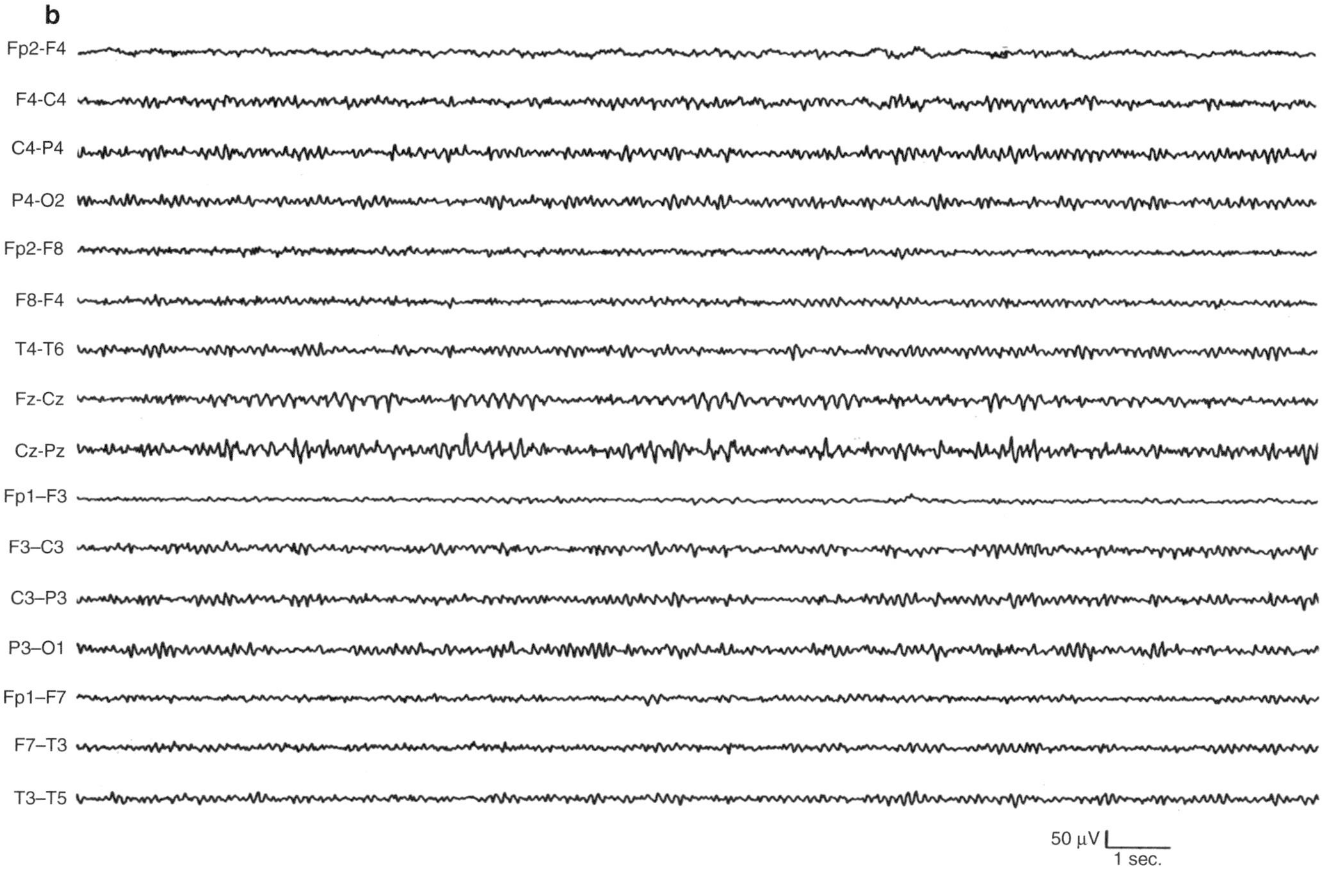

Fig. 12.5 (continued)

resemblance to epileptiform activity. In fact, spikes and other paroxysmal EEG patterns do not automatically indicate epilepsy or even pathology. In clinical practice, EEG "overreading" does more damage than "underreading." For instance, EEGs in patients diagnosed with psychogenic non-epileptic seizures were frequently read as "showing epilepsy." Overread patterns included wicket spikes, hypnagogic hypersynchrony, hyperventilation-induced slowing, or most commonly simple fluctuations of sharply contoured background rhythms or fragmented alpha activity [19]. The fact that BEVs are rarely identified in routine EEG recordings has probably contributed to make them a controversial discovery. BEVs prevalence varies across literature studies, with an overall prevalence ranging from 0.07% for subclinical rhythmic electrographic discharges of adults (SREDA) to 1.85% for small sharp spikes [20].

BEVs can be divided into two groups: rhythmic epileptiform patterns and the "benign" spikes. Rhythmic epileptiform patterns include midline theta rhythms, rhythmic mid-temporal discharges, and subclinical rhythmic electrographic discharges of adults. "Benign" spikes consist of wicket spikes, 14- and 6-Hz positive bursts, phantom spikes and waves, and small sharp spikes.

12.2.1 Midline Theta Rhythm

The midline theta rhythm is recorded in both children and adults during wake and drowsiness. It consists of trains of rhythmic theta activity (from 5 to 7 Hz) over the midline central head region and may have a smooth, sinusoidal, arciform, spiky, or mu-like morphology (Fig. 12.7). In addition, the duration of this pattern varies and tends to wax and wane, typically lasting from 4 to 20 seconds. The midline theta rhythm displays variable reactivity to eye opening, alerting, and limb movements [1, 2].

Initially described by Ciganek et al. in 1961, the midline theta rhythm was thought to be an "EEG symptom of temporal lobe epilepsy" [21], whereas later studies

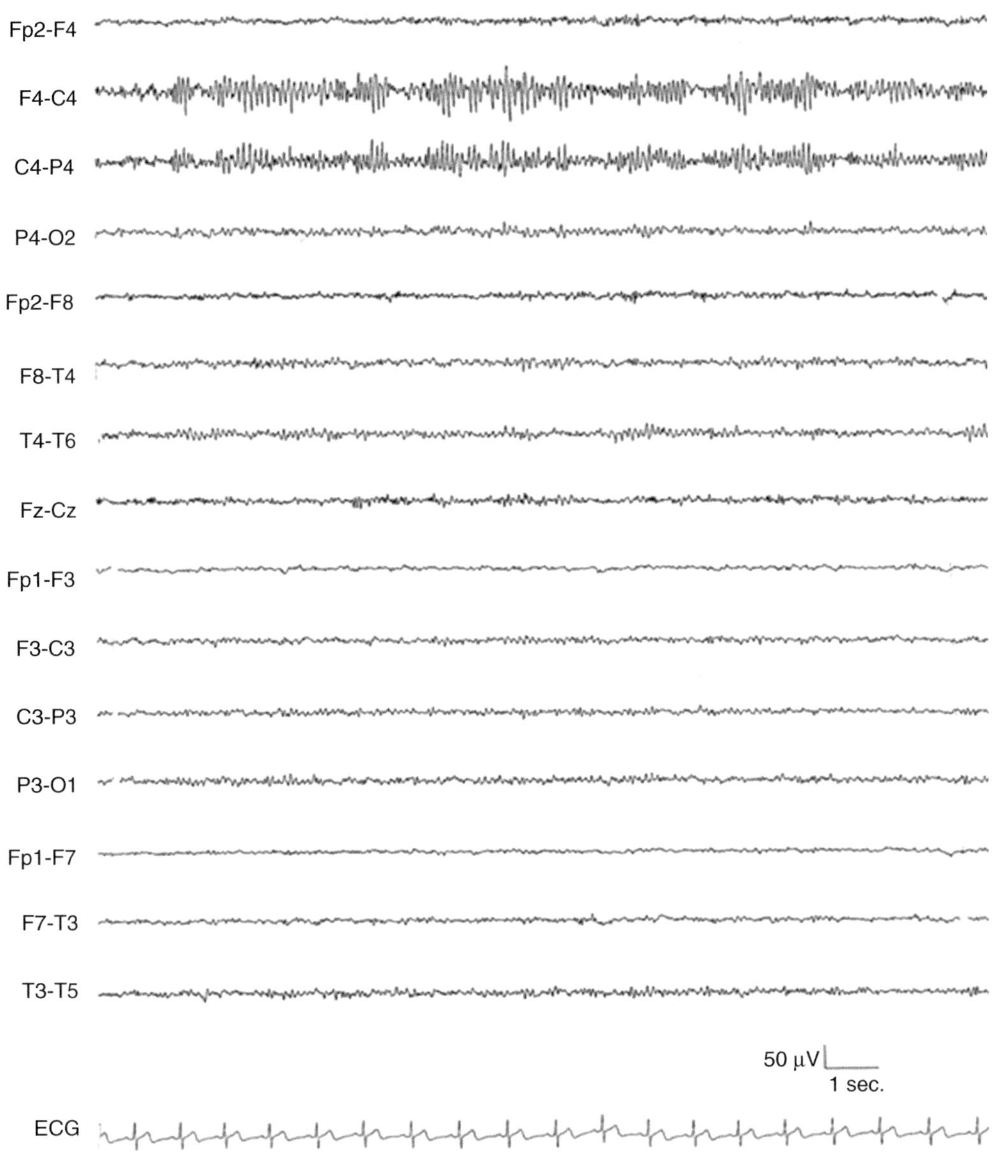

Fig. 12.6 (M, 42 years) The patient underwent a neurosurgical intervention for a right frontal meningioma. The absence of the bone in a small scalp area, normally representing the major resistive element between the cortex and the scalp electrode, leads to the appearance of a spiky irregular activity that remains localized over the area concerned. The breach rhythm is composed of intermixed beta, alpha, and theta frequencies and can have an arch-shaped or a slow and sharp morphology

found the pattern to represent a nonspecific variant of theta activity, not clearly associated with a seizure disorder [22].

Previous studies analyzed the relation between the midline theta rhythm and mental tasks, concluding that the appearance of this rhythm is related to mental activity even during sleep: it is more frequent during rapid eye movement (REM) and stage 1 of non-REM (NREM) sleep and is related to dream images during slumber. This pattern has also been related to certain personality traits: if well represented, it correlates with a lower anxiety score (on the Manifest Anxiety Scale), a higher score on the extrovertive scale (Maudsley Personality Inventory), and a lower score on the nevrotic scale [23].

12.2.2 Rhythmic Theta Bursts of Drowsiness or Rhythmic Mid-temporal Discharges or Psychomotor Variant

Rhythmic mid-temporal discharges (RMTD) are recorded in adolescents and young adults, with reported occurrences varying from 0.1 to 2%. They occur during relaxed wakefulness and drowsiness [1].

RMTD consist of trains of mixed frequency activities, alternating with a monophasic and regular theta (5–6 Hz) activity with an occasionally interposed double-frequency activity (10–12 Hz) [24] (Fig. 12.8a, b).

Located predominately over the temporal head regions, RMTD are usually maximal over the mid-temporal regions.

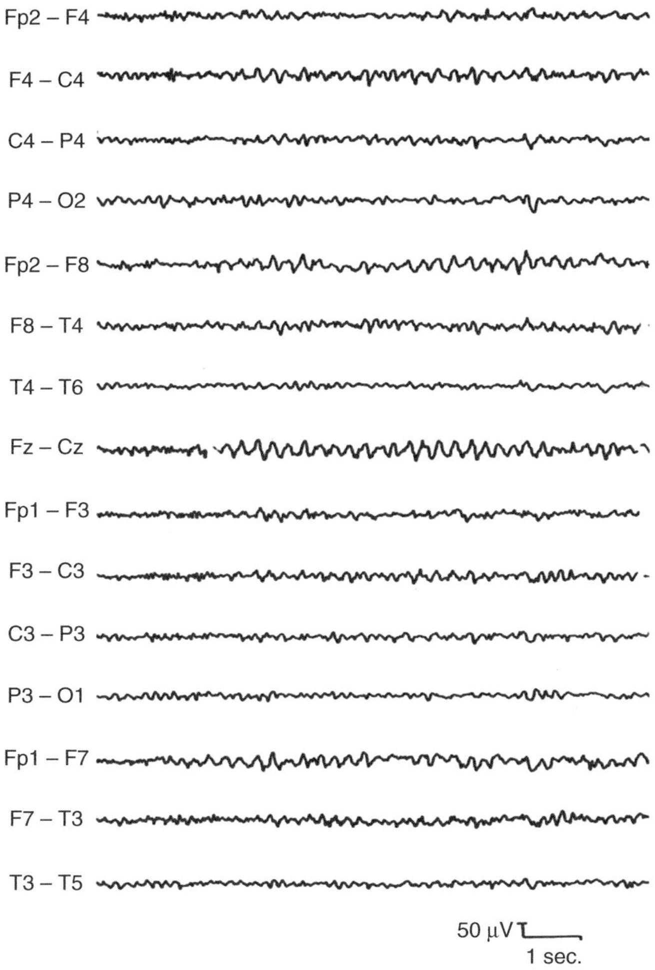

Fig. 12.7 (M, 40 years) The midline theta rhythm consists of trains of rhythmic theta activity over the midline central head region, of a variable duration lasting 4–20 s. The rhythm tends to wax and wane, and it may have a smooth, sinusoidal, arciform, or spiky morphology

They can occasionally spread to the parasagittal and occipital head regions. The origin from the posterior inferior temporal cortex has been suggested [25].

RMTD may occur unilaterally, bilaterally, or synchronously over the two hemispheres, and their amplitude may gradually fluctuate. The regular, rhythmic trains of theta activity classically increase in amplitude at onset and decrease at the end of the discharge. The discharges may have a sharpened, notched, or flat-topped appearance. Each train of activity lasts some seconds and rarely exceeds 1 min. RMTD do not change in relation to stimulus [1, 2].

RMTD were originally called "psychomotor variants" [26] because of their resemblance to ictal activity during complex partial seizures over the temporal lobe (previously referred to as psychomotor seizures). Today, RMTD are considered a relatively nonspecific finding and do not suggest a seizure tendency [27, 28]. They can be differentiated from ictal discharges by their monomorphic pattern which does not evolve in frequency or morphology, their short duration of only a few seconds, their possible bilateral appearance, and finally the lack of disrupted background EEG activity.

Differential diagnosis with Chatrian's theta rhythm. Chatrian's theta pattern consists of burst of waves at 3–5 Hz [29]. It is considered a highly specific sign of temporal epilepsy and has the same value as isolated temporal spikes or spike-waves for its diagnosis (Fig. 12.9).

This theta pattern is believed to be specific for sclerosis of the anterior median temporal cortex, and it presents ipsilaterally to the lesion, localized on the anterior temporal region in one hemisphere. It involves a spiky rhythmic activity starting from the inner side of the temporal lobe and recorded over its external face as a slightly sharpened activity [30] with an arciform morphology.

Differential diagnosis with the ring 20 EEG pattern. Classic chromosome 20 syndrome is a rare structural chromosomal mutation characterized by mental retardation, behavioral problems, epilepsy, and no definite dysmorphic features. High levels of mosaicism have been shown to correlate with a lower age of symptom onset and a more severe cognitive impairment [31, 32].

EEG recordings of these patients show frequent bursts or long trains of theta waves, with a peak at 5 Hz. The theta bursts may occur on both temporal lobes, or may shift from one temporal lobe to the other or spread to the parasagittal regions (Fig. 12.10). This activity is characterized by a sharp-contoured appearance combined with large portions of normal-appearing EEG tracings [33].

The bursts of theta activity are not associated with any clinical modification. The complete absence of delays in reaction times, subjective symptoms, and cognitive impairment during the theta wave bursts probably indicates a non-epileptic nature of this pattern, so that the activity could be interpreted as non-epileptogenic patterns of uncertain significance.

12.2.3 Subclinical Rhythmic Electrographic Discharges of Adults

Subclinical rhythmic electrographic discharge of adults (SREDA) is the rarest benign epileptiform variant. It is frequently reported in adults over the age of 50, with a prevalence of 0.7% of patients arriving at the EEG laboratory [34–36].

SREDA may appear in relaxed wake or drowsiness, and there is one reported case occurring during REM sleep [37]. It can be elicited by hyperventilation or intermittent photic stimulation.

SREDA consists of a rhythmic-sustained theta pattern (with a range of 4–7 Hz) combined with a double-frequency activity (10–12 Hz). Frequency analysis, using both the conventional fast Fourier transform (FFT) and time-frequency, mapping with the Wigner FFT variant, has demonstrated that the SREDA consists of a complex mixture of multiple rapidly shifting frequencies with little spatial or temporal correlation [38].

SREDA is typically widespread and in the majority of cases is maximal over the parietal and posterior temporal head regions. It is normally bisynchronous and symmetrical, but is asymmetric or unilateral in less than 0.05% of patients.

SREDA is characterized by sharply contoured, arch-shaped, or sinusoidal waveforms. It can appear in two different ways, beginning abruptly, like a paroxysm, or starting shortly after a single high-amplitude sharp or slow wave component. The discharge can end brusquely or can gradually vanish into the background EEG activity [24]. It typically lasts 40–80 s but may be less than 10 s or more than 5 min.

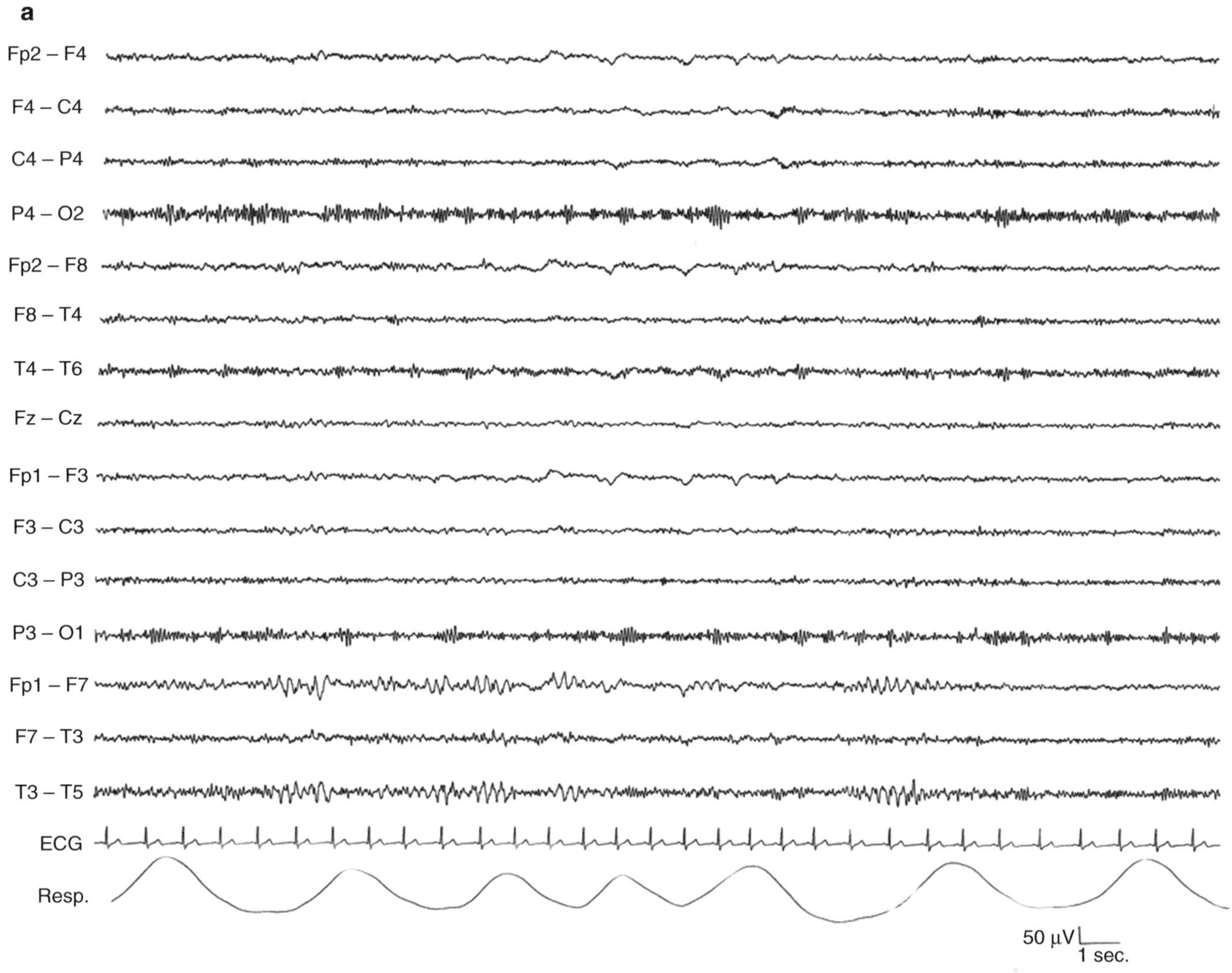

Fig. 12.8 (**a**) (F, 32 years) and (**b**) regular rhythmic trains of theta activity appearing over the left mid-temporal regions, increasing in amplitude at the onset of the discharge and decreasing at its end. EEG frequency spectroscopy (Fig. 12.8b) graphically represents in peaks all the frequencies composing the global background activity. In this example the global rhythm can be divided into peaks of all multiples of a principal background rhythm (2.5, 5, 10, and 15 Hz), demonstrating that the theta rhythm shown in the EEG trace simply consists of a variant rhythm of the background activity itself. In fact, rhythmic mid-temporal discharges typically consist of mixed frequencies, alternating a monophasic and regular theta (5–6 Hz) activity with an occasionally interposed double frequency discharge (10–12 Hz). They may occur unilaterally, bilaterally, or synchronously over the two hemispheres

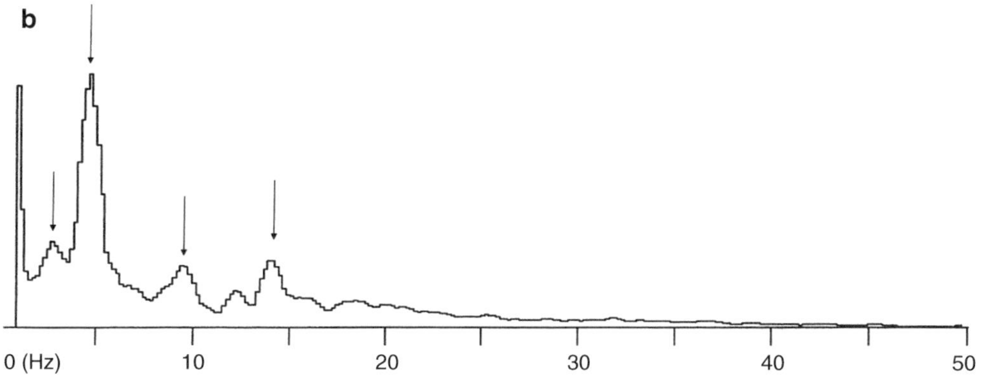

Fig. 12.8 (continued)

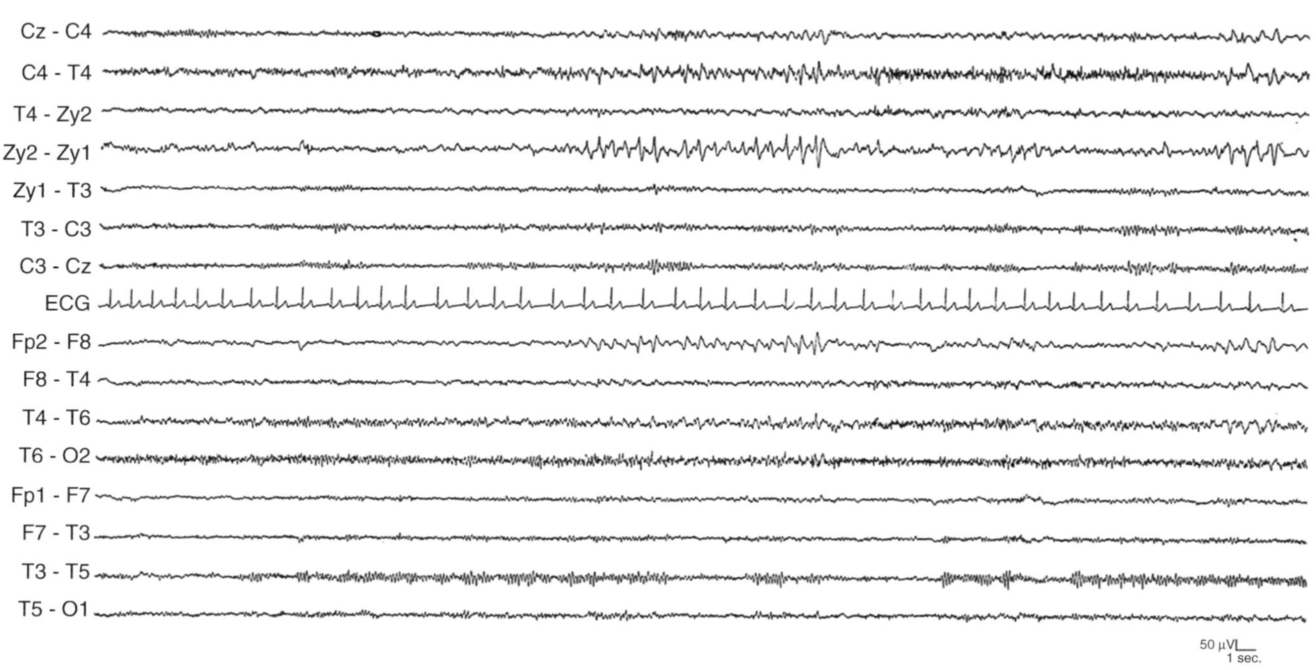

Fig. 12.9 (F, 35 years) In this tracing electrodes were placed according to the 10–20 International System, following a bipolar montage and adding zygomatic electrodes placed over the zygomatic notch in the posterior portion of the cheek, 2 cm beyond the tragus [45]. The figure shows how patients with sclerosis of the anterior temporal region cortex, recorded during a temporal lobe epileptic event, may show a spiky, sharpened, or arciform rhythmic theta activity on the EEG tracing, localized over the anterior temporal region, ipsilaterally to the lesion

Like rhythmic theta bursts of drowsiness, the SREDA can be misinterpreted as an ictal epileptiform discharge (Clinical Case n°1—Fig. 12.11a, b). If tested by the EEG technologist, patients with a SREDA pattern will have no alteration in their level of consciousness, unlike most patients with widespread electrographic ictal activity. In addition, there is no slowing of background EEG activity following SREDA, which instead is very frequent in postictal recordings.

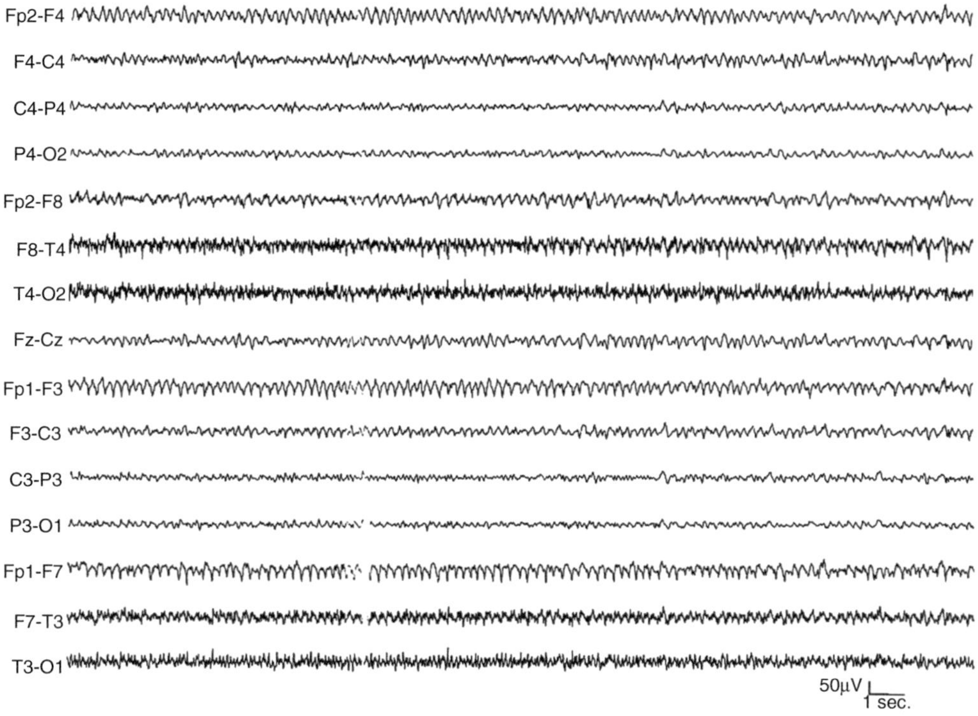

Fig. 12.10 (F, 33 years, mental retardation) An EEG recording of a patient with classic chromosome 20 syndrome. This patient's traces frequently show trains of theta activity, which can be localized (in this case over the frontal regions) or with a generalized pattern characterized by a sharp-contoured morphology. Epochs with this appearance are combined with large portions of normal-appearing EEG tracings

12.2.4 Wicket Spikes or Wicket Rhythms

Seen predominately in adults over 30 years of age, wicket spikes are relatively rare, having an incidence of 0.9%. They have been reported to be more common in patients with cerebrovascular diseases [39], whereas they are not associated with epilepsy.

Wicket spikes are present during the awake portion of the recording, but are often masked by background EEG activity, so that they are better appreciated during drowsiness and light sleep. They have also been reported to occur during REM sleep [40].

They can manifest as monophasic paroxysmal waves or in clusters with a frequency of 6–11 Hz. They may morphologically resemble an arciform/mu rhythm, being composed of a negative sharper component of the waveform and a variable amplitude, ranging from 60 to 200 µV.

Wicket spikes are usually recorded over the anterior or mid-temporal head regions and can appear bilaterally or unilaterally (Fig. 12.12a, b). For these reasons, an isolated wicket waveform can be misinterpreted as a temporal lobe discharge. To differentiate them it is advisable to follow these criteria:

1. There is no slow wave component following wicket spikes.
2. They tend to occur in trains, so when a wicket spike occurs in isolation, it should be compared to a succession of spikes with a similar morphology to those of the train.
3. They do not disrupt the background activity [24].

12.2.5 14- and 6-Hz Positive Bursts

14- and 6-Hz positive bursts more frequently appear in children and adolescents, with a peak incidence between the ages of 13 and 14 years. The incidence of this benign variant declines with age.

Such bursts are most commonly recorded during drowsiness and light non-REM sleep. They are recognized as a common pattern in asymptomatic individuals, with a prevalence of 10–58% of normal subjects. Positive bursts have no epileptogenic significance. They have been described in various pathologies as in comatose patients with acute hepatic failure, and most prominently in Reye's syndrome, metabolic- or anoxia-induced comas and in head traumas [41, 42].

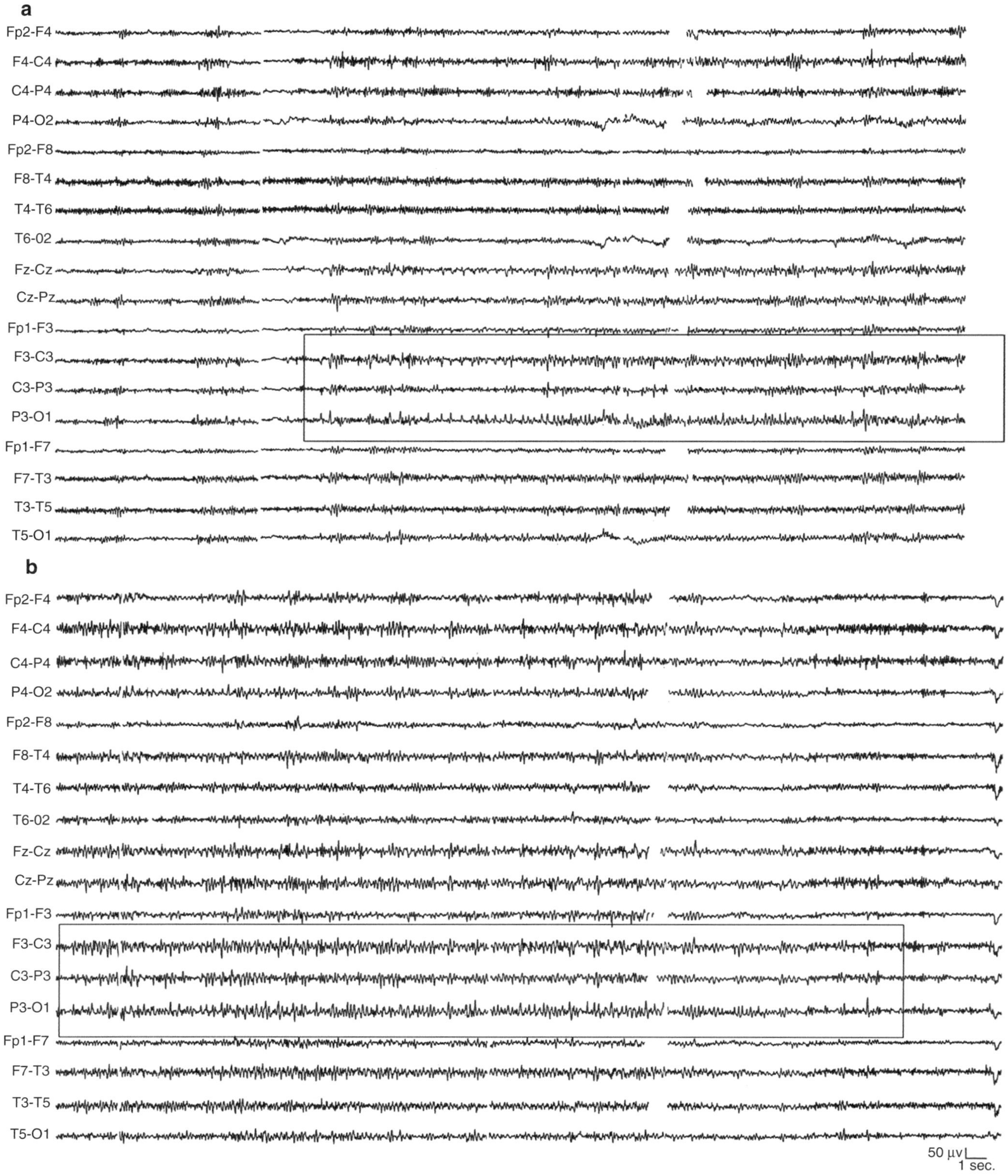

Fig. 12.11 (**a**, **b**) (M, 69 y) A 69-year-old man was admitted to a neurological service for progressive worsening of daily somnolence since the age of 49 years and the recent onset of episodes characterized by an abrupt impairment of awareness. These episodes occurred many times per day, had a brief duration (few seconds), and were not followed by confusion or other neurological signs. During sleep he had snoring and apneas. The EEG recording showed a sustained train of sharply contoured theta activity, interposed by background activity, which remains unmodified both during and after the discharge (Fig 12.11a and b). It begins and vanishes gradually and is localized over the left frontoparietal leads. This EEG activity was misinterpreted as a subclinical left temporal seizure. The patient was diagnosed with focal epilepsy in the context of a chronic cerebral vasculopathy and was started on carbamazepine with worsening of the episodes in terms of frequency and duration. He was hospitalized again and repeated an EEG recording, showing the same focal rhythmic pattern, now recognized as SREDA. He was diagnosed with obstructive sleep apnea syndrome and carbamazepine was withdrawn. Now he has been seizure-free for 5 years, he is on treatment with C-PAP and can drive his car

14- and 16-Hz positive bursts consist of chains of rhythmic waves with a faster component of 14 Hz (range of 13–17 Hz) which resembles a sleep spindle in morphology and a slower 6-Hz (range of 4–7 Hz) wave. 14-Hz and 6-Hz bursts can occur separately or within the same burst, bisynchronously or independently [24] (Fig. 12.13). Usually the bursts are visible symmetrically over the parieto-temporal areas, even though their predominance may shift from side to side. They are arch-shaped with a spiky component, positive on the surface, alternating with a smooth surface-negative rounded waveform. These discharges are low in voltage, usually less than 75 μV on a referential montage. Positive bursts have a brief duration lasting from 1 to 2 s.

12.2.6 Phantom Spikes and Waves or 6-Hz Spikes and Waves

The phantom spike and wave discharges (also named 6-Hz spike and wave bursts) are brief (lasting 1–2 s), low-voltage, bilateral spike-wave complexes. They have a repetition rate of 6 Hz with a range of 5–7 Hz. They occur during wakeful-

a

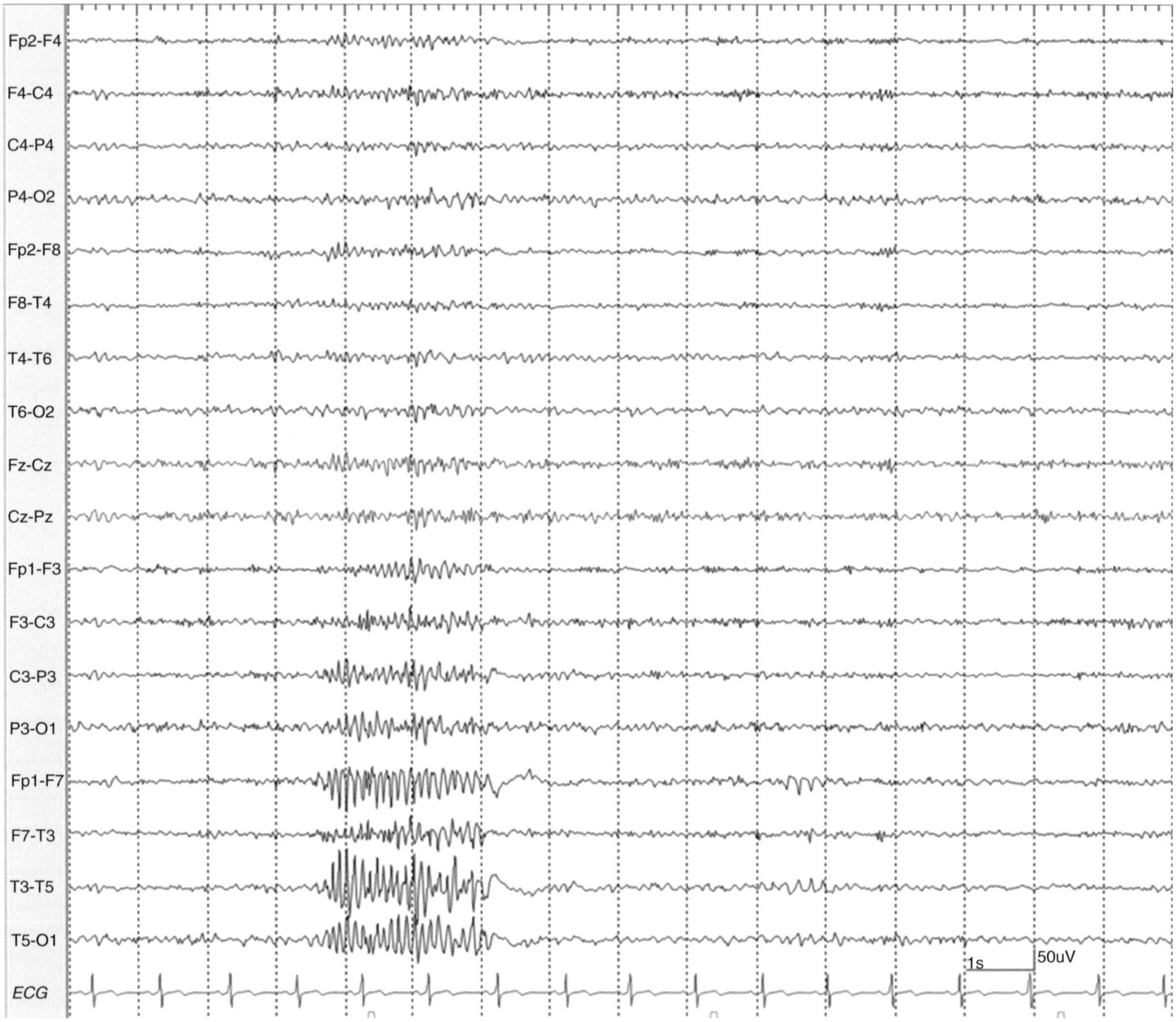

Fig. 12.12 (**a**) (F, 43 years) and (**b**) (F, 25 years). Wicket spikes are most frequently appreciated during drowsiness or light sleep. They present as clusters of arciform waves, being composed of a negative sharper component of the waveform and a variable amplitude (ranging from 60 to 200 μV). They may vary in frequency, ranging from 6 (Fig. 12.12b) to 11 Hz (Fig. 12.12a). Wicket spikes are usually recorded over the anterior or mid-temporal head regions, and can be present bilaterally or unilaterally

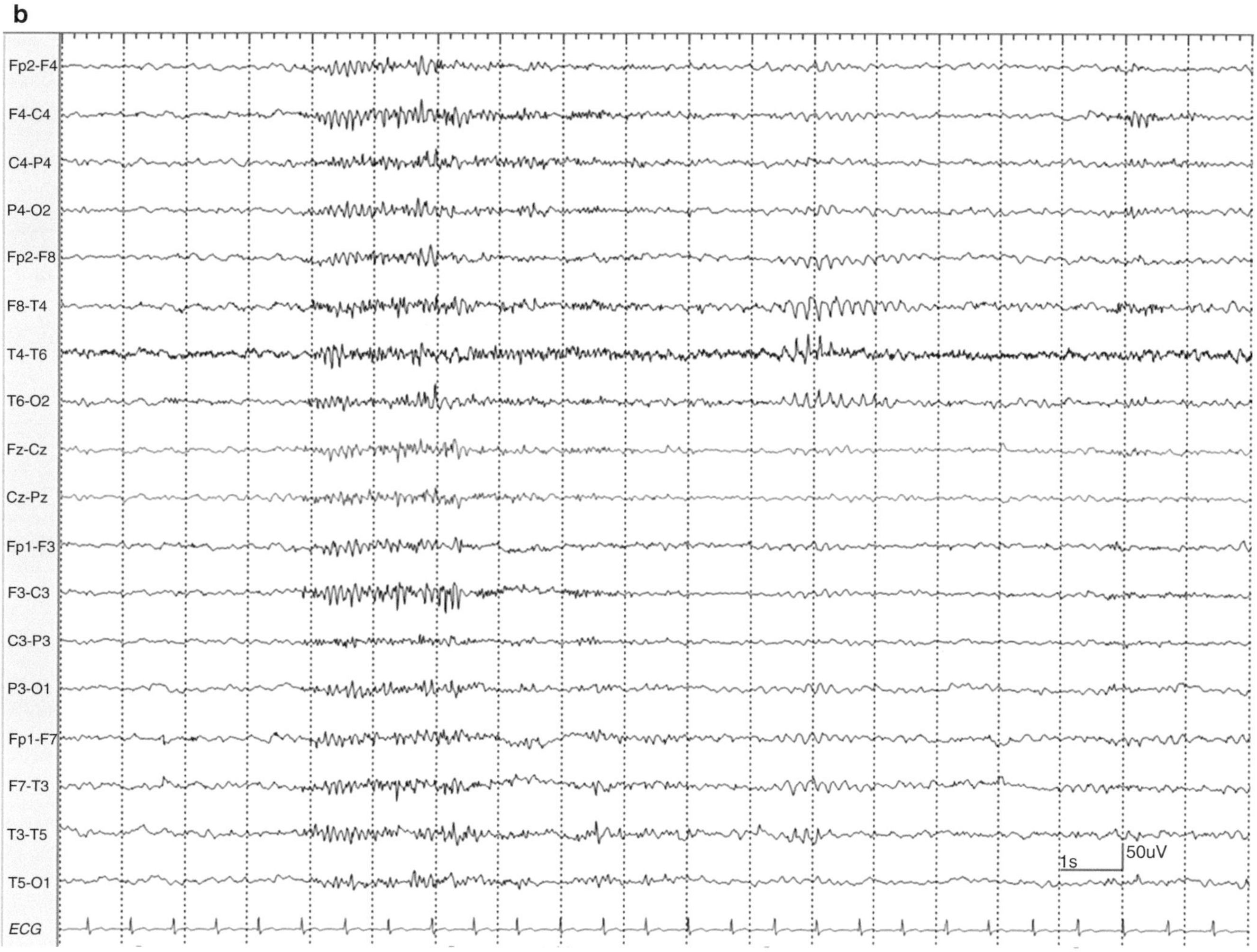

Fig. 12.12 (continued)

ness and mild drowsiness and are most prominent over the anterior or posterior head regions. Phantom spike and wave discharges can appear in both adolescents and adults and usually have a diffuse, bilateral, synchronous distribution. This type of rhythm is called "phantom" due to its short duration and the fleeting quality of the spike, that is, smaller in amplitude and shorter than the slow wave component of the pattern [1].

Sometimes it can be difficult to distinguish the 6-Hz spike and wave discharge from epileptic activities. For this reason, it is important to bear in mind that the benign 6-hz spike and wave bursts tend to disappear during sleep, are not high in amplitude, and have a monomorphic morphology [1] (Clinical Case n°2—Fig. 12.14).

12.2.7 Small Sharp Spikes

Small sharp spikes (SSS) are isolated, fast (less than 50 ms), low-amplitude (less than 50 μV) spikes occurring during drowsiness and light sleep. During the past decades, SSS have also been described as "benign epileptiform transients of sleep" [43] or "benign sporadic sleep spikes." SSS consist of single monophasic or diphasic spikes; when diphasic, they have an abrupt ascending limb and a steep descending limb. They may exhibit a subtle following slow wave. SSS are usually seen in the frontotemporal areas and mainly occur in adults either unilaterally or bilaterally; when bilateral, they can appear independently or (rarely) synchronously [1] (Fig. 12.15).

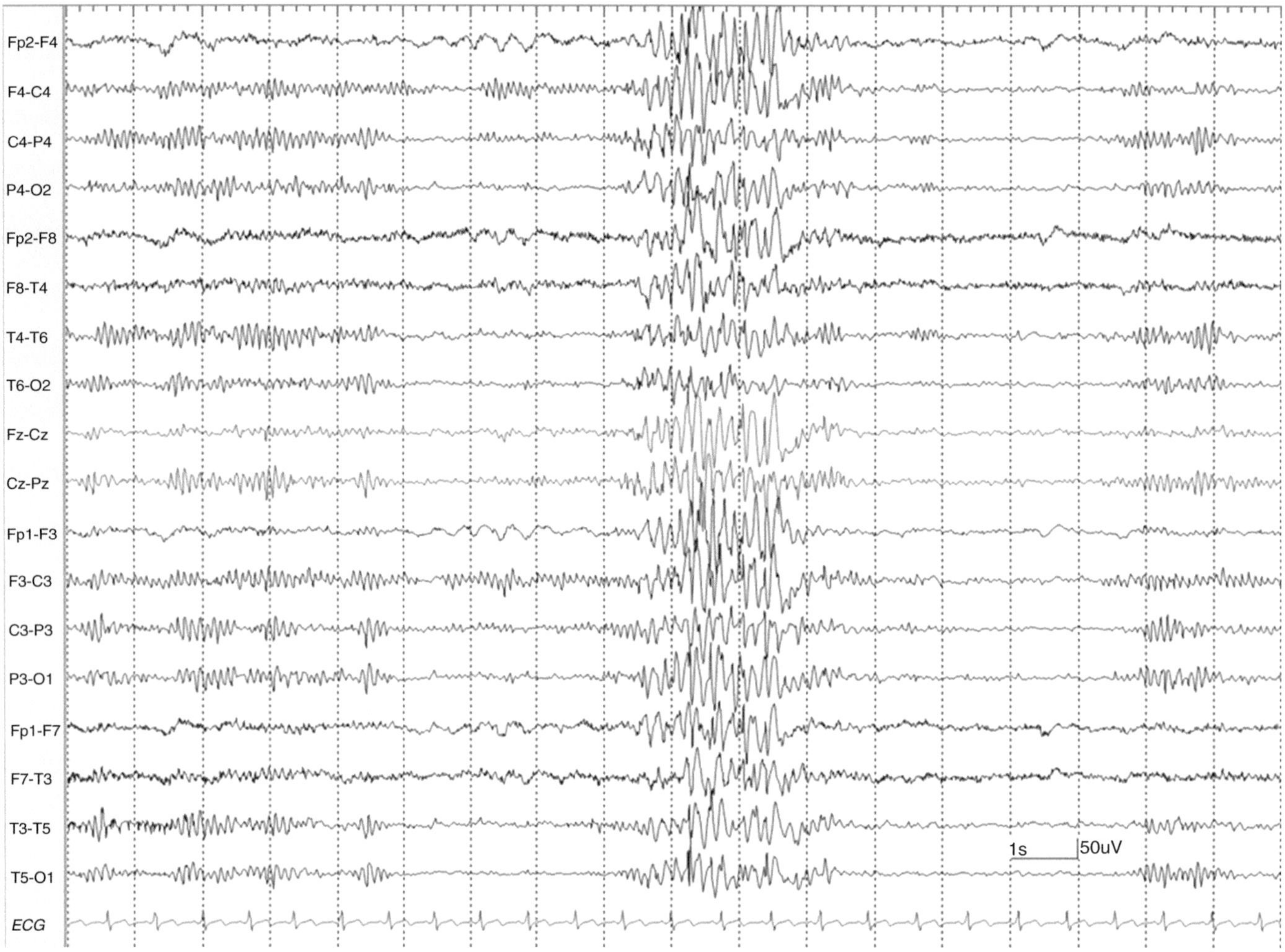

Fig. 12.13 (F, 20 y) 14- and 6-Hz positive bursts are short (lasting 1 or 2 s) trains of rhythmic waves with a faster component of 14-Hz and slower 6-Hz waves. These two components can occur separately or within the same burst, bisynchronously or independently. Usually the bursts can be seen symmetrically over parieto-temporal areas, even though their predominance may shift from side to side. They are arch-shaped with a spiky component, positive on the surface, alternating with a smooth surface-negative rounded waveform

12.3 Conclusion

Distinguishing normal EEG variants that could resemble epileptiform discharges from pathological activities is a challenge for electroencephalographers, especially for the novice EEG reader. It is essential to avoid over reading of non-epileptic sharp patterns because a misdiagnosis of epilepsy may have serious clinical consequences. For example, it may result in an antiepileptic treatment which is not only useless, but also expensive and sometimes harmful.

As we have seen in this chapter, not all sharply contoured EEG transient potentials are associated with clinical seizures. All of these normal variants have basic features that need to be committed to memory with the aim of avoiding mistakes. Some simple tips may serve to distinguish epileptiform activity from a benign EEG variant: an abnormal EEG rhythm is usually bi- or triphasic, asymmetrical, generally followed by a slow wave, and can be clearly distinguished from the background activity by its abrupt change in polarity. On the other hand, an EEG physiological variant is usually monophasic, symmetrical, not followed by a slow wave, and is part of the background rhythm itself [44] (Take-Home Message Box, Fig. 12.16).

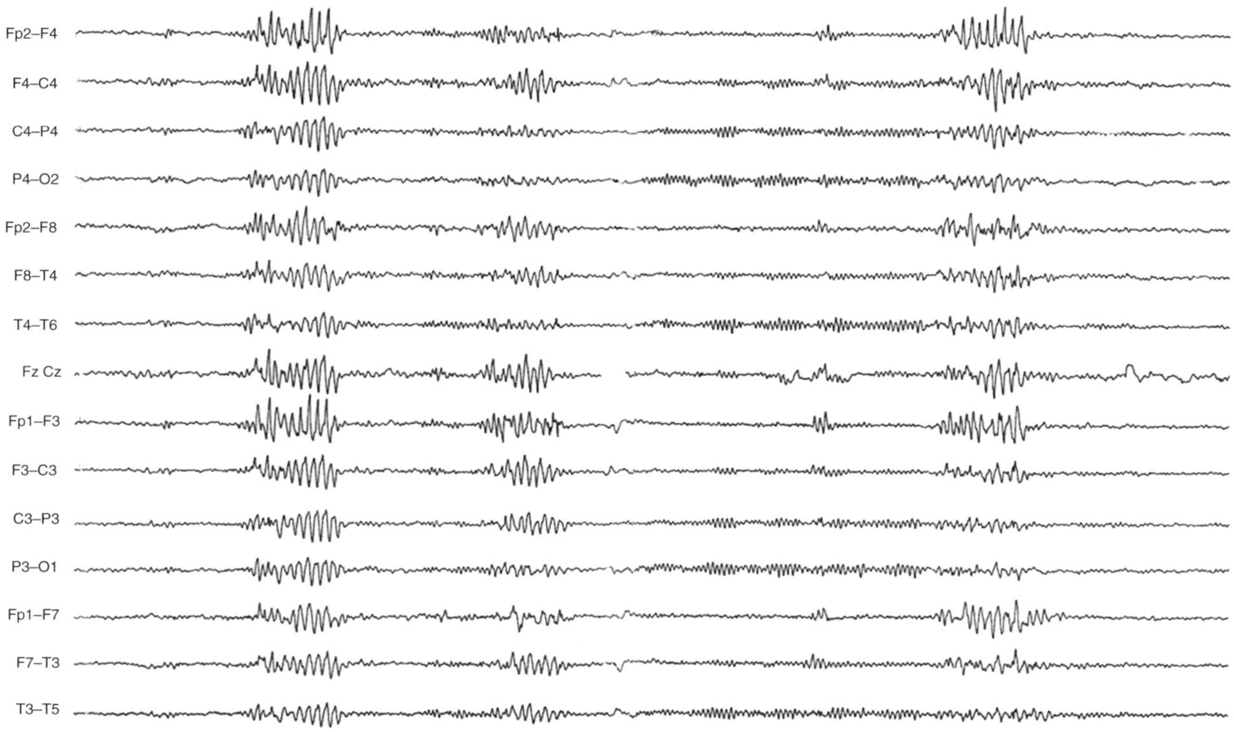

Fig. 12.14 (F, 21 years) While moving from a clinostatic to orthostatic position, an 11-year-old girl had an episode of brief loss of consciousness, with no postictal confusion. Almost 2 months later, while standing up, she suddenly fell down, not losing contact, and rapidly got up. She underwent tests to investigate these episodes, including an EEG, which contained some epileptiform patterns. She was then treated with carbamazepine for several years. During a follow-up EEG (reported here), the trace showed brief, low-voltage, monomorphic spike-wave complexes, with a repetition rate of 6 Hz. They were bilateral and synchronous, most prominent over the anterior or posterior head regions. They occurred during wakefulness and drowsiness and disappeared during sleep. The pattern was recognized as typical phantom spike-and-wave discharges. Her therapy was then stopped, and she did not present with any further episode (the first probably could have been interpreted as syncopal event)

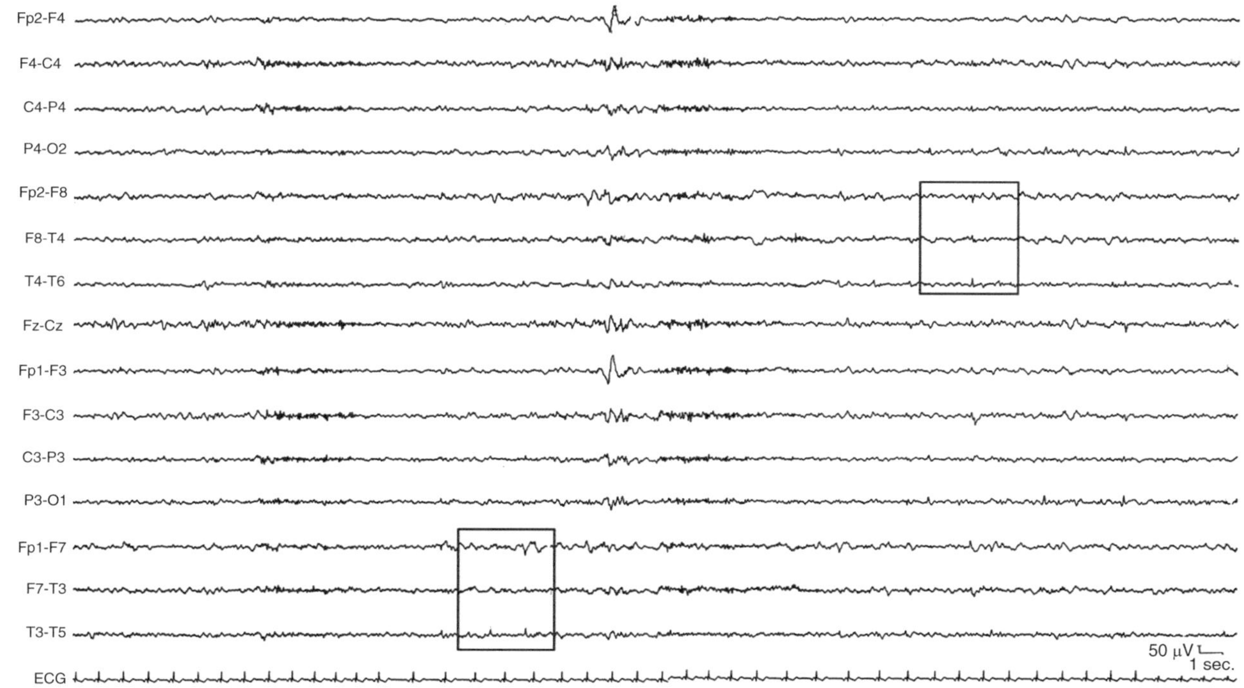

Fig. 12.15 (F, 35 years) Small sharp spikes (SSS) are isolated, fast (less than 50 ms), low-amplitude (less than 50 μV) spikes occurring during drowsiness and light sleep. They may have a subtle following slow wave. SSS are usually seen over the frontotemporal regions, either unilaterally or bilaterally. Figure 12.15 shows SSS coexisting with but independent from some paroxysmal activity

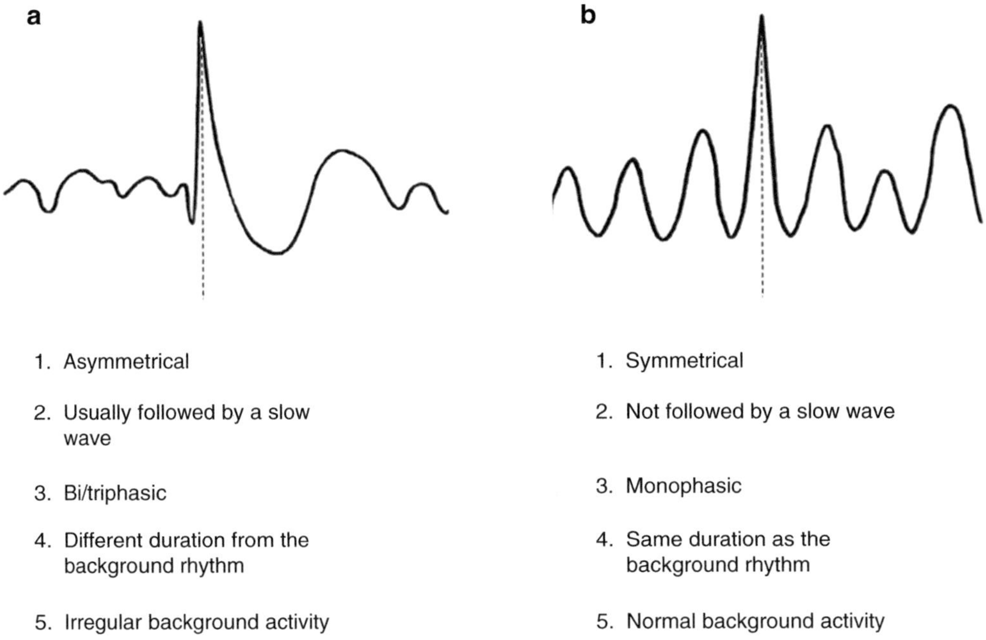

Fig. 12.16 Spike morphology: differential diagnosis between epileptiform transient (**a**) and sharp normal EEG transient (**b**)

Acknowledgments We thank our EEG technicians, especially Lara Alvisi, for the technical assistance in carrying out the EEG studies. We are also grateful to Elena Zoni for the help in editing the figures.

References

1. Westmoreland BF. Benign electroencephalography variants and patterns of uncertain clinical significance. In: Ebersole JS, Pedley TA, editors. Current practice of clinical electroencephalography; 2003. p. 235–245.
2. Gastaut H, Gastaut J-L. Les Activités EEG spontanées. In: Encycl. Méd. Chi., Paris, Neurologie. I7031. 1980;A20:10.
3. Goodwin J. The significance of alpha variants in the EEG, and their relationship to an epileptiform syndrome. Am J Psychiatr. 1947;104:369–79.
4. Pitot M, Gastaut Y. Les rythmes postereurs a 4 cycles/seconde. Rev Neurol. 1956;94:189–91.
5. Gastaut H, Poire R, Regis H. Les activites EEG lentes posterieures. In: Gauthier-Villars, editor. Les activites electriques cerebrales spontanees et evoquees chez l'homme. Paris; 1967. p. 133–234.
6. Doose H, Baier WK. Theta rhythms in the EEG: a genetic trait in childhood epilepsy. Brain and Development. 1988;10(6):347–54.
7. Gastaut H, Dongier M, Jest C. Confrontations entre les donnees de l' EEG et des examens psychologiques: existence d'ondes lentes posterieures. In: Masson et Cie, editor. Conditionnement et Reactivite en EEG. Paris; 1957. p. 286–287.
8. Aird R, Gastaut Y. Occipital and posterior EEGraphic rhythms. Electroencephalogr Clin Neurophysiol. 1959;11:637–56.
9. Gastaut Y. Un signe EEG peu connu: les pointes occipitales survenant pendant l'overture des yeux. Rev Neurol. 1951;84:640–3.
10. Evans C. Spontaneous excitation of the visual cortex: lambda waves. Electroencephalogr Clin Neurophysiol. 1953;5:69–74.
11. Gastaut H, Terzian H, Gastaut Y. Le Rythme rolandique en arceau. Mars Med. 1952;89:296–310.
12. Kellaway P. Orderly approach to visual analysis: elements of the normal EEG and their characteristics in children and adults. In: Ebersole JS, Pedley TA, editors. Current practice of clinical electroencephalography, 3rd ed. 2003. p. 100–159.
13. Schoppenhorst M, Brauer F, Freund G, et al. The significance of coherence estimates in determining central alpha and mu activities. Electroencephalogr Clin Neurophysiol. 1980;48(1):25–33.
14. Fischgold H, Pertuiset B, Arfel G. Quelques particularités électroencéphalographiques au niveau des brèches et des volets neurochirurgicaux. Rev Neurol. 1952;86:126–32.
15. Farnarier G, Mattei JP, Naquet R. The mu rhythm of the vertex and its reactivity: an infrequent observation. Electroencephalogr Clin Neurophysiol. 1980;10(4):357–65.
16. Cobb WA, Guiloff RJ, Cast J. Breach rhythm: the EEG related to skull defects. Electroencephalogr Clin Neurophysiol. 1979;47:251–71.
17. Van Doorn J, Cherian PJ. Breach rhythm related to a solitary skull lesion caused by multiple myeloma. BMJ Case Rep. 2009;2009:bcr2007129528.
18. Brigo F, Cicero R, Fiaschi A, et al. The breach rhythm. Clin Neurophysiol. 2011;122(11):2116–20.
19. Benbadis SR, Tatum WO. Overinterpretation of EEGs and misdiagnosis of epilepsy. J Clin Neurophysiol. 2003;20(1):42–4.
20. Santoshkumar B, Chong JJ, Blume WT, et al. Prevalence of benign epileptiform variants. Clin Neurophysiol. 2009;120(5):856–61.
21. Ciganek L, Zohuar A, Grunert V. Some peculiarities of sleep activity in the EEG in children. Cesk Neurol. 1961;24:166–71.
22. Mokran V, Ciganek L, Kabatnik Z. Electroencephalographic theta discharges in the midline. Eur Neurol. 1971;5:288–93.
23. Inanaga K. Frontal midline theta rhythm and mental activity. Psychiatry Clin Neurosci. 1998;52(6):555–66.
24. Mushtaq R, Van Cott AC. Benign EEG variants. Am J Electroneurodiagnostic Technol. 2005;45(2):88–101.
25. Lin YY, Wu ZA, Hsieh JC, et al. Magnetoencephalographic study of rhythmic mid-temporal discharges in non-epileptic and epileptic patients. Seizure. 2003;12(4):220–5.
26. Gibbs FA, Rich CL, Gibbs EL. Psychomotor variant type of seizure discharge. Neurology. 1963;13(12):991–8.
27. Klass DW, Westmoreland BF. Non epileptogenic epileptiform electroencephalographic activity. Ann Neurol. 1985;18(6):627–35.

28. Hughes JR. Two forms of the 6/sec spike and wave complex. Electroencephalogr Clin Neurophysiol. 1980;48:535–50.
29. Chatrian GE. Etude ectroencephalographique et electrocorticographique du rythme theta local des epilepsies temporalis. Rev Neurol. 1953;88:384–6.
30. Gastaut H, Santanelli P, Salinas MJ. Une activite EEG intercritique specifique d'une variete particuliere d'epilepsie temporale. Le rythme theta temporal epileptique. Rev EEG Neurophysiol. 1985;15:113–20.
31. Hirose G. Ring (20) Chromosome epileptic syndrome. Brain Nerve. 2015;67(5):585–97.
32. Elens I, Lagae L. Ring Chromosome 20 syndrome: electroclinical description of six patients and review of the literature. Epilepsy Behav. 2012;23(4):409–14.
33. Canevini MP. Chromosome 20 ring: a chromosomal disorder associated with a particular electroclinical pattern. Epilepsia. 1998;39(9):942–51.
34. Dash GK, Radhakrishnan A. What does "subclinical rhythmic electrographic discharge of adults" in EEG signify? J Clin Neurophysiol. 2013;30(3):255–60.
35. Miller CR, Westmoreland BF, Klass DW. Subclinical Rhythmic EEG Discharge of Adults (SREDA): further observations. Am J EEG Technol. 1985;25(4):217–24.
36. Westmoreland BF, Klass DW. Unusual variants of subclinical rhythmic electrographic discharge of adults (SREDA). Electroencephalogr Clin Neurophysiol. 1997;102(1):1–4.
37. Fleming WE, Avidan A, Malow BA. Subclinical rhythmic electrographic discharge of adults (SREDA) in REM sleep. Sleep Med. 2004;5(1):77–81.
38. O'Brien TJ, Sharbrough FW, Westmoreland BF, et al. Subclinical rhythmic electrographic discharges of adults (SREDA) revisited: a study using digital EEG analysis. J Clin Neurophysiol. 1998;15(6):493–501.
39. Krauss GL, Abdallah A, Lesser R, et al. Clinical and EEG features of patients with EEG wicket rhythms misdiagnosed with epilepsy. Neurology. 2005;64(11):1879–83.
40. Gélisse P, Kuate C, Coubes P, et al. Wicket spikes during rapid eye movement sleep. J Clin Neurophysiol. 2003;20:345–50.
41. Yamada T, Tucker RP, Kooi KA. Fourteen and six c/sec positive bursts in comatose patients. Electroencephalogr Clin Neurophysiol. 1976;40(6):645–53.
42. Yamada T, Young S, Kimura J. Significance of positive spike burst in Reye syndrome. Arch Neurol. 1977;34(6):376–80.
43. White JC, Langston JW, Pedley TA. Benign epileptiform transients of sleep. Clarification of the small sharp spike controversy. Neurology. 1977;27(11):1061–8.
44. Gloor P. The EEG and differential diagnosis of epilepsy. In: Van Duijn H, Donker DN, Van Huffelen AC, editors. Current concepts in clinical neurophysiology, vol. 1977. The Hague: Trio; 1977. p. 9–21.
45. Sindrup E, Thygesen N, Kristen O, et al. Zygomatic electrodes: their use and value in complex partial epilepsy. In: Dam M, Gram L, Penry JK, editors. Advances in epileptology. The XIIyh epilepsy international symposium, New York; 1981. p. 313–318.

13 Pathological EEG Patterns

Oriano Mecarelli

13.1 Changes in Background Rhythms

Regarding the EEG background abnormalities, it is overall necessary to consider the amplitude reduction or the poor synchronization of the physiological rhythms, the unilateral or bilateral slowings and the reduced or absent reactivity to eye opening or alerting.

Many healthy subjects have constitutionally low-amplitude EEG tracings, while others show a poorly appreciable posterior alpha rhythm (low-amplitude or desynchronized tracings), in relation to anxiety or to the non-relaxing registration environment [1]. These patterns are not to be considered as abnormal, unless they are observed monolaterally. The amplitude of the posterior alpha rhythm may be asymmetrical in the two hemispheres, with a lower voltage in the dominant hemisphere [2, 3]. However, this difference usually does not exceed 20%. An asymmetry of the posterior alpha rhythm is considered to be abnormal when its difference is greater than 50% - or more - when compared to contralateral side, and when the abnormality is localized in the side where the amplitude is lower. Unilateral attenuation or absence of the alpha rhythm usually occurs in lesions of the occipital cortex and of the anterior ventral thalamus; posterior subcortical lesions may also induce the absence of alpha reactivity to eye opening (Bancaud phenomenon). In Chap. 9 it has been already explained which EEG features should not be interpreted as pathological: the slow or fast variants of the normal background rhythm, the changes correlated with age or with the variations in the level of awareness, etc.

O. Mecarelli (✉)
Department of Human Neurosciences, Sapienza University of Rome, Rome, Italy
e-mail: oriano.mecarelli@uniroma1.it

13.2 Slowings

EEG slowings include all types of activity with a frequency less than the alpha band (i.e. theta and delta bands). Slow-wave abnormalities can be defined in multiple features, considering the *localization* (focal or regional vs. diffuse), the *morphology* (mono- or polymorphic), the *rhythmicity* (irregular vs. rhythmic), the *amplitude* (low or high voltage), and the *continuity* (intermittent/subcontinuous vs. continuous).

Diffuse, non-specific EEG slowings can be observed in many pathological conditions that include consciousness disorders of various etiology, cerebral inflammations, neurodegenerative processes, post-ictal status, metabolic and toxic disorders, etc. In these cases, EEG recording is important because, on the basis of the extent of the slowings and their reactivity to external stimuli, deductions can be made on the severity of the underlying pathology and also to express prognostic indications. Hypersynchronous diffuse slowings may be induced by drowsiness or be the result of hyperventilation (see Chap. 13) and not necessarily, therefore, represent a pathological pattern.

EEG slowings can also be *focal*, when localized in a restricted area of the scalp, and these are highly correlated with localized structural brain lesions, such as tumors, intraparenchymal hematoma, stroke, encephalitic focus, etc. In these cases, the characteristics of the slowing sequences (delta or theta frequency, duration, morphology, amplitude) and their correlation with the clinical symptomatology are very important for a correct interpretation. EEG slow changes induced by the abovementioned structural brain lesions probably reflect alterations in the cortical function caused by direct or indirect local neuronal network dysfunction. Though the electrographic pattern is important for prognostic purposes, EEG is generally not useful in distinguishing among different types of brain lesions. The EEG slowings that tend to repeat periodically or rhythmically will be described later in this chapter. Figure 13.1 shows examples of diffuse and focal slowings.

O. Mecarelli (ed.), *Clinical Electroencephalography*, https://doi.org/10.1007/978-3-030-04573-9_13

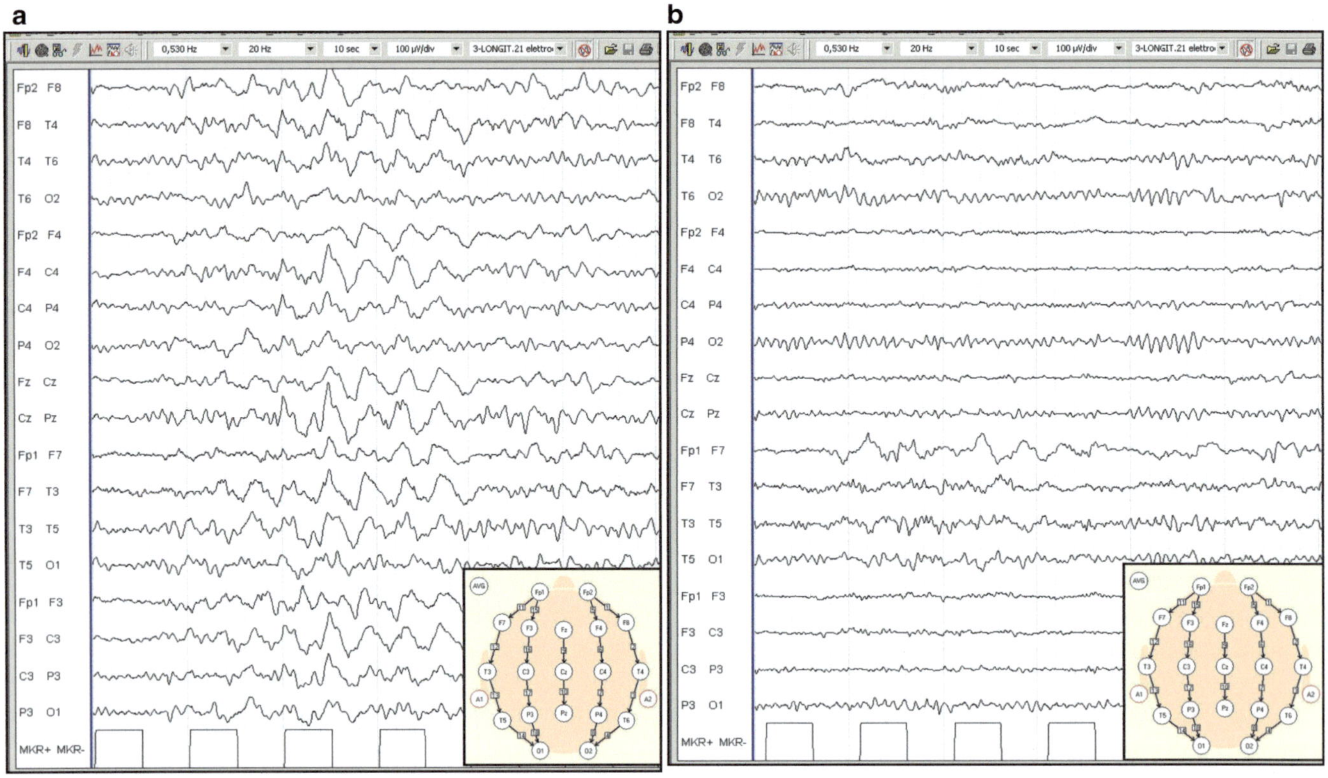

Fig. 13.1 (**a**) Burst of diffuse monomorphic delta waves. (**b**) Sequence of focal polymorphic delta waves in the left fronto-temporal region

13.3 Epileptiform Abnormalities

First of all, it must be reminded that there is still a terminology confusion regarding the definition of the epileptic abnormalities among electroencephalographers. Not all those who interpret and report an EEG use the same terms or give them similar meaning. Often, we do not give identical meanings to terms like "discharge", "interictal", "ictal", and "subclinical". For example, some electroencephalographers still use the term "irritative" (a term to be nowadays discouraged) to indicate an EEG transient that may be correlated with epilepsy. The various editions of IFCN glossary often derives from compromise choices between the various positions, and it is more universally accepted; it focuses the attention on the morphology of EEG graphoelements, without interpreting them in relation to the clinical aspects. Therefore, the principal characteristics of epileptiform EEG abnormalities, as described in the revised glossary of IFNC, will be described here [4].

The term epileptiform pattern (synonyms: interictal epileptiform discharge, epileptiform activity) refers to interictal transients distinguishable from the background activity, with—but not exclusively—spiky morphology. Even the term paroxysm indicates a graphoelement phenomenon with a sudden onset and abrupt termination, clearly distinguished from the background activity. During routine EEG recordings in the laboratory, the majority of epileptic patients do not experience a seizure. Consequently, the interictal epileptiform discharges are the main tool in defining a specific diagnosis. The ictal activity is then referred to the seizure EEG patterns, consisting of: a) repetitive epileptiform EEG discharges, with relatively abrupt onset and termination, lasting several seconds; b) electrodecremental period (usually with superimposed fast activity); c) fast paroxysmal activity. The epileptiform EEG discharges have a characteristic frequency with spatiotemporal evolution (i.e., gradual change in frequency, amplitude, morphology and location). When the seizure EEG pattern is related to concurrent clinical symptoms, the term electroclinical seizure can be used; when the seizure EEG pattern is, instead, without clinical correlates, it should be referred to as electrographic or subclinical seizures. However, always consider that the demonstration of a clinical correlation with the seizure EEG pattern may not be always possible. The sporadic epileptiform discharges (nonrhythmic and nonperiodic) can be quantified and categorized as follows: "abundant", ≥1/10 s; "frequent", <1/10 s ≥1/min; "occasional", <1/min ≥1/h; "rare", <1/h [5, 6].

The epileptiform graphoelements, according to revised glossary of IFCN 2017 [4], are described as follows:

- Spike: a transient with pointed peak, clearly distinguished from the background activity, and with a duration from 20 to less than 70 ms (1/50–1/14 s). Amplitude is variable, but typically >50 μV. As regards to morphology, the spike can be mono- or multiphasic, with a dominant negative component.
- Polyspike complex: a sequence of two or more spikes.
- Sharp wave: an epileptiform transient clearly distinguished from the background activity, with pointed peak and a duration of 70–200 ms (1/14–1/5 s). Usually, the sharp wave (di-triphasic) has a variable amplitude (100–200 μV): the main component is negative and the ascending phase is steeper when compared to the descending phase. The term "sharp wave" does not apply to vertex sharp transients of sleep, lambda waves, positive occipital sharp transients of sleep and sharp transients poorly distinguished from the background activity.
- Spike-and-Slow-Wave complex (SSWc): single or multiple epileptiform patterns consisting of a spike and an associated following slow wave, clearly distinguished from the background activity. Based on the frequency, it is necessary to distinguish the classical (typical) SSWc at 3 Hz from the slow (atypical) SSWc at 1.5–2.5 Hz.
- Polyspikes-and-slow-wave complex: an epileptiform pattern consisting of two or more spikes associated with one or more slow waves.
- Sharp-and-slow-wave complex: an epileptiform pattern (single or multiple) consisting of a sharp wave and an associated following slow wave, clearly distinguished from the background activity.

The characteristics of various types of epileptiform abnormalities are showed in Figs. 13.2, 13.3, 13.4, 13.5 and 13.6.

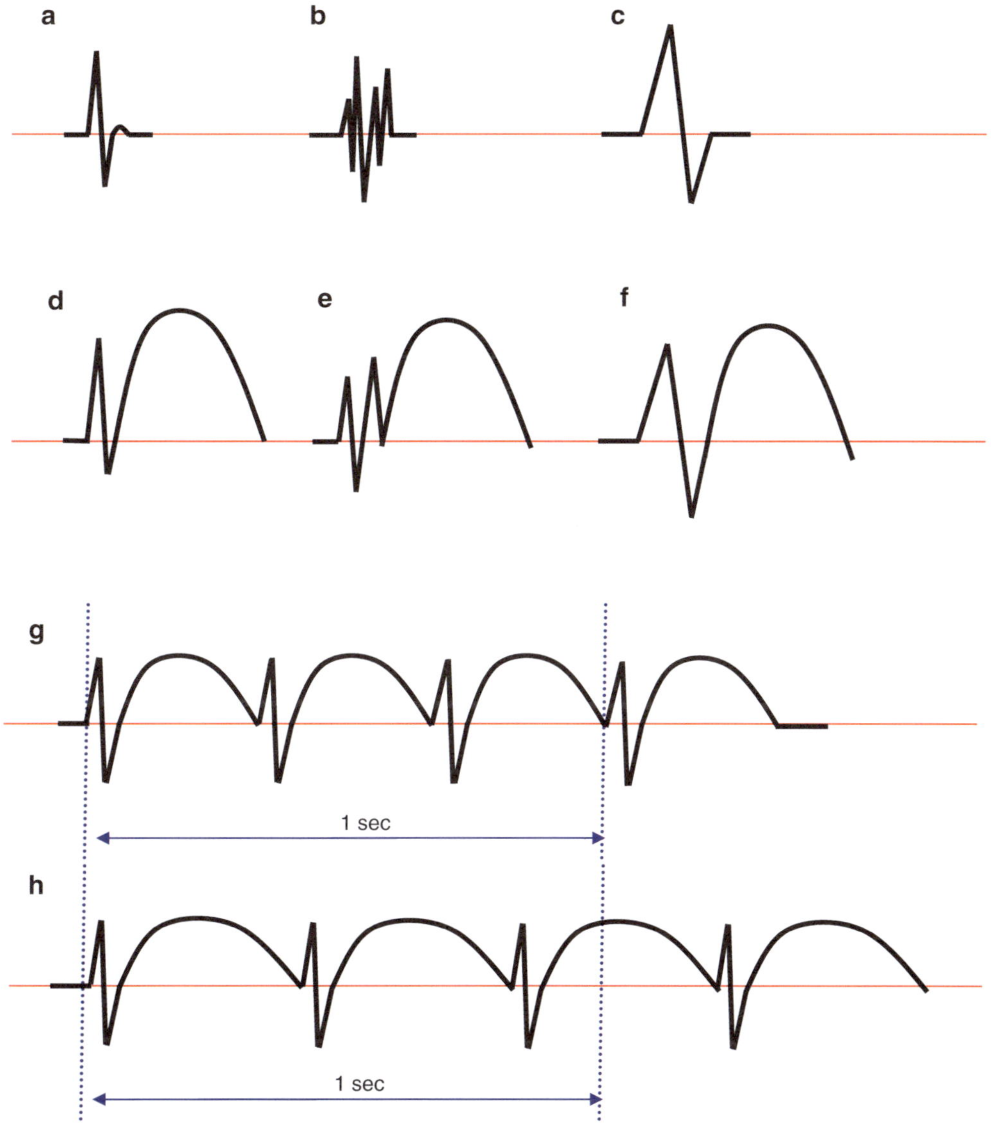

Fig. 13.2 Graphic representation of epileptiform abnormalities: (**a**) spike, (**b**) polyspikes (**c**) sharp wave, (**d**) Spike-and-Slow-Wave complex (SSWc), (**e**) polyspikes-and-slow-wave complex, (**f**) sharp-and-slow-wave complex, (**g**) typical SSWc (3 Hz), (**h**) atypical slow SSWc (<3 Hz)

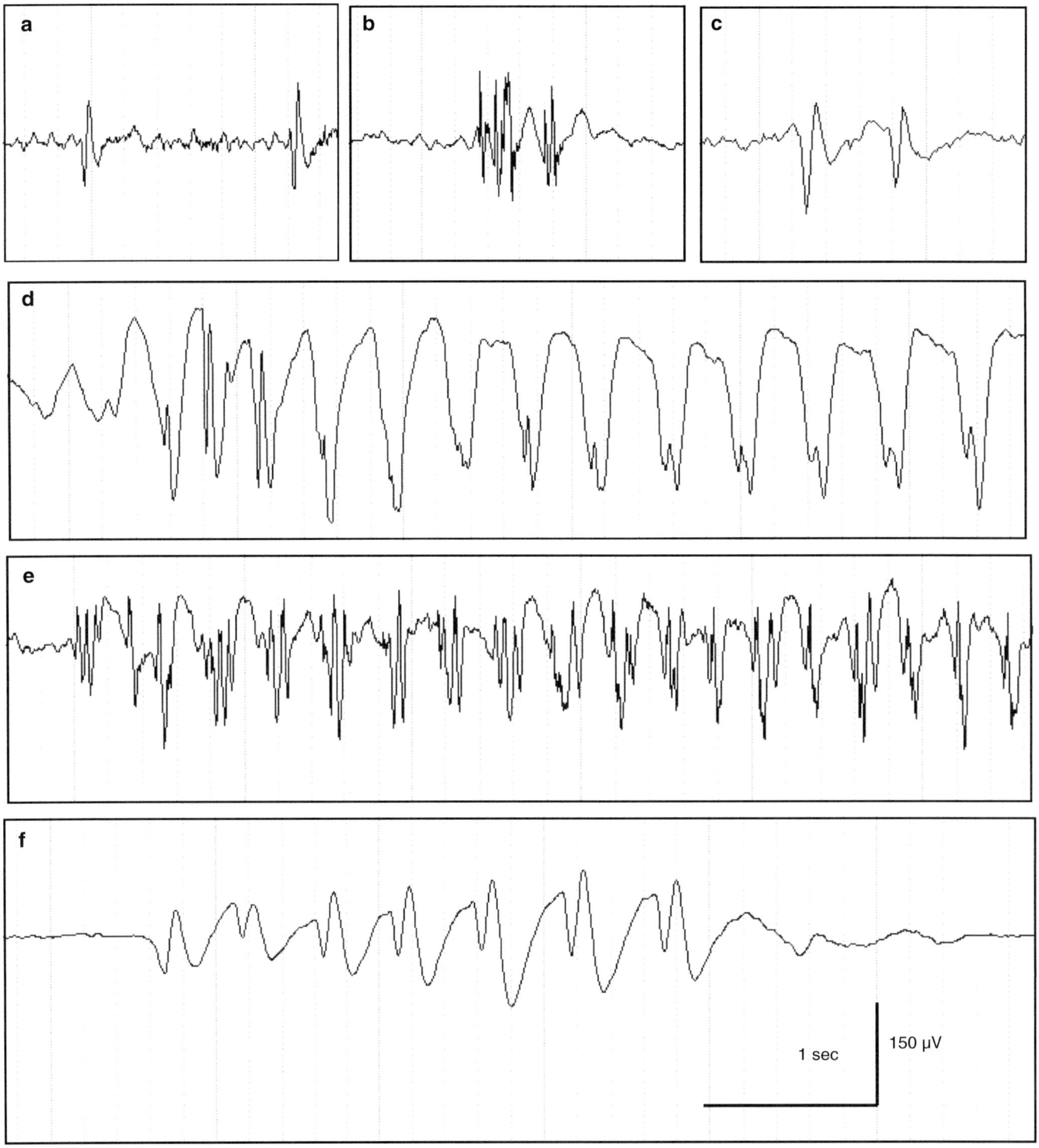

Fig. 13.3 Raw EEG examples of epileptiform abnormalities (**a**, **b**, **c**, **d**, **e**, **f** in Fig. 13.2)

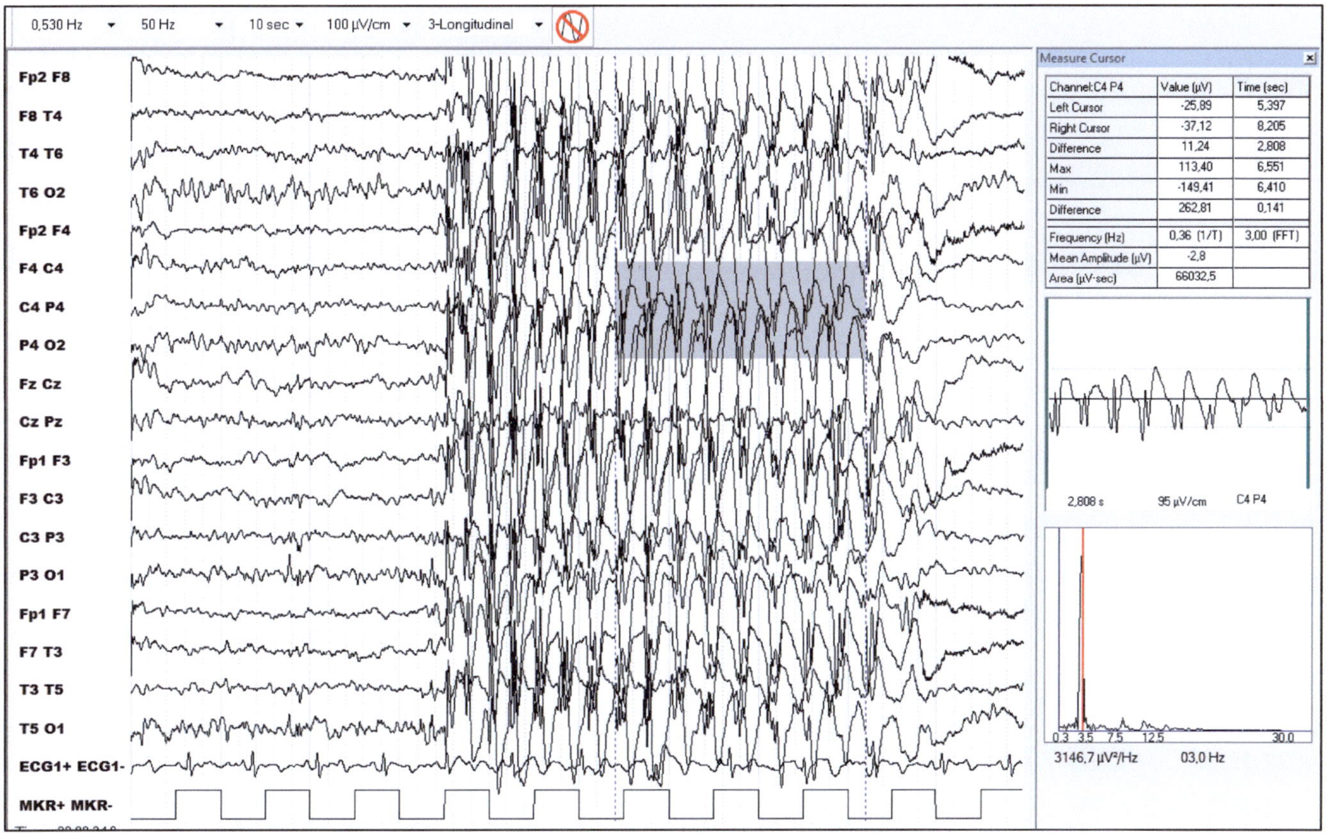

Fig. 13.4 Typical discharge of Spike-and-Slow-Wave complexes (SSWc) at 3 Hz in a child with absence seizures

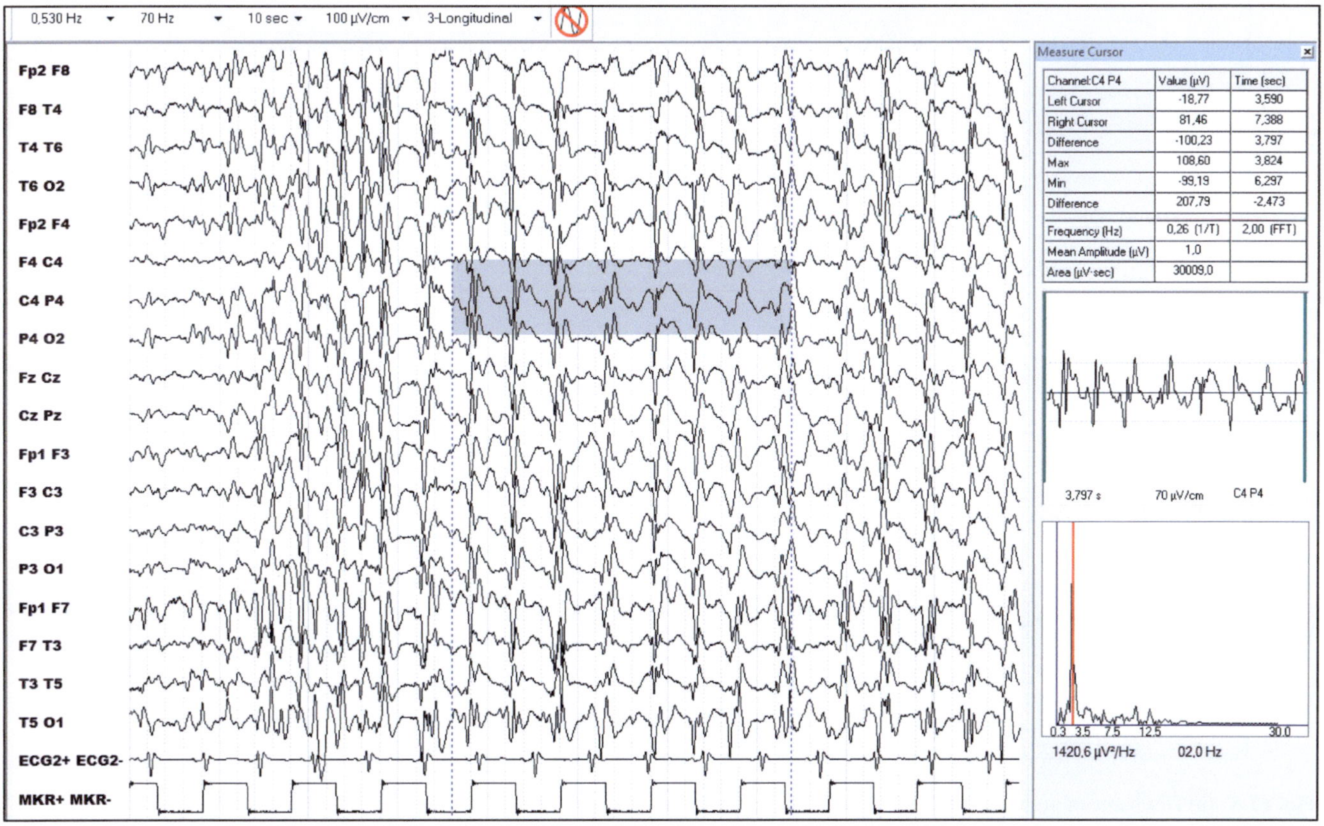

Fig. 13.5 Atypical discharge of spike-and-slow-wave complexes, at 2 Hz, in a patient with Lennox-Gastaut syndrome

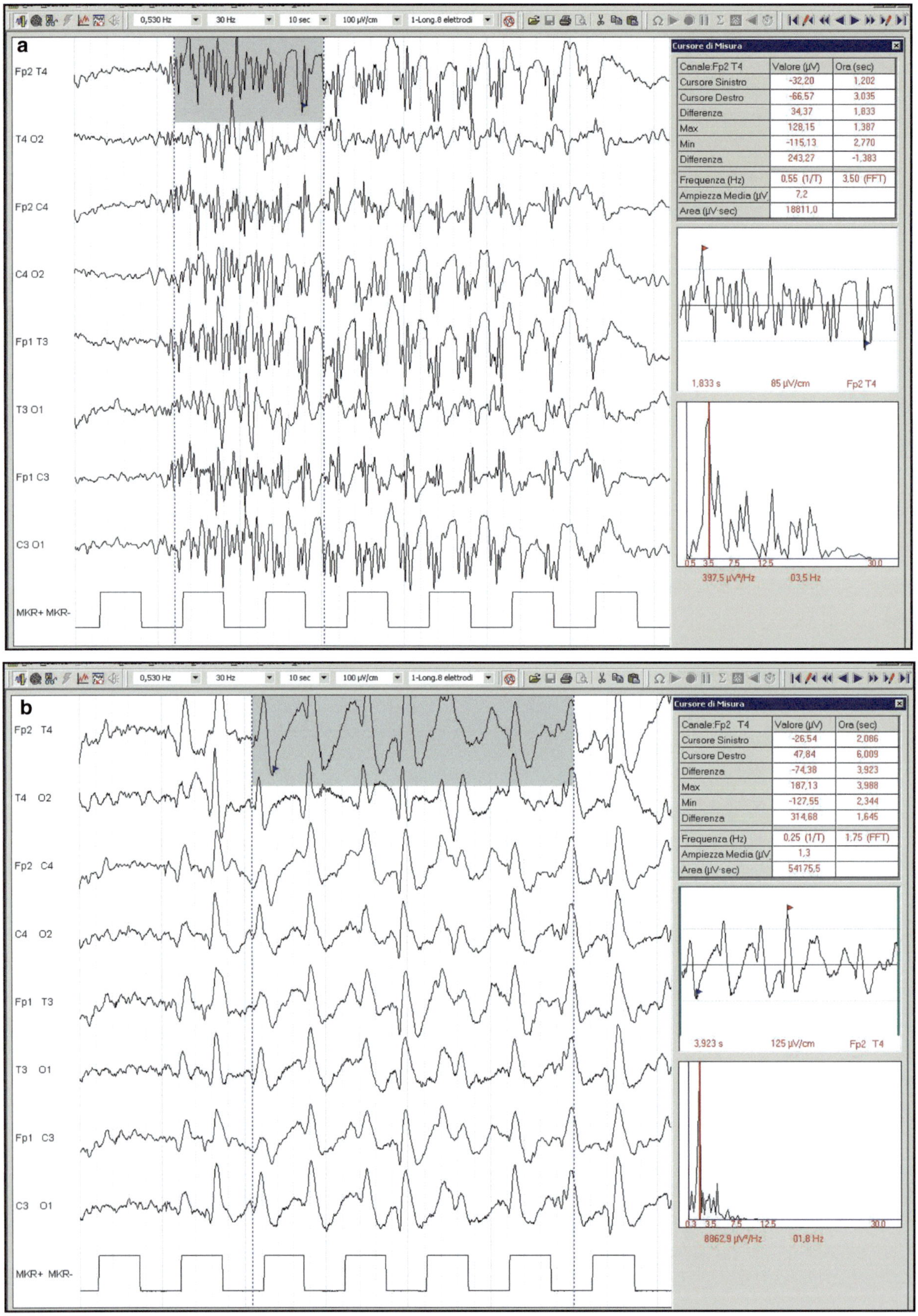

Fig. 13.6 (**a**) Discharge of polyspike-and-slow-wave complexes and (**b**) discharge of sharp-wave and slow-wave complexes

13.4 Periodic and Rhythmic Patterns

13.4.1 Periodic Patterns

According to the revised glossary of IFCN [4], the term *periodic* is applied to EEG waves or complexes occurring in a sequence or intermittently, at an approximately regular rate or intervals (generally of one to several seconds). When the waves or complexes occur at random or non-regular intervals, the *quasiperiodic* (preferable than *pseudoperiodic*) term is used, defined as having a period varying by 25–50% from one cycle to the next. The distinction between periodic and quasiperiodic is to be applied only if determined by quantitative computer analysis.

For *Periodic Discharges* (PDs), we mean the repetition of a waveform with a relatively uniform morphology and duration, with a quantifiable inter-discharge interval between consecutive waveforms and a recurrence of waveform at nearly regular intervals.

According to the old terminology [5, 7, 8] periodic EEG patterns have been classified in diffuse and lateralized. The diffuse periodic discharges included the Periodic Short-Interval Diffuse Discharges (PSIDDs) and the Periodic Long-Interval Diffuse Discharges (PLIDDs).

PSIDDs are represented by diffuse graphoelements (spikes, polyspikes, sharp waves, etc.) occurring periodically at inter-discharge interval of 0.5–4 s, and they are more frequently associated to anoxic encephalopathy. A subset of PSIDDs may be considered the Triphasic Waves (TWs). TWs are actually defined as high-amplitude (>70 μV) positive sharp transients, preceded and followed by relatively low-amplitude negative waves. TWs are usually bilateral (with an anteroposterior or a posteroanterior lag) and they have a repetition rate of about 1–>2 Hz. TWs occur in sequences and can be induced or regressed by alerting or noxious stimuli. They are non-specific, since they can be found in various metabolic and degenerative encephalopathies, usually in comatose patients. TWs may decrease with sleep and after intravenous benzodiazepines [4]. Recently, Alkhachroum et al. [9] have prospectively studied 92 patients with Generalized Periodic Discharges (GPDs) to assess the reliability of electroencephalographers to differentiate triphasic from non-triphasic periodic discharges, as well as to report seizure association with the two EEG patterns. The results of the study indicate a strong inter-rater agreement and that GPDs of triphasic morphology confer less risk of seizures when compared with GPDs without triphasic morphology. PLIDDs refer to repetitive polymorphic waveforms separated by intervals of 4–20 s of duration. PLIDDs are the hallmark finding of Subacute Sclerosing PanencEphalitis (SSPE).

Always according to the old nomenclature, the best-known periodic lateralized pattern is represented by the Periodic Lateralized Epileptiform Discharges (PLEDs). Typically, PLEDs waveform contains sharp or spike-like features bi-triphasic; the amplitude is variable (100–300 μV) and the duration is between 100 and 400 ms. When PLEDs are present, they are represented almost thoroughly in the EEG tracing, approximately every 1–4 s. The word *lateralized* is used in place of the word *focal*, in consideration that the PLEDs spread across a whole hemisphere. Furthermore, Reiher et al. [10] proposed a subclassification of PLEDs in two major groups: *PLEDs-proper*, defined as simply configured and uniform discharges; *PLEDs-plus*, with accompanying low-amplitude rhythmic fast activity between the periodisms. The few literature data show that clinical seizures are more frequent in patients with PLEDs-plus, but this finding still remains controversial.

PLEDs that occur in both hemispheres simultaneously—but asynchronous or independent—are termed (according to old terminology) Bilateral Independent Periodic Lateralized Epileptiform Discharges (BIPLEDs). PLEDs and BIPLEDs are associated with multiple etiologies (stroke, infections, tumor, etc.) and they are, in general, considered an interictal pattern, usually resistant to the treatment with antiepileptic drugs [11]. However, there are also significant evidences that PLEDs are sometimes ictal or simply just postictal. The wide variety of etiologies that determine the PLEDs and their electrographic heterogeneity suggests considering these findings as a continuum between interictal and ictal phases [8, 12]. Electrographic features of periodic lateralized discharges may help to determine the seizure risk in patients with acute structural lesions. PLEDs with sharply contoured morphology and/or with overlying a fast activity are related with a higher risk of seizures during continuous EEG monitoring, whereas a blunt delta morphology is at the lowest seizures risk [13].

In 2013, the American Clinical Neurophysiology Society (ACNS) published a new standardized terminology of periodic and rhythmic EEG patterns, to be used in the critically ill patients and continuous EEG monitoring. The main purpose is to avoid terms with clinical connotations and to completely define the terms to maximize inter-rater reliability. In the new definition of the periodic patterns, the term "epileptiform" has then been avoided, as it is an interpretative term, since periodic patterns may be - or may be not - associated with clinical seizures. According to this new nomenclature [6], Periodic Discharges (PDs) are considered as Generalized (GPDs), Lateralized (LPDs), Bilateral Independent (BIPDs), or Multifocal (MfPDs).

The GPDs refer to any bilateral bisynchronous and symmetric pattern. GPDs may be predominant in frontal, occipital or midline regions. The pattern predominance is defined where the amplitude of the pattern is at least 50% greater than that in the other derivations. The LPDs include focal, regional and hemispheric patterns; BIPDs refer to the presence of two independent/asynchronous lateralized patterns, one in each hemisphere; MfPDs refer to the presence of at least three independent lateralized patterns with at least one in each hemisphere. For the description of LPDs, it is important to specify: - if the patterns are purely unilateral or bilateral and synchronous, but clearly more prominent on one side (unilateral vs. bilateral asymmetric); - the lobe or lobes mostly involved. For BIPDs and MfPDs, it is necessary to specify: - symmetric vs. asymmetric (asymmetric when the pattern is clearly more prominent on one side); - lobes mostly involved in both hemispheres.

Examples of periodic generalized and focal patterns are shown in Figs. 13.7 and 13.8.

13.4.2 Rhythmic Patterns

The term *rhythmic* is applied to regular waves occurring at a constant period and of relatively uniform morphology (old term discouraged: monomorphic).

13.4.2.1 Rhythmic Delta Activity

Rhythmic Delta Activity (RDA) is represented by a repetition of rhythmic slow signals (≤4 Hz) without interval between the consecutive waves. When the RDA occurs in bursts (usually lasting no longer than a few seconds) and it is interrupted by an interval, it is defined as Intermittent Rhythmic Delta Activity (IRDA). IRDA are classified in FIRDA, OIRDA, or TIRDA.

Frontal Intermittent Rhythmic Delta Activity (FIRDA) is characterized by bursts of fairly regular and sinusoidal waves at 1.5–2.5 Hz, synchronously in the frontal areas of the two hemispheres, occasionally unilateral. This rhythmic activity is associated with non-specific encephalopathies and, in older

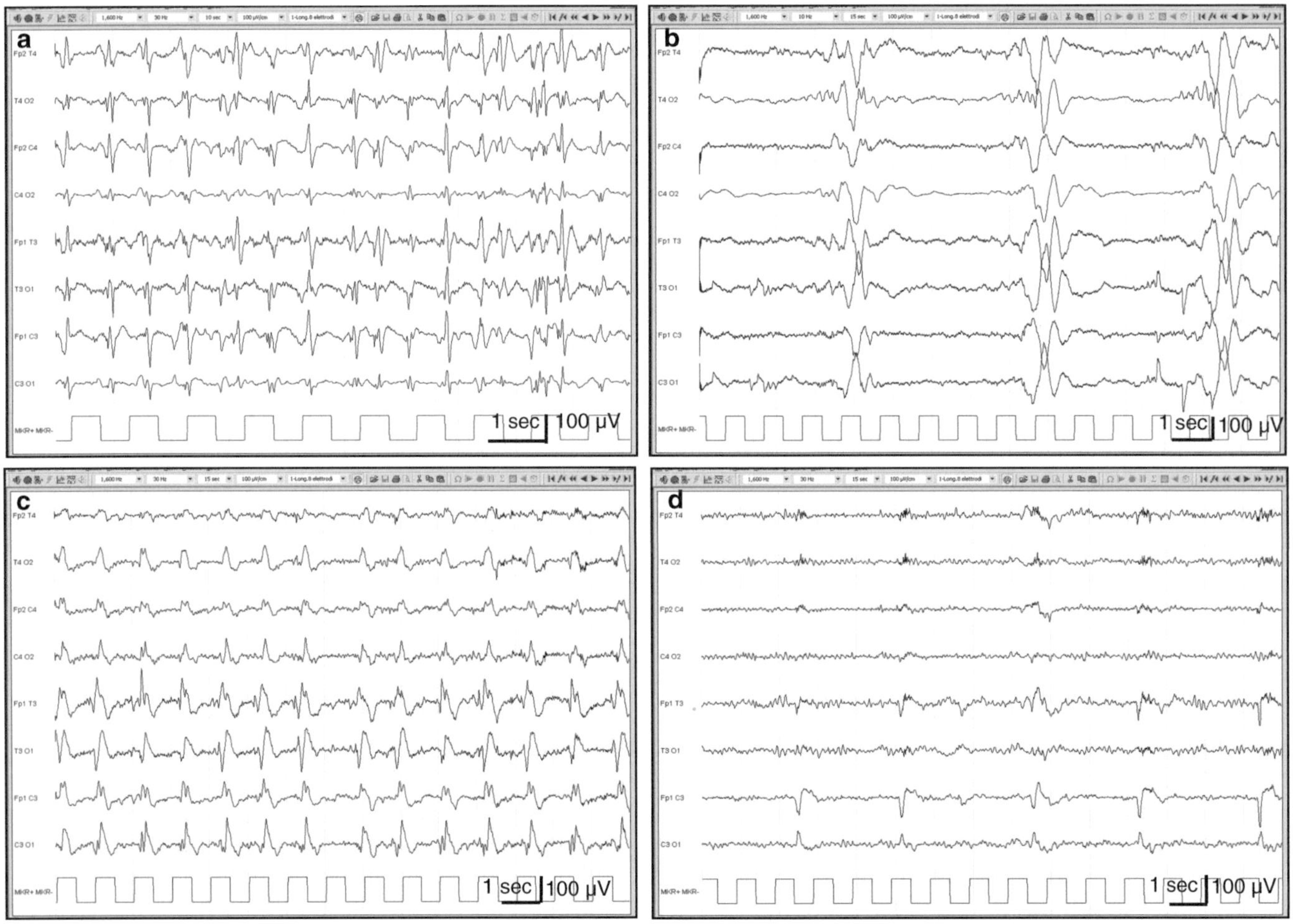

Fig. 13.7 (**a**) Generalized Periodic Discharges (GPDs) with triphasic morphology (diffuse triphasic waves (TWs)) in a patient with hepatic encephalopathy; (**b**) Periodic Long-Interval Diffuse Discharges (PLIDDs) in a patient with subacute sclerosing panencephalitis; (**c**) Lateralized Periodic Discharges (LPDs) in left hemisphere, with tendency of contralateral diffusion, in a patient with massive left hemorrhage; (**d**) LPDs localized in left centro-temporal region in a patient with a homolateral ischemic stroke

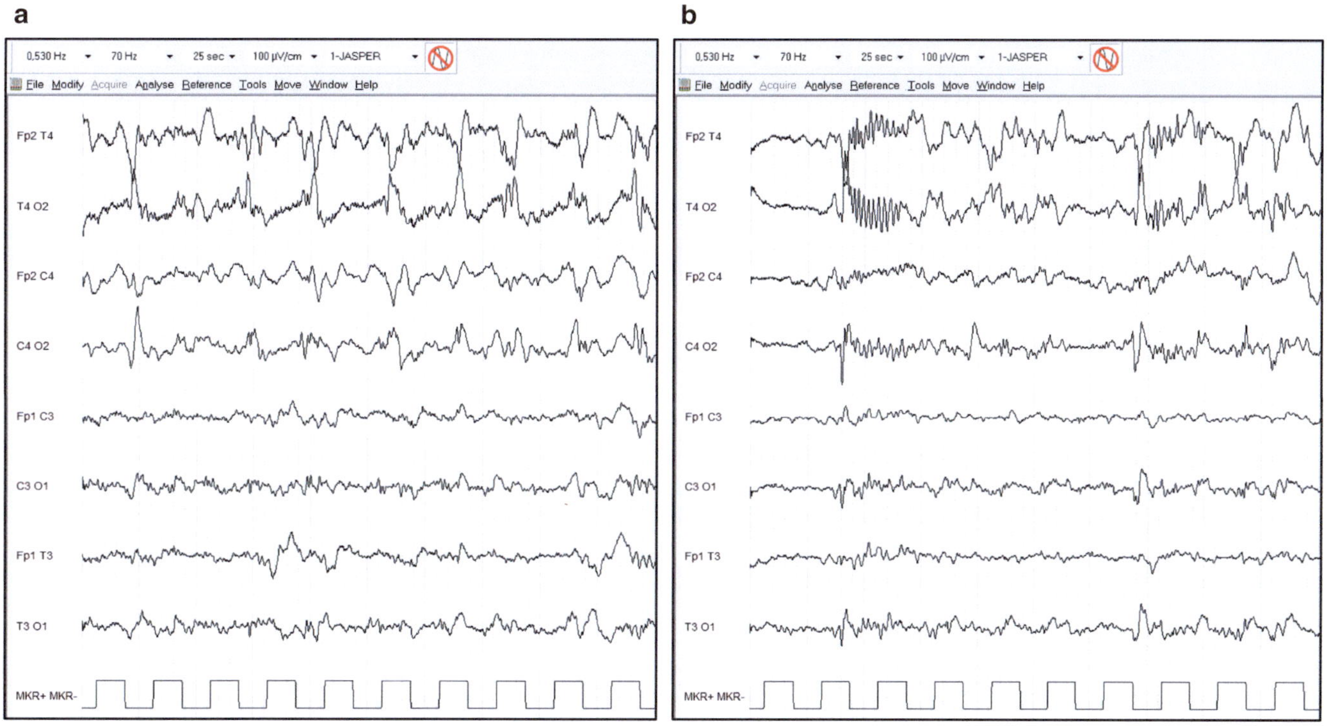

Fig. 13.8 Periodic Lateralized Epileptiform Discharges (PLEDs, new terminology: LPDs) proper (**a**) and plus (**b**), during continuous EEG monitoring in a patient with herpetic encephalitis

patients, hyperventilation response may mimic the appearance of FIRDA (Fig. 13.9a). Occipital Intermittent Rhythmic Delta Activity (OIRDA) is represented by bursts of regular slow waves at 2–3 Hz in the occipital areas of one or both hemispheres. This abnormal pattern, frequently blocked or attenuated by eye opening, is observed more frequently in children than in adults, associated or not with generalized epilepsies (Fig. 13.9b) [14]. In younger patients, a pattern that mimics OIRDA is hyperventilation-induced occipital slowings. Temporal Intermittent Rhythmic Delta Activity (TIRDA) represents an EEG pattern characterized by short sequences (unilateral or bilateral) of rhythmic delta activity at 1–3.5 Hz, recorded predominantly in the anterior temporal regions. TIRDA occurs more frequently during drowsiness and light sleep and it is associated with temporal lobe epilepsy [15].

13.4.2.2 Stimulus-Induced Rhythmic, Periodic, or Ictal Discharges

This EEG pattern was first described by Hirsch et al. [16] in critically ill patients. Stimulus-Induced Rhythmic, Periodic, or Ictal Discharges (SIRPIDs) are rhythmic-, periodic-, or ictal-appearing EEG discharges of sharp transients, elicited by alerting stimuli (auditory, sensory, or noxious stimulation). SIRPIDs may be of variable duration, lateralized or generalized. In the ACNS nomenclature, the SI prefix indicates "Stimulus Induced," and the pattern elicited may be GPDs (SI-GPDs), LPDs (SI-LPDs), and SI-RDA [6]. The relation between SIRPIDs and clinical seizures is unclear and this phenomenon usually represents an electrographic pattern without a clinical correlate. However, there are some reports that demonstrate the ictal nature of SIRPIDs [17, 18]. A recent multicenter retrospective study [19] has shown that SIRPIDs occurred in 10.3% of critically ill patients submitted to EEG and they were associated with other EEG patterns indicative of a poor prognosis. However, in this study, SIRPIDs were not independently associated with in-hospital mortality. A prospective study of Alsherbini et al. [20] found a 19% incidence of SIRPIDs on continuous EEG monitoring during coma, most often as rhythmic delta activity, generalized or lateralized. This study used a standard stimulation protocol and showed a moderate inter-rater agreement. Although the clinical significance of this pattern remains to be clarified, patients with SIRPIDs had more severe brain injuries and poor prognosis (Fig. 13.10). The main quantitative

a

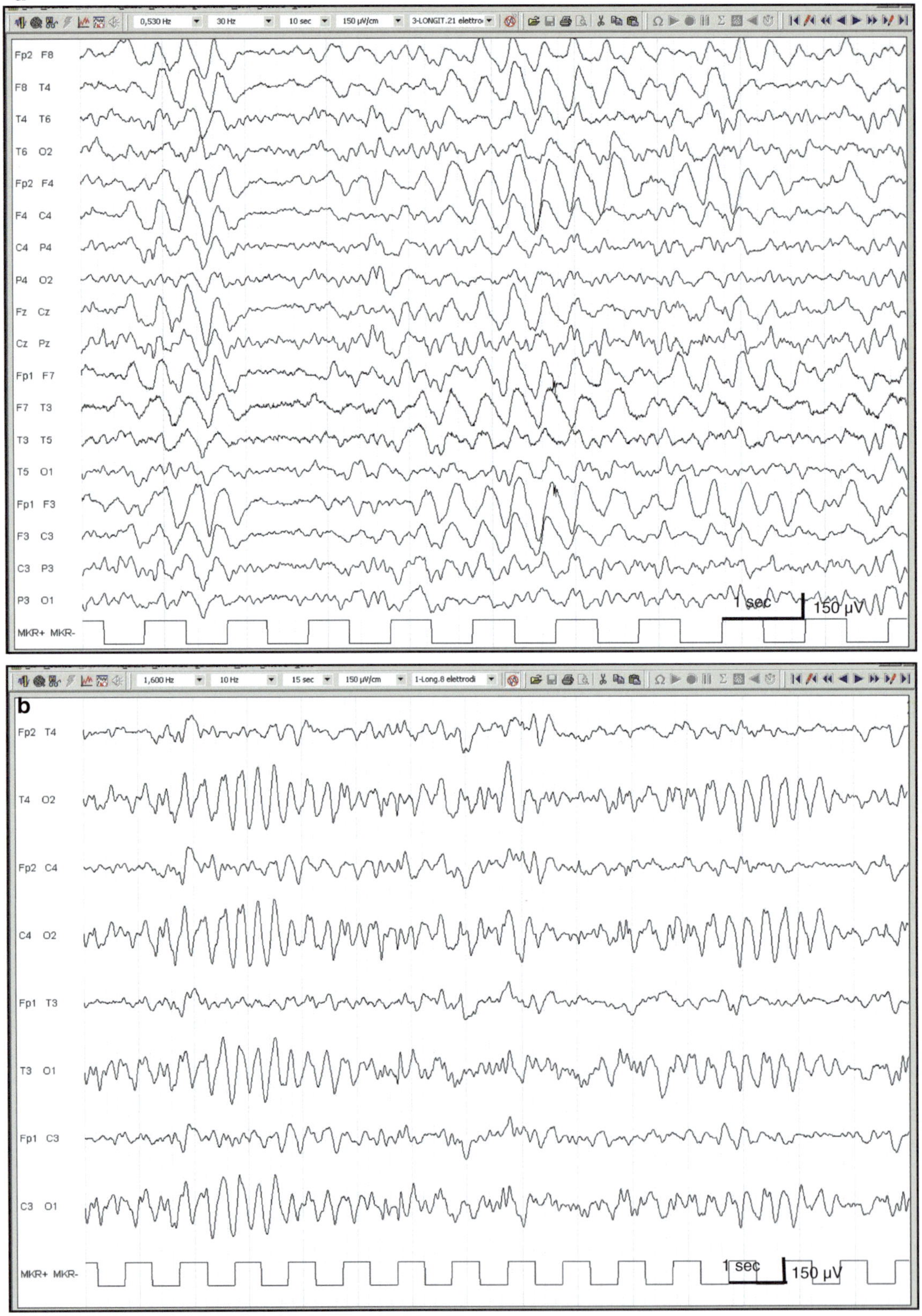

Fig. 13.9 (**a**) Bursts of Intermittent Rhythmic Delta Activity (IRDA), predominantly in frontal areas (Frontal Intermittent Rhythmic Delta Activity, FIRDA) in an old patient with dysmetabolic encephalopathy; (**b**) sequences of regular delta waves in the occipital areas (Occipital Intermittent Rhythmic Delta Activity, OIRDA) in a child with absence epilepsy

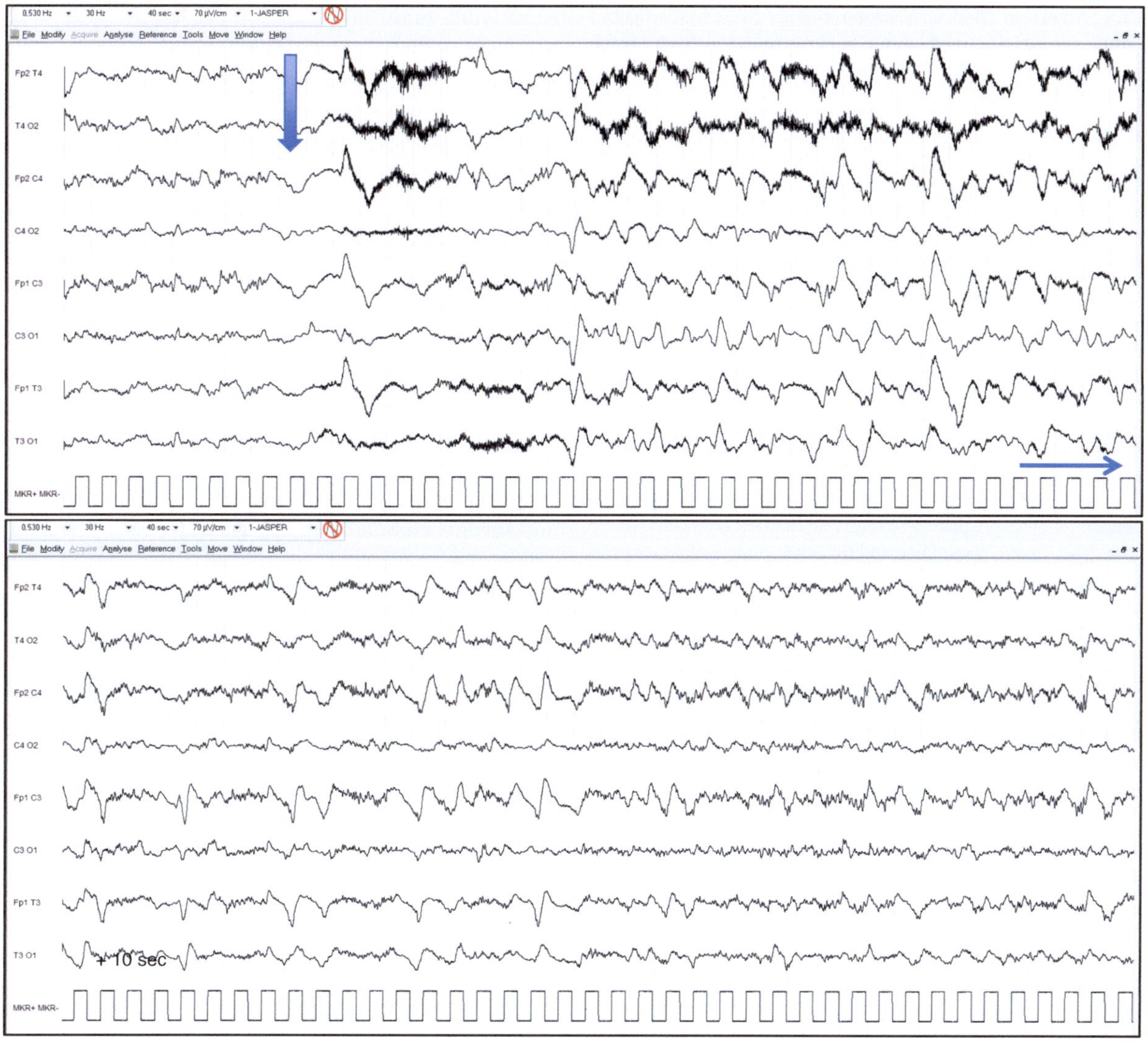

Fig. 13.10 Stimulus-Induced Diffuse Rhythmic Delta Activity (SI-RDA) in a comatose post-traumatic patient with poor outcome. Acoustic stimulus (arrow) induces a prolonged discharge of slow diffuse activity, with sometimes sharp morphology

characteristics of periodic and rhythmic patterns are detailed in note 1.[1]

[1]Main quantitative characteristics of periodic and rhythmic EEG patterns (evaluated on first 30 min of recording or each 24-h period) are as follows [4, 6]:

(a) Prevalence: percent of record that includes the pattern:

- Continuous: >90%
- Abundant: 50–89%
- Frequent: 10–49%
- Occasional: 1–9%
- Rare: <1%

(b) Duration: typical duration of pattern if not continuous:

- Very long: ≥1 h
- Long: 5–59 min
- Intermediate duration: 1–4.9 min
- Brief: 10–59 s
- Very brief: <10 s

(c) Frequency: rate per second (e.g., 1/s, 2/s, etc.).
(d) Number of phases: number of baseline crossings of the typical discharges (apply only to PDs and epileptiform abnormalities).
(e) Sharpness: (categories: spiky, sharp, sharply contoured, blunt).
(f) Amplitude absolute (of PDs, epileptiform pattern, and RDA):measured from peak to trough (very low, <20 μV; low, 20–49 μV; medium, 50–199 μV; high: ≥200 μV).
(g) Polarity: specify for the phase with the greatest amplitude. Applies only to PDs and epileptiform pattern (categories: positive; negative; dipole, horizontal/tangential; unclear).
(h) Spontaneous or stimulus-induced (specify type of stimulus).
(i) Evolving or fluctuating: evolving is defined by at least two unequivocal, sequential changes in frequency, morphology, or location; fluctuating is defined as ≥3 changes, not more than 1 min apart, in frequency, morphology, or location, but not qualifying as evolving.
(j) Plus (+): additional feature which renders the pattern more ictal-appearing than the usual term without the plus.

Table 13.1 American Clinical Neurophysiology Society's proposed nomenclature for periodic or rhythmic patterns (adapted from Hirsch et al. J Clin Neurophysiol 2013; 30: 1–27)

Main term 1	Main term 2
Generalized (G): any bilateral, bisynchronous, and symmetric pattern, even with restricted field	Periodic Discharges (PDs): repetition of waveform—with relatively uniform morphology and duration—at nearly regular intervals, with a quantifiable interdischarge interval between consecutive waveforms
Lateralized (L): unilateral and bilateral (synchronous but asymmetric) patterns	Rhythmic Delta Activity (RDA): repetition of a waveform with relatively uniform morphology and duration, and without an interval between consecutive waveforms
Bilateral Independent: two independent (asynchronous) L patterns (one in each hemisphere)	Spike-and-Slow-Wave or Sharp-and-Slow- Wave Complex (SSWc): spike, polyspike or sharp wave followed by a slow wave in a regularly and alternating pattern, without an interval between one complex and the next
Multifocal (Mf): at least three independent L patterns (at least one in each hemisphere)	

Table 13.2 Old and new terms proposed for Periodic or Rhythmic EEG Patterns (adapted from Hirsch et al. J Clin Neurophysiol 2013; 30: 1–27)

Old term	New term
Periodic Lateralized Epileptiform Discharges (PLEDs)	Lateralized Periodic Discharges (LPDs)
Bilateral Independent Epileptiform Discharges (BIPLEDs)	Bilateral Independent Periodic Discharges (BIPDs)
Generalized Periodic Epileptiform Discharges (GPEDs)	Generalized Periodic Discharges (GPDs)
Triphasic Waves (TW), most of record	GPDs continuous 2/s (with triphasic morphology)
Frontal Intermittent Rhythmic Delta Activity (FIRDA)	occasionally frontally predominant brief 2/s GRDA (fGRDA) (if 1–10% of record)
Stimulus-Induced Rhythmic, Periodic or Ictal Discharges (SIRPIDs)	Stimulus-Induced Generalized Periodic Discharges (SI- GPDs); Stimulus-Induced Lateralized Periodic Discharges (SI-LPDs); Stimulus-Induced Rhythmic Delta Activity (SI-RDA)

The main term proposed for periodic and rhythmic pattern and the comparison between the old and new terminologies are described in Tables 13.1 and 13.2.

13.5 Attenuation/Suppression and Electrocerebral Inactivity

The attenuation, suppression, or total loss of EEG activity may be considered as the expression of the reduced or absent cortical neuronal metabolic function, due to reversible or irreversible brain injuries of multiple etiologies. This EEG pattern may vary in degree and duration, until electrocerebral inactivity (terms discouraged: electrocerebral silence, flat, or isoelectric EEG) is reached, typical of brain death.

Short periods of EEG attenuation/suppression, either diffuse or localized, may precede an epileptic seizure onset and be its first EEG sign, useful also for locating purposes. In comatose subjects, it is sometimes possible to clearly distinguish short periods (0.5–4 s) of flattening of the tracing, followed by a change in the preexisting background activity. This feature, described as Episodic Low-Amplitude Events (ELAEs), is generally of poor prognostic significance [21]. A clearly evident alternation of periods of attenuation/suppression of the tracing and of bursts of EEG activity at various morphology and amplitude is defined as "burst-suppression" pattern. This pattern is a observed in various and severe cerebral diseases, but it also may be of iatrogenic origin (i.e., excessive sedative/anesthetic level). When the periods of attenuation/suppression are excessively prolonged, alternated with short bursts of residual activity, the finding is defined as "suppression-burst" pattern (Fig. 13.11).

According to Standardized Critical Care EEG Terminology of ACNS [6] and to the revised glossary of terms most commonly used by clinical electroencephalographers of IFCN [4], the "attenuation" is defined as the continuous or nearly continuous amplitude reduction of the EEG background activity <50%, with period of lower voltage ≥10 μV; the term "suppression" indicates, instead, that the period of lower voltage is <10 μV. On the basis of its characteristics, background activity is classifiable into five main categories:

- *Continuous*: background activity not interrupted by periods of attenuation/suppression.
- *Nearly continuous*: background activity continuous, but with occasional (≤10% of the record) periods of attenuation/suppression (spontaneous or stimulus-induced).
- *Discontinuous*: periods of attenuation/suppression consisting of 11–49% of the record.
- *Burst-attenuation/burst-suppression*: >50% of the record is attenuated/suppressed.[2]
- Suppression: entirety of the recording is suppressed (<10 μV).

[2]Burst-suppression is a pattern characterized by paroxysmal burst of theta-delta wave with intermixed sharp and faster waves, alternating with periods of attenuation or suppression. In this case, it is necessary to specify the typical duration of bursts and interburst intervals, the sharpest component of a typical burst, and the presence or absence of *highly epileptiform bursts*. The term "highly epileptiform burst" describes a situation where >50% of bursts contain multiple epileptiform discharges or rhythmic potentially ictal pattern at a rate of 1/s or faster.

Bursts within burst-attenuation or burst-suppression pattern must average more than 0.5 s and can last up to 30 s.

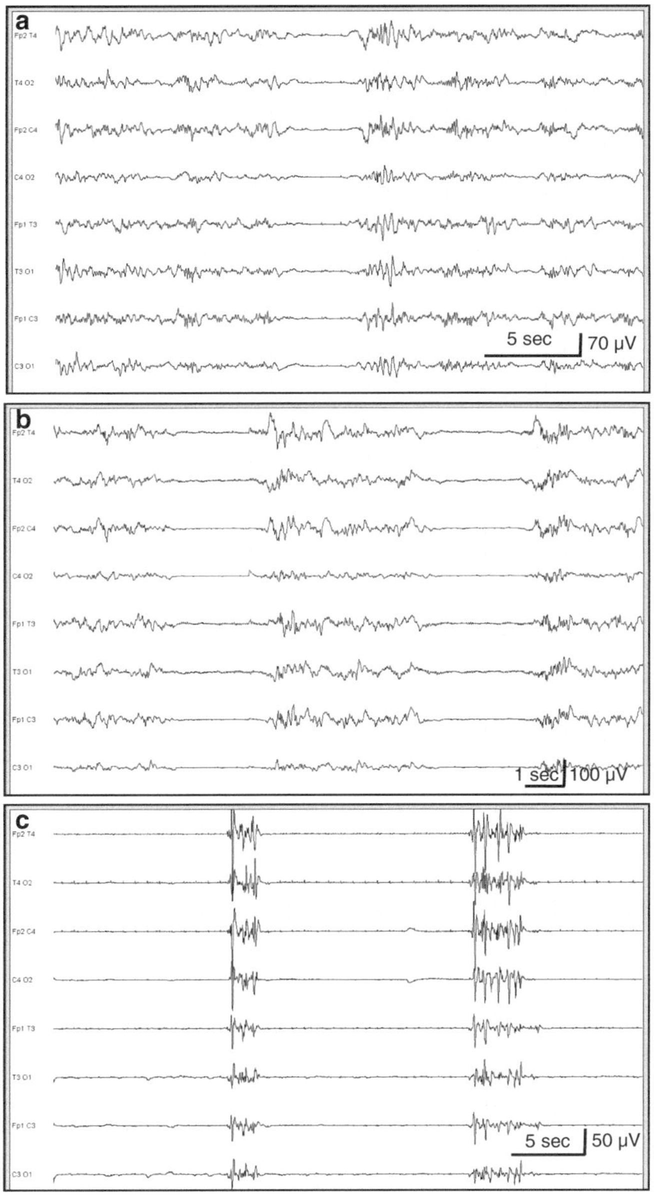

Fig. 13.11 (**a**) Short periods of EEG attenuation in a comatose patients; (**b**, **c**) patterns of burst-suppression and suppression-burst, respectively, of iatrogenic origin

References

1. Cooper R, Binnie C, Billings R. Techniques in clinical neurophysiology. EEG phenomenology. Amsterdam: Elsevier; 2003. p. 169–221.
2. Libenson MH. Visual analysis of the EEG: wakefulness, drowsiness and sleep. In: Libenson MH, editor. Practical approach to electroencephalography. Philadelphia, PA: Saunders Elsevier; 2010. p. 5–30.
3. Krishnan V, Chang BS, Schomer DL. Normal EEG in wakefulness and sleep: adults and elderly. In: Schomer DL, Lopes da Silva FH, editors. Niedermeyer's electroencephalography. Basic principles, clinical applications, and related fieds, 7th ed. New York: Oxford University Press; 2018. p. 202–228.
4. Kane N, Acharya J, Benickzy S, et al. A revised glossary of terms most commonly used by clinical electroencephalographers and updated proposal for the report format of the EEG findings. Revision 2017. Clin Neurophysiol Pract. 2017; 2: 170–85.
5. Noachtar S, Binnie C, Ebersole J, Mauguiere F, Sakamoto A, Westmoreland B. A glossary of terms most commonly used by clinical electroencephalographers and proposal for the report form for the EEG findings. Electroenceph Clin Neurophysiol Suppl. 1999; 52: 21–41.
6. Hirsch LJ, LaRoche SM, Gaspard N, et al. American Clinical Neurophysiology Society's standardized critical care EEG terminology: 2012 version. J Clin Neurophysiol. 2013; 30: 1–27.
7. Brenner RP, Schaul N. Periodic EEG patterns: classification, clinical correlation, and pathophysiology. J Clin Neurophysiol. 1990; 7: 249–67.
8. Chong DJ, Hirsch LJ. Which EEG patterns warrant treatment in the critically ill? Reviewing the evidence for treatment of periodic epileptiform discharges and related patterns. J Clin Neurophysiol. 2005; 22: 79–91.
9. Alkhachroum AM, Al-Abri H, Sachdeva A, et al. Generalized periodic discharges with and without triphasic morphology. J Clin Neurophysiol. 2018; 35: 144–50.
10. Reiher J, Rivest J, Grand'Maison F, Leduc CP. Periodic lateralized epileptiform discharges with transitional rhythmic discharges: association with seizures. Electroencephalogr Clin Neurophysiol. 1991; 78: 12–7.
11. Pohlmann-Eden B, Hoch DB, Cochius JI, Chiappa KH. Periodic lateralized Epileptiform discharges—a critical review. J Clin Neurophysiol. 1996; 13: 519–30.
12. Witsch J, Frey HP, Schmidt JM, et al. Electroencephalographic periodic discharges and frequency-dependent brain tissue hypoxia in acute brain injury. JAMA Neurol. 2017; 74: 301–9.
13. Newey CR, Sahota P, Hantus S. Electrographic features of lateralized periodic discharges stratify risk in the interictal-ictal continuum. J Clin Neurophysiol. 2017; 34: 365–9.
14. Watemberg N, Linder I, Dabby R, Blumkin L, Lerman-Sagie T. Clinical correlates of Occipital Intermittent Rhythmic Delta Activity (OIRDA) in children. Epilepsia. 2007; 48: 330–4.
15. Di Gennaro G, Quarato PP, Onorati P, Colazza GB, et al. Localizing significance of temporal intermittent rhythmic delta activity (TIRDA) in drug-resistant focal epilepsy. Clin Neurophysiol. 2003; 114: 70–8.
16. Hirsch LJ, Claassen J, Mayer SA, Emerson RG. Stimulus-induced Rhythmic, Periodic, or Ictal Discharges (SIRPIDs): a common EEG phenomenon in the critically ill. Epilepsia. 2004; 45: 109–23.
17. Hirsch LJ, Pang T, Claassen J, et al. Focal motor seizures induced by alerting stimuli in critically ill patients. Epilepsia. 2008; 49: 968–73.
18. Kaplan PW, Duckworth J. Confusion and SIRPIDs regress with parenteral lorazepam. Epileptic Disord. 2011; 13: 291–4.
19. Braksick SA, Burkholder DB, Tsetsou S, et al. Associated factors and prognostic implications of stimulus-induced rhythmic, periodic, or ictal discharges. JAMA Neurol. 2016; 73: 585–90.
20. Alsherbini KA, Plancher JM, Ficker DM, et al. Stimulus-induced rhythmic, periodic, or Ictal discharges in coma—incidence and interrater reliability of continuous EEG after a standard stimulation protocol: a prospective study. J Clin Neurophysiol. 2017; 34: 375–80.
21. Rae-Grant AD, Strapple C, Barbour PJ. Episodic low-amplitude events: an under-recognized phenomenon in clinical electroencephalography. J Clin Neurophysiol. 1991; 8: 203–11.

14 Activation Procedures

Oriano Mecarelli

14.1 Hyperventilation

HyperVentilation (HV)–or overbreathing (synonym)–is the first described EEG activation procedure, always used in clinical EEG laboratories; it is recommended as part of the standard EEG recording by the most prestigious international guidelines [1, 2]. The procedure is easy to perform and very safe [3, 4] and, in most cases, is able to induce the appearance of interictal or ictal epileptiform discharges [5]. Gibbs and colleagues already described in 1935 that HV was able to determine the appearance of a 3 Hz SW discharge, associated with absence seizure [6].

This method consists of seriated acts of deep and regular breathing, performed for a minimum of 3 min at a rate of about 18–20 breaths per minute, with the EEG recording lasting at least 1–2 min after cessation of overbreathing [1, 2]. In special cases, it is necessary to continue the recording even for longer periods after stopping HV. A recent large-scale study [5] showed that HV prolonged for 5 min increased the diagnostic yield of HV (16% of seizures and 30% of interictal EEG abnormalities triggered by HV occurred after 3 min of HV) and that 99% of patients who are able to hyperventilate for 3 min can complete a 5 min HV, without additional adverse events.

Adult subjects generally ensure a good cooperation in HV execution, even though the technician should give very precise and comprehensible instructions and supervise carefully that the procedure is carried out appropriately. The EEG technician should, therefore, ask the subject to breathe faster than normal (with deep inhalation, prolonged and intense exhalation, with semi-open mouth), and he should always write down an assessment of the quality of patient's efforts, throughout the HV procedure.

HV can be normally carried out in children older than 5–6 years; younger children generally indeed perform HV discontinuously and irregularly and the manoeuvre could therefore be useless or even counterproductive. It should also be remembered that, in very young children, EEG changes similar to those obtained with HV are observed during prolonged crying. Finally, the technician should inform the subject that, during the HV test, he sometimes might experience symptoms, such as tingling limbs, dizziness and blurred vision, but these should not prevent the continuation of the test, being these mostly negligible and transitory.

HV is contraindicated in severe cardiac or pulmonary diseases, recent stroke or myocardial infarction, intracerebral or subarachnoid haemorrhage, hyperviscosity state, sickle cell anaemia, uncontrolled hypertension, severe carotid stenosis and Moyamoya disease [7]. Contraindication should however be evaluated in each case, and chronic cardiovascular and respiratory diseases in older patients do not always exclude the possibility of HV execution.

14.1.1 Normal EEG Changes Induced by HV

The characteristic EEG response to HV, most evident in children and young subjects, consists in a slowing of posterior dominant background rhythm and in a fluctuating, bilaterally synchronous, slow activity. The slowings induced by HV are dominant posteriorly in children and anteriorly in adolescents and young subjects (Fig. 14.1), the incidence and magnitude of these slowings depending on the efforts during the test and on age. The age of subjects is an important factor for the magnitude of HV response, since the most evident EEG slowings are observed between 8 and 12 years. Approximately 10% of young adults and 70% of children show a physiological response to HV [7], with a remarkable interindividual variability. After HV interruption, EEG generally returns to basal conditions in <30 up to 60 s; sometimes, especially in children, the tracing does not revert to baseline, because the subject continues actually to hyperventilate, even if discontinuously. Very often, in children, HV causes the appearance of

O. Mecarelli (✉)
Department of Human Neurosciences, Sapienza University of Rome, Rome, Italy
e-mail: oriano.mecarelli@uniroma1.it

O. Mecarelli (ed.), *Clinical Electroencephalography*, https://doi.org/10.1007/978-3-030-04573-9_14

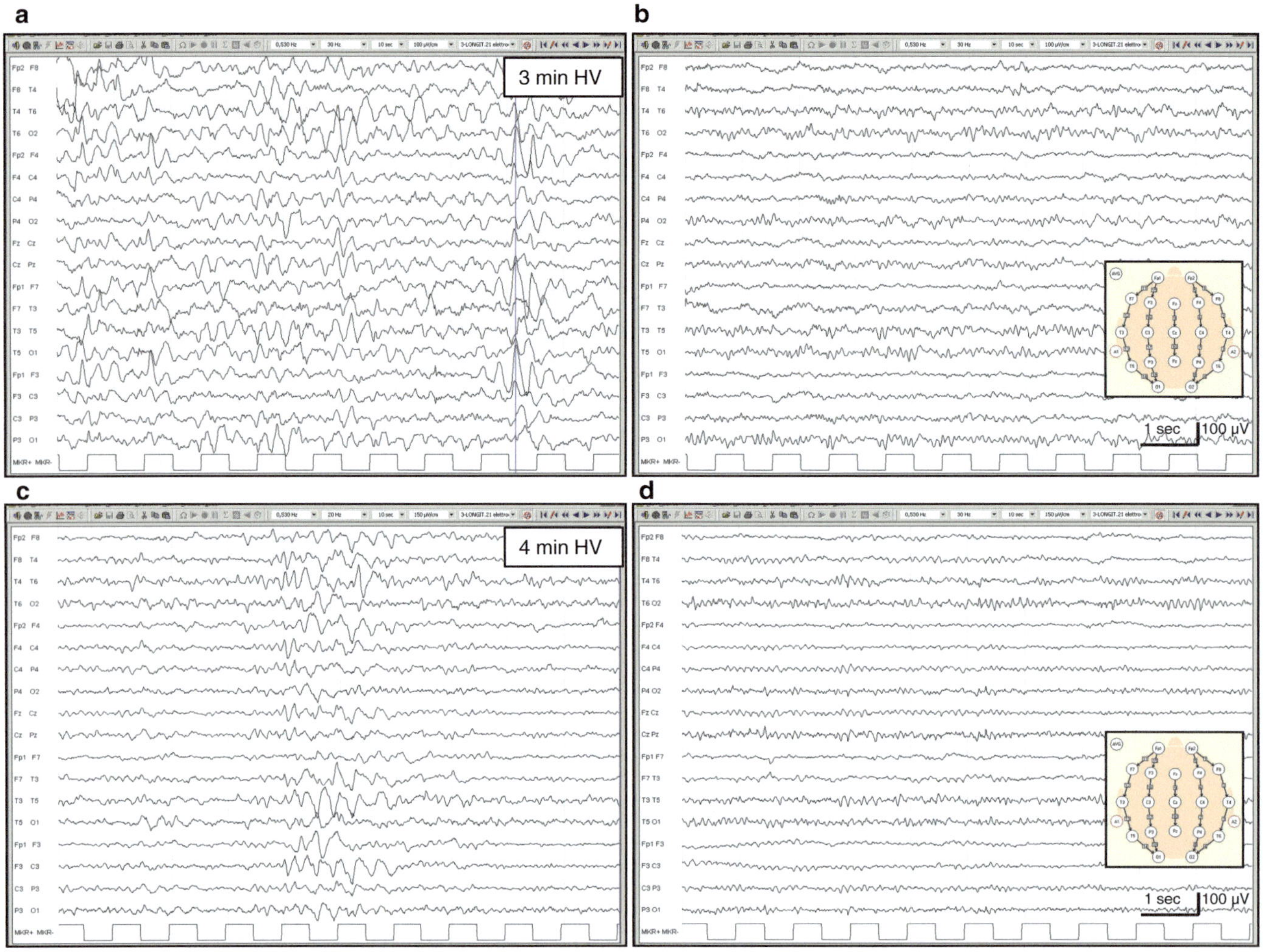

Fig. 14.1 Physiological EEG changes induced by HyperVentilation (HV). Sequences of delta slowings, dominant posteriorly, after 3-min HV, in a 7-year-old child (**a**); basal reverting of EEG recording 30 s after HV end (**b**). Burst of delta waves dominant anteriorly after 4 min of HV in an 18-year-old subject (**c**), with EEG return to basal condition after 20-s HV end (**d**)

a slow (2–5 Hz) high-amplitude hypersynchronous activity, even with paroxysmal morphology (*HV-Induced High-Amplitude Rhythmic Slowing, HIHARS*), which generally promptly disappears at the interruption of the test (within 30–60 s) (Fig. 14.2). Children with HIHARS sometimes present altered responsiveness and automatisms during the test, but these symptoms are not correlated with epileptic typical discharges [8–10]. Other relevant factors in determining the EEG slowings are the blood glucose level (hypoglycaemia can induce delta waves during HV, particularly if it is less than 80 mg/dL) and the upright position, as compared to the reclining position [11].

Diffuse intermittent rhythmic delta activity during HV may be also observed in young adults with recurrent vasovagal syncope. These distinctive EEG changes, a common finding in syncope patients, should not therefore be confused with any abnormal slow pattern or epileptiform activity [12] (Fig. 14.3).

14.1.2 Abnormal EEG Changes Induced by HV

The EEG changes elicited - or increased - by the HV can be represented by focal and/or diffuse slowings and by epileptiform abnormalities (Figs. 14.4 and 14.5). Classically, HV is considered to be the more effective activation test in the majority of cases (80–90%) of untreated generalised epilepsy with absences of childhood. In these cases, HV induces the appearance of typical diffuse SSW discharges at 3 Hz, related or not to clinical seizures [5, 7, 10, 11]. Furthermore, HV may activate atypical SSW discharges in approximately 50% of patients with symptomatic generalised epilepsy who are able to perform the procedure correctly. Focal epileptic seizures can also be triggered by a correctly performed HV, even though in significantly lower percentages (seizures originating from the temporal lobe are more easily activated by HV compared to the frontal ones) [13]. Beyond the facilitation of electroclinical discharges,

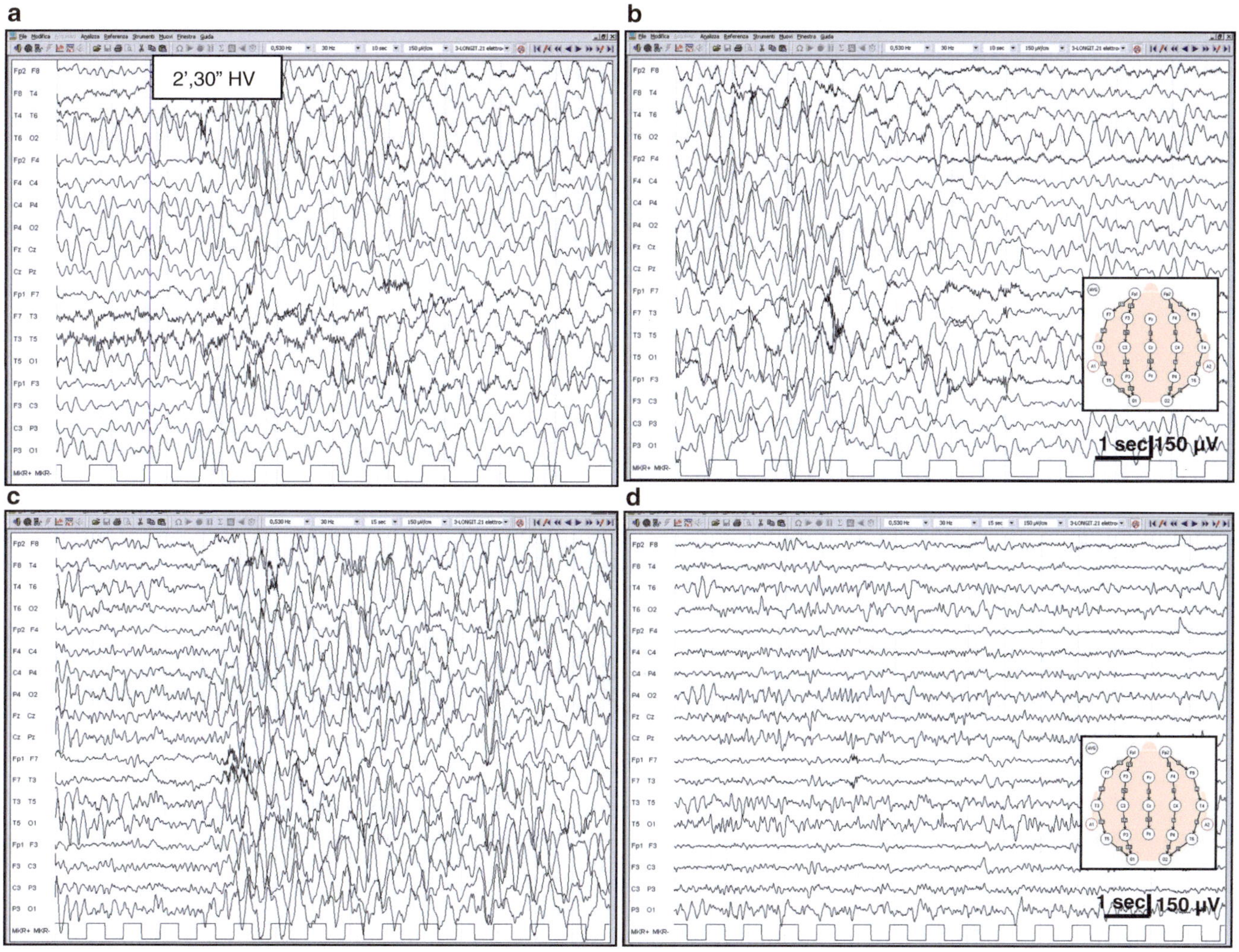

Fig. 14.2 Two examples of hyperventilation-induced high-amplitude rhythmic slowing, in a 6-year-old (**a**, **b**) and 7-year-old child, respectively (**c**, **d**). In (**b**) a gradual reappearance of normal background activity 40 s after the HV stop is observed, while in **d** the EEG normalisation is earlier, 30 s after the end of the activation procedure

HV may also increase interictal epileptic abnormalities already present in the baseline tracing, or allow identification of previously unreported epileptic foci [3, 4]. Focal epilepsies are relatively resistant to HV activation in adolescent and adults and, in these cases, a 5 min HV is recommended [7]. However, some studies report contrasting views regarding the utility and effectiveness of HV in this type of epilepsy. The existing literature describes a yield of 6–11% in focal epilepsies and a recent population-based study found that the yield of activation-related epileptiform abnormalities accounted for 7.9% on the first EEG, higher in children and in generalised seizure types [14].

HV can be avoided if abundant epileptiform activity on the pre-HV baseline EEG is already present. The technician should consider that, during the HV, an epileptic seizure (generalised or focal) might occur. In this event, he will try to continue the recording and to test the level of consciousness of the subject. The ideal solution in these cases is always to start a video-EEG registration, if available in the laboratory.

For the clinical interpretation of HV-induced slow EEG changes, a few simple guidelines should be followed. HV-induced slowings should be considered abnormal when the slowings are significantly asymmetrical (2:1 ratio) or with superimposed spikes and when the slowings persist for several minutes after the command to stop hyperventilation.

In children with Moyamoya disease it was reported, about 5 min after HV cessation, a "re-buildup" of slow waves, in correspondence with a decrease of cerebral blood flow. In this view, HV should be avoided in patients with Moyamoya syndrome [15].

Finally, HV is very effective (as other suggestive manoeuvres) to activate Psychogenic Non-Epileptic Seizures (PNES). According to Abubakr et al. [16], more than one-third of patients with PNES may have events precipitated by

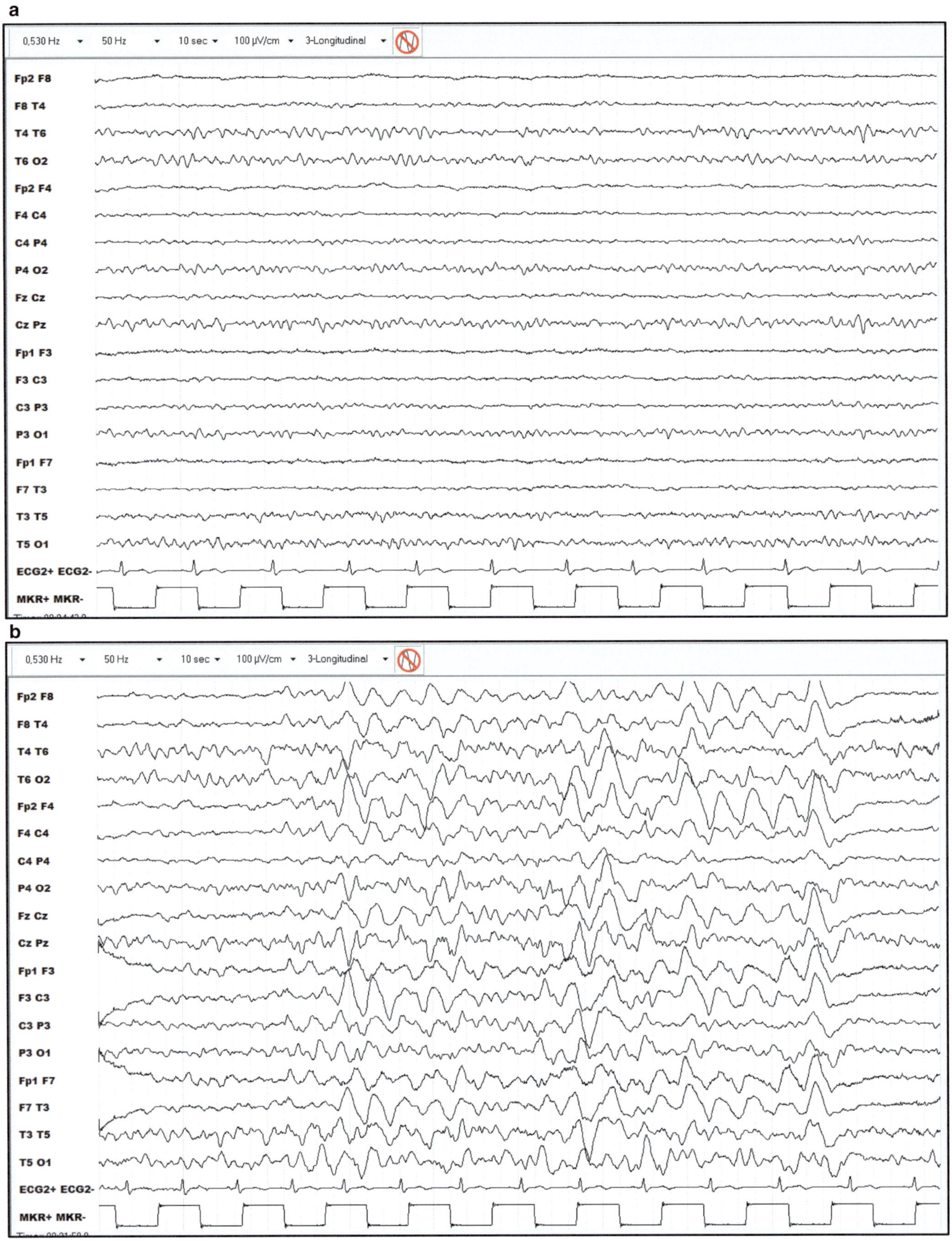

Fig. 14.3 Normal basal EEG (**a**) and slow diffuse hypersynchrony after 3-min hyperventilation (**b**) in an 18-year-old subject with recurrent neurally mediated syncopes

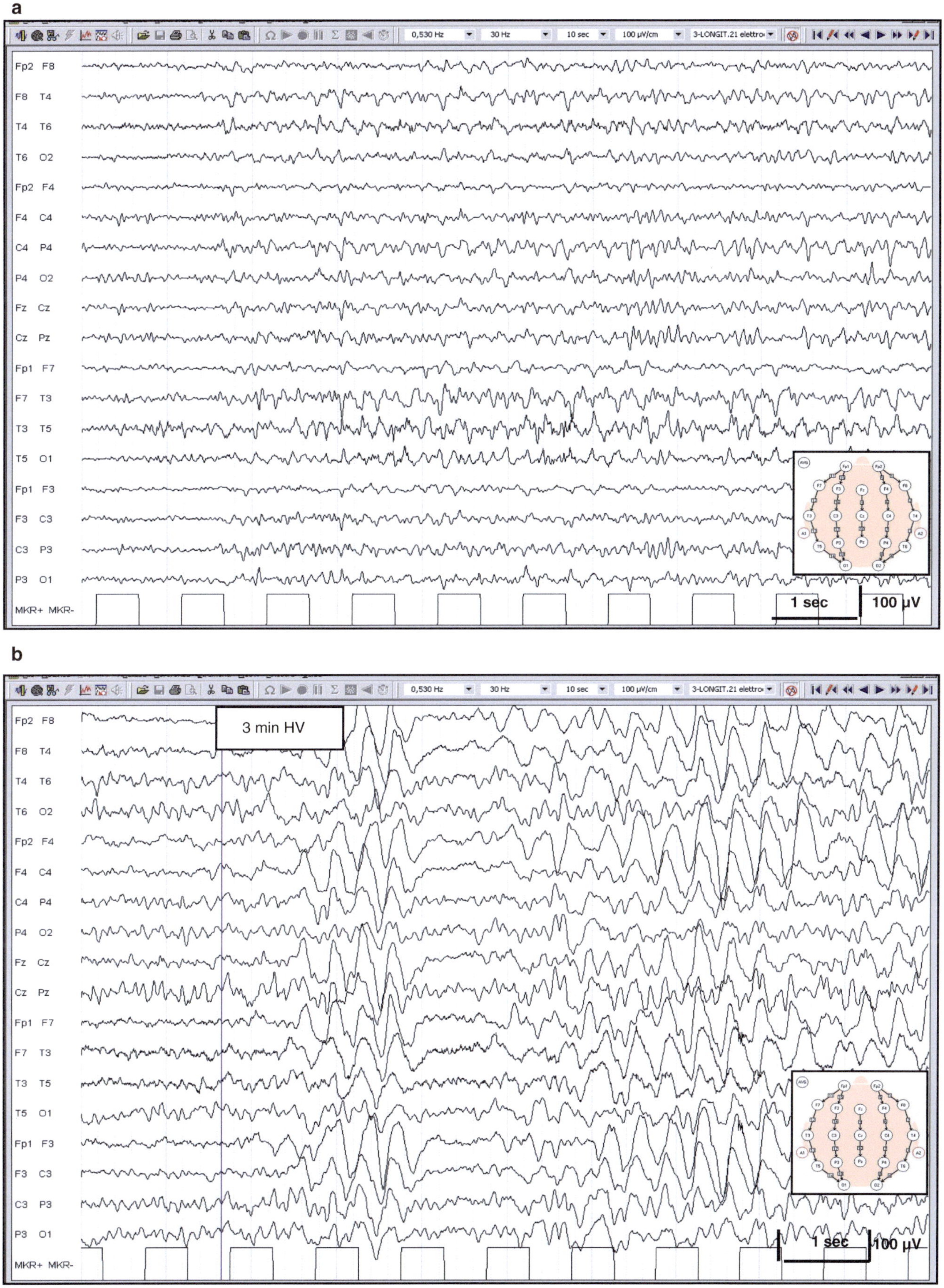

Fig. 14.4 (**a**) Focal hyperventilation-induced slowings in the left anterior temporal region in a 48-year-old patient with a brain tumour. (**b**) Diffuse and rhythmic high-amplitude delta activity dominant anteriorly, in a 26-year-old patient with generalised genetic epilepsy on antiepileptic treatment

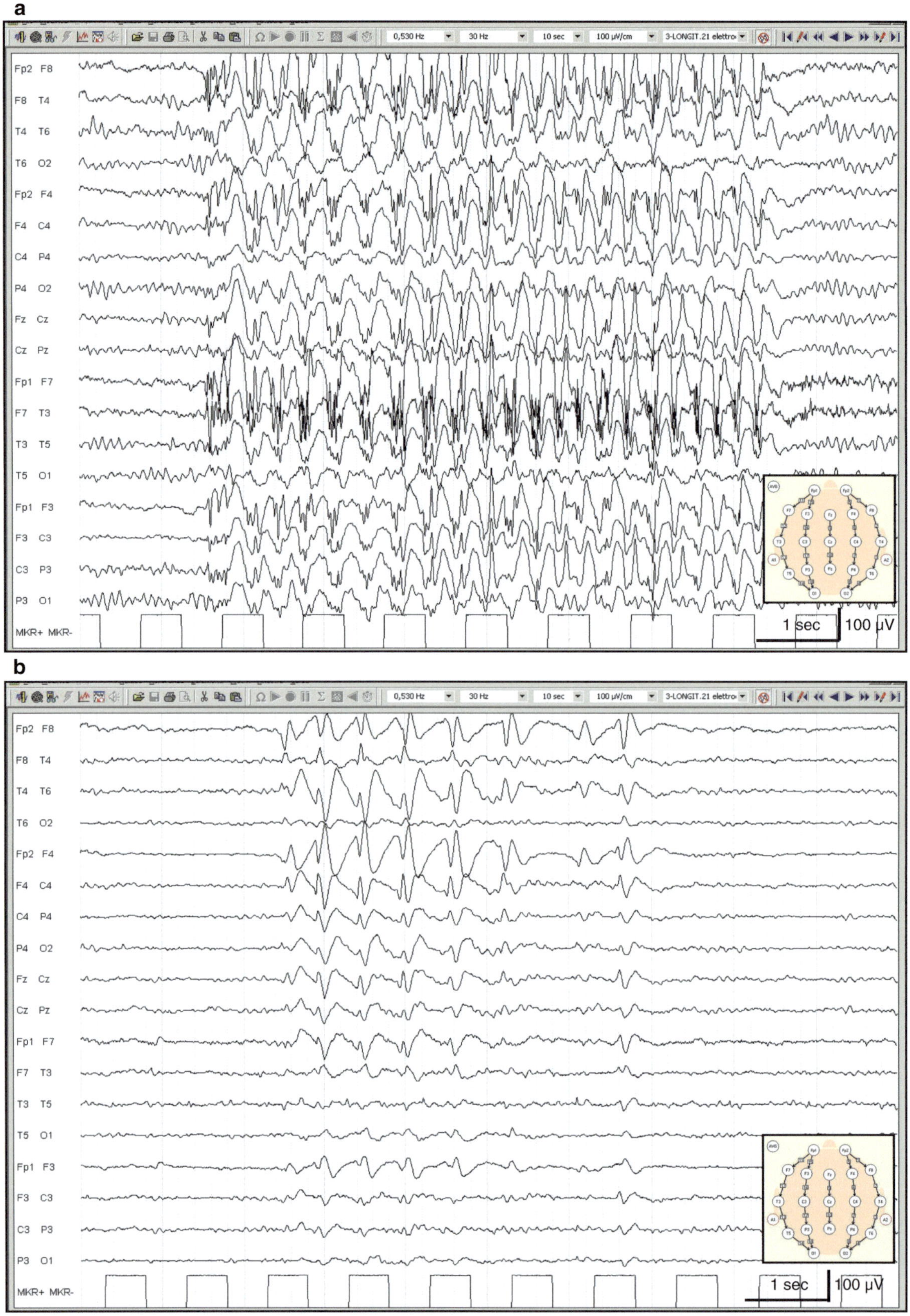

Fig. 14.5 Epileptic hyperventilation-induced abnormalities. (**a**) Generalised discharge of spike- and polyspike-and-wave complexes at 3 Hz in a 16-year-old adolescent 150 sec after the beginning of the procedure; typical discharge is correlated with absence seizure. (**b**) Interictal hyperventilation-induced focal discharge of sharp wave-and-slow wave complexes in a 36-year-old adult with right frontotemporal post-traumatic lesion and focal epilepsy

Table 14.1 HyperVentilation (HV): modality of execution and synthesis of EEG changes

Hyperventilation	Methods and activated EEG pattern
Patient	Sitting or reclining position; relaxed environment
Modality of execution (breath)	Deep inhalation and prolonged and intense exhalation, with semi-open mouth; 18–20 breaths per minute
Duration procedure	3–5 min
Normal EEG changes	Slowing alpha rhythm Diffuse slowings (>in posterior regions in children; >in anterior regions in young): – Variable entity (depending on the age, individual characteristics, etc.) – EEG return to baseline within <30 up to 60 s
Abnormal EEG changes	Focal and/or diffuse slowings not justified by age and of considerable entity Relevant asymmetries EEG return to baseline very late Epileptiform abnormalities (interictal or ictal): >Generalised (>SW discharges at 3 Hz), more rarely focal

HV. In these cases, the absence of EEG abnormalities is essential to clarify the non-epileptic origin of the behavioural manifestations [17].

Table 14.1 synthetizes the modality of execution of HV and the various EEG changes induced by this activation procedure.

14.1.3 Pathophysiological Changes Induced by HV

In healthy individuals, the primary effect of HV is a decrease in carbon dioxide (CO_2) in the alveolar area. CO_2 is present in small quantities in the air we breathe, but it is also produced by metabolic activity and eliminated through the lungs. When blood CO_2 increases (e.g. as in the case of physical activity), the brainstem breath centres induce an increase in lung ventilation to eliminate the CO_2 excess. This mechanism can be stimulated voluntarily increasing the frequency of breaths/minute. In this case, blood pCO_2 reduces from the normal values of 40 mmHg to 20–30 mmHg (hypocapnia); furthermore, the CO_2 reacts with the fluids to form carbonic acid, with a consequent increase in the pH of 0.20 units (alkalosis). Achenbach-Ng et al. [18] have studied the changes in blood gases and EEG in healthy adult subjects before, during and after HV. The mean pCO_2 reduced to 18 mmHg from the baseline during HV and recovered in 7 min. The mean pO_2 increased to 7 mmHg during HV and reduced to 25 mmHg below baseline 5 min after the end of HV. The changes of EEG median power frequency showed marked variability; on average, the median frequency dropped 1 Hz during HV and returned to baseline within 2 min of normal breath resumption. The changes in pCO_2 and blood pH determine a cerebral vasoconstriction, with a consequent reduction of blood flow (minimum 30%) and hypoxia while, at the peripheral level, there is a vasodilatation with decreased blood pressure, less blood return to the brain, slower elimination of brain CO_2 and restoration of normal carbon dioxide pressure (Fig. 14.6). Studies performed by transcranial Doppler [19, 20] have confirmed a reduction of up to 50–60% of cerebral blood flow during HV in the middle cerebral artery (Fig. 14.7). According with these studies, the decrease of the pCO_2 and the reduction of cerebral blood flow during HV are the fundamental factors inducing EEG slowings. It should be added that the decrease of cerebral flow does not only provoke the reduction of the concentration of O_2, but also induce a decrease in the glycaemic rate, both mechanisms responsible of the EEG activation. In addition to the blood flow decrease, hypoxia is also determined for the Bohr effect, the phenomenon whereby oxyhemoglobin increases in alkalosis conditions its affinity for O_2, which is then exchanged with higher difficulty to the tissues. Hypoxia can then lead to a greater nerve cell anaerobic glycolysis, as it results from the increase of the lactate/pyruvate ratio and, therefore, from the tissue acidity.

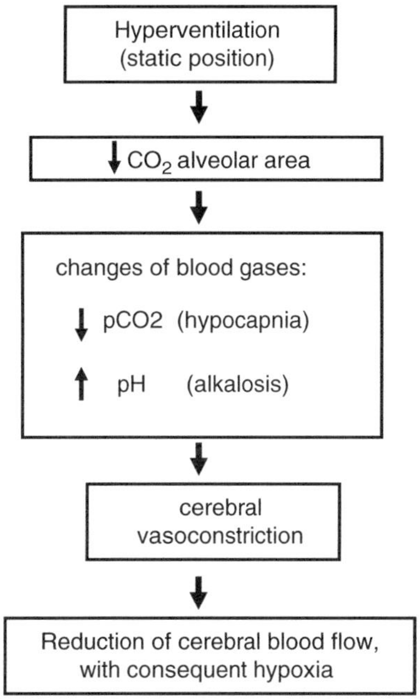

Fig. 14.6 Hyperventilation-induced metabolic and vascular changes, according to the theory of cerebral hypoxia

The theory of cerebral hypoxia is still the most accredited as the fundamental cause of the appearance of EEG abnormalities during forced HV, but it is not free from criticism and it is not universally accepted.

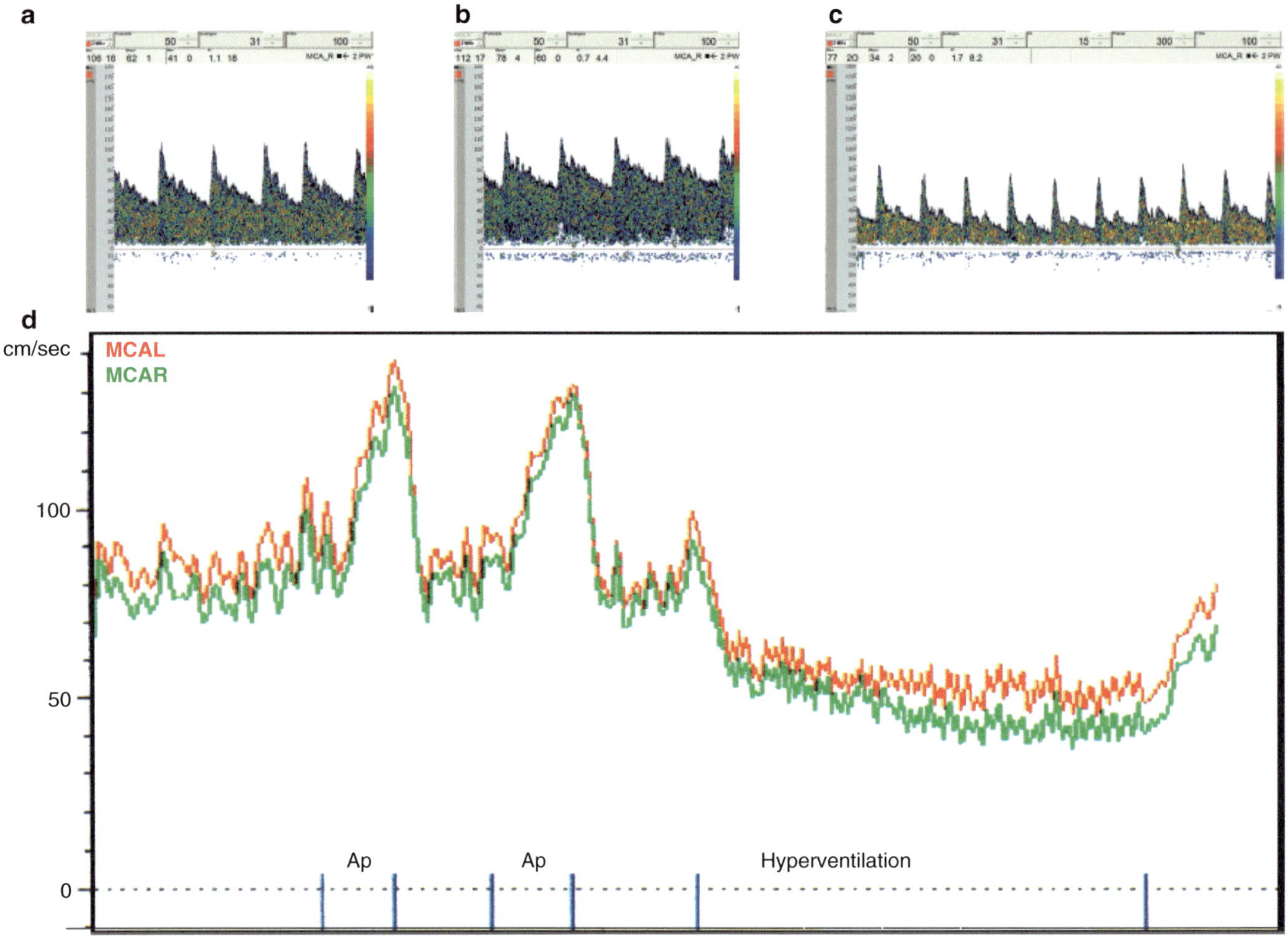

Fig. 14.7 Transcranial Doppler showing variations of cerebral blood flow velocities in the middle cerebral artery during apnea (Ap, **a**, **b**) and hyperventilation (**c**). Apnea induces vasodilation with increase of blood flow velocities. Hyperventilation induces vasoconstriction with the reduction of blood flow velocities. In **d** the throughout middle cerebral artery monitoring during two apnea trials (Ap) and a hyperventilation is shown. Note the green and red lines indicating blood flow mean flow velocities changes (cm/sec) in the left middle cerebral artery (MCAL) and in the right middle cerebral artery (MCAR).

Van der Worp et al. [21] compared, in healthy subjects, EEG changes and mean cerebral artery flow during hypocapnia (induced by voluntary hyperventilation) and during progressive normobaric hypoxia. The slow activity increase was less pronounced during hypoxia in comparison with HV-induced hypocapnia, while the blood flow velocities were reduced in the case of hyperventilation and increased in hypoxia. Consequently, according to these authors, EEG changes observed during hyperventilation must be attributed to factors other than to cerebral hypoxia. In this regard, it should be furthermore noted that during HV cerebral O_2 consumption not only is not reduced (as we would expect considering vasoconstriction), but it rather tends to increase; oxidative phosphorylation processes are adequate, as shown by normal ATP and phosphocreatine values and, therefore, there should be no need to activate the anaerobic glycolysis; increase in the lactate/pyruvate ratio may be the consequence of the stimulation of the phosphofructokinase due to blood alkalosis, rather than the increased use of anaerobic glycolysis. In normal adult subjects, HV-induced cerebral hypoxia is generally unable to determine appreciable changes in electrical activity, probably for the rapid establishment of physiological compensatory mechanisms. On the other hand, in children and adolescents, there are usually changes in the electrocortical patterns, more relevant when the subject is young, even in the absence of specific pathologies. This is probably related to a more pronounced lowering of the pCO_2, to a more rapid and vigorous decrease in cerebral flow (due to the immaturity of the vascular response to CO_2) and to a different sensitivity of the CNS itself to CO_2, depending on age.

With regard to the cerebral structures responsible for EEG changes onset during forced HV, it seems that hypocapnia inhibits the mesencephalic reticular ascending system, causing the diffuse EEG slowings, due to the predominance of non-specific thalamic projection system [22]. It was also hypothesised that, due to a specific reduction of blood flow at the diencephalic level, an increase in the activity of the non-specific thalamic nuclei could be determined, resulting in cortical hyperexcitability. It should also be highlighted that a potential link between thalamocortical networks, HV and absence epileptic seizures exists. In particular, it has been shown that the non-specific thalamic projecting system appears to be critically involved in both SW discharges and HV-triggered cortical activity patterns [10].

Finally, pathophysiological modifications induced by HV (hypocapnia and alkalosis) cannot be compared to those occurring as a result of elevated breathing during physical exercise (hyperpnea). Compensatory hyperpnea during physical exercise is associated with the increased metabolic demands and high CO_2 elimination is matched by high CO_2 production. In this case, blood pCO_2 is relatively stable and pH does not significantly change. Furthermore, muscle activity determines the production of lactic acid that contributes to the blood pH lowering. As a matter of fact, during physical activity, even though hyperpnea is determined, an accentuation of the SW discharges at 3 Hz in children with absence epilepsy has not been observed [23] and, therefore, sport practice should not be discouraged.

14.2 Intermittent Photic Stimulation

According to a revised glossary [24], the Intermittent Photic Stimulation (IPS) or Photic Stimulation (PS, synonymous) is an EEG activation procedure consisting of the presentation of intermittent flashes of light to the eyes. The first pioneering studies on the effects of visual stimuli on human EEG were carried out in 1934 by Adrian and Matthews [25]; subsequently, the stimulation method was developed by Walter et al. [26] and it became routinary used in standard EEG from the 1950s [7, 27, 28]. Since IPS is performed with different methods all over the world, several publications have been recently designed in an attempt to standardise the technical procedure and the interpretation of results [29, 30].

14.2.1 Methodology

IPS should be performed in a room with dimmed lighting, because the sensitivity to photostimulation increases in ambient conditions of reduced illumination. Several factors have been considered as the cause of this phenomenon: adaptation to the dark, pupils dilatation, higher contrast between the flash and the dim light of the environment, etc. The procedure should be performed before the HV, or at least 3 min after stopping HV, when both HV-related EEG and metabolic changes have resolved [2], with a patient in a sitting position. In order to have the patient more relaxed, the EEG recording with IPS should be performed with the subject lying on a bed. However, IPS should always be carried out while the patient is awake after a normal night sleep.

The equipment required to perform IPS consists of a preferably circular lamp (about 13 cm in diameter), placed at least 30 cm from the patient's face with an angle of 13°. The subject should be sitting comfortably, with the head slightly reclined, and he should fix on the centre of the lamp. The flash intensity should be at least 0.7 Joule (preferably 1 Joule).

The test is more effective when executed on the subject with the eyes closed, apparently paradoxical phenomenon for the interposition of the eyelids between the light source and the eyes. In reality, this situation seems to facilitate the appearance of the paroxysmal response to IPS, since the eyelids act as light diffusers and behave like selective filters for the wavelengths of the visible light spectrum, which gives rise to the perception of red. Not surprisingly, considering the different susceptibility of photosensitive epileptic patients to different colours, red is the most incriminating colour (at wavelengths of 660–720 nm) than blue or white, at the same overall intensity.

Normally, IPS should be however performed in three eye conditions, with separate trains of flashes of 5 s duration each during eye closure, eyes closed and eyes open, and with a 5 s rest time between each flashes train. If there is not enough time, it is preferable to apply each flash frequency for 7 s, after the closure of eyes on command.

According to the most recent recommendations [30], the IPS must be carried out as follows: stimulation sequence including in ascending order the frequencies of 1—2—8—10—15—18—20—25—40—50—60 Hz. When the patient is not sensitive, all the frequencies stimulations are done and the IPS can be stopped when 60 Hz is reached (the global duration of IPS procedure is 330 s). If there is a Photo Paroxysmal Response (PPR) to a specific frequency (*lower threshold*), the authors recommend skipping the remaining frequencies of the ascending series, starting again with IPS at higher 60 Hz frequency and going down (60—50—40—25—…) until a PPR again occurs (*upper threshold*). In this case, the duration of the IPS will be obviously shorter in time. The lower and the upper thresholds should be determined to prevent seizure occurrence and, when they have been identified, further stimulations should not be attempted.

In our EEG laboratory, to shorten the IPS recording time, flash frequencies described earlier are applied for 5 s with eyes open and for another 5 s after closing the eyes, with an interstimulus interval of 7 s. Therefore, if all the photic stimulation trains are executed in an increasing direction and the photoparoxysmal response does not appear, IPS should last a total of 180 s.

Table 14.2 Methodology for Intermittent Photic Stimulation (IPS)

IPS	Methods
Environment	Dimly lit room
Patient	Sitting position, head slightly reclined Fixing the centre of the lamp
Photic stimulator	Circular lamp (13 cm diameter) Intensity of flash: at least 0.7 Joule Viewing distance: 30 cm; angle: 13 degrees
Standard IPS procedure	*Flash frequencies*: 1-2-8-10-15-18-20-25-40-50-60 Hz *Eye conditions*: Eye closure, eyes closed, eyes open (5 s IPS and 5 s rest times, for each eye condition)
Appearance of PR	Lower threshold: appearance of PPR at a certain frequency In this case: skip the remaining of the series, start again with 60 Hz and go down (60-50-40-25...) until PPR again occurs (upper threshold)

During IPS, the technicians should apply the electrodes for monitoring eye movements and myoclonia of the limbs and face and a simultaneous video recording could be helpful or mandatory for a precise clinical correlation. For more sophisticated studies on individual photosensitivity, the following more extensive flash frequencies can be used: 1-2-6-8-9-10-13-15-18-20-23-25-30-40-50-60 Hz; the retest of photosensitive patients with these frequencies can allow to determine with higher accuracy the photosensitivity range.

The EEG technician, for the risk assessment, must have all the clinical information about the patient and must be alert to stop the IPS immediately upon the appearance of a photoparoxysmal response, since prolonged stimulation can trigger an epileptic seizure. Furthermore, it is helpful to previously describe the stimulation procedure to the patient, especially if naive, also explaining possible risks. It would also be important, for the patient or the family members, to sign the informed consent, especially in cases where the risk of triggering a seizure is higher. Table 14.2 summarises the methodology for IPS.

14.2.2 IPS-Induced EEG Changes

14.2.2.1 Photic Driving Response

The Photic Driving Response (PDR) consists of a physiological response to IPS, characterised by the appearance of a rhythmic posterior activity, with a frequency identical - or harmonically related - to that of the photic stimulus [24]. This response is time-locked to the light stimulus; it can be symmetrical or asymmetric (even up to 50%) and of variable morphology according to the stimulation frequency (Fig. 14.8). PDR is usually more evident in older children and in young adults, and its amplitude is higher in children and in elderly people in respect to adults. An abnormal PDR to low frequencies (less than 5 Hz) is observed in patients with severe diffuse encephalopathy, such as progressive myoclonic epilepsy, mitochondrial encephalopathy, ceroid lipofuscinoses and Creutzfeldt-Jakob disease. Changes in PDR, of poor clinical value, are also observed in various neuropsychiatric disorders: in patients with Alzheimer's disease and schizophrenia a decrease in PDR has been reported, whereas an increase has been observed in migraine and major depression [11].

14.2.2.2 Photomyogenic Response

The Photo Myogenic Response (PMR) (also called incorrectly 'photomyoclonic response') is a non-cerebral response characterised by the appearance of brief repetitive muscle spikes in the anterior regions of the head, induced by IPS (>at 8–20 Hz) and it should be considered as a physiological electromyographic artifact. The incidence of PMR is low (0.1–0.8%) and the muscular activity often increases gradually in amplitude as stimulation continues, ceasing promptly when the stimuli are stopped. Frequently, PMR is associated with flutter of the eyelids and vertical oscillations of the eyeballs, sometimes also with myoclonic jerks involving the face and the head [24]. PMR occurs less commonly in children than in adults and it seems to be correlated with muscular tension (Fig. 14.9).

14.2.2.3 Photoparoxysmal Response

The Photo Paroxysmal Response (PPR), also called incorrectly 'photoconvulsive response', is an abnormal response to IPS characterised by the appearance of epileptiform abnormalities.

The PPR has been classified into four phenotypically different types (Waltz criteria) [31]:

- Type 1, focal occipital spikes time-locked to the flashes.
- Type 2, parieto-occipital spikes with a biphasic slow wave.
- Type 3, parieto-occipital spikes with a biphasic slow wave and spread to the frontal region.
- Type 4, generalised spike-and-slow-wave or polyspike-and-slow-wave complexes.

Figures 14.10 and 14.11 show the different types of PPRs.

Only the more generalised spike-and-wave responses (type 3 and 4 PPRs) show a strong association with epilepsy, and they may continue after the end of visual stimuli for a few seconds. There are two types of PPRs: self-limited, which ceases before or when the IPS stops, and prolonged (or self-sustaining), which continues even after the flashes stop. The generalised prolonged and self-sustaining responses show a strong association with epilepsy and patients with a prolonged PPR more often have spontaneous epileptiform abnormalities on EEG than the patients with self-limited response [7].

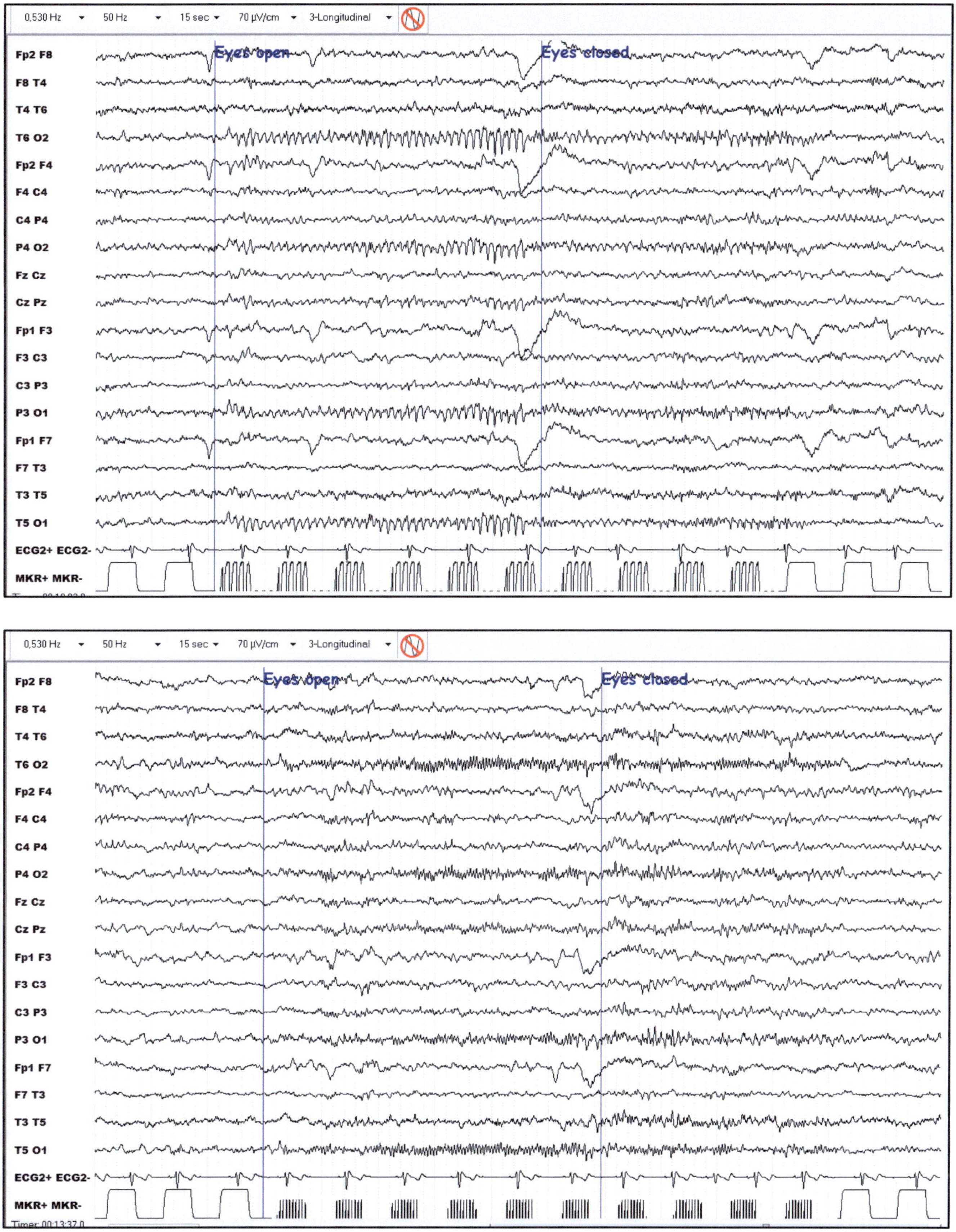

Fig. 14.8 Occipital Photic Driving Response (PDR) in a 19-year-old subject, at 8 Hz (upper) and 18 Hz (bottom)

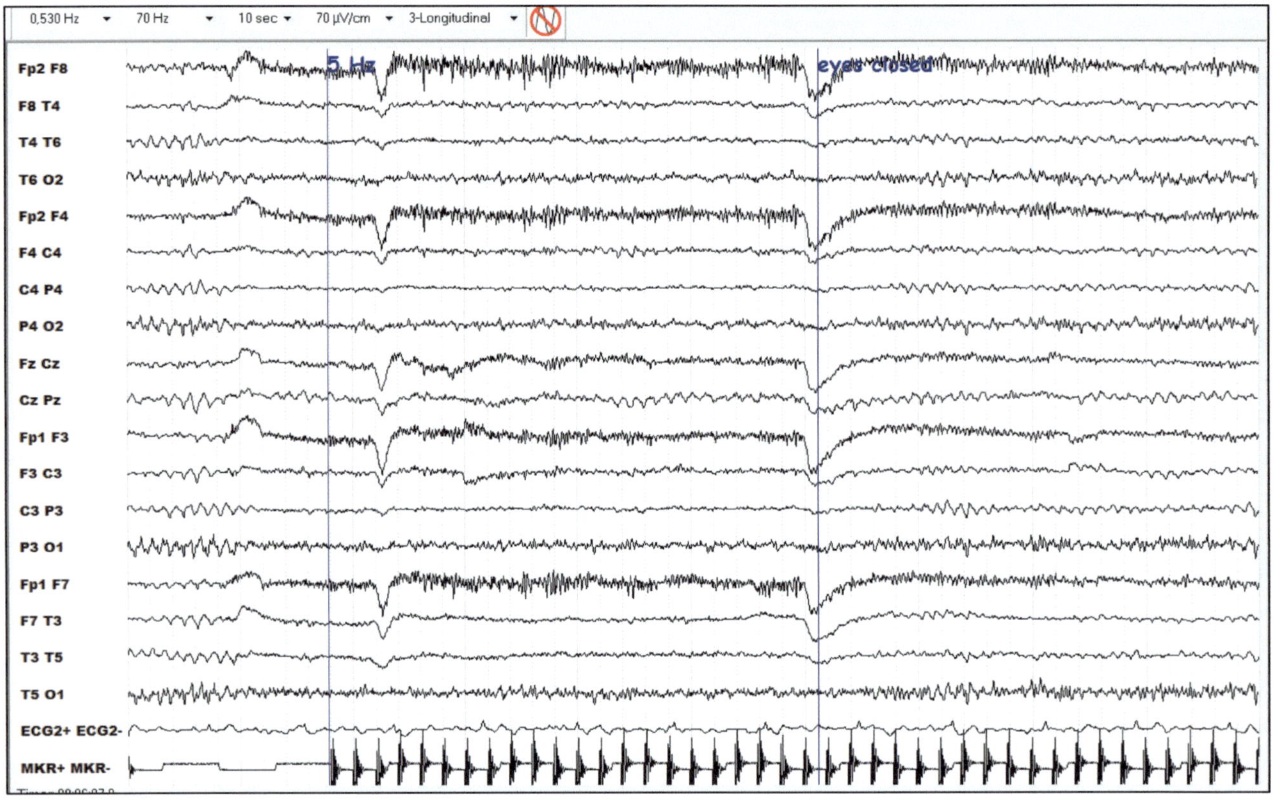

Fig. 14.9 Frontally Photo Myogenic Response (PMR) in a 35-year-old subject

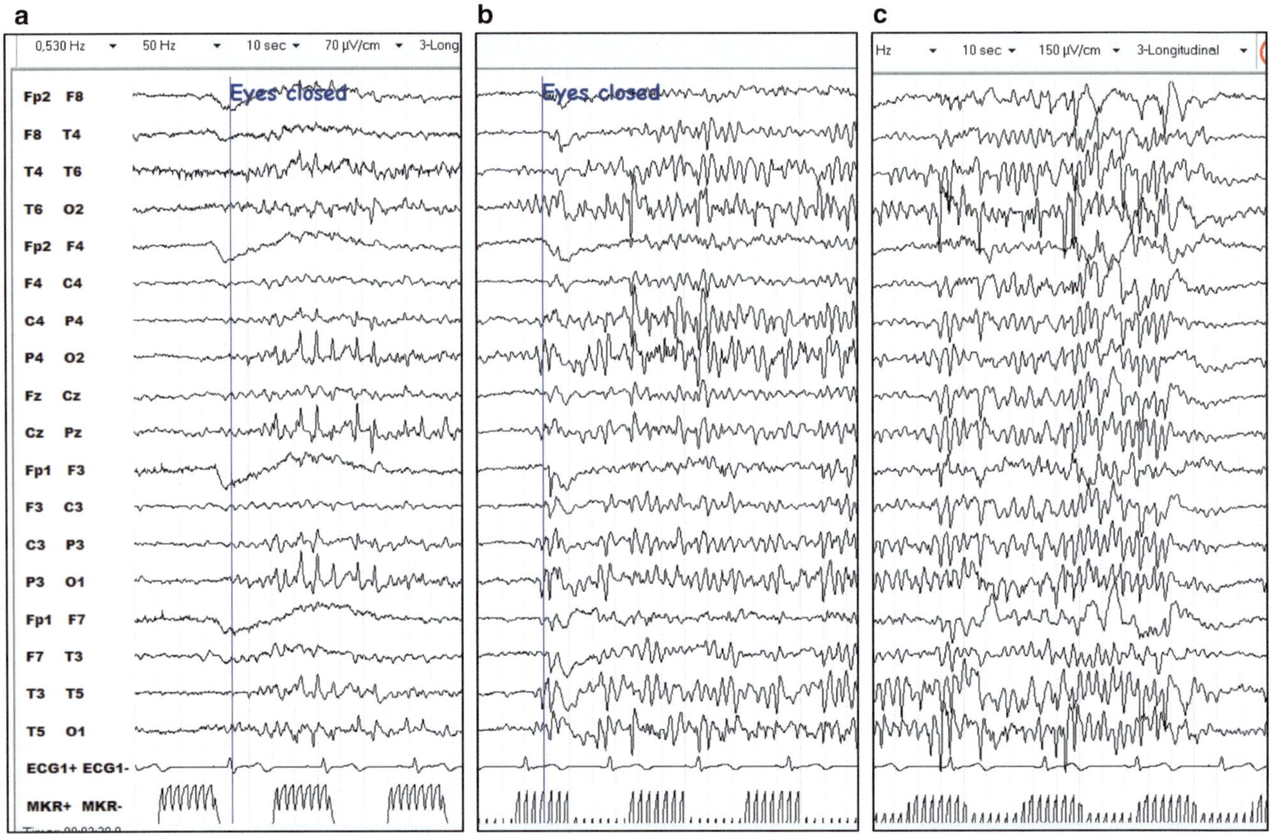

Fig. 14.10 Photo Paroxysmal Response (PPR) of type 1 (a), type 2 (b) and type 3 (c), according to Waltz criteria [31]

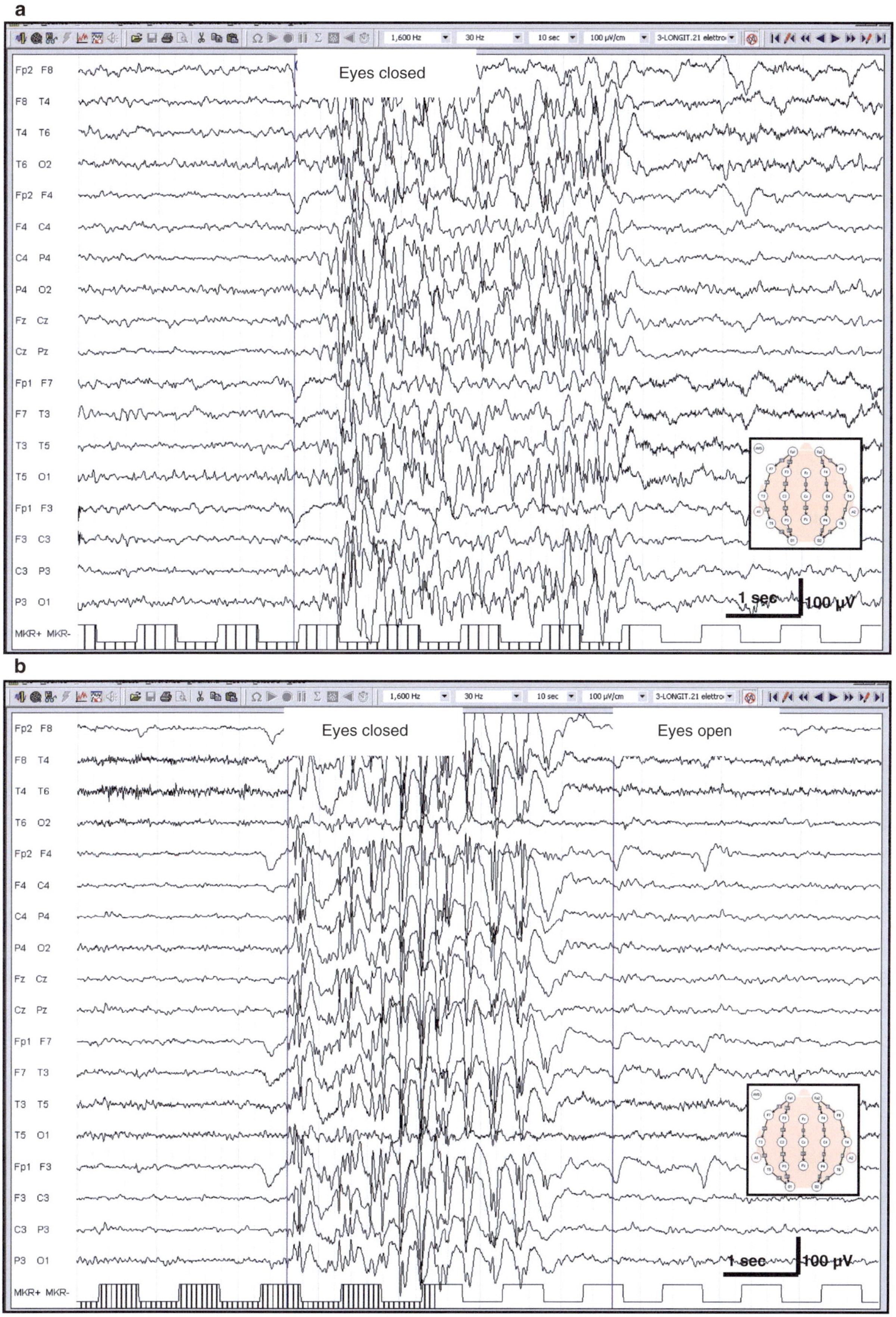

Fig. 14.11 Two examples of Photo Paroxysmal Response (PPR) type 4, in (**a**) self-limited and in (**b**) self-sustaining

Table 14.3 EEG patterns induced by IPS

Photic Driving Response (PDR)	– Time-locked to light stimulus – Same frequency or harmonically related to stimuli
PhotoMyogenic Response (PMR)	Repetitive muscle spikes over anterior regions (electromyographic response)
PhotoParoxysmal Response (PPR) Different types (Waltz criteria)	Epileptiform abnormalities induced by IPS 1. Focal occipital spikes time-locked to light stimuli 2. Parieto-occipital spikes and slow waves 3. Parieto-occipital spikes and slow waves, spreading to frontal regions 4. Generalised spike- or polyspike-and-slow-wave complexes – Self-limited – Prolonged/self-sustaining

Table 14.3 summarises the physiological and pathological EEG changes induced by Intermitten Photic Stimulation (IPS).

Occasionally, an epileptic seizure may occur in the laboratory during the IPS, particularly in a patient with evident photosensitivity, if IPS is not promptly stopped. The ictal manifestations that may be induced by IPS are absence seizures, tonic or tonic-clonic seizures and myoclonia, especially of the eyelids or limbs. Sometimes, during IPS, the patient with photosensitivity shows a negative myoclonus. As hyperventilation, IPS may also provoke psychogenic, non-epileptic seizures.

The PPRs in epileptic patients with photosensitivity are elicited by a broad range of flash frequencies, but those within the range of 10–20 Hz are the most provocative (in particular 18 Hz).

The prevalence of photosensitivity varies substantially among studies, also depending on age and gender, being highest in adolescents and in females [5, 11, 27].

In healthy children the prevalence of PPR has been reported in 1.3–8% of subjects, but higher percentages are reported in older studies that include EEG patterns non-characteristic of PPR [32]. In healthy adults examined with EEG—as aircrew candidates—PPR is identified in 0.4–0.7% up to 2.2% [28, 33, 34]. The variability of PPR prevalence in healthy subjects depends mostly on the methods of IPS and their definition.

The PPR has been also described as incidental finding in patients with other neurologic diseases (neurodegenerative disorders, migraine, etc.), but without a history of epilepsy. PPRs in non-epileptic persons rarely evolve into epilepsy [35].

Among Persons With Epilepsy (PWE), PPR is evident within a range of 0.6–5.5%, with a high prevalence in generalised genetic epilepsies of white people [5, 11, 36]. In patients with a generalised PPR, the likelihood of having epilepsy ranges approximately from 70 to 90% [37] and the likelihood of having seizures induced by IPS (photosensitivity epilepsy) is 60% [38]. The age of onset of the PPR is between 8 and 25 years, with a female predominance and a decline in IPS sensitivity after the age of 30. The PPR is a genetic trait and the epilepsies most strongly associated with photosensitivity are juvenile myoclonic epilepsy (up to 90%), generalised genetic epilepsy with tonic-clonic seizures (percentages variable from 8% to 20%) and eyelid myoclonia with absences (Jeavons syndrome) [39–41]. Waltz et al. in 1992 [31] highlighted that PPRs type 4 were present in a high proportion of the asymptomatic siblings of patients with epilepsy and recent studies have started identifying specific genes that convey risk for PPR [11]. Recent evidence points to CHD2 as a novel gene implicated in photosensitive epilepsy [42].

A high incidence of photosensitivity has also been reported in patients with progressive myoclonic epilepsies [43] and neuronal ceroid lipofuscinosis. Focal epilepsy is rarely associated with a PPR, but this pattern elicited by IPS has been described in some patients with temporal or occipital lobe epilepsy [44]. In this regard, recent studies have suggested that the Jeavons syndrome may be generated in the occipital areas [41, 45].

In patients with IPS-induced seizures, a clinical focal onset is actually often provable, due to the appearance of simple or complex visual symptoms (illusions or hallucinations). Visual symptoms are usually accompanied and/or followed by deviation of eyes and head on one side, or eyelids myoclonic jerks. Subsequently, spread of the epileptic discharge towards the limbic structures determines the appearance of automatisms typical of the temporal lobe epilepsy, with epigastric symptoms and loss of awareness.

The pathophysiological mechanisms underlying photosensitivity have been studied, but not yet fully clarified. Several studies have suggested that PPRs are triggered from the hypersyncronised visual cortex [46]. Patients with idiopathic occipital photosensitive epilepsy show increased Visual Evoked Potential (VEP) amplitude and abnormal latencies for high-contrast visual stimuli, suggesting a failure of cortical gain control (the gain control is the mechanism by which a biological system dynamically adjusts its sensitivity to the inputs) [47, 48]. In addition, patients with idiopathic generalised epilepsy have demonstrated less saturation of the VEP response amplitudes, thus reflecting an abnormality in neuronal gain control, possibly due to reduced GABAergic inhibition [49].

On the other hand, the hyperexcitability of the occipital cortex alone cannot fully explain the clinical and EEG correlates of photosensitivity (motor symptoms associated with generalised epileptiform discharges). Current data indicate indeed that photosensitivity is the expression of an alteration of the visual system not limited to the occipital cortex, but extended also to the parietal and premotor cortex. Studies conducted using EEG in combination with functional Magnetic Resonance Imaging (fMRI) have described the metabolic and hemodynamic consequences of IPS in control subjects and in patients with PPR [50, 51]. IPS led to a significant activation of the visual cortex and, 3 s before the PPR onset, the cortical activation was also found in the parietal and in the premotor cortex [52]. In patients with eyelid myoclonus with absences (Jeavons syndrome), it have been demonstrated that visual system alterations involve a circuit encompassing the occipital cortex and the cortical/subcortical system physiologically involved in the motor control of eye closure and eye movements [41]. Furthermore, studies combining Transcranial Magnetic Stimulation (TMS) of motor cortex or visual stimulation of occipital cortex have demonstrated that the PPR is due to abnormal visuomotor interactions [53, 54]. Subsequently, the PPR is due to the hyperexcitability of occipital cortex that affects other regions via network interactions.

Finally, Vaudano et al. [55] studied the hemodynamic correlations of the alpha rhythm in photosensitivity epileptic patients, in comparison to patients without photosensitivity and healthy controls. The authors used EEG-fMRI to investigate if the fluctuations in the alpha rhythm were correlated with changes in the Blood Oxygenation Level-Dependent (BOLD) signal in cortical and subcortical regions. Whole brain functional connectivity was evaluated for two thalamic nuclei (posterior and medio-dorsal). In photosensitive patients the alpha-related BOLD changes decrease in the occipital, sensory-motor, anterior cingulate and supplementary motor cortices in comparison with other groups. Furthermore, the same brain regions showed abnormal connectivity with thalamus only in epileptic photosensitive patients. These results demonstrate that the cortical-subcortical network generating the alpha oscillation is different in persons with epilepsy and photosensitivity.

14.3 Other Methods of Visual Stimulation

14.3.1 Pattern Stimulation

A remarkable number of photosensitive patients are sensitive not only to IPS, but also to geometric patterns. The incidence of paroxysmal discharges induced by patterns varies widely across studies (from 5% to 72%) depending on the spatial and temporal characteristics of visual pattern and stimulation protocol [11, 56]. However, there have also been reported patients responding to these pattern, but not to IPS. The most activating geometric pattern consists of parallel lines or stripes with sharp edges, black-and-white and high-contrasted (Fig. 14.12) [29]. The stimulation can be performed with eyes open, in ambient light with a monitor

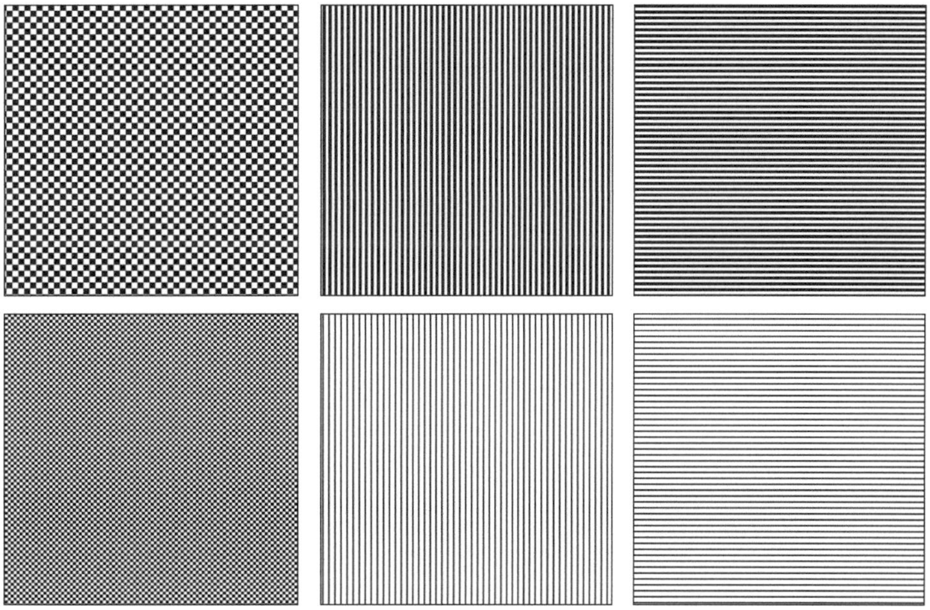

Fig. 14.12 Examples of geometric pattern used for the pattern stimulation

connected to an electronic grating generator, positioned 1 m from the patient's eyes. Each pattern is presented for 10 s, in oscillatory (optimal oscillation frequency, 15–20 Hz) or stationary modality, at spatial frequencies between 0.5 and 6 cycles/degree. Pattern sensitivity occurs in various epileptic syndromes, but according to Radhakrishnan et al. [57], it is a readily distinguishable subtype of the visually provoked reflex epilepsies.

14.3.2 Low-Luminance Visual Stimulation

The Low-Luminance Visual Stimulation (LLVS) is performed only with eyes open, with luminance ranging between 10 and 30 cd/m² [29]. The combination of low-luminance flickering at 18 Hz with red light and pattern modality has been reported as particularly useful for activating PPR [58]. For this stimulation, three different patterns can be used (dot pattern, vertical grating, or horizontal grating) with spatial frequency of 2 cycles/degree; a red strobo-filter can be used to produce a red flicker at >600 nm wavelength [29]. The importance of flickering colour/pattern was demonstrated in the famous Pokémon incident in Japan in December 1997. In this case, a TV cartoon containing a 4 s red/blue sequence flickering at 12 Hz elicited simultaneous seizures in 685 children; 76% of them had never presented a seizure before.

14.3.3 Fixation-Off Sensitivity

Fixation-Off Sensitivity (FOS) is a rare phenomenon induced by the elimination of central vision/fixation. FOS is characterised by continuous posterior or diffuse epileptiform discharges that appear 1–3 s after eye closure, persist throughout the EEG recording with eye closed and disappear immediately with eye opening (Fig. 14.13) [59, 60]. A definite diagnosis of FOS requires a demonstration that the epileptiform abnormalities also occur by impending central vision and fixation using Frenzel lenses or by placing a sheet of white paper 20 cm in front of the subject (with eyes open, but without fixation). The

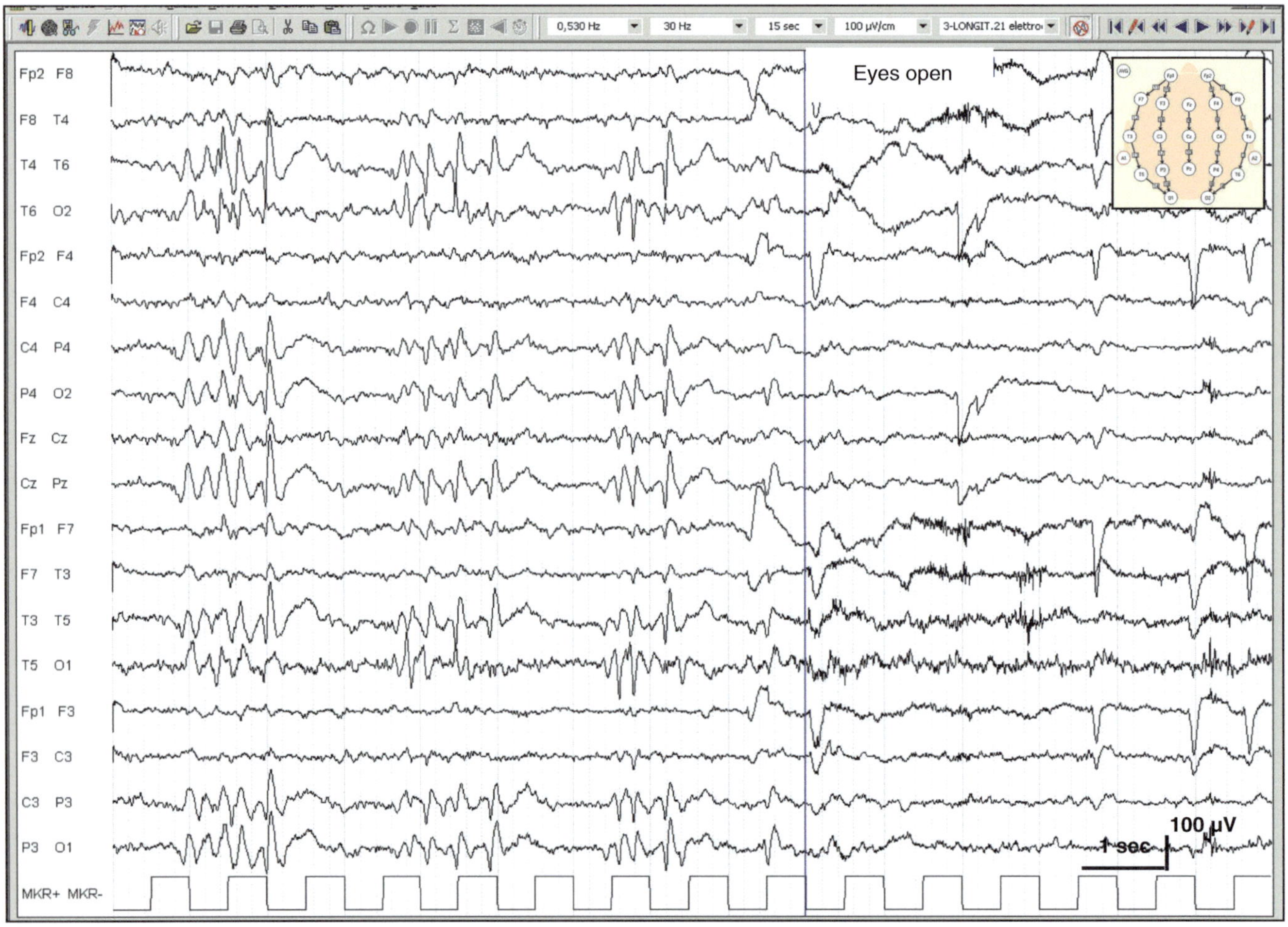

Fig. 14.13 Fixation-Off Sensitivity (FOS) phenomenon in a 26-year-old patient with focal epilepsy. With eyes closed, subcontinuous epileptiform abnormalities in the posterior regions of both hemispheres, without clinical correlates appear. Epileptiform activity immediately disappears with eyes opening

epileptiform abnormalities (spike, spike and wave, sharp wave) can be registered in patients without clinical epileptic seizures, but most commonly FOS is associated with occipital idiopathic childhood epilepsies or with focal or generalised symptomatic epilepsies. fMRI studies showed a correlation between posterior FOS and a focal activation of both extrastriate temporo-occipital and also of the frontal lobe regions [61]. Low-frequency repetitive TMS (rTMS) reduce FOS-related focal epileptiform activity [62]. In conclusion, based on the knowledge acquired so far, FOS seems to be the expression of the occipital hyperexcitability, but the exact mechanisms underlying this phenomenon remains somewhat obscure.

14.4 Sleep and Sleep Deprivation

According to American Clinical Neurophysiology Society [1], sleep EEG recording should be performed whenever possible, even if not alternatively with the awake recording. As a matter of fact, there are evidences that sleep EEG helps make a better classification of an epileptic syndrome that helps for the diagnosis in patients with suspected epilepsy [5]. The sleep recording should include wakefulness, drowsiness and at least 40 min of sleep [2].

It is well known that some types of epileptic seizures can be closely related to the sleep-wake rhythm and that it is common to observe, in sleep EEG, the appearance of epileptic abnormalities that are not present in the awake recording. Moreover, in patients with epileptiform abnormalities in the awake EEG, the increase or spatial change of the abnormal features (focal vs multifocal or diffuse pattern) can be observed during the sleep EEG. Sleep, therefore—like hyperventilation and photostimulation—can be considered a method of EEG activation, easy to perform and completely harmless.

In patients who previously had a normal standard awake EEG, the recording during sleep has a variable diagnostic yield percentage, from 11% to 92%; this wide variability is due to the differences in study design, the specific characteristics of patient population, etc. In summary, from the evidences in the literature review, it can be argued that sleep may activate Interictal Epileptiform Discharges (IEDs) in about 30% of persons with epilepsy, mostly in those with epilepsies sleep-related or with seizures at awakening.

Prolonged night-time recordings in patients with epilepsy have shown that not all the sleep stages are equally in activating EEG abnormalities, but that the most important information is obtained from the early stages (N1–N2) and from awakening, while the stages N3 and R are the less activating. For this reason, it is generally sufficient to record in the EEG laboratory only a brief (40–60 min) period of daytime sleep, allowing to record N1 and N2 sleep stages and awakening (afternoon nap).

The evaluation of the effect of the various stages of sleep on IEDs, focal or generalised is particularly interesting. The focal IEDs most commonly increase at sleep onset; they reach the maximum of their activity in N2 stage (with tendency to multifocal or diffuse spread) and then fall in R sleep to levels lower than seen in wakefulness, remaining well localised (Fig. 14.14). This influence of sleep on focal IEDs is evident in the epilepsy with centro-temporal spikes; in this type of epilepsy, rolandic spikes have the maximal activity in N1 and N2 sleep and appear to be related to sleep spindle synchronisation. In addition, the diffuse IEDs, characteristic of the genetic generalised epilepsies, usually increase in N sleep (>in stages N1 and N2). Typically, spike rates increase with sleep onset, continue to increase during sleep progression, diminish sharply in R sleep and increase in the morning after awakening. During the N sleep, the generalised IEDs often become more disorganised, with shorter bursts of polyspikes, at quasi-periodic recurrence ('fragmented' epileptiform activity) (Fig. 14.15) [63, 64]. In the R stage, the discharges are instead rare and quite similar to those of the awake state. Closely related to the sleep-wake rhythm are the generalised IEDs of the juvenile myoclonic epilepsy; in this type of epilepsy, the IEDs are often only observed at sleep onset and at awakening, disappearing completely during the course of sleep. Moreover, the provoked and early awakening seems to be more activating on IEDs than spontaneous awakening.

In summary, both focal and generalised IEDs appear to be activated by N sleep and inhibited by R sleep. During N sleep, the EEG synchronisation processes are particularly active (involving the thalamocortical circuits) and the same hypersynchronous oscillations of cortical neurons that determine the appearance of sleep spindles, K complexes and slow hypersynchronous EEG activity can therefore facilitate the IEDs appearance. Conversely, increased brainstem excitatory inputs in R sleep depolarize the thalamocortical cells and induce EEG desynchronisation, being responsible also for the inhibition of IEDs [64].

Studies on the microstructure of sleep have shown that there is an association between IEDs recurrence during N sleep and different phases of Cyclic Alternating Pattern (CAP). CAP is considered a marker of sleep instability and IEDs are activated mostly during the phase A, while phase B exerts a powerful and prolonged inhibitory action. The NCAP period represents instead an intermediate stationary level. Both in generalised and focal epilepsies, the IEDs and seizures have an onset in correlation with the phase A of CAP. The only exception is the epilepsy with centro-temporal spikes of childhood, in which the frequency of discharges does not show any significant modification by comparing the two phases of the CAP and the CAP and NCAP period [65–67].

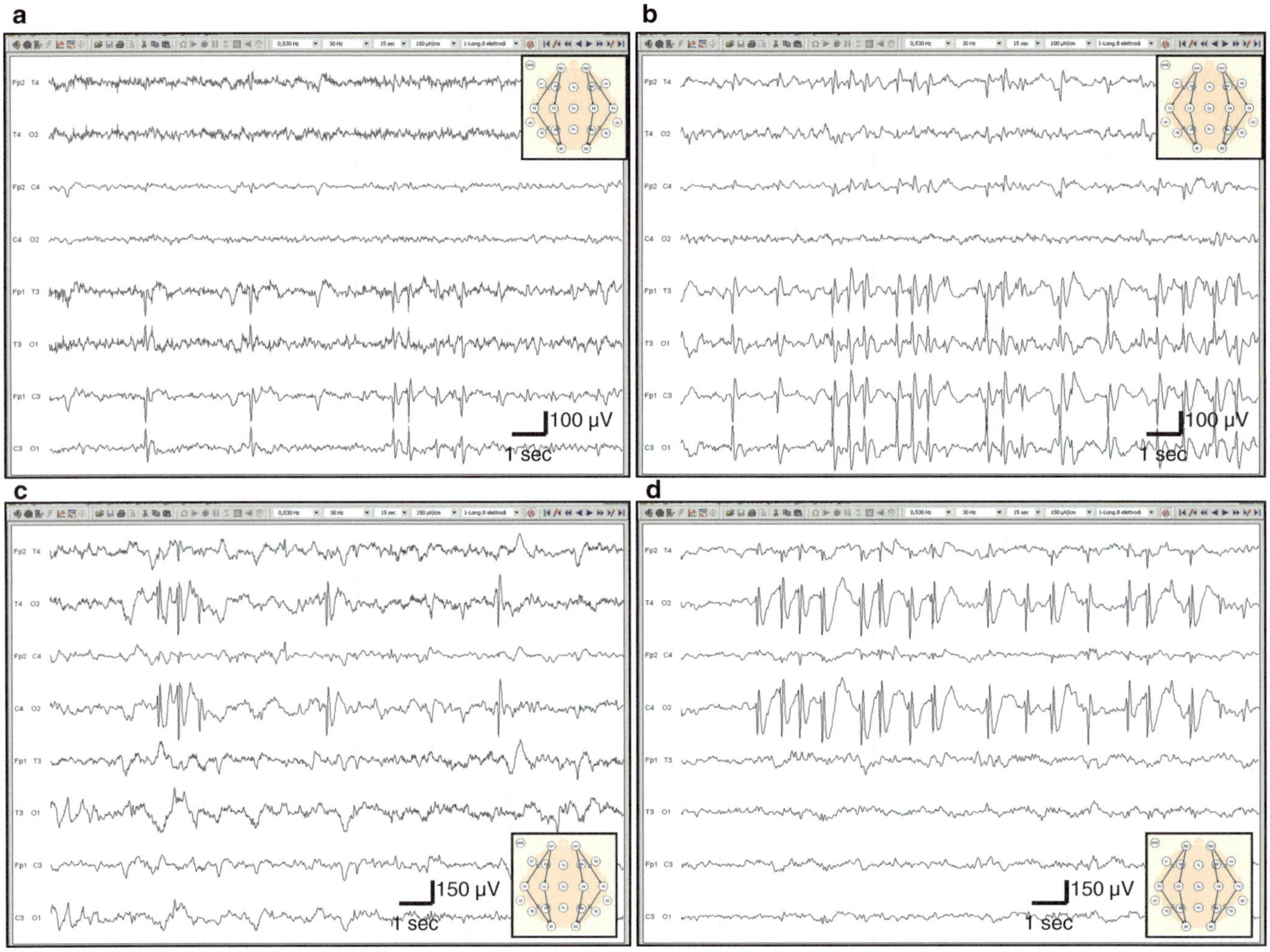

Fig. 14.14 Two examples of sleep-induced focal epileptic activity increase during N2 stage. Top: focal centro-temporal spikes during wake (**a**) in an 8-year-old child and their increase during sleep, with tendency to contralateral anterior regions diffusion (**b**). Bottom: right occipital epileptiform abnormalities in an awaken 6-year-old child (**c**) and their increase during light sleep (**d**)

Another EEG activating method, closely related to mechanisms of induction of sleep, is the so-called Sleep Deprivation (SD). Loss of nocturnal sleep is one of the major trigger for epileptic seizures, both in the healthy and epileptic people. In the 18–24% of epileptic adults, seizures are elicited by sleep deprivation and about 30–70% of persons with epilepsy having a nonsignificant standard EEG patterns show a pathological EEG activation after a long and forced awake period [68, 69]. Since it has been described that EEG recordings after SD do not show particular abnormalities in healthy subjects and in patients with neurological disorders other than epilepsy, this activating procedure is considered specific for persons with epilepsy, already diagnosed or only suspected.

However, the diagnostic yield of SD is still under discussion, also because the numerous studies carried out on this topic have been conducted with different methods, in patients with different types of epilepsy and, sometimes, also treated with antiepileptic drugs.

The SD method varies significantly from one centre to another, with length of sleep deprivation ranging from 3 to 36 h and the duration of EEG recording ranging from 30 min to 24 h.

In our laboratory, EEG recording in adults is usually performed early in the morning, after a total night-time sleep deprivation, while children are generally woken up early at night, with only partial deprivation (6–8 h). The EEG recording (as prolonged as possible) includes a quiet awake period, followed by falling asleep and recording at least N1–N3 stages; after waking up, both IPS and HV are performed (the SD accentuates the response both to photostimulation and to hyperventilation) (Fig. 14.16).

While most of the literature studies used 24 h of SD, some studies confirmed the activating effect of partial SD as

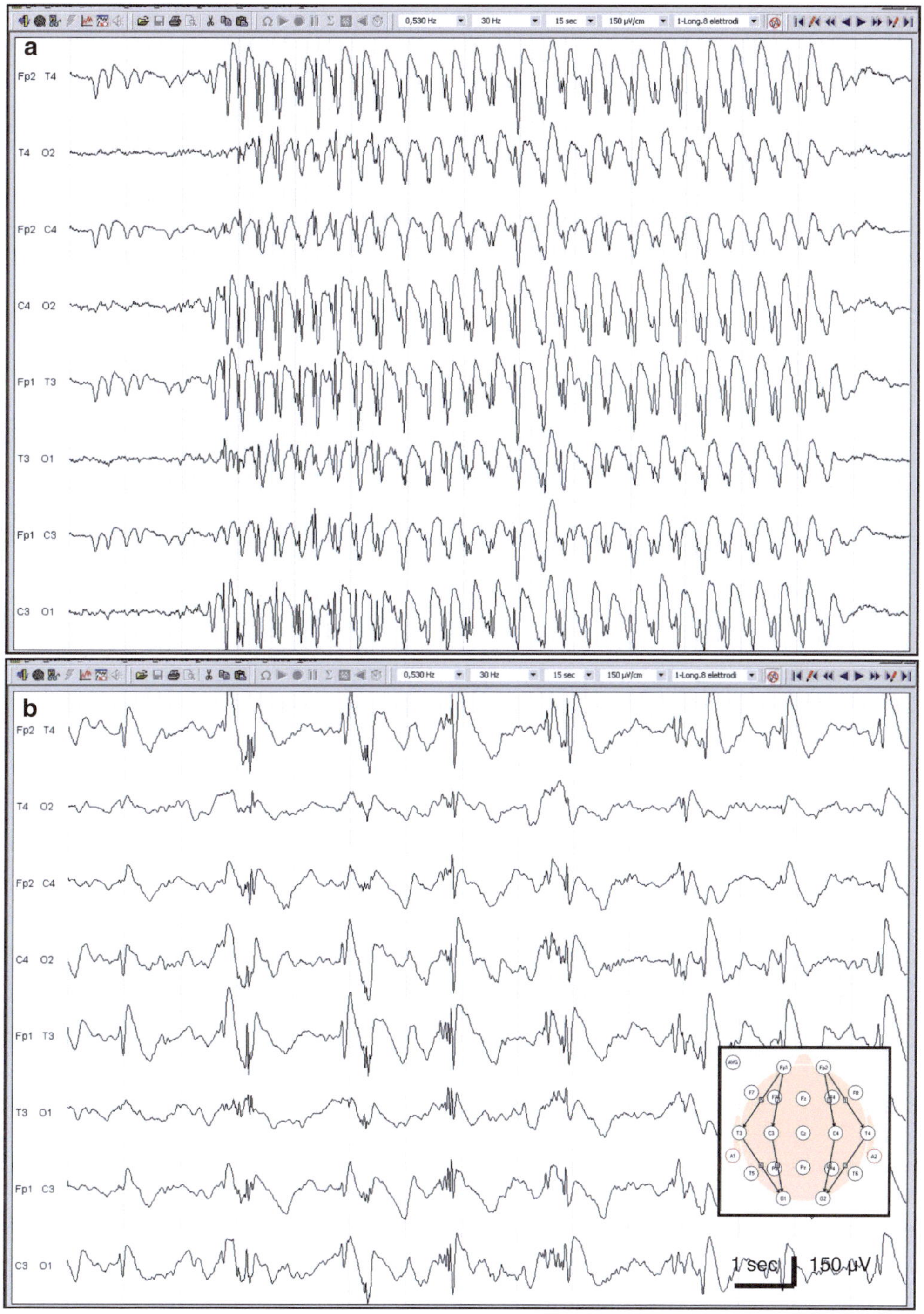

Fig. 14.15 Typical discharge of spike-and-wave complexes at 3 Hz in an awake adolescent with generalised epilepsy with absences (**a**). During N2 stage of sleep (**b**), the epileptic activity is organised in brief bursts of polyspikes-and-wave complexes, at quasi-periodic recurrence

well [5, 70, 71]. Giorgi et al. [72] evaluated the role of a simple SD-EEG protocol in a wide population of de novo patients with suspected epileptic seizures; the protocol consisted of waking up at 2:00 a.m. and EEG monitoring from 8:00 until 10:30 a.m. The authors report 91.1% specificity for epilepsy diagnosis and showed IEDs in 41.2% of all patients. According to authors, the IEDs yield in SD-EEG is higher than in second routine EEG for focal epilepsies. Nevertheless, these results are not confirmed by Renzel et al. [73] who studied patients with suspected epilepsy with an EEG after 24 h SD and comparing the results with those of a previous routine EEG. The overall sensitivity is of 25%, superior in patients with idiopathic generalised epilepsy, compared to patients with focal epilepsies (65% vs. 17%). Recently, Baldin et al. [11] found that in their population-based study, the yield on the first sleep EEG was 16.45%, consistent with a previous literature studies, and that it did not differ between generalised and focal seizure types.

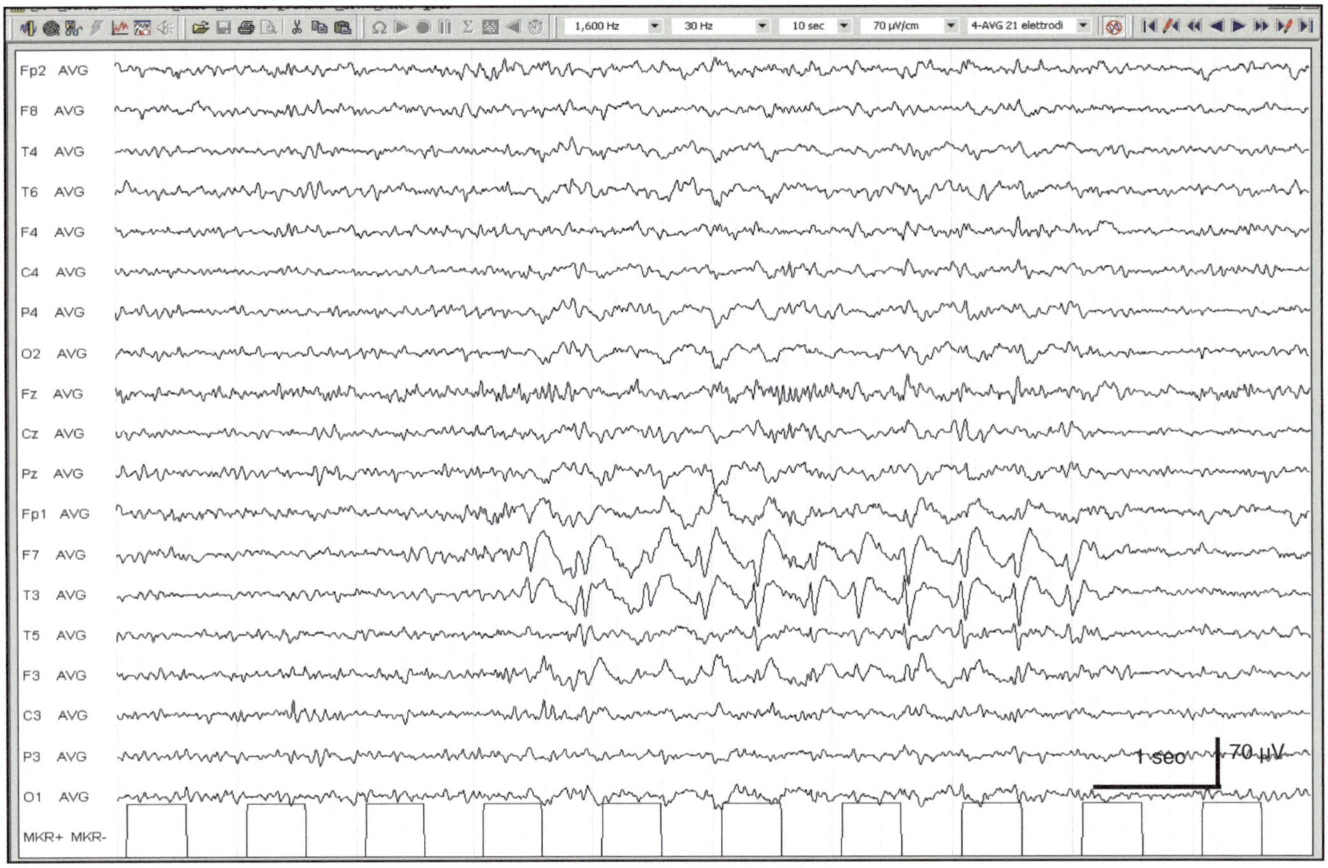

Fig. 14.16 A 25-year-old patient with temporal lobe epilepsy. Basal EEG without remarkable abnormalities. During hyperventilation, after 24-h sleep deprivation, clear focal epileptiform abnormalities in left temporal region appear

It is still debated whether the EEG activation induced by SD is merely due to the drowsiness and sleep (consequent of SD) or whether SD per se has an activating effect [64, 74]. Using transcranial magnetic stimulation, Badawy et al. [75] have demonstrated that cortical excitability increased at short and long interstimulus interval in patients with epilepsy after SD. In the generalised epilepsies, these changes were significant in both hemispheres while, in focal epilepsies, they were localised in the seizure focus hemisphere.

Finally, the results of studies on drug-induced sleep are conflicting [5] and it is preferable to obtain a natural sleep. In agitated and fearful children, it is however sometimes necessary to use a mild sedation, classically with chloral hydrate or with alternative sedatives such as dexmedetomidine, hydroxyzine or melatonin [71, 76].

14.5 Other Stimulation

Specific activation procedures can be applied to patients with reflex epilepsy, from auditory or somatosensory stimuli to more complex stimuli such as eating, reading, writing, etc. (see Chap. 28 on Reflex Epilepsy). Repetitive acoustic stimulation through click trains can trigger epileptic abnormalities both in patients with focal epilepsy (especially of the temporal lobe) and, more rarely, with generalised epilepsy [77]. Moreover, acoustic stimulation is extremely effective in all those cases in which the level of alertness is fluctuating. For these reasons, it would be useful that each EEG machine is equipped also with a sound stimulator. It is also known that, in some types of epilepsy, reflex seizures can be triggered by listening to particular musical pieces, songs and other structured sound sources; therefore, in the laboratory, an instrument for the reproduction of such stimuli should always be available. The application of somatosensory stimuli at the extremities of the limbs can induce the appearance on the EEG of the epileptiform graphoelements both in children with benign epilepsy with centro-temporal spikes as well as in non-epileptic persons.

Each stimulus (i.e. finger tapping) should be administered 5–10 times with an interstimulus interval of 2 s. In epileptic children with centro-temporal spikes, it should be observed on the scalp, after stimulation of tibial or median nerves, the giant somatosensory evoked potentials (giant SEPs), due to a hyperexcitability of primary somatosensory and motor cortices.

These features are recorded also in progressive myoclonic epilepsies and in cortical reflex myoclonus [11, 78–80].

Acknowledgments I am grateful to Dr. Patrizia Pulitano for her help in selecting and editing the EEG figures.

References

1. Flink R, Pedersen B, Guekht AB, et al. Guidelines for the use of EEG methodology in the diagnosis of epilepsy. Acta Neurol Scand. 2002;106:1–7.
2. Sinha SR, Sullivan L, Sabau D, et al. American Clinical Neurophysiology Society Guideline 1:minimum technical requirements for performing clinical electroencephalography. J Clin Neurophysiol. 2016;33:303–7.
3. Kane N, Grocott L, Kandler R, Lawrence S, Pang C. Hyperventilation during electroencephalography:safety and efficacy. Seizure. 2014;23:129–34.
4. Craciun L, Varga ET, Mindruta I, et al. Diagnostic yeld of five minutes compared to three minutes hyperventilation during electroencephalography. Seizure. 2015;30:90–2.
5. Tatum WO, Rubboli G, Kaplan PW, et al. Clinical utility of EEG in diagnosing and monitoring epilepsy in adults. Clin Neurophysiol. 2018;129:1056–82.
6. Gibbs F, Davis H, Lennox W. The electro-encephalogram in epilepsy and in conditions of impaired consciousness. Arch Neurol Psychiatry. 1935;34:1133–48.
7. Mendez OE, Brenner RP. Increasing the yield of EEG. J Clin Neurophysiol. 2006;23:282–93.
8. Lum LM, Connolly MB, Farrel K, Wong PK. Hyperventilation-induced high-amplitude rhythmic slowing with altered awareness: a video-EEG comparison with absence seizures. Epilepsia. 2002;43:1372–8.
9. Barker A, Ng J, Rittey CD, Kandler RH, Mordekar SR. Outcome of children with hyperventilation-induced high-amplitude rhythmic slow activity with altered awareness. Dev Med Child Neurol. 2012;54:1001–5.
10. Salvati KA, Beenhakker MP. Out of thin air: hyperventilation-trigger seizures. Brain Res;2017 (online).
11. Shafi MM, Westover MB. EEG activation methods. In: Schomer DL, Lopes da Silva Eds FH, editors. Niedermeyer's electroencephalography. Basic principles, clinical applications, and related fields. 7th ed. Oxford: Oxford University Press;2018. p. 247–65.
12. Mecarelli O, Pulitano P, Vicenzini E, Vanacore N, Accornero N, De Marinis M. Observations on EEG patterns in neurally-mediated syncope: an inspective and quantitative study. Neurophysiol Clin. 2004;34:203–7.
13. Guaranha MSB, Garzon E, Buchpiguel CA, Tazima S, Yacubian EMT, Sakamoto AC. Hyperventilation revisited: physiological effects and efficacy on focal seizure activation in the era of video-EEG monitoring. Epilepsia. 2005;46:69–75.
14. Baldin E, Hauser WA, Buchhalter JR, Hesdorffer DC, Ottman R. Utility of EEG activation procedures in epilepsy: a population-based study. J Clin Neurophysiol. 2017;34:512–9.
15. Dlamini N, Goyal S, Jarosz J, Hampton T, Siddiqui A, Hughes E. Paroxysmal episodes, "re-buildup" phenomenon and Moyamoya disease. Epileptic Disord. 2009;11:324–8.
16. Abubakr A, Iteayni I, Wambacq I. The efficacy of routine hyperventilation for seizure activation during prolonged video-electroencephalography monitoring. J Clin Neurosci. 2010;17:1503–5.
17. Benbadis SR, Johnson K, Anthony K, et al. Induction of psychogenic non-epileptic seizures without placebo. Neurology. 2000;55:1904–5.
18. Achenbach-Ng J, Siao TC, Mavroudakis N, Chiappa KH, Kiers L. Effects of routine hyperventilation on PCO2 and PO2 in normal subjects: implications for EEG interpretations. J Clin Neurophysiol. 1994;11:220–5.
19. Duarte J, Markus H, Harrison MJG. Changes in cerebral blood flow as monitored by transcranial Doppler during voluntary hyperventilation and their effect on the electroencephalogram. J Neuroimg. 1995;5:209–11.
20. Yamatani M, Konishi T, Murakami M, Okuda T. Hyperventilation activation on EEG recording in children with epilepsy. Pediatr Neurol. 1995;13:42–5.
21. Van der Worp HB, Wienecke GH, Van Huffelen AC. Quantitative EEG during progressive hypocarbia and hypoxia. Hyperventilation-induced EEG changes reconsidered. Electroencephalogr Clin Neurophysiol. 1991;79:335–41.
22. Patel VM, Maulsby RL. How hyperventilation alters the electroencephalogram: a review of controversial viewpoints emphasizing neurophysiological mechanisms. J Clin Neurophysiol. 1987;4:101–20.
23. Esquivel E, Chaussain M, Plouin P, Ponsot G, Arthuis M. Physical exercise and voluntary hyperventilation in childhood absence epilepsy. Electroencephalogr Clin Neurophysiol. 1991;79: 127–32.
24. Kane N, Acharya J, Benickzy S, et al. A revised glossary of term most commonly used by clinical electroencephalographers and uptated proposal for the report format of the EEG findings. Revision 2017. Clin Neurophysiol Practice. 2017 ;2:170–85.
25. Adrian E, Matthews B. The Berger rhythm: potential changes from the occipital lobes in man. Brain. 1934;57:355–85.
26. Walter W, Dovey V, Shipton H. Analysis of the electrical response of the human cortex to photic stimulation. Nature. 1946;158:540–1.
27. Kasteleijn-Nolst Trenité DG. Photosensitivity in epilepsy. Electrophysiological and clinical correlates. Acta Neurol Scand Suppl. 1989;125:3–149.
28. Kasteleijn-Nolst Trenité DG. Intermittent photic stimulation as an activation method for electroencephalographic screening of aircrew applicants. Epilepsy Behav. 2005;6:21–6.
29. Rubboli G, Parra J, Seri S, Takahashi T, Thomas P. EEG diagnostic procedures and special investigations in the assessment of photosensitivity. Epilepsia. 2004;45:35–9.
30. Kasteleijn-Nolst Trenité DG, Rubboli G, Hirsch E, et al. Methodology of photic stimulation revisited: updated European algorithm for visual stimulation in the EEG laboratory. Epilepsia. 2012;53:16–24.
31. Waltz S, Christen H-J, Doose H. The different patterns of the photoparoxysmal response – a genetic study. Electroencephalogr Clin Neurophysiol. 1992;82:138–45.
32. Doose H, Gerken H. On the genetics of EEG anomalies in childhood (1)-(IV). Photoconvulsive reaction. Neuropediatrics. 1973;4:162–71.
33. Trojaborg W. EEG abnormmalities in 5.893 jet pilot applicants registered in a 20-year period. Clin EEG Electroenceph. 1992;23:72–8.
34. Gregory RP, Oates T, Merry RT. Electroencephalogram epileptiform abnormalities in candidates for aircrew training. Electroencephalogr Clin Neurophysiol. 1993;86:75–7.
35. So EL, Ruggles KH, Ahmann PA, Olson KA. Prognosis of photoparoxysmal response in nonepileptic patients. Neurology. 1193;43:1719–22.
36. De Graaf AS, Lombard CJ, Claasen DA. Influence of ethnic and geographic factors on the classic photoparoxysmal response in the electroencephalogram of epilepsy patients. Epilepsia. 1995;36:210–23.
37. Jayakar P, Chiappa KH. Clinical correlations of photoparoxysmal responses. Electroencephalogr Clin Neurophysiol. 1990;75:251–4.
38. Kasteleijn-Nolst Trenité DG, Guerrini R, Binnie CD, et al. Visual sensitivity and epilepsy: a proposed terminology and classification for clinical and EEG phenomenology. Epilepsia. 2001;42: 692–701.

39. Stephani U, Tauer U, Koeleman B, Pinto D, Neubauer BA, Lindhout D. Genetics of photosensitivity (photopharoxysmal response): a review. Epilepsia. 2004;45(s1):19–23.
40. Viravan S, Go C, Ochi A, Akiyama T, Carter Snead O, Otsubo H. Jeavons syndrome exisisting as occipital cortex initiating generalized epilepsy. Epilepsia. 2011;5:1273–9.
41. Vaudano AE, Ruggieri A, Tondelli M, et al. The visual system in eyelid myoclonia with absences. Ann Neurol. 2014;76:412–27.
42. Galizia EC, Myers CT, Leu C, et al. CDH2 variants as a risk factor for photosensitivity in epilepsy. Brain. 2015;138:1198–207.
43. Rubboli G, Meletti S, Gardella E, et al. Photic reflex myoclonus: a neurophysiological study in progressive myoclonic epilepsies. Epilepsia. 1999;40:50–8.
44. Guerrini R, Dravet C, Genton P, et al. Idiopathic photosensitive occipital lobe epilepsy. Epilepsia. 1995;36:883–91.
45. Giraldez BG, Serratosa JM. Jeavons syndrome as an occipital cortex initiated generalized epilepsy: further evidence for a patient with a photic-induced occipital seizure. Seizure. 2015;32:72–4.
46. Wilkins AJ, Bonanni P, Porciatti V, Guerrini R. Physiology of human photosensitivity. Epilepsia. 2004;45:7–13.
47. Porciatti V, Bonanni P, Fiorentini A, Guerrini R. Lack of cortical contrast gain control in human photosensitive epilepsy. Nat Neurosci. 2000;3:259–63.
48. Siniatchkin M, Moeller F, Shepherd A, Siebner H, Stephani U. Altered cortical visual processing in individuals with a spreading photoparoxysmal EEG response. Eur J Neurosci. 2007;26:529–36.
49. Tsai JJ, Norcia AM, Ales JM, Wade AR. Constrast gain control abnormalities in idiopathic generalized epilepsy. Ann Neurol. 2011;70:574–82.
50. Chiappa KH, Hill RA, Huang-Hellinger F, Jenkins BG. Photosensitive epilepsy studied by functional magnetic resonance imaging and magnetic resonance spectroscopy. Epilepsia. 1999;40(Suppl 4):3–7.
51. Hill RA, Chiappa KH, Huang-Hellinger F, Jenkins BG. Hemodynamic and metabolic aspects of photosensitive epilepsy revealed by functional magnetic resonance imaging and magnetic resonance spectroscopy. Epilepsia. 1999;40:912–20.
52. Moeller F, Siebner HR, Ahlgrimm N, et al. fMRI activation during spike and wave discharges evoked by photic stimulation. Neuroimage. 2009;48:682–95.
53. Strigaro G, Falletta L, Varrasi C, et al. Overactive visuomotor connections underlie the photoparoxysmal response. A TMS study. Epilepsia. 2015;56:1828–35.
54. Suppa A, Rocchi L, Li Voti P, et al. The photoparoxysmal response reflects abnormal early visuomotor integration in the human motor cortex. Brain Stimul. 2015;8:1151–61.
55. Vaudano AE, Ruggieri A, Avanzini P, et al. Photosensitive epilepsy is associated with reduced inhibition of alpha rhythm generating networks. Brain. 2017;140:981–97.
56. Fisher RS, Harding G, Erba G, Barkley GL, Wilkins A. Photic- and pattern-induced seizures:a review for the Epilepsy Foundation of America Working Group. Epilepsia. 2005;46:1426–41.
57. Radhakrishnan K, St.Louis EK, Johnson JA, McClelland RL, Westmoreland BF, Klass DW. Pattern-sensitive epilepsy:electroclinical characteristics, natural hystory, and delineation of the epileptic syndrome. Epilepsia. 2005;46:48–58.
58. Takahashi T, Nakasato N, Yokoyama H, et al. Low-luminance isual stimuli compared with stroboscopic IPS in eliciting PPR in photosensitive patients. Epilepsia. 1999;40(Suppl 4):44–9.
59. Koutroumanidis M, Tsatsou K, Sanders S, et al. Fixation-off sensitivity in epilepsies other than the idiopathic epilepsies of childhood with occipital paroxysms: a 12 year clinical-videoEEG study. Epileptic Disord. 2009;11:20–36.
60. Brigo F, Rossini F, Stefani A, et al. Fixation-off sensitivity. Clin Neurophysiol. 2013;124:221–7.
61. Krakow K, Baxendale SA, Maguire EA, et al. Fixation-off sensitivity as a model of continuous epileptiform discharges: electroencephalographic, neuropsycological, and functional MRI findings. Epilepsy Res. 2000;42:1–6.
62. Mecarelli O, Gregori B, Gilio F, et al. Effects of repetitive transcranial magnetic stimulation in a patient with fixation-off sensitivity. Exp Brain Res. 2006;173:180–4.
63. Shouse MN, da Silva AM, Sammaritano M. Circadian rhythm, sleep, and epilepsy. J Clin Neurophysiol. 1996;13:32–50.
64. Foldvary-Schaefer N, Grigg-Damberger M. Sleep and epilepsy: what we know, don't know, and need to know. J Clin Neurophysiol. 2006;23:4–20.
65. Parrino L, Halasz P, Tassinari CA, Terzano MG. Cap, epilepsy and motor events during sleep: the unifying role of arousal. Sleep Med Rev. 2006;10:267–85.
66. Bruni O, Novelli L, Luchetti A, et al. Reduced NREM sleep instability in benign childhood epilepsy with centro-temporal spikes. Clin Neurophysiol. 2010;121:665–71.
67. Giorgi FS, Maestri M, Guida M, et al. Cyclic alternating pattern and interictal epileptiform discharges during morning sleep after sleep deprivation in temporal lobe epilepsy. Epilepsy Behav. 2017;73: 131–6.
68. Ellingson RJ, Wilken K, Bennett DR. Efficacy of sleep deprivation as an activation procedure in epilepsy patients. J Clin Neurophysiol. 1984;1:83–101.
69. Degen R, Degen HE. Sleep and sleep deprivation in epileptology. Epilepsy Res Suppl. 1991;2:235–60.
70. Leach JP, Stephen LJ, Salveta C, Brodie MJ. Wich electroencephalography (EEG) for epilepsy? The relative usefulness of different EEG protocols in patients with possible epilepsy. J Neurol Neurosurg Psychiatry. 2006;77:1040–2.
71. Gustafsson G, Brostrom A, Ulander M, Vrethem M, Svanborg E. Occurrence of epileptiform discharges and sleep during EEG recordings in children after melatonin intake versus sleep deprivation. Clin Neurophysiol. 2015;126:1493–7.
72. Giorgi FS, Perini D, Maestri M, et al. Usefulness of a simple sleep-deprived EEG protocol for epilepsy diagnosis in de novo subjects. Clin Neurophysiol. 2013;124:2101–7.
73. Renzel R, Baumann CR, Poryazova R. EEG after sleep deprivation is a sensitive tool in the first diagnosis of idiopathic generalized but not focal epilepsy. Clin Neurophysiol. 2016;127:209–13.
74. Fountain NB, Kim JS, Lee SI. Sleep deprivation activates epileptiform discharges independent of the activating effects of sleep. J Clin Neurophysiol. 1998;15:69–75.
75. Badawy RAB, Curatolo JM, Newton M, Bercovic SF, Macdonnell RAL. Sleep deprivation increases cortical excitability in epilepsy. Neurology. 2006;67:1018–22.
76. Khrishnan V, Chang BS, Schomer DL. Normal EEG in wakefulness and sleep: adults and elderly. In: Schomer DL, Lopes da Silva FH, editors. Niedermeyer's electroencephalography. Basic principles, clinical applications, and related fields. 7th ed. Oxford: Oxford University Press;2018. p. 202–28.
77. Hogan T, Sundaram M. Rhythmic auditory stimulation in generalized epilepsy. Electroencephalogr Clin Neurophysiol. 1989;72:455–8.
78. De Marco P, Tassinari CA. Estreme somatosensory evoked potential (ESEP): an EEG sign forecasting the possible occurrence of seizures in children. Epilepsia. 1981;22:569–75.
79. Hitomi T, Ikeda A, Matsumoto R, et al. Generators and temporal succession of giant somatosensory evoked potentials in cortical reflex myoclonus: epilcortical recording from sensorimotor cortex. Clin Neurophysiol. 2006;117:1481–6.
80. Visani E, Canafoglia L, Rossi Sebastiano D, et al. Giant SEPs and SEP-recovery function in Unverricth-Lunborg disease. Clin Neurophysiol. 2013;124:1013–8.

15 Polygraphic Techniques

Lara Alvisi, Francesca Bisulli, Laura Licchetta, and Paolo Tinuper

Polygraphy is a method of electrophysiological investigation that allows the simultaneous recording and acquisition of several physiological, bioelectrical, and non-electrical parameters (signals), for short or long periods, correlating them with cerebral electrical activity. Polygraphy has therefore become the ideal and indispensable tool for the evaluation of patients who need a differential diagnosis for a sleep disorder (polysomnography (PSG)), for movement disorder, or for suspected epilepsy with episodes during waking and/or sleep. The acquisition of physiological parameters is allowed by the polygraph, which transforms the data captured from the patient into traces displayed on the monitor of the digital device.

15.1 Polygraphy Room

The laboratory where polygraphy is carried out requires specific features:

- *Patient preparation room*, equipped with cabinets for the storage of materials and adequately ventilated for the montage of collodion electrodes; appropriate suction systems in case collodion is used. Collodion, the glue used to fix the electrodes, is highly flammable and volatile; therefore it is necessary to mount the electrodes in a room equipped both with compressed air and with an exhaust air ventilation system designed to guarantee at least 14 changes of air per hour and without trigger sources.
- *Recording room*, i.e. the room where the patient will stay during the recording. It must be partially soundproof and far from the common areas to ensure better silence, away from sources of electrical and magnetic interference (elevators, operating theaters, etc.) to avoid interference and sources of artifacts that may compromise the quality of the recording and cause possible interpretative errors. Also, the room must be air-conditioned, with dimmable lighting, bed, armchair, and a locker for personal effects. This room must be equipped with a closed-circuit television system to monitor the patient (Fig. 15.1).
- *Control room*, where the technician observes the recording. Here is are the polygraph used for data acquisition, the control panel for audio and video control, and all the specific instruments. This room must have the connection for the instrumentation and be communicating and adjoining the patient room to facilitate the timely intervention of the technical staff (Fig. 15.2).
- *Room dedicated to data processing and storage*, it can be shared with other clinical neurophysiology laboratories (Fig. 15.3).
- In case the recording is performed in an outpatient setting or during hospitalization, but is of short duration, it can be performed in electroencephalography laboratories. These rooms require the presence of the technician close to the patient, and the available space must be such as to allow easy movement for the correct montage of the electrodes and for any assistance maneuvers.

15.1.1 Equipment

The instruments used for the acquisition of polygraphic data are digital. The paramount task of the neuro-pathophysiology technician is to correctly set the sampling frequency as this defines the bandwidth of the acquired signals. The high-pass filter, expressed in Hz (also called time constant if expressed in seconds), and the low-pass filter, also expressed in Hz, are set to the sole end of reading the signal displayed on the monitor.

L. Alvisi (✉) · F. Bisulli · L. Licchetta · P. Tinuper
IRCCS Istituto delle Scienze Neurologiche di Bologna, Bologna, Italy

Department of Biomedical and Neuromotor Sciences, University of Bologna, Bologna, Italy
e-mail: lara.alvisi@unibo.it

O. Mecarelli (ed.), *Clinical Electroencephalography*, https://doi.org/10.1007/978-3-030-04573-9_15

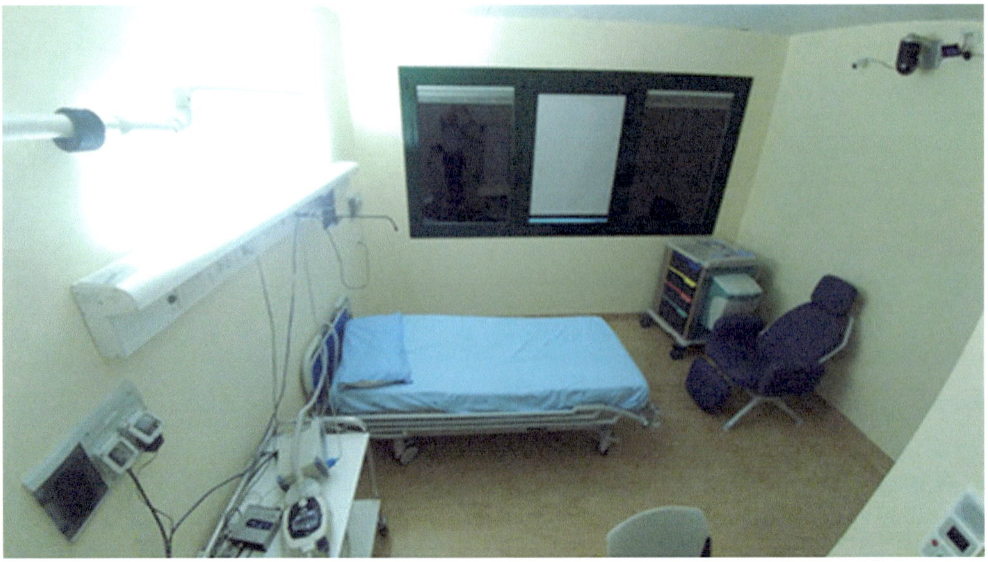

Fig. 15.1 Recording room

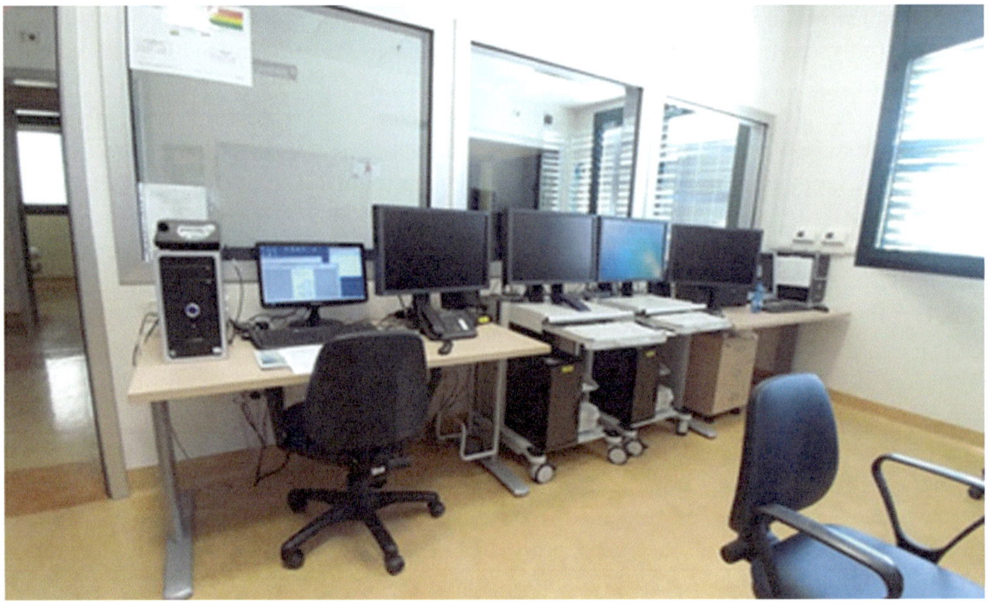

Fig. 15.2 Control room

15.2 Polygraphic Parameters

The biological parameters that can be recorded with polygraphy can be observed directly as bioelectrical signals or in other physical forms non-electrical in nature. The electrical parameters, naturally occurring as potential difference, can be detected directly with the electrodes. The non-electrical parameters, instead, in order to be recorded, must be converted into electrical signals using special "transducers" or other dedicated instruments.

15.2.1 Capturing Signals with Electrodes

In polygraphy the most used electrodes for capturing the signal are the cup electrodes that come with a central hole and a rim. A very thin, flexible cable, insulated with silicone or PVC, connects the electrode to the connector. The electrode must be mounted on previously degreased and dried skin after having filled the inside with conductive paste and having fixed it with a plaster. The plaster, if previously pierced at the electrode hole, will facilitate the

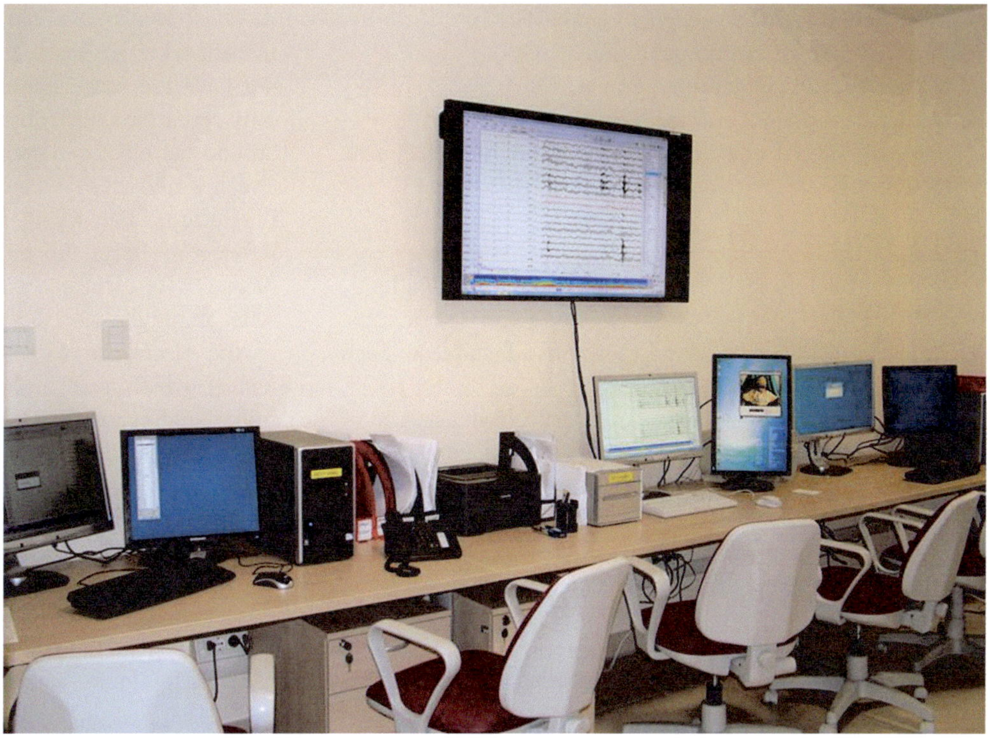

Fig. 15.3 Data processing room

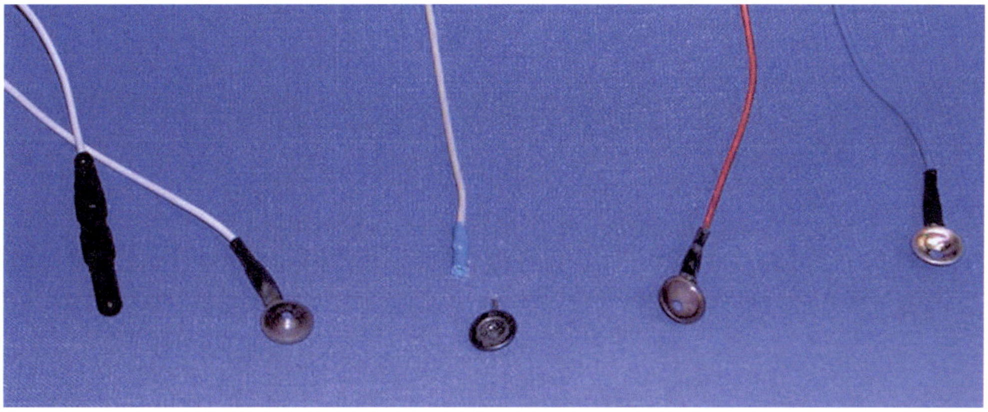

Fig. 15.4 Cup electrodes, from left to right: sintered electrode, single-use AgCl electrode, Ag-AgCl electrode, gilded-silver electrode

technician in inserting additional electroconductive gel, if necessary.

Commonly used electrodes have a variable diameter, between 3 and 10 mm depending on the size of the area to be explored, and can be in silver covered with a layer of silver chloride (AgCl), in gilded silver, or "single use" consisting of a plastic support with a layer of AgCl (Fig. 15.4).

The silver chloride electrode is the "ideal" electrode, but it needs continuous maintenance because the AgCl layer covering the silver electrode wears out in a short time resulting in the polarization of the electrode and causing possible artifacts in signal acquisition.

The gold electrodes have a greater "electrode noise" but require little maintenance. In both cases, a very accurate cleansing and appropriate sterilization are necessary after each use, making sure to remove any gel and glue residue. Moreover, an accurate drying and a periodic chlorination are important. The single-use electrodes with AgCl layer are very stable, and with low "electrode noise", they guarantee maximum safety for the patient and the operators. Once the recording has been completed, the cup is extracted and disposed of in the appropriate containers, while it is ensured that no grease or glue remains on the cable (Fig. 15.4).

15.2.2 Bioelectrical Parameters

The biological signals that are most frequently acquired during polygraphy recording are:

- Brain activity: electro-encephalogram (EEG).
- Eye movements: electro-oculogram (EOG).
- Muscle activity: electro-myogram (EMG).
- Cardiac activity: electro-cardiogram (ECG).
- Sympathetic skin response: sympathetic skin response (SSR).

15.2.2.1 EEG

For short recording sessions (2–3 h) and compliant patients, it is possible to use pre-wired electrodes on Lycra caps, available in different sizes and therefore adaptable to each patient.

For longer recordings the use of cup electrodes is recommended with the following procedure for montage:

- Clean the area of the scalp where the electrode is to be placed with a rigid shaft cotton swab soaked in abrasive paste, following the International 10–20 System (Fig. 15.5).
- Fix the electrode containing conductive paste on the scalp with gauze soaked in collodion, and then dry with compressed air (Fig. 15.6). During this procedure it is important to do not use a blow dryer or other equipment that might develop sparks that would be a source of ignition because collodion is highly flammable.

  As an alternative, there are nowadays both electroconductive and adhesive pastes that are easy to handle and that do not have the same limitations of use as collodion. The only precaution for its use is to not exceed in the quantity around the electrode because, being also electroconductive, it would act as if the surface of the electrode increased in size and, when drying, it would act as if it were reduced. After some days the product tends to dry completely; therefore the electrode must be removed and replaced.
- After fixing the electrodes, check the contact impedances of the electrodes with a dedicated device (impedance meter), which must be less than 10 kΩ (Fig. 15.7). It is important to verify that the impedances are all equal, especially between the two electrodes of a bipolar derivation to avoid the overlap of the network signal and the distortion of the bioelectrical signal. The EEG recording procedure with electrodes attached with the collodion ensures excellent stability and durability so that the recordings can last several days. In case contact impedances are high and in any case, on the following days, if the recording continues, it is possible, through a bevel needle, to pierce the gauze covering the electrode and introduce more gel. The electrodes will then be removed using a collodion remover (in case collodion is used) or simply water (in case of latest-generation adhesive pastes and electro-conductors).

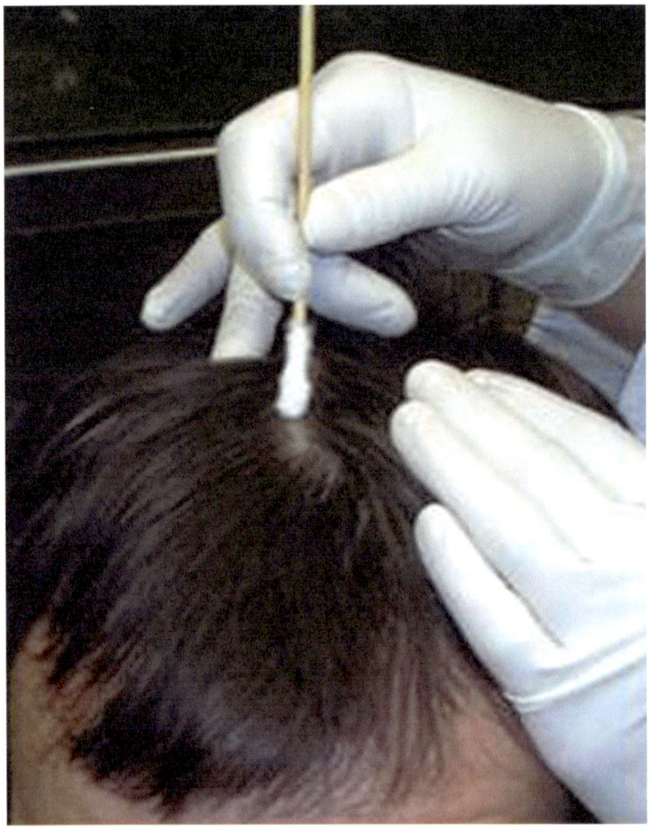

Fig. 15.5 Preparation of the scalp with a rigid shaft cotton swab soaked in abrasive paste

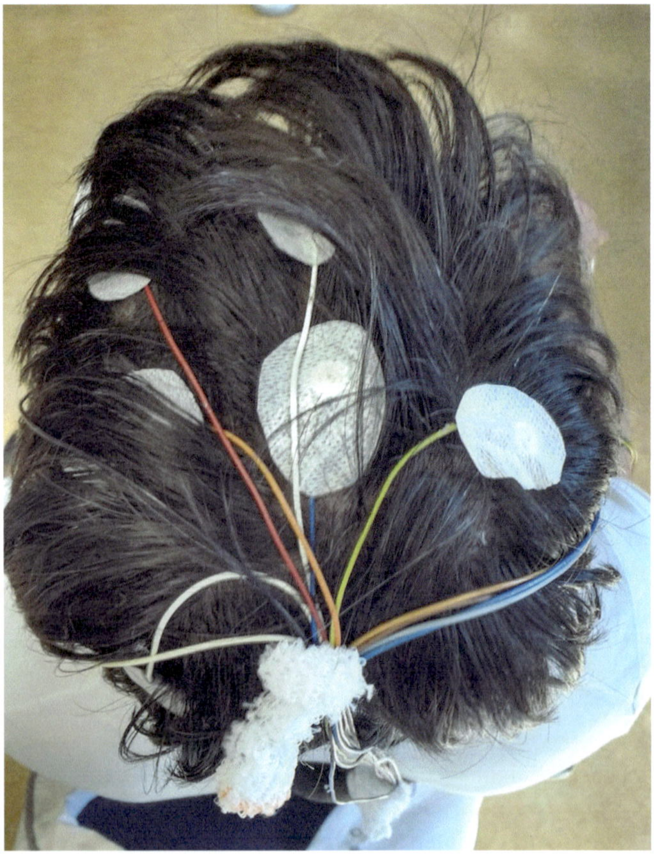

Fig. 15.6 Electrode placement

According to the raccommendation of the American Academy of Sleep Medicine in order to stage sleep correctly are necessary at least three EEG derivations including the following leads: frontal, central, and occipital (Fig. 15.8) [1].

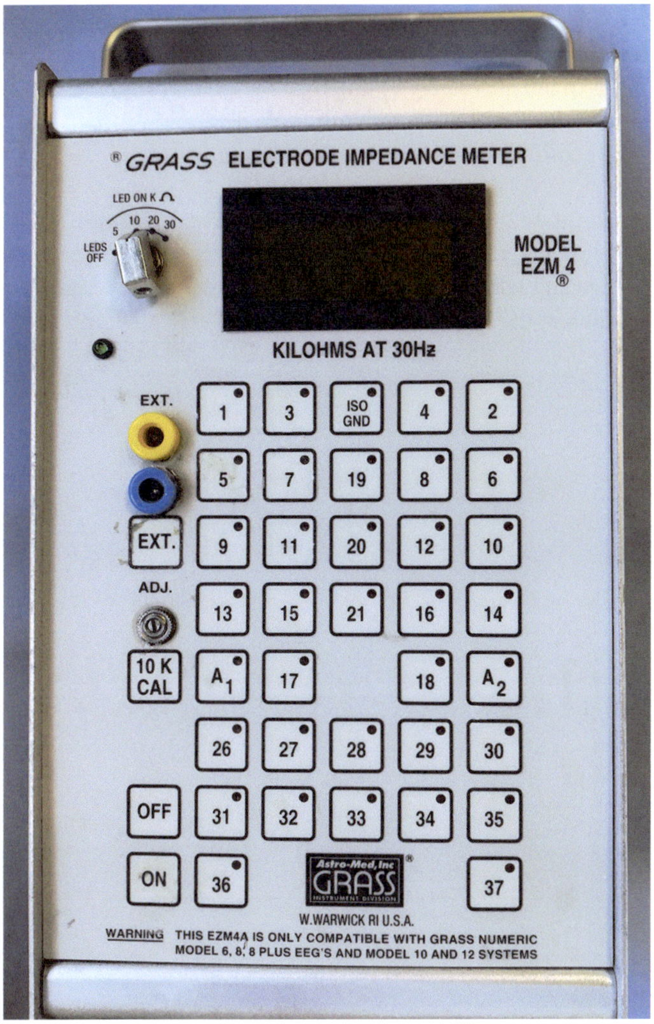

Fig. 15.7 Impedance meter to measure contact impedances

Technical box: the signal captured from the scalp is processed by an AC preamplifier; on visualization a high-pass filter is set at 0.3 Hz (time constant 0.5 s) and a low-pass filter at 35 or 70 Hz.

Technical tip: the electrode from the mastoid process could be moved 3–4 cm upward to reduce the ECG artifact.

15.2.2.2 EOG

EOG is necessary for the identification of eye movements and uses the potential difference between cornea (electropositive) and retina (electronegative). This corneo-retinal potential generates an electric dipole with the cornea facing forward, and still, the distribution of the charges has its maximum positive potential at the center of the eye, with a tendency to decrease as one moves away from it (Fig. 15.9). When the eye globe moves, it generates a potential that is proportional to the movement: if the globe moves upward, it makes the upper part of the eye more positive, and if the globe moves downward, it makes the undereye area more positive.

When the globe moves sideways, it makes the side of the eye toward which the cornea moves more positive.

Eye movements cause the artifacts that are most frequently found in frontal and frontotemporal derivations of the EEG and that often pose doubts about their origin.

For their recording, cup electrodes filled with conductive paste are required. These are fixed with a hypoallergenic plaster after having slightly degreased the skin.

Possible eye movements:

- Eye opening and closure.
- Vertical movements.
- Lateral movements.
- Oblique and rotational movements.

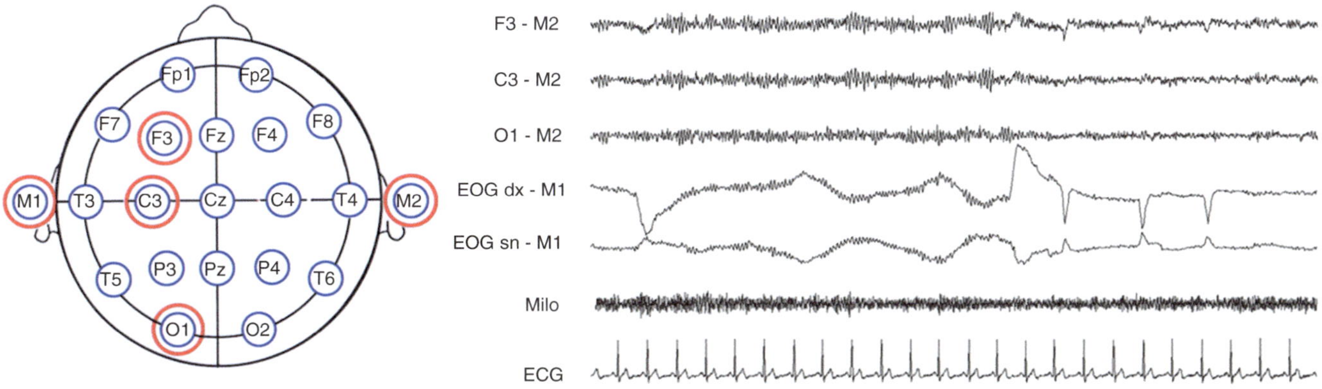

Fig. 15.8 Mounting of the electrodes on the scalp as recommended by the AASM for sleep scoring

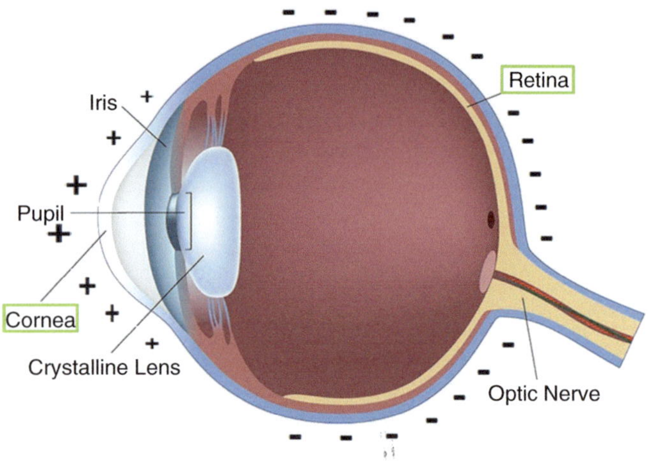

Fig. 15.9 Electrical discharges location in the retina and cornea

- Blinking and flutter.
- Slow movements when falling asleep.
- Nystagmus.

On EEG the artifacts related to eye movements are more evident on the frontopolar and frontal leads (Fig. 15.10).

Since the correct identification of eye movements, both horizontal and vertical are essential for sleep staging. In order to unequivocally distinguish the EOG from EEG diffusion and other artifact activities, two derivations are used.

According to AASM there are two options:

1. Right-M2 EOG and left-M2 EOG: where the right EOG is mounted 1 cm above the external canthus of the right eye and left EOG is mounted 1 cm under the external canthus of the left eye (Fig. 15.11).

Fig. 15.10 Electrical potential on EEG derivations provoked by eye movements

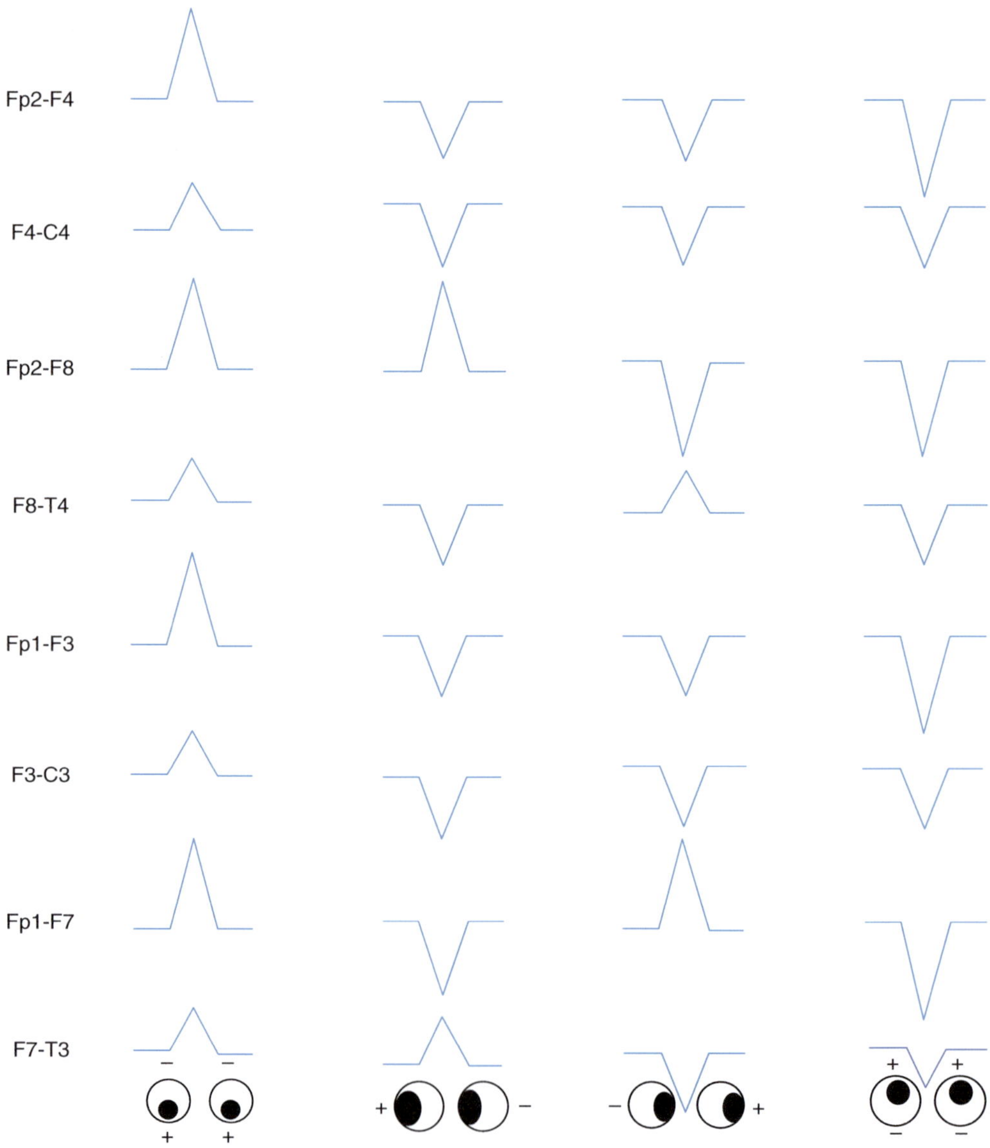

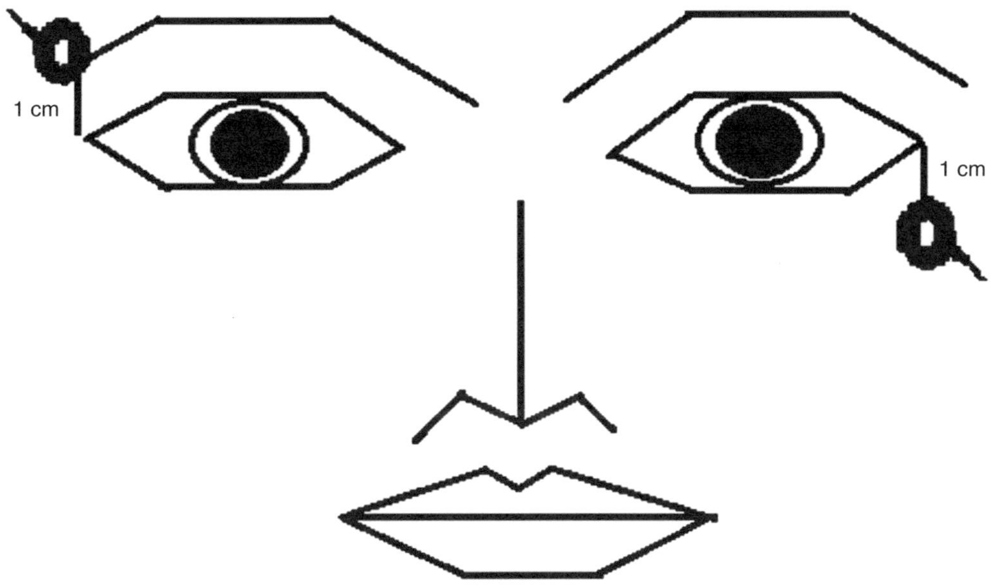

Fig. 15.11 AASM recommendations for monitoring eye movements for sleep scoring, first option

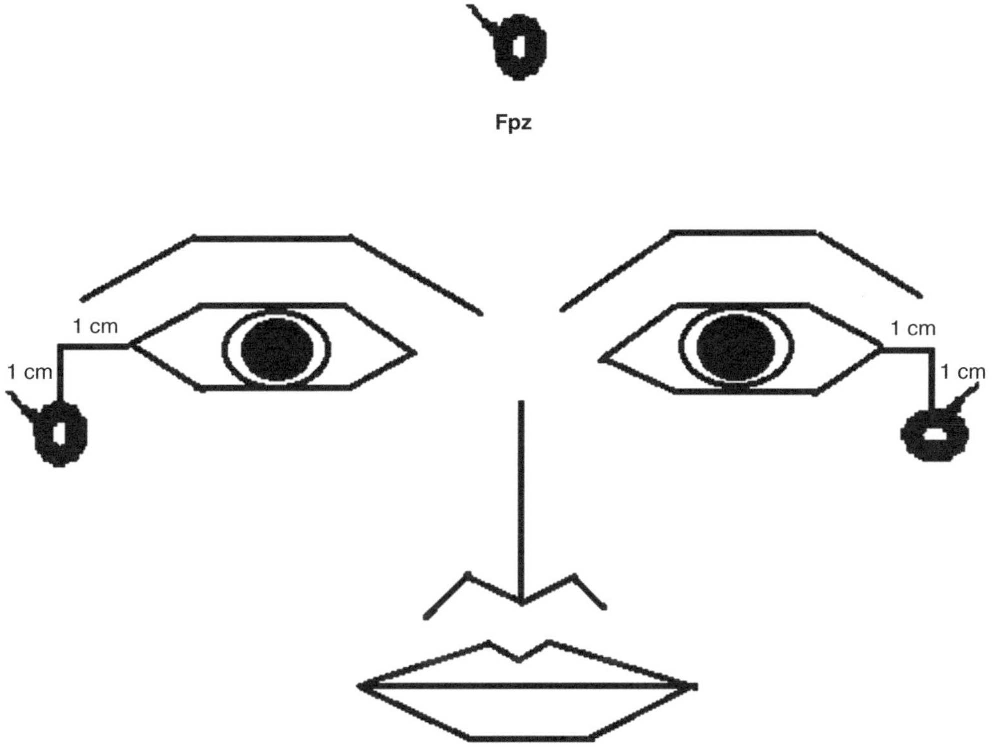

Fig. 15.12 AASM recommendations for monitoring eye movements for sleep scoring, second option

2. Right-Fpz EOG and left-Fpz EOG: where the right EOG is mounted 1 cm out and 1 cm under the external canthus of the right external canthus and left EOG 1 cm under and out the left external canthus; whereas Fpz is mounted following the instructions of the International 10–20 System (Fig. 15.12).

To record the horizontal movements of the eyes, the two electrodes must be fixed at 1 cm to the right of the external canthus of the right eye and 1 cm to the left of the external canthus of the left eye, respectively, referred to each other (Fig. 15.13).

To record the vertical movements of the eyes, the two electrodes must be fixed as follows: one at 1 cm below the median axis of the eye and the second 1 cm above the median axis of the same eye, relating them to each other (Fig. 15.14).

Finally, to record both horizontal and vertical movements, place an electrode 1 cm above the external canthus of the right eye and the second electrode at 1 cm below the external canthus of left eye canthus, relating them to each other.

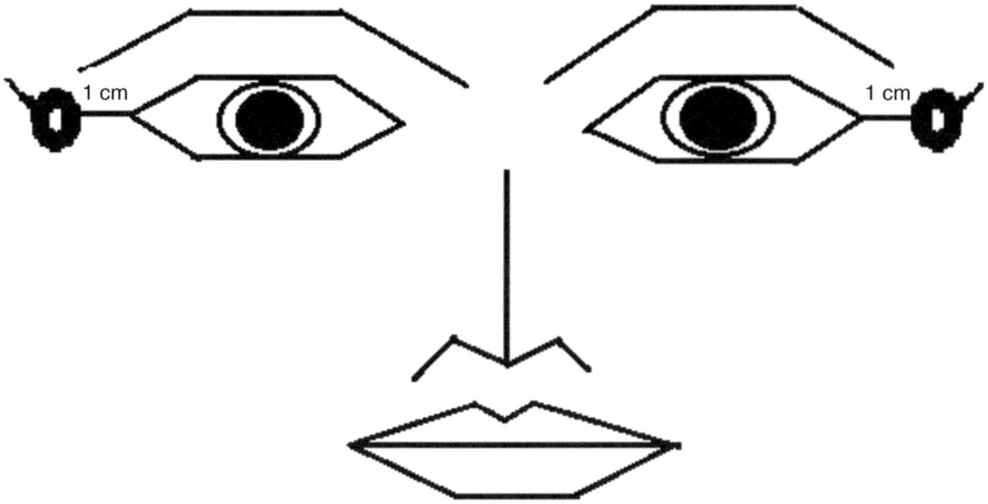

Fig. 15.13 Electrode placement to record horizontal eye movements

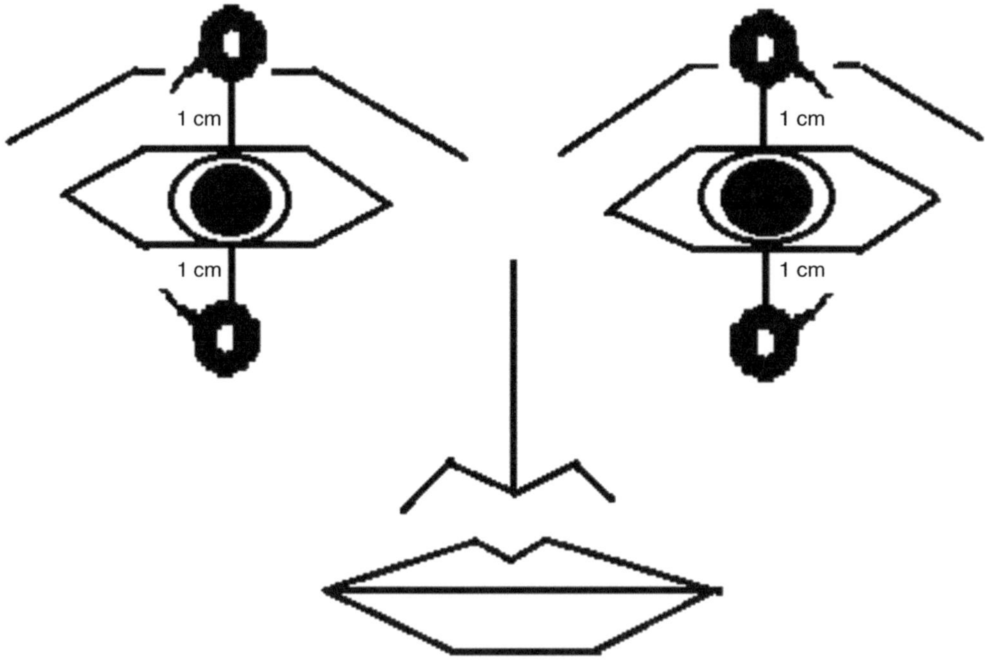

Fig. 15.14 Electrode placement to record vertical eye movements

It should be noted that all these three methods, using a single derivation (i.e., two electrodes are derived from each other), allow the easy detection of eye movements. However, using a single trace for EOG, it is difficult to distinguish ocular movements from EEG activities and/or artifacts. Therefore the use of two traces should be preferred.

Conversely, if the first electrode (positioned 1 cm above the external canthus of the right eye) and the second electrode (positioned 1 cm below the external canthus of the left eye), are derived from either M1 or M2, the eye movements will always be in opposition phase, while EEG and artifact activities will always be in phase (Fig. 15.15).

> *Technical box*: EOG signals are processed with an AC preamplifier. To display the signal, a high-pass filter is set at 0.3 Hz (time constant 0.5 s), and a low-pass filter is set at over or equal to 10 Hz.

15.2.2.3 EMG

With polygraphy the activity of all superficial muscles can be acquired.

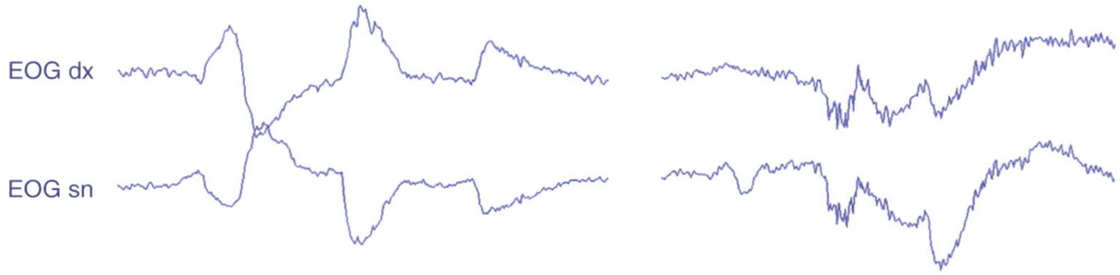

Fig. 15.15 Two traces for EOG to distinguish the ocular movements from EEG activities and/or artifacts

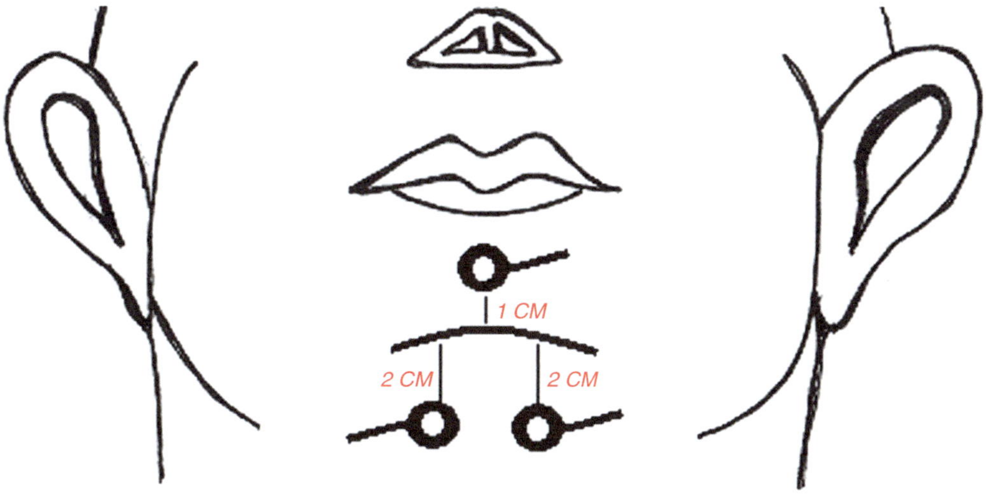

Fig. 15.16 Electrode placement to record mylohyoid muscle activity

Technical tip: to capture the signal, cup electrodes of variable size, filled with conductive paste, are used depending on the district to be investigated. The electrodes should be placed on the skin at the chosen muscle belly at a distance of about 2 cm from each other, so as to avoid creating a single field between them. After having cleaned the skin with a rigid shaft cotton swab soaked in degreasing paste, the electrodes must be fixed with a hypoallergenic plaster.

For sleep scoring the activity of the mylohyoid muscle needs to be recorded. It is useful in identifying the various stages of sleep and is indispensable for the identification of REM atonia.

Technical tip: to capture the activity of the mylohyoid muscle, three electrodes are placed 2 cm below the lower edge of the jaw, one 2 cm to the right, and one 2 cm to the left, while the third reference electrode is placed at the center of the chin 1 cm above the edge of the jaw (Fig. 15.16).

To record the activity of the tibial muscle for scoring periodic limb movements in sleep, the muscle belly must be identified by making the patient perform a dorsiflexion of the foot, and then carefully degrease the skin with the rigid shaft cotton swab soaked in abrasive paste. Once this task has been completed, the cup electrode must be filled with an electroconductive paste and fixed with a hypoallergenic plaster. The use of a bigger plaster is recommended to fix the cable wiring it around itself to guarantee the stability of the electrodes even if small tractions occur. Both legs should be monitored for the presence of the leg movements, and separated channels for each leg are strongly preferred.

Technical box: very fast frequencies of muscle activity are processed with an AC preamplifier, setting a high-pass filter at 30 Hz (time constant 0.005 s) to cut low frequencies and a low-pass filter at 90 Hz (or OFF) to view high frequencies.

For a good visualization of the signal, sensitivity must be regulated by making the patient perform a maximal effort with the recorded muscle.

For polygraphic studies aimed at the accurate characterization of specific motor phenomena and to highlight a possible correlation with the cortical electrical activity (see Chap. 15. Rubboli), EMG traces must be sampled at, at least, 2 kHz.

15.2.2.4 ECG

ECG is a high-potential signal (measured in millivolt) that can be captured in almost all parts of the body. It is 100-fold higher than the signal generated by the brain activity.

Technical tip: the derivation that allows a good morphological representation is D2, which is obtained by placing an electrode on the right clavicle and the other on the left axillary line at the level of the seventh rib. Standard disposable adhesive electrodes for ECG or cup electrodes can be used. At this point, the skin must be degreasevd as needed for the other parameters described above before the electrode is positioned (Fig. 15.17).

Technical box: the signal is sent to an AC preamplifier, with a high-pass filter at 0.5 Hz (time constant 0.3 s), low-pass filter at 60 Hz, and sampling frequency greater than or equal to 100 Hz. For particular studies of the QRS, it is necessary to use much higher sampling rates.

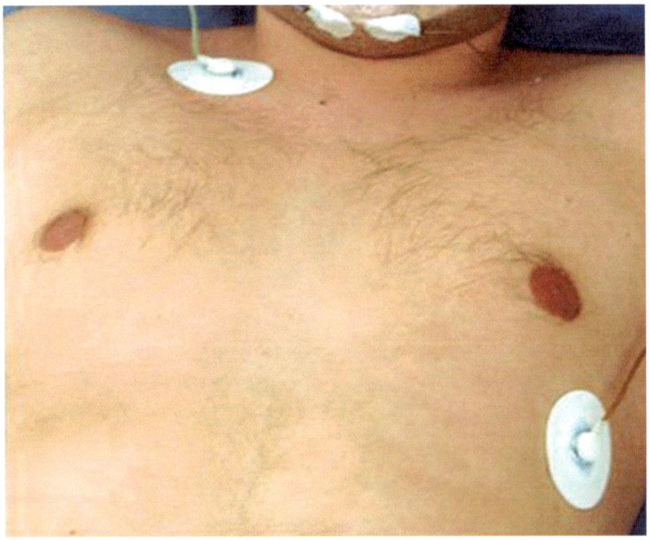

Fig. 15.17 D2 derivation to monitor ECG activity

The monitoring of an ECG trace is fundamental as it is decisive in the identification of artifacts and is useful in highlighting any alterations of the cardiac rhythm related or not to modifications of the EEG pattern. Alterations in cardiac rhythm are common during seizures, and tachycardia is seen in up to 64% of temporal lobe seizures (Fig. 15.18) [2]. Ictal bradyarrhythmias (IB), including ictal asystole (IA), are rare but potentially serious occurrences. Ictal asystole has been proposed as a possible mechanism behind sudden unexplained death in epilepsy (SUDEP) [2]. Definitive diagnosis relies upon capturing an episode of ictal bradyarrhythmias/ictal asystole, either through combined EEG/ECG recording or through the use of an implantable loop recorder (Fig. 15.19).

The combined EEG/ECG recording is also useful in detecting changes in underlying activity related to primary changes in cardiac rhythm, such as in the case of syncope (see Chap. 33, Fig. 1), that could not be interpreted or could be confused with activity of cortical origin.

15.2.2.5 SSR

The sympathetic skin response (SSR) is a transient variation of the electrical potential at the skin level. It is a somatosympathetic reflex with three components, i.e., spinal, bulbar, and suprabulbar, that originates from the synchronous activation of the eccrine sweat glands in response to a discharge of postganglionic sympathetic nerve fibers.

The SSR can be spontaneous, i.e., provoked by internal stimuli such as deep breathing or emotional reactions or evoked by external stimuli, such as electrical or magnetic stimulation.

Generally, the answer consists of a wave with a first positive component followed by a negative one: the first is the expression of the sweat gland and its innervation, while the second is still unclear (Fig. 15.20).

The amplitude of the wave is closely related to the patient's age (over 60 years of age it is found only in 50% of the subjects), emotional reactions, and the temperature of the environment and of the skin.

The frequency of spontaneous SSR increases during NREM sleep phases and then disappears in REM sleep. It can be evoked by external stimuli only in wakefulness or early NREM sleep stages that cause EEG arousal. Recording this parameter is useful in the study of sleep or peculiar diseases and is possible only in some laboratories.

SSR abnormalities have been reported in 66–83% of diabetic patients, familial amyloid polyneuropathy, patients with distal small fiber peripheral neuropathy, hereditary motor and sensory neuropathy type I, hereditary sensory autonomic neuropathy type IV, entrapment neuropathies, alcoholic subjects, scleroderma, and Sjogren's disease.

SSR is abnormal in 45–67% of patients with chronic renal failure and autonomic dysfunction; studies on Parkinson

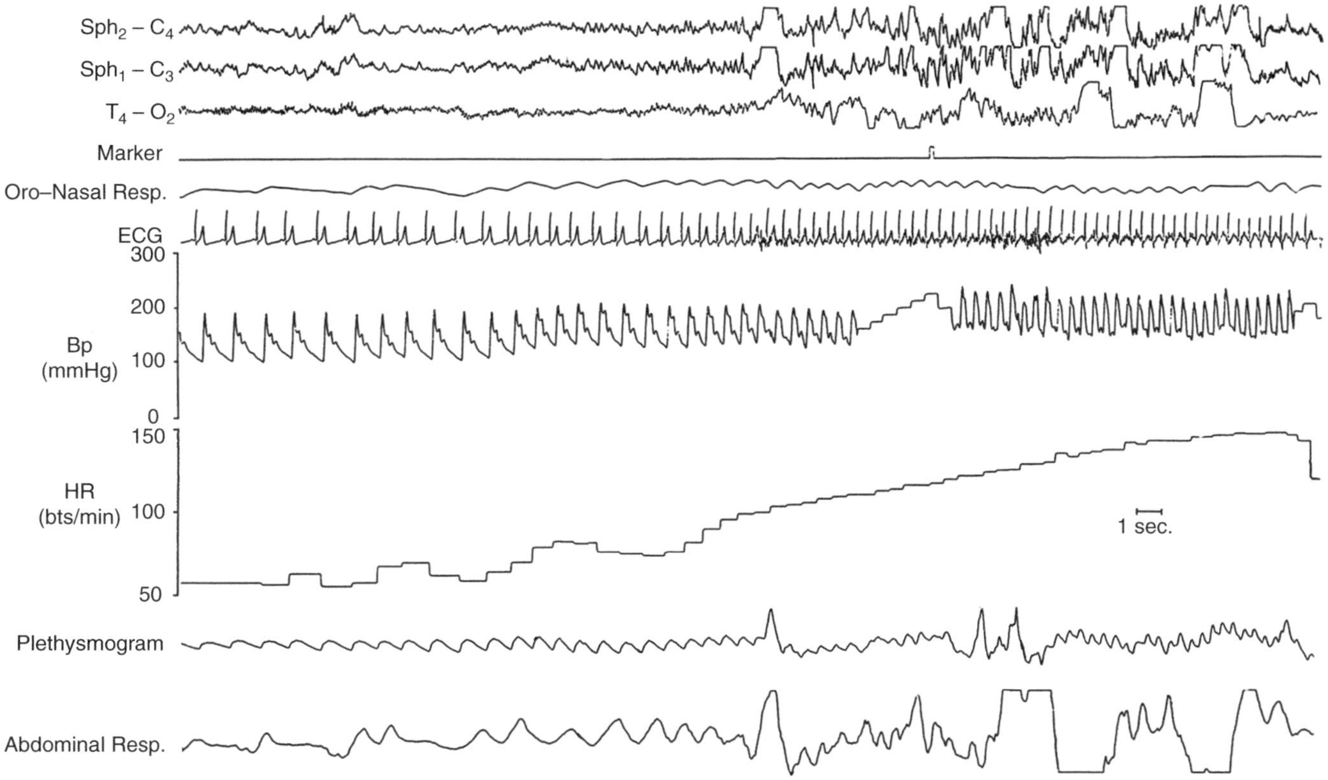

Fig. 15.18 Ictal polygraphic recording of a right temporal lobe seizures associated with an increased blood pressure associated with tachycardia. Plethysmogram showed a signal of decreased amplitude (Sph 2 = right sphenoidal, Sph 1 = left sphenoidal)

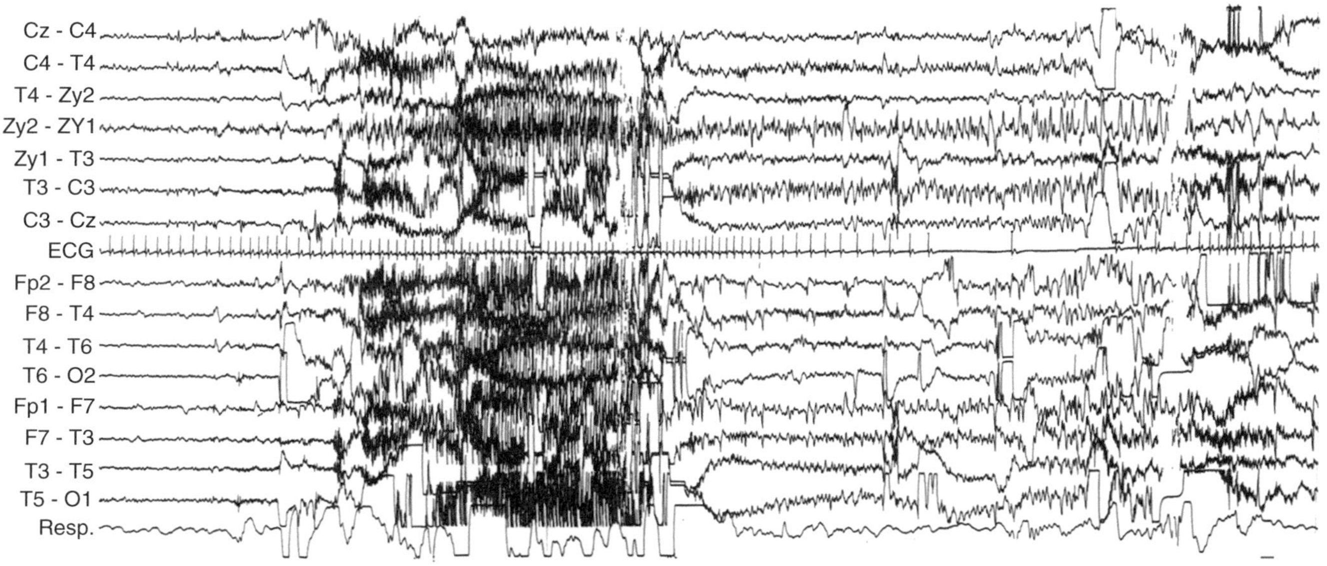

Fig. 15.19 Polygraphic recording of a left temporal seizure. After 40 s from seizure onset, a progressive slowing cardiac rhythm till became evident complete asystole (Zy2 = right zygomatic, Zy1 = left zygomatic)

disease have shown qualitative and quantitative SSR abnormalities, including loss of response. Absent or abnormal SSR has been found in multiple system atrophy, with longer latency and smaller amplitude of the responses [3].

Technical tip: the electrodes should be fixed to the palm or sole of the foot (active electrode) and the other one to the back of the hand or foot, respectively (reference electrode) (Fig. 15.21). The cup electrodes must be applied following the same instructions described above for the other parameters. Also in this case, to eliminate any external interference, it is very important that the contact impedances of the two recording electrodes are equal to each other.

Technical box: the setting of the AC channel must have a bandwidth with a high-pass filter at 0.3 Hz (time constant 0.5 s) and a low-pass filter at 30 Hz; the sensitivity must be set to 0.5 mV/cm and the sampling frequency to 60 Hz.

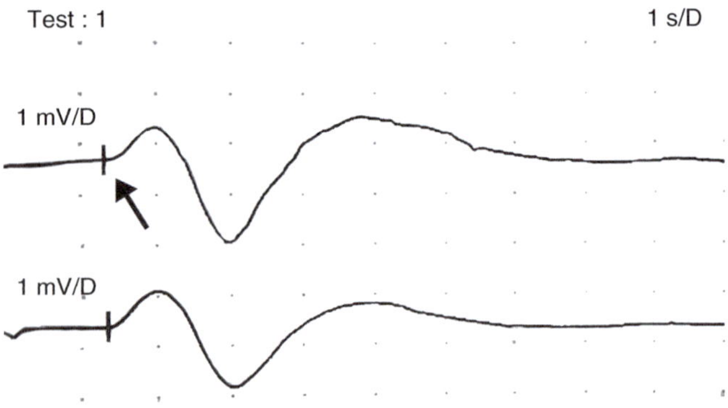

Fig. 15.20 SSR response

15.3 Non-electrical Parameters

The non-electrical parameters that are most frequently acquired during polygraphy recording are:

- Breathing: oronasal flow, thoracic activity, abdominal activity, intraesophageal pressure.
- Noise.
- Identification of body position.
- Pulse oximetry.
- Plethysmogram.

As already mentioned above, in order to polygraphically document non-electrical signals, it is necessary to transform them into electrical signals using special transducers and/or dedicated and validated instruments.

The function of the transducer is to be influenced by the physical quantity to be measured and the ability to process the acquired information in order to make it available to the technician.

15.3.1 Breathing

During polygraphic or EEG recordings, the respiratory activity is often observed in order to complete the study of autonomic functions. In fact, the concurrent study of many parameters related to breathing leads to selective and targeted diagnoses in conjunction with critical events, in the detection of daytime hypersomnias, and in the definition of syndromes with particular respiratory conditions.

15.3.1.1 Oronasal Flow

The oronasal flow is monitored using thermistors and/or thermocouples and/or cannula airflow sensors.

Thermistors (in combination with a battery-powered Wheatstone bridge) are resistors whose resistance varies with temperature changes during inhalation and exhalation

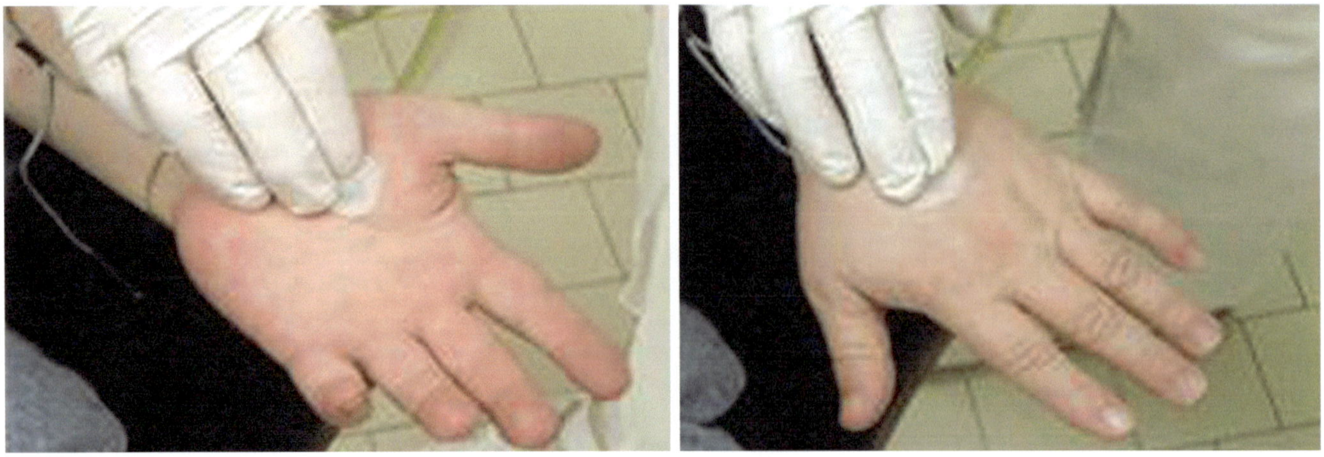

Fig. 15.21 Placement and mounting of electrodes to detect SSR on the hand

at the nostrils and mouth. At the output of the Wheatstone bridge, a potential difference that is proportional to the variations in resistance, i.e., to the change in flow, is generated (Fig. 15.22).

Thermocouples are "active" transducers made up of two conductors of different materials: if the junctions are placed at different temperatures, an electrical signal is developed that is proportional to the variations in the temperature of the airflow during inhalation and exhalation. The pairs of materials generally used are iron-constantan, copper-constantan, nickel-chromium, and nickel-aluminum (Figs. 15.23 and 15.24).

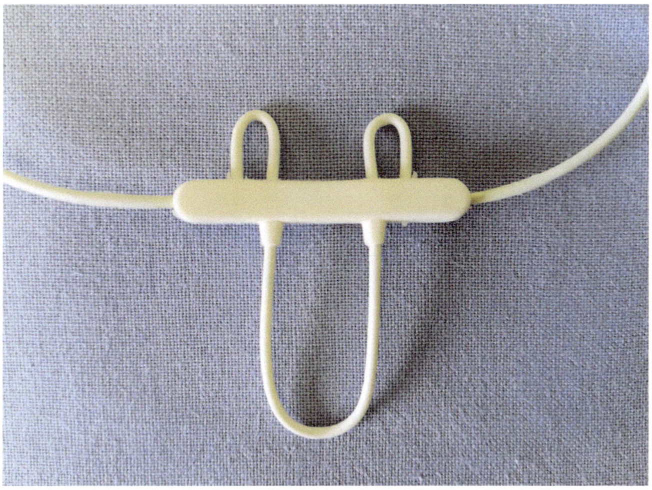

Fig. 15.22 Thermistor for the detection of oronasal flow

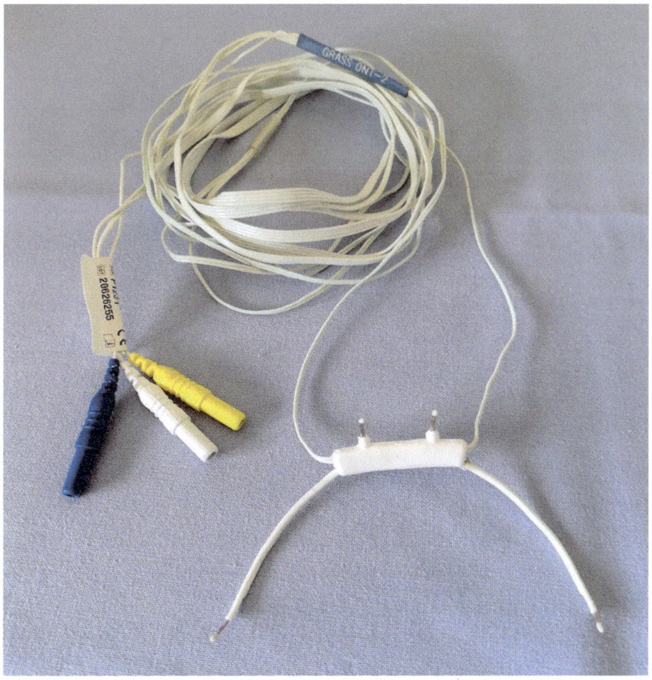

Fig. 15.23 Thermocouples for the detection of oronasal flow

These transducers must be fixed with a hypoallergenic plaster under the nostrils to ensure stability during the entire duration of the recording.

These are practical and inexpensive systems that provide only a qualitative measure; they do not detect flow limitations and are not particularly accurate in detecting hypopneas as they are affected by temperature variations in the environment.

A more reliable system consists of the pressure transducer with an oronasal cannula. This method transforms the depression that is created in the cannula during inhalation and the positive pressure during exhalation into an electrical signal. This system is therefore not affected by temperature variations, is very reliable in the detection of hypopneas and limitations of flow, and allows the detection of noise, which is useful for the diagnosis of snoring (Fig. 15.25).

15.3.1.2 Thoracic and Abdominal Activity

Transducers with piezoelectric crystal sensors or bands for inductive plethysmography are used to detect the movements of the chest and abdomen.

Piezoelectric transducers are "active," reliable, practical, robust, and inexpensive and can be used on any polygraph but only allow qualitative measurements.

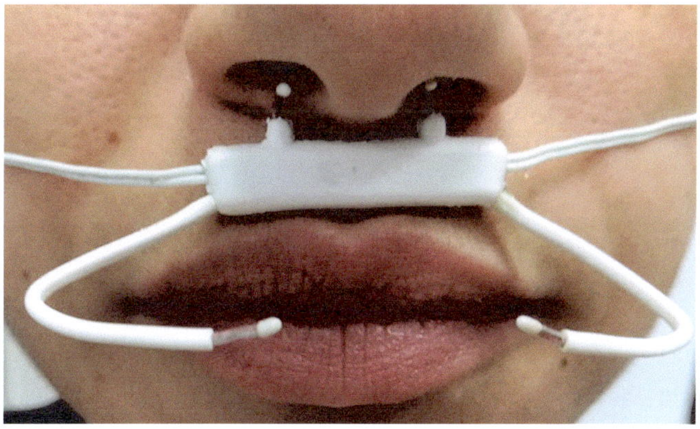

Fig. 15.24 Mounting procedure of the thermocouples transducer

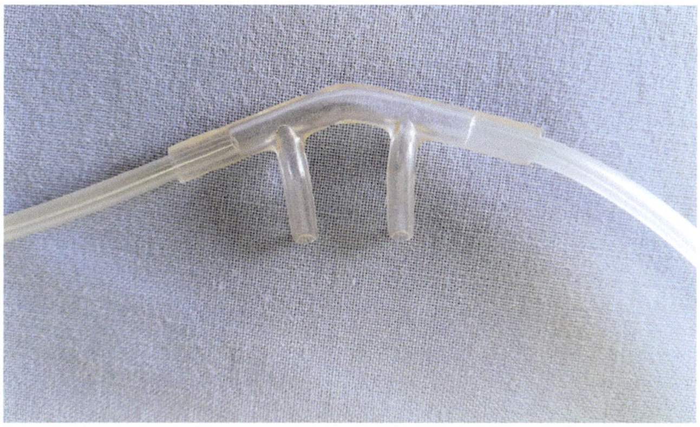

Fig. 15.25 Pressure transducer with oronasal cannula

The sensor is connected to elastic straps that, when wound around the chest or abdomen, solicit the crystal during expansion and contraction. This stress causes the crystal to produce a significant potential for stress (Fig. 15.26). On the midline the following must be applied: the thoracic sensor on the mammillary line and the abdominal sensor on the umbilical line (Fig. 15.27).

The inductive plethysmography bands allow semiquantitative recordings but require a special transducer. The elastic bands consist of two or more wires of Teflon-insulated coils (Fig. 15.28).

Technical box: the electrical signals at the output of these transducers require bipolar or polygraphic inputs at the patient's end. The setting of the AC channel must include a high-pass filter at 0.1 Hz (time constant 1.6 s) and low-pass filter at 5 Hz.

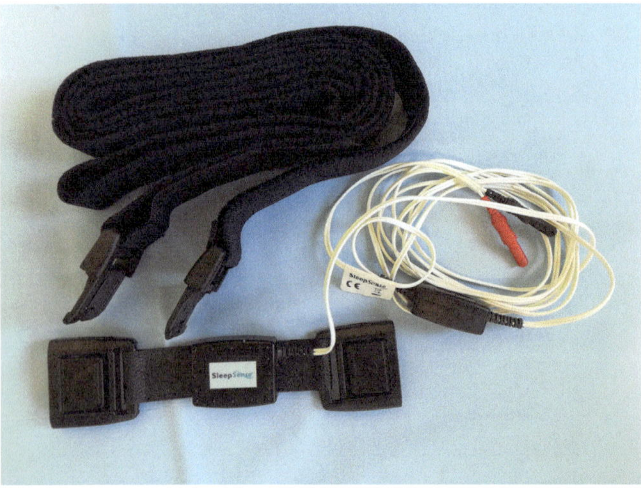

Fig. 15.26 Piezoelectric transducer

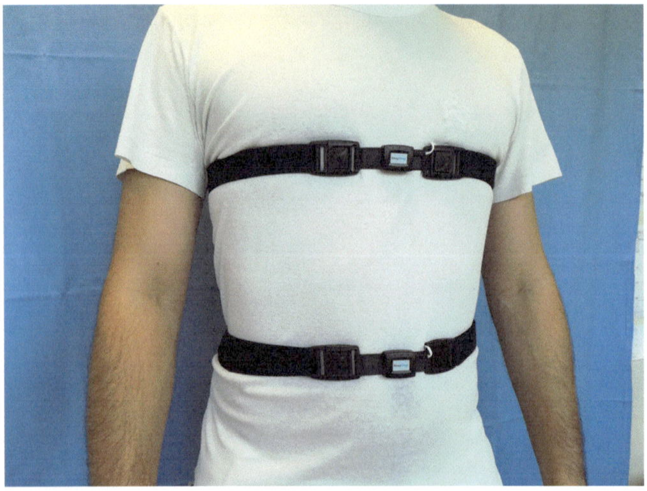

Fig. 15.27 Landmark for piezoelectric transducer

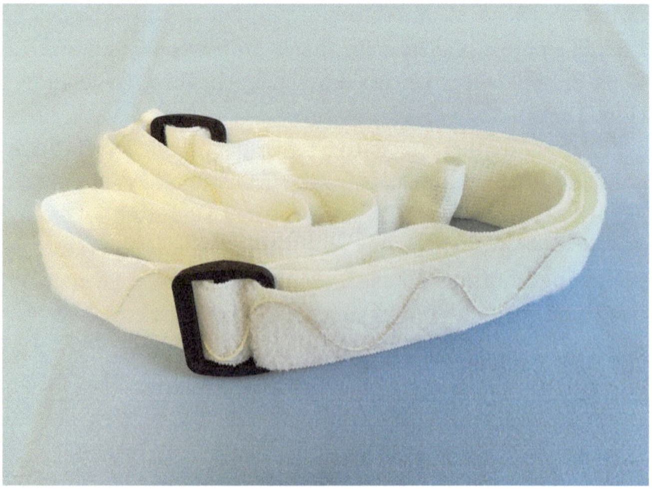

Fig. 15.28 Inductive plethysmography band

By convention, in polygraphy, the derivations of the respiratory activity must be set so that inhalation coincides with a deflection of the trace downward and exhalation upward.

To obtain semiquantitative values, in addition to the inductive plethysmography bands, you must use the polygraph channels with DC input, performing a starting calibration and setting the low-pass filter at 5 Hz.

15.3.1.3 Endoesophageal Pressure

The respiratory effort can be recorded with a specific transducer; it is placed in the esophagus in order to detect the positive or negative pressure at that site.

This recording method, used in the past for the study of OSA, has been gradually abandoned due to its invasive nature and is currently reserved for selected cases.

Technical box: the transducer transmits the intrathoracic pressure variations and in turn transforms them into proportional electrical signals. Since this is a quantitative method, it is necessary, before starting the recording, to perform a calibration on a sample pressure signal and to use a channel in DC mode, setting the low-pass filter to 15 Hz. Since the pressure exerted by inhalation is negative, the trace will deflect downward and then return to a value of 0 during exhalation.

15.3.2 Noise

The recording of the snoring noise produced by the upper airways involves the use of microphones with different operating principles and application methods depending on the environmental conditions in which the recording is performed

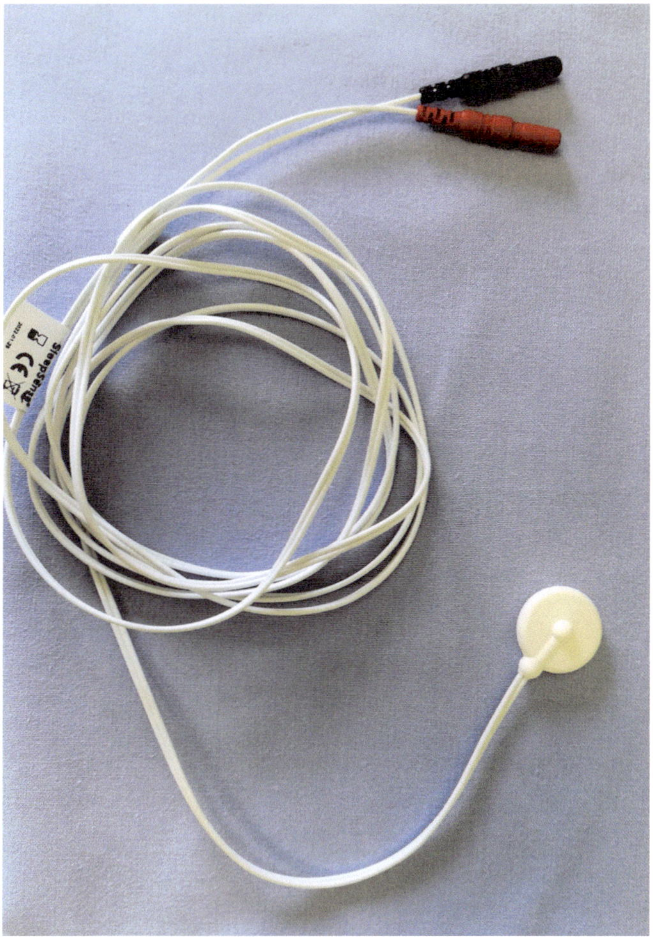

Fig. 15.29 Tracheal microphone

(Fig. 15.29). The microphone is therefore a transducer that, when hit by a sound wave, starts vibrating and generates a potential difference at the output.

The piezoelectric microphones have a light, compact structure and are small in size.

The landmark is identified by placing the fingers on the trachea and asking the patient to speak; the microphone will be placed where greater vibrations are felt immediately above the jugular fossa, using an appropriately shaped hypoallergenic plaster (Fig. 15.30).

> *Technical box*: the microphone outputs must be inserted in the recording head with a bipolar or polygraph input. The setting of the AC channel must include a high-pass filter at 30 Hz (time constant 0.005 s) and a low-pass filter at 90 Hz or OFF.

If the cannula is used to detect the oronasal flow, and the transducer has been set up, snoring can also be detected.

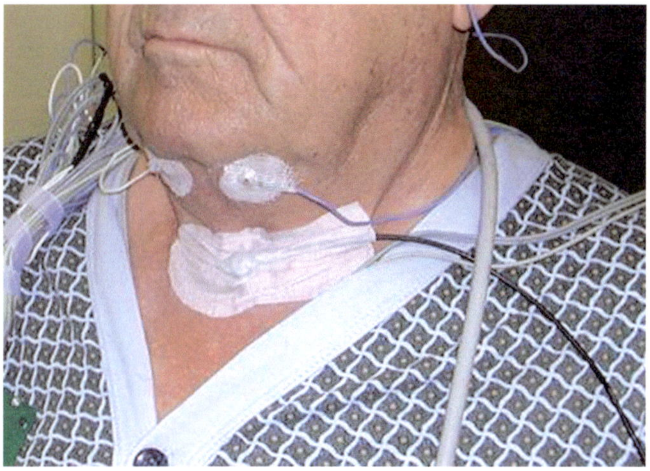

Fig. 15.30 Microphone positioned with a specific-shaped plaster

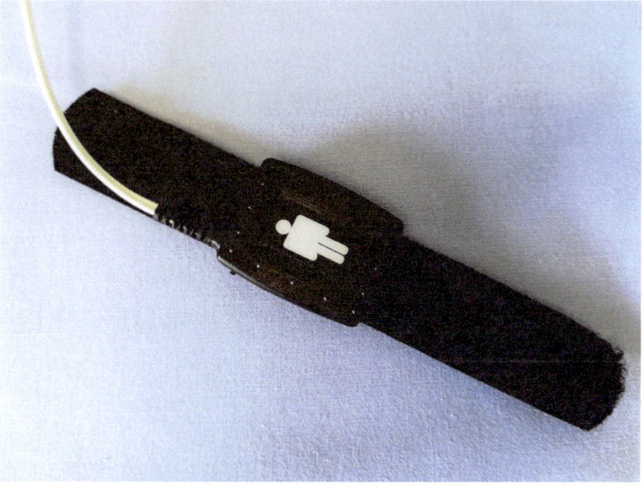

Fig. 15.31 Position transducer

This parameter is often acquired in the study of snoring in OSA patients but can also be used for the characterization of other disorders that are challenging for the diagnosis (groaning).

15.3.3 Body Position

When the respiratory events need to be correlated with the type of decubitus, it becomes necessary to document the patient's body position. For this purpose, special position transducers are used that must be fixed at the sternum (Fig. 15.31).

The supine position, in fact, predisposes the sleeper to airway collapse and to reduce lung volume and has long been known to exacerbate OSA; indeed, some affected person experience obstructive events exclusively when sleeping on their backs [4].

Technical box: there are position transducers that work in AC, and their output produces more potential variations depending on the position, or in DC, whose output has an electric potential that is proportional to the state of the transducer. In case of AC position transducers, the signal must be sent to a bipolar input by setting a high-pass filter to 10 Hz (time constant 0.02 s) and a low-pass filter to 50 Hz. With the transducer in DC, the electrical output potential must be sent to a DC input by setting a low-pass filter to 0.5 Hz.

Also in this case, before beginning the recording, it is necessary to perform a calibration of the trace by manually simulating the various body positions with the transducer.

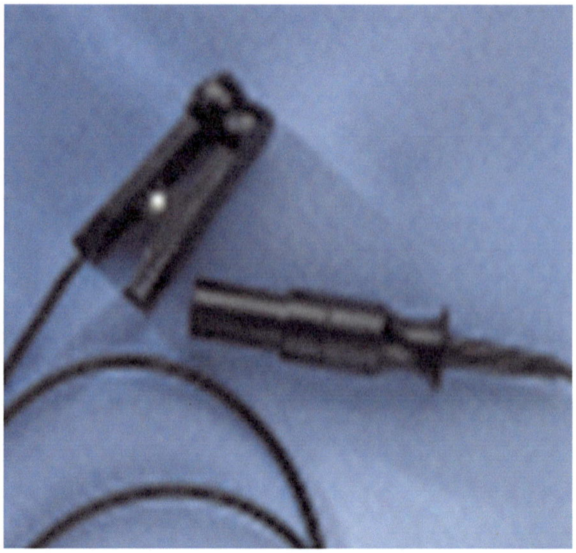

15.3.4 Pulse Oximetry

To document the severity of an apneic patient, it is essential to monitor the saturation of oxygen (blood bound hemoglobin, SaO2) through pulse oximetry (oximeter). The oximeter consists of a specific probe and a processing system. The probe consists of a photoemitter and a photoreceiver that captures the light that passes through the earlobe or the finger (Fig. 15.32).

Technical tip: in the case of the ear, it is a clip, while in the case of the finger, in addition to the clips, there are strip probes where the sensor is placed on the top and the end of the finger; the part that emits light should be placed on the fingernail while the detector on the opposite side. The sensor must then be wrapped with adhesive tape but not excessively tight (Fig. 15.32).

Technical box: a computerized system processes the light signal captured by the photoreceiver, proportional to blood-related hemoglobin, transforming it into percentage values ranging from 0% to 100%. To be able to use an instrument external to the polygraph, it is necessary that the first one is equipped with an analogue output and a sample signal for the calibration.

The signal of the analogue output of the oximeter must be sent to a DC input by setting a low-pass filter at 2 Hz.

15.3.5 Plethysmogram

It is a system for evaluating peripheral volumes and is used to highlight vasoconstriction and vasodilation. The system

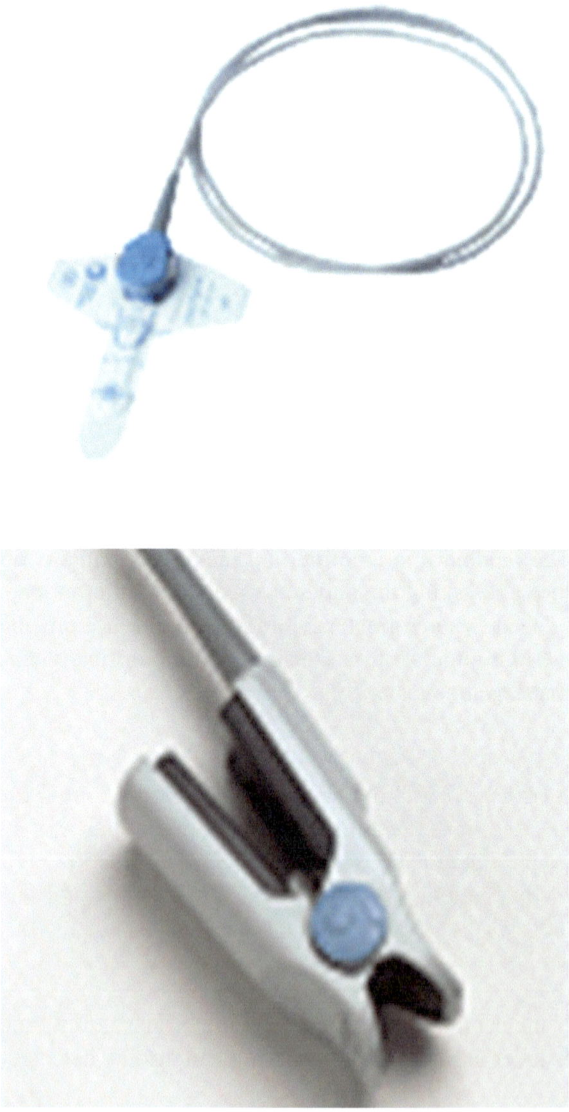

Fig. 15.32 Pulse oximetry transducer

consists of a probe that is fixed to a finger, consisting of a photoemitter and a photoreceiver that, in turn, has the task of capturing the reflected light and sending the signal to a specific transducer, producing an electrical output signal (Fig. 15.33). The attenuated pulse amplitude of plethysmogram is the consequence of peripheral vasoconstriction related by sympathetic tone activation due to different causes (ictal tachycardia, sleep apnea, REM sleep, etc.) (Fig. 15.18). Whereas an increased amplitude could be related to a peripheral vasodilatation (Fig. 15.34).

In principle, it has been used to detect all forms of respiratory events and cardiovascular event risk associated with sleep apnea. Peripheral arterial tonometry can be used to assess cardiovascular risk by measuring endothelial function during sleep-disordered breathing episodes. Arousals terminating sleep apnea events are accompanied by attenuated pulse amplitude. This decrease is due to peripheral vasoconstriction caused by sympathetic tone activation. If pulse rate also is analyzed, probability analysis can be used to distinguish between slow-wave sleep and rapid eye movement (REM) sleep [5].

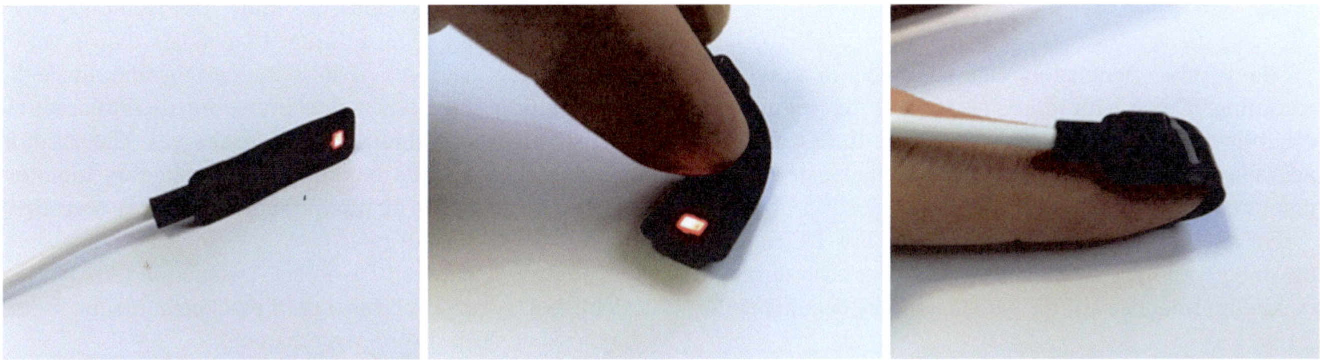

Fig. 15.33 Plethysmogram transducer

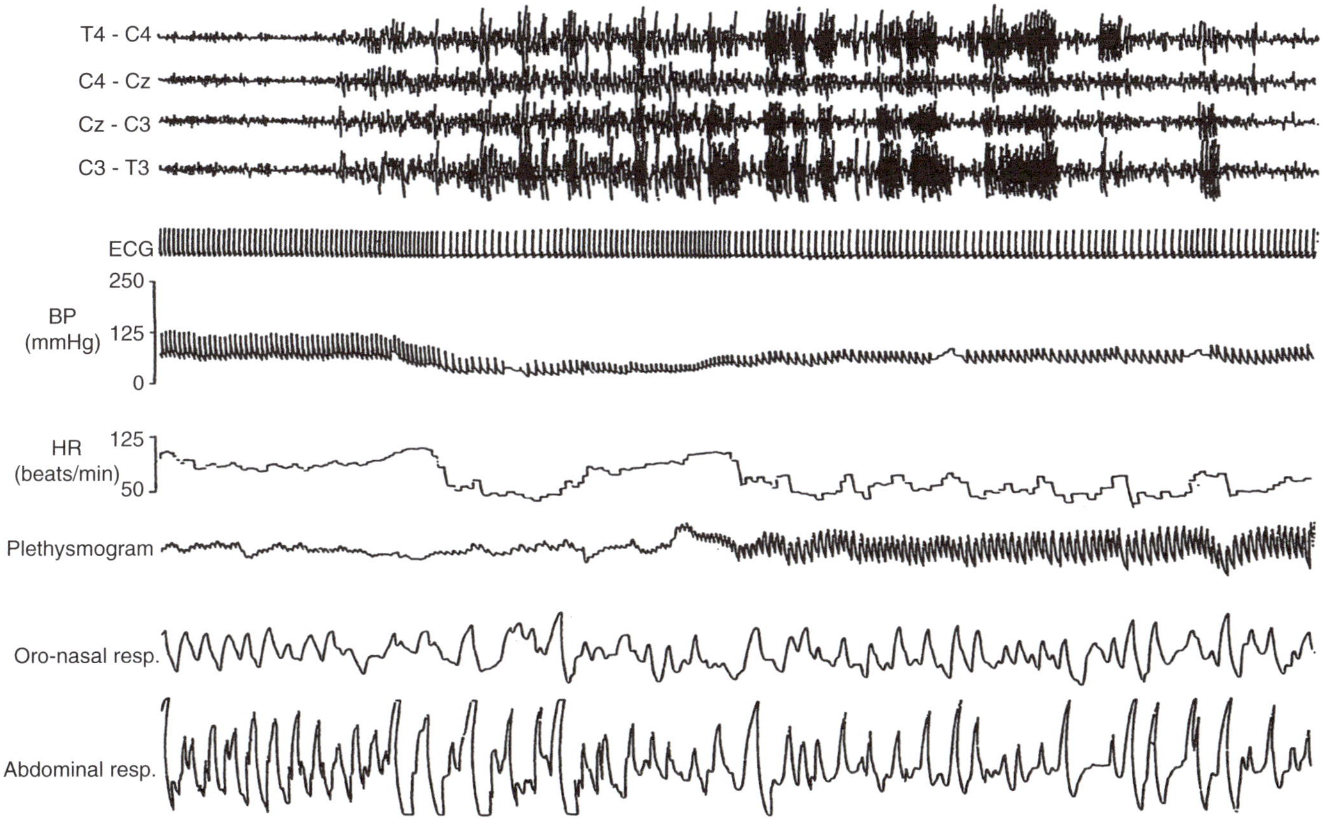

Fig. 15.34 Ictal polygraphic recording on a compressed scale. After seizure onset there was a sudden and sustained blood pressure fall associated with bradycardia. A plethysmogram showed a signal of increased amplitude

Actually it is used almost exclusively in laboratories specialized in the study of cardiovascular reflexes. In the epileptological field, it was used to study autonomic changes during focal seizures [2].

Technical box: to display the trace, a bipolar or polygraph input and an AC preamplifier are used, setting a high-pass filter at 0.3 Hz (time constant 0.5) and a low-pass filter at 30 Hz.

Many other parameters can be added to polygraphic recording. Those with more specific use that require dedicated devices are esophageal pH, penile tumescence, capnography, body temperature (internal and external), and noninvasive blood pressure.

For these signals it is necessary to use DC inputs of the polygraph by setting the low-pass filter according to the maximum frequency of the parameter to be documented.

15.4 Ambulatory Monitoring

Ambulatory monitoring combines the extended recording time of V-EEG-PSG with the convenience of recording in a patient's home. There are several products on the market that allow patients to be monitored at home via portable recording devices, some of which include video monitoring. Patients and their bed partners are instructed to keep an activity log to document events. The indications for ambulatory monitoring in the differential diagnosis of nocturnal events are not established. This monitoring technique appears promising for evaluating interictal epileptiform activity during sleep. Depending on the sophistication of the video recordings, ambulatory monitoring can identify some cases of epileptic seizures, NREM arousal disorders, RBD, rhythmic movement disorder, panic disorder, and dissociative disorder. This type of monitoring is convenient as it does not require the constant presence of a professional, and on average it is less expensive than laboratory recordings. On the other hand, the absence of a professional excludes the possibility of making adjustments to the device if needed and does not allow the technologist to interact with the patient in order to evaluate their level of consciousness. The lack of this datum might complicate the interpretation stage when discriminating rhythmic activities that might look similar to ictal discharges. The addition of synchronized video recordings to ambulatory monitoring has potential for facilitating correlation between EEG activity and clinical events.

The American Sleep Disorders Association (ASDA) has established a four-level standard of practice guideline for the diagnosis of sleep-disordered breathing:

- Level I: attended cardiorespiratory polysomnography with at least 7 signals.
- Level II: unattended, at-home cardiorespiratory polysomnography with at least seven signals (Fig. 15.35).
- Level III: unattended portable sleep apnea testing with at least four signals including airflow, respiratory effort, oxygen saturation, ECG, or heart rate or pulse rate (Fig. 15.36).
- Level IV: unattended one or two signal recording, such as actigraphy or oximetry (Fig. 15.37) [6].

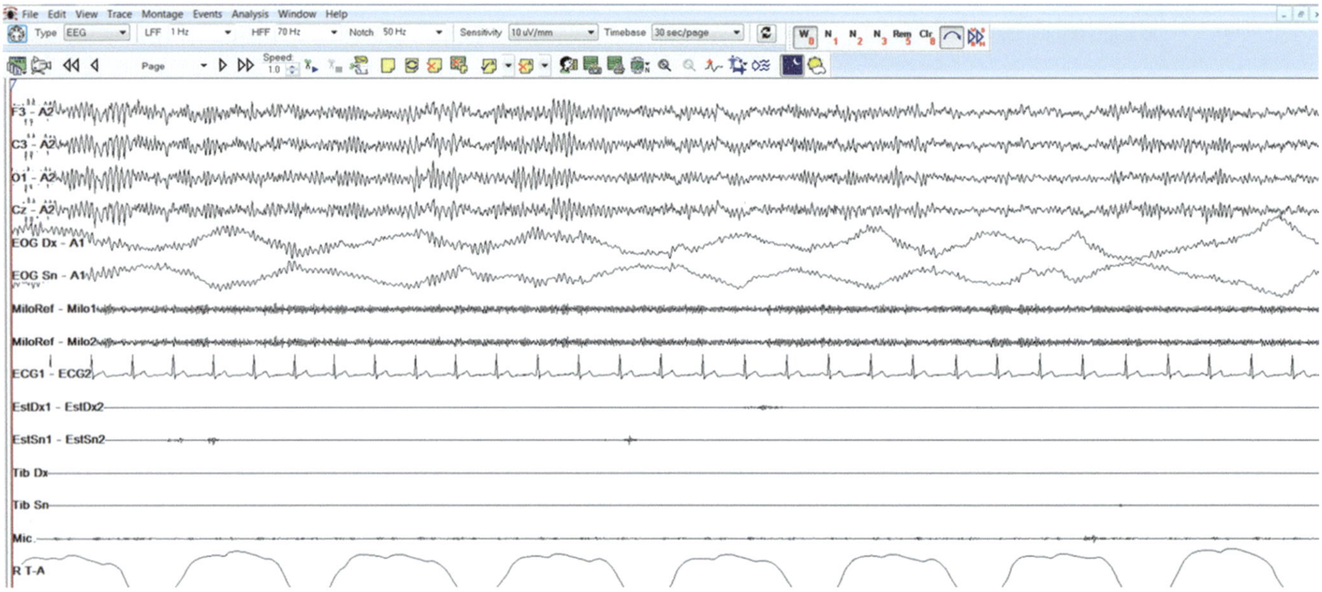

Fig. 15.35 Traces of a level II cardiorespiratory polysomnography

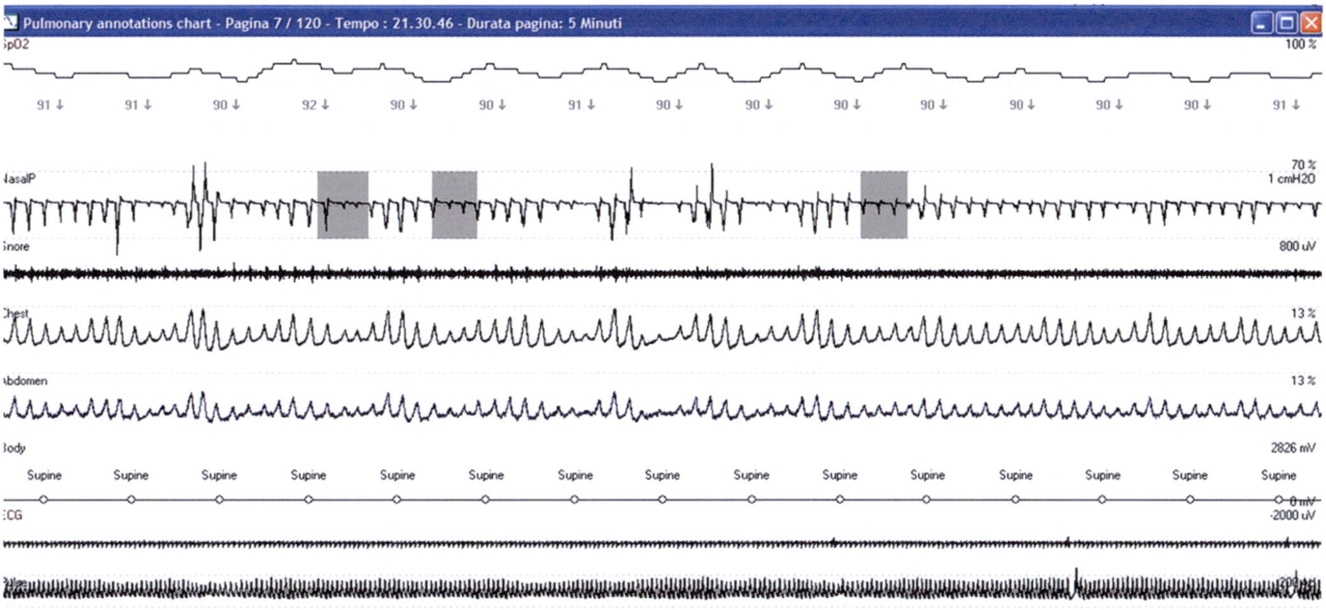

Fig. 15.36 Traces of a level III portable sleep apnea testing

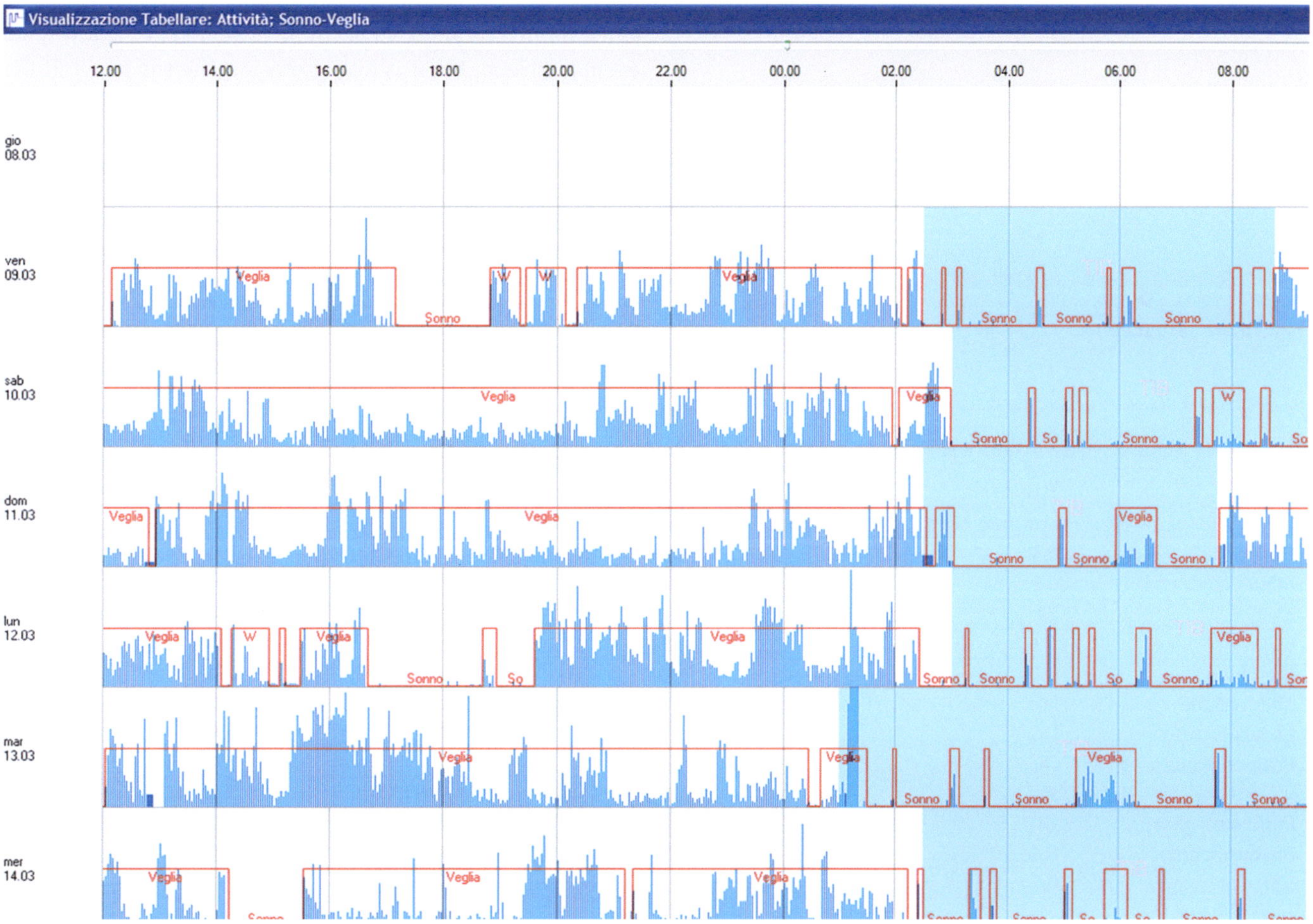

Fig. 15.37 Level IV recording of an actigraphy

15.4.1 Actigraph

It is a dynamic system used for restless legs syndrome, for the evaluation of the effectiveness of its treatment, and for the diagnosis of parasomnias, insomnia, and sleep-induced seizures. It is nothing more than a motor activity recorder of the size of a wristwatch made up of a ceramic bar and a piezoelectric transducer that generates an electrical signal whenever it senses any acceleration. It is equipped with a watchband; it is applied to the wrist, generally of the dominant limb, or to the ankle but sometimes in both the upper or lower limbs (Fig. 15.38).

It offers the advantage of providing monitoring for protracted periods (days or weeks), and it is useful for the follow-up of patients receiving pharmacological treatment; it has the disadvantage of not providing information on the type of movement, and during the recording it is not possible to detect possible malfunctions [7].

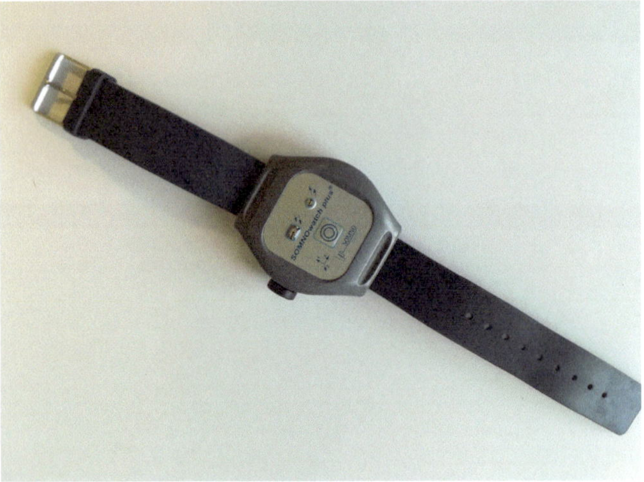

Fig. 15.38 Actigraphy

15.5 Conclusion

In this excursus on polygraphic parameters, we have considered an ideal digital polygraph, characterized by maximum versatility and therefore by the possibility to set a specific sampling frequency for each channel. If the polygraph has a single digital-analogue converter for all channels, the sampling frequency to be selected will be that of the signal with the highest frequency. In the Summary Table (Table 15.1), the values of the filters to be set can be considered as reference even if they are random because with the new digital systems it is possible to modify them until a good representation of the signal is obtained without affecting the acquired signal. We have also intentionally left out the audio-video recording of the patient synchronized with the track, considering that this has become an integral part of every modern polygraphic equipment. Nowadays video-polygraphy is not only a fundamental and irreplaceable instrument in every situation that requires an accurate evaluation of semi-motor events in sleep, but it is also a precious means to avoid frequent major interpretative errors of polygraphic traces.

Acknowledgments We would like to thank Dr. Federica Provini, Dr. Ezechiele Foschini, Dr. Francesco Mignani, and Dr. Giuseppe Loddo for providing us with images and for their valuable suggestions. Thanks to Prof. Pietro Cortelli and Dr. Giorgio Barletta, working in the autonomic nervous system laboratory, for their helpful collaboration. We also would like to thank Dr. Cecilia Baroncini for the accurate translation of the text and Massimo Armaroli and Elena Zoni for figure editing.

Table 15.1 Summary table of filter and sampling frequency setting for each polygraphic parameter

	Passa Alto		Passa Basso	Filtro Notch	Sampling rate
	Low freq. (Hz)	C.T. (s)	High freq. (Hz)		
EEG	0.3	0.5	260	OUT	200–256
EOG	0.3	0.5	235	IN	200–256
EMG	30	0.005	290	OUT	200–256
ECG	0.3	0.5	260	OUT	200–256
Breathing	0.1	1.6	215	IN	200–256
Mycrophone	30	0.005	290	OUT	200–256
Esophageal pressure	DC		215	IN	200–256
Position transducer	DC		20.5	IN	200–256
	10	0.02	250	OUT	200–256
Pulse oximetry	DC		22	IN	200–256
Plethysmogram	0.3	0.5	230	IN	200–256
SSR	0.3	0.5	30	IN	200–256

References

1. Berry RB, Brooks R, Gamaldo CE, et al. The AASM manual for the scoring of sleep and associated events. Rules, terminology and technical specification.Version 2.1; 2014.
2. Tinuper P, Bisulli F, Cerullo A, et al. Ictal bradycardia in partial epileptic seizures. Autonomic investigation in three cases and literature review. Brain. 2001;124:2341–71.
3. Vetrugno R, Liguori R, Cortelli P, et al. Sympathetic skin response basic mechanisms and clinical applications. Clin Auton Res. 2003;13:256–70.
4. Kryger M, Roth T, Dement WC. Principles and practice of sleep medicine. 6th ed. Philadelphia, PA: Elsevier; 2017.
5. Grote L, Zou D. Pulse wave analysis during sleep. In: Kryger M, Roth T, Dement WC, editors. Principles and practice of sleep medicine. 6th ed. Philadelphia, PA: Elsevier; 2017. p. 1624–32.
6. Malow BA. Neurologic monitoring techniques. In: Kryger M, Roth T, Dement WC, editors. Principles and practice of sleep medicine. 6th ed. Philadelphia, PA: Elsevier; 2016. p. 1588–97.
7. Stone KL, Israel SA. Actigraphy. In: Kryger M, Roth T, Dement WC, editors. Principles and practice of sleep medicine. 6th ed. Philadelphia, PA: Elsevier; 2017. p. 1671–8.

16 Polygraphic Investigations and Back-Averaging Techniques in the Study of Epileptic Motor Phenomena

Guido Rubboli, Carlo Alberto Tassinari, and Elena Gardella

16.1 Introduction

The term *polygraphy* refers to the simultaneous recording of multiple physiologic measures. The main aim of polygraphic monitoring is to correlate behavioral manifestations with changes occurring in a set of physiologic parameters. Therefore, to obtain the maximum yield from a polygraphic study, it is necessary to tailor it to the clinical problem that is going to be investigated by selecting the parameters that are relevant to the nature and the characteristics of this specific clinical manifestation [1, 2].

In epileptology, polygraphic investigations (PI) can be extremely useful to detect subtle and unnoticed clinical manifestations, to define the clinical characteristics of different epileptic conditions, to describe the semiology of epileptic seizures contributing to the syndromic diagnosis, to evaluate the clinical relevance of some paroxysmal activity (ictal? interictal? subclinical?), to clarify the physiopathogenetic mechanisms of epileptic phenomena, and to monitor and evaluate the effects of drugs.

As a general methodological approach, it is advisable that before a PI is set up, the epileptic phenomena that are the subject of the investigation have been previously evaluated.

with the usual video-EEG (or other) recordings. Indeed, the PI complemented with video recording is intended to document what has been collected on anamnestic data or observed by previous investigations. Consequently, various parameters will be associated to EEG recording, to evaluate the muscular activity (electromyogram, usually with surface electrodes), the respiratory and cardiac functions, the degree of performance or responsiveness, and other parameters that might be relevant for the specific clinical condition that has to be investigated [1].

In addition video-polygraphy can be of paramount importance in the differential diagnosis of non-epileptic manifestations or when both non-epileptic and epileptic phenomena are combined in the same patient [3, 4].

The aim of this chapter is to illustrate the usefulness of polygraphic recording in the detection and characterization of epileptic motor phenomena. In addition we will introduce some concepts on the contribution of computerized techniques such as back-averaging of the polygraphic signal to further describe some epileptic motor phenomena and to obtain valuable information on their underlying pathophysiological mechanisms.

16.2 Polygraphic Features of Epileptic Motor Manifestations

Motor manifestations often represent one of the most overt clinical phenomena of an epileptic seizure. PI with recording of surface EMG activity can be helpful to identify and characterize the type of motor events, the pattern of muscular activation, and the temporal correlation with changes of the EEG activity; in addition they can be a very effective tool to identify even subtle and apparently subclinical muscular manifestations such as mild contractions or sporadic muscle twitches that can be missed by the observer.

Therefore PI with surface EMG recording can be crucial to identify and to define different types of motor phenomena that can occur either isolated or in various combinations, to constitute the clinical manifestations of the different types of epileptic seizures.

G. Rubboli (✉)
Danish Epilepsy Center, Filadelfia/University of Copenhagen, Dianalund, Denmark
e-mail: guru@filadelfia.dk

C. A. Tassinari
University of Bologna, Bologna, Italy

E. Gardella
Danish Epilepsy Center, University of Southern Denmark, Dianalund, Denmark

O. Mecarelli (ed.), *Clinical Electroencephalography*, https://doi.org/10.1007/978-3-030-04573-9_16

16.2.1 Myoclonus

Myoclonus is defined as positive myoclonus when it is characterized by a massive, shock-like muscular contraction that involves one or more body segments [5]. It appears in the EMG as a brief burst of muscular potentials (Fig. 16.1a) synchronous on agonist and antagonist muscles, with or without an EEG correlate. The opposite phenomenon, a "negative" myoclonus, is a brief interruption of a tonic muscular contraction (Fig. 16.1b), sometimes clinically indistinguishable from the positive myoclonus [6]. Negative myoclonus is defined as an interruption of tonic muscular activity lasting <500 ms without evidence of preceding positive myoclonia [5]. When associated with a paroxysmal EEG event, a negative myoclonus is defined as "epileptic negative myoclonus" (Fig. 16.1c) [7–9]. Polygraphic recordings can be crucial to identify negative myoclonus and sometimes to distinguish it from positive myoclonus. In epileptic negative myoclonus, the interruption of the muscular activity occurs synchronously on agonist and antagonist muscles; when epileptic negative myoclonus is focal, involving one or both limbs on the same side of the body, it is usually associated with a contralateral EEG spike located in the centroparietal region [9]. Epileptic negative myoclonus has been recognized as a seizure type by the Task Force of the International League Against Epilepsy on Classification and Terminology [5].

16.2.2 Spasms

A spasm is characterized by a massive and slow contraction reaching a climax and progressively decreasing, more often involving axial and proximal muscular groups. PI with multiple EMG channels have shown that epileptic spasms may occur with complex patterns of muscular activation, recruiting cranial as well as limb and axial muscles (Fig. 16.2) [10, 11]. Spasms can be devoid of any EEG correlate or they can be associated with an EEG flattening, with a diffuse low-voltage fast activity [12] or with a slow wave [11, 13].

16.2.3 Tonic Contractions

The polygraphic feature of a tonic contraction is a slow, sustained contraction maintained over time that involves several muscular groups and that is usually associated with fast-recruiting EEG activity.

16.2.4 Clonic Contractions

Clonic contractions are characterized by a series of muscle jerks, whose amplitude, symmetry, frequency, and topography can vary, and that are often associated with contralateral EEG epileptic paroxysms [12].

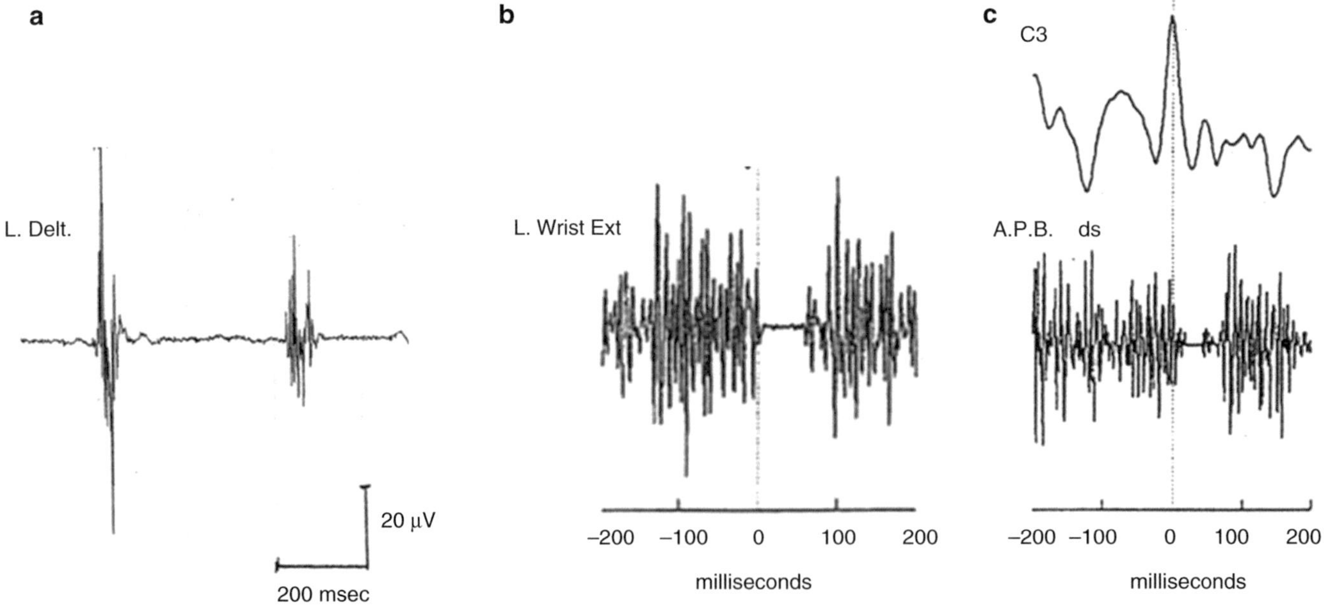

Fig. 16.1 (**a**) Two positive myoclonia in the left deltoid. (**b**) Negative myoclonus in the left wrist extensor in an outstretched left upper limb. Negative myoclonus requires a tonic contraction to be detected (the vertical marker is positioned at the onset of the EMG silent period). (**c**) Epileptic negative myoclonus in the right abductor pollicis brevis. The onset of the EMG silent period is time-locked to the peak of the spike in C3

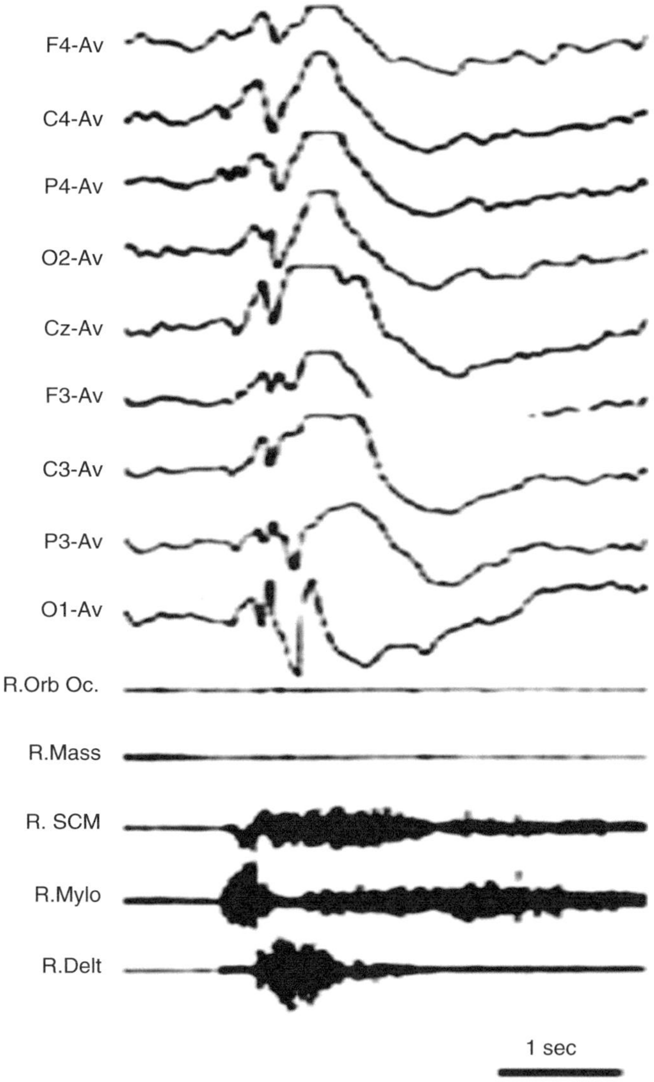

Fig. 16.2 Epileptic spasm. A massive and slow contraction reaching a climax and progressively decreasing involves the proximal limb muscles and the sternocleidomastoideus. The spasm is associated with a slow wave encompassing a spike. *R.* right, *Mass* masseter, *SCM* sternocleidomastoideus, *Mylo* mylohyoideus, *Delt* deltoid

16.2.5 Atonic Phenomena

The main feature of atonic phenomena is a sudden global or focal loss of muscular tone that corresponds in the EMG to an abrupt flattening and that can be related to different types of EEG epileptic abnormalities such as generalized spike- or polyspike-and-wave discharges, diffuse fast rhythmic spikes (Fig. 16.3), bilateral synchronous fast waves intermixed with slow waves, or no EEG changes at all [2, 12]. PI can be helpful to document the combination of myoclonic and atonic phenomena in conditions such as myoclonic-astatic epilepsy [14].

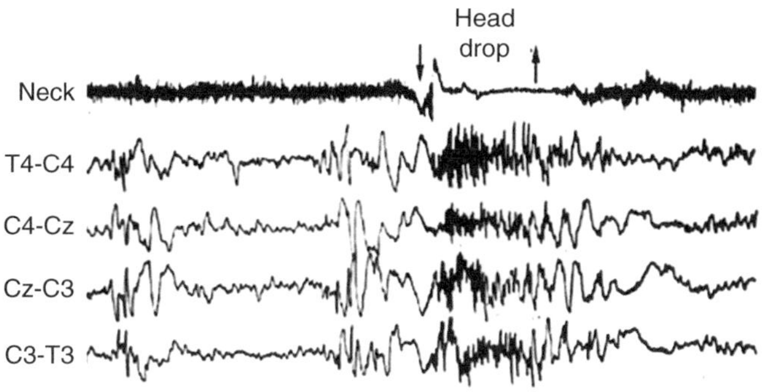

Fig. 16.3 Polygraphic recording of an atonic seizure showing the abrupt loss of muscular tone in the neck muscles, corresponding in the EMG to an abrupt flattening that clinically results in a head drop. The muscular atonia is associated with diffuse fast rhythmic spikes in the EEG

16.3 Polygraphic Patterns in Different Types of Epileptic Seizures or Syndromes

16.3.1 Generalized Tonic-Clonic Seizures

The manifestations of generalized tonic-clonic seizures consist of a more or less stereotyped sequence of motor phenomena [15, 16]. At seizure onset there is an initial tonic phase of sustained muscular contraction lasting 10–20 s and involving all skeletal muscles that corresponds clinically to a flexion involving the whole body, followed by a longer extension phase. Then a diffuse vibratory contraction follows, eventually evolving to massive clonic manifestations that progressively slow down until the seizure ends. The clonic manifestations are usually brief. PI have shown that few seconds after the last clonic jerk, often a new tonic contraction can occur, involving mainly facial and masticatory muscles. In the EEG, the initial phase is usually associated with a desynchronization, sometimes preceded by generalized bursts of polyspike-and-waves and followed by a recruiting rhythm. During the evolution of the seizure, the recruiting rhythm starts to be intermixed with slow waves of decreasing frequency and increasing amplitude that at a certain point correspond to the fragmentation of the tonic massive contraction and to the appearance of the clonic manifestations. The end of the motor manifestations is associated with a flattening of the EEG activity lasting several seconds.

16.3.2 Tonic Seizures

The tonic seizures are characterized clinically by muscular tonic contraction, lasting about 5–20 s, and accompanied by

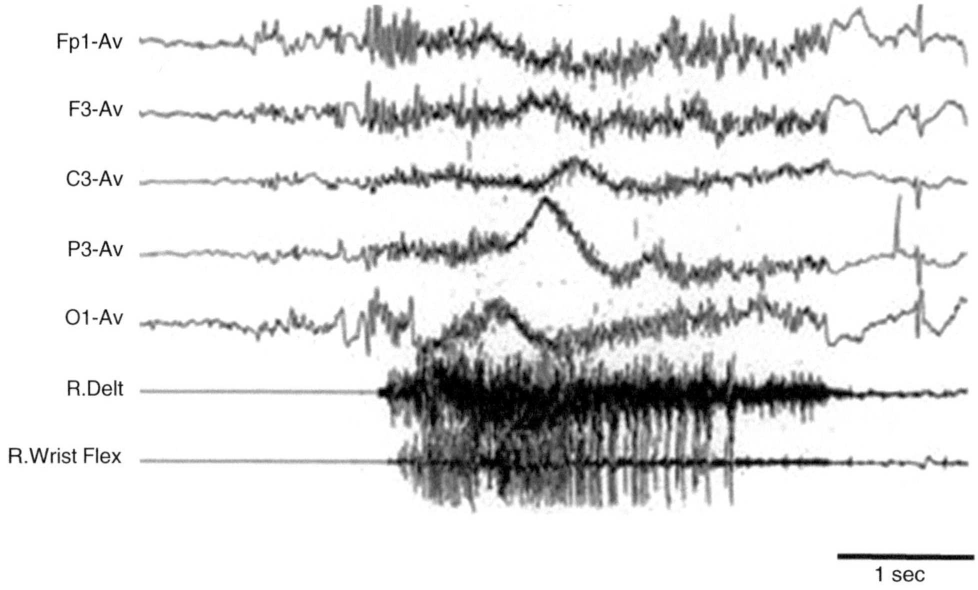

Fig. 16.4 Polygraphic recording of a tonic seizure, characterized by a muscular tonic contraction in the recorded muscles associated with rhythmic fast activity (around 20 Hz) in the EEG. *R.* right, *Delt* deltoid, *Wrist Flex* wrist flexor

impairment of consciousness, involving, with varying degrees of intensity, mainly muscles of the head, trunk, limb girdles, and, to a lesser extent, legs [17–19]. PI can show different EEG patterns such as (a) flattening of the tracing, (b) fast activity (around 20 Hz) of progressively increasing amplitude (Fig. 16.4), and (c) recruiting rhythmic discharge at about 10 Hz, sometimes of high amplitude from the onset. In the EMG channels, the tonic contraction is associated with an interference pattern in all muscles involved by the seizure. In short tonic seizures, the EMG activity is maximal at the onset and then decreases; in longer seizures, the intensity of the EMG activation progressively increases reflecting the increasing intensity of the contraction. In global tonic seizures, an axial preponderance of the muscular activation is evident. An asymmetric tonic contraction or a massive myoclonia at the end of the tonic muscular activity can be observed. Autonomic changes, such as modifications of heart and respiration rate, vasomotor phenomena, mydriasis, and positive electrodermogram responses are additional features of tonic seizures [18].

16.3.3 Myoclonic Absences

The distinguishing features of myoclonic absences are (a) appearance of a generalized 3 c/s spike-and-wave discharge lasting up to several seconds and (b) myoclonic jerks associated with spike-wave complexes, particularly evident in the upper limbs that, a few seconds after the onset of the EEG epileptic activity, are superimposed to a progressively increasing tonic muscular contraction, maximal at the shoulders that clinically results in the abduction and elevation of the arms (Fig. 16.5) [20, 21]. Detailed analysis of the EEG-EMG correlations has shown that the positive transient of the 3 c/s spike-and-wave complex is time-locked to the appearance of the myoclonic jerks. The myoclonic bursts are followed by a brief (60–120 ms) silent period that fragments the tonic contraction [21, 22].

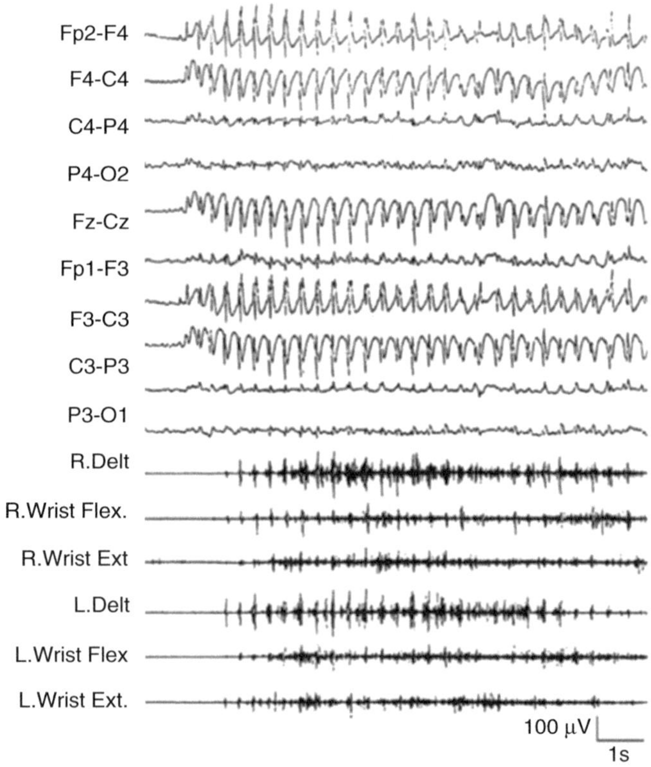

Fig. 16.5 Myoclonic absence seizure. The main feature of this seizure type are (a) generalized 3 c/s spike-and-wave discharge lasting up to several seconds; (b) myoclonic jerks time-locked to the spike-wave complexes, more prominent in the upper limbs that, a few seconds after the onset of the EEG epileptic activity, are superimposed to a progressively increasing tonic muscular contraction, maximal at the shoulders that clinically results in the abduction and elevation of the arms. *R.* right, *Delt* deltoid, *Wrist Flex* wrist flexor, *Wrist Ext* wrist extensor

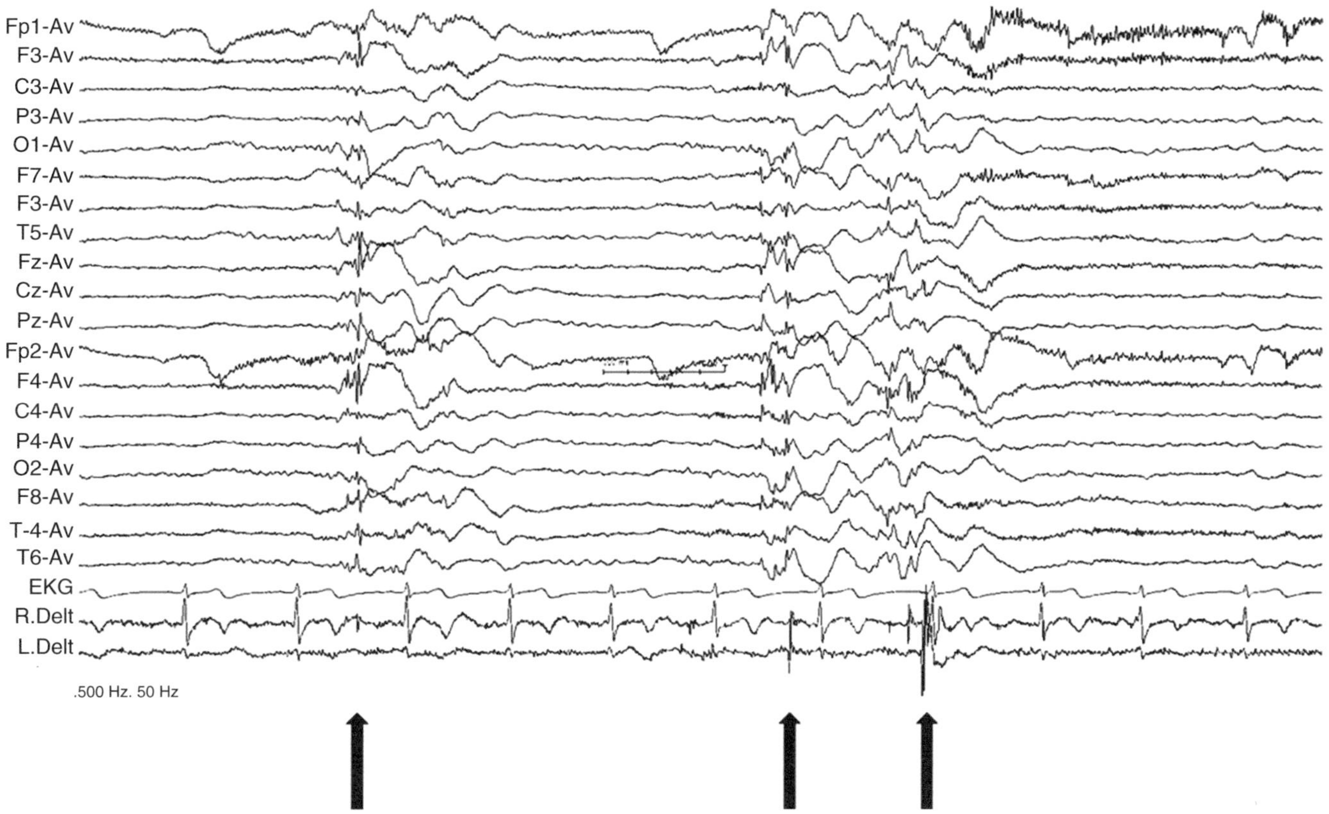

Fig. 16.6 Myoclonic jerks in juvenile myoclonic epilepsy. The myoclonic jerks, indicated by the arrows, are associated with a generalized polyspike-wave discharge. *R.* right, *L.* left, *Delt* deltoid

16.3.4 Juvenile Myoclonic Epilepsy

The polygraphic signature of juvenile myoclonic epilepsy are short bursts of myoclonic jerks—particularly at the upper limbs—associated with polyspike-and-wave complexes at a frequency of 3–3.5 c/s (Fig. 16.6) [23]. Computerized analysis of the polygraphic signal has demonstrated that the myoclonic bursts are correlated to a cortical positive potential encompassed in the polyspike rhythm of the polyspike-wave complex [24].

16.3.5 Epilepsia Partialis Continua

PI in epilepsia partialis continua has shown more or less rhythmic myoclonic EMG potentials whose EEG correlate can be variable, such as slow focal abnormalities, focal paroxysmal discharges, or no evident paroxysmal activity [25]. In some patients, a clinical picture resembling epilepsia partialis continua, characterized by frequent, subcontinuous jerks, evident when the patient maintains a posture or a tonic contraction, can be caused by subcontinuous epileptic negative myoclonia (i.e., brief lapses of the muscular activity time-locked to paroxysmal EEG activity). In these cases, PI are crucial for the correct diagnosis.

16.3.6 Progresive Myoclonus Epilepsies

Progressive myoclonus epilepsies (PMEs) are a group of rare inherited diseases featuring a combination of myoclonus, seizures, and variable degrees of neurological and cognitive impairment. Despite extensive investigations, a large number of PMEs remain undiagnosed. PI can be helpful in the diagnostic process either in the initial phase for differential diagnosis or to detect distinguishing features in the different forms of PMEs.

The main polygraphic feature of progresive myoclonus epilepsies is myoclonus, either at rest or during action that is characterized by EMG potentials of short duration (20–30 ms), which are synchronous on agonist and antagonist muscles (Fig. 16.7) [27]. At rest, erratic myoclonic twitches can occur asynchronously in different muscular groups. In action myoclonus the EMG potentials are of high amplitude and are followed by an EMG silent period lasting 40–120 ms (rarely up to 300 ms). The myoclonic EMG bursts and the silent periods are inconstantly related to EEG spike-and-waves and polyspike-and-waves (Fig. 16.7). In Unverricht-Lundborg disease, myoclonic seizures are characterized by generalized myoclonia, predominant proximally in the upper limbs, with varying rhythm and associated with generalized, symmetrical polyspikes or polyspike-and-waves [28, 29].

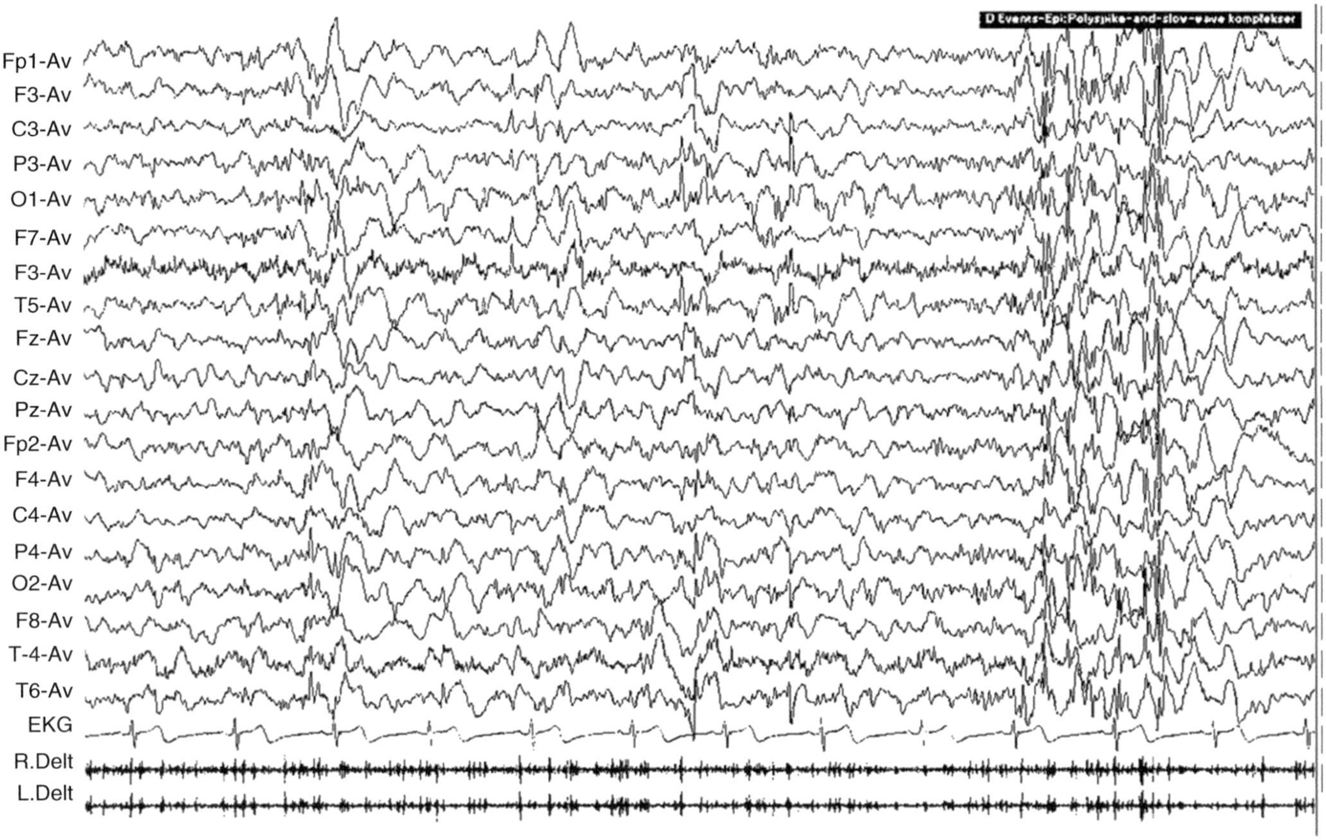

Fig. 16.7 Polygraphic tracing in progressive myoclonus epilepsy with *KCNC1* mutation [26]. The recording at rest shows subcontinuous myoclonic potentials, intermingled with negative myoclonia in both deltoids. The myoclonic EMG bursts and the silent periods are inconstantly related to EEG spike-and-waves and polyspike-and-waves. *R.* right, *L.* left, *Delt.* deltoid

PIs in Lafora disease show abundant, asymmetrical, asynchronous, subtle myoclonia at rest, diffuse to all muscular groups, usually without an EEG correlate [27, 30, 31]. Rarer forms of PMEs, such as sialidosis [32]; ceroid neuronal lipofuscinosis [33]; PMEs associated with *SCARB2* mutations [34], with ASAH1 mutations [35], and with *GOSR2* mutations [36, 37]; and rhythmic myoclonia, clinically resembling a tremor, i.e., "cortical tremor" [38], have been shown, by means of computerized technique of the EEG-EMG signals, to be associated with a rhythmic cortical potential at the same frequency of the myoclonus in the contralateral central regions [39, 40]. In PMEs, visual stimuli and intermittent photic stimulation can be extremely effective in eliciting fast polyspikes and polyspike-and-waves associated with massive myoclonic jerks, i.e., "photic reflex myoclonus" (Fig. 16.8) or even in precipitating myoclonic seizures [41].

16.4 Some Reflections on EEG-EMG Correlations in Epileptic Seizures

The relationships between the features of the epileptic EEG discharges and the associated EMG event can indeed be variable. In fact, based on polygraphic recordings, we can recognize:

1. Seizure types in which there is a strict, time-locked association between the EEG paroxysmal event and the related clinical/EMG phenomenon, such as juvenile myoclonic epilepsy [24], positive and negative myoclonus of epileptic nature [6, 42], photic-induced myoclonus [41], and certain epileptic action myoclonus [27, 43]. In these conditions, a proper analysis, supported by computerized techniques, can show a very precise correlation between the EEG epileptic abnormality, or even to some component of it, and the EMG manifestations.
2. Seizure types in which similar EEG patterns can result in different clinical phenomena. Examples are "tonic" and "atonic" seizures which both can feature rhythmically repeated spikes in the EEG (Figs. 16.3 and 16.4). Similarly with positive and negative myoclonus, we can speculate that "tonic" and "atonic" seizures with apparently "similar" expression on the EEG are indeed related to different positive or negative components of the EEG discharge possibly reflecting different functional and anatomical networks.
3. Seizure types in which the ictal EEG features and the motor event are concomitant but without a strict temporal correlation. Examples of this possibility are represented by tonic seizures (Fig. 16.4), spasms (Fig. 16.2), or even the complex albeit stereotyped motor patterns that can be observed

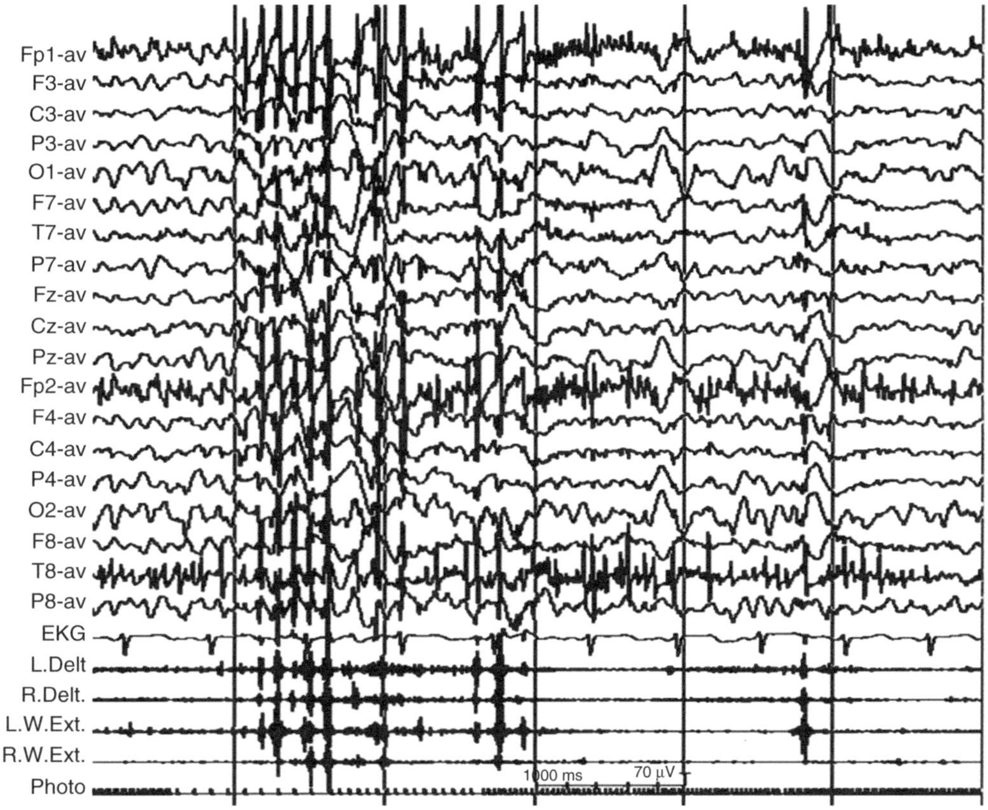

Fig. 16.8 Photic reflex myoclonus in a photosensitive patient. Intermittent photic stimulation elicits generalized spike-wave discharges associated with myoclonic jerks in the upper limbs. *L.* left, *R.* right, *EKG* electrocardiogram, *Photo* intermittent photic stimulation, *Delt.* deltoid, *Wrist Ext.* wrist extensor

in some focal epilepsies. In these instances, the epileptic event in the cortex represents the "trigger" that releases a cascade of motor sequences. In fact, in both tonic seizures and spasms, the muscular manifestations outlast the end of the EEG discharge and encompass some "archaic" motor patterns, such as a startle reaction in tonic seizures [44]. These observations have led to the hypothesis that in certain seizures, the motor semiology results from the activation of genetically determined archaic functional motor systems, such as the central pattern generators [45].

4. Seizure types that seem to result from the combination of different seizures. The best example are myoclonic absences which are characterized by (1) 3 c/s spike-and-wave discharges, almost undistinguishable from the pattern of Childhood Absence Epilepsy; (2) a positive transient encompassed in the spike-wave complex that is associated with rhythmic myoclonias; and (3) a tonic contraction as in tonic seizures (as described by [46]).

16.5 Back-Averaging Techniques Applied to the Analysis of Polygraphic Signals

The introduction of computer-assisted techniques for the collection and the processing of the polygraphic signal has increased the yield of PI. In epilepsy, these techniques have been applied in particular to the analysis of EEG and EMG signals, simultaneously collected, to extract information not obtainable with standard PI. One of the most widespread techniques is back-averaging of the EEG activity triggered by a muscular event.

Back-averaging techniques have been introduced mainly to detect eventual brain electrical potentials associated with an involuntary movement and to study their temporal correlation and their topographic distribution over the scalp. The first description of a temporal correlation between a paroxysmal EEG abnormality and a myoclonic contraction dates back to Grinker [47]. However, by commenting on these data, Dawson [48] recognized that although the two phenomena (EEG abnormality and myoclonic contraction) appeared closely related, their exact temporal relationship could not be determined. It was Shibasaki and Kuroiwa [49] who introduced a method based on the technique of "summation" of neurophysiological signals introduced by Dawson [50]. By using this approach, it was possible to identify cortical events, hidden in the background activity, associated with a muscular phenomenon, to determine their spatial distribution over the scalp, and to establish the temporal relations between the two events. These techniques were called "back-averaging" or "jerk-locked averaging" methods, as they used as trigger for the summation or "averaging" procedure of the related EEG activity, the muscle potential associated with a positive myoclonia (myoclonic jerk) (Fig. 16.9). Later on, techniques that use as trigger an abrupt interruption of muscle contraction, i.e., a negative myoclonus, such as in asterixis, have been introduced (Fig. 16.9). These latter methods have been

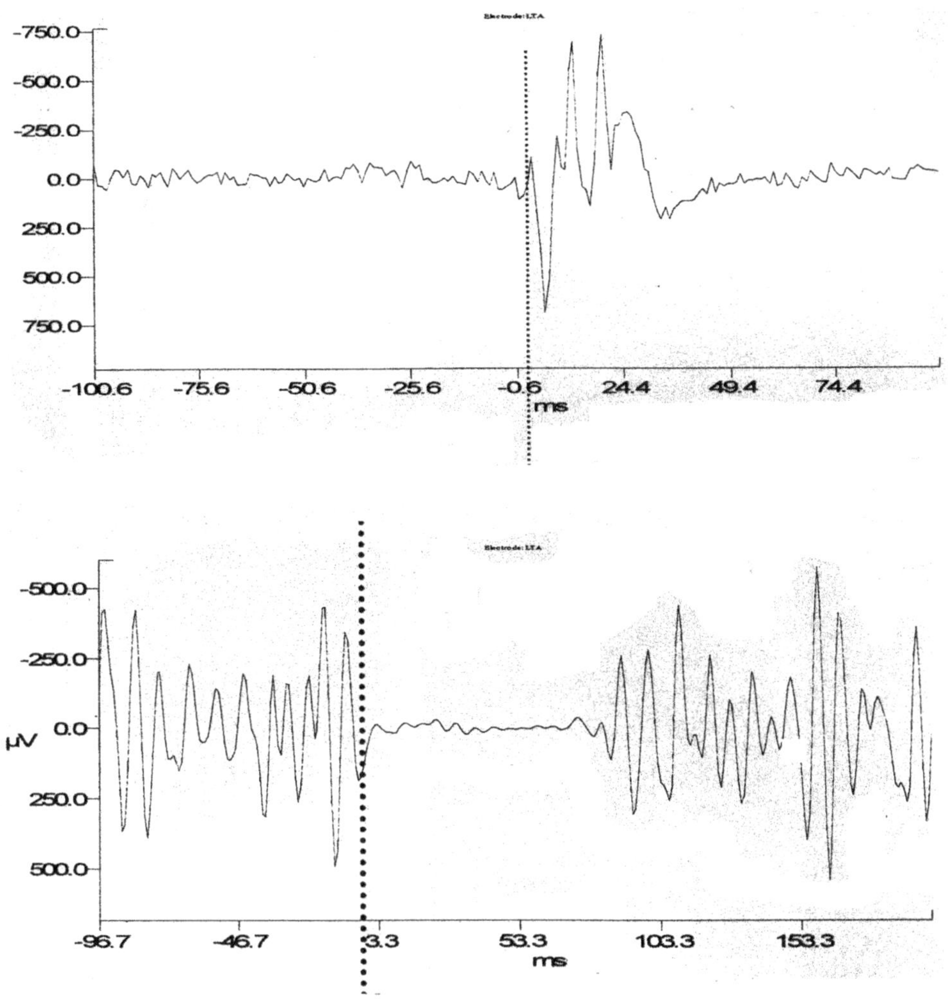

Fig. 16.9 Back-averaging applied to the study of positive and negative myoclonus. Upper trace: In positive myoclonus, the marker (vertical line) for the triggering of the averaging procedure is positioned at the onset of the myoclonic burst. Lower trace: In negative myoclonus, the marker (vertical line) for the averaging procedure is positioned at the onset of the muscular silent period

labelled as "silent period-locked averaging," i.e., summation procedures related to the silent period [51].

The fundamental principle on which the back-averaging techniques of EEG-EMG activity are based is that the electric activity due to "noise" or unrelated to the muscular phenomenon progressively cancels out until it approaches to zero with the process of averaging. On the contrary, the electric brain activities related to the muscular phenomenon add up to a constant latency and will appear, after the process of averaging, as a well-defined signal, distinct from the underlying activity. An important requirement for the muscular phenomenon to act as a "trigger" is that this phenomenon has a rapid and well-defined onset (Fig. 16.9) [52]. Therefore the motor disturbances that are best suitable for this type of analysis and that have been more extensively investigated with these techniques are the myoclonic phenomena.

16.5.1 Back-Averaging Applications to the Study of Myoclonus

By using "jerk-locked averaging," Shibasaki and Kuroiwa [49] were able to demonstrate the existence of a premyoclonic EEG potential, not identifiable by visual inspection of the polygraphic tracing. Moreover, this procedure proved equally effective in defining the temporal relationships between the cortical potential and the myoclonic event even when a paroxysmal activity associated with myoclonus was already evident in the polygraphy. The demonstration of an EEG activity temporally correlated with the myoclonic phenomenon is considered one of the main criteria in the definition of cortical myoclonus, either positive or negative [6]. Therefore, the "jerk-locked averaging" as well as the "silent period-locked averaging" methods can be extremely useful in demonstrating a cortical origin of a myoclonic event.

In this section, we illustrate the EEG and EMG features associated with the different types of myoclonus and the yields provided by computer-assisted techniques.

16.5.1.1 EMG correlates of Positive and Negative Myoclonus

The EMG features of positive cortical myoclonus can be variable. Myoclonic potentials consist of short burst (≤50 ms) of EMG activity, usually synchronous in agonist and antagonist muscles. This EMG activity can be focal, affecting a single muscle, but more often it involves many adjacent muscles.

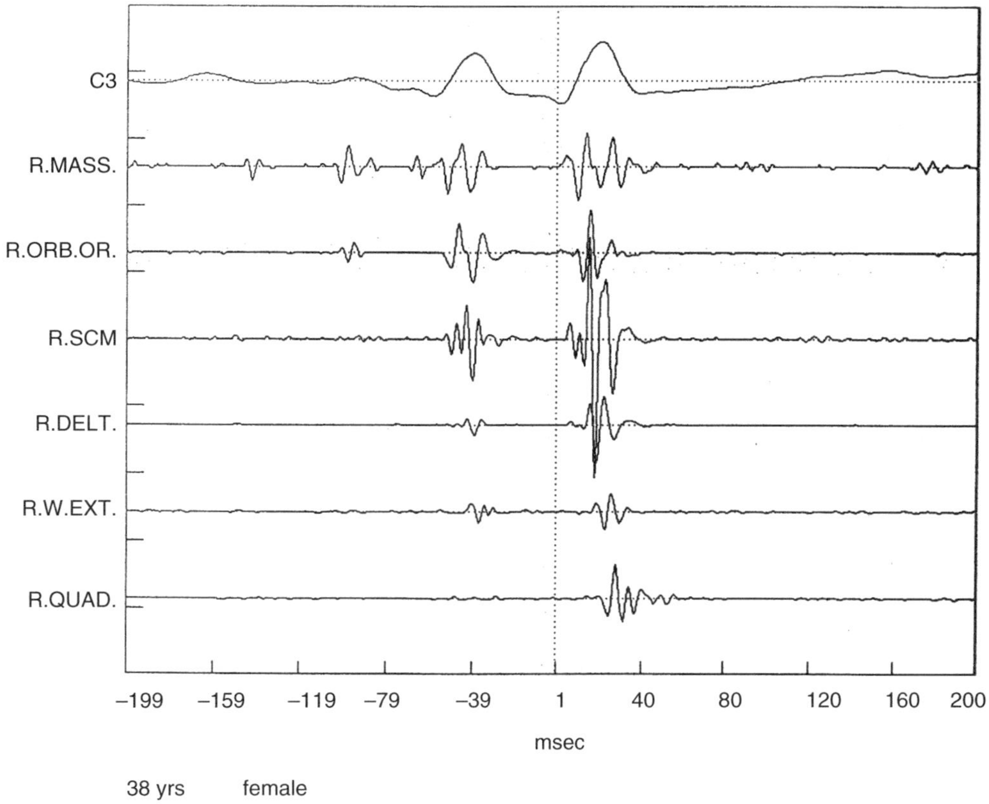

Fig. 16.10 Myoclonic bursts in photic reflex myoclonus. The myoclonic jerks in the right side of the body are related to low-amplitude EEG potentials in the left central region (C3). The different muscles are activated according to a rostro-caudal pattern, and the latency of activation of the different muscles from the EEG potential is consistent with a propagation according to fast-conducting corticospinal pathways. *R.* right, *Mass* masseter, *Orb. Or.* orbicularis oris, *SCM* sternocleidomastoideus, *Delt.* deltoid, *Wrist Ext.* wrist extensor, *Quad.* quadriceps

PI can also show that this type of myoclonus is propagated to different muscle groups with a rostro-caudal pattern and the speed of propagation corresponds to that of the large myelinated motor axons (Fig. 16.10) [6, 53, 54]. Cortical myoclonus can be irregular as well as rhythmic or pseudorhythmic, such as in the so-called cortical tremor or familial cortical tremor with epilepsy and sometimes also in corticobasal degeneration [38, 55, 56]. Frequently, the cortical myoclonus is sensitive to stimuli of various kinds, such as tendon stretching or other somatosensory stimulations, such as maintaining a posture, or active or passive movement. In epileptic positive myoclonus, such as in epilepsia partialis continua, the EMG potentials may be very short and with a very abrupt onset (less than 50 ms) (Fig. 16.11). Myoclonic activities observed in myoclonic absence seizures have peculiar features, as already outlined, such as rhythmic EMG potentials at the same frequency of the spike-wave discharge, superimposed to a tonic activity of progressively increasing amplitude (Fig. 16.5) [21]. This tonic contraction can mask the myoclonus and make the clinical manifestation complex. Each myoclonus is followed by a silent period, with a duration ranging from 60 to 120 ms, which interrupts the tonic EMG activity.

Subcortical positive myoclonus sometimes can be difficult to distinguish from cortical positive myoclonus. Common neurophysiological features of the subcortical myoclonus are a less abrupt onset and often a longer duration. For example, myoclonus of Creutzfeldt-Jakob disease is generally not stimulus-sensitive and occurs subcontinuously and quasi-periodically, with intervals varying between 0.6 and 1.5 s. It is often associated with postures or dystonic movements in the affected limb. The duration of each EMG phenomenon is similar or slightly longer than that of cortical myoclonus. It should be noted that, in more advanced stages of the disease, patients may also show a myoclonus undistinguishable from the typical reflex cortical myoclonus. In some cases of subcortical reflex myoclonus, the pattern of muscular recruitment indicates an initial activation of the muscles related to the nuclei of the VII and XI cranial nerves, and then the myoclonic bursts spread rostrally and caudally. This has led to the hypothesis of the existence of a generator of myoclonic activity at the level of the reticular formation of the brain stem, subserved by fast-conducting reticulospinal pathways [57]. Myoclonia featuring these characteristics is labelled as reflex reticular myoclonias.

The EMG correlates of negative myoclonic phenomena can be variable as well. To identify such phenomena, it is necessary that the subject maintains a tonic contraction in the affected muscular districts. The interruption of the interferential EMG activity due to the negative myoclonus is expressed clinically by a sudden cessation of the muscle contraction, causing a postural lapse or interfering with the execution of a motor task [58]. The longer the duration of the EMG silent period, the more clinically evident and disturbing will be the negative myoclonus. A form of stimulus-sensitive cortical negative myoclonus has been described [59].

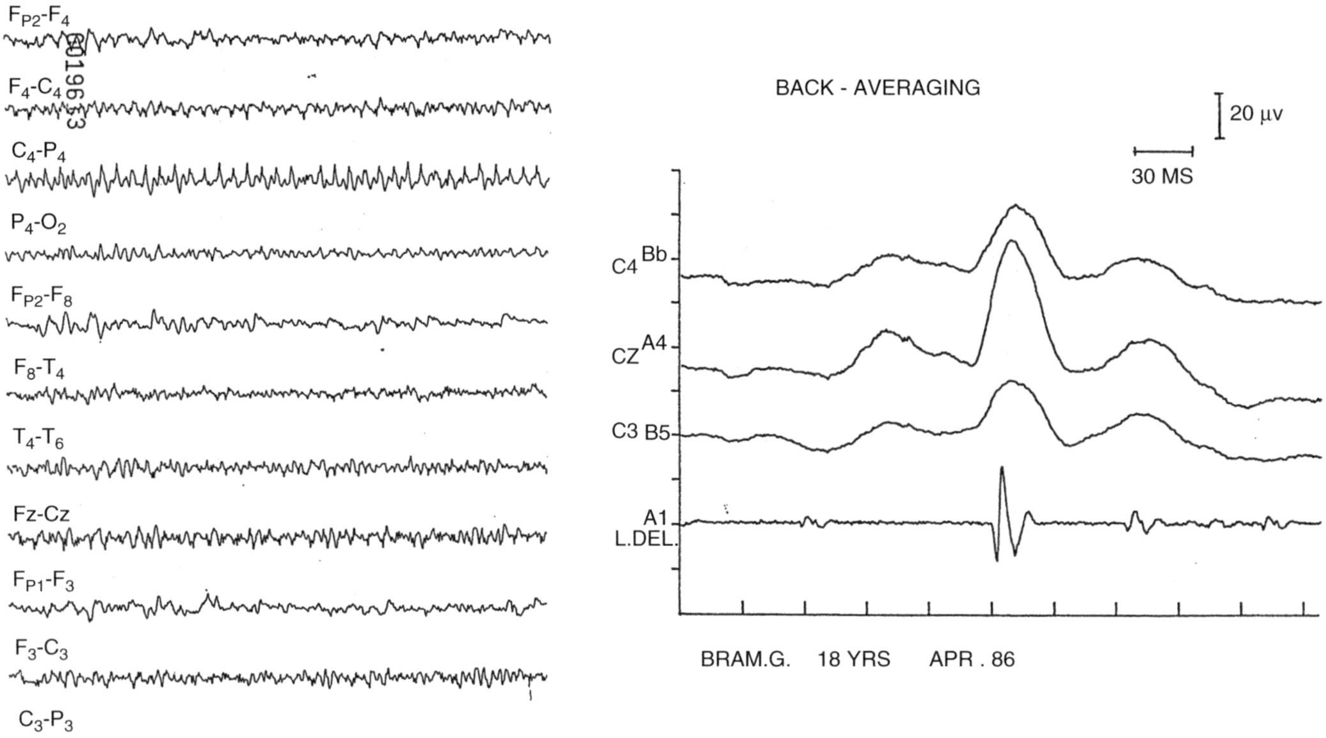

Fig. 16.11 Left: EEG tracing of a patient with epilepsia partialis continua with rhythmic myoclonia at the left upper limb. The EEG shows rhythmic spikes in the right centroparietal leads. Right: back-average of 20 myoclonic jerks in the left deltoid showing a time-locked correlation between the muscular bursts and the EEG potential (that has higher amplitude over Cz). *Delt.* deltoid, *L.* left

Epileptic negative myoclonus (ENM) is characterized by the occurrence of a silent period both on the agonist and antagonist muscle, without being preceded by a positive myoclonia, time-locked to an EEG epileptic discharge [9]. ENM duration can be extremely variable (up to 400 ms).

The subcortical negative myoclonus tends to be rhythmic, and if bilateral, often synchronous between the two sides. Also in this type of negative myoclonus, the EMG silent period is detectable both on agonist and antagonist [60]. Asterixis, probably the most common type of subcortical negative myoclonus, can be relatively rhythmic at a frequency of 6–11 Hz, with silent periods lasting from 50 to 200 ms.

Finally, there are conditions, such as postanoxic myoclonus and progresive myoclonus epilepsies, in which action myoclonus is characterized by a variable combination of positive and negative myoclonic phenomena, inconstantly associated with an EEG correlate (Fig. 16.7) [43].

16.5.1.2 EEG Correlates of Positive and Negative Myoclonus

The demonstration of an EEG potential time-locked to the myoclonic phenomenon is one of the main criteria for the definition of cortical myoclonus. In some epileptic conditions, polygraphic recording can show a clear correlation between an EEG paroxysmal activity and the myoclonic EMG burst. Typical examples are myoclonic absences, where myoclonias are related to the positive transient encompassed in the spike-wave complex. The latencies between the positive transient and the onset of myoclonus is about 15–40 ms, for the most proximal muscles, and of 50–70 ms, for the most distal muscles ([21, 22]). In juvenile myoclonic epilepsy, there is a clear association between the polyspike rhythm of the polyspike-wave complex and the myoclonic jerk (Fig. 16.12). The analysis of this correlation showed a predominantly frontal distribution of the myoclonus-related EEG potential; the myoclonic volley propagates to various muscular segments with a rostrocaudal pattern via fast corticospinal pathways (Fig. 16.12) [24]. In conditions with cortical myoclonus in which standard PIs do not show an overt myoclonus-related EEG event, jerk-locked averaging can unveil the cortical correlate and can provide a measure of the latency between the EEG potential and the EMG myoclonic burst, which ranges between 20 and 40 ms for the muscles of the hand and of the lower limbs, respectively (Fig. 16.13) [61]. It has also been shown that the topography of the premyoclonic potential on the scalp may vary in relation to the muscle affected by myoclonus, respecting the somatotopia of the motor homunculus [53, 61].

In the study of photic reflex myoclonus (Fig. 16.8), a peculiar form of reflex myoclonus induced by visual stimuli,

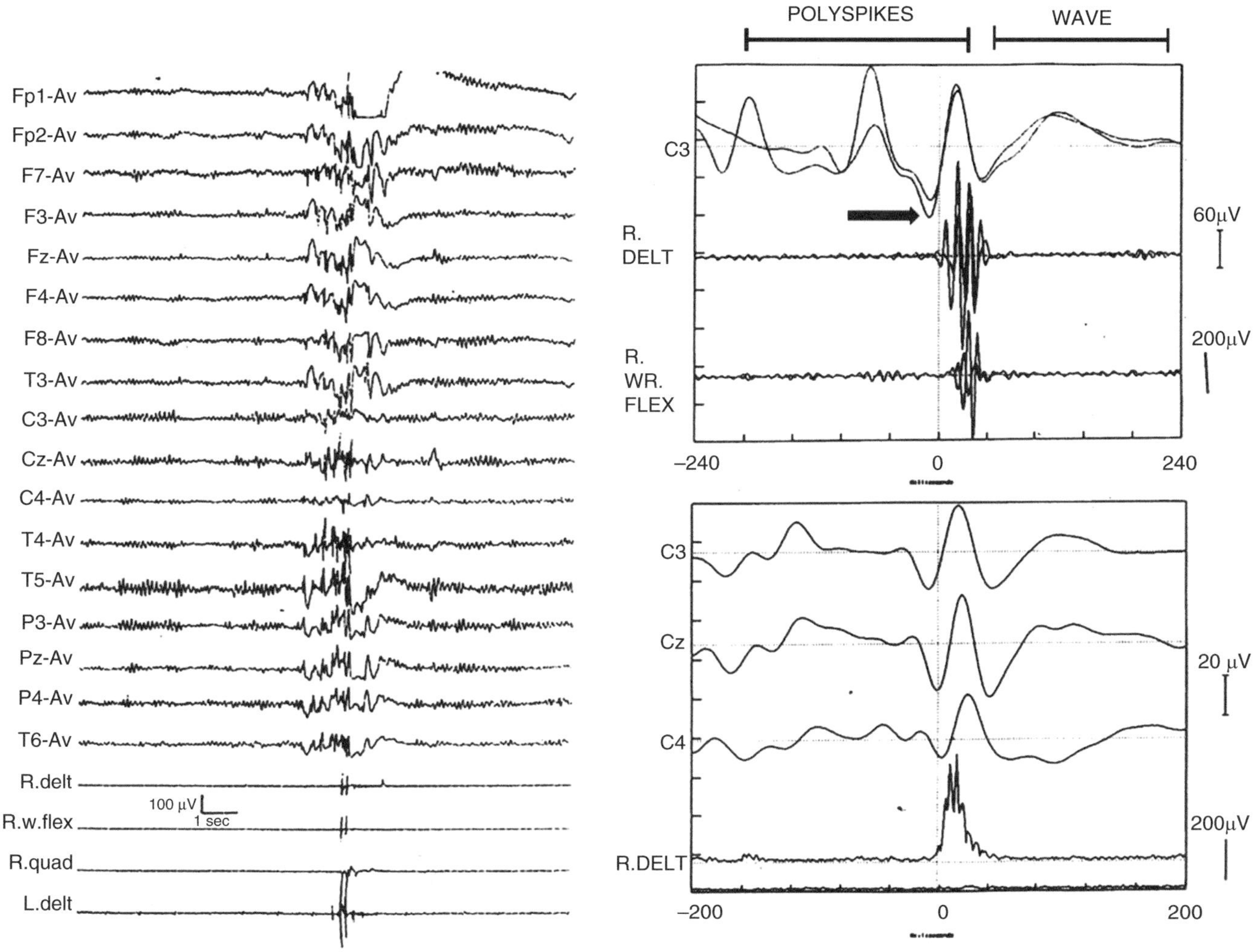

Fig. 16.12 Left: polygraphic recording of a myoclonic jerk in a patient with juvenile myoclonic epilepsy. Right, upper panel: the relationship between the positive transient (arrow) encompassed in the polyspike discharge (indicated by a horizontal line above the figure) and the myoclonus in the muscles of the right upper limb is shown. Right, lower panel: jerk-locked average of 20 myoclonias showing the relationship between the EEG potential and the myoclonic event. The EEG potential in C3 (related to the myoclonia in the right deltoid) anticipated of about 10 ms, the EEG potential in C4. *Delt* deltoid, *Wrist Flex* wrist flexor, *R* right

jerk-locked averaging of the EEG-EMG signals has shown that the visual stimulus activates first the visual cortex and then the cortical excitation propagates (with a latency of about 10 ms), probably via occipito-frontal pathways, to the motor cortex, where a myoclonic volley originates recruiting various muscular districts, according to a rostro-caudal pattern, with latency of recruitment compatible with direct, fast-conducting corticospinal pathways, as observed in other forms of cortical myoclonus (Fig. 16.10) [41, 62]. In action myoclonus [53], photic reflex myoclonus [41], and juvenile myoclonus epilepsy [24], the analysis of bilateral, apparently synchronous, myoclonic jerks showed that there is a brief interval, of about 10 ms, between the myoclonia of the two sides, corresponding to a similar interval between the respective EEG correlates (Fig. 16.12). This data suggests that the cortical myoclonic activity originates in one hemisphere and spreads, probably via transcallosal fibers, to the contralateral one.

The "jerk-locked averaging" techniques can also be very useful in demonstrating either the absence of a myoclonus-related EEG potential or the absence of a temporal relationship between the muscular and the EEG event [57]. These aspects, associated with somatosensory evoked potentials of normal amplitude, are compatible with a subcortical myoclonus.

16.5.2 Averaging Techniques to Study Negative Motor Phenomena

PI associated with "silent period-locked averaging" techniques are crucial to demonstrate the existence of a negative muscular phenomenon and to detect possible EEG correlates. Ugawa et al. [51], by using this method, showed that asterixis in the upper limbs may be, in some cases, devoid of a clear cortical potential, whereas in other conditions it may be associated with an EEG potential in the contralateral central regions. In postanoxic myoclonus, Lance and Adams [63] found a relationship between the onset of the EMG silent period and the onset of the slow wave of the spike-wave complex. In ENM, "spike-averaging" techniques, where the average is performed using the peak of ENM-related spike as the trigger, have shown that the EMG silent period is related to the ENM-related spikes (Fig. 16.14) [42, 64] or to the slow wave of a spike-wave complex [65]. Further studies have shown that the negative phenomenon occurs when the epileptic activity spreads to frontal (Fig. 16.15) or parietal (Fig. 16.16) inhibitory areas (Fig. 16.17) [9, 42, 64, 67]. Recent data, obtained by intracerebral electrical stimulation combined with averaging techniques of the EMG signal triggered by the electrical stimulus in patients undergoing presurgical evaluation for drug-resistant epilepsies, showed the differential role of premotor, supplementary motor, primary motor, and parietal areas in producing positive or negative myoclonic phenomena. Interestingly, these investigations demonstrated that, regardless the intensity of the electrical stimulation, primary/premotor cortex originates mainly positive myoclonia, whereas supplementary motor cortex originates only negative myoclonia. Stimulation of the parietal cortex could elicit either positive or negative phenomena depending on the stimulus intensity [66]. These findings are in agreement with evidences showing the existence of negative motor areas encompassed in the supplementary motor cortex and in the inferior frontal gyrus [68, 69].

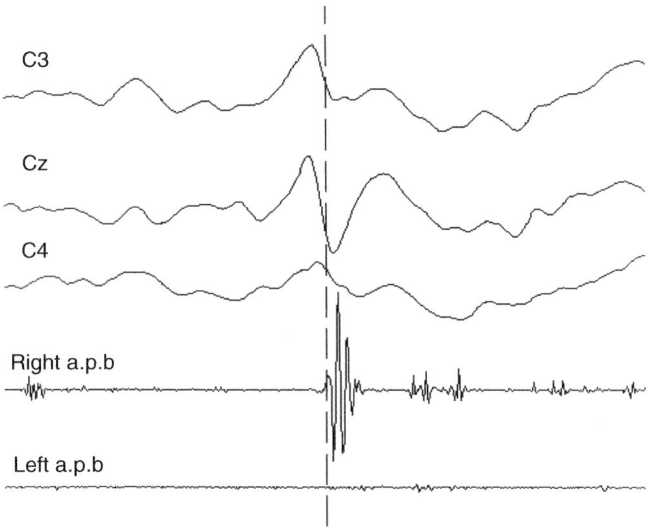

Fig. 16.13 Jerk-locked average of 25 myoclonias in the right abductor pollicis brevis (APB) in a patient with progressive myoclonus epilepsy. A low-amplitude potential in the contralateral central regions, not visible in the polygraphic tracing, is correlated with the myoclonia. *R.* right, *L.* left, *A.P.B.* abductor pollicis brevis

16.6 Conclusions

Back-averaging techniques offer several advantages, such as the possibility to demonstrate a cortical correlate, even of low amplitude, not detectable by visual inspection of the PI,

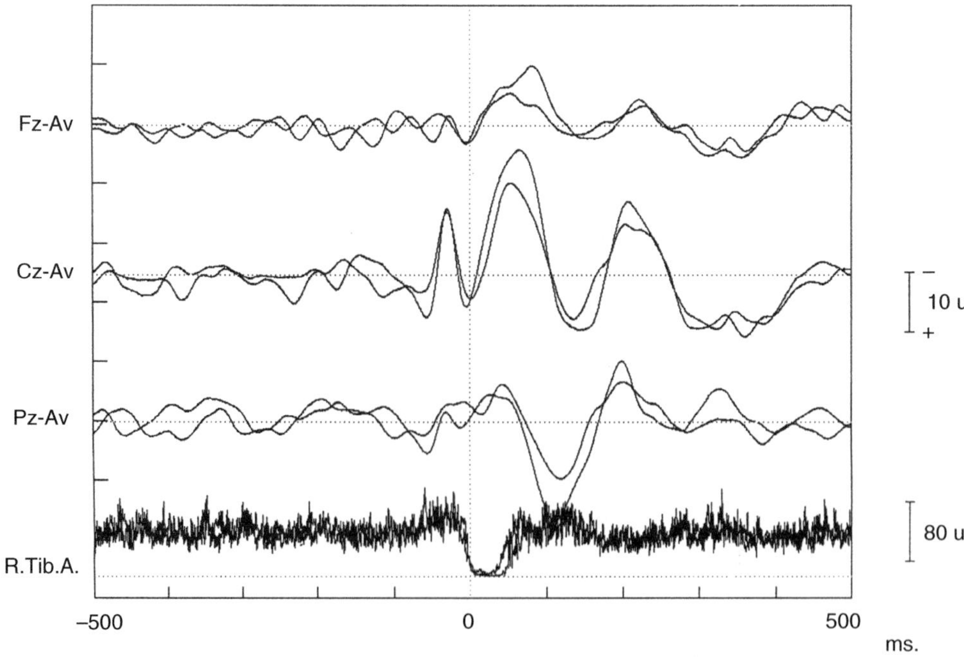

Fig. 16.14 Silent period locked average of 20 epileptic negative myoclonias in the right anterior tibialis (R. Tib. A.—rectified EMG) in a patient with benign partial epilepsy of infancy. The onset of the muscular silent period of the epileptic negative myoclonus is correlated with the peak of spike in Cz, and it precedes the onset of the slow wave

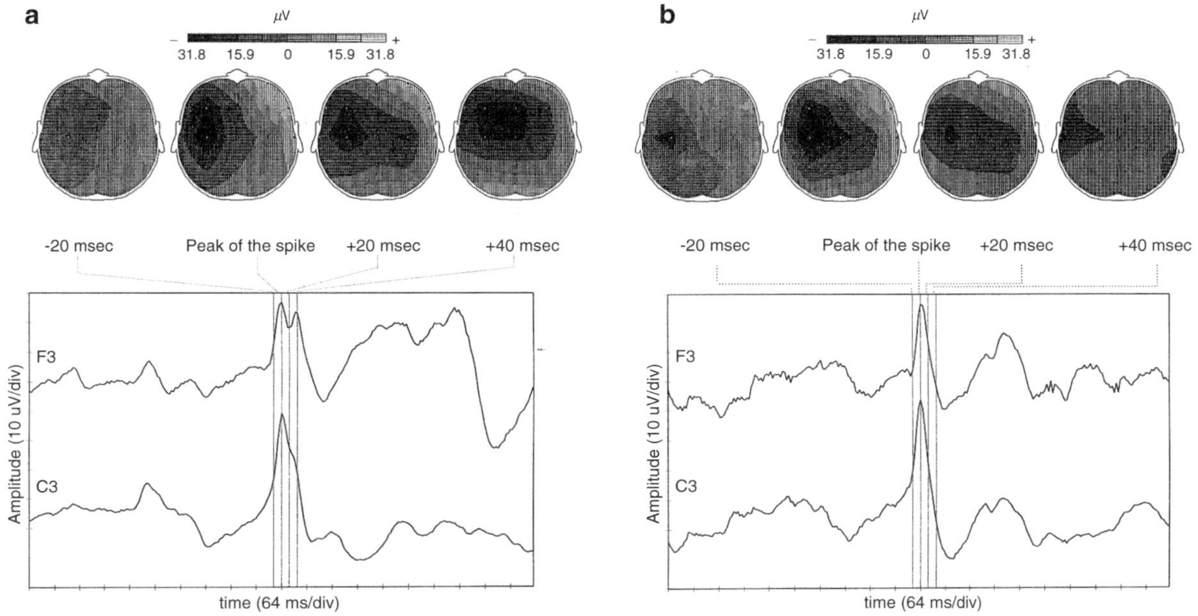

Fig. 16.15 Topographic analysis and spike-averaging of spikes associated with epileptic negative myoclonia (**a**) and spikes nonassociated with epileptic negative myoclonia (**b**). Each averaged spike is the result of the averaging of 20 individual spikes. In (**a**), the averaged spike associated with epileptic negative myoclonus has a second component (evident on F3) distributed over the frontal regions, which is absent in the spike non associated with epileptic negative myoclonus (see also [42])

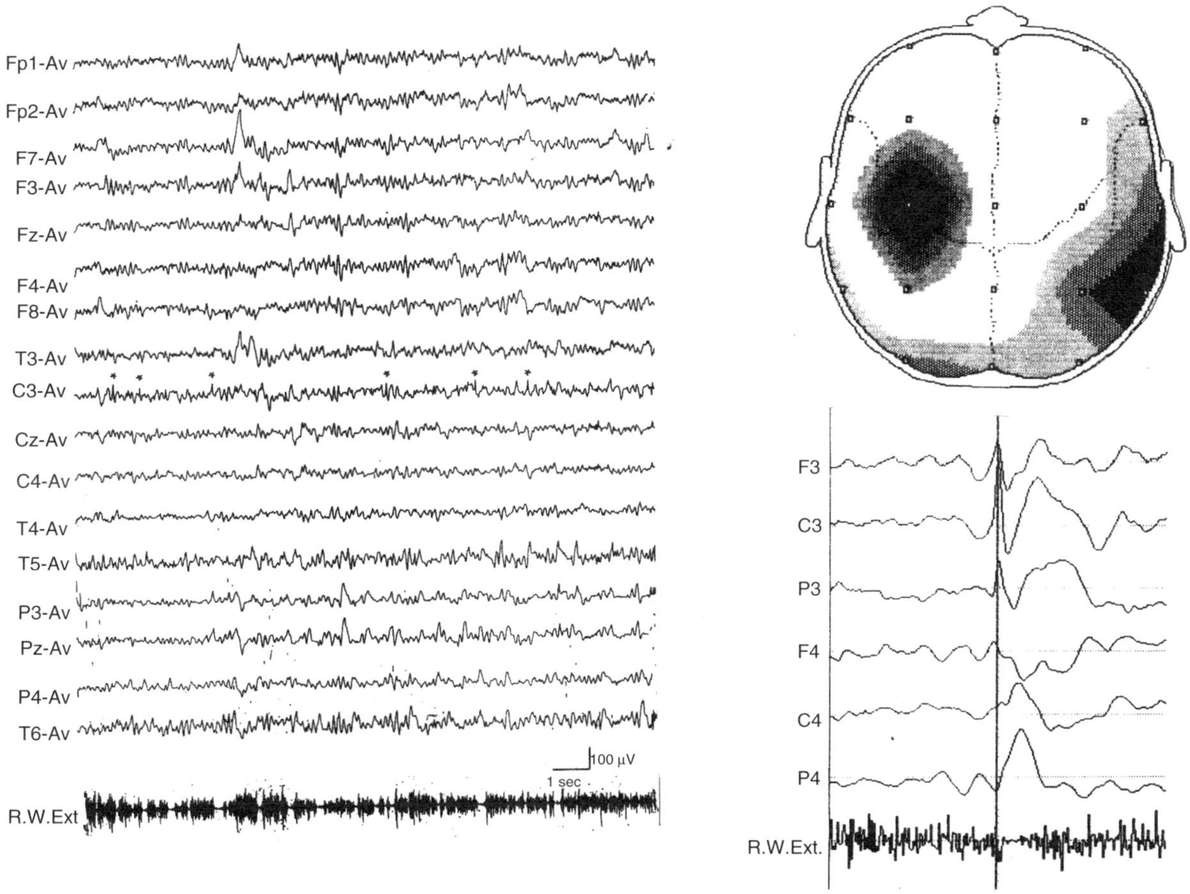

Fig. 16.16 Left: Polygraphic recording in a patient with focal epilepsy associated with left parietal dysplasia and epileptic negative myoclonus in the right wrist extensor (R. Wrist Ext.) The epileptic negative myoclonia is associated with low-amplitude spikes in C3. Right: back-average of 30 epileptic negative myoclonia showing a clear correlation with a low-amplitude sharp spike in C3 (as shown by the topographic map)

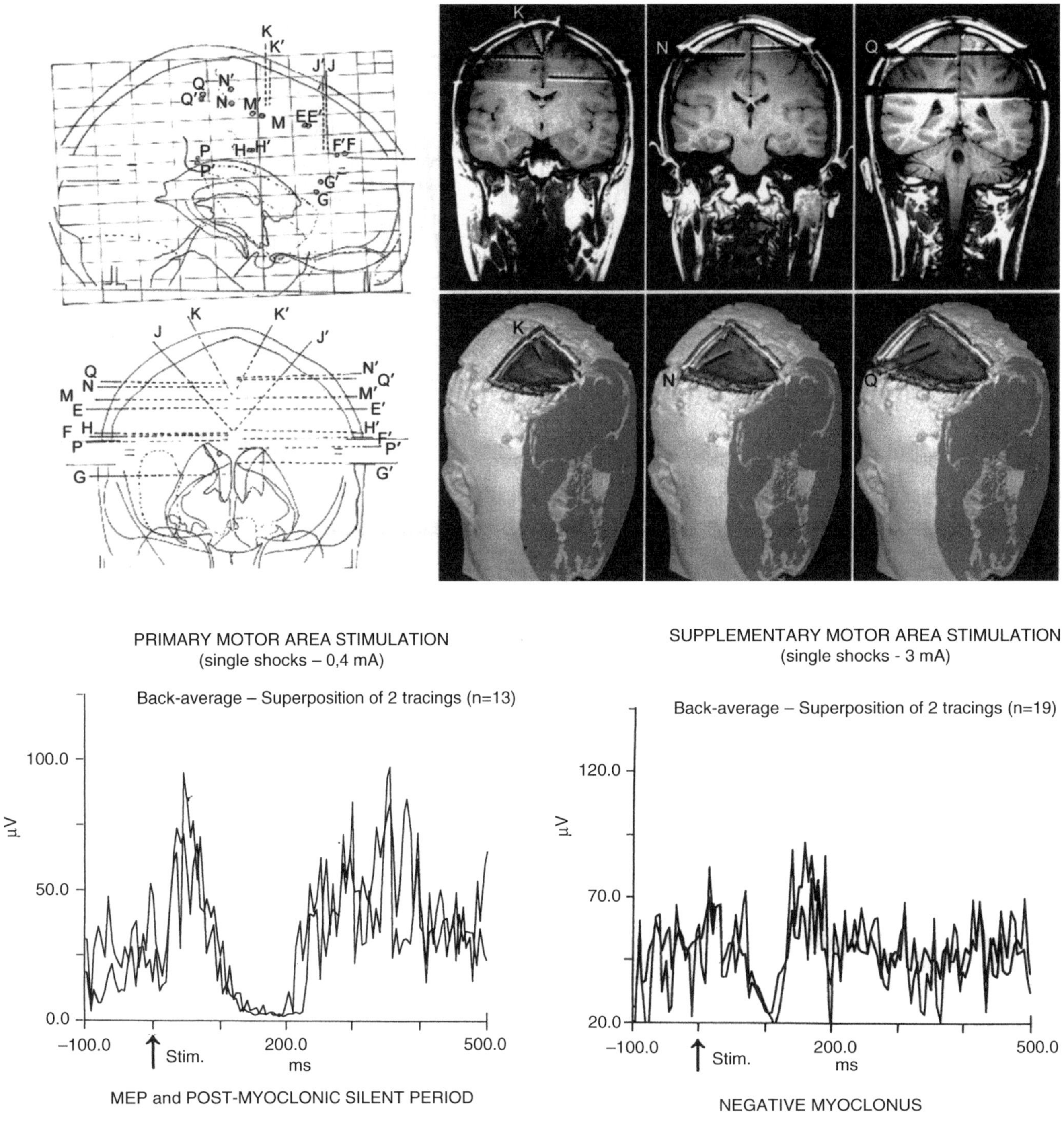

Fig. 16.17 Upper panel: stereo-electroencephalographic scheme (left) and localization of the electrodes in the brain MRI (right). The stereo-EEG electrodes explore the primary motor region (external N electrode), the supplementary motor area (internal electrode K), and parietal cortex (external Q electrode). Lower panel. Left: the electrical stimulation with low-intensity stimuli of the primary motor cortex produces a motor evoked potential (MEP) followed by a post-myoclonic silent period. Right: the electrical stimulation with high-intensity stimuli of the supplementary motor area produces a negative myoclonus. The trigger for the averaging of the EMG signal was the electrical stimulus delivered for intracranial electrical stimulation. EMG tracing rectified from the deltoid muscle contralateral to the electrical stimulation (see also [66])

of a EMG contraction, and to analyze precisely the temporal relationships between the cortical and the muscular phenomena. These techniques have some limits such as a relative arbitrariness in the identification of the onset of the "trigger" event and difficulties in the analysis of rhythmic myoclonic activities, particularly at high frequency. However, if correctly performed and interpreted, they can be useful to investigate the pathophysiological mechanisms of some motor disorders and to orient the diagnostic work-up with possible treatment implications.

References

1. Tassinari CA, Rubboli G. Polygraphic recordings. In: Engel J, Pedley TA, editors. Epilepsy. A comprehensive textbook. Philadelphia: Wolters Kluwer—Lippincott Williams & Wilkins; 2008. p. 873–94.
2. Tassinari CA, Cantalupo G, Rubboli G. Polygraphic recording of epileptic seizures. In: Panayiotopoulos CP, editor. The atlas of epilepsies. Berlin: Springer; 2010. p. 723–40.
3. d'Orsi G, La Selva L, Specchio LM. Video-polygraphy in Rett syndrome. Pediatr Neurol. 2014;50:e5. https://doi.org/10.1016/j.pediatrneurol.2013.07.006.
4. Gardella E, Becker F, Møller RS, Schubert J, Lemke JR, Larsen LH, et al. Benign infantile seizures and paroxysmal dyskinesia caused by an *SCN8A* mutation. Ann Neurol. 2016;79:428–36.
5. Blume WT, Lüders HO, Mizrahi E, Tassinari C, van Emde Boas W, Engel J Jr. Glossary of descriptive terminology for ictal semiology: report of the ILAE task force on classification and terminology. Epilepsia. 2001;42:1212–8.
6. Tassinari CA, Rubboli G, Shibasaki H. Neurophysiology of positive and negative myoclonus. Electroencephalogr Clin Neurophysiol. 1998;107:181–95.
7. Guerrini R, Dravet C, Genton P, Bureau M, Roger J, Rubboli G, et al. Epileptic negative myoclonus. Neurology. 1993;43:1078–83.
8. Tassinari CA, Regis H, Gastaut H. A particular form of muscular inhibition in epilepsy: the related epileptic silent period (RESP). Proc Aust Assoc Neurol. 1968;5:595–602.
9. Tassinari CA, Rubboli G, Parmeggiani L, et al. Epileptic negative myoclonus. In: Fahn S, et al., editors. Negative motor phenomena, vol. 67. Philadelphia: Lippincott-Raven; 1995. p. 181–97.
10. Bisulli F, Volpi L, Meletti S, et al. Ictal pattern of EEG and muscular activation in symptomatic infantile spasms: a videopolygraphic and computer analysis. Epilepsia. 2002;43:1559–63.
11. Fusco L, Vigevano F. Ictal clinical electroencephalographic findings of spasms in west syndrome. Epilepsia. 1993;34:671–8.
12. Gastaut H, Tassinari CA. Epilepsies. In: Remond A, editor. Handbook of electroencephalography and clinical neurophysiology, vol. 13A. Amsterdam: Elsevier; 1975.
13. Gobbi G, Bruno L, Pini A, Giovanardi Rossi P, Tassinari CA. Periodic spasms: an unclassified type of epileptic seizures in childhood. Dev Med Child Neurol. 1987;29:766–75.
14. Dragoumi P, Chivers F, Brady M, Craft S, Mushati D, Venkatachalam G, et al. Epilepsy with myoclonic-atonic seizures (Doose syndrome): when video-EEG polygraphy holds the key to syndrome diagnosis. Epilepsy Behav Case Rep. 2015;5:31–3.
15. Drury I, Henry TR. Ictal patterns in generalized epilepsy. J Clin Neurophysiol. 1993;10:268–80.
16. Gastaut H, Broughton R. Epileptic seizures: clinical and electrographic features. Springfield: Charles C Thomas; 1972.
17. Chatrian GE, Lettich E, Wilkus RJ, Vallarta J. Polygraphic and clinical observations on tonic-autonomic seizures. In: Broughton R, editor. Henri Gastaut and the Marseilles School's contribution to the neurosciences. EEG Suppl 35. Amsterdam: Elsevier; 1982. p. 101–24.
18. Gastaut H, Roger J, Ouachi S, Timsit M, Broughton R. An electroclinical study of generalized epileptic seizures of tonic expression. Epilepsia. 1963;4:15–44.
19. Gastaut H, Roger J, Soulayrol R, Tassinari CA, Regis H, Dravet C. Childhood epileptic encephalopathy with diffuse slow spike-waves (otherwise known as "petit mal variant") or Lennox syndrome. Epilepsia. 1966;7:139–79.
20. Tassinari CA, Lyagoubi S, Santos V, et al. Etude des decharges de pointes ondes chez l'homme, II—Les aspects cliniques et electroencephalographiques des absences myocloniques. Rev Neurol. 1969;121:379–83.
21. Tassinari CA, Rubboli G, Gardella E, Michelucci R. Epilepsy with myoclonic absences . In: SJ Wallace, K Farrell, editors. Epilepsy in children, 2nd ed. Arnold, London, 2004: p.189–194.
22. Tassinari CA, Lyagoubi S, Gambarelli F, et al. Relationships between EEC discharge and neuromuscular phenomena. Electroencephal Clin Neurophysiol. 1971;31:176.
23. Janz D. In: Lugaresi E, Pazzaglia P, Tassinari CA, editors. The natural history of primary generalized epilepsies with sporadic myoclonias of the "impulsive petit mal" type. Bologna: Aulo Gaggi; 1973. p. 55–61.
24. Panzica F, Rubboli G, Franceschetti S, et al. Cortical myoclonus in Janz syndrome. Clin Neurophysiol. 2001;112:1803–9.
25. Thomas JE, Thomas JR, Klass DW. Epilepsia partialis continua. A review of 32 cases. Arch Neurol. 1977;34:266–75.
26. Oliver KL, Franceschetti S, Milligan CJ, Muona M, Mandelstam SA, Canafoglia L, et al. Myoclonus epilepsy and ataxia due to KCNC1 mutation: analysis of 20 cases and K+ channel properties. Ann Neurol. 2017;81:677–89.
27. Avanzini G, Shibasaki H, Rubboli G, Canafoglia L, Panzica F, Franceschetti S, Hallett M. Neurophysiology of myoclonus and progressive myoclonus epilepsies. Epileptic Disord. 2016;18(S2):11–27.
28. Crespel A, Ferlazzo E, Franceschetti S, Genton P, Gouider R, Kälviäinen R, et al. Unverricht-Lundborgh disease. Epileptic Disord. 2016;18(S2):28–37.
29. Tassinari CA, Bureau-Paillas M, Dalla Bernardina B, Grasso E, Roger J. Etude electroencephalographique de la dyssynergie cerebelleuse myoclonique avec epilepsie (syndrome de Ramsay-Hunt). Rev EEG Neurophysiol. 1974;4:407–28.
30. Roger J, Gastaut H, Boudouresques J, Toga M, Dubois D, Lob H. Epilepsie myoclonique progressive avec corps de Lafora. Etude clinique et polygraphique. Controle anatomique ultra-structural. Rev Neurol. 1967;116:197–212.
31. Tassinari CA, Bureau-Paillas M, Dalla Bernardina B, et al. La maladie de Lafora. Rev EEG Neurophysiol. 1978;8:107–22.
32. Canafoglia L, Franceschetti S, Uziel G, Ciano C, Scaioli V, Guerrini R, et al. Characterization of severe action myoclonus in sialidoses. Epilepsy Res. 2011;94:86–93.
33. Canafoglia L, Gilioli I, Invernizzi F, Sofia V, Fugnanesi V, Morbin M, et al. Electroclinical spectrum of the neuronal ceroid lipofuscinoses associated with *CLN6* mutations. Neurology. 2015;85:316–24.
34. Rubboli G, Franceschetti S, Berkovic SF, Canafoglia L, Gambardella A, Dibbens LM, et al. Clinical and neurophysiologic features of progressive myoclonus epilepsy without renal failure caused by *SCARB2* mutations. Epilepsia. 2011;52:2356–63.
35. Rubboli G, Veggiotti P, Pini A, Berardinelli A, Cantalupo G, Bertini E, et al. Spinal muscular atrophy associated with progressive myoclonic epilepsy: a rare condition caused by mutations in *ASAH1*. Epilepsia. 2015;56:692–8.
36. Boissé Lomax L, Bayly MA, Hjalgrim H, Møller RS, Vlaar AM, Aaberg KM, et al. 'North Sea' progressive myoclonus epilepsy: phenotype of subjects with *GOSR2* mutation. Brain. 2013;136:1146–54.
37. Dibbens LM, Rubboli G. *GOSR2*: a progressive myoclonus epilepsy gene. Epileptic Disord. 2016;18(S2):111–4.
38. Ikeda A, Kakigi R, Funai N, Neshige R, Kuroda Y, Shibasaki H. Cortical tremor: a variant of cortical reflex myoclonus. Neurology. 1990;40:1561–5.
39. Brown P, Farmer SF, Halliday DM, Marsden J, Rosenberg JR. Coherent cortical and muscle discharge in cortical myoclonus. Brain. 1999;122:461–72.
40. Panzica F, Varotto G, Canafoglia L, Rossi Sebastiano D, Visani E, Franceschetti S. EEG-EMG coherence estimated using time-varying autoregressive models in movement-activated myoclonus in patients with progressive myoclonic epilepsies. Conf Proc IEEE Eng Med Biol Soc. 2010;2010:1642–5.

41. Rubboli G, Meletti S, Gardella E, et al. Photic reflex myoclonus: a neurophysiological study in progressive myoclonus epilepsies. Epilepsia. 1999;40(Suppl 4):50–8.
42. Rubboli G, Parmeggiani L, Tassinari CA. Frontal inhibitory spike component associated with epileptic negative myoclonus. Electroencephalogr Clin Neurophysiol. 1995;95:201–5.
43. Tassinari CA, Coccagna G, Mantovani M, Bernardina BD, Roger J. Polygraphic study of dyssynergia cerebellaris myoclonica (Ramsay-hunt syndrome) and of the intention myoclonus (Lance-Adams syndrome) during sleep. Eur Neurol. 1973;9:105–20.
44. Ikeno T, Shigematsu H, Miyakoshi M, Ohba A, Yagi K, Seino M. An analytic study of epileptic falls. Epilepsia. 1985;26:612–21.
45. Tassinari CA, Rubboli G, Gardella E, Cantalupo G, Calandra-Buonaura G, Vedovello M, et al. Central pattern generators for a common semiology in fronto-limbic seizures and in parasomnias. A neuroethologic approach. Neurol Sci. 2005;26(Suppl 3):s225–32.
46. Ikeda A, Nagamina T, Kunieda T, Yazawa S, Ohara S, Taki W, et al. Clonic convulsion caused by epileptic discharges arising from the human supplementary motor area as studied by subdural recording. Epileptic Disord. 1999;1:21–6.
47. Grinker RR, Serota H, Stein SI. Myoclonic epilepsy. Arch Neurol Psych. 1938;40:968–80.
48. Dawson GD. The relation between the electroencephalogram and muscle action potentials in certain convulsive states. J Neurol Neurosurg Psychiatry. 1946;9:5–22.
49. Shibasaki H, Kuroiwa Y. Electroencephalographic correlates of myoclonus. Electroencephalogr Clin Neurophysiol. 1975;39:455–63.
50. Dawson GD. A summation technique for the detection of small evoked potentials. Electroencephalogr Clin Neurophysiol. 1954;6:65–84.
51. Ugawa Y, Shimpo T, Mannen T. Physiological analysis of asterixis: silent period locked averaging. J Neurol Neurosurg Psychiatry. 1989;52:89–92.
52. Barrett G. Jerk-locked averaging: technique and application. J Clin Neurophysiol. 1992;9:495–508.
53. Brown P, Day BL, Rothwell JC, et al. Intrahemispheric and interhemispheric spread of cerebral cortical myoclonic activity and its relevance to epilepsy. Brain. 1991;114:2333–51.
54. Shibasaki H, Hallett M. Electrophysiological studies of myoclonus. Muscle Nerve. 2005;31:157–74.
55. Gardella E, Tinuper P, Marini C, et al. Autosomal dominant early-onset cortical myoclonus, photic-induced myoclonus, and epilepsy in a large pedigree. Epilepsia. 2006;47:1643–9.
56. Lu CS, Ikeda A, Terada K, et al. Electrophysiological studies of early stage corticobasal degeneration. Mov Disord. 1998;13:140–6.
57. Hallett M, Chadwick D, Adam J, Marsden CD. Reticular reflex myoclonus: a physiologic type of human post-hypoxic myoclonus. J Neurol Neurosurg Psychiatry. 1977;40:253–64.
58. Rubboli G, Tassinari CA. Negative myoclonus. An overview of its clinical features, pathophysiological mechanisms, and management. Neurophysiol Clin. 2006;36:337–46.
59. Shibasaki H, Ikeda A, Nagamine T, Mima T, Terada K, Nishitani N, et al. Cortical reflex negative myoclonus. Brain. 1994;117:477–86.
60. Shibasaki H. Overview and classification of myoclonus. Clin Neurosci. 1995;3:189–92.
61. Shibasaki H, Yamashita Y, Kuroiwa Y. Electroencephalographic studies of myoclonus. Myoclonus-related cortical spikes and high amplitude somatosensory evoked potentials. Brain. 1978;101:447–60.
62. Shibasaki H, Neshige R. Photic cortical reflex myoclonus. Ann Neurol. 1987;22:252–7.
63. Lance JW, Adams RD. The syndrome of intention or action myoclonus as a sequel to hypoxic encephalopathy. Brain. 1963;86:111–36.
64. Noachtar S, Holthausen H, Luders HO. Epileptic negative myoclonus. Subdural EEG recordings indicate a postcentral generator. Neurology. 1997;49:1534–7.
65. Parmeggiani L, Seri S, Bonanni P, Guerrini R. Electrophysiological characterization of spontaneous and carbamazepine-induced epileptic negative myoclonus in benign childhood epilepsy with centro-temporal spikes. Clin Neurophysiol. 2004;115:50–8.
66. Rubboli G, Mai R, Meletti S, et al. Negative myoclonus induced by cortical electrical stimulation in epileptic patients. Brain. 2006;129:65–81.
67. Baumgartner C, Podreka I, Olbrich A, et al. Epileptic negative myoclonus: an EEG- single-photon emission CT study indicating involvement of premotor cortex. Neurology. 1996;46:753–8.
68. Lim SH, Dinner D, Pillay P, et al. Functional anatomy of the human supplementary sensorimotor area: results of extraoperative electrical stimulation. Electroencephalogr Clin Neurophysiol. 1994;91:179–93.
69. Luders HO, Lesser RP, Morris HH, Dinner DS, Hahn J. Negative motor responses elicited by stimulation of the human cortex. In: Wolf P, Dam M, Janz D, Dreifuss FE, editors. Advances in epileptology, vol. 16. New York: Raven Press; 1987. p. 229–31.

Ambulatory EEG

17

Marianna Brienza, Chiara Davassi, and Oriano Mecarelli

17.1 Ambulatory EEG Equipment

NJ Holter introduced, for the first time in the early 1960s, the concept of a portable long-term recording device into the field of cardiology. Based on the analogy of the two techniques, the long-term Ambulatory-EEG (A-EEG) monitoring is often improperly called the "Holter-EEG" [1].

However, the continuous recording of cerebral bioelectric activity is more complex, due to the need for a multichannel amplification and recording system. The possibility to record ambulatory EEG was described for the first time in 1975 by Ives and Woods [2]. Easy handling and lightweight systems were introduced in 1979, allowing to record four EEG channels on cassette tape recorders for 24 h. The recorded analog signals could then be easily revised on a video at a speed of up to 60 times the real one, so that 24 h of recording could be checked in 24 min. Subsequently, in 1983, an eight-channel recording system was developed, equipped with a digital display and an "event-marking" device, enabling the patient to enter a signal during the EEG acquisition, to allow a better electro-clinical association [3, 4].

By that time, the review unit was able to quickly search for the signalled events, using the marker. From the late 1980s, systems with 16 or more channels were introduced as well as polygraphic systems (EEG, ECG, EOG, EMG, etc.), able to store up to 24–48 h of recording. Finally, in 1996, the first portable digital recorders were introduced.

Nowadays, systems for A-EEG are exclusively digital, allowing the visualisation of up to 32 channels. The acquisition unit is independent, small in size and powered by several AA or rechargeable batteries. The EEG-recorded signals are stored on a flash memory card of 2–4 GB, capable of storing up to 2–4 days of continuous data. Factors that influence the duration of the recording and the quantity of memory required are the sampling rate of the EEG signal (128, 256 or 512 Hz), the number of bits used for digitisation of the signal (8, 12 or 16 bit resolution) and the number of recording channels (up to 21 channels or more).

The most modern portable systems for A-EEG also have the possibility to be integrated in a digital audio-video recording system (Fig. 17.1). They are also equipped with a graphic display that allows programming, impedance check and online visualisation of the trace.

The review system consists of a dedicated computer on which the recorded signals can be transferred for later off-line analysis and storage. The recorded EEG (usually of 24 h duration) can be read at a scrolling speed range between 10 and 60 times the real one (for a "reading" time varying between 144 and 24 min for a 24-h A-EEG).

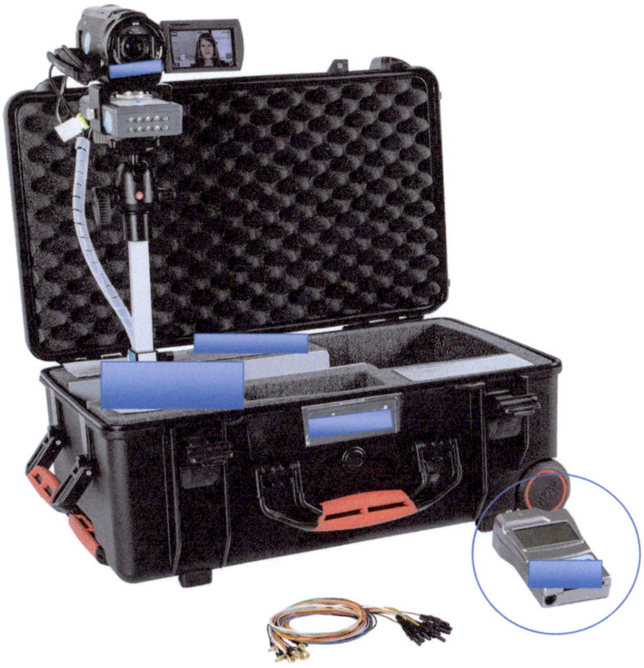

Fig. 17.1 An example of A-EEG wireless recording system (weight 200 g) synchronised with a video camera

M. Brienza · C. Davassi · O. Mecarelli (✉)
Department of Human Neurosciences, Sapienza University of Rome, Rome, Italy
e-mail: oriano.mecarelli@uniroma1.it

O. Mecarelli (ed.), *Clinical Electroencephalography*, https://doi.org/10.1007/978-3-030-04573-9_17

The EEG trace is usually displayed on a monitor, but it can also be printed on paper, entirely or by selection. Moreover, the recorded material can be stored and used for later processing (quantification of epileptic activity, quantitative analysis of selected periods, etc.). The quality of the recorded signal and its reformatting possibility are similar to the ones of a standard digital electroencephalograph.

17.1.1 Electrode Placement and Instructions for the Patient

The electrodes used for A-EEG recordings must guarantee a reliable adherence to the skin for many hours; they also should cause the minimum discomfort to the patient. Electrodes usually applied on the scalp are Ag cup electrodes, attached with gauze pads soaked in collodion (quickly dried with cold air) or with adhesive pastes (like EC2).

The main disadvantage of this type of montage is that it is fixed and it cannot be rechecked or modified during the entire recording. A-EEG system can record a limited number of channels so that routine EEG electrodes applied are also limited (at least Fp1, Fp2, C3, C4, T3, T4, O1, O2, G1 and G2). For polygraphic recordings, cup electrodes are used for EOG, ECG and EMG, and specific transducers and sensors are used for nasal and thoracic pneumogram (PNG), pulse oximetry, etc.

Electrodes must be accurately attached to the skin and the wires must also be locked into the junction section to the cup. Grouping the wires together can be useful, and this vigilance is important to minimise the risk of traction or rupture of the cable, the appearance of artifacts and the unreliability of the trace. Once the electrode positioning is completed, skin-electrode impedances must be checked and the reliability of the recording must be verified before the patient leaves the laboratory. To this purpose, simply connect the portable recorder, with its cable, to the central unit; the EEG trace will be displayed online on the computer monitor so that the correct application and reliability of every single electrode can be verified. Generally, before letting the patient out, a recording is made for a short period of time with eyes closed, and many laboratories also carry out routine activation patterns, like hyperpnea and photic stimulation, just like a standard EEG. Finally, a soft hairnet should be put on the head to stabilise the montage and the patient is instructed about the correct use and care of the equipment. A-EEG recording usually does not limit the patient's daily activities, even though it is preferable to suggest avoiding excessive physical activity, that could cause artifacts, and any action that could create traction of the wires or pressure to the head. The patient will be asked to fill in a clinical diary, taking note of any type of activity, symptoms, treatment taken, sleep time, wake-up time, etc. The recording device is also equipped with a specific "event-marking" button which should be pushed by the patients and/or his observers in case of clinically relevant symptoms.

17.1.2 Clinical Utility of Ambulatory EEG

There are several clinical indications for A-EEG monitoring and, although they mainly concern the management of the epileptic disorders, they are not limited to this field. The principal indications are as follows:

- *Recording of a seizure*. For this purpose, A-EEG is useful when the frequency of the ictal events is high (preferably daily), to improve the probability of detection. The recording of a seizure can supply important information both in the case of an already diagnosed epileptic syndrome and when a differential diagnosis with non-epileptic disorders is necessary (psychogenic seizures, syncopes, parasomnias, etc.) [5]. Psychogenic Non-Epileptic Seizures (PNES) are common in patients with epilepsy and, in this case, A-EEG can help to discriminate epileptic seizures from other paroxysmal episodes. In the case of syncope, a contextual ECG recording is useful to better characterise the cause of the loss of consciousness. Furthermore, it would be advisable to obtain a simultaneous video-audio recording, to make a better electro-clinical correlation of the ictal events. There is also evidence to support that A-EEG is more likely to capture events than a sleep-deprived EEG [6].
- *Quantification of epileptic abnormalities*. A-EEG allows quantification of ictal and interictal epileptiform activity, both focal and generalised, allowing the definition of objective parameters, as the total number of discharges/h, total discharge duration/h, average, minimum and maximum duration, etc. such data can then be graphically represented for better visualisation and analysis of the circadian distribution of the epileptic discharges (Fig. 17.2) [7, 8].
- *Recording of subclinical epileptic abnormalities*. Many patients with epilepsy show epileptic abnormalities without clinical correlation, both ictal and interictal, that are not always highlighted by a standard EEG. A-EEG also allows the identification of epileptic discharges whose duration is not long enough to determine a clinical manifestation. A-EEG is also helpful when the patient does not remember the seizures or cannot describe them (paediatric patients or patients with cognitive disorders). In particular, absence seizures may be so brief that the patient is even unaware of them; patients with focal seizures with consciousness impairment may often be amnesic from their seizures [7, 9].

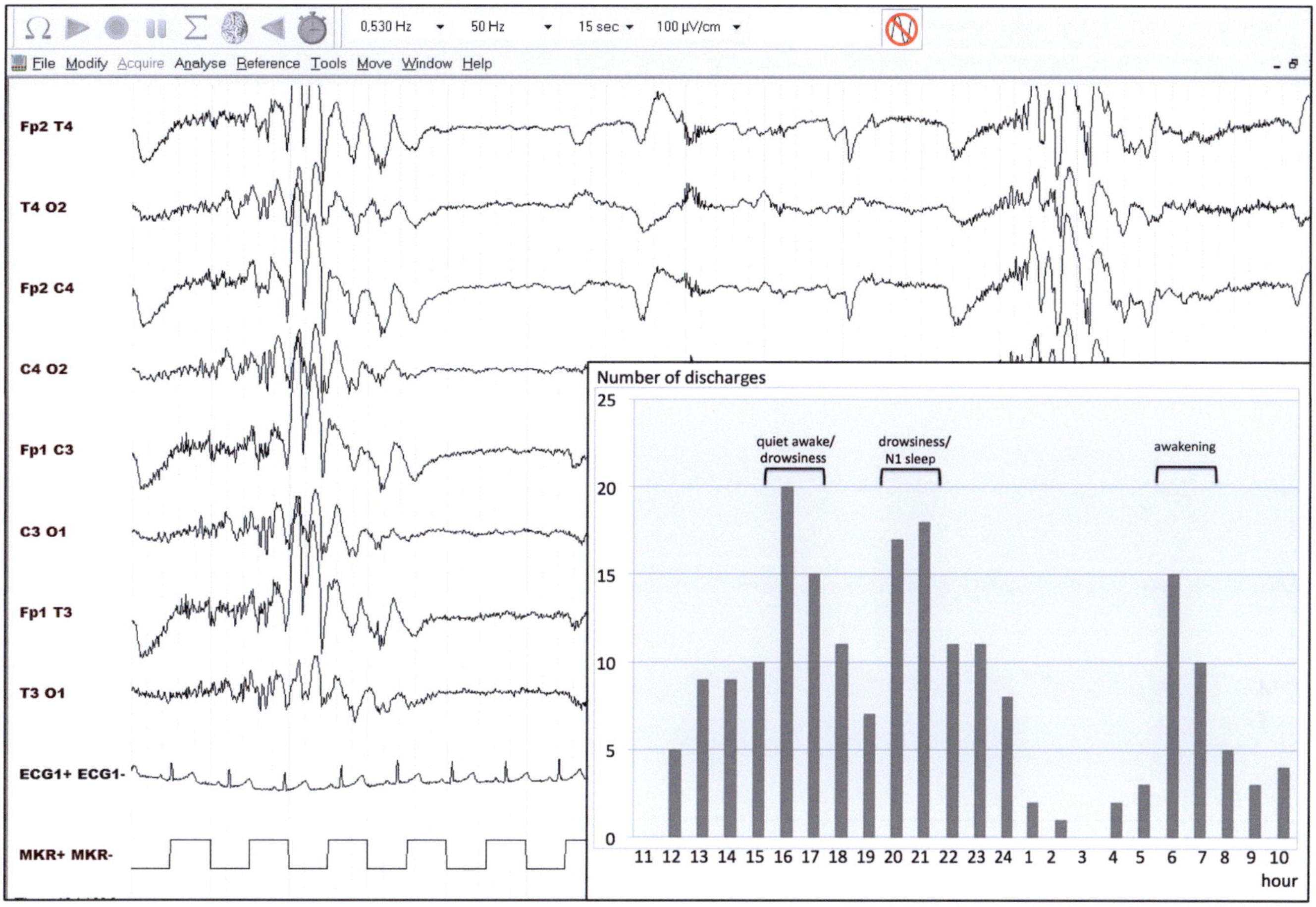

Fig. 17.2 A-EEG of a patient with frequent epileptic generalised discharges. The box shows the quantification of the discharges during the 24 h recording, in relation to wake and sleep stages

- *Evaluation of sleep activating effect*. Sleep (nocturnal or diurnal) represents a trigger for the appearance of epileptic abnormalities, both ictal and interictal, especially in the early stages of NREM sleep and during the awakening and, in such cases, A-EEG is the most common and simple tool to record them. It is important for the diagnosis of particular conditions in which standard outpatient EEG does not often reveal specific information. Emblematic examples include epileptic syndromes in which EEG abnormalities appear almost exclusively during sleep (i.e. childhood epilepsy with centrotemporal spikes, Landau-Kleffner syndrome, epileptic encephalopathy with continuous spike-and-wave during sleep, autosomal dominant nocturnal frontal lobe epilepsy) (Fig. 17.3). Furthermore, A-EEG plays an important role in the differential diagnosis between seizures and nocturnal non-epileptic paroxysmal events [9–11].
- *Monitoring of drug therapy effects*. Execution of EEG monitoring during the various phases of antiepileptic therapy (titration, maintenance, adjustment, withdrawal) is useful to evaluate the effectiveness of the drugs administered to the patient. It may occur that a drug controls the clinical symptoms, without causing the disappearance or reduction of the epileptiform abnormalities [12]. Drugs can also cause neurophysiological effects indicating neurotoxicity (slowing of background activity when awake, excessive sleepiness, sleep macrostructure disorganisation, etc.) that A-EEG can indeed document. Lastly, before therapy withdrawal, an A-EEG recording can be useful in providing additional information on the real absence of interictal epileptic abnormalities. This is of significant importance, as it has been observed that the presence of epileptic discharges, before or during antiepileptic drugs withdrawal, may attain up to a 100% prediction of seizure relapse in particular groups [13].

Furthermore, A-EEG is very helpful when it is impossible to perform a standard outpatient EEG, due to the poor cooperation of special categories of patients, such as those suffering from autistic disorders, or in case of serious disability that impedes the patients to visit the laboratory (Fig. 17.4).

The request to the caregiver to take a home video recording, even just with a mobile phone, may further help the interpretation of the recording, obtaining a "rudimentary" video -EEG and allowing a better electro-clinical correlation [14].

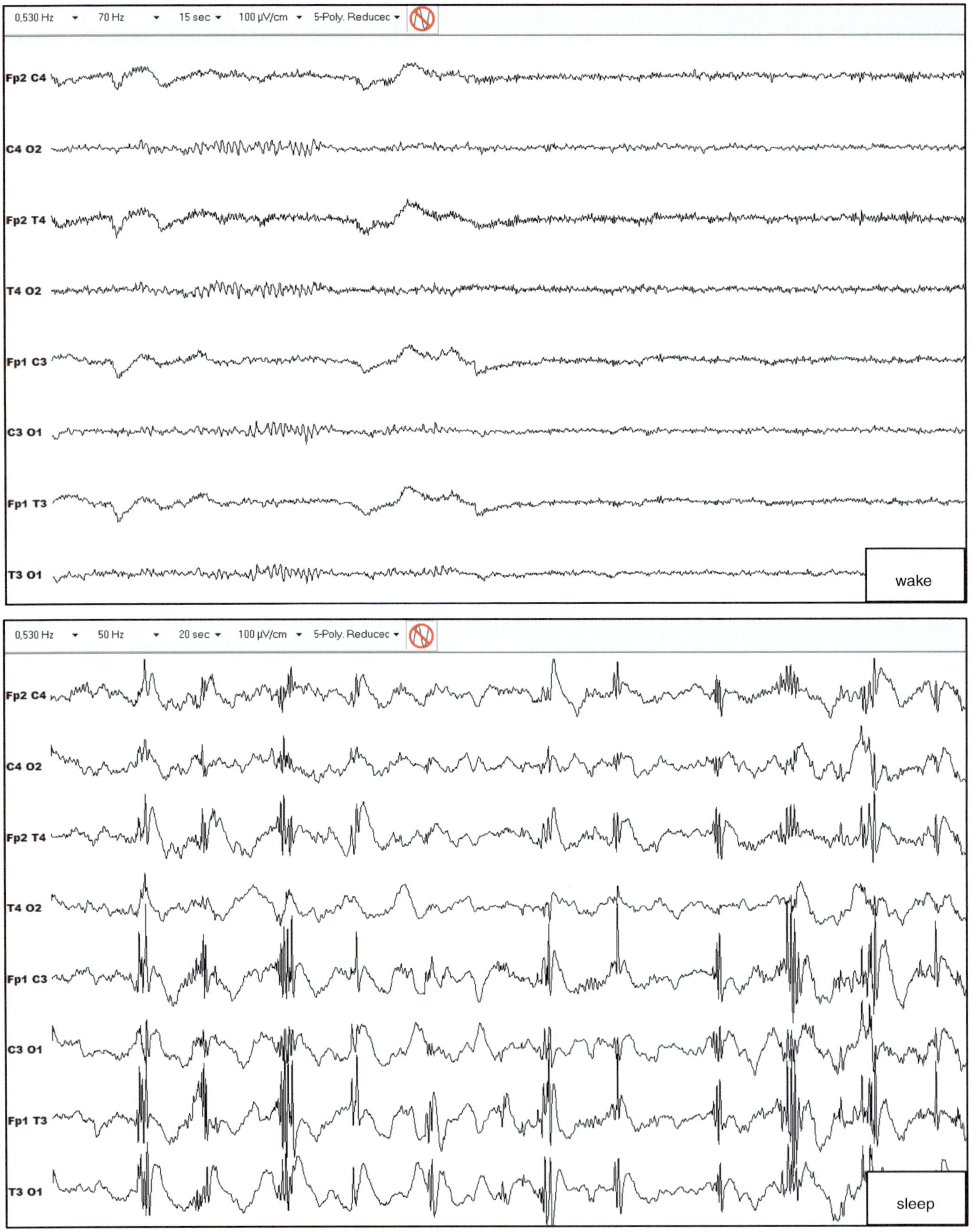

Fig. 17.3 An 18-year-old autistic patient, with focal to bilateral tonic-clonic epileptic seizures. The A-EEG recording shows no epileptic activity during wake. As the patient falls asleep, subcontinuous polyspike-and-wave discharges appear, with a prevalence on the left hemisphere

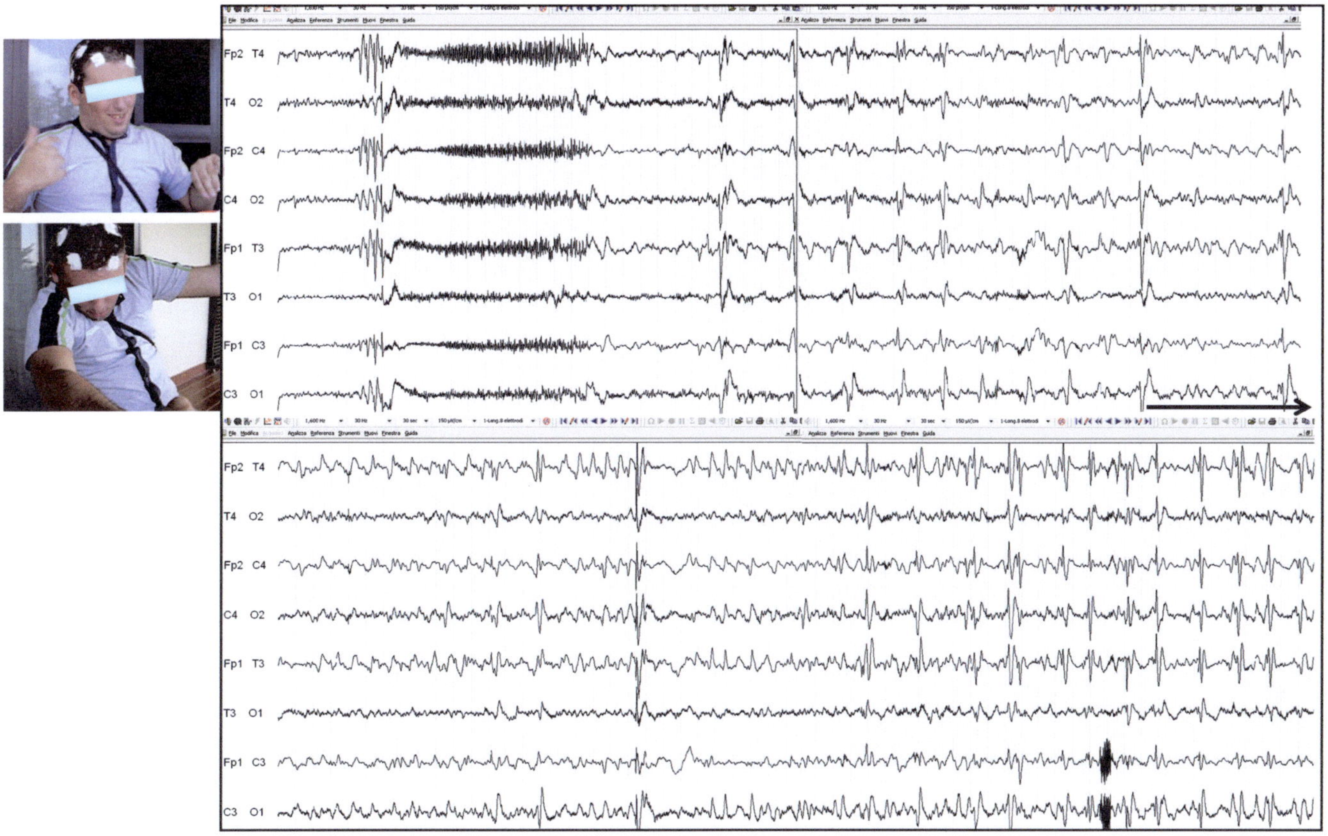

Fig. 17.4 A 24-year-old patient with severe epileptic encephalopathy and behavioural disturbances. The absence of collaboration does not allow an outpatient standard EEG recording. With the A-EEG it was possible to obtain a reliable home recording of a tonic-clonic seizure, supplied with a video performed by the caregiver. This video, together with the annotation on the diary, allowed to make an electro-clinical correlation, even without a video-EEG synchronised recording

Besides being useful in epilepsy management A-EEG is also used in other fields, including the study of sleep disorders. As a matter of fact, an advantage of A-EEG is that it is suitable for an entire night of sleep recordings at home, giving patients the comfort of sleeping in their own bed. The recording of polygraphic parameters (ECG, EOG, EMG, PNG, etc.) allows quite a suitable assessment of sleep disturbances (i.e. sleep breathing disorders, parasomnias, dyssomnias) [15].

Finally, when necessary, A-EEG equipment may be used for prolonged recordings or even for monitoring in particular environments (operating rooms, intensive care units, etc.). In these cases very small recording units are preferred, powered by batteries and not requiring to be connected to the power grid, that can be easily moved with the patient without interrupting the recording.

17.1.3 Limitations and Pitfalls

Listed above were the main and undeniable A-EEG advantages; however, its limitations and pitfalls must not be ignored:

- Artifacts. In an A-EEG recording, artifacts are inevitable, especially during wake. The most frequently observed arise from masticatory activity, muscular activity, pressure on the electrodes, traction on the cables, drying of the conductive paste, total or partial detachment of one or more electrodes and peculiar activities carried out by the patient. When artifactual graphoelements are particularly abundant and continuous, they may also invalidate the entire recording, making it impossible to detect potential abnormalities (Figs. 17.5 and 17.6).
- The number of applicable electrodes is limited and the montage is fixed and unchangeable during the recording: this may represent a limitation in defining a focal abnormal activity. For this purpose, a tailored montage of the available electrodes can be useful, as well as the use of special electrodes.
- Accurate association between the symptoms reported and the recorded EEG pattern is not always easy, although this is partially solvable with annotations on the clinical diary, pushing on the event-marking button and performing a home video recording.

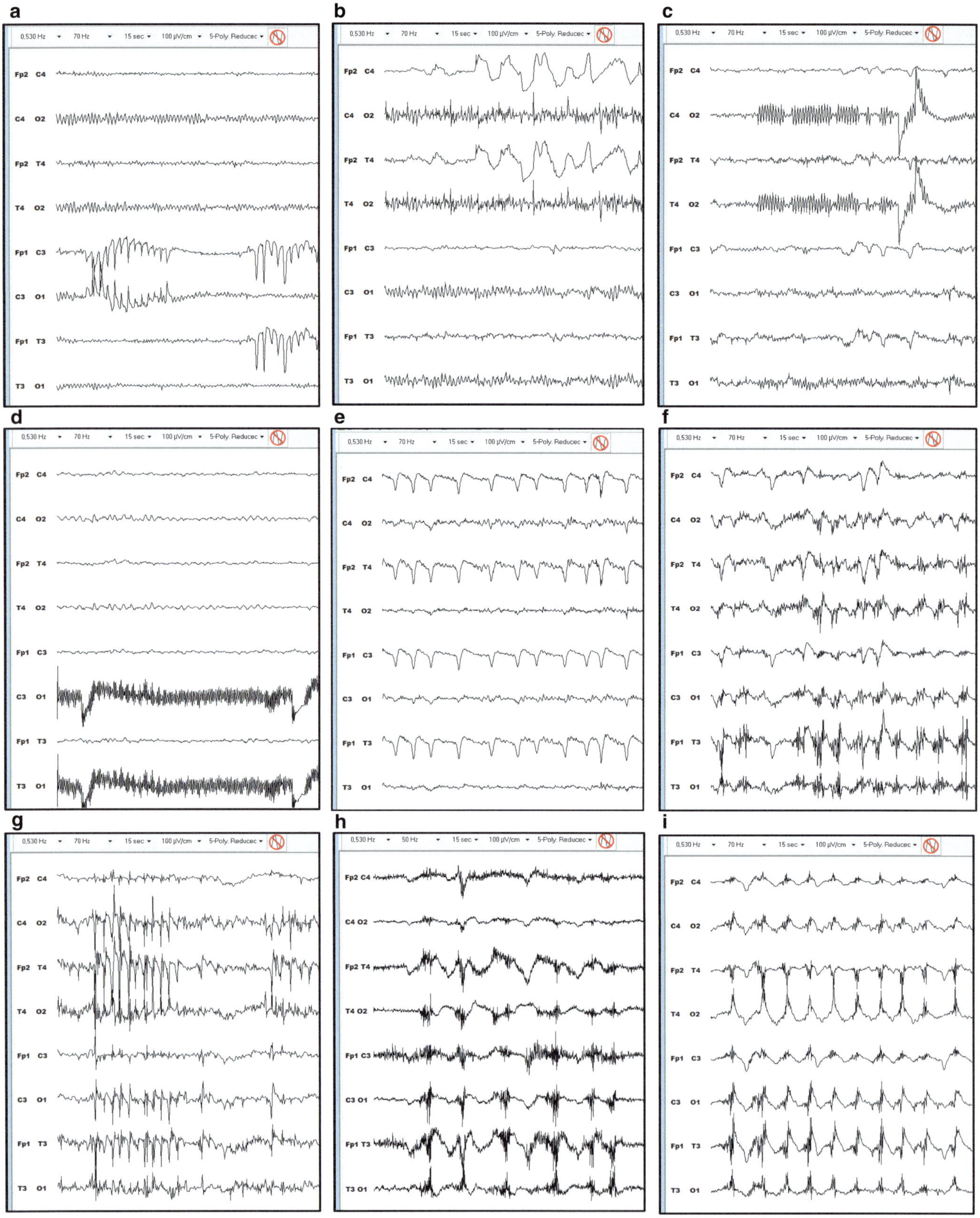

Fig. 17.5 Examples of artifacts observable during A-EEG. (**a**) Pressure on C3 and Fp1 electrodes; (**b**) bad skin-electrode contact on Fp2 and muscle activity on O2; (**c**, **d**) partial and total disconnection of, respectively, O2 and O1 electrodes; (**e**) repetitive blinking; (**f**) bitemporal muscular contraction; (**g**–**i**) different chewing artefacts

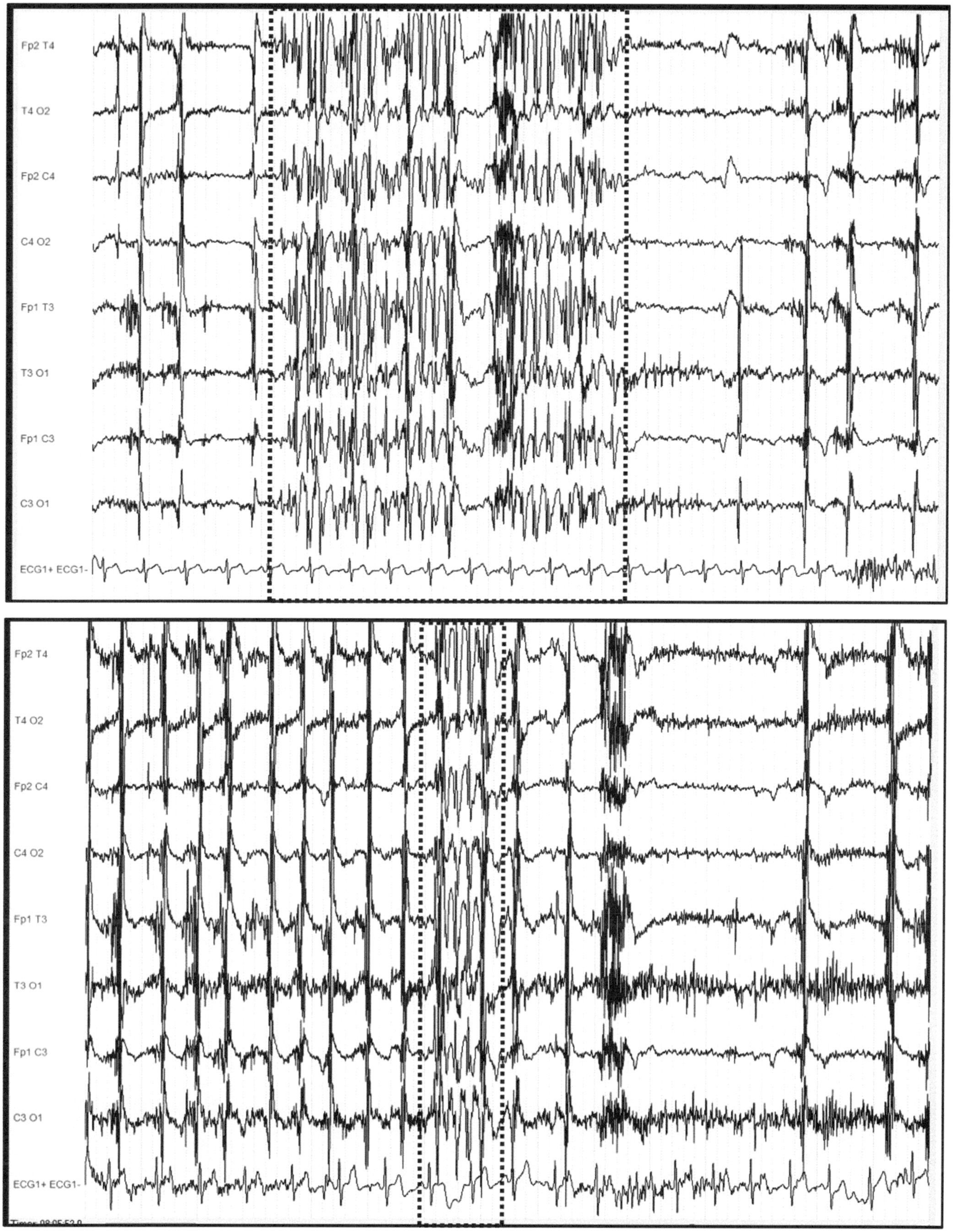

Fig. 17.6 Examples of epileptic diffuse discharges (dotted line) partially obscured by chewing artifact during eating

In conclusion, after more than 40 years since its introduction, A-EEG is an important tool in neurophysiological diagnosis, with undoubtable usefulness in many clinical conditions, epilepsy above all. However, this technique should not be requested as a substitute for standard EEG, but it should be considered as an additional neurophysiological test, to be performed just in selected clinical conditions, not clarified by an outpatient standard EEG.

References

1. Holter NJ. New method for hearth studies. Science. 1961;134:1214–20.
2. Ives JR, Woods JF. Four-channel 24 hour cassette recorder for long-term EEG monitoring of ambulatory patients. Electroencephalogr Clin Neurophysiol. 1975;39:88–92.
3. Ebersole JS, Leroy RF. An evaluation of ambulatory, cassette EEG monitoring: II. Detection of interictal abnormalities. Neurology. 1983;33:8–18.
4. Ebersole JS, Leroy RF. Evaluation of ambulatory cassette EEG monitoring: III. Diagnostic accuracy compared to intensive inpatient EEG monitoring. Neurology. 1983;33:853–60.
5. Faulkner HJ, Arima H, Mohaed A. The utility of prolonged outpatient ambulatory EEG. Seizure. 2012;21:491–4.
6. Lawley A, Evans S, Manfredonia F, Cavanna AE. The role of outpatient ambulatory electroencephalography in the diagnosis and management of adults with epilepsy or nonepileptic attack disorder: a systematic literature review. Epilepsy Behav. 2015;53:26–30.
7. de Feo MR, Mecarelli O, Ricci G, Rina MF. The utility of ambulatory EEG monitoring in typical absence seizures. Brain Dev. 1991;13:223–7.
8. Nuwer MR, Emerson RG, Hahn CD. Principles and techniques for long-term EEG recording (epilepsy monitoring unit, intensive care unit, ambulatory). In: Schomer DL, Lopes da Silva FH, editors. Niedermeyer's electroencephalography. Basic principles, clinical applications, and related fields. 7th ed. Oxford: Oxford University Press; 2011. p. 781–98.
9. Waterhouse EJ. New horizons in ambulatory electroencephalography. IEEE Eng Med Biol Mag. 2003;22:74–80.
10. Hussain N, Gayatri N, Blake A, et al. Ambulatory electroencephalogram in children: a prospective clinical audit of 100 cases. J Pediatr Neurosci. 2013;8:188–91.
11. Ontiveros S, Novy J, Jequier-Gygax M, Rossetti AO. Yield of outpatient sleep EEG for epileptiform alterations' detection in children. J Clin Neurophysiol. 2016;33:72–5.
12. Pro S, Vicenzini E, Pulitano P, Li Voti P, Zarabla A, Randi F, Mecarelli O. Effects of levetiracetam on generalized discharges monitored with ambulatory EEG in epileptic patients. Seizure. 2009;18:133–8.
13. Koepp MJ, Farrell F, Collins J, Smith S. The prognostic value of long-term ambulatory electroencephalography in antiepileptic drug reduction in adults with learning disability and epilepsy in long-term remission. Epilepsy Behav. 2008;13:474–7.
14. Schomer DL. Ambulatory EEG telemetry: how good is it? J Clin Neurophysiol. 2006;23:294–305.
15. Fry JM, DiPhillipo MA, Curran K, Golberg R, Baran AS. Full polysomnography in the home. Sleep. 1998;21:635–42.

18 Video-Electroencephalography (Video-EEG)

Laura Tassi, Valeria Mariani, Veronica Pelliccia, and Roberto Mai

18.1 General Indications

The epilepsies represent a wide expression of dysfunction of both a part and the whole brain. The classification and the optimization of the subsequent "ideal" treatment are mostly based on syndromic and etiological assessment.

Consisting in a neurological heterogeneous disease, anatomical, clinical, and neurophysiological elements are complementary and necessary to estimate the diagnosis and to propose the most adequate treatment and to advise, when possible, a long-term prognosis.

Frequently clinical ictal symptomatology, both subjective and objectivable, is identified by a retrospective anamnestic detailed investigation during outpatient counseling, and most part of the neurophysiological assessment is based on a routinely brief interictal EEG. In specific cases an exhaustive neuroradiological evaluation is also indicated.

The study and knowledge of epilepsies began before the end of 1900, based only on clinical diagnosis and on eventual autoptic confirmations. Only since 1929, Berger, inventing the EEG, gives the scientific world the possibility of recording the electrical activity of the brain [1].

Since 1937, Gibbs and Gibbs and Lennox have been the firsts to describe the pathological changes associated with epilepsy [2–5].

From the 1950s, 8 up to 16 channel hardwired recordings became possible, and the EEG turned out to be an integral part of the routine clinical practice. Only in the 1970s the first use of CCTV linked to analogue EEG appeared and in the 1980s was introduced for the first long-term monitoring.

Between 1990 and 2005, analogue EEG was gradually replaced by digital recordings, subsequently digital EEG with simultaneous video for both standard recordings and telemetry, and ambulatory monitoring was widely used [6–8].

Over the years Video-EEG has allowed an enormous improvement in the knowledge of ictal clinical modifications and their correlation with the contextual modifications of the EEG.

Its utilization allows to:

1. Diagnose.
2. Quantify.
3. Evaluate.

The diagnosis in the definition of the epilepsies is essential for the following therapeutic decision (Fig. 18.1). On the basis of the diagnosis, the necessary exams to better delineate it and the essential therapies and the timing of the follow-up can be indicated [9–12].

The presence of pathological interictal abnormalities in a standard EEG predicts a high risk of recurrence following a first seizure as well as in patients with controlled epilepsy may predict a higher risk of seizure relapse following modification of the pharmacological treatment. Moreover Video-EEG helps classify seizure type (focal or generalized), making easier to choose the drug treatment.

The Video-EEG is necessary and indispensable in the differential diagnosis between epileptic seizures and non-epileptic paroxysmal manifestations or disorders of cardiovascular origin [13–18].

Furthermore Video-EEG permits the definition of the type of seizure in the presurgical work-up; seizures can be observed and quantified, as well as interictal abnormalities, during both sleep and wakefulness. Their presence will be useful to define the prognosis and eventually modify the therapy. Continuous Video-EEG monitoring is a useful adjunct to diagnosing and quantifying seizures, especially in critically ill patients.

Comparing the quality and usefulness of information obtained from Video-EEG monitoring with that from careful routine EEG, intensive monitoring was found to be far superior to the routine EEG examination as an aid to precise diagnosis of seizure disorders. The routine EEG recorded seizures

L. Tassi (✉) · V. Mariani · V. Pelliccia · R. Mai
"Claudio Munari" Epilepsy Surgery Centre, Niguarda Hospital, Milan, Italy
e-mail: laura.tassi@ospedaleniguarda.it

O. Mecarelli (ed.), *Clinical Electroencephalography*, https://doi.org/10.1007/978-3-030-04573-9_18

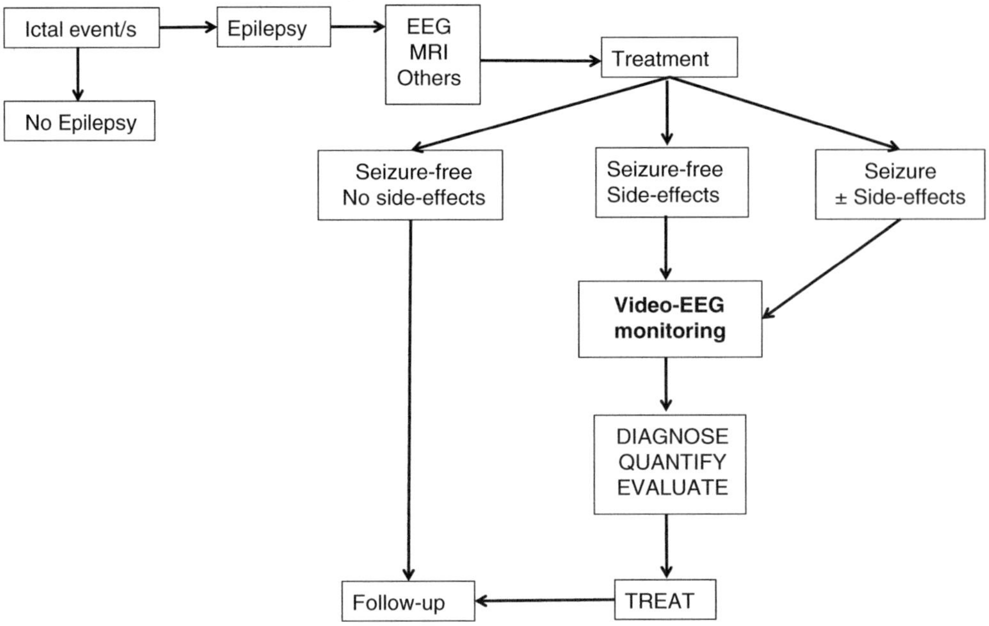

Fig. 18.1 Flowchart concerning utility, indication, and goals of the long-term monitoring with the Video-EEG

in only 7% of patients, while with Video-EEG, following careful withdrawal of antiepileptic drugs (AEDs), seizures were recorded in 70% of patients. Moreover Video-EEG revealed that 60% of patients for whom the routine EEG study had recorded only one seizure type actually suffered from two or more. Clinical diagnosis was afterward changed in the majority (84%) of the patients [8].

The ILAE recommends long-term Video-EEG when there is diagnostic uncertainty to classify seizure type or epilepsy syndrome, quantify seizures, and evaluate electro-clinical seizure characteristics prior to epilepsy surgery [19]. Clinical usefulness of Video-EEG varies widely (19–75%) depending on how utility is defined and on the patient selection [20, 21]. Only video monitoring may be helpful [22], but not sufficient in confirming a definitive diagnosis separate from EEG recording [19].

18.2 Methodology

Video-electroencephalography (Video-EEG) is the combined, contemporary recording of the EEG and the clinical behavior of the patient. It allows correlating the clinical signs and symptoms, already acquired in the past clinical history of the patient [22], with the eventual EEG modifications. In the clinical practice, Video-EEG is particularly useful not only to analyze and visualize seizures but also paroxysmal repetitive or isolated, episodic events. The comprehensive characterization of the clinical manifestations of the seizures and the analysis of associated EEG modifications is essential to diagnose and differentiate epilepsy and is crucial in the clinical presurgical work-up of the patient. The digital EEG and the computed-assisted technologies make possible to record for a long time, increasing exponentially the possibility to catch one or more ictal episodes. The further advantage of 24-h recordings is mandatory to observe and analyze seizures occurring exclusively during nocturnal sleep or at the awakening, identifying interictal abnormalities more expressed during sleep, and discriminate epileptic seizures from other paroxysmal episodes during sleep. The recording of EEG signals and other polygraphic parameters (e.g., different muscles, cardiac and respiratory activity, eye movements) with clinical manifestations allows a more accurate diagnosis.

18.3 Indications and Limits

The Video-EEG goal is implementing video with EEG, increasing the diagnostic yield beyond EEG alone when events are recorded [23], with similar sensitivity when the two modalities are compared (Chen et al., 2008).

Detection of ictal events and/or interictal abnormalities is increased if standard EEGs are extended up to 60 min compared to routine 30-min studies [24].

Only 19% of interictal abnormalities were identified after 30 min, and longer recording times increased event capture rate by 30% [24].

Brief Video-EEG, lasting less than 24 h [25], is emerging as a less costly and resource-demanding technique in comparison to long-term monitoring (LTM) with Video-EEG and can differentiate among epilepsy and other paroxysmal disorders in more than 50% [26, 27]. In selected outpatient, short-term Video-EEG with induction may be used to diagnose psychogenic non-epileptic seizures (PNES) avoiding Video-EEG [28].

Polygraphy during Video-EEG may be used as a dynamic adapted short-term diagnostic test, tailored to a patient-specific clinical process.

Video-EEG is indicated in the following situations:

- *Identification, differentiation, classification, and characterization of ictal events.*
- The first aim is recording fits and to characterize the episodes from clinical and electrical point of view and collecting the data to classify. Achieving the right diagnosis allows choosing the right treatment. It is possible to discriminate epileptic from non-epileptic paroxysmal episodes and also to recognize minor, frequently underdiagnosed, epileptic seizures. Finally, it gives the opportunity to quantify the epileptic seizures and to establish the relationship with the sleep-wake cycle.
- *Identification and analysis of interictal EEG abnormalities and ictal patterns.*
- It is particularly helpful when there is a diagnostic question (epilepsy or other types of non-epileptic paroxysmal episodes) or when the interictal abnormalities are infrequent. Interictal abnormalities can be assessed, and patients during status epilepticus can be monitored for both seizures and discharges, indicating treatment adjustments.
- *Presurgical work-up for drug-resistant epilepsies.*
- During the presurgical work-up, it is often mandatory to record and analyze clinical and neurophysiological features of the seizures. It is essential to carefully describe the seizure semiology, considering the chronological occurrence of symptoms and signs. The clinical description has to be related with EEG modifications, and electroclinical correlations permit to formulate a localizing hypothesis of the epileptogenic zone and its diffusion to close or distant cortical areas. Finally, Video-EEG gives the opportunity to identify polymorphic seizures and their EEG seizure onset and the corresponding anatomical localization. Consequent diagnostic exams (i.e., invasive recordings, direct epilepsy surgery or exclusion from a surgical treatment) are scheduled on these bases.

18.4 Technical Features

18.4.1 Electrodes

The same electrodes as during the routine EEG are used. Electrodes for long-term monitoring must carefully be placed according to the 10–20 International System (Fig. 18.2), considering different head dimension, also in young children. In particular cases an increased number of the recording electrodes can be placed according to 10–10 International System [29–32].

Disk gold-plated electrodes should be applied with collodion/gauze for effective long-term results, possibly with a hole in top, permitting a periodic refilling with electrode conductant. It is also preferable to collect together the cables with the patch, limiting movement artifacts. Needle electrodes are not recommended for long-term recordings [33].

Other type of electrodes can be added, in particular sphenoidal, used to record interictal and ictal activity close to the mesial or anterior aspects of the temporal lobe. Other locations, such as nasoethmoidal, supraoptic, and auditory canal electrode positions, have also been used to better record focal discharges; however, being indications for these placements not well defined, these electrodes are not recommended for routine use.

Nasopharyngeal locations should not be used in long-term monitoring because of the resultant irritation and the demonstrate superiority of other electrode positions.

Surface electromyography (EMG) makes available an excellent noninvasive possibility of recording the electrical activity from muscles, using this information to gain a better insight into valuable information to the clinician. Furthermore, the EMG electrodes can be easily time-locked to the EEG trace recorded, improving the diagnostic utility of Video-EEG recordings. The information obtained from surface EMG recordings aided the differentiation of clinical events during Video-EEG monitoring in 7.5%, increasing the diagnosis rate [34].

18.4.2 Maintenance

Every electrode should be checked every single day or when artifacts appear, so that contact deterioration can be detected and corrected. Impedance should be checked periodically and if recording characteristics change. Refilling of the electrodes with conductant gel should be performed as necessary to maintain low impedance.

18.4.3 EEG Amplifiers

New amplifiers being of small dimension is possible to fix them to the patient's body, even in very little children, with an appropriate equipment, reducing the electromagnetic and muscular artifacts. In the digital EEG system, the EEG signal is analyzed with different sampling frequencies, but generally twice the maximum analogic sampling frequency.

18.4.4 Montage

Montages should be appropriate for the specific patient and corrected during the LTM, on the basis of the abnormalities.

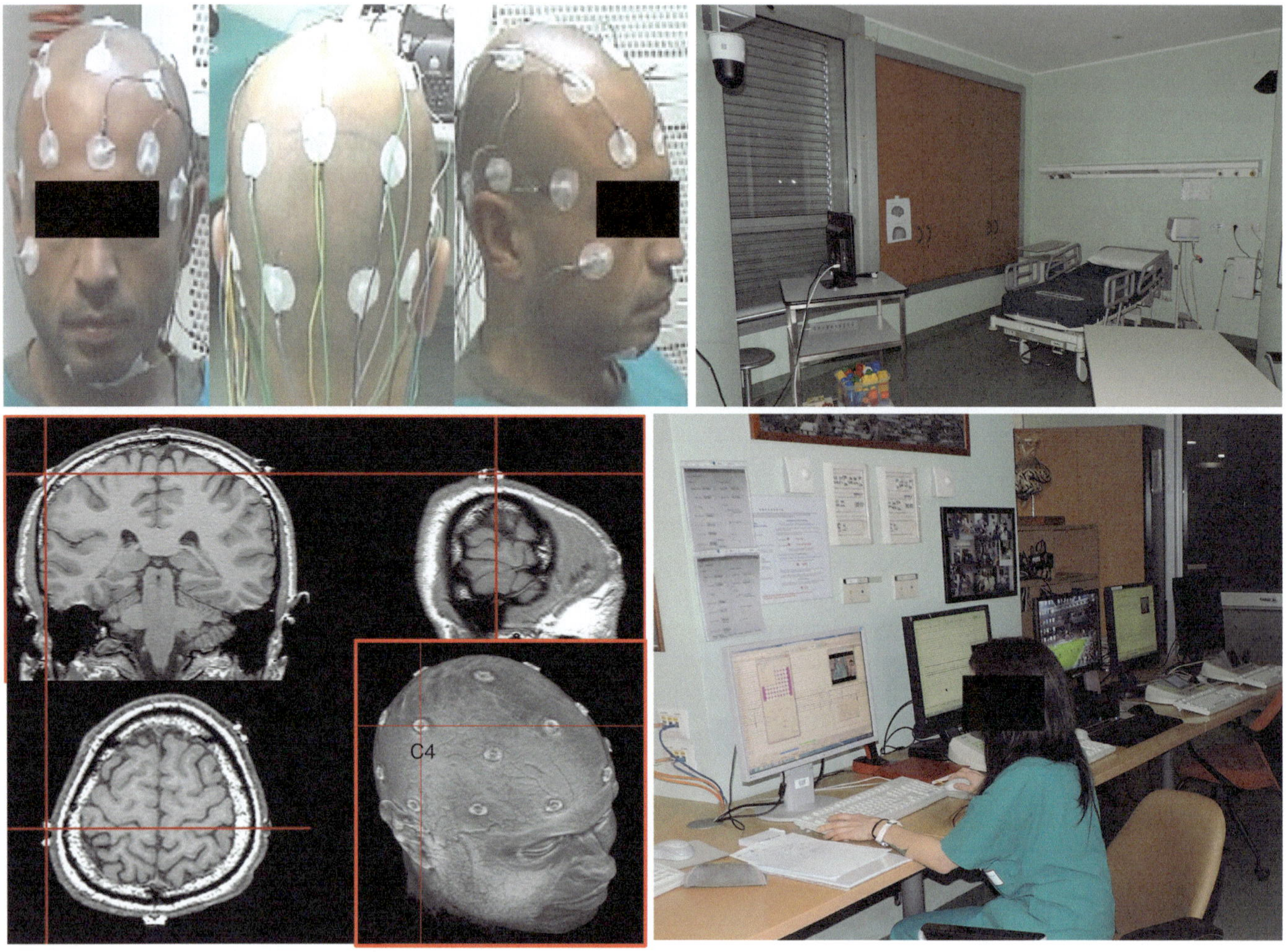

Fig. 18.2 Upper right: a room for prolonged video-EEG long-term monitoring. Upper left: a collodion montage after accurate measurement and the correspondent location of the electrodes on the MRI (lower left). Lower right: control room with direct access to the recording rooms

Simultaneous ECG and polygraphic channels recording are recommended, since cardiac arrhythmias or spontaneous movements may produce artifacts mimicking pathological EEG modifications (Fig. 18.3). The choice of ECG, electrooculogram (EOG), EMG position, or respiration may be indicated for particular clinical situations, reflecting the event semiology.

The digital signal is acquired with a referential montage allowing personal modification of the settings, choosing monopolar or bipolar montages. The modern Video-EEG systems utilize digital formats for both video and EEG signals, giving the possibility to interpret the EEG using different montages.

A longitudinal and a transversal montages are strongly recommended. In reviewing Video-EEG recording, it is also advantageous to modify the filters and reduce the artifacts, adapting them to the current clinical situation. Filters must be modified carefully in order to avoid strong and false conversion of the electrical activity.

18.4.5 Online Computed Analysis

To date, some EEG systems recognize automatically the seizures and/or interictal abnormalities [35, 36]. These systems are based on different algorithms analyzing EEG modifications, and, depending on the duration, they try to discriminate between seizures and interictal activity. Computer recognition programs have not been perfected and are subject to a variable amount of false-negative and false-positive error. The selected EEG components are automatically stored, and the technicians or the epileptologists can confirm or deny the automatic classification.

18.4.6 Video Recordings

Video recordings are carried out using a closed-circuit television camera. Cameras are both black and white and color; infrared are useful and necessary to recording during noctur-

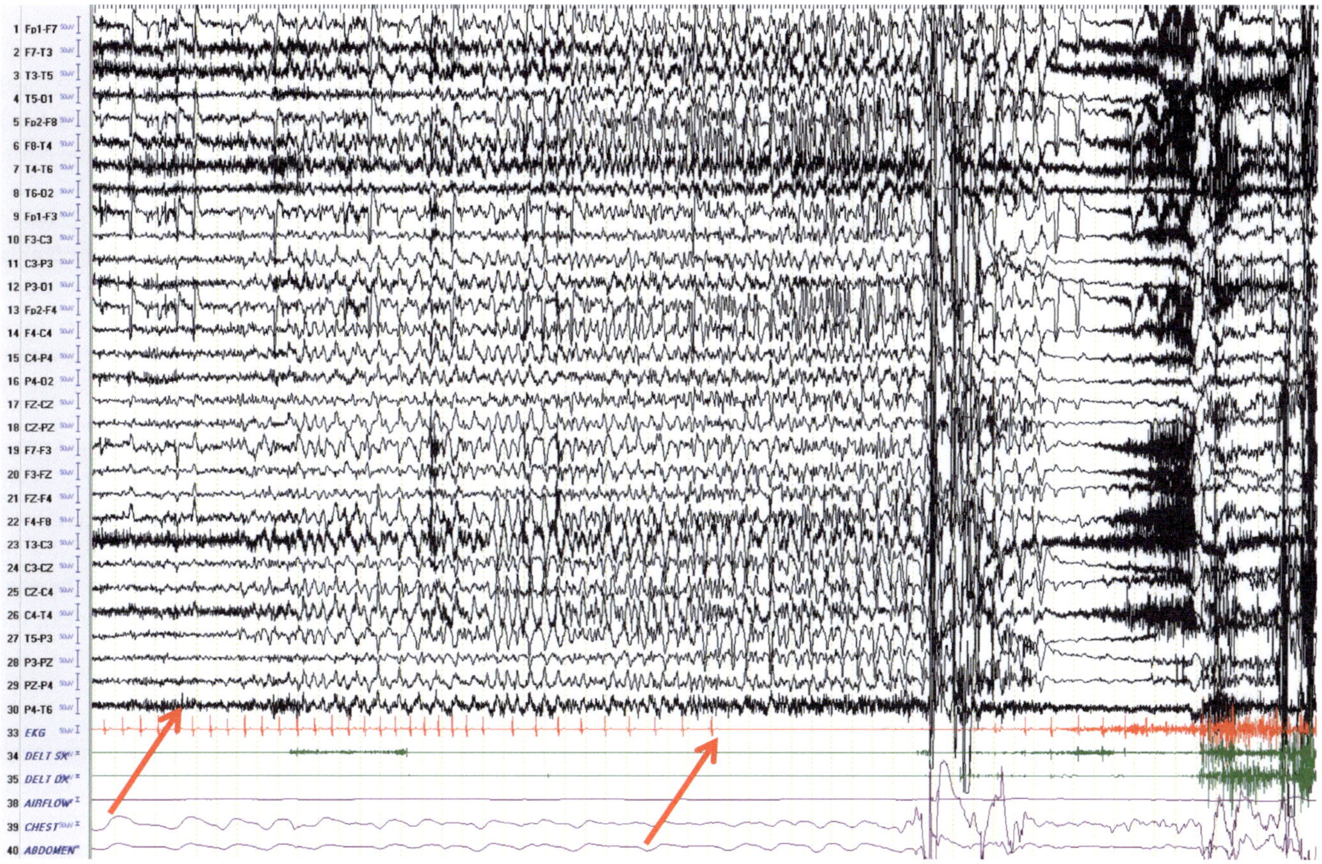

Fig. 18.3 Video-polygraphic recording of a focal seizure starting on the right temporal region (left arrow) rapidly involving the contralateral temporal lobe. The right arrow indicates the onset of a cardiac arrest (13 s) after a bradycardia, induced by the focal seizure. Timescale 60 s/page

nal sleep. The perfect synchronization in between video and EEG is mandatory to follow the onset and the development of the seizures and to compare EEG modifications with clinical events.

Appropriate lightings permit to frame correctly the total body image of the patient; in particular cases only a part of the patient should be monitored (e.g., the face for subtle periocular myoclonic jerks). Off-line visualization with zooming allows reviewing carefully significant details of the body. It could be useful to utilize two different cameras: one for the entire patient body and the other one concentrating on a detailed part of the body, depending on the clinical symptomatology.

Well-trained nurses in conjunction or in alternative with monitoring expert technologists are responsible for patient safety; they are also responsible for the integrity of the recording, and the facilities have to be designed for giving easy access to patients and to facilitate examination and eventual provision of first aid.

They also have to enumerate number and duration of seizures every day and to refer to the physician notification. Measures should be taken if number, duration, or severity of seizures observed is excessive.

Providing continuous surveillance permits to detail video and/or EEG changes, to be reviewing, as it could be time-consuming to carefully review off-line all the LTM.

Particular attention must be paid to audio recording and the lights. Different microphone types such as omnidirectional, unidirectional, or cardioid may be utilized. It's worth to remember that during the patient's testing, the operator should have a normal tone of voice in order to not cover the patient voice, encouraging him/her to explain subjective sensations. It remains necessary to avoid echoes (or Doppler effect) when opening the room door or the volume of the recording device is too high.

Into the recording room, it is often advantageous to add a spotlight focused on patient's face. Using colored sheets (green or light blue) permits a better contrast with patient's skin, making more identifiable little face and/or body movements.

18.4.7 Activation Techniques

During EEG recordings the use of activation procedures is routinely employed, to elicit or intensify interictal epileptiform abnormalities (IEA) and/or clinical events. They may be useful in patients where the diagnosis of epilepsy is suspected and has already been made or when the type of seizure or syndrome remains unclear [37].

Hyperventilation (HV) and intermittent photic stimulation (IPS) are routine activation procedures to enhance the possibility of detecting EEG abnormalities, especially in peculiar epilepsy syndromes [38]. Sleep is probably the most powerful modulator of seizures and IEA [39–41]. Sleep, amplifying the diagnostic yield, can be recorded physiologically during the nighttime or after sleep deprivation [42] or drug-induced [43].

Hyperventilation is by far the oldest activation used during EEG [40] and worldwide utilized [44] having few or none adverse effect [45, 46]. It should be performed for a minimum of 3 min, [47]; HV is helpful to distinguish epilepsy syndromes, especially absences frequently HV-induced [48]. In psychogenic non-epileptic seizures (PNES), HV is a method for eliciting ictal events [45, 46] in more than one-third (37%) of patients [49] (Fig. 18.4b, c).

Interictal abnormalities can be elicited or increased by HV in more than 12% of patients [46, 50] particularly prolonging HV to 5 min [45].

Most of the seizures (>85%) elicited by HV are absences and, in some rare cases, myoclonic seizures [45, 46], while in focal seizures the efficacy is less tough and more inconstant [41, 51].

Intermittent photic stimulation has to be performed in a room with low-level lighting, placing the lamp at least 30 cm from the patient's eyes. Photosensitivity (paroxysmal epileptiform response) is age-dependent phenomena, highest in late childhood and early adolescence, and more common in females, inducing myoclonias, absences, eyelid fluttering, and "cognitive impairment" [52]. The middle frequencies, in between 10 and 20 Hz, are most provoking, with a risk of provoking generalized tonic-clonic seizure.

These phenomena are rarely present in focal epilepsies, except those originating into the occipital lobe [53–55].

Relationships between sleep (spontaneous, drug-induced, and after sleep deprivation), seizures, and sleep cycles were identified longtime ago [56, 57] (Fig. 18.4a, c). IEA may be triggered in approximately one-third of patients, up to 90% of epilepsies activated by sleep or awakening [58–60]. Sleep deprivation (24 h) is an accepted practice adopted by European and American societies [47]. Drug-induced sleep as an activating technique is still debating [43, 61–66].

Reading, talking, writing, mental arithmetic counting, and manipulating objects are considered specific activation methods in patients with reflex epilepsy, even if patients may have normal EEG during the procedure (;Koutroumanidis M, Koepp MJ, Richardson MP, Camfield C, Agathonikou A, Ried S,et al. The variants of reading epilepsy. A clinical and video-EEG study of 17patients with reading-induced seizures. Brain 1998;121:1409–27. [67]). In reflex epilepsy associated with photosensitivity, television and electronic games may play a role [68, 69].

18.4.8 Testing the Patient during Seizures

Trained staffs into the epilepsy monitoring unit (EMU) must accurately supervise the patient, during all the Video-EEG monitoring, in order to notify, record, and examine the clinical events; the quality of both video and EEG must be guaranteed during all the recording time. Seizures can be detected by supervising staff, or by the patient himself, with the handy push button or verbally warning. Patients must be trained to warn speaking or using the push button, immediately after the onset of subjective manifestation, if any. The supervising personnel should have access to a screening, investigating seizure types and frequency and the cognitive status.

During and after every ictal events, it is mandatory to:

- Take care of the patient, avoiding dangerous behavior.
- Help the patient describing the subjective feelings.
- Observe the patient carefully, describing verbally the neurological functions, testing the level of consciousness, the language, the muscle tone, and eventual deficit of the visual field.

Ictal and postictal testing is a cardinal element to approach an accurate diagnosis associated with the Video-EEG recording. Every EMU should have a protocol for testing patients systematically. The battery is devoted to demonstrate the semiologic features, occurring during both ictal and postictal periods. Furthermore, there are items reminding about patient safety, observing and reporting very discrete changes not evident on video recordings (pallor, flushing, sweating, piloerection, and sialorrhea). All the tests must be adaptive to the dynamics of the individual seizures.

Additional specifics for testing individuals with suspected non-epileptic events should be an integral part of the same protocol (e.g., hand drop, resistance to passive eye opening, arm or leg elevation, etc). Once back to the baseline, patient must be asked whether the event was typical and its severity [70–72].

18.4.9 Pharmacological Treatment

Antiepileptic drugs (AED) are often tapered to reduce the duration sufficient to record ictal events during long-term Video-EEG monitoring, especially during presurgical evaluation, using different seizure provocative methods [7, 73–78]. More than half of EMUs reduced or completely withdrawn one or more antiepileptic drugs (AEDs) in 75–100% of patients, even if fast AED reduction is considered less safe. Complete AED discontinuation was associated with three times increased necessary rescue therapy during LTM and double risk of having bilateral tonic-clonic seizures. Many factors can influence the strategy of AED

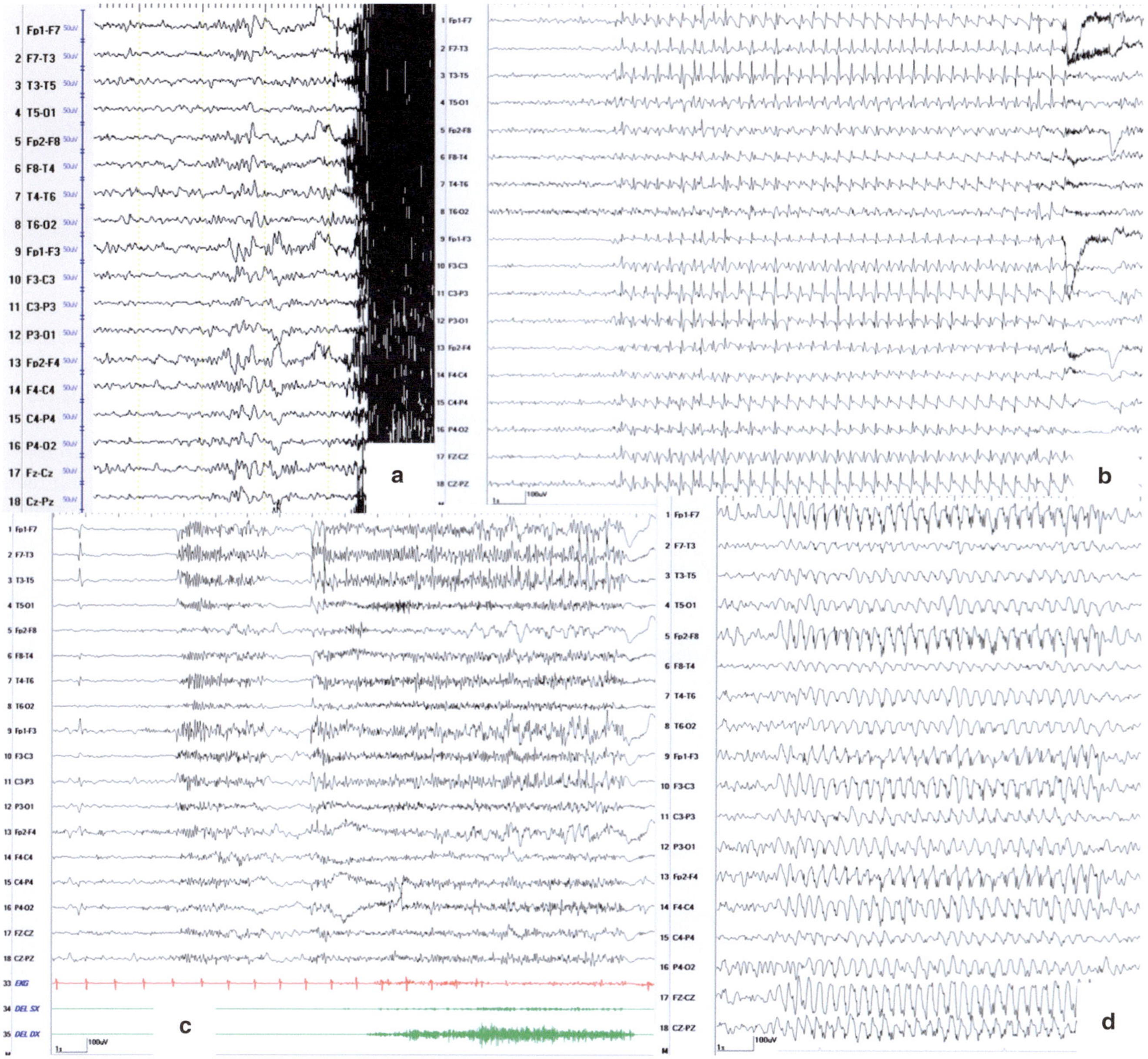

Fig. 18.4 Ictal discharges occurring during sleep (**a**, **c**) and hyperventilation (**b**, **d**). (**a**) Seizure arising for sleep in a 24-year-old female, having hypermotor seizures sleep-related. No discharges are evident before artifacts cover the EEG. (**c**) Tonic seizure during sleep in a 45-year-old patient suffering from a Lennox-Gastaut syndrome. The onset of the discharge is characterized by a burst of fast activity followed by a fast tonic generalized component. On the clinical point of view, the patient opened his eyes and slightly moved both the superior limbs as indicated by the polygraphy. (**b**, **d**) Generalized spike and wave discharges during or at the very end of the hyperventilation

tapering/withdrawal as seizure frequency and type, past history of status epilepticus, and seizure clusters [79]. More than half of EMUs performed tapering/withdrawal of AEDs before the admission. No specific protocols of AEDs are available. Drug monitoring is performed at very different intervals [80, 81].

A recent study pointed out fast AED tapering reduces significantly LTM duration compared to slow, without inducing serious adverse events [82].

18.4.10 Safety

Patients are vulnerable to potential injury during all the LTM in Video-EEG, being observed for the whole recording time by competent personnel in only 80% of the EMU, having the pharmacological treatment quite always withdrawn. Ictal events are potentially dangerous leading to serious injury or death [83–88]. It is therefore recommended to have safety protocols [19], lacking in more than 20% of the EMU, particularly concerning bilaterale tonic-clonic seizures, status epilepticus and clustering episodes, postictal psychosis, and related injuries.

Every EMU must have guidelines for patients in and out of bed, with adequate levels of nursing to provide quality care, after a formal educational program [89]. Protocol for the management of cardiac arrest and prompt access to intensive care unit should be required. The prevalent complications were status epilepticus in about 80%, injuries in more than 70%, and postictal psychoses (67%).

Prevention consists of bed protections in 96% of EMUs, but antisuffocation pillows are employed in only 21%, and environmental protections in monitoring rooms and in bathrooms are present in less than 35% of EMUs.

Most of the EMUs introduced standardized procedures to ensure patients' safety also after being discharged, consisting of inhospital stay for AED reintroduction and/or protocols for contacting on-call patient's physicians [90–92].

18.4.11 Guidelines for Video-EEG Monitoring Laboratory

Signed informed consent prior to admission was requested in the majority of the EMUs, containing also a screening investigating epilepsy features and possible comorbidities.

Each patient should be scheduled with the following data:

- Personal clinical data.
- Detailed clinical history containing hypothesis about and suggestions in order to focus the ictal testing, identifying facilitating factors, prevent injuries.
- Sequential number, detailed daily diary of monitoring (recorded hours, provoking events, AED posology, number of ictal events).
- Type of EEG recording (i.e. standard EEG, EEG during sleep, EEG after sleep deprivation).
- Informed consent of the patient or tutors.

The placement of the electrodes should be performed in a special room with a suction hood. Collodion should be dried slowly to make a film over the electrode, preventing the jelly drying out. This may be facilitated by the use of pressured air using a compressor.

A collodion montage required about 30–40 min, in a collaborating patient. The recording quality must be verified daily, with adding of conductive paste. As generally the acquisition is in monopolar, special attention must be paid to the ground and reference electrodes.

Patients must be educated to observe some simple rules:

- Warn about every kind of presumable ictal subjective feeling, verbally speaking or with the handy push button.
- Do not touch the electrodes.
- Do not chew candies or chewing gum because the relevant artifacts induced.
- Do not cover the face with newspapers and books.
- Do not sleep with bedsheets or blankets.
- Do not move into the room without warning the personnel.
- Minimize the use of mobile phone.

18.4.12 Storage

Storage of the whole Video-EEG recordings is not useful and technically not advisable. Interictal basal stimulations (HV, IPS, etc.) and sleep and wakening recordings may be stored without the conjoint video.

All video and audio monitoring data and the associated EEG recordings should be saved until appropriately analyzed and reduced by trained personnel or by expert epileptologists. A partial data reduction can be performed online erasing data containing no episodes. If a clinically significant event has occurred, the video and EEG data should be retained for later analysis.

When a behavioral episode is considered clinically relevant, video-recorded data should be copied onto a durable medium for long-term storage. About 5 min before and after the end of the clinical event must be included.

18.4.13 Report

The final report of a Video-EEG recording should consist of different principal parts [33, 93–95].

Firstly a brief statement about the clinical pathology requiring a LTM, including a brief summary of the anamnestic data, a review of current medications, and other comorbidities, should be declared. The purpose of the LTM (diagnostic study, presurgical evaluation, control after drugs modification/introduction) has to be clearly stated.

The technological aspects of the recording (number of channels, type, and location of electrodes, eventual polygraphy) should be documented. Activation procedures (HV, IPS, drug injection, suggestion, sleep deprivation) have to be fully described. The reduction of medications, especially those intended to increase or decrease the incidence of seizures, should be described.

Interictal findings as a description of the neurophysiological data at first (at rest, during sleep, during activation techniques) should be described, including a report concerning waking and sleeping EEG patterns. Then a precise description about the degree and location of interictal pathological slowing and spiking abnormalities, explaining the frequency of occurrence, the topographic distribution, and the eventual propagation, should be reported (Fig. 18.5).

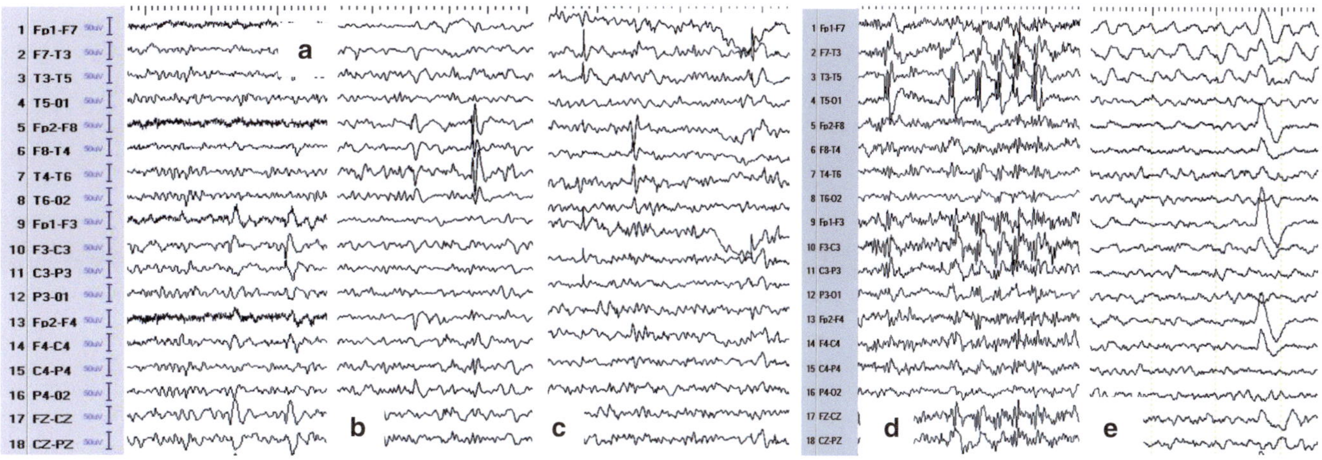

Fig. 18.5 Interictal epileptiform abnormalities. (**a**) Sharp waves located in the precentro-central region on the left side (maximum C3). (**b**) Sharp waves and spike and waves into the right temporal lobe. (**c**) Asynchronous spike and waves on both temporal regions. (**d**) During sleep, runs of spiking activity well localized on the temporo-occipital regions on the left side. (**e**) Continuous delta polymorphic activity in the left temporal territories, not related to a recent seizure

Video-EEG aims to record behaviors, and great importance is due to the description of ictal events.

On the clinical point of view, a precise account is needed about the patient behavior, including the activity immediately preceding the episode, then the features of the very onset (warned by the patient or signaled by the personnel), the chronological evolution of ictal symptoms and signs and the termination of the episode, and finally ictal and postictal behaviors. All the neurological functions are to be reported, including responsiveness, time-space orientation, language, memory, visual and motor function.

Once identified the first clinical signs or symptoms, the preceding and/or contemporary EEG modifications are to be reported including a brief description of background activity and interictal discharges preceding the clinical event and then morphology, location, evolution, and the eventual spread, including postictal changes.

All the former are to be included into the conclusions. An interpretation is required, stating the overall impressions, the clinical significance, and the electrographic and behavioral correlations being an interpretive synthesis rather than a reiteration of the description. A conceivable diagnosis has to be stated and associated with a proposed treatment.

In the presurgical Video-EEG monitoring, a hypothesis on the location of the epileptogenic zone would be detailed, including further surgical possibilities, with or without invasive recordings (Fig. 18.6).

18.5 Conclusion

The field of EEG associated with video recordings has witnessed a dramatic development during the last decades, now fully used as an "online" monitoring of neurological functions with its excellent temporal resolution.

Long-term monitoring of scalp and synchronized Video-EEG recordings studies are well-established tools in the localization of the epileptogenic region for identification of potential candidates for surgery. The advent of digital EEG with digital storage has allowed maximizing the information and reducing artifacts. These changes have revolutionized the way in which EEG is performed and interpreted.

The most common indications for Video-EEG recordings for EMU admissions are:

- Differential diagnosis.
- Presurgical evaluation.
- Characterization of seizure types.

The evaluation is essential to determine whether individuals with drug-resistant epilepsy are candidates for epilepsy surgery and which are the requested exams, to define a diagnosis in cases in which a psychogenic origin is suspected, to delineate and eventually modify the current pharmacological treatment (during status epilepticus or in specific epileptic syndromes).

Monitoring in a specialized EMU is safer, more efficient, and more effective; the appropriate use of this specialized evaluation can lead to an early and more correct diagnosis in many clinical circumstances.

In the past the diagnosis of epilepsy was based upon a thorough history and physical examination that can be misleading [21].

When standard EEG recordings are unrevealing, additional methods of EEG recordings can enhance its usefulness, and long-term Video-EEG is able to document the relationship between the ictal semiology and the EEG, synchronizing signals from multiple generators including at least EEG, ECG, and EMG.

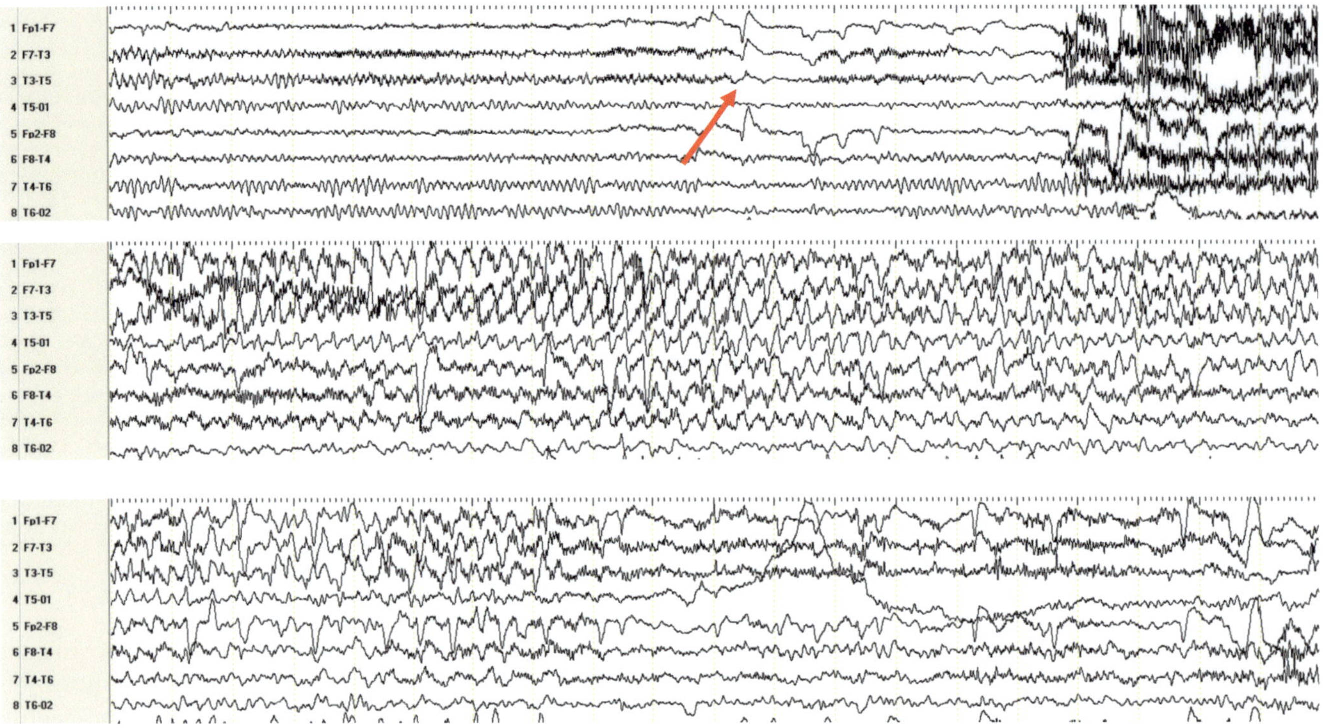

Fig. 18.6 Focal seizure on the left temporal lobe, during wakening. The red arrow shows the onset of the discharge with a flattening on the left temporal channels, while on the right side, the background activity is continuing. Then, intermingled with the artifacts, a theta activity is growing up, on the left side, slowing down during the following seconds and stopping in the third part of the EEG

The EMU evaluation is currently considered the gold standard test for the definitive diagnosis of epilepsy and seizure-like events, for eventual indication to proceed to epilepsy surgery and for the management of critical patients.

At least 4–7 days of recording are needed to store a sufficient number of seizures, but sometimes longer recordings are necessary, varying on the base of the indication for the EMU study: seizures are by their nature intermittent and periodic [96–99]. Well-trained interdisciplinary teams are needed to adequately address the clinical questions [89].

Furthermore we have to remember LTM Video-EEG is a high time-consuming methodology and the full management cost of the noninvasive diagnostic stage is not remunerative [100].

References

1. Berger H. Uber das Elektrenkephalogramm des Menschen. Archiv für Psychiatrie und Nervenkrankheiten. 1929;87:527–70.
2. Adrian ED, Matthews BHC. The Berger rhythm, potential changes from the occipital lobe in man. Brain. 1934;57:345–59.
3. Gibbs FA, Gibbs EL, Lennox WG. Electroencephalographic classification of epileptic patients and control subjects. Arch Neurol (Chicago). 1943;50:111–28.
4. Gibbs FA, Gibbs EL. Clinical and pharmacological correlates of fast activity in electroencephalography. J Neuropsychiatr. 1962;3(Suppl 1):73–8.
5. Vannemreddy P, Stone JL, Slavin KV. Frederic Gibbs and his contributions to epilepsy surgery and electroencephalography. Neurosurgery. 2012;70(3):774–82.
6. Burgess RC. Design and evolution of a system for long-term electroencephalographic and video monitoring of epilepsy patients. Methods. 2001;25:231–48.
7. Engel J Jr, Burchfield J, Ebersole J, et al. Long term monitoring for epilepsy. Report of an IFCN Committee. Electroencephalogr Clin Neurophysiol. 1993;87:437–58.
8. Perry TR, Gumnit RJ, Gates JR, Leppik IE. Routine EEG vs. intensive monitoring in the evaluation of intractable epilepsy. Public Health Rep. 1983;98(4):384–9.
9. Appleton RE, Beirne M. Absence epilepsy in children: the role of EEG in monitoring response to treatment. Seizure. 1996;5:147–8.
10. Asan E, Pawlak C, Shah A, et al. The diagnostic value of initial video-EEG monitoring in children—review of 1000 cases. Epilepsy Res. 2005;66:129–35.
11. Ghougassian DF, d'Souza W, Cook MJ, O'rien TJ. Evaluating the utility of inpatient video-EEG monitoring. Epilepsia. 2004;45(8):928–32.
12. Mohan KK, Markand ON, Salanova V. Diagnostic utility of Video-EEG monitoring in paroxysmal events. Acta Neurol Scand. 1996;47(Suppl 1):26–30.
13. Benbadis SR, Agrawal V, Tatum WO. How many patients with psychogenic nonepileptic seizures also have epilepsy? Neurology. 2001;57:915–7.
14. Devinsky O, Gazzola D, LaFrance WC. Differentiating between nonepileptic and epileptic seizures. Nat Rev Neurol. 2011;7:210–20.
15. Mostacci B, Bisulli F, Alvisi L, et al. Ictal characteristics of psychogenic nonepileptic seizures: what we have learned from video/EEG recordings—a literature review. Epilepsy Behav. 2011;22:144–53.

16. Popkirov S, Jungilligens J, Grönheit W, Wellmer J. Diagnosing psychogenic nonepileptic seizures: video-EEG monitoring, suggestive seizure induction and diagnostic certainty. Epilepsy Behav. 2017;73:54–8.
17. Reuber M. Psychogenic nonepileptic seizures: answers and questions. Epilepsy Behav. 2008;12:622–35.
18. Shih JJ, Spector AR, Taha FA, et al. Clinically significant bradyarrhythmias in video-EEG patients. Seizure. 2011;20:225–30.
19. Velis D, Plouin P, Gotman J, da Silva FL, ILAE DMC Subcommittee on Neurophysiology. Recommendations regarding the requirements and applications for long-term recordings in epilepsy. Epilepsia. 2007;48(2):379–84.
20. Alving J, Beniczky S. Diagnostic usefulness and duration of the inpatient long-term video-EEG monitoring: findings in patients extensively investigated before the monitoring. Seizure. 2009;18:470–3.
21. Deacon C, Wiebe S, Blume WT, McLachlan RS, Young GB, Matijevic S. Seizure identification by clinical description in temporal lobe epilepsy: how accurate are we? Neurology. 2003;61:1686–9.
22. Beniczky SA, Fogarasi A, Neufeld M, et al. Seizure semiology inferred from clinical descriptions and from video recordings. How accurate are they? Epilepsy Behav. 2012b;24:213–5.
23. Cascino GD. Clinical indications and diagnostic yield of video-electroencephalographic monitoring in patients with seizures and spells. Mayo Clin Proc. 2002;77:1111–20.
24. Burkholder DB, Britton JW, Rajasekaran V, Fabris RR, Cherian PJ, Kelly-Williams KM, et al. Routine vs extended outpatient EEG for the detection of interictal epileptiform discharges. Neurology. 2016;86:1524–30.
25. Bubrick EJ, Yazdani S, Pavlova MK. Beyond standard polysomnography: advantages and indications for use of extended 10–20 EEG montage during laboratory sleep study evaluations. Seizure. 2014;23:699–702.
26. Tallawy HN, Fukuyama H, Kader AA, Kamel NF, Badry R. Role of short-term out patient video electroencephalography in diagnosis of paroxysmal disorders. Epilepsy Res. 2010;88:179–82.
27. Tinuper P, Grassi C, Bisulli F, Provini F, Plazzi G, Zoni E, et al. Split-screen synchronized display. A useful video-EEG technique for studying paroxysmal phenomena. Epileptic Disord. 2004;6:27–30.
28. Benbadis SR, O'Neill E, Tatum WO, et al. Outcome of prolonged video-EEG monitoring at a typical referral epilepsy center. Epilepsia. 2004;45:1150–3.
29. Acharya JN, Hani A, Cheek J, et al. American Clinical Neurophysiology Society Guideline 2: Guidelines for standard electrode position nomenclature. J Clin Neurophysiol. 2016;33:308–11.
30. Buelow JM, Privitera M, Levisohn P, et al. A description of current practice in epilepsy monitoring units. Epilepsy Behav. 2009;15:308–13.
31. Klem GH, Lüders HO, Jasper HH, Elger C. The ten-twenty electrode system of the International Federation. The International Federation of Clinical Neurophysiology. Electroencephalogr Clin Neurophysiol Suppl. 1999;52:3–6.
32. Sharbrough F, Chatrian G-E, Lesser RP, Lüders H, Nuwer M, Picton TW. American Electroencephalographic Society guidelines for standard electrode position nomenclature. J Clin Neurophysiol. 1991;8:200–2.
33. American Clinical Neurophysiology Society. Guideline twelve: guidelines for long-term monitoring for epilepsy. Am J Electroneurodiagnostic Technol. 2008;48:265–86.
34. Hill AT, Briggs BA, Seneviratne U. Simultaneous recordings of EEG and electromyographic polygraphy increases the diagnostic yield of Video-EEG monitoring. J Clin Neurophysiol. 2014;31:203–7.
35. Gotman J. Computer analysis during intensive monitoring of epileptic patients. Electroencephalogr Clin Neurophysiol. 1987;67(2):120–33.
36. Gotman J. Automatic detection of seizures and spikes. J Clin Neurophysiol. 1999;16:130–40.
37. Tatum WO, Rubboli G, Kaplan PW, Mirsatari SM, Radhakrishnan K, Gloss D, Caboclo LO, Drislane FW, Koutroumanidis M, Schomer DL, Kastelijn-Nolst Trenite D, Cook M, Beniczky S. Clinical utility of EEG in diagnosing and monitoring epilepsy in adults. Clin Neurophysiol. 2018;129:1056–82.
38. Mendez OE, Brenner RP. Increasing the yield of EEG. J Clin Neurophysiol. 2006;23:282–93.
39. Beniczky S, Guaranha MS, Conradsen I, Singh MB, Rutar V, Lorber B, et al. Modulation of epileptiform EEG discharges in juvenile myoclonic epilepsy: an investigation of reflex epileptic traits. Epilepsia. 2012a;53:832–9.
40. Gibbs EL, Gibbs FA. Diagnostic and localizing value of electroencephalographic studies in sleep. J Nerv Ment Dis. 1947;26:336–76.
41. Guaranha MS, da Silva Sousa P, de Araujo-Filho GM, Lin K, Guilhoto LM, Caboclo LO, et al. Provocative and inhibitory effects of a video-EEG neuropsychologic protocol in juvenile myoclonic epilepsy. Epilepsia. 2009;50:2446–55.
42. Degen R. A study of the diagnostic value of waking and sleep EEGs after sleep deprivation in epileptic patients on anticonvulsive therapy. Electroencephalogr Clin Neurophysiol. 1980;49:577–84.
43. Degen R, Degen HE. A comparative study of the diagnosis value of drug-induced sleep EEGs and sleep EEGs following sleep deprivation in patients with complex partial seizures. J Neurol. 1981;225:85–93.
44. Binnie CD, Stefan H. Modern electroencephalography: its role in epilepsy management. Clin Neurophysiol. 1999;110:1671–97.
45. Craciun L, Varga ET, Mindruta I, Meritam P, Horvath Z, Terney D, et al. Diagnostic yield of five minutes compared to three minutes hyperventilation during electroencephalography. Seizure. 2015;30:90–2.
46. Kane N, Grocott L, Kandler R, Lawrence S, Pang C. Hyperventilation during electroencephalography: safety and efficacy. Seizure. 2014;23:129–34.
47. Sinha SR, Sullivan L, Sabau D, San-Juan D, Dombrowski KE, Halford JJ, et al. American Clinical Neurophysiology Society Guideline 1: Minimum technical requirements for performing clinical electroencephalography. J Clin Neurophysiol. 2016;33:303–7.
48. Koutroumanidis M, Aggelakis K, Panayiotopoulos CP. Idiopathic epilepsy with generalized tonic-clonic seizures only versus idiopathic epilepsy with phantom absences and generalized tonic-clonic seizures: one or two syndromes? Epilepsia. 2008;49:2050–62.
49. Abubakr A, Ifeayni I, Wambacq I. The efficacy of routine hyperventilation for seizure activation during prolonged video-electroencephalography monitoring. J Clin Neurosci. 2010;17:1503–5.
50. Angus-Leppan H. Seizures and adverse events during routine scalp electroencephalography: a clinical and EEG analysis of 1000 records. Clin Neurophysiol. 2007;118:22–30.
51. Jonas J, Vignal JP, Baumann C, Anxionnat JF, Muresan M, Vespignani H, et al. Effect of hyperventilation on seizure activation: potentiation by antiepileptic drug tapering. J Neurol Neurosurg Psychiatry. 2011;82:928–30.
52. Kasteleijn-Nolst Trenite DG, Guerrini R, Binnie CD, Genton P. Visual sensitivity and epilepsy: a proposed terminology and classification for clinical and EEG phenomenology. Epilepsia. 2001;42:692–701.
53. Ricci S, Vigevano F. Occipital seizures provoked by intermittent light stimulation: ictal and interictal findings. J Clin Neurophysiol. 1993;10:197–209.

54. Shiraishi H, Fujiwara T, Inoue Y, Yagi K. Photosensitivity in relation to epileptic syndromes: a survey from an epilepsy center in Japan. Epilepsia. 2001;42:393–7.
55. Wolf P, Goosses R. Relation of photosensitivity to epileptic syndromes. J Neurol Neurosurg Psychiatry. 1986;49:1386–91.
56. Kellaway P, Frost JD Jr, Crawley JW. Time modulation of spike-and-wave activity in generalized epilepsy. Ann Neurol. 1980;8:491–500.
57. Steriade M, Amzica F. Sleep oscillations developing into seizures in corticothalamic systems. Epilepsia. 2003;44(Suppl 12):9–20.
58. Nickels K, Wirrell E. Electrical status epilepticus in sleep. Semin Pediatr Neurol. 2008;15:50–60.
59. Pratt KL, Mattson RH, Weikers NJ, Williams R. EEG activation of epileptics following sleep deprivation: a prospective study of 114 cases. Electroencephalogr Clin Neurophysiol. 1968;24:11–5.
60. Vaughn BV, D'Cruz OF. Sleep and epilepsy. Semin Neurol. 2004;24:301–13.
61. Gustafsson G, Brostrom A, Ulander M, Vrethem M, Svanborg E. Occurrence of epileptiform discharges and sleep during EEG recordings in children after melatonin intake versus sleep-deprivation. Clin Neurophysiol. 2015;126:1493–7.
62. Leach JP, Stephen LJ, Salveta C, Brodie MJ. Which electroencephalography (EEG) for epilepsy? The relative usefulness of different EEG protocols in patients with possible epilepsy. J Neurol Neurosurg Psychiatry. 2006;77:1040–2.
63. Malow BA, Passaro E, Milling C, et al. Sleep deprivation does not affect seizure frequency during inpatient video-EEG monitoring. Neurology. 2002;59:1371–4.
64. Roupakiotis SC, Gatzonis SD, Triantafyllou N, Mantouvalos V, Chioni A, Zournas C, et al. The usefulness of sleep and sleep deprivation as activating methods in electroencephalographic recording: contribution to a long-standing discussion. Seizure. 2000;9:580–4.
65. Rowan AJ, Veldhuisen RJ, Nagelkerke NJ. Comparative evaluation of sleep deprivation and sedated sleep EEGs as diagnostic aids in epilepsy. Electroencephalogr Clin Neurophysiol. 1982;54:357–64.
66. Wassmer E, Carter PF, Quinn E, McLean N, Welsh G, Seri S, et al. Melatonin is useful for recording sleep EEGs: a prospective audit of outcome. Dev Med Child Neurol. 2001;43:735–8.
67. Koepp MJ, Caciagli L, Pressler RM, Lehnertz K, Beniczky S. Reflex seizures, traits, and epilepsies: from physiology to pathology. Lancet Neurol. 2016;15:92–105.
68. Harding GF, Jeavons PM, Edson AS. Video material and epilepsy. Epilepsia. 1994;35:1208–16.
69. Quirk JA, Fish DR, Smith SJ, Sander JW, Shorvon SD, Allen PJ. First seizures associated with playing electronic screen games: a community-based study in Great Britain. Ann Neurol. 1995;37:733–7.
70. Beniczky S, Neufeld M, Diehl B, et al. Testing patients during seizures: a European consensus procedure developed by a joint taskforce of the ILAE—Commission on European Affairs and the European Epilepsy Monitoring Unit Association. Epilepsia. 2016;57:1363–8.
71. Shih JJ, Fountain NB, Herman ST, Bagic A, Lado F, Arnold S, Zupanc ML, Riker E, Labiner DM. Indications and methodology for video-electroencephalographic studies in the epilepsy monitoring unit. Epilepsia. 2018;59:27–36.
72. Touloumes G, Morse E, Chen WC, Gober L, Dente J, Lilenbaum R, Katzenstein E, Pacelli A, Johnson E, Si Y, Sivaraju A, Grover E, Khozein R, Cunningham C, Hirsch LJ, Blumenfeld H. Human bedside evaluation versus automatic responsiveness testing in epilepsy (ARTiE). Epilepsia. 2016;57(1):e28–32.
73. Haut SR, Swick C, Freeman K, et al. Seizure clustering during epilepsy monitoring. Epilepsia. 2002;43:711–5.
74. Marciani MG, Gotman J, Andermann F, et al. Patterns of seizure activation after withdrawal of antiepileptic medication. Neurology. 1985;35:1537.
75. Marks DA, Katz A, Scheyer R, et al. Clinical and electrographic effects of acute anticonvulsant withdrawal in epileptic patients. Neurology. 1991;41:508.
76. So N, Gotman J. Changes in seizure activity following anticonvulsant drug withdrawal. Neurology. 1990;40:407.
77. Thomas P, Valton L, Genton P. Absence and myoclonic status epilepticus precipitated by antiepileptic drugs in idiopathic generalized epilepsy. Brain. 2006;129:1281–92.
78. Zhou D, Wang Y, Hopp P, et al. Influence on ictal seizure semiology of rapid withdrawal of carbamazepine and valproate in monotherapy. Epilepsia. 2002;43:386–93.
79. Cox FME, Reus EEM, Visser GH. Timing of first event in inpatient long-term video-EEG monitoring for diagnostic purposes. Epilepsy Res. 2017;129:91–4.
80. Guld AT, Sabers A, Kjaer TW. Drug taper during long-term video-EEG monitoring: efficiency and safety. Acta Neurol Scand. 2017;135:302–7.
81. Kobulashvili T, Hofler J, Dobesberger J, Ernst F, Ryvlin P, Cross HJ, Braun K, Dimova P, Francione S, Hecimovic H, Helmstaedter C, Kimiskidis VK, Lossius MI, Malmgren K, Marusic P, Steinhoffmm BJ, Boon P, Craiu D, Delanty N, Fabo D, Gil-Nagel A, Guekht A, Hirsch E, Kalviainen R, Mameniskiene R, Ozkara C, Seeck M, Rubboli G, Krsek P, Rheims S, Trinka E. Current practices in long-term video-EEG monitoring services: a survey among partners of the E-PILEPSY pilot network of reference for refractory epilepsy and epilepsy surgery. Seizure. 2016;38:38–45.
82. Kumar S, Ramanujam B, Chandra PS, Dash D, Mehta S, Anubha S, Appukutan S, Rana MK, Tripathi M. Randomized controlled study comparing the efficacy of rapid and slow withdrawal of antiepileptic drugs during long-term video-EEG monitoring. Epilepsia. 2018;59:460–7.
83. Noe KH, Drazkowski JF. Safety of long-term video-electroencephalographic monitoring for evaluation of epilepsy. Mayo Clin Proc. 2009;84:495–500.
84. Rheims S, Ryvlin P. Patients' safety in the epilepsy monitoring unit. Curr Opin Neurol. 2014;27:213–8.
85. Sauro KM, Wiebe N, Macrodimitris S, et al. Quality and safety in adult epilepsy monitoring units: a systematic review and meta-analysis. Epilepsia. 2016;57:1754–70.
86. Shafer PO, Buelow J, Ficker DM, et al. Risk of adverse events on epilepsy monitoring units: a survey of epilepsy professionals. Epilepsy Behav. 2011;20:502–5.
87. Spritzer SD, Riordan KC, Berry J, et al. Fall prevention and bathroom safety in the epilepsy monitoring unit. Epilepsy Behav. 2015;48:75–8.
88. van Griethuysena R, Hofstraa WA, van der Salma SMA, Bourez-Swarta MD, de Weerda AW. Safety and efficiency of medication withdrawal at home prior to long-term EEG video-monitoring. Seizure. 2018;56:9–13.
89. Stecker M, Stecker M. The effect of education on nurses' assessments in an epilepsy monitoring unit. Can J Neurosci Nurs. 2012;34:23–32.
90. Labiner DM, Bagic AI, Herman ST, Fountain NB, Walczak TS, Gumnit RJ. Essential services, personnel, and facilities in specialized epilepsy centers—revised 2010 guidelines. Epilepsia. 2010;51:2322–33.
91. Ryvlin P, Nashef L, Lhatoo SD, et al. Incidence and mechanisms of cardiorespiratory arrests in epilepsy monitoring units (MORTEMUS): a retrospective study. Lancet Neurol. 2013;12:966–77.
92. Rubboli G, Beniczky S, Claus S, Canevini MP, Kahane P, Stefan H, van Emde Boas W, Velis D, Reus E, Gil-Nagel A, Steinhoff BJ, Trinka E, Ryvlin P. A European survey on current practices

in epilepsy monitoring units and implications for patients' safety. Epilepsy Behav. 2015;44:179–84.
93. Blume WT, Luders HO, Mizrahi E, et al. Glossary of descriptive terminology for ictal semiology: report of the ILAE taskforce on classification and terminology. Epilepsia. 2001;42:1212–8.
94. Flink R, Pedersen B, Guekht AB, et al. (ILAE Commission Report). Guidelines for the use of EEG methodology in the diagnosis of epilepsy. Acta Neurol Scand. 2002;106:1–7.
95. Shafer PO, Buelow JM, Noe K, et al. A consensus-based approach to patient safety in epilepsy monitoring units: recommendations for preferred practices. Epilepsy Behav. 2012;25: 449–56.
96. Gazzola DM, Thawani S, Agbe-Davies O, et al. Epilepsy monitoring unit length of stay. Epilepsy Behav. 2016;58:102–5.
97. Herman ST, Abend NS, Bleck TP, et al. Consensus statement on continuous EEG in critically ill adults and children, part II: personnel, technical specifications, and clinical practice. J Clin Neurophysiol. 2015;32:96–108.
98. Struck AF, Cole AJ, Cash SS, et al. The number of seizures needed in the EMU. Epilepsia. 2015;56:1753–9.
99. Zarkou S, Grade M, Hoerth MT, et al. Indeterminate EMU admissions: does repeating the admission help? Epilepsy Behav. 2011;20:706–8.
100. Marras CE, Canevini MP, Colicchio G, Guerrini R, Rubboli G, Scerrati M, Spreafico R, Tassi L, Lo Russo G, Tinuper P. Health Technology Assessment report on the presurgical evaluation and surgical treatment of drug-resistant epilepsy. Epilepsia. 2013;54(Suppl 7):49–58.

Invasive EEG

19

Laura Tassi

19.1 General Indications

Surgical exeresis in patients suffering from drug-resistant epilepsies can be performed on the solely basis of noninvasive evaluation, but still many require more precise information from intracranial EEG (iEEG) studies. About 35% of the operated patients (Fig. 19.1) across the world underwent iEEG evaluation prior to surgical resection, even if recent advances in noninvasive imaging techniques generally tend to reduce this percentage; this trend is partially counterweight by the increasingly complex cases being considered for surgical candidacy.

Proceeding with iEEG recordings is managed by the analysis of all noninvasive data including subjective and objectivable seizure semiology, interictal and ictal scalp-EEG patterns, structural MRI, and functional imaging. On this basis the epileptologist can generate a reasonable hypothesis (or hypotheses) concerning the site(s) of seizure onset and the possible region that needs be resected or disconnected, as the epileptogenic zone (EZ) results correctly defined. When noninvasive hypothesis is either inconclusive or divergent, iEEG recordings became mandatory to better define the location and extent of the EZ and its relationships to critical functional cortex. Undefined setups commonly arise when the overall location of the EZ may be evident, but its exact extent and/or involvement of high-functioning surrounding cortex remains unclear. Divergences are not uncommon and occur when noninvasive evaluation reveals discrepancies between clinical, anatomical (if any), neurophysiological, and functional imaging data. As iEEG consists in a surgical procedure, it should be indicated only when the hypothetical localization of the EZ is consistent with a forthcoming surgical procedure and/or a correct individualization of the EZ: a multifocal, not localized or lateralized EZ should be a major contraindication to the invasive procedure.

19.2 Introduction

Independently from the methodologies, all iEEGs share common recording features based on physical principles: being very close to and/or within the source permits a very high spatial resolution [1]. However, we have to keep in mind that [2], whatever the exploration, only a small portion of brain tissue can be sampled by each electrode, making invasive recording "blind" if the electrodes are placed in wrong areas or in insufficient numbers. As it is possible to miss a source even in close proximity to an electrode, it is advisable to sample the selected targeted areas with a large number of electrodes located on a clear hypothesis on the anatomo-functional network(s) involved at seizure onset and during seizure propagation.

The epileptologist guides the placement of electrodes, applying the anatomo-electro-clinical correlations, a very critical step since an error at this stage may lead to inappropriate placement of intracranial electrodes and the information obtained will likely be inadequate or even misleading.

iEEG recordings should not be used as an "exploratory procedure", always asking the question if a more precise definition of EZ will be able to transform the surgical strategy and outcome.

Within this background, the MRI-negative patients present the commonest justification for iEEG studies, even if, in cases in which the MRI reveals a discrete lesion consistent with focal cortical dysplasia (FCD), tuberous sclerosis, or benign developmental glioneuronal tumors, some epilepsy surgery centers prefer to explore the patient as the EZ could be more extensive [3–5].

It remains unclear the role of iEEG in other discrete lesional substrates such as acquired vascular lesions or Sturge-Weber syndrome and polymicrogyria [6]; some

L. Tassi (✉)
"Claudio Munari" Epilepsy Surgery Centre, Niguarda Hospital, Milan, Italy
e-mail: laura.tassi@ospedaleniguarda.it

O. Mecarelli (ed.), *Clinical Electroencephalography*, https://doi.org/10.1007/978-3-030-04573-9_19

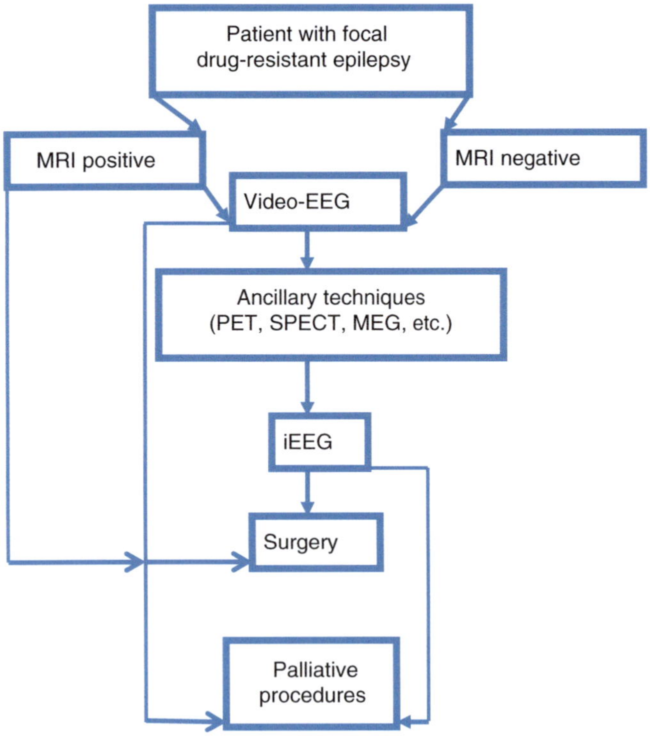

Fig. 19.1 Surgical flow chart: different option are depending on different clinical characteristics

	SEEG	SDE
Contacts N°	+	-
Explored area	-	+
Location Accuracy	+	-
Complications	-	+
Functional mapping	-	+
Bilateral iEEE	+	-
Deep EZ	+	-
Pts already operated	+	-
Pts <2 years	-	+
Recording duration	+	-
Tailored strategy	+	-
One hosp. stay	-	+
Time-consuming	+	-

Fig. 19.2 A outline for understanding advantages and limits of the two methodologies. Abbreviations: *SEEG* stereo-EEG, *SDE* subdural electrodes, *iEEG* invasive EEG, *EZ* epileptogenic zone, *PTS* patients

studies promote extending the resection to the lesional cortex and/or beyond the anatomic lesion to achieve higher rates of seizure freedom, but others plain in favor of a not complete involvement of the malformative cortex in generating ictal discharges. In some cases such as where the MRI lesion can be hemispheric but other noninvasive data suggest that seizures arise from only a restricted region, iEEG may allow focal successful resections. In deep-seated cortical malformation, as periventricular nodular heterotopia, SEEG remains the gold standard for exploring both the nodules and the overlying cortex [7].

19.3 Methodologies

Depending on the variable experience at each center, the choice of a methodology is conducted, and there is considerable mutability in their usage and protocols across epilepsy surgery centers worldwide.

Several different methods are available to perform iEEG studies. The study can be achieved during surgery (electrocorticography, ECoG) or extraoperatively following surgical implantation of electrodes; the latter is, based on the type of electrodes, employing subdural electrodes (SDE) or stereotactically implanted intracerebral electrodes, stereo-EEG (SEEG) (Fig. 19.2). While grids and strips of subdural electrodes provide a large coverage over only the surface of the cerebral cortex, they are quite always implanted in only one hemisphere and do not reach deeper brain structures particularly the bottom of the sulci. By comparison, depth intracerebral electrodes can enable bilateral contemporary monitoring of superficial and deep cortical structures, but only the most superficial or deeper contacts will be within the cortical gray matter.

SDE are circular plate, while SEEG electrodes have a cylindrical shape (Fig. 19.3). The diameter of subdural plate electrodes is between 1.2 and 3 mm, while the diameter of depth electrodes is 0.8–1.2 mm with 2.00 or 2.5 mm height. The distance between the centers of two adjacent electrodes (subdural or depth) is often 3 and 5–10 mm. The total area of the brain enclosed with electrodes can be in the range of 1–15 mm^2.

In few centers the approaches with combined subdural/depth EEG are chosen in particular pre-definite conditions.

Each technique has advantages, limitations, and risks with little data comparing the value of each invasive method in specific substrates, clinical scenarios, and age groups.

19.4 The Epileptogenic Zone: Meaning and Definition

To define the EZ (the hypothetical minimum cortical area required to be resected or disconnected in order to stop the patient's seizures), iEEG is considered to be the gold standard. Intracranial recordings should allow precisely defining and then removing different cortical areas and each one with

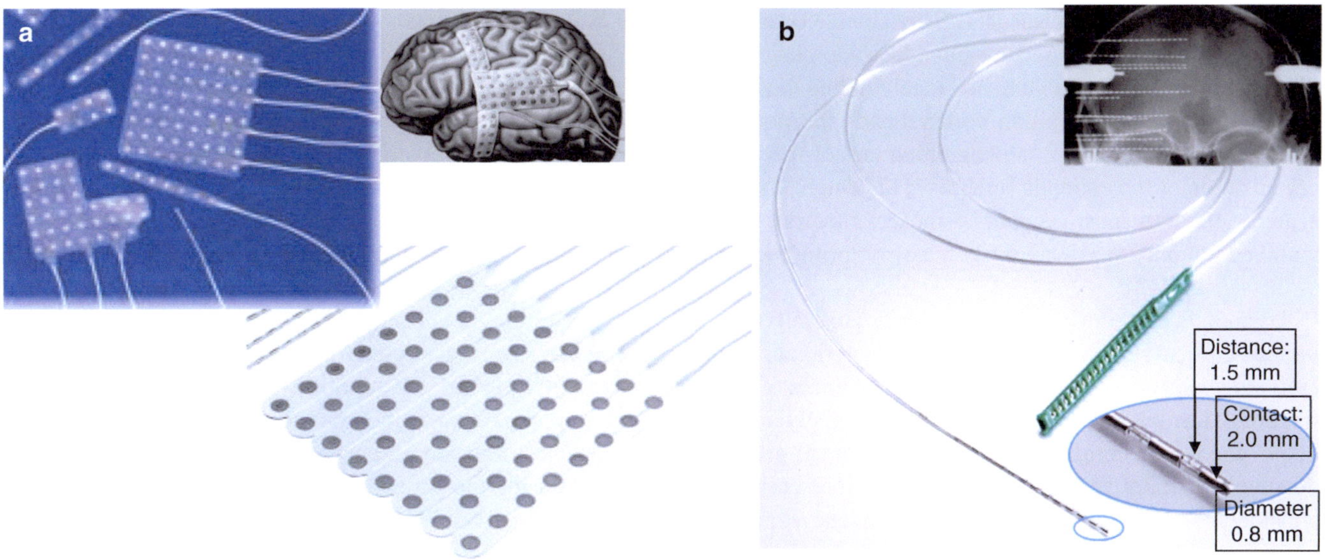

Fig. 19.3 The two principal methods for iEEG: subdural electrodes (**a**) and stereo-EEG intracerebral electrodes (**b**)

dissimilar and strategic meanings. The old Bancaud EZ characterization underlined and described diverse cortical areas, not exactly superimposable excepted few cases, and completely patient-related. The lesional area was delineated as the region in which were existing a large amount of slow waves and the background activity is absent; the irritative area where spikes, spikes and waves are numerous and repeated. The high functional areas were identified by both functional examination (fMRI, MEG) and the results of the intracranial electrical stimulations. Considering all the precedent, defining the location and extension of the epileptogenic area is a puzzling procedure. The epileptologist have to take into account not only the presence of interictal paroxysms, the onset and propagation of the discharges during the spontaneous seizures, and the results of the electrical stimulations but also incorporate all the precedents as well as the nature and topography of any lesion [8, 9].

The ictal clinical signs and symptoms may reflect either the function or the dysfunction (in a positive or negative sense), or a simple propagation both cortical and subcortical of the ictal discharges, or the involvement of a neuronal network. Consequently, defined on the basis of anatomo-electro-clinical correlations, the EZ should be delineated in different ways, as the cortical area(s) in which ictal discharges originate, or whose removal is sufficient to cure the patient, or coincident with the anatomical lesion, or, finally, the brain area responsible for the symptomatogenic zone.

Since the beginnings, the ambiguities and complexity of iEEG patterns were well recognized [10], and their use in synthesizing the EZ or the epileptogenic network is often based on empirical criteria and individual experience. The challenge in an individual case is to identify the minimum amount of tissue to remove and balance between a bigger resection for seizure control and smaller and consequently less dangerous, resection strategies.

Ictal patterns may differ in terms of morphology, shape, and rapidity on the different iEEG methods. Depending on the mean of exploration, the electrode polarity, and the position, they require slightly dissimilar conceptualization and a 3D scheme of the involved volume to be resected.

Abnormal interictal EEG data and seizure onsets, both on the subdural and depth electrodes, depending on the underlying pathology, can vary the spatial relationship between the lesion and the cortical surface and the correct placement of the electrodes [11].

Defining the region(s) in which ictal discharges originate and from which propagate (the epileptogenic zone) accurately is the strongest justification for iEEG recordings. This cortical area could be considered as the region showing the opening transformation from the interictal state. Different patterns are commonly observed during the initial phase including focal low-voltage fast activity in the gamma bands, spike/polyspikes or runs of spikes, flattening and delta brush [10, 12–15]. Very high-frequencies modifications or slow (DC) shifts can be observed but needing a modification of the conventional filters. The presence of a localized low-voltage fast activity seems to be the most important positive prognostic factor [16].

Many variables can influence the morphologies of ictal discharges, reflecting a variety of EEG transition mechanisms, modulating the brain involved structure, as the underlying substrate, age, the type and the distance from the EZ of the recording electrodes, and the eventual withdrawal of antiepileptic medication.

However, if the first clear ictal EEG change occurs after the clinical onset of the seizure, the electrode placement is likely incorrect and not able to accurately define the EZ.

The "European" definition comprehends the notion the EZ represents the "site of the beginning and of the primary organization of the epileptic seizures" [17] emphasizing that a great attention must be paid to those structures that are involved not only at seizure onset but also during the course of the seizure [18].

Hypothetically the surgical resection generally should include cortical regions with "significant" interictal potential epileptogenicity, in order to maximize the chances of seizure freedom. Ideally it is considered as "potentially epileptogenic" the region entitled "irritativa area", for the great incidence of interictal spikes and sharp waves, presenting with considerable variation in morphology, frequency, and distribution, being a poor prognostic value if persisting after resection [2, 19, 20].

A second region is usually identified, defined as "lesional area" [21], characterized by a suppressed activity or a focal attenuation of background, and considered by the neurophysiological point of view, a "functional deficit zone."

19.5 Subdural Electrodes and Combination of Subdural/Depth Electrodes

19.5.1 Surgical Technique

Subdural and depth electrodes are generally made of platinum-iridium. The electrodes are shaped as rounds 4–5 mm in diameter and spaced 5–10 mm apart. They are secured in silastic strips (4–8 contacts) or square/rectangular grids (20–64 contacts); the option of special configuration may aid placement in particular regions [22].

The electrodes are implanted following a vast craniotomy, but strips may be placed via burr holes. Following the removal of the bone and the opening of a dural flap, they are placed directly on the cortex or slid in the basal or interhemispheric aspect of the brain.

A brief SDE recording may be accomplished at the end of the implantation with the aim to check the electrodes work or the abnormalities extend beyond the coverage permitting to modify the electrode positioning. A dural flap is then wrapped around the cables; a dural graft may be required to guarantee adequate seal. Cables for each electrode are then tunneled under the scalp to minimize risk of leaking and secured. Images of the cortex and the overlying electrodes help to define electrode placement but an MRI or a coregistered CT scans determine the actual location extra-operatively [23, 24].

19.5.2 Recordings

Chronic iEEG recordings are generally performed both during wakefulness and sleep, the main aim being to record spontaneous seizures. The recording software should allow to record simultaneously at least 128 channels, with a minimal sampling rate of 200–256 Hz; higher rates of 1024–2048 are required to permit signal analysis and research protocols. The reference is chosen among one of the contacts distant from the expected EZ. Recordings are displayed using bipolar montages, but referential or special configurations focused on restricted areas of interest may be added. Additional scalp electrodes may be used to provide information on the regions unexplored by the intracranial electrodes or help for sleep stage scoring.

Decreasing the antiepileptic medications, having in mind the risks of activating atypical seizures, may augment seizure recording chance. Spontaneous seizures are usually captured over 1–10 days; the longer periods of up to a month may occasionally be accepted.

As soon as one or more spontaneous seizures are acquired, medications are restored before the functional mapping with the electrical cortical stimulation.

19.5.3 Strong Points and Limits

SDE permit sampling of large areas of the hemispheric surface; coverage over the convexity is generally easier than interhemispheric or basal or mesial cortices. SDE are also largely suited especially for mapping functional regions, chiefly the motor and language cortex on the convexity. They can be used in all ages and are mostly well tolerated both in adults and children. Some trajectories (basal or interhemispheric) are difficult to manage, since the neurosurgeon tries to avoid veins and deflection of the electrodes [22], particularly in patients already undergone to surgery since the dura adherence. The surgery eventually planned is inevitably performed at the end of the monitoring.

A combined depth/SDE implantation can be suitable [25] in particular situation, as the necessity to cover large brain surface, or the need for precise mapping, or the evaluation of deep-seated anatomical lesion [26–29], even in the pediatric population [30], particularly in children with widespread or hemispheric cortical malformations.

19.5.4 Risks

General complications include wound infection, cerebrospinal fluid leak, intracranial bleeding, or symptomatic pneumocephalus [31–34], with a very rare risk of permanent neurological deficit or death. In a recent review comprehending a total of

2542 patients (52–95 subdural electrodes during 5–17 days) [35], neurologic infections were reported in 2.3%, bone or skin infections in 3.0%, intracranial hemorrhage in 4%, and augmented intracranial pressure in 2.4%. Less than 3.5% of patients required additional surgical procedure(s) for management of these adverse events. Risks are slightly higher in reoperated children [33] without a significant concern [36].

19.6 Stereo-EEG

19.6.1 Surgical Technique

The SEEG methodology belonging to Talairach and Bancaud [21, 37–39] employs only intracerebral depth electrodes, with a much larger number compared to the use of SDE/depth electrodes. Based on anatomo-electro-clinical correlations, the planning of electrodes insertion aims at verifying the hypothesis of localization of the EZ and studying not only the origin of ictal discharges but also their propagation and the organization of the whole epileptogenic network. As every patient is unique, each exploration is tailored (Figs. 19.4 and 19.5).

SEEG electrodes (platinum and iridium) are flexible, semirigid or rigid wires or catheters, generally with a diameter of less than 1 mm. Each electrode contains several contacts disposed at regular intervals along the wire. Between 5 and 20 electrodes are implanted per patient under general anesthesia during several hours, inserted through a burr hole, and placed (sometimes after a angiography is acquired and coregistered with 3D MRI) either with or without a stereotactic frame. The actual position of the electrodes is

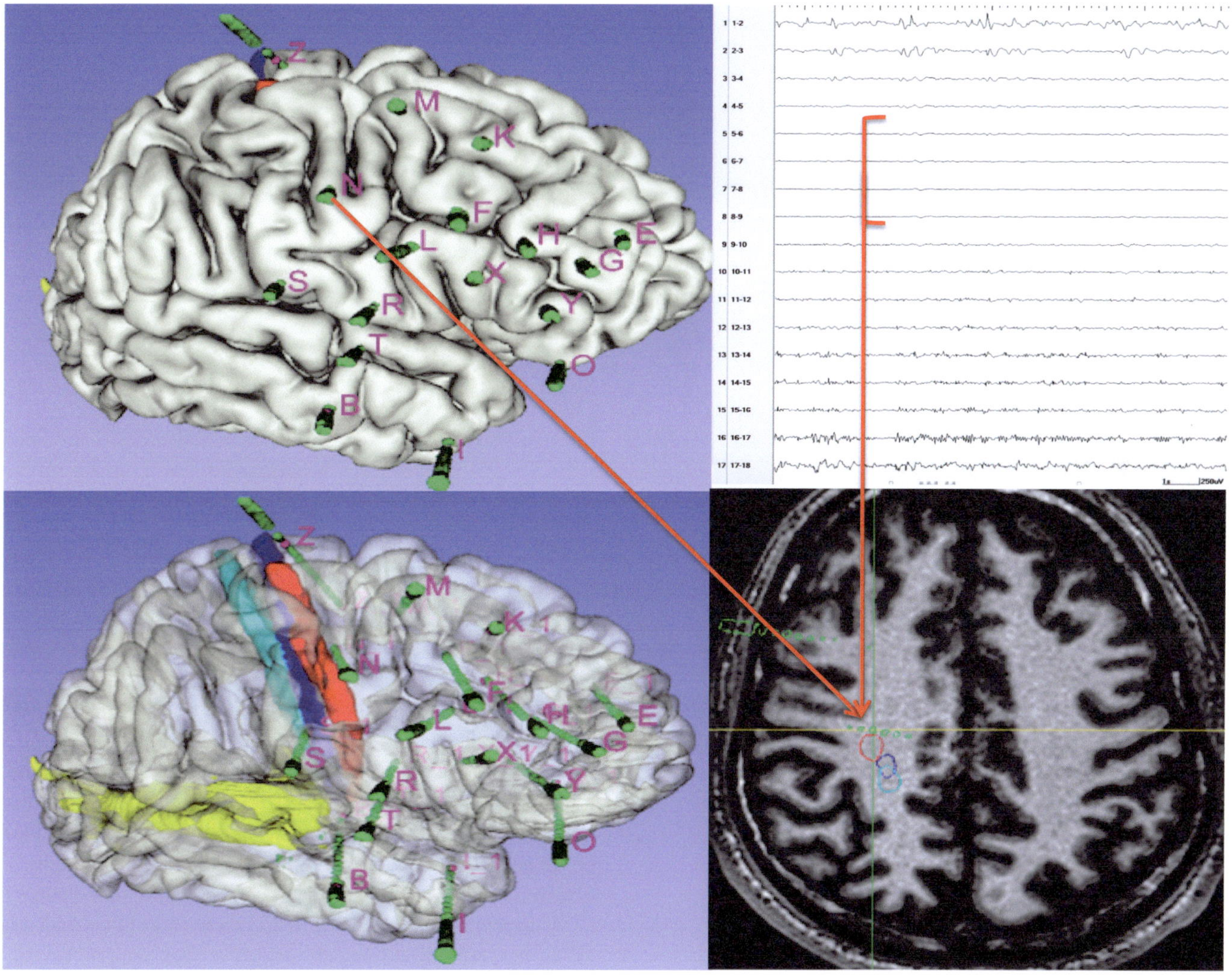

Fig. 19.4 Pial surface reconstruction of a stereo-EEG schema in a patient suffering from a right frontotemporal epilepsy (top left). Each electrode is labeled with a capital letter. Electrode N is exploring the central cingulate region with the mesial contacts (1 is deepest one) and the motor strip with the lateral leads (faded schema, lower left) in which in red and blue, the pyramidal tracts appears. In light blue the corticothalamic tract and in yellow the visual radiations. The bipolar recordings (top right) show the very small amplitude of the contacts lying in the white matter (arrow). The axial MRI (lower right) permits the actual verification of the position of each contact

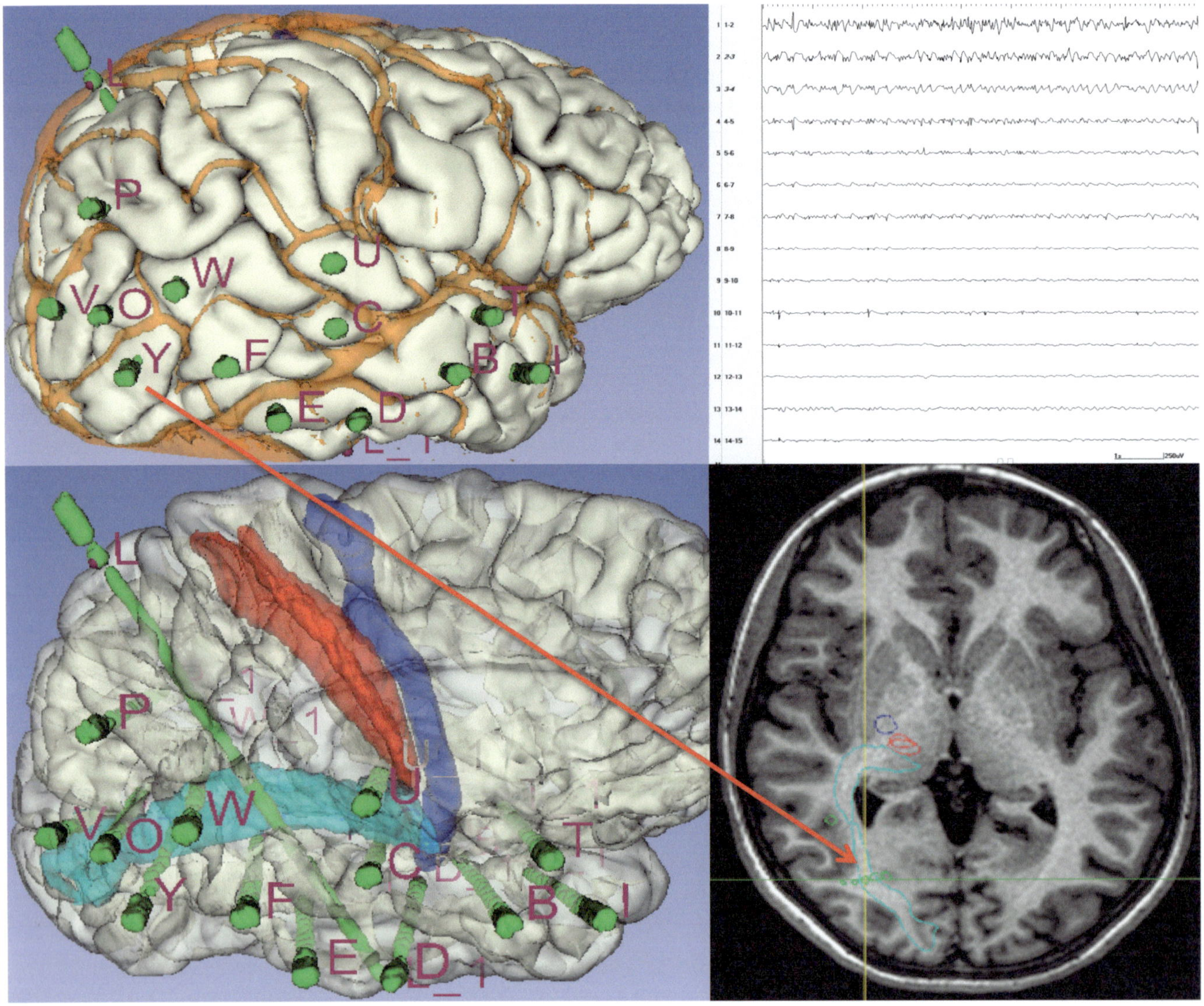

Fig. 19.5 Patient with a temporo-parieto-occipital right exploration (top left, with vessels). Electrode Y appears very close to the visual radiation (light blue, lower left)

reconstructed using CT or MRI, or directly visualized on MRI. A brief recording may be performed at the end of the surgical procedure to verify electrode integrity and the cortical targeting. SEEG recordings are performed during wakefulness and sleep, with the main aim to record spontaneous seizures. In children, the duration of the recordings may vary from 1 to 21 days [40–42].

19.6.2 Recordings

The monitoring system should allow to record simultaneously at least 128 EEG channels in each patient, with a minimum sampling rate of 200–256 Hz; 512 Hz (or above) is needed to assess higher frequencies and research projects. The reference is chosen as far as possible from the EZ, possibly in the white matter. SEEG channels are displayed in bipolar recordings, canceling the influence of the external reference.

Because the number of channels can easily exceed 100, being beyond the limits of adequate visual resolution, a restricted montage should be chosen in between the most pathological contacts. Adjunctive scalp electrodes can provide information on the regions unexplored by the intracerebral electrodes, or to help sleep stage scoring. An additional polygraphy is assessed depending on the clinical characteristics of the patient.

A correct interpretation of SEEG recordings is an available 3D surface reconstruction permitting the placement of the electrodes in the multiplanar MRI [43]. Electrodes are removed either under general (in children) or without any anesthesia in the operating room (or at the bedside with little discomfort), and resective surgery is performed in a second step.

Recently and more and more regularly, a radio-frequency SEEG-guided thermocoagulation (THC) can be performed as a therapeutic option to "burn" limited well-defined cortical areas, previously identified by the iEEG recordings. The methodology offers a negligible possibility of rendering seizure-free to the patient, except those related to nodular heterotopy, even in bilateral cases [44]. In patients in whom conventional resective surgery is not feasible for a multifocality or a epileptogenic zone located into high-functioning cortical areas [45], THC can be considered as an alternative palliative therapeutic option, even if only with the goal of interrupting the pathological network.

19.6.3 Strong Points and Limits

SEEG can be accomplished without large craniotomies, providing a sampling of all cortical areas, simultaneously recording all cortical areas potentially involved in the onset, propagation, and clinical manifestations [17, 46–48].

The placement of a sufficient number of SEEG electrodes after a very careful analysis of all the noninvasive data permits to formulate one or more hypotheses concerning the site(s) of seizure onset and the pathways of preferential ictal spread. An adequate depth electrode placement must result from a suitable balance between the need to map cortical regions, the anatomical constraints, and the risks of parenchymatous damage. SEEG monitoring is feasible and safe, even in children less than 3 years of age [40, 41].

SEEG is suited to record from all structures particularly deep and intrasulcal regions. SEEG as a surgical procedure must be proposed only when it seems reasonable to lead to a satisfactory surgical outcome and is not indicated when a diffuse, bilateral, and multifocal epilepsy is suspected. Also, severe cognitive or behavioral disturbances that do not allow long-term monitoring and an age less than 2 years represent contraindication to perform a SEEG study.

19.6.4 Risks

The morbidity using stereo-EEG is predominantly related to hemorrhagic or infectious complications, varying from 0 to 7.5%. Only two studies reported specifically the risks of SEEG in children: the procedure also appears safe in this age group [40, 41]. Generally speaking the complication rate appears lower than in adults.

19.7 Intraoperative Electrocorticography (ECoG)

19.7.1 Technique

An ECoG recording is performed during 10–30 min before beginning the resection; briefer recordings are possible at the end to guide an eventual enlargement [49]. SDE or depth electrodes are used for as a collection of individual wire-tipped electrodes, permitting also a direct stimulation. The methodology appears to be useful only for recording over the hemispheric convexity. All agents used in general anesthesia have effects on epileptiform discharges [50].

19.7.2 Strong Points and Limits

The only advantage of ECoG is providing intracranial EEG data during the resective surgery, recordings can be conducted prior to, during, and at the end of resection to ensure that all regions revealing non-pathological activities.

The number of channels is forcedly restricted, and ECoG generally provides only interictal data with unpredictable effects of anesthesia.

These intracranial recordings can be very useful in a subset of patients with focal cortical dysplasia or in the MRI-negative cohort, with focal continuous epileptiform discharges [51, 52]. ECoG gives the possibility to extend the resection during the surgical procedure with a reported 95% of patients with good surgical outcome [53, 54] without an increased neurological morbidity.

19.7.3 Electrical Stimulations (ES)

The principles of ES are similar in the different employed methodologies: protocols and equipment are specifically used by individual centers. The cortical mapping is performed after almost a spontaneous seizure is acquired.

The duration of ES sessions also varies spreading across several days. The approved safe diagnostic stimulation of the human brain is a constant current rectangular biphasic pulse generator.

Generally speaking with SDE and ECoG, ES is generally performed using 50 Hz pulses; infrequently 1 Hz may be used especially to differentiate primary motor from supplementary cortex. For the most part, pulse durations are maintained constant at 0.3 ms during trains for 0.5–10 s, starting with a low intensity, increasing in 0.5–1.0 mA increments until an electro-clinical modification occurs. The maximum intensity depends on the utilized stimulator.

A EEG recording is carried out to identify after-discharges and their location and extent.

With SEEG electrodes, ES are performed either at low (LFES, 1–12 Hz; pulse width, 1–3 ms; 0.2–10 mA; duration, 30–40 s) (Fig. 19.6) or high frequency (HFES, 50–60 Hz; pulse width, 0.1–3 ms; 0.2–5 mA; duration, 3–10 s). LFES is preferred when studying the motor cortex to avoid unpleasant motor signs, while in visual, sensory, auditory, language, and insular cortices, HFES must be applied cautiously to avoid disabling sensations [55, 56]. Some cerebral structures as mesio-temporal lobe structures or FCD type II, are more prone to develop a seizure when stimulated.

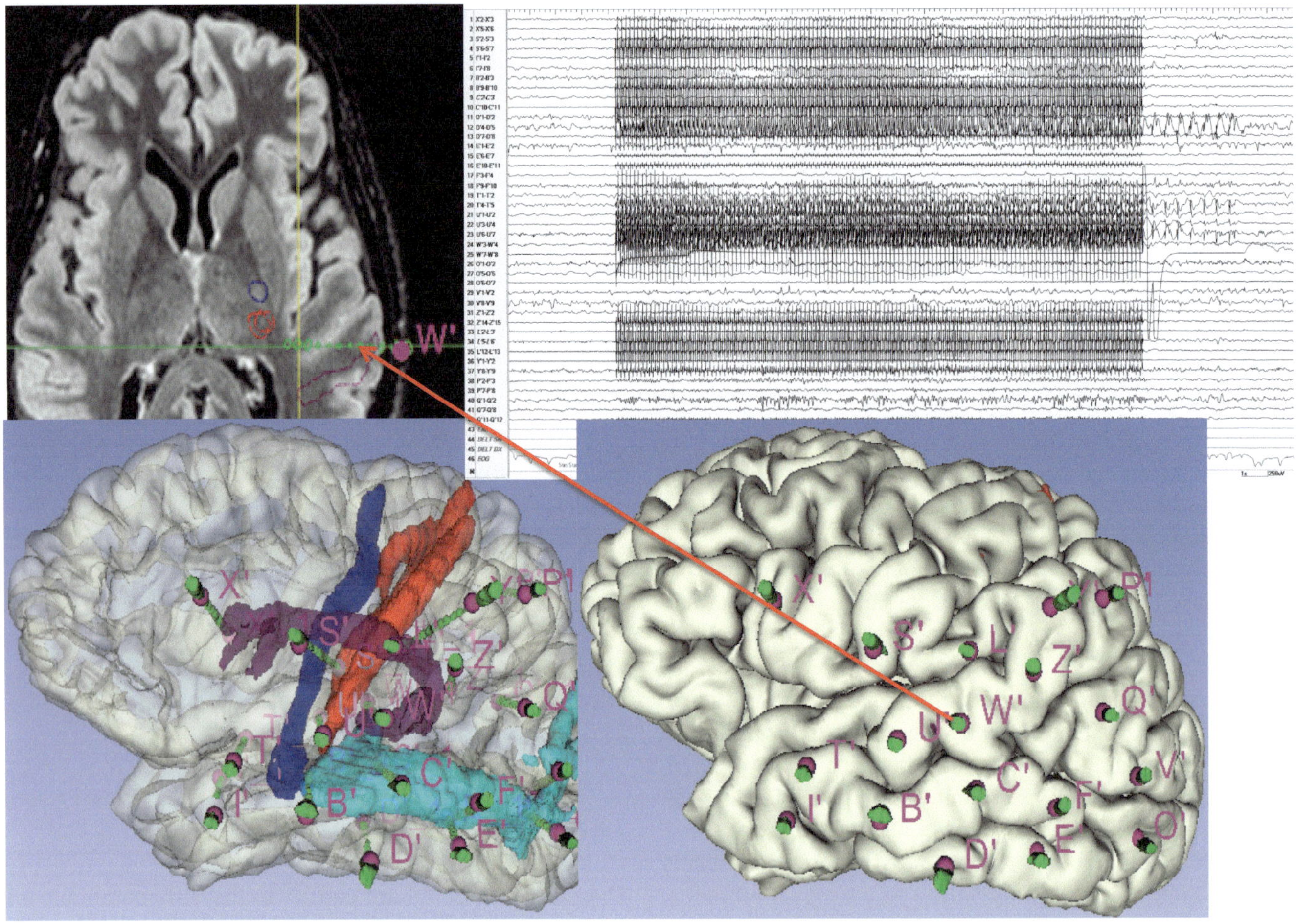

Fig. 19.6 A low-frequency stimulation (6 Hz, top right) inducing a language deficit into the Wernicke's area (external contacts of electrode W′, lower right), in which the arcuate fasciculus is recognizable (purple, lower left)

Stimulation paradigms are quite different for older children or adults and younger children, probably because immature cortex and nonmyelinated nerve fibers require different pulse characteristics in order to be activated [57]. ES in this age group thus requires stimuli with longer pulse duration applied at higher intensities to elicit responses.

The general limitations of ES are related to concerns of current spread and false and negative findings and the necessary cooperation of the patient.

Subdural electrodes overlying vessels or sulci may give false-negative responses as ES during SEEG may miss a precise functional map.

ES are safe and these parameters shown to produce no structural damage [58].

ES can produce a number of clinical responses (for a review, see [59–61]), especially true for subjective manifestations [62].

Area 6 can also be tested by documenting inability to initiate/sustain bilateral alternating movements. In bilingual subjects, languages may have distinct representations [63].

Clinical responses elicited without electrical modifications suggest the presence of functioning cortex under the electrode, while an after discharge without clinical effect indicates absence of critical function under the electrode [57].

19.8 Conclusion

Nowadays iEEG persists as the best practice in order to define the EZ and its related cortices. However, the assessment about the employed methodology is primarily determined by both the center experience and the economic possibilities.

No iEEG strategy should be proposed in the absence of data to guide the implantation, and an extremely accurate evaluation of all the noninvasive tests must be taken into account, especially video-EEG long-term recordings and neuroradiological data.

In very recent years, SEEG methodology has expanded very considerably at the major epilepsy surgery centers previously using SDE, suggesting that SEEG might offer specific benefits through its approach to accurately localizing the epileptogenic zone. SEEG could be considered the most malleable methodology to explore syndromes and very different cases. However, considering its total dependence on the experience of the epileptologist and the mutual two-way collaboration with the surgeon, it should be reserved for second level centers with a long experience. Moreover, SEEG appears to be a unique tool for the in vivo investigation of human networks and to reach very deep-seated regions (Bulacio et al., 2016).

Nevertheless it is important to emphasize that regardless of the iEEG strategy, the final surgical resection needs to be guided by a comprehensive consideration of other data including anatomo-electro-clinical data and considering the limitations of all the technologies used.

References

1. von Ellenrieder N, Beltrachini L, Muravchik CH. Electrode and brain modeling in stereo-EEG. Clin Neurophysiol. 2012;123(9):1745–54.
2. Gloor P. Contributions of electroencephalography and electrocorticography to the neurosurgical treatment of the epilepsies. Adv Neurol. 1975;8:59–105.
3. Englot DJ, Berger MS, Barbaro NM, et al. Factors associated with seizure freedom in the surgical resection of glioneuronal tumors. Epilepsia. 2012;53(1):51–7.
4. Giulioni M, Rubboli G, Marucci G, et al. Seizure outcome of epilepsy surgery in focal epilepsies associated with temporomesial glioneuronal tumors: lesionectomy compared with tailored resection. J Neurosurg. 2009;111(6):1275–82.
5. Thom M, Blumcke I, Aronica E. Long-term epilepsy-associated tumors. Brain Pathol. 2012;22(3):350–79.
6. Maillard LG, Tassi L, Bartolomei F, Catenoix H, Dubeau F, Szurhaj W, Kahane P, Nica A, Marusic P, Mindruta I, Chassoux F, Ramantani G. Stereoelectroencephalography and surgical outcome in polymicrogyria-related epilepsy: a multicentric study. Ann Neurol. 2017;82(5):781–94.
7. Mirandola L, Mai RF, Francione S, Pelliccia V, Gozzo F, Sartori I, Nobili L, Cardinale F, Cossu M, Meletti S, Tassi L. Stereo-EEG: diagnostic and therapeutic tool for periventricular nodular heterotopia epilepsies. Epilepsia. 2017;58(11):1962–71.
8. Kahane P, Landré E, Minotti L, Francione S, Ryvlin P. The Bancaud and Talairach view on the epileptogenic zone: a working hypothesis. Epileptic Disord. 2006;8(Suppl 2):S16–26.
9. Najm IM, Tassi L, Sarnat HB, Holthausen H, Russo GL. Epilepsies associated with focal cortical dysplasias (FCDs). Acta Neuropathol. 2014;128(1):5–19.
10. Jayakar P. Chronic intracranial EEG monitoring in children: when, where and what? J Clin Neurophysiol. 1999;16(5):408–18.
11. Herberhold T, Pieper T, KudernatschM PB, Hartlieb T, Weber K, Eitel H, Getzinger T, Holthausen H, Winkler P, Blümcke I, Staudt M. Invasive pre-surgical epilepsy diagnostics in children: the advantage of depth electrodes combined with subdural grids in the evaluation of focal cortical lesions. Klinische Neurophysiologie. 2014;45:01.
12. Fisher RS, Webber WR, Lesser RP, Arroyo S, Uematsu S. High frequency EEG activity at the start of seizures. J Clin Neurophysiol. 1992;9:441–8.
13. Ikeda A, Terada K, Mikuni N, Burgess RC, Comair Y, Taki W, Hamano T, Kimura J, Luders HO, Shibasaki H. Subdural recordings of ictal DC shifts in neocortical seizures in humans. Epilepsia. 1996;37(7):662–74.
14. Perucca P, Dubeau F, Gotman J. Intracranial electroencephalographic seizure-onset patterns: effect of underlying pathology. Brain. 2014;137:183–96.
15. Schiller Y, Cascino GD, Sharbrough FW. Chronic intracranial EEG monitoring for localizing the epileptogenic zone: an electro-clinical correlation. Epilepsia. 1998;39(12):1302–8.
16. Singh S, Sandy S, Wiebe S. Ictal onset on intracranial EEG: do we know it when we see it? State of the evidence. Epilepsia. 2015;56(10):1629–38.
17. Munari C, Bancaud J. The role of stereo-electro-encephalography (SEEG) in the evaluation of partial epileptic patients. In: Porter RJ, Morselli PL, editors. The epilepsies. London: Butterworths; 1987. p. 267–306.
18. Bartolomei F, Bettus G, Stam CJ, Guye M. Interictal network properties in mesial temporal lobe epilepsy: a graph theoretical study from intracerebral recordings. Clin Neurophysiol. 2013;124(12):2345–53.
19. Ajmone-Marsan C. Preoperative electroencephalographic localization of large epileptogenic zones in the frontal and temporal lobes. Can J Neurol Sci. 1991;18(4 Suppl):564–5.
20. Lieb JP, Joseph JP, Engel J Jr, Walker J, Crandall PH. Sleep state and seizure foci related to depth spike activity in patients with temporal lobe epilepsy. Electroencephalogr Clin Neurophysiol. 1980;49(5–6):538–57.
21. Bancaud J, Talairach J, Bonis A, Schaub C, Szikla G, Morel P, Bordas-Ferer M. La stéréoencéphalographie dans l'épilepsie. Informations neuro-physio-pathologiques apportées par l'investigation fonctionnelle stéréotaxique. Paris: Masson; 1965.
22. Bekelis K, Radwan TA, Desai A, Moses ZB, Thadani VM, Jobst BC, Bujarski KA, Darcey TM, Roberts DW. Subdural interhemispheric grid electrodes for intracranial epilepsy monitoring: feasibility, safety, and utility: clinical article. J Neurosurg. 2012;117(6):1182–8.
23. Serra C, Huppertz HJ, Kockro RA, Grunwald T, Bozinov O, Krayenbühl N, Bernays RL. Rapid and accurate anatomical localization of implanted subdural electrodes in a virtual reality environment. J Neurol Surg A Cent Eur Neurosurg. 2013;74(3):175–82.
24. Taimouri V, Akhondi-Asl A, Tomas-Fernandez X, Peters JM, Prabhu SP, Poduri A, Takeoka M, Loddenkemper T, Bergin AM, Harini C, Madsen JR, Warfield SK. Electrode localization for planning surgical resection of the epileptogenic zone in pediatric epilepsy. Int J Comput Assist Radiol Surg 2013.
25. Bulacio JC, Jehi L, Wong C, Gonzalez-Martinez J, Kotagal P, Nair D, Najm I, Bingaman W. Long-term seizure outcome after resective surgery in patients evaluated with intracranial electrodes. Epilepsia. 2012;53(10):1722–30.
26. Bouthillier A, Surbeck W, Weil AG, Tayah T, Nguyen DK. The hybrid operculo-insular electrode: a new electrode for intracranial investigation of perisylvian/insular refractory epilepsy. Neurosurgery. 2012;70(6):1574–80.
27. Nespeca M, Wyllie E, Luders H, Rothner AD, Hahn J, Awad I, Dinner DS, Morris HH, Cruse R, Erenberg G, Kotagal P, Kanner A, Estes ML. EEG recording and functional localization studies with subdural electrodes in infants and young children. J Epilepsy. 1990;3:107–24.
28. Surbeck W, Bouthillier A, Weil AG, Crevier L, Carmant L, Lortie A, Major P, Nguyen DK. The combination of subdural and depth electrodes for intracranial EEG investigation of suspected insular (perisylvian) epilepsy. Epilepsia. 2011;52(3):458–66.
29. Wellmer J, von der Groeben F, Klarmann U, Weber C, Elger CE, Urbach H, Clusmann H, von Lehe M. Risks and benefits of invasive

epilepsy surgery workup with implanted subdural and depth electrodes. Epilepsia. 2012;53(8):1322–32.
30. Taussig D, Dorfmüller G, Fohlen M, Jalin C, Bulteau C, Ferrand-Sorbets S, Chipaux M, Delalande O. Invasive explorations in children younger than 3 years. Seizure. 2012;21(8):631–8.
31. Burneo JG, Steven DA, McLachlan RS, Parrent AG. Morbidity associated with the use of intracranial electrodes for epilepsy surgery. Can J Neurol Sci. 2006;33(2):223–7.
32. Johnston JM Jr, Mangano FT, Ojemann JG, Park TS, Trevathan E, Smyth MD. Complications of invasive subdural electrode monitoring at St. Louis Children's Hospital, 1994-2005. J Neurosurg. 2006;105(5 Suppl):343–7.
33. Musleh W, Yassari R, Hecox K, Kohrman M, Chico M, Frim D. Low incidence of subdural gridrelated complications in prolonged pediatric EEG monitoring. Pediatr Neurosurg. 2006;42(5):284–7.
34. Vale FL, Pollock G, Dionisio J, Benbadis SR, Tatum WO. Outcome and complications of chronically implanted subdural electrodes for the treatment of medically resistant epilepsy. Clin Neurol Neurosurg. 2013;115(7):985–90.
35. Arya R, Mangano FT, Horn PS, Holland KD, Rose DF, Glauser TA. Adverse events related to extraoperative invasive EEG monitoring with subdural grid electrodes: a systematic review and meta-analysis. Epilepsia. 2013;54(5):828–39.
36. Vadera S, Jehi L, Gonzalez-Martinez J, Bingaman W. Safety and long term seizure free outcomes of subdural grid placement in patients with a history of prior craniotomy. Neurosurgery. 2013;73(3):395–400.
37. Bancaud J, Talairach J, Geier S, Scarabin JM. EEG et SEEG dans les tumeurs cérébrales et l'épilepsie. Paris: Edifor; 1973. p. 351.
38. Talairach J, Bancaud J. Stereotaxic approach to epilepsy. Methodology of anatomofunctional stereotaxic investigations. Progr Neurol Surg. 1973;5:297–354.
39. Talairach J, Bancaud J, Szikla G, Bonis A, Geier S. Approche nouvelle de la neurochirurgie de l'épilepsie. Méthodologie stéréotaxique et résultats thérapeutiques. Neurochirurgie. 1974;20(Suppl 1):1–240.
40. Cossu M, Schiariti M, Francione S, et al. Stereoelectroencephalography in the presurgical evaluation of focal epilepsy in infancy and early childhood. J Neurosurg Pediatr. 2012;9:290–300.
41. Dorfmüller G, Ferrand-Sorbets S, Fohlen M, Bulteau C, Archambaud F, Delalande O, Chipaux M, Taussig D. Outcome of surgery in children with focal cortical dysplasia younger than 5 years explored by stereo-electroencephalography. Childs Nerv Syst. 2014;30(11):1875–83.
42. Fohlen M, Jalin C, Soufflet C, Bulteau C, Dorfmuller G, Oliver V, Delalande O. Electrophysiological investigations in childhood epilepsy surgery. Neurochirurgie. 2008;54:347–52.
43. Cardinale F, Cossu M, Castana L, Casaceli G, Schiariti MP, Miserocchi A, Fuschillo D, Moscato A, Caborni C, Arnulfo G, Lo Russo G. Stereoelectroencephalography: surgical methodology, safety, and stereotactic application accuracy in 500 procedures. Neurosurgery. 2013;72(3):353–66.
44. Cossu M, Fuschillo D, Cardinale F, Castana L, Francione S, Nobili L, Lo Russo G. Stereo-EEGguided radio-frequency thermocoagulations of epileptogenic grey-matter nodular heterotopy. J Neurol Neurosurg Psychiatry. 2014;85:611–7.
45. Guénot M, Isnard J, Catenoix H, Maguiére F, Sindou M. SEEG-guided RF-thermocoagulation of epileptic foci: a therapeutic alternative for drug-resistant non-operable partial epilepsies. Adv Tech Stand Neurosurg. 2011;36:61–78.
46. Kahane P, Dubeau F. Intracerebral depth electrodes encephalography (stereoelectroencephalography). In: Ebersole JE, editor. Current practice of clinical encephalography. 4th ed; 2014.
47. Kahane P, Francione S. Stereoencephalography. In: Lüders HO, editor. Textbook of epilepsy surgery. London: Informa Healthcare; 2008. p. 649–58.
48. Kahane P, Minotti L, Hoffmann D, Lachaux JP, Ryvlin P. Invasive EEG in the definition of the seizure onset zone: depth electrodes. In: Rosenow F, Lüders HO, editors. Handbook of clinical neurophysiology, Presurgical assessment of the epilepsies with clinical neurophysiology and functional imaging, vol. 3. Amsterdam: Elsevier BV; 2004. p. 109–33.
49. Chui J, Manninen P, Valiante T, Venkatraghavan L. The anesthetic considerations of intraoperative electrocorticography during epilepsy surgery. Anesth Analg. 2013;117(2):479–86.
50. Bindra A, Chouhan RS, Prabhakar H, Dash HH, Chandra PS, Tripathi M. Comparison of the effects of different anesthetic techniques on electrocorticography in patients undergoing epilepsy surgery—a bispectral index guided study. Seizure. 2012;21(7):501–7.
51. Jayakar P, Dunoyer C, Dean P, Ragheb J, Resnick T, Morrison G, Bhatia S, Duchowny M. Epilepsy surgery in patients with normal or non-focal MRI scans: integrative strategies offer long-term seizure relief. Epilepsia. 2008;49(5):758–64.
52. Palmini A, Gambardella A, Andermann F, Dubeau F, da Costa JC, Olivier A, Tampieri D, Gloor P, Quesney F, Andermann E, et al. Intrinsic epileptogenicity of human dysplastic cortex as suggested by corticography and surgical results. Ann Neurol. 1995;37(4):476–87.
53. Gelinas JN, Battison AW, Smith S, Connolly MB, Steinbok P. Electrocorticography and seizure outcomes in children with Lesional epilepsy. Childs Nerv Syst. 2011;27(3):381–90.
54. Tripathi M, Garg A, Gaikwad S, Bal CS, Chitra S, Prasad K, Dash HH, Sharma BS, Chandra PS. Intra-operative electrocorticography in lesional epilepsy. Epilepsy Res. 2010;89(1):133–41.
55. Fish DR, Gloor P, Quesney FL, et al. Clinical responses to electrical brain stimulation of the temporal and frontal lobes in patients with epilepsy. Pathophysiological implications. Brain. 1993;116:397–414.
56. Kahane P, Tassi L, Francione S, et al. Electroclinical manifestations elicited by intracerebral electric stimulation "shocks" in temporal lobe epilepsy. Neurophysiol Clin. 1993;23:305–26.
57. Jayakar P, Resnick TJ, Duchowny MS, Alvarez LA. A safe and effective paradigm to functionally map the cortex in childhood. J Clin Neurophysiol. 1992;9(2):288–93.
58. Gordon B, Lesser RP, Rance NE, et al. Parameters for direct cortical electrical stimulation in the human: histopathologic confirmation. Electroencephalogr Clin Neurophysiol. 1990;75:371–7.
59. Balestrini S, Francione S, Mai R, Castana L, Casaceli G, Marino D, Provinciali L, Cardinale F, Tassi L. Multimodal responses induced by cortical stimulation of the parietal lobe: a stereo-electroencephalography study. Brain. 2015;138(Pt 9):2596–607.
60. Chassagnon S, Minotti L, Krémer S, Hoffmann D, Kahane P. Somatosensory, motor and reaching/grasping responses to direct electrical stimulations of the human cingulate motor areas. J Neurosurg. 2008;109:593–604.
61. Selimbeyoglu A, Parvizi J. Electrical stimulation of the human brain: perceptual and behavioral phenomena reported in the old and new literature. Front Hum Neurosci. 2010;4:46.
62. Lobel E, Kahane P, Leonards U, Grosbras MH, Lehericy S, Le Bihan D, Berthoz A. Localization of the human frontal eye fields: anatomical and functional findings from fMRI and intracerebral electrical stimulation. J Neurosurg. 2001;95:804–15.
63. Lucas TH 2nd, GM MK 2nd, Ojemann GA. Functional separation of languages in the bilingual brain: a comparison of electrical stimulation language mapping in 25 bilingual patients and 117 monolingual control patients. J Neurosurg. 2004;101(3):449–57.

Electromagnetic Source Imaging, High-Density EEG and MEG

20

Sándor Beniczky and Praveen Sharma

20.1 Introduction

Epilepsy is one of the commonest chronic neurologic diseases affecting about 65 million people worldwide [1]. Its overall prevalence and annual incidence are 5–8/1000 and 0.45/1000 population, respectively, and it is also associated with two to five times elevated risk of death [2, 3]. Despite availability of many antiepileptic drugs with different mechanism of actions, about 30% of patients remain refractory to the medical treatment, and half of the drug-resistant patient may achieve remission by surgery if appropriately chosen [4]. The aim of epilepsy surgery should be the seizure freedom with no or minimum functional loss, by removal of epileptogenic zone which is a focal area of the brain responsible for onset of seizure as well as its clinical features.

Describing the location of the observed abnormalities is an essential aspect of the clinical evaluation, and it is specified in the EEG and MEG reports. Traditionally, in the visual interpretation of EEG recordings, the location of the peak negativity on the scalp is reported as the location of the abnormality. This is determined by spotting the electrodes(s) where negative phase reversal occurs in bipolar montages or where the negative (upwards) deflection has the highest amplitude in referential montages. However, the scalp negativity is not necessarily located over the cortical source—it can be over a different lobe and even on the side opposite to the source (false lateralization).

Case: This is the case of a 42-year-old right-handed male patient with focal epileptic seizures since the age of 13 years. He has tried seven antiepileptic drugs but has not become seizure-free (has 2–4 seizures per week). The seizures start with a relatively long (20–50 s) period with staring and motor arrest, followed by unilateral (left hand) or bimanual automatisms. The patient is not responsive during the seizures and has ictal and postictal aphasia. Aura has not been reported. MRI was unrevealing. The epileptiform EEG discharges (Fig. 20.1) showed negative phase reversal in the left anterior temporal region. However, electric source imaging indicated location of the source in the left orbitofrontal region, and this was confirmed by intracranial recordings (SEEG). The patients were operated and have been seizure-free for 2 years. The histopathological examination showed type II focal cortical dysplasia (FCD).

In this chapter, we explain how to circumvent this problem in clinical practice, with focus on the presurgical evaluation. We start by explaining basic phenomena of how epileptiform discharges are generated in the brain, and how they are recorded at the surface of the scalp, by EEG electrodes and by MEG sensors. We emphasize the importance of assessing the distribution of voltage topographies (both the negative and positive potentials) and magnetic field (flux) maps, since this is the cornerstone of any source imaging technique. We explain the steps of source imaging, the basic principles of estimating the source and the importance of high spatial sampling (high-density EEG and MEG). We reviewed the published evidence on localization accuracy and clinical utility of electromagnetic source imaging (EMSI). The reader will become familiar with the advantages, clinical added value and the limitations of EMSI methods.

In spite of the compelling evidence published on the accuracy of EMSI, surprisingly few centres integrate these methods into

S. Beniczky (✉)
Department of Clinical Neurophysiology, Aarhus and Danish Epilepsy Centre, Dianalund, Denmark

Department of Clinical Neurophysiology, Aarhus University Hospital, Aarhus, Denmark
e-mail: sbz@filadelfia.dk

P. Sharma
Department of Neurology, King George's Medical University, Lucknow, India

O. Mecarelli (ed.), *Clinical Electroencephalography*, https://doi.org/10.1007/978-3-030-04573-9_20

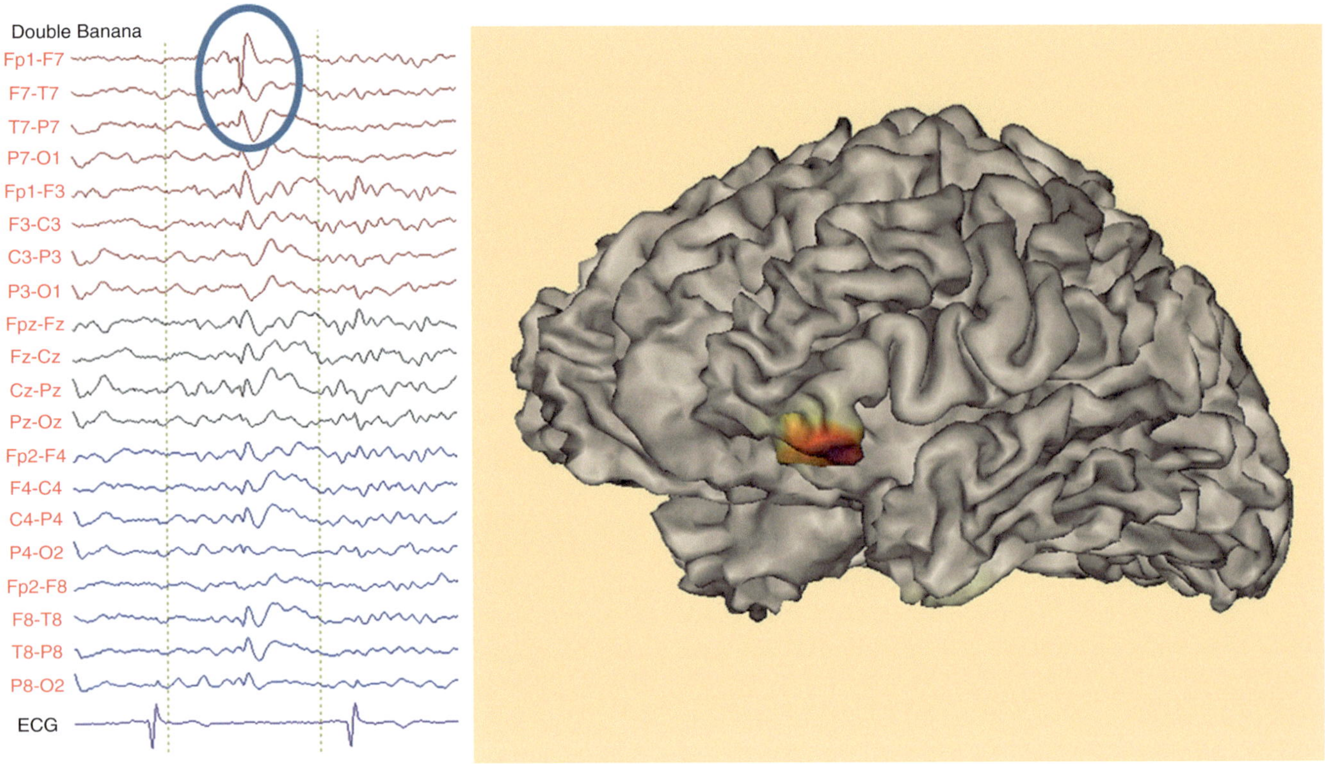

Fig. 20.1 EEG (longitudinal bipolar montage) and source imaging (distributed source model, 3D image of the brain seen from the left side) of the epileptiform discharge in the patient described in the case box

their armamentarium [5]. While other neuroimaging methods experience a rapid development of novel methods implemented in the daily clinical practice, the EEG community seems to be ultraconservative: in most centres EEGs are read exactly as five decades ago, and signal analysis is rarely a part of the formal training in EEG. The goals of this chapter are to demystify source imaging, to promote a paradigm shift in localization (from seeking phase reversals to assessing topographic maps) and to encourage use of EMSI in the presurgical evaluation of patients with drug-resistant focal epilepsy.

20.2 Cortical Generators of Epileptiform Discharges

EEG involves recording of electrical activity of the brain which is conducted passively through the volume of extracellular space (volume conduction) to the electrodes, at the surface of the scalp. There is physical physiological barrier of membranes around the brain; along with containing spaces and skull bone, they all attenuate conducted electric signals markedly before reaching scalp. There should be about 10 cm^2 area of the brain activated to generate current of a magnitude to be recorded over the scalp [6]. Postsynaptic potentials that occur synchronously in a large number of dendrites with parallel orientation generate electric currents in the extracellular space that, by summation, become large enough to cross through skull so that it can be recorded over the scalp. Cerebral cortex has vertically oriented pyramidal neurons (perpendicular to the cortical surface) with the cell body lying in layers IV and V. Apical dendrites of these neurons run parallel to each other towards the surface; in other words, they are arranged like palisades. Thus, extracellular spaces around them are arranged parallel to each other, and currents passing through them may summate to be large enough to cross physiological barriers and can be recorded over scalp. Such dendrodendritic synapses can be excitatory or inhibitory, producing excitatory or inhibitory postsynaptic potentials, respectively (EPSP and IPSP). Generally, excitatory synapses that participate in generating epileptiform discharges are located superficially (near the surface) and inhibitory synapses in deeper part (near the cell body). Thus, an EPSP would produce local negative potential in extracellular space, and since it is near the cortical surface, it would produce a dipole with negative pole towards surface and (through return currents) positive pole in the depth (near the cell body). On the contrary, an IPSP from a synapse close to the cell body would produce local positive potential in the extracellular space, but since it is deeper in location, again the resulting dipole will have negative pole towards the surface (Fig. 20.2). Thus, in both scenarios, imaginary dipole would have negative pole towards the surface.

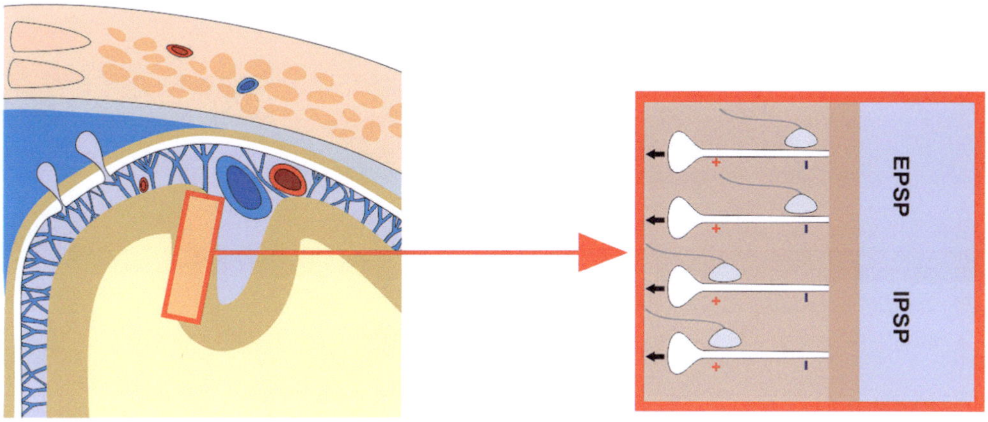

Fig. 20.2 Cortical generators of EEG signals. Excitatory postsynaptic potentials (EPSP) close to the cortical surface and inhibitory postsynaptic potentials (IPSP) close to the cell body generate currents in the extracellular space, with specific orientation (negative at the cortical surface and positive towards the white matter)

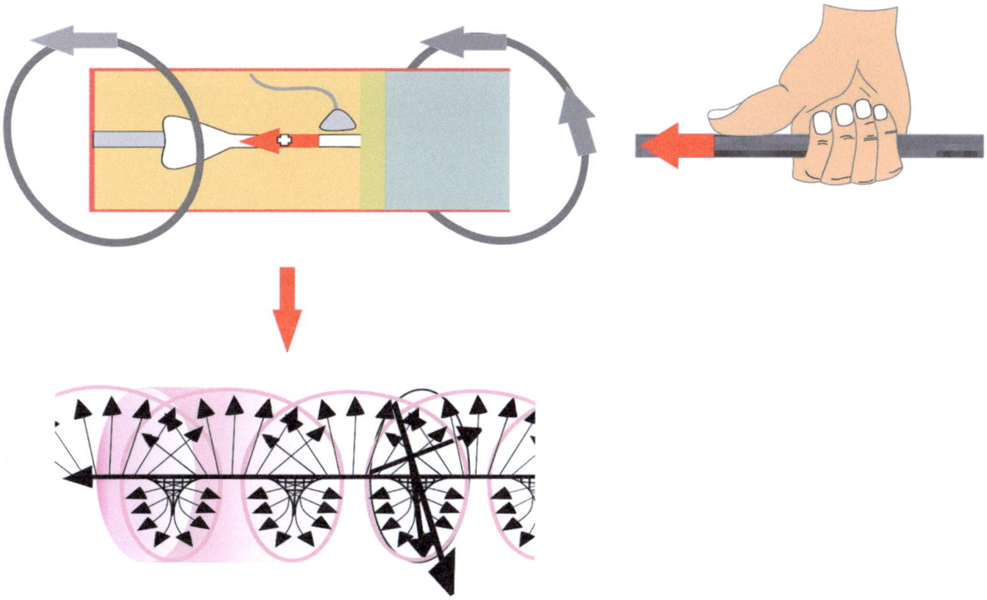

Fig. 20.3 The current in the apical dendrites generates magnetic field around the axis of the pyramidal neurons. The red arrow indicates the direction of the intracellular positive charges (according to the right-hand rule, this is the right thumb). The grey arrow indicates the direction of the induced magnetic field (fingers 2–5, according to the right-hand rule)

The electric current inside thc apical dendrites (positive charges moving from the cortical surface towards the cell body) generates magnetic field around the axis of the pyramidal neurons (Fig. 20.3). The relationship between the direction of the current and the magnetic field is given by the right-hand rule: the thumb indicates the direction of the intracellular positive charges, and fingers 2–5 indicate the direction of the magnetic field (Fig. 20.3).

20.3 Topographic Maps

Digital EEG recordings made possible visualization of the distribution of negative and positive electric potentials on the surface of the scalp, using topographic maps (synonyms: voltage maps, amplitude maps) [7, 8]. Similarly, for MEG, magnetic flux maps visualize the magnetic fields intersecting the scalp, distinguishing between the two directions of the magnetic field (towards the brain and departing from the brain).

The values of the potentials on the scalp, at locations situated between the electrodes, are estimated using interpolation and, for the points outside the electrodes, using extrapolation of the values measured from the recording electrodes. Topographic maps are two- or three-dimensional representations of the head or scalp. The distribution of the potentials on the scalp, at the point in time indicated by the position of the cursor in the waveform, is displayed using colour codes (usually blue for negative and red for the positive potentials). The deeper the nuance is, the larger the amplitude of the signal it depicts. In addition, isoelectric lines visualize the steps (gradient) between the peak-negative and the peak-positive values. The closer the isoelectric lines are to each other in a certain area, the steeper the voltage gradient in that area.

Inspection of topographic maps provides a more accurate picture about the electric signal than evaluating only the

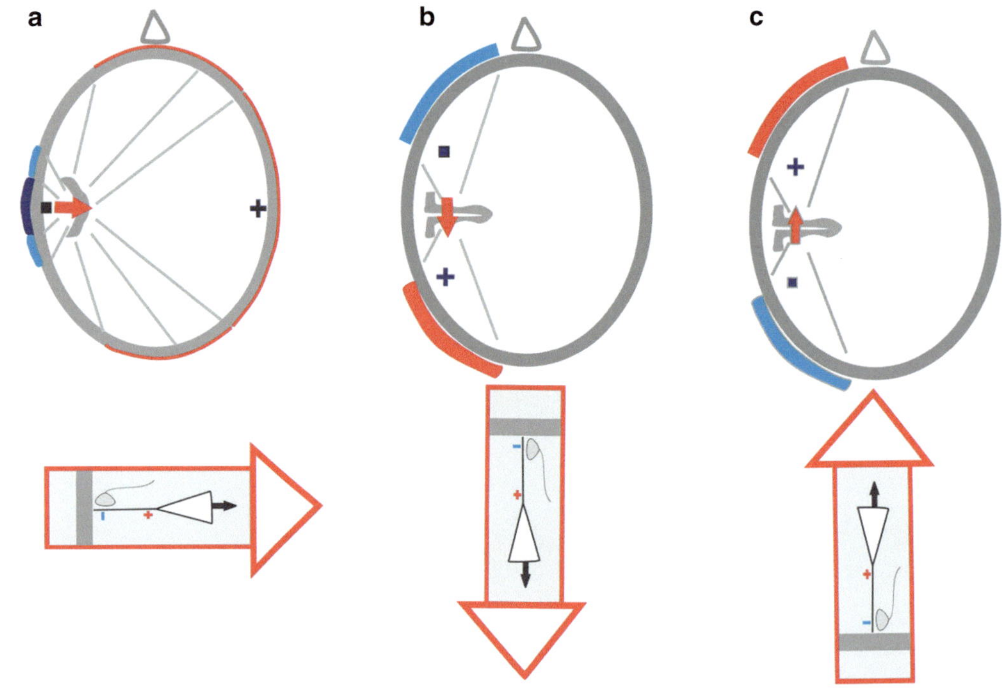

Fig. 20.4 Schematic representation of currents volume-conducted from the cortical generators to the scalp (head seen from the top; the grey triangle symbolizes the nose). (**a**) The cortical generator has a radial orientation (the cortex is parallel with the scalp). (**b, c**) The cortical generator has a tangential orientation (the cortex is perpendicular to the scalp). (**b**) Corresponds to the posterior and (**c**) to the anterior wall of the central sulcus. The blue and red colours on the surface indicate the topographic distribution of the negative and the positive charges, respectively. The red arrows under the head plots indicate the orientation of the neurons in the cortical generators. Note that in case of radially oriented source, the peak scalp negativity is located above the source. Yet, when the orientation is tangential, the source is away from the peak scalp negativity (in between the peak negativity and peak positivity)

morphology of the waveform. For inspection of the topographic maps, it is essential to understand how location and orientation of the cortical generator determines the distribution of the negative and positive potentials on the scalp. Most importantly, one needs to distinguish between cortical sources that are parallel to the surface of the scalp and those that are perpendicular to it (cortical wall of a sulcus). The schematic drawings in Fig. 20.4 illustrate this.

When the cortical area generating the signal is parallel to the scalp surface (radial orientation of the source), there is a short distance between the generator and the scalp. As we described above, for epileptiform discharges, the negative polarity is towards the cortical surface. Thus, for radially oriented sources, signals of negative polarity, volume-conducted to the scalp, have large amplitude and are recorded in a relatively circumscribed area of the scalp, lying above the source. Positivity volume conducts in the opposite direction, where the distance from the cortical generator to the scalp is longer. Therefore, the positive potentials are widely distributed on the scalp and have a lower amplitude (Figs. 20.4a and 20.5a).

When the cortical area generating the signal is located in the cortical wall of a sulcus, it is perpendicular to the scalp surface (tangential orientation of the source). In this case, there are similar distances from the source to the areas on the scalp, where the negative and the positive potentials will be volume-conducted to (Fig. 20.4b, c), and the topographic map will have a distribution that is clearly distinguishable from the ones generated by radial sources. For tangential sources, both a positive and a negative pole, of similar amplitude and area, will be visible on the scalp (Fig. 20.4b, c). As opposed to radial sources, for tangential orientation, the source is not just under the negative pole; the source is in between the negative pole and the positive poles, where the voltage maps have the steepest gradient (Fig. 20.5b). One can estimate this by connecting the negative and positive maxima with a straight line. The source is located under the area where the isoelectric lines are closest to each other, on the line connecting the positive and the negative maxima (Fig. 20.5b). In addition, the polarity helps in distinguishing between the sources situated in the adjacent walls of a sulcus. Since negativity volume conducts in the direction of the cortical surface, and the positivity in the opposite direction (towards the underlying white matter), the location of the negative and positive poles is distinguished between anterior and posterior (or inferior and superior) walls of a gyrus (Fig. 20.4b, c).

For radially oriented sources, spotting the location of peak negativity on the scalp (where the phase reversal is seen in a bipolar montage) approximates the location of the

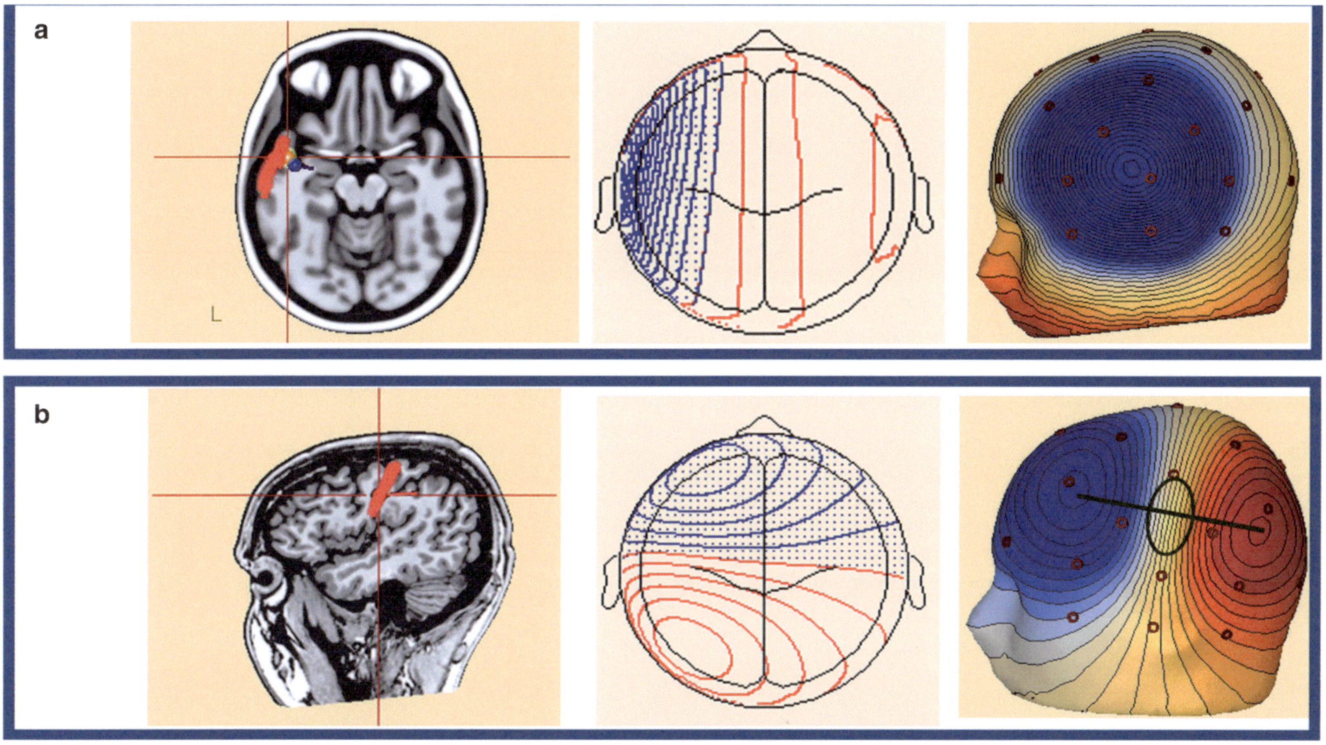

Fig. 20.5 Topographic (voltage) maps corresponding to sources with radial (**a**) and tangential (**b**) orientation of the cortical source, symbolized by the area marked in red on the MRIs. In the voltage maps, blue depicts negative and red depicts positive potentials on the scalp. Isoelectric lines are in black colour. In case of radial orientation (**a**), the source is under the peak negativity. For tangential orientation (**b**), the source is in between the negative and positive poles. Connect these poles by a straight line (in green in **b**). The area where the isoelectric lines are closest to each other (green ellipse) is over the source

source, since it is in the cortical area lying under the peak negativity. However, this is not true for tangentially oriented source. Thus, spotting only the area of the scalp with peak negativity (as in the traditional reading of EEG) does not convey information enough for estimating the location, since it either can originate from a radially oriented source just under the scalp peak negativity or from a tangentially oriented source, situated away from the scalp peak negativity. However, inspecting the location and distribution of both the negative and the positive potentials on the scalp clearly distinguishes between the two orientations, and the location of the source can be estimated as described above.

One needs to keep in mind that due to the low conductivity of the skull, there will be a blurring (smearing) of the potentials on a larger area on the scalp, compared to the brain.

Voltage maps are independent of the recording reference electrode. For a proper visualization of the negative and positive potentials, voltage maps need to be constructed from signals re-montaged using common average reference.

Propagation of electrical activity from one cortical area to the other is reflected by changes in time of the topographic maps. Thus, constructing sequential voltage maps, corresponding to the points in time of the spike's ascending slope, is informative about the propagation of the activity.

The same principles apply for magnetoencephalography: the location and the orientation of the cortical generators determine the recorded magnetic flux maps on the surface of the scalp (Fig. 20.6). Using the right-hand rule, one can determine the direction of the magnetic fields (fingers 2–5) generated by the intracellular flow of positive charges (thumb). When the source is perfectly radial, the magnetic field rotates around it and remains within the scalp, without being measurable on the surface. However, when the source has a tangential orientation, the magnetic signals can be measured at the surface of the scalp. Thus MEG is "blind" to the perfectly radial sources. Fortunately, the brain is not a cubistic design with perfectly radial and perfectly tangential orientations. In reality, most cortical generators have both radial and tangential cortex. It has been estimated that less than 5% of the brain has an orientation that is close (within 15°) to perfectly radial orientation; thus the insensitivity of MEG to radial dipoles does not reduce significantly the sensitivity of MEG for signals from the brain [9]. The colour codes in magnetic flux maps depict the direction of the magnetic field: blue indicates towards the brain, and red indicates the opposite direction. In the vast majority of cases, spikes can be detected both by EEG and MEG. In such cases, interpretation of the topographic maps (voltage maps and magnetic flux maps) leads to the same result (Fig. 20.7).

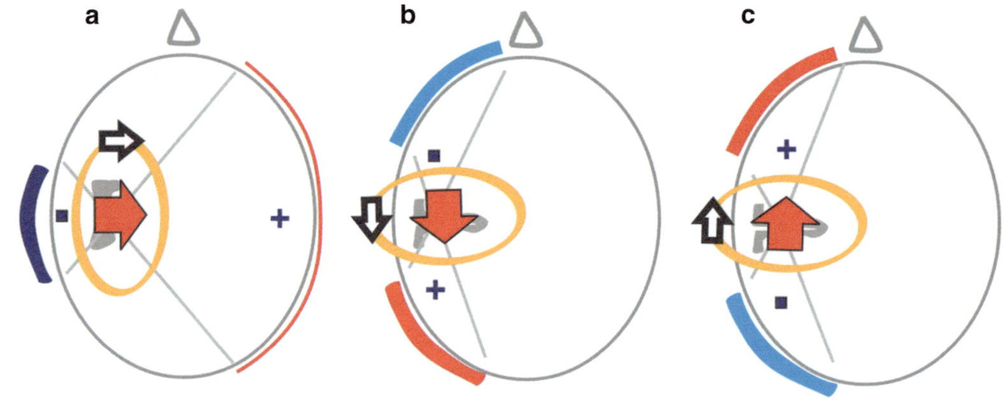

Fig. 20.6 Schematic representation of magnetic fields induced by different cortical generators (head seen from the top; the grey triangle symbolizes the nose). (**a**) The cortical generator has a radial orientation (the cortex is parallel with the scalp). (**b**, **c**) The cortical generator has a tangential orientation (the cortex is perpendicular to the scalp). (**b**) Corresponds to the posterior and (**c**) to the anterior wall of the central sulcus. The red arrow indicates the intracellular direction of the positive charges, the yellow circle symbolizes the induced magnetic field, and the black arrow indicates its direction. The blue and the red surfaces indicate the topographic distribution of the negative and of the positive charges, respectively

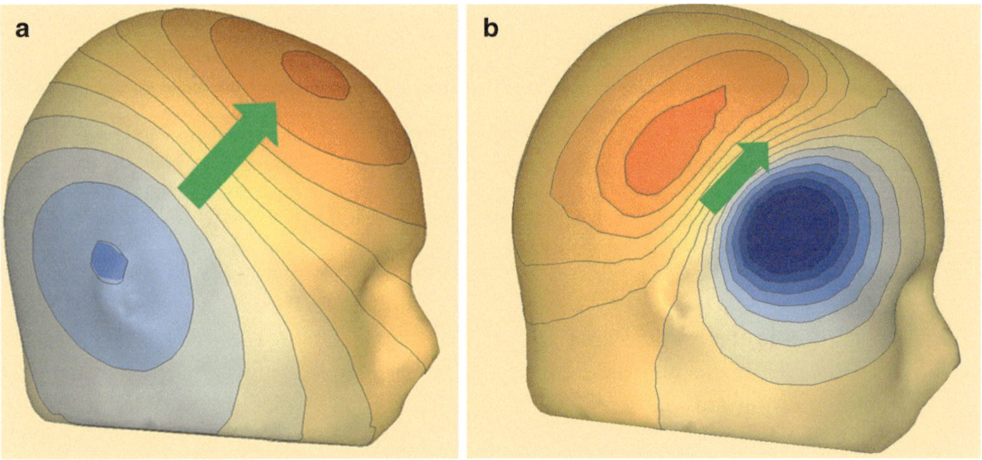

Fig. 20.7 Topographic maps: voltage map (**a**) and magnetic flux maps (**b**) of a source in the right parietal operculum. The green arrow indicates the intracellular flow of positive charges. Note that in case of a perfectly radial generator, the generated field is totally contained within the scalp, and magnetic signals cannot be recorded at the surface

20.4 Source Reconstruction

Knowing the anatomy of the subject and the conductivity of the tissues between the source and the recording electrodes, one can accurately determine the signal on the scalp generated by a cortical area in the brain. This is the forward problem. However, the clinical setting is the opposite: we record signals on the scalp, and we need to determine where it is generated (inverse problem). However, this is underdetermined: the number of unknowns exceeds the number of the measured data. There are multiple sources/combination of sources in the brain that give the same topographic map at the surface. Therefore, the inverse problem does not have one single solution, but multiple, possible solutions, and one needs to impose additional constrains. Different source imaging methods (inverse solutions) use different types of constrains. Solving the forward problem generates a realistic head model, used in advanced methods of source imaging.

20.4.1 Forward Solution

Its computation depends upon the space geometry (head shape) and conducting properties of the space elements (brain, CSF, skull, scalp). There are two types of head models used for this purpose: first, spherical head model which assumes the head as a closed sphere with uniform volume conduction property of the contents inside but it is not so in reality; hence source localization accuracy by this model is limited [7]. Second, the realistic head model takes real shape of head into account as multilayered shell along with anisotropic properties of different brain tissues and the volume conduction property of each layer. So, the realistic head model which is based on the individual's own high-resolution MRI provides better solution. Still, the computation of scalp potential from knowledge of a source location within the brain is difficult owing to nonhomogeneous shape of the brain and different conductivities of structures within the head like the brain, cerebrospinal fluid, meninges, etc. as well as anisotropic properties of brain tissue itself. Till now, there is no technique which can accurately image conductivities of various tissues or components of the head, though there are methods to minimize the uncertainty of the conductivity differences among tissues. The methods commonly used to compute in realistic head models are boundary element method (BEM) wherein triangulations of interfaces between compartments of the brain with equal isotropic properties are used, finite element model (FEM) wherein individual anisotropic conductivities of each element are used by a process of tessellation of the brain and finite difference method (FDM) where conducting volume is divided in cubic grids of different conductivities [10–12]. Due to the complexities involved in realistic head models, new methods to compute source from spherical head models are also evolving. Ideally, realistic head models are calculated using the patients' own MRI, but when this is not possible, age-matched template models can be used.

20.4.2 Inverse Solution

The oldest method for source modelling is the dipole fitting (Fig. 20.8), and it is still commonly used in clinical practice. It is assumed under this model that a scalp topographic map at a given time point is produced by single equivalent current dipole (ECD). This is the "equivalent" of many tiny dipoles, around the ECD; thus the model represents the "centre of gravity" of the source. Here, the best-fitting single dipole to explain the topographic map at a given time point is compared with the measured voltage map to extract the best location of the source [13]. Further dipole modelling is done for each subsequent topographic map with different distribution than the previous one (spatio-temporal model).

Another strategy is to scan the whole brain volume for possible sources. Here, it is assumed that the recorded topography is produced by multiple sources in the cortex so numerous dipoles are fitted in given time frame. Subsequently, that block of data is used to identify source location by method of least square fit (least number of dipoles explaining the voltage map) [14]. Methods used for this purpose are multiple signal classification (MUSIC), multiple signal classification recursively applied (RAP-MUSIC) and beamformer. Erroneous calculation of the location and number of dipoles to explain scalp potential may affect the result.

Distributed source models (linear inverse solutions) have gained much acceptance in clinical practice (Fig. 20.9). Here, the assumption is that multiple sources can be simultaneously active across many locations at any given time point. So, a priori assumption on number of dipoles is avoided. This model creates image of cerebral activity at each point of a 3D grid, and each point is considered as a mini dipole with a fixed position that is projected to the scalp. However, the strength of the activity at these solution points varies, to model the recorded topography. Since there are many distributions of cortical currents that can explain the recorded data, further assumptions are required to produce best source location. One of these assumptions is that neighbouring neurons are more likely to be active during electrical discharge from a

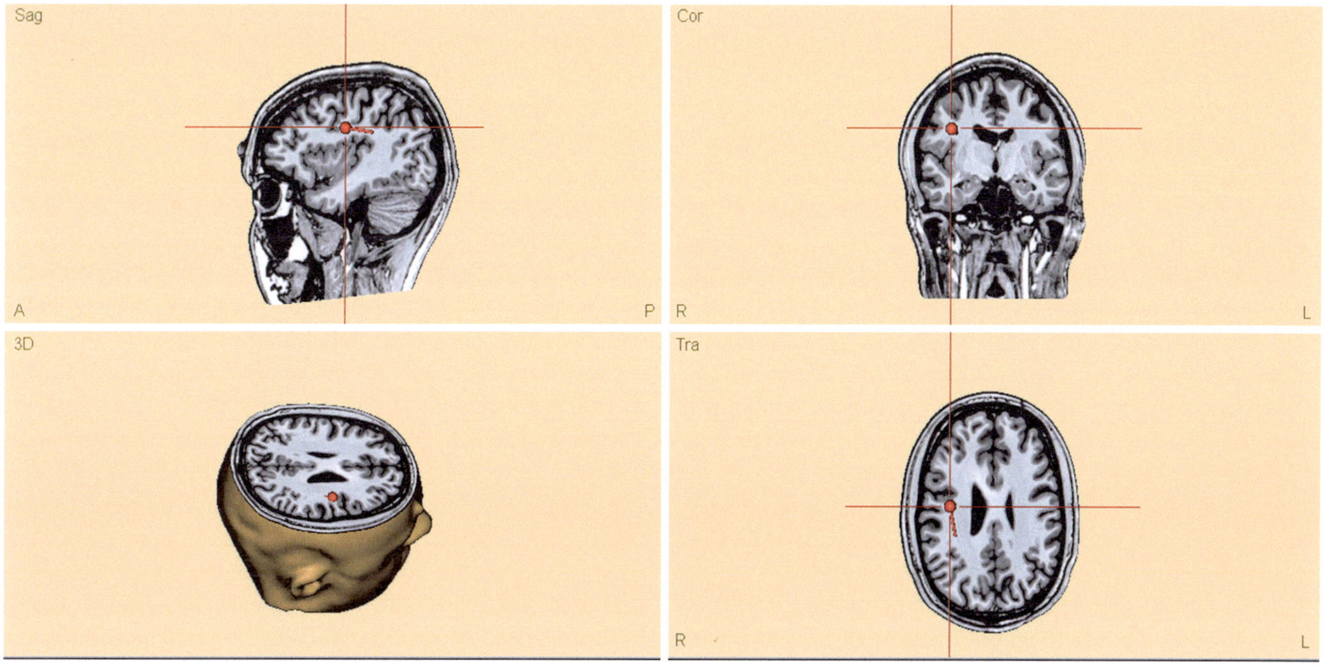

Fig. 20.8 Equivalent current dipole (ECD) of a source in the right precentral region

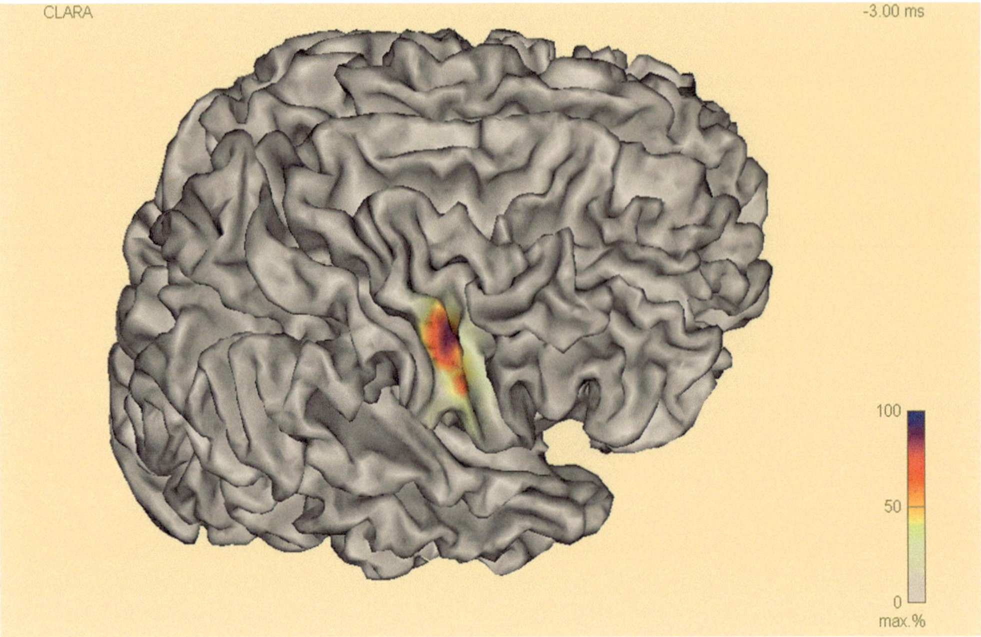

Fig. 20.9 Distributed source model (CLARA) displayed on an inflated cortex, to visualize also current distribution in the sulci (the same patient as in Fig. 20.8)

focus so the solution will include strengths of neighbour regions. This assumption model is used in low-resolution electromagnetic tomography (LORETA). Other examples of distributed source models are minimum norm, weighted minimum norm, LAURA (local autoregressive average), EPIFOCUS and CLARA. Source maximum is considered as the location of focus in distributed source models [15–19].

20.5 High-Density EEG (HD-EEG) Recordings

Although topographic maps visualize the electric potentials covering the whole surface of the scalp, these values are estimated from the recording electrodes. A low number of recording electrodes mean that a larger part of the topographic map is merely estimated (using interpolation and extrapolation); thus the accuracy is lower. Hence, increasing the number and the density of electrodes increases the accuracy of source imaging.

It is important to emphasize that not only the number of electrodes matters but also their distribution. Since volume conduction occurs in all directions, one has to sample also from the inferior part of the head. An uneven spatial sampling (higher density of electrodes in certain areas of the scalp) distorts the topographic map and (in consequence) leads to errors in source imaging, even when electrodes are placed more densely around the hypothetical focus.

The original EEG electrode array, the so-called 10-20 system [20], did not cover the inferior part of the temporal lobe; thus the first step in improving the array is extending it with the electrodes in the inferior temporal chain [21]. Placing electrodes at 10% of the distances, using the modified combinatorial nomenclature [22], gives an evenly distributed array of 64 electrodes, further improving the spatial sampling of EEG recordings.

It has been debated how many electrodes one needs for accurate ESI. Clinical studies on accuracy of ESI recorded with HD arrays, and the down-sampling to lower densities, showed that the accuracy increased significantly up to an array of 63–64 electrodes [23, 24]. Although the accuracy increased further to 123–128 electrodes, this was not significant. Theoretically, to reconstruct the distribution of the electric potentials on the scalp, one needs a spatial sampling with interelectrode distance of 2–3 cm [25].

Although the accuracy of ESI increases when using HD-EEG, this should not discourage clinicians in doing ESI based on low-density (LD) arrays, when HD-EEG recordings are not available. Although the spatial sampling is lower, the advantage of LD array is that it is tolerated well by patients for long-term recordings. Reasonable results (i.e. comparable with the conventional functional neuroimaging methods) have been obtained with LD arrays.

There are commercially available systems for HD-EEG recordings, using arrays with interelectrode distances <2 cm, even spatial distribution, which cover the inferior parts of the head too (cheek and neck). These characteristics optimize the accuracy of the reconstructed electric potentials on the scalp (Fig. 20.10). Application of these arrays (electrode nets) on the head is not more time-consuming than classical electrode caps, especially when saline-based (sponge) electrodes are used. However, this makes possible recordings of relatively limited time (up to 2 h). Longer recordings (including long-term monitoring) are also possible using electrode

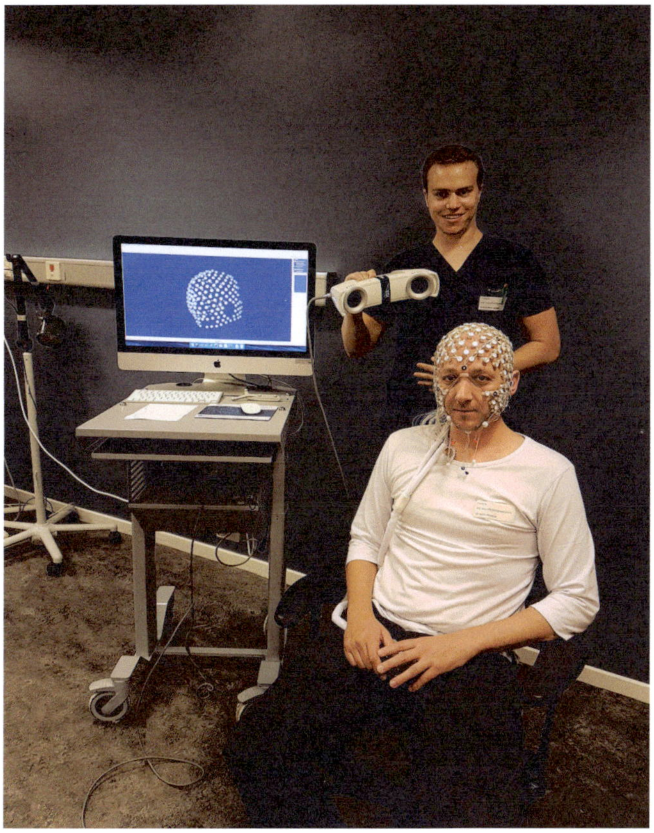

Fig. 20.10 High-density EEG recording using an array of 256 evenly distributed electrodes, covering the inferior part of the head too. The 3D position of the electrodes is rapidly measured using an optical scanner

gel, the disadvantage being the prolonged time for electrode setup. The high input impedance of the amplifiers (1000 MΩ) allows for higher electrode impedance, without increasing the level of noise.

Measuring the positions of the EEG electrodes, in three dimensions (3D), further increases the accuracy of source imaging, allowing precise co-registration of the electrode array with the MRI of the patient [21]. There are several methods for measuring 3D electrode positions, based on ultrasound, infrared light (Fig. 20.10), photographic analyses (photogrammetry), 3D LASER scanners or using MR-visible scalp electrodes [21].

20.6 Magnetoencephalography (MEG) Recordings

MEG records magnetic signals from the brain. In Sect. 2 we explained how the intracellular electric currents in the apical dendrites of the pyramidal neurons generate magnetic fields, and in Sect. 3 we explained how the position and orientation of the cortical generator determine the distribution of the magnetic fields on the scalp.

The neuro-magnetic signals originating in the brain penetrate the skull without being significantly distorted (as opposed to EEG signals that are distorted by the anatomical layers). For source imaging, this is an important advantage. However, the neuro-magnetic signals are very small, and therefore they are easily distorted by the magnetic signals in the environment, including the Earth's magnetic field. To circumvent this problem, MEG is recorded in shielded rooms (made of aluminium and mu-metal) that attenuate the magnetic noise from the environment. Systems using active shielding are available.

MEG records the magnetic signals using superconducting sensors with extremely low resistance. This is achieved by cooling the sensors to very low temperatures. To further process the weak recorded signals, these are amplified. Superconductive quantum interference devices (SQUIDS) convert the weak magnetic signals to high-amplitude voltages.

Various MEG equipment are available. Typically, they have a high spatial sampling, and the array consists of magnetometers, gradiometers or a combination of them. Ideally, MEG is co-registered with EEG (MEEG).

20.7 Methodological Steps of Source Imaging

The methodology of source imaging (Fig. 20.11) includes the following steps:

1. *Identification of the epileptiform discharges.* Most often these are visually identified by trained experts. One can use a single spike or an average of several spikes as template, to conduct automated pattern search for identifying further spikes in the recording, belonging to the same type of spike. Semiautomated systems for spike identification have been reported and validated [26]. Averaging spikes belonging to the same type (same cluster), having the same scalp topography, increases the signal-to-noise ratio and hence improves the accuracy of source imaging [27, 28]. Since the single (i.e. not averaged) discharges are distorted by noise, we do not recommend performing source imaging of individual discharges.
2. *Segmentation and co-registration.* For computing the realistic, individual head model, the MRI is segmented for the different conductive tissues, and this is co-registered in space with the 3D positions of the recording electrodes.
3. *Assessment of intra-spike propagation and determining the time points for the analysis.* The spike waveform can be the results of activity in several, sequentially activated cortical areas, including some temporal overlap between them. Inspection of the topographic maps, corresponding

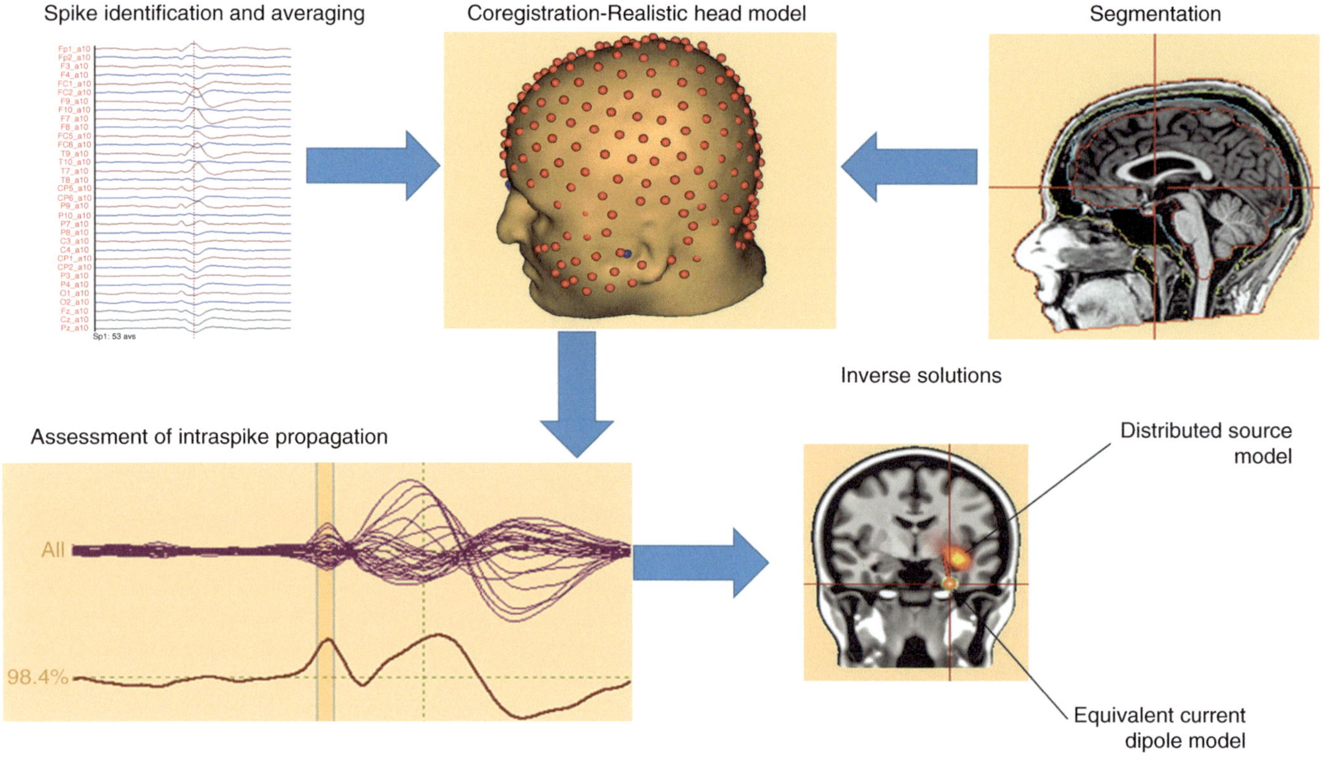

Fig. 20.11 Flowchart of the methodological steps of source imaging

to the time points on the ascending slope of the averaged spike waveform (sequential maps), helps in assessing whether the signal originates from propagation of activity from one cortical area to the other, since this implies corresponding changes in the recorded topography. The earliest stable topography corresponds to the onset. Alternatively, one can use algorithms for assessment of propagation and identification of the onset (principal component analysis; microstate segmentation method, based on cluster analysis) [7]. Ideally, signals are analysed both at onset and at the peak [29]. A more simplistic approach is to analyse the signals at the middle one-third of the ascending slope, since this gives accurate results in most of the cases [30].

4. *Inverse solutions*. It is recommended to use at least two types of inverse solutions, belonging to different groups of algorithms (see Sect. 4.2), to estimate the source of the signals.

20.8 Evidence from Clinical Validation Studies

Routine interictal EEG record may be normal in 50% cases, and by prolonged recording and incorporation of provocative measures like sleep deprivation, its yield can be increased to 70–80% [31]. Still, 20–30% would be normal interictal EEGs where source analysis would not be possible. It has been proven that high-density (>60 electrodes) EEG recording is better for the electric source imaging but the studies, including ictal source imaging, with low-density electrodes, have also shown good localization results in terms of concordance with structural and functional neuroimaging and accuracy [32–34]. It is recommended that 19-electrode scalp EEG recording according to the standard 10-20 system along with inferior temporal chain of 6 electrodes as per IFCN standard should be the minimum for the electric source imaging. As stated earlier, source analysis from the interictal EEG data gives location about the irritative zone which may not correlate seizure onset zone in each case; moreover, spike analysis may represent propagated electrical activity as the electrical activity can reach other parts of the brain within milliseconds [35]. These points pose a theoretical challenge to the correct localization of seizure focus by source analysis from the interictal EEG data. However, studies show high accuracy in determining seizure onset zone by ESI from interictal scalp EEG [36–42]. It is generally accepted that simultaneous intracranial EEG recording with source imaging from scalp-recorded interictal EEG can solve this issue, but such studies are technically difficult and studies about concordance between ESI focus and intracranial EEG done at different time points have shown good correlation [43–45]. Studies on electric source imaging from ictal scalp EEG are less in number but seem to be more promising as there is very little chance to fail to record an ictus electrographically and rarely ictal pattern, unanalyzable for the ESI, is encountered (e.g. electrodecrement without recognized pattern). The available ictal source imaging studies show results as good as they are for the interictal ESI [46, 47].

There is significant heterogeneity among clinical studies in terms of parameters of assessment of accuracy and adaptation of different models of inverse solution and head model for forward solution. The accuracy standard used in studies is multidisciplinary team decision, complete seizure freedom which is score 1 as per Engel outcome scale or score 2 (rare seizures) on Engel outcome scale or concordance with intracranial EEG recording, varying from study. Since seizure freedom after epilepsy surgery gives incontrovertible truth of the localization of epileptogenic zone in the resected region of the brain, source localization in relation to resected brain region and seizure outcome status can be used to calculate accuracy measures of ESI [33]. We made literature search in Medline to find studies of interictal as well as ictal ESI with seizure outcome data and analyse pooled data to ascertain accuracy with standard set as follows:

1. True positive: Those with ESI source concordant with resected area and seizure outcome Engel 1
2. False positive: Those with ESI source concordant with resected area but seizure outcome not Engel 1
3. False negative: Those with ESI source not concordant with resected area but Engel outcome 1
4. True negative: Those with ESI source not concordant with resected area and seizure outcome not Engel 1

Out of the 104 studies, 29 observational prospective studies were scanned for the surgery and outcome data. Finally, 18 studies were selected which had data to analyse at least 1 parameter seizure outcome as per abovesaid standard. Two studies were included despite not fulfilling strictly to the abovesaid criteria. (1) The data about surgery was available, but outcome was assessed as per the concordance with MRI lesion and decision of multidisciplinary team to operate or not operate [32]. This study was important as it provided ictal ESI with higher number of cases. (2) Seizure outcome data were given as the best seizure outcome (Engel 1 or 2) [48]. Those cases with seizure outcome data of less than 1 year were excluded from the analysis. Results showed that overall sensitivity of the electric source imaging was 81% (63–91%); specificity was 49.5% (25–77%) (Fig. 20.12), positive likelihood ratio, 1.4, and negative likelihood ratio, 0.36 (Fig. 20.13); and diagnostic odds ratio was 4.3 (Fig. 20.14). There was gross variability in specificity data, possibly due to small number of true negative cases making it less reliable, but sensitivity was reproducible in almost all studies. We need to have more studies with seizure outcome data adopting uniform definition of the outcome standard.

20.9 Limitations and Future Direction

The accuracy of source imaging depends on the spatial sampling (number and distribution of electrodes/sensors), appropriate head model, accuracy of co-registration, the choice of analysis time point in the signal and the inverse solution model which are still not perfect, and new models are evolving. All these factors limit the spatial resolution of source imaging. Interictal EEG being normal despite active epilepsy is another limitation of the method. Although patients evaluated for epilepsy surgery have seizures recorded during long-term video-EEG monitoring, there is higher risk of incorrect source imaging of ictal signals, due to artefacts causing less signal-to-noise ratio. Clinical studies, prospectively including a substantial number of patients and following a strict and uniform design of diagnostic studies, are still required for optimizing source imaging.

Nevertheless, the already published data provide compelling evidence for the accuracy of these methods. Source imaging has not yet been widely implemented in the clinical practice. We hope this chapter, explaining the basic principles using a language accessible for clinicians and reviewing the published evidence, will help to spread the use of these methods.

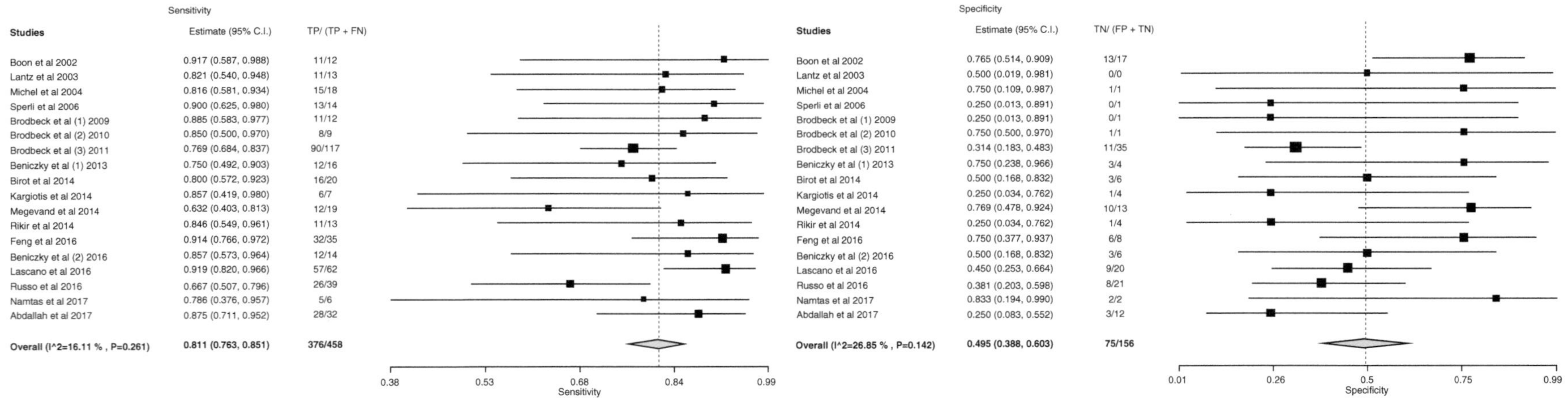

Fig. 20.12 Sensitivity and specificity of source imaging, inferred from the included studies

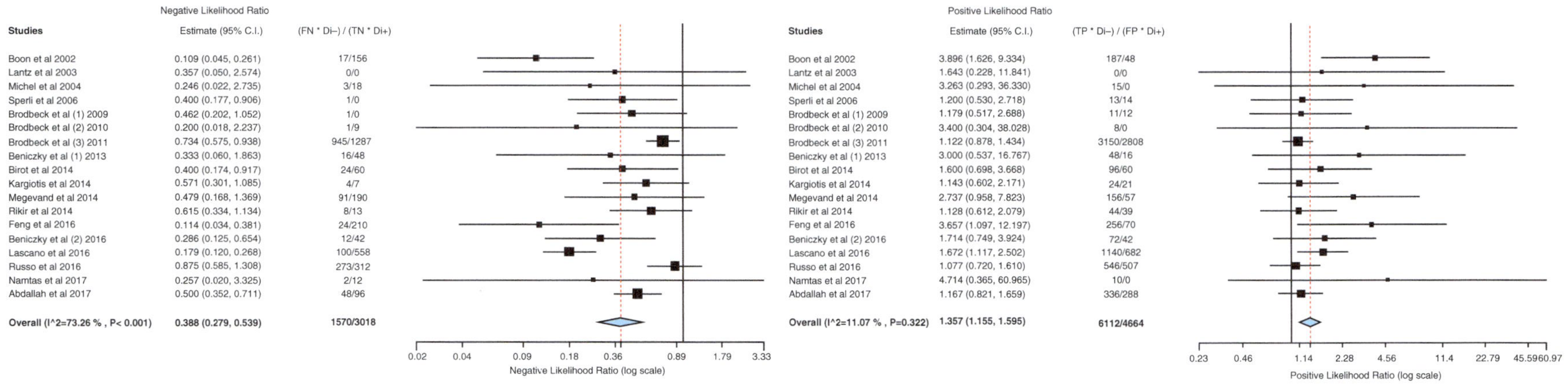

Fig. 20.13 Negative and positive likelihood ratios of source imaging, inferred from the included studies

Studies	Estimate (95% C.I.)	(TP * TN) / (FP * FN)
Boon et al 2002	35.750 (3.465, 368.829)	143/4
Lantz et al 2003	4.600 (0.072, 292.287)	0/0
Michel et al 2004	13.286 (0.441, 399.812)	15/0
Sperli et al 2006	3.000 (0.081, 111.781)	0/1
Brodbeck et al (1) 2009	2.556 (0.068, 95.874)	0/1
Brodbeck et al (2) 2010	17.000 (0.446, 648.202)	8/0
Brodbeck et al (3) 2011	1.528 (0.664, 3.515)	990/648
Beniczky et al (1) 2013	9.000 (0.717, 113.016)	36/4
Birot et al 2014	4.000 (0.575, 27.819)	48/12
Kargiotis et al 2014	2.000 (0.090, 44.350)	6/3
Megevand et al 2014	5.714 (1.163, 28.069)	120/21
Rikir et al 2014	1.833 (0.121, 27.797)	11/6
Feng et al 2016	32.000 (4.373, 234.180)	192/6
Beniczky et al (2) 2016	6.000 (0.671, 53.681)	36/6
Lascano et al 2016	9.327 (2.621, 33.198)	513/55
Russo et al 2016	1.231 (0.408, 3.712)	208/169
Namtas et al 2017	18.333 (0.536, 627.204)	10/0
Abdallah et al 2017	2.333 (0.437, 12.454)	84/36
Overall (I^2=22.78 % , P=0.184)	**4.302 (2.503, 7.394)**	2420/972

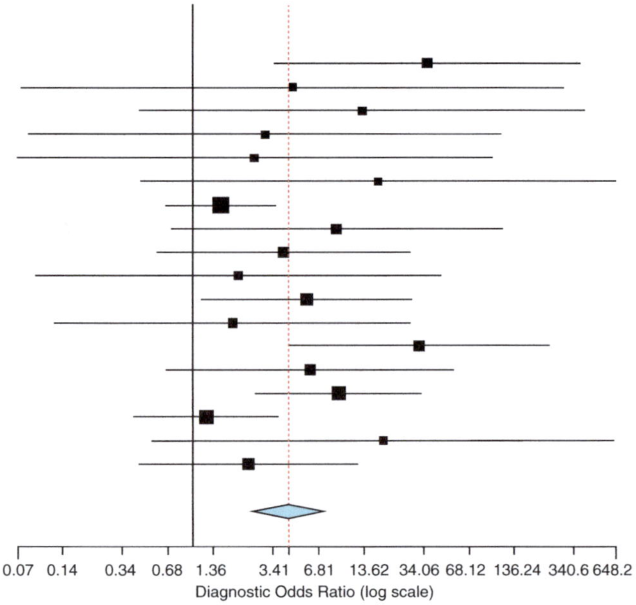

Fig. 20.14 Odds ratio for source imaging, inferred from the included studies

References

1. Thurman DJ, Beghi E, Begley CE, Berg AT, Buchhalter JR, Ding D, Hesdorffer DC, Hauser WA, Kazis L, Kobau R, Kroner B, Labiner D, Liow K, Logroscino G, Medina MT, Newton CR, Parko K, Paschal A, Preux PM, Sander JW, Selassie A, Theodore W, Tomson T, Wiebe S, ILAE Commission on Epidemiology. Standards for epidemiologic studies and surveillance of epilepsy. Epilepsia. 2011;52(suppl 7):2–26.
2. Neligan A, Bell GS, Shorvon SD, Sander JW. Temporal trends in the mortality of people with epilepsy: a review. Epilepsia. 2010;51:2241–6.
3. Ngugi AK, Kariuki SM, Bottomley C, Kleinschmidt I, Sander JW, Newton CR. Incidence of epilepsy: a systematic review and meta-analysis. Neurology. 2011;77:1005–12.
4. de Tisi J, Bell GS, Peacock JL, McEvoy AW, Harkness WF, Sander JW, Duncan JS. The long-term outcome of adult epilepsy surgery, patterns of seizure remission, and relapse: a cohort study. Lancet. 2011;378:1388–95.
5. Mouthaan BE, Rados M, Barsi P, Boon P, Carmichael DW, Carrette E, Craiu D, Cross JH, Diehl B, Dimova P, Fabo D, Francione S, Gaskin V, Gil-Nagel A, Grigoreva E, Guekht A, Hirsch E, Hecimovic H, Helmstaedter C, Jung J, Kalviainen R, Kelemen A, Kimiskidis V, Kobulashvili T, Krsek P, Kuchukhidze G, Larsson PG, Leitinger M, Lossius MI, Luzin R, Malmgren K, Mameniskiene R, Marusic P, Metin B, Özkara C, Pecina H, Quesada CM, Rugg-Gunn F, Rydenhag B, Ryvlin P, Scholly J, Seeck M, Staack AM, Steinhoff BJ, Stepanov V, Tarta-Arsene O, Trinka E, Uzan M, Vogt VL, Vos SB, Vulliémoz S, Huiskamp G, Leijten FS, Van Eijsden P, Braun KP, E-PILEPSY consortium. Current use of imaging and electromagnetic source localization procedures in epilepsy surgery centers across Europe. Epilepsia. 2016;57:770–6.
6. Tao JS, Ray A, Hawes-Ebersole S, Ebersole JS. Intracranial EEG substrate of scalp EEG interictal spikes. Epilepsia. 2005;46:669–76.
7. Michel CM, Murray MM, Lantz G, Gonzalez S, Spinelli L, Grave de Peralta R. EEG source imaging. Clin Neurophysiol. 2004;115:2195–222.
8. Scherg M, Ille N, Bornfleth H, Berg P. Advanced tools for digital EEG review: virtual source montages, whole-head mapping, correlation, and phase analysis. J Clin Neurophysiol. 2002;19:91–112.
9. Hillebrand A, Barnes GR. A quantitative assessment of the sensitivity of whole-head MEG to activity in the adult human cortex. NeuroImage. 2012;16:638–50.
10. He B, Musha T, Okamoto Y, Homma S, Nakajima Y, Sato T. Electric dipole tracing in the brain by means of the boundary element method and its accuracy. IEEE Trans Biomed Eng. 1987;34:406–14.
11. Lemieux L, McBride A, Hand JW. Calculation of electrical potentials on the surface of a realistic head model by finite differences. Phys Med Biol. 1996;41:1079–91.
12. Miller CE, Henriquez CS. Finite element analysis of bioelectric phenomena. Crit Rev Biomed Eng. 1990;18:207–33.
13. Ebersole JS, Hawes-Ebersole S. Clinical application of dipole models in the localization of epileptiform activity. J Clin Neurophysiol. 2007;24:120–9.
14. Achim A, Richer F, Saint-Hilaire JM. Methodological considerations for the evaluation of spatio-temporal source models. Electroencephalogr Clin Neurophysiol. 1991;79:227–40.
15. Fuchs M, Wagner M, Kohler T, Wischmann HA. Linear and nonlinear current density reconstructions. J Clin Neurophysiol. 1999;16:267–95.
16. Kaiboriboon K, Luders HO, Hamaneh M, Turnbull J, Lhatoo SD. EEG source imaging in epilepsy—practicalities and pitfalls. Nat Rev Neurol. 2012;8:498–507.
17. Michel CM, de Peralta RG, Lantz G, Andino SG, Spinelli L, Blanke O. Spatiotemporal EEG analysis and distributed source estimation in presurgical epilepsy evaluation. J Clin Neurophysiol. 1999;16:239–66.
18. Plummer C, Harvey AS, Cook M. EEG source localization in focal epilepsy: where are we now? Epilepsia. 2008;49:201–18.
19. Plummer C, Wagner M, Fuchs M, Harvey AS, Cook MJ. Dipole versus distributed EEG source localization for single versus averaged spikes in focal epilepsy. J Clin Neurophysiol. 2010;27:141–62.
20. Jasper HH. The ten-twenty electrode system. Electroencephalogr Clin Neurophysiol. 1958;16:371–5.

21. Seeck M, Koessler L, Bast T, Leijten F, Michel C, Baumgartner C, He B, Beniczky S. The standardized EEG electrode array of the IFCN. Clin Neurophysiol. 2017;128:2070–7.
22. American Electroencephalographic Society. Guideline thirteen: guidelines for standard electrode position nomenclature. J Clin Neurophysiol. 1994;11:111–3.
23. Luu P, Tucker DM, Englander R, Lockfeld A, Lutsep H, Oken B. Localizing acute stroke- related EEG changes: assessing the effects of spatial undersampling. J Clin Neurophysiol. 2001;18:302–17.
24. Lantz G, Grave de Peralta R, Spinelli L, Seeck M, Michel CM. Epileptic source localization with high density EEG: how many electrodes are needed? Clin Neurophysiol. 2003a;114:63–9.
25. Gevins A, Brickett P, Costales B, Le J, Reutter B. Beyond topographic mapping: towards functional- anatomical imaging with 124- channel EEGs and 3- D MRIs. Brain Topogr. 1990;3:53–64.
26. Scherg M, Ille N, Weckesser D, Ebert A, Ostendorf A, Boppel T, Schubert S, Larsson PG, Henning O, Bast T. Fast evaluation of interictal spikes in long-term EEG by hyper-clustering. Epilepsia. 2012;53:1196–204.
27. Wennberg R, Cheyne D. EEG source imaging of anterior temporal lobe spikes: validity and reliability. Clin Neurophysiol. 2014;125:886–902.
28. Wennberg R, Cheyne D. Reliability of MEG source imaging of anterior temporal spikes: analysis of an intracranially characterized spike focus. Clin Neurophysiol. 2014;125:903–18.
29. Mălîia MD, Meritam P, Scherg M, Fabricius M, Rubboli G, Mîndruţă I, Beniczky S. Epileptiform discharge propagation: analyzing spikes from the onset to the peak. Clin Neurophysiol. 2016;127:2127–33.
30. Lantz G, Spinelli L, Seeck M, de Peralta Menendez RG, Sottas CC, Michel CM. Propagation of interictal epileptiform activity can lead to erroneous source localizations: a 128-channel EEG mapping study. J Clin Neurophysiol. 2003b;20:311–9.
31. Smith SJM. EEG in the diagnosis, classification and management of patients with epilepsy. J Neurol Neurosurg Psychiatry. 2005;76(Suppl II):ii2–7.
32. Boon P, D'Have M, Vanrumste B, Van Hoey G, Vonck K, Van Walleghem P, Caemaert J, Achten E, De Reuck J. Ictal source localization in presurgical patients with refractory epilepsy. J Clin Neurophysiol. 2002;19:461–8.
33. Brodbeck V, Spinelli L, Lascano AM, Wissmeier M, Vargas MI, Vulliemoz S, et al. Electroencephalographic source imaging: a prospective study of 152 operated epileptic patients. Brain. 2011;134:2887–97.
34. Sperli F, Spinelli L, Seeck M, Kurian M, Michel CM, Lantz G. EEG source imaging in pediatric epilepsy surgery: a new perspective in presurgical workup. Epilepsia. 2006;47:981–90.
35. Alarcon G, Guy CN, Binnie CD, Walker SR, Elwes RD, Polkey CE. Intracerebral propagation of interictal activity in partial epilepsy: implications for source localization. J Neurol Neurosurg Psychiatry. 1994;57:435–49.
36. Brodbeck V, Spinelli L, Lascano AM, Pollo C, Schaller K, Vargas MI, Wissmeyer M, Michel CM, Seeck M. Electrical source imaging for presurgical focus localization in epilepsy patients with normal MRI. Epilepsia. 2010;51:583–91.
37. Gavaret M, Badier JM, Marquis P, Bartolomei F, Chauvel P. Electric source imaging in temporal lobe epilepsy. J Clin Neurophysiol. 2004;21:267–82.
38. Gavaret M, Badier JM, Marquis P, McGonigal A, Bartolomei F, Regis J, Patrick C. Electric source imaging in frontal lobe epilepsy. J Clin Neurophysiol. 2006;23:358–70.
39. Lantz G, de Peralta RG, Spinelli L, Seeck M, Michel CM. Epileptic source localization with high density EEG: how many dipole modelling of scalp EEG. Clin Neurophysiol. 2007;118:2344–61.
40. Leijten FS, Huiskamp G. Interictal electromagnetic source imaging in focal epilepsy: practices, results and recommendations. Curr Opin Neurol. 2008;21:437–45.
41. Lascano AM, Perneger T, Vulliemoz S, Spinelli L, Garibotto V, Korff CM, Vargas MI, Michel CM, Seeck M. Yield of MRI, high-density electric source imaging (HD-ESI), SPECT and PET in epilepsy surgery candidates. Clin Neurophysiol. 2016;127:150–5.
42. Megevand P, Spinelli L, Genetti P, BrodbecK V, Momjian S, Schallar K, Michel CM, Vulliemoz S, Seeck M. Electric source imaging of interictal activity accurately localizes the seizure onset zone. J Neurol Neurosurg Psychiatry. 2014;85:38–43.
43. Abdallah C, Maillard LG, Rikir E, Jonas J, Thiriaux A, Gavaret M, Bartolomei F, Colnat-Coulbois S, Vignal JP, Koessler L. Localizing value of electrical source imaging: frontal lobe malformations of cortical development and negative MRI related epilepsies are the best candidates. Neuroimage Clin. 2017;16:319–29.
44. Merlet I, Gotman J. Dipole modeling of scalp electroencephalogram epileptic discharges: correlation with intracerebral fields. Clin Neurophysiol. 2011;112:414–30.
45. Rikir E, Koessler L, Gavaret M, Bartolomei F, Colnat-Coulbois S, Vignal JP, Vespignani RG, Maillard LG. Electrical source imaging in cortical malformation–related epilepsy: a prospective EEG-SEEG concordance study. Epilepsia. 2014;55:918–32.
46. Beniczky S, Rosenzweig I, Scherg M, Jordanov T, Lanfer B, Lantz G, Larsson PG. Ictal EEG source imaging in presurgical evaluation: high agreement between analysis methods. Seizure. 2016;43:1–5.
47. Nemtsas P, Birot G, Pittau F, Michel CM, Schaller K, Vulliemoz S, Kimiskidis VK, Seeck M. Source localization of ictal epileptic activity based on high-density scalp EEG data. Epilepsia. 2017;58:1027–36.
48. Feng R, Hu L, Pan L, Wu J, Lang L, Jiang S, Gu X, Guo J, Zhou L. Application of 256-channel dense array electroencephalographic source imaging in presurgical workup of temporal lobe epilepsy. Clin Neurophysiol. 2016;127:108–16.

Simultaneous Recording EEG and fMRI

21

Stefano Meletti

Abbreviation

BECTS	Benign epilepsy with centro-temporal spikes
BOLD	Blood oxygen level dependent
DMN	Default mode network
GLM	General linear model
HRF	Haemodynamic response function
icEEG	Intracranial EEG
IED	Interictal epileptiform discharge
SPM	Statistical parametric mapping
SWD	Spike and wave discharge

21.1 Neural Basis of BOLD Signal and Rationale of Simultaneous Recording EEG and fMRI

Today, functional neuroimaging methods allow mostly non-invasive in vivo visualization of cerebral activity. However, to infer brain functions using these methods, it is important to recognize their limitations. The main limitation is that the method with the best spatial accuracy, i.e. blood oxygen level-dependent functional magnetic resonance imaging (BOLD fMRI), is based on haemodynamic changes in active areas and therefore able to provide only indirect information on neural activity, based on the phenomenon of "neurovascular coupling", i.e. the relationship that exists between neural activity at cellular (neuronal and glial) and subcellular (neurotransmitters, chemical and electrical channels) levels and cerebral blood flow changes. Understanding neurovascular coupling is crucial in order to use this technique correctly in human diseases.

As the acronym indicates, the BOLD signal detected in fMRI is dependent on the level of blood oxygenation. The signal recorded from the scanner is T2*, the transverse relaxation time (T2) plus the component related to the local variations in magnetic susceptibility due to the variations in deoxyhaemoglobin (Hb) concentration. In 1992, two different groups simultaneously demonstrated a BOLD signal increase (up to 5%) in human sensory areas during functional activation [1, 2]. In fact, significant variations in Hb occur in capillaries and venules draining blood from activated functional areas. Arteriolar vasodilatation produces an increase in cerebral blood flow, with delivery of fresh arterial blood, which increases the oxyhaemoglobin/deoxyhaemoglobin (HbO/Hb) concentration ratio, overcompensating for the oxygen consumption. BOLD fMRI studies are currently carried out considering the 3–5% BOLD increase 4–6 s after the stimulus. This latency between neural activity and BOLD signal is an intrinsic limitation of BOLD fMRI, further complicated by the inhomogeneity of this latency in different brain regions [3], which can be marked in diseases affecting cerebrovascular reactivity.

Despite its intrinsic limitations, BOLD fMRI is the best available tool for brain mapping. To compensate for its poor temporal resolution, simultaneous acquisition of electrophysiological data is a perfect integration. EEG, independently of the number of channels, allows online recording of cerebral activity with virtually real temporal resolution. This direct window onto the cerebral processes is an unbeatable feature of the EEG, intrinsically impossible using pure imaging tools. For this reason, the combination of the high temporal resolution of EEG and the high spatial resolution of fMRI offers a powerful integration of the respective complementary strengths of both methods.

However, while both methods, fMRI and EEG, can detect in vivo cerebral activity associated with sensory, motor or cognitive tasks, it still has to be demonstrated that the neural activity recorded by the two methods is exactly the same. To obtain the two signals from the exact same region, Logothetis et al. [4] used micro-coil coaxial intracerebral electrodes implanted in the monkey's occipital cortex. Using this sophisticated approach, they demonstrated that visual stimulation causes an almost simultaneous increase in BOLD

S. Meletti (✉)
Department of Biomedical, Metabolic, and Neural Science, OCSAE Hospital, University of Modena and Reggio Emilia, Modena, Italy
e-mail: stefano.meletti@unimore.it

O. Mecarelli (ed.), *Clinical Electroencephalography*, https://doi.org/10.1007/978-3-030-04573-9_21

signal and electrophysiological activity. Then, they showed that the BOLD signal is associated with synaptic activity of local field potentials, rather than with output activity due to multiunit spiking activity. Other studies in monkeys confirmed the BOLD-local field potential correlation [5].

21.2 EEG-fMRI in Epilepsy

EEG is an important tool for the investigation of patients with epilepsy. It can help to diagnose and classify epilepsy and localize sources of epileptic activity. However, EEG is characterized by a number of disadvantages. The EEG has low spatial resolution with a limited ability to detect epileptic activity from deep brain structures and is characterized by the inverse problem with ambiguous source solutions for a given spatiotemporal distribution of a cerebral current [6]. In contrast, fMRI is characterized by high spatial resolution, is equally sensitive to signals of deep and superficial brain structures and represents a measurement of whole-brain haemodynamic changes. By combining EEG with fMRI, it is possible to detect BOLD signal changes associated with ictal and interictal epileptiform discharges (IEDs) obtained from the scalp EEG, even if deep brain structures are involved in their generation. In the last 20 years, EEG-correlated fMRI studies have been used to delineate epileptic networks noninvasively [7]. Studies were carried out both in adult and children with epilepsy (for clinical reviews, see refs. [8–10]). These multimodal data integration studies may be called EEG-informed fMRI, EEG-correlated fMRI or simply EEG-fMRI because the EEG temporal dynamics is taken as surrogate for haemodynamic fluctuations.

Briefly, an EEG-fMRI study consists of the following steps (Fig. 21.1). Firstly, electrodes and an amplifier/recorder system that are MR compatible are needed. Silver or gold electrodes can be used, and optical transmission of the amplified EEG outside the scanner room is recommended. Secondly, it must be ensured that the patient is comfortable and remains as immobile as possible during the necessarily long scanning session; the session can be long to ensure that the patient has a sufficient number of epileptic events recorded. fMRI scanning while recording the EEG results in large artefacts in the EEG. These can be removed by software after the scanning session to recover a clean EEG and allow one to mark the time of epileptic events.

Finally, a mathematical model of what the BOLD signal should be at the voxels involved in the epileptic event is build. Also, to obtain the most accurate results, it is noteworthy to consider carefully any possible confounds that can explain the variance of the BOLD signal (see Figs. 21.1 and 21.2).

If a voxel is involved in the event, its time course should change as a result of each event in a predictable fashion. In the general linear model (GLM) framework, a mathematical representation of each electrophysiological-derived event is convolved with a haemodynamic kernel, commonly the canonical haemodynamic response function (HRF) [11], resulting in a regressor of an effect of interest [12]. Statistical inferences on the estimated GLM parameters are then made to find the voxels at which the BOLD signal fluctuations are significantly correlated with the EEG-derived regressor. Such voxels, which show a significant BOLD signal change related to the marked epileptic events in the EEG, represent either the brain areas that take part in its generation or brain areas that are involved as a consequence of the event.

21.3 EEG Artefacts due to Recording in the MR Scan

The major physical effect underlying the MR environment-related EEG data degradation is due to the application of time-varying magnetic fields or by movement of the conducting circuit (in our case formed by the EEG wires, electrodes, patient and EEG amplification system) in a static magnetic field. Time-varying magnetic field gradients, used for the MR signal spatial encoding, produce large changes in the magnetic flux over short time periods, creating voltages at the amplifier inputs that appear as artefacts one to three orders of magnitude larger than the EEG signal [13]. Such artefacts represent the most significant effect corrupting the EEG data simultaneously acquired with fMRI. Given the repetitive nature of the gradient switching sequence, they can be removed [13]. However, changes in the conductive circuit geometry or position relative to the magnetic field, due to head movements or system vibrations, combined with the gradient temporal variation, can lead to random fluctuations in the induced voltages, which represent a real challenge for the artefact correction [14].

The second most significant effect corrupting EEG data is the pulse artefact, which results from the quasi-periodic motion and blood flow (Hall effect) linked to the cardiac cycle [15, 16]. Because its temporal and spatial characteristics are similar across repeated cardiac cycles, a commonly used pulse artefact correction method involves the computation of an artefact template by averaging the waveform at each lead across multiple cardiac cycles [13]. However, in general, this correction is more problematic than the gradient artefact correction given the variability of the artefact waveform over time and space [16]. Moreover, the amplitude and spatial variability of this artefact increase with the strength of

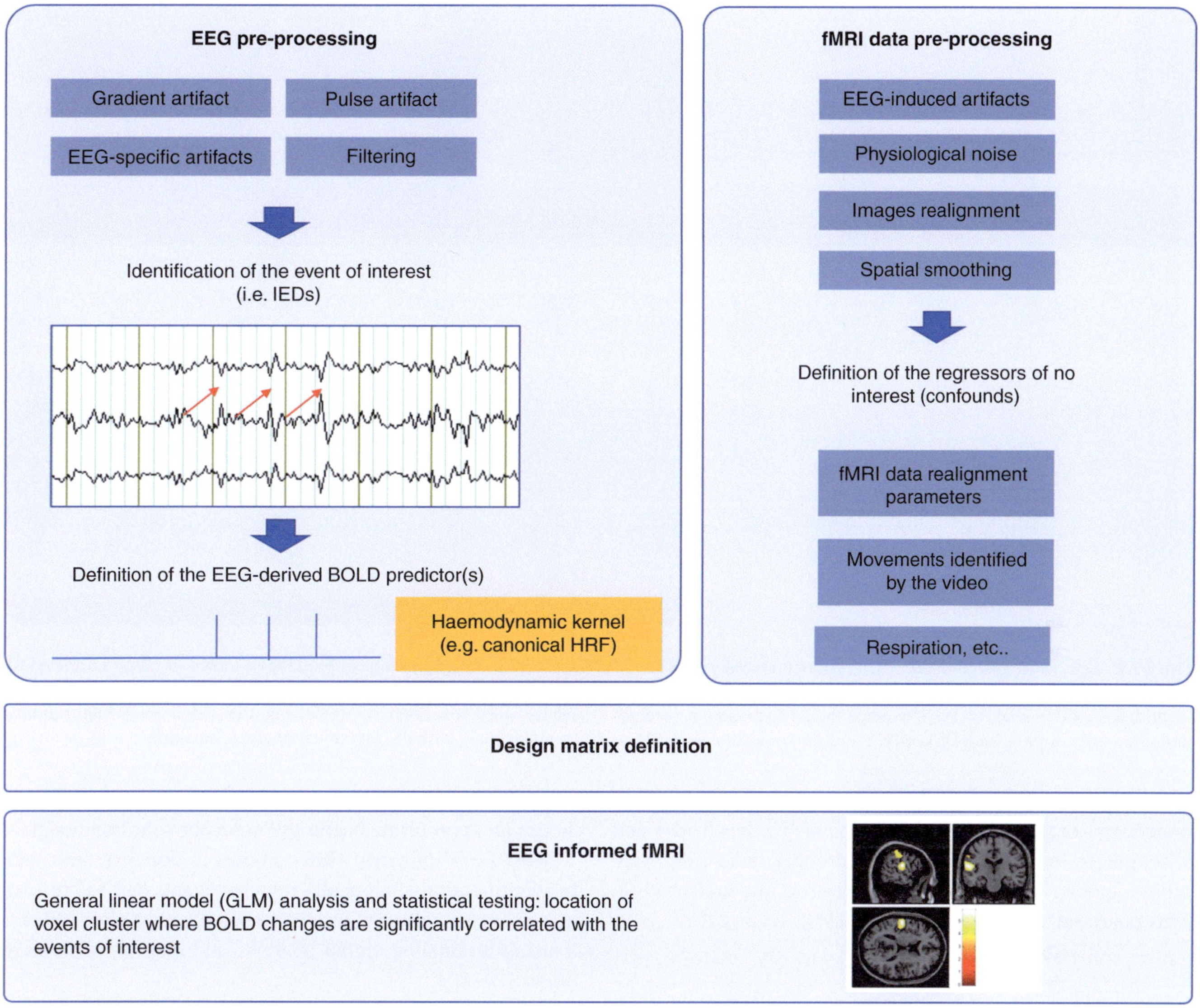

Fig. 21.1 Exemplificative pipeline of an EEG-fMRI study in epilepsy, where interictal epileptiform discharges (IEDs) are used to map brain areas showing significant BOLD changes related to spike generations

the static magnetic field, making its correction even more difficult at higher fields.

To limit both the pulse- and MR acquisition-related artefacts, useful data acquisition strategies such as limiting the area inside the conductive circuit, twisting the wires and mechanically restricting the motion of the head (e.g. vacuum cushion) have been proposed. Even after gradient and pulse artefact correction, EEG data may remain contaminated, especially when there is motion during the acquisition. Therefore, the identification and/or quantification of EEG phenomena may be compromised. For example, inappropriate pulse artefact correction may lead to spurious delta/theta activity, while inappropriate gradient artefact correction may lead to spurious high-frequency activity.

21.4 MRI Artefacts due to EEG Equipment

fMRI data degradation caused by the presence of the EEG recording system conducting wires and electrodes is a relatively minor effect when compared to the degradation of scalp EEG data, at simultaneous acquisitions [16]. It results from magnetic susceptibility effects, which lead to signal dropout and geometric distortion, as well as from the perturbation of the radio-frequency fields, which may cause local signal changes and a global reduction in the signal-to-noise ratio. The impact of such effects on fMRI data quality depends on the strength of the magnetic field and the number of electrodes.

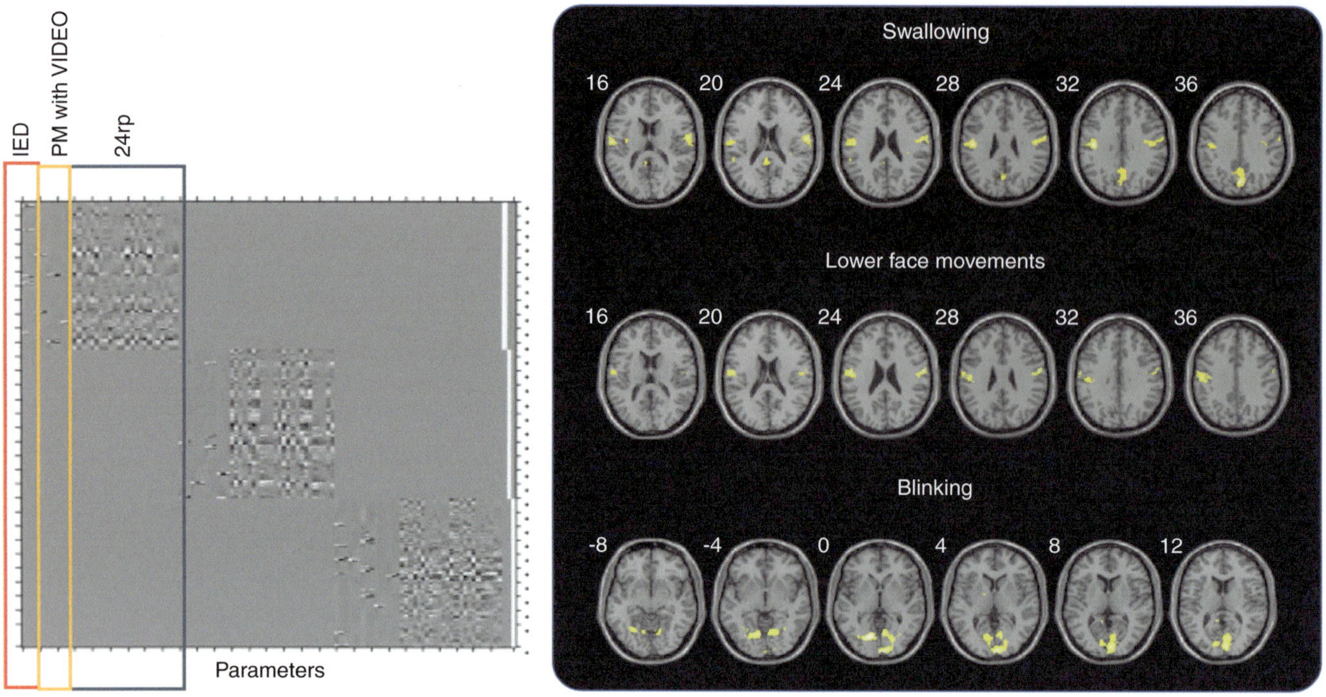

Fig. 21.2 *Left*: SPM design matrix. IED, interictal paroxysmal activities, the event of interest (red box); the patient's face/cranial movements identified by video analysis (yellow box); the 24 realignment parameters (blue box). *Right*: the BOLD effect of different spontaneous facial movements and physiological blinking is shown ($p < 0.05$ corrected for multiple comparisons; red: positive BOLD responses). These confounds were identified by reviewing the video recording acquired simultaneously with the functional image acquisition

Finally, a note must be on safety. The increased amount of material brought into the magnetic field (i.e. electrodes and wires) leads to shielding requiring stronger radio-frequency pulses leading to an increased absorption rate and heating. This poses safety issues (i.e. burns) [17].

21.5 Modelling the EEG Signal to Inform fMRI Analysis

EEG phenomena can be categorized as either isolated events with varying durations (i.e. epileptic spikes, epileptic seizures, EEG band power change time-locked to a stimulus or task) or continuously varying (e.g. spontaneous fluctuations in EEG alpha-band power during awake rest). EEG-fMRI studies have been performed according to the type of brain activity being addressed: epileptic or non-epileptic spontaneous activity and cognitive, sensory and motor functions. The reader can refer to recent extensive reviews on the types of EEG signal used to inform fMRI and to the different strategies of data analysis methods [18, 19].

In EEG-fMRI studies of spontaneous epileptic activity, the EEG is used to indicate the occurrence of events of interest in relation to the fMRI time series, and the experimenter's challenge is to accurately represent the epileptiform activity to build a model of the associated BOLD signal changes and choose an appropriate haemodynamic convolution model.

Most EEG-informed fMRI studies in epilepsy start with the identification of clinically relevant events on EEG recordings either visually by an electroencephalographer [20–23] or using automated signal analysis and classification techniques [24–27].

In the GLM framework, IEDs are commonly represented as (zero-duration) stick functions at the time of spikes [28, 29] (see Figs. 21.3 and 21.4).

IEDs with different electroclinical characteristics are modelled as separate effects, reflecting the modelling assumption of distinct generators [30, 31]. Formaggio et al. [24] used an independent component analysis (ICA) on EEG data to find potential IED generators, which were back-projected to the EEG channel space to obtain the IED-related EEG signals (IED-EEG). Assuming that scalp EEG signals represent a linear mixture of neuronal activities originated from independent sources, ICA can be used to unmix the signal into statistically independent subcomponents [32, 33].

Investigations of BOLD fluctuations related to ictal event (seizures) [34–39] are fewer than interictal studies due to methodological and practical concerns (patient safety, relative paucity of events and seizure-related motion); see

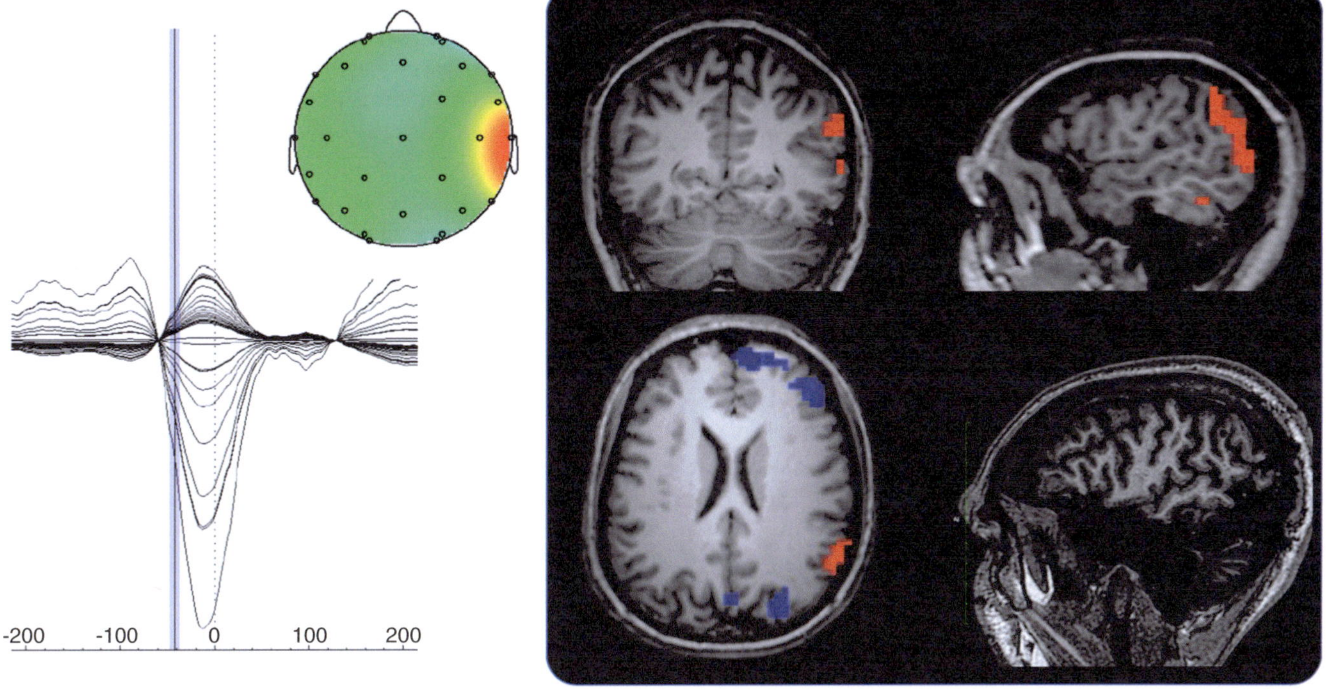

Fig. 21.3 *Left*: butterfly plot and voltage map of the average of 72 spikes in a 32-year-old man with a MRI-negative right temporal lobe epilepsy. *Right*: BOLD results are displayed using a threshold of $p < 0.05$ corrected for multiple comparisons and displayed on the patient's T1 images. BOLD signal increases were detected in the right temporo-parietal junction and posterior lateral temporal cortex. Also decreases in BOLD signal were detected in distant areas, involving the occipital and fronto-polar cortex. The patient is seizure free at 8 months post-surgery (the cortectomy encompassed voxels with BOLD signal increments)

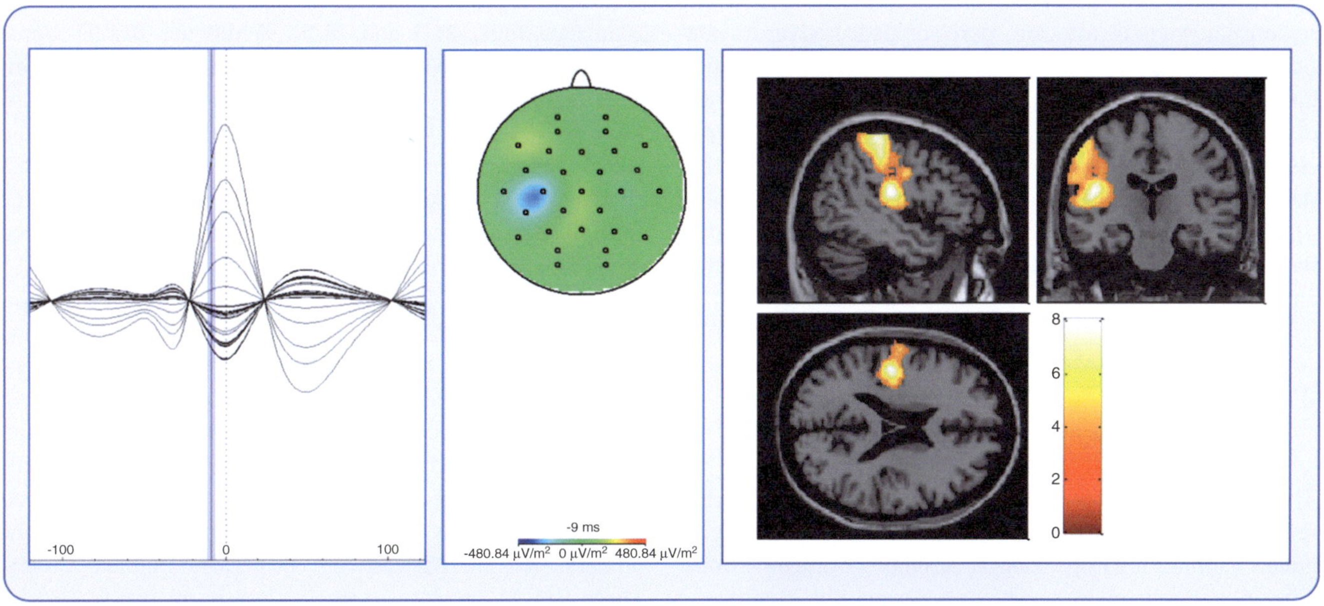

Fig. 21.4 *Left*: butterfly plot and voltage map of the average of 152 left rolandic spikes in a 13-year-old boy with benign epilepsy with centro-temporal spikes (BECTS). *Right*: BOLD results are displayed using a threshold of $p < 0.05$ corrected for multiple comparisons. BOLD signal increases were detected in left pericentral and insular cortex

Chaudhary et al. [40] for a recent review on the topic. Despite both being markers of epileptogenicity, ictal and interictal discharges are most likely to be generated by different neuronal populations, through different cellular and network mechanisms [41]. Consequently, their BOLD correlates may have a different physiological meaning [42].

Ictal events are often represented as boxcar functions with the duration of the clinical event [35, 42]. Arguing that such an approach does not account for ictal dynamics, more complex models of ictal BOLD changes have been proposed [38, 39, 43]. For example, Donaire et al. [43] divided the preictal, ictal and postictal periods into a sequence of 10 s boxcar functions. Tyvaert et al. [42] used sequential full-width at half-maximum 2 s gamma functions peaking around the ictal EEG onset as regressors of interest, in independent GLMs. Donaire et al. [43] and Tyvaert et al. [42] found a good agreement between the location of the earliest positive BOLD changes and the clinically inferred seizure onset zone (SOZ). Thornton et al. [38] partitioned each seizure into up to three phases, namely, early ictal (first EEG changes), clinical onset and late ictal (onset of high amplitude low frequency), each represented by a boxcar function. This group found greater concordance between the most significant BOLD clusters and the seizure onset zone (defined by icEEG), for the early ictal phase, which is not surprising because the ictal activity is likely to start at the seizure onset zone. See Fig. 21.5 for a personal case study of ictal-related BOLD changes investigating this approach [36].

In summary, different representations of interictal (and ictal) activity have been related to BOLD changes within regions known to be affected; more sophisticated representations have been leading to better results, but no study so far has identified an optimal approach conclusively, in large part due to the limitations of the "gold standard". For example, electroclinical information derived from scalp EEG has limited sensitivity and intracranial EEG has limited spatial sampling. A potentially more promising approach is to compare the BOLD maps with the area of resection, in light of surgical outcomes [44, 45].

21.6 Variability of the Haemodynamic Response Function

The most uncertain part of the analysis of EEG-fMRI data relates to the choice of the HRF in creating the model. A so-called canonic HRF, peaking at around 5 s after neuronal activation, has been used commonly in cognitive studies and in epilepsy. It was shown, however, that the HRF can have different shapes and latencies and that it may be important to use different HRFs to ensure the optimal uncovering of BOLD responses [46–48].

Various studies reported morphological differences in the HRF associated with epileptic discharges, when compared to that observed for sensory and cognitive events in the healthy brain [30, 48–51]. Differences across subjects, brain regions [46, 48], age and discharge frequency [52] have also been reported. Such findings do not necessarily imply a systematically abnormal HRF, since they only report that different HRFs are estimated from data in different conditions, when particular EEG-fMRI integration models are assumed (which can be close/far from the real physiology). An important caveat is that neurovascular coupling may be altered in epilepsy patients due to the presence of a structural lesion with implications for detection, localization, shape and sign of the HRF. However, the few studies in focal epilepsy assessing the statistical significance of such deviations within individual subjects have found weak effects [53]. A compromise between allowing HRF of almost arbitrary shape and the canonical form to account for variations in response onset is obtained by adding temporal and dispersion derivatives [54].

21.7 The Negative BOLD Response

The meaning of the decreased BOLD signal related to interictal spikes and ictal events has not been elucidated yet. Interictal- and ictal-related BOLD responses usually show increases (so-called positive BOLD response) in brain regions generating the ictal activity. Intriguingly, also negative BOLD signal changes (negative BOLD response) have been observed in most of the patients, usually remote from the epileptogenic zone (see Figs. 21.3 and 21.5). While the BOLD signal increases have been related to an increased neuronal and synaptic activity, the significance of the negatively BOLD response is less understood [55, 56]. Epileptic spike-related BOLD decreases remain unexplained because epileptic discharges are a marker of neuronal hyperexcitability, while BOLD decreases are thought to mainly reflect decreased blood flow linked to decreased neuronal activity [57].

Regional BOLD changes negatively correlated with epileptic activity have been observed in focal and generalized epilepsies [22, 29, 48, 58, 59]. In generalized epilepsies, commonly widespread spike-related BOLD decreases have been detected in the cortex [59–63]. Several groups consistently demonstrated the following pattern: activation of the thalamus and of mesial frontal regions as well as the cerebellum and prominent negative BOLD response involving the bilateral frontal, parietal and posterior cingulate cortex. These BOLD decreases were in close correspondence with the default mode network (DMN) [64], a network that is active when normal subjects are at rest and deactivated when they engage in a task. In the context of spike and wave discharges, this lifting of the default mode network was

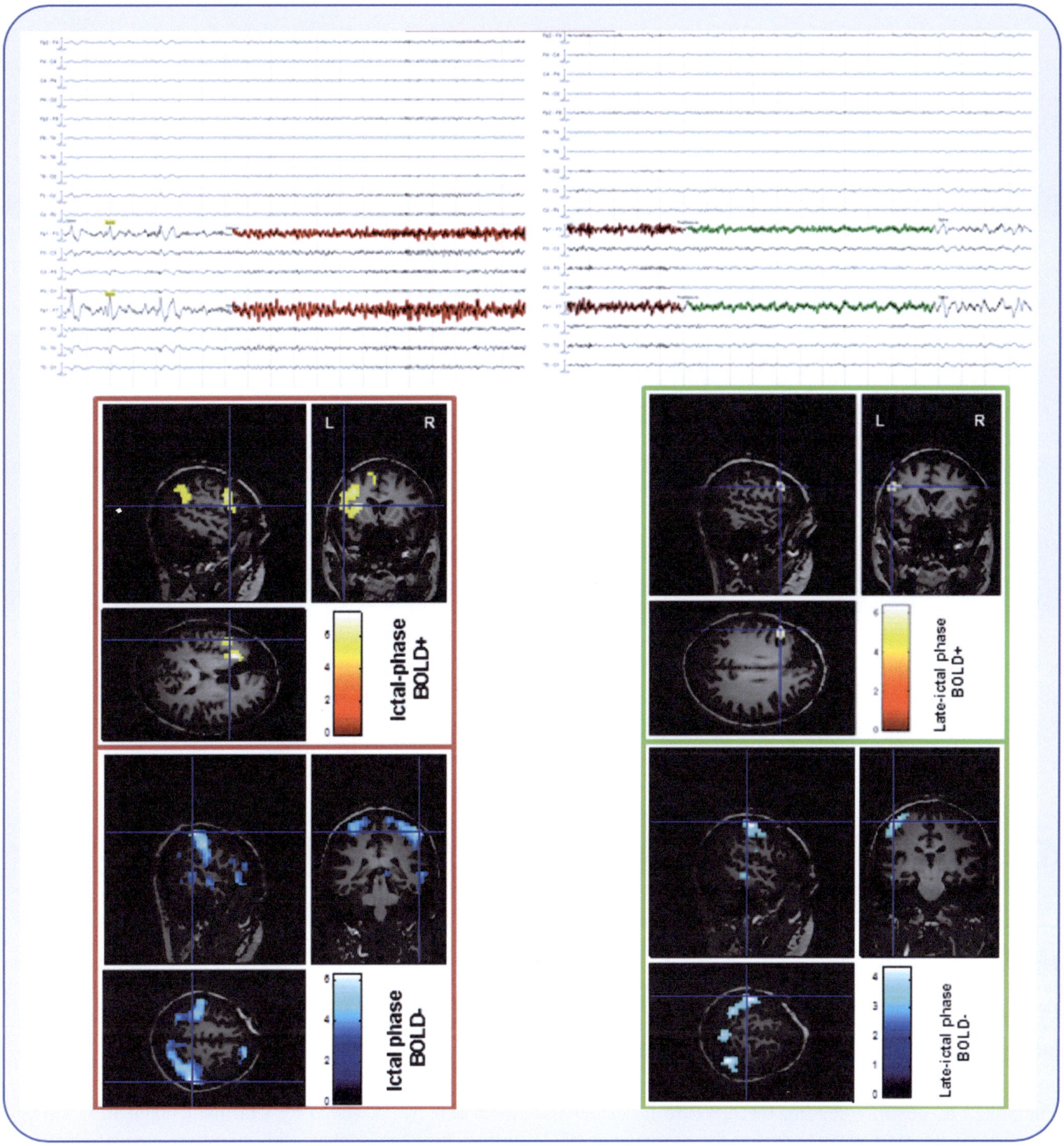

Fig. 21.5 *Left upper panel*: representative page of the EEG recorded during fMRI data acquisition showing a single clinical seizure (initial part of the ictal phase, underlined in red) characterized by low-voltage fast activity on the left anterior frontal leads (Fp1, F3 and F7 electrodes on scalp EEG). The EEG trace is shown in bipolar montage. *Left lower panel*: results of canonical GLM, SPM{T} ($p < 0.05$ corrected for multiple comparisons; red, positive BOLD responses; blue, negative BOLD responses) showing a BOLD signal increase over the left dorsolateral prefrontal cortex (crosshair at the global maxima) plus a smaller cluster in the ipsilateral temporo-parietal cortex. A strong negative BOLD response was detected at the bilateral central cortex (global maxima at the crosshair, right central cortex, BA4) and right cuneus. Results were overlaid on the patient's T1 scan. L = Left; R = right. *Right upper and lower panels* show the BOLD signal changes related to the second half of the seizures (late ictal, green). Note the BOLD signal increase is less pronounced, while the negative BOLD response is still present

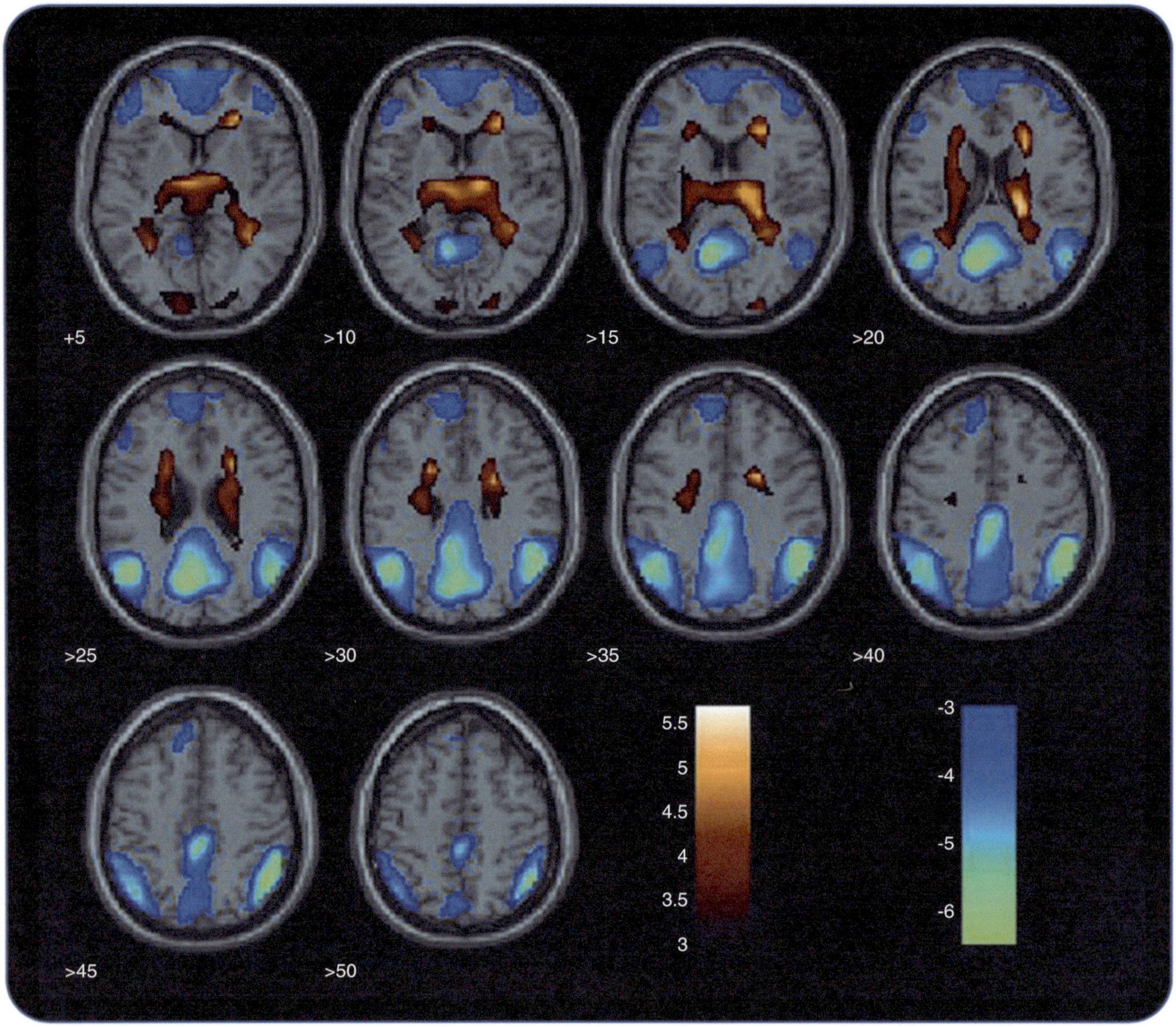

Fig. 21.6 BOLD changes related to 3 Hz generalized spike and waves in childhood and juvenile absence epilepsy. The results of second-level random effect group analysis of 15 patients with the HRF model starting at the absence onset are shown. Axial sections (MNI coordinates) display BOLD fMRI changes at $p < 0.001$ uncorrected. Increases in BOLD signal (red) were seen bilaterally in the thalamus, cerebellum and anterior cingulate gyrus, while BOLD decreases (blue) were mainly localized bilaterally in the medial prefrontal cortex, lateral parietal cortex, middle and posterior cingulate gyrus and precuneus (adapted from ref. 63)

interpreted as possibly causing the decrease in awareness experienced by most patients during the generalized EEG spike and wave discharge [59] (Fig. 21.6).

Recently, Fahoum et al. [65] investigated the intracranial neurophysiological correlates of runs of distant interictal epileptic discharges on default mode network. They observed that during spikes, regions of the DMN showing a decreased BOLD signal had a reduction in gamma frequencies paralleled by an increase in the EEG content of lower (<30 Hz) frequencies. We observed a similar relationship, between intracranial EEG and BOLD signal for the ictal events in the motor cortex [36]. In this case, we have shown that the neuronal activity measured by ictal intracranial EEG strongly differs between regions with seizure-related positive (prefrontal cortex) and negative BOLD (motor areas) response. The epileptogenic zone showed an increased BOLD signal during focal seizures that was characterized by a marked increase of power in frequencies ranging from 10 up to about 200 Hz. On the contrary, the distant ictal negative BOLD response correlated with increase in icEEG beta-frequencies. These findings are concordant with the ones recently reported by Fahoum at al [65]. and extend the role of lower frequencies as neurophysiological counterpart of the negative BOLD response to ictal events and to the motor system.

Schridde et al. [66] argued that a sustained BOLD decrease does not unequivocally imply decreased neuronal activity or cerebral blood flow. In fact, it can also result from increased neuronal activity depending on the complex interplay between haemodynamic and metabolism. In summary, a number of explanations for epilepsy-related BOLD decreases have been offered, which may be explored further using simultaneous icEEG-fMRI data recorded in humans, with its exquisite local sensitivity [67–69].

21.8 Sensitivity and Reproducibility in Epilepsy Studies

A limitation of EEG-fMRI recordings relies in the need of recording a sufficient number of IED to allow a statistical analysis feasible. Scalp EEG-fMRI depends on epileptiform events to be captured during recording sessions to detect associated BOLD changes. However, recordings lasting 20–30 min have low sensitivity to capture epileptiform activity, unless in cases with frequent IEDs. This is possibly related to the fact that at least 6–10 cm^2 area of the brain is required to be activated to produce an IED to be captured on scalp EEG [70, 71] and epileptiform events that are of smaller magnitude may remain undetected.

It has been shown that in adults 30% of cases showed no clear IED during studies; in another 30% of cases where IED has been identified and modelled, there has been no significant BOLD change which reflects limitations in the modelling of the fMRI signal [29]. In order to improve the sensitivity of technique, Grouiller et al. have suggested the construction of topographic maps from IEDs recorded during long-term video-EEG monitoring [72]. In turn these topographic maps are correlated with the EEG recorded during fMRI and used to evaluate BOLD changes associated with epileptic activity. This approach has increased sensitivity of EEG-fMRI to around 80% [45, 72, 73].

In order to increase the sensitivity, it is recommended also to consider forms of physiological noise to explain unknown variance in fMRI data. Several approaches attempted to characterize motion in the design matrix to improve sensitivity [74, 75]. The cardiac pulse, respiration and head and face movements, such as swallowing or eyeblinks, all are source of variance in fMRI data and represent possible confounds in the analysis (see Figs. 21.1 and 21.2).

As concern with the reproducibility of EEG-fMRI results, it was shown recently that scanning with a 3 T (3 Tesla) magnet was more sensitive than scanning with 1.5 T, a finding that is not surprising but was confirmed [76]. In the same study, the reproducibility of EEG-fMRI studies was demonstrated, making one more confident in clinical applicability. In Fig. 21.7, it is shown the reproducibility of BOLD signal changes in two EEG-fMRI studies performed 12 months apart in a 13-year-old boy with atypical BECTS.

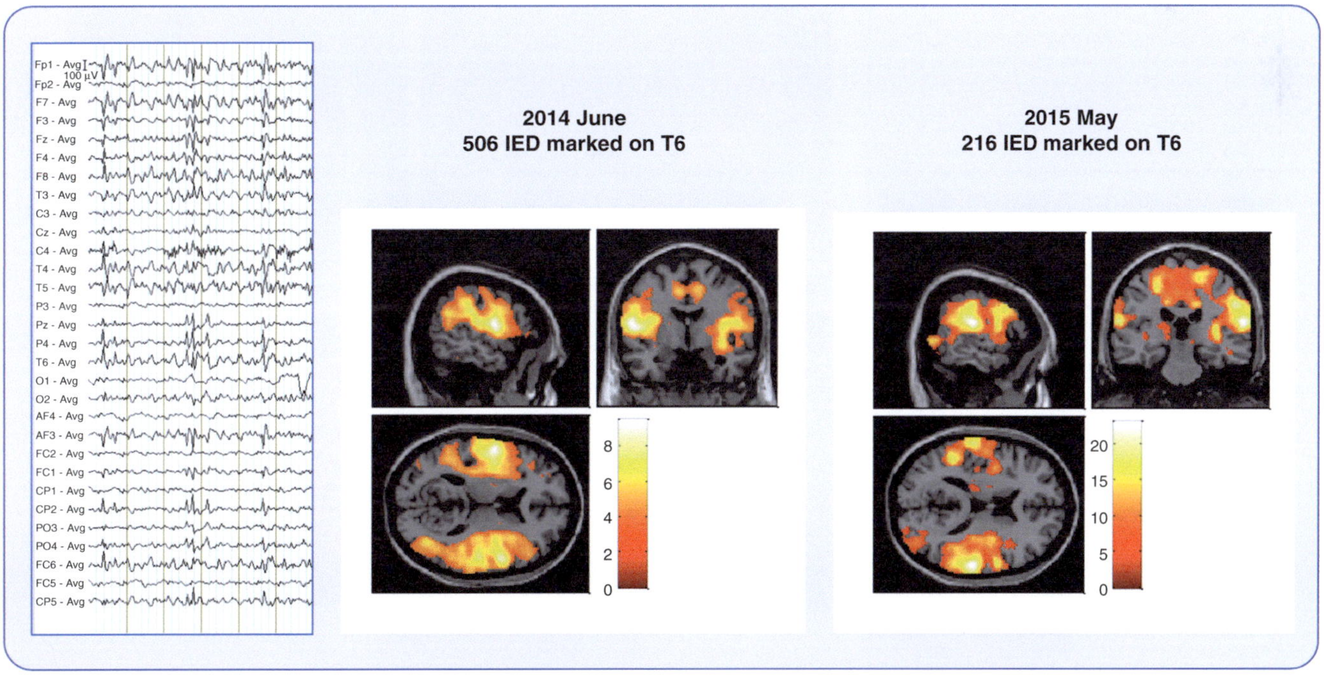

Fig. 21.7 The reproducibility of BOLD signal changes in two EEG-fMRI studies performed 12 months apart in a 13-year-old boy with atypical BECTS and electrical status epilepticus during sleep (ESES) is shown. A bilateral fronto-insular-temporal involvement is evident plus mesial frontal cortex and cingulate gyrus. BOLD results are displayed using a threshold of $p < 0.001$ uncorrected

21.9 EEG-fMRI in Children and Adolescents

In the last 15 years, several EEG-fMRI studies have been performed in children with different epilepsy forms [9]. The general pipeline and analysis methods do not differ with respect to adults. However, EEG-fMRI recordings in children are challenging due to a lack of cooperation, especially if the children are young or mentally disabled, which can often be the case with epilepsy patients. For this reason, it is necessary to minimize anxiety, so that the child will agree to enter the scanner and remain inside the scanner for the duration of the recording and to ensure that the child stays motionless throughout the entire examination (30 min on average). Some groups have used sedation in children undergoing EEG-fMRI recordings [52, 77–81]. These authors used chloral hydrate (50 mg/kg body weight) as sedative agent. By comparing haemodynamic changes in epilepsy patients with and without sedation, these groups were unable to describe significant effects of chloral hydrate on the results of EEG-fMRI maps [52, 77, 82]. In non-sedated children (usually older and without mental retardation), the anxiety can be minimized, if parents or someone familiar to the child stays in the MR room during data acquisition, if EEG-fMRI is simulated first to allow the child to get used to conditions of the test and if external stimulation (video- and audiotapes) is used before the test to distract the child [83]. However, even well-prepared children move extensively (head and body movements) during data acquisition. To reduce the effect of head motion on EEG-fMRI results, different algorithms have been developed to improve quality and sensitivity of fMRI analysis (see previous sections).

Jacobs et al. underscored the impact of age on the spike-related BOLD signal changes and demonstrated that children with focal lesional epilepsy show deactivations more frequently than activations in the epileptogenic zone compared to adults [52]. The shape of the HRF was different, especially in young children, where it peaked significantly later than the typical HRF in older children and adults. We and other groups have demonstrated that the BOLD changes related to IEDs in idiopathic childhood epilepsies, BECTS and occipital lobe epilepsies [50, 51] are maximized using noncanonical HRF (see Fig. 21.8). Despite these differences however, EEG-fMRI studies in children have been successful in elucidating the networks underlining several epileptic disorders like West syndrome [79], Lennox-Gastaut syndrome [81, 84], electrical status epilepticus during sleep [80], ring-20 epilepsy [33], eyelid myoclonia with absences and photosensitive epilepsies [85–87].

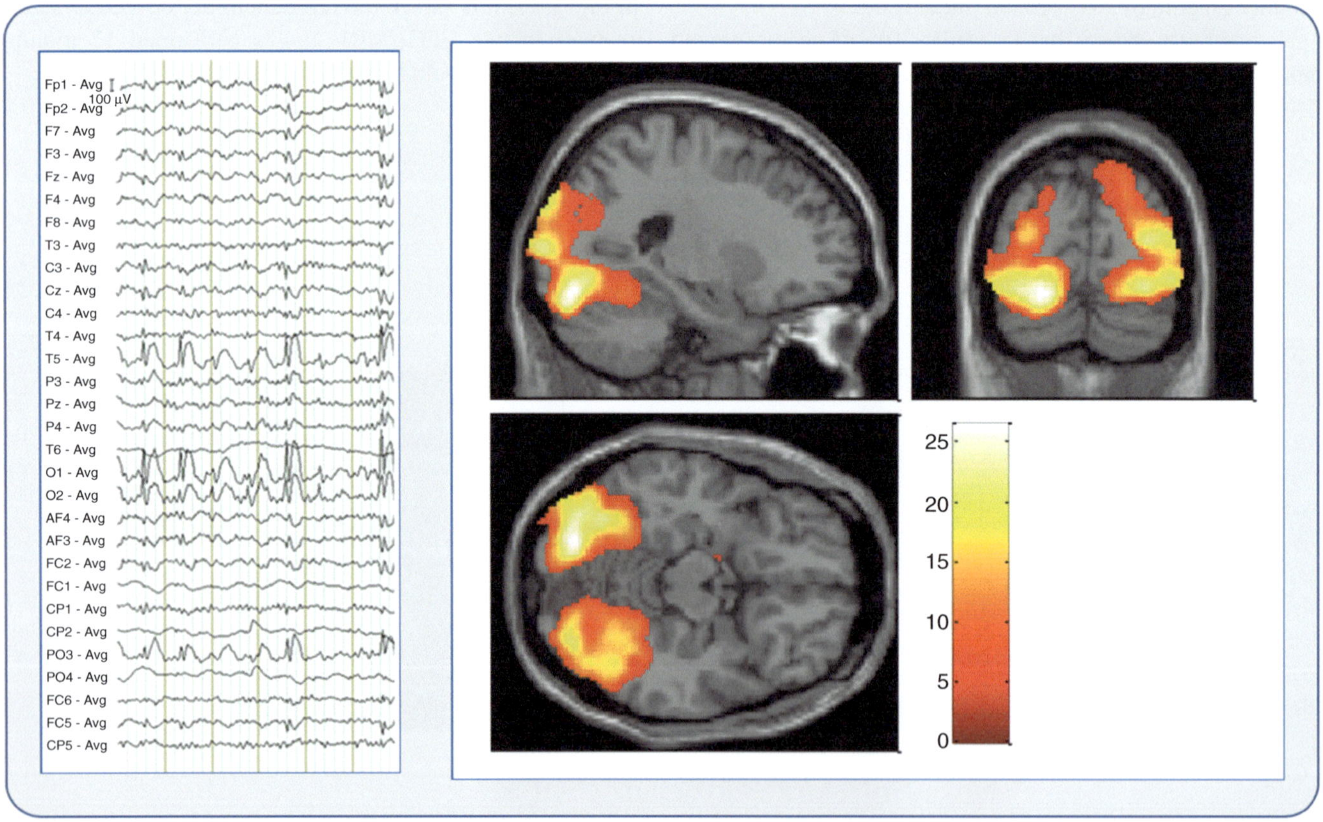

Fig. 21.8 *Left*: temporo-occipital spike and waves in the eye-closed condition in a 10-year-old girl with idiopathic childhood occipital lobe epilepsy (ICOE). These spikes recorded during fMRI scanning were the event of interest to model the BOLD effect. *Right*: BOLD results are displayed using a threshold of $p < 0.05$ corrected for multiple comparisons. BOLD signal increases were detected bilaterally in temporo-occipital cortex (a full description of BOLD changes in this patient population can be found in ref. [51])

21.10 Clinical Utility of EEG-fMRI Studies

As reported in previous sections, EEG-fMRI has been a fruitful research tool that contributed to the understanding of epileptic networks in several conditions, especially in idiopathic epilepsies and epileptic encephalopathy. However, its main clinical implications rely on its capability to add useful information to delineate the epileptogenic zone in focal epilepsy, in particular in the presurgical diagnostic workup. From this point of view, Pittau et al. reported that spike-related BOLD changes were present and concordant in patients with active EEG, and more specific localization of the epileptic focus was gained from EEG/fMRI in half of the patients who were scanned, when compared with scalp EEG alone [58, 88]. IED-related BOLD localization has been found to be more specific than scalp EEG for localizing invasively defined epileptic focus [89]. It has also shown that widespread and discordant IED-related BOLD changes are associated with poor postsurgical outcome [20, 44, 90], thus showing promise as a technique to predict surgical outcome noninvasively. Coan et al. have shown that localization of IED-related BOLD changes within 2 cm of the epileptogenic zone/area of surgical resection has a positive predictive value of 78% and negative predictive value of 81% [45]. Recently, Khoo et al. [91] retrospectively studied 37 consecutive patients who underwent stereo-EEG (SEEG) and EEG-fMRI that resulted in significant haemodynamic responses: 77% had at least 1 study with primary cluster concordant with the seizure onset zone. Discriminant analysis showed that the seizure onset zone was predictable with high confidence (>90%) if the primary cluster was highly significant and if the next significant cluster was much less significant or absent [91].

Mapping seizure-related BOLD changes using EEG-fMRI [34–40, 42] (see also Sect. 5) has offered an alternative to ictal SPECT in principal. Due to the rarity and unpredictability of seizures, most studies have only been case reports during interictal EEG-fMRI studies. However, following specific selection criteria based on seizure frequency and seizure types, the UCL group has published the largest ictal case series showing that seizure onset-related BOLD maps have the highest degree of concordance with independently defined invasive and/or noninvasive seizure onset zone, providing localization at sub-lobar level [34]. Moreover, EEG-fMRI was able to separate ictal onset, propagation and preictal-related BOLD changes [34, 92].

One relevant issue in the interpretation of BOLD imaging, especially in a presurgical clinical setting, is related to the fact that interictal and seizure-related maps show a multiplicity of BOLD clusters. Therefore, a number of concordance schemes have been developed [23, 31, 34, 37, 91] based on the location of statistically most significant or clinically most relevant cluster and by means of sophisticated statistical methods (i.e. dynamic causal modelling). These multiple clusters are seen in the epileptogenic zone, seizure propagation-related areas, symptomatogenic zone as well as resting state areas, which is more consistent with network involvement as opposed to mere spatial zone delineation [93].

Overall, these studies indicate that noninvasive spike- and seizure-related BOLD localization provided by scalp EEG-fMRI can be useful for guiding clinical decision and to assist implantation of intracranial electrodes in patients who require invasive evaluation prior to surgery. The exploration of the relationship between simultaneously recorded BOLD and intracranial EEG measures of network dynamics may provide useful insights for future treatment options, especially for epilepsy surgery.

References

1. Ogawa S, Tank DW, Menon R, Ellermann JM, Kim SG, Merkle H, Ugurbil K. Intrinsic signal changes accompanying sensory stimulation: functional brain mapping with magnetic resonance imaging. Proc Natl Acad Sci U S A. 1992;89:5951–5.
2. Kwong KK, Belliveau JW, Chesler DA, Goldberg IE, Weisskoff RM, Poncelet BP, et al. Dynamic magnetic resonance imaging of human brain activity during primary sensory stimulation. Proc Natl Acad Sci U S A. 1992;89:5675–9.
3. Chang C, Thomason ME, Glover GH. Mapping and correction of vascular hemodynamic latency in the BOLD signal. NeuroImage. 2008;43:90–102.
4. Logothetis NK, Pauls J, Augath M, Trinath T, Oeltermann A. Neurophysiological investigation of the basis of the fMRI signal. Nature. 2001;412:150–7.
5. Issa EB, Papanastassiou AM, DiCarlo JJ. Large-scale, high-resolution neurophysiological maps underlying FMRI of macaque temporal lobe. J Neurosci. 2013;33:15207–19.
6. Michel CM, Murray MM, Lantz G, Gonzalez S, Spinelli L, Grave de Peralta R. EEG source imaging. Clin Neurophysiol. 2004;115:2195–222.
7. Laufs H. A personalized history of EEG-fMRI integration. NeuroImage. 2012;62:1056–67.
8. Gotman J, Pittau F. Combining EEG and fMRI in the study of epileptic discharges. Epilepsia. 2011;52(Suppl. 4):38–42.
9. Moeller F, Stephani U, Siniatchkin M. Simultaneous EEG and fMRI recordings (EEG-fMRI) in children with epilepsy. Epilepsia. 2013;54:971–82.
10. van Graan LA, Lemieux L, Chaudhary UJ. Methods and utility of EEG-fMRI in epilepsy. Quant Imaging Med Surg. 2015;5:300–12.
11. Logothetis NK. The underpinnings of the BOLD functional magnetic resonance imaging signal. J Neurosci. 2003;23:3963–71.
12. Worsley KJ, Friston KJ. Analysis of fMRI time-series revisited—again. NeuroImage. 1995;2:173–81.
13. Allen PJ, Josephs O, Turner R. A method for removing imaging artifact from continuous EEG recorded during functional MRI. NeuroImage. 2000;12:230–9.
14. Ritter P, Becker R, Freyer F, Villringer A. EEG quality: the image acquisition artefact. In: Mulert C, Lemieux L, editors. EEG-fMRI physiological basis, technique, and applications. Berlin: Springer; 2010.
15. Ives JR, Warach S, Schmitt F, Edelman RR, Schomer DL. Monitoring the patient's EEG during echo planar MRI. Electroencephalogr Clin Neurophysiol. 1993;87:417–20.
16. Mullinger K, Bowtell R. Combining EEG and fMRI. Methods Mol Biol. 2011;711:303–26.

17. Lemieux L, Allen PJ, Franconi F, Symms MR, Fish DR. Recording of EEG during fMRI experiments: patient safety. Magn Reson Med. 1997;38:943–52.
18. Murta T, Leite M, Carmichael DW, Figueiredo P, Lemieux L. Electrophysiological correlates of the BOLD signal for EEG-informed fMRI. Hum Brain Mapp. 2015;36:391–414.
19. Abreu R, Leal A, Figueiredo P. EEG-informed fMRI: a review of data analysis methods. Front Hum Neurosci. 2018;12:29. https://doi.org/10.3389/fnhum.2018.00029.. eCollection 2018
20. An D, Fahoum F, Hall J, Olivier A, Gotman J, Dubeau F. Electroencephalography/functional magnetic resonance imaging responses help predict surgical outcome in focal epilepsy. Epilepsia. 2013;54:2184–94.
21. Flanagan D, Badawy RA, Jackson GD. EEG-fMRI in focal epilepsy: local activation and regional networks. Clin Neurophysiol. 2014;125:21–31.
22. Moeller F, Tyvaert L, Nguyen DK, LeVan P, Bouthillier A, Kobayashi E, et al. EEG-fMRI: adding to standard evaluations of patients with nonlesional frontal lobe epilepsy. Neurology. 2009;73:2023–30.
23. Vaudano AE, Avanzini P, Tassi L, Ruggieri A, Cantalupo G, Benuzzi F, et al. Causality within the epileptic network: An EEG-fMRI study validated by intracranial EEG. Front Neurol. 2013;14(4):185. https://doi.org/10.3389/fneur.2013.00185.. eCollection 2013
24. Formaggio E, Storti SF, Bertoldo A, Manganotti P, Fiaschi A, Toffolo GM. Integrating EEG and fMRI in epilepsy. NeuroImage. 2011;54:2719–31.
25. Liston AD, De Munck JC, Hamandi K, Laufs H, Ossenblok P, Duncan JS, Lemieux L. Analysis of EEG-fMRI data in focal epilepsy based on automated spike classification and signal space projection. NeuroImage. 2006;31:1015–24.
26. Marques JP, Rebola J, Figueiredo P, Pinto A, Sales F, Castelo-Branco M. ICA decomposition of EEG signal for fMRI processing in epilepsy. Hum Brain Mapp. 2009;30:2986–96.
27. Sharma NK, Pedreira C, Centeno M, Chaudhary UJ, Wehner T, França LG, et al. A novel scheme for the validation of an automated classification method for epileptic spikes by comparison with multiple observers. Clin Neurophysiol. 2017;128:1246–54.
28. Al-Asmi A, Benar CG, Gross DW, Khani YA, Andermann F, Pike B, et al. fMRI activation in continuous and spike-triggered EEG-fMRI studies of epileptic spikes. Epilepsia. 2003;44:1328–39.
29. Salek-Haddadi A, Diehl B, Hamandi K, Merschhemke M, Liston A, Friston K, et al. Hemodynamic correlates of epileptiform discharges: an EEG-fMRI study of 63 patients with focal epilepsy. Brain Res. 2006;1088:148–66.
30. Jacobs J, Levan P, Moeller F, Boor R, Stephani U, Gotman J, Siniatchkin M. Hemodynamic changes preceding the interictal EEG spike in patients with focal epilepsy investigated using simultaneous EEG-fMRI. NeuroImage. 2009;45:1220–31.
31. Vulliemoz S, Rodionov R, Carmichael DW, Thornton R, Guye M, et al. Continuous EEG source imaging enhances analysis of EEG-fMRI in focal epilepsy. NeuroImage. 2010;49:3219–29.
32. Makeig S, Westerfield M, Jung TP, Enghoff S, Townsend J, Courchesne E, Sejnowski TJ. Dynamic brain sources of visual evoked responses. Science. 2002;295:690–4.
33. Vaudano AE, Ruggieri A, Vignoli A, Avanzini P, Benuzzi F, Gessaroli G, et al. Epilepsy-related brain networks in ring chromosome 20 syndrome: an EEG-fMRI study. Epilepsia. 2014;55(3):403–13.
34. Chaudhary UJ, Carmichael DW, Rodionov R, Thornton RC, Bartlett P, Vulliemoz S, et al. Mapping preictal and ictal haemodynamic networks using video-electroencephalography and functional imaging. Brain. 2012;135:3645–63.
35. Meletti S, Vignoli A, Benuzzi F, Avanzini P, Ruggieri A, et al. Ictal involvement of the nigrostriatal system in subtle seizures of ring chromosome 20 epilepsy. Epilepsia. 2012;53:156–60.
36. Meletti S, Vaudano AE, Tassi L, Caruana F, Avanzini P. Intracranial time-frequency correlates of seizure-related negative BOLD response in the sensory-motor network. Clin Neurophysiol. 2015;126:847–9.
37. Murta T, Leal A, Garrido MI, Figueiredo P. Dynamic causal modelling of epileptic seizure propagation pathways: a combined EEG-fMRI study. NeuroImage. 2012;62:1634–42.
38. Thornton RC, Rodionov R, Laufs H, Vulliemoz S, Vaudano A, Carmichael D, et al. Imaging haemodynamic changes related to seizures: comparison of EEG based general linear model, independent component analysis of fMRI and intracranial EEG. NeuroImage. 2010;53:196–205.
39. Tyvaert L, LeVan P, Dubeau F, Gotman J. Noninvasive dynamic imaging of seizures in epileptic patients. Hum Brain Mapp. 2009;30:3993–4011.
40. Chaudhary UJ, Duncan JS, Lemieux L. Mapping hemodynamic correlates of seizures using fMRI: a review. Hum Brain Mapp. 2013;34:447–66.
41. De Curtis M, Avanzini G. Interictal spikes in focal epileptogenesis. Prog Neurobiol. 2001;63:541–67.
42. Tyvaert L, Hawco C, Kobayashi E, LeVan P, Dubeau F, Gotman J. Different structures involved during ictal and interictal epileptic activity in malformations of cortical development: An EEG-fMRI study. Brain. 2008;131:2042–60.
43. Donaire A, Bargallo N, Falcon C, Maestro I, Carreno M, Setoain J, et al. Identifying the structures involved in seizure generation using sequential analysis of ictal-fMRI data. NeuroImage. 2009;47:173–83.
44. Thornton R, Vulliemoz S, Rodionov R, Carmichael DW, Chaudhary UJ, Diehl B, et al. Epileptic networks in focal cortical dysplasia revealed using electroencephalography-functional magnetic resonance imaging. Ann Neurol. 2011;70:822–37.
45. Coan AC, Chaudhary UJ, Grouiller F, Campos BM, Perani S, De Ciantis A, et al. EEG-fMRI in the presurgical evaluation of temporal lobe epilepsy. J Neurol Neurosurg Psychiatry. 2016;87:642–9.
46. Benar CG, Gross DW, Wang Y, Petre V, Pike B, Dubeau F, Gotman J. The BOLD response to interictal epileptiform discharges. NeuroImage. 2002;17:1182–92.
47. Bagshaw AP, Aghakhani Y, Benar CG, Kobayashi E, Hawco C, Dubeau F, et al. EEG-fMRI of focal epileptic spikes: analysis with multiple haemodynamic functions and comparison with gadolinium-enhanced MR angiograms. Hum Brain Mapp. 2004;22:179–92.
48. Grouiller F, Vercueil L, Krainik A, Segebarth C, Kahane P, David O. Characterization of the hemodynamic modes associated with interictal epileptic activity using a deformable model-based analysis of combined EEG and functional MRI recordings. Hum Brain Mapp. 2010;31:1157–73.
49. Moeller F, Siebner HR, Wolff S, Muhle H, Boor R, Granert O, et al. Changes in activity of striato-thalamo-cortical network precede generalized spike wave discharges. NeuroImage. 2008;39:1839–49.
50. Masterton RA, Harvey AS, Archer JS, Lillywhite LM, Abbott DF, Scheffer IE, Jackson GD. Focal epileptiform spikes do not show a canonical BOLD response in patients with benign rolandic epilepsy (BECTS). NeuroImage. 2010;51:252–60.
51. Meletti S, Ruggieri A, Avanzini P, Caramaschi E, Filippini M, Bergonzini P, et al. Extrastriate visual cortex in idiopathic occipital epilepsies: the contribution of retinotopic areas to spike generation. Epilepsia. 2016;57:896–906.
52. Jacobs J, Hawco C, Kobayashi E, Boor R, LeVan P, Stephani U, et al. Variability of the hemodynamic response as a function of age and frequency of epileptic discharge in children with epilepsy. NeuroImage. 2008;40:601–14.
53. Lemieux L, Laufs H, Carmichael D, Paul JS, Walker MC, Duncan JS. Noncanonical spike-related BOLD responses in focal epilepsy. Hum Brain Mapp. 2008;29:329–45.
54. Friston KJ, Fletcher P, Josephs O, Holmes A, Rugg MD, Turner R. Event-related fMRI: characterizing differential responses. NeuroImage. 1998;7:30–40.
55. Shmuel A, Yacoub E, Pfeuffer J, Van de Moortele PF, Adriany G, Hu X, et al. Sustained negative BOLD, blood flow and oxygen

consumption response and its coupling to the positive response in the human brain. Neuron. 2002;36:1195–210.
56. Pittau F, Fahoum F, Zelmann R, Dubeau F, Gotman J. Negative BOLD response to interictal epileptic discharges in focal epilepsy. Brain Topogr. 2013;26:627–40.
57. Shmuel A, Augath M, Oeltermann A, Logothetis NK. Negative functional MRI response correlates with decreases in neuronal activity in monkey visual area V1. Nat Neurosci. 2006;9:569–77.
58. Benar CG, Grova C, Kobayashi E, Bagshaw AP, Aghakhani Y, Dubeau F, Gotman J. EEG-fMRI of epileptic spikes: concordance with EEG source localization and intracranial EEG. NeuroImage. 2006;30:1161–70.
59. Gotman J, Grova C, Bagshaw A, Kobayashi E, Aghakhani Y, Dubeau F. Generalized epileptic discharges show thalamocortical activation and suspension of the default state of the brain. Proc Natl Acad Sci U S A. 2005;102:15236–40.
60. Hamandi K, Salek-Haddadi A, Laufs H, Liston A, Friston K, Fish DR, et al. EEG-fMRI of idiopathic and secondarily generalized epilepsies. NeuroImage. 2006;31:1700–10.
61. Salek-Haddadi A, Lemieux L, Merschhemke M, Friston KJ, Duncan JS, Fish DR. Functional magnetic resonance imaging of human absence seizures. Ann Neurol. 2003;53:663–7.
62. Bai X, Vestal M, Berman R, Negishi M, Spann M, Vega C, et al. Dynamic time course of typical childhood absence seizures: EEG, behavior, and functional magnetic resonance imaging. J Neurosci. 2010;30:5884–93.
63. Benuzzi F, Mirandola L, Pugnaghi M, Farinelli V, Tassinari CA, Capovilla G, et al. Increased cortical BOLD signal anticipates generalized spike and wave discharges in adolescents and adults with idiopathic generalized epilepsies. Epilepsia. 2012;53:622–30.
64. Raichle ME, MacLeod AM, Snyder AZ, Powers WJ, Gusnard DA, Shulman GL. A default mode of brain function. Proc Natl Acad Sci U S A. 2001;98:676–82.
65. Fahoum F, Zelmann R, Tyvaert L, Dubeau F, Gotman J. Epileptic discharges affect the default mode network—fMRI and intracerebral EEG evidence. PLoS One. 2013;8:e68038.
66. Schridde U, Khubchandani M, Motelow JE, Sanganahalli BG, Hyder F, Blumenfeld H. Negative BOLD with large increases in neuronal activity. Cereb Cortex. 2008;18:1814–27.
67. Carmichael DW, Thornton JS, Rodionov R, Thornton R, McEvoy AW, et al. Feasibility of simultaneous intracranial EEG-fMRI in humans: a safety study. NeuroImage. 2010;49:379–90.
68. Carmichael DW, Vulliemoz S, Rodionov R, Walker M, Rosenkranz K, et al. Simultaneous intracranial EEG-fMRI in humans suggests that high gamma frequencies are the closest neurophysiological correlate of BOLD fMRI. In: 19th Annual Meeting & Exhibition of the International Society for Magnetic Resonance in Medicine. Montreal. 2011.
69. Vulliemoz S, Carmichael DW, Rosenkranz K, Diehl B, Rodionov R, et al. Simultaneous intracranial EEG and fMRI of interictal epileptic discharges in humans. NeuroImage. 2011;54:182–90.
70. Tao JX, Ray A, Hawes-Ebersole S, Ebersole JS. Intracranial EEG substrates of scalp EEG interictal spikes. Epilepsia. 2005;46:669–76.
71. Ray A, Tao JX, Hawes-Ebersole SM, Ebersole JS. Localizing value of scalp EEG spikes: a simultaneous scalp and intracranial study. Clin Neurophysiol. 2007;118:69–79.
72. Grouiller F, Thornton RC, Groening K, Spinelli L, Duncan JS, Schaller K, et al. With or without spikes: localization of focal epileptic activity by simultaneous electroencephalography and functional magnetic resonance imaging. Brain. 2011;134:2867–86.
73. Elshoff L, Groening K, Grouiller F, Wiegand G, Wolff S, Michel C, Stephani U, Siniatchkin M. The value of EEG-fMRI and EEG source analysis in the presurgical setup of children with refractory focal epilepsy. Epilepsia. 2012;53:1597–606.
74. Friston KJ, Ashburner J, Frith C, Poline JB, Heather JD, Frackowiak RSJ. Spatial registration and normalization of images. Hum Brain Mapp. 1995;3:165–89.
75. Lemieux L, Salek-Haddadi A, Lund TE, Laufs H, Carmichael D. Modelling large motion events in fMRI studies of patients with epilepsy. Magn Reson Imaging. 2007;25:894–901.
76. Gholipour T, Moeller F, Pittau F, Dubeau F, Gotman J. Reproducibility of interictal EEG-fMRI results in patients with epilepsy. Epilepsia. 2011;52:433–42.
77. Jacobs J, Kobayashi E, Boor R, Muhle H, Wolff S, Hawco C, Dubeau F, Jansen O, Stephani U, Gotman J, Siniatchkin M. Hemodynamic responses to interictal epileptiform discharges in children with symptomatic epilepsy. Epilepsia. 2007;48:2068–78.
78. Moeller F, Siebner H, Wolff S, Muhle H, Boor R, Granert O, et al. EEG-fMRI in children with untreated childhood absence epilepsy. Epilepsia. 2008;49:1510–9.
79. Siniatchkin M, van Baalen A, Jacobs J, Moeller F, Moehring J, Boor R, et al. Different neuronal networks are associated with spikes and slow activity in hypsarrhythmia. Epilepsia. 2007;48:2312–21.
80. Siniatchkin M, Groening K, Moehring J, Moeller F, Boor R, Brodbeck V, et al. Neuronal networks in children with continuous spikes and waves during slow sleep. Brain. 2011;133:2798–813.
81. Siniatchkin M, Coropceanu D, Moeller F, Boor R, Stephani U. EEG-fMRI reveals activation of brainstem and thalamus in patients with Lennox-Gastaut syndrome. Epilepsia. 2011;52:766–74.
82. Moehring J, Coropceanu D, Galka A, Moeller F, Wolff S, et al. Improving sensitivity of EEGfMRI studies in epilepsy: the role of sleep-specific activity. Neurosci Lett. 2011;505:211–5.
83. Centeno M, Tierney TM, Perani S, Shamshiri EA, StPier K, Wilkinson C, et al. Optimising EEG-fMRI for localisation of focal epilepsy in children. PLoS One. 2016;11(2):e0149048. https://doi.org/10.1371/journal.pone.0149048.. eCollection 2016
84. Pillay N, Archer JS, Badawy RA, Flanagan DF, Berkovic SF, Jackson G. Networks underlying paroxysmal fast activity and slow spike and wave in Lennox-Gastaut syndrome. Neurology. 2013;81:665–73.
85. Vaudano AE, Ruggieri A, Tondelli M, Avanzini P, Benuzzi F, Gessaroli G, et al. The visual system in eyelid myoclonia with absences. Ann Neurol. 2014;76:412–27.
86. Moeller F, Muthuraman M, Stephani U, Deuschl G, Raethjen J, Siniatchkin M. Representation and propagation of epileptic activity in absences and generalized photoparoxysmal responses. Hum Brain Mapp. 2013;34:1896–909.
87. Vaudano AE, Ruggieri A, Avanzini P, Gessaroli G, Cantalupo G, et al. Photosensitive epilepsy is associated with reduced inhibition of alpha rhythm generating networks. Brain. 2017;140:981–97.
88. Pittau F, Dubeau F, Gotman J. Contribution of EEG/fMRI to the definition of the epileptic focus. Neurology. 2012;78:1479–87.
89. van Houdt PJ, de Munck JC, Leijten FS, Huiskamp GJ, Colon AJ, Boon PA, Ossenblok PP. EEG-fMRI correlation patterns in the presurgical evaluation of focal epilepsy: a comparison with electrocorticographic data and surgical outcome measures. NeuroImage. 2013;75:238–48.
90. Thornton R, Laufs H, Rodionov R, Cannadathu S, Carmichael DW, Vulliemoz S, et al. EEG correlated functional MRI and postoperative outcome in focal epilepsy. J Neurol Neurosurg Psychiatry. 2010;81:922–7.
91. Khoo HM, Hao Y, von Ellenrieder N, Zazubovits N, Hall J, Olivier A, et al. The hemodynamic response to interictal epileptic discharges localizes the seizure-onset zone. Epilepsia. 2017;58:811–23.
92. Vaudano AE, Carmichael DW, Salek-Haddadi A, Ramp S, Stefan H, Lemieux L, Koepp MJ. Networks involved in seizure initiation. A reading epilepsy case studied with EEG-fMRI and MEG. Neurology. 2012;79:249–53.
93. Laufs H. Functional imaging of seizures and epilepsy: evolution from zones to networks. Curr Opin Neurol. 2012;25:194–200.

Part II

Pathological EEG Patterns

22 Abnormal Neonatal Patterns

Massimo Mastrangelo, Barbara Scelsa, and Francesco Pisani

22.1 Abnormal Neonatal EEG

The distinctive features of the neonatal electroencephalogram (EEG), the development of the behavioral states and of the EEG patterns from 27 weeks of conceptional age (CA) to the end of the neonatal period have been described in the first part of this Manual. Particular attention has been devoted to the development of the EEG features as a function of the different stages of the central nervous system development.

This chapter is dedicated to the description of the most characteristic artifacts and the abnormal EEG findings in the neonatal age. As in the previous chapter, we have emphasized the iconographic material, taken from EEG recordings carried out within the daily clinical practice of the authors at Buzzi Hospital in Milan (Pediatric Neurology Unit and Neonatal Intensive Care Unit) and at University Hospital of Parma (Pediatric Neurophysiology Lab and Neonatal Intensive Care Unit). The caption of the figures will report the anamnestic, clinical, and instrumental data related to the clinical cases described, in order to underline and confirm the importance of a complete integration among clinical, neurophysiological, and neuroimaging data in the approach of newborns with neurological impairments.

22.2 Introduction

In the previous chapter, it has already been emphasized that the EEG, together with the clinical and neuroimaging data, has both a diagnostic and an early prognostic meaning in the neonatal age [1, 2]. It is clear how the EEG allows an essential evaluation of the degree of development and functionality of the central nervous system (CNS), becoming one of the actions of a multispecialistic management of a newborn with neurological and possibly systemic diseases.

The current neonatal neurology assumes the need to integrate the information acquired by EEG recordings with both the clinical and neuroradiological findings at the same time, especially for the "abnormal EEG pattern," before giving a prognosis. This integrated approach through the three points of observations (clinical, neurophysiological, and anatomomorphological) allows to provide the clinician and the neonatologist, in this context, with important information to correctly manage the pathology in progress.

22.3 Extra Cerebral Artifacts

In Figs. 22.1–22.18, a series of images related to newborns with and without neurological pathology are shown. In the caption of each single image, the symbol "A" indicates tracings with artifacts, the gestational age ("GA") expressed in weeks, and the age at the time the study was carried out (CA); finally, the type of artifact and the location is described.

For the visual analysis and interpretation of the EEG recording, it is essential to distinguish the electrical activity coming from the brain and from the extracerebral artifacts [3]. Although frequently extracerebral artifacts are easily identifiable, there are some artifacts that may not be recognized as such, thus leading to false-positive recognition of pathological findings, which can result in erroneous interpretation of the recording and consequently lead to an incorrect clinical management of the newborn.

There are artifacts secondary to the technical-instrumental characteristics of the recording ("technical artifacts") and artifacts secondary to physiologic manifestations of the child ("biological or physiological artifacts"). As for the "technical artifacts" related to the recording conditions, in addition to the faulty contact of the electrode (Figs. 22.1 and 22.2), to field problems related to the electrode wire itself or to the EEG connection cable (Fig. 22.10), and to the presence of alternating current (Fig. 22.1), it is known that in Neonatal

M. Mastrangelo (✉) · B. Scelsa
Pediatrics Department, V.Buzzi Children Hospital, ASST Fatebenefratelli Sacco, Milan, Italy
e-mail: massimo.mastrangelo@asst-fbf-sacco.it

F. Pisani
Medicine and Surgery Department, Parma University, Parma, Italy

O. Mecarelli (ed.), *Clinical Electroencephalography*, https://doi.org/10.1007/978-3-030-04573-9_22

Intensive Care Units, there are often several monitors and other devices, including infusion pumps and mechanical ventilators (Figs. 22.3 and 22.4), which can interfere with the acquisition of the EEG signal. The "biological or physiological artifacts" are instead related to the patient. Several examples of artifacts spreading to the scalp are illustrated: the electrical signal generated from the electrocardiogram (EKG, Fig. 22.9); more or less massive or rhythmical muscle contractions (Fig. 22.12); diffuse or segmental tremors at low, medium, or high frequency (Figs. 22.13–22.16); the anterior fontanel pulsations (Fig. 22.5) or of the caregiver who carries it; eye movements (Fig. 22.8); suction and hiccup (Figs. 22.11, 22.12, 22.17, and 22.18); sweating (Figs. 22.5 and 22.13); movements caused by parents rocking the newborn (Figs. 22.6 and 22.7).

The presence of the EEG technician, appropriately trained for the newborn management, appears essential in the definition and elimination of technical artifacts. On several occasions, however, physiological artifacts cannot be eliminated, but they must nevertheless be identified and described in the report that accompanies the recording. Furthermore, polygraphy helps to distinguish artifact from an activity of cerebral origin: the eye movements (Fig. 22.8) and the rhythmic deflection of the QRS cardiac complex are detected on the EEG traces with the same deflection (Fig. 22.9), the eye artifact is generally irregular and of high amplitude, the EKG artifact is rhythmic and of high frequency, and the breathing movements detected by the pneumogram and the rhythmic activity produced by the ventilator machines generally induce a slow rhythmic deflection (Figs. 22.3 and 22.4). On the other hand, rocking the newborn causes a slow and intermittent, but irregular, sinusoidal activity on the EEG traces (Figs. 22.6 and 22.7). Sucking, especially when the baby's head is rotated with the temporal electrode close to the bed, can result in a double artifact, with rapid activity due to muscle contraction and slow rhythmic activity linked to the movement of the mandibular segment (Figs. 22.1 and 22.12).

The simultaneous video recording is an important technological acquisition, above all for the possibility to review offline what happened during the recording [4], but this cannot absolutely exclude the visual monitoring of the recording in progress. Therefore, once the child is prepared for the recording, the EEG technician must check the characteristics of the recording and is responsible for the recording that he provides to the physician for the final interpretation.

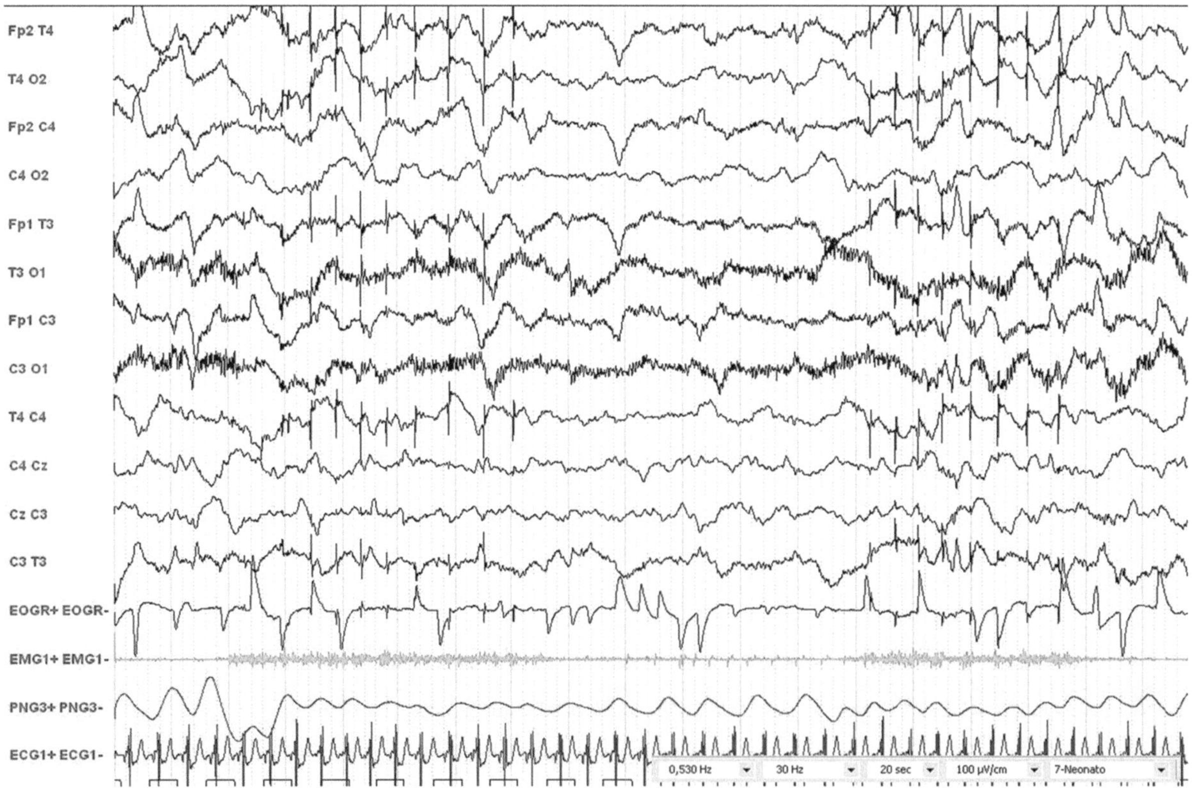

Fig. 22.1 40 weeks GA, 40.2 weeks CA. Healthy newborn. Wakefulness, open eyes. Sucking artifact in T4 and T3: rhythmic fast spikes strictly related to the rhythmic contraction of mylohyoid muscle in EMG channel. Low-voltage fast activity muscle artifact in O1 and less evident in Fp1–Fp2. Alternating current artifact (50 Hz) of variable amplitude involving left side electrodes (mostly O1) and Fp2, produced by high skin-electrode interface impedance

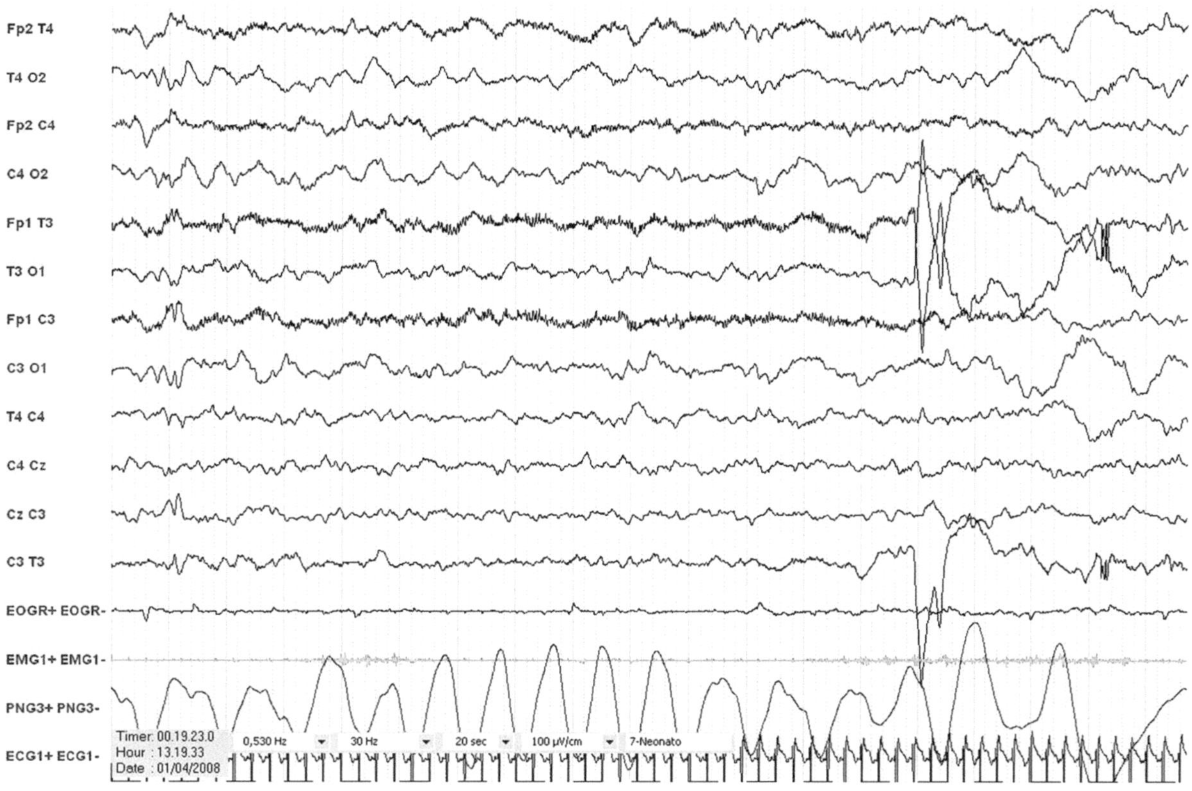

Fig. 22.2 39 weeks GA, 39.4 weeks CA. Healthy newborn. Wakefulness, open eyes. Artifact in T3 with fast spike >high amplitude and sharp slow wave produced by unstable T3 electrode: abnormal cable-electrode connection. Artifact in Fp1–Fp2 with fast continuous and low-voltage activity produced by frontal muscle contraction

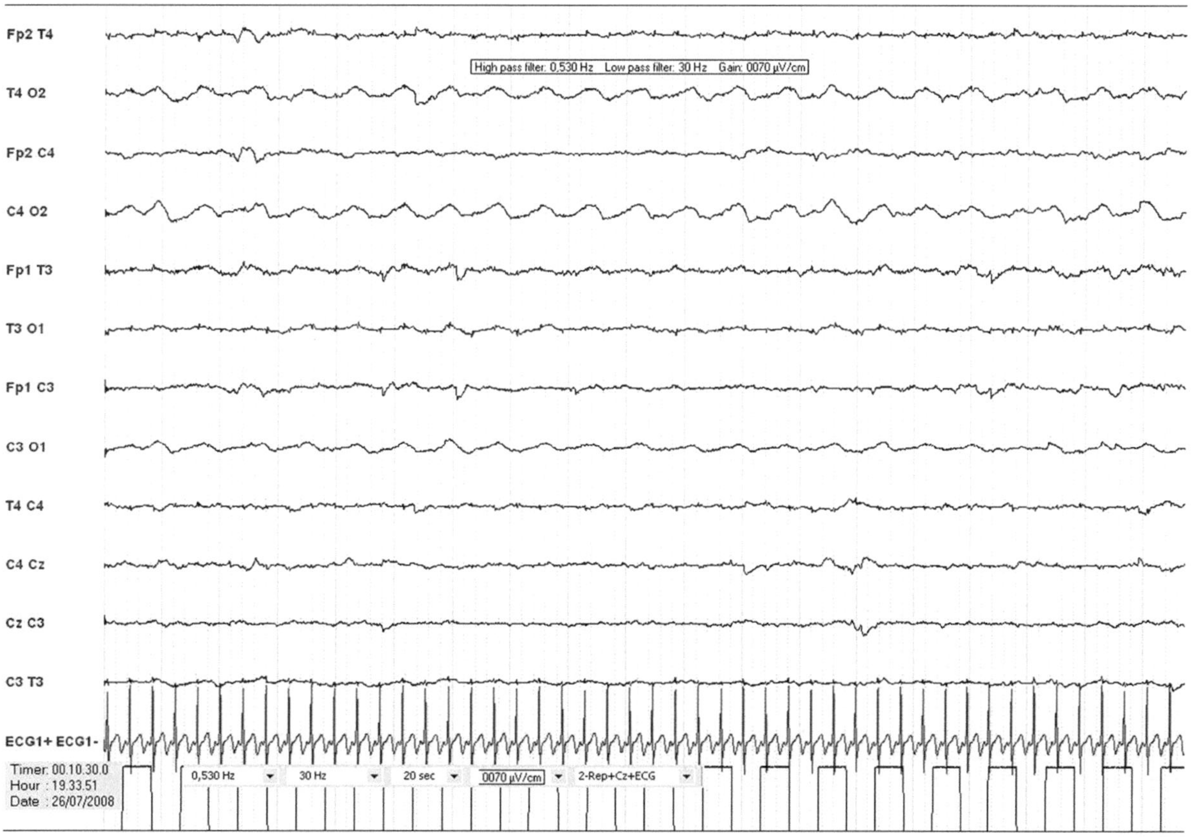

Fig. 22.3 32 weeks GA, 33.1 weeks CA. Coma in newborn affected by intraventricular grade IV hemorrhage. Constantly inactive tracing. Artifact in O2 and less evident in O1: slow and rhythmic activity, synchronous with head movements and with mechanical ventilation. Low-voltage EKG artifact in several leads

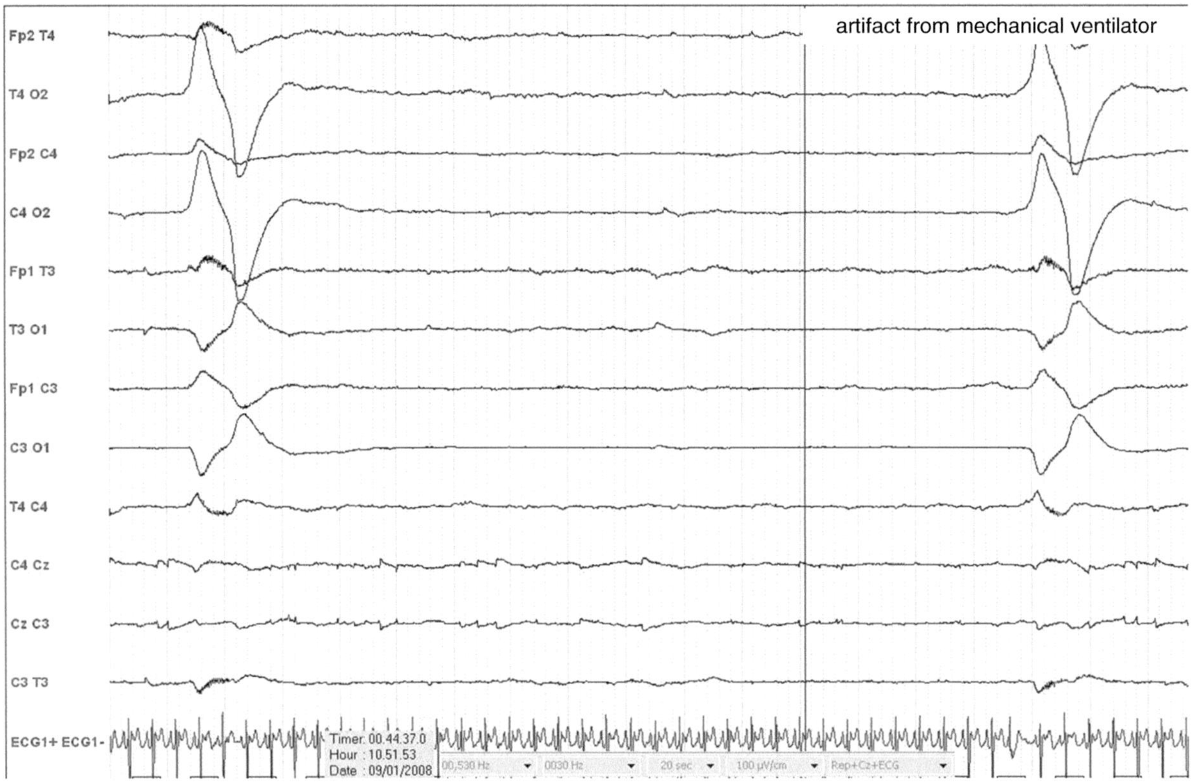

Fig. 22.4 27 weeks GA, 42.3 weeks CA. Coma in newborn after prolonged cardiac arrest. Mechanical ventilation. Constantly inactive tracing. Complex artifacts: short sequence of low-voltage fast activity (frequency over 25 Hz) superimposed on a diphasic and high-amplitude slow deflection. The same artifact repeats after 14 s related to the trigger of the mechanical ventilation system

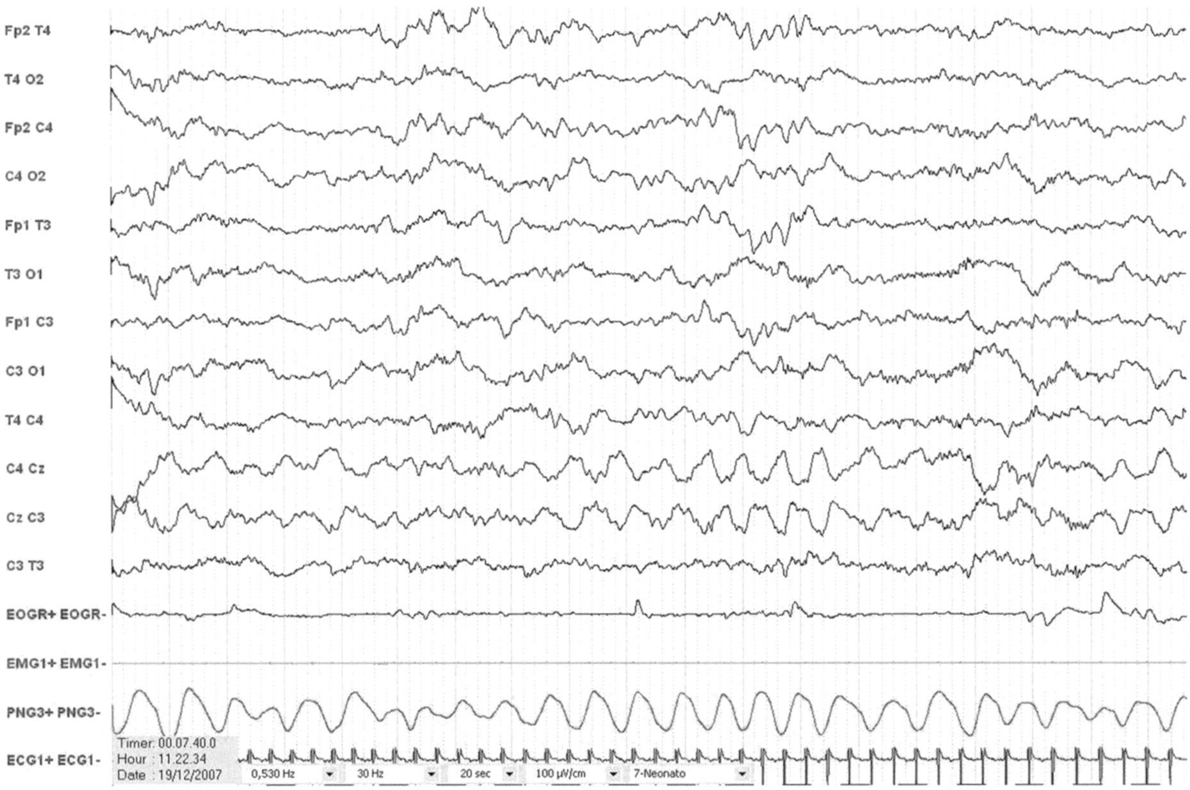

Fig. 22.5 36 weeks GA, 38.3 weeks CA. Healthy newborn. Cz artifact with rhythmic deflections having the same frequency of abdominal respiration and reflecting increasing/decreasing impedance in an unstable electrode, partially placed near the anterior fontanel. Tracé alternant (quiet sleep) is the EEG pattern in this newborn, while polygraphic parameters (presence of eye movements and irregular respiration) are consistent with active sleep. Moreover a very slow deflection artifact is present in all leads, due to excessive sweating

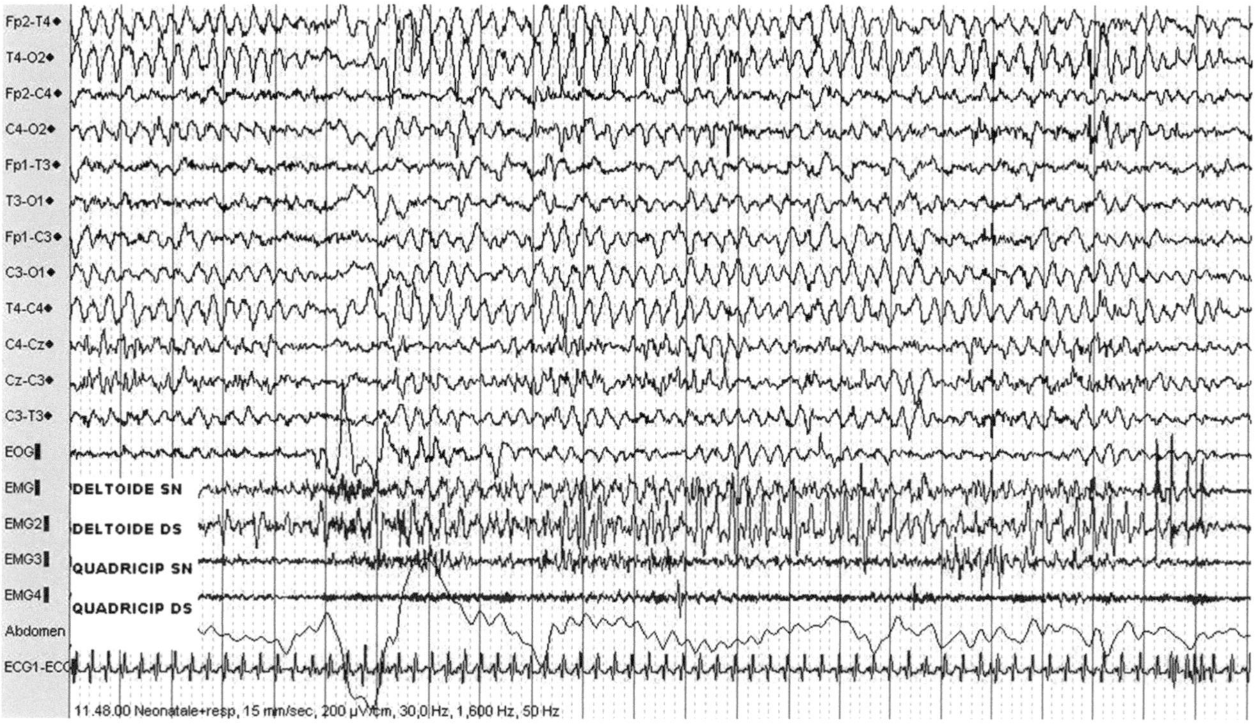

Fig. 22.6 40 weeks GA, 40.3 weeks CA. Healthy newborn. The infant is difficult to console. Artifacts in all leads more prominent in T4, C4, and C3 with high-voltage rhythmic activity, mimicking the same fluctuation frequency of polygraphic electrodes (EMG and abdominal transducer) produced by parent's rocking of the child

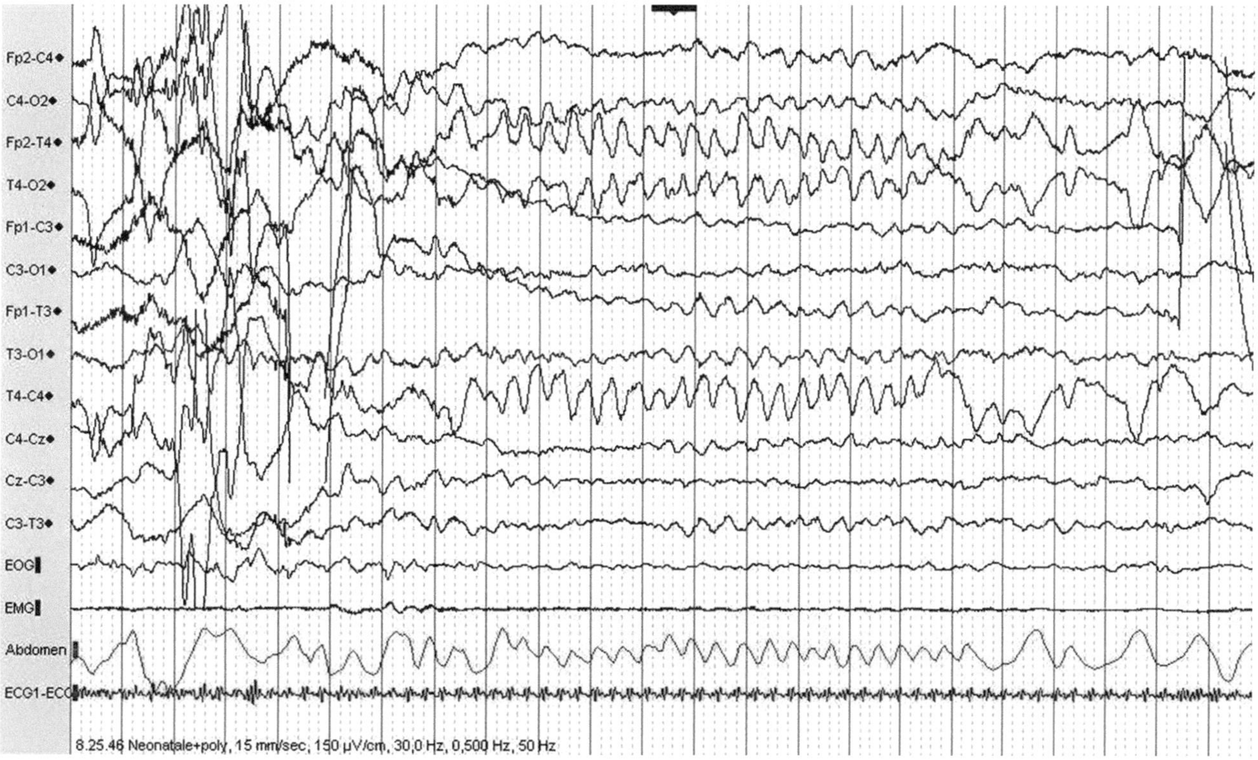

Fig. 22.7 38 weeks GA, 39 weeks CA. Awake, difficult to console. Same rocking artifact only in T4 which results in electrode instability. In the right side of the figure, T4 electrode "pop" is recognized by irregular high-voltage slow waves

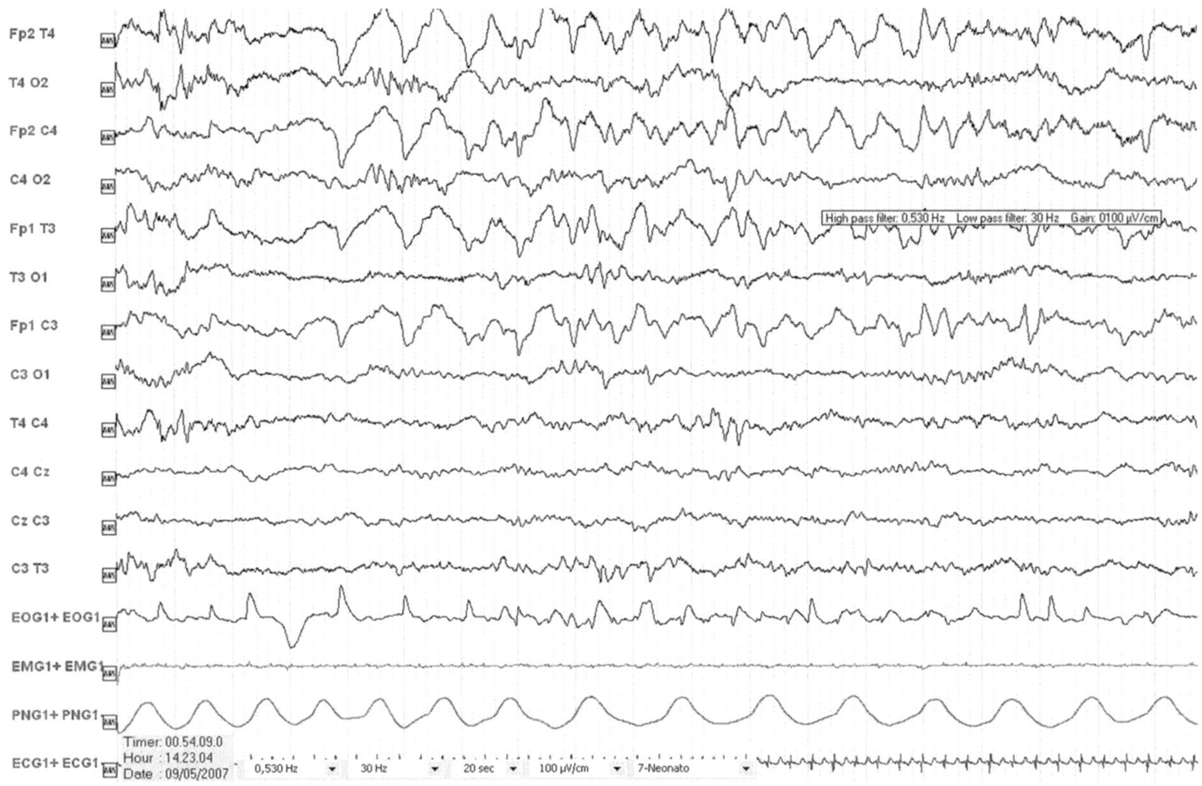

Fig. 22.8 39 weeks GA, 39.2 weeks CA. Healthy newborn. Quiet alert, open eyes. Ocular movement artifacts limited to Fp1 and Fp2 (placed too low in the forehead): slow and sharp polymorphic deflections, synchronous with eye movements detected by electrooculogram

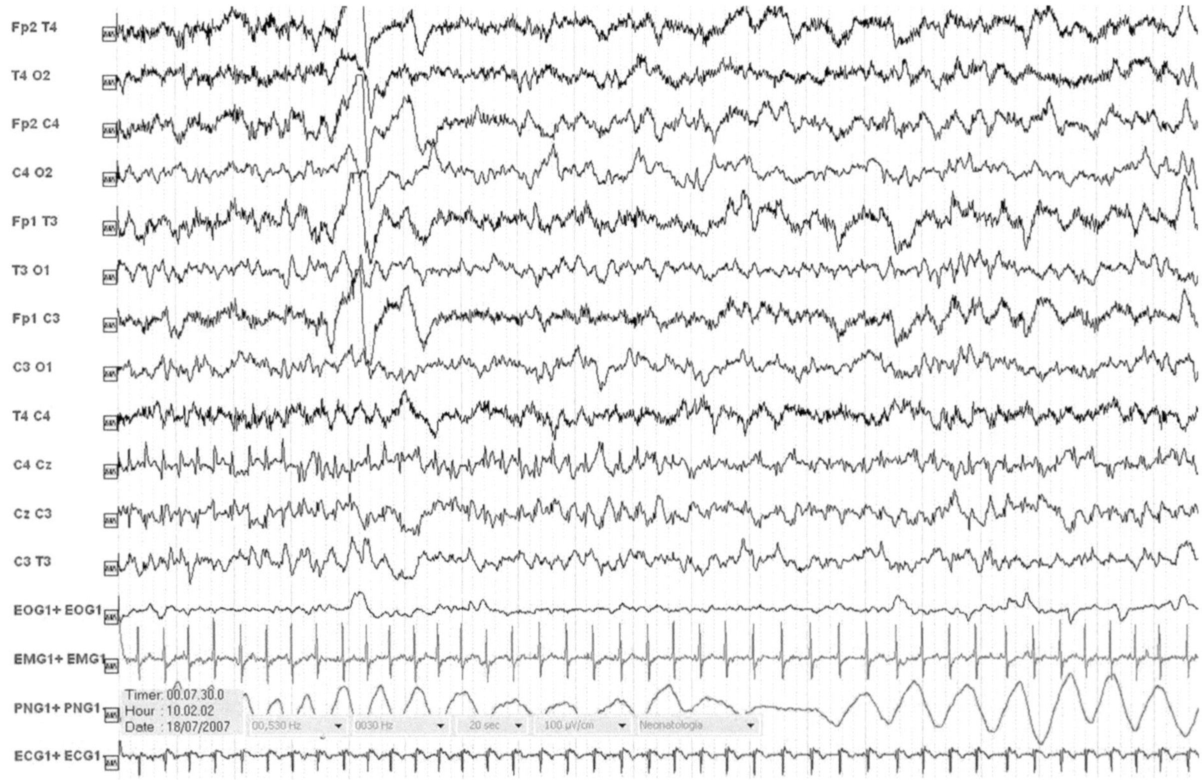

Fig. 22.9 36 weeks GA, 38.5 weeks CA. Healthy newborn. Quiet alert, eyes open and closed. Cz artifact in which EKG complex is recognized even in mylohyoid muscle. In Fp1, Fp2, and T4 fast low-voltage activity produced by muscles. High-voltage vertical deflection produced by eye movements in Fp1 and Fp2

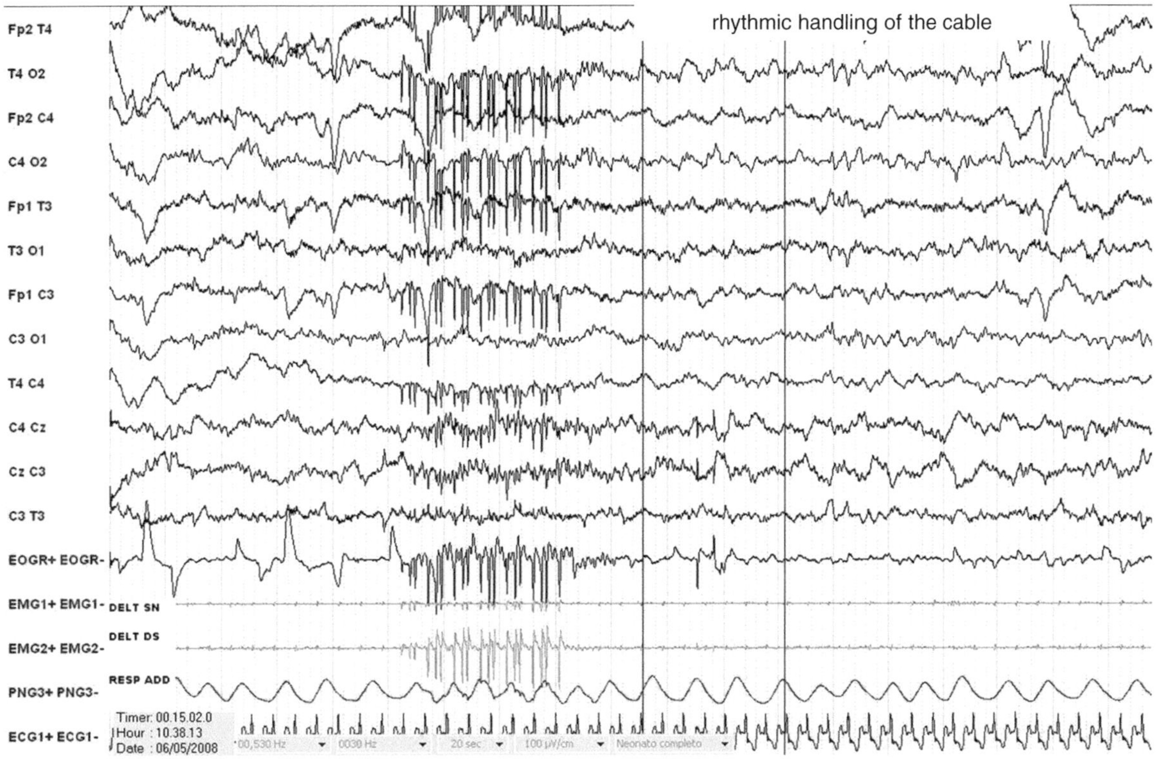

Fig. 22.10 38 weeks GA, 40 weeks CA. Healthy newborn. Quiet alert, open eyes. Electromagnetic field artifacts in all recording leads induced by rhythmic handling of the cable connecting to the head-box. NB: Potentials recognized in EMG channels (right and left deltoid muscles) are not the expression of child movements

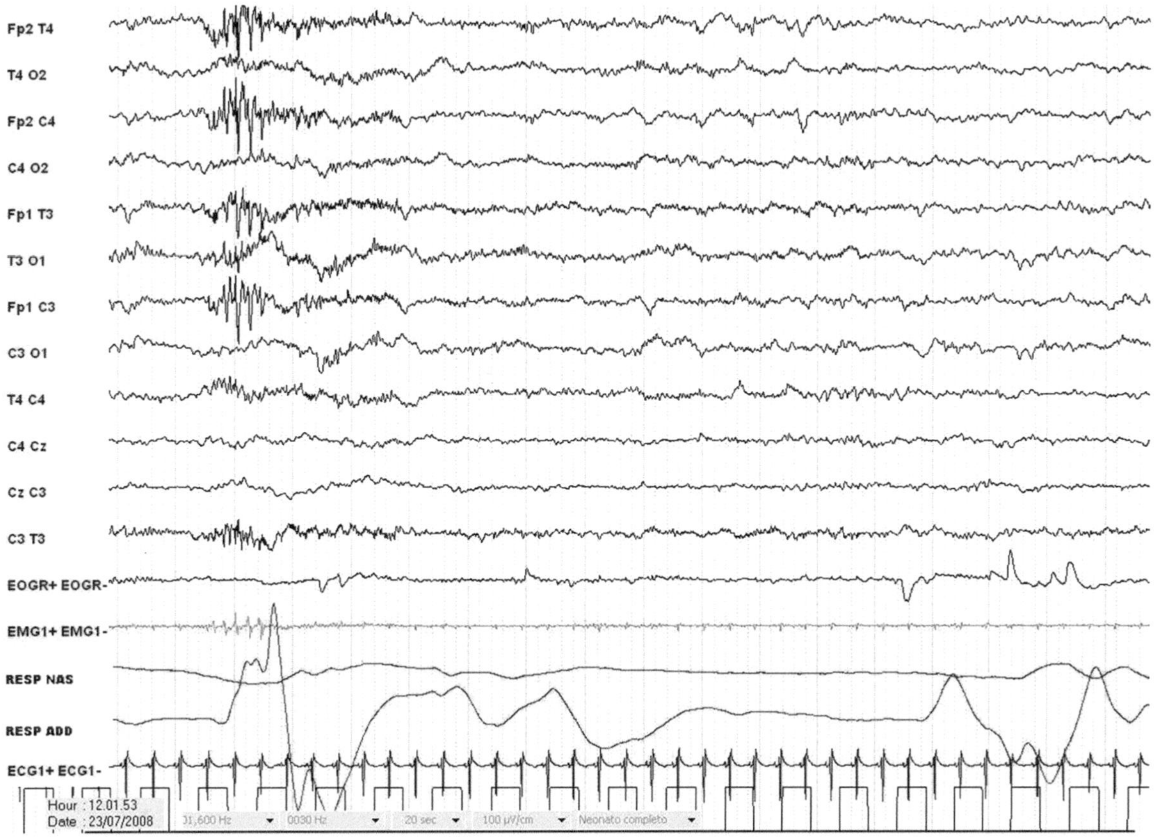

Fig. 22.11 36 weeks GA, 38 weeks CA. Healthy newborn. Active sleep after quiet sleep. Complex artifacts induced by hiccup, represented by a high-voltage deflection in the abdominal respiration channel. Five rhythmic chest contractions are recorded simultaneously in EMG1 (mylohyoid muscle); they produce an interfering fast low-voltage muscular activity intermingled with single rhythmic spike waves induced by chest movements

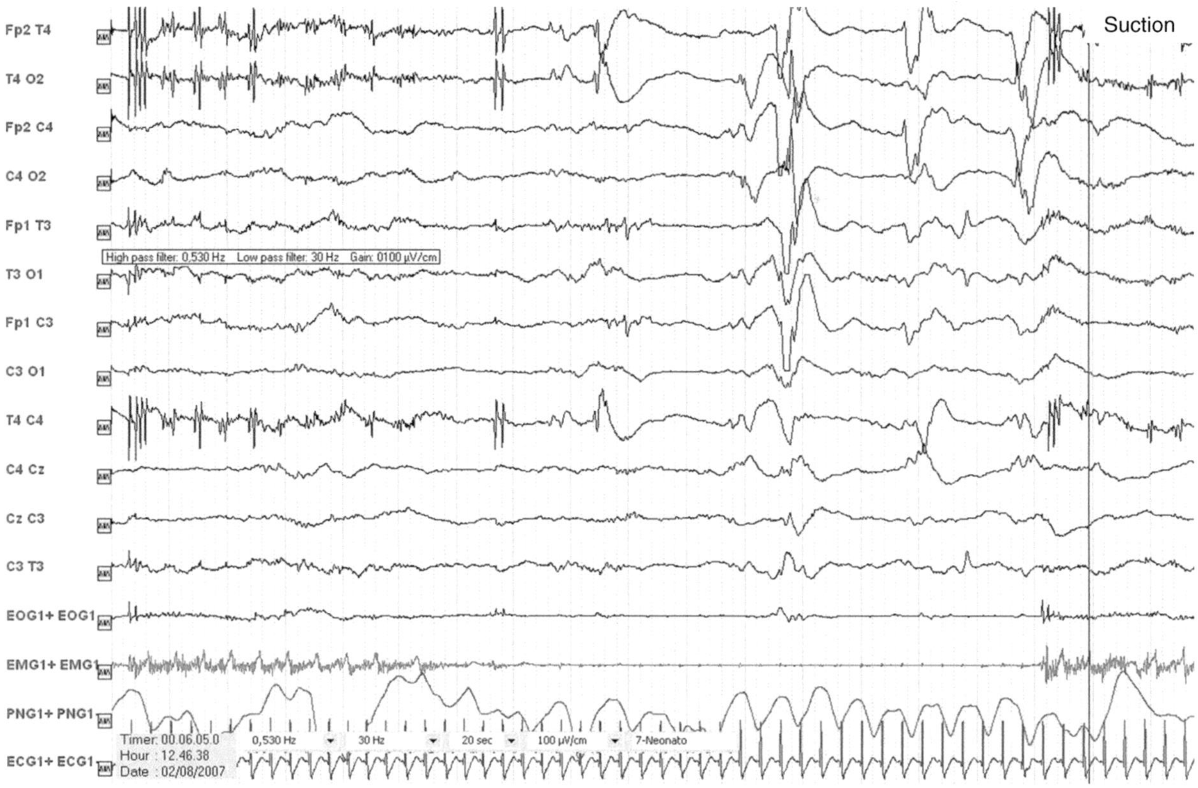

Fig. 22.12 31 weeks GA, 31.5 weeks CA. Intraparenchymal fronto-temporal hemorrhage in the right hemisphere. In wakefulness T4 artifact (less evident in T3) produced by sucking (see mylohyoid muscle in EMG1) with rhythmic muscular spike superimposed to an interfering activity of 6-s duration, occurring again with the same morphology after 11 s. In T4 it is also present a slow and high-voltage spike-wave complex of cerebral origin evidence of intraparenchymal injury

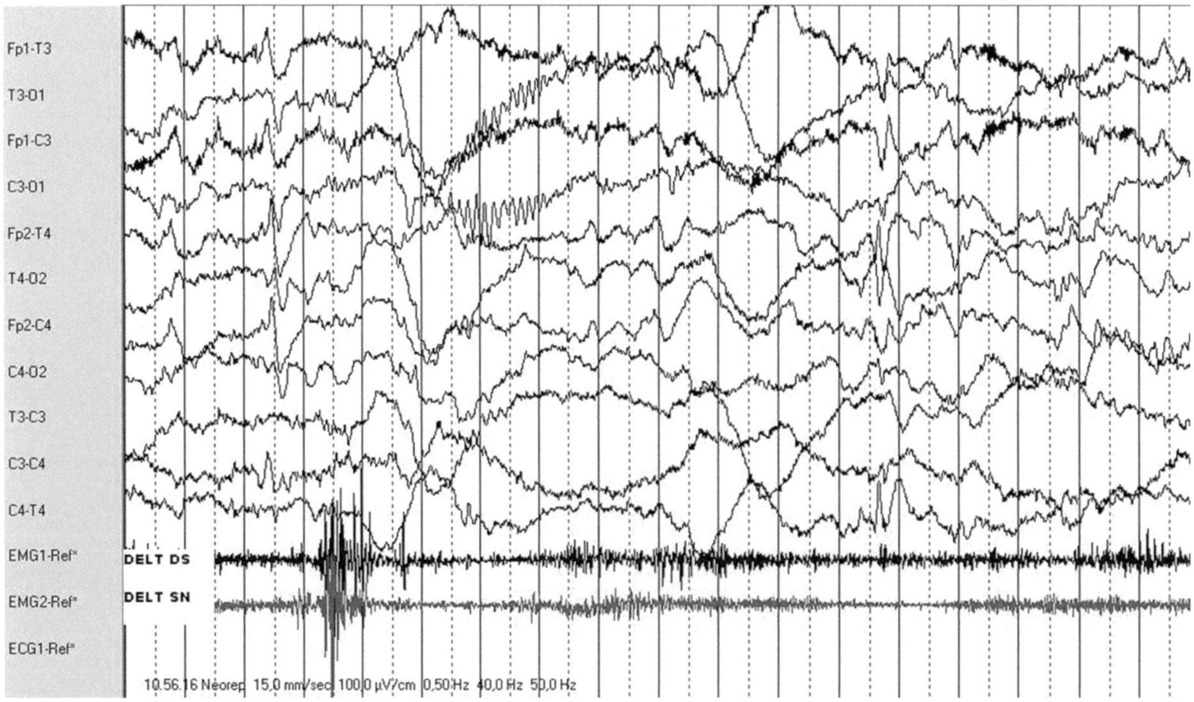

Fig. 22.13 40.4 weeks GA, 41 weeks CA. Healthy newborn with jitteriness, awake. O2 artifact in which a rhythmic 7 Hz oscillation, induced by shaking limbs tremor, produces rhythmic oscillation of the head. It is overlapping with an interfering fast low-voltage activity originating in muscles, more evident on the left side, induced by jitteriness that produces in the right and left side increased and sustained hypertonus of deltoid muscles. Moreover a very slow deflection artifact is present in all leads, due to excessive sweating

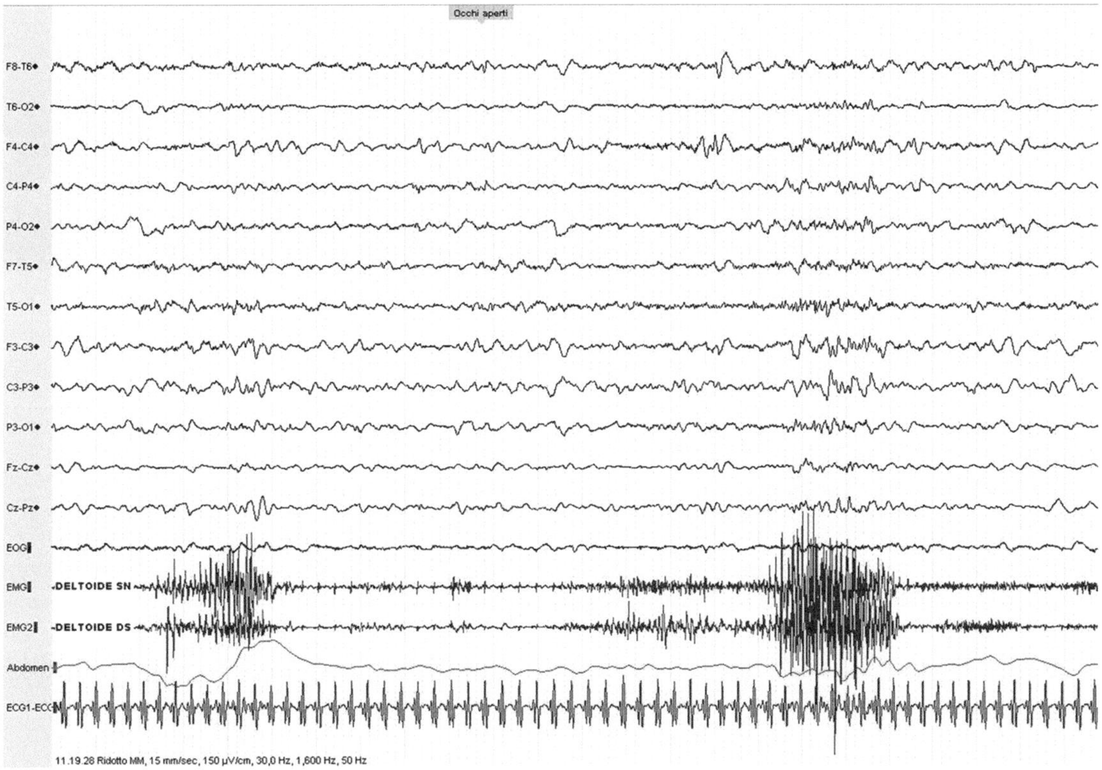

Fig. 22.14 40 weeks GA, 40.3 weeks CA. Healthy newborn, tremulousness. Quiet alert. Two high-frequency short runs of tremors in deltoid muscles. Increased low-voltage fast activity over temporal and frontal regions. On the left side electrodes, a 9 Hz fast and rhythmic activity synchronous with head movement induced by tremor

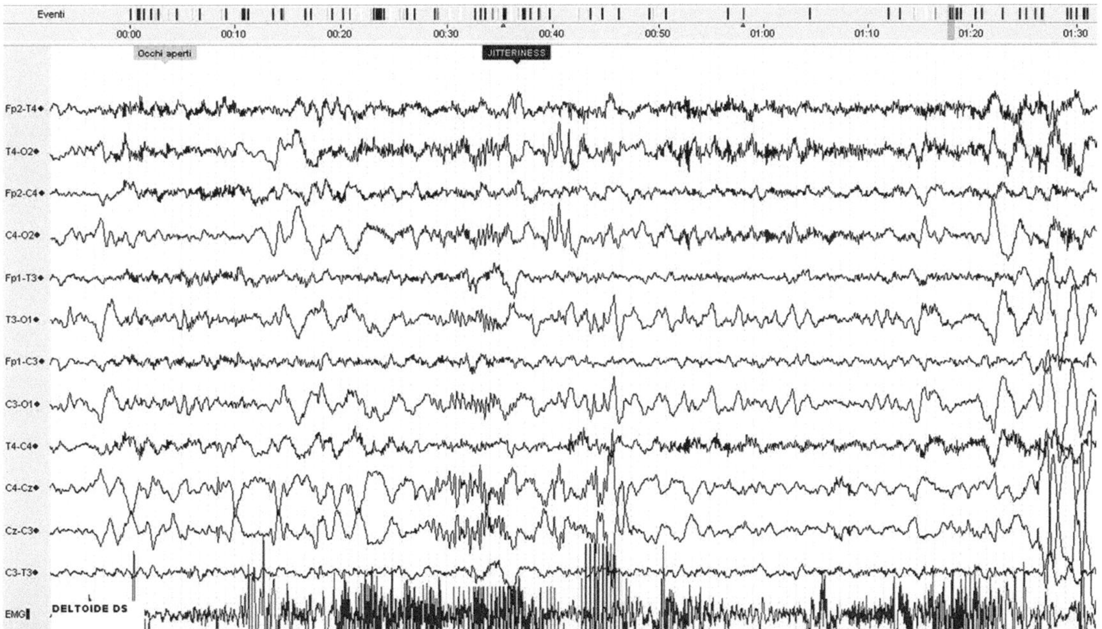

Fig. 22.15 33.2 weeks GA, 37 weeks CA. Healthy newborn. Awake, open eyes. Jitteriness. In Cz, O1, and O2, the protracted and rhythmic high-frequency movements of the four limbs, spreading to the scalp, induce a 10–18 Hz rhythmic activity synchronous with the movements. This activity intermingled with the interfering and generalized low-voltage activity originating from the muscles, produced by the generalized hypertonus shown on muscular polygraphy, unrelated to jitteriness

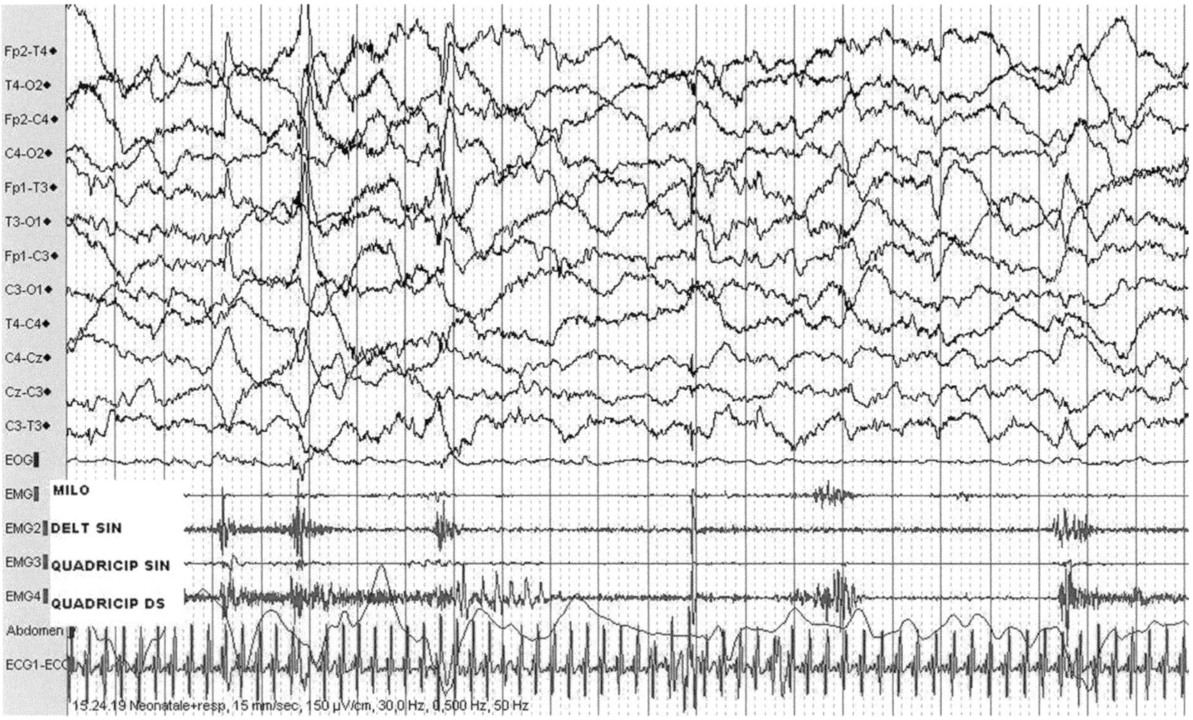

Fig. 22.16 39 weeks GA, 39.6 weeks CA. Healthy newborn. Active alert. Several paroxysmal non-epileptic jerks are distinguished in the polygraphic leads: myoclonia, spasm, and spasm with protracted tonic contraction. Polymorphic artifacts are associated over the scalp, in which is constantly present a vertical signal deflection expression of the paroxysmal movement onset and followed by return to baseline, depending on the features of the different movements

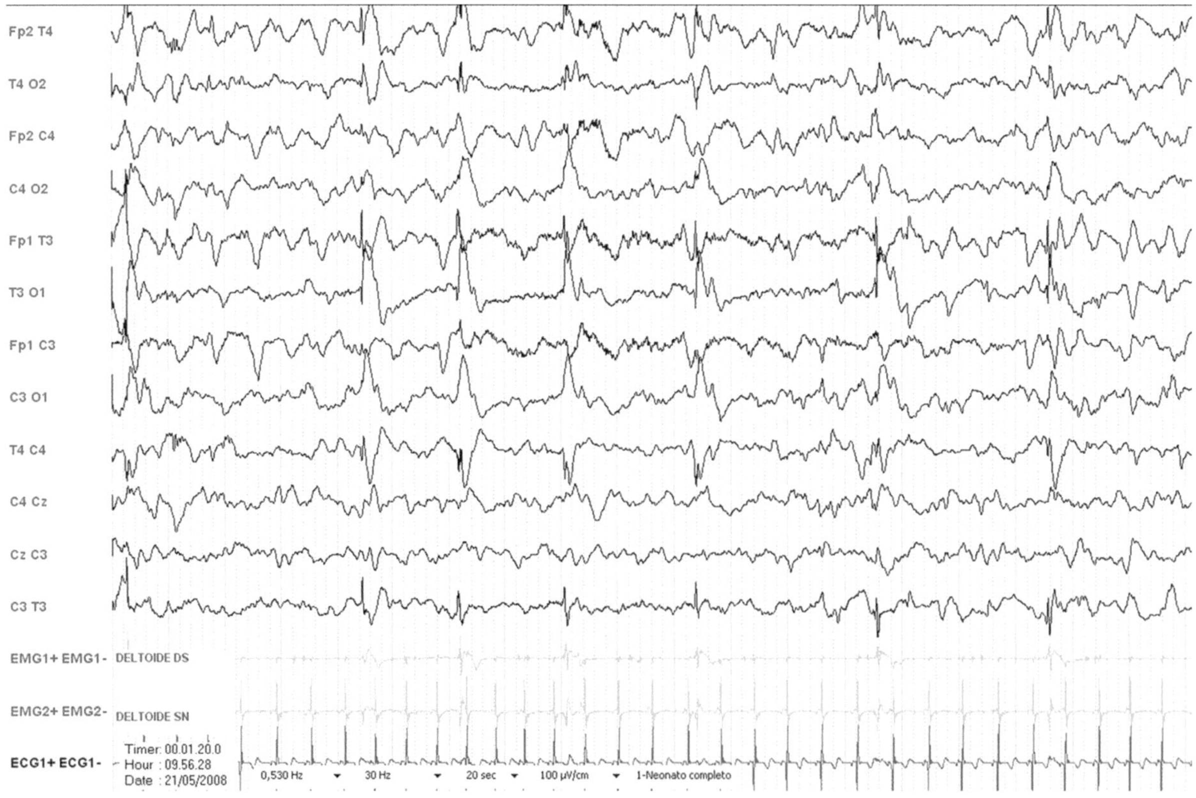

Fig. 22.17 40 weeks GA, 41 weeks CA. Brother of a patient with undiagnosed congenital encephalopathy. At birth arthrogryposis of the limbs and drowsiness. Beginning on the 1st day of life massive contraction of superior limbs and hiccup. In the figure drowsiness and theta-delta mixed background activity, without significant asymmetry. Polygraphic recordings of deltoid muscles permit to detect bilateral high frequency contractions. Seven events are recorded in 18 s coinciding with an anterior and temporal bilateral artifact over the scalp. This artifact is characterized by a vertical fast deflection followed by an angular slow wave

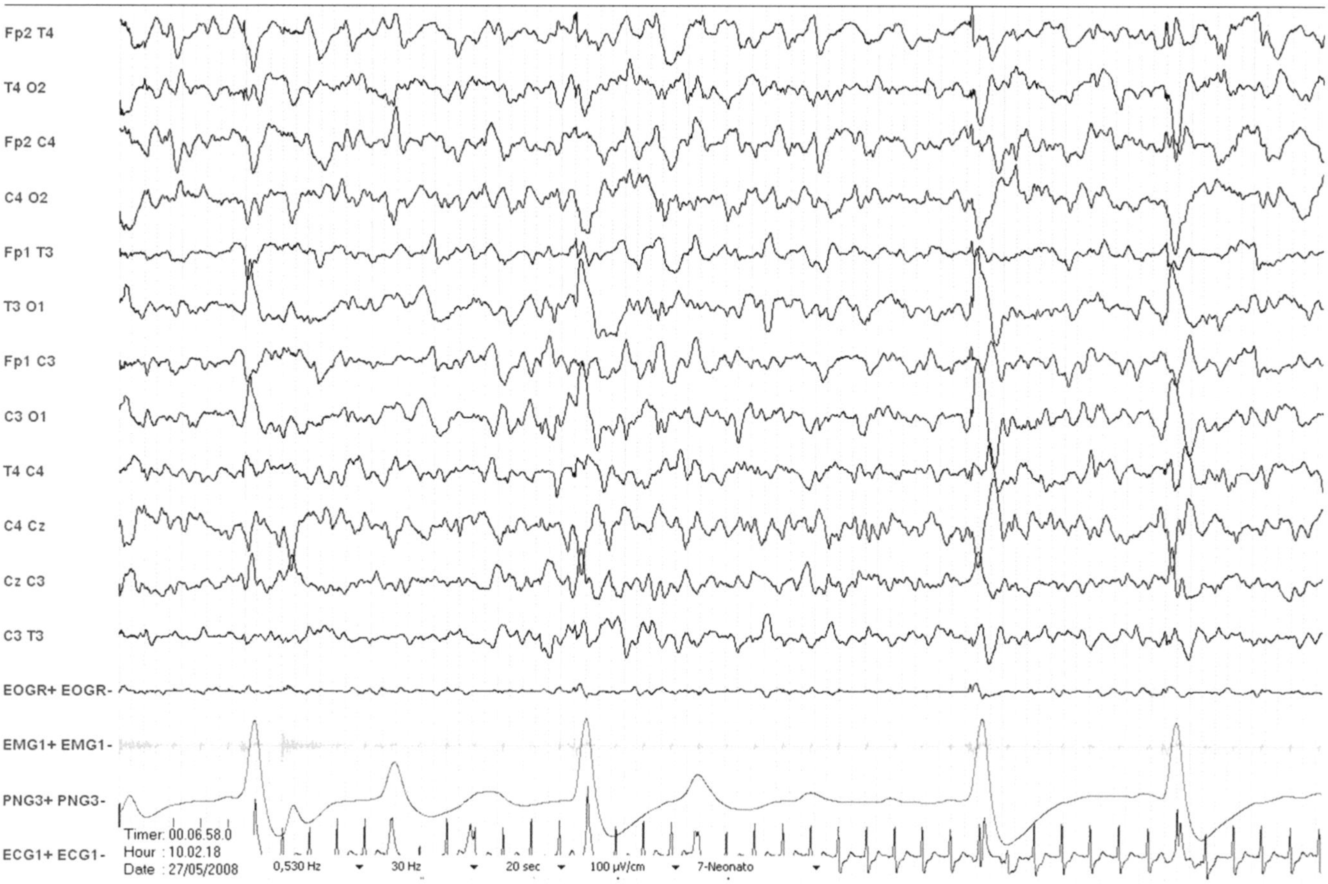

Fig. 22.18 40.6 weeks GA, 42 weeks CA (same child shown in the previous figure). After 1 week, same clinical conditions. It is shown how the superior limb muscle contraction during sleep, identified in mylohyoid muscle lead, is strictly related to an abdominal contraction (4 events in 18 s), detectable in PNG3 (abdominal respiration). A similar artifact is detected over the scalp: high-voltage negative deflection, more evident in O1, directly associated with a slight vertical deflection

22.4 The Abnormal EEG Recording: Historical References

The French school of Dreyfus-Brisac [5, 6] and Monod [7] should be acknowledged for the interest and the development of electroencephalography in newborns. Later, many other authors have tried defining and systematizing the characteristics of the EEG abnormalities. Given the practical intentions of this Handbook, should be cited above all Lombroso [8], Stockard-Pope et al. [9], Ferrari et al. [10], Mizrahi et al. [11], André et al. [12], and Hrachovy and Mizrahi [3]. There is a concordance among the authors about the opportunity to subdivide the abnormalities into four main categories:

- Abnormal features of development (Box 22.1)
- Abnormal features of the underlying background activity (Box 22.2)
- Abnormal EEG patterns/transients (Box 22.3)
- Ictal epileptic discharges (Box 22.4)

The severity of the abnormalities detected on the EEG generally correlates with the severity of neurological damage. However, the time elapsed between the clinical event and the time of recording should be considered. Indeed, the abnormalities are more significant close to the clinical event and then tend to be less evident moving away from it. Nevertheless, either their persistence, worsening, or slow regression represents a sign of severity related to the underlying brain pathology. To delineate the evolution of the abnormalities, several recordings are needed (see the following paragraph on the approach methodology to the abnormal recording).

Lombroso [8, 13] describes in detail the characteristics of the abnormal EEG features and of the ictal epileptic patterns in the preterm and in the full-term newborns. Stockard-Pope and coll. [9] provide a broad framework, with a corresponding iconography, of the four main categories, examining constantly the clinical significance of the EEG abnormalities. However, they suggest a "classification system" that seems excessively difficult to apply; therefore, it is scarcely used in neonatal electroencephalography labs. Ferrari and coll. [10], after describing both the normal and the abnormal EEG patterns in different CAs, compared to the other authors, identify the peculiar EEG patterns subdividing them into three main categories: the first includes extremely pathological activity, the second moderately pathological activity, and the third normal or mildly abnormal activity. This classification has a clear relation with the clinical picture, thus being the tool to include the EEG features in the clinical context. In the summary table of their work, the authors highlight the different types of recordings and the different "abnormal transients" in the previously mentioned three main categories. André et al. [12] underline the need for a precise neonatal EEG terminology to achieve homogeneity and interobserver agreement in the analysis of normal and abnormal EEG recordings. Mizrahi et al. [11] and Hrachovy and Mizrahi [3] emphasize the patterns of uncertain meaning and, with respect to the background EEG activity, differentiate the generalized abnormal feature from the focal ones. In the chapter dedicated to neonatal seizures, they provide an exhaustive exposition of neonatal seizures, with a significant iconography illustrating seizures in different clinical conditions.

The interested reader is invited to refer to the abovementioned works and to the recommended references at the end of this chapter for further information.

22.5 Methodological Approach

The EEG examiner's knowledge of the "normal" features, taking into account the individual variability and the extraneurological conditions that can modify these features, is the essential condition to face the "abnormal" EEG with its related questions. It has also been emphasized how the visual analysis of the EEG recording involves the observation and the spatial and temporal definition of specific characteristics of both the "EEG features" of the background activity and the "typical graphoelements" of each specific CA.

Once the neurological clinical condition and the behavioral state of the newborn have been delineated, the EEG allows to acquire essential information to answer the questions that together contribute to define the three fundamental points in the management of a pathological newborn: the diagnostic definition, the therapeutic approach, and the prognostic definition. Are there signs of CNS diffuse or focal injury? Are clinical or electrical seizures present? Are there any significant elements suggestive of a specific etiology? What is the effectiveness of a given therapy? When did the brain injury occur? What is the evolution of the acute event? [14].

The answer to these questions relies on the assessment of an abnormal background pattern and its relation with the CA, the lack of age-specific features, the presences of abnormalities in spatial and temporal EEG organization along with the identification of abnormal features (slow, focal, and/or diffuse), epileptic and/or non-epileptic paroxysmal abnormalities, the possible presence of ictal discharges, and finally the detection of EEG graphoelements suggestive for specific etiologies.

With respect to therapeutic behavior, the presence of specific patterns can lead to an etiological and symptomatic therapeutic treatment. In case of use of sedative drugs (midazolam, thiopental sodium, phenobarbital), the EEG characteristics allow to establish the optimal therapeutic dosage of drugs, in particular in relation to the characteristics of the ictal paroxysmal abnormalities or suppression-burst pattern. Only the EEG allows the recognition of electrical-only seizures or minimal clinical signs (i.e., electro-clinical dissociation) that might suggest therapeutic modification. In the presence of well-defined electro-clinical seizures, isolated or recurrent up to the epilepticus status, the EEG allows to evaluate the efficacy of the anticonvulsant therapy. In the hypoxic-ischemic encephalopathy, the EEG or the more commonly used amplitude-integrated EEG (aEEG) has become an important tool for the diagnosis and for the hypothermic treatment. (Discussing the aEEG characteristics is beyond the purpose of the present chapter.)

Moreover, with respect to the prognostic significance, it is only with the repetition of the EEG recordings over time, evaluating the evolution of what was found in the previous examinations that it is possible to provide some preliminary prognostic information.

Lastly, it is well known that most epileptic seizures in the neonatal period are symptomatic of an acute brain injury [2, 14]. However, in recent years, the huge expansion in genetics techniques allowed to define etiological diagnosis. Regarding the genetically determined cellular mechanisms causing nonstructural acute symptomatic neonatal seizures, three main neonatal epileptic conditions are defined: neonatal genetic epilepsies, early-onset encephalopathy, and early-onset epileptic encephalopathy [15–18, 30]. Interestingly, however, the phenotypical spectrum associated with variations in each gene can vary widely. In the majority of cases there is a spectrum of clinical manifestations, which can be associated with a wide range of phenotypic severity. For example, mutations in KCNQ2 gene have been associated with both self-limited neonatal-onset epilepsies and neonatal-onset epileptic encephalopathies [17]. Therefore, a clear-cut genotype–phenotype correlations is not always possible [16, 18].

In view of the above and according to literature [14, 19–29], it is considered useful to propose some "operational considerations."

22.5.1 EEG Recording

- It must be performed under all clinical conditions in which CNS involvement is suspected. EEG-polygraphy is essential for the definition of the behavioral states and must be individualized according to the clinical events to be documented. For the definition of the paroxysmal events, either epileptic or non-epileptic, video-EEG recording is strongly recommended. The first recording must be carried out as soon as possible and must last at least 45–60 min in the suspicion of epileptic seizures, if possible, before the anticonvulsant treatment and in hypoxic-ischemic encephalopathy in the first 6 h of life to prescribe cooling therapy.
- Long-term monitoring (24–48–72 hours) or repeated recordings in the short run are strongly suggested in the evidence of a documented or suspected status epilepticus. Moreover, also in case of subclinical or suspected seizures, it is useful to perform an EEG recording in an appropriate time in order to capture the ictal event, possibly with a video-EEG recording.
- The subsequent EEG or long-term monitoring must be performed in relation to the different peculiar clinical pictures, following the evolution of the symptoms. For the long-term prognostic definition, it is essential to evaluate clinical signs and symptoms following the acute brain injury together with the different short-term and long-term evolution of EEG patterns.

Only after the acquisition of such a methodological approach it will be possible to take into consideration the characteristics of the abnormal EEGs findings.

22.6 Essential Terminology

According to the indications of Lombroso [13], Stockard-Pope et al. [9], Ferrari et al. [10] and Mizrahi et al. [11], Andrè et al. [12], and Hrachovy et al. [3], we consider useful to report the most frequent definitions regarding the description of pathological EEG patterns.

Box 22.1: Abnormalities of the Behavioural States Organization and of the Developmental Pattern

Abnormalities of the behavioural states organization and of the developmental pattern.

Unrecognizable behavioral states: persistent absence of a recognizable sleep and waking cycle in a newborn of at least 34 weeks of CA (Figs. 22.19 and 22.20)[1].

Development of the behavioral sleep states: REM sleep state lasts 50% of the sleep cycle in a newborn at term, whereas NREM sleep state lasts about 30–40%, and the rest is occupied by indeterminate sleep. There is an intra- and interindividual variation of approximately 20–30%.

Abnormal development of the sleep-wake cycling: in the pathological cases, during NREM sleep state, the presence of an abnormal ratio between trace alternant (TA) and continuous high-voltage slow activity can be observed, with persistency of TA beyond the 7th to 8th weeks after birth; abnormalities of the onset of the REM sleep state do not bear a great clinical importance; however the presence of a REM pattern in the beginning of sleep should be carefully evaluated.

Dysmaturity (external dyschronism): electrical EEG pattern where the developmental physiological features in both sleep and wakefulness states are immature for the stated CA. A dyschronism of 3 or more weeks is suggestive of persistent brain dysfunction and is often associated with other EEG abnormalities (Figs. 22.21, 22.22, 22.23, 22.24, 22.25, 22.26, 22.27, 22.28 and 22.29).

Dysmaturity (internal dyschronism): electrical pattern where the physiological features of the NREM sleep state are immature for the stated CA and consistent with a lower CA, while the wake EEG has a normal background activity. It is considered abnormal a dyschronism of 3 or more weeks, and in this case other electrical abnormalities are usually present (Figs. 22.23–22.27).

Interhemispheric asynchrony: it is defined as pathological when the EEG activity is still asynchronous for more than 75% at a CA over 30 weeks (Figs. 22.26 and 22.27).

[1]For all the figures, the following EEG recording parameters were utilized: time base 15 mm/s, sensitivity 70/150 mcV/cm, high-pass filter 0.5/1.6 Hz, low-pass filter 30/70 Hz. Otherwise, parameters are indicated (in italics).

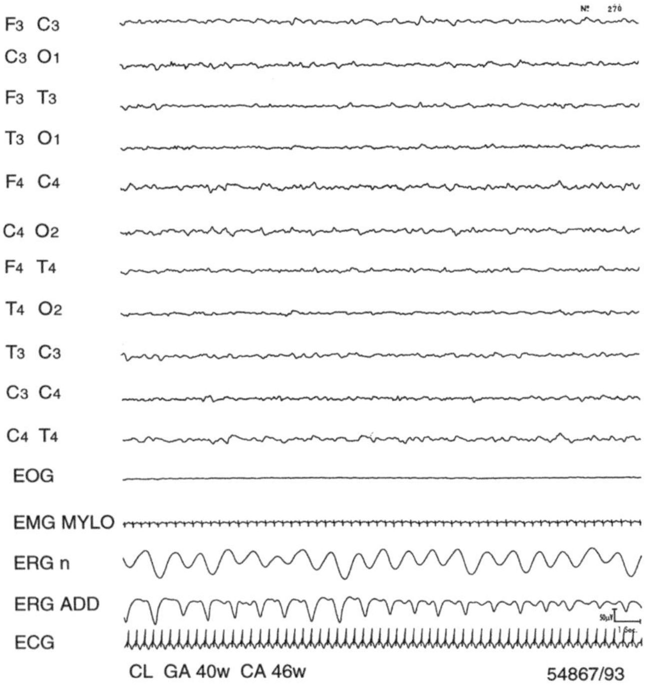

Fig. 22.19 See Fig. 22.20 caption

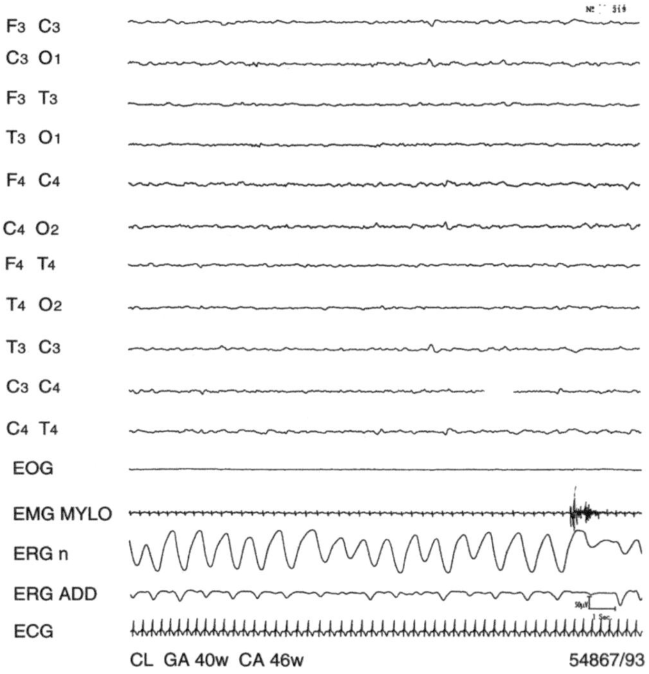

Fig. 22.20 40 weeks GA, 46 weeks CA. At 40 weeks CA, cesarean section was performed 30 h after pre-labor rupture of membranes. Maternal and newborn hyperpyrexia. Comatose newborn with AED's resistant status epilepticus, followed by recurrent seizures for a week. At 6 weeks of age **low voltage** (less than 30 mcV) **and undifferentiated tracing** throughout long-lasting EEG recording. In Fig. 22.19 polygraphic parameters are suggestive for a NREM sleep state, while those in this figure are suggestive for a REM sleep state: EEG background remains identical, undifferentiated, also during awake state. This condition is related to a **complex encephalopathy with combined etiology** (post-infective, anoxic hyschemic, intraventricular, and intraparenchymal hemorrhages). Brain MRI confirmed the etiological conclusions and documented severe and extensive lesions. Follow-up: severe neurocognitive impairment, spastic apostural tetraparesis with AED's resistant epilepsy (12 years old)

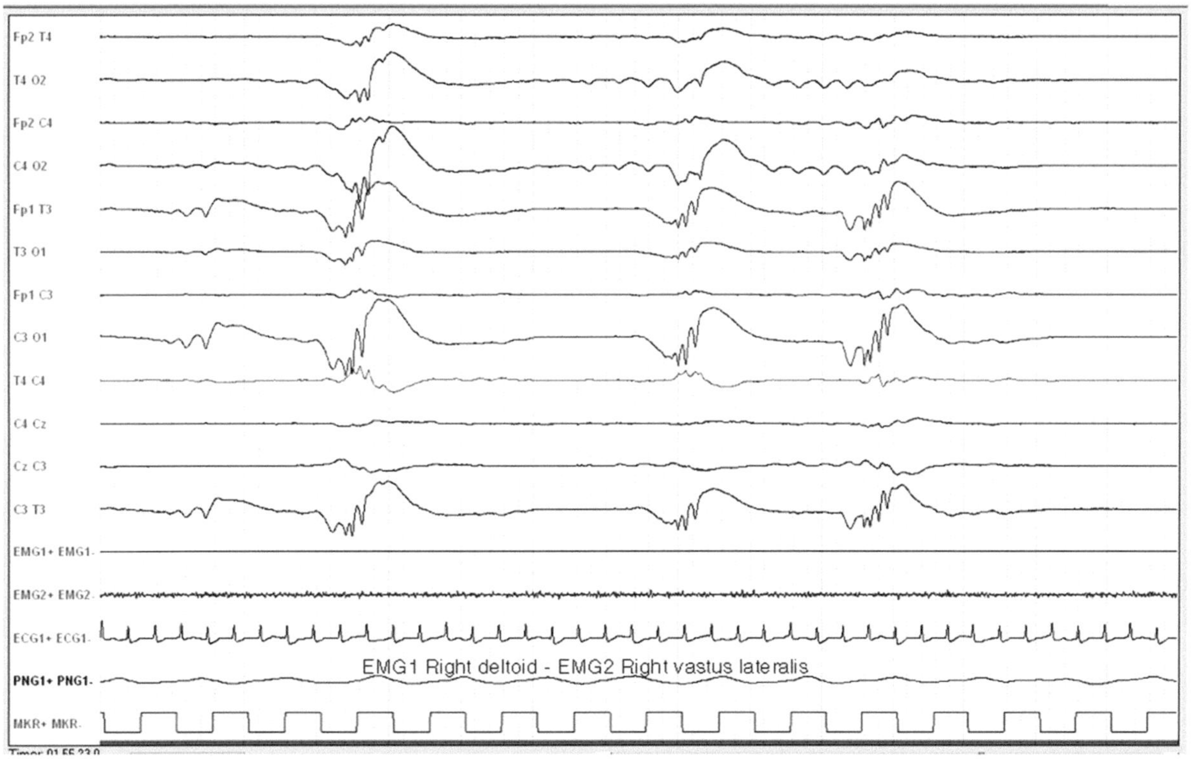

Fig. 22.21 30.3 weeks GA, 31 weeks CA. Cesarean section for pre-eclampsia. **Pathological delta brushes with discontinuous activity and temporal and occipital delta waves, synchronous on the two sides, with superimposed theta activity**. Follow-up: moderate motor and intellectual impairment (22 months old)

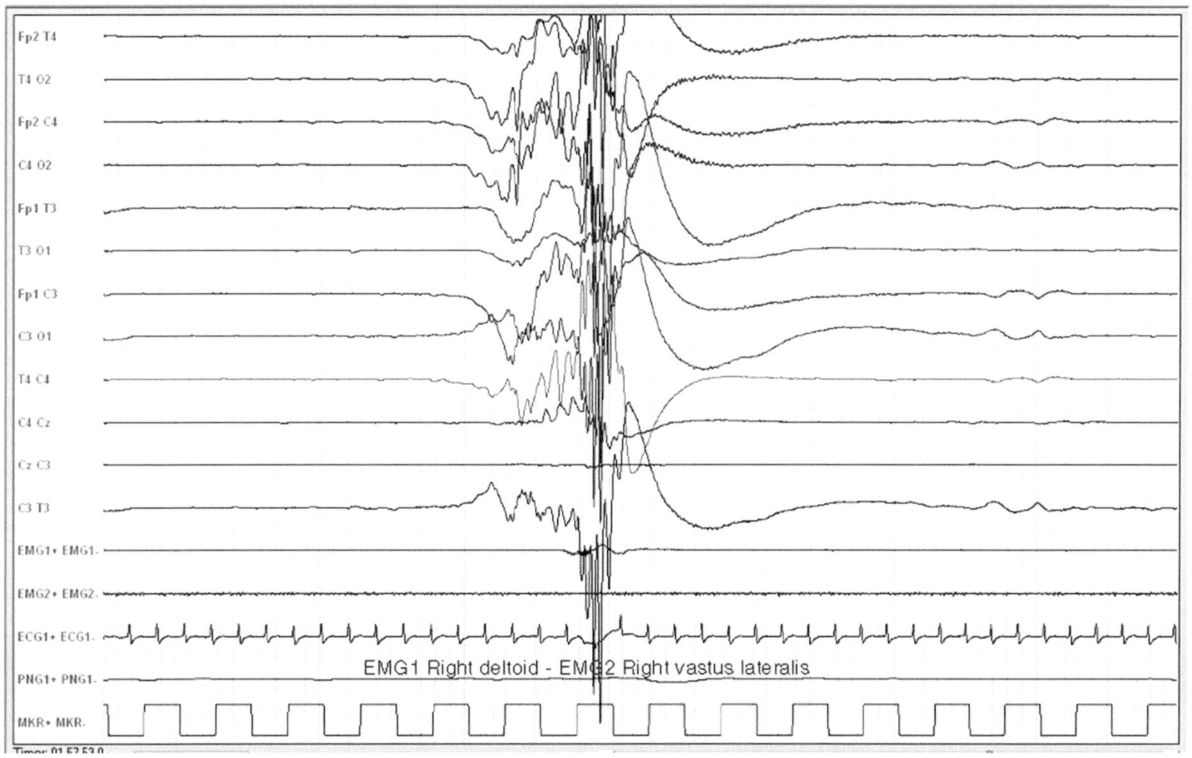

Fig. 22.22 28 weeks GA, 28.6 weeks CA. Twin pregnancy, pre-labor rupture of membranes. **External dyschronism**. During quiet sleep, discontinuous background activity **with high-amplitude delta wave superimposed by rapid and spiky rhythms. The burst begins with theta activity and is followed by very high-voltage very slow wave transient**. Synchronous low-voltage delta activity on the central regions is seen in the interburst period. Follow-up: normal brain ultrasound; normal psychomotor development (8 months old)

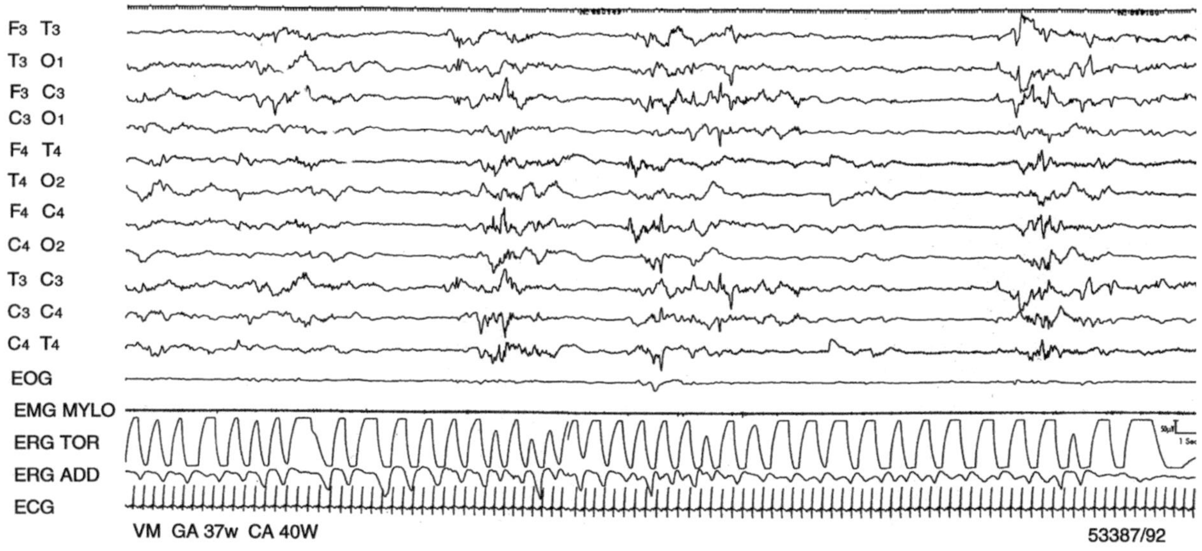

Fig. 22.23 37.6 weeks GA, 40 weeks CA. Pregnancy not monitored. Normal delivery at 37.6 weeks. Hypotonia and reduced alertness in the first 3 weeks of life. In the first week, the EEG (not shown) is characterized by immature pattern for the reported CA in all states of sleep and wakefulness. At 40 weeks CA in tracé alternant sleep, the bursts are rich in sharp elements, although exceedingly asynchronous for age. Interburst intervals have significant low voltage. **External dyschronism**

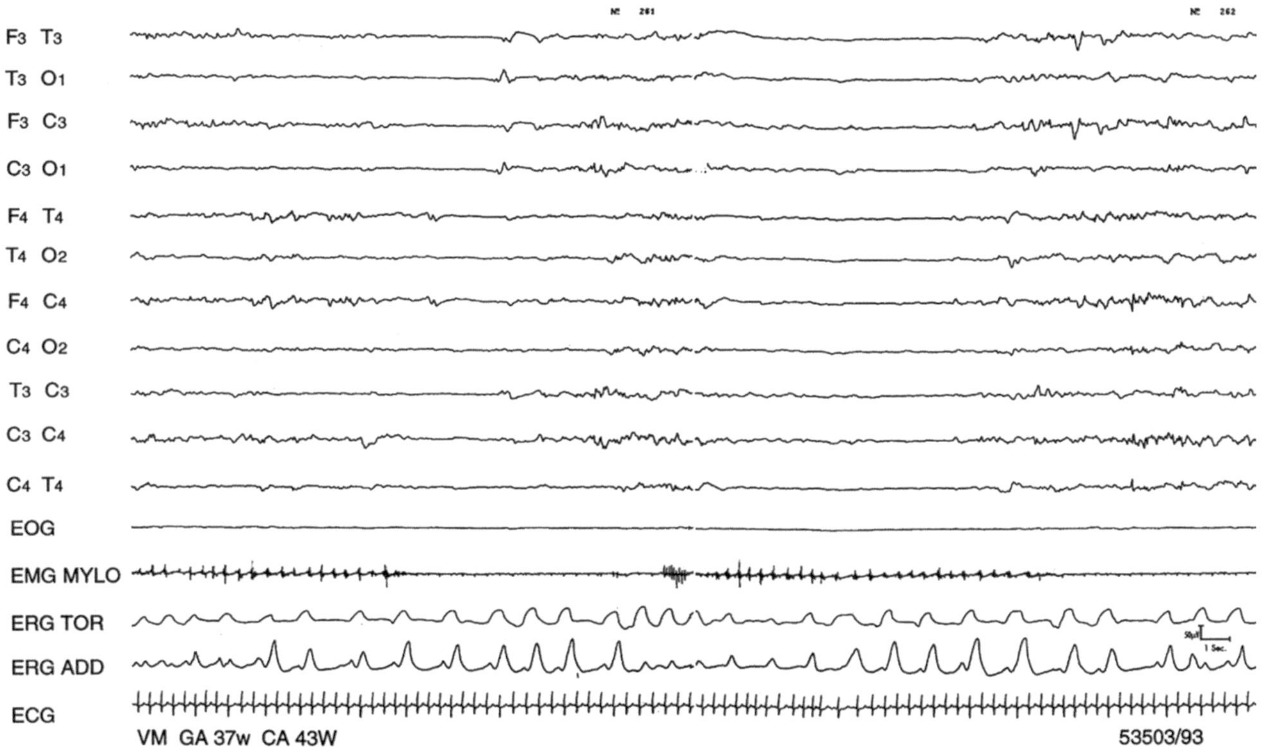

Fig. 22.24 37.6 weeks GA, 43 weeks CA (same child as the previous figure). Progressive decline of reactivity and spontaneous motility. Three weeks later in quiet sleep, significant decrease of burst amplitude and increase of low-voltage interburst intervals. The external dyschronism is evolving to a **low voltage depressed background activity** (undifferentiated EEG). Brain MRI: cortical and subcortical atrophy, bilateral lesions of white matter, result of **prenatal chronic hypoxia**. Follow-up: at 4 months West syndrome, severe neurocognitive impairment

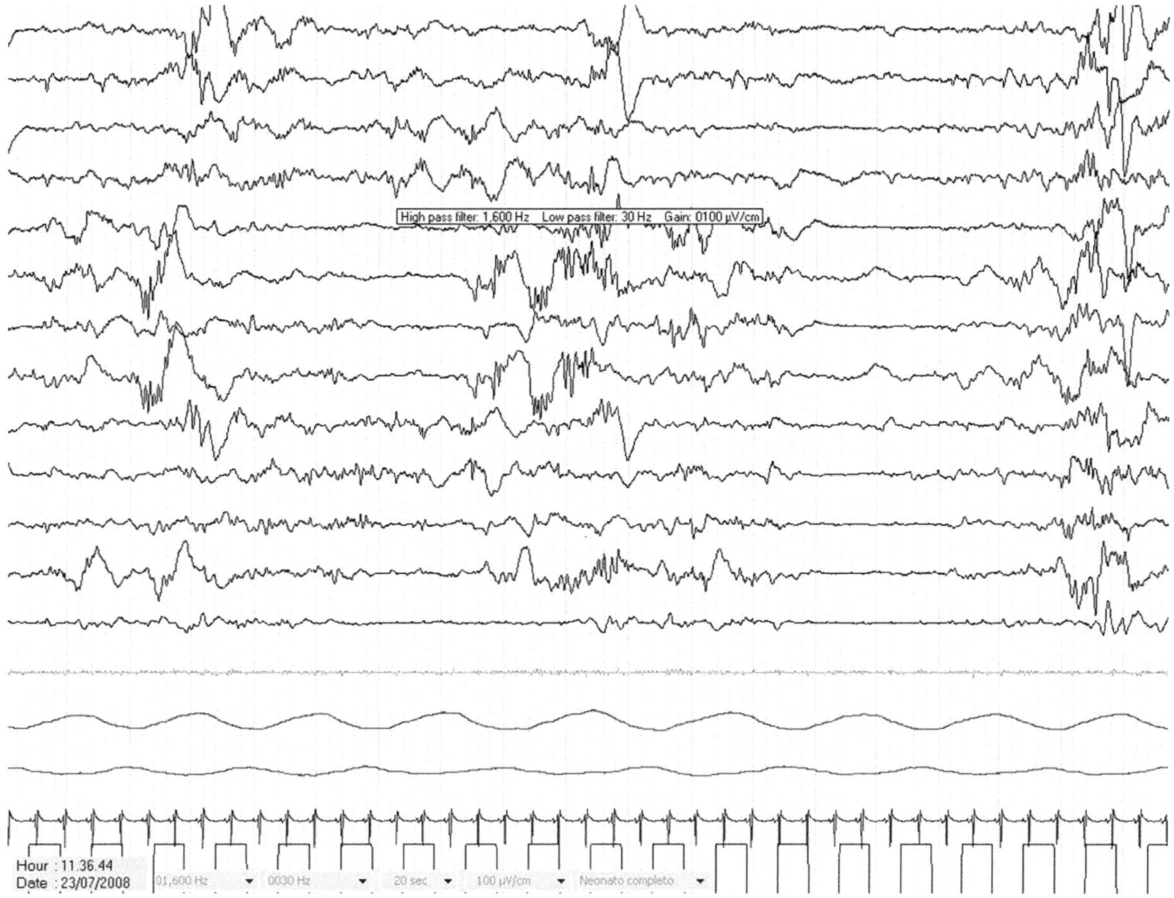

Fig. 22.25 36.6 weeks GA, 37.4 weeks CA. Uneventful pregnancy and delivery. On the 5th day of life prolonged (non-epileptic) cyanotic event. In quiet sleep asynchronous tracé alternant pattern, persistence of delta brushes and bursts with exceedingly sharp grapho-elements, and low-voltage interburst intervals. Dysmaturity (**internal dyschronism**). Normal cerebral ultrasound. Follow-up: normal neurodevelopment at 4 months of age

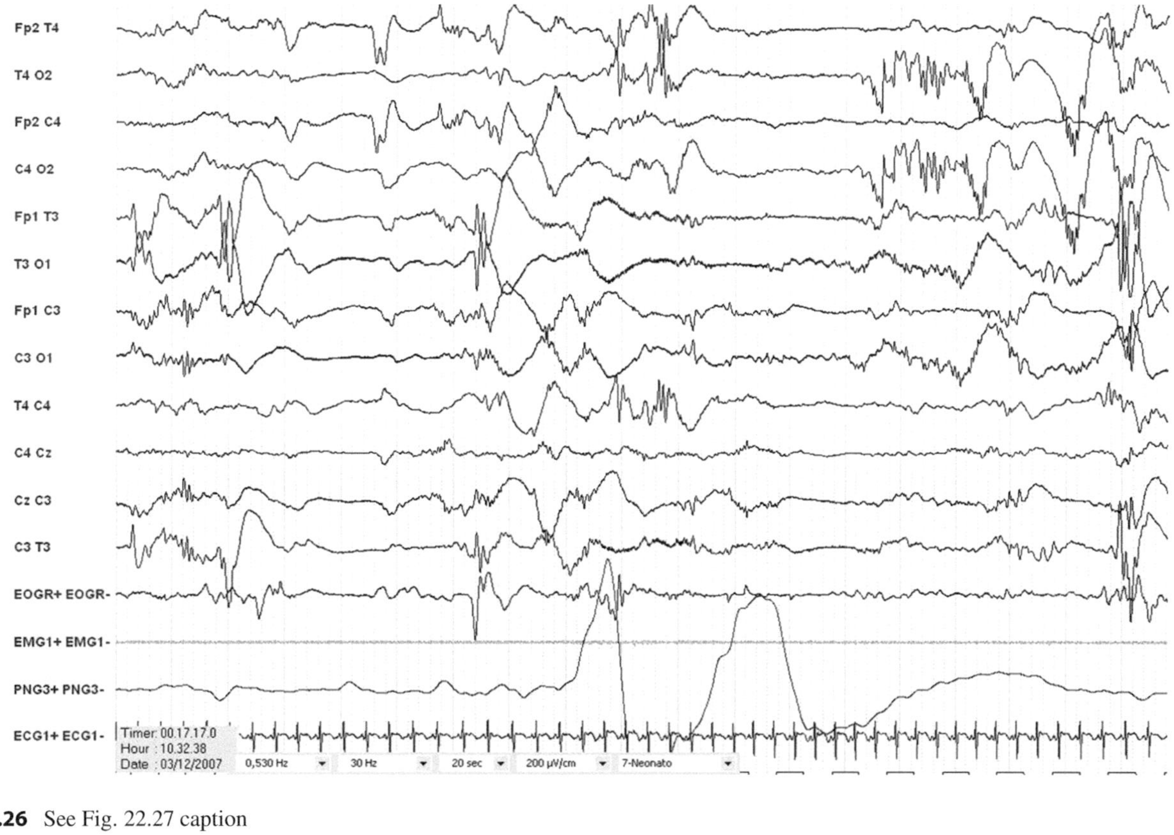

Fig. 22.26 See Fig. 22.27 caption

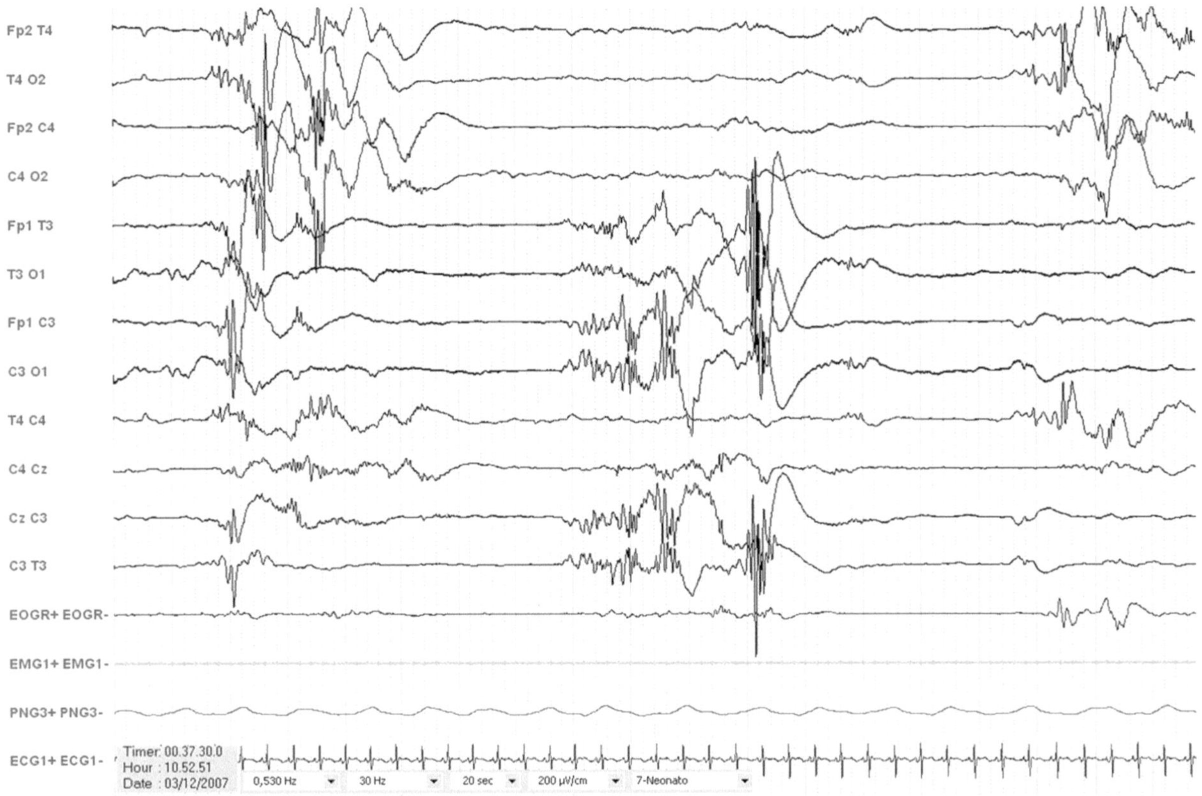

Fig. 22.27a 28 weeks GA, 32 weeks CA. **Intraventricular hemorrhage and tetraventricular hydrocephalus** occurring 5 days after birth. The newborn is lethargic. At 4 weeks of life (Fig. 22.26), active sleep with significant **interhemispheric asynchrony** of electrical activity and of inactive intervals. Multifocal spikes and polyspike-slow waves with an amplitude of 200–600 mcV, predominant in left and right temporal region. In Fig. 22.27 quiet sleep with substantial increase of inactive segments and **interhemispheric asynchrony**. Abnormal discharges with enhanced amplitude. The tracing can be defined as dysmature (**external dyschronism**), but it is highly suggestive of a multifocal injuries in consideration of discharges strictly focal and repetitive in the temporal regions. Brain MRI: tetraventricular hydrocephalus. Follow-up: ventriculoperitoneal shunt, normal electro-clinical conditions at 11 months

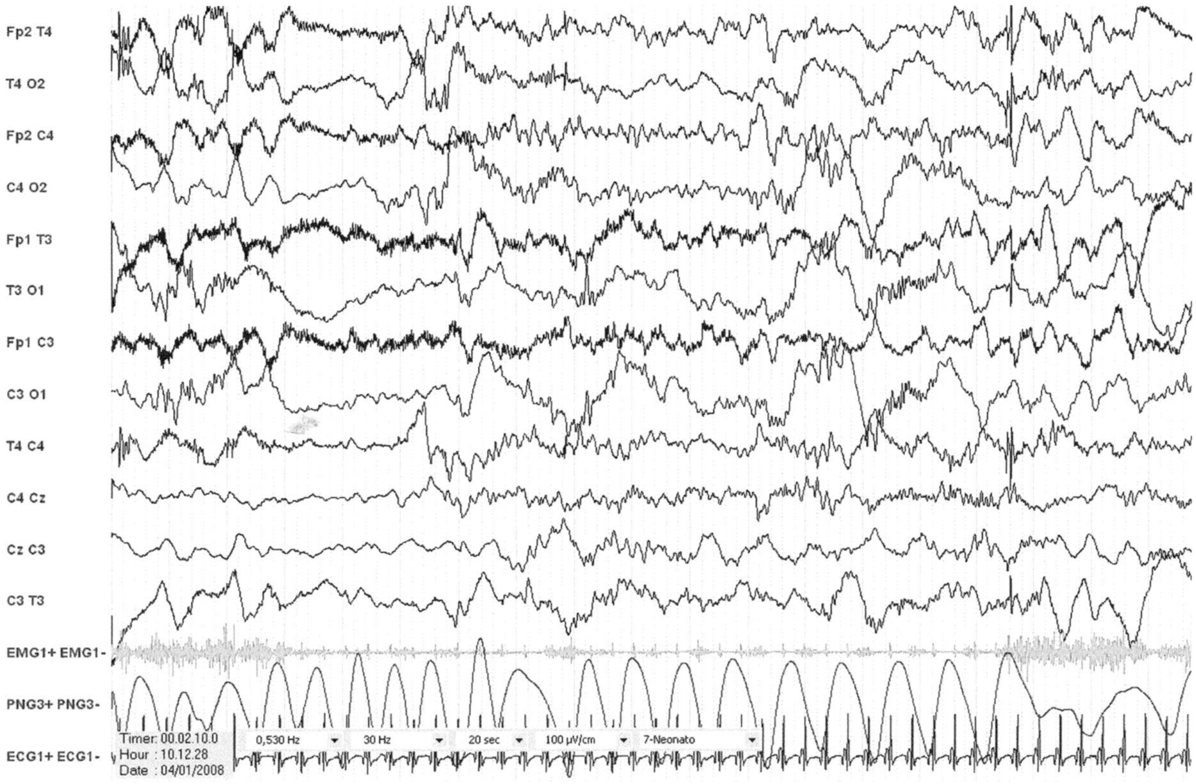

Fig. 22.27b 27 weeks GA, 40.4 weeks CA. **Prematurity** with low birth weight 517 g (small for gestational age—SGA). Cerebral ultrasound: persistent periventricular parenchymal echogenicity. Irritability and wake/sleep cycle alteration. Awake EEG shows, besides the associated muscle activity, several artifacts, diffuse and transient (4 s) attenuation of the background, **external dischronism** (present also during quite sleep with prolonged bilateral asynchronous flattening of the background)

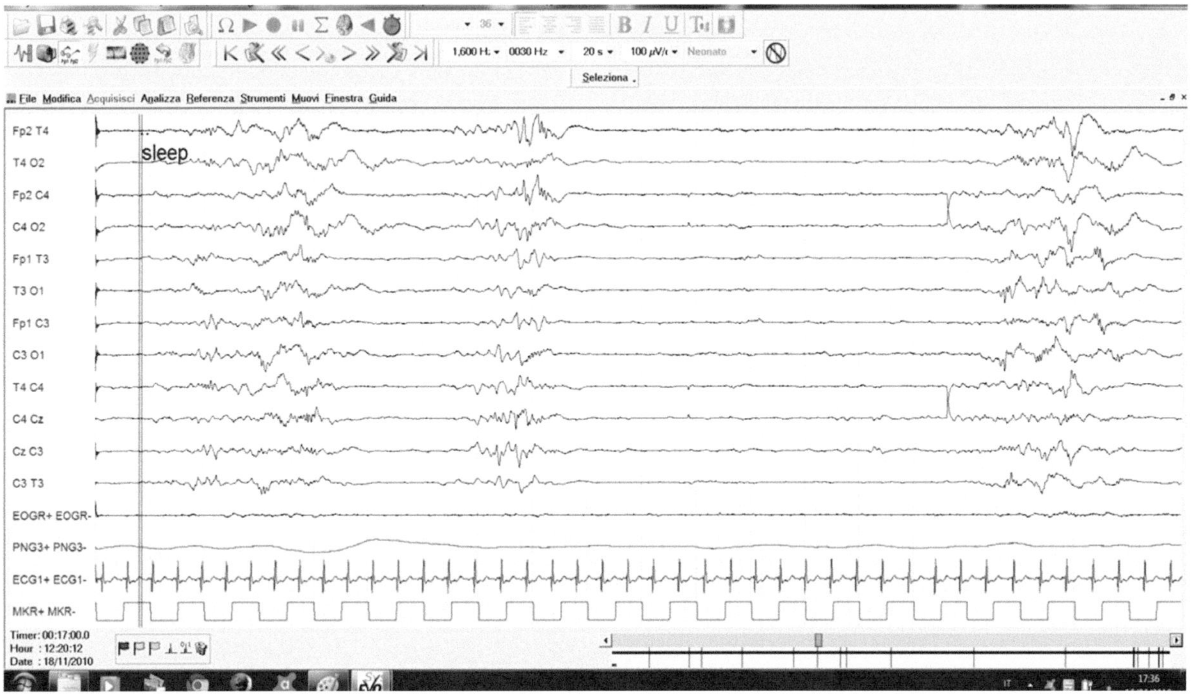

Fig. 22.28 38 weeks GA, 38.5 weeks CA. Pregnancy complicated by polyhydramnios from the 32nd week GA. Uneventful spontaneous delivery. The newborn is hypotonic and hyporeactive, with feeding difficulties. During quite sleep, the **EEG background is quite discontinuous** with bursts (3–8 s) characterized by delta-theta high-voltage and beta slow-voltage activities with intermixed sharp waves asymmetrical between the two hemispheres separated by periods (3–10 s) of marked generalized voltage attenuation

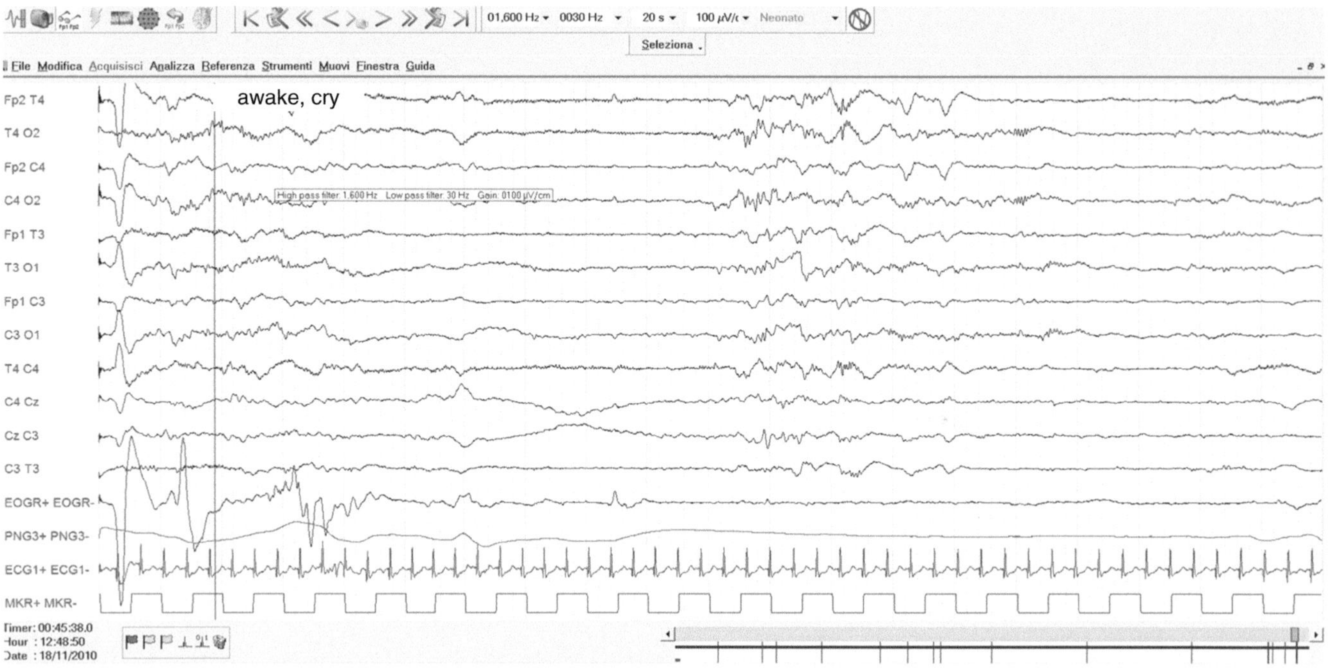

Fig. 22.29 Same newborn and same recording of Fig. 22.28. While awake, the baby is crying with open eyes. The **EEG pattern is discontinuous** and similar to what shown during quite sleep; however the bursts are longer. CGH array disclosed a 2.4 Mb de novo deletion in 9q34.11, containing STXBP1 and SPTAN1. **STXBP1 and SPTAN1 neonatal encephalopathy**. Follow-up: epileptic spasms at 2 months, easily controlled by GVG. Severe neurocognitive impairment, without epilepsy at 4 years

Box 22.2: Background EEG Activity Abnormalities

Inactive or isoelectric EEG: cerebral activity constantly lower than 5 mcV and unreactive to somatosensory stimuli (Figs. 22.30 and 22.31).

Suppression-burst EEG pattern: characterized by low-voltage intervals of inactivity (voltage <5 mcV) of variable length, usually longer than 10 s, separated by bursts of high-amplitude (rarely of low voltage) activity of 0.5 up to 10 s in duration. This pattern (Figs. 22.32, 22.33, 22.34, 22.35, 22.36, 22.37 and 22.38) must be distinguished from the discontinuous EEG pattern of the very preterm newborn. In some cases there is a continuum between very discontinuous EEG pattern and suppression-burst EEG pattern (Figs. 22.28, 22.29, 22.39, 22.40, and 22.41).

Persistent low-voltage activity (undifferentiated): EEG activity constantly between 5 mcV and 30 mcV; usually the voltages are modestly higher in the active sleep state compared to the wakefulness and the quiet sleep state (*rapid eye movements*) (Figs. 22.19 and 22.20).

Persistent asymmetry: persistent asymmetry of voltage higher than 50% between homologous regions of the two hemispheres or clear asymmetry of background features between the two hemispheres in all behavioral states: the typical physiological EEG transients of each conceptional week are either reduced or absent in the hemisphere with the lowest activity (Figs. 22.42, 22.43 and 22.44).

Diffuse delta activity: persistent and diffuse high-amplitude delta waves, scarcely reactive to external stimuli.

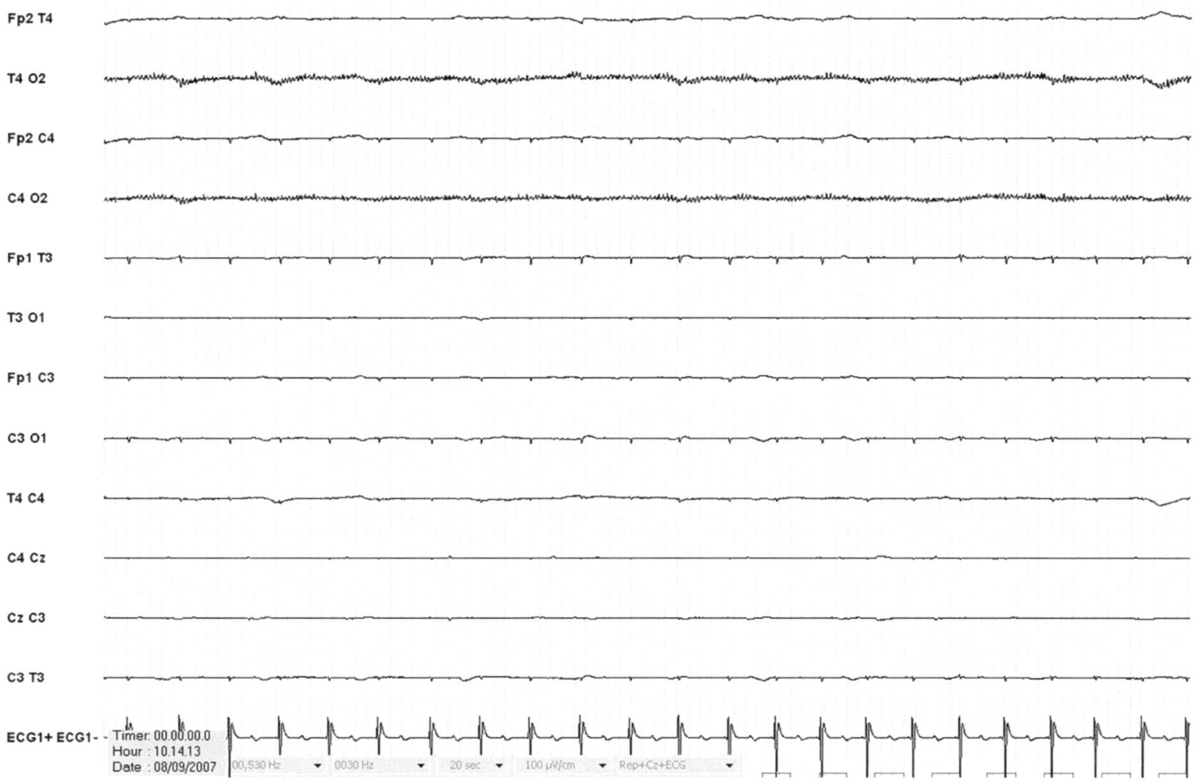

Fig. 22.30 40 weeks GA; 40 weeks CA. Uneventful pregnancy, spontaneous delivery, with shoulder engagement in the expulsive phase >**acute transitory hypoxic ischemic encephalopathy**. Birth weight gr 3770, Apgar score 1-3-5 (at 1′-5′-10′), pH 6.8, BE-22 mmol/L. At 10 h after birth, the newborn is still comatose, unreactive, with severe hypotonia and absence of spontaneous motility, mechanically ventilated in hypothermia treatment. **Inactive tracing** (amplitude constantly less than 5 mcV), not reactive to stimulation. In the first 12 h isolated symptomatic epileptic seizures. Normal brain MRI at 7 and 30 days. Follow-up: normal psychomotor development associated with brachial plexus palsy

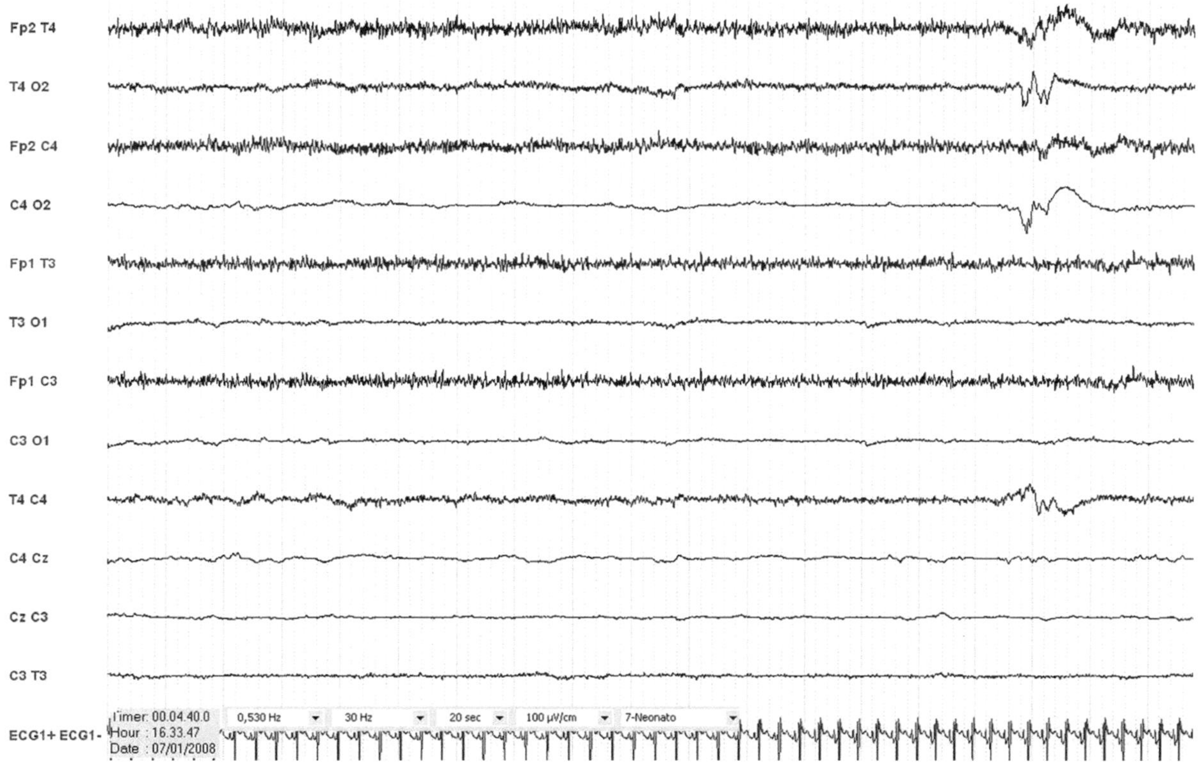

Fig. 22.31 Same case of Figs. 22.66 and 22.41 weeks CA. Three days after the above examination a prolonged heart arrest occurred. Unreactive coma, mechanically ventilated. **Inactive tracing** (amplitude constantly less than 5 mcV), not reactive to stimulation. Few isolated erratic delta and sub-delta slow waves (40–80 mcV) rarely occur, intermingled with slow spikes (up to 80 mcV) or short runs of sharpened theta activity. **Post-anoxic coma**. The next day the newborn died

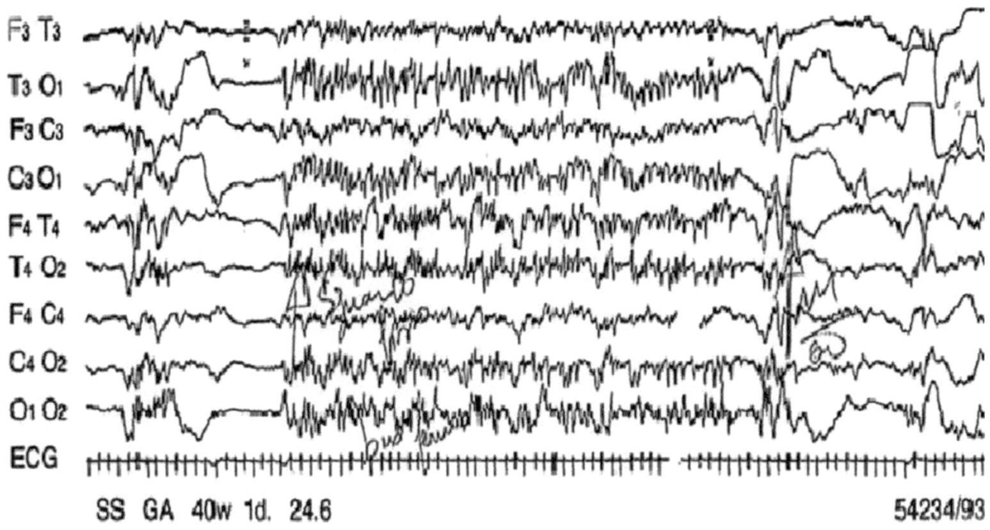

Fig. 22.32 40 weeks GA. Uneventful pregnancy and delivery. On the 1st day, the newborn is lethargic and hyporeactive. Atypical suppression-burst EEG pattern (1–3 s inactive periods intermingled with 1–2 s bursts of slow waves, spike, and sharp-wave activity, up to 250 mcV). In the middle of the figure, **electrical seizure with fast activity that arises from the posterior region, clinically associated with staring**. **Neonatal epileptic encephalopathy B6 deficiency related**. Vit B6 150 mg EV therapy led to seizures control and disappearance of suppression-burst pattern (not shown). Follow-up: mild neurocognitive impairment, normal brain MRI. Remission of epilepsy with chronic B6 therapy (8 years old)

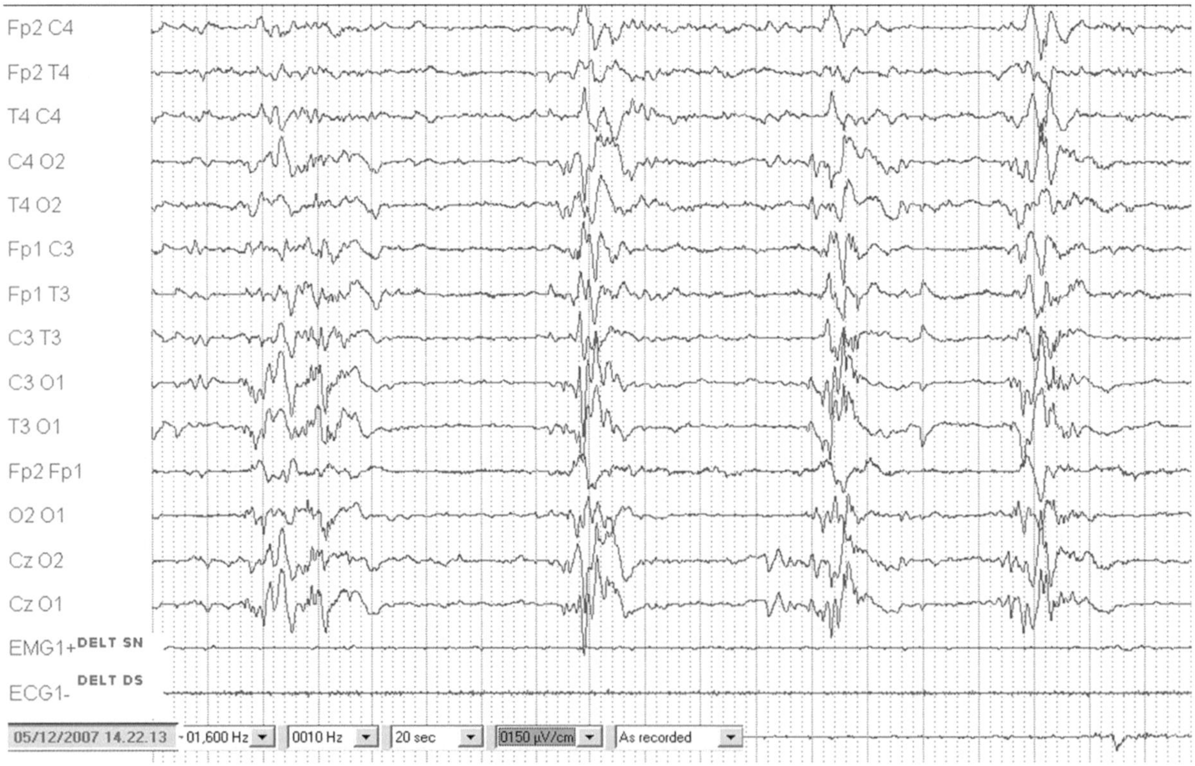

Fig. 22.33 40 weeks GA, 41.4 weeks CA. Uneventful pregnancy and delivery. Recurrent focal right clonic seizures and series of focal spasms from the 2nd day of life, resistant to B6, LZP, and PB IV. In between the seizures, the newborn is hypotonic and hyporeactive. **Asymmetrical suppression-burst** EEG pattern with high-voltage spikes and polyspikes, more evident in left regions. **Neonatal encephalopathy related to repetitive seizure recurrence.** Seizures were controlled by GVG (105 mg/kg/die) therapy, with disappearance of the suppression-burst pattern. Focal clonic right seizures recurred at 1 year old; the brain MRI showed a dysplastic left parieto-occipital lesion. Follow-up: slow progressive neurocognitive impairment associated with AED's resistant epilepsy (12 months old). (Dott. ML Carpanelli courtesy)

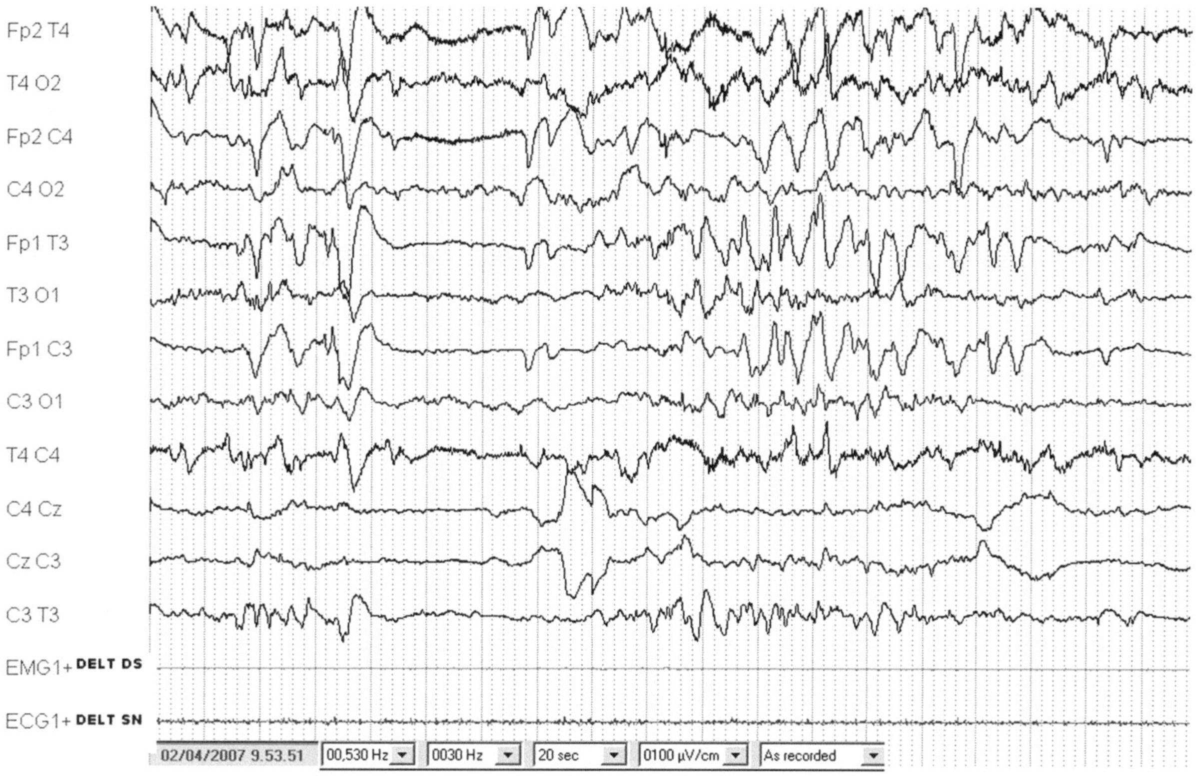

Fig. 22.34 See Fig. 22.35 caption

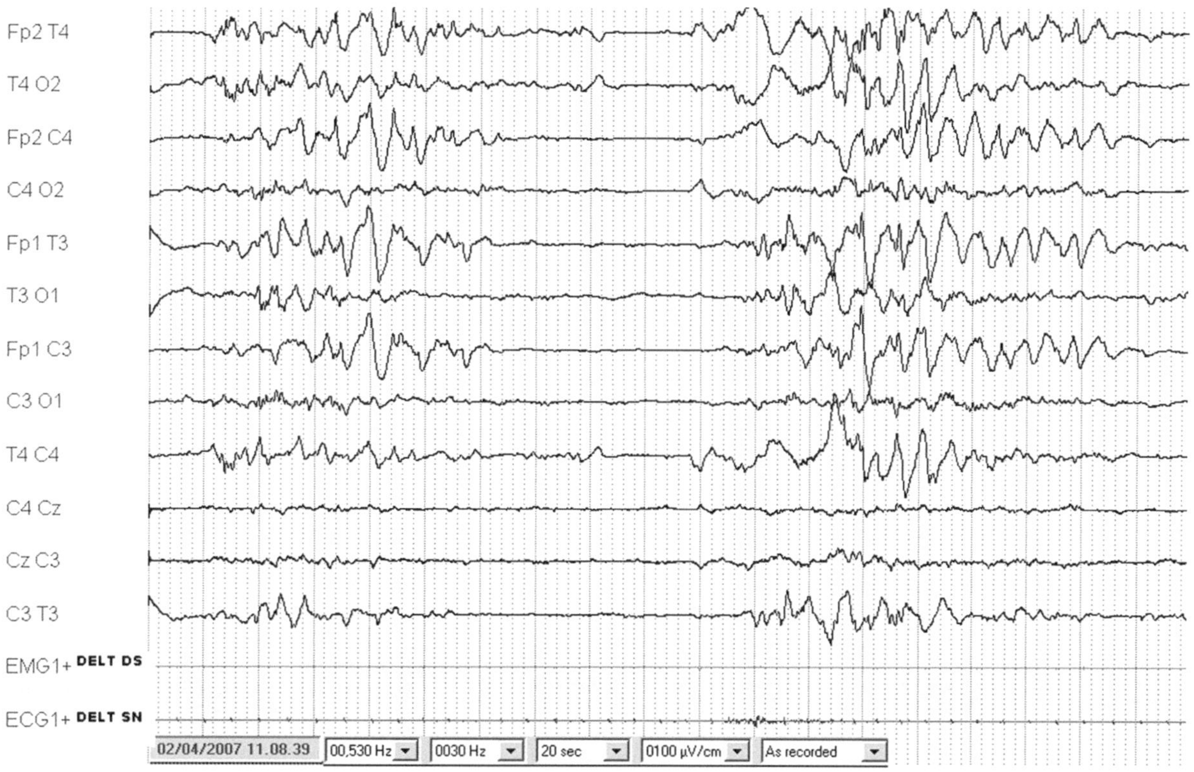

Fig. 22.35 40 weeks GA. Decrease fetal movements starting the day before delivery in an otherwise uneventful pregnancy. Acute hypoxia lasting a minimum of 24 h. Asphyxia at birth. Recurrent seizures in the first 13 days. On the 21st day of life, during PB therapy, **suppression-burst** EEG pattern: interburst bilateral intervals of 3–5 s, "inactive" (below 5–10 mcV), are intermingled with bilateral 4–10 s bursts of delta sharp slow waves mixed with spikes, up to 300 mcV. In wakefulness (Fig. 22.34) compared to sleep (Fig. 22.35), interburst intervals are shorter, and burst activity is longer; however the suppression-burst pattern is unchanged throughout the recording. **Post-anoxic neonatal encephalopathy with suppression- burst.** Brain MRI at 7 and 25 days of life: diffuse cortical-subcortical lesions due to anoxic-ischemic damage. Follow-up: West syndrome at 3 months with severe neurocognitive impairment (12 months old)

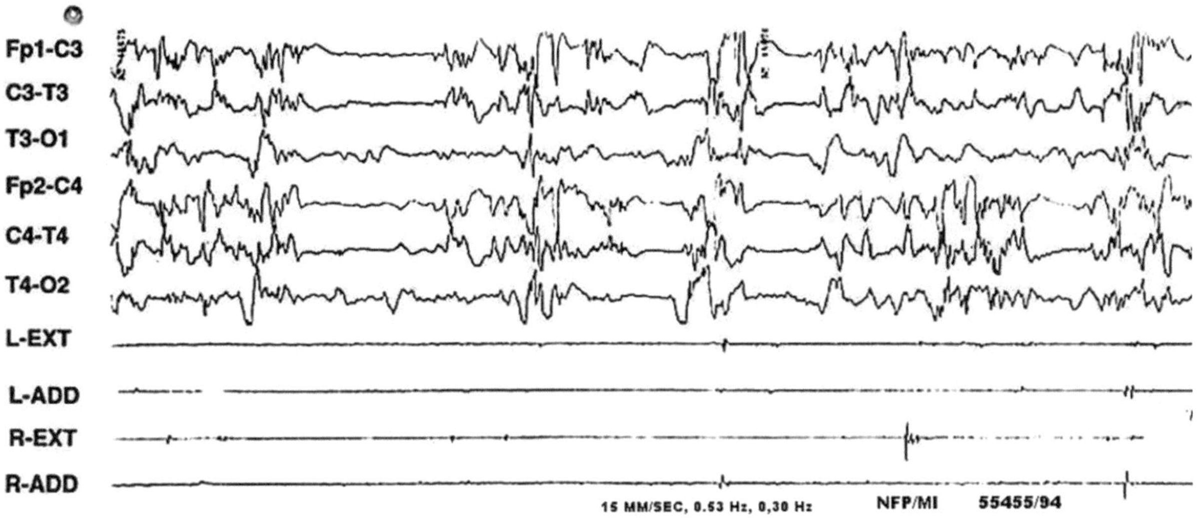

Fig. 22.36 38.4 weeks GA, 40 weeks CA. Uneventful pregnancy and delivery. In the 1st day of life, the newborn is lethargic and hyporeactive. Myoclonic jerks and spasms are referred. On the 9th day **asymmetric/asynchronous suppression-burst pattern**: 2–5 s inactive intervals are intermingled with bilateral 2–5 s asynchronous bursts, with delta and theta broad slow wave activity, up to 350 mcV, mixed with spikes and sharp waves. The bursts appear generally asynchronous between the two hemispheres, and the electrical activity within the bursts is consistently asynchronous. The polygraphy documents the presence of non-epileptic erratic myoclonies. **Early myoclonic encephalopathy due to non-ketotic hyperglycinemia**. Normal brain MRI, hyperammonemia, and high glycine levels both in blood and cerebrospinal fluid. Follow-up: tonic epileptic spasms and severe neurocognitive impairment in the first 3 months followed by continuous non-epileptic segmental erratic myoclonus. Died at 16 years old

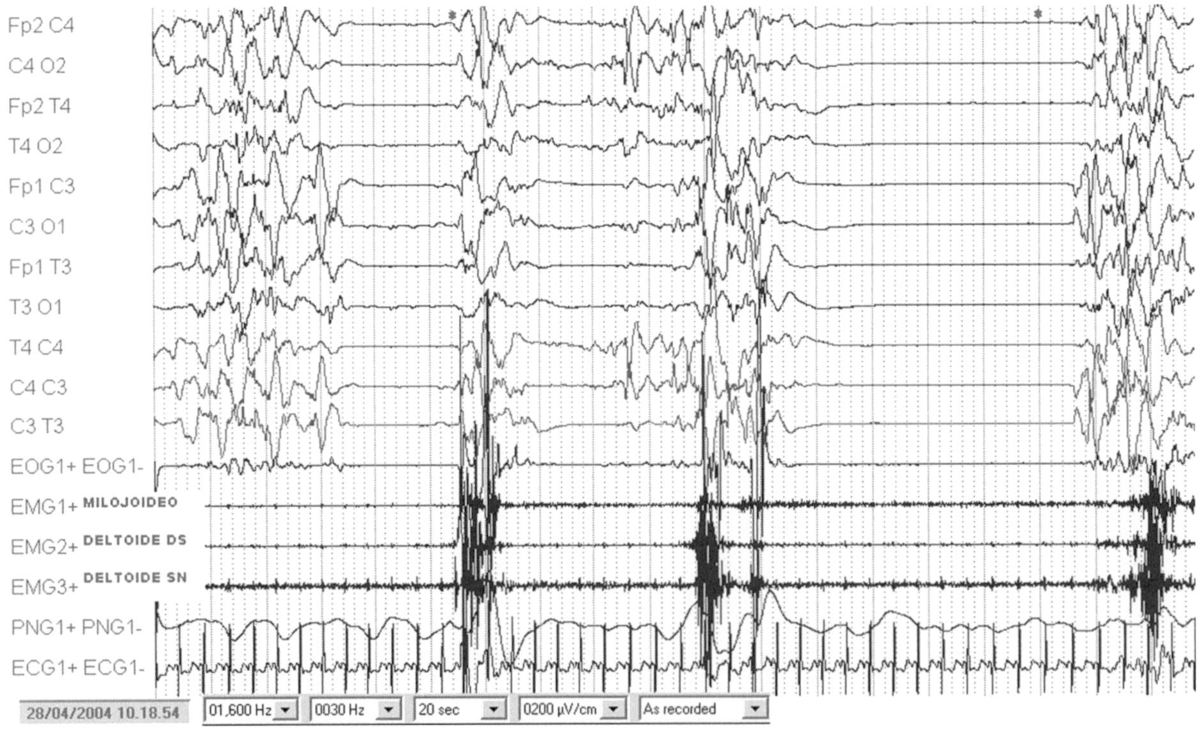

Fig. 22.37 39 weeks GA, 42 weeks CA. Uneventful pregnancy and delivery. Since the 1st day of life, the newborn is hypotonic and hyporeactive with spasms, isolated and in sequence tonic spasms, bilateral independent focal motor clonic seizures, resistant to DZP, PB, and PHT. At 21 days of life, **suppression-burst pattern with undifferentiated trace in wakefulness and sleep**. Two to five seconds flat traces (less than 10 mcV) are regularly interspersed with 2–5 s bilateral bursts of slow waves, spikes, and polyspike-slow wave complexes, up to 400 mcV. The bursts are often associated with clinic spasms and tonic spasms (recorded in polygraphy). **Early infantile epileptic encephalopathy (EIEE)**, presumed genetic in nature (Brain MRI, blood and urinary metabolic screening were normal). Follow-up: AED's resistant epilepsy > West syndrome > Lennox Gastaut syndrome with severe neurocognitive impairment (36 months old)

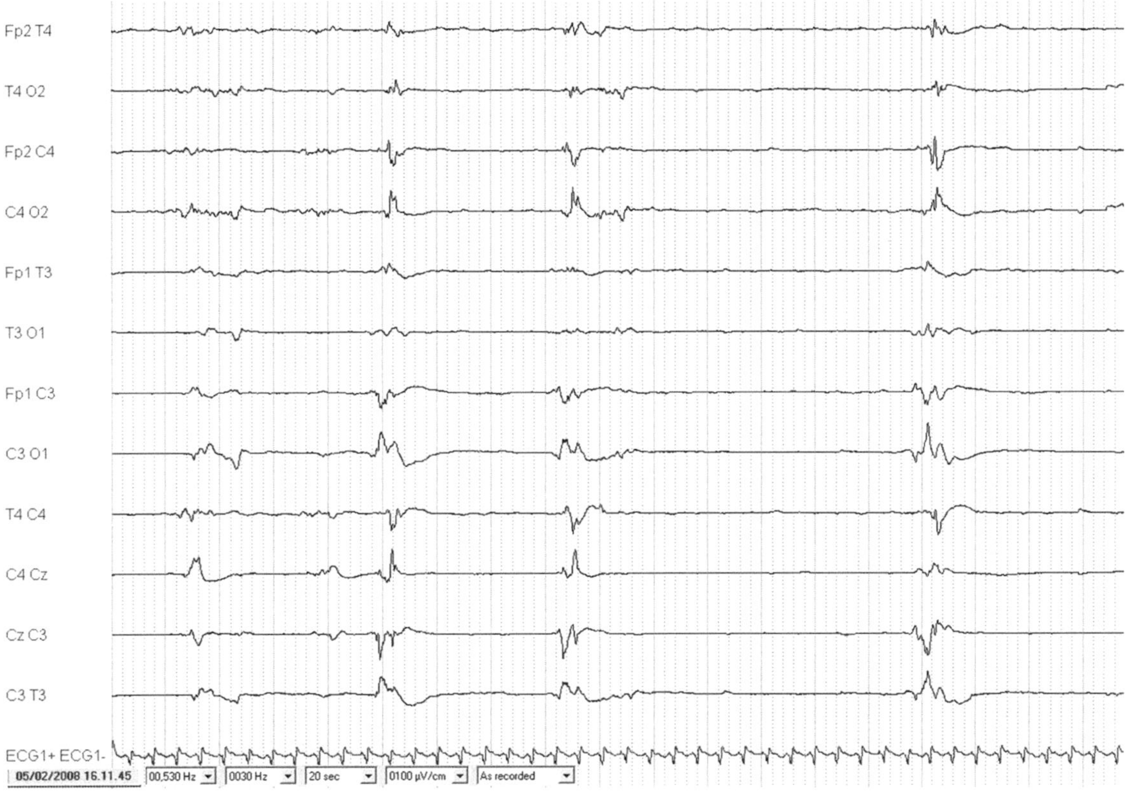

Fig. 22.38 40 weeks GA, 43.3 weeks CA. Uneventful pregnancy and delivery. At 22 days of life ***Streptococcus beta-haemolyticus* type B encephalitis associated with convulsive > electrical status epilepticus. Induced thiopental sodium coma with infraclinical multifocal recurrent seizures with electro-clinical dissociation and severely abnormal background activity**. Follow-up: severe neurocognitive impairment > West syndrome at 6 months > developmental encephalopathy with AED's resistant epilepsy > died at 3 years old. At 24 days of life: **suppression-burst EEG pattern** during thiopental sodium therapy with 5 mg/kg/h: 2–5 s flat periods (less than 10 mcV) are regularly intermingled with 2–5 s bilateral short (1–2 s) bursts of theta and/or delta slow waves, with superimposed spikes and/or polyspikes high as 50–150 mcV. Slow wave complexes, up to 400 mcV

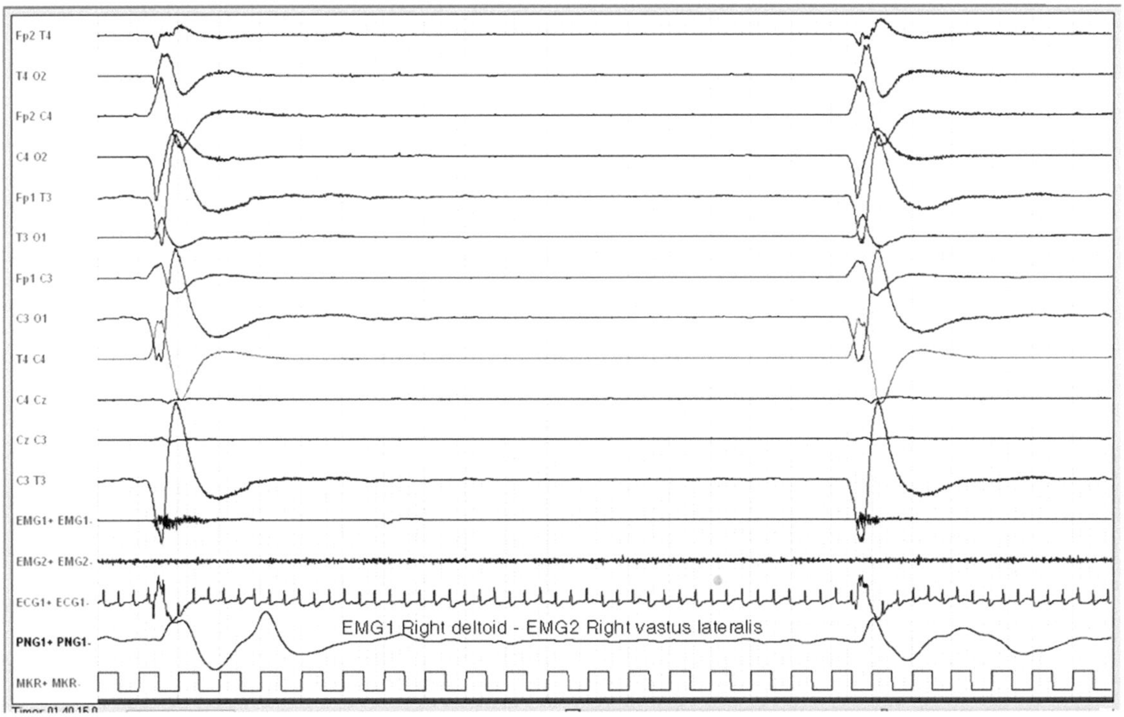

Fig. 22.39 26 weeks GA; 26.3 weeks CA. In the 2nd day of life **bilateral intraventricular hemorrhage** of severe degree. **Pathological discontinuous background activity with periodic high amplitude, biphasic delta waves with a smooth and acute shape**. Interburst intervals are flat, without electrical activity. *Time base: 10 mm/s*. Follow-up: mild intellectual disability, spastic diplegia (5 years old)

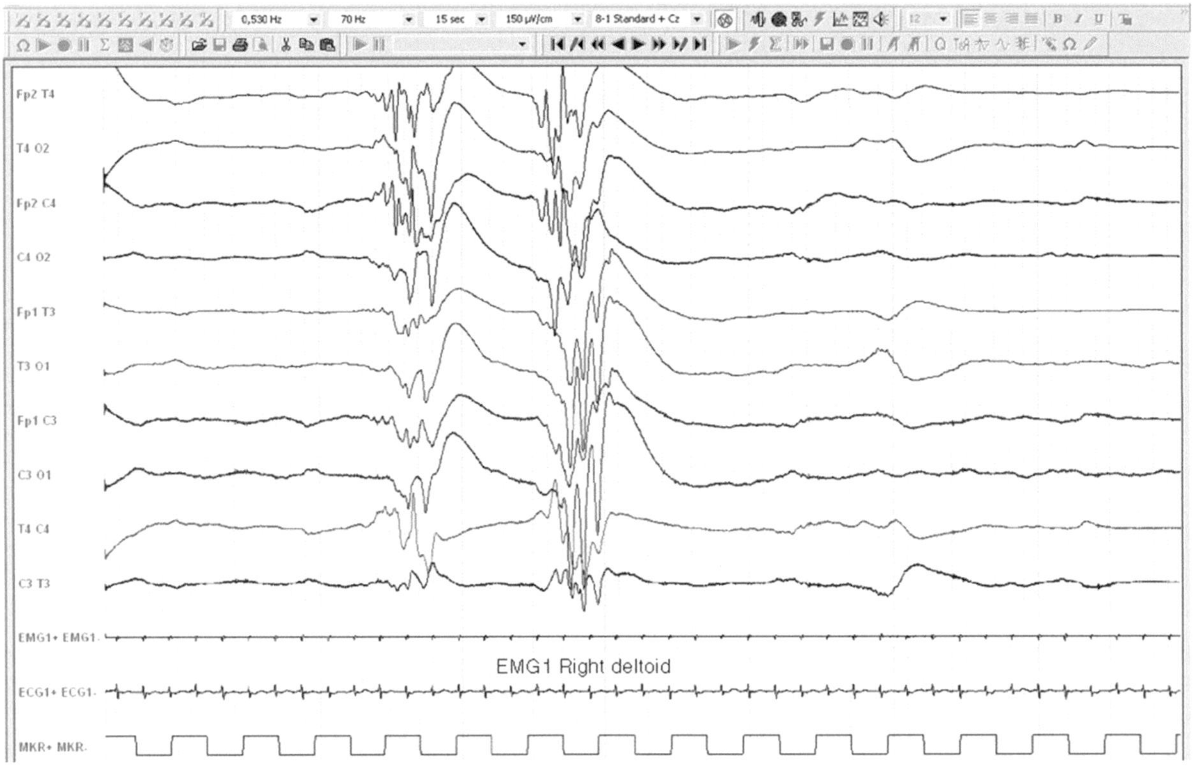

Fig. 22.40 26 weeks GA; 26.3 weeks CA. Uneventful pregnancy, prelabor rupture of membranes with caesarian section. **Bilateral intraventricular hemorrhage**. Diffuse, high-voltage theta bursts. **Pathological discontinuous tracing**. The bursts are followed by high-voltage very slow wave transients**.** The interburst interval is variable. Follow-up: mild intellectual disability with minimal motor impairment (3 years old)

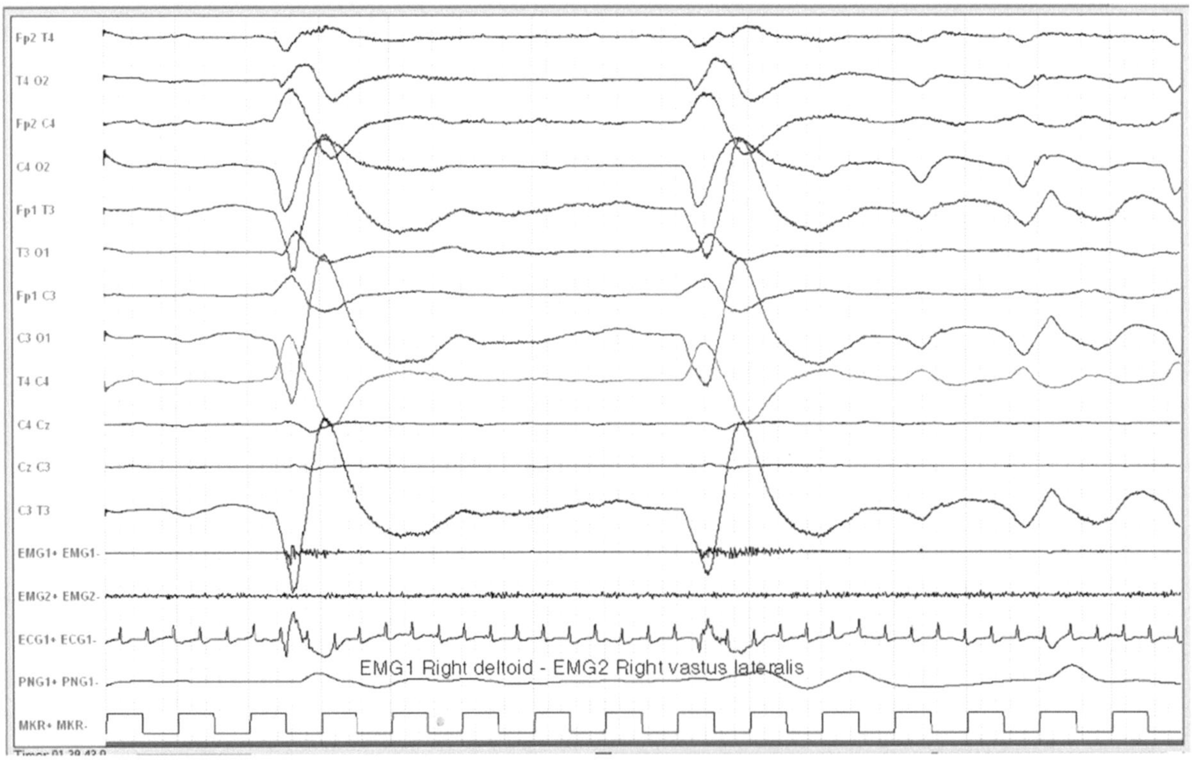

Fig. 22.41 26.4 weeks GA, 27 weeks CA. Prematurity related to cesarean section performed for IUGR. Brain ultrasound: intraventricular hemorrhage of III–IV degree. Discontinuous background activity. **High amplitude, biphasic delta waves more evident on the left temporal region**. Interburst interval with bilateral, positive, very slow waves. Absent delta brushes and theta temporal sequences. Follow-up: at 14 months hyperactivity and mild neurocognitive impairment

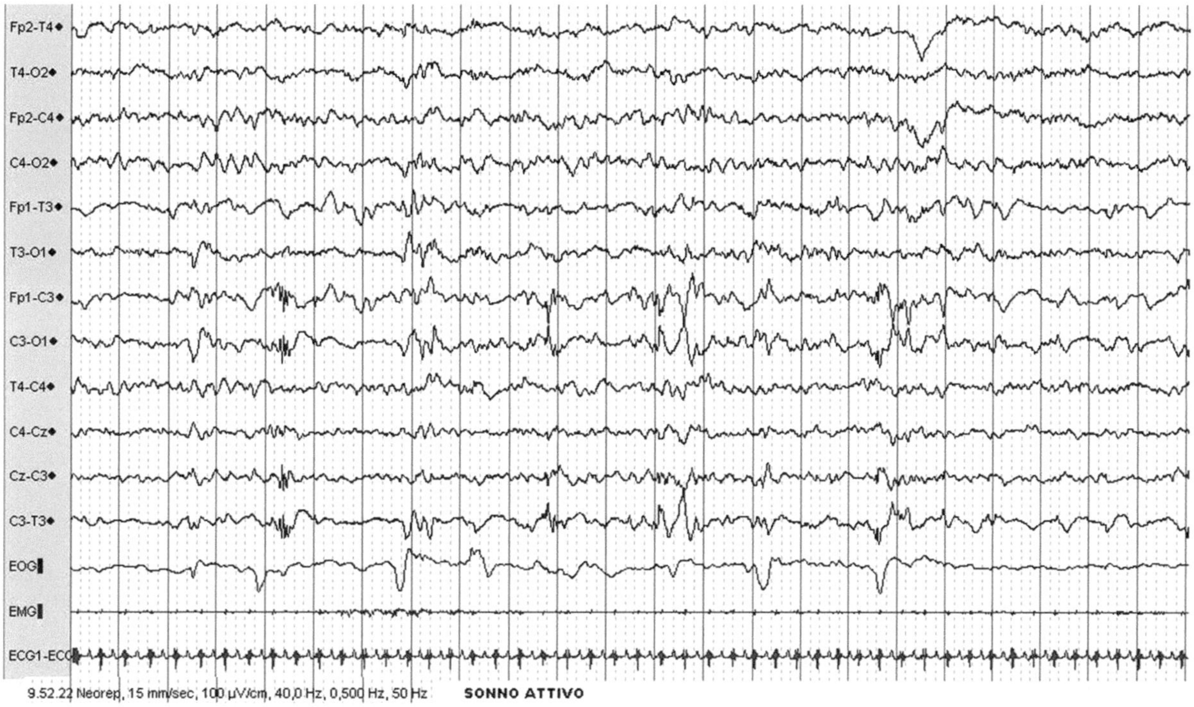

Fig. 22.42 See Fig. 22.43 caption

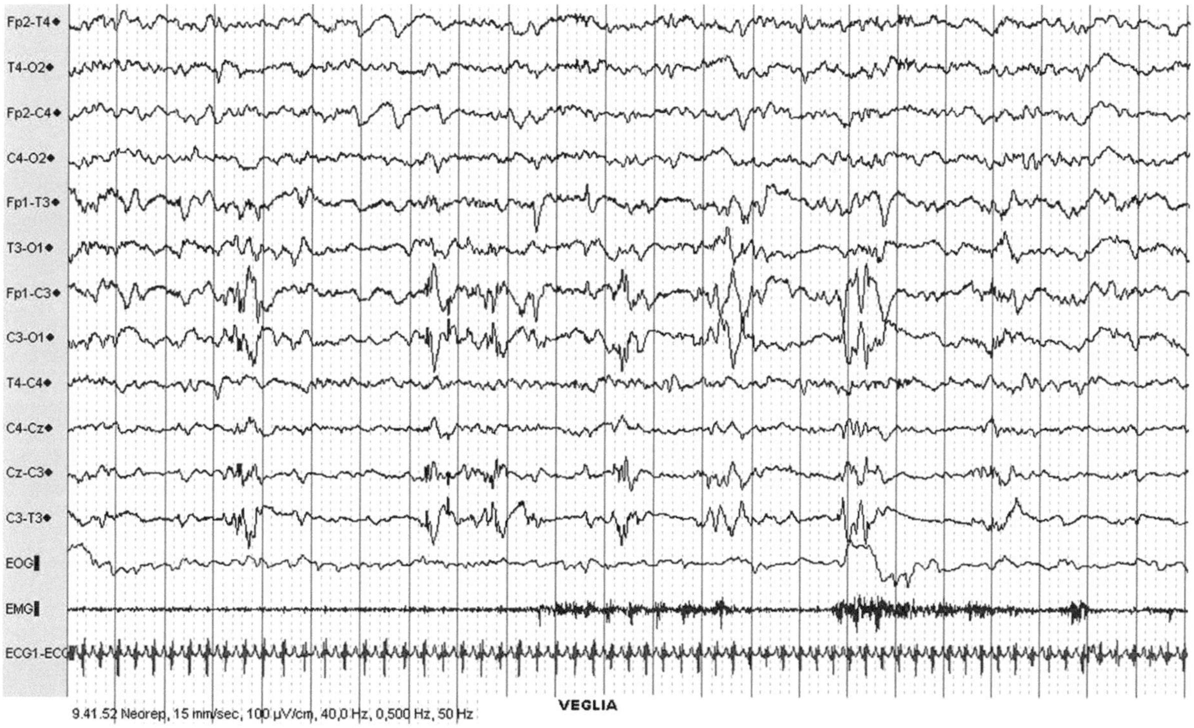

Fig. 22.43 36 weeks GA, 43 weeks CA. Uneventful pregnancy and delivery, the mother is a factor V Leiden mutation carrier. At birth asymmetric spontaneous movements (reduced in right side). Background activity is normal in the right side during wakefulness. Pattern characterized by **constant interhemispheric voltage asymmetry of background activity in the left hemisphere; slow theta-delta activity with superimposed spikes and polyspikes up to 200 mcV**. These EEG characteristics are observed both during wakefulness (Fig. 22.43) and during active sleep (Fig. 22.42). Brain MRI: hyschemic arterial infarction in the left median cerebral artery territory—factor V Leiden mutation heterozygosity. Follow-up: right-side pyramidal hemisyndrome, mild neurocognitive impairment (18 months old)

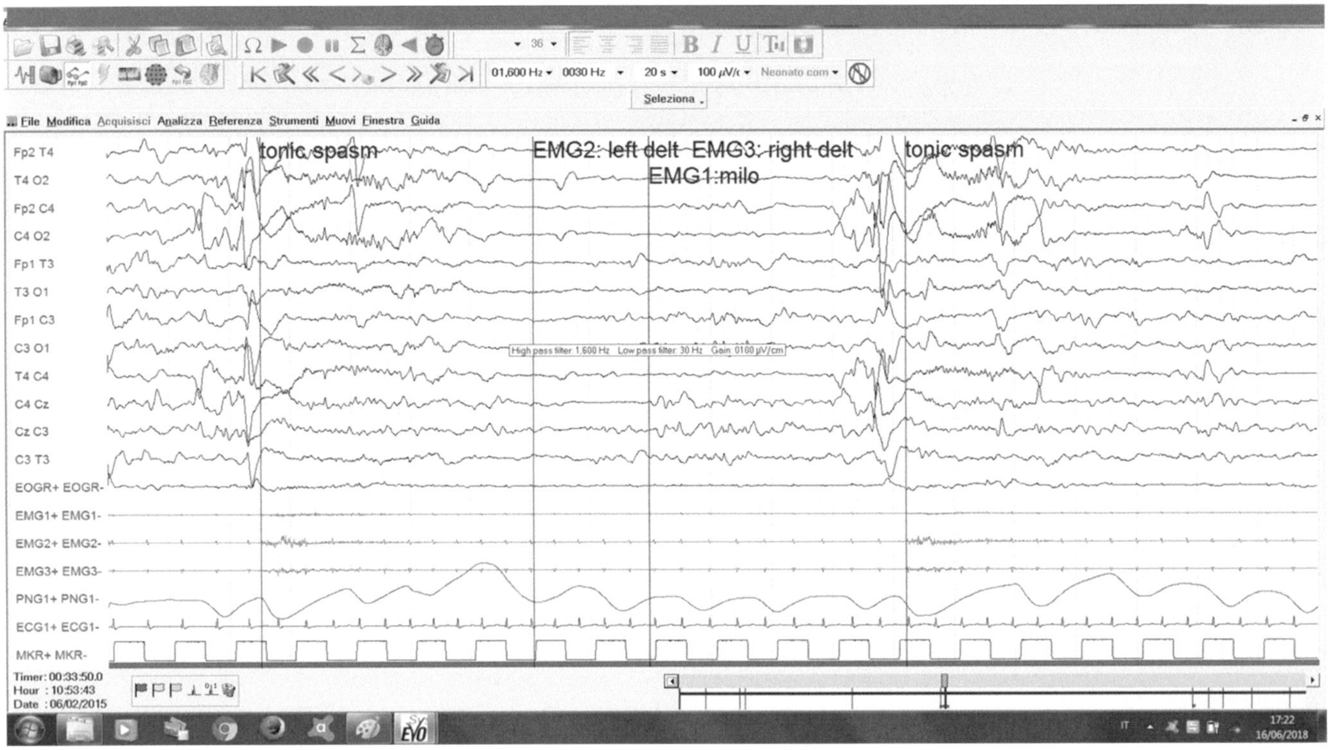

Fig. 22.44 40.6 weeks GA, 43.5 weeks CA. Uneventful pregnancy, till the last week, when the mother referred jerky repetitive fetal movements; urgent cesarean section due to oligohydramnios. Neonatal left arm and leg clonic seizures from the 1st day of life. **Neonatal focal symptomatic epilepsy**. Series of spasms in the second and third week of life. In therapy with PB 4 mg/kg/die, PHT 19 mg/kg/die. **Asymmetrical suppression-burst EEG pattern with high-voltage slow spike followed by high-voltage slow wave more evident in the right hemisphere, associated with a tonic spasm evident in the EMG channel. After the tonic spasm, a short run of alpha slow-voltage activity is evident in the right posterior region**. Two electro-clinical events are shown. Brain MRI: **right hemisphere polymicrogyria**

Box 22.3: Abnormal EEG Pattern/Transients

Positive rolandic sharp waves (PRSWs): they can be identified in the rolandic regions (phase reversal in C3 and C4): they are physiological if isolated, with onset between 28 and 32 weeks of CA, bilateral and asynchronous, with an amplitude lower than 150 mcV; if frequent, repetitive, unilateral, and of high amplitude, they can be expression of a focal hemorrhage or white matter injury (Fig. 22.45).

Positive temporal sharp waves (PTSWs): temporal sharp waves that according to morphology, polarity and frequency can represent underlying focal brain injury (Figs. 22.46, 22.47, and 22.48).

Spikes or sharp waves (frontal, temporal, central, occipital): recurrent spikes or sharp waves in the frontal, temporal, central, or occipital regions. They are usually single, bilateral, synchronous, and asynchronous between homologous regions of the two hemispheres (Figs. 22.45 and 22.47).

Multifocal slow sharp waves: multiple foci of high-amplitude slow waves, abundant and recurrent with an irregular rhythmicity. They can be associated with underlying diffuse brain injury (Fig. 22.49).

Focal rhythmic activity (at the vertex and/or in variable regions): the presence of rhythmic activity in beta, alpha, theta, or delta frequency, in short runs, superimposed to a normal background activity, is an unusual pattern in healthy newborns (Figs. 22.50 and 22.51).

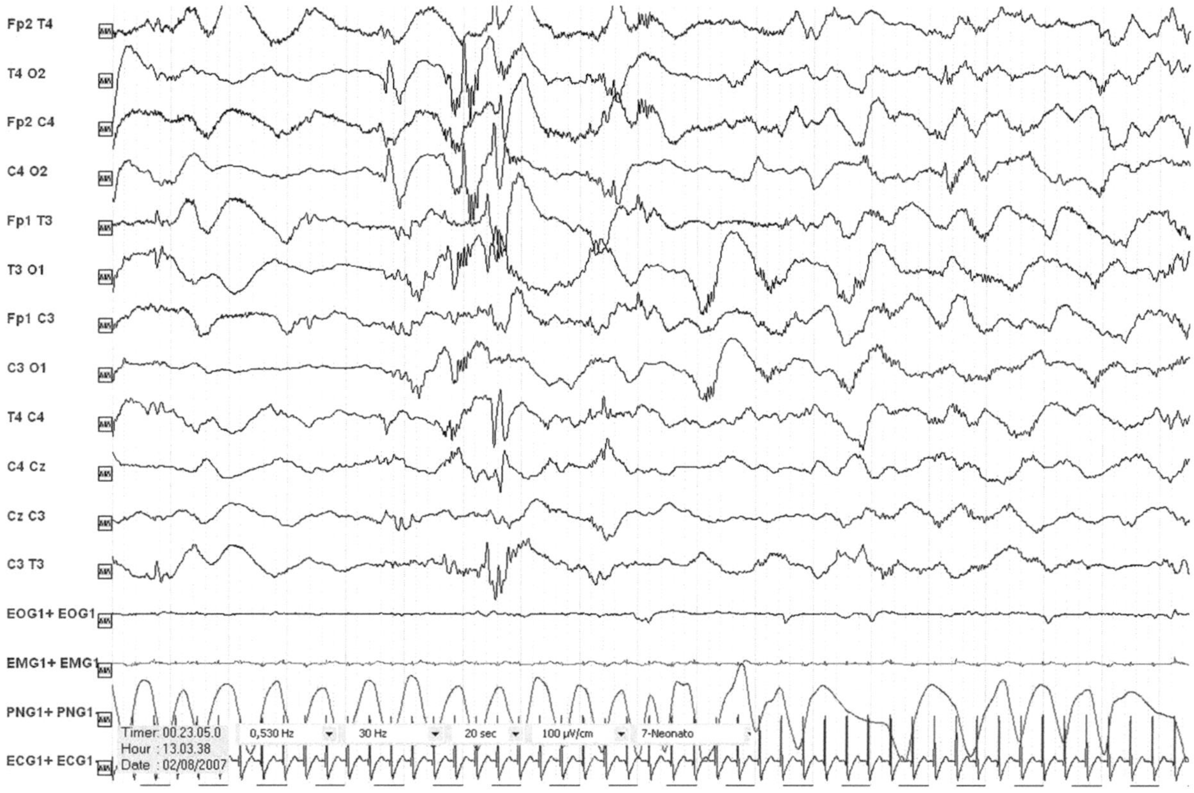

Fig. 22.45 31.2 weeks GA, 32 weeks CA. Uneventful pregnancy; at 31 weeks GA, fetal growth arrest with abnormal blood flows; the baby born through a cesarean section in **fetal distress with IUGR** (1280 g). Intubated and ventilated with surfactant replacement. Brain ultrasound: high echogenicity within right temporoparietal regions. Brain MRI: right hemisphere intraparenchymal hemorrhagic injury. During active sleep normal activity in the left hemisphere. In the right side, in occipital and central regions, spike, slow spike, and polyspike activity is present, within a right background activity with short periods of posterior flattening. **Multifocal slow spike activity associated with constant background asymmetry**

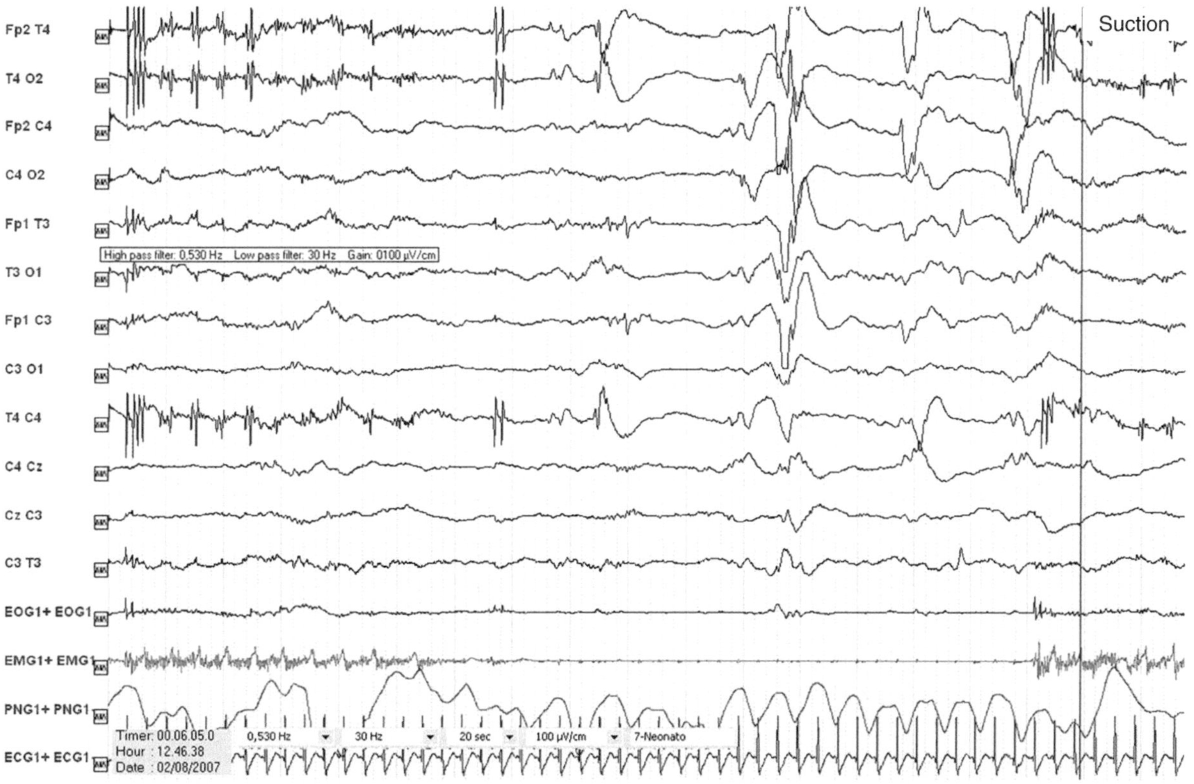

Fig. 22.46 Same newborn as in Fig. 22.45 Quite alert. Besides artifacts in T4, notice the positive slow- and low-voltage spike intermingled with a high-amplitude slow wave, followed by focal and isolated slow spikes in the frontotemporal region. **Positive temporal sharp waves (PTSWs)**

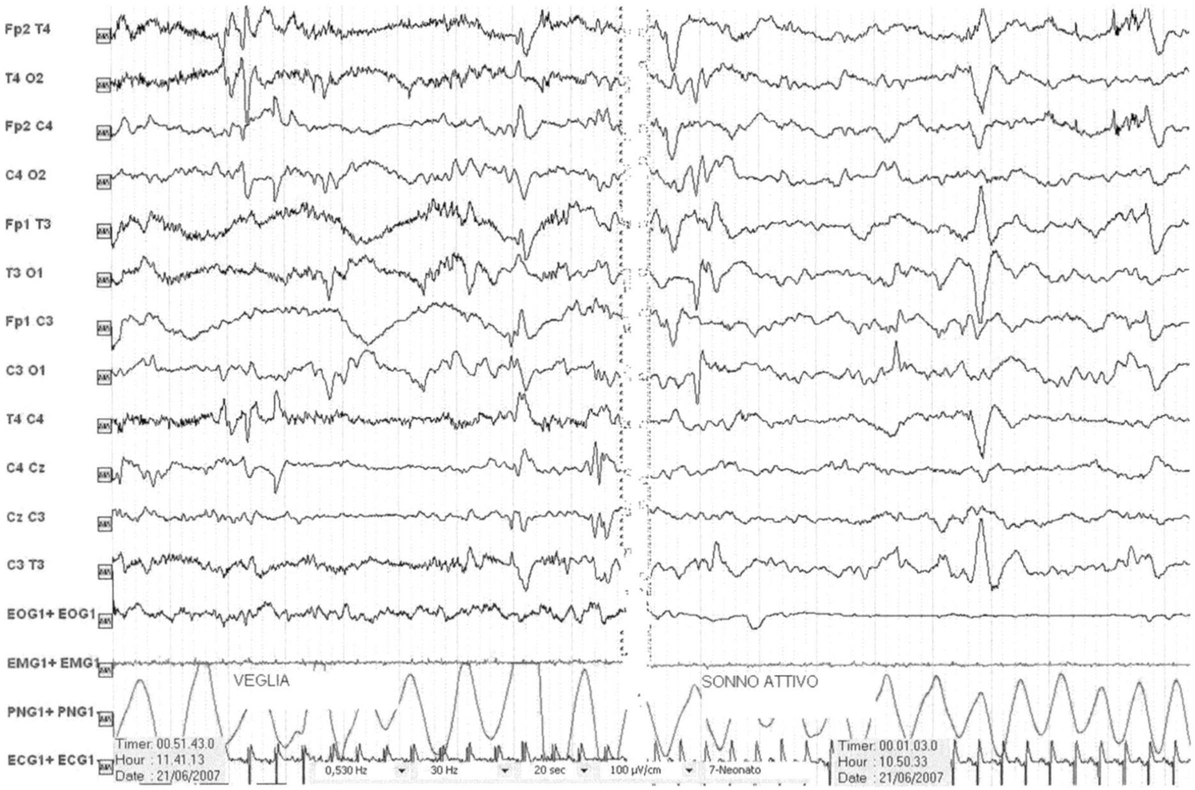

Fig. 22.47 36 weeks GA, 36.4 weeks CA. Urgent cesarean section due to fetal movements reduction in the last 48 h. At birth the newborn is hypotonic and hyporeactive. In the 1st day of life brisk, synchronous and asynchronous, erratic movements. **Prenatal hypoxic ischemic injury-hyperalert.** During wakefulness (in the left side of the image) normal background activity with superimposed right temporal slow wave and slow spikes high up to 250 mcV; during active sleep (right side) bilateral positive temporal slow spikes high up to 300 mcV are present. **Positive temporal sharp waves (PTSWs)**. Follow-up: normal development (8 months old)

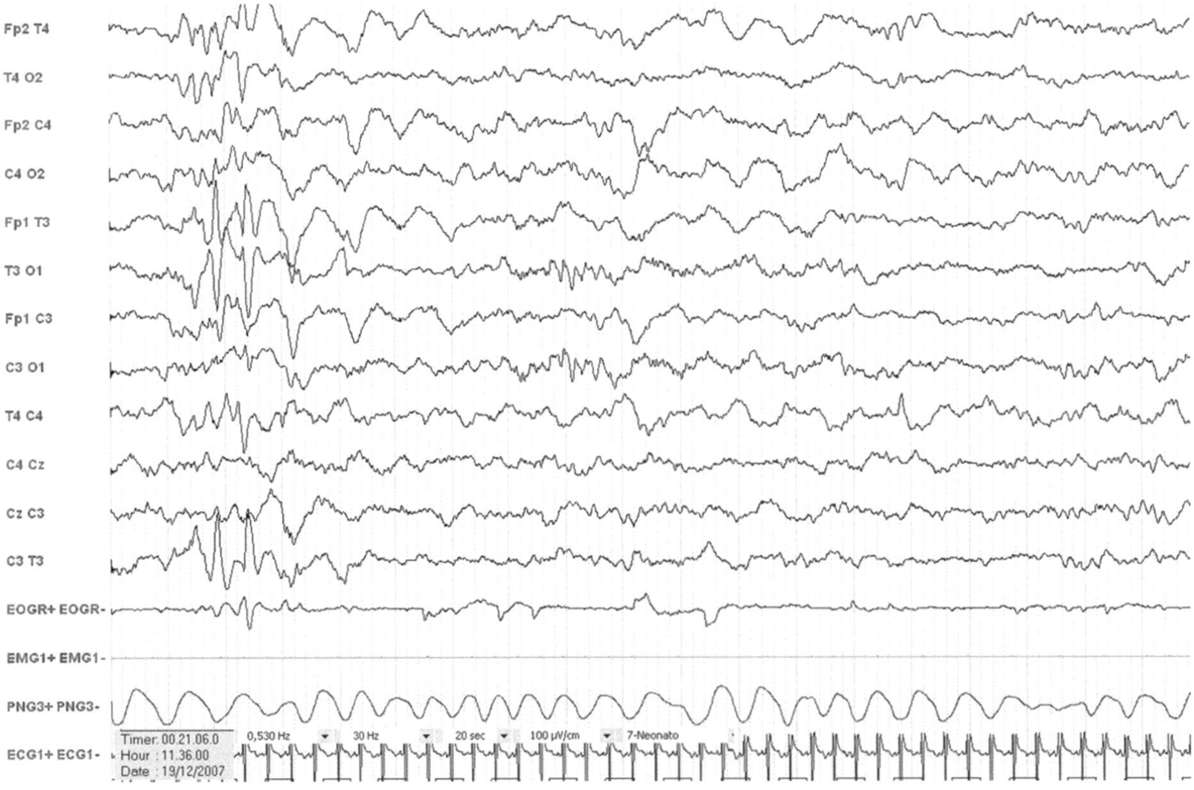

Fig. 22.48 38.4 weeks GA, 39.4 weeks CA. Fetal ascites. Normal delivery and perinatal period. 8 days of life, active sleep: **sequence of two-three phase-reversal high-voltage slow spikes in the left temporal region**. Background activity is normal for age. Brain MRI: mega-cisterna magna, **peritrigonal multiple micro-hemorrhagic lesions in the left hemisphere**. Follow-up: normal development (7 months old)

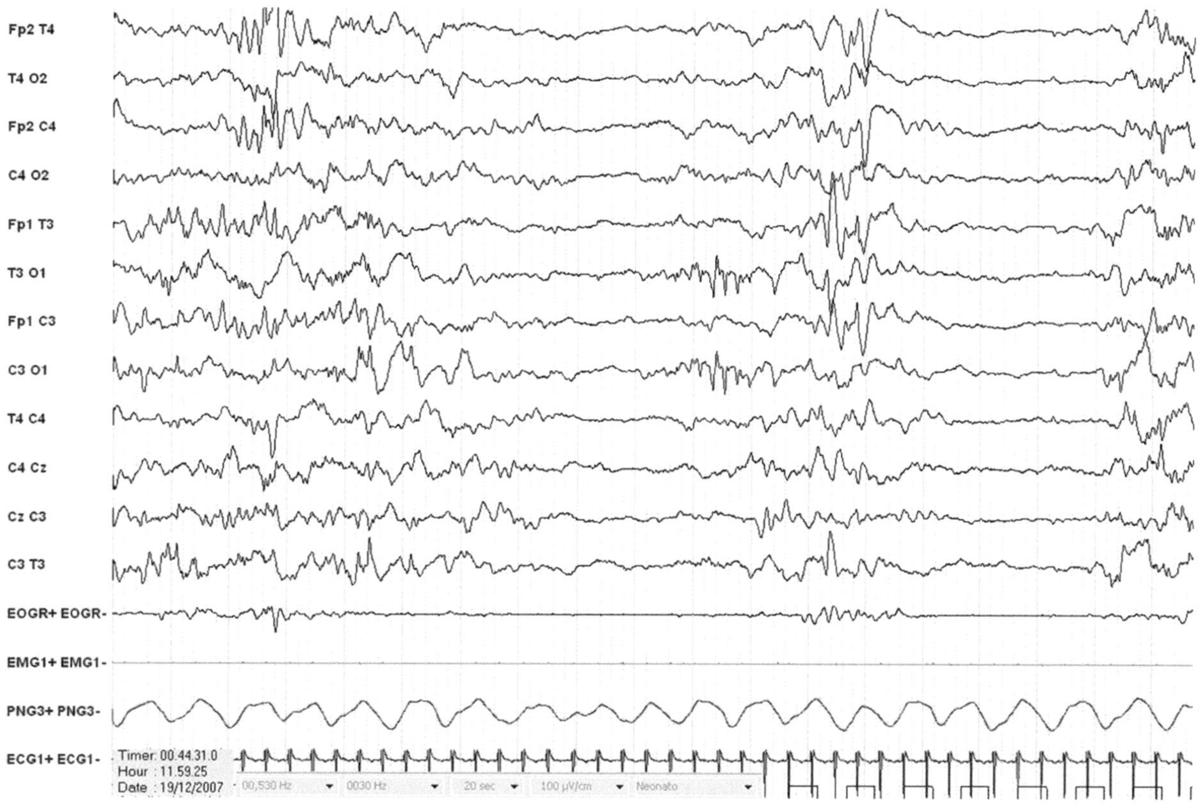

Fig. 22.49 Same newborn and same tracing as in Fig. 22.48. During quite sleep the tracè alternant pattern is quite discontinuous and asynchronous for the CA (**internal dyschronism**) with low-amplitude inter-burst interval. In addition **multifocal polymorphic slow spike** with voltage within 80–200 mcV, expressed independently in the left posterior frontal right and left regions

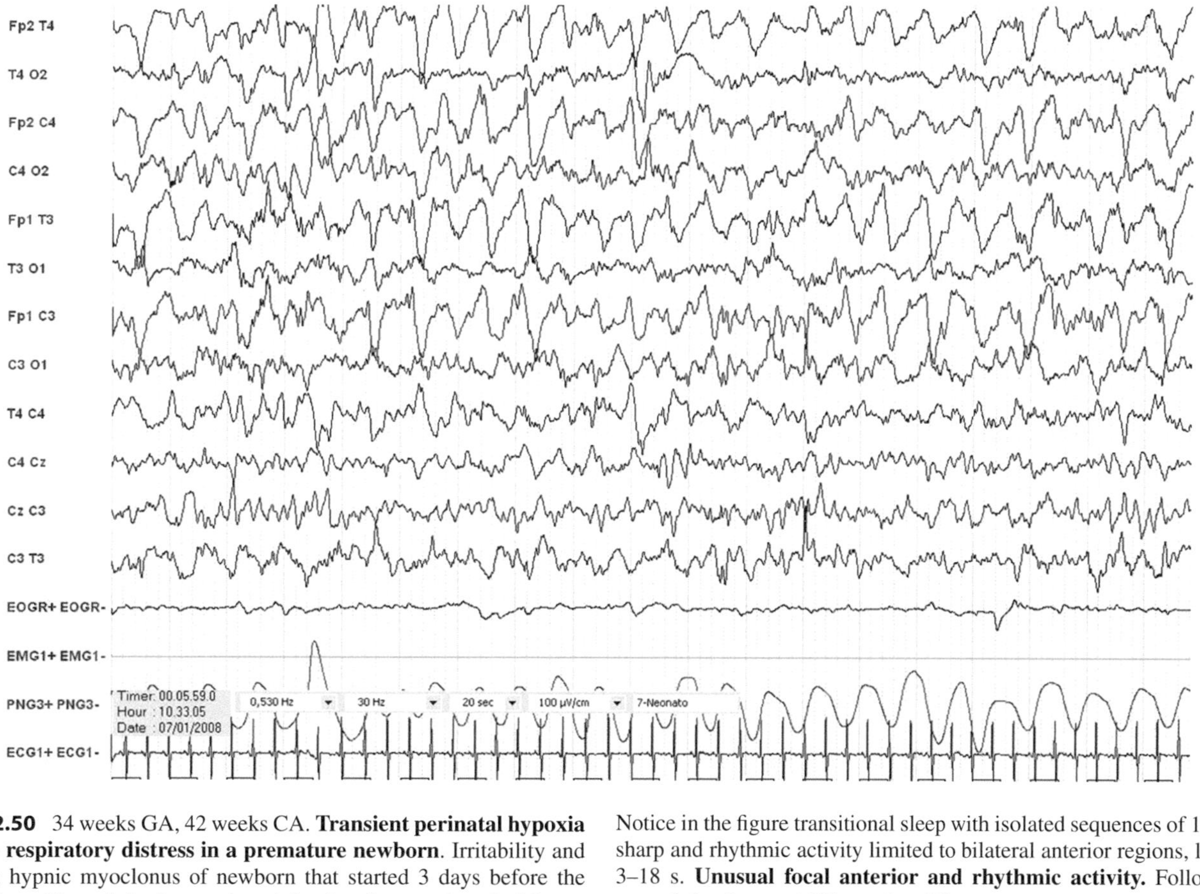

Fig. 22.50 34 weeks GA, 42 weeks CA. **Transient perinatal hypoxia due to respiratory distress in a premature newborn**. Irritability and benign hypnic myoclonus of newborn that started 3 days before the recording. Normal background activity in sleep and wakefulness. Notice in the figure transitional sleep with isolated sequences of 1–2 Hz sharp and rhythmic activity limited to bilateral anterior regions, lasting 3–18 s. **Unusual focal anterior and rhythmic activity.** Follow-up: normal development (30 months old)

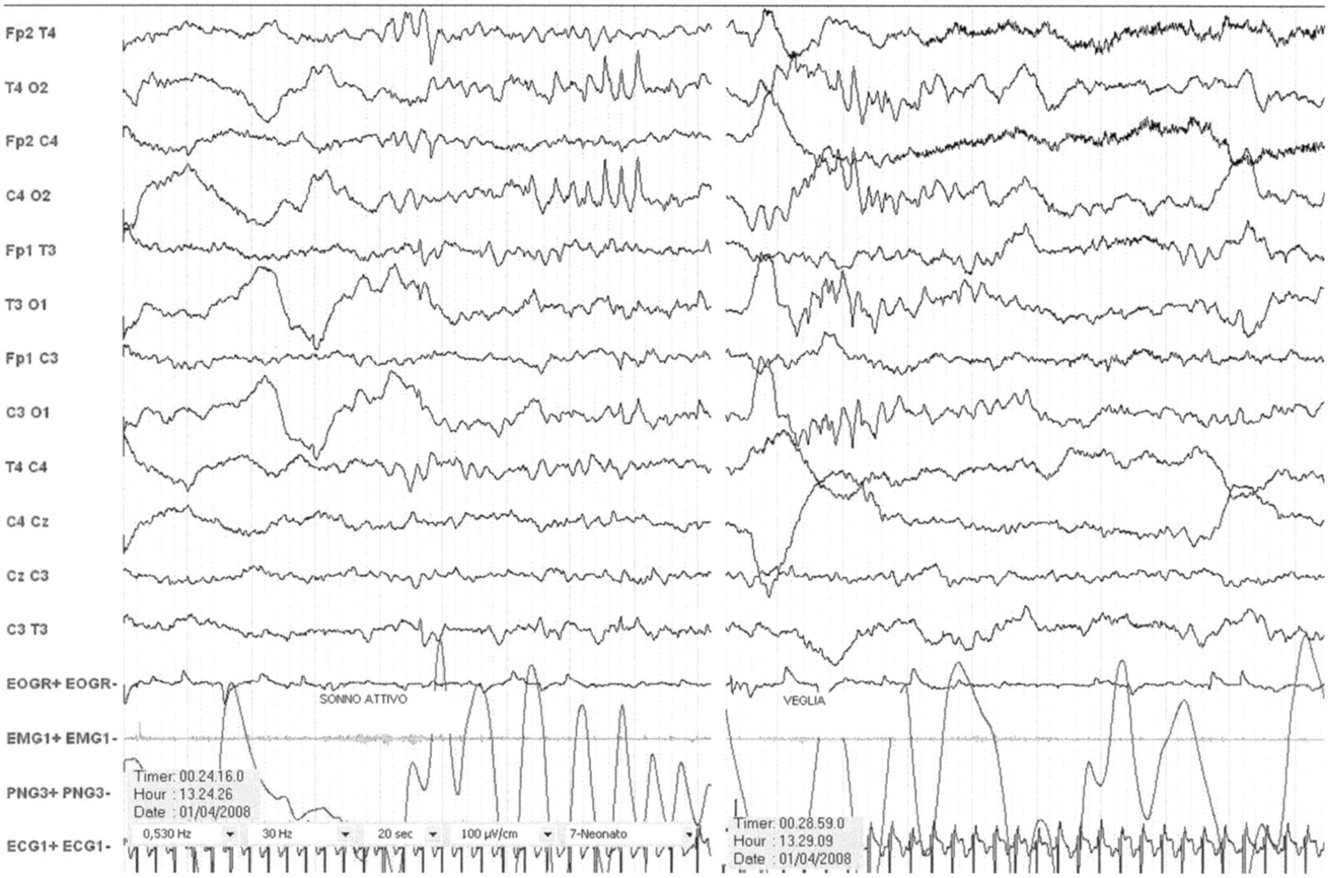

Fig. 22.51 GA 38 weeks, CA 41 weeks. Uneventful pregnancy and delivery. **Irritability at 3 weeks of life**. EEG recording include normal cycles of wake, tracé alternant in quiet sleep and active sleep. In active sleep in O2 (left side of the figure) and during awake state in O1 (right side of the picture), 2–4 s sequences of sharp theta and bilateral (asynchronous) activity with an amplitude up to 120 mcV. **Unusual focal and rhythmic posterior activity**. Follow-up: normal neurodevelopment at 6 months of age

Box 22.4: Ictal Epileptic Abnormalities

Focal or unifocal: sequence of high-amplitude sharp waves with a focal onset, with a range frequency between 5 and 10 Hz, monorhythmic, with sudden onset and end, usually related to clinical focal seizures (Figs. 22.38, 22.52, 22.53, 22.54, 22.55, 22.66, and 22.67).

Focal pseudo-beta-alpha-theta-delta: ictal EEG pattern characterized at the beginning by a low-amplitude rapid electrical activity faster than 12 Hz followed by a frequency reduction up to 4–7 Hz and then up to 0.5–3 Hz with a focal localization (Figs. 22.54, 22.55, and 22.56).

Multifocal activity associated with a pathological background: Multifocal ictal sequence with a synchronous or independent onset with either a fast or variable frequency (sometime with a slow rhythm). An abnormal background activity of low voltage is constantly associated during the inter-ictal periods and with a suppression-burst pattern in the most severe cases (Figs. 22.56, 22.57, 22.58, 22.59, 22.60, 22.61, 22.62, 22.63, and 22.64).

Ictal activities of low frequency associated with a low-voltage background EEG activity: they are characterized by sharp waves at 1 Hz with either focal or multifocal and independent localizations (Figs. 22.58, 22.59, and 22.65).

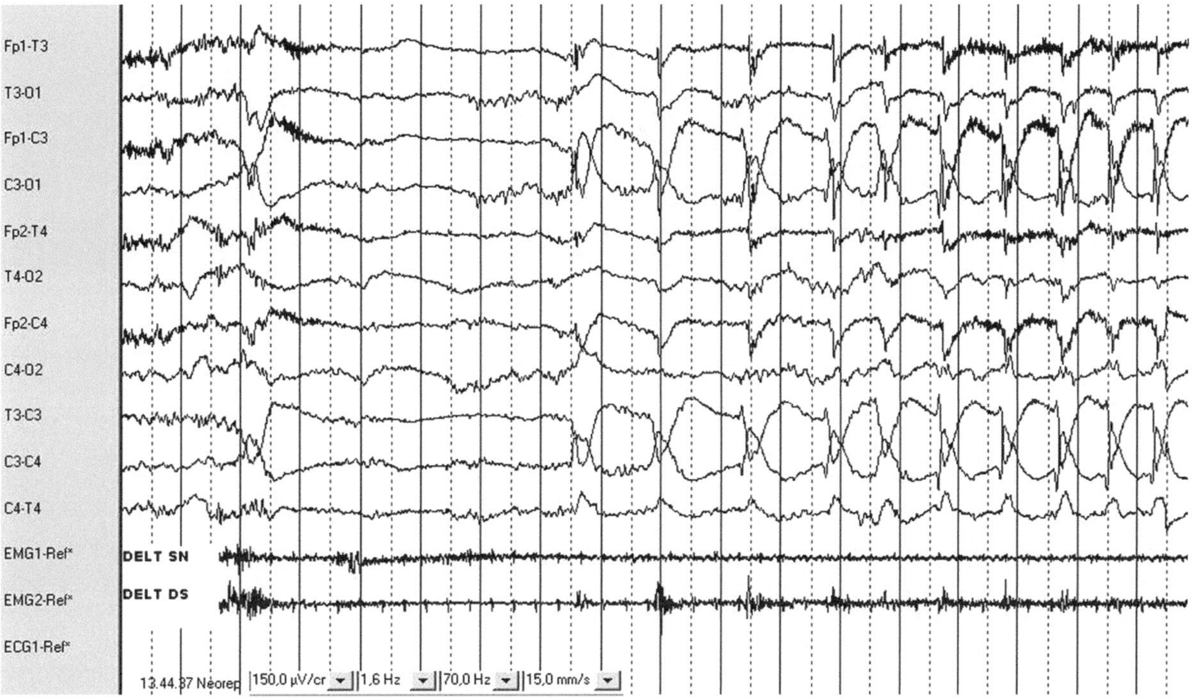

Fig. 22.52 See Fig. 22.53 caption

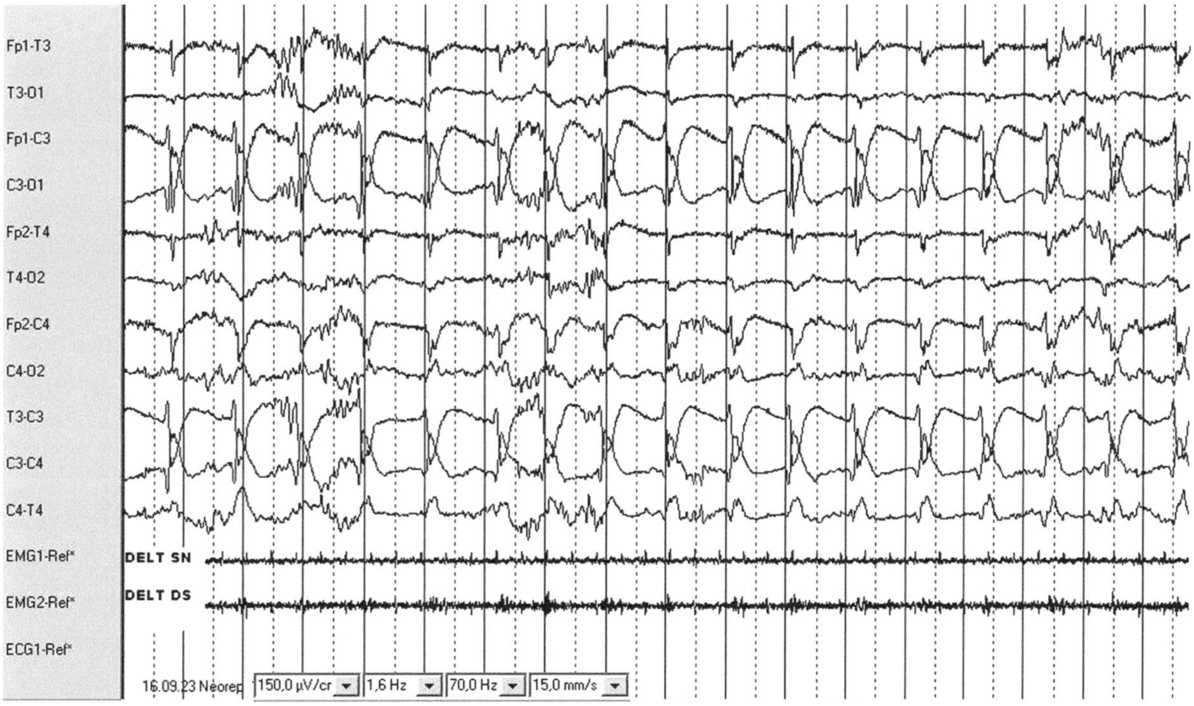

Fig. 22.53 35 weeks GA, 35 weeks CA: Tuberous sclerosis suspected during prenatal ultrasound due to the presence of cardiac rhabdomyomas. At birth the newborn is hypotonic and hyporeactive. Brain ultrasound investigation: multiple periventricular echodensities. On the 3rd day of life, recurrent short (lesser than 1 min) focal proximal right arm clonic seizures associated with staring. **Unifocal (left fronto central) ictal EEG pattern** (the first consecutive 40 s of a seizure are shown in Figs. 22.52 and 22.53): after 5 s EEG flattening associated with a brief bilateral arms contraction seizure discharge arise from the left posterior areas with alpha-like activity lasting less than 2 s, followed by repetitive rhythmic (1/s) spike and high-voltage (up to 180 mcV) slow wave complexes in the fronto-central region. EMG polygraphy of the right deltoid channel shows the rhythmic proximal jerks strictly associated with the spike-slow wave complexes. The seizures (aware, clonic focal motor) end spontaneously in 1–3 min. During the EEG recording (110 min), 14 similar electro-clinical seizures were recorded. Brain MRI: several cortical tubers (the most evident in the left rolandic region). **Focal neonatal symptomatic (tuberous sclerosis complex) epilepsy**. Follow-up: West syndrome at fourth months followed by Lennox Gastaut syndrome with severe neurocognitive impairment (24 months of age)

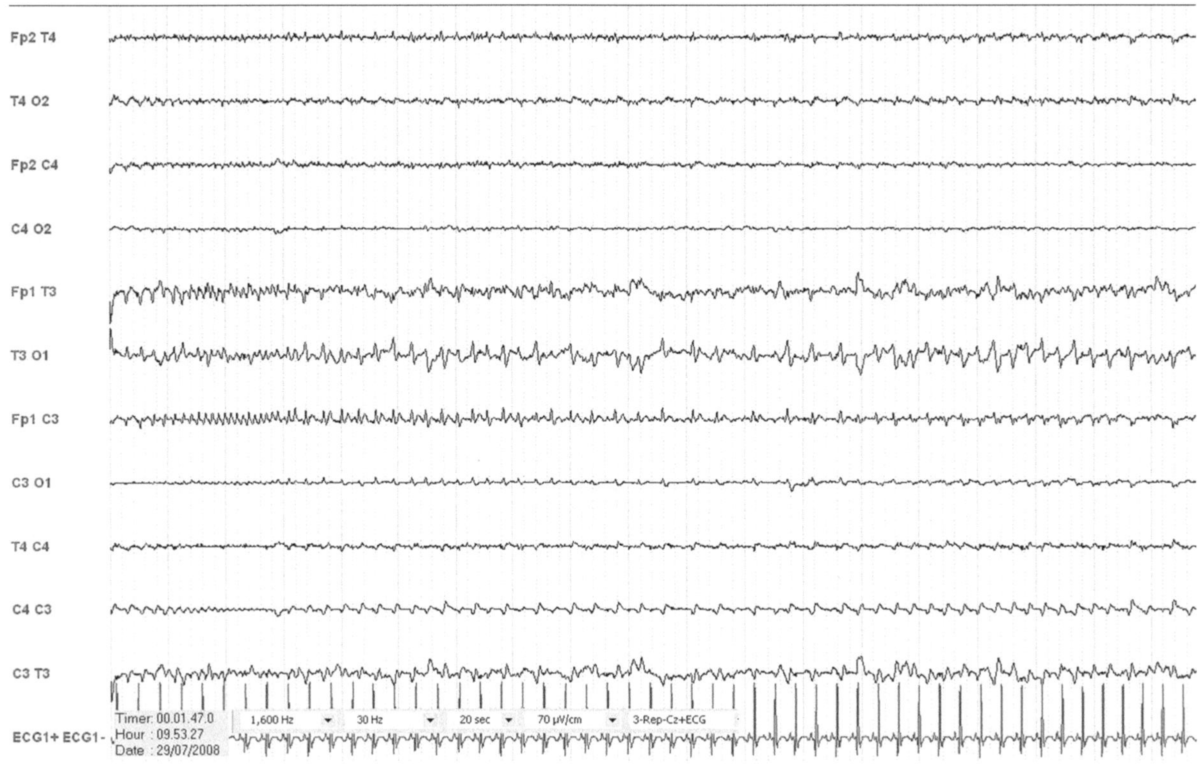

Fig. 22.54 See Fig. 22.55 caption

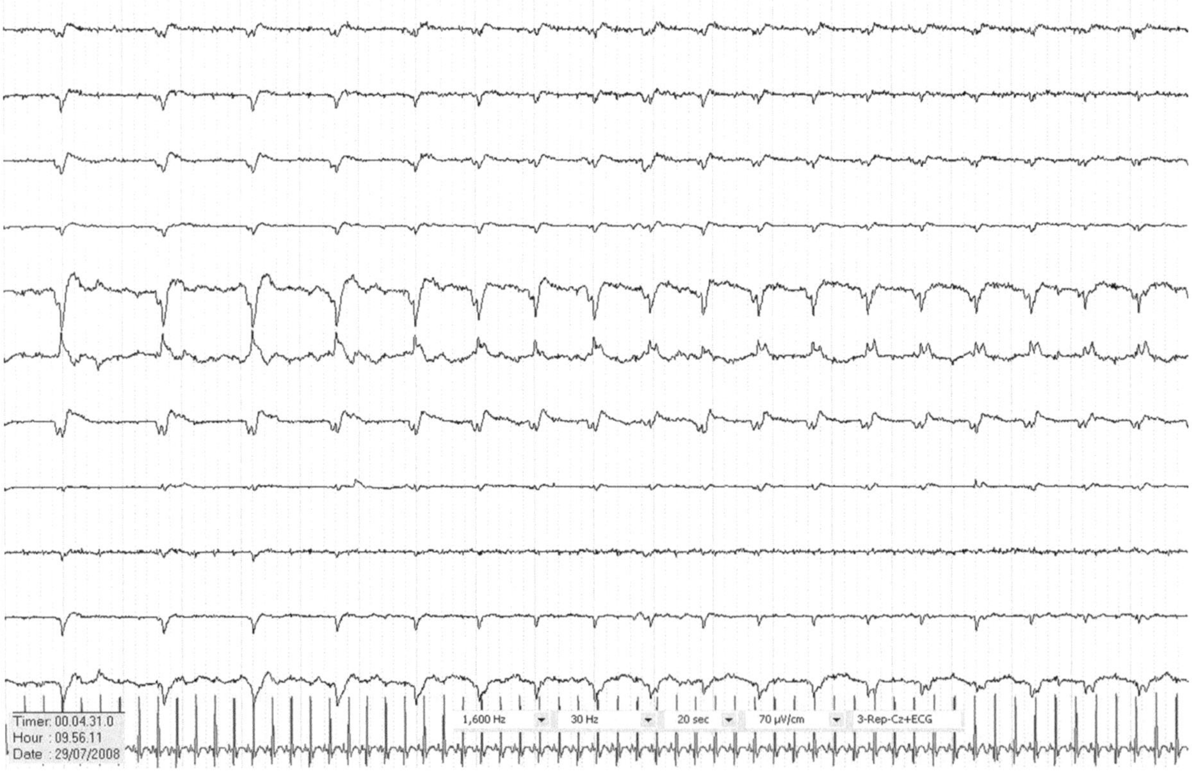

Fig. 22.55 35 weeks GA, 35.3 weeks CA. Pregnancy complicated by maternal-fetal Rh-isoimmunization. Uneventful delivery. Birth weight 2750 g, Apgar score 8–9. After 7 min deteriorating of general condition: pH 6.9, BE-19 mmol/L, CO_2 43 mmHg, lactic acid 24 mmol/L, glycemia 37 mg/dL, Hb 4.5 g/dL. At 3 days of life, the newborn became hypotonic and hyporeactive. The EEG background activity is constantly lower than 30 mcV, and **repetitive infraclinical seizure discharges characterized by left alpha > beta and sharpened theta activity** (Fig. 22.54) **evolving to rhythmic slow spikes and slow wave complexes** higher in the right hemisphere. The discharge seems to spread to the right hemisphere; however it is more likely an electrical signal diffusion. **Low voltage undifferentiated tracing. Cerebral cortical-subcortical anoxia due to isoimmunization.** Brain MRI (4 days): cortical and subcortical malacic lesions involving gray and with matter basal ganglia and midbrain nuclei. Follow-up: severe dystonic–hypotonic quadriparesis associated with static encephalopathy with abnormal social interaction. (24 months old)

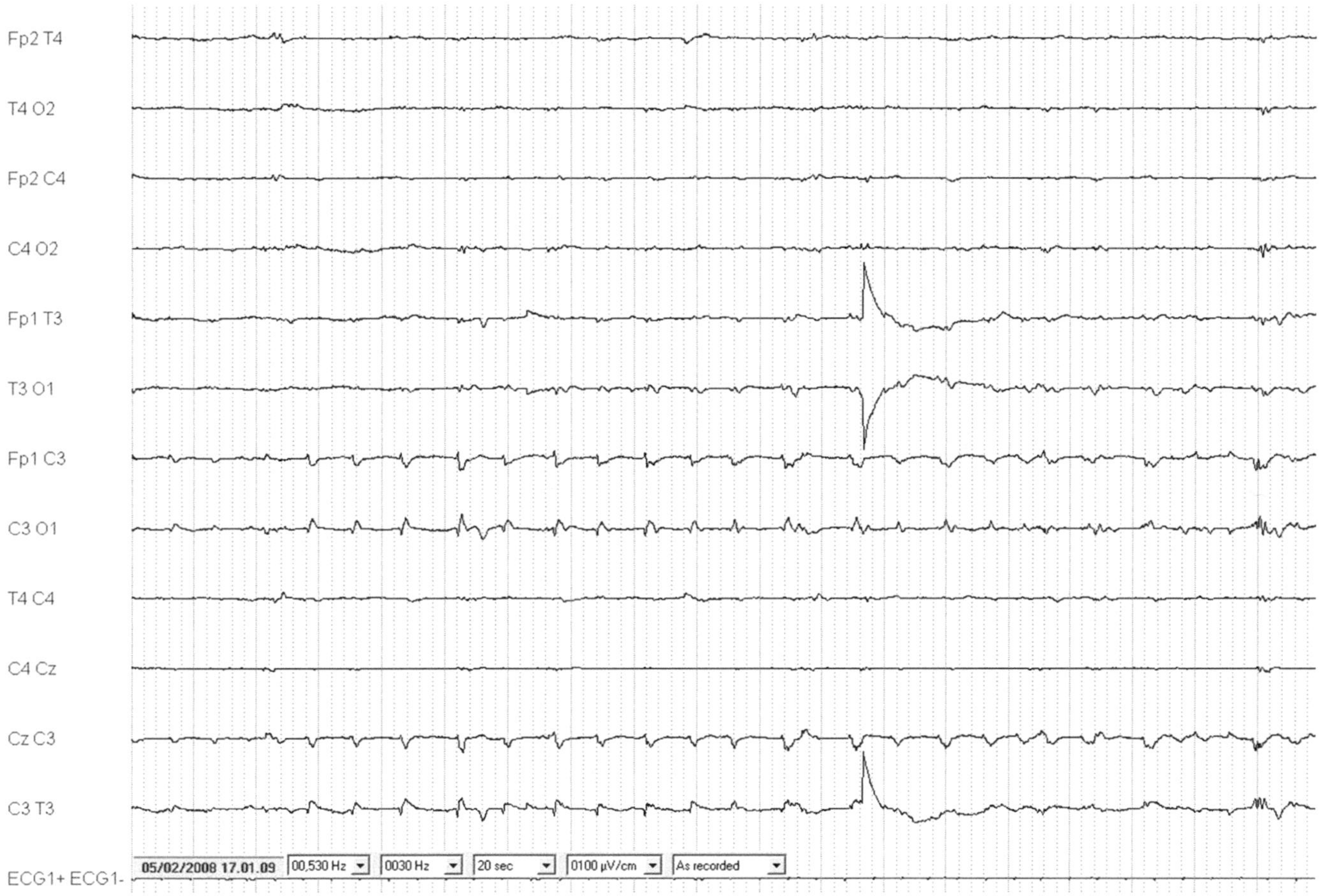

Fig. 22.56 40 weeks GA, 43.3 weeks CA. Uneventful pregnancy and delivery. At 22 days of life ***Streptococcus beta-haemolyticus* type B encephalitis associated with convulsive > electrical status epilepticus. Induced thiopental sodium coma with infraclinical multifocal recurrent seizures with electro-clinical dissociation and severely abnormal background activity**. Follow-up: severe neurocognitive impairment >West syndrome at 6 months >developmental encephalopathy with AED's resistant epilepsy >died at 3 years old. 1 h after thiopental sodium therapy reduction to 2.5 mg/kg/h, electrical focal (C3) seizure activity recurs, characterized by rhythmic (1/s) low-amplitude (lesser than 40 mcV) slow spikes

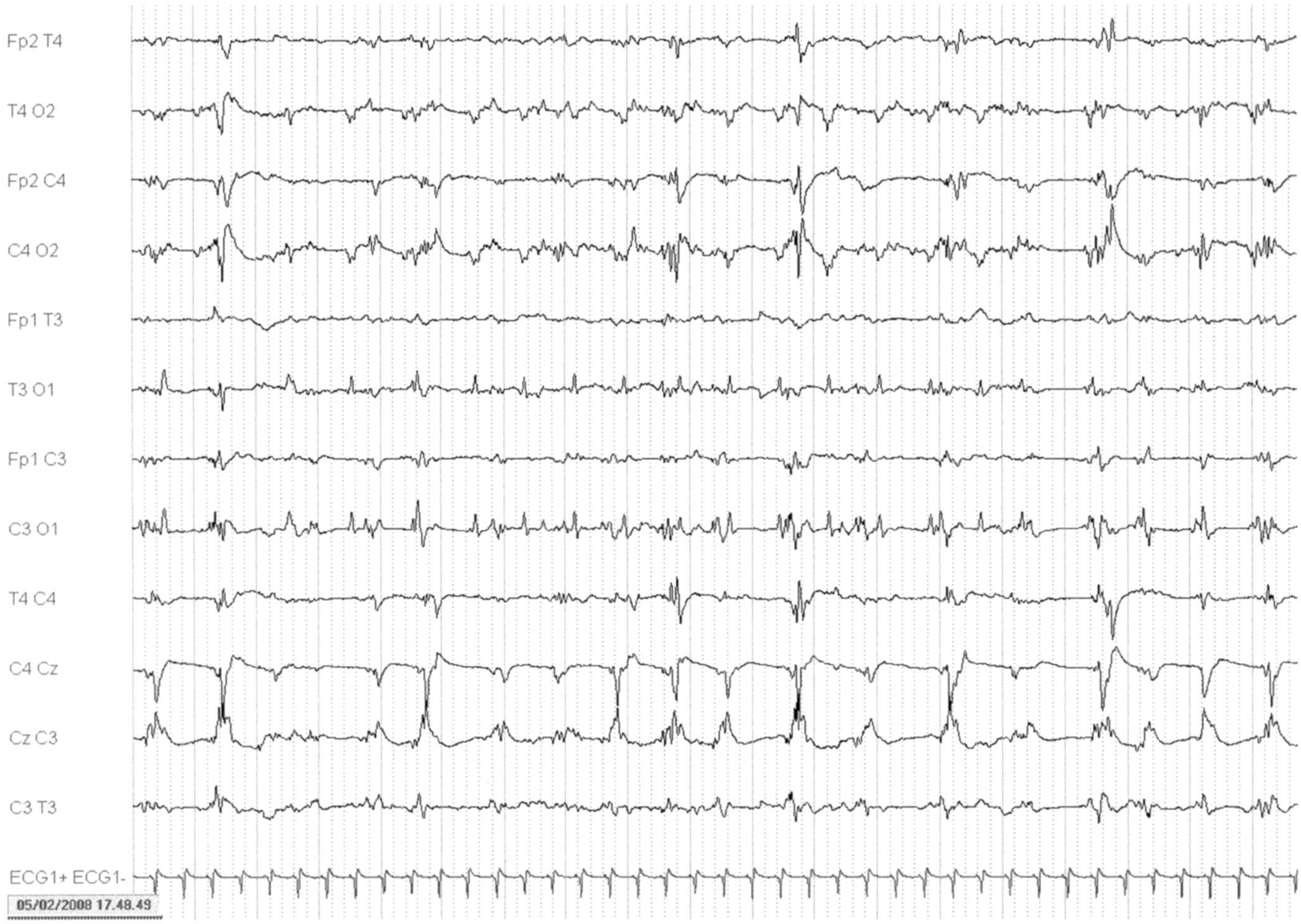

Fig. 22.57 40 weeks GA, 43.3 weeks CA. Uneventful pregnancy and delivery. At 22 days of life ***Streptococcus beta-haemolyticus*** **type B encephalitis associated with convulsive > electrical status epilepticus. Induced thiopental sodium coma with infraclinical multifocal recurrent seizures with electro-clinical dissociation and severely abnormal background activity**. Follow-up: severe neurocognitive impairment >West syndrome at 6 months >developmental encephalopathy with AED's resistant epilepsy >died at 3 years old. Eighteen minutes later, **bilateral independent electrical seizures** arise from occipital, left and right, and central region with different morphology: rhythmic slow spikes (left occipital), rhythmic polyspike complexes (right occipital), rhythmic slow spike, and slow wave complexes high as 130 mcV

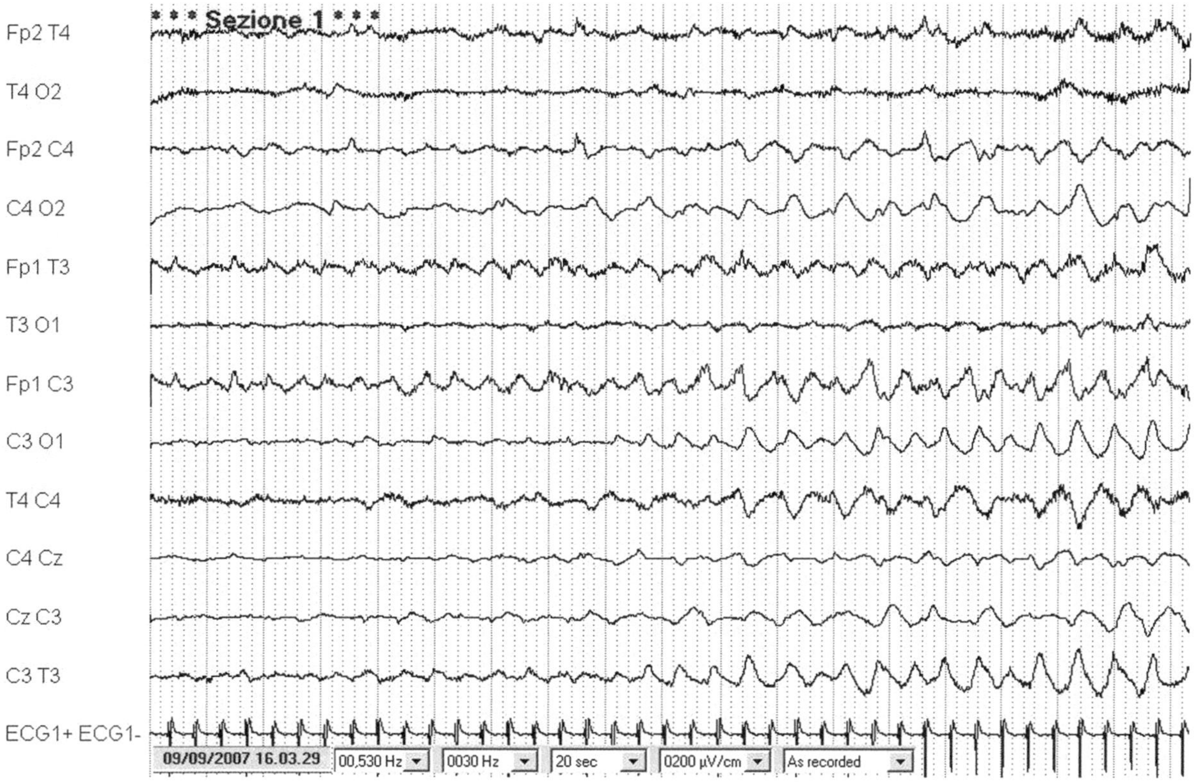

Fig. 22.58 See Fig. 22.59 caption

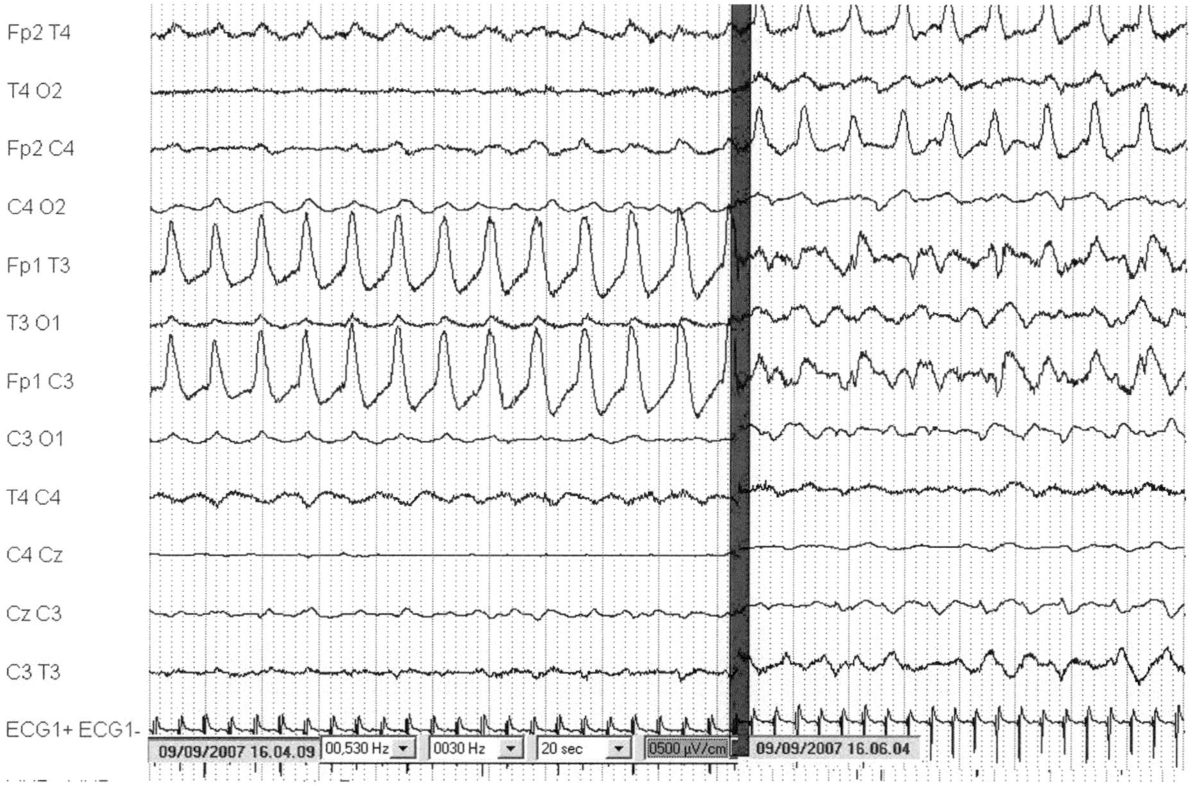

Fig. 22.59 Same newborn as in Fig. 22.30 40 h after, mechanical ventilation, and hypothermia treatment: **Acute transitory hypoxic ischemic encephalopathy**. Within a constantly low-voltage tracing (amplitude between 5 and 30 mcV), in Fig. 22.58 infraclinical ictal sharpened delta activity high up to 300 mcV in the fronto-central left region, with diffusion to the adjacent region. After 40 s, in Fig. 22.59 (in the left side of the image), a seizure infraclinical discharge characterized by sharpened delta activity high up to 600 mcV is present in the frontal region. Two minutes after (right side of the image) the seizure abates in the left region, becoming focal in the right anterior region. **Multifocal and low-voltage/slow-frequency discharges superimposed on a low-voltage background activity**

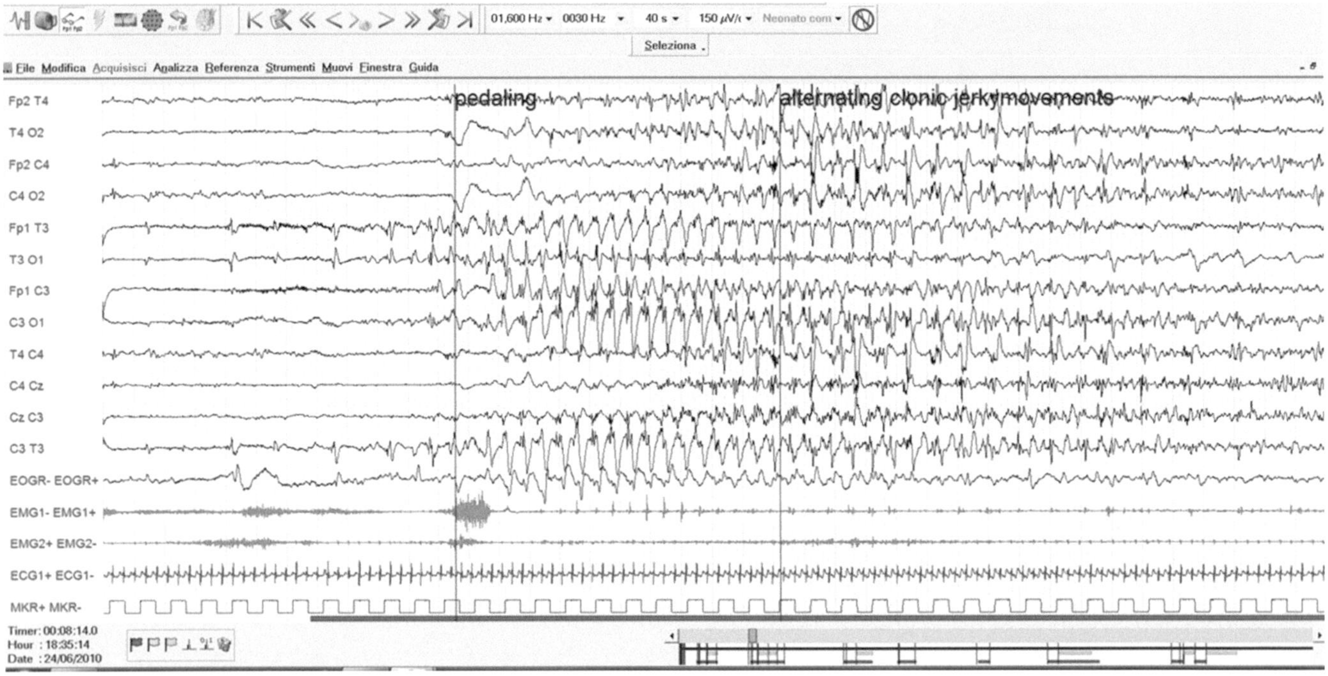

Fig. 22.60 39 weeks GA, 42.3 weeks CA. Pregnancy complicated by fetal growth retardation; cesarean section due to breech presentation, 2540 g (SGA), APGAR: 4-7-10. Relative macrocephaly. At birth the newborn is hypotonic and hyporeactive. Transient hypoglycemia in the first 2 days of life. From the 3rd day of life repetitive AED's resistant polymorphic seizures (clonic bilateral asynchronous, oral automatisms, spasms, and pedaling of the legs). The newborn is comatose. The background activity is depressed. **Two independent seizures arise from the left and then on the right hemisphere evolving with polyspikes-wave rhythmic complexes associated with pedaling of the legs and clonic jerks of the right and then left deltoid (see EMG polygraphy)**. The focal bilateral seizures end in 1 min followed by a flat trace (not shown). *Time base 7.5 mm/s*

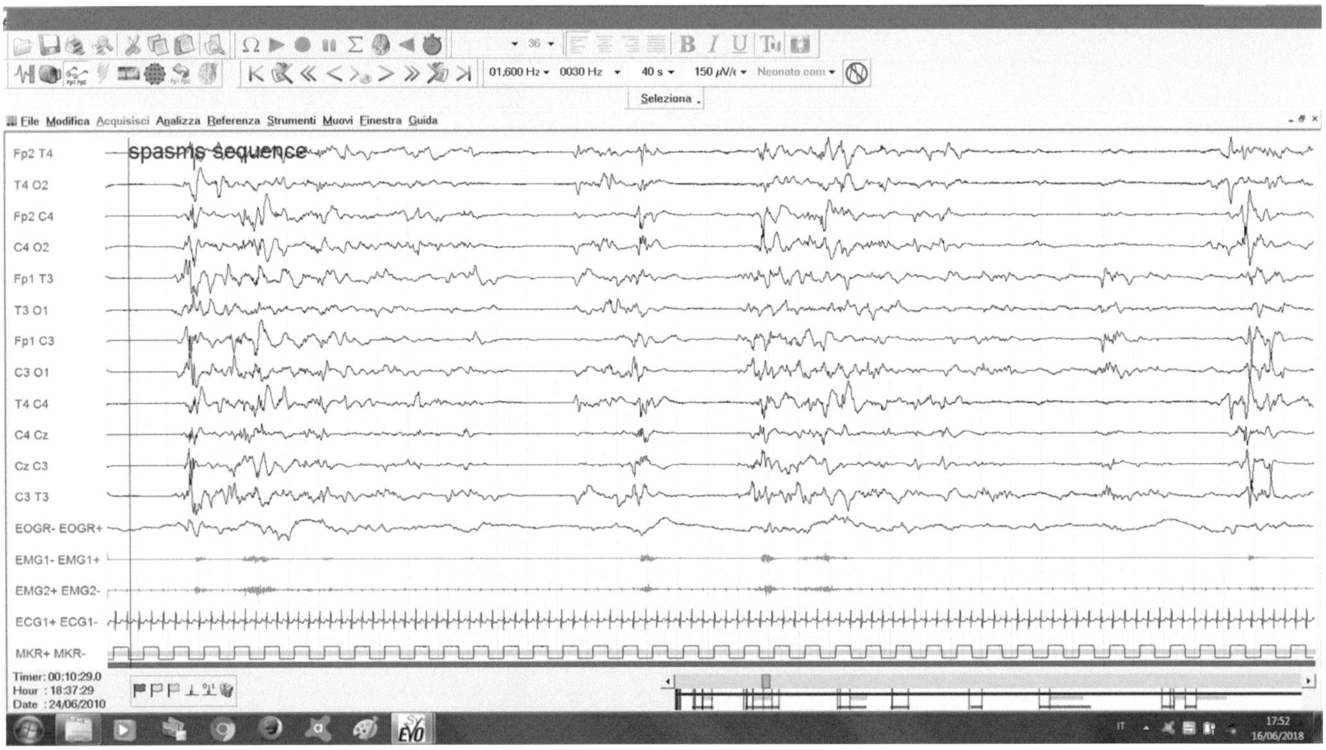

Fig. 22.61 Same newborn and same recording of Fig. 22.60). **A sequence of spasms** occurs 40 s after the end of the seizure shown in this figure. The spasms, clearly documented by EMG polygraphy, are symmetrical, associated with a bilateral high-voltage polyspikes slow wave complex and recur within an ictal suppression-burst pattern, with flat periods lasting 4–8 s. PHT high-dosage i.v. therapy, with blood levels above 20 mcg/mL, controlled the seizures with disappearance of the suppression-burst pattern. Brain MRI and extended metabolic blood and cerebrospinal fluid analysis were normal. Genes panel analysis for early onset epileptic encephalopathy (EOEE) detected a **SCN2A causative de novo mutation**. **Neonatal genetic epilepsy within a condition of Early Onset Epileptic Encephalopathy (EOEE)**. *Time base 7.5 mm/s*

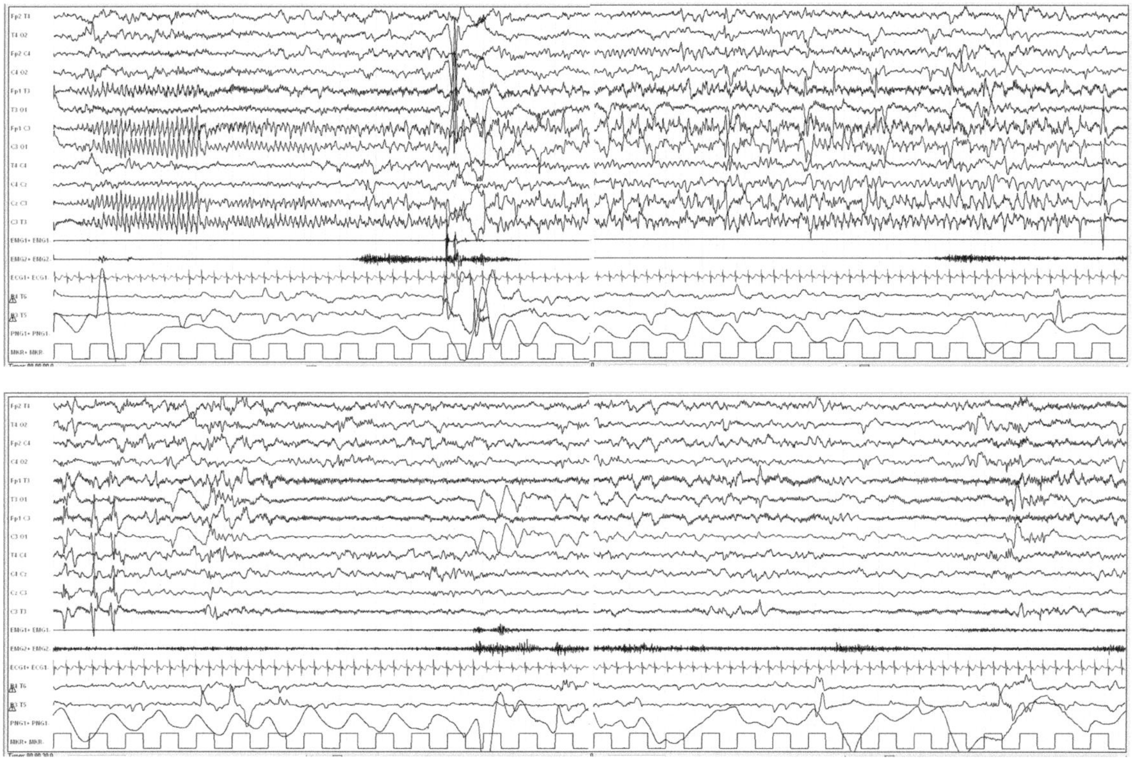

Fig. 22.62 39 weeks GA, 39.2 weeks CA. Uneventful pregnancy and delivery. Outborn. Referred apneic seizures in the first 2 days of life, then transferred in our hospital. In the figures **electro-clinical seizures** arose either **from the left** (or the right) central regions with slow >high voltage, fast, rhythmic sharp waves activity. Then abruptly evolved to rhythmic slower activity with sharply contoured theta activity intermixed with spikes. Post-ictal background activity is asymmetrical and excessively discontinuous for CA. The electrical seizure **tends to spread to the contralateral side**. The clinical component was characterized by oral automatism followed by asymmetrical tonic posturing, bradypnea, and tonic eye deviation. Brain MRI and extended metabolic blood and cerebrospinal fluid analysis were normal. Genes panel analysis for early onset epileptic encephalopathy (EOEE) detected a **KCNT1 causative de novo mutation, as the cause of a neonatal onset malignant migrating focal seizures syndrome**. *Time base 10 mm/s*

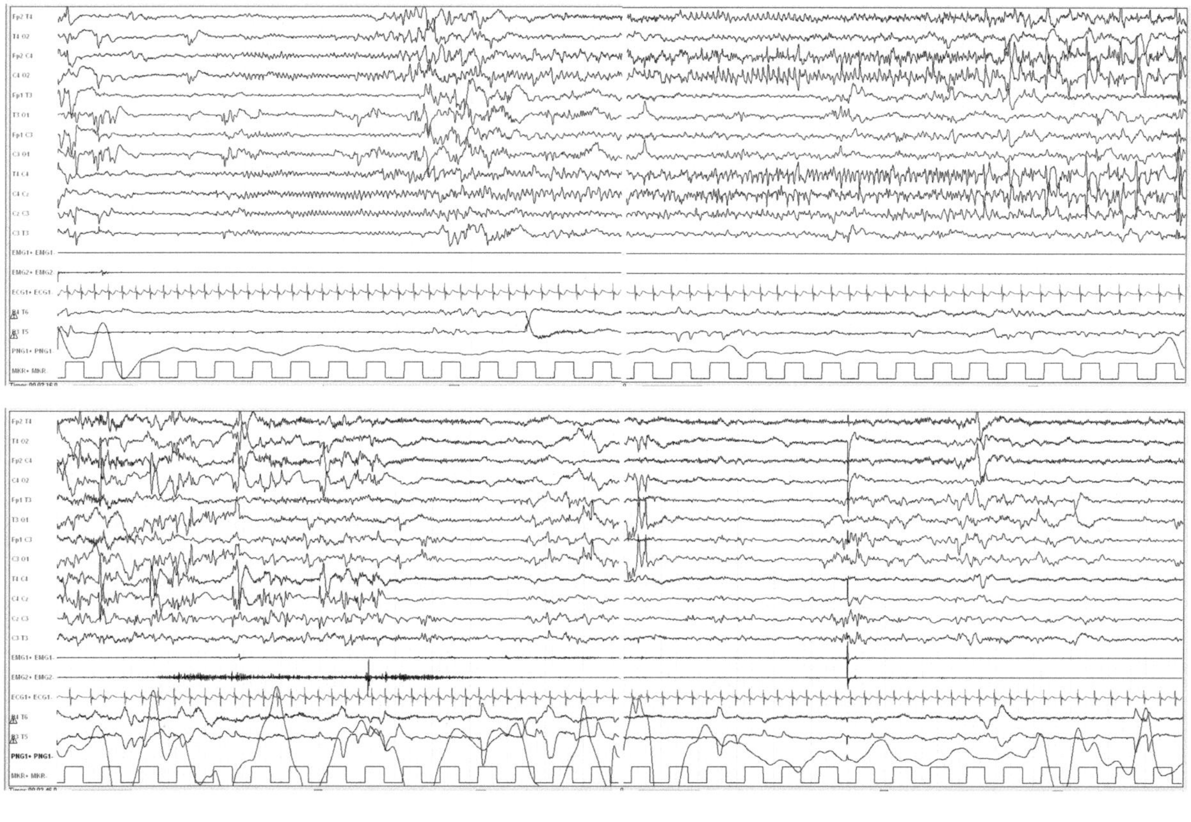

Fig. 22.63 Same newborn and same recording of Fig. 22.62. The same ictal pattern arose from the right hemisphere. *Time base 10 mm/s*

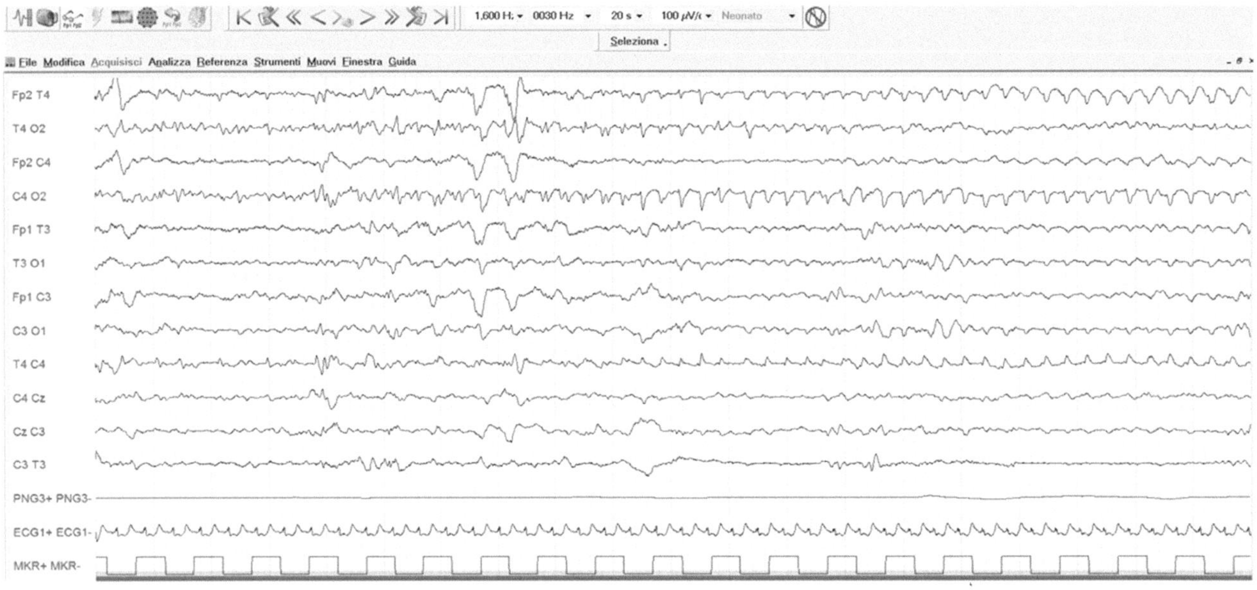

Fig. 22.64 38 weeks GA, 40 weeks CA. Normal pregnancy and delivery. In the 1st day of life, bilateral asynchronous focal clonic seizures and oral-buccal-lingual seizures occurred, controlled after PB and PHT iv therapy. The newborn, however, was lethargic and hyporeactive. **During a long-lasting EEG monitoring during all the night, 14 infraclinical electrical-only seizures (1–3 min) were detected**. In the figure a seizure discharge, characterized by rhythmic theta sharp activity evolves on the right hemisphere from the posterior to the temporal region and then to the centro-temporal region of the left hemisphere with a similar but asynchronous pattern between the two hemispheres. Brain MRI and extended metabolic blood and cerebrospinal fluid analysis were normal. The pattern is suggestive for a neonatal symptomatic epilepsy, presumed genetic in nature, as **malignant migrating focal seizures**

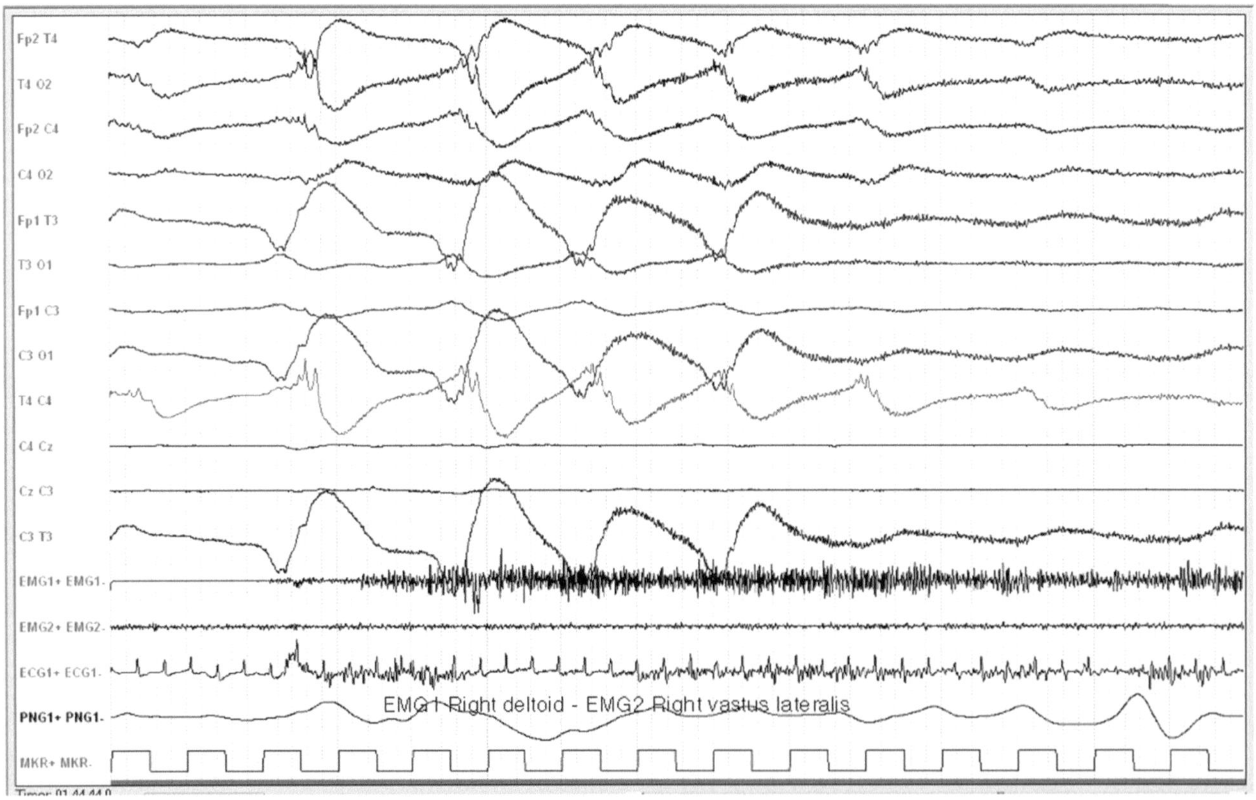

Fig. 22.65 28 weeks GA, 28.3 weeks CA. Prematurity: after a normal pregnancy, urgent cesarean section for maternal reasons. The newborn was unreactive and lethargic. **Prolonged infraclinical sequences of bilateral, synchronous, very slow, high-amplitude delta waves, more pronounced in the temporal areas**, which are smooth and are associated with slow-voltage rhythmic sharpened theta activity. The sequences described might be epileptic in nature. Follow-up: normal brain ultrasound, normal psychomotor development (16 months)

22.7 Iconography of the Abnormal EEG

The following information in the caption of each single image report: the acronym P stands for pathological trace, GA for gestational age, expressed in weeks, and CA for the conceptional age, expressed in weeks. In summary a short comment of the pathology is also provided to define the clinical condition for which the examination has been performed.

Regarding the iconography shown, in Figs. 22.21, 22.22, 22.27, 22.39–22.41, and 22.65 peculiar pathological findings of the premature tracing are reported. In Figs. 22.19, 22.20, 22.30–22.37 inactive and suppression-burst patterns have a completely different clinical evolution, to testify how these patterns, associated generally with unfavorable prognosis, could have a different evolution in relation to different clinical conditions. In Figs. 22.42–22.44, 22.52, 22.53, 22.66, and 22.67, the constantly asymmetric pattern, relative to both the underlying activity and the critical abnormalities, is related to a structural, congenital, or acquired focal etiology. In Figs. 22.38, and 22.54–22.59, it is emphasized how the characteristics of the critical discharge can be modified according to the severe alteration of the underlying background activity. In Figs. 22.45–22.51, the abnormalities with spike and/or sharp wave morphology, focal or multifocal, require an extreme caution in interpretation, and they must be constantly correlated with the characteristics of the basic activity of the recording. Figures 22.23–22.27, with regard to discontinuity (with external and internal dyschronism) and to asynchrony, show that a careful evaluation of the clinical picture is necessary. The evolution of the electrical pattern must be also taken into account to provide an adequate, diagnostic and prognostic judgment. Similarly, Figs. 22.50 and 22.51 show rhythmic activities at a variable location for which caution is required with respect to an interpretation of "normal" or "abnormal" finding. In Figs. 22.28, 22.29, and 22.60–22.64 are reported peculiar features both of the background activity and ictal activity related to genetic conditions, documented or suspected.

All the children, whose iconography has been reported, have been evaluated personally by at least one of the authors.

Acknowledgments A heartfelt thanks to the EEG technicians of the Pediatric Neurology Unit: Teresa Iuorno, Carlo Landoni, Debora Meroni, Francesca Tabarelli and Gaetano Turi, for their competence and sensitivity repeatedly expressed in the management of newborns and in the acquisition of EEG recordings; to Alfredo Radaelli for his valuable collaboration in the editorial organization of the work; to the colleagues of the Neonatology and Neonatal Intensive Care of the Buzzi Hospital Milan directed by Dr G. Lista, for the useful collaboration in everyday practice.

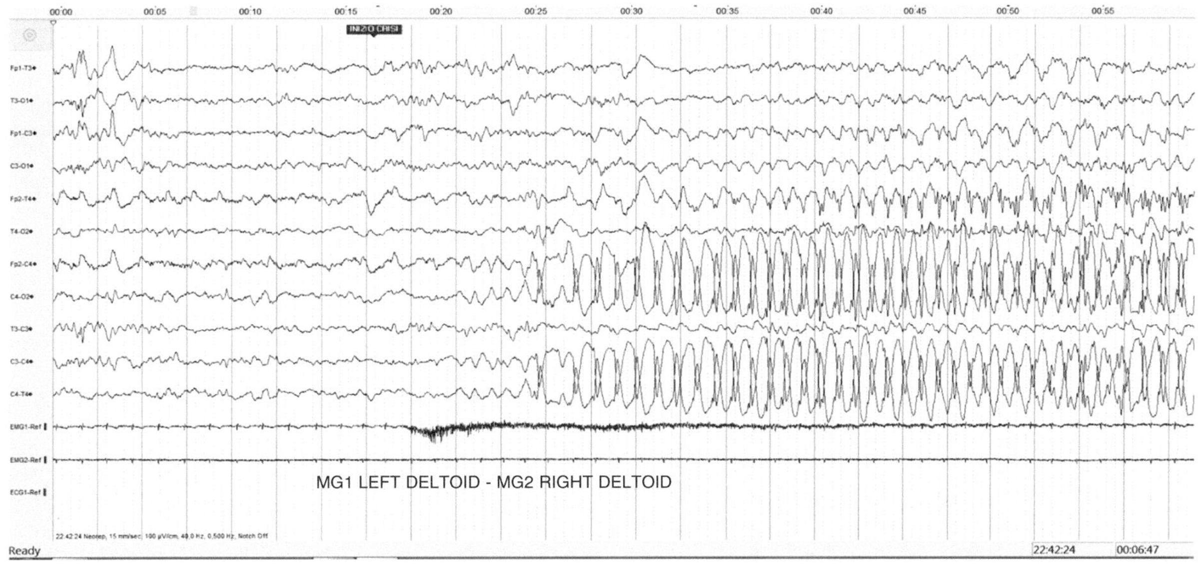

Fig. 22.66 39 weeks GA, 39.1 weeks CA. Normal pregnancy and delivery (2530 g, SGA), Apgar score 9–10. Thirty six hours after birth repetitive bilateral jerks with stiffening are referred by the nurse. An **electro-clinical focal motor tonic > clonic seizure** is recorded during the EEG performed 1 h after, an emergency. Right central rhythmic slow waves are followed by rhythmic spike-slow wave complexes high up to 250 mcV at increasing frequency with diffusion to the right temporal region: clinically the EMG polygraphy hyperactivity on the left deltoid documents the initial stiffening of the left arm. Rhythmic jerks of the left limbs follow (not shown)

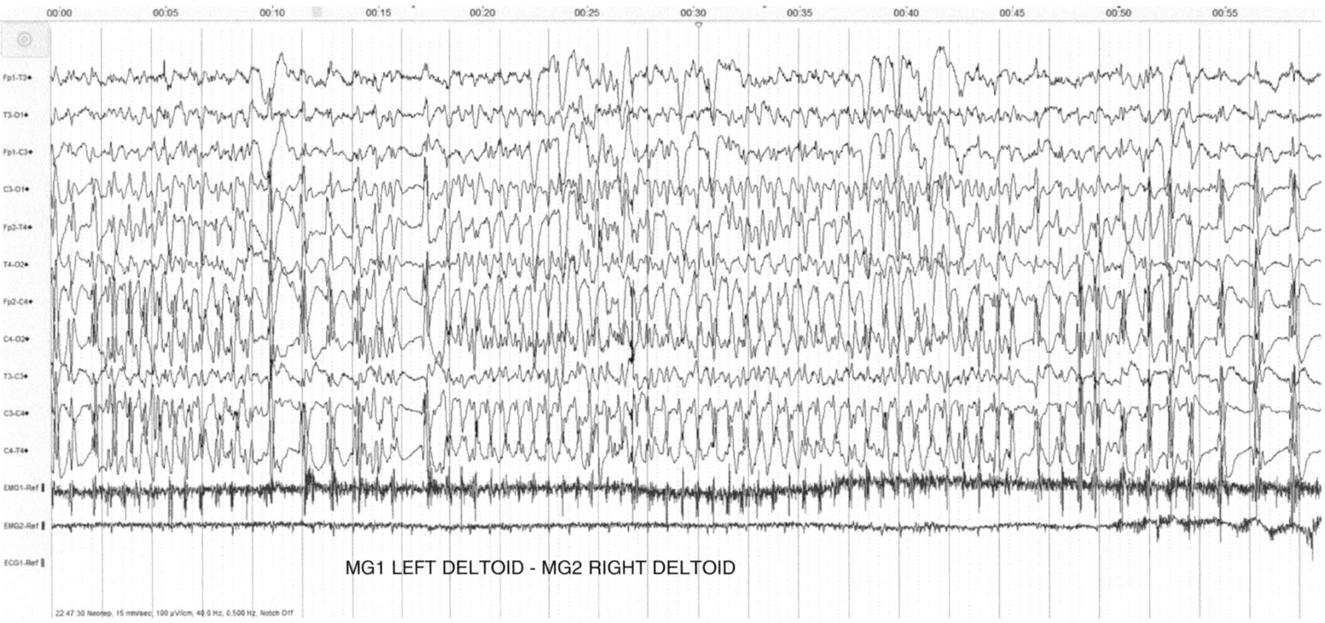

Fig. 22.67 Same newborn and same recording of Fig. 22.67). Five minutes later the ictal pattern modifies: the seizure spreads to the centro-occipital left region; polyspike-slow wave complexes are followed by transient (1 s) flattening and beta fast low-amplitude activity arises in the right occipital region; high-frequency clonic jerks of left limbs persist strictly related to the polyspikes/slow wave and spike/wave complexes. The seizure ends spontaneously within 30 s. Twenty-five minutes later a second similar seizure was recorded: after PB loading dose, 20 mg/kg, i.v. seizures never recurred. Background activity is normal in the left hemisphere. Brain ultrasound and MRI: **middle cerebral artery territory infarction**. Follow-up: normal motor and neurocognitive development at 4 years, without epilepsy, despite a poroencephalic cyst in the abovementioned region

References

1. Lamblin MD, André M, Auzoux M, et al. Indications of electroencephalogram in the newborn. Arch Pediatr. 2004;11(7):829–33.
2. Lamblin MD, de Villepin-Touzery A. EEG in the neonatal unit. Neurophysiol Clin. 2015;45:87–95.
3. Hrachovy RA, Mizrhai EM. Atlas of neonatal electroencephalography. 4th ed. New York, NY: Springer Publishing Company; 2015.
4. Tsuchida TN. Diagnostic yield of continuous video EEG for neonatal seizures. Pediatr Neurol Briefs. 2015;29(8):63.
5. Dreyfus-Brisac C, Samson-Dreyfus D, Fischgold H. Activité électrique cerebrale du prematuré et du nouveau-né. Ann Pediatr. 1955;31:1–7.
6. Dreyfus-Brisac C. The electroencephalogram of the premature infant. World Neurol. 1962;3:5–15.
7. Monod N, Dreyfus-Brisac C. Le tracé paroxistique chez le nouveau- né. Rev Neurol. 1962;106:129–30.
8. Lombroso CT. Neonatal polygraphy in full term and premature infants: a review of normal and abnormal findings. J Clin Neurophysiol. 1985;2:105–55.
9. Stockard-Pope JE, Wener SS, Bickford R. Atlas of neonatal electroencephalography. 2nd ed. New York, NY: Raven; 1992.
10. Ferrari F, Biagioni E, Cioni G. Neonatal electroencephalography. In: Levene MI, Chervenak FA, Whittle M, editors. Fetal and neonatal neurology and neurosurgery. 3rd ed. London: Churchill Livingston; 2001. p. 155–80.
11. Mizrhai EM, Hrachovy RA, Kellaway P. Atlas of neonatal electroencephalography. 3rd ed. Philadelphia, PA: Lippincott Williams & Wilkins; 2004.
12. André M, Lamblin MD, d'Allest AM, et al. Electroencephalography in premature and full-term infants. Developmental features and glossary. Neurophysiol Clin. 2010;40:59–124.
13. Lombroso CT. Neonatal electroencephalography. In: Niedermeyer E, Lopes da Silva F, editors. Electroencephalography: basic principles, clinical applications and related field. Munich: Urban & Schwartzenberg; 1982. p. 725–62.
14. Mizrahi EM, Kellaway P. Diagnosis and management of neonatal seizures. Philadelphia, PA: Lippincott-Raven; 1998.
15. Mastrangelo M, Peron A, Spaccini L, et al. Neonatal suppression-burst without epileptic seizures: expanding the electroclinical phenotype of STXBP1-related, early-onset encephalopathy. Epileptic Disord. 2013;15:55–61.
16. Shellhaas RA, Wusthoff CJ, Tsuchida TN, et al. Profile of neonatal epilepsies: characteristics of a prospective US cohort. Neurology. 2017;89:893–9.
17. Spagnoli C, Salerno GG, Iodice A, et al. KCNQ2 encephalopathy: a case due to a de novo deletion. Brain Dev. 2018;40:65–8.
18. Axeen EJT, Olson HE. Neonatal epilepsy genetics. Semin Fetal Neonatal Med. 2018;23(3):197–203.
19. Sarnat HB, Sarnat MS. Neonatal encephalopathy following fetal distress. A clinical and electroencephalographic study. Arch Neurol. 1976;33:696–705.

20. Tharp BR, Cukier F, Monod N. Valeur prognostique de l'EEG du prématuré. Rev EEG Neurophysiol. 1977;7:386–91.
21. Holmes G, Rowe J, Hafford J, et al. Prognostic value of the electro- encephalogram in neonatal asphyxia. Electroencephalogr Clin Neurophysiol. 1982;53:60–72.
22. Takeuchi T, Watanabe K. The EEG evolution and neurological prognosis of neonates with perinatal hypoxia. Brain Dev. 1989;11:115–20.
23. Holmes G, Lombroso C. Prognostic value of background patterns in the neonatal EEG. J Clin Neurophysiol. 1993;10:323–52.
24. Watanabe K, Hayakawa F, Okumura A. Neonatal EEG: a powerful tool in assessment of brain damage in preterm infants. Brain Dev. 1999;21:361–72.
25. Plouin P. Intéret de l'électroencéphalogramme vidéo en néonatologie. Arch Pediatr. 2000;7:332–3.
26. Tsuchida TN, Wusthoff CJ, Shellhaas RA, et al. American clinical neurophysiology society standardized EEG terminology and categorization for the description of continuous EEG monitoring in neonates: report of the American Clinical Neurophysiology Society critical care monitoring committee. J Clin Neurophysiol. 2013;30:161–73.
27. Wusthoff CJ. Diagnosing neonatal seizures and status epilepticus. J Clin Neurophysiol. 2013;30:115–21.
28. Pisani F, Pavlidis E. The role of electroencephalogram in neonatal seizure detection. Expert Rev Neurother. 2018;18:95–100.
29. Nagarajan L. Neonatal seizures, current management and future challenges. London: Mac Keith Press; 2016.
30. Melani F, Mei D, Pisano T, et al. CDKL5 gene-related epileptic encephalopathy: electroclinical findings in the first year of life. Dev Med Child Neurol. 2011;53(4):354–60.

23 Early-Onset Epileptic Encephalopathies

Marina Trivisano and Nicola Specchio

23.1 Introduction

Early myoclonic epilepsy (EME) and Ohtahara syndrome (OS) or early infantile epileptic encephalopathy (EIEE) are the earliest presenting within the age-dependent epileptic encephalopathy syndromes. These are electro-clinical syndromes, defined by their clinical features and electroencephalographic findings [1, 2].

These two entities share many features, including age at presentation, a similar electroencephalographic pattern, intractable seizures, and poor prognosis. Tonic seizures and focal motor seizures are frequently observed in both syndromes. Differentiating between the two conditions can be difficult, especially early in their course. As far as considerable clinical overlap between these conditions can occur [2], these two conditions have been conceptualized as part of the same continuum of disease.

EME and EIEE are traditionally distinguished according to different types of seizures, differences in the pattern of suppression-burst, and aetiologies. Specifically, in its original form, Ohtahara syndrome is thought to result mostly from structural malformations, whereas EME is associated with metabolic abnormalities [3].

New understandings of the genetic and pathophysiologic mechanisms underlying these diseases revealed further similarities between them. Both syndromes frequently seem associated with conditions that lead to abnormal neuronal migration, possibly leading to both structural brain abnormalities and a functional disconnection between the cortex and the deep brain and brainstem [4]. The prominence of brainstem abnormalities in both syndromes similarly indicates a disconnection between the cortex and subcortical structures [4].

M. Trivisano · N. Specchio (✉)
Rare and Complex Epilepsy Unit, Department of Neuroscience and Neurorehabilitation, Bambino Gesù Children's Hospital, Rome, Italy
e-mail: nicola.specchio@opbg.net

23.2 Ohtahara Syndrome

Ohtahara syndrome or early infantile epileptic encephalopathy (EIEE) was firstly described by Ohtahara in 1976, who named it "early infantile epileptic encephalopathy with suppression-burst" [5]. Ohtahara syndrome starts early in infancy, within the first 3 months of age and often within the first 2 weeks [6]. Ohtahara syndrome can result from a variety of aetiologies, but the majority of cases have been associated with structural brain abnormalities [7–10]. Cases related to genetic mutations and metabolic abnormalities have also been reported, although at least some of these cases also exhibited associated structural malformations [7]. Even in some cases when no structural lesions were evident on imaging, post-mortem examinations demonstrated evidences of a migration disorder or dysgenesis not previously appreciated on neuroimaging [7, 10].

A variety of structural malformations have been associated with Ohtahara syndrome, including hemimegalencephaly, agenesis of the corpus callosum, and porencephaly. Hypoxic injury, cortical dysplasia, and cerebral migration disorders are also frequently described [7, 9].

Among metabolic disorders, non-ketotic hyperglycinemia, cytochrome C oxidase deficiency, pyridoxine dependency, and carnitine palmitoyltransferase deficiency are the most frequently associated with Ohtahara syndrome [11–13].

Underlying genetic mutations have been increasingly reported with Ohtahara syndrome. Mutations in the syntaxin-binding protein 1 (STXBP1) gene, for example, have been described in Ohtahara syndrome since 2008 [14]. A variable proportion of patients, ranging from 10% to 38% with Ohtahara syndrome, might be caused by STXBP1 genetic variants [14]. Similarly, mutations of the ARX gene have also been associated with Ohtahara syndrome [15, 16]. Finally, mutations in the mitochondrial glutamate carrier family 25 (SLC25A22) gene have been identified as cause of Ohtahara syndrome.

Epilepsy onset is within the first 3 months of age and often within the first 2 weeks [6]. Infants acutely develop

O. Mecarelli (ed.), *Clinical Electroencephalography*, https://doi.org/10.1007/978-3-030-04573-9_23

tonic spasms that can be either generalized or lateralized, can occur both isolated or in clusters, and are independent from the sleep cycle. Spasms typically last up to 10 s and can occur hundreds of times per day [6, 17]. One third of patients with Ohtahara syndrome might also develop other seizure types, most commonly focal motor seizures, hemiconvulsions, or focal to bilateral tonic-clonic seizures [6, 17].

The prognosis is universally poor. Only anecdotal evidence supports the use of specific antiepileptic drugs in these conditions. Phenobarbital, valproate, pyridoxine, zonisamide, and benzodiazepines have all demonstrated limited effects in seizure control in Ohtahara syndrome [18]. Adrenocorticotropic hormone therapy also exerts limited efficacy and may be particularly beneficial in cases of Ohtahara syndrome that progress to West syndrome [17]. The correction of underlying metabolic disorders may lead to a more favourable outcome. In particular, patients with Ohtahara syndrome have been reported to do relatively well after the correction of underlying pyridoxine deficiencies or biotinidase deficiencies [12]. Cases with structural abnormalities such as hemimegalencephaly or cortical dysplasia can benefit from surgery with focal resection or hemispherectomy [19].

The most specific EEG feature is the suppression-burst (SB). This pattern is characterized by high-voltage bursts alternating with almost flat suppression phases at an approximately regular rate [1, 5] (Fig. 23.1).

It should be stressed that distinguished features of SB in Ohtahara syndrome are similar in both waking and sleeping states and regular appearance of periodicity [20]. This finding has critical importance for the diagnosis of this syndrome [20]. SB pattern differs definitely from the periodic type of hypsarrhythmia where it becomes remarkable in sleep (Figs. 23.2 and 23.3).

23.3 Early Myoclonic Encephalopathy

Early myoclonic encephalopathy (EME) can be associated with structural, metabolic, and genetic abnormalities. As in Ohtahara syndrome, also in the pathogenesis of EME seems to be involved a diffuse dysfunction which particularly involves brainstem and white matter, leading to deafferentation and hyperexcitability of the cortex [4].

Focal structural abnormalities are not frequently observed, while progressive, diffuse cortical atrophy – suggestive of an underlying metabolic or degenerative disorders [17] – has been reported in most cases [3].

Metabolic abnormalities are frequently associated with EME, particularly non-ketotic hyperglycinemia. Cases have also been reported in association with D-glyceric acidemia, propionic aciduria, molybdenum cofactor deficiency, pyridoxine deficiency (Fig. 23.4), methylmalonic acidemia, sulphite oxidase deficiency, Menkes disease, Zellweger syndrome, and CDG disorders (Fig. 23.5) [21, 22].

Pathologic findings in early myoclonic encephalopathy include demyelination, multifocal spongy changes in the white matter, imperfect lamination of the deep cortical layers, perivascular concentric bodies, and astrocytic proliferation [4]. Autopsy findings revealed prevalent white matter abnormalities and brainstem pathology [4, 10]. The presence

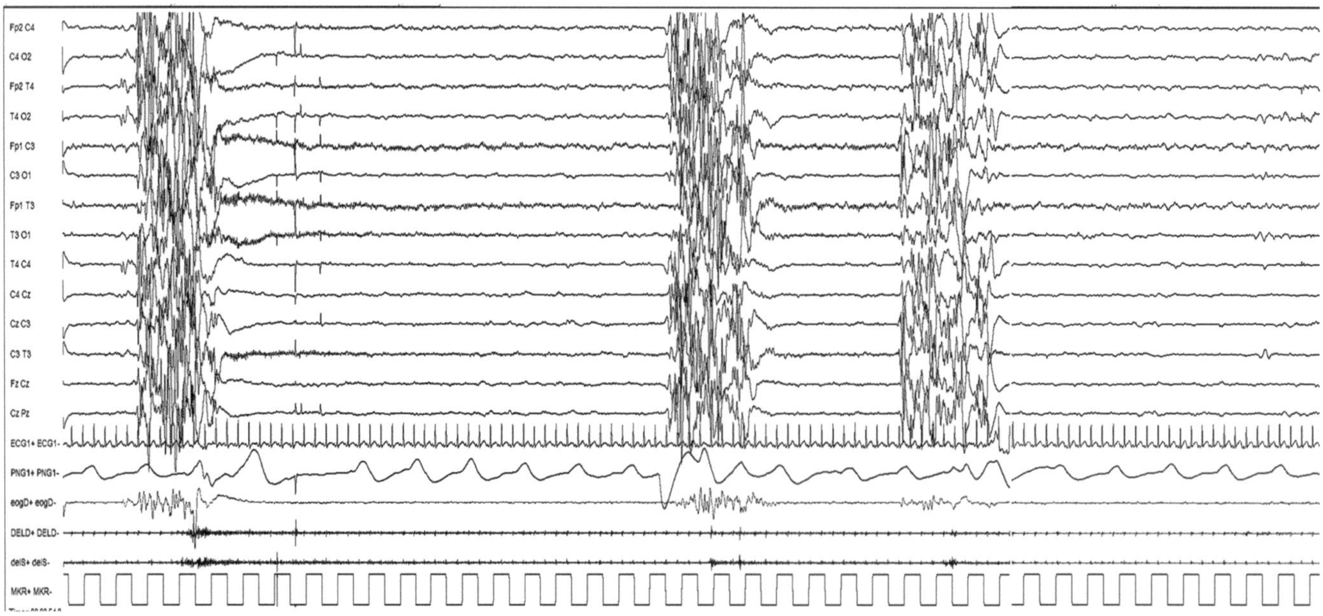

Fig. 23.1 Suppression-Burst pattern in a patient 1 month old boy with hypoxic-ischemic damage at birth. The EEG pattern is characterized high voltage bursts of spikes alternating with almost flat suppression phases at an approximately regular rate

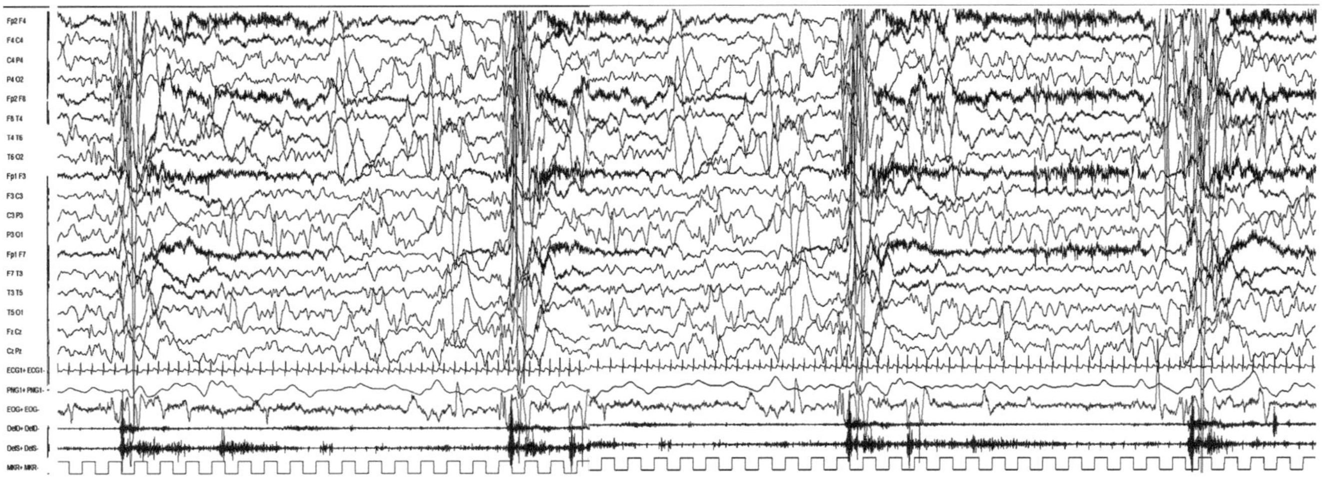

Fig. 23.2 Epileptic spasms in a 4 months old boy with STXBP1 gene mutation during awake state. Documentation of tonic-spasms

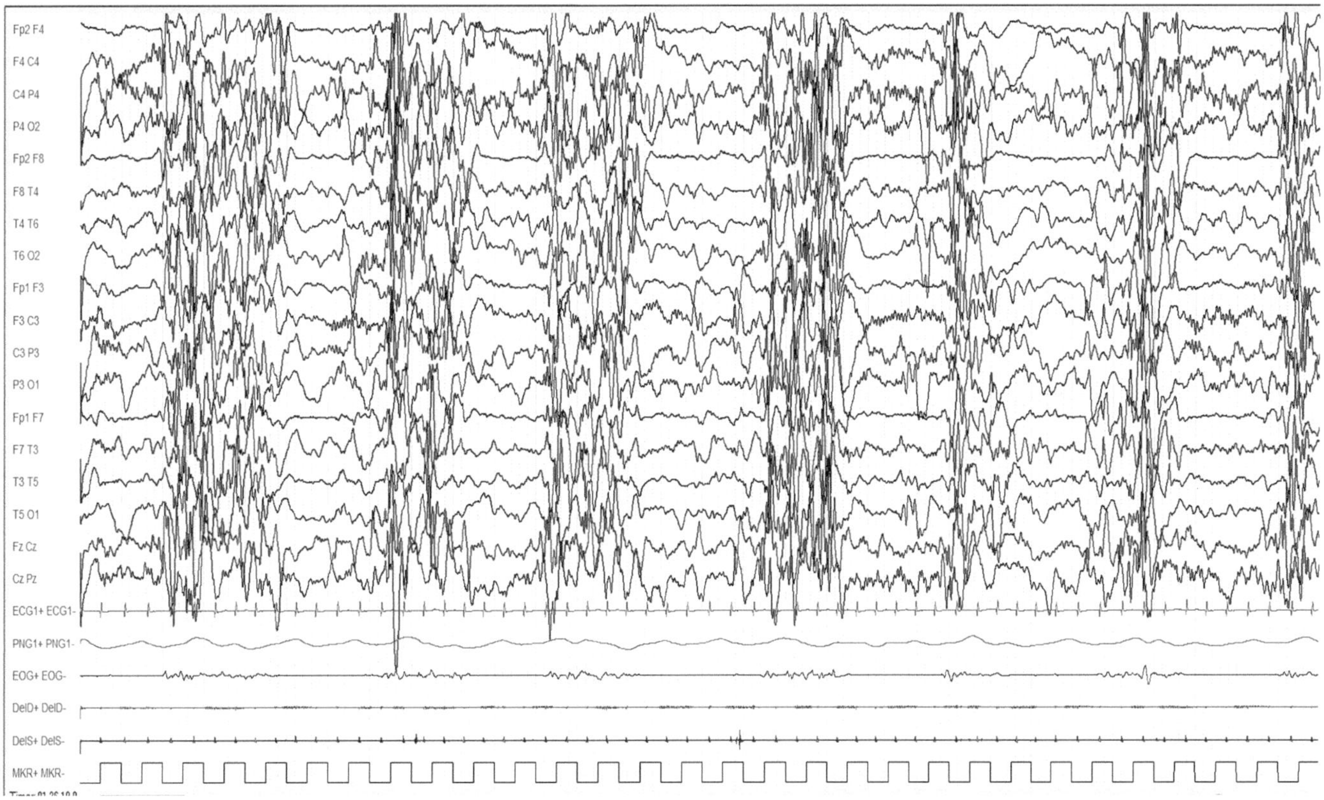

Fig. 23.3 Sleep EEG in a patient with STXBP1 gene mutation during sleep state. It's evident an increasing of epileptiform abnormalities, grouped in bursts of diffuse poly-spikes, intermingled with suppression of cerebral activities

of numerous spiny neurons dispersed in the white matter has also been reported, which is suggestive of impaired neuronal migration and apoptosis [11]. Also a dysfunction of basal ganglia and thalami has been documented [10].

Dealing with genetic aetiology, in 2009, EME was reported in association with a mutation of the verba erythroblastic leukaemia viral oncogene homologue 4 (ErbB4 gene), which is involved in the migration of interneurons to the cortex [23]. This genetic abnormality is consistent with the persistence of spiny neurons in the white matter on pathologic examination and of the functional deafferentation described by Hirose et al. [4]; both of them seem to indicate impaired neuronal migration to the cortex, suggesting a degree of "cortical isolation" in the brains of these patients [4].

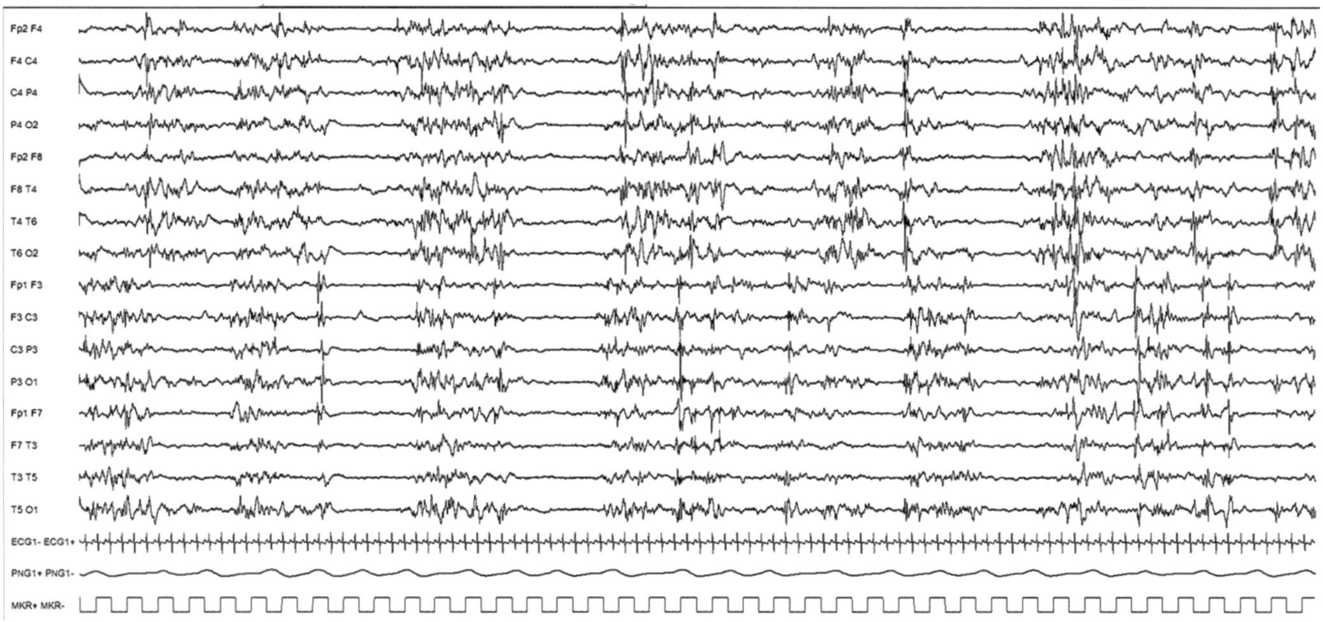

Fig. 23.4 Suppression-burst with multifocal epileptiform abnormalities in a patient with pyridoxine-deficiency encephalopathy

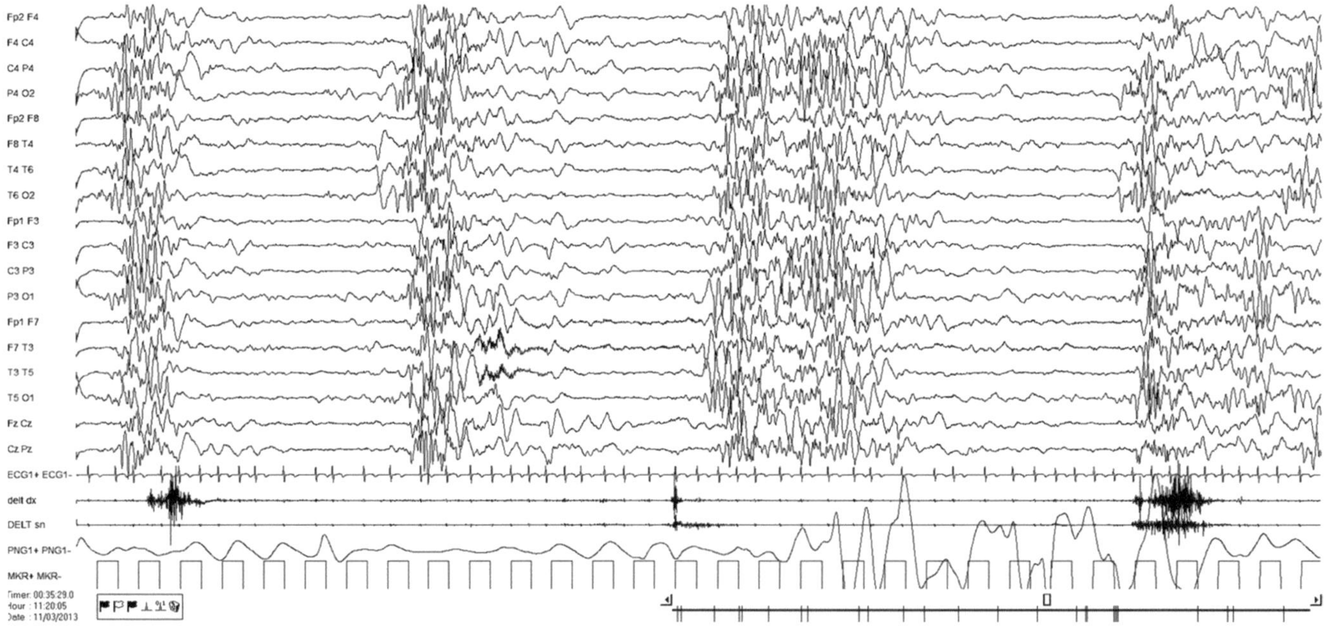

Fig. 23.5 EEG during awake state of a 6 month old boy with suppression-burst pattern due to CDG type 1 disorder due to ALG11 mutation. EEG indicates typical suppression burst pattern that can be observed in both Ohtahara syndrome and early myoclonic encephalopathy

23.4 Other Early-Onset Epileptic Encephalopathies due to Specific Genetic Aetiology

23.4.1 CDKL5-Related Epileptic Encephalopathy (OMIM 300672)

Early infantile epileptic encephalopathy type 2 (EIEE2, OMIM #300672) is an X-linked dominant severe neurologic disorder characterized by onset of seizures in the first months of life and severe global developmental delay resulting in mental retardation and poor motor control [24]. The epilepsy course has been distinguished into three successive stages: (stage I) early epilepsy (onset 1–10 weeks) with normal interictal EEG despite frequent convulsive seizures, (stage II) epileptic encephalopathy with infantile spasms and hypsarrhythmia, and (stage III) refractory epilepsy with tonic seizures and myoclonia [25]. Interictal EEG in this last phase is characterized by a marked

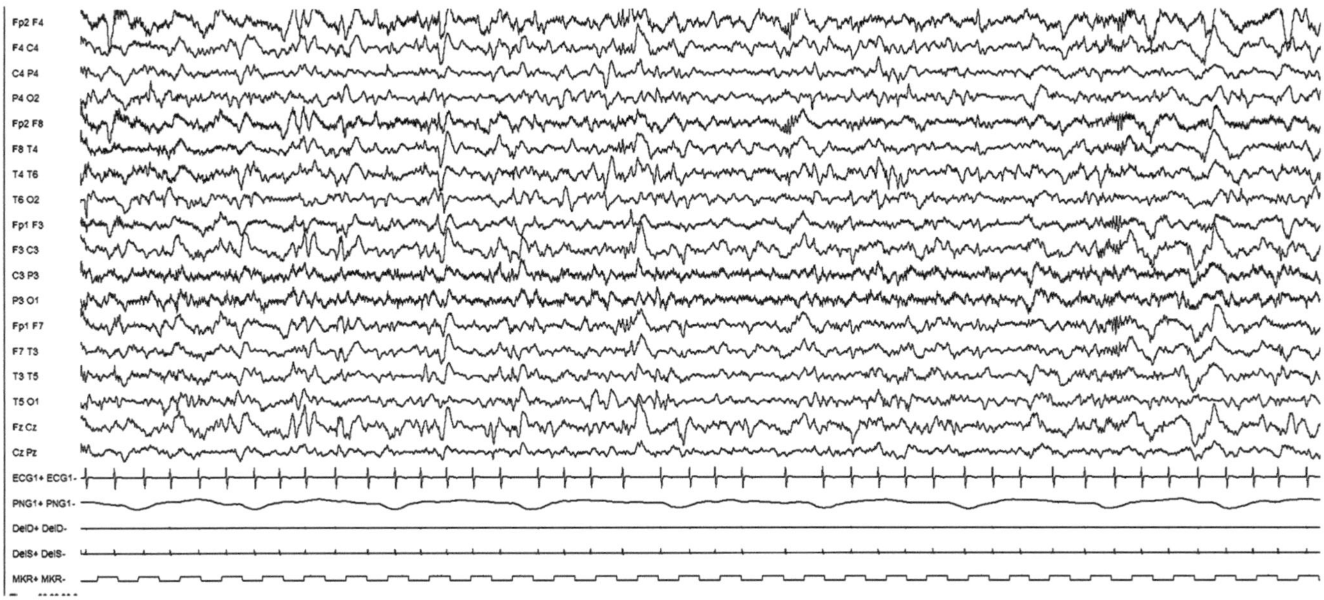

Fig. 23.6 Interictal EEG of a 8 years old girls with CDKL5-related encephalopathy. Bilateral epileptiform abnormalities are intermingled with brief phases of flattening of cerebral activity

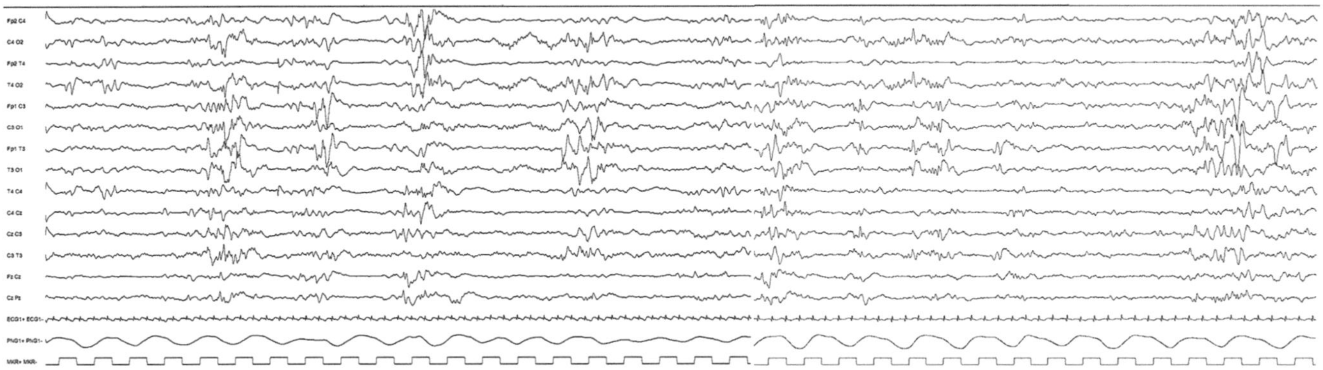

Fig. 23.7 Multifocal epileptiform abnormalities intermingled with diffuse suppression of cerebral activity in a patient with KCNQ2 at onset

slowing down of background activity and multifocal abnormalities (Fig. 23.6). The phenotypes associated with CDKL5 mutations range from a mild form with controlled epilepsy and ability to walk to a severe form with absolute microcephaly and poor motor development. Genotype-phenotype correlation is not still defined even if a relationship between severity and the type of CDKL5 mutation, depending on whether the catalytic domain is impaired or not, has been reported [24, 25].

23.4.2 KCNQ2-Related Epileptic Encephalopathy (OMIM 613720)

KCNQ2-related epileptic encephalopathy type 7 (OMIM #613720) is a neonatal-onset epilepsy characterized by daily seizures, predominantly tonic and drug-resistant, associated with intellectual disability [26]. Seizure onset is between 1 and 4 days of age with daily tonic asymmetric, focal, and clonic seizures. EEG is characterized by multifocal epileptiform abnormalities intermingled with disuse suppression of cerebral activity (Fig. 23.7).

Most patients reach seizure control within the first year of life and remain seizure-free thereafter; however, cognitive deterioration of variable degree remains evident. Sodium channel blockers, especially carbamazepine and phenytoin are the drugs of choice for effective seizure control [27].

23.4.3 SCN2A-Related Epileptic Encephalopathy (OMIM 613721)

Early infantile epileptic encephalopathy type 11 (EIEE11, OMIM #613721) is a recently recognized syndrome caused by de novo SCN2A missense variants. Epilepsy onset is reported within the first 3 months of life [28] About 40% of patients have an identifiable epilepsy syndrome, i.e. Ohtahara syndrome or epilepsy of infancy with migrating focal seizures (EIMFS) [28, 29]. The remaining patients have

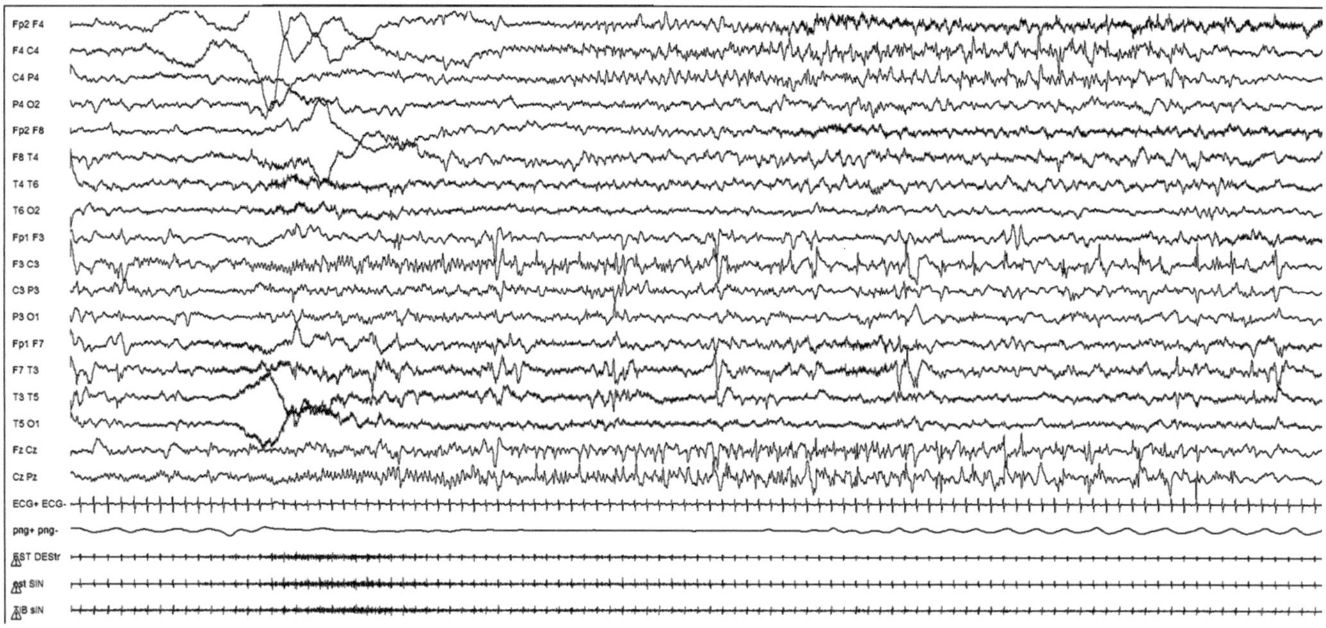

Fig. 23.8 Bilateral indipendent epileptiform abnormalities over left and right frontal regions in a 1 month old girl with early-onset epileptiform encephalopathy due to SCN2A mutation

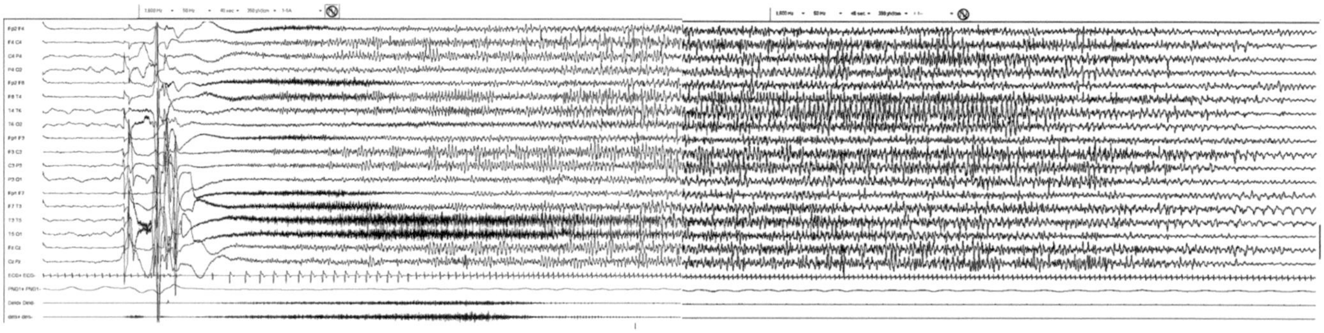

Fig. 23.9 Ictal EEG of a 4 months old boy with SCN8A mutation. Tonic seizure with diffuse onset, consisting of a flattening of cerebral activity, later on recruiting and increasing in amplitude. The ECG trace, shows an ictal bradicardia as one of the first signs of seizure

unclassifiable epilepsies. The predominant seizure types in these are focal (Fig. 23.8), tonic, and tonic-clonic seizures or spasms. Initial EEGs shows a suppression-burst pattern in one third of cases and multifocal spikes in the majority of the remaining cases [28].

Regardless of the epileptic syndrome, all patients present with intellectual disability, being severe in about two third of cases [28]. Sodium channel blockers, especially carbamazepine and phenytoin, are the drugs of choice for effective seizure control [30].

23.4.4 SCN8A-Related Epileptic Encephalopathy (OMIM 614558)

Early infantile epileptic encephalopathy type 13 (EIEE13, OMIM #614558) is a recently recognized syndrome caused by de novo SCN8A missense variants. Epilepsy starts before 18 months of age and is intractable and is associated with developmental impairment, usually severe, and pyramidal and extrapyramidal signs [31]. Also in SCN8A developmental and epileptic encephalopathy, it has been reported an improvement with sodium channel-blocking antiepileptic drugs [30].

Interictal EEG at epilepsy onset is reported normal in 35% patients and with discrete slowing and infrequent epileptiform abnormalities in 40%. More rarely hypsarrhythmia has been described. All patients develop during the following years a progressive slowing of background activity and multifocal epileptiform abnormalities, mainly over the temporo-parieto-occipital regions [31]. Multiple seizure types occur, including focal seizures, generalized seizures, and epileptic spasms [31]. Ictal bradycardia is frequently reported, mainly in tonic seizures (Fig. 23.9).

References

1. Beal JC, Cherian K, Moshe SL. Early-onset epileptic encephalopathies: Ohtahara syndrome and early myoclonic encephalopathy. Pediatr Neurol. 2012;47:317–23.
2. Djukic A, Lado FA, Shinnar S, Moshé SL. Are early myoclonic encephalopathy (EME) and the Ohtahara syndrome (EIEE) independent of each other? Epilepsy Res. 2006;70:S68–76.
3. Murakami N, Ohtsuka Y, Ohtahara S. Early infantile epileptic syndromes with suppression-bursts: early myoclonic encephalopathy vs. Ohtahara syndrome. Jpn J Psychiatry Neurol. 1993;47:197–200.
4. Hirose M, Haginoya K, Yokoyama H, et al. Functional cortical deafferentation from the subcortical structures in a patient with early myoclonic encephalopathy: a functional neuroimaging study. Epilepsia. 2010;51:699–702.
5. Ohtahara S, Ishida T, Oka E, Yamatogy Y, Inoue H. On the specific age-dependent epileptic syndromes: the early-infantile epileptic encephalopathy with suppression-burst. No To Hattatsu. 1976;8:270–80.
6. Ohtahara S. Seizure disorders in infancy and childhood. Brain and Development. 1984;6:509–19.
7. Miller SP, Dilenge ME, Meagher-Villemure K, O'Gorman AM, Shevell MI. Infantile epileptic encephalopathy (Ohtahara syndrome) and migrational disorder. Pediatr Neurol. 1998;19:50–4.
8. Trinka E, Rauscher C, Nagler M, et al. A case of Ohtahara syndrome with olivary-dentate dysplasia and agenesis of the mamillary bodies. Epilepsia. 2001;42:950–3.
9. du Plessis AJ, Kaufmann WE, Kupsky WJ. Intra-uterine onset myoclonic encephalopathy associated with cerebral cortical dysgenesis. J Child Neurol. 1993;8:164–70.
10. Spreafico R, Angelini L, Binelli S, Granata T, Rumi V, Rosti D, Runza L, Bugiani O. Burst suppression and impairment of neocortical ontogenesis: electroclinical and neuropathologic findings in two infants with early myoclonic encephalopathy. Epilepsia. 1993;34(5):800–8.
11. Williams AN, Gray RG, Poulton K, Ramani P, Whitehouse WP. A case of Ohtahara syndrome with cytochrome oxidase deficiency. Dev Med Child Neurol. 1998;40:568–70.
12. Singhi P, Ray M. Ohtahara syndrome with biotinidase deficiency. J Child Neurol. 2011;26:507–9.
13. Castro-Gago M, Blanco-Barca MO, Gómez-Lado C, Eirís-Puñal J, Campos-González Y, Arenas-Barbero J. Respiratory chain complex I deficiency in an infant with Ohtahara syndrome. Brain and Development. 2009;31:322–5.
14. Saitsu H, Kato M, Mizuguchi T, et al. De novo mutations in the gene encoding STXBP1 (MUNC18-1) cause early infantile epileptic encephalopathy. Nat Genet. 2008;40:782–8.
15. Kato M, Saitoh S, Kamei A, et al. A longer polyalanine expansion mutation in the ARX gene causes early infantile epileptic encephalopathy with suppression-burst pattern (Ohtahara syndrome). Am J Hum Genet. 2007;81:361–6.
16. Eksioglu YZ, Pong AW, Takeoka M. A novel mutation in the Aristaless domain of the ARX gene leads to Ohtahara syndrome, global developmental delay, and ambiguous genitalia in males and neuropsychiatric disorders in females. Epilepsia. 2011;52:984–92.
17. Ohtahara S, Yamatogi Y. Ohtahara syndrome: with special reference to its developmental aspects for differentiating from early myoclonic encephalopathy. Epilepsy Res. 2006;70:S58–67.
18. Ohno M, Shimotsuji Y, Abe J, Shimada M, Tamiya H. Zonisamide treatment of early infantile epileptic encephalopathy. Pediatr Neurol. 2000;23:341–4.
19. Komaki H, Sugai K, Sasaki M, et al. Surgical treatment of a case of early infantile epileptic encephalopathy with suppression bursts associated with focal cortical dysplasia. Epilepsia. 1999;40:365–9.
20. Fusco L, Pachatz C, Di Capua M, Vigevano F. Video-EEG aspects of early-infantile epileptic encephalopathy with suppression-bursts (Ohtahara syndrome). Brain and Development. 2001;23:708–14.
21. Lee WT. Disorders of amino acid metabolism associated with epilepsy. Brain and Development. 2011;33:745–52.
22. Aukett A, Bennett MJ, Hosking GP. Molybdenum cofactor deficiency: an easily missed inborn error of metabolism. Dev Med Child Neurol. 1988;30:531–5.
23. Backx L, Ceulemans B, Vermeesch JR, Devriendt K, Van Esch H. Early myoclonic encephalopathy caused by a disruption of the neuregulin-1 receptor ErbB4. Eur J Hum Genet. 2009;17:378–82.
24. Bahi-Buisson N, Villeneuve N, Caietta E, Jacquette A, Maurey H, Matthijs G, Van Esch H, Delahaye A, Moncla A, Milh M, Zufferey F, Diebold B, Bienvenu T. Recurrent mutations in the CDKL5 gene: genotype-phenotype relationships. Am J Med Genet A. 2012;158A(7):1612–9.
25. Bahi-Buisson N, Kaminska A, Boddaert N, Rio M, Afenjar A, Gérard M, Giuliano F, Motte J, Héron D, Morel MA, Plouin P, Richelme C, des Portes V, Dulac O, Philippe C, Chiron C, Nabbout R, Bienvenu T. The three stages of epilepsy in patients with CDKL5 mutations. Epilepsia. 2008;49(6):1027–37.
26. Weckhuysen S, Mandelstam S, Suls A, et al. KCNQ2 encephalopathy: emerging phenotype of a neonatal epileptic encephalopathy. Ann Neurol. 2012;71:15–25.
27. Pisano T, Numis AL, Heavin SB, Weckhuysen S, Angriman M, Suls A, Podesta B, Thibert RL, Shapiro KA, Guerrini R, Scheffer IE, Marini C, Cilio MR. Early and effective treatment of KCNQ2 encephalopathy. Epilepsia. 2015;56(5):685–91.
28. Wolff M, Johannesen KM, UBS H, Masnada S, Rubboli G, Gardella E, Lesca G, Ville D, Milh M, Villard L, Afenjar A, Chantot-Bastaraud S, Mignot C, Lardennois C, Nava C, Schwarz N, Gérard M, Perrin L, Doummar D, Auvin S, Miranda MJ, Hempel M, Brilstra E, Knoers N, Verbeek N, van Kempen M, Braun KP, Mancini G, Biskup S, Hörtnagel K, Döcker M, Bast T, Loddenkemper T, Wong-Kisiel L, Baumeister FM, Fazeli W, Striano P, Dilena R, Fontana E, Zara F, Kurlemann G, Klepper J, Thoene JG, Arndt DH, Deconinck N, Schmitt-Mechelke T, Maier O, Muhle H, Wical B, Finetti C, Brückner R, Pietz J, Golla G, Jillella D, Linnet KM, Charles P, Moog U, Õiglane-Shlik E, Mantovani JF, Park K, Deprez M, Lederer D, Mary S, Scalais E, Selim L, Van Coster R, Lagae L, Nikanorova M, Hjalgrim H, Korenke GC, Trivisano M, Specchio N, Ceulemans B, Dorn T, Helbig KL, Hardies K, Stamberger H, de Jonghe P, Weckhuysen S, Lemke JR, Krägeloh-Mann I, Helbig I, Kluger G, Lerche H, Møller RS. Genetic and phenotypic heterogeneity suggest therapeutic implications in SCN2A-related disorders. Brain. 2017;140(5):1316–36.
29. Howell KB, McMahon JM, Carvill GL, Tambunan D, Mackay MT, Rodriguez-Casero V, Webster R, Clark D, Freeman JL, Calvert S, Olson HE, Mandelstam S, Poduri A, Mefford HC, Harvey AS, Scheffer IE. SCN2A encephalopathy: a major cause of epilepsy of infancy with migrating focal seizures. Neurology. 2015;85(11):958–66.
30. Barker BS, Ottolini M, Wagnon JL, Hollander RM, Meisler MH, Patel MK. The SCN8A encephalopathy mutation p.Ile1327Val displays elevated sensitivity to the anticonvulsant phenytoin. Epilepsia. 2016;57(9):1458–66.
31. Gardella E, Marini C, Trivisano M, Fitzgerald MP, Alber M, Howell KB, Darra F, Siliquini S, Bölsterli BK, Masnada S, Pichiecchio A, Johannesen KM, Jepsen B, Fontana E, Anibaldi G, Russo S, Cogliati F, Montomoli M, Specchio N, Rubboli G, Veggiotti P, Beniczky S, Wolff M, Helbig I, Vigevano F, Scheffer IE, Guerrini R, Møller RS. The phenotype of SCN8A developmental and epileptic encephalopathy. Neurology. 2018;91(12):e1112–24.

Epileptic Encephalopathies of Infancy and Childhood

24

Mario Brinciotti and Maria Matricardi

24.1 Introduction

Epilepsies associated with encephalopathy or cerebral damage were defined in the past with the term *epileptic encephalopathies*. Recently this concept has been deeply revised, restricting the criterion of inclusion to the forms in which the epilepsy itself is responsible of brain dysfunctions with mental and neurologic decline [1–4]. This implies that some syndromes, once included in this chapter, according to the new definition, are no longer considered today. Incidence and prevalence of these epilepsies are generally low, and many syndromes are included in the National Register of Rare Diseases of several countries in order to provide specific supports and related health services to patients. The electro-clinical features are often influenced by the underlying processes of brain maturation and therefore by age (some forms are typically age-dependent); in addition, some syndromes present a clear continuity with evolution from one type to another. The etiology is variable, often characterized by brain structural damage, although the role of genetic factors has recently been emphasized in some forms [5, 6].

The prognosis is variable, depending on clinical features and underlying etiology, but it is generally unfavorable both for seizure outcome and neurocognitive development.

24.2 West Syndrome

It is the most common epileptic encephalopathy in the first 2 years of life, with incidence ranging from 2.2 to 4.5 per 10,000 live births, very similar among different ethnic groups [7–10]. The onset occurs within the 1st year of life, usually between 3 and 12 months, with a peak at 5 months in 90% of cases. The electro-clinical feature is characterized by a triad: (a) infantile spasms, (b) typical EEG pattern (*hypsarrhythmia*), and (c) developmental arrest or psychomotor delay with intellectual impairment. In many cases, it is preceded by other types of seizures, especially partial, or by Ohtahara syndrome [11, 12].

The etiology is variable, often linked to infectious during pregnancy (rubella, toxoplasmosis, cytomegalovirus, etc.), severe pre-perinatal anoxic-ischemic encephalopathies, neurocutaneous diseases (tuberous sclerosis, neurofibromatosis), cerebral malformations (microgyria, pachygyria, heterotopias, etc.), and chromosomal abnormalities (trisomy 21). Recently, genetic studies based on complementary cytogenetic and genomic approaches provided evidence for the involvement of de novo mutations in children with infantile spasms of unknown etiology [6, 13].

Infantile spasms are a well-defined type of epileptic seizure, originally described by West [14], characterized by a brief axial contraction. They may be typical (anti-flexion of the head and simultaneous flexion of the limbs on the trunk) or atypical (in extension, asymmetric, asynchronous) and usually tend to repeat in cluster, with rapid succession for several minutes, almost always stereotypic [15–17].

Some clinical variants of spasms (tonic, atonic) have been recently described in some patients [18, 19]. Infantile spasms may be found in other epileptic encephalopathies other than West syndrome, such as Lennox-Gastaut syndrome, epilepsy with myoclonic-atonic seizures, Dravet syndrome, and epilepsy of infancy with migrating focal seizures [20]. The appearance of spasms can be preceded, accompanied, and followed by other types of seizures, especially focal.

M. Brinciotti (✉)
Department of Human Neurosciences, Neurophysiopathology - Epilepsy Centre (C.I.M.S.), Sapienza University of Rome, Rome, Italy
e-mail: mario.brinciotti@uniroma1.it

M. Matricardi
Department of Human Neurosciences, Epilepsy Centre (C.I.M.S.), Sapienza University of Rome, Rome, Italy
e-mail: maria.matricardi@uniroma1.it

O. Mecarelli (ed.), *Clinical Electroencephalography*, https://doi.org/10.1007/978-3-030-04573-9_24

Hypsarrhythmia is the typical interictal EEG feature of West syndrome and occurs in two-thirds of patients. It is characterized by a disorganized high-amplitude background activity with a chaotic mixture of arrhythmic and asynchronous slow and sharp waves of high-voltage, multifocal spikes and polyspikes, interspersed with short periods of low voltage (Fig. 24.1). This pattern may be present in wakefulness or be more evident during non-REM sleep, generally associated with poor or absent representation of physiological figures such as spindles and K-complexes (Fig. 24.2). In sleep, epileptic anomalies tend to be grouped in short sequences; the track then becomes discontinuous in deep sleep. The hypsarrhythmia can be atypical, and several variants have been reported [21], among which an asymmetric or unilateral one can be found especially in patients with unilateral or clearly prevailing brain damage in a hemisphere (Figs. 24.3, 24.4, and 24.5). Ictal EEG, corresponding to the spasms, shows paroxysmal generalized slow waves followed by a brief period (1–2 s) of diffuse voltage attenuation, sometimes associated with rapid activity.

In about 3% of cases, West syndrome is preceded by Ohtahara syndrome [11, 12, 22], and the hypsarrhythmia represents a progressive transition from a previous pattern of suppression-brust (Figs. 24.6 and 24.7). Over one-third of patients suffering from West syndrome evolve to a Lennox-Gastaut syndrome, usually after 2–4 years of age [23, 24]; in these cases, the hypsarrhythmia is followed by an intermediate phase characterized by multifocal epileptic anomalies with subsequent appearance of typical generalized slow spike-and-wave complexes.

24.3 Dravet Syndrome

Initially described as severe myoclonic epilepsy in infancy by Dravet [25], it has a rare incidence, probably less than 1 in 30/40,000 [26, 27]. Even if the etiology is not completely clarified, the high family incidence of both epilepsy and febrile convulsions and the finding of genetic mutations in about 80% of patients, especially for SCN1A and PCDH19

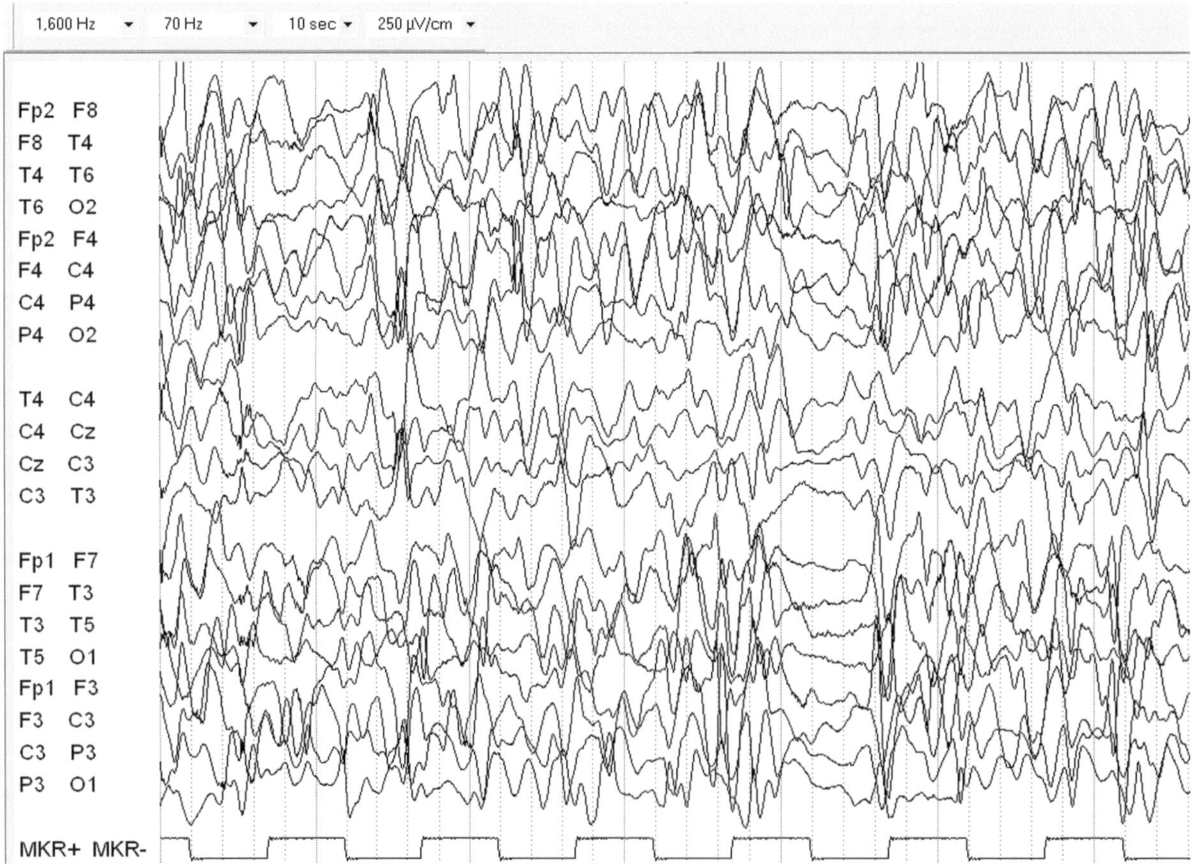

Fig. 24.1 Hypsarrhythmia (awake EEG). Disorganized high-amplitude background activity with a chaotic mixture of arrhythmic and asynchronous slow and sharp waves of high-voltage, multifocal spikes and polyspikes, with short periods of diffuse low voltage

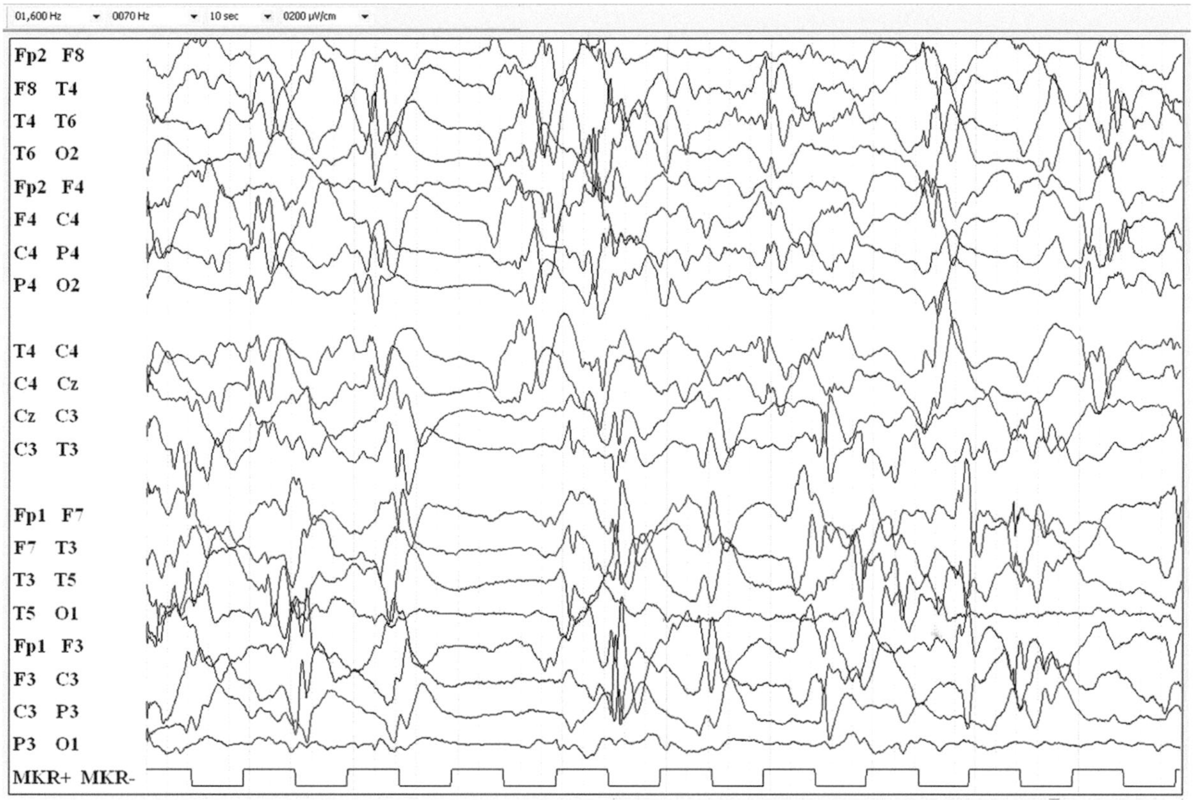

Fig. 24.2 Hypsarrhythmia (sleep EEG). Poor representation of physiological elements. Spikes, sharp waves, slow waves, and atypical synchronous and asynchronous spike-wave complexes, sometimes grouped in irregular sequences tending to diffusion, with short periods of diffuse low voltage

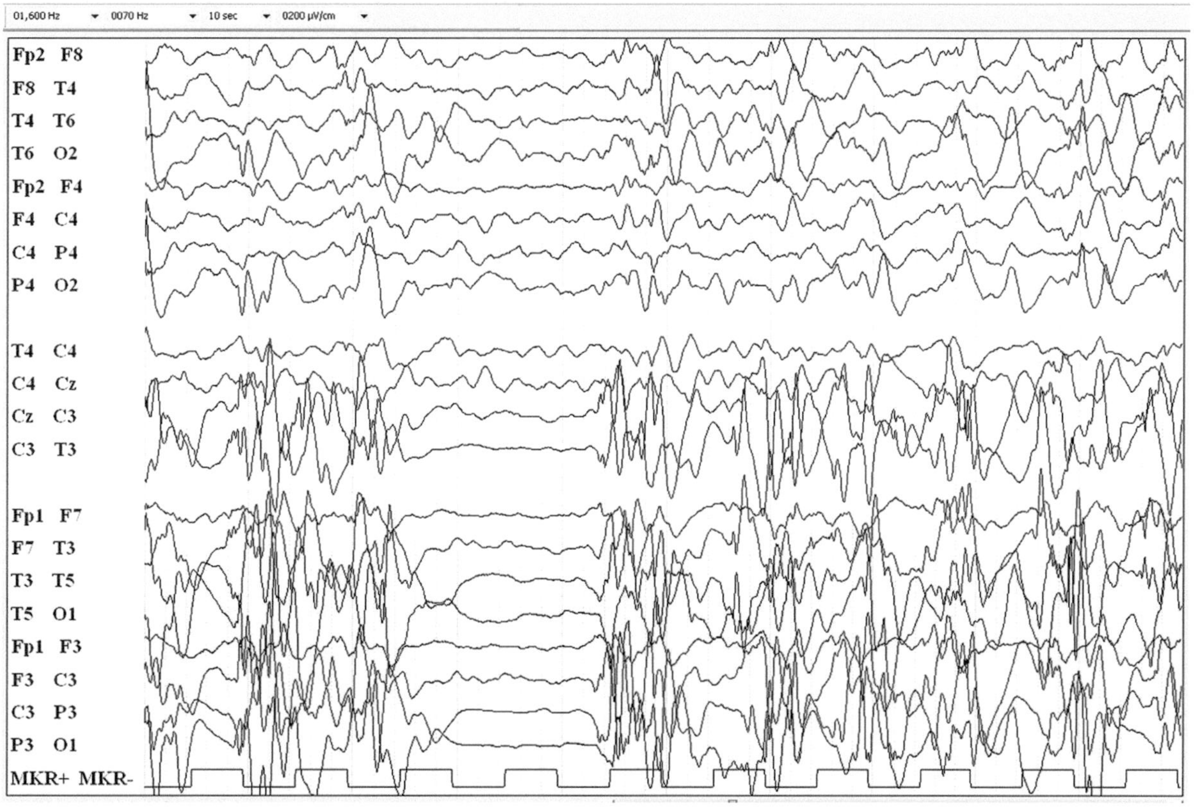

Fig. 24.3 Hemi-hypsarrhythmia (awake EEG). Asymmetrical EEG with hypsarrhythmic pattern on the left hemisphere and a better organized background activity on the right

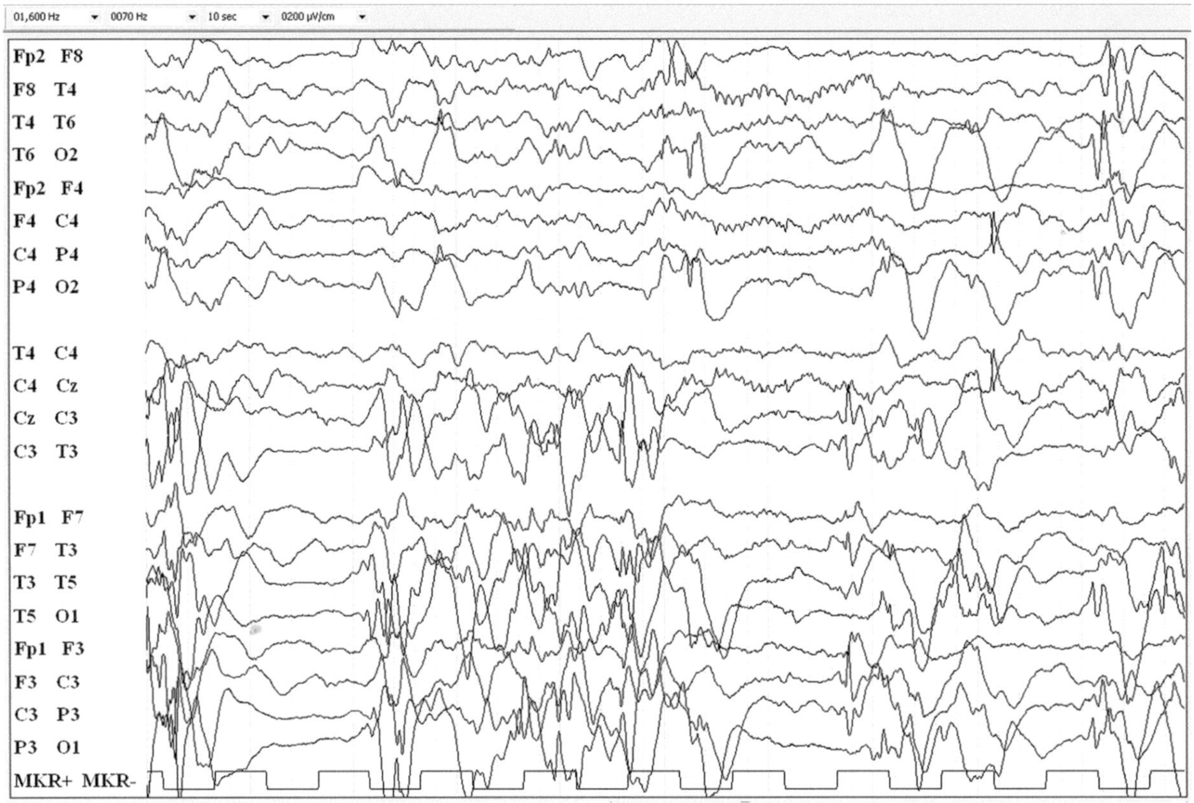

Fig. 24.4 Hemi-hypsarrhythmia (sleep EEG; same patient of Fig. 24.3). The EEG asymmetry persists with hypsarrhythmic pattern on the left and occurrence of delta activity and epileptic anomalies in the right posterior areas, inscribed on background activity however better organized and with well-represented physiological elements (note the presence of the spindles)

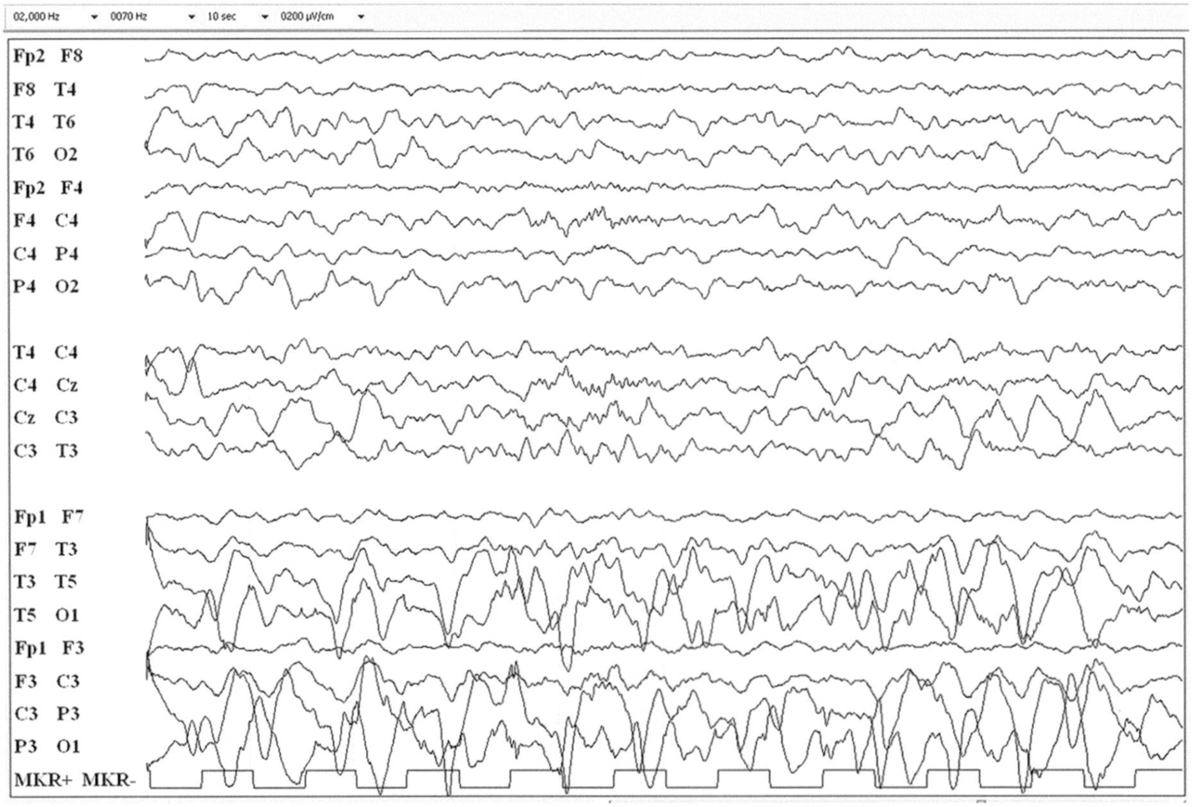

Fig. 24.5 Evolution of hemi-hypsarrhythmic pattern (same patient of Figs. 24.3 and 24.4—sleep EEG recorded after 16 months from the previous ones). Hypsarrhythmic pattern is no longer evident, whereas interhemispheric asymmetry persists, with slower and wider activity in the left posterior regions and the absence of the physiological elements on the left hemisphere

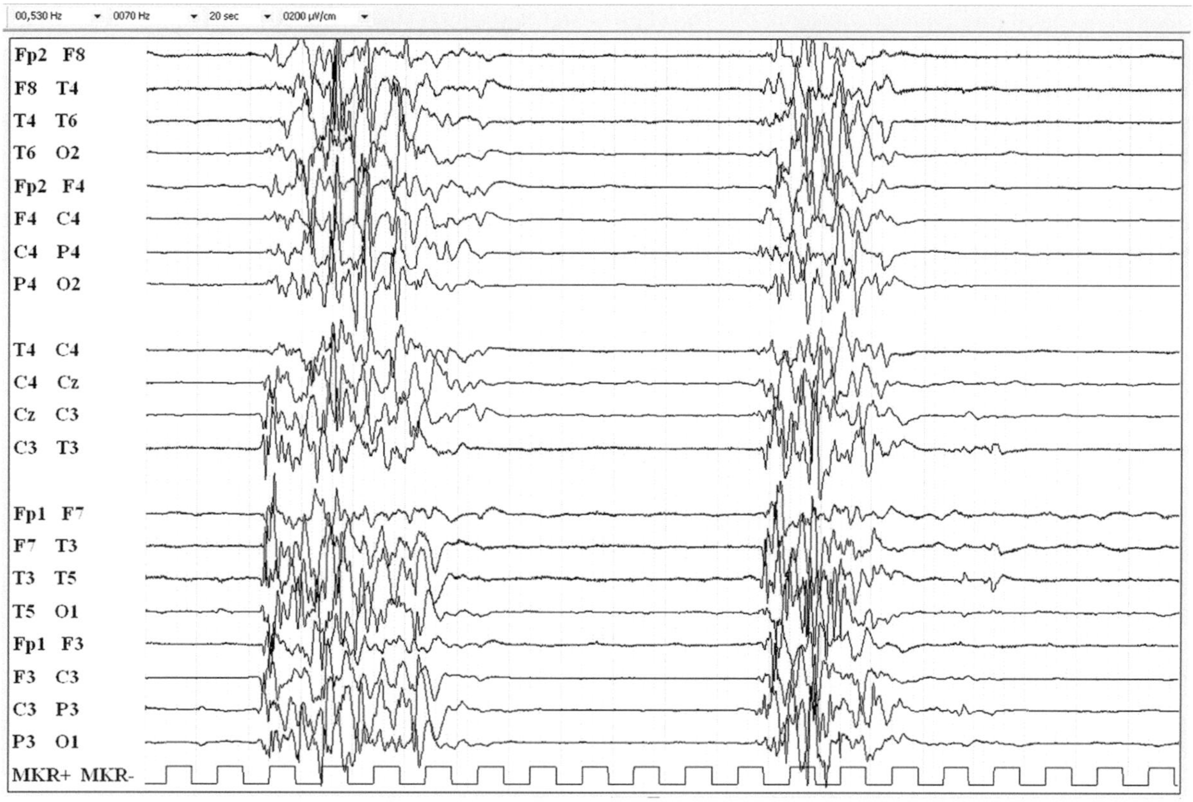

Fig. 24.6 Suppression-burst (awake EEG). Brief bursts (2–4 s) of spikes, sharp waves, slow waves, and atypical spike-wave complexes on diffuse low-voltage EEG

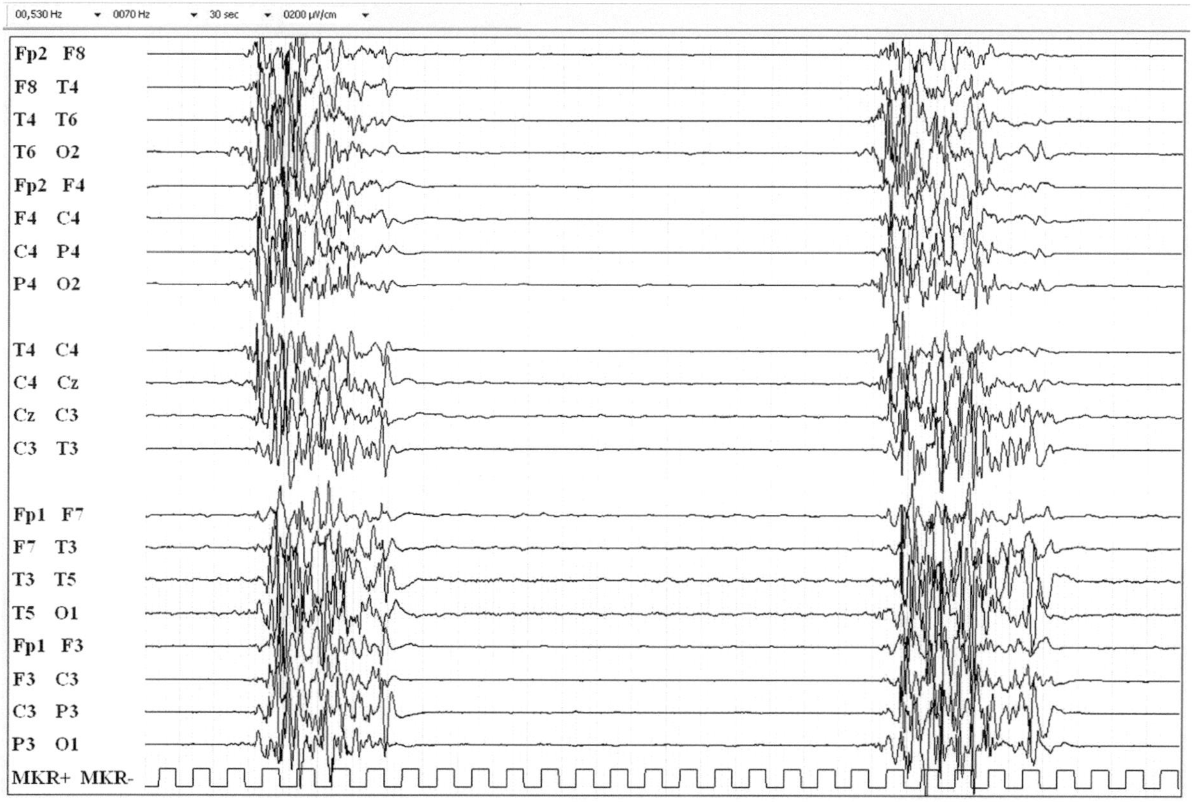

Fig. 24.7 Suppression-burst (sleep EEG). Longer periods of low-voltage interposed among epileptic discharges

genes, identify a causal role in genetic factors [28]. The clinical onset occurs within the 1st year of life (between 5 and 8 months) with a generalized or unilateral clonic seizure, even prolonged, often associated with fever, which tends to recur. Subsequently, other seizure types appear [29]: (1) Generalized tonic-clonic seizures and/or unilateral clonic seizures, often evolving to status. (2) Myoclonic seizures usually start between the ages of 1 and 5 years, with massive jerks involving all muscles, particularly the axial ones. (3) Atypical absences occur isolated or accompanied by myoclonic component such as rapid eyelid myoclonia. Episodes of *obtundation status* have been reported in 30–40% of patients [30, 31], consisting of consciousness' impairment, variable in intensity, associated with segmental and erratic myoclonus. (4) Focal seizures occur in 43–79% of patients [31–33], with motor signs or more complex semiology, including prominent autonomic symptoms, and with or without secondary generalization. (5) Tonic seizures are unusual. The presence of seizure-triggering factors (slight temperature variations, hot baths, photo and pattern sensitivity, environmental light, physical exercise, emotions, etc.) is a characteristic feature of this syndrome [29]. Developmental delay, cognitive deficits, and behavioral disturbances are common and usually start progressively from the 2nd year of life. Even if no regression is observed after 5 years in the stabilization stage, the evolution is however unfavorable in all cases, with constant intellectual impairment (severe in 60%) often associated with behavioral disturbances and psychosis [29].

The EEG at the onset shows normal background activity during wakefulness and normal organization of physiologic patterns during sleep. A peculiar 4–5 Hz rhythmic theta activity may be recorded over the rolandic areas and the vertex in some cases, starting at the end of the 1st year of life and persisting throughout the follow-up [34, 35]. Afterward, the interictal EEG shows both generalized and focal (more often, multifocal) epileptic abnormalities (spike, polyspikes, spike-wave and polyspike-wave complexes) accentuated by sleep [36]. Photoparoxysmal responses (PPR) may be induced by intermittent light stimulation (ILS) and/or pattern stimulation in 26–40% of cases [36, 37], even at an early stage, representing an unusual finding at this age. The background activity, initially normal, tends to gradually deteriorate over time [36, 37].

The ictal abnormalities are characterized by generalized spike-wave complexes and/or fast polyspikes, diffuse or

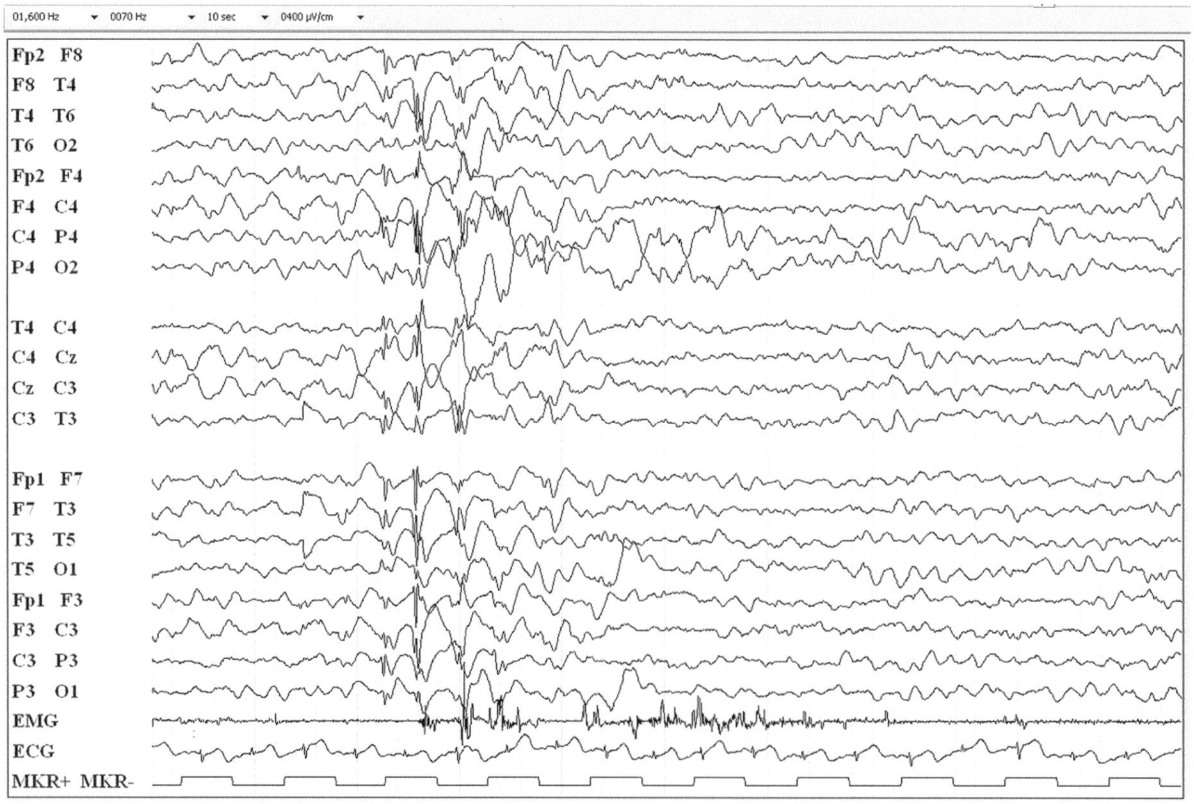

Fig. 24.8 Polygraphic EEG during non-REM sleep (*EMG* right deltoid muscle). Generalized spike-wave and polyspike-wave complexes associated with proximal myoclonia of the upper limbs

involving mainly the frontocentral regions, often associated with focal and multifocal fast spikes or polyspikes [36, 37]. Paroxysms vary according to seizure type:

- Myoclonic seizures are associated with brief bursts of generalized spike-wave and polyspike-wave complexes or fast polyspikes, mainly involving the frontocentral regions especially at onset (Fig. 24.8).
- Atypical absences coincide with generalized, often irregular, spike-wave complexes.
- Focal seizures are accompanied by spikes, sharp waves, spike-wave complexes, and polyspike-wave complexes tending to transmission or generalization.

24.4 Lennox-Gastaut Syndrome

Lennox-Gastaut syndrome is one of the most severe epileptic encephalopathies of childhood [38, 39]. The incidence is low (only 0.6% of all new-onset epilepsies), but, due to its poor treatability, its prevalence varies from 1 to 10% of all childhood epilepsies [40, 41]. The etiology is symptomatic in 75% of cases, with considerable heterogeneity with respect to the type of lesion [40]. The onset is between 2 and 6 years of age, often in children with previous West syndrome or other forms of severe epilepsy and episodes of status epilepticus. The diagnosis is based on a characteristic triad of electro-clinical signs [38–42]:

(a) *Multiple seizure types*: atypical absences, tonic seizures especially during sleep, tonic and atonic drop attacks with fall, and more rarely myoclonic seizures
(b) *Specific (but not pathognomonic) EEG abnormalities*: interictal slow spike-wave complexes (<3 Hz) and paroxysmal fast activity (PFA), consisting of bursts of diffuse fast rhythms, during non-REM sleep
(c) *Cognitive impairment*: intellectual slowing/regression and behavioral problems

The interictal EEG during wakefulness and sleep shows typical slow spike-wave complexes at 1.5–2.5 Hz. These abnormalities consist most often of a sharp wave (70–200 ms), followed by a sinusoidal slow wave (300–500 ms) of high voltages (200–800 μV) or, less often, by a spike (duration <70 ms) or polyspikes followed by a slow wave. These abnormalities are generally diffused, prevailing in the frontal areas (Fig. 24.9), synchronous and symmetrical, but sometimes may be arrhythmic, asynchronous, or prevalent

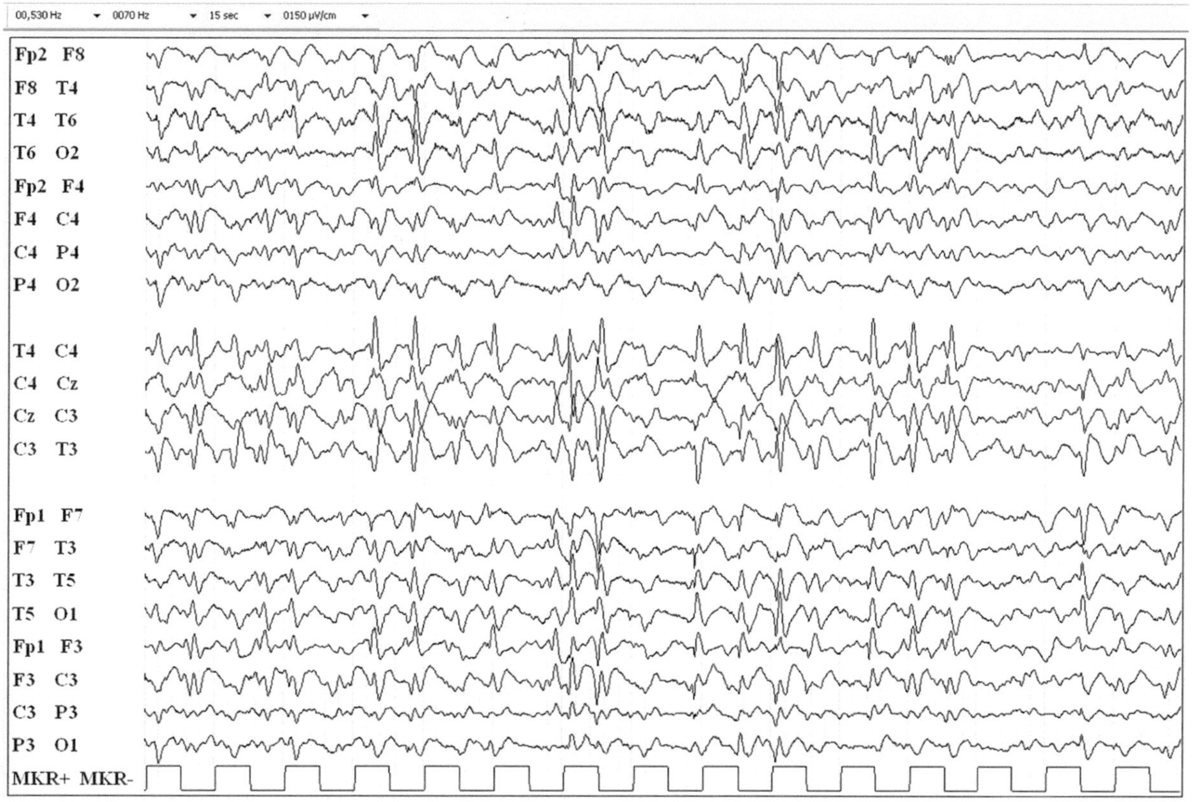

Fig. 24.9 Awake EEG. Generalized 2–2.5 Hz spike-wave complexes of high amplitude on poorly organized background activity

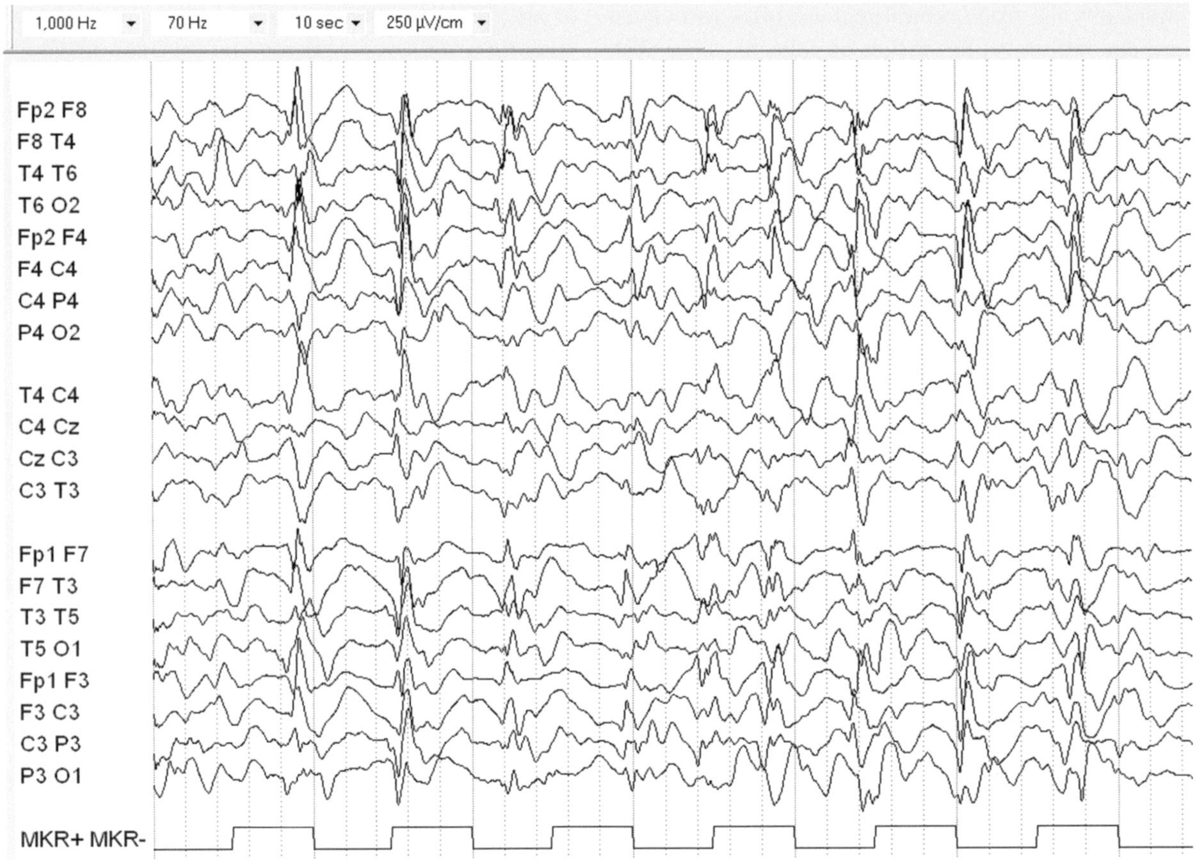

Fig. 24.10 EEG during non-REM sleep. Slow (1.5–2 Hz) spike-wave complexes of high voltage, more synchronous and symmetrical than waking state

in a hemisphere. Hyperventilation and intermittent photic stimulation (IPS) have little influence on this paroxysmal activity. Usually, spike-wave complexes increase during non-REM sleep and become more synchronous, symmetrical, and slower (Fig. 24.10). Focal or multifocal abnormalities (spikes, spike-waves, polyspikes, slow waves, and focal bursts of rapid rhythms) may also be found in the awake state and tend to become bisynchronous during sleep. These focal abnormalities are more common in patients with structural brain lesions and are nonspecific, depending on the underlying pathology.

The background EEG activity appears disorganized and slowed, with the posterior alpha rhythm poorly structured or absent. The slowdown of background activity may be moderate to severe, and its degree correlates with the severity of cognitive impairment.

The sleep EEG is also poorly structured, with alterations of the cyclic architecture and a lesser representation of physiological elements (vertex waves, spindles, K-complexes). During non-REM sleep, periods of electrodecremental activity alternated with periods of irregular high-amplitude sharp and slow activity may also be observed [39].

The ictal EEG varies according to seizure type:

- Tonic seizures, required for the diagnosis [38], may be associated with four types of ictal patterns [39]: (a) diffuse desynchronization; (b) discharge of PFA, progressively increasing in amplitude; (c) initial flattening followed by PFA; and (d) rhythmic discharge at 10–15 Hz of high amplitude from the beginning. The typical pattern of PFA is characterized by brief sequences (from 2 to 10 or more seconds in duration) of rapid rhythmic activity (10–25 Hz), sometimes preceded by a brief burst of slow spike-wave complexes (Fig. 24.11).
- Atypical absences are accompanied by generalized discharges of slow spike-wave complexes at 2–2.5 Hz of high voltage.
- Atonic seizures are associated with bursts of irregular spike-wave and/or polyspike-wave complexes, polyspikes, or rapid rhythms.
- Drop attacks constitute the third most common seizure types. The falling seizures may be pure atonic, myoclonic-atonic, myoclonic, and tonic and may involve the whole body or just the head (head drop) [39]. The EEG correlates of drop/falling seizure are heterogeneous. During atonic or myoclonic-atonic seizures, the ictal EEG shows diffuse polyspike-and-wave complexes, with loss of tone related to the wave of complex.

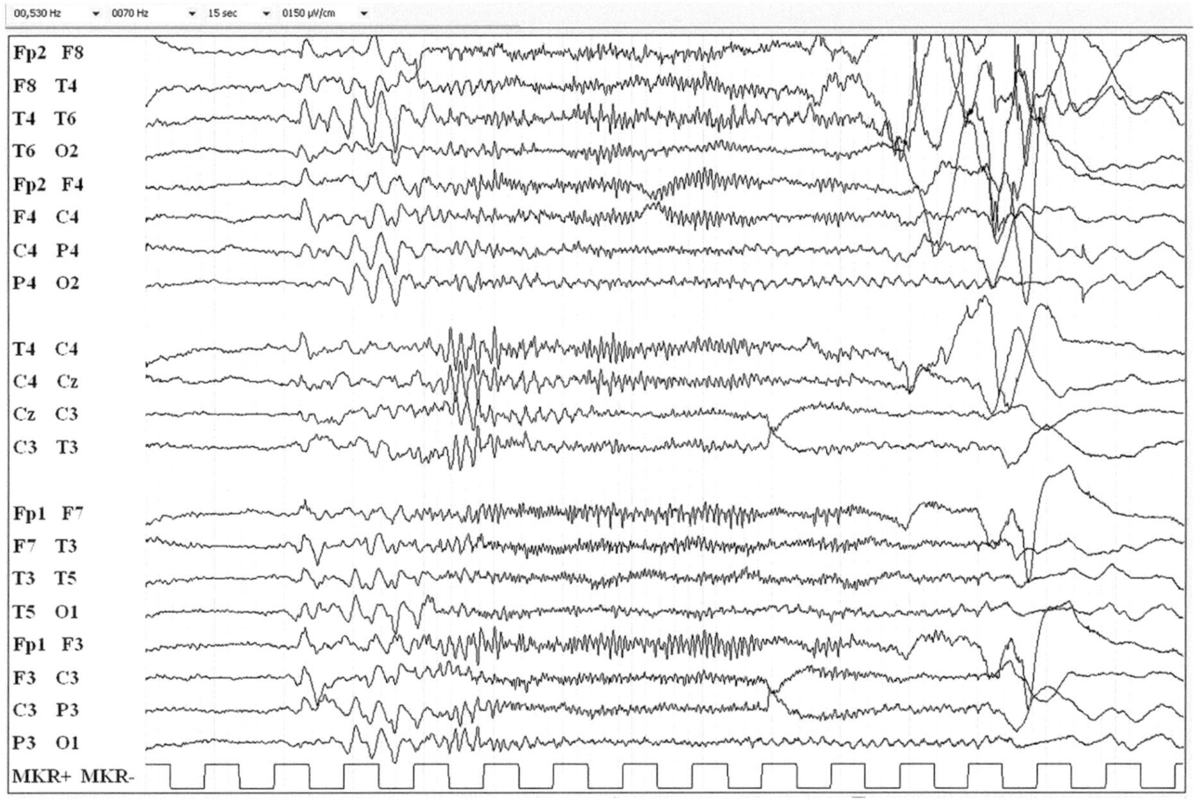

Fig. 24.11 Ictal EEG during non-REM sleep. Sequence of recruiting rhythms at 10–15 Hz, dominant in anterior regions, clinically associated with tonic seizure

Myoclonic drop attacks are accompanied by bursts of polyspikes or polyspike-wave complexes. Brief tonic seizure may produce only desynchronization of the EEG activity.

– Status epilepticus is common in these patients, and it can be convulsive (tonic status) or nonconvulsive (atypical absence status) [39]. The EEG during status epilepticus is similar to the interictal EEG, with diffuse slow spike-wave complexes more persistent.

The long-term outcome of Lennox-Gastaut syndrome is generally poor for the persistence of pharmacoresistant epilepsy and cognitive deficits. The typical EEG pattern of slow spike-wave complexes persists in more than one-third of adult patients, whereas in the remaining ones, the diffuse discharges are replaced by focal or multifocal epileptic abnormalities [43, 44].

24.5 Epilepsy with Myoclonic-Astatic Seizures (Doose Syndrome)

It is a generalized epilepsy syndrome of young children characterized by multiple seizure types, predominantly myoclonic, astatic, and myoclonic-astatic seizures, as well as generalized tonic-clonic, absence, myoclonic absence, and tonic seizures [45–48].

The incidence is not known, while the prevalence is estimated to be between 1 and 2% of all epilepsies of infancy and childhood. The onset occurs between 2 and 5 years of age in children, especially males (74%) [45, 46]. At the beginning, psychomotor development is normal in 84% of cases (with a slight delay, prevalent in language, in the remaining ones). In more than half of the cases, the onset is characterized by generalized tonic-clonic or clonic seizures, even prolonged and repeated, which precede the appearance of typical myoclonic-astatic and myoclonic seizures [45–48]. Myoclonic-astatic seizures consist of sudden massive myoclonic contractions, followed by brief and abrupt loss of muscle tone with fall (*drop attack*). Repeated and protracted episodes of status epilepticus occur in about 36% of patients, accompanied by intellectual deterioration especially of some functions (praxis and language). The unfavorable epilepsy outcome, especially with the appearance of tonic seizures, is constantly associated with progressive global intellectual impairment [45–48]. At the onset, the interictal EEG during waking may show abnormal 4–7 Hz rhythms prevailing in the central areas. Afterward, generalized epileptic abnormalities appear: bilateral, synchronous and symmetrical, regular

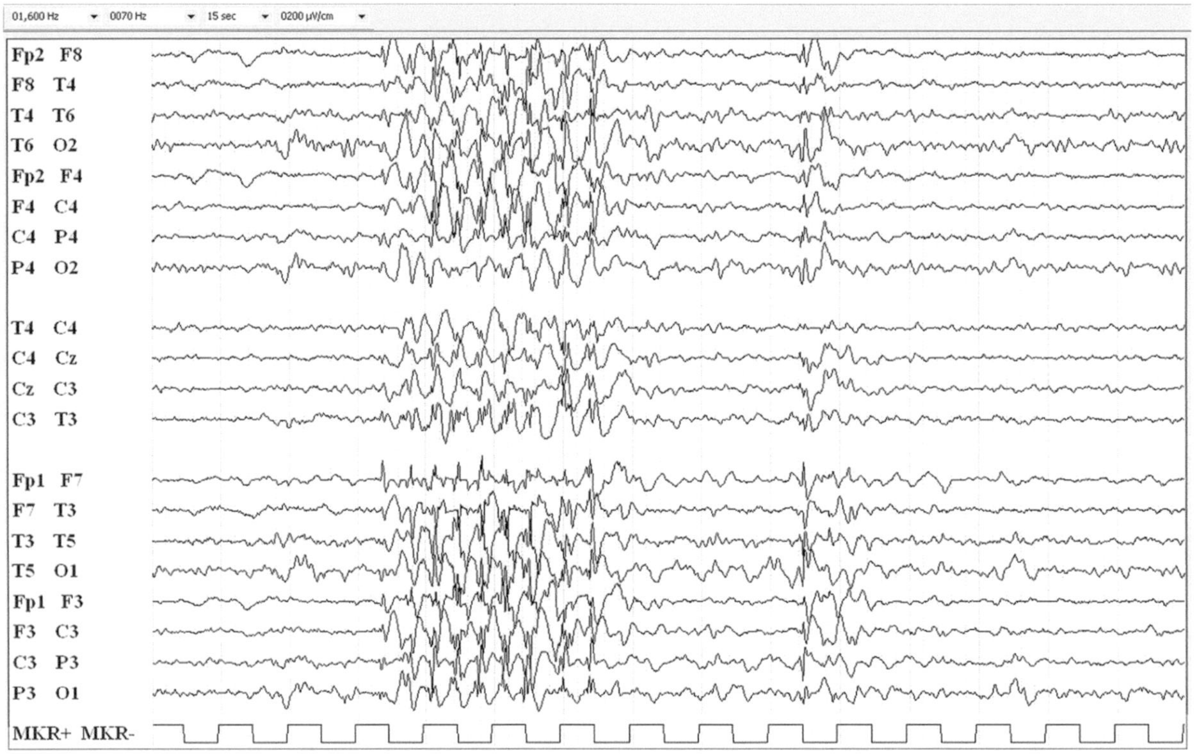

Fig. 24.12 Awake EEG. Short discharge of bilateral synchronous and symmetrical spike-wave and polyspike-wave complexes at 2–3 Hz of high voltage

or more often irregular, spike-wave and polyspike-wave complexes at 2–3 Hz of wide voltage (Fig. 24.12), often more evident during non-REM sleep phases (Fig. 24.13).

The ictal EEG shows bursts of generalized spike or polyspikes-and-wave complexes; in the atonic seizures, the spike-and-wave morphology was characterized by a positive-negative-deep-positive wave followed by a large negative slow wave [45].

24.6 Progressive Myoclonic Epilepsies

This name indicates a heterogeneous group of neurodegenerative disorders distinguished by etiology but brought together by clinical symptomatology and unfavorable prognosis [49–52]. Clinical feature includes a triad of signs common to all forms: myoclonic seizures, tonic-clonic seizures, and progressive neurological dysfunctions (especially, ataxia and dementia). Their incidence is rare, and the onset varies from adolescence to adulthood. Based on their relative frequency, five forms are considered as major (Lafora disease, Unverricht-Lundborg disease, myoclonus epilepsy with ragged-red fibers or MERRF, neuronal ceroid lipofuscinosis, sialidosis-galactosialidosis) compared to other rare or sporadic ones [49–52] (Table 24.1).

Lafora disease is the most common form in childhood (estimated prevalence, less than 1/1,000,000). It is a genetically heterogeneous disease caused by mutations of the genes EPM2A for laphorine (22–58% of cases) and EPM2B for malin (35–72%) [49–53]. The pathological picture is characterized by typical cytoplasmic inclusions consisting of accumulations of polyglucosans (bodies of Lafora) both in the nervous system (especially cerebral and cerebellar cortex) and in extracerebral parenchyma (the skin, muscles, and liver) [49–52]. The onset occurs between 6 and 19 years, more frequently during adolescence, with generalized tonic-clonic or clonic-tonic-clonic seizures and massive and/or segmental myoclonia. Myoclonus, often associated with negative myoclonus, may be spontaneous as well as intentional, or of action, and tends to rapid progression. About half of the patients have occipital lobe seizures with transient amaurosis or visual hallucinations. The course is characterized by a rapid deterioration of movement (ataxia, extrapyramidal stiffness) and mental disorders (dementia, behavior disorders), accompanied by a progressive increase in intensity and frequency of seizures and myoclonia [49–53]. The interictal EEG at the onset can detect generalized polyspikes and polyspike-wave complexes inscribed on a well-organized background activity both in wakefulness and in sleep. Isolated erratic myoclonia, not associated with evident EEG abnormalities, can be documented with polygraphic recordings. As the disease develops,

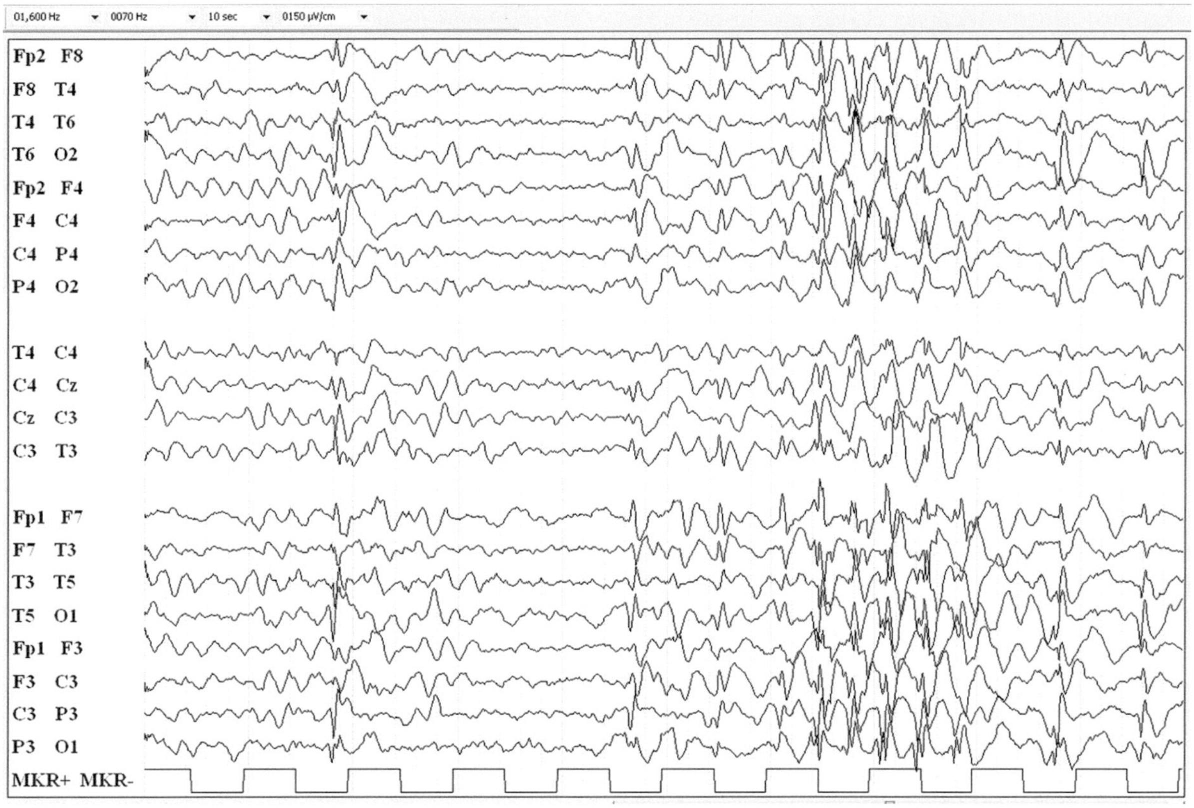

Fig. 24.13 EEG during non-REM sleep. Spikes and spike-wave and polyspike-wave complexes at 2–4 Hz, of high voltage, bilateral, synchronous and symmetrical, isolated, and in sequence, evident in drowsiness

Table 24.1 Progressive myoclonic epilepsies: hereditary transmission and involved genes

Main forms	Transmission	Chromosome	Gene
Lafora disease	AR	6q24	EPM2A (laforin)
	AR	6p22	EMP2B (malin)
Unverricht-Lundborg disease	AR	21q22.3	EPM1 (cystatin B)
MERRF	Maternal	mt-DANN	tRNA $^{\text{Lys (8344, 8356, 8363, 8361)}}$ tRNA $^{\text{Phe (611)}}$
MERRF-MELAS	Maternal	mt-DANN	tRNA $^{\text{Leu (pos. 3243)}}$ ND5 $^{\text{(13042)}}$
Neuronal ceroidolipofuscinosis			
– Late infantile (Jansky-Bielschowsky)	AR	11p15.5	CLN2
– Juvenile (Spielmeyer-Vogt-Sjogren)	AR	16p	CLN3
Sialidosis			
– Type 1	AR	6p21.3	Neuraminidase
– Type 2	AR	6p21.3	Neuraminidase
– Galactosialidosis	AR	20q13.1	PPCA
Rare forms			
Dentatorubro-Pallido-Luysiana atrophy	AD	12p13.31	B 37 (athrophin)
Gangliosidosis GM2	AR	15q23-q24	HEXA
Gaucher disease type III	AR	1p21	Glucocerebrosidase
Hallervorden-Spatz disease	AR	20p13-p12.3	Pank-2
Juvenile Huntington's disease	AD	4p16.3	Huntingtin

AD autosomal dominant, *AR* autosomal recessive, *MERRF* myoclonus epilepsy with ragged-red fibers, *MELAS* mitochondrial encephalomyopathy, lactic acidosis, and stroke-like episodes the background activity becomes slower and disorganized, the physiological elements of sleep tend to disappear, while the epileptic anomalies become more active, with generalized or bi-frontal spike-wave and polyspike-wave complexes, almost constantly associated with focal epileptic anomalies, located mainly in the occipital regions. At this stage, myoclonia and negative myoclonus become increasingly frequent and can be well documented by suitable polygraphic recordings (Figs. 24.14 and 24.15). IPS evokes PPR, both interictal and ictal, often throughout the course of the disease (Fig. 24.16). As in the other forms of this group, the prognosis is unfavorable with progressive deterioration and death after 2–10 years from the onset of symptoms.

Unverricht-Lundborg disease is a rare progressive myoclonic epilepsy, found mainly in Mediterranean and Baltic countries (in Finland, estimated incidence of 1/20,000) [54]. It is an autosomal recessive disease, caused by mutations of the EPM1 gene for cystatin B. It starts, insidiously, in the second infancy or adolescence (in 86% of the cases between 9 and 13 years) with action myoclonus, characteristically more evident after the awakening, associated with clonic or clonic-tonic-clonic seizures during sleep. Myoclonus gradually becomes invalidating due to its severe interference on motor activity, especially in the execution of complex praxies. Generally in this phase there is also a cerebellar ataxia of variable entity. The disease progresses by alternating periods of remission, to periods of worsening with increased frequency of myoclonia and epileptic seizures. Gradually, a mild to moderate degree of cognitive impairment occurs. The EEG at onset shows a normal organization of the background activity which subsequently presents a modest slowing of the posterior alpha rhythm. Later on, sequences of delta activity appear which become progressively more and more evident. Spike-wave and polyspike-wave discharges are occasionally associated with massive myoclonia, whereas the action myoclonus is never accompanied by EEG anomalies. In 90% of patients, ILS evokes a PPR. With the progression of the disease, epileptic abnormalities tend to decrease, while the slowing and disorganization of the background activity become increasingly evident.

MERRF syndrome is a progressive myoclonic epilepsy with maternal transmission, due to a mutation in the tRNA of the mitochondrial lysine [55]. It begins in children or young adults, and the complete clinical picture includes myoclonic

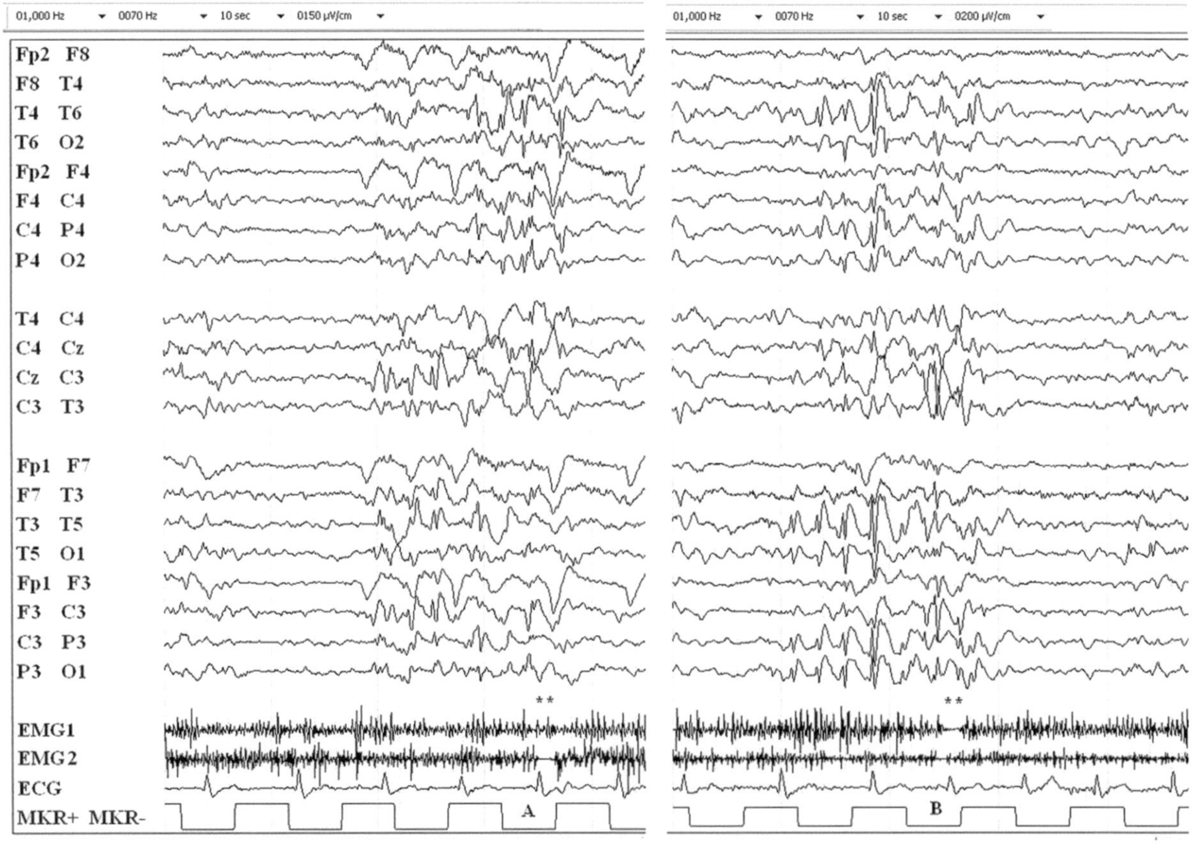

Fig. 24.14 Polygraphic EEG in wakefulness (*EMG 1* right deltoid muscle, *EMG 2* left deltoid muscle). Two episodes of negative myoclonus (**) evident during antigravity contraction of the arm muscles, both left (*A*) and right (*B*), associated with rapid spikes, polyspikes, and spike-wave complexes in frontocentral regions contralateral to the interested limb. Note the simultaneous presence of spikes and spike-wave complexes in the posterior regions, prevalent on the left (the patient reported short episodes of amaurosis and visual hallucinations)

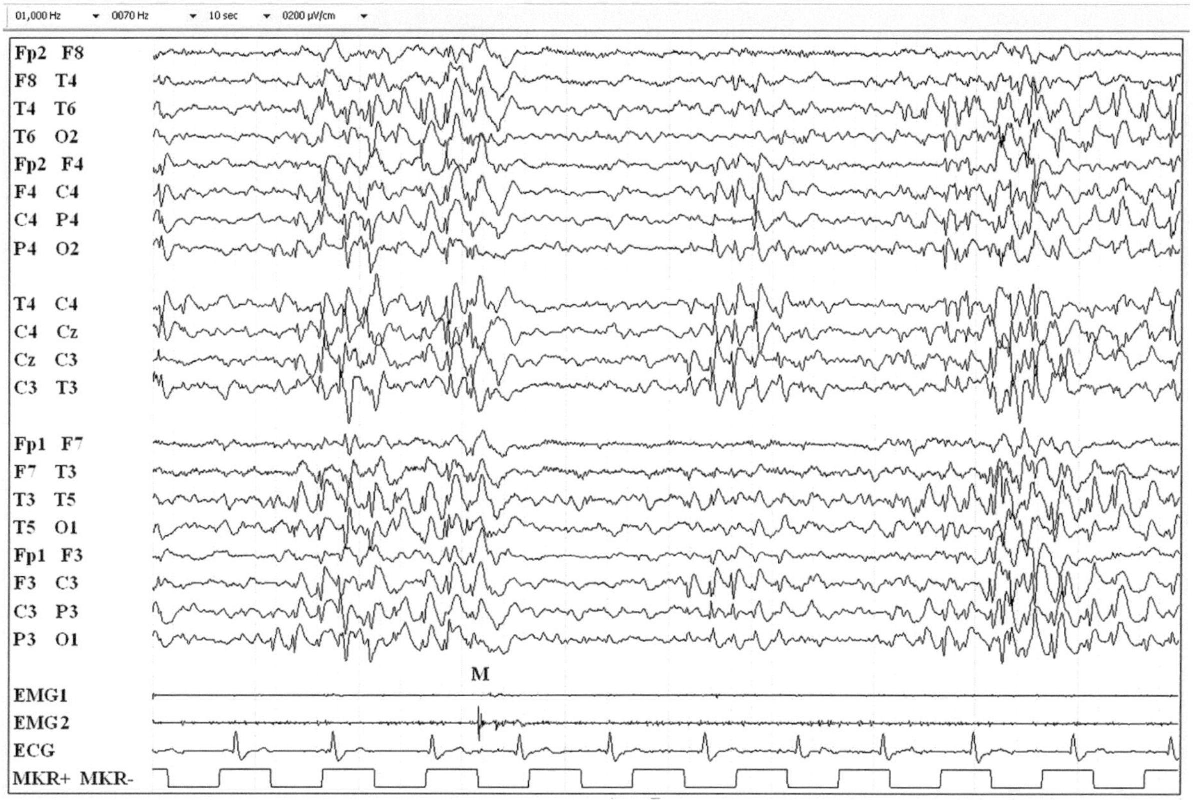

Fig. 24.15 Polygraphic EEG in wakefulness (*EMG 1* right deltoid muscle, *EMG 2* left deltoid muscle; same patient of Fig. 24.14). Isolated myoclonus (*M*) in the upper left limb, recorded under conditions of basic muscle relaxation

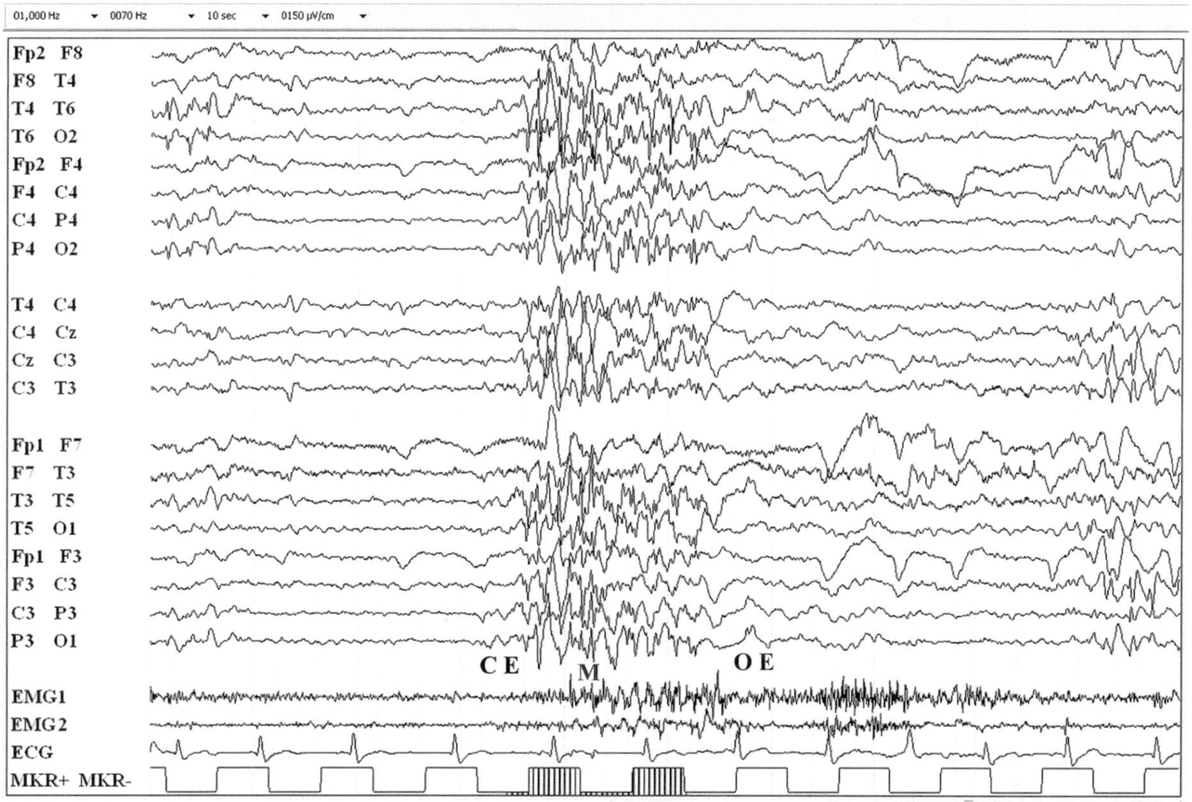

Fig. 24.16 Polygraphic EEG during ILS (*EMG 1* right deltoid muscle, *EMG 2* left deltoid muscle, *CE* closed eyes, *OE* open eyes, *M* myoclonus; same patient of Figs. 24.14 and 24.15). Photoparoxysmal response characterized by a generalized sequence of spikes, polyspikes, and spike-wave and polyspike-wave complexes, synchronous and symmetrical, associated with axial and limb myoclonia

seizures, ataxia, muscular hyposthenia, dysarthria, optic atrophy, nystagmus, short stature, gradual hearing loss, and progressive mental deterioration. Clinical findings and progression are very variable, and many patients can be asymptomatic even for a long time.

The *neuronal ceroid lipofuscinoses* represent the most common form of lysosomal disease in childhood. They are genetically heterogeneous multisystem diseases in which the malfunctioning of lysosomes causes a progressive storage of characteristic lipopigments [56]. Patients present drug-resistant myoclonic seizures, progressive retinopathy with consequent loss of visual function, cerebellar ataxia, cognitive and global deterioration, and premature death.

Sialidoses are lysosomal storage diseases with autosomal recessive inheritance. The overall incidence is estimated at 1/4,200,000 live births. There are three main forms: (a) *sialidosis type 1*, also known as "cherry-red spot syndrome and myoclonus," generally normomorphic; (b) *sialidosis type 2*, which includes also complex facial dysmorphias, bone dysplasias, and psychomotor retardation; (c) *gangliosidosis*. The onset is variable, generally between 5 and 25 years, with progressive difficulty in walking, loss of visual acuity, which initially prevails on the chromatic vision, night blindness, corneal opacity, and, in some cases, nystagmus. Progressive multifocal myoclonus usually starts in the second decade of life, associated with seizures and ataxia, especially in sialidosis [57].

24.7 Landau-Kleffner Syndrome

Originally described by Landau and Kleffner in 1957 [58] as "syndrome of acquired aphasia with convulsive disorder," Landau-Kleffner syndrome is characterized by a progressive language dysfunction (verbal and/or auditory agnosia) associated with epileptic seizures, although not constantly (70–80% of cases). The onset is from 3 to 8 years (mean age of onset 4.8 years) in children with previously normal psychomotor and language development [59, 60]. Language regression is generally gradual and subtle but in some patients may be sudden and rapid. Behavior disorders with attention deficit and/or hyperactivity may coexist [59]. In 70–80% of patients, seizures of different types occur: focal seizures, secondarily generalized tonic-clonic seizures, absences, or atonic seizures [59, 60]. The interictal awake EEG shows spikes, sharp waves, and spike-wave complexes located at temporal or temporo-occipital regions, often bilateral, symmetrical, or asymmetric (Fig. 24.17). Sometimes the anomalies may be

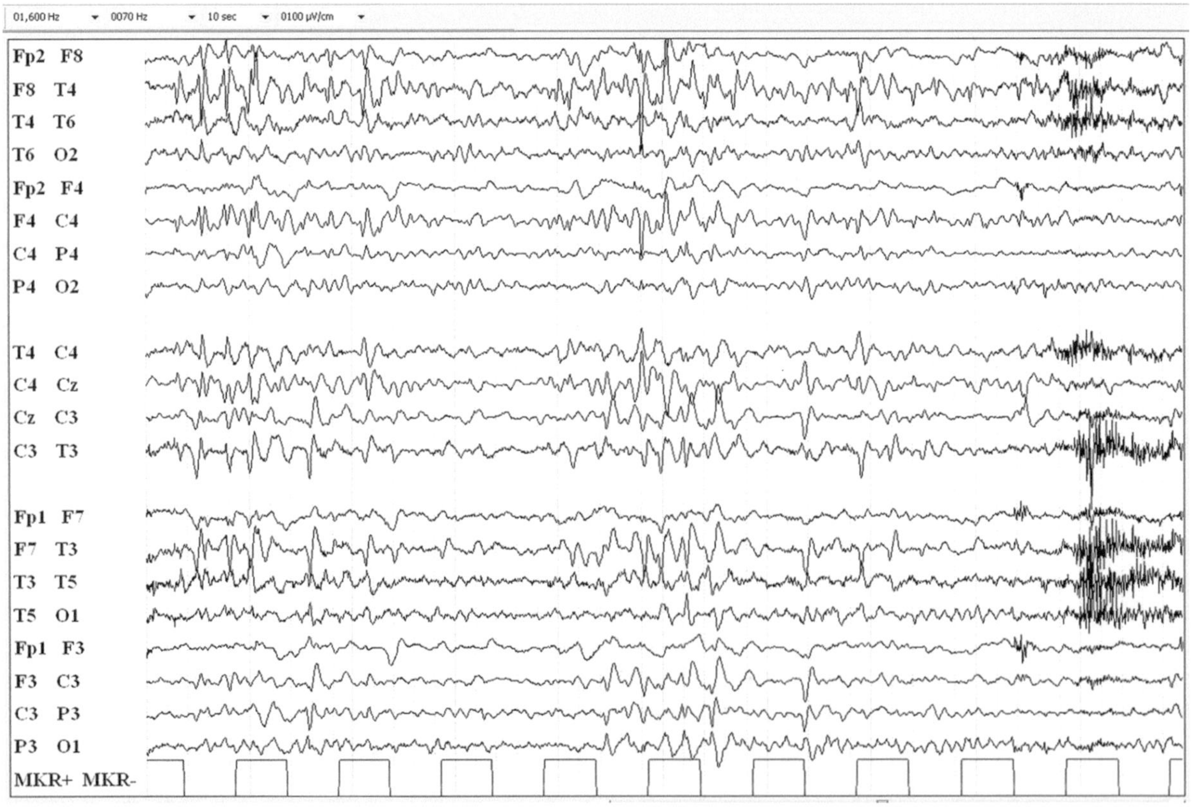

Fig. 24.17 Awake EEG. Spikes, sharp waves, and atypical spike-wave complexes dominant in the anterior temporal areas of both hemispheres

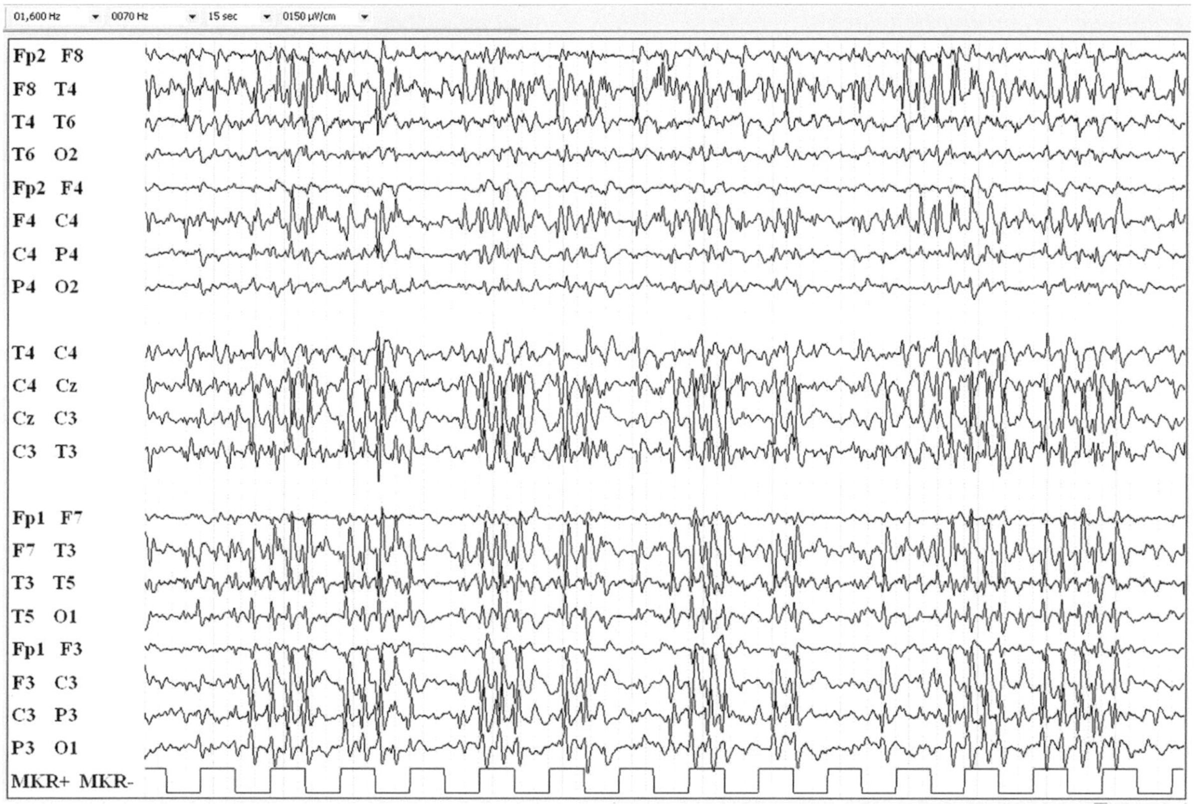

Fig. 24.18 EEG during non-REM sleep (same patient of Fig. 24.17). Sub-continuous spikes, sharp waves, and atypical spike-wave complexes at 3–5 Hz of high voltage on the anterior temporal regions of both hemispheres, with slight tendency to spread to the contiguous areas on the left

multifocal, but a clear prevalence in the temporal regions is always evident. The EEG becomes typical in sleep [59–61], due to the increase of epileptic anomalies, continuous or subcontinuous during non-REM sleep, clearly localized or dominant in temporal regions, with maximal amplitude in posterior temporal and/or parietal electrodes (Fig. 24.18). The ictal EEG has no peculiar features but correlates with seizure type. Background activity and sleep macro-architecture are usually normal. The prognosis of these patients is variable [62, 63]; seizures are generally controlled by therapy, and the EEG anomalies tend to resolve after some years, but this positive outcome of the epilepsy is not always associated with an equally favorable evolution of the language; usually, more or less serious language disorders persist even after the disappearance of the EEG anomalies [59–63].

24.8 Electrical Status Epilepticus During Slow Sleep

The main characteristic of this syndrome (electrical status epilepticus during slow sleep—ESES) is the strong activation of epileptic anomalies during non-REM sleep, with spike-wave complexes occurring for more than 85% of the duration of non-REM phases [64, 65]. This pattern tends to repeat every night for longer or shorter periods of time (months or years). No epidemiological data are available, but it is considered a rare condition (incidence of 0.5% on over 12,000 children studied over a 10-year period). Three types of clinical manifestations are associated with this EEG pattern:

– *Seizures of different type.* The age at onset varies from a few months to 12 years, with a peak around 4–5 years. Seizures may occur in children with normal psychomotor development as well as in those with signs of pre-existing brain damage. In about half of the patients, the first episode consists of a unilateral epileptic seizure during nighttime sleep. Ictal manifestations may be both focal and generalized, and about 60% of patients have multiple seizure types (clonic, tonic-clonic, focal motor, and/or with complex semiology), but there are never tonic seizures in sleep. At the beginning the seizure frequency is generally low, but it tends to increase when the typical EEG pattern arises. ESES generally occurs 1 or 2 years after the first seizure and is often associated with the appearance of other types of attacks (especially, atypical absences and drop attacks).

- *Deterioration of neuropsychological functions.* The appearance of the EEG pattern is accompanied by a progressive and often severe impairment of neuropsychological functions, with particular involvement of the language. Serial evaluations show a progressive reduction of the cognitive level both global and sectorial, with low scores especially in memory, attention, ability of orientation, and space-time organization. The functional profile is however variable from case to case, and behavioral disorders may appear with hyperactivity, aggressiveness, and psychotic manifestations.
- *Movement disorders.* The appearance of ESES interferes with the control of the motor action both at the cortical and cerebellar level (dyspraxia, dystonia, ataxia). Unilateral deficits, sometimes transient or fluctuating, and negative myoclonus may also occur.

  The EEG in wakefulness does not show any specific aspects before, during, and after the ESES phase; there may be both generalized and focal epileptic anomalies, with the latter being more often located in the anterior regions. Predictive signs of the imminent onset of an ESES are considered: (a) the appearance of 2–3 Hz spike-wave complexes in short generalized discharges, apparently subclinical, (b) a greater tendency to the diffusion of focal anomalies, and (c) increased seizure frequency and appearance of other types of attacks.

  The EEG during sleep typically presents continuous or sub-continuous epileptic activity (spike-wave index between 85 and 100%) during all non-REM phases. The anomalies are characterized by high-voltage synchronous and symmetrical spike-wave complexes, diffuse, often dominant in the anterior regions (Fig. 24.19). Although the anomalies are widespread, in many patients there is a clear prevalence in some areas, with consequent changes in the clinical picture: anomalies prevalent in the temporal regions of one or both hemispheres involve a greater interference on the language, while those dominant in the frontal regions are more frequently associated with the development of psychosis, especially in the autistic spectrum.

  The ESES abruptly disappears during the REM phases; short discharges of diffuse spike-wave complexes or focal anomalies, mainly frontal, may persist. The cyclic alternating pattern of the non-REM and REM phases is discreetly conserved, but the microstructural organization and architecture of sleep are globally altered, which might have further adverse effects on cognitive function [64–66]. The presence of an ESES may be suspected by short

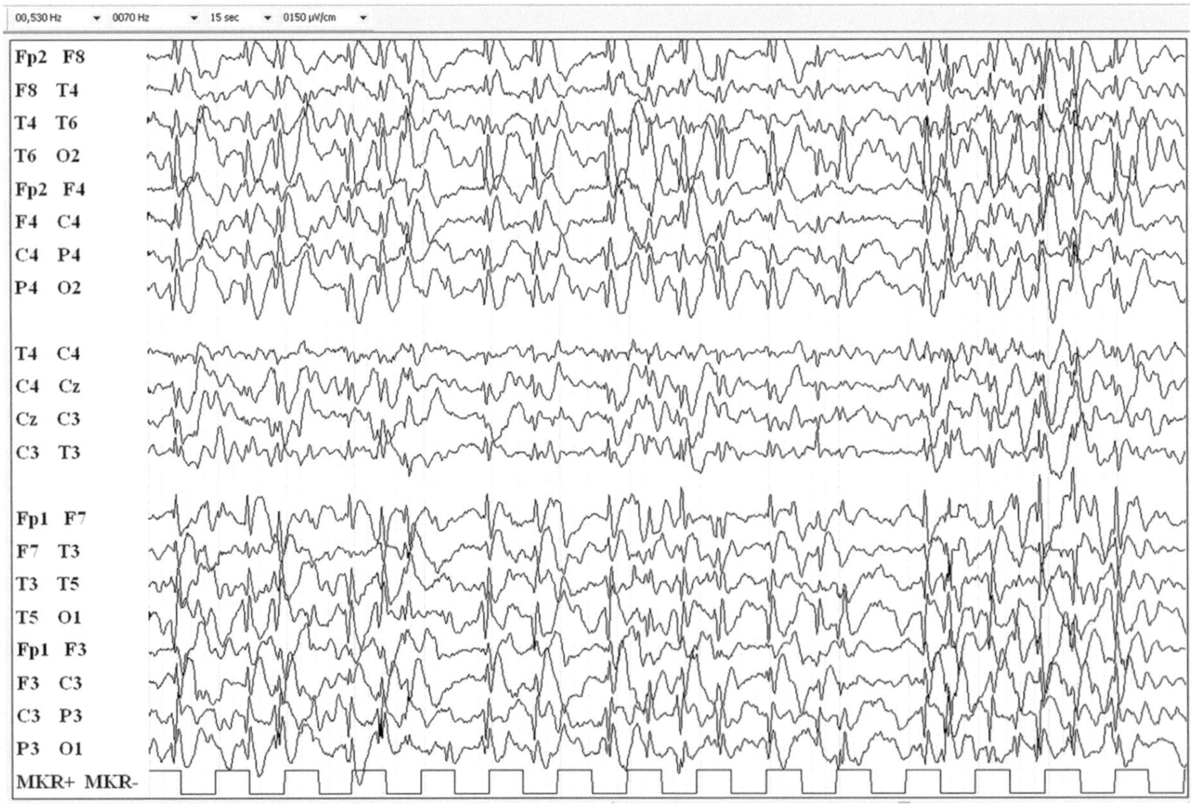

Fig. 24.19 EEG during non-REM sleep. Sub-continuous generalized 2–4 Hz spike-wave complexes of high voltage

EEG during sleep, but nocturnal sleep recording is generally essential to confirm the diagnosis and to better outline the prognosis. Although the long-term outcome of seizures and ESES is generally favorable, greater cautiousness must be placed in assessing the overall prognosis in individual patient. Indeed, the remission of ESES is generally associated with improvement of cognitive function, attention, language, and behavior, but in about half of the cases, serious neuropsychological and/or motor deficits may persist.

References

1. Berg AT, Berkovic SF, Brodie MJ, Buchhalter J, Cross H, van Emde Boas W, et al. Revised terminology and concepts for organization of seizures and epilepsies: report of the ILAE Commission on Classification and Terminology, 2005–2009. Epilepsia. 2010;51:676–85.
2. Engel J. A proposed diagnostic scheme for people with epileptic seizures and with epilepsy: report of the ILAE task force on classification and terminology. Epilepsia. 2001;42:796–803.
3. Dulac O. Epileptic encephalopathy. Epilepsia. 2001;42(Suppl 3):23–6.
4. Capovilla G, Wolf P, Beccaria F, Avanzini G. The history of the concept of epileptic encephalopathy. Epilepsia. 2013;54(Suppl 8):2–5.
5. Michaud JL, Lachance M, Hamdan FF, Carmant L, Lortie A, Diadori P, et al. The genetic landscape of infantile spasms. Hum Mol Genet. 2014;23(18):4846–58.
6. Epi4K Consortium; Epilepsy Phenome/Genome Project, et al. De novo mutations in epileptic encephalopathies. Nature. 2013;501(7466):217–21.
7. Sidenvall R, Eeg-Olofsson O. Epidemiology of infantile spasms in Sweden. Epilepsia. 1995;36:572–4.
8. Ludvigsson P, Olafsson E, Siguroardottir S, Hauser WA. Epidemiologic features of infantile spasms in Iceland. Epilepsia. 1994;35:802–5.
9. Trevathan E, Murphy CC, Yeargin-Allsopp M. The descriptive epidemiology of infantile spasms among Atlanta children. Epilepsia. 1999;40:748–51.
10. Lee WL, Ong HT. Epidemiology of West syndrome in Singapore. Brain and Development. 2001;23(7):584–5.
11. Ohtahara S, Yamatogi Y. Epileptic encephalopathies in early infancy with suppression-burst. J Clin Neurophysiol. 2003;20:398–407.
12. Ohtahara S, Yamatogi Y. Ohtahara syndrome: with special reference to its developmental aspects for differentiating from early myoclonic encephalopathy. Epilepsy Res. 2006;70(Suppl 1):S58–67.
13. Wirrell EC, Shellhaas RA, Joshi C, Keator C, Kumar S, Mitchell WG. Pediatric Epilepsy Research Consortium. How should children with West syndrome be efficiently and accurately investigated? Results from the National Infantile Spasms Consortium. Epilepsia. 2015;56(4):617–25.
14. West WJ. On a peculiar form of infantile convulsions. Lancet. 1841;1:724–5.
15. Guzzetta F, Dalla Bernardina B, Guerrini R. Progress in epileptic spasms and West syndrome. 1st ed. Montrouge: John Libbey Eurotext; 2007.
16. Lee YJ, Berg AT, Nordli DR Jr. Clinical spectrum of epileptic spasms in children. Brain and Development. 2015;37(1):37–48.
17. Lux AL, Osborne JP. A proposal for case definitions and outcome measures in studies of infantile spasms and West syndrome: consensus statement of the West Delphi group. Epilepsia. 2004;45(11):1416–28.
18. De Menezes MA, Rho JM. Clinical and electrographic features of epileptic spasms persisting beyond the second year of life. Epilepsia. 2002;43(6):623–30.
19. Xue J, Qian P, Li H, Yang H, Liu X, Zhang Y, et al. Atonic elements combined or uncombined with epileptic spasms in infantile spasms. Clin Neurophysiol. 2017;128(1):220–6.
20. Caraballo RH, Fortini S, Reyes G, Carpio Ruiz A, Sanchez Fuentes SV, Ramos B. Epileptic spasms in clusters and associated syndromes other than West syndrome: a study of 48 patients. Epilepsy Res. 2016;123:29–35.
21. Hrachovy RA, Frost JD Jr. Infantile spasms. Handb Clin Neurol. 2013;111:611–8.
22. Kobayashi K, Inoue T, Kikumoto K, Endoh F, Miya K, Oka M, et al. Relation of spasms and myoclonus to suppression-burst on EEG in epileptic encephalopathy in early infancy. Neuropediatrics. 2007;38(5):244–50.
23. Riikonen R. Long-term outcome of patients with West syndrome. Brain and Development. 2001;23:683–7.
24. Lux AL, Osborne JP. The influence of etiology upon ictal semiology, treatment decisions and long-term outcomes in infantile spasms and West syndrome. Epilepsy Res. 2006;70S:S77–86.
25. Dravet C. Les epilepsies graves de l'enfant. Vie Med. 1978;8:543–8.
26. Hurst DL. Epidemiology of severe myoclonic epilepsy of infancy. Epilepsia. 1990;31(4):397–400.
27. Yakoub M, Dulac O, Jambaqué I, Chiron C, Plouin P. Early diagnosis of severe myoclonic epilepsy in infancy. Brain and Development. 1992;14(5):299–303.
28. Marini C, Scheffer IE, Nabbout R, Suls A, De Jonghe P, Zara F, et al. The genetics of Dravet syndrome. Epilepsia. 2011;52(Suppl 2):24–9.
29. Dravet C. The core Dravet syndrome phenotype. Epilepsia. 2011;5(Suppl 2):3–9.
30. Dalla Bernardina B, Capovilla G, Chiamenti C, Trevisan E, Colamaria V, Fontana E. Cryptogenic myoclonic epilepsies of infancy and early childhood: nosological and prognostic approach. In: Wolf P, Dam M, Janz D, Dreifuss FE, editors. Advances in epileptology, vol. 16. New York: Raven Press; 1987. p. 175–80.
31. Dravet C, Bureau M, Oguni H, Fukuyama Y, Cokar O. Severe myoclonic epilepsy in infancy (Dravet syndrome). In: Roger J, Bureau M, Dravet C, Genton P, Tassinari CA, Wolf P, editors. Epileptic syndromes in infancy, childhood and adolescence. 4th ed. London: John Libbey Eurotext Ltd; 2005. p. 89–113.
32. Oguni H, Hayashi K, Awaya Y, Fukuyama Y, Osawa M. Severe myoclonic epilepsy in infants—a review based on the Tokyo Women's medical university series of 84 cases. Brain and Development. 2001;23:736–48.
33. Ragona F, Brazzo D, De Giorgi I, Morbi M, Freri E, Teutonico F, et al. Dravet syndrome: early clinical manifestations and cognitive outcome in 37 Italian patients. Brain and Development. 2010;32:71–7.
34. Dalla Bernardina B, Capovilla G, Gattoni MB. Epilepsie myoclonique grave de la première année. Rev EEG Neurophysiol. 1982;12:21–5.
35. Ohki T, Watanabe K, Negoro K, Aso K, Haga Y, Kasai K, et al. Severe myoclonic epilepsy in infancy: evolution of seizures. Seizure. 1997;6:219–24.
36. Bureau M, Dalla Bernardina B. Electroencephalographic characteristics of Dravet syndrome. Epilepsia. 2011;52(Suppl 2):13–23.
37. Dravet C, Bureau M, Guerrini R, Giraud N, Roger J. Severe myoclonic epilepsy in infants. In: Roger J, Bureau M, Dravet C, Dreifuss FE, Perret A, Wolf AP, editors. Epileptic syndromes in

infancy, childhood and adolescence. 2nd ed. London: John Libbey Eurotext Ltd; 1992. p. 75–88.
38. Arzimanoglou A, French J, Blume WT, Cross JH, Ernst JP, Feucht M, et al. Lennox-Gastaut syndrome: a consensus approach on diagnosis, assessment, management, and trial methodology. Lancet Neurol. 2009;8(1):82–93.
39. Markand ON. Lennox-Gastaut syndrome (childhood epileptic encephalopathy). J Clin Neurophysiol. 2003;20(6):426–41.
40. Camfield PR. Definition and natural history of Lennox-Gastaut syndrome. Epilepsia. 2011;52(Suppl 5):3–9.
41. Trevathan E, Murphy CC, Yeargin-Allsopp M. Prevalence and descriptive epidemiology of Lennox-Gastaut syndrome among Atlanta children. Epilepsia. 1997;38:1283–8.
42. Bourgeois BF, Douglass LM, Sankar R. Lennox-Gastaut syndrome: a consensus approach to differential diagnosis. Epilepsia. 2014;55(Suppl 4):4–9.
43. Ferlazzo E, Nikanorova M, Italiano D, Bureau M, Dravet C, Calarese T, et al. Lennox-Gastaut syndrome in adulthood: clinical and EEG features. Epilepsy Res. 2010;89(2–3):271–7.
44. Kerr M, Kluger G, Philip S. Evolution and management of Lennox-Gastaut syndrome through adolescence and into adulthood: are seizures always the primary issue? Epileptic Disord. 2011;13(Suppl 1):S15–26.
45. Doose H. Myoclonic-astatic epilepsy. Epilepsy Res Suppl. 1992;6:163–8.
46. Guerrini R, Aicardi J. Epileptic encephalopathies with myoclonic seizures in infants and children (severe myoclonic epilepsy and myoclonic-astatic epilepsy). J Clin Neurophysiol. 2003;20(6):449–61.
47. Kilaru S, Bergqvist AGC. Current treatment of myoclonic astatic epilepsy: clinical experience at the Children's Hospital of Philadelphia. Epilepsia. 2007;48(9):1703–7.
48. Oguni H, Fukuyama Y, Tanaka T, Hayashi K, Funatsuka M, Sakauchi M, et al. Myoclonic-astatic epilepsy of early childhood—clinical and EEG analysis of myoclonic-astatic seizures, and discussions on the nosology of the syndrome. Brain and Development. 2001;23(7):757–64.
49. Chan EM, Andrade DM, Franceschetti S, Minassian B. Progressive myoclonus epilepsies: EPM1, EPM2A, EPM2B. Adv Neurol. 2005;95:47–57.
50. Shahwan A, Farrell M, Delanty N. Progressive myoclonic epilepsies: a review of genetic and therapeutic aspects. Lancet Neurol. 2005;4(4):239–48.
51. Girard JM, Turnbull J, Ramachandran N, Minassian BA. Progressive myoclonus epilepsy. Handb Clin Neurol. 2013;113:1731–6.
52. Franceschetti S, Michelucci R, Canafoglia L, Striano P, Gambardella A, Magaudda A, et al. Collaborative LICE study group on PMEs. Progressive myoclonic epilepsies: definitive and still undetermined causes. Neurology. 2014;82(5):405–11.
53. Franceschetti S, Gambardella A, Canafoglia L, Striano P, Lohi H, Gennaro E, et al. Clinical and genetic findings in 26 Italian patients with Lafora disease. Epilepsia. 2006;47(3):640–3.
54. Hyppönen J, Äikiä M, Joensuu T, Julkunen P, Danner N, Koskenkorva P, et al. Refining the phenotype of Unverricht-Lundborg disease (EPM1): a population-wide Finnish study. Neurology. 2015;84(15):1529–36.
55. Bindoff LA, Engelsen BA. Mitochondrial diseases and epilepsy. Epilepsia. 2012;53(Suppl 4):92–7.
56. Nita DA, Mole SE, Minassian BA. Neuronal ceroid lipofuscinoses. Epileptic Disord. 2016;18(Suppl 2):73–88.
57. Franceschetti S, Canafoglia L. Sialidoses. Epileptic Disord. 2016;18(Suppl 2):89–93.
58. Landau WM, Kleffner FR. Syndrome of acquired aphasia with convulsive disorder in children. Neurology. 1957;7:523–30.
59. Caraballo RH, Cejas N, Chamorro N, Kaltenmeier MC, Fortini S, Soprano AM. Landau-Kleffner syndrome: a study of 29 patients. Seizure. 2014;23(2):98–104.
60. Stefanatos G. Changing perspectives on Landau-Kleffner syndrome. Clin Neuropsychol. 2011;25(6):963–88.
61. Massa R, de Saint-Martin A, Hirsch E, Marescaux C, Motte J, Seegmuller C, et al. Landau–Kleffner syndrome: sleep EEG characteristics at onset. Clin Neurophysiol. 2000;111(Suppl 2):S87–93.
62. Robinson RO, Baird G, Robinson G, Simonoff E. Landau–Kleffner syndrome: course and correlates with outcome. Dev Med Child Neurol. 2001;43:243–7.
63. Rotenberg J, Pearl PL. Landau–Kleffner syndrome. Arch Neurol. 2003;60:1019–21.
64. Scheltens-de Boer M. Guidelines for EEG in encephalopathy related to ESES/CSWS in children. Epilepsia. 2009;50(Suppl 7):13–7.
65. Tassinari CA, Rubboli G, Volpi L, Meletti S, d'Orsi G, Franca M, et al. Encephalopathy with electrical status epilepticus during slow sleep or ESES syndrome including the acquired aplasia. Clin Neurophysiol. 2000;111(Suppl 2):S94–S102.
66. Scholtes FB, Hendriks MP, Renier WO. Cognitive deterioration and electrical status epilepticus during slow sleep. Epilepsy Behav. 2005;6:167–73.

25 Focal "Idiopathic" Epilepsies of Infancy

Elena Gardella and Gaetano Cantalupo

25.1 Introduction

Under the old term of focal "idiopathic" epilepsies of infancy are comprised a group of epilepsy conditions characterized by *focal (or localization-related)-onset seizures* and a relatively "benign" course. These conditions account for about the 20% of children with nonfebrile seizures.

The term "idiopathic epilepsy" means that epilepsy is not subtended by a detectable structural brain abnormality and probably is due to a genetically determined propensity to a certain type of seizures, EEG abnormalities, and evolution. Furthermore the term "idiopathic," from the Greek word "idios" ("self" or "proper"), points to the fact that epilepsy is not a manifestation of another disease, but it represents the disease in itself. In fact, this group of epilepsies arose in children without any other neurological or cognitive impairment, seizures are likely to be controlled with appropriate antiepileptic therapy (or even do not need drug treatment), and the seizure propensity is ultimately self-limited, since they are expected to have a spontaneous and definitive remission before adulthood. After the seizure onset, the neuropsychological development of these children is usually normal, but may present a transient or even long-lasting impairment. Therefore, the term "benign," often used in connection with this group of epilepsy syndromes, is not considered appropriate any longer and has been recently replaced by the term "self-limited" (ILAE Commission for Classification and Terminology [1]).

Three electro-clinical syndromes recognized by the International League Against Epilepsy (ILAE) (1989) [2] are Rolandic epilepsy (RE), Early-Onset Epilepsy with Occipital Paroxysms (Panayiotopoulos Syndrome) and Late-Onset Childhood Epilepsy with Occipital Paroxysms (Gastaut Type). Within each entity, although focal, seizures and EEG abnormalities usually affect asynchronously homologous regions in both hemispheres, thus leading to quite homogeneous and reproducible clinical and EEG features. This suggests that seizure propensity does not involve a single focus but primarily involves a particular system (e.g., the autonomic system in Panayiotopoulos syndrome or the sensorimotor system in Rolandic epilepsy); thus the term "system epilepsies" was proposed to unify all "idiopathic" epilepsies [3]. All those entities have been considered part of a spectrum of an age-related genetically determined focal "seizure susceptibility syndrome" (Panayiotopoulos et al. 2008).

Part of this spectrum are also some less frequent epilepsies with specific inter-ictal focal EEG patterns (e.g., with vertex spikes-and-waves during sleep or with giant somatosensory evoked spikes) or nonfebrile self-limiting seizure conditions, not requiring a diagnosis of epilepsy (benign familial and non-familial infantile seizures).

25.2 Rolandic Epilepsy (or Benign Childhood Epilepsy with Centrotemporal Spikes)

Rolandic epilepsy (RE), or self-limited epilepsy with centrotemporal spikes, formerly also called benign childhood epilepsy with centrotemporal spikes (BECTS), is the most common non-lesional focal epilepsy of childhood, accounting for about the 15% of nonfebrile focal epilepsies in otherwise normal children. The epilepsy onset peaks at the range of age 7–10 years.

Seizures typically are focal motor and occur from sleep, presenting with orofacial motor signs, specifically tonic or

E. Gardella (✉)
Department of Clinical Neurophysiology, Danish Epilepsy Centre - Filadelfia, Dianalund, Denmark

University of Southern Denmark, Odense, Denmark
e-mail: elga@filadelfia.dk

G. Cantalupo
Child Neuropsychiatry, University of Verona, Verona, Italy

O. Mecarelli (ed.), *Clinical Electroencephalography*, https://doi.org/10.1007/978-3-030-04573-9_25

clonic contractions of one side of the face, mainly involving the oropharyngeal muscles, with guttural sounds, drooling (sialorrhea), swallowing, and in some cases speech arrest (anarthria). Somatosensory symptoms are also frequent, if the children are specifically asked, mainly consisting of unilateral paresthesia of the tongue, lips, gums, and inner cheek [4–7]. The lower limb is affected only in 8% of children, and in a minority of cases, postictal dysarthria, Todd's paresis, or exceptionally hemiplegia may persist for a few minutes [6, 8]. Other seizure types, with associated autonomic, motor, and visual manifestations, have been described [8].

Less frequently generalized tonic-clonic seizures are observed, particularly in younger children [8].

The seizure frequency is generally low, with half having fewer than five attacks in their life [5].

Some degrees of stable or intermittent neuropsychological deficits are quite common and may be related to the marked accentuation of the interictal epileptic abnormalities during sleep, which in very few children may lead to an atypical evolution consisting with encephalopathy with status epilepticus during sleep (ESES/CSWS see below).

25.2.1 Interictal EEG

The EEG background is well organized both during wakefulness and sleep.

The interictal epileptiform abnormalities have a characteristic morphology and topography. They are slow, dysphasic, and high-voltage spikes (100–300 μV), often followed by a slow wave; in some cases, the centrotemporal spikes can be of small voltage (Fig. 25.1a). They may be sporadic or occur in clusters and may be unilateral or bilateral and synchronous or asynchronous in the centrotemporal (Rolandic) regions. Their maximal amplitude is halfway between the central (C3/C4) and the mid-temporal (T3/T4) electrodes (Fig. 25.1a, b), corresponding to the lower central electrodes (C5/C6), in case of a montage with supplementary EEG derivations [9].

The orientation of the dipole of the spikes is perpendicular to the cortex within the Rolandic fissure (sagittal dipole) with anterior positivity (Fig. 25.1b). Integrated localization techniques (high-resolution EEG, MEG, source analysis, and fMRI) localize the generator of the Rolandic spikes in the lower part of the sensorimotor cortex, revealing two dis-

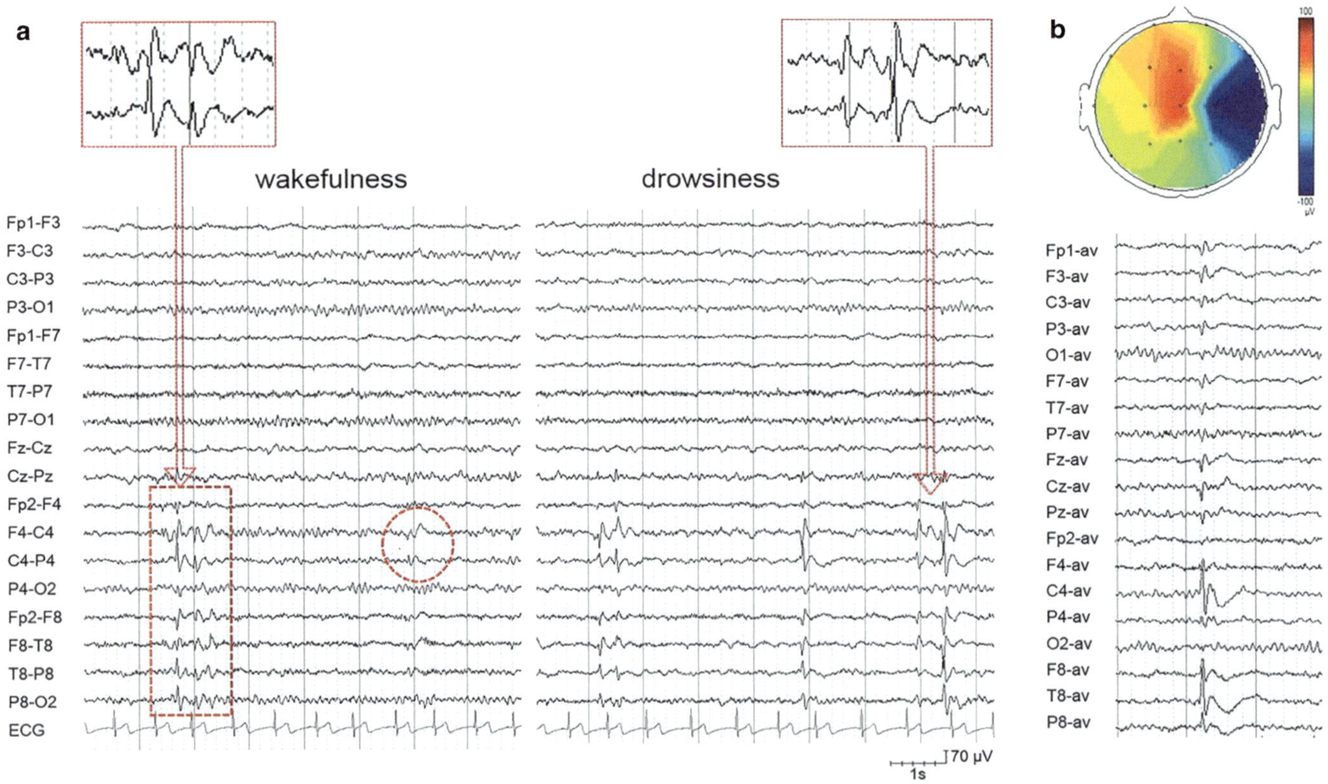

Fig. 25.1 Interictal EEG during wakefulness and drowsiness in a patient with Rolandic epilepsy. The characteristic slow, dysphasic spike-and-slow wave complexes show maximum in the centrotemporal (Rolandic) regions (maximal amplitudes C4 and T8). (**a**) The typical high-voltage spikes alternate sometimes to some small-voltage ones (circle). The spikes become more frequent during drowsiness, when a discrete focal rhythmic slow activity can also appear. (**b**) The map of amplitude corresponding to the negative peak of the spike shows the maximum of negativity in the mid-temporal regions with anterior positivity (sagittal dipole) *(EEG band-pass filter 1–70 Hz)*

tinct sources, one in the postcentral and the other in the precentral cortex [10].

The presence of a very fast EEG component (ripples) on top of the Rolandic spikes predicts a worst clinical outcome and need of a chronic pharmacologic treatment [11]. Focal rhythmic slow activity is occasionally observed in the region epileptic focus (Figs. 25.1 and 25.3).

The centrotemporal spikes are not affected by eye opening/closure, hyperventilation (HV), or photic stimulation (PS) but can be evoked or suppressed by protrusion of the tongue [12, 13].

Spikes in other areas and multifocal spikes can be seen from the first EEG recording or during evolution [4] (Fig. 25.2). The presence of multifocal spikes does not seem to correlate with the seizures frequency or semiology.

During drowsiness and NREM sleep is observed an accentuation of the epileptiform abnormalities, without changes in the morphology (Fig. 25.3). Sleep may also activate independent centrotemporal spikes over the other hemisphere or generalized spike-wave discharges that would argue against a structural cause. Sleep recording in these

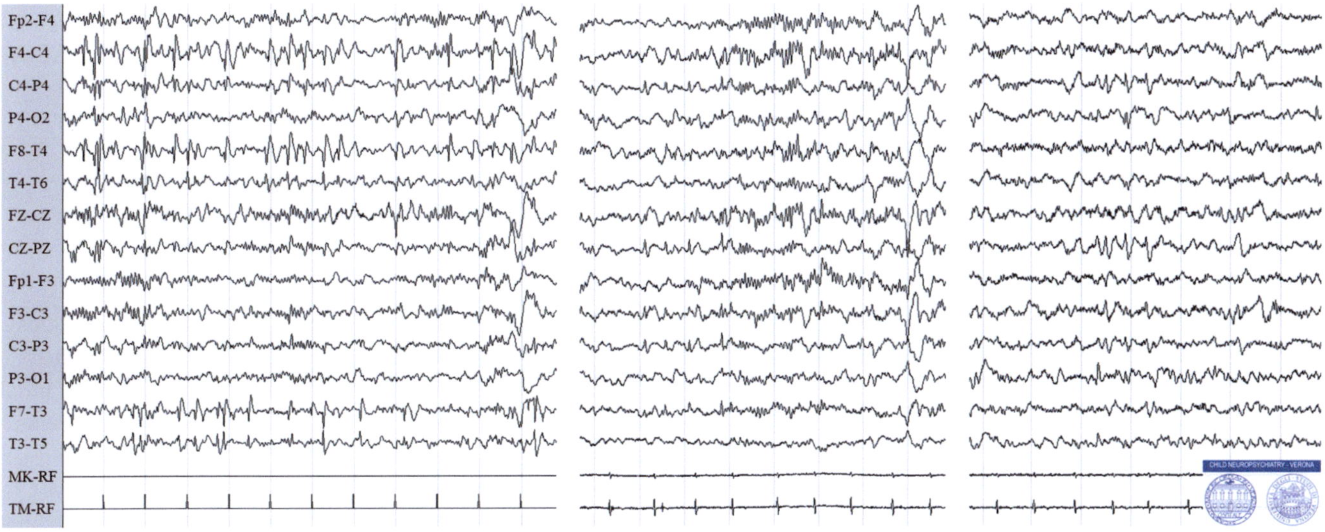

Fig. 25.2 Left panel: during sleep, stage N2, frequent and high-amplitude focal spike-and-waves, asynchronous on centrotemporal region of both hemispheres, can be observed in a patient with Rolandic epilepsy during the active phase (by age 7 years). In the middle and right panel, two EEGs from the same patient, during N2 sleep, at 9 and 10 years old, respectively (during the initial remission phase), in which small focal spikes or spike-and-waves are evident on central and vertex region. Please note that in the right panel, the spike component became longer in duration ("slow spikes" or "sharp waves") but with the same topographical distribution

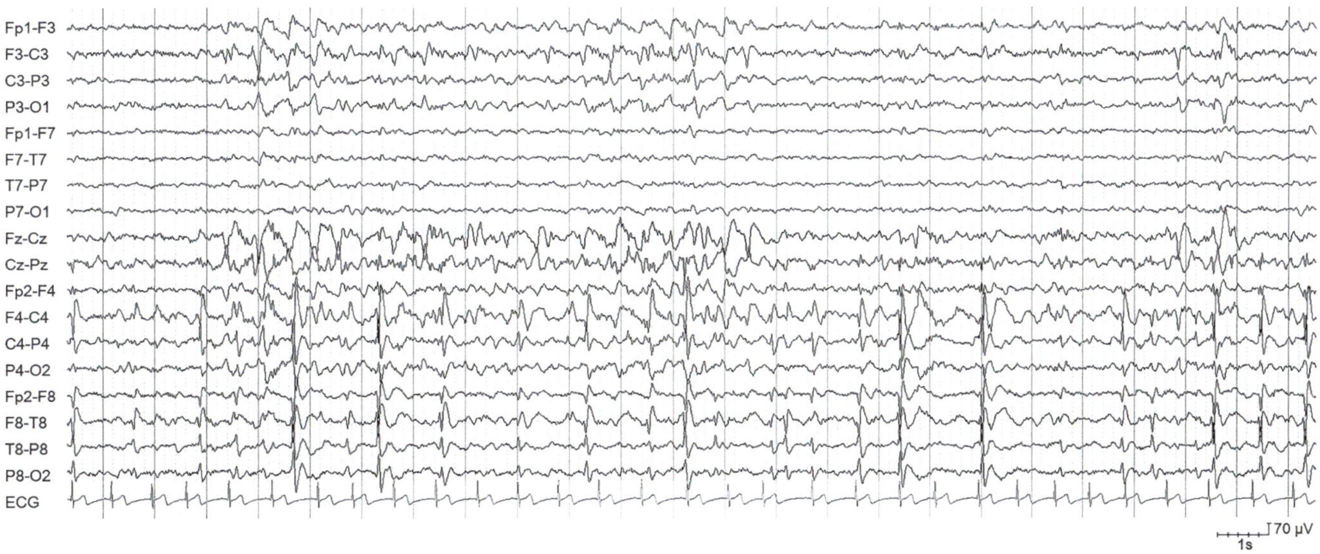

Fig. 25.3 Interictal EEG during sleep in a child with Rolandic epilepsy (same patient as in Fig. 25.1), where the right centrotemporal spikes and the intermixed rhythmic slow activity are accentuated. During N2 sleep some centrotemporal spikes and focal slow activity appear also in the left hemisphere, synchronously and asynchronously *(EEG band-pass filter 1–70 Hz)*

children is therefore highly recommended because typical EEG findings may only be seen during sleep [14].

Generalized spike-wave discharges are rare during wakefulness and do not occur during sleep, but are not infrequent during drowsiness [4, 8].

There is no correlation between amount of the interictal spikes and the frequency or severity of the seizures. Anyway, atypical EEG features (spike morphology or location, abnormal background, etc.) have been associated with a higher percentage of learning and behavioral disabilities [15]. The EEG renormalization occurs usually later than clinical remission [16].

25.2.2 Ictal EEG

Given the low seizure frequency and their preferential nocturnal occurrence, ictal EEG recordings are rare.

The ictal EEG pattern is generally characterized by fast rhythms in the Rolandic regions, contralateral to the motor manifestations, progressively increasing in amplitude and evolving to a spike- or polyspike-and-slow wave pattern (Fig. 25.4) with or in most cases without diffuse spreading and secondary generalization [17]. In the late part of a seizure, the ictal spikes show a maximum of positivity at the mid-temporal EEG derivations. That means, a reversal of the interictal dipole is observed, which has maximum negativity in the central and medial-temporal derivations [18].

25.2.3 Atypical Evolution

In a few patients with RE, a severe neuropsychological impairment may occur and become persistent for years. This is an age-related condition, associated with a peculiar EEG pattern, characterized by the striking activation of epileptic abnormalities during non-REM sleep, which may became almost continuous during NREM sleep. This condition is known as encephalopathy with status epilepticus during slow sleep (ESES) [19] or with continuous spike and waves during sleep (CSWS) (see [20], for a review).

Different patterns of EEG distribution have been described (diffuse, hemispheric, focal) (for a review, see [21]) (Fig. 25.5). The reasons why some children develop this EEG pattern are still not understood. In some cases, certain antiepileptic drugs seemed to be responsible [22]. The remission is spontaneous before puberty, but the cognitive recovery is not always complete [23].

25.3 Early-Onset Epilepsy with Occipital Paroxysms (Panayiotopoulos Syndrome)

The "early-onset" variant of the childhood occipital epilepsy, also called Panayiotopoulos syndrome (COE-PS), has a prevalence of about 5% in children with an afebrile focal seizure. The peak age of onset is 3–6 years, and the spontaneous remission is up to 3 years.

Seizures are infrequent; only a few children report to have had more than ten seizures in total. COE-PS seizures are usually prolonged (average duration 5–90 min) and sleep related, about 70% occurring out of sleep and 13% upon awakening [24].

The hallmark of the COE-PS is the prolonged autonomic seizures (nausea, retching and vomiting, pallor/flushing, pupillary dilatation, and hypersalivation) with emesis (70–

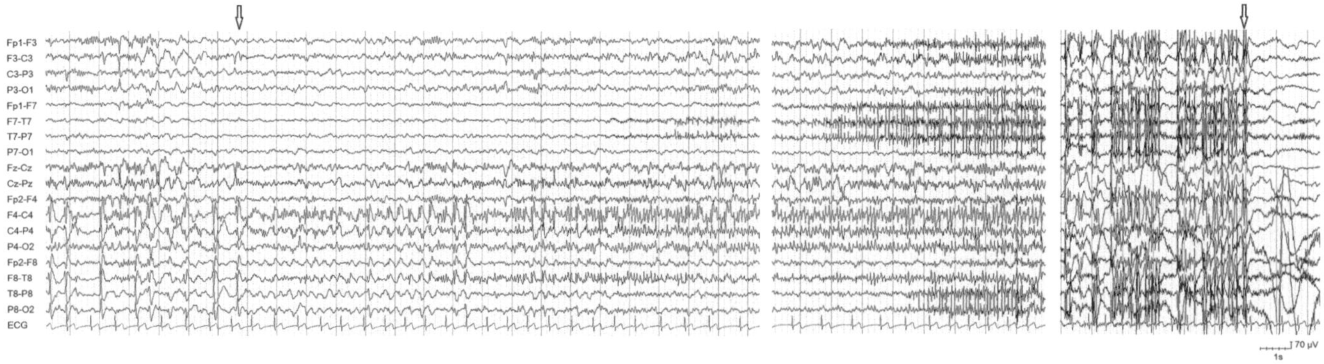

Fig. 25.4 Rolandic epilepsy. EEG recordings of a focal seizure with onset during sleep, characterized by myoclonia around the mouth and in the left part of the face, arousal and anartria. The duration of the seizure is 1 min and 2 s. On the EEG, the seizure starts with an arrest of the interictal epileptiform abnormalities consisting of trains of high-amplitude Rolandic spikes (left arrow) and with the appearance of a rhythmic 12–14 Hz activity on the right centro-frontotemporal regions, progressively increasing in amplitude with intermixed spike-and-slow waves. The right arrow indicates the seizure end *(EEG band-pass filter 1–70 Hz)*

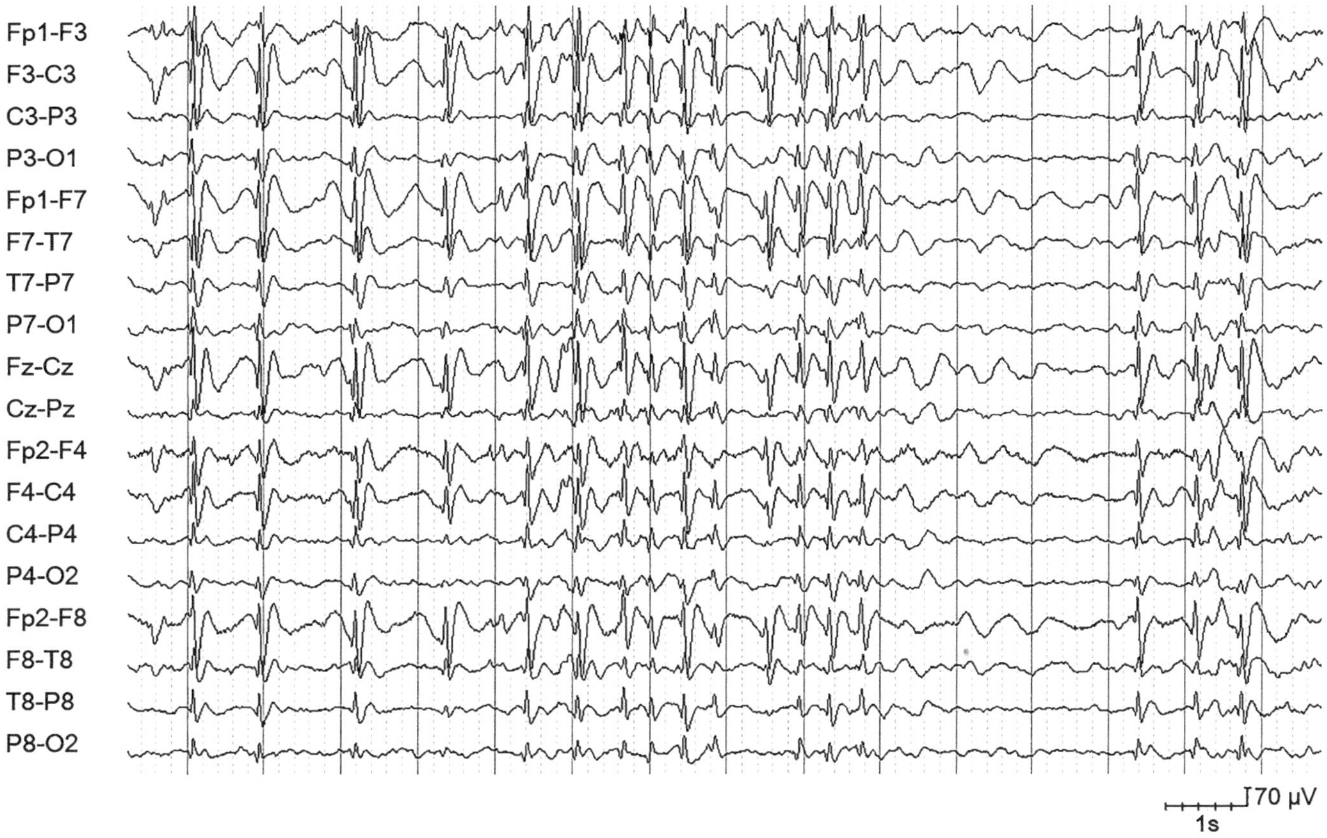

Fig. 25.5 Girl with Rolandic epilepsy, aged 9 years and 3 months, having had a few focal clonic seizures during sleep with onset at the age of 6 years and 9 months. Previous EEG showed infrequent epileptiform abnormalities in the Rolandic regions. She developed cognitive stagnation/regression from the age of 7.5 years. Twenty-four hours EEG recordings show almost continuous diffuse spike-and-slow waves (frontal predominance) during NREM sleep, consistent with the diagnosis of ESES/CSWS *(EEG band-pass filter 1.6–70 Hz)*

80%), up to autonomic status epilepticus. Impairment of consciousness and motor manifestations (deviation of the eyes, hemi-clonic or tonic-clonic manifestations) can also occur. Visual symptoms are very rare.

Many children also present syncope-like seizures characterized by sudden loss of consciousness and flaccidity [25].

25.3.1 Interictal EEG

The first routine EEG is normal in 66–85% of children [26]. The EEG background is generally normal also at follow-up but can show focal or diffuse slowing postictally.

Interictal EEG abnormalities show a great variability, ranging from completely normal EEG (21%) to focal spikes (any site) or even brief generalized discharges. The most common localization is in the occipital regions (Fig. 25.6a); anyway, "apparently" extra-occipital spikes are the only interictal abnormalities in about a third of cases, shifting from side to side and from one region to another in the same patient. However, it is important to note that apparently frontal spikes represent actually a fast spread of occipital spikes toward anterior regions (Fig. 25.7), as demonstrated by computer-aided analysis (Leal phenomenon [27]).

High-voltage and diffuse (Fig. 25.8a) or multifocal sharp-slow-wave complexes are seen in up to 90% of children at some point in their follow-up, particularly in drowsiness or sleep. Repetitive small-voltage spikes or sharp-wave discharges ("clone-like") are also present.

The epileptiform abnormalities are inhibited by eye opening in a minority of cases (Fig. 25.6a), can be induced by photic stimulation (Fig. 25.6b), and are typically markedly activated during sleep or only occur in sleep (Fig. 25.8b). The sensitivity of the sleep EEG ranges from 80 to 100%; therefore sleep EEG recording is considered mandatory [26, 28].

The frequency and location of the spike-wave discharges do not correlate with the severity of the clinical manifestations and prognosis. The EEG normalization

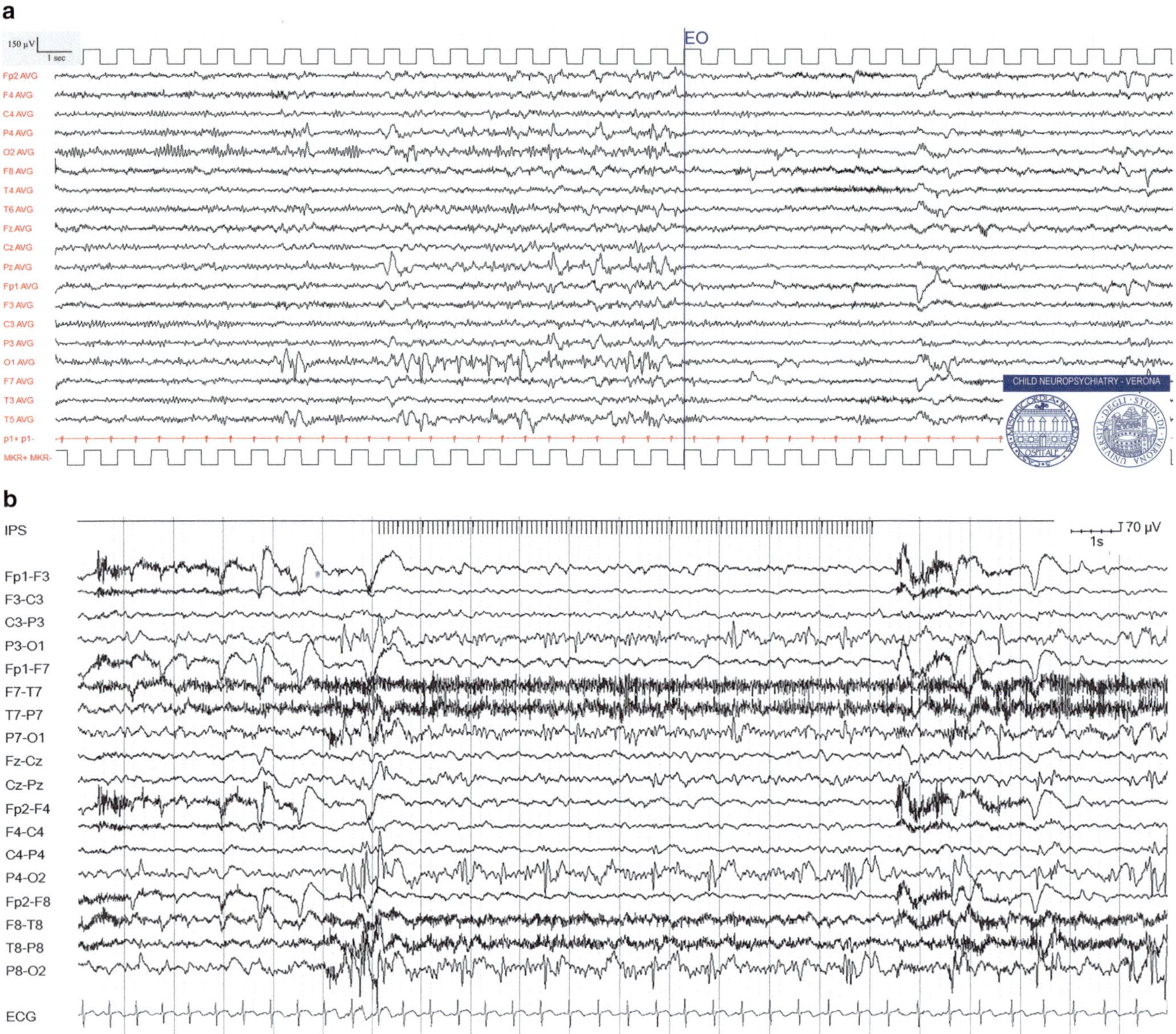

Fig. 25.6 (**a**) Typical focal posterior spike-and-waves (in this case more evident on the left occipital channels) in a case of focal idiopathic occipital epilepsy, inhibited by eye opening (EO) (**b**) In another patient, with eye closure sensitivity, the intermittent photic stimulation induces an occipital photoparyoxysmal response

can occur up to 7 years after clinical remission [29], and often interictal EEG abnormalities only disappear by adolescence.

25.3.2 Ictal EEG

Seizures are typically sleep related, and the ictal EEG onset can occur several minutes prior to the clinical onset [24, 30].

The seizure-onset zone is variable, either in a wide posterior region or in the frontotemporal regions, usually consisting of rhythmic theta waves, intermixed by small spikes and spike-and-slow waves, followed by a fast rhythm spreading to both hemispheres.

25.3.3 Atypical Evolution

As in the case of RE, in a minority of patients with COE-PS, an atypical evolution to encephalopathy with status epilepticus during sleep (ESES/CSWS) can occur, with impairment of cognitive and/or motor function.

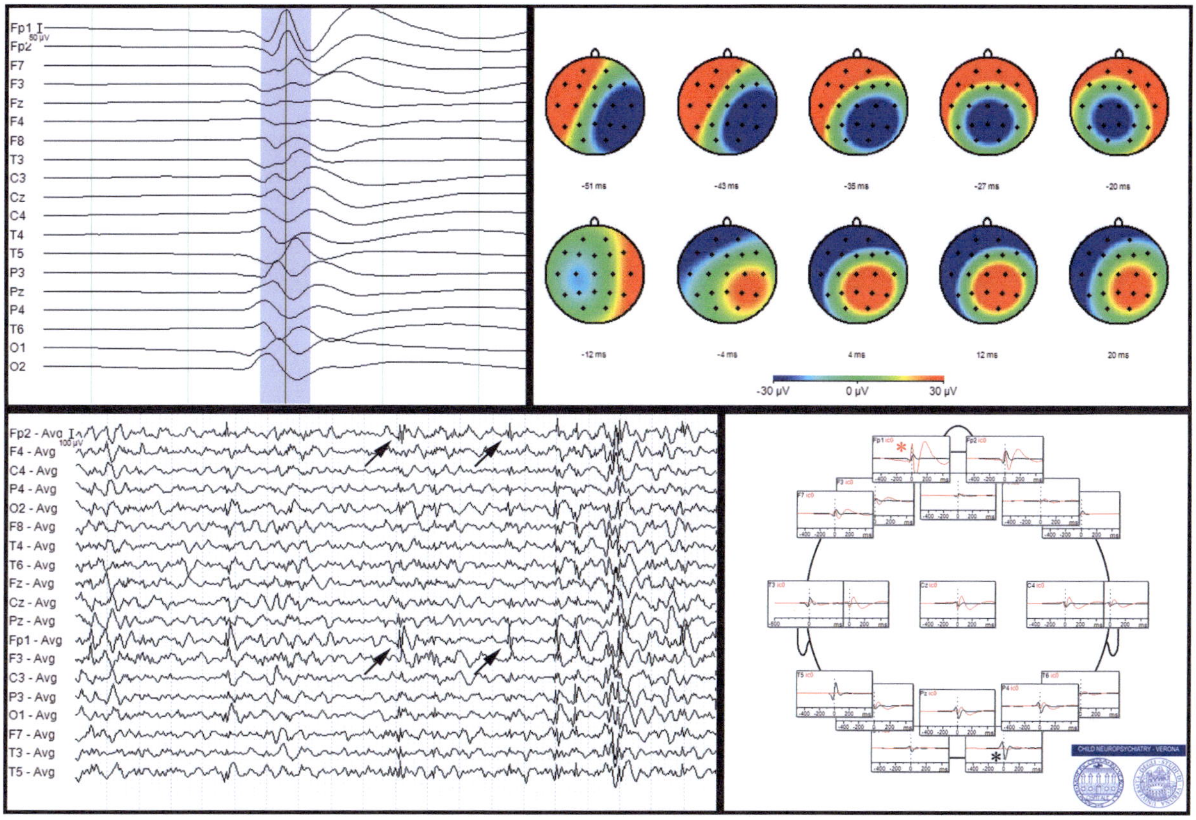

Fig. 25.7 Diffuse spike-and-wave during sleep in a patient with COE-PS. In this case the paroxysmal abnormalities are of higher amplitude and more evident on frontopolar channels (arrows), erroneously suggesting a frontal origin, representing instead a propagation of posterior abnormalities, as demonstrated by Leal et al. [27]. Actually, spike-averaging—centered on the frontopolar peak of the spike—demonstrates a negative transient on right posterior channels constantly preceding by 30 ms (peak-to-peak) the anterior one (upper line, left panel; blue-shaded area extends from −50 ms to 50 ms around 0). On the right—upper line—ten consecutive scalp voltage maps at 8 ms intervals showing the evolution from −51 ms to 20 ms across 0 line. In the lower right panel, the two principal components of the spike-and-wave complex, computed by independent component analysis (ICA) decomposition (Makeig et al. 1996), are overlaid, the red one representing the frontopolar component peaking at time 0 on Fp1 (red asterisk), while the black one is the earlier posterior component (black asterisk)

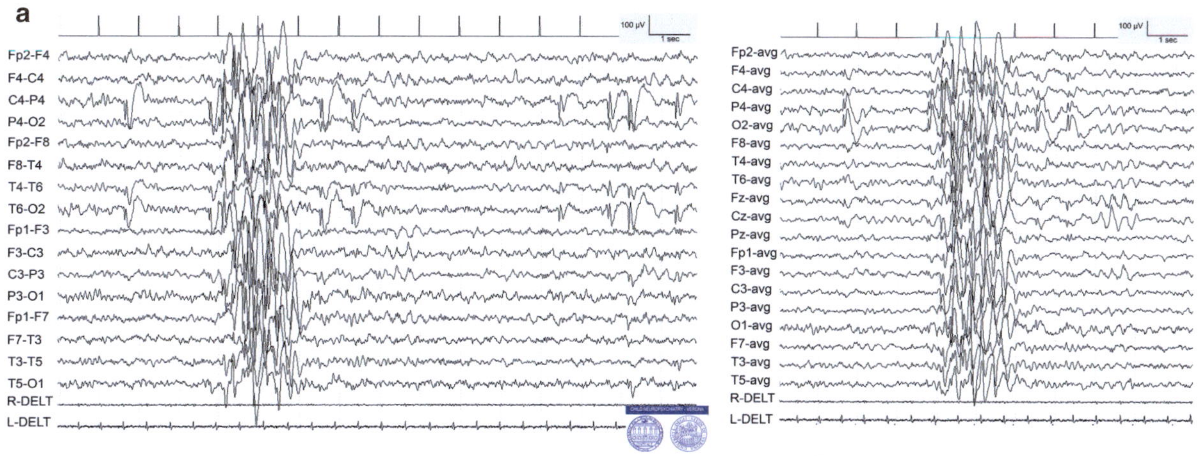

Fig. 25.8 (**a**) Drowsiness and sleep EEG findings in patients with COE-PS (same patient ads in Fig. 25.6b), showing frequent, high-amplitude 2–3 Hz spike/sharp-and-slow-wave complexes (SW) in the posterior quadrants, isolated or in short trains. The SW appears on eye closing (EC) (left panel) and is accentuated during NREM sleep (right panel) *(EEG band-pass filter 1–70 Hz, notch filter 50 Hz)*. (**b**) Typical focal posterior SW in a case of focal idiopathic occipital epilepsy (same patient ads in Fig. 25.6a). In this case, paroxysmal abnormalities are more evident on the right occipital channels, isolated or in brief sequences, sometimes organized in discharges with bilateral diffusion, constituting brief bouffées (bursts) of diffuse irregular SW complexes. Please note the different shape of the abnormalities in bipolar (left panel) and monopolar (right panel) montages

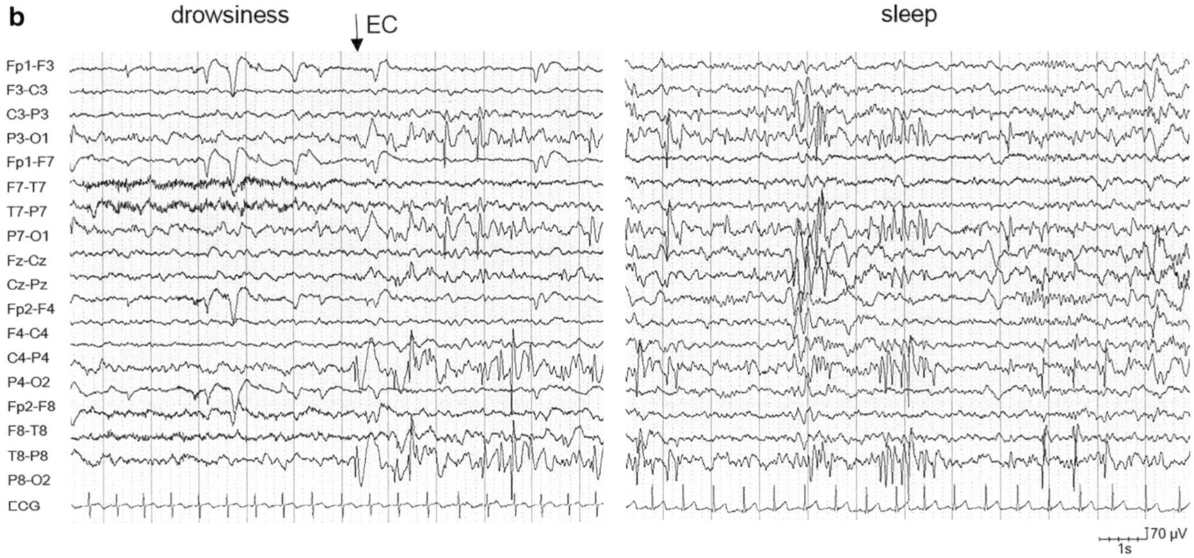

Fig. 25.8 (continued)

25.4 Late-Onset Childhood Epilepsy with Occipital Paroxysms (Gastaut Type)

The childhood occipital epilepsy of Gastaut (COE-G) is a purely occipital and probably genetic epilepsy syndrome, including the idiopathic photosensitive occipital lobe epilepsy, as a less common form with uncertain prognosis [31].

The peak age of onset is 7–8 years, and the clinical course is considered benign, although full epilepsy remission is lower than for RE and for COE-PS [32].

Most seizures occur during wakefulness, and their duration might be up to 15 min, though typically brief (<2 min). Seizure starts with visual symptoms (mainly simple hallucinations), followed by eye and head deviation and hemiconvulsions in 34–45% of case, sometimes alternating sides [33, 34]. Infrequently (11–15% of cases), visual aura can be followed by temporal lobe symptoms [34, 35].

The ictal symptoms of the occipital lobe seizures in COE-G are grossly similar to those in occipital epilepsies of structural origin. Therefore, recognizing the typical EEG pattern and ictal semiology of COE-G is important for their differential diagnosis.

In a minority of children, at any time during epilepsy course, may also occur absences associated with 3-Hz generalized spike-and-slow waves (<15%) or Rolandic seizures (<6%) [33, 36].

25.4.1 Interictal EEG

The background activity is normal. The interictal EEG abnormalities consist of high-amplitude occipital spikes, not associated with focal background slowing, occurring either as a single potential or in long rhythmic clusters with a peak of negativity on O1–O2.

In up to 60% of the children with COE-G, occipital spikes are bilateral synchronous and asynchronous [33], suggesting a diffuse occipital hyper-excitability (Fig. 25.9).

The epileptiform abnormalities are accentuated by eye closure and by drowsiness (Fig. 25.9) and sleep (Fig. 25.10). Fixation-off sensitivity is present in more than 90% of children with COE-G [34].

In about 24–38% of COE-G patients have been also reported centrotemporal spikes and brief bursts of generalized spike-and-slow waves [33, 34], more irregular than those observed in idiopathic generalized epilepsies.

Photosensitivity occurs in 11–15% [33, 34] of children (Fig. 25.9). The effect of sleep can result both in an accentuation of the epileptiform activity (Fig. 25.10), which in some children appears only during drowsiness and light sleep, and less frequently in an attenuation of the abnormalities. In addition, the centrotemporal spikes and generalized spike-waves occur typically during sleep [34].

Hyperventilation has no significant effect on the focal epileptiform abnormalities but can facilitate the occurrence of generalized spike-wave discharges.

Conversely, in structural occipital lobe epilepsy, the occipital spikes are often unilateral and are associated with focal background slowing [37, 38]; photosensitivity and fixation-off sensitivity are not expected.

25.4.2 Ictal EEG

In children with COE-G, the seizures occur typically during sleep and might be very prolonged. Typically, the ictal dis-

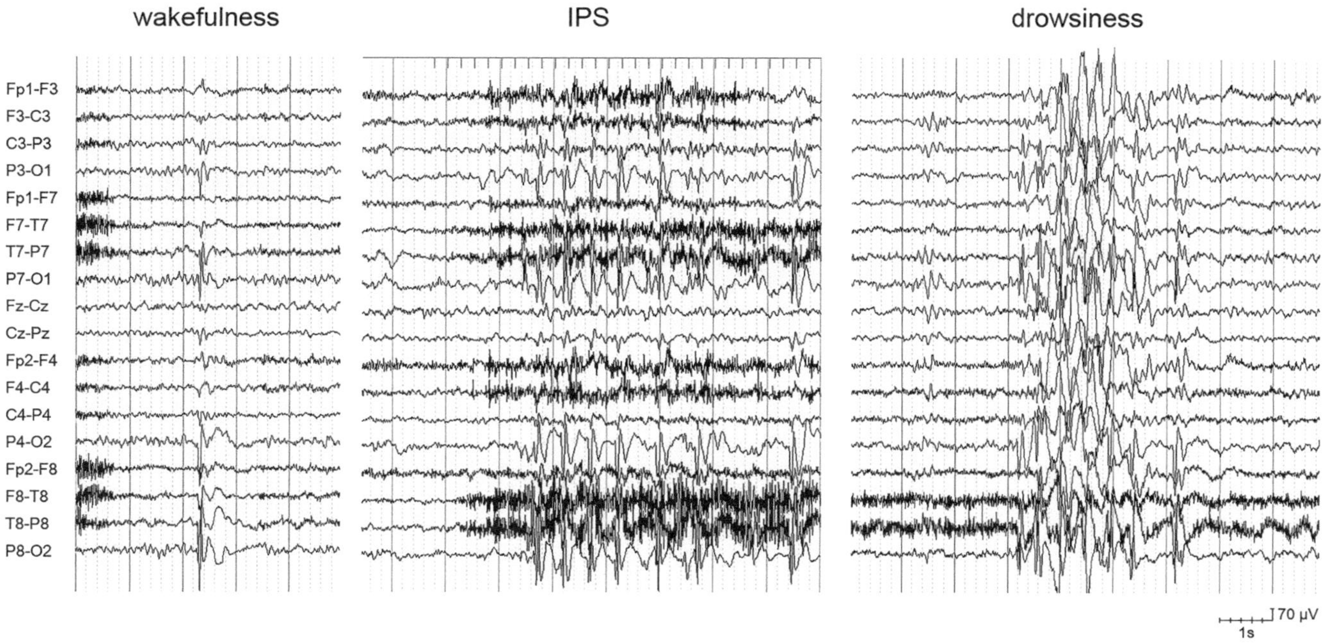

Fig. 25.9 In a patient with childhood occipital epilepsy of Gastaut (COE-G), the EEG during wakefulness showed isolated high-amplitude spike/sharp-and-slow-wave complexes (SW). The intermittent photic stimulation (IPS) induces an occipital photoparyoxysmal response, limited to the stimulus train. During drowsiness brief bursts of diffuse irregular SW complexes appeared, as observed in RE and COE-PS *(EEG band-pass filter 1–70 Hz)*

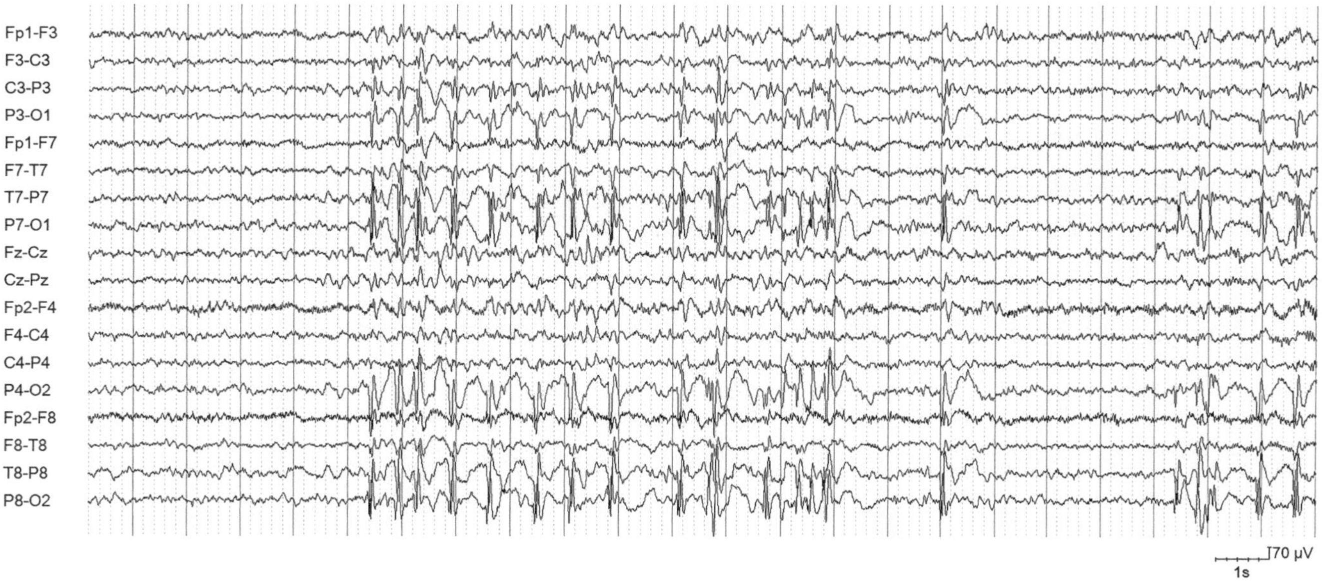

Fig. 25.10 Marked accentuation of the epileptiform abnormalities in the occipito-parieto-post-temporal regions in patients with COE-G (same patient ads in Fig. 25.9). The spike-and-slow-wave complexes appear isolated or in short trains *(EEG band-pass filter 1–70 Hz)*

charge consists of rhythmical fast spikes limited in the occipital lobe of one of both sides. The amplitude of the ictal occipital spikes is usually smaller than the one of the interictal occipital spikes (Fig. 25.11) [34]. In COE-G the pattern of EEG propagation is slow and suprasylvian, leading to hemiconvulsions.

In contrast, structural occipital lobe epilepsy frequently has a fast ictal propagation to the supplementary motor areas

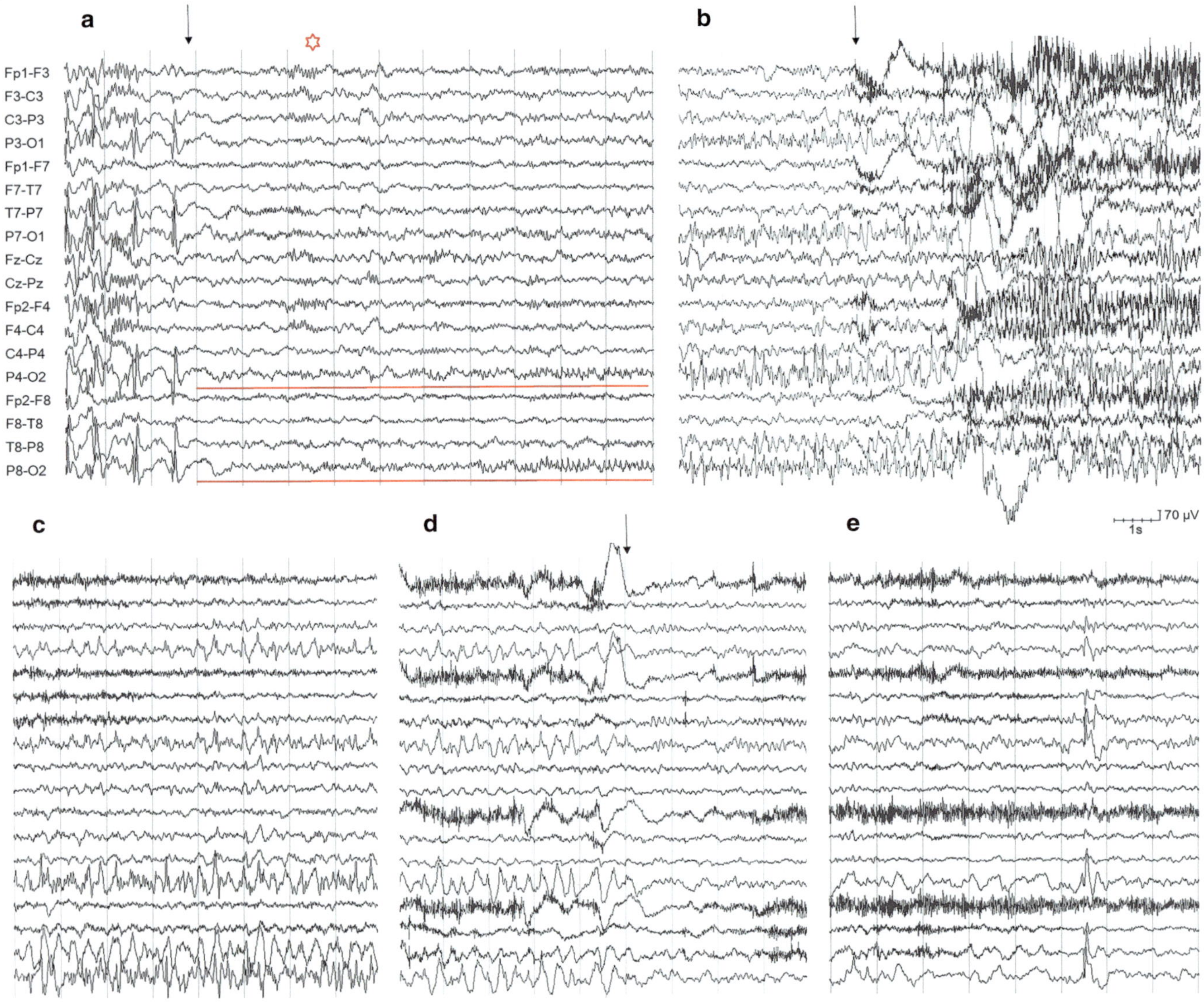

Fig. 25.11 A typical focal seizure in a patient with COE-G. (**a**) The seizure occurs out of N2 sleep, where there were very frequent, high-voltage 1 Hz spike-and-slow-wave complexes (SW) bilaterally in the posterior regions (occipital predominance). At seizure onset (arrow), the interictal epileptiform abnormalities stop abruptly, and a rhythmic low-voltage activity appears in the right occipito-post-temporal regions. Notably, in the anterior regions, the spindles are physiologically represented during the first part of the seizure (star). In this phase no evident clinical manifestations are observed. (**b**) The focal epileptiform discharge is gradually increasing in amplitude and spreading to the contralateral occipito-post-temporal regions. After 1 min and 22 s from seizure onset (arrow), the child wakes up crying and saying that he can't see; the eyes are deviated to the left. The amplitude of the ictal occipital spikes is smaller than the one of the interictal occipital spikes (see panels **a** and **e**). (**c**, **d**) The propagation of the ictal discharge remains confined to the occipito-post-temporal regions (right side prevalence). Fear, crying, and blindness still persist. A theta-delta component of increasing amplitude becomes more and more evident, intermixed to the focal rhythmic spikes. The seizure abruptly stops after 8 min and 9 s (arrow, panel **d**). (**e**) A postictal EEG slowing in the right posterior quadrant (max occipital: see P4-O_2/P8-O_2) is evident; a few minutes after seizure ends, the interictal SW appears in the posterior quadrants bilaterally (max in the right occipital region). The child experiences a gradual recovery of vision *(EEG band-pass filter 1–70 Hz)*

or an infra-sylvian propagation, mimicking temporal lobe seizures [35, 37, 38].

25.5 Other "Minor" Localization-Related Self-Limited Genetic Epilepsies

Other less defined and probably rare self-limiting epilepsy condition, described in otherwise normal children, are the "benign focal epilepsy with extreme somatosensory evoked potential" (ESEP) and the "benign infantile focal epilepsy with midline spikes and waves during sleep" (BIMSE).

The benign focal epilepsy with ESEP was described by de Marco and Tassinari in 1981 [39].

Initially, patients show only high-voltage ESEP elicited from the tapping on the feet, on an otherwise normal EEG. With variable delay, spontaneous interictal spikes

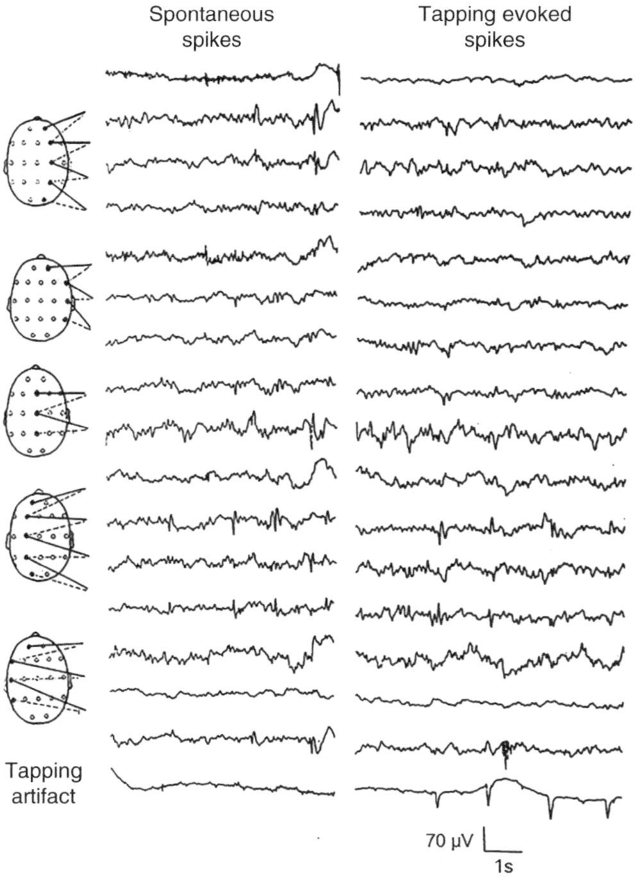

Fig. 25.12 Patients with ESEP showing spontaneous high-voltage spikes in the right centro-parietal and left centro-frontal and midline regions, asynchronously (left panel), and high-voltage spikes in the left centro-parietal elicited from the tapping on the right feet (right panel) *(Courtesy of Dr. Guido Rubboli)*

appear in the parietal and midline regions (same regions as ESEP), initially only during sleep (Fig. 25.12).

After 5 months to 2 years from the appearance of the spontaneous spikes, these patients have a few focal motor seizures (versive type), usually in clusters, mainly during wakefulness. Seizures might evolve to a generalized tonic-clonic phase or to status epilepticus and remit spontaneously after circa 1 year from their onset. ESEP and EEG abnormalities usually persist for several years. Accordingly with the idea of a spectrum, ESEP can be found also in patients with RE and BIMSE.

BIMSE was described by Capovilla and colleagues in 2000. The frequency of this condition is unknown, probably rare. The age of onset peaks between 16 and 20 months. All children have favorable outcomes, and the majority of them do not need to be chronically treated.

Seizure is sporadic, sometimes in clusters, and occurs mainly while awake. They are characterized by cyanosis, staring, and rare automatisms or lateralizing motor signs (duration 1–5 min).

The typical EEG pattern consists of spike followed by a bell-shaped slow-wave, localized in the mid-frontal regions, only present during sleep (Fig. 25.13) [40].

25.6 Non-familial and Familial Benign Infantile Seizures (Watanabe-Vigevano Syndrome)

Non-familial and familial benign infantile seizures (BIS/BFIS) represent a benign age-related idiopathic condition with focal seizures during early infancy, in otherwise normal infants [41, 42].

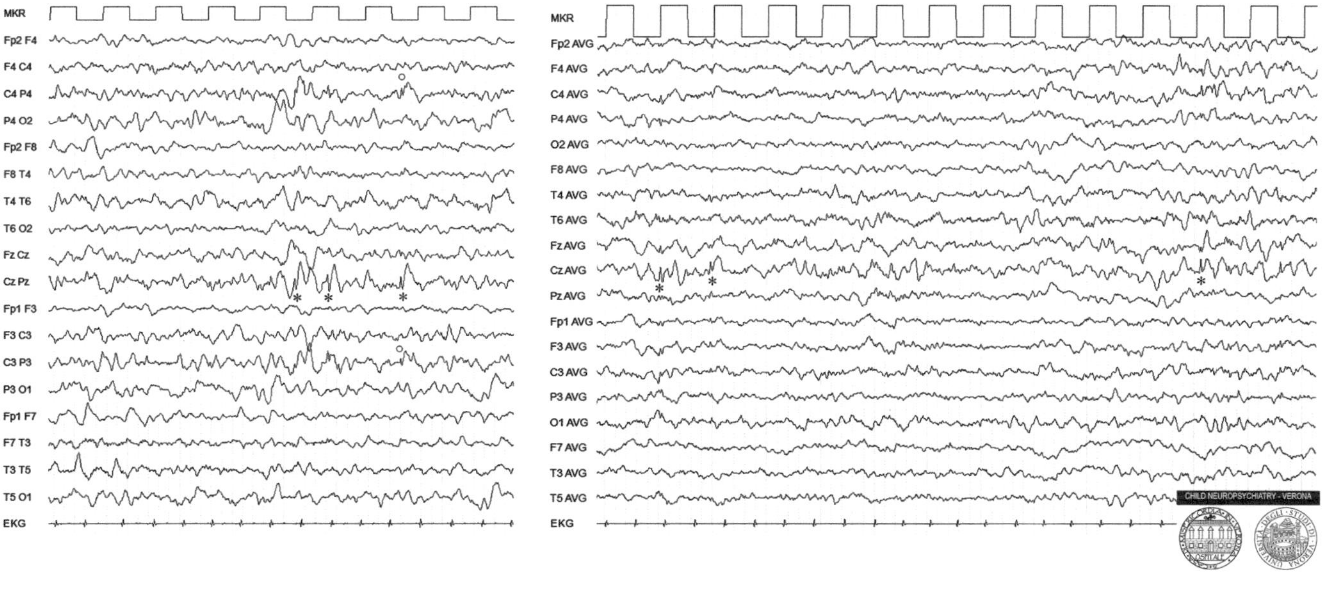

Fig. 25.13 Small spikes followed by a bell-shaped slow-wave, evident on the midline region (Cz-Pz channel, see asterisks), sometime with diffusion to centro-parietal channels of both hemispheres (circles). On the right panel are other examples of "Capovilla's spikes" (asterisks) in a monopolar average-reference montage

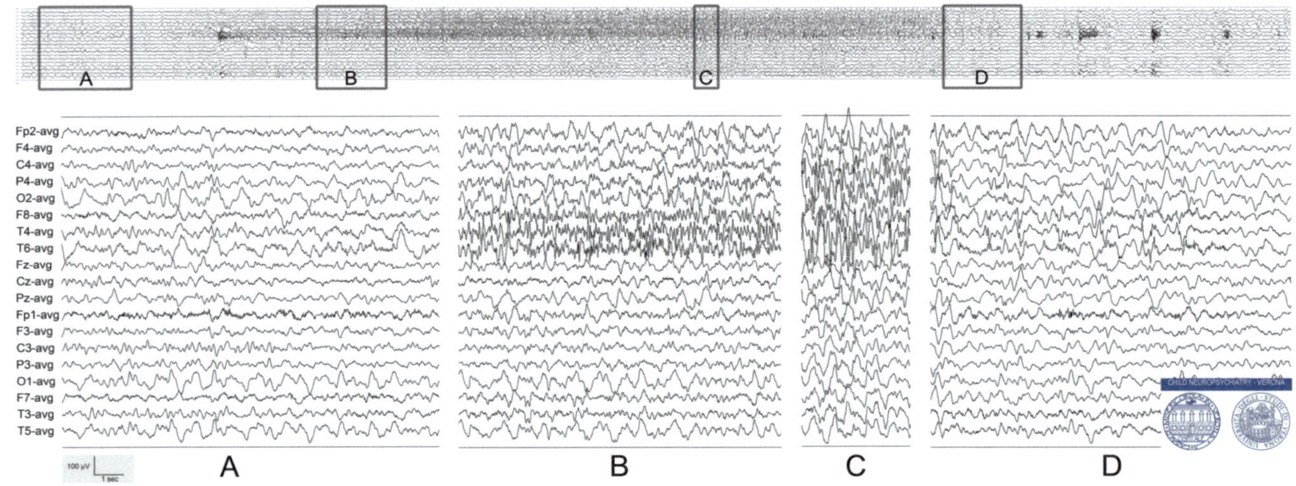

Fig. 25.14 A typical focal seizure in a patient carrying a mutation of PRRT2 gene, occurring during sleep. In the upper line is the entire evolution of the seizure, while in the lower line, four details are shown, corresponding to the four rectangles of the upper line and accordingly labeled. In (**a**) the seizure onset is visible as a low-amplitude fast activity on temporal region, superimposed to the slow background (arrowhead), increasingly becoming more evident over T6 (arrow); the paroxysmal discharge progressively involves all temporal channels (**b**), then the entire right hemisphere (**c**), ending within 3 min from seizure onset with a mild right hemisphere slowing (**d**)

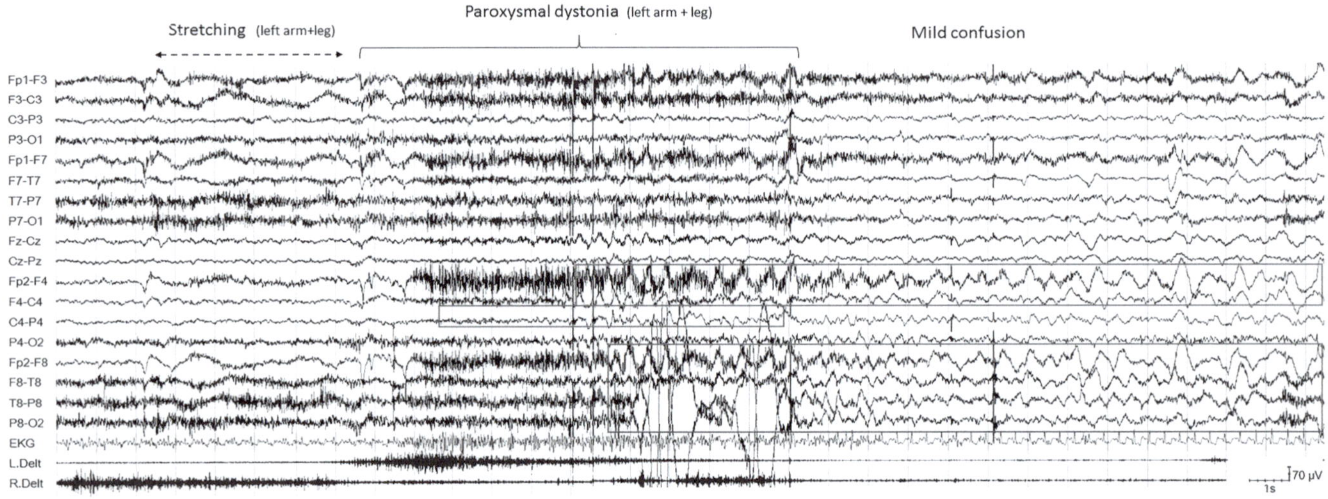

Fig. 25.15 This 14-year-old boy with BFIS developed brief but frequent episodes (several every day) of paroxysmal dystonia elicited by the abrupt onset of a voluntary movement or by stretching. He denied any impairment of consciousness during the episodes. Conversely, the video-EEG recordings documented a mild subconfusion during and after the episode of PD, together with an EEG correlate and a prolonged delta activity in the frontal regions, suggesting an ictal-cortical event. This further confirms the importance of ictal video-EEG recordings for the proper assessment of paroxysmal motor events in these patients [45]

Age of seizure onset ranges from 3 to 20 months (4–7 months in familial form). Seizures are predominantly diurnal in clusters for 1–3 days. The ictal symptoms are motor arrest/staring, eye and head deviation, simple automatisms and hemi-clonic jerks, and sometimes progression to a generalized tonic-clonic seizure. The seizures frequency is very low, and the response to anticonvulsive medication is prompt. A spontaneous seizure offset is expected before the age of 2 years.

About 20% of patients with BIFS might develop paroxysmal kinesigenic dyskinesia (PKD) after puberty; this combination of symptoms is called ICCA (infantile convulsions and paroxysmal choreoathetosis, [43]). Mutations in *PRRT2* have been identified as the major cause of BFIS and of ICCA [44]. Recently a causative association with *SCN8A* mutation, BFIS, and ICCA has been also described [45].

25.6.1 Interictal and Ictal EEG

The interictal EEG is usually normal. The ictal EEG is characterized by a variable side and site of onset (either frontal, temporal, parietal, or occipital), even among seizures of the same patient. EEG shows focal, low-amplitude fast activity, intermixed with spikes, with spreading to the neighboring areas or diffusely (Fig. 25.14).

The video-EEG recording of the episodes of PKD is rare; anyway these manifestations are generally assumed to be a subcortical event. Anyway, in a patient with SCN8A-ICCA, PKD turned out having an EEG correlate, suggesting an epileptic nature of the phenomenon is also possible (Fig. 25.15).

References

1. Scheffer IE, Berkovic S, Capovilla G, et al. ILAE classification of the epilepsies: position paper of the ILAE Commission for Classification and Terminology. Epilepsia. 2017;58:512–21.
2. Commission on Classification and Terminology of the International League Against Epilepsy. Proposal for revised classification of epilepsies and epileptic syndromes. Epilepsia. 1989;30:389–99.
3. Wolf P. Basic principles of the ILAE syndrome classification. Epilepsy Res. 2006;70(Suppl 1):S20–6.
4. Dalla Bernardina B, Sgro V, Fejerman N. Epilepsy with centrotemporal spikes and related syndromes. In: Roger J, Bureau M, Dravet CH, Genton P, Tassinari CA, Wolf P, editors. Epileptic syndromes in infancy, childhood and adolescence. Montrouge: John Libbey Eurotext; 2005.
5. Loiseau P, Beaussart M. The seizures of benign childhood epilepsy with rolandic paroxysmal discharges. Epilepsia. 1973;14:381–9.
6. Panayiotopoulos CP, Bureau M, Caraballo R, Dalla Bernardina B, Valeta T. Idiopathic focal epilepsies in childhood. In: Bureau M, Genton P, Dravey C, et al., editors. Epileptic syndrome in infancy, childhood and adolescence. Montrouge: John Libbey Eurotext; 2012a.
7. Panayiotopoulos CP, Michael M, Sanders S, et al. Benign childhood focal epilepsy: assessment of established and newly recognized syndromes. Brain. 2012b;131:2264–86.
8. Fejerman N, Caraballo R. Benign focal epilepsies in infancy, childhood and adolescence. London: John Libbey Eurotext; 2007.
9. Legarda S, Jayakar P, Duchowny M, et al. Benign rolandic epilepsy: high central and low central subgroups. Epilepsia. 1994;35:1125–9.
10. van der Meij W, Huiskamp GJ, Rutten GJ, et al. The existence of two sources in rolandic epilepsy: confirmation with high resolution EEG, MEG and fMRI. Brain Topogr. 2001;13:275–82.
11. van Klink NEC, van 't Klooster MA, FSS L, et al. Ripples on rolandic spikes: a marker of epilepsy severity. Epilepsia. 2016;57:1179–89.
12. Dalla Bernardina B, Sgrò V, Caraballo R, Fontana E, et al. Sleep and benign partial epilepsies of childhood: EEG and evoked potentials study. Epilepsy Res Suppl. 1991;2:83–96.
13. Veggiotti P, Beccaria F, Gatti A, et al. Can protrusion of the tongue stop seizures in Rolandic epilepsy? Epileptic Disord. 1999;1:217–20.
14. Koutroumanidis M, Arzimanoglou A, Caraballo R, et al. The role of EEG in the diagnosis and classification of the epilepsy syndromes: a tool for clinical practice by the ILAE Neurophysiology Task Force. Epileptic Disord. 2017;19:305–437.
15. Metz-Lutz MN, Filippini M. Neuropsychological findings in Rolandic epilepsy and Landau-Kleffner syndrome. Epilepsia. 2006;47:71–5.
16. Arzimanoglou A, Guerrini R, Aicardi J. Aicardi's epilepsy in children. Philadelphia: Lippincott Williams& Wilkins; 2004.
17. Dalla Bernardina B, Tassinari CA. EEG of a nocturnal seizure in a patient with benign epilepsy of childhood with rolandic spikes. Epilepsia. 1975;16:497–501.
18. Gutierrez AR, Brick JF, Bodensteiner J. Dipole reversal: an ictal feature of benign partial epilepsy with centrotemporal spikes. Epilepsia. 1990;31:544–8.
19. Patry G, Lyagoubi S, Tassinari CA. Subclinical electrical status epilepticus induced by sleep in children. Arch Neurol. 1971;24:242–52.
20. Tassinari CA, Cantalupo G, Dalla Bernardina B, et al. Encephalopathy related to status epilepticus during slow sleep (ESES) including Landau-Kleffner syndrome. In: Bureau M, Genton P, Dravet C, et al., editors. Epileptic syndromes in infancy, childhood and adolescence. London: John Libbey Eurotext Ltd; 2012.
21. Gardella E, Cantalupo G, Larsson P, et al. EEG features in ESES. Epileptic Dis; in press.
22. Guerrini R, Belmonte A, Genton P. Antiepileptic drug-induced worsening of seizures in children. Epilepsia. 1998;39(S.3):S2–S10.
23. Bölsterli BK, Gardella E, Pavlidis E, et al. Remission of encephalopathy with status epilepticus (ESES) during sleep renormalizes regulation of slow wave sleep. Epilepsia. 2017;58:1892–901.
24. Specchio N, Trivisano M, Di Ciommo V, et al. Panayiotopoulos syndrome: a clinical, EEG, and neuropsychological study of 93 consecutive patients. Epilepsia. 2010;51:2098–107.
25. Koutroumanidis M, Ferrie CD, Valeta T, Sanders S, Michael M, Panayiotopoulos CP. Syncope-like epileptic seizures in Panayiotopoulos syndrome. Neurology. 2012;79:463–7.
26. Sanders S, Rowlinson S, Manidakis I, et al. The contribution of the EEG technologists in the diagnosis of Panayiotopoulos syndrome (susceptibility to early onset benign childhood autonomic seizures). Seizure. 2004;13:565–73.
27. Leal AJ, Ferreira JC, Dias AI, Calado E. Origin of frontal lobe spikes in the early onset benign occipital lobe epilepsy (Panayiotopoulos syndrome). Clin Neurophysiol. 2008;119(9):1985–91.
28. Tata G, Guveli BT, Dortcan N, et al. Panayiotopoulos syndrome and symptomatic occipital lobe epilepsy of childhood: a clinical and EEG study. Epileptic Disord. 2014;16:197–202.
29. Lada C, Skiadas K, Theodorou V, et al. A study of 43 patients with Panayiotopoulos syndrome, a common and benign childhood seizure susceptibility. Epilepsia. 2003;44:81–8.
30. Panayiotopoulos CP. The EEG in Panayiotopoulos syndrome is a multifocal EEG. In: Panayiotopoulos CP, editor. Panayiotopoulos syndrome, a common and benign childhood epileptic syndrome. London: John Libbey Eurotext; 2002.
31. Guerrini R, Dravet C, Genton P, et al. Idiopathic photosensitive occipital lobe epilepsy. Epilepsia. 1995;36:883–91.
32. Caraballo RH, Koutroumanidis M, Panayiotopoulos CP, Fejerman N. Idiopathic childhood occipital epilepsy of Gastaut: a review and differentiation from migraine and other epilepsies. J Child Neurol. 2009;24:1536–42.
33. Caraballo R, Fontana E, Darra F, et al. Childhood absence epilepsy and electroencephalographic focal abnormalities with or without clinical manifestations. Seizure. 2008;17:617–24.
34. Gastaut H, Zifkin BG. Benign epilepsy of childhood with occipital spike and wave complexes. In: Andermann F, Lugaresi E, editors. Migraine and epilepsy. Boston: Butterworths; 1987. p. 47–81.
35. Panayiotopoulos CP. Visual phenomena and headache in occipital epilepsy: a review, a systematic study and differentiation from migraine. Epileptic Disord. 1999;1:205–16.
36. Wakamoto H, Nagao H, Fukuda M, et al. Idiopathic childhood occipital epilepsy of Gastaut: report of 12 patients. Pediatr Neurol. 2011;44:183–6.
37. Salanova V, Andermann F, Olivier A, et al. Occipital lobe epilepsy: electroclinical manifestations, electrocorticography, cortical

stimulation and outcome in 42 patients treated between 1930 and 1991. Surgery of occipital lobe epilepsy. Brain. 1992;115: 1655–80.
38. Williamson PD, Thadani VM, Darcey TM, et al. Occipital lobe epilepsy: clinical characteristics, seizure spread patterns, and results of surgery. Ann Neurol. 1992;31:3–13.
39. De Marco P, Tassinari CA. Extreme somatosensory evoked potential (ESEP): an EEG sign forecasting the possible occurrence of seizures in children. Epilepsia. 1981;22:569–75.
40. Capovilla G, Beccaria F, Montagnini A. 'Benign focal epilepsy in infancy with vertex spikes and waves during sleep'. Delineation of the syndrome and recalling as 'benign infantile focal epilepsy with midline spikes and waves during sleep' (BIMSE). Brain and Development. 2006;28:85–91.
41. Vigevano F, Fusco L, Di Capua M, et al. Benign infantile familial convulsions. Eur J Pediatr. 1992;151:608–12.
42. Watanabe K, Yamamoto N, Negoro T, et al. Benign complex partial epilepsies in infancy. Pediatr Neurol. 1987;3:208–11.
43. Szepetowski P, Rochette J, Berquin P, et al. Familial infantile convulsions and paroxysmal choreoathetosis: a new neurological syndrome linked to the pericentromeric region of human chromosome 16. Am J Hum Genet. 1997;61:889–98.
44. Heron SE, Grinton BE, Kivity S, et al. PRRT2 mutations cause benign familial infantile epilepsy and infantile convulsions with choreoathetosis syndrome. Am J Hum Genet. 2012;90:152–60.
45. Gardella E, Becker F, Møller RS, et al. Benign infantile seizures and paroxysmal dyskinesia caused by an SCN8A mutation. Ann Neurol. 2016;79:428–36.

Non-age-Related Focal Epilepsies

26

Guido Rubboli and Elena Gardella

26.1 Introduction

The term "focal seizures" refers to seizures in which the semiology at seizure onset indicates, or is compatible with, the initial activation of a limited region of cortex of a cerebral hemisphere [1]. In 2017, the Commission for Classification and Terminology of the International League Against Epilepsy (ILAE) has issued two position papers, the first presenting a revised operational classification of seizure types [2] and the second proposing a revised framework for the Classification of the Epilepsies, that is designed to work along with the classification of seizure types [3].

In the new proposal [2], focal seizures are optionally classified as "aware" or "impaired awareness" seizures, replacing the former labels "simple" and "complex," respectively, for the definition of the impairment of consciousness. Importantly, the "impaired awareness" definition should be used to classify a seizure when awareness is impaired at any time during the seizure, not only at seizure onset. If awareness cannot be assessed or information are lacking, this level of classification should be omitted. The next step after the assessment of awareness is the definition of the seizure as "motor" or "non-motor" based on the evidence of motor components, or their absence, at seizure onset. Then further items for additional semiological characterization are listed [2]. Regarding secondarily generalized seizures, the proposed term is "focal to bilateral tonic-clonic seizures," in order to restrict "generalized" to seizures of generalized onset in the context of generalized epilepsies [2]. After the classification of the seizure type, the following step should be to define the epilepsy type and, whenever possible, the epilepsy syndrome [3]. This latter proposal applies to all ages and it has a major focus on etiology [3]. Focal epilepsies include unifocal and multifocal disorders as well as seizures involving one hemisphere. Variable seizure types can be observed including focal aware seizures, focal impaired awareness seizures, focal motor seizures, focal non-motor seizures, and focal to bilateral tonic-clonic seizures. Interictal EEG typically can be helpful to detect focal epileptiform discharges, but the diagnosis has to be clinical, complemented by EEG findings.

A new group of Combined Generalized and Focal Epilepsies is admitted, as there are patients who can present with both generalized and focal seizures. As above, the diagnosis is clinical, supported by EEG findings. Of course, ictal recordings can be very helpful, but they are not mandatory. In the interictal EEG both generalized epileptic discharges and focal abnormalities can be detected.

Dravet syndrome and Lennox-Gastaut syndrome are examples of these combined forms of epilepsies [3].

In this chapter we will illustrate the EEG features of focal epilepsies according to localization criteria, which still are among the common criteria used in clinical practice [4–6]. Therefore we will discuss the EEG features of focal epilepsies originating from the temporal, frontal, parietal, and occipital lobes, thus using essentially an anatomical classification criterion to define epileptic disorders that in some instances can be included in a syndromic framework, as, for example, for mesial temporal lobe epilepsy associated with mesial temporal sclerosis, sleep-related hypermotor epilepsy, or autosomal dominant lateral temporal lobe epilepsy with auditory features. This type of "anatomical" classification is based largely on the data provided by the epilepsy surgery centers and by neuroimaging techniques, in particular MRI, whose advent has extremely enhanced the possibility to identify in vivo small brain alterations of potentially epileptogenic significance. This type of classification is particularly useful when a surgical approach is considered, even though the identification of the lobe is often not sufficient,

G. Rubboli (✉)
Danish Epilepsy Center, Filadelfia/University of Copenhagen, Dianalund, Denmark
e-mail: guru@filadelfia.dk

E. Gardella
Danish Epilepsy Center, University of Southern Denmark, Dianalund, Denmark

O. Mecarelli (ed.), *Clinical Electroencephalography*, https://doi.org/10.1007/978-3-030-04573-9_26

but further data (generally provided by both scalp and intracranial video-EEG recordings, by accurate morphological and functional neuroimaging studies, by a neuropsychological assessment) are necessary to define more precisely the epileptogenic area. An aspect that may limit the clinical utility of this classification criterion is the evidence that some types of seizures originate from epileptogenic networks that extend beyond the boundaries of a given lobe, such as seizures from the perirolandic region, insular seizures, or seizures from the temporal-parietal-occipital carrefour. Moreover, this type of classification defines essentially, with some exceptions (an example is mesial temporal epilepsy associated with mesial temporal sclerosis, as mentioned above), seizure types rather than syndromic entities.

In this chapter we will review the scalp EEG features of the main forms that can be classified in the four subtypes listed above, namely, temporal, frontal, parietal, and occipital epilepsies, without dealing with the intracranial EEG findings, which are beyond the scope of this chapter. We will also describe the EEG features of two other forms of focal epilepsy non-age-related such as epilepsy with gelastic seizures and Rasmussen's syndrome.

26.2 Temporal Lobe Epilepsy

Temporal lobe epilepsies (TLEs) include a group of epileptic conditions with focal seizures originating from temporal lobe structures, and they represent the most common form of the adult focal epilepsies. In 1964, Falconer [7] suggested that TLEs are not a single and uniform pathological entity but that there are several types of TLEs, with distinct clinical and prognostic characteristics. From the etiological point of view, we can identify (a) TLEs associated with mesial temporal sclerosis; (b) TLEs associated with structural lesions (e.g., low-grade glioneuronal tumors, astrocytomas, hamartomas, xantoastrocytomas, cavernous angiomas, vascular malformations, dysplasias, neuroepithelial dysembryoplastic tumors) that can lie in both mesial and neocortical temporal structures; and (c) cryptogenic TLE, not associated with identifiable structural abnormalities. The incidence of cryptogenic TLE is difficult to establish, because the results of the histological study on the surgical specimens obtained in patients operated for drug-resistant TLEs vary between the different centers and because the incidence of genetically transmitted TLEs has not yet been defined. In the surgical series of patients with drug-resistant TLEs, however, studies performed on histological samples have reported a negativity of the pathological study only in 2–10% of patients. Regarding focal epilepsies associated with genetic mutations, in recent years, two conditions have been identified whose ictal semiology suggests involvement of temporal structures: autosomal dominant lateral temporal epilepsy, associated with known genetic mutations (see below), and autosomal dominant mesial temporal epilepsy, whose genetic background is still undetermined.

Although seizures originate from the mesial structures of the temporal lobe in the majority of cases, about 10% of patients with TLE have seizures arising from the lateral neocortex [8]. Therefore, based on the site of onset in the temporal lobe of the ictal discharges, two types of TLEs are recognized:

(a) Mesial temporal lobe epilepsy (MTLE)
(b) Lateral neocortical temporal lobe epilepsy (LNTLE)

The differential diagnosis between MTLE and LNTLE is based on anamnestic, clinical, neurophysiological, and neuroradiological data. The characteristics of the interictal and ictal EEG are not sufficient per se for distinguishing the two forms. In fact, various ictal EEG patterns have been described, but their specificity in distinguishing the mesial forms from the lateral ones remains controversial.

26.2.1 Mesial Temporal Lobe Epilepsy (MTLE)

The real incidence of the MTLE is not established, either because the criteria for the recognition of this form have been outlined only recently or because mainly patients with drug-resistant MTLE are extensively investigated allowing a precise diagnosis, whereas the diagnostic assessment is usually limited in MTLEs adequately controlled by drugs, and this probably reduces the diagnostic accuracy in a proportion of patients. The most common finding in drug-resistant MTLE is the sclerosis of mesial temporal lobe structures (MTS), with inclusion of the hippocampus; other structures that may be involved are the amygdala, the entorhinal cortex, and the parahippocampal gyrus. An association between MTS and prolonged febrile convulsions or other insults (traumas, infections) in childhood is reported in about 2/3 of the patients. The pathophysiological mechanisms of MTLE associated with MTS and the neuropathological consequences on seizures remain mostly unresolved [9]. Typically, when MTLE with MTS is diagnosed, a typical course of the disease can be retrospectively recognized, including early prolonged febrile seizures, a latent period, onset of focal seizures in mid-to-late childhood, auras that may initially occur in isolation, and periods of seizure remission during adolescence or early adulthood. Then the condition progresses, associating elaborated seizures, drug resistance, and cognitive, mainly memory, disorders of variable severity [10].

MTLE can be associated also with other lesions such as, for example, tumors, vascular malformations, cavernous angioma, focal cortical dysplasias, and neuroepithelial dysembryoplastic tumors, located in the mesial temporal regions. However, there are no diagnostic criteria that can allow a reliable distinction of the MTLEs associated with the different etiologies based on the EEG features.

26.2.1.1 Interictal EEG Features

The interictal EEG may be normal or with nonspecific alterations. A recent study has reported that 47.1% of standard scalp EEG recordings were normal or had nonspecific features, though sleep deprivation improved the yield [11]. Indeed, a sufficiently prolonged waking or sleep EEG (Fig. 26.1) is likely to reveal epileptic spikes or slow spikes associated with a slow wave, more frequently in the anterior or middle temporal leads (Fig. 26.2). It is not uncommon that spikes with both topographies are observed in the same patient. Surface-negative anterior temporal spikes or sharp waves occur in more than 90% of patients [12] and usually predict the side of seizure onset. Asynchronous epileptic abnormalities in bilateral temporal derivations have been reported in one-third of the patients in long-term EEG recordings and particularly during sleep [13]. The EEG may also demonstrate focal slowing, which can occur in the form of temporal intermittent rhythmic delta activity often ipsilateral to seizure onset.

26.2.1.2 Ictal Clinical EEG Semiology

Ictal clinical semiology shows several features suggesting the involvement of mesial temporal lobe structures. Subjective manifestations at seizure onset, i.e., the "aura," have been reported in up to 90% of the patients [12]. The most common and typical aura is an epigastric sensation that from the abdomen spreads up to the head; other subjective manifestations are fear, "deja vu," "jamais vu," and pseudovertiginous sensa-

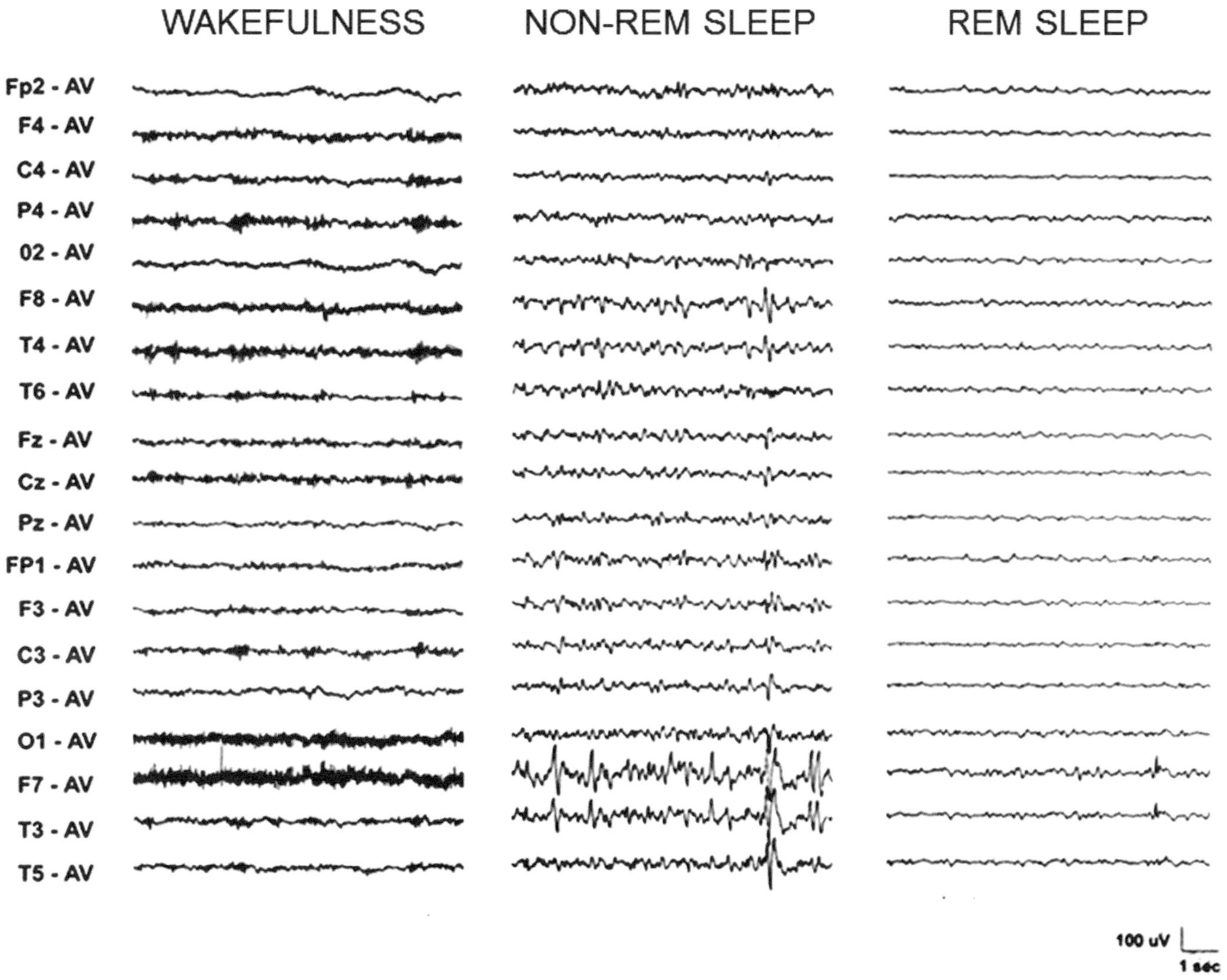

Fig. 26.1 Interictal EEG in a patient with left mesial temporal lobe epilepsy associated with left mesial temporal sclerosis. Left panel: the wakefulness EEG does not show abnormalities. Middle panel: during non-REM sleep, high amplitude spikes appear in the left temporal channels, occasionally spreading to the homo- and contralateral hemisphere. Right panel: in REM sleep, the epileptic abnormalities show a lower amplitude, and they are distributed focally only on the left frontotemporal leads

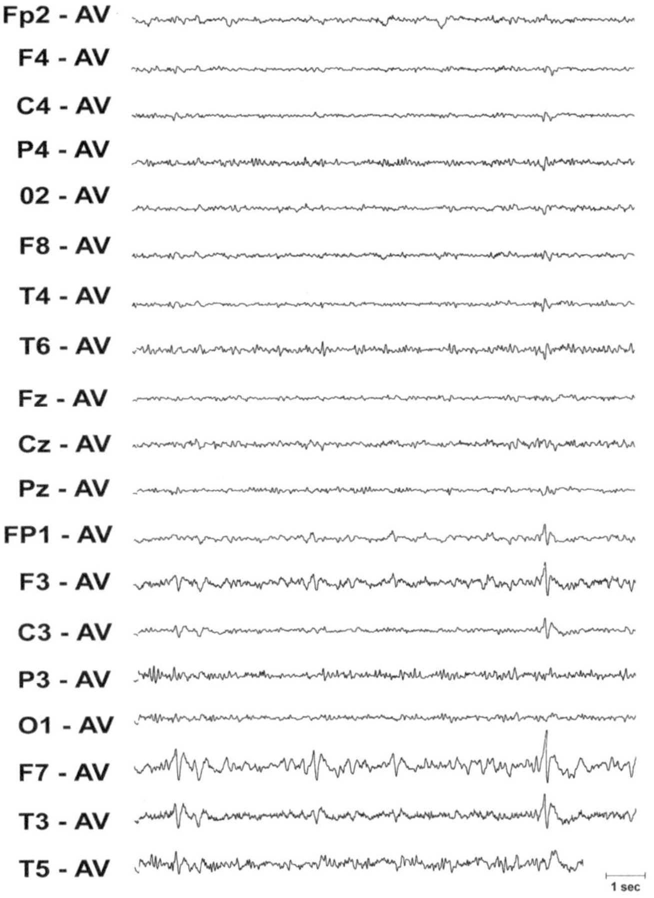

Fig. 26.2 The interictal EEG in a patient with left mesial temporal epilepsy associated with vascular malformation of the left hippocampus shows spikes followed by a slow wave in the left anterior temporal leads, with occasional spread to the ipsilateral hemisphere

tions; later in the evolution of the seizure, olfactory, gustatory, and visual hallucinations may appear. Objective phenomena are the arrest of the ongoing activities, staring, oro-alimentary automatisms (chewing, licking, swallowing, lip smacking, teeth grinding), gestural automatisms usually ipsilateral to the side of seizure onset, and elementary vocalizations. Some clinical manifestations have been particularly investigated for their possible lateralizing significance: in addition to the gestural automatisms mentioned above, an early eye-version and head turning tends to occur ipsilaterally to the ictal discharge, while the occurrence of a unilateral tonic or dystonic posture occurs to the arm contralateral to the epileptic activity. Other manifestations that can be part of the ictal semiology may be language disorders (ictal aphasia, verbalizations, language arrest), ictal vomiting, and enuresis. In the postictal phase, a language disorder suggests the involvement of the hemisphere dominant for language. A motor deficit, contralateral to the side of the ictal discharge, can be observed. However, attention has to be paid in interpreting these latter signs as localizing or lateralizing for the seizure-onset zone, since they might occur also due to an ipsilateral or contralateral spread of the ictal discharge. Confusion, disorientation, and, sometimes, the persistence of automatic semifinalistic movements or oro-alimentary automatisms are common in in the postictal phase.

The ictal EEG is frequently characterized by a rhythmic activity at 5–9 Hz, preceded sometimes by a brief flattening of the electrogenesis that can affect all EEG leads (as a diffuse “arrest reaction”) or focused on frontotemporal/mid-temporal leads [14]. The seizure onset can be characterized also by an abrupt arrest of the frontotemporal interictal spikes and slow-wave activity, followed by a flattening of the electrogenesis. The rhythmic activity tends to be lateralized to the side of the epileptic focus, mainly in the temporal leads, and then it spreads to the suprasylvian ipsilateral regions and possibly contralaterally (Fig. 26.3a). Frequently, the EEG tracing is partially masked by rhythmic muscular artifacts caused by chewing automatisms. In the postictal phase, a slow, theta-delta activity is common, often predominant on the side of seizure onset (Fig. 26.3b). Abnormalities of the heart rhythm, either tachycardia or bradycardia, and even asystolia, have been described during MTLE seizures [15].

26.2.2 Lateral Neocortical Temporal Lobe Epilepsy (LNTLE)

LNTLE is considered less common than MTLE. It is often associated with structural abnormalities in the lateral neocortex even though forms without any evidence of cortical lesions have been documented as well [16]. A genetic form of LNTLE is the autosomal dominant lateral temporal epilepsy (ADLTE) otherwise labelled as autosomal dominant partial epilepsy with auditory features (ADPEAF). The onset of ADLTE can be at any age, although more often in young adults, and it is characterized by focal seizures, with or without impairment of consciousness, with prominent auditory features or other symptoms, such as aphasia, suggesting a lateral temporal onset, that can eventually evolve to tonic-clonic seizures [17, 18]. Patients with this form of epilepsy have normal neurological and cognitive status, MRI is unremarkable, and they belong to families where one or more members show a similar phenotype with evidence of autosomal dominant transmission. Several reports have demonstrated that ADLTE is associated with leucine-rich glioma inactivated 1 (LGI1) gene mutations [19, 20]. However, a considerable proportion of families, more than 50%, does not carry any LGI1 abnormality. Recently, mutations of the

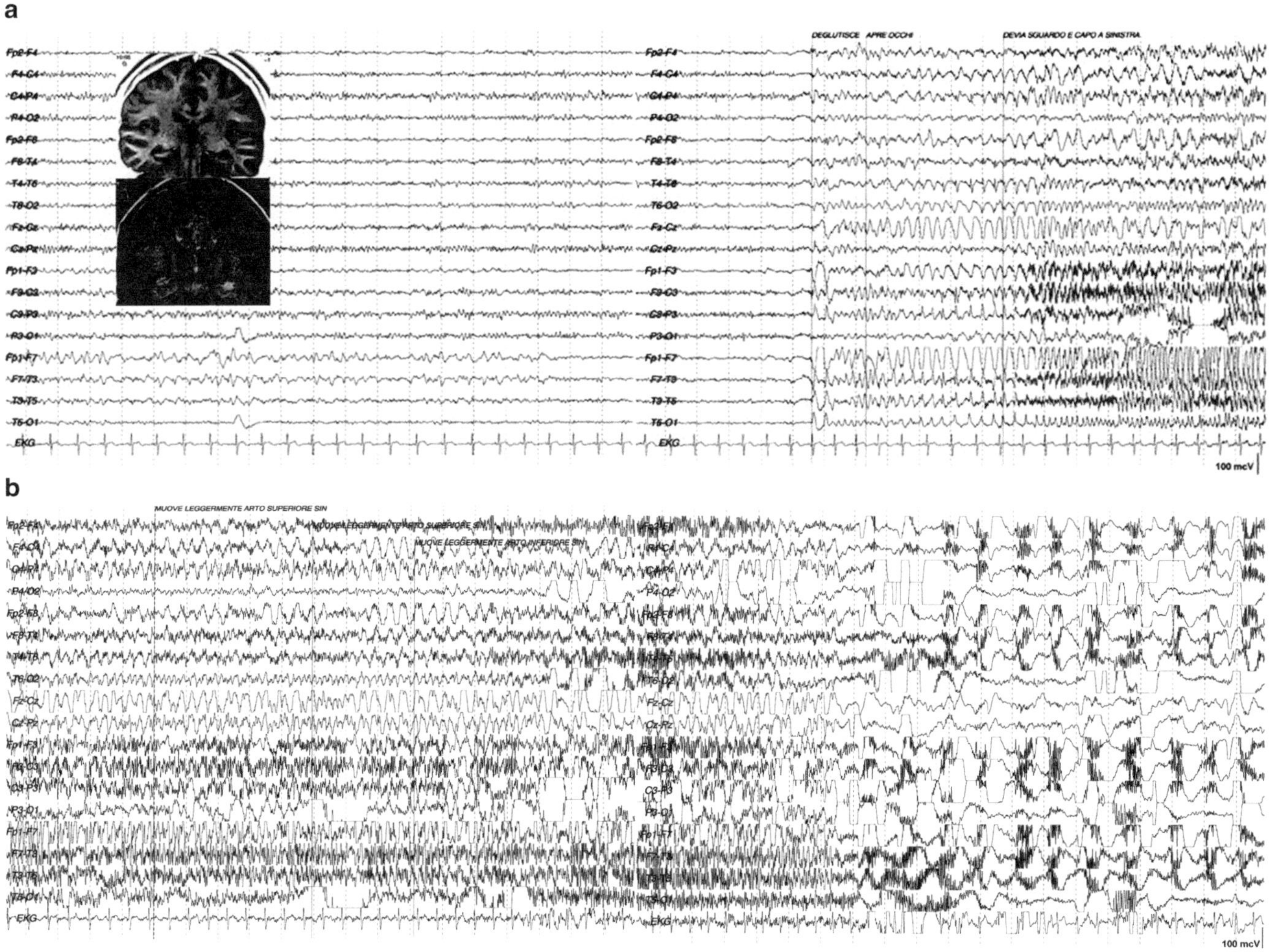

Fig. 26.3 (**a**) Ictal EEG in the same patient as in Fig. 26.2. At seizure onset, an abrupt interruption of the interictal abnormalities in the left temporal derivations is followed by a flattening of the EEG activity for a few seconds. Then a rhythmic theta activity appears in the left temporal derivations, that, after slowing down for a few seconds, is followed by a recruiting rhythm of spikes that tend to spread contralaterally. In the insert, RMN images showing a vascular malformation in the left hippocampus. (**b**) The evolution of seizure in (**a**) is shown. The ictal discharge has greater amplitude in the left hemisphere EEG channels, and then it stops abruptly to be followed by a widespread slow activity with rhythmic muscular artifacts superimposed, due to oro-alimentary automatisms

reelin (RELN) and MICAL-1 genes have been shown to cause ADTLE in a subset of patients [21–23].

26.2.2.1 Interictal EEG Features

The interictal EEG shows spikes more often in the mid-temporal EEG channels, sometimes associated with slow waves. Asynchronous contralateral epileptic abnormalities occur less frequently than in the MTLE.

26.2.2.2 Ictal Clinical EEG Semiology

The seizure duration tends to be shorter than in MTLE. Cephalic, vertiginous, auditory, or visual auras seem to be more common than in mesial-onset seizures. The clinical onset can often be represented by staring, and then unilateral gestural automatisms ipsilateral to the EEG discharge, inconstantly associated with a contralateral dystonic posture, can occur. Visual hallucinatory phenomena (e.g., macropsia, micropsia, palinopsia) occur when the epileptic activity involves the temporo-parieto-occipital and inferotemporal cortices [16]. An auditory hallucinatory-illusory semiology is the most typical auditory aura in ADTLE. The auditory sensations can be elementary such as "whistle or hissing" or more complex like "whispers, voices, or music"; in some patients, the seizures can be triggered by environmental noises. Motor manifestations, in particular clonic phenomena contralateral to the discharge and versions of the eyes and of the head, can appear during the seizure evolution.

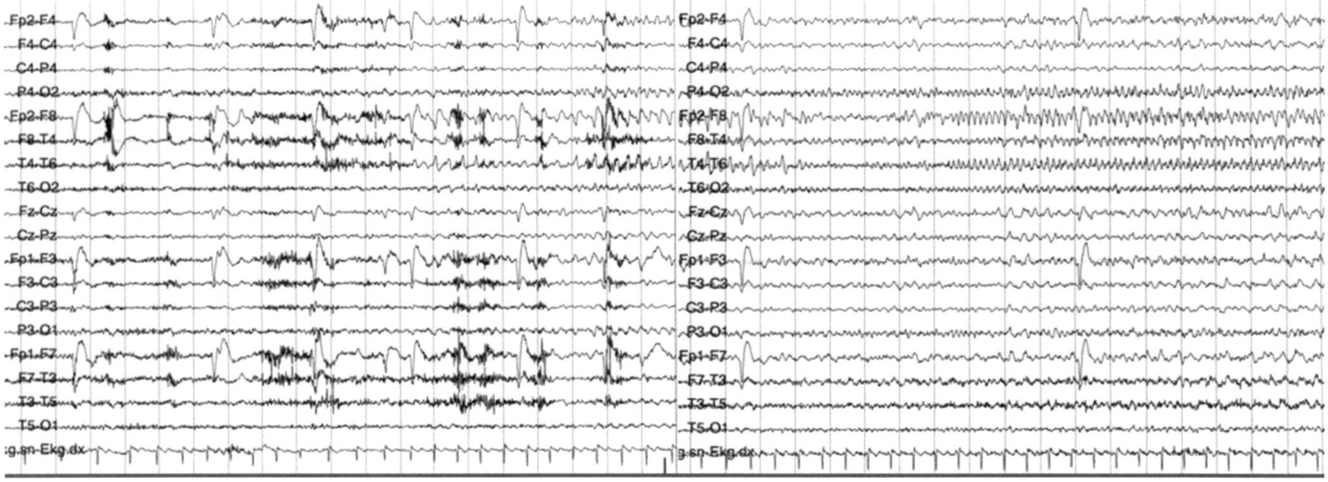

Fig. 26.4 Ictal EEG in a lateral neocortical temporal lobe seizure. Clinically, the patient does not report any aura, she loses consciousness suddenly, and she displays rhythmic automatic movements first of both upper limbs and then also of the lower ones. The EEG shows initially sharp waves in the right temporal regions, which progressively accelerate until they are organized into a rhythmic discharge that tends to remain confined to the right temporal derivations

At seizure onset, the ictal EEG may show a lateralized theta/delta rhythmic activity, corresponding to the side of the focus, distributed over the temporal derivations or on all the derivations of one hemisphere. The morphology is often irregular and polymorphic; it can become more regular during seizure evolution (Fig. 26.4). An activity of rhythmic spikes preceding the theta activity has been also described. In some instances, no clear lateralization of the discharge is recognizable. During the seizure evolution, the ictal discharge, when lateralized, can remain confined to the temporal regions, or it can spread to ipsilateral fronto-central derivations. The ictal discharge is relatively shorter as compared to MTLE. Postictal slowing may be encountered in 70% of seizures; however its lateraling significance is debated, since some studies concluded that it is less consistent than seizure onset in reflecting the site and side of seizure onset [14], in contrast, with other reports showing that a consistent postictal slowing was a very reliable lateralizing finding [12].

26.3 Frontal Lobe Epilepsies

Frontal lobe epilepsy (FLE) is the second most common form of focal epilepsy in adulthood [24]. Seizures originating in frontal lobe structures may display bizarre and polymorphic features (Fig. 26.5), and the differential diagnosis with other paroxysmal non-epileptic motor manifestations that can occur both in wakefulness and sleep (i.e., parasomnias) or with psychogenic seizures can be challenging.

A peculiar form of frontal lobe epilepsy is the autosomal dominant nocturnal frontal lobe epilepsy (ADNFLE), recently labelled as sleep-related hypermotor epilepsy (SHE) [25]. SHE is related to mutations of genes encoding subunits of the neuronal acetylcholine receptor (nAChR); recently other genes (*KCNT1*, *DEPDC5*) have been shown to be associated with a SHE phenotype. SHE is characterized by sleep-related seizures with extremely variable semiological features, ranging from minimal motor phenomena ("paroxysmal arousal") (Fig. 26.6) to asymmetric tonic motor manifestations and to prominent hyperkinetic motor behaviors (Figs. 26.5 and 26.7). The diagnosis of SHE generally requires video-EEG recordings of the seizures to document the stereotype in the same patient of the ictal semiology and possible associated EEG-polygraphic modifications [26].

Frontal lobe seizures can be distinguished in [24]:

– Focal motor clonic seizures: they can be devoid of other accompanying manifestations, and, in this case, consciousness can be preserved. This seizure type is related to the involvement of the primary motor cortex.
– Asymmetric tonic seizures: these seizures arise from the involvement of the supplementary motor area (SMA). SMA seizures can feature a subjective symptomatology that includes sensory phenomena, bilateral, contralateral, or ipsilateral (such as tingling, skin numbness, "pressure," etc.), that has led some authors to label this area as "supplementary sensorimotor area" [27]. Common motor manifestations are tonic postures with sudden onset, classically with abduction of the extended limb contralateral to the ictal discharge, and elevation of the flexed upper limb ipsilateral to the epileptic discharge; the lower limb, contralateral to the seizure focus, can be either extended, stiff, or flexed at the hip. These manifestations can be associated with vocalizations or language arrest. The seizure can end with clonic contractions in the hand or in the

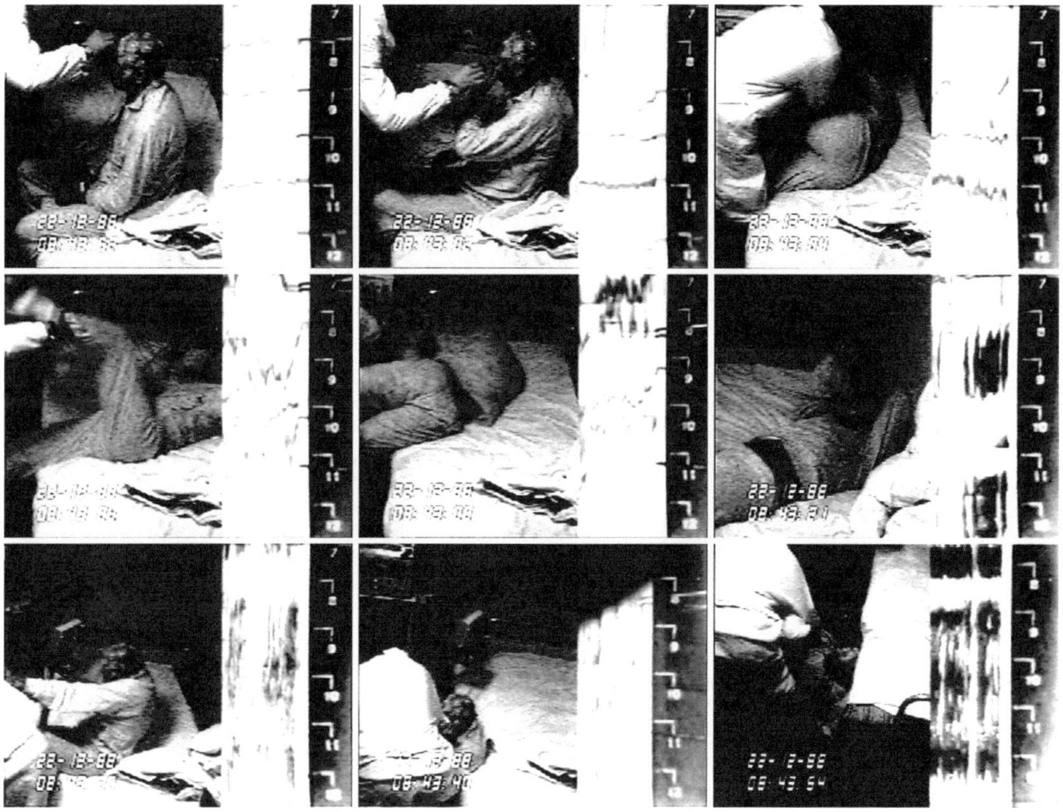

Fig. 26.5 Frontal lobe seizure with hyperkinetic motor manifestations. The patient presents complex movements, such as grabbing of his neck; grasping of the examiner, associated with violent kicking movements; and the tendency to pronate his body over the bed; these phenomena are associated with loud vocalizations. At the end of the seizure, the recovery is quick, without postictal confusion

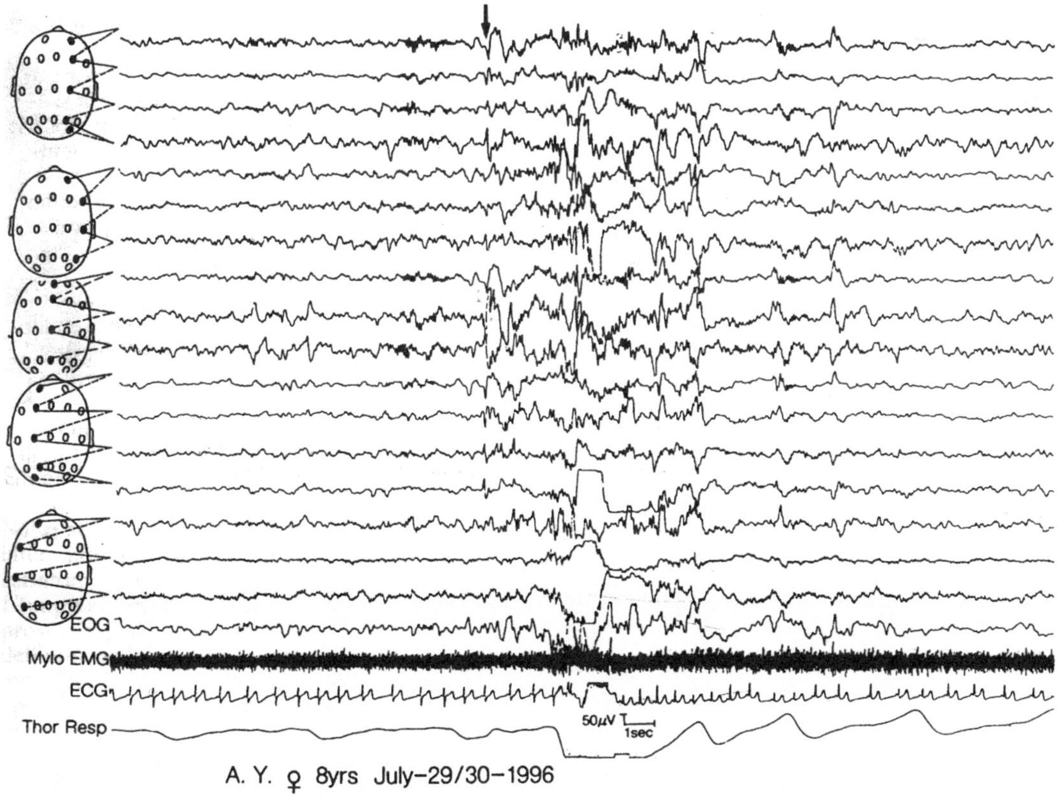

Fig. 26.6 Patient with sleep-related hypermotor epilepsy. EEG during a "paroxysmal arousal," characterized by a sudden movement of the limbs and the head, followed by recovery of sleep. Such episodes could occur several times per night. The EEG shows a high amplitude spike (arrow) in the anterior frontal leads, followed by low-amplitude fast activity

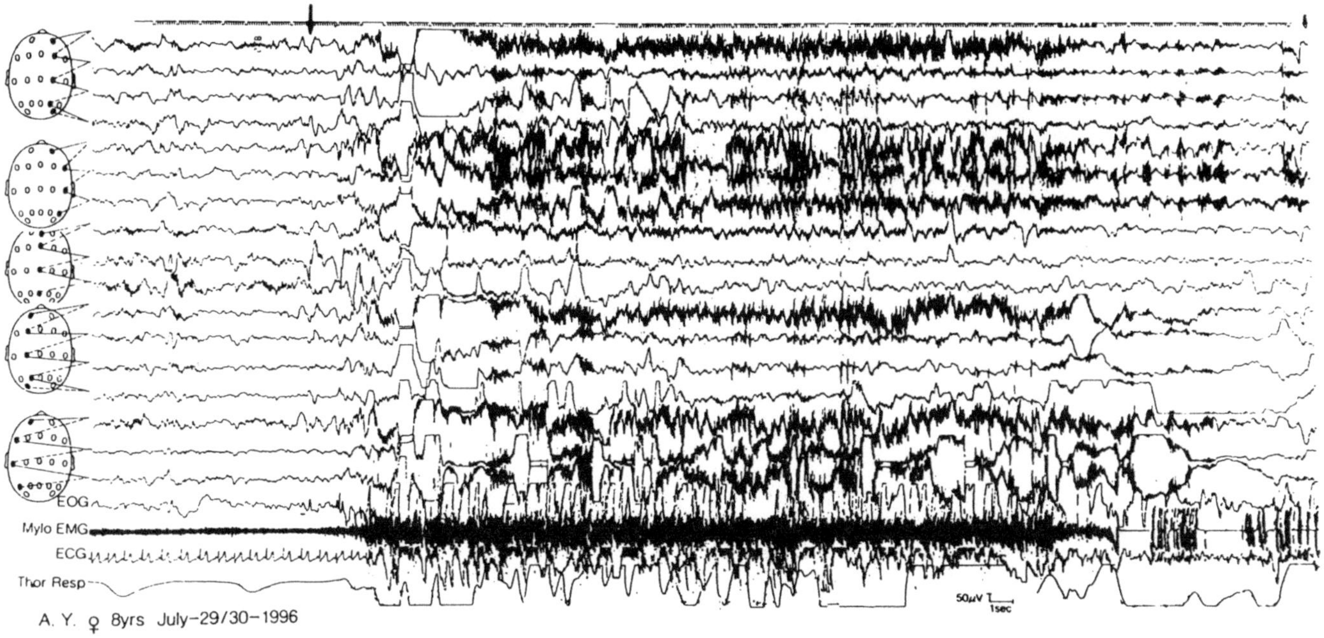

Fig. 26.7 Same patient as in Fig. 26.7. Hyperkinetic motor seizure clinically characterized by sitting abruptly on the bed with a frightened expression, moaning, grasping behavior toward the persons around, uncoordinated movements of the limbs, and flexion-extension of the trunk, with partially maintained consciousness; at the end of the seizure, the patient recovers immediately without postictal confusion. The EEG shows a sharp wave in the right frontal regions, followed by a low-amplitude fast activity, rapidly masked by artifacts

face, contralateral to the ictal discharge, or sometimes with a secondary generalization. Other not uncommon semiologies, such as the assumption of tonic or symmetrical limb postures of the limbs, athetoid-like movements of the upper limbs, and alternating motor activity of the lower limbs, can be observed. Finally, inhibitory motor phenomena (like negative myoclonia, postural lapses, and inhibitory seizures) can occur as well. The duration of SMA seizures is usually short, and they may occur in clusters either during the day or during the night. Consciousness is often preserved.

- Hyperkinetic motor seizures: they are characterized by prominent motor, often bizarre, activities, generally not associated with tonic components. The semiology of these events is peculiar, and it is considered relatively specific of seizures originating from the frontal lobe. Some data however have shown that a similar phenomenology can also be observed in seizures with temporal lobe onset and then spreading to frontal areas [28]. Hyperkinetic frontal seizures generally occur in clusters, most often during nocturnal sleep; the seizures are brief, with an abrupt onset, without postictal confusion, and they are characterized by complex, bizarre, frenetic motor automatisms (such as grasping, pedaling, kicking, uncoordinated movements of the limbs, and pelvic thrusting). Intense vocalizations and screaming can accompany the motor manifestations (Figs. 26.5 and 26.7). Despite the apparent chaotic and polymorphic motor activity, stereotypic semiological patterns can be identified in a given patient [29]. During the evolution of the seizure, variation of ictal semiology can result from the spreading of the epileptic activity to other frontal or extra-frontal areas. A recent hypothesis has proposed that the complex motor semiology featured by frontal lobe seizures may result from the release, provoked by the cortical epileptic activity (which would act as a "trigger"), of genetically determined, archaic motor sequences organized as central patterns generators, located at a subcortical or spinal level [30, 31].
- Frontal "absence" seizures: the semiology of these seizures can be very similar to those of typical absences. The EEG picture is characterized by diffuse spikes-and-waves, showing various degree of asymmetry, which is related to a secondary bisincrony mechanism (see below).
- Fronto-opercular seizures: they are characterized by profuse drooling, orofacial dyspraxia, and facial clonic twitches.

26.3.1 Interictal and Ictal EEG Features

Focal interictal epileptiform abnormalities or focal paroxysmal fast activity is seen in 40–60% of EEGs in patients with FLE. Discharges may be localized to the midline or appear as bifrontal or bilateral discharges. False localization of frontal lobe seizures to the temporal regions or when the focus is in mesial frontal cortices may also occur [32]. Focal repetitive epileptiform abnormalities highly predict lateral FLE [33]. In a study of patients with FLE and TLE, interictal rhythmic midline activity was observed in up to 48% of patients with FLE, whereas 62% of those patients lacked interictal abnormalities [34]. The analysis of the postictal EEG can provide valuable lateralizing and localizing information (such as lateralized or regional slow activity or lateralized or regional spikes) in about 40% of FLE patients [35]. In postoperative scalp EEG performed 2 months after surgery, the persistence of residual epileptic spikes during wakefulness and sleep predicted poor seizure outcome [36].

In patients with or without a structural lesion, generalized interictal epileptiform discharges can depend on a mechanism of secondary bilateral synchrony [37]. This EEG pattern is observed more frequently when the focus is in the antero-mesial regions, and it is characterized by a lead, visible in the EEG, of the epileptic activity from a focal cortical site that is followed by a bilateral, synchronous, relatively symmetrical, more or less irregular paroxysmal spike-wave activity (Fig. 26.8). The rapid bilateral spread occurs most probably through callosal fibers. The appearance of secondary bilateral synchrony is often associated with pharmacoresistance and sometimes with a modification of the ictal semiology, with seizures that start to feature falls or tonic contractions, or occurrence during wakefulness. During sleep, a rhythm of diffuse polyspikes can be observed.

In a non negligible proportion of patients, both interictal and ictal EEGs can be uninformative or even misleading. In fact, in these instances, some authors have stated that the correct diagnosis can be reached with certainty only with invasive EEG recordings, in particular when the seizures originate in fronto-mesial or fronto-orbitary regions. On the contrary, when the seizure focus is in the convexity of the frontal lobe, the EEG can provide both localizing and lateralizing information. A focal beta activity suggesting seizure onset in the dorsolateral prefrontal cortex has been reported in about 25% of FLE patients, and it is predictive of excellent seizure outcome after surgery [38–40]. A seizure focus in the mesial frontal region can show either no interictal abnormalities or multifocal epileptiform discharges [41, 42].

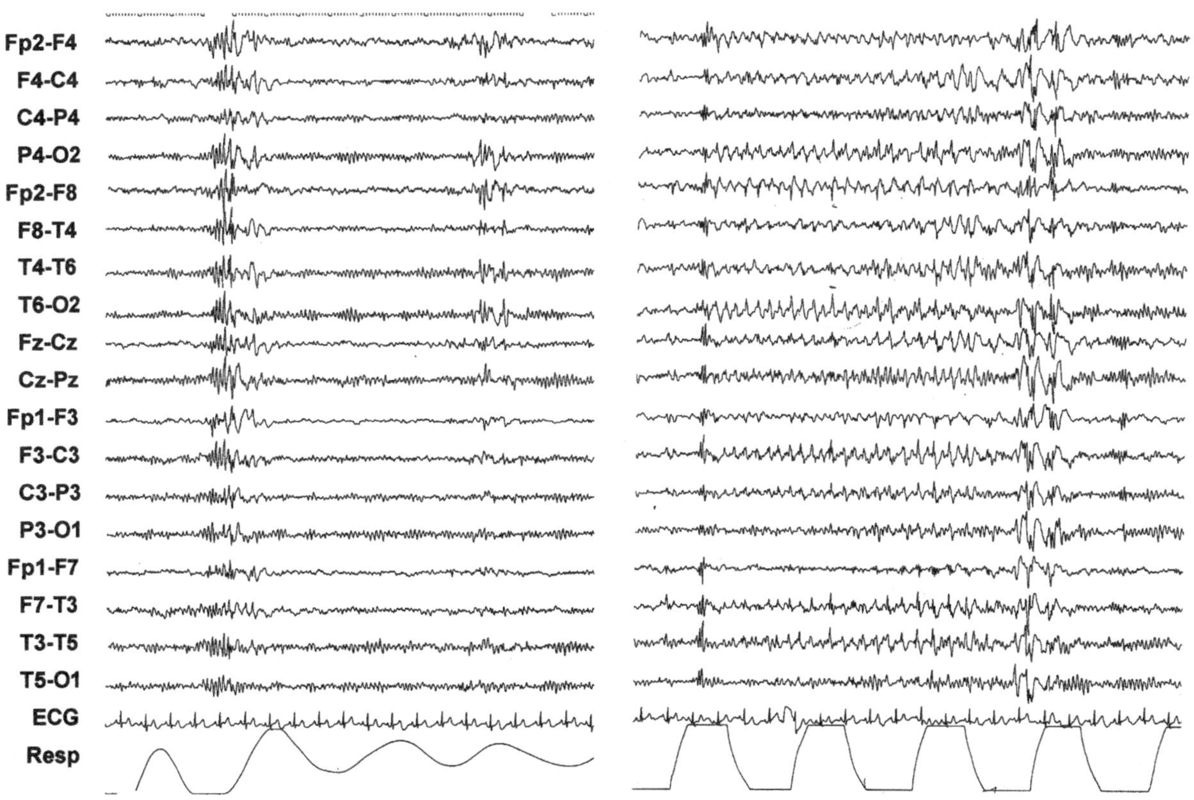

Fig. 26.8 Secondary bilateral synchronism in patients with cryptogenic drug-resistant focal epilepsy with right frontal lobe seizures. The interictal discharge shows a very brief lead in the right frontal channel, then a rapid bilateral spread follows, and a rhythmic spike-wave activity predominant anteriorly and on the right follows (right panel)

In FLE, ictal EEG is nonlocalizing in more than 50% of patients. EEG patterns such as bilateral attenuation, bilateral theta and delta activity, and generalized epileptiform activity may be encountered without providing lateralizing information. In other instances, localization is hindered by ictal-related massive artifacts. In general, the diagnostic yield of long-term scalp EEG in patients with FLE is often limited compared to patients with TLE, in particular due to the difficulty of recording paroxysmal activity from mesial and basal cortical areas, as mentioned above. In patients submitted to surgical treatment, the absence of generalized EEG signs was associated with seizure freedom after surgery [43]; conversely generalized or nonlocalized ictal EEG patterns predicted seizure recurrence [44]. Other studies however did not confirm these findings [45], and this might depend on different sample sizes and different methodologies.

26.4 Occipital Lobe Epilepsies

Seizures in occipital lobe epilepsies (OLE) are characterized by both subjective and objective signs and symptoms, some of which depend on the initial involvement of the occipital lobe, while others depend on the spreading of the epileptic activity anteriorly to regions located superiorly and/or inferiorly to the Sylvian fissure or contralaterally through the splenium of the corpus callosum [46]. Elementary visual hallucinations (such as bright flashes, "spots" in the visual field, and geometric, sometimes colored, shapes), both stationary and moving, represent the most common semiological symptoms of the involvement of the primary visual cortex; if lateralized in the visual field, they are related to a contralateral epileptic activity. Unilateral or bilateral amaurosis and sensations of eye movements are also often reported. Other clinical manifestations can be an ocular deviation, both tonic and clonic, sometimes with a version of the head toward the same side. The lateralization of the ocular version can be both ipsilateral and contralateral to the epileptic activity. A forced blinking or an eyelid "flutter" at seizure onset is also consistent with an occipital onset [46]. Other signs observed in occipital seizures are vomiting combined with other vegetative symptoms.

As already mentioned, the possibilities of a propagation of the epileptic discharge to other cortical regions are relatively frequent; therefore, the appearance, during the seizure evolution, of sensory and auditory phenomena suggests the diffusion of the epileptic activity to somatosensory or auditory cortices, while motor manifestations are indicative of the activation of both lateral motor areas (such as clonic phenomena, in the case of spread to the primary motor cortex) and mesial motor areas (tonic contractions when SMA is involved); finally, the appearance of automatisms typical of anterior TLE indicates the propagation of the seizure activity to the anterior temporal lobe structures.

26.4.1 Interictal and Ictal EEG

The interictal EEG can show a modification of the occipital alpha rhythm, often fragmented and with lower amplitude on the side of the focus. In OLE associated with posterior structural lesions, the posterior background activity can be frequently interrupted or replaced by slow abnormalities (e.g., in case of tumors) or fast activities (in the case of focal cortical dysplasias). In OLE, well-defined interictal epileptic discharges over the occipital EEG leads occur in less than 20% of patients. Furthermore, like other extratemporal lobe epilepsies, they may falsely localize to the temporal (especially posterior temporal) region [47]. When IED are observable, they appear as spike-wave-like complexes, sometimes with irregular morphology, in brief runs located in posterior leads, with tendency to spread anteriorly [48] (Fig. 26.9).

In the ictal EEG, it may be difficult to identify the first ictal modifications (particularly when the epileptic discharge originates from the basal or mesial structures of the occipital lobes); then, during the course of the seizure, the epileptic activity can become more evident, appearing as a low-amplitude fast activity that can evolve progressively into a well-structured rhythmic discharge (Fig. 26.10). In general, however, a well-formed ictal rhythm is localized infrequently to one occipital lobe, and some studies have reported the ictal EEG as nonlocalizing in up to 90% of patients [49], at variance with a study in patients with lesional OLE who underwent surgery, in whom ictal EEG provided a correct localization of the lesion in 13 out of 16 postsurgery seizure-free patients and in 5 out of 10 nonseizure-free patients [50]. Patients with OLE who have undergone intracranial EEG have shown a rapid propagation from the occipital lobe to the temporal lobe or even to the frontal lobe [51].

26.5 Parietal Lobe Epilepsies

Parietal lobe epilepsies (PLE) appear to be the least represented in surgical series; in fact, in the original report of the Montreal School, they did not exceed 5% of cases [52]. Parietal seizures are characterized by both objective and subjective manifestations. The most common subjective symptoms include paresthetic sensations (like tingling, skin numbness, itching), not always lateralized [53, 54]. Other symptoms can be disturbances of the body image, vertiginous sensations (due to the involvement of the temporal-parietal cortex), gustatory sensations (due to activation of the parietal operculum) [54], and inhibitory motor phenomena (appearing as focal atonic seizures). Ictal painful phenomena are rarely described, and they are thought to depend on the involvement of both cortico-thalamic circuits and primary and secondary sensory areas. Objective manifestations can be a language disturbance, in the case of the involvement of

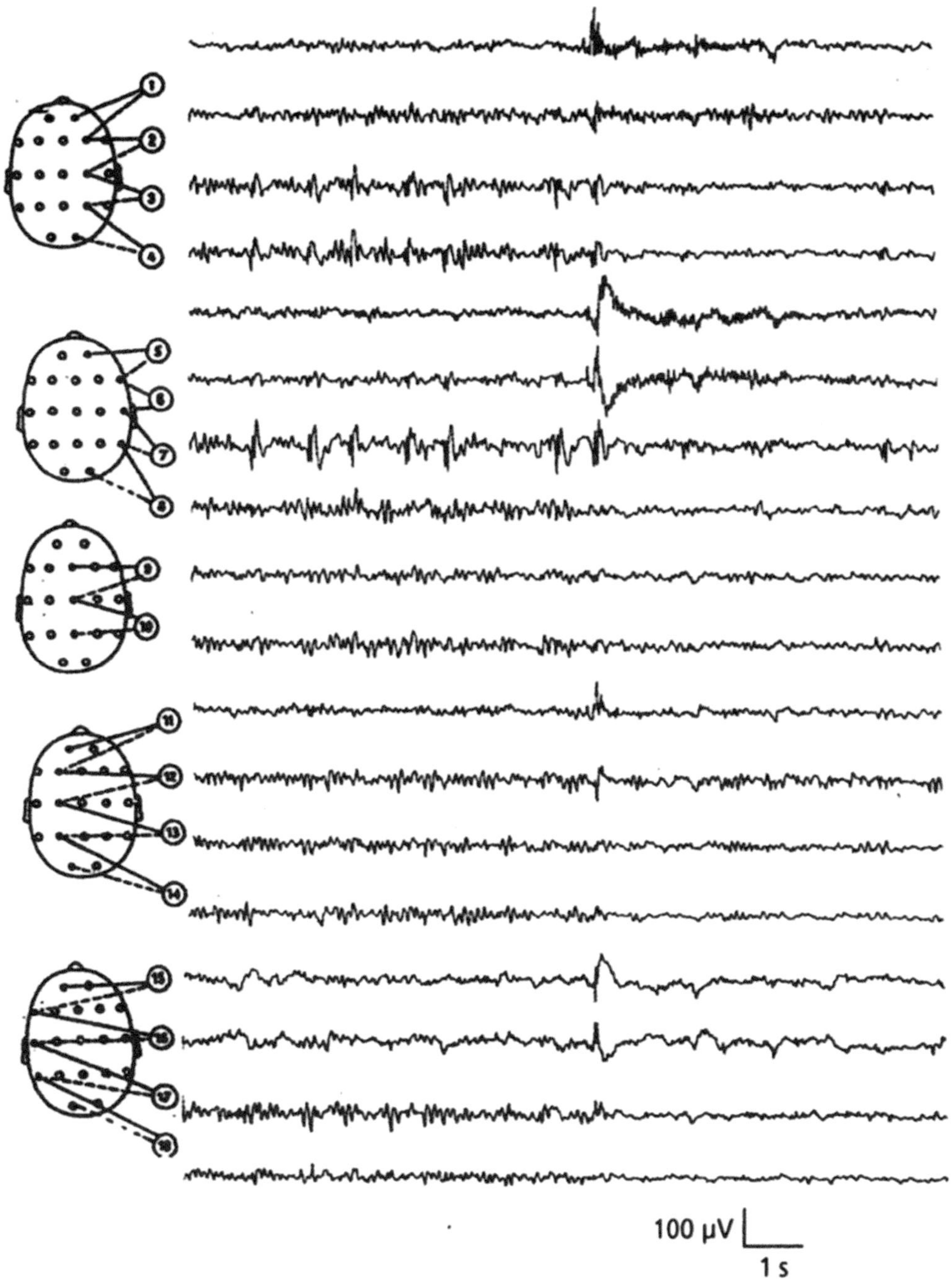

Fig. 26.9 Interictal EEG in a patient with cryptogenic occipital epilepsy with complex ictal visual hallucinatory manifestations in the left visual hemifield. The EEG shows spike- or polyspike-waves in the right posterior (temporo-parieto-occipital) quadrant, attenuated by eye opening

the antero-inferior parietal areas of the dominant hemisphere, or manifestations that depend on the cortical areas (frontal, temporal, occipital) in which the epileptic activity has propagated. In general, parietal seizures are followed by a brief postictal phase.

26.5.1 Interictal and Ictal EEG Features

Interictal epileptiform discharges in epilepsies originating within the posterior quadrant, including the parietal lobe, may be inconsistently observed, and some reports suggest that lateralized discharges are detected in less than 15% of cases [55]. When interictal/ictal EEGs are insufficient to determine the site of onset, correlation of the available EEG data with an eventual structural lesion demonstrated by neuroimaging methods and with ictal clinical manifestations can orient the diagnosis. When interictal epileptiform abnormalities are encountered in PLE, they are often bilateral, or they can be falsely localizing (often to the temporal region). Interictal epileptiform discharges can appear as spikes (Fig. 26.11) and/or slow waves; the morphology of the EEG abnormality can also be related to the type and extent of the underlying epileptogenic lesion. A sleep EEG can be helpful

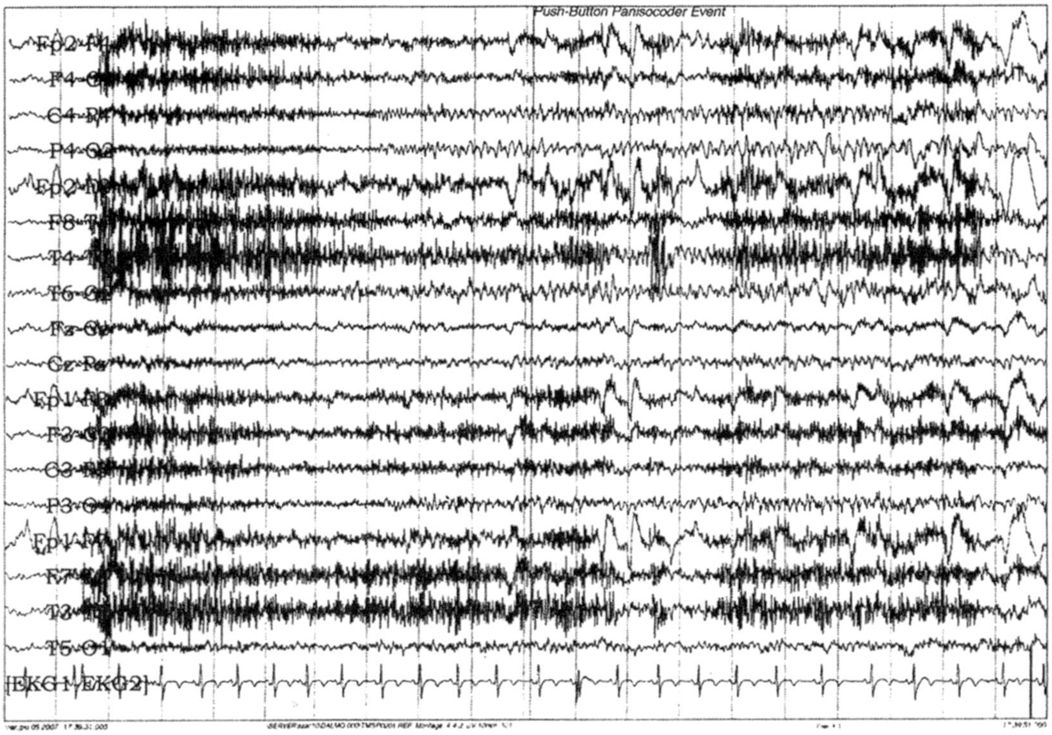

Fig. 26.10 Ictal EEG in a patient with right occipital epilepsy associated with right occipital dysplasia. The seizures are characterized by brief elementary visual hallucinations ("spots, luminous dots") in the left visual hemifield, without impairment of consciousness. The EEG shows a brief flattening in C4-P4 and P4-O2, followed by a brief discharge of low-voltage fast activity, followed by a rhythmic theta that remains confined in the right posterior derivations

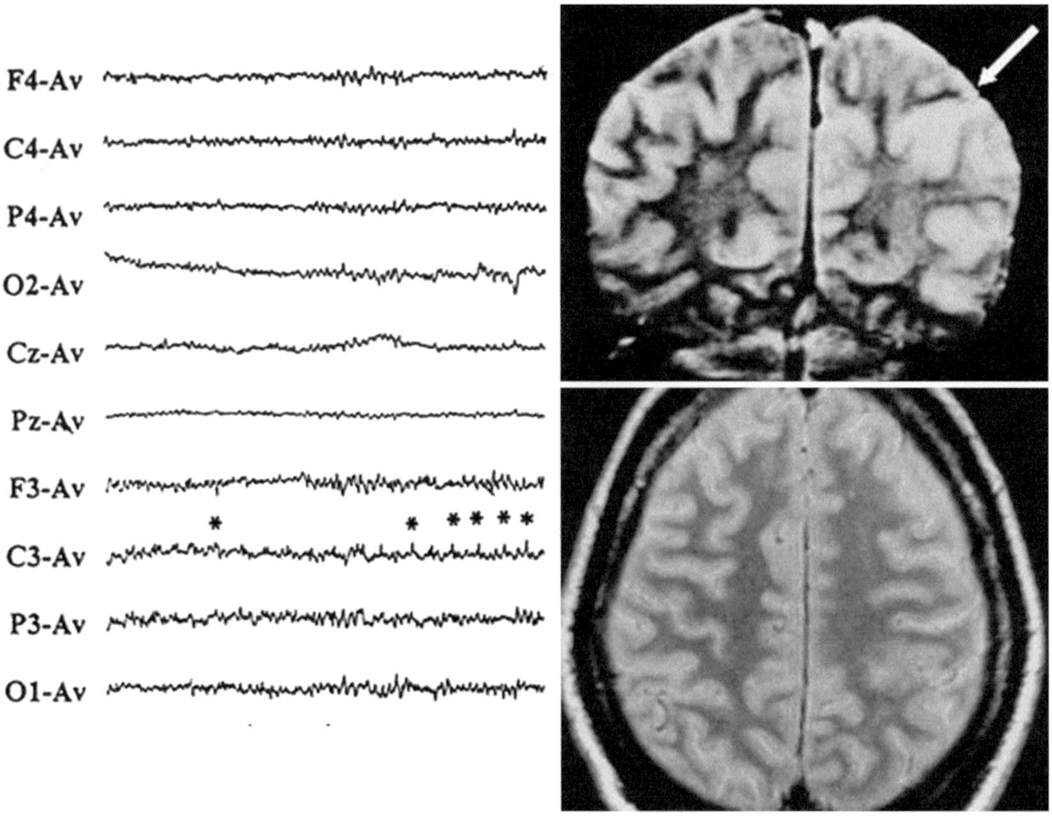

Fig. 26.11 Left panel: interictal EEG in a patient with drug-resistant focal epilepsy associated with left parietal focal cortical dysplasia. The EEG shows small amplitude spikes (asterisks) in the left central (C3) region. Right panel: coronal (above) and axial (below) MRI images showing a focal cortical dysplasia in the left parietal cortex

to detect epileptiform abnormalities and their location; in some instances, however, sleep may favor diffusion and bilateralization of the discharge. Less than 10% of ictal EEGs can provide localizing information; in this case, the EEG at seizure onset can show a focal low-voltage discharge.

26.6 Epilepsy with Gelastic Seizures

Epilepsy with gelastic seizures is a type of epilepsy in which the seizures are characterized by laughter as prominent sign (from the Greek word "gelastikos"). This epilepsy type is rare (0.1–0.2% of epilepsies in childhood), and it is slightly preponderant in males. Epilepsy onset can be at any age but most commonly occurs in the first 3–4 years of age. The seizures usually start with laughter, generally described as "empty," not amused, without emotional content; laughter appears suddenly, without any triggering factor. Patients may sometimes report a premonitory sensation, difficult to describe. Laughter is of short duration (less than 1 min), and it is followed by impairment of consciousness, lateral movements of the head or eyes, and gestural and sometimes oro-alimentary automatisms (such as lip smacking). The duration of the seizures can vary from a few seconds to a few minutes. Patients, especially those in pediatric age, may present other types of ictal phenomena such as abrupt atonic phenomena (appearing as "drop attacks") or clear convulsive manifestations. Such manifestations may also occur independently from gelastic seizures, as an additional seizure type [56].

From the pathophysiological point of view, gelastic seizures are related to the involvement of the hypothalamic structures, the temporal regions, or the frontal areas. Hypothalamic tumors, usually a hamartoma or an astrocytoma, both of which are slow-growing lesions, are relatively common causes of gelastic epilepsy. The association "epilepsy with gelastic seizures with hypothalamic hamartoma" is often characterized by the occurrence of precocious puberty (generally before the age of 10 years). In adolescence, learning and behavioral disorders may also appear, and they may worsen during the course of the disease [56, 57].

A correct diagnosis requires an accurate description of the episodes that excludes also that sudden and inappropriate laughter is not due to behavioral or emotional disorder problems. Video-EEG recording of the seizures can be extremely useful for the recognition of this condition.

EEG may show focal or generalized abnormalities such as spikes, sharp waves, or slow spike-waves [57]. Brain MRI is crucial to detect small lesions, especially when they are located in the hypothalamus.

Epilepsy with gelastic seizures can be refractory to antiepileptic drugs. A surgical or radiotherapeutic approach can be considered in cases with a hypothalamic lesion. The treatment of precocious puberty is carried out by hormonal therapy. Behavioral or learning disorders show poor response to medical therapy, whereas improvement after surgical or radiotherapy treatment of hypothalamic hamartoma can be observed. In general, a surgical treatment of the hypothalamic lesion is associated, both in children and adults, with the best prognosis for the seizures and for the cognitive-behavioral disorders.

26.7 Rasmussen's Syndrome

Rasmussen's syndrome is a rare disease (one to two cases per million) that is caused by a progressive inflammatory process that begins in a circumscribed area of the cerebral cortex and then spreads to neighboring areas of the same hemisphere and eventually, during the evolution, contralaterally [58]. As a consequence of the inflammatory process, a progressive neuronal depletion associated with gliosis occurs, which clinically results in the appearance of neurological deficits. Although Rasmussen's syndrome is diagnosed in children before 10 years of age, cases with onset in juvenile or adult age have also been reported [58]. The clinical manifestations are related to the cortical areas that are affected by the inflammatory process. During the evolution of the disease, the neuroinflammatory pathology progressively extends to other cortical areas worsening the neurological picture. A typical evolution is the progression of the inflammation to involve a whole hemisphere (Fig. 26.12), although the speed of progression may differ from patient to patient, varying from a few weeks or months to several years. The slower modality of progression seems to affect adolescents or adults [59]. Typical clinical manifestations are [58, 59]:

- Epilepsy: generally epileptic seizures are the first manifestation of the disease. Focal motor seizures are observed when the motor cortex is affected, and the ictal motor manifestations can occur (sub)continuously, resulting in epilepsia partialis continua. In case of involvement of the temporal lobe, the patient can present with temporal lobe seizures with impairment of consciousness. The epileptic discharge can also spread homo- and contralaterally, evolving eventually to a secondary generalization. With the progression of the disease, seizures become more frequent, more intense, and less responsive to antiepileptic treatment.
- Neurological deficits. The most frequent are (a) hemiparesis with possible sensory deficits, in case of involvement of the motor cortex and of the adjacent somatosensory cortex; (b) hemianopia when the visual areas of one hemisphere are affected; (c) language disorders resulting from

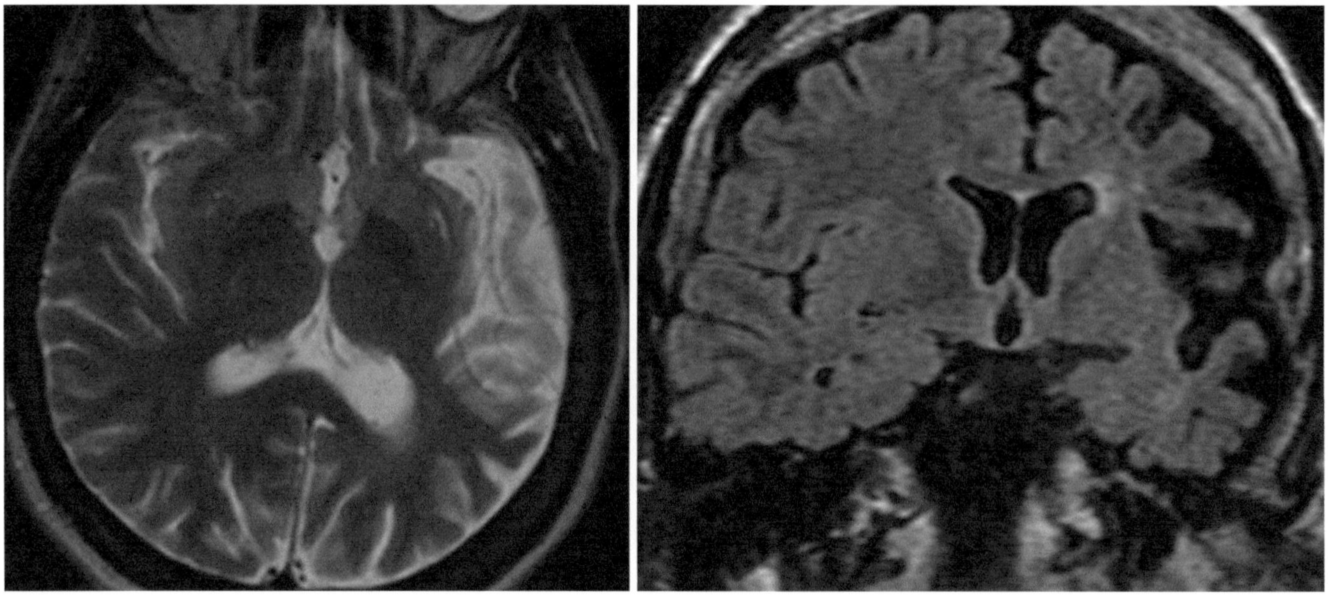

Fig. 26.12 Brain MRI in a patient with Rasmussen's syndrome showing a marked atrophy of the left hemisphere

the involvement of language areas; and (d) memory disorders and cognitive impairment.

From the pathophysiological point of view, an autoimmune process underlies Rasmussen's syndrome, although in most cases it is not possible to identify the agent or the event that has triggered the abnormal immune response.

The EEG picture can vary accordingly to the stage of the disease. In general, an asymmetry of electrogenesis with slowing or irregularity of the background activity in the affected side is observed. Initially the epileptiform interictal abnormalities are focal, and then, during the course of the disease, they tend to spread to both hemispheres (Fig. 26.13). With the evolution of the clinical picture, multifocal epileptiform activities located in the same hemisphere, and, sometimes, bisynchronous paroxysmal discharges appear. In the advanced stages of Rasmussen's syndrome, the ictal EEG can show a unilateral localization, although with multifocal onset.

Neuroimaging studies can provide essential elements for diagnosis. In particular, brain MRI can demonstrate the progression of brain damage, toward a marked brain hemiatrophy.

The treatment aims to contrast the ongoing autoimmune process, by using steroids, immunosuppressants, immunoglobulins, and plasmapheresis, sometimes in association and for long periods of time. Generally an early treatment achieves better results; however, considering the potential side effects of these treatments, careful monitoring is necessary, particularly in the pediatric age. Unfortunately, antiepileptic therapy, often with multiple drugs in combination, is not able to control seizures completely. The surgical removal or disconnection of extensive cortical areas and sometimes of an entire hemisphere can be an alternative treatment option that can lead to better seizure control and that can stop the progression of the disease. The extension of the surgical exeresis depends on the duration, on the rapidity of the evolution and extension of the brain damage, on the age of the patient, and on the neurological status.

26.8 Conclusions

In this chapter we have outlined the main clinical and EEG features of focal epilepsies classified according to localization criteria. Indeed, a standard scalp EEG is still the most useful and easily available test when evaluating focal epilepsies, either for the diagnosis or for the management of the patient in the follow-up. When standard EEG recordings with activation methods are unrevealing, the employment of additional methods of EEG recordings, such as sleep EEG, can enhance its capability of capturing an abnormality, or when the clinico-EEG correlations are necessary, long-term video-EEG can provide essential information for the diagnosis, for classification purposes, and eventually for treatment decisions, in particular when the surgical treatment is an option. More sophisticated methods for EEG recording and analysis, such as source localization and high-density EEG, complemented with multimodal imaging methods, have renewed the interest in EEG, and they will further expand the amount of information on the functioning of the brain that this "old" technique can offer to us.

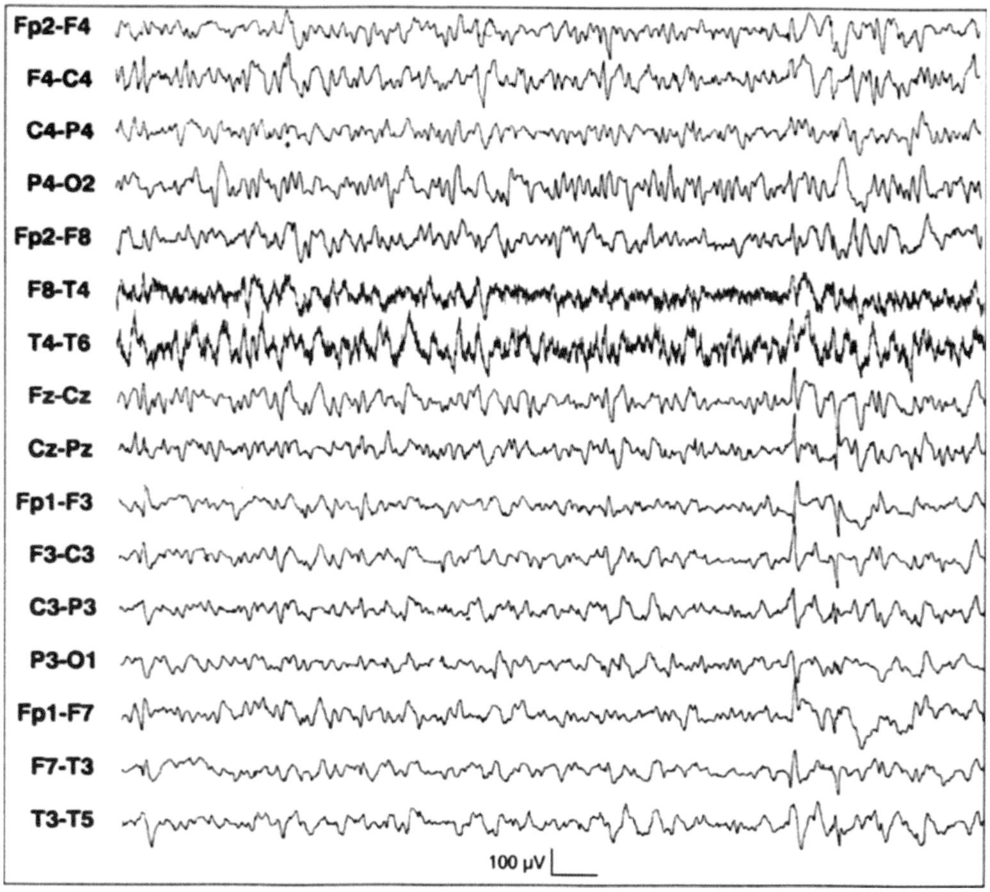

Fig. 26.13 Same patient as in Fig. 26.12. The interictal EEG shows a generalized slowing of the background activity with abundant irregular theta-delta abnormalities intermixed, clearly predominant in the left hemisphere where occasional high amplitude spikes are observed. Time scale: 1 s

References

1. Blume WT, Luders HO, Mizrahi E, Tassinari CA, van Emde Boas W, Engel J. Glossary of descriptive terminology for ictal semiology: report of the ILAE Task Force on Classification and Terminology. Epilepsia. 2001;42(9):1212–8.
2. Fisher RS, Cross JH, French JA, Higurashi N, Hirsch E, Jansen FE, et al. Operational classification of seizures types by the International League Against Epilepsy: Position paper of the ILAE Commission for Classification and Terminology. Epilepsia. 2017;58:522–30.
3. Scheffer IE, Berkovic S, Capovilla G, Connolly MB, French J, Guilhoto L, et al. ILAE classification of the epilepsies: position paper of the ILAE Commission for Classification and Terminology. Epilepsia. 2017;58:512–21.
4. Michelucci R., Rubboli G., Tinuper P. L'EEG nelle epilessie. Atlante interattivo. Lega Italiana Contro l'Epilessia. QBGroup; 2007.
5. Tatum WO, Rubboli G, Kaplan PW, Mirsatari SM, Radhakrishnan K, Gloss D, et al. Clinical utility of EEG in diagnosing and monitoring epilepsy in adults. Clin Neurophysiol. 2018;129:1056–82.
6. Williamson PD, Engel J. Anatomic classification of focal epilepsies. In: Engel J, Redley TA, editors. Epilepsy. A comprehensive textbook. 2nd ed. Philadelphia: Wolters Kluwer; Lippincott, Williams & Wilkins; 2008. p. 2465–77.
7. Falconer MA, Serafetinides EA, Corsellis JA. Etiology and pathogenesis of temporal lobe epilepsy. Arch Neurol. 1964;10:233–48.
8. Schramm J, Kral T, Grunwald T, Blumcke I. Surgical treatment for neocortical temporal lobe epilepsy: clinical and surgical aspects and seizure outcome. J Neurosurg. 2001;94:33–42.
9. Hamelin S, Depaulis A. Revisiting hippocampal sclerosis in mesial temporal lobe epilepsy according to the "two-hit" hypothesis. Rev Neurol (Paris). 2015;171(3):227–35.
10. Baulac M. MTLE with hippocampal sclerosis in adult as a syndrome. Rev Neurol. 2015;171:259–66.
11. Dericioglu N, Colpak AI, Ciger A, Saygi S. The yield of preoperative sequential routine scalp EEGs in patients who underwent anterior temporal lobectomy for mesial temporal sclerosis. Clin EEG Neurosci. 2010;41:166–9.
12. Williamson P, French JA, Thadani VM, et al. Characteristics of medial temporal lobe epilepsy II. Interictal and ictal scalp electroencephalography, neuropsychological testing, neuroimaging, surgical results and pathology. Ann Neurol. 1993;34:781–7.
13. Tatum WO. Mesial temporal lobe epilepsy. J Clin Neurophysiol. 2012;29:356–65.
14. Ebersole JS, Pacia S. Localization of temporal lobe foci by ictal EEG patterns. Epilepsia. 1996;37:386–99.
15. Rubboli G, Bisulli F, Michelucci R, et al. Sudden falls due to seizure-induced cardiac asystole in drug-resistant focal epilepsy. Neurology. 2008;70:1933–5.
16. Wieser HG. Semiology of neocortical temporal lobe epilepsy. In: Williamson PD, Siegel AM, Roberts DW, Thadani VM, Gazzaniga MS, editors. Neocortical epilepsies, Advances in neurology, vol. 84. Philadelphia: Lippincott Williams & Wilkins; 2000. p. 201–14.
17. Michelucci R, Poza JJ, Sofia V, de Feo MR, Binelli S, Bisulli F. Autosomal dominant lateral temporal epilepsy: clinical spectrum, new epitempin mutations, and genetic heterogeneity in seven European families. Epilepsia. 2003;44:1289–97.

18. Ottman R, Risch N, Hauser WA, Pedley TA, Lee JH, Barker-Cummings C, et al. Localization of a gene for partial epilepsy to chromosome 10q. Nat Genet. 1995;10:56–60.
19. Kalachikov S, Evgrafov O, Ross B, Winawer M, Barker-Cummings C, Martinelli Boneschi F, et al. Mutations in LGI1 cause autosomal-dominant partial epilepsy with auditory features. Nat Genet. 2002;30:335–41.
20. Morante-Redolat JM, Gorostidi-Pagola A, Piquer-Sirerol S, Sáenz A, Poza JJ, Galán J, et al. Mutations in the LGI1/Epitempin gene on 10q24 cause autosomal dominant lateral temporal epilepsy. Hum Mol Genet. 2002;11:1119–28.
21. Dazzo E, Fanciulli M, Serioli E, Minervini G, Pulitano P, Binelli S, et al. Heterozygous reelin mutations cause autosomal-dominant lateral temporal epilepsy. Am J Hum Genet. 2015;96:992–1000.
22. Dazzo E, Rehberg K, Michelucci R, Passarelli D, Boniver C, Vianello Dri V, et al. Mutations in MICAL-1cause autosomal-dominant lateral temporal epilepsy. Ann Neurol. 2018;83:483–93.
23. Michelucci R, Pulitano P, Di Bonaventura C, Binelli S, Luisi C, Pasini E, et al. The clinical phenotype of autosomal dominant lateral temporal lobe epilepsy related to reelin mutations. Epilepsy Behav. 2017;68:103–7.
24. Williamson PD, Spencer DD, Spencer SS, Novelly RS, Mattson RH. Complex partial seizures of frontal lobe origin. Ann Neurol. 1985;18:497–504.
25. Tinuper P, Bisulli F, Cross JH, Hesdorffer D, Kahane P, Nobili L, et al. Definition and diagnostic criteria of sleep-related hypermotor epilepsy. Neurology. 2016;86:1834–42.
26. Provini F, Plazzi G, Tinuper P, Vandi S, Lugaresi E, Montagna P. Nocturnal frontal lobe epilepsy. A clinical and polygraphic overview of 100 consecutive cases. Brain. 1999;122:1017–31.
27. Luders HO. Supplementary sensorimotor area. Philadelphia: Lippincott Raven; 1996.
28. Nobili L, Cossu M, Mai R, et al. Sleep-related hyperkinetic seizures of temporal lobe origin. Neurology. 2004;62(3):482–5.
29. Gardella E, Rubboli G, Tassinari CA. Ictal grasping: prevalence and characteristics in seizures with different semiology. Epilepsia. 2006;47(Suppl 5):59–63.
30. Tassinari CA, Rubboli G, Gardella E, et al. Central pattern generators for a common semiology in fronto-limbic seizures and in parasomnias. A neuroethologic approach. Neurol Sci. 2005;26(Suppl 3):s225–32.
31. Tassinari CA, Cantalupo G, Högl B, Cortelli P, Tassi L, Francione S, et al. Neuroethological approach to frontolimbic epileptic seizures and parasomnias: the same central pattern generators for the same behaviours. Rev Neurol. 2009;165:762–8.
32. Verma A, Radtke R. EEG of partial seizures. J Clin Neurophysiol. 2006;23:333–9.
33. Foldvary N, Klem G, Hammel J, Bingaman W, Najm I, Luders H. The localizing value of ictal EEG in focal epilepsy. Neurology. 2001;57:2022–8.
34. Beleza P, Bilgin O, Noachtar S. Interictal rhythmical midline theta differentiates frontal from temporal lobe epilepsies. Epilepsia. 2009;50:550–5.
35. Whitehead K, Gollwitzer S, Millward H, Wehner T, Scott C, Diehl B. The additional lateralizing and localizing value of the postictal EEG in frontal lobe epilepsy. Clin Neurophysiol. 2016;127:1774–80.
36. Di Gennaro G, De Risi M, Quarato PP, Sparano A, Mascia A, Grammaldo LG, et al. Prognostic significance of serial postoperative EEG in extratemporal lobe epilepsy surgery. Clin Neurophysiol. 2012;123:2346–51.
37. Blume WT, Pillay N. Electrographic and clinical correlates of secondary bilateral synchrony. Epilepsia. 1985;26:636–41.
38. Liava A, Francione S, Tassi L, Lo Russo G, Cossu M, Mai R, et al. Individually tailored extratemporal epilepsy surgery in children: anatomo-electro-clinical features and outcome predictors in a population of 53 cases. Epilepsy Behav. 2012;25:68–80.
39. Worrell GA, So EL, Kazemi J, O'Brien TJ, Mosewich RK, Cascino GD, et al. Focal ictal beta discharge on scalp EEG predicts excellent outcome of frontal lobe epilepsy surgery. Epilepsia. 2002;43:277–82.
40. Zakaria T, Noe K, So E, Cascino GD, Wetjen N, Van Gompel JJ, et al. Scalp and intracranial EEG in medically intractable extratemporal epilepsy with normal MRI. ISRN Neurol. 2012; https://doi.org/10.5402/2012/942849.
41. Bautista RE, Spencer DD, Spencer SS. EEG findings in frontal lobe epilepsies. Neurology. 1998;50:1765–71.
42. Vadlamudi L, So EL, Worrell GA, Mosewich RK, Cascino GD, Meyer FB, et al. Factors underlying scalp-EEG interictal epileptiform discharges in intractable frontal lobe epilepsy. Epileptic Disord. 2004;6:89–95.
43. Janszky J, Jokeit H, Schulz R, Hoppe M, Ebner A. EEG predicts surgical outcome in lesional frontal lobe epilepsy. Neurology. 2000;54:1470–6.
44. Jeha LE, Najm I, Bingaman W, Dinner D, Widdess-Walsh P, Luders H. Surgical outcome and prognostic factors of frontal lobe epilepsy surgery. Brain. 2007;130:574–84.
45. Ferrier CH, Engelsman J, Alarcon G, Binnie CD, Polkey CE. Prognostic factors in presurgical assessment of frontal lobe epilepsy. J Neurol Neurosurg Psychiatry. 1999;66:350–6.
46. Blume WT, Wiebe S. Occipital lobe epilepsies. In: Williamson PD, Siegel AM, Roberts DW, Thadani VM, Cazzaniga MS, editors. Neocortical epilepsies, Advances in neurology, vol. 84. Philadelphia: Lippincott Williams and Wilkins; 2000. p. 173–87.
47. Usui N, Mihara T, Baba K, Matsuda K, Tottori T, Umeoka S, et al. Early seizure propagation from the occipital lobe to medial temporal structures and its surgical implication. Epileptic Disord. 2008a;10:260–5.
48. Williamson PD, Thadani VM, Darcey TM, Spencer DD, Spencer SS, Mattson RH. Occipital lobe epilepsy: clinical characteristics, seizure spread patterns, and results of surgery. Ann Neurol. 1992;31:3–13.
49. Lee SK, Kim JY, Hong KS, Nam HW, Park SH, Chung CK. The clinical usefulness of ictal surface EEG in neocortical epilepsy. Epilepsia. 2000;41:1450–5.
50. Kun Lee S, Young Lee S, Kim DW, Soo Lee D, Chung CK. Occipital lobe epilepsy: clinical characteristics, surgical outcome, and role of diagnostic modalities. Epilepsia. 2005;46:688–95.
51. Usui N, Mihara T, Baba K, Matsuda K, Tottori T, Umeoka S, et al. Posterior cortex epilepsy secondary to ulegyria: is it a surgically remediable syndrome? Epilepsia. 2008b;49:1998–2007.
52. Rasmussen T. Cortical resection in the treatment of focal epilepsy. In: Purpura DP, Penry JK, Walter RD, editors. Neurosurgical management of the epilepsies. New York: Raven Press; 1975. p. 139–54.
53. Siegel AM, Williamson PD. Parietal lobe epilepsy. In: Williamson PD, Siegel AM, Roberts DW, Thadani VM, Cazzaniga MS, editors. Neocortical epilepsies, Advances in neurology, vol. 84. Philadelphia: Lippincott Williams and Wilkins; 2000.
54. Sveinbjornsdottir S, Duncan JS. Parietal and occipital lobe epilepsy: a review. Epilepsia. 1993;34:493–521.
55. Salanova V, Andermann F, Rasmussen T, Olivier A, Quesney LF. Parietal lobe epilepsy. Clinical manifestations and outcome in 82 patients treated surgically between 1929 and 1988. Brain. 1995;118:607–27.
56. Striano S, Striano P, Sarappa P, Boccella C. The clinical spectrum and natural history of gelastic epilepsy-hypothalamic hamartoma syndrome. Seizure. 2005 Jun;14(4):232.
57. Harvey AS, Freeman JL. Epilepsy in hypothalamic hamartoma: clinical and EEG features. Semin Pediatr Neurol. 2007;14(2):60–4.
58. Dubeau F, Andermann F, Wiendl H, Amit B-O. Rasmussens's encephalitis (chronic focal encephalitis). In: Engel J, Pedley T, editors. Epilepsy: a comprehensive textbook. Philadelphia: Lippincott Williams and Wilkins; 2008. p. 2439–53.
59. Hart Y, Andermann F. Rasmussen's syndrome. In: Roger J, et al., editors. Epileptic syndromes in infancy, childhood and adolescence. 4th ed. Montrouge: John Libbey Eurotext Ltd; 2005. p. 537–54.

Genetic Generalized Epilepsies

27

Aglaia Vignoli and Maria Paola Canevini

Genetic generalized epilepsies (GGE) are a cluster of epilepsy syndromes, diagnosed and classified according to clinical features and electroencephalographic (EEG) characteristics, the etiology has a known or presumed genetic defect, and seizures are the core symptom of the disorder.

Since hereditary predisposition seems to be the only identified cause of GGE, the ILAE Task Force on Classification has recently suggested to remove the term "idiopathic" from the International Classification and to replace it with the term "genetic," due to increasing recognition and discovery of the genes involved in many of these epilepsies, including those with monogenic (with inherited or de novo pathogenic variants) or complex (polygenic with or without environmental factors) inheritance [1].

The majority of GGE individuals are reported as sporadic, with no family history [2]. Indeed, this is consistent with complex inheritance believed to underlie GGE, so that different genetic mechanisms such as polygenic transmission, multifactorial etiology, and other factors have been encompassed. Mutated DNA sequences in genes encoding for ion channels or neurotransmitter receptors have been identified in GGE, but genotype-phenotype correlations are poor, arguing for additional factors determining the effect of a genetic predisposition, such as epigenetic factors [3].

In addition, several copy-number variants (CNVs) have been discovered to be associated to generalized epilepsies as risk alleles. The most frequently identified CNVs, each found in approximately 1% of GGE, are 15q13.3, 15q11.2, and 16p13.11 [4].

These syndromes, accounting for 15–20% of all epilepsies, are defined by an age-related onset and specific clinical features [5]. The most common electro-clinical syndromes recognized by the International League Against Epilepsy (ILAE) [1] are childhood absence epilepsy (CAE), juvenile absence epilepsy (JAE), juvenile myoclonic epilepsy (JME), and generalized tonic-clonic seizures alone (GTCSa).

According to the current ILAE definition [1], GGE patients are required to be intellectually unimpaired, with standard magnetic resonance imaging (MRI) of the brain showing no abnormalities. Structural differences between GGE and healthy controls were observed only with volume detection techniques (reductions in whole brain and in other areas (especially in the thalamus-cortical networks)) [6].

The defining EEG characteristic of GGE is typical generalized, bisynchronous, and symmetric activity with spike-wave (SW) or polyspike-wave (PSW) discharges.

EEG research has focused on the origin of generalized SW discharges, as they remain a core sign of GGE. Many studies support the corticoreticular theory proposed by Gloor [7], which indicates that these generalized SWs could be generated by an interplay between the thalamus and a hyperexcitable cortex. Studies on animal models began to support the cortical focus theory [8, 9]. Recently, several EEG-functional MRI (fMRI) studies, EEG source analysis, MEG, PET, and TMS have suggested that generalized SW discharges and seizures have cortical onset and the thalamus has an essential role in the recruitment of the network comprising determine an activation in the frontal, parietal and occipital cortex and the default-mode network [10]. The involvement of thalamus-cortical networks, including frontal cortex, putamen, amygdala, and supplementary motor area (SMA), has been also demonstrated by functional connectivity studies [11, 12].

The diagnosis of GGE is based on clinical and EEG findings. The clinical criteria are:

– Seizure types: typical absences (TAs), myoclonic and generalized tonic-clonic seizures (GTCS) alone or in combination.

Electronic Supplementary Material The online version of this chapter (https://doi.org/10.1007/978-3-030-04573-9_27) contains supplementary material, which is available to authorized users.

A. Vignoli (✉) · M. P. Canevini
Department of Health Sciences, Epilepsy Center—Child and Adolescent Neurology and Psychiatry, University of Milan, Milan, Italy
e-mail: aglaia.vignoli@unimi.it

O. Mecarelli (ed.), *Clinical Electroencephalography*, https://doi.org/10.1007/978-3-030-04573-9_27

- No etiologic factor could be found with the exception of genetic predisposition.

Besides, EEG criteria of GGEs are the following [13]:

- Normal background activity.
- Normal sleep organization with bilateral and symmetrical sleep patterns.
- Presence of interictal abnormalities such as generalized spikes, or polyspikes, generalized SW and PSW discharges at 3 Hz, or more.
- Increase of interictal abnormalities in slow sleep and no abnormalities during rapid eye movement sleep.
- Ictal discharges are generalized at their onset, bilateral, symmetrical, and synchronous.

In some clinical conditions, these criteria will not strictly apply:

- The background activity will be markedly slowed in the wake of a GTCS; such slowing may be found hours and in some cases days after the seizure.
- The ictal and interictal abnormalities are usually of higher voltage over the frontal and vertex areas; sometimes they can be slightly asymmetrical; however, whenever the discharges are irregular in their morphology or in their frequency, or are slower than 2.5 Hz, or constantly asymmetrical, the diagnosis of GGE must be reappraised.

Photosensitivity is not one of the core features of the syndrome; however during EEG, 20–30% of patients could present a photoparoxystic response, especially when at younger age and in the absence of therapy [14].

In adult patients interictal abnormalities may show an irregular morphology. Nonlocalizing abnormalities may occur, usually spikes over the fronto-central areas [13].

The occurrence of focal discharges constantly recorded in the same region should make the suspicion of a structural abnormality, as well as the hemispheric predominance of the discharges or its fragmentation during the evolution of the seizure.

The first EEG, ideally with video recording and performed before starting treatment, should be sufficiently long and include more than one hyperventilation (HV) session if needed. Sleep EEG recording should be recommended, and partial sleep deprivation the night before almost guarantees the natural occurrence of sleep and contributes to maximal activation in combination with the effects of drowsiness and light sleep, and of HV and intermittent photic stimulation (IPS), after provoked awakening. Basic EMG recording should be always required, with at least bilateral deltoid muscles and pneumogram, in order to demonstrate hesitation or interruption in breath effort and myoclonic jerks. All recordings should be individualized according to clinical information/questions [15].

27.1 Childhood Absence Epilepsy (CAE)

CAE is the most common type of childhood-onset epilepsy syndrome, occurring in neurologically normal children, between the age of 4 and 10 years, with a peak at 5–7 years. Girls are affected greater than boys [16]. Pathogenic variants of SLC2A1 leading to autosomal dominant GLUT1 deficiency account for up to 1% of cases, increasing to 10% of those with absence seizures starting before the age of 4 years [5].

The hallmark of the syndrome is the presence of TAs, characterized by sudden arrest of voluntary activities, although semi-voluntary preictal behaviors may persist for a few seconds after seizure onset. TAs usually last for 10–20 s and are typically associated with severe loss responsiveness. Staring or upward drifted eyes, with eyelid blinking, are common features. TAs may be associated with oroalimentary, gestural, or speech automatisms that are related to the duration of seizures, being present in up to 95% of those longer than 16 s [17]. Clonic movements of the eyelids or face, head turning, autonomic changes, and reduction of muscle tone can occur but are mild and do not persist throughout the seizure. TAs may be interrupted by sudden auditory stimuli (calling a child's name or clapping of hands). Offset is also sudden with resumption of the preictal activities as though the latter were never interrupted. There are no postictal symptoms [15].

GTCS are not expected early in the active absence phase. Their early occurrence may indicate a poor prognosis [18–20].

27.1.1 EEG Features

Background EEG activity is normal for age. In 13–20% of children with TAs, an occipital intermittent rhythmic delta activity (around 3 Hz) [21] (Fig. 27.1) can occur, which enhances with HV and sometimes evolves into the generalized SW discharges associated. This hallmark is related to a good prognosis, according to Loiseau [22].

The characteristic feature of the interictal and ictal EEG is a 3–4 Hz generalized symmetric SW discharge. Onset is bilateral synchronous, but regional (usually frontal or occipital), bilateral, or lateralized onsets are not infrequent, without a constant side in the same or subsequent recordings.

Centro-temporal spikes and waves similar to those usually recorded in children with benign epilepsy with centro-temporal spikes have been reported by Dalla Bernardina et al. in 14% of 119 children with TAs [23].

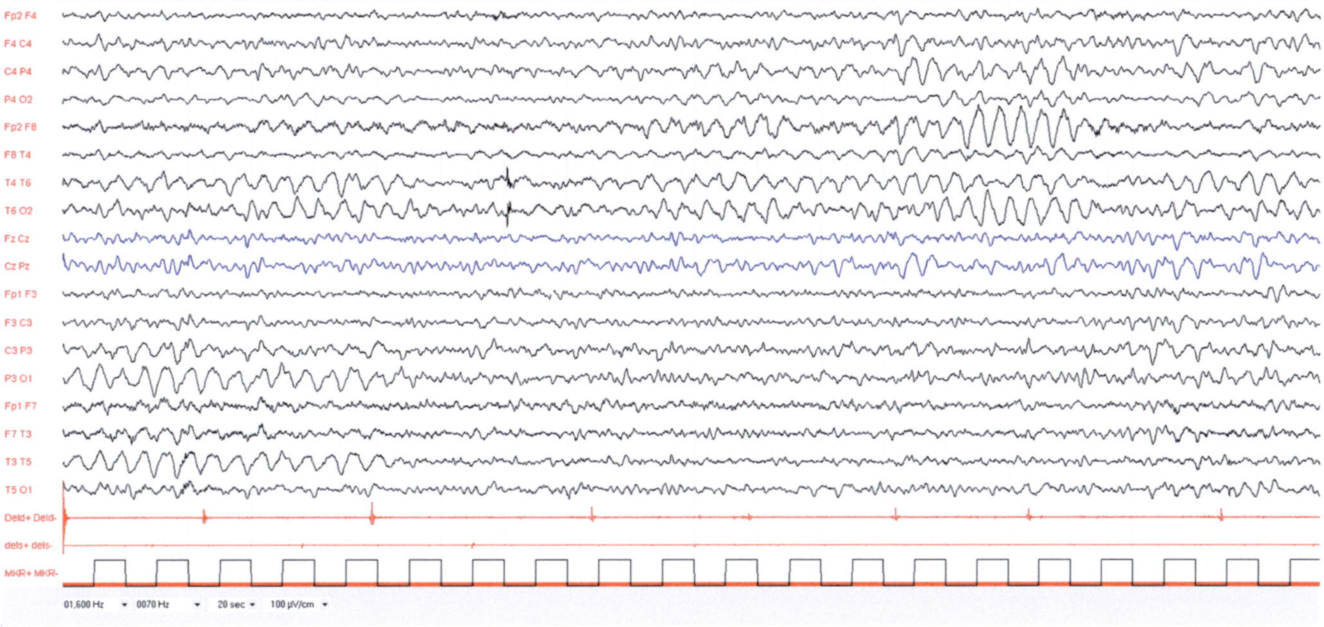

Fig. 27.1 Occurrence of trains of delta activity over the posterior region of both hemispheres, independently, in a 7-year-old girl with CAE

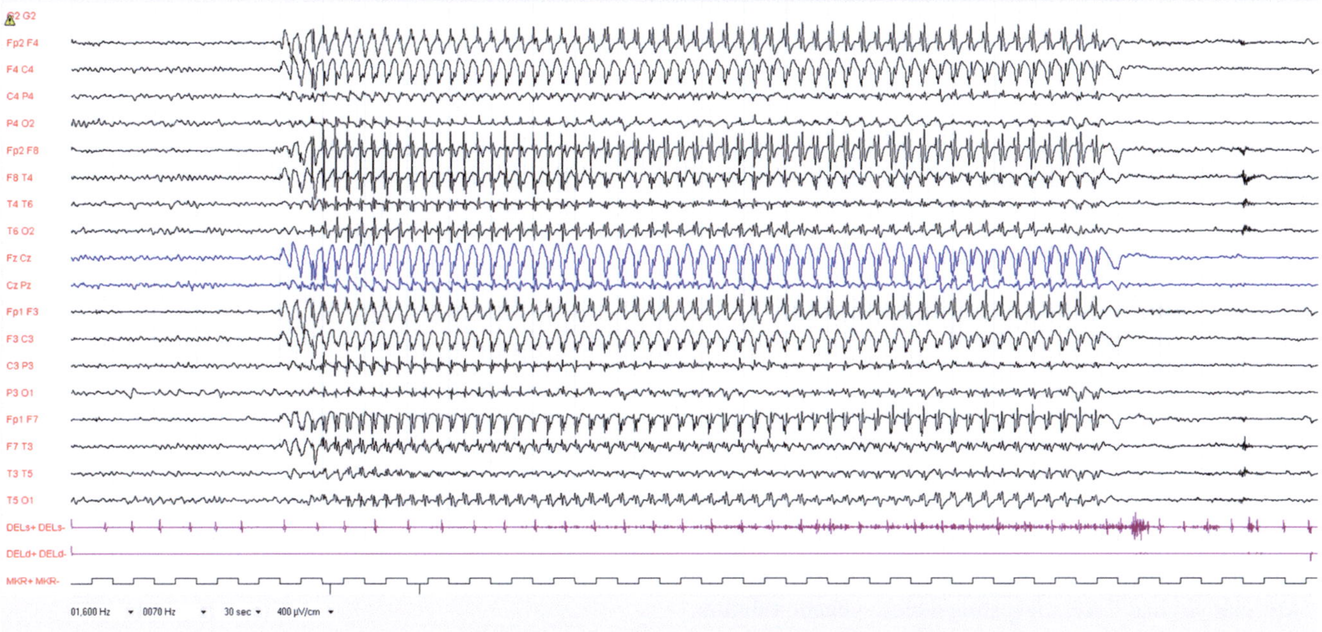

Fig. 27.2 Ictal recording of a typical absence seizure in a 5-year-old boy: 3 Hz spike and wave discharge lasts up to 20 s. Note the abrupt onset and end of the discharge. The boy does not answer to the acoustic stimulus (MRK) produced by the technician

In untreated children with CAE, absences are expected to occur during or immediately after HV. HV should be performed twice or more if the diagnostic suspicion of CAE is high.

Even though IPS can provoke TAs, nevertheless, when TAs are constantly related to IPS or specific visual patterns, CAE diagnosis cannot be performed [24, 25].

Sleep recordings show normal organization; paroxysmal discharges increase in frequency in NREM sleep (stages 2 and 3). Generalized SW discharges during drowsiness and sleep may be more frequent and brief than in wakefulness and may acquire a clear polyspike component, although less than in juvenile myoclonic epilepsy (JME).

Focal discharges may become more apparent during sleep [15].

EEG features of absence in CAE are shown in Figs. 27.2 and 27.3.

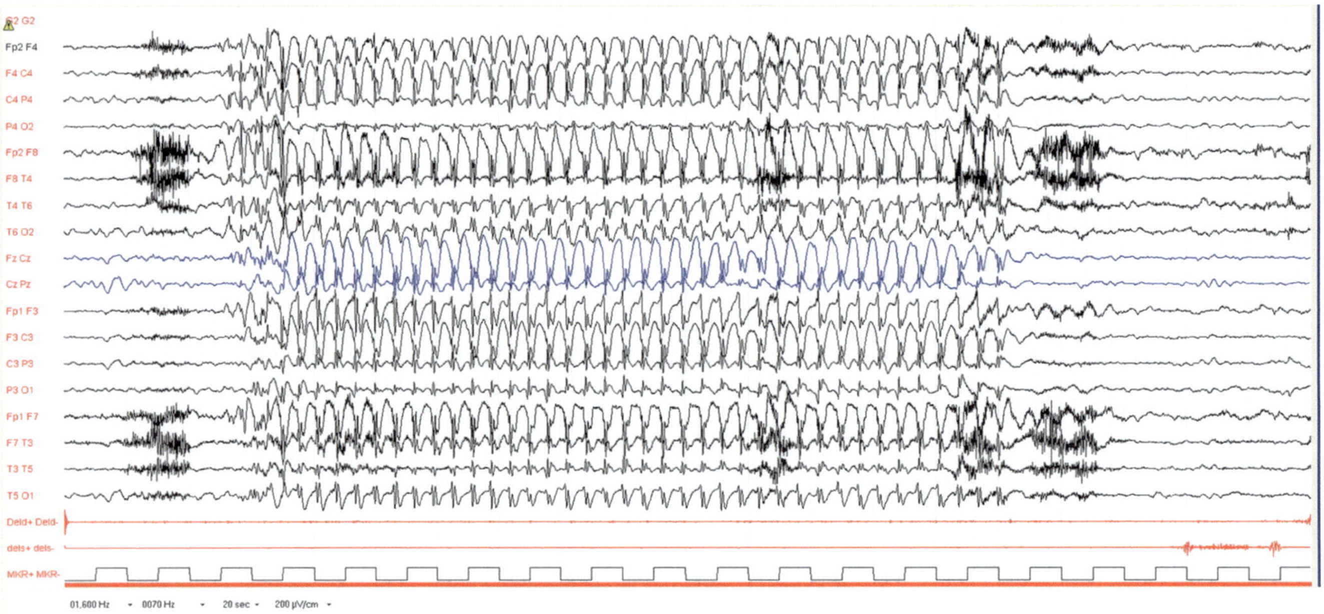

Fig. 27.3 Typical absence in an 8-year-old girl with CAE: the 3 Hz spike and wave discharge is preceded by bilateral spikes over the frontal regions

When absences continue in adulthood, generalized SW discharges tend to become irregular in their morphology, and, even when patients are correctly tested during the seizure, a complete loss of awareness cannot be clearly demonstrated. Adult patients with TAs generally report a sensation of dizziness or a vague woolliness in relation to the ictal event.

27.2 Juvenile Absence Epilepsy (JAE)

Age of seizure onset is usually around puberty (range 10–17 years with a peak at 10–12 years) [22]. Compared to CAE and JME, where a female preponderance is widely accepted, there are no sex difference in JAE [26].

A family history is frequent. Marini et al. [27] found a low phenotypic concordance within families with JAE (10%) compared to other GGE syndromes. Thirty-one percent of JAE relatives had CAE suggesting a close genetic relation.

The absences in JAE show the same characteristics of absences in CAE, but absences with retropulsive movements are less common, and often loss of consciousness is less pronounced than in CAE. The seizure frequency is lower than in CAE, with clinical absences occurring less frequently than every day, mostly sporadically. Clusters of absences at awakening are a possible occurrence. The majority of patients also have GTCS [28], and it may be that the diagnosis is often missed if absences are the only seizure type. The occurrence of GTCS often precedes absences more often than in CAE. Most frequently, patients experience GTCS at awakening [26].

Association with myoclonic seizures is more common than in CAE, probably of the order of 15–20% [29].

Few studies describe the clinical characteristics of seizures in JAE; in one video-based study [30] in three patients with JAE during absences, language functions were less rapidly abolished, consciousness was less severely impaired, and HV stopped later than in CAE.

In our personal series of patients with JAE, during absences awareness was only partially impaired and corresponded to an increasing latency between stimulus and response for discharges lasting more than 5 s [31].

It is not infrequent to record absence status in patients with JAE, precipitated by drug withdrawal or related to inappropriate treatment (especially carbamazepine) [32]. As in all GGE, other precipitating factors are sleep deprivation, abnormal lifestyle, and premenstrual period.

27.2.1 EEG Features

Background EEG activity is usually normal. The characteristic feature of the interictal and ictal EEG is symmetric generalized SW discharge, often prevalent on the frontal regions. The SW frequency is usually faster than 3 Hz (3.5–4 Hz), the first complex of a group sometimes being even faster. The slow wave could be preceded by two or three spikes. The generalized SW discharges could show fragmentation more than in CAE.

Sleep recordings show normal organization; paroxysmal discharges increase in frequency in NREM sleep and decrease in REM.

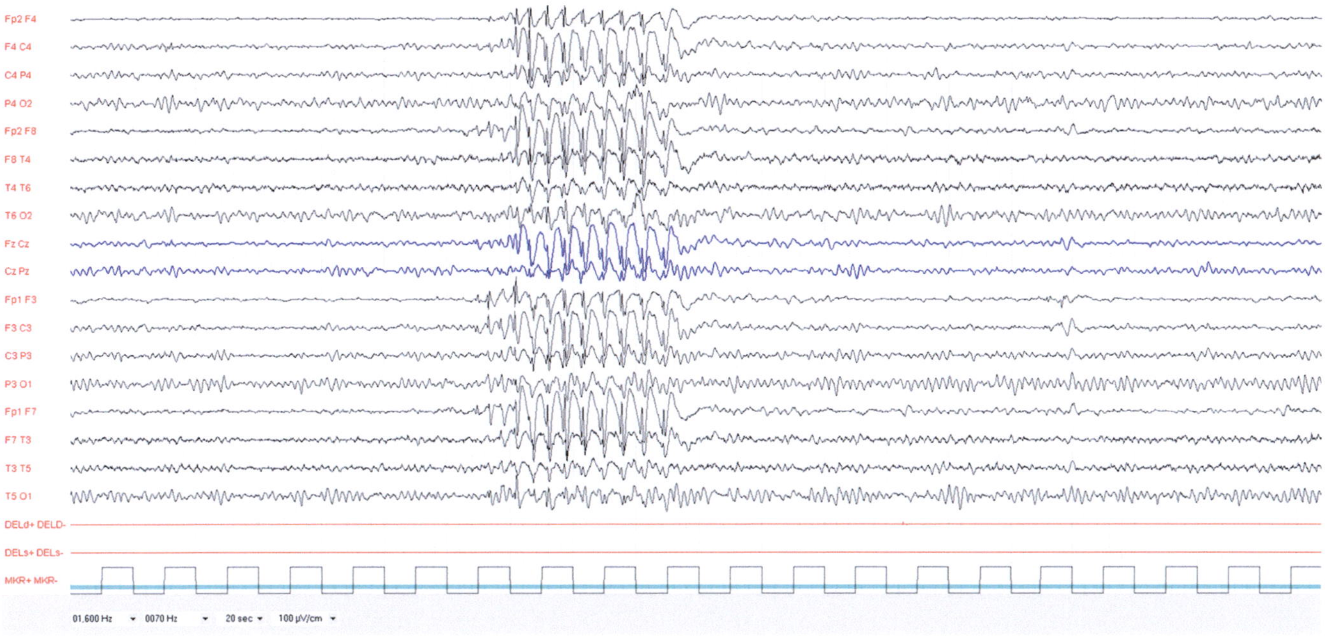

Fig. 27.4 Ictal discharge occurring during HV in an 18-year-old boy with JAE; note that absences are usually shorter than in CAE. At the onset of the ictal discharge, polyspikes followed by 3 Hz spike and waves

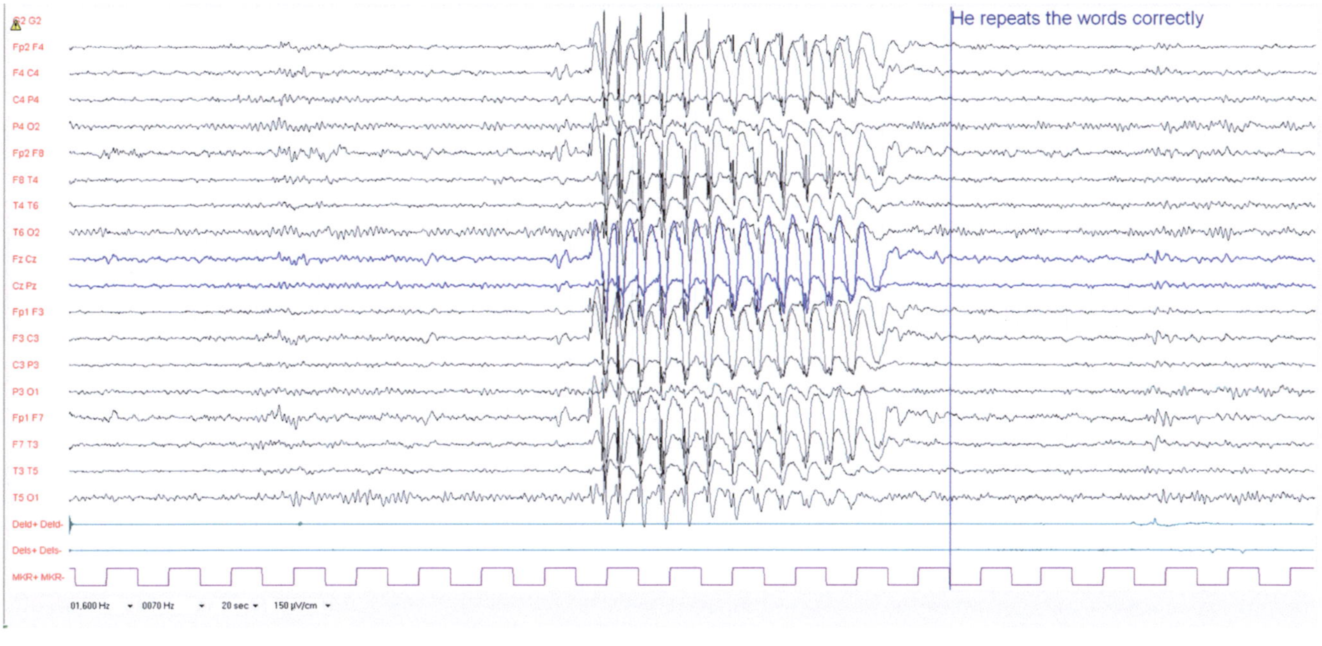

Fig. 27.5 Awareness can be preserved during absences in JAE, like in this 16 year old boy with 3 Hz ictal discharge with frontal predominance

EEG features of absences in JAE are shown in Figs. 27.4 and 27.5.

27.3 Juvenile Myoclonic Epilepsy (JME) (Janz Syndrome)

JME has been described by Janz and Christian in 1957 [33].

JME is a very common form of epilepsy (5–10% of all epilepsies) and one of the most frequent forms of GGE [34]. A family history of epilepsy is found in one third of cases. From a genetic point of view, though, JME appears very heterogeneous. Two main susceptibility genes (GABRA1 and EFHC1) and many other genes have been found in families with JME, and microdeletions in 15q13.3, 15q11.2, and 16p13.11 also contribute risk to JME, but research is still ongoing [35].

The seizure onset is clearly age-related, with a range between the ages of 8 and 26 and a mean age of 14. Even if JME has an equal sex distribution, myoclonic jerks occur sooner in girls than in boys, which can reflect different hormonal developments.

In the most typical cases, patients are usually referred following the first GTCS, which had been preceded by isolated jerks for several months. This first major seizure could be precipitated by provoking factors (e.g., sleep deprivation) [36]. When accurately investigated, the patients report that after waking up in the morning, they experience unprovoked jerks, mainly in the upper limbs, causing them to drop whatever they hold (generally the coffee cup, the toothbrush, or the razor). The jerks can present in clusters with an increasing course; sometimes they can escape to the attention of onlookers, but they can also make the patient fall, without loss of consciousness [37].

In the majority of patients, myoclonic jerks predominate on the upper limbs, grossly symmetric, even if they can be felt to be asymmetric or unilateral [38] or their amplitude can be dependent on the degree of tonic contraction of the arm involved (patients often report that jerks affect prominently their dominant limb) [36]. Myoclonic jerks infrequently involve the lower limbs, causing a sudden fall, after which the patient promptly recovers his balance [33].

Myoclonic jerks can be precipitate by lack of sleep and sudden provoked awakening, excessive alcohol intake and, in some patients, photic stimulation, eye closure [38, 39], and poor adherence to antiepileptic drugs [40].

Mental tasks that imply manual activity and decision-making may also trigger seizures, evoking a relationship between JME and certain reflex epilepsies [41] and can be attributed to hyperexcitability of distinctive brain networks [42].

Rarely myoclonic jerks occur in status with a full preservation of consciousness, being facilitated by acute drug withdrawal or by intake of inadequate drug (see below).

Most patients (80–95%) present myoclonic jerks and rare GTCS, which usually follow a longer series of jerks, with increasing amplitude and frequency, until myoclonic jerks melt into the initial tonic phase of the GTCS (Fig. 27.6). GTCS are not very frequent in the natural course of JME (one or two per year), but they can cluster over a short period during adolescence. They may be invalidating in noncompliant or mistreated patients, especially when lifestyle is grossly abnormal [36].

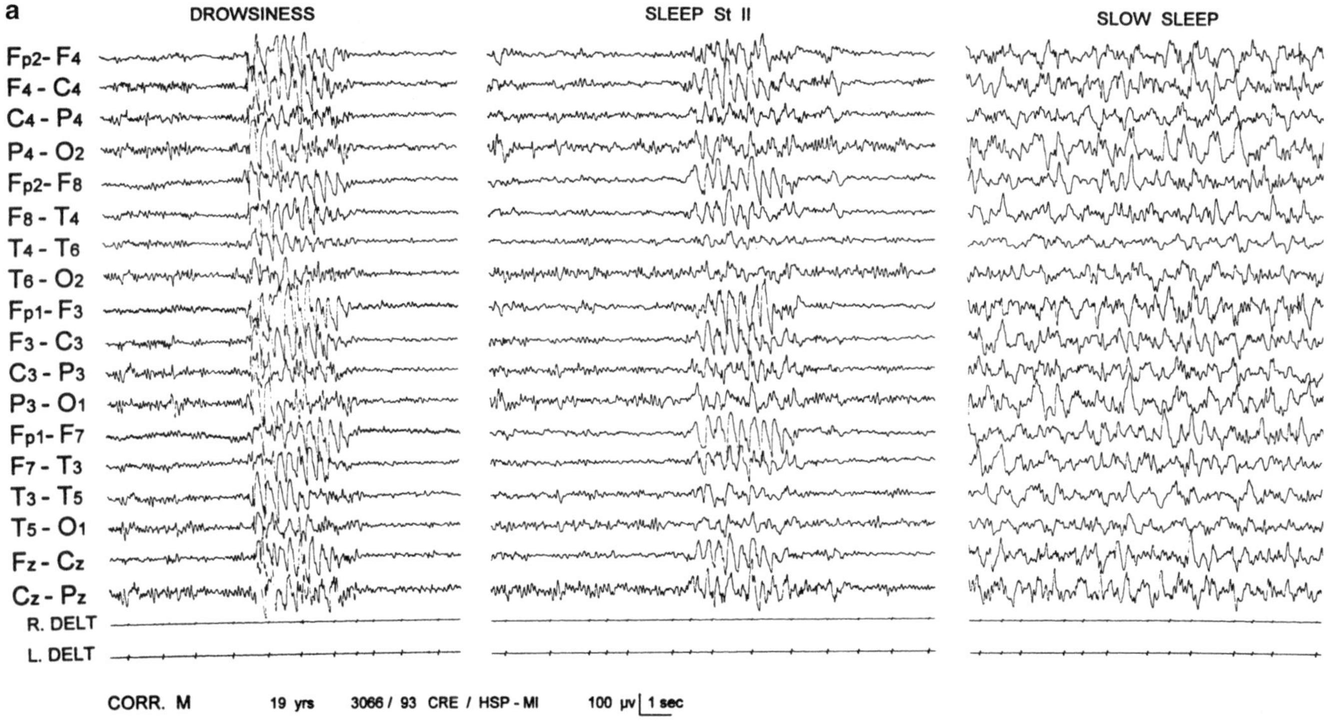

Fig. 27.6 A 19-year-old patient with JME. EEG recording after sleep deprivation. Panel (**a**): during drowsiness and sleep stage 2, sharp and slow wave discharges without clinical correlate. During slow sleep, rare slow abnormalities intermingled with slow background activity. Panel (**b**): 15 min after awakening myoclonic jerks at upper limbs, both at rest and during HV. Panel (**c**): After the myoclonic jerks, ictal recording of a generalized tonic-clonic seizure. EEG showed sharp and slow wave complexes at 3.5 Hz. Panel (**d**): EEG showed fast spike activity at 10 Hz, correlated to the tonic phase of the seizure; after 75 s from the onset, sharp wave discharges associated to the clonic phase of the seizure. Panel (**e**) At the end of the seizure, diffuse slow activity which progressively disappeared

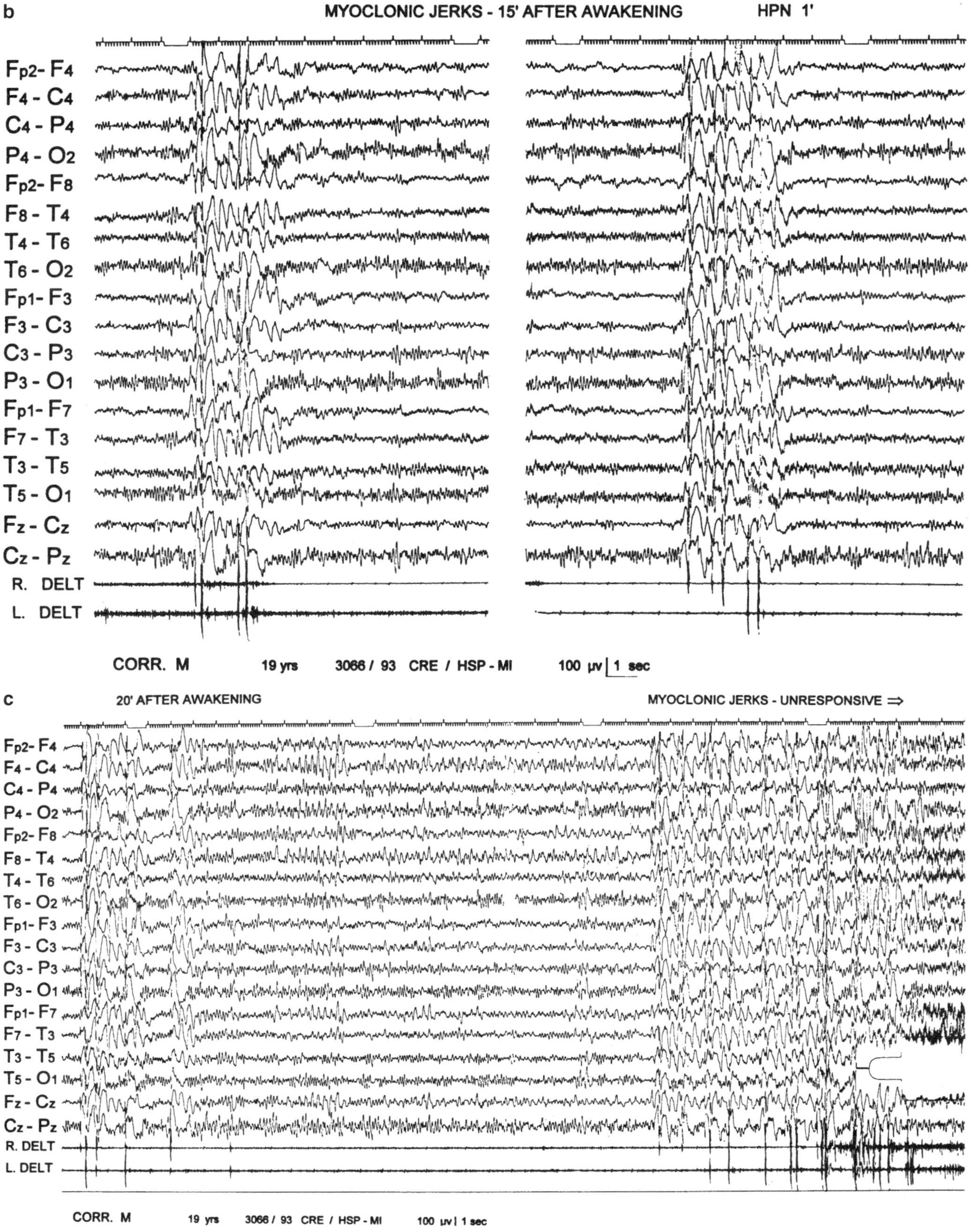

Fig. 27.6 (continued)

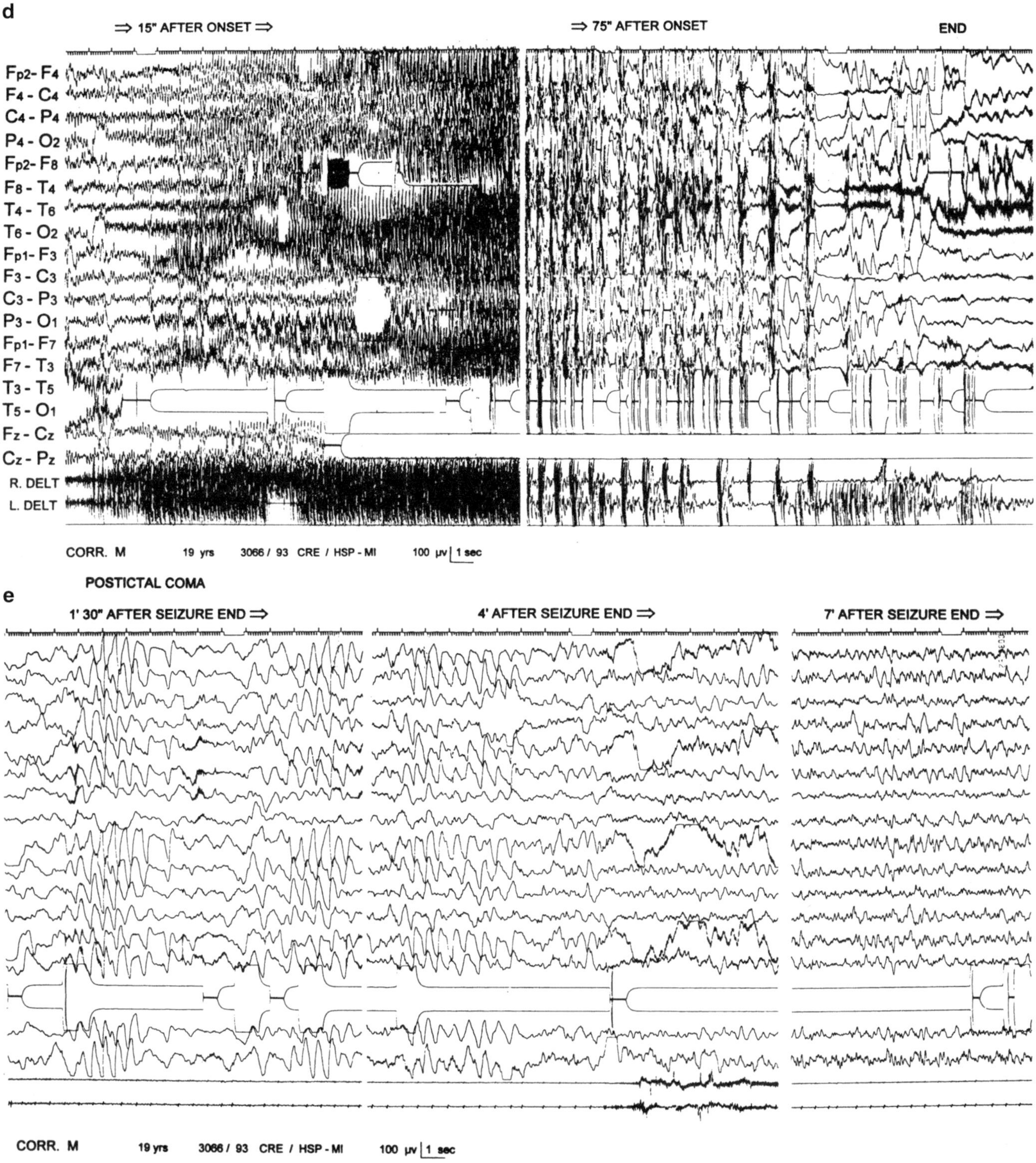

Fig. 27.6 (continued)

Asymmetric semeiological features, such as asymmetric myoclonic jerks and asymmetric evolution of GTCS, can be observed [43].

Patients with JME may also experience TAs with mild impairment of consciousness, as found in JAE [44].

27.3.1 Neurophysiology

Diagnosis of JME should be confirmed by an ictal recording, easily obtained by polygraphic video-EEG performed after a nocturnal sleep deprivation, before starting treatment. The characteristic EEG trait is bilateral, synchronous, symmetric PSW discharges, that precede (about 20 ms) a myoclonic jerk recorded on polygraphic surface EMG deltoids. The amplitude of spikes is typically increasing and is maximal over the frontal areas (Fig. 27.7). Slow waves often precede or follow the polyspikes, resulting in a PSW complex that lasts longer than myoclonic jerks, around 2–4 s. The number of spikes appears to be correlated to the intensity of the jerks [36]. Back averaging of myoclonic jerks shows the characteristics of cortical myoclonus [45].

Interictal EEG recordings show normal background activity during wakefulness and sleep. Interictal generalized PSW may have anterior prevalence. Focal epileptiform discharges can be detected in the course of the disease [46].

In 30% of JME patients, especially in females, IPS determines PSW discharges sometimes associated with myoclonic jerks. This photosensitivity provoked in EEG laboratory in most of the cases does not correspond to a clinical problem in natural ambience.

27.4 Epilepsy with Generalized Tonic-Clonic Seizures Alone (GTCSa)

Although the clinical characteristics of this syndrome are not broadly described yet, this epileptic syndrome has been considered even in the new classification [1]. Epilepsy with GTCS alone includes the previously called "epilepsy with grand mal on awakening" (EGMA) listed in the 1989 classification besides other forms of IGE with GTCS, even if less well-defined entities.

Range of epilepsy onset is between ages 9 and 24 years, with a peak around puberty.

A slight male preponderance has been reported in some series [47], but sex distribution seems to be equal.

There is a family history of febrile convulsions and epilepsy [48].

Main seizure type is GTCS, but many patients have in addition minor generalized seizures, either absence or myoclonic or both, which can precede or follow the convulsive seizure. Seizure frequency is generally low [49].

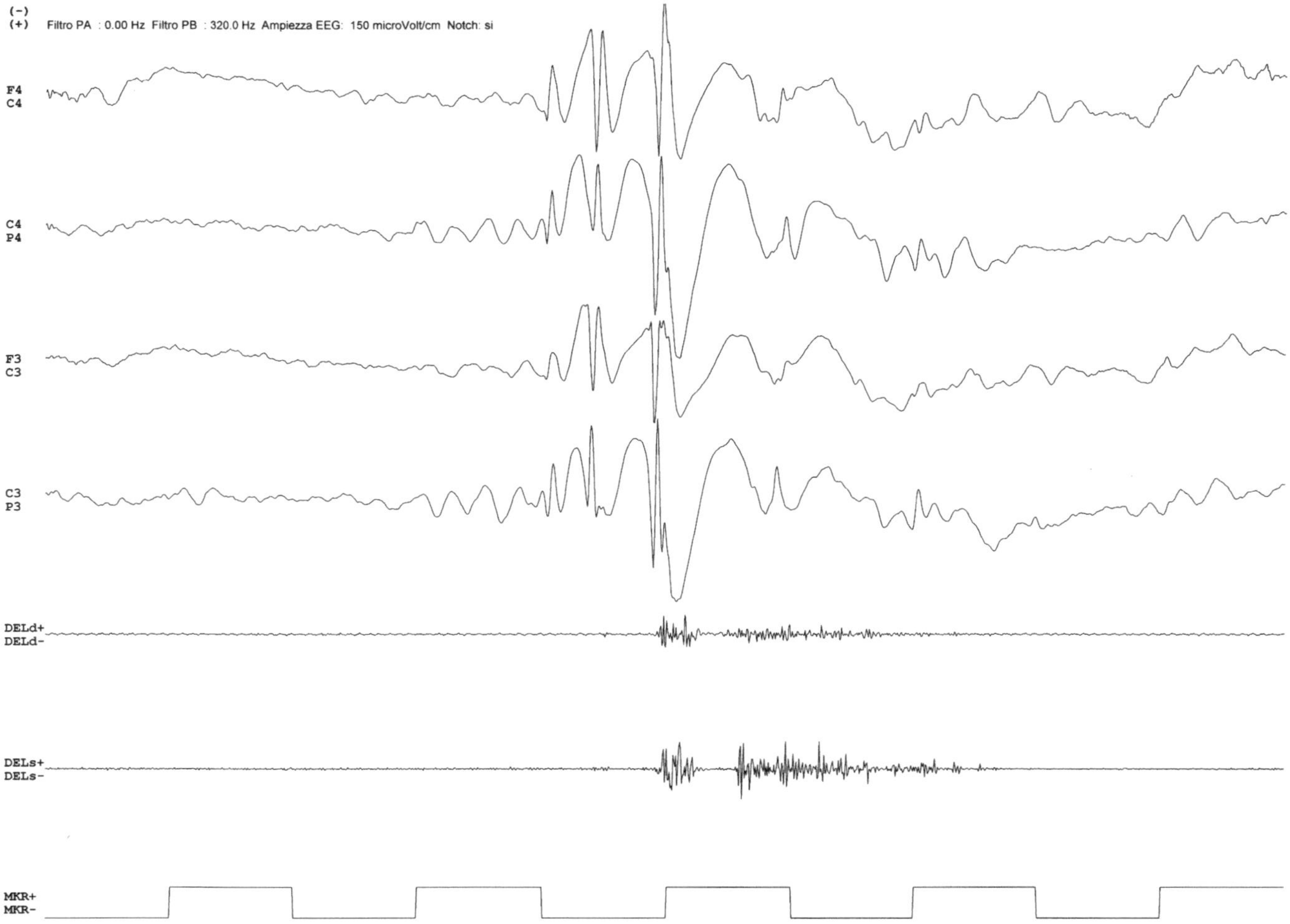

Fig. 27.7 Polyspike-wave discharges have a prominent amplitude on bilateral frontal regions. The polyspike component is related to the occurrence of myoclonic jerks

The clear majority of seizures in GTCS alone occur either in the 2 h after awakening (regardless of the time of the day) or in the second peak, during the evening relaxation phase [50].

EEG characteristics include occurrence of generalized SW and PSW activity. In order to confirm the diagnosis, since routine EEG can be uninformative, sleep-deprived recordings increase the opportunity of SW/PSW detection. It is recommended to provide a registration that includes awakening from a sleep period, where SWs are more probably be recorded. Focal abnormalities are extremely rare. In contrast with focal syndromes with convulsive seizures during sleep, GTCS alone is one of the epileptic syndromes that are related to photosensitivity.

27.5 Eyelid Myoclonia with/Without Absences (EMA) (Jeavons Syndrome)

The 2010 revised ILAE Report on Terminology and Classification recognized an additional type of absence seizures characterized by special features: eyelid myoclonia with absence (EMA) [51]. These seizures have been reported also in the recent ILAE classification of seizures [52], but a distinct syndrome has not been identified among the epilepsy syndromes [1]. Indeed, patients with EMA show very peculiar seizure features, which deserve a distinct description.

Moreover, recent studies demonstrated that the clinical genetics of EMA is suggestive of complex inheritance with shared genetic determinants overlapping with both classical GGE and GEFS+ [53].

Seizures in EMA are characterized as prominent jerking of the eyelids with upward deviation of the eyes, often triggered by eye closure, and retropulsion of the head. Impairment of awareness may be brief and subtle. Independent absence or myoclonic seizures may occur in some patients, triggered by HV or IPS or even spontaneously. Onset occurs in childhood (peak 6–8 years), with a female predominance (M:F = 1:3–4) [15].

The ictal EEG pattern for EMA has been described as 3–6 Hz generalized PSW complexes with occasional paroxysmal bursts in the occipital regions, which can precede the generalized discharges [54] (Fig. 27.8). It is unclear whether Jeavons syndrome should be classified as a type of absence epilepsy or as a myoclonic epilepsy, given its prominent eyelid myoclonia.

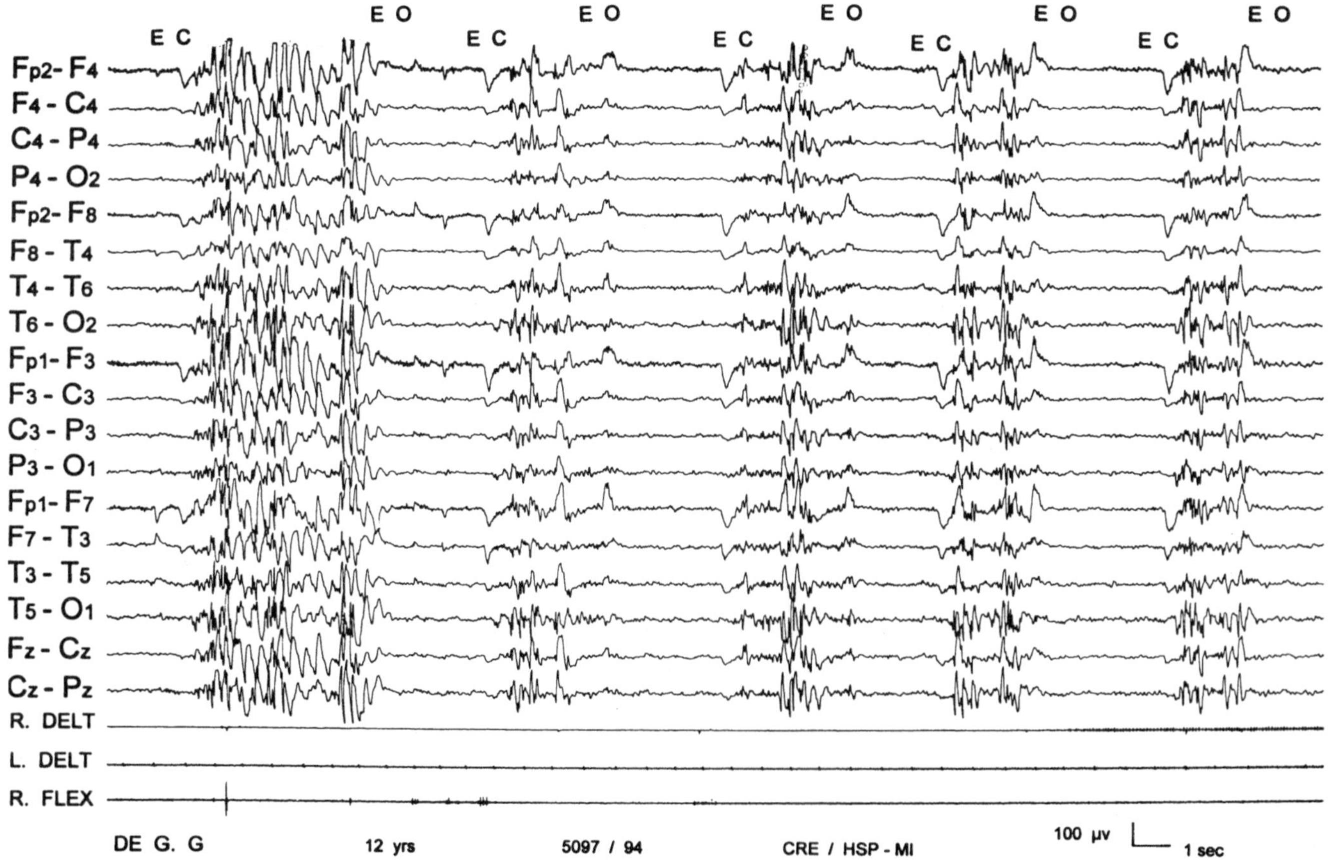

Fig. 27.8 Eyelid myoclonia without absence in a 12-year-old girl. Note that the discharge is characterized by polyspikes occurring at eye closure (EC), which disappear at eye opening (EO)

EMA can occur both in genetic and in symptomatic epilepsies. The genetic form is referred to as Jeavons syndrome, and EMA in this syndrome usually occurs following eyelid closure; all patients are photosensitive [39].

The distinctive feature of seizures in EMA has been recently studied by fMRI: alterations of the anatomo-functional properties of the visual system were demonstrated, involving a circuit encompassing the occipital cortex and cortical/subcortical systems physiologically activated in the motor control of eye closure and eye movements [55].

The outcome and prognosis for Jeavons syndrome is poorly understood. There is some evidence that GTCS, either light-induced or spontaneous, will occur in most patients over the long term [56]. Jeavons syndrome is thought to be a lifelong disorder, resistant to medical treatment [53].

27.6 Lifestyle and Drugs Can Influence EEG in GGE

In patients with GGE, lifestyle recommendations are mandatory: the sleep-wake rhythm must be regulated, and circumstances that can interfere with normal sleep and cause precocious awakening in the morning should be avoided. Alcohol intake should be restricted and permitted only in small quantities.

Even if easily controlled by AED therapy in most cases, JME should be considered a lifelong condition since relapses are very common after drug withdrawal, and only a third of the patients can remain off medication [33].

Choosing the appropriate drug can be challenging in patients with GGE; although valproate is still considered the drug of choice in JME, it should be possibly avoided in women in childbearing potential. Levetiracetam can be a therapeutic option in these patients [57], together with topiramate [58] and zonisamide [59].

The use of lamotrigine in JME is still controversial, as worsening in seizure frequency and severity has been reported with this drug, as well as with carbamazepine and vigabatrin, which can increase the occurrence of jerks and of subclinical interictal discharges.

27.7 Conclusion

In order to distinguish GGE from other forms of epilepsies, strict clinical and EEG criteria have been proposed by the ILAE classification; however, clinical experience shows that these criteria are not fulfilled by all patients all of the time. Epileptic conditions considered as representative of GGE are a heterogeneous group, and their clinical and EEG correlates may vary slightly, due to many factors, such as age, interfering drugs, time of the day, and state of vigilance.

References

1. Scheffer IE, Berkovic S, Capovilla G, Connolly MB, French J, Guilhoto L, et al. ILAE classification of the epilepsies: position paper of the ILAE Commission for Classification and Terminology. Epilepsia. 2017;58(4):512–21. https://doi.org/10.1111/epi.13709.
2. Ottman R. Genetic epidemiology of epilepsy. Epidemiol Rev. 1997;19:120–8.
3. Kobow K, Blümcke I. Epigenetics in epilepsy. Neurosci Lett. 2018;667:40–6. https://doi.org/10.1016/j.neulet.2017.01.012.
4. Scheffer IE, Mefford HC. Epilepsy: beyond the single nucleotide variant in epilepsy genetics. Nat Rev Neurol. 2014;10(9):490–1. https://doi.org/10.1038/nrneurol.2014.146.
5. Mullen SA, Berkovic S, ILAE Genetics Commission. Genetic generalized epilepsies. Epilepsia. 2018;59:1148–53. https://doi.org/10.1111/epi.14042.
6. Nuyts S, D'Souza W, Bowden SC, Vogrin SJ. Structural brain abnormalities in genetic generalized epilepsies: a systematic review and meta-analysis. Epilepsia. 2017;58(12):2025–37. https://doi.org/10.1111/epi.13928.
7. Gloor P. Generalized cortico-reticular epilepsies. Some considerations on the pathophysiology of generalized bilaterally synchronous spike and wave discharge. Epilepsia. 1968;9(3):249–63.
8. Polack PO, Mahon S, Chavez M, Charpier S. Inactivation of the somatosensory cortex prevents paroxysmal oscillations in cortical and related thalamic neurons in a genetic model of absence epilepsy. Cereb Cortex. 2009;19(9):2078–91. https://doi.org/10.1093/cercor/bhn237.
9. Meeren H, van Luijtelaar G, Lopes da Silva F, Coenen A. Evolving concepts on the pathophysiology of absence seizures: the cortical focus theory. Arch Neurol. 2005;62(3):371–6.
10. Wolf P, Beniczky S. Understanding ictogenesis in generalized epilepsies. Expert Rev Neurother. 2014;14(7):787–98. https://doi.org/10.1586/14737175.2014.925803.
11. Norden AD, Blumenfeld H. The role of subcortical structures in human epilepsy. Epilepsy Behav. 2002;3(3):219–31.
12. Luo C, Li Q, Xia Y, Lei X, Xue K, Yao Z, et al. Resting state basal ganglia network in idiopathic generalized epilepsy. Hum Brain Mapp. 2012;33(6):1279–94. https://doi.org/10.1002/hbm.21286.
13. Roger J, Bureau M, Ferrer-Vidal LO, Daurella LO, Saltarelli A, Genton P. Clinical and electroencephalographic characteristics of idiopathic generalized epilepsies. In: Malafosse A, Genton P, Hirsch E, et al., editors. Idiopathic generalized epilepsies: clinical, experimental and genetic aspects. London: John Libbey; 1994.
14. Kasteleijn-Nolst Trenite DGA, Hirsch E, Takahashi T. Photosensitivity, visual induced seizures and epileptic syndromes. In: Roger J, Bureau M, et al., editors. Epileptic syndromes in infancy, childhood and adolescence. London: John Libbey; 2002.
15. Koutroumanidis M, Arzimanoglou A, Caraballo R, Goyal S, Kaminska A, Laoprasert P, et al. The role of EEG in the diagnosis and classification of the epilepsy syndromes: a tool for clinical practice by the ILAE Neurophysiology Task Force (Part 1). Epileptic Disord. 2017;19(3):233–98. https://doi.org/10.1684/epd.2017.0935.
16. Loiseau P. Absence epilepsy. In: Roger J, Dravet C, Bureau M, Dreifuss FE, Wolf P, editors. Epileptic syndromes in infancy, childhood and adolescence. London: John Libbey; 1992.
17. Penry JK, Porter RJ, Dreifuss RE. Simultaneous recording of absence seizures with video tape and electroencephalography. A study of 374 seizures in 48 patients. Brain. 1975;98(3):427–40.
18. Trinka E, Baumgartner S, Unterberger I, Unterrainer J, Luef G, Haberlandt E, Bauer G. Long-term prognosis for childhood and juvenile absence epilepsy. J Neurol. 2004;251(10):1235–41.
19. Grosso S, Galimberti D, Vezzosi P, Farnetani M, Di Bartolo RM, Bazzotti S, et al. Childhood absence epilepsy: evolution and prognostic factors. Epilepsia. 2005;46(11):1796–801.

20. Callenbach PM, Bouma PA, Geerts AT, Arts WF, Stroink H, Peeters EA, et al. Long-term outcome of childhood absence epilepsy: Dutch Study of Epilepsy in Childhood. Epilepsy Res. 2009;83(2–3):249–56. https://doi.org/10.1016/j.eplepsyres.2008.11.011.
21. Cobb W. EEG interpretation in clinical medicine. Part B. In: Remond A, editor. Handbook of electroencephalography and clinical neurophysiology. Amsterdam: Elsevier; 1976.
22. Loiseau P, Duche B. Childhood absence epilepsy. In: Duncan JS, Panayiotopoulos CP, editors. Typical absences and related epileptic syndromes. Edinburgh: Churchill Livingstone; 1995.
23. Dalla Bernardina B, Sgrò V, Fejerman N. Epilepsy with centro-temporal spikes and related syndromes in:. “Epileptic syndromes in infancy, childhood and adolescence”, Roger J, Bureau M, Dravet CH, Genton P, Tassinari CA, Wolf P (John Libbey, London, 2002.
24. Hirsch E, Blanc-Platier A, Marescaux C. What are the relevant criteria for a better classification of epileptic syndromes with typical absences? In: Malafosse A, Genton P, Hirsch E, Marescaux C, Broglin D, Bernasconi R, editors. Idiopathic generalized epilepsies: clinical experimental and genetic aspects. London: John Libbey; 1994.
25. Panayiotopoulos CP. Absence epilepsies. In: Engel J, Pedley TA, editors. Epilepsy. A comprehensive textbook. Philadelphia: Lippincott-Raven; 1997.
26. Gelisse P, Wolf P, Inoue Y. Juvenile absence epilepsy. In: Bureau M, Genton P, Dravet C, Delgado-Escueta A, Tassinari CA, Thomas P, Wolf P, editors. Epileptic syndromes in infancy, childhood and adolescence. 5th ed. London: John Libbey Eurotext; 2012.
27. Marini C, Scheffer IE, Crossland KM, Grinton BE, Phillips FL, McMahon JM, et al. Genetic architecture of idiopathic generalized epilepsy: clinical genetic analysis of 55 multiplex families. Epilepsia. 2004;45(5):467–78.
28. Wolf P, Inoue Y. Therapeutic response of absence seizures in patients of an epilepsy clinic for adolescents and adults. J Neurol. 1984;231:225–9.
29. Wolf P, Inoue Y. Juvenile absence epilepsy. In: Roger J, Bureau M, Dravet CH, et al., editors. Epileptic syndromes in infancy, childhood and adolescence. London: John Libbey; 2002.
30. Panayiotoupolos CP, Obeid T, Waheed G. Differentiation of typical absence seizures in epileptic syndromes. Brain. 1989;112:1039–56.
31. Sgrò V, Canevini MP, Lastrico A, Guidolin L, Vignoli A, Saltarelli A, et al. Assenze tipiche: analisi elettroclinica di 37 pazienti con epilessia-assenza dell’infanzia o dell’adolescenza. Aggiornamenti in Epilettologia. Boll Lega It Epil. 1995;91/92:97–9.
32. Thomas P, Valton L, Genton P. Absence and myoclonic status epilepticus precipitated by antiepileptic drugs in idiopathic generalized epilepsy. Brain. 2006;129(Pt 5):1281–92.
33. Janz D, Christian W. Impulsiv petit mal. Dtsch Z Nervenheilk. 1957;176:346–86.
34. Yacubian EM. Juvenile myoclonic epilepsy: challenges on its 60th anniversary. Seizure. 2017;44:48–52. https://doi.org/10.1016/j.seizure.2016.09.005.
35. Delgado-Escueta AV, Koeleman BP, Bailey JN, Medina MT, Durón RM. The quest for juvenile myoclonic epilepsy genes. Epilepsy Behav. 2013;28(Suppl 1):S52–7. https://doi.org/10.1016/j.yebeh.2012.06.033.. Review
36. Thomas P, Genton P, Gelisse P, Medina M, Serafini A. Juvenile myoclonic epilepsy. In: Bureau M, Genton P, Dravet C, Delgado-Escueta A, Tassinari CA, Thomas P, Wolf P, editors. Epileptic syndromes in infancy, childhood and adolescence. London: John Libbey; 2012.
37. Janz D, Cristian W. Impulsive Petit Mal (traduction anglaise par P Genton). In: Malafosse A, Genton P, Hirsch E, Marescaux C, Broglin D, Bernasconi R, editors. Idiopathic generalized epilepsies: clinical, experimental and genetic aspects. London: John Libbey; 1994.
38. Canevini MP, Mai R, Di Marco C, Bertin C, Minotti L, Pontrelli V, et al. Juvenile myoclonic epilepsy of Janz: clinical observations in 60 patients. Seizure. 1992;1(4):291–8.
39. Striano S, Capovilla G, Sofia V, Romeo A, Rubboli G, Striano P, et al. Eyelid myoclonia with absences (Jeavons syndrome): a well-defined idiopathic generalized epilepsy syndrome or a spectrum of photosensitive conditions? Epilepsia. 2009;50(Suppl 5):15–9. https://doi.org/10.1111/j.1528-1167.2009.02114.x.
40. Kasteleijn-Nolst Trenité DG, Schmitz B, Janz D, Delgado-Escueta AV, Thomas P, Hirsch E, et al. Consensus on diagnosis and management of JME: from founder’s observations to current trends. Epilepsy Behav. 2013;28(Suppl 1):S87–90. https://doi.org/10.1016/j.yebeh.2012.11.051.
41. Inoue Y, Seino M, Kubota H, Yamakaku K, Tanaka M, Yagi K. Epilepsy with praxis-induced seizures. In: Wolf P, editor. Epileptic seizures and syndromes. London: John Libbey; 1994.
42. Vollmar C, O’Muircheartaigh J, Barker GJ, Symms MR, Thompson P, Kumari V, et al. Motor system hyperconnectivity in juvenile myoclonic epilepsy: a cognitive functional magnetic resonance imaging study. Brain. 2011;134.(Pt 6:1710–9. https://doi.org/10.1093/brain/awr098.
43. Park KI, Lee SK, Chu K, Lee JJ, Kim DW, Nam H. The value of video-EEG monitoring to diagnose juvenile myoclonic epilepsy. Seizure. 2009;18(2):94–9. https://doi.org/10.1016/j.seizure.2008.07.001.
44. Canevini MP, Sgrò V, Canger R. Le assenze nell’epilessia mioclonica giovanile. Boll Lega It Epil. 1995;91/92:39–42.
45. Panzica F, Rubboli G, Franceschetti S, Avanzini G, Meletti S, Pozzi A, et al. Cortical myoclonus in Janz syndrome. Clin Neurophysiol. 2001;112(10):1803–9.
46. Lombroso CT. Consistent EEG focalities detected in subjects with primary generalized epilepsies monitored for two decades. Epilepsia. 1997;38:797–812.
47. Janz D, Wolf P. Epilepsy with Grand Mal on awakening. In: Engel J, Pedley TA, editors. Epilepsy a comprehensive textbook. Philadelphia: Lippincott-Raven; 1997.
48. Unterberger I, Trinka E, Luef G, Bauer G. Idiopathic generalized epilepsies with pure grand mal: clinical data and genetics. Epilepsy Res. 2001;44(1):19–25.
49. Camfield P, Camfield C. Idiopathic generalized epilepsy with generalized tonic-clonic seizures (IGE-GTC): a population-based cohort with >20 year follow up for medical and social outcome. Epilepsy Behav. 2010;18(1–2):61–3. https://doi.org/10.1016/j.yebeh.2010.02.014.
50. Janz D. Epilepsy with grand mal on awakening and sleep-waking cycle. Clin Neurophysiol. 2000;111(Suppl 2):S103–10.
51. Berg AT, Berkovic SF, Brodie MJ, Buchhalter J, Cross JH, van Emde Boas W, et al. Revised terminology and concepts for organization of seizures and epilepsies: report of the ILAE commission on classification and terminology, 2005–2009. Epilepsia. 2010;51(4):676–85. https://doi.org/10.1111/j.1528-1167.2010.02522.x.
52. Fisher RS, Cross JH, French JA, Higurashi N, Hirsch E, Jansen FE, et al. Operational classification of seizure types by the International League Against Epilepsy: position paper of the ILAE Commission for Classification and Terminology. Epilepsia. 2017;58(4):522–30. https://doi.org/10.1111/epi.13670.
53. Sadleir LG, Vears D, Regan B, Redshaw N, Bleasel A, Scheffer IE. Family studies of individuals with eyelid myoclonia with absences. Epilepsia. 2012;53(12):2141–8. https://doi.org/10.1111/j.1528-1167.2012.03692.x.
54. Tenney JR, Glauser TA. The current state of absence epilepsy: can we have your attention? Epilepsy Curr. 2013;13(3):135–40. https://doi.org/10.5698/1535-7511-13.3.135.
55. Vaudano AE, Ruggieri A, Tondelli M, Avanzini P, Benuzzi F, Gessaroli G, et al. The visual system in eyelid myoclonia with

absences. Ann Neurol. 2014;76(3):412–27. https://doi.org/10.1002/ana.24236.
56. Giannakodimos S, Panayiotopoulos CP. Eyelid myoclonia with absences in adults: a clinical and video-EEG study. Epilepsia. 1996;37:36–44.
57. Tomson T, Marson A, Boon P, Canevini MP, Covanis A, Gaily E, Kälviäinen R, Trinka E. Valproate in the treatment of epilepsy in girls and women of childbearing potential. Epilepsia. 2015;56(7):1006–19. https://doi.org/10.1111/epi.13021.
58. Bourgeois BF. Chronic management of seizures in the syndromes of idiopathic generalized epilepsy. Epilepsia. 2003;44(Suppl 2):27–32.
59. Marinas A, Villanueva V, Giráldez BG, Molins A, Salas-Puig J, Serratosa JM. Efficacy and tolerability of zonisamide in idiopathic generalized epilepsy. Epileptic Disord. 2009;11(1):61–6. https://doi.org/10.1684/epd.2009.0239.

Reflex Seizures and Reflex Epilepsies

28

Salvatore Striano and Pasquale Striano

28.1 Introduction to Reflex Seizures and Reflex Epilepsies

Reflex seizures represent the 4–7% of all epileptic seizures. Most of these are visually induced seizures (about 1/4000 of the population and about 5% of people with epileptic seizures, with higher prevalence in females and in the adolescence. However, rate widely differs among studies, between 1 and 10%). The multiplication of artificial light stimulations in the modern environment has greatly increased the possibility of clinical expression of this phenomenon [1].

Provoked epilepsy is defined as an epilepsy in which a specific systemic or environmental factor is the predominant cause of the seizures and in which there are no gross causative neuroanatomic or neuropathologic changes. Some "provoked epilepsies" will have a genetic basis and some an acquired basis, but in many no inherent cause can be identified. The reflex epilepsies are included in this category (which are usually genetic) as well as the epilepsies with a marked seizure precipitant. The most part of RS have been already described in the pre-EEG era and are traditionally identified on the basis of the provoking stimulus [2–6] (Table 28.1).

RS can be either generalized or focal, with or without impairment of consciousness, and may be genetically inherited or acquired, idiopathic, cryptogenic, or supported by a brain lesion. Therefore, with reference to the classifications of the epileptic syndromes of the International League

Table 28.1 List of reflex epileptic seizures

1. Induced by simple stimuli
1.1 Visual-induced epilepsy
1.1.1 Photosensitive epilepsy
1.1.2 Television-induced epilepsy
1.1.3 Pattern-induced epilepsy
1.1.4 Video game-induced epilepsy
1.1.5 On closing the eyes epilepsy
1.1.6 Visual exploratory epilepsy
1.1.7 Scotosensitive epilepsy
1.2 Somatosensory evoked epilepsy
1.2.1 Movement-induced epilepsy
1.2.2 Startle-induced epilepsy
1.2.3 Toothbrushing epilepsy
1.2.4 Amputees' epilepsy
1.2.5 Auricular epilepsy
1.2.6 Rubbing epilepsy
2. Induced by complex stimuli
2.1.1 Eating epilepsy
2.1.2 Hot water epilepsy
2.1.3 Water-immersion epilepsy
3. Induced by higher cerebral functions
3.1 Language-induced epilepsy
3.1.1 Reading epilepsy
3.1.2 Writing (graphogenic) epilepsy
3.1.3 Speaking-induced epilepsy
3.2 Musicogenic epilepsy
3.2.1 Voice-induced epilepsy
3.2.2 Music-playing epilepsy
3.2.3 Singing epilepsy
3.2.4 Telephone-induced epilepsy
3.3. Epilepsia arithmetices
3.3.1 Game-induced epilepsy
3.3.2 Decision-making epilepsy
3.3.3 Thinking epilepsy
3.3.4 Praxis-induced epilepsy
3.4 Lies-induced epilepsy ("Pinocchio" syndrome)
4. With self-induced seizures
4.1 Photosensitive epilepsy with self-induced seizures
4.1.1 Sunflower epilepsy

From Striano and Striano (2009)

S. Striano
Department of Neurological Sciences, Epilepsy Centre, Federico II University, Naples, Italy

P. Striano (✉)
Pediatric Neurology and Muscular Diseases Unit, Department of Neurosciences, Rehabilitation, Ophthalmology, Genetics, Maternal and Child Health, "G. Gaslini" Institute, University of Genoa, Genoa, Italy

O. Mecarelli (ed.), *Clinical Electroencephalography*, https://doi.org/10.1007/978-3-030-04573-9_28

Against Epilepsy (ILAE), reflex epilepsies can be recognized, with different frequencies, both among generalized and focal epileptic syndromes and both among idiopathic and symptomatic forms [7]. In the report of the ILAE in 2010 [8], radical changes have been proposed in terms and concepts for the classification of seizures and syndromes. However, RE are taken as a whole list of other electroclinical syndromes and epilepsies as a *miscellanea* "with less age-specific relationship."

28.2 Epileptic Seizures and Reflex Epilepsy Related to Visual Stimuli

Photosensitivity, the propensity to produce epileptic seizures in response to light stimuli, is a frequent phenomenon and can be found in a wide range of epilepsies and may express with a lot of seizure types [9]. Photosensitivity is present in nearly all patients with *eyelid myoclonia with absences* (EMA, see below), and, however, it is very frequent in *idiopathic generalized epilepsies* (IGEs), in particular in *juvenile myoclonic epilepsy* (JME), with about 30% of patients (40–45% of girls) showing, at least during a part of the natural course of the disease, this finding. Photosensitivity is also found in some idiopathic focal epileptic syndromes, and in some symptomatic generalized epilepsies, in particular in progressive myoclonic ones (Lafora disease, Unverricht-Lundborg disease, ceroid lipofuscinosis, etc.); photosensitivity may be also present, as an early but transient finding, in some patients with severe myoclonic epilepsy in infancy (or Dravet syndrome). The most frequently found EEG pattern is the photoparoxysmal response (PPR), usually easily provoked in laboratory with intermittent light stimulation (IPS), even if, in some cases, geometrical patterns are necessary to induce PPR (*pattern-induced seizures*) (Fig. 28.1). Overall, seizures induced by intermittent light stimulation (ILS) are

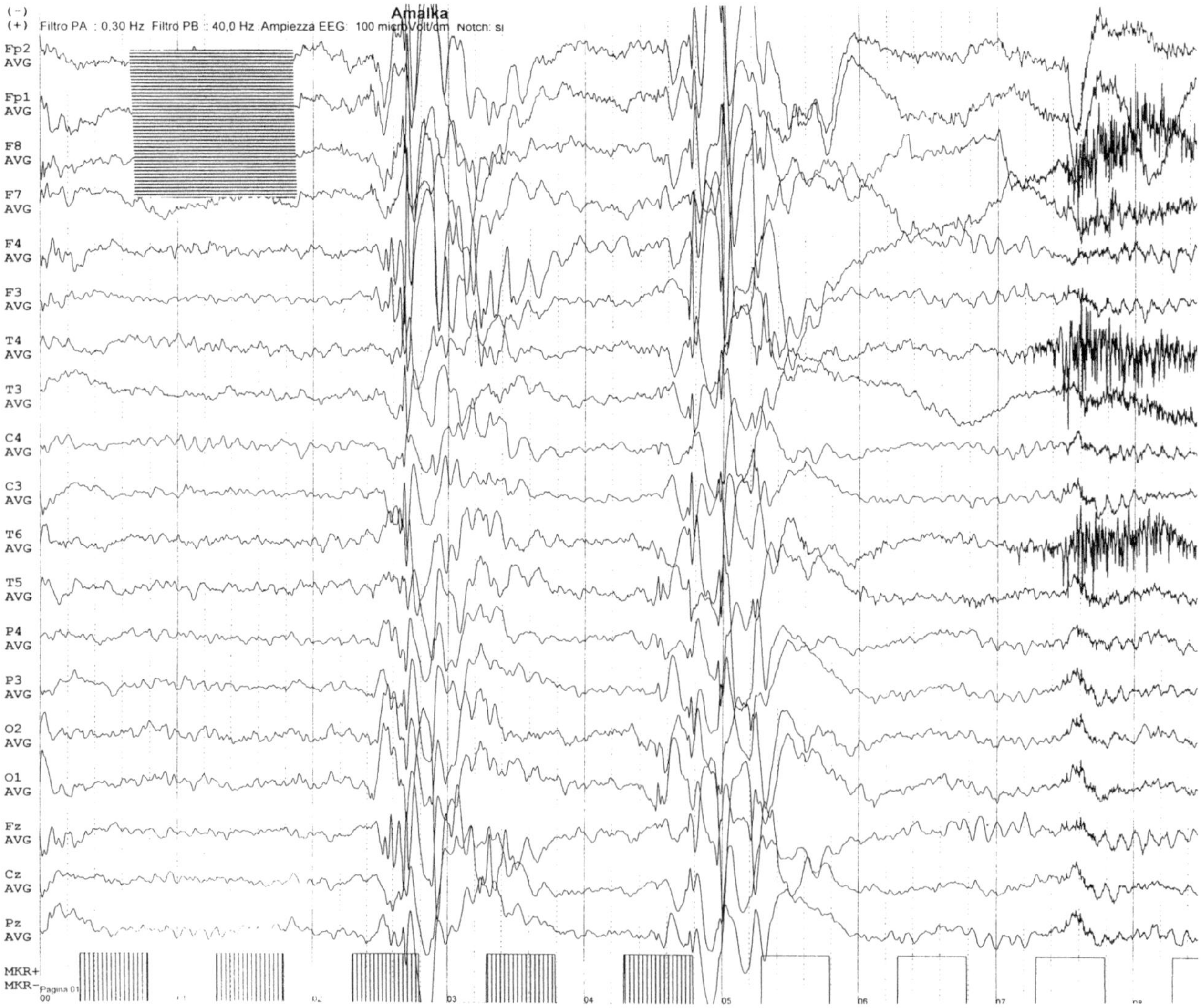

Fig. 28.1 *Pattern sensitivity*: generalized polyspike discharges, concomitant to proximal myoclonies, induced by the interposition of a geometric pattern during ILS

present in about 5% of patients with epilepsy, and the trait is genetically determined, with a higher expression in certain age groups (7–19 years) and in the female sex.

Light-induced seizures are rarely produced by a natural light stimulation, with the exception of EMA [10, 11] (Figs. 28.2 and 28.3) and in some cases of *self-induced seizures*. In eyelid myoclonia, followed or not by a brief absence, seizures are triggered by eye closure in a bright-lighted environment and by IPS. In self-induction the patient is able to trigger seizures with some maneuvers, e.g., looking at the sun and waving a hand over his eyes, jumping behind a shutter, and so on. Sometimes, the patient seems to be magnetically attracted by the light (*sunflower syndrome*, [12]), provoking the seizure. Anecdotally, seizures are triggered by natural flickering light such as rays of sunlight filtering through the trees or reflected by the waves of the sea or snow. Recently environmental risks represented by the proliferation of wind turbines have been evaluated. In the recent decades, the development of artificial light stimulation (stroboscopic light, television, video games, and so on) has enormously increased the occurrence of seizures, sometimes creating an epidemic condition, as occurred in Japan in December 1997, when several hundred children developed seizures while watching a Pokemon cartoon [13, 14]. These seizures are usually clinical and EEG generalized in type

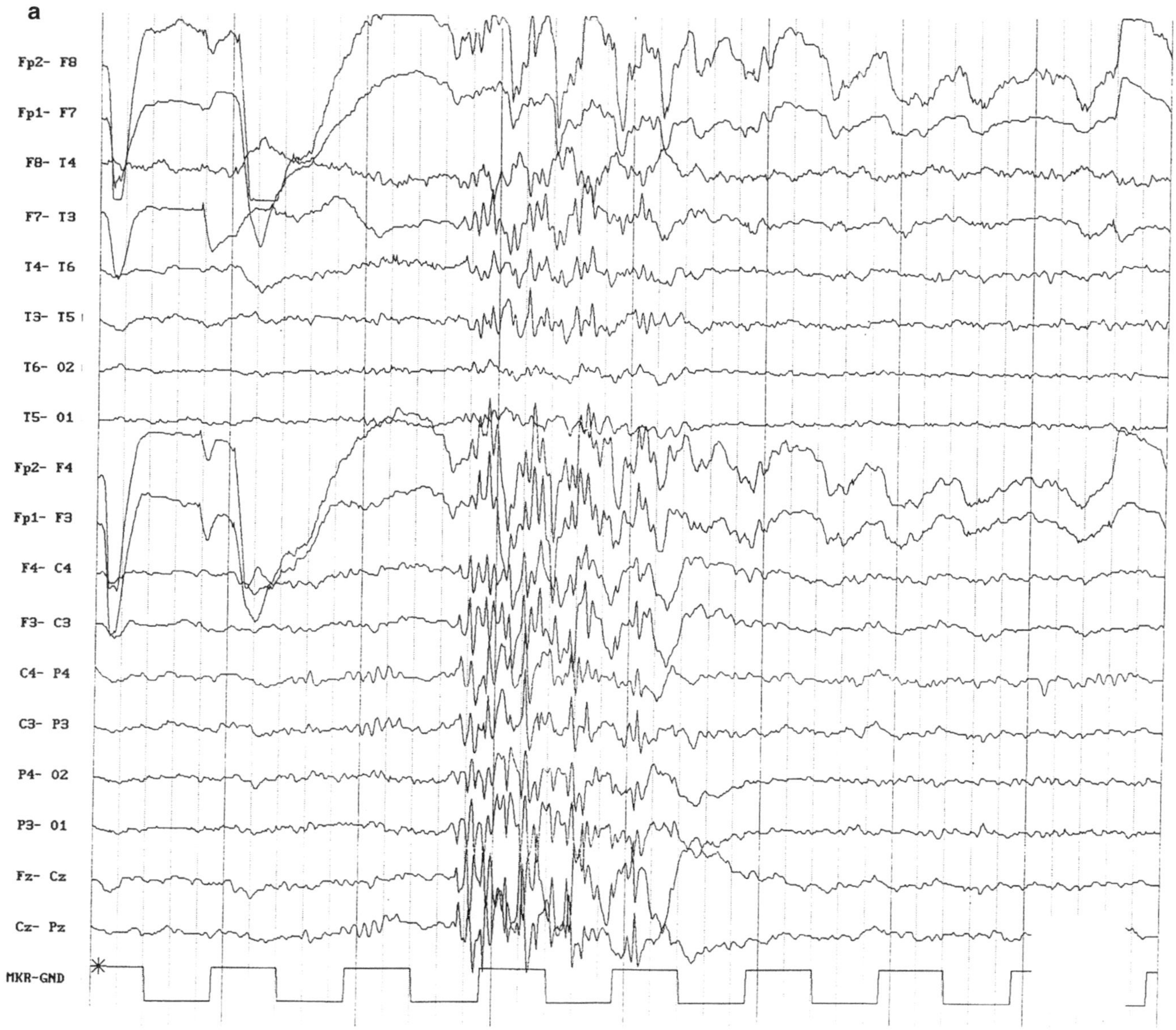

Fig. 28.2 (**a**) *EMA:* eyelid myoclonia followed by a brief absence at eye closure. (**b**) *EMA:* generalized polyspike discharge followed by a brief spike-wave sequence at about 3 Hz concomitant to ILS

b

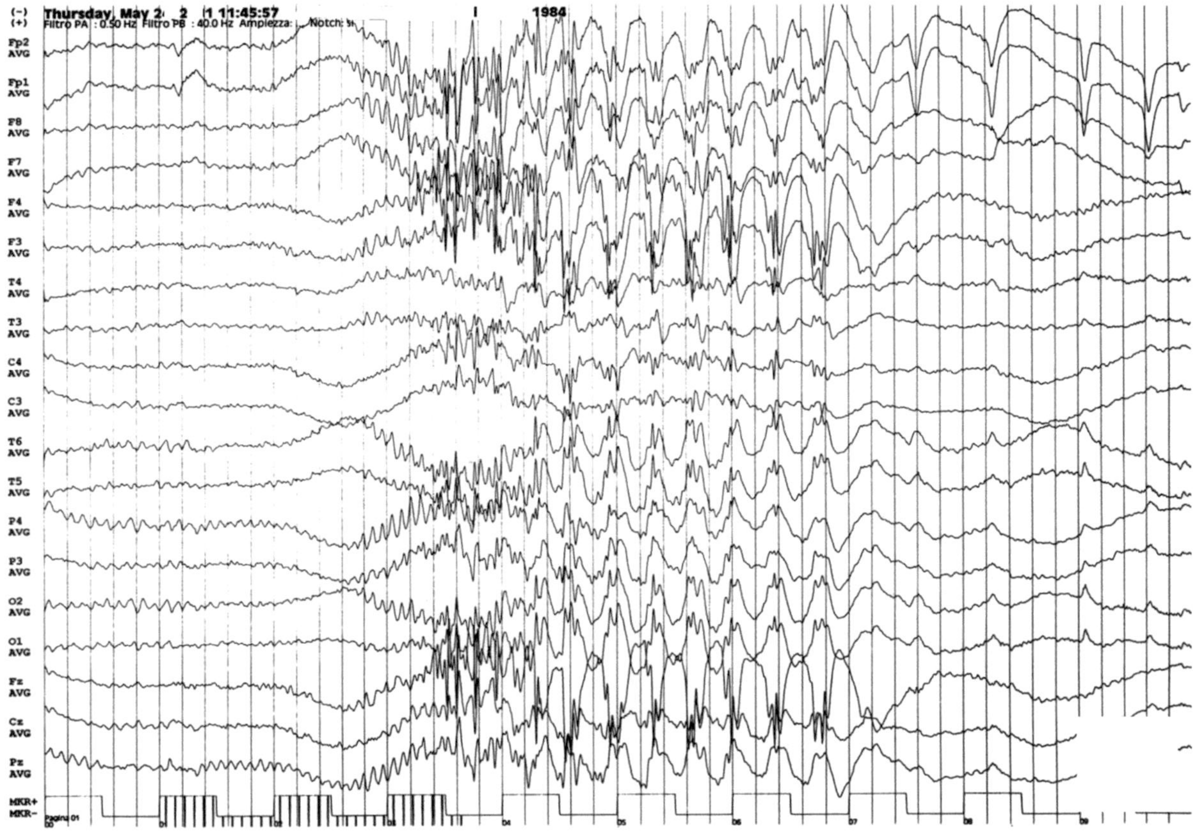

Fig. 28.2 (continued)

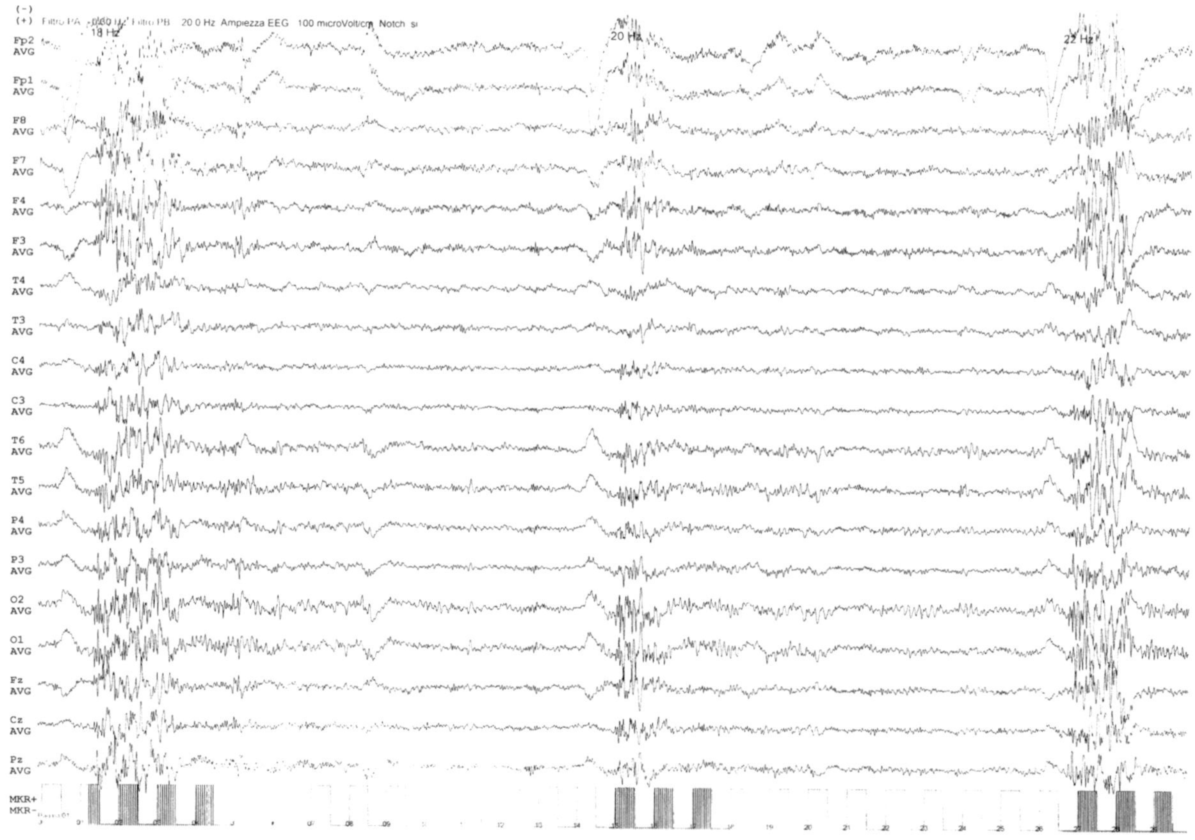

Fig. 28.3 *EMA:* eyelid myoclonias induced by ILS at various stimulation rates. Myoclonus may not be always followed by the absence

(absence, myoclonus, tonic-clonic seizures), more rarely with occipital onset featuring an IPOLE. Focal extra-occipital seizures caused by visual stimulation are exceptional [15]. In idiopathic occipital epilepsy, "Gastaut-type" EEG paroxysmal activities are related to keeping eyes closed rather than the closure of the eyes (diagnostic criterion for EMA and frequent phenomenon in idiopathic generalized epilepsies). The occipital paroxysmal activity is also present while keeping the eyes open in total darkness and with maneuvers that eliminate central fixation, e.g., wearing Frenzel glasses, and also in the presence of light. This phenomenon has been described as *fixation-off sensitivity* (FOS) [16]; generally there are not any other evident clinical manifestations. These patients are not sensitive to IPS. Rarely the patient has seizures only due to FOS (Fig. 28.4). Sometimes these are seizures induced by exceptional triggers, and, according to the ILAE's classification proposal, the diagnosis of epilepsy is not indicated.

28.3 Reflex Epilepsy Calculation or Other Higher-Level Cortical Processes and by Complex Motor Performances

First described as epilepsia arithmetices [17], this form of epilepsy, that is always idiopathic in nature and generalized in type, is characterized by seizures (most often myoclonic but also typical absence and tonic-clonic) triggered by mental calculation or by various types of board games (board game epilepsy, card game epilepsy, chess-induced epilepsy, and so on) or by other complex mental processes (thinking epilepsy), with the pressure to decide (decision-making epilepsy) (Fig. 28.5). Probably seizures triggered by complex spatial tasks, motor ideation, and complicated movements (praxis-induced epilepsy) share similar mechanism of induction [18]. Ictal EEG and clinical pattern is typical of idiopathic generalized epilepsies, but focal or asymmetrical features (clinical or EEG) are sometimes described. Interictal

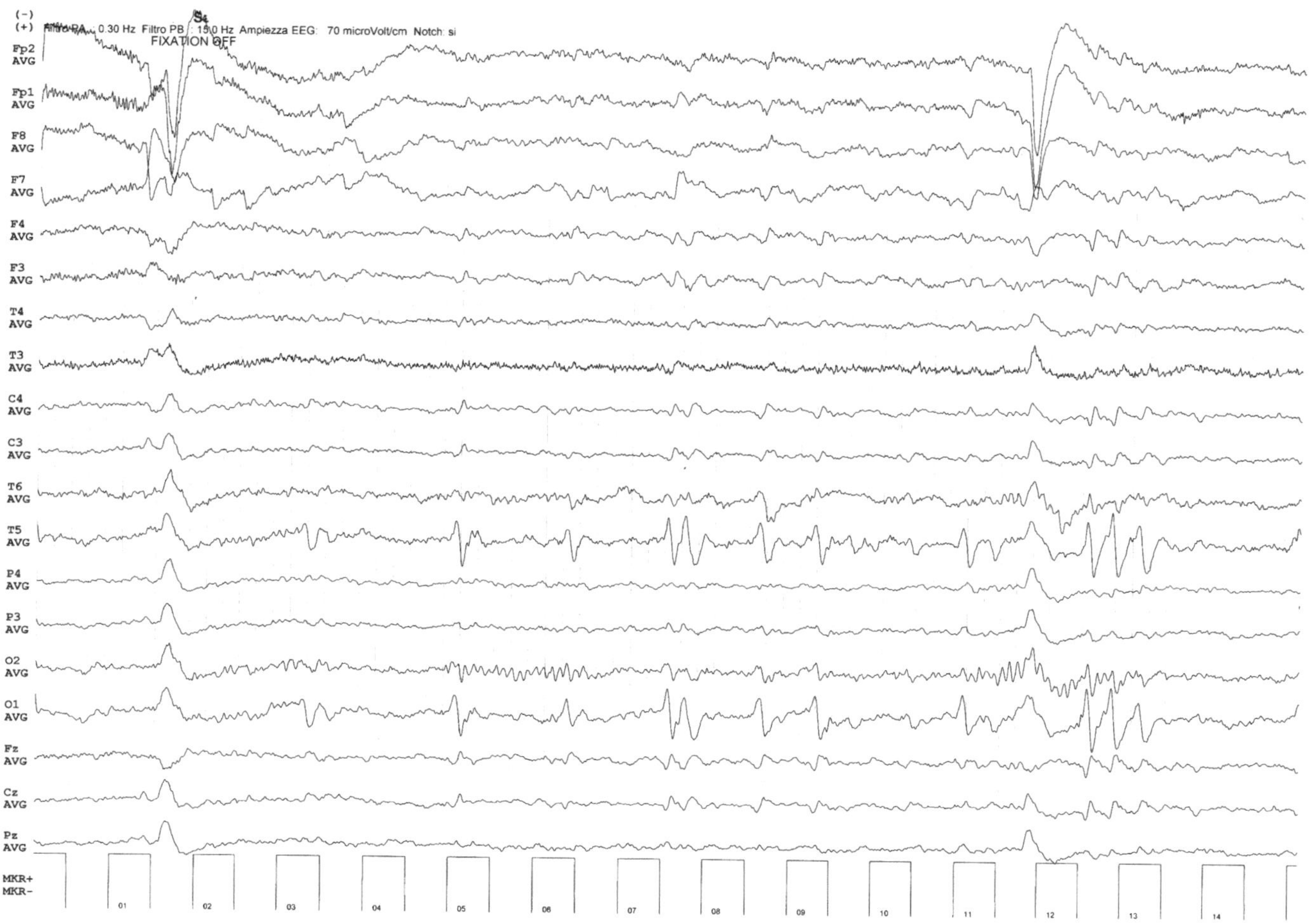

Fig. 28.4 *Fixation-off sensitivity:* patient with open eyes. Paroxysmal activity on the left occipital areas provoked by the loss of central fixation (obtained simply by placing a blank paper in front of the patient's eyes). This EEG finding is usually found in patients with benign "Gastaut-type" occipital epilepsy, where it is typically caused by keeping eyes closed and with open eyes in total darkness; there is no photosensitivity

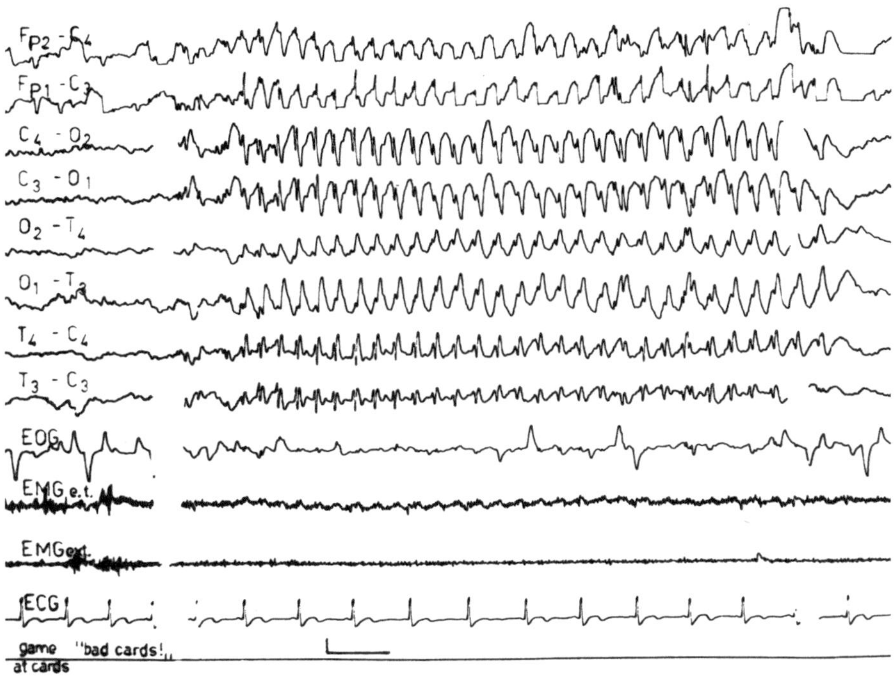

Fig. 28.5 *Epilepsia arithmetices:* typical absence caused by playing cards. This patient had repetitive absences during complex sequential calculations

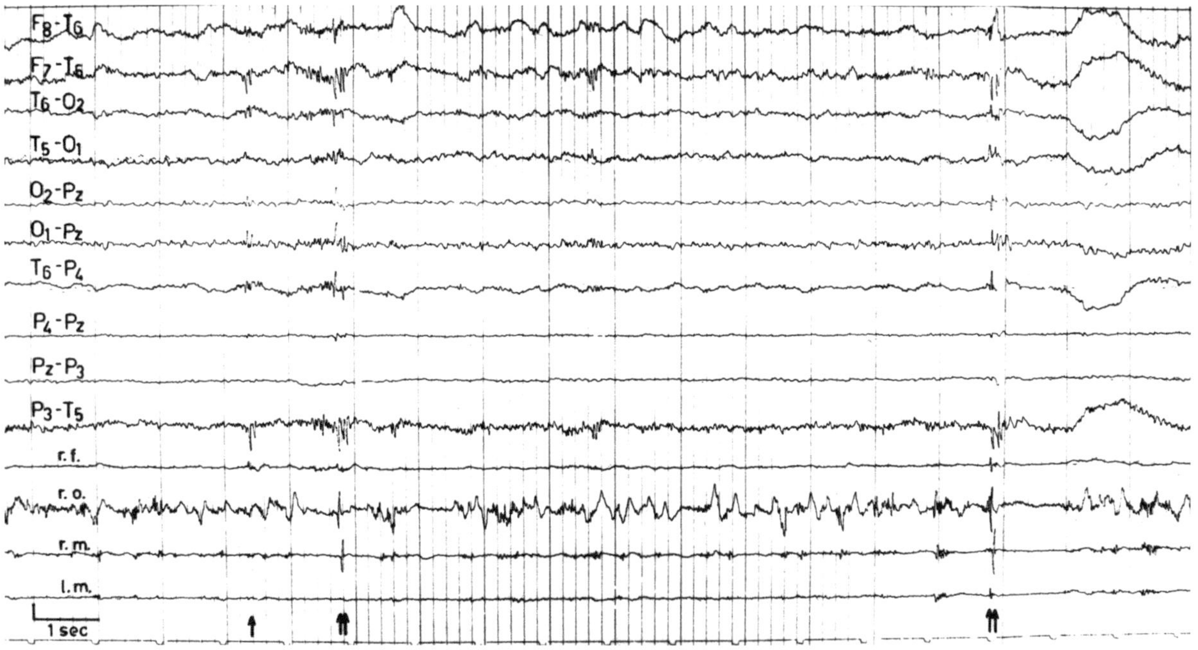

Fig. 28.6 *Primary reading epilepsy:* myoclonias of the jaw (rm, EMG right masseter) and perioral (ro, EMG right orbicularis oris) concomitant to spikes on the posterior temporal left areas while reading aloud. Occasional generalized seizures if the patient insists on reading

focal spikes in specific cortical regions (parietal, frontal, occipital) may occasionally be present.

28.4 Primary Reading Epilepsy

Reading epilepsy is a distinct form of reflex epilepsy in which almost all seizures are precipitated by reading and are characterized by a clicking sensation or actual jerks in the jaw or in the tongue (Fig. 28.6). If the patient continues to read, generalized seizures may occur, always preceded by a clicking sensation or actual jerks. Reading aloud is generally more effective than mental reading in triggering jaw clicking, and sometimes the difficulty of reading the text is more effective than the content itself [19]. Despite its rarity, it is one of the few forms of reflex epilepsy specifically described by ILAE Classification as a focal idiopathic epilepsy syndrome with onset in late adolescence. The boundaries with generalized myoclonic epilepsies (in particular with perioral myoclonias) remain blurred, even if SPECT seems to confirm the focal nature of these crises.

28.5 Startle Epilepsy

The effective stimulus, in this particular form, is represented by the proprioceptive afferents linked to the startle, activating a frontal focus [20]. Functional neuroimaging techniques confirm that startle-induced seizures could be generated by the interaction of a mesial frontoparietal network, involving the supplementary motor area, perirolandic cortex, and precuneus [21]. Such involvement of the frontal cortex has also been confirmed by a macaque model (frontal lobe epilepsy, sudden stimuli able to give a startle response activate the frontal focus and induce seizure, the curarization of the animal prevents the reaction and the activation of the focus). So, various stimuli, provided they are sudden and unexpected, and therefore able to induce a startle response, can be effective; most often it is a sudden noise. The proprioceptive afferents resulting from the startle reaction activate an epileptic focus of the motor or supplementary motor area, generally inducing a tonic or hemitonic or atonic focal seizure (Fig. 28.7). Patients have usually large brain lesions, mostly perinatal hypoxic injury (Liddle syndrome, congenital hemiparesis), and frequently they show also enhanced startle reaction (syncinésie-sursaut) [22]. This type of provocation is particularly frequent even in Down syndrome. At least in some cases, even the *movement-induced epilepsy* recognizes a similar mechanism of triggering. Ricci et al. [23] described a rare infantile condition, in neurologically normal children, age-related and self-limited, characterized by myoclonus with generalized spikes and polyspikes-wave caused by sudden acoustic or tactile stimuli (*reflex myoclonic epilepsy in infancy*).

28.6 Eating Epilepsy

Eating-induced seizures are reported quite frequently, even if patients with seizures exclusively triggered by eating (eating epilepsy) are rare. Reproduction of these seizures in the EEG is often difficult, since the effective stimulus is frequently complex and requires the complete sequence of having a meal rather than the individual components (sight of food, proprioceptive, olfactive, or gustative stimulations, chewing, salivation, gastric distension) of eating [24]; moreover, artifacts from chewing often obscure EEG activity. Ictal semiology may differ from a patient to another. The seizures are generally focal, more often complex focal, but, especially in patients with diffuse cerebral damage (and/or with spontaneous seizures too), generalized seizures may coexist, in particular atypical absences [25]. Amygdala seems to play an important role as an integrative center, particularly in temporo-mesial focal seizures; in other patients, the activation of a perirolandic focus is also possible, as demonstrated by stereo-EEG studies. These seizures may be supported by different lesional etiologies [26] (Fig. 28.8), such as malformation of cortical development (MCD). Indeed, as explained above, only few patients have epilepsy characterized only by this type of seizure

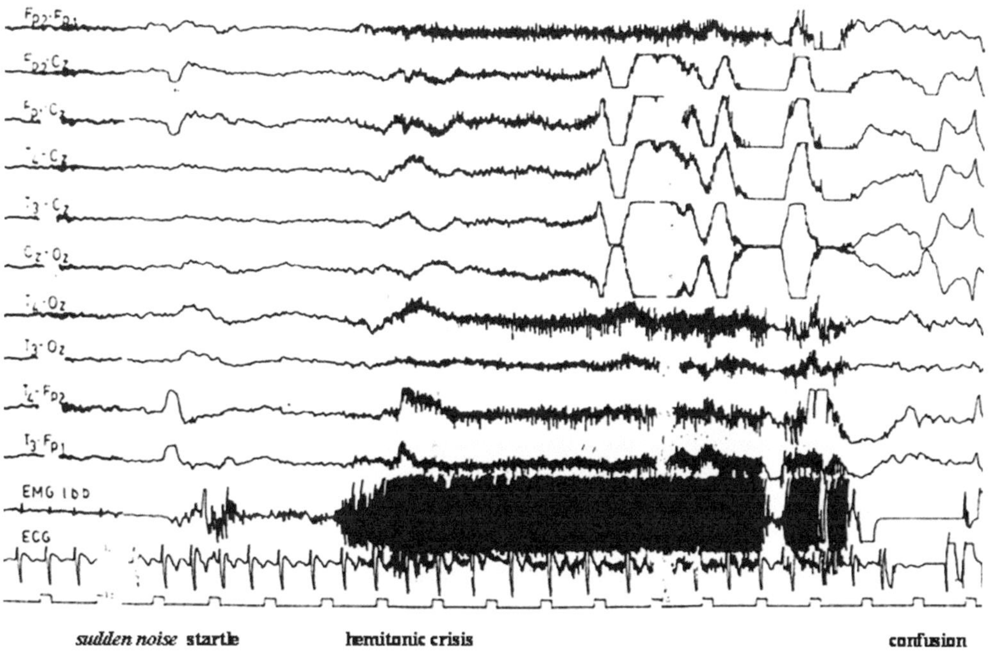

Fig. 28.7 *Startle epilepsy*: patient with periventricular leukomalacia due to perinatal hypoxic-ischemic injury. Seizure triggered by a startle provoked by a sudden noise. After the startle response (surface EMG of left brachial biceps [lbb]) occurs, a tonic-clonic seizure followed by a brief postictal confusion. EMG artifacts obscure the EEG tracing

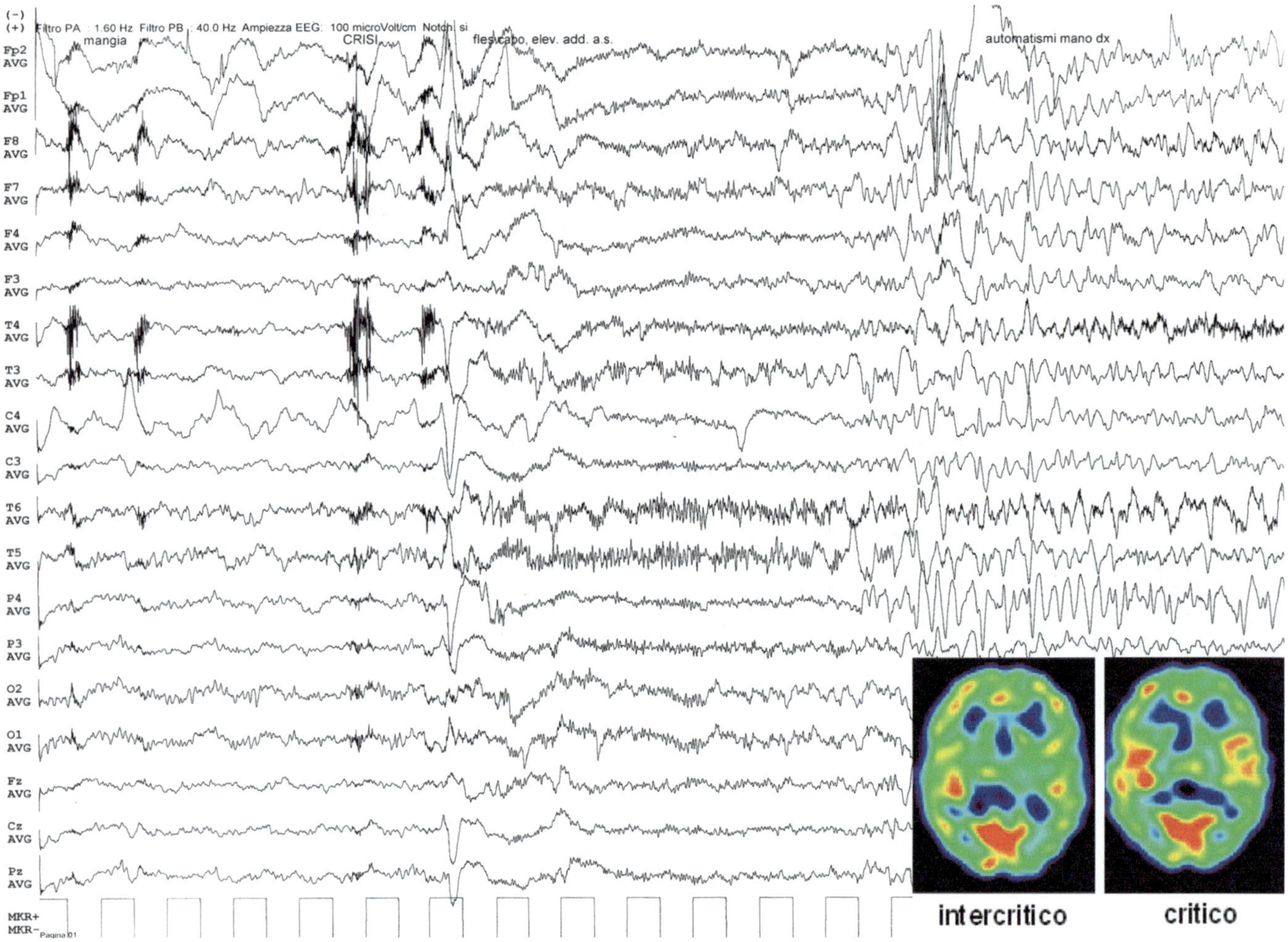

Fig. 28.8 *Eating-induced epilepsy:* ictal recording of focal impaired awareness seizure triggered by eating in a patient with left perisylvian polymicrogyria. After sudden fall of the head, a bitemporal ictal recruitment rhythm appears, more evident on the left, followed by irregularly diffused slow waves. The FDG shows bitemporal hypermetabolism (courtesy Dr. Pappatà)

(eating epilepsy). Curiously, a high incidence of eating epilepsy, with familial clusters in most cases, has been described in Sri Lanka. However, in these cases, the role of specific eating habits cannot be excluded; among them, bulky meals rich in carbohydrates have been postulated as possible triggering factors [27, 28].

28.7 Musicogenic Epilepsy

An intriguing trigger for seizure induction is listening to the music (musicogenic epilepsy, [29]). This form of RE has been anecdotally reported in the pre-EEG era, but little more than a hundred observations are reported in literature [30]. There is a case in which a specific type of music or only a particular song—and only that—is effective. These particular forms have been described primarily in music lovers. The effective stimulus appears to be very complex, associating strong emotional feelings to the specific sensorial and perceptive factors; the latency between exposition to the music and the seizure onset can be of some minutes during which the stimulation must continue. Besides music, there have been reports of seizures induced by recitation or singing (singing epilepsy) or playing (music-playing epilepsy), thinking or dreaming about music, but also by "non-musical" sounds as hearing a human voice (voice-induced epilepsy), listening to the radio, phoning (telephone-induced seizure), and listening to mewing of a cat, croaking of a frog, or crowing of a rooster.

Seizures are typically focal impaired awareness seizures of the temporal lobe (right temporal lobe more often), as demonstrated by EEG recordings and SPECT imaging (right temporal or bilateral hyperperfusion) [31]; secondary generalization is possible, and focal onset aware seizures are just few. Rarely the epilepsy is symptomatic: these cases probably should be classified in the lateral temporal lobe epilepsies with auditory features [32]. Seizures induced by sudden noises should be distinguished: the effective trigger is constituted by the afferents related to the startle (epilepsy startle, see above) or by emotional stimuli.

28.8 Hot Water Epilepsy

In *hot water epilepsy (or bath epilepsy, water-immersion epilepsy)*, seizures are triggered by contact or immersion in hot water. These seizures are very rare in Western literature, with episodic cases described in symptomatic epilepsies; on the other hand, this type of epilepsy is singularly frequent in southern of India, probably in relation to the peculiar habits of pouring hot water (40–50°) over the head. This form of geographically specific reflex epilepsy is age-related, more frequent in males, usually self-limited, and frequently familial. History is suggestive of febrile convulsions in a large number of patients [33]. Hot water-induced seizures are difficult to study because of the technical difficulty due to this singular trigger, but they seem to be focal impaired awareness seizures, with gaze staring, fear, irrelevant speech, visual and auditory hallucinations, complex automatism, and possible secondary generalization. Some patients experience a sensation of intense pleasure and continue to wash until the seizure comes. It has been suggested a mechanism of "hyperthermic kindling," reproduced in adult rats, by repeated exposition of the head to hot water [34], in the presence of a genetic predisposition. We recall the possibility of hot water-induced seizures in *severe myoclonic epilepsy of infancy (SMEI)*, linked to the extreme sensibility to body temperature elevation in this syndrome, in particular in the early stages of life.

28.9 Other Unusual Seizure Triggers

Occasionally seizures may be elicited by particular stimulations such as skin friction (*rubbing epilepsy*), touching or tapping, toothbrushing (*toothbrushing epilepsy*), and stimulation of external ear conduct (*auricular epilepsy*). In most cases the effective stimulus is limited to a specific skin area or regions, particularly the head and back. Sometimes touch-induced seizures may be induced by cutaneous self-stimulation [35, 36]. In other case, seizures are induced by movement involving one particular joint or a group of joint and exceptionally by simple ideation of the movement. Semiology of seizures varies from myoclonic jerks to somatomotor or somatosensorial focal seizures with Jacksonian propagation, in some cases with secondary generalization. Usually the seizures are brief and frequently followed by a refractory period [37, 38]. Usually these reflex seizures are linked to brain lesions of various types (clastic, dysplastic, inflammatory as in Rasmussen syndrome) involving the parietal and sensorimotor cortex or supplementary motor area, but also temporal lobe may be involved [39]. Interestingly, seizures may sometimes follow a peripheral lesion, typically after stimulating the stump in an amputee (*amputees' reflex epilepsy*), suggesting an increase of excitability in the corresponding brain area. Lastly, a unique intriguing case of symptomatic temporal epilepsy with seizures triggered by lying has been reported with the evocative name of Pinocchio syndrome [40], and a case of lesional reflex epilepsy associated with the thought of food has been described by El Bouzidi et al. [41].

28.10 Reflex Seizures in Patients with Malformations of Cortical Development

MRI has allowed in vivo demonstration of MCDs as a frequent and often refractory cause of epilepsy. The MCDs are intrinsically highly epileptogenic lesions [42], able to create abnormal connections with other cortical or subcortical structures. Therefore, it is likely that patients with MCDs could manifest seizures triggered by different kinds of stimulations. Anecdotic observations of different types of reflex seizures provoked by different triggers in patients with MCDs are reported in literature, but the attention to these reflex seizures has been generally scarce [43]. A small series of patients with video-EEG documentation is reported by Palmini et al. [44]. In all these observations, patients showed both reflex and more frequent spontaneous seizures; in two cases, self-induction has also been reported. As for spontaneous seizures, also reflex seizures are drug-resistant in these patients. Likely, more attention would demonstrate that these reflex seizures are not infrequent and that their careful observation may provide an opportunity for exploring both excitatory and inhibitory influences of these lesions on epileptogenic networks. The development of reflex seizures is also reported in patients with slow-growing tumors, where epileptogenicity is probably related to peritumoral tissue abnormalities. Modification of local connectivity (disruption of "small-world networks," [45]) can explain some unusual types of triggering seizures as in Pinocchio syndrome or in eating thought-induced seizures (see above).

28.11 Conclusions

The study of RE is an interesting field of research that has always aroused curiosity in epileptologists. The possibility of reproducing seizures in laboratory, of analyzing the characteristics of effective stimulus, and of studying the progression of clinical signs and EEG discharges, has greatly contributed to the understanding of some basic pathophysiological mechanisms. A further contribution came from the availability of functional neuroimaging techniques (fMRI, SPECT, PET) and from their fusion with EEG, which has allowed also morpho-functional correlations. All these have led to open new opportunities in the identification of brain areas and networks involved in triggering and development of seizures and of epileptogenesis [46]. Furthermore the recognition of provocative stimuli may contribute to the management of epilepsy. Finally, in the last decades, the proliferation of a lot of types of artificial light stimulation has greatly increased the number of patients with seizures induced by visual stimulation, making photosensitive epilepsy a topic of great relevance: an example is the research of equipment and software with lower risk for seizure induction.

References

1. De Bittencourt PRM. Photosensitivity: the magnitude of the problem. Epilepsia. 2004;45:30–4.
2. Dreyfuss FE. Classification of reflex epilepsies and reflex seizure. In: Zifkin BG, Andermann F, Beaumanoir A, Rowan AJ, editors. Reflex epilepsies and reflex seizures, Advances in neurology, vol. 75. Philadelphia: Lippincott-Raven Publisher; 1998. p. 5–13.
3. Gastaut H. Synopsis and conclusions of the international Colloquium on reflex seizures and epilepsies. In: Beaumanoir A, Gastaut H, Naquet R, editors. Reflex seizures and reflex Epilepsies. Geneva: Editions Médicine et Hygiéne; 1989. p. 497–507.
4. Merlis JK. Reflex epilepsy. In: Vinken PJ, Bruyn GW, editors. Handbook of clinical neurology, The epilepsies, vol. 15. New York: Elsevier; 1974. p. 440–56.
5. Panayiotopoulos CP. The epilepsies. In: Seizure, syndromes and management. Oxfordshire: Bladon Med Publisher; 2005.
6. Ritaccio AL. Reflex seizures. Neurol Clin. 1994;12:57–83.
7. Striano S, Meo R, Bilo L, Perrone M. An attempt to classify reflex seizures in accordance to the recent proposals for classification of epilepsies. In: Beaumanoir A, Gastaut H, Naquet R, editors. Reflex seizures and reflex epilepsies. Geneva: Editions Médicine et Hygiéne; 1989. p. 489–93.
8. Berg AT, Berkovic SF, Brodie MJ, Buchhalter J, Cross JH, van Emde Boas W, Engel J, French J, Glauser TA, Mathern GW, Moshé SL, Nordli D, Plouin P, Scheffer IE. Revised terminology and concepts for organization of seizures and epilepsies: report of the ILAE Commission on Classification and Terminology, 2005–2009. Epilepsia. 2010;5:676–85.
9. Guerrini R, Genton P. Epileptic syndromes and visually induced seizures. Epilepsia. 2004;45(1):14–8.
10. Jeavons PM. Nosological problems of myoclonic epilepsies in childhood and adolescence. Dev Syndrom Med. 1977;19:3–8.
11. Striano S, Capovilla G, Sofia V, Romeo A, Rubboli G, Striano P, Kasteleijn-Nolst Trenité D. Eyelid myoclonia with absences (Jeavons syndrome): a well-defined idiopathic generalized syndrome or a spectrum of photosensitive conditions? Epilepsia. 2009;50(5):15–9.
12. Ames FR, Saffer D. The sunflower syndrome. J Neurol Sci. 1983;59:1–11.
13. Ishida S, Yamashita Y, Matsuishi T, Ohshima M, Ohshima H, Kato H, Maeda H. Photosensitive seizures provoked while viewing "pocket monsters," a made-for-television animation program in Japan. Epilepsia. 1998;39:1340–4.
14. Takada H, Aso K, Watanabe K, Okumura A, Negoro T, Ishikawa T. Epileptic seizures induced by animated cartoon, "Pocket Monster". Epilepsia. 1999;40:997–1002.
15. Kasteleijn-Nolst DGA, Guerrini R, Binnie CD, Genton P. Visual sensitivity and epilepsy: a proposed terminology and classification for clinical and EEG Phenomenology. Epilepsia. 2001;42:692–701.
16. Panayiotopoulos CP. Fixation-off, scotosensitive, and other visual related epilepsies. In: Zifkin BG, Andermann F, Beaumanoir A, Rowan AJ, editors. Reflex epilepsies and reflex seizures, Advances in neurology, vol. 75. Philadelphia: Lippincott-Raven Publisher; 1998. p. 139–57.
17. Ingvar DH, Nyman GE. Epilepsia arithmetices: a new psychologic trigger mechanism in a case of epilepsy. Neurology. 1962;12:282–7.
18. Inoue Y, Zifkin BG. Praxis induction and thinking induction: one or two mechanisms? A controversy. In: Wolf P, Inoue Y, Zifkin B, editors. Reflex epilepsies: progress in understanding. Esher: John Libbey Eurotext; 2004. p. 41–55.
19. Stella L, Fels A, Pillo G, Fragassi N, Buscaino GA, Striano S. "Primary reading epilepsy". Clinical and EEG study of a case and characteristics of the effective stimulus. Acta Neurol. 1983;5:426–31.
20. Bancaud J, Talairach J, Bonis A. Physiopathogenies des épilepsies-sursaut (a propos d'une épilepsie de l'aire motrice supplementaire). Rev Neurol. 1967;117:441–53.
21. Fernández S, Donaire A, Maestro I, Seres E, Setoain X, Bargalló N, Rumià J, Boget T, Falcón C, Carreño M. Functional neuroimaging in startle epilepsy: involvement of a mesial frontoparietal network. Epilepsia. 2011;52:1725–32.
22. Alajouanine T, Gastaut H. La syncinésie-sursaut et l'épilepsie sursaut à déclenchement sensorial ou sensitive inopié. Les faits anatomo-cliniques (15 observations). Rev Neurol. 1955;93:29–41.
23. Ricci S, Cusmai R, Fusco L, Vigevano F. Reflex myoclonic epilepsy in infancy: a new age-dependent idiopathic epileptic syndrome related to startle reaction. Epilepsia. 1995;36:342–8.
24. Cirignotta F, Marcacci G, Lugaresi E. Epileptic seizures precipitated by eating. Epilepsia. 1977;18:445–9.
25. Loreto V, Nocerino C, Striano P, D'Aulos F, Boccella P, Striano S. Eating epilepsy: heterogeneity of ictal semiology: the role of video-EEG monitoring. Epileptic Disord. 2000;2:93–8.
26. Manyam SC, Kung DH, Rhodes RB, Newmark ME, Friedman ED. Unilateral opercular lesion and eating-induced seizures. Epileptic Disord. 2010;12:309–13.
27. Nagaraja D, Chand RP. Eating Epilepsy. Clin Neurol Neurosurg. 1984;86:95–9.
28. Senanayake N. Familial eating epilepsy. J Neurol. 1990;237:388–91.
29. Critchley M. Musicogenic epilepsy. Brain. 1937;60:13–27.
30. Pittau F, Tinuper P, Bisulli F, Naldi I, Cortelli P, Bisulli A, Stipa C, Cevolani D, Agati R, Leonardi M, Baruzzi A. Videopolygraphic and functional MRI study of musicogenic epilepsy. A case report and literature review. Epilepsy Behav. 2008;13:685–92.
31. Gelisse P, Thomas P, Padovani R, Hassan-Sebbag N, Pasquier J, Genton P. Ictal SPECT in a case of pure musicogenic epilepsy. Epileptic Disord. 2003;5:133–7.
32. Michelucci R, Gardella E, de Haan GJ, Bisulli F, Zaniboni A, Cantalupo G, Tassinari CA, Tinuper P, Nobile C, Nichelli P, Kasteleijn-Nolst Trenité DG. Telephone-induced seizures: a new type of reflex epilepsy. Epilepsia. 2004;45(3):280–3.
33. Satishachndra P, Shivaramakrishana A, Kaliaperumal VG, Schoenberg BS. Hot-water epilepsy: a variant of reflex epilepsy in southern India. Epilepsia. 1988;29:52–6.
34. Ullal GR, Satishandra P, Shankar SK. Hypertermic seizures: an animal model for hot water epilepsy. Seizure. 1996;5:221–8.
35. Guerrini R, Genton P, Dravet C, Viallat D, Bureau M, Horton EJ, Roger J. Compulsive somatosensory self-stimulation inducing epileptic seizures. Epilepsia. 1992;33:509–16.

36. Striano S, Meo R, Bilo L, Ruosi P, Soricellis M, Estraneo A, Caporella A. The use of EEG activating procedures in epileptology. Acta Neurol (Naples). 1992;47:275–89.
37. Biraben A, Doury E, Scarabin JM. Motor reflex Epilepsy induced by touch and movement. In: Wolf P, Inoue Y, Zifkin B, editors. Reflex epilepsies: progress in understanding. Esher: John Libbey Eurotext; 2004. p. 135–42.
38. Deonna T. Reflex seizures with somatosensory precipitation. In: Zifkin BG, Andermann F, Beaumanoir A, Rowan AJ, editors. Reflex epilepsies and reflex seizures, Advances in neurology, vol. 75. Philadelphia: Lippincott-Raven Publisher; 1998. p. 193–206.
39. Hsieh CY, Chiou NJ, Wu YJ, Tsai JJ, Huang CW. Somatosensory rub evoked reflex epilepsy of a temporal lobe origin. Neurol Sci. 2011;32(2):297–9.
40. Sellal F, Chevalier Y, Collard M. “Pinocchio syndrome”: a peculiar form of reflex epilepsy? Neurol Neurosurg Psychiat. 1993;56:963.
41. El Bouzidi K, Duncan S, Whittle IR, Butler CR. Lesional reflex Epilepsy associated with the thought of food. Neurology. 2010;74:710–2.
42. Palmini A. Electrophysiology of the focal cortical dysplasias. Epilepsia. 2010;51(1):23–6.
43. Palmini A, Halàsz P, Scheffer IE, Takahashi Y, Jimenez AP, Dubeau F, Andermann F, Rosenow F, Fritsch B. Malformations of cortical development as a cause of reflex seizures: neurobiological insights. In: Wolf P, Inoue Y, Zifkin B, editors. Reflex epilepsies: progress in understanding. Esher: John Libbey Eurotext; 2004. p. 143–56.
44. Palmini A, Halàsz P, Scheffer I, Takahashi Y, Perez-Jimenez A, Dubeau F, Andermann F, Paglioli-Neto E, da Costa JC, Rosenow F, Fritsch B. Reflex seizures in patients with malformations of cortical development and refractory epilepsy. Epilepsia. 2005;46:1224–34.
45. Douw L, van Dellen E, de Groot M, Heimans JJ, Klein M, Stam CJ, Reijneveld JC. Epilepsy is related to theta band brain connectivity and network topology in brain tumor patients. BMC Neurosci. 2010;23:103.
46. Gotman J, Pittau F. Combining EEG and fMRI in the study of epileptic discharges. Epilepsia. 2011;52(4):38–42.

Photosensitivity and Epilepsy

29

Dorothee Kasteleijn-Nolst Trenite

29.1 Introduction

Intermittent photic stimulation (IPS) is a routine provocation method with stroboscopic light flashing between 2 and 60 Hz to diagnose epilepsy. It can easily be repeated in a standardized manner to evaluate the seizure threshold in an individual patient over time and with different AEDs. With IPS or any other provocative visual stimulus (striped patterns, computer screen, etc.), the EEG may show regular or irregular polyspike or spike-and-wave activity starting or maximum over the temporo-parieto-occipital areas with or without generalization: these visually evoked epileptiform EEG reactions are called photoparoxysmal responses or PPR [1].

About 3–5% of epilepsy patients will show PPR; in adolescents PPR can even be found up to 10% [2], and females are more affected than males (greater prevalence and sensitivity to a wider range of flash frequencies) [3]. About 10% of PPR-positive patients were found also recently in first-seizure patients (children 14% and adults 5%) and predominant with generalized epileptiform discharges [4]. A specific subgroup are the patients with Dravet syndrome: 40% will show PPR as early as the age of 1 year, and there is no sex difference [5].

IPS is most effective with an intensity of 1 J/flash and a flash frequency between 10 and 30 Hz [6]. Deep red monochromatic flashing light (~600 nm) as is used in cartoons has proven to be very provocative [7].

Striped patterns with high contrast and a spatial frequency of 4 cycli per degree give PPRs in about 30% of IPS-sensitive patients [8]. Only in specialized laboratories these patterns are tested in photosensitive patients [9]. It is however a readily recognized subtype of photosensitivity; patients suffer differently from environmental stimuli [10].

See for further details the EU guidelines of 2012, published at the ILAE website under guidelines for diagnosis [11].

Below, important issues related to visual sensitivity will be highlighted and examples given.

29.2 Important Issues

29.2.1 Why Do We Use Intermittent Photic Stimulation? How Was It Discovered to Be a Valuable Tool in Epilepsy Diagnostics and Research?

After the finding of Hans Berger [12] in the late 1920s of spontaneous occipital rhythm—alpha waves—being blocked by eye opening as well as by light from a torch, the British Adrian and Matthews started experimenting with *flickering* light in 1934: hereto they used an illuminated opal glass bowl with a rotating sectored disc to produce flickering light of up to 25 flashes/s [13]. Photic driving was shown with harmonics and subharmonics. It took more than 10 years though before Walter et al. in 1946 described that flickering lights could evoke epileptiform discharges [14]. He also developed the first electronic photostimulator, and from then on it became more and more common in Europe and the USA to use intermittent photic stimulation (IPS) in EEG diagnostics; this was certainly helped by the observation of Cobb in 1947 that IPS could evoke clinical seizures (absences) in epilepsy patients in the laboratory [15]. On the market came a variety of gas-filled strobe lights (mainly xenon), which emitted bright flashes of short duration (15 or 30 μs) to prevent retinal damage [16].

Thanks to society and personal meetings and publications, the enthusiasm of the modulation of the EEG traces by IPS was spreading through the English and French speaking community: neurophysiologist in different centers in the USA, Canada, Western Europe, and South Africa studied

D. Kasteleijn-Nolst Trenite (✉)
Department of Neurosurgery and Epilepsy, University Medical Center Utrecht, Utrecht, The Netherlands

Faculty of Medicine and Psychology, Nesmos Department, Sapienza University, Rome, Italy
e-mail: d.kasteleijn@umcutrecht.nl; dkasteleijn@planet.nl; Dorothee.Kasteleijn@uniRoma1.it

O. Mecarelli (ed.), *Clinical Electroencephalography*, https://doi.org/10.1007/978-3-030-04573-9_29

intensively in the 1950s and 1960s the effect of IPS on the EEG traces in healthy volunteers (adults and children), psychiatric patients, alcoholics, patients with different kinds of brain damage and headaches, and those with known epilepsy or family with epilepsy. It was a fascinating time of exploring reactions of the brain to visual stimuli: asymmetries, localization, and spreading of (poly)-spike-and-wave discharges related to flash frequencies, light intensities, and color and eye conditions were registered. This is still valid today [17].

IPS methodology was considered soon to be in particular valuable for diagnosing epilepsy: Melsen showed in 1959 IPS-evoked epileptiform discharges in 16/565 (2.8%) of patients with suspected epilepsy and confirmation of the epilepsy in 110/445 (24.7%) and in 24/356 (6.7%) of those with symptomatic epilepsy (13% with temporal lobe seizures) [18]. It did not take therefore long that IPS became a routine method in EEG diagnostics. And until today it offers an excellent way of dealing with and learning more about not only photosensitive epilepsy but also epilepsy in general. PPR is common in syndromes like JME (30–40%) [19] and Dravet syndrome (40%) [5]. In Dravet syndrome PPRs can occur already at the age of 1 and predict a less favorable outcome [5].

29.2.2 Photomyoclonic, Photoconvulsive, and Photoparoxysmal Responses: How to Use the Respective Terms Nowadays?

Gastaut and Naquet performed photo-metrazol provocation tests (combination of epileptogenic metrazol injections—used at the time predominantly in animal studies—and IPS) in Marseille, France, in the early 1950s and found "frontal spikes" occurring in normal persons and even more prominent in alcoholic, neurotic, and psychiatric patients [20, 21]. They considered these photomyoclonic responses as a frontopolar recruiting response of muscular origin. Bickford et al. repeated these studies in Rochester, Minnesota, in 72 patients with an already known positive response to IPS with or without metrazol [22]. Based on their experiences, they dissected the EEG responses into those with a predominant myoclonic symptomatology (photomyoclonic) versus absence type (photoconvulsive). Included in the epileptogenic photomyoclonic responses was however the Gastaut type of myogenic responses. It is thus not surprising that Bickford et al. found both types of responses in the same patients.

Our current use of the terms is the following:

1. Photomyoclonic (or photomyogenic) reactions—as originally considered by Gastaut and Remond—are myogenic potentials locked to the flash that build up in intensity as the stimulus continues and cease as soon as the flashing stops. Usually frontal EEG leads are involved, although some spreading can be seen. During these *myogenic* potentials, eye and face muscles twitch, while the patient is fully aware of it. It is considered as very annoying. It can be evoked in a minority of normal adults, especially when they are close to the lamp; it has ***no** relation with epilepsy.*
2. Photoconvulsive reactions. The word "convulsive" suggests an evoked tonic-clonic convulsion, which is rare if stimulation is done according to the European guidelines [11, 23]. *No current term anymore.*
3. Photoparoxysmal reactions = epileptiform EEG reactions evoked by IPS or other visual stimuli [1, 11]. This term "photoparoxysmal" or PPR includes the older term photoconvulsive and comprises thus all epileptiform EEG responses to IPS, regardless of the type of clinical sign (myoclonic jerking of eyelids or arms; absences and focal seizures) or symptom (pain in the eyes, dizziness, loss of awareness, headache).

29.2.3 Photoparoxysmal Responses (PPRs) Outlasting the Stimulus or Not: Is It Relevant?

Driving and photomyoclonic responses are linked to the stimulus and unrelated to epilepsy. PPRs are often seen to be outlasting the stimulus train combined with clinical symptomatology. PPR can also occur in patients without epilepsy [24]. It is therefore not surprising that Reilly and Peters hypothesized in 1973 that outlasting the stimulus is a key factor for the diagnosis of epilepsy [25]. They indeed found a strong relationship between PPRs (focal and generalized) outlasting the stimulus train and having clinical epilepsy. Their methodology was such as to stimulate with a Grass PS2 to the max according to the author, i.e., with separate trains of 5 s flashing at 6, 10, and 14 Hz as well as continuous flashing between 1 and 20 Hz for a duration of 20 s. Out of a total of 132 pediatric and adult patients with any type of reaction to IPS (photomyoclonic, flash dependent, or PPR), 54 showed a prolonged PPR, 56 showed a self-limited PPR, and 7 had both self-limited and prolonged PPRs.

Later studies by Jayakar and Chiappa [26] (1990) and Puglia et al. [27](1992), addressing this same issue, led to the conclusion that outlasting the stimulus train of the PPR (prolonged response) was not a predictor for clinical epilepsy by itself. Only if there was spontaneous epileptiform activity in the EEG, the likelihood of having sustained PPRs was indeed higher ("confounding factor of the Reilly and Peters study") (see Fig. 29.1). It was also stressed that timing of switching off of the photostimulator by the technician determines whether or not PPR outlasts the stimulus ("technical artifact") (Fig. 29.1).

Interestingly, short-lasting afterdischarges at normal driving responses ("flicker responses") have been documented by Mundy-Castle in 1953 [28]. This strengthens the fact that outlasting the stimulus train of a PPR by a few milliseconds does not necessarily have an additional meaning.

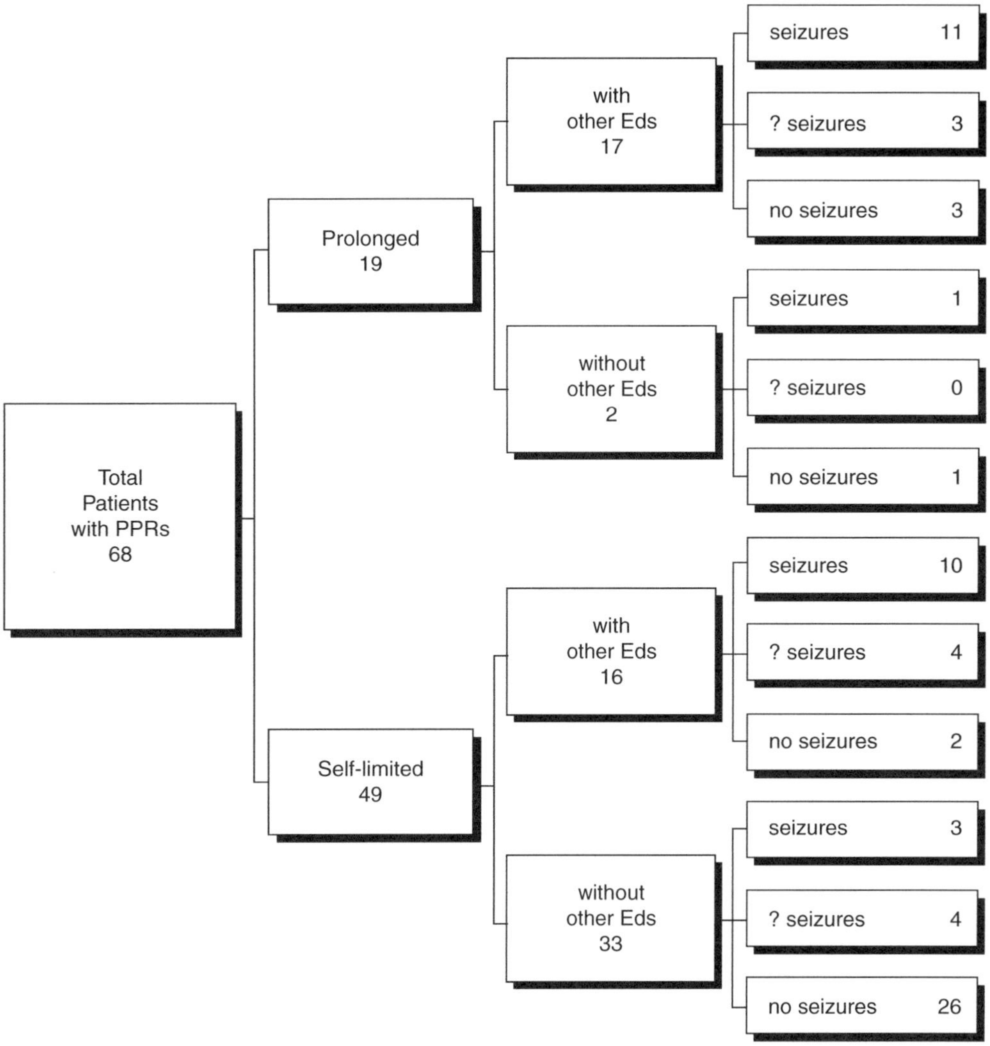

Fig. 29.1 Overview of results for patients with PPRs. *EDs* = epileptiform discharges (Fig. 3 from Puglia et al., 1992, reference 27)

29.2.4 Does a PPR Equals a Seizure?

There is a strong link between PPR and seizure signs and symptoms:

1. Observational studies as early as 1953 described in detail the overall spectrum of clinical signs and symptoms *during* a PPR, namely, myoclonic jerks in the arms, head, eyelids, or upper limbs; speech arrest; and turning of the eyes to the left or right side or a GTCS after head-turning to the left with buildup of occipital epileptiform activity on the right side with generalization afterward [16].

   In a later observational study, 27/36 (75%) photosensitive patients showed clinical signs during PPRs with a duration between 0.5 and 8 s [29]. Only when the PPR lasted at least 2 s, loss of consciousness was found. Symptoms were also common: 25/36 (69%) complained about dizziness, pain in the head/eyes, or queer feeling in the stomach during the PPR. They recognized that these complaints were equal to those felt at the onset of visually induced seizures in daily life.

   A more recent video-controlled study revealed clinical signs in *all* patients with a generalized PPR. Myoclonus was observed in all 29 patients: eyelid myoclonia was observed in all; many also exhibited myoclonus of the head, arms, or body. Loss of consciousness was noted in three patients (33%). Six (67%) showed asymmetrical signs, and three manifested both right- and left-sided signs [30].
2. A statistically significant linear trend can be found between those patients with a history of triggered seizures and a greater sensitivity to IPS (chi-square test for linear trends, $p < 0.05$) [3]. The Birmingham Group followed 50 patients, where 67% of those who continued to have seizures still showed a PPR [31].

Thus, PPRs are in fact seizure manifestations by itself. Not all people showing PPRs necessarily will experience GTCS and/or need treatment. Children need in general more protection: Fallah and Nair [32] showed that PPRs without clear concomitant clinical symptomatology, still in 50% caused delay in a simple motor task, equal to spontaneous generalized epileptiform discharges [33]. Having a PPR is thus not only an indication of having increased risk of provoked and spontaneous seizures, but also of transitory cognitive impairment.

The likelihood of having seizures in daily life depends on the duration of PPR and amount of flash frequencies that produce a PPR, so-called photosensitivity range. If, for example, a PPR can be evoked between 2 and 60 Hz, disco lights, TV screens, and sunlight flickering through trees will all be provoking and leading to seizures (and thus the diagnosis of epilepsy).

29.2.5 Does Photosensitivity Mean "Automatically" that the Patient Has Genetic Generalized Epilepsy (Formerly Known as Idiopathic Generalized Epilepsy)?

One of the first IPS-evoked clinical symptoms [15] was an absence seizure, and from then on much emphasis has been placed on the relationship of photosensitivity/PPR and idiopathic generalized epilepsies (IGE): not only in childhood absence epilepsy but also in juvenile myoclonic epilepsy (JME), high prevalence rates of PPR (30% of patients) were especially found [19]. Photosensitivity has been noticed also as an important characteristic of the severe myoclonic epilepsy of childhood or Dravet syndrome since its first description [34]. Both are generalized types of epilepsy.

With all this emphasis on generalized epilepsy, one wonders if PPR can be found in focal epilepsies as well. PPRs were reported in patients with occipital and temporal lobe epilepsy, even with ictal focal seizure symptomatology during the PPR [35–38]. Recently, an overview is made of studies published between 1983 and 2016 in patients with a PPR with documented epilepsy diagnoses [39]. Fifteen clinical studies (5 prospective) could be analyzed. A total of 955 patients (55% female) from 10 different countries revealed that focal epilepsy was found in 159 (17%) of all patients. Benbadis et al. remarked in 1996 that even a temporal focus can be the driver in photosensitive temporal lobe in IPS-evoked seizures [38].

The presence of a PPR means thus not necessarily the patient *must* have the diagnosis of IGE or encephalopathy, but can be focal epilepsy.

29.2.6 Is any Type of Photostimulator Appropriate?

The answer is clearly no! We have recently shown in Bambino Gesu, Rome, Italy, that the use of a specific type of photic stimulator was necessary to reveal the epileptic cause of the reported complaints with as consequence new diagnoses and different treatment options (blue lenses; AEDs) [40]. The Grass PS 2 or PS 33 has been the golden standard since the 1960s (see Fig. 29.2).

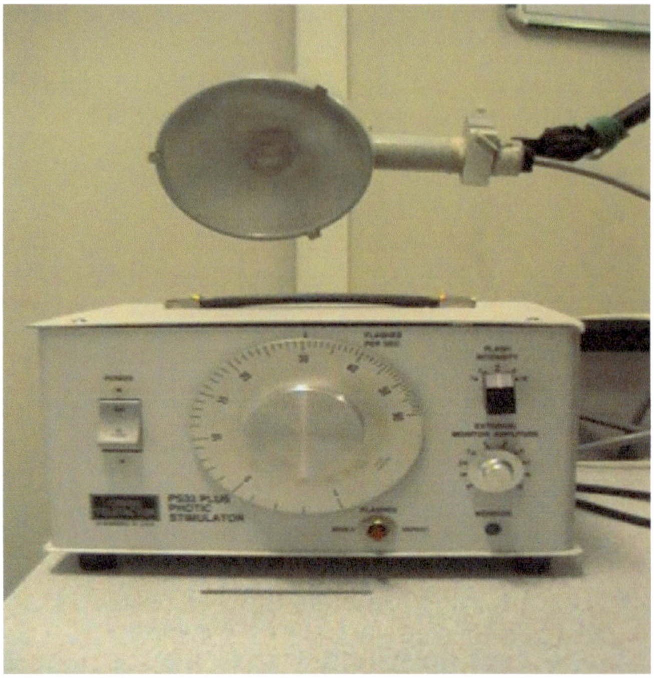

Fig. 29.2 The gold standard photostimulator Grass PS 33

These round high-quality xenon gas lamps produce white diffuse light of 10 μs with an intensity of 1 J at flash frequencies ranging from 0.5 up to 60 Hz. The EEG response to IPS depends mainly on the relative brightness of the flickering light and the total number of retinal cells being stimulated [40]. Original LED lamp technology (first developed for the EEG machine by Nihon Kohden) has taken over the gas-filled lamps: this meant much less intensity of the flash, flash frequencies only up to 20 or 30 Hz, and rectangular shape (less stimulation of the retina). Currently developed modern LED lamps, such as the Lifelines stimulator, equal the old Grass gas-filled lamp [41].

Just diminishing the distance between the eyes and the lamp will only increase the area of the retina stimulated, but not the total brightness. If the lamp is too close to the face, unwanted photomyoclonic reactions occur, besides anxiety and limited observation of the patient.

The advice is thus to use a round, modern LED lamp at a distance of 30 cm to the nasion (see guidelines) [11].

29.2.7 Why Testing Different Eye Conditions with IPS?

Photosensitive patients are most sensitive when flashing starts precisely at the act of eye closure (see Fig. 29.3).

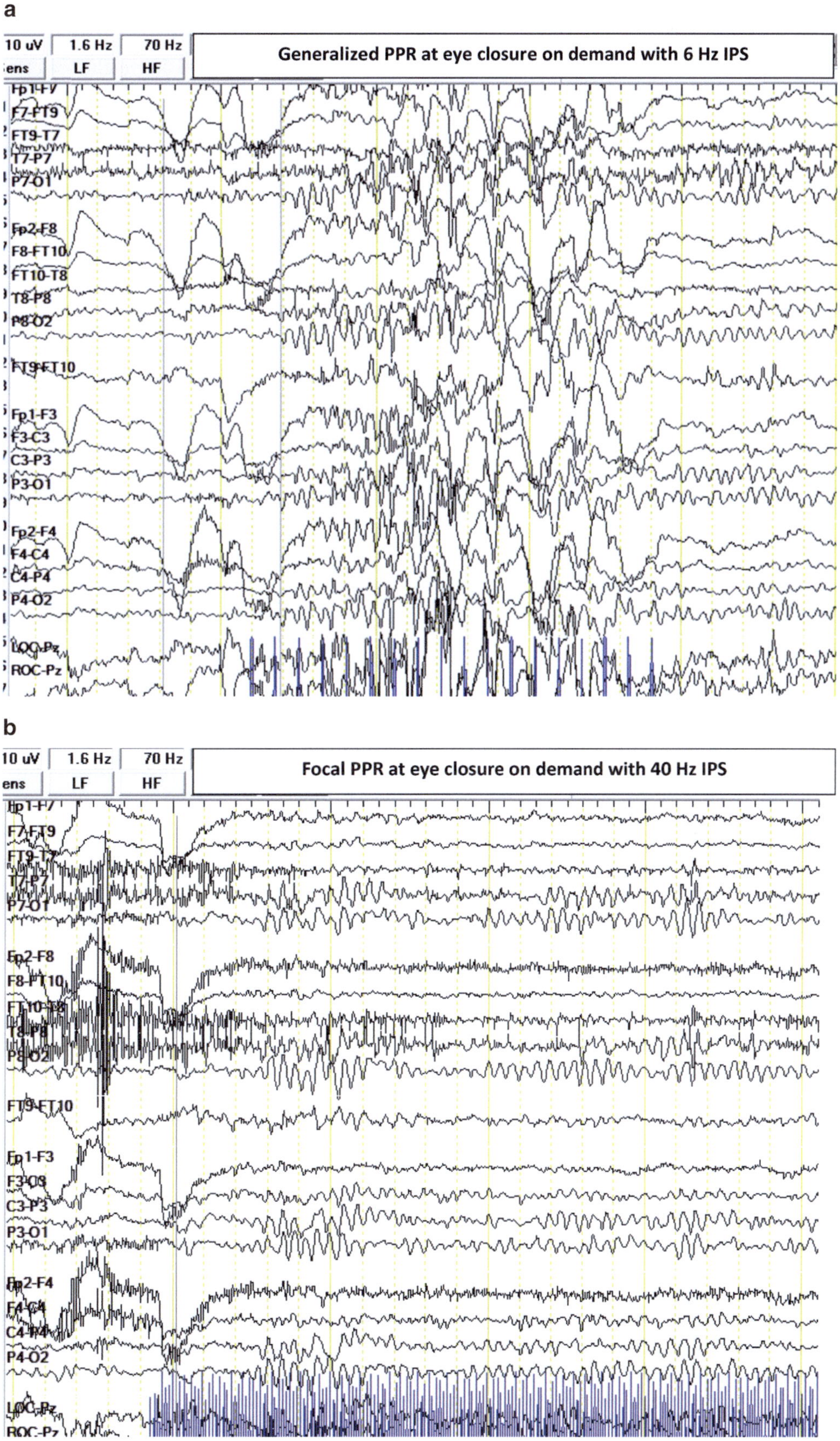

Fig. 29.3 (**a**) A 23-year-old female with generalized PPR at eye closure with IPS 6 Hz. (**b**) The same 23-year-old female with focal PPR at eye closure with IPS 40 Hz

The best explanation for this is that just after eye closure, a so-called alpha squeak occurs, and combined with the spiky higher voltage alpha, the PPR can more easily develop (see Fig. 29.4). It is shown by Vaudano et al. very recently that the alpha rhythm of photosensitive patients has reduced inhibition [42]. Ninety percent of the photosensitive patients will show their sensitivity at this eye closure act [3]. The second most sensitive eye condition during IPS is eyes closed (80% of photosensitive patients), related with the alpha waves again. With eyes open the likelihood of discovering a PPR is much less: about 65%. With eyes open, fixation plays an inhibiting role, and spontaneous blinks do not produce alpha squeaks. Furthermore, especially in children there is the likelihood that they do not look into the center of the lamp and have only part of the retina being stimulated. About 10% of patients will be unrecognized as being photosensitive when IPS at eye closure is not performed. The best method is to ask the patient "close your eyes as soon as the flickering light starts." Alternatively, ask them to close their eyes and start stimulating just exactly at that moment (Fig. 29.4).

29.2.8 How Can You Be Sure that a Patient Is Photosensitive?

When a patient has a history of seizures provoked by flashing lights (sunlight through the trees, discotheque, episodes in TV program or movie) or striped patterns (clothes,

a

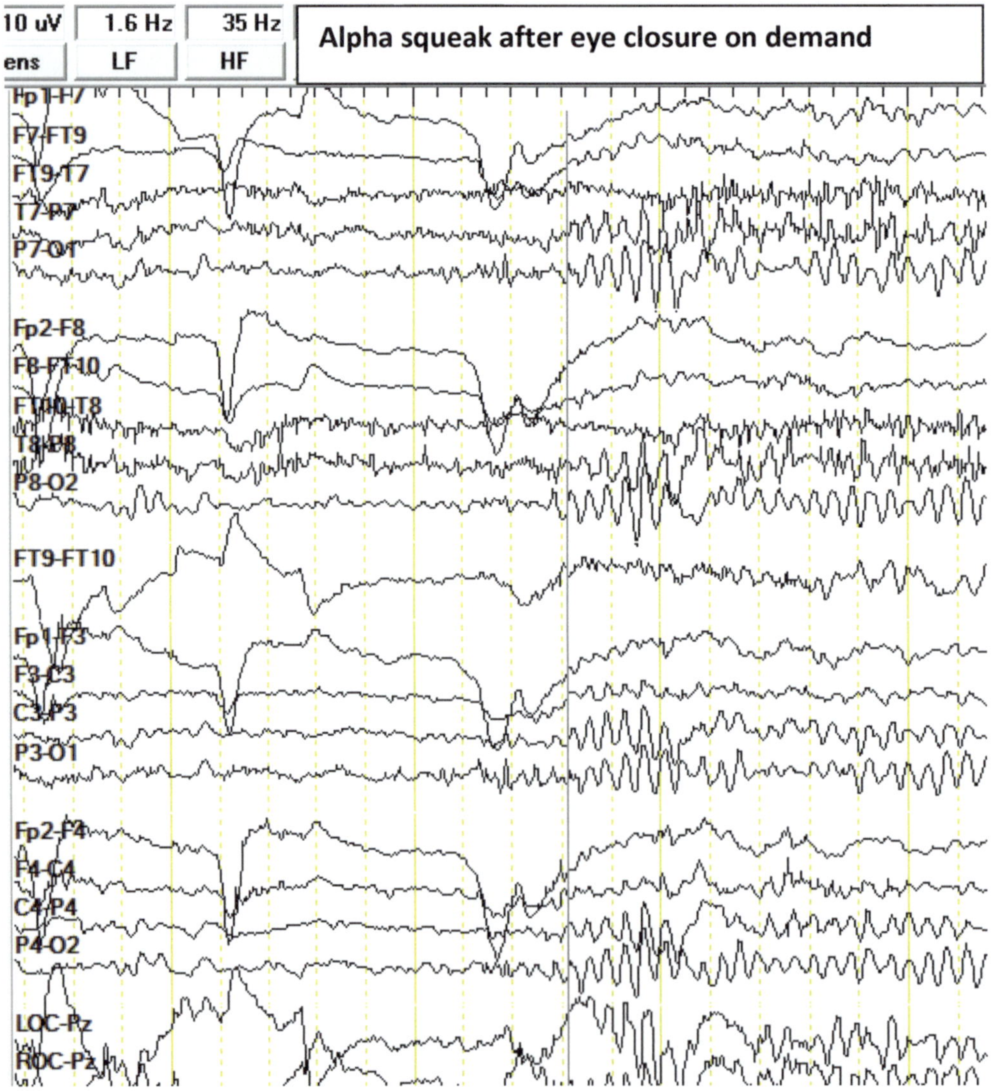

Fig. 29.4 (**a**) The same 23-year-old female as in Fig. 29.2 with alpha squeak after eye closure on demand. (**b**) The same 23-year-old female patient with eyes closed IPS 10 Hz: first a driving response is seen, and then a transitioning is seen to a generalized PPR

b

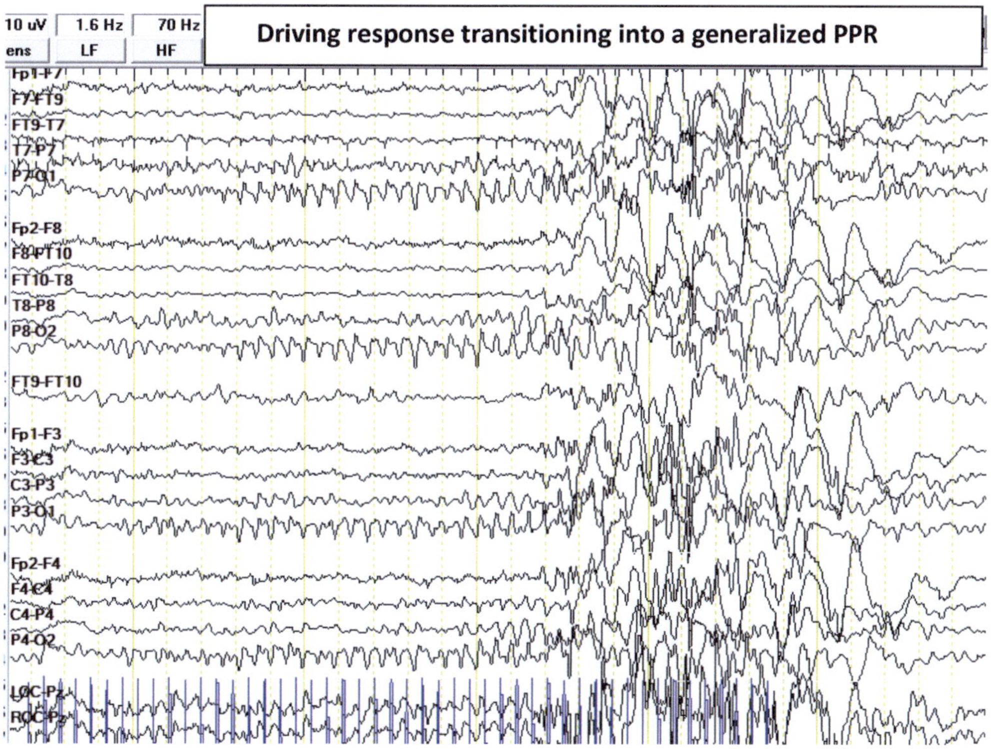

Fig. 29.4 (continued)

Table 29.1 Example of a patient with lower thresholds of 10 and 18, respectively, for eye closure and eyes closed and open and higher thresholds of 40, 30, and 20 Hz, respectively, for the eye closure condition, eyes closed and open
See for details: ref. [11]

Methodology
Identifying the photosensitivity ranges in three eye conditions

Flash frequency in Hz	1	2	8	10	15	18	20	25	40	50	60
Eye closure	-	-	V	+					+	V	-
Eyes closed	-	-	-	-	V	+		+	-	-	-
Eyes open	-	-	-	-	-	+	+	-	-	-	-

	Ranges	
Eye closure :	**10–40 Hz**	**– = no epileptiform activity**
Eyes closed :	**18–25 Hz**	**V = focal epileptiform activity**
Eyes open :	**18–20 Hz**	**+ = generalized epileptiform activity**

curtains, etc.), the EEG will show a PPR, and photosensitivity is confirmed [3]. However, when it is unclear whether the seizures are related with visual stimuli (large variety of screens and patterns in the surrounding) or patient/caregivers do not notice his/her visually induced seizures, standardized IPS with determination of flash sensitivity ranges helps in identifying a photosensitive patient [11]. Determination of ranges (lower and upper threshold of sensitivity) allows safe and repeated photic stimulation. Knowing that most patients are sensitive between 10 and 30 Hz and more with eye closure than with eyes closed and open, occurrence of PPRs should follow this paradigm (see Table 29.1).

In other words, when an epileptiform reaction is, for example, seen at 5 Hz with eyes open and at 30 Hz during eye closure only, these are spontaneous discharges and not PPRs. Patients with spontaneous discharges can certainly be photosensitive—about 40% of Dravet patients are photosensitive. Proper IPS testing is thus also of importance in children with many spontaneous discharges and known to have Dravet syndrome [43]. Flashing at very low frequencies detects/confirms furthermore encephalopathic epilepsies like Lafora disease and ceroid lipofuscinosis [44].

29.2.9 Use of PPR Ranges in Evaluation of Epileptogenic Threshold and Treatment

One of the big advantages of photosensitivity is that standardized repeated IPS assessments are possible allowing evaluation of age effects (maximum expression during puberty), colored glasses, and anti-epileptic drugs (acute and in steady state). Photosensitivity can be monitored thus on an individual level by determining the photosensitivity ranges before and after drug treatment. Diminishment of range equals an anti-epileptic protective effect. It is not necessary to have a complete abolishment of photosensitivity to yet establish a clinically important effect. AED dosages can even be titrated using the photosensitivity ranges [6]. Many patients, especially children, can be adequately treated with a relatively low dosage of an anti-epileptic drug. During adolescence, the prescribed dosage usually needs to be raised, partly because of the greater body weight and partly due to the natural increase in photosensitivity around puberty. The PPR ranges help you with making such decisions. Therapy should be maintained at least until after puberty. IPS in the laboratory can similarly help to predict the relapse rate after partial and total withdrawal of the drug. Early withdrawal of VPA gives a high risk of seizure recurrence as has been documented [45, 46] with even in some cases status epilepticus as result (personal comment).

29.3 Conclusions

Photic stimulation is still today an important tool to diagnose (photosensitive) epilepsy and to evaluate treatment. Recently, Parisi et al. have advocated to recognize the intricate relationship between migraine and photosensitivity; visual stimuli can provoke migraine, and in families with migraine, photosensitivity is very frequently found [47, 48].

Photic stimulation needs certainly be done with care to get the maximum of information needed without making it too uncomfortable for the patient, let alone provoking GTCS. In the guidelines advice can be found on how to achieve that (see website ILAE under guidelines for diagnosis) [11].

Acknowledgement *Conflict of Interest*: none.

References

1. Kasteleijn-Nolst Trenité DG, Guerrini R, Binnie CD, Genton P. Visual sensitivity and epilepsy: a proposed terminology and classification for clinical and EEG phenomenology. Epilepsia. 2001;42:692–701.
2. Clement MJ, Wallace SJ. A survey of adolescents with epilepsy. Dev Med Child Neurol. 1990;32(10):849–57.
3. Kasteleijn-Nolst Trenite DG. Photosensitivity in epilepsy. Electrophysiological and clinical correlates. Acta Neurol Scand Suppl. 1989;125:3–149.
4. Taoufiqi FZ, Mounach J, Satte A, Ouhabi H, El Hessni A. IPS interest in the EEG of patients after a single epileptic seizure. Neurosci J. 2016:5050278.
5. Verbeek NE, Kasteleijn-Nolst Trenité DGA, Wassenaar M, van Campen JS, Gunning B, de Weerd A, Knoers N, Spetgens W, Gutter T, Leijten F, Brilstra EH. Relevance of seizure precipitants and especially photosensitivity in children with Dravet syndrome. Clin Neurophysiol. 2017;128(2):323–30.
6. Harding GFA, Jeavons M. Photosensitive epilepsy. London: MacKeith Press; 1994.
7. Takahashi T, Nakasato N, Yokoyama H, Tsukahara Y. Low luminance visual stimuli compared to stroboscopic IPS in eliciting PPR in photosensitive patients. Epilepsia. 1999;40(Suppl 4):44–9.
8. Wilkins A, Andermann F, Ives J. Proceedings: stripes, complex cells and seizures. Electroencephalogr Clin Neurophysiol. 1975;39(4):428.
9. Brinciotti M, Matricardi M, Pelliccia A, Trasatti G. Pattern sensitivity and photosensitivity in epileptic children with visually induced seizures. Epilepsia. 1994;35(4):842–9.
10. Radhakrishnan K, St Louis EK, Johnson JA, McClelland RL, Westmoreland BF, Klass DW. Pattern-sensitive epilepsy: electroclinical characteristics, natural history, and delineation of the epileptic syndrome. Epilepsia. 2005;46(1):48–58.
11. Kasteleijn-Nolst Trenité D, Rubboli G, Hirsch E, Martins da Silva A, Seri S, Wilkins A, Parra J, Covanis A, Elia M, Capovilla G, Stephani U, Harding G. Methodology of photic stimulation revisited: updated European algorithm for visual stimulation in the EEG laboratory. Epilepsia. 2012;53(1):16–24.
12. Berger H. Das Elektrenkephalogramm des Menschen. Nova Acta Leopoldina. 1938;6:173–309.
13. Adrian ED, Matthews BHC. The Berger rhythm: potential changes from the occipital lobes of man. Brain. 1934;57:355–85.
14. Walter WG, Dovey VJ, Shipton H. Analysis of the electrical response of the human cortex to photic stimulation. Nature. 1946;158(4016):540.
15. Cobb S. Photic driving as a cause of clinical seizures in epileptic patients. Arch Neurol Psychiatr. 1947;58(1):70.
16. Bickford RG, Daly D, Keith HM. Convulsive effects of light stimulation in children. AMA Am J Dis Child. 1953;86(2):170–83.
17. Tatum WO, Rubboli G, Kaplan PW, Mirsatari SM, Radhakrishnan K, Gloss D, Caboclo LO, Drislane FW, Koutroumanidis M, Schomer DL, Kasteleijn-Nolst Trenite D, Cook M, Beniczky S. Clinical utility of EEG in diagnosing and monitoring epilepsy in adults. Clin Neurophysiol. 2018;129(5):1056–82.
18. Melsen S. The value of photic stimulation in the diagnosis of epilepsy. J Nerv Ment Dis. 1959;128(6):508–19.
19. Wolf P, Goosses R. Relation of photosensitivity to epileptic syndromes. J Neurol Neurosurg Psychiatry. 1986;49(12):1386–91.

20. Gastaut H. Photo-metrazol activationElectroencephalogr Clin Neurophysiol. 1952;4(3):271–4.
21. Naquet R, Gastaut Y. Radiation of specific photic and radiated responses during cerebral diseases; diagnostic value of photo-cardiazol stimulation in man. Riv Neurol. 1951;21(4):318–26.
22. Bickford RG, Sem-Jacobsen CW, White PT, Daly D. Some observations on the mechanism of photic and photometrazol activation. Electroencephalogr Clin Neurophysiol. 1952;4(3):275–82.
23. Angus-Leppan H. Seizures and adverse events during routine scalp electroencephalography: a clinical and EEG analysis of 1000 records. Clin Neurophysiol. 2007;118(1):22–30.
24. Herrlin KM. EEG with photic stimulation: a study of children with manifest or suspected epilepsy. Electroencephalogr Clin Neurophysiol. 1954;6:573–89.
25. Reilly EL, Peters JF. Relationship of some varieties of electroencephalographic photosensitivity to clinical convulsive disorders. Neurology. 1973;23(10):1050–7.
26. Jayakar P, Chiappa KH. Clinical correlations of photoparoxysmal responses. Electroencephalogr Clin Neurophysiol. 1990;75(3):251–4.
27. Puglia JF, Brenner RP, Soso MJ. Relationship between prolonged and self-limited photoparoxysmal responses and seizure incidence: study and review. J Clin Neurophysiol. 1992;9(1):137–44.
28. Mundy-Castle AC. The clinical significance of photic stimulation. Electroencephalogr Clin Neurophysiol. 1953;5(2):187–202.
29. Kasteleijn-Nolst Trenité DGA, Binnie CD, Meinardi H. Photosensitive patients: symptoms and signs during intermittent photic stimulation and their relation to seizures in daily life. J Neurol Neurosurg Psychiatry. 1987;50:1546–9.
30. Piccioli M, Vigevano F, Buttinelli C, Kasteleijn-Nolst Trenité DG. Do videogames evoke specific types of epileptic seizures? Epilepsy Behav. 2005;7(3):524–30.
31. Fylan F, Edson AS, Harding GF. Clinical significance of EEG abnormalities during photic stimulation in patients with photosensitive epilepsy. Epilepsia. 1999;40(3):370–2.
32. Fallah A, RamachandranNair R. Does photoparoxysmal response in children represent provoked seizure? Evidence from simultaneous motor task during EEG. Clin Neurol Neurosurg. 2009;111(2):147–50.
33. Kasteleijn-Nolst Trenité DG, Smit AM, Velis DN, Willemse J, van Emde Boas W. On-line detection of transient neuropsychological disturbances during EEG discharges in children with epilepsy. Dev Med Child Neurol. 1990;32(1):46–50.
34. Dravet C, Bureau M, Oguni H, et al. Severe myoclonic epilepsy in infancy (Dravet syndrome). 4th ed. London: John Libbey Eurotext. 2005. p. 200.
35. Guerrini R, Dravet C, Genton P, Bureau M, Bonanni P, Ferrari AR, Roger J. Idiopathic photosensitive occipital lobe epilepsy. Epilepsia. 1995;36:883–91.
36. Hennessy MJ, Binnie CD. Photogenic partial seizures. Epilepsia. 2000;41:59–64.
37. Lee CY, Jeon JY, Cho YW, Moon HJ. A case of temporal onset partial seizure induced by photic stimuli. J Epilepsy Res. 2014;4(1):18–20.
38. Benbadis SR, Gerson WA, Harvey JH, Lüders HO. Photosensitive temporal lobe epilepsy. Neurology. 1996;46(6):1540–2.
39. Kasteleijn-Nolst Trenité DG, Genton P, Brandt C, Reed RC. The 'Photosensitivity Model' is (also) a model for focal (partial) seizures. Epilepsy Res. 2017;133:113–20.
40. Specchio N, Kasteleijn-Nolst Trenité DG, Piccioli M, Specchio LM, Trivisano M, Fusco L, Buttinelli C, Vigevano F. Diagnosing photosensitive epilepsy: fancy new versus old fashioned techniques in patients with different epileptic syndromes. Brain and Development. 2011;33(4):294–300.
41. Kasteleijn-Nolst Trenité DGA, Carr B, Stefano S. New LED photic stimulators can effectively replace the Grass xenon gold standard for intermittent photic stimulation (IPS) Poster presentation ILAE congress Barcelona. 2017. Article submitted.
42. Vaudano AE, Ruggieri A, Avanzini P, Gessaroli G, Cantalupo G, Coppola A, Sisodiya SM, Meletti S. Photosensitive epilepsy is associated with reduced inhibition of alpha rhythm generating networks. Brain. 2017;140(4):981–97.
43. Specchio N, Pontrelli G, Serino D, Trivisano M, Cappelletti S, Terracciano A, Vigevano F, Fusco L. Occipital seizures induced by intermittent photic stimulation in Dravet syndrome. Seizure. 2014;23(4):309–13.
44. Kasteleijn-Nolst Trenité D, Mastrangelo M, Spalice A, Parisi P. Photosensitivity as an early marker of epileptic and developmental encephalopathies. Epilepsia. 2018;59(5):1086–7.
45. Matricardi M, Brinciotti M, Benedetti P. Outcome after discontinuation of antiepileptic drug therapy in children with epilepsy. Epilepsia. 1989;30(5):582–9.
46. Ambrosetto G, Tassinari CA. Photosensitivity related to valproate withdrawal. J Neurol Neurosurg Psychiatry. 1987;50:1709–10.
47. Papetti L, Nicita F, Parisi P, Spalice A, Villa MP, Kasteleijn-Nolst Trenité DG. "Headache and epilepsy"—how are they connected? Epilepsy Behav. 2013;26(3):386–93.
48. Piccioli M, Parisi P, Tisei P, Villa MP, Buttinelli C, Kasteleijn-Nolste Trenité DGA. Ictal headache and visual sensitivity. Cephalalgia. 2009;29:194–203.

Febrile Seizures and Febrile Status Epilepticus

30

Nicola Specchio and Giusy Carfi' Pavia

30.1 Introduction

Febrile seizures (FS) are nosological entities that affect 2–5% of children aged 6 months to 5 years [1, 2]. In most cases, these seizures are isolated or sporadic, of short duration, and with no focal semiological features; in such cases they are defined as simple febrile seizures. However, a febrile seizure that lasts more than 15 min, which has focal signs, or that recurs within 24 h is defined as "complex" febrile seizure [2, 3]. Prolonged febrile seizure (PFS) is therefore a particular type of complex febrile seizure. PFS are events that last more than 10–15 min (there is debate about which is the cutoff to be considered): according to some authors, it would be more appropriate to consider 10 min, but for the risk assessment of status epilepticus or response to treatment, 15 min seems a most appropriate benchmark [4, 5]. In case the duration exceeds 30 min, the more appropriate definition is febrile status epilepticus (FSE). FSE occurs in approximately 5% of children with ongoing febrile seizures and in about 25% of all status epilepticus in childhood. There are reports concerning the possible association of PFS/FSE and hippocampal lesions, which might justify the subsequent onset of temporal lobe epilepsy [6].

30.2 EEG in FS and FSE

Electroencephalogram (EEG) is not indicated in the routine evaluation of simple febrile seizures; on the other hand, the role of EEG in children with complex febrile seizures including febrile status epilepticus is not well-known [7]. One of the most remarkable findings in EEGs done within 1 week after febrile status epilepticus is focal slowing. The acute EEG findings after prolonged febrile seizures reveal abnormal activity in at least one third of cases across different series. Usually what is seen in those cases is slowing of background activity with wide amplitude over bilateral posterior regions (Fig. 30.1). Even if it has been estimated that about one third of patients with prolonged febrile seizures might develop epilepsy in the future, this has not been correlated with the presence of slowing at EEG, which therefore do not confer any added risk.

In old series it has been reported that focal slowing at EEG might be of added value in predicting the subsequent development of epilepsy [8] even if this is not completely clarified [9]. Moreover, in both reported series, the follow-up was limited to less than 5 years (Fig. 30.2).

Regarding the possible association with temporal lobe epilepsy, it is likely that the previous mentioned series had no sufficient follow-up in order to ascertain whether an initial abnormal EEG was predictive of subsequent temporal lobe epilepsy [10].

The FEBSTAT study [11] is a multicenter study that is prospectively identifying children with febrile status epilepticus. The children have both an MRI and EEG along with additional studies performed at baseline and at 1 year as well as if they develop epilepsy and are being followed long term. These EEGs are being interpreted by two readers blinded to the clinical histories and outcomes.

Consensus is reached on the findings in all studies. Early findings [12] confirm that focal slowing is a common finding with a frequency similar to that reported in the older series. Correlations between EEG findings and the MRI as well as the long-term outcomes are inconsistent. The study is adequately powered to eventually address the question of the relationship between prolonged febrile seizures and subsequent mesial temporal sclerosis and mesial temporal lobe epilepsy as well as the predictive value of the EEG for short- and long-term outcomes. The physiological mechanisms underlying the slowing are unknown.

A small portion of children at the age of 3 years and below with EEG was recorded soon after a febrile status epilepticus

N. Specchio (✉) · G. C. Pavia
Rare and Complex Epilepsy Unit,
Department of Neuroscience and Neurorehabilitation,
Bambino Gesù Children's Hospital, Rome, Italy
e-mail: nicola.specchio@opbg.net

O. Mecarelli (ed.), *Clinical Electroencephalography*, https://doi.org/10.1007/978-3-030-04573-9_30

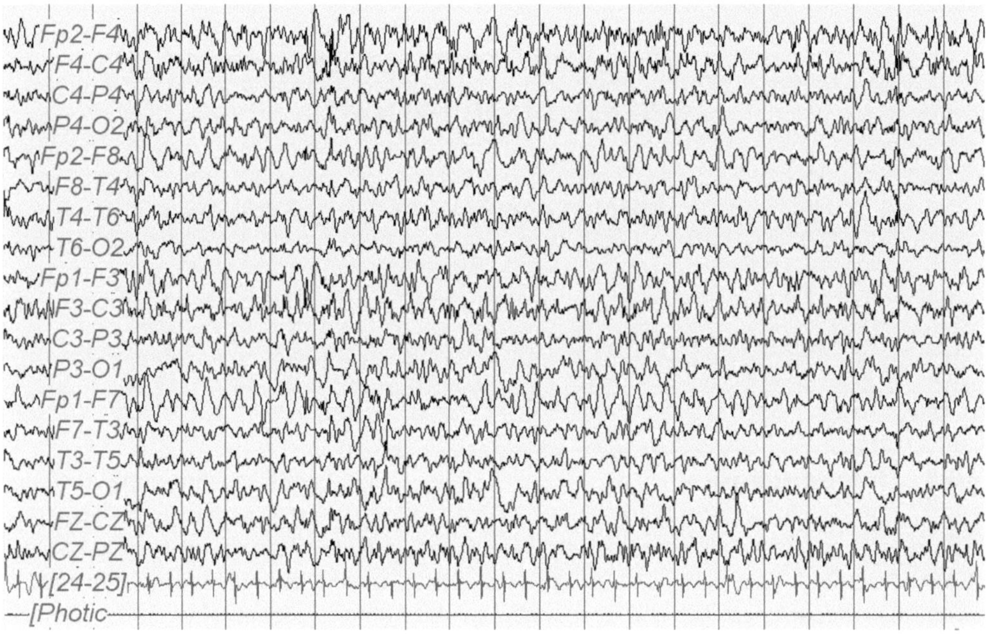

Fig. 30.1 Post-ictal EEG in a patient with complex febrile seizures (buccal midazolam was administered 30 min before the EEG). Background activity is slightly slow. Over frontal and fronto-temporal left regions some theta-delta waves are evident

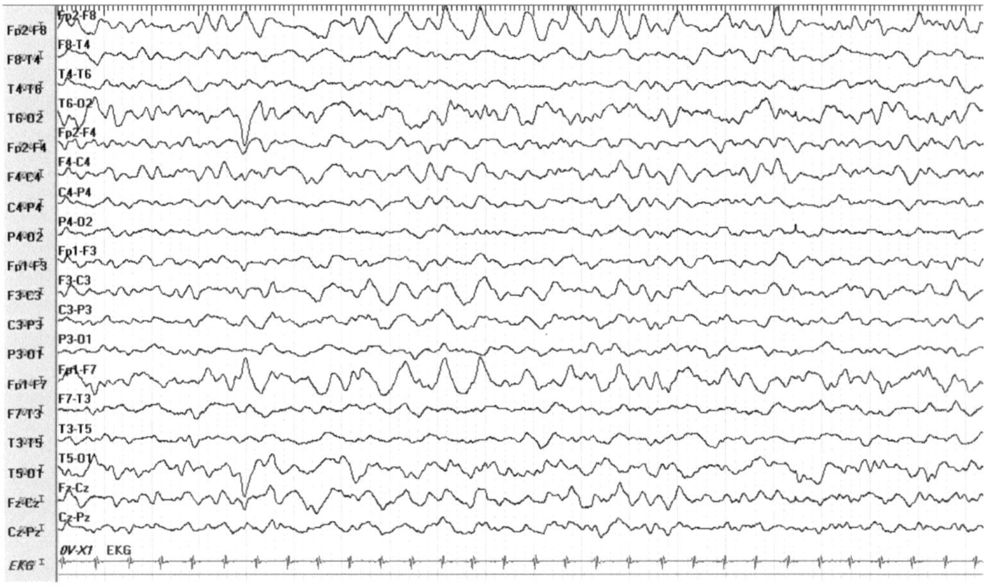

Fig. 30.2 Post-ictal EEG of a patient with simple febrile seizure. Rare slow waves are evident over frontal bilateral regions

revealed epileptiform discharges [13]. The clinical significance of these interictal epileptiform discharges is not clear. According to Yucel et al., detection of epileptiform activity is less common in the first week following the prolonged febrile convulsion [14]. The most common type of epileptiform activity to observe in the older children are bursts of generalized spike-wave discharges, although an association with centrotemporal spikes has also been noted [15]. Frantzen et al. reported that generalized spike-wave discharges did not usually appear in the acute EEG, but were found on follow-up, on average 16 months after the febrile convulsion [9]. It is possible that the occurrence of spikes indicates a genetic susceptibility. The long-term value of the early EEG findings after prolonged febrile seizures is not yet known, but the data so far suggest that the focal slowing is not associated with pre-existing focal structural lesions since it is only present for a short period of time. These data suggest that it might be important to correlate the findings with experimentally induced febrile status [16]. The precise relation between the focal slowing and epilepsy is uncertain. Studies to date were underpowered and lacked sufficient follow-up to rigorously assess the risk of focal slowing for the development of epilepsy. In addition the best studies were performed decades ago, long before the advent of MR, so the relationship with

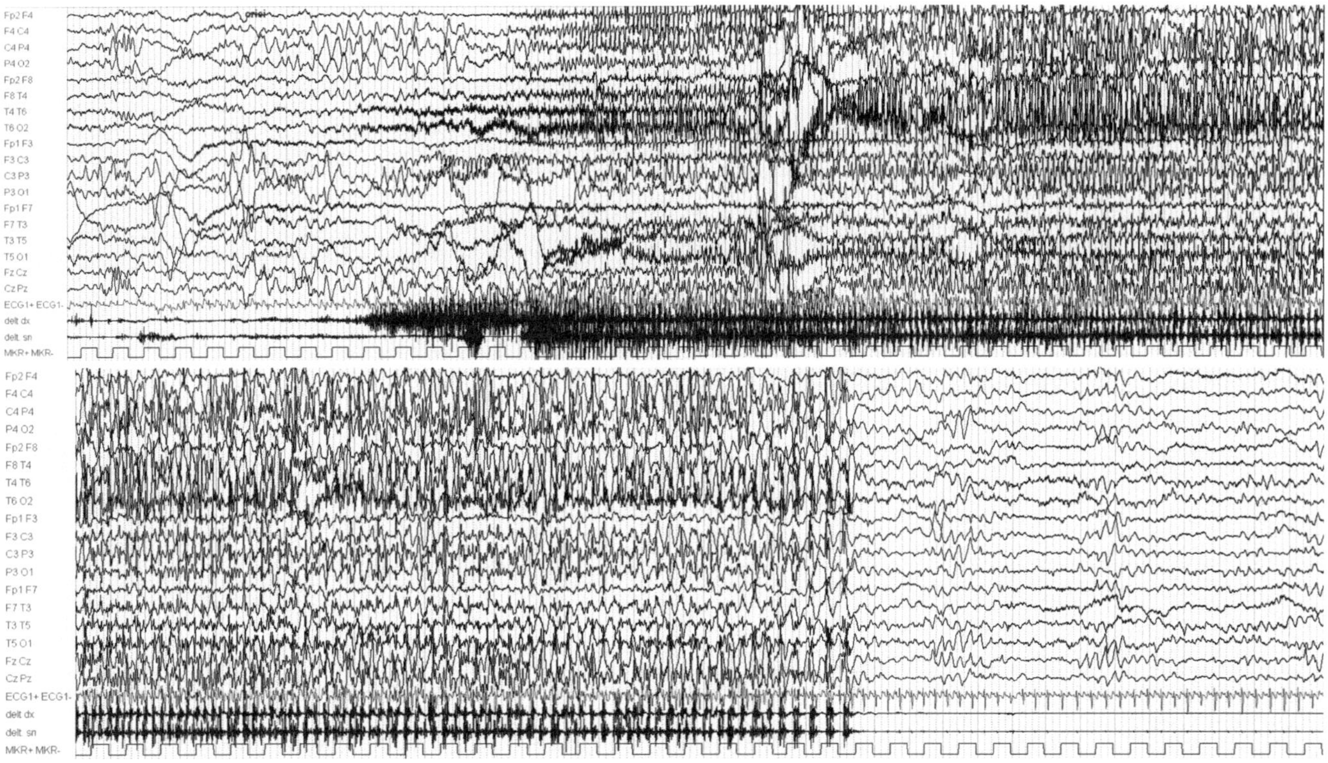

Fig. 30.3 EEG counterpart of a simple febrile seizure in a 2 years old patient. The EEG shows a diffuse attenuation of cerebral activity followed by repetitive spikes more prominent over left frontal region. The EMG trace show a bilateral hypertonus at beginning followed by clonic jerks

mesial temporal sclerosis, if any, is undetermined. Completion of existing prospective clinical studies, refinement of the existing animal models for febrile seizures to better match the clinical characteristics observed in children, and correlation between the two may help to accelerate our understanding of this very interesting phenomenon. Figure 30.3 shows an ictal recording of a simple febrile seizure.

30.3 Other Conditions with Seizures Induced by Fever

Febrile infection-related epilepsy syndrome (FIRES) is a catastrophic epileptic encephalopathy with refractory status epilepticus (SE) in developmentally normal children [17] without a diagnostic biologic marker. FIRES is characterized by the development of seizures in healthy children few days after a short febrile illness that rapidly exacerbated into a SE or a cluster of seizures, followed by a chronic drug-resistant epilepsy and cognitive function deficit [18].

Since most of the patients presented with seizures immediately following a febrile episode, an autoimmune mechanism has been considered. Different antibodies have been investigated in patients with FIRES with negative results; therefore up to now there are no evidence to support that autoantibodies are the etiology of FIRES. Furthermore, poor response to immunotherapy has been reported. FIRES is likely to represent an immune-inflammatory-mediated epileptic encephalopathy rather than an autoimmune process [19]. The syndrome invariably begins with a febrile illness, most commonly a minor upper respiratory tract infection or a gastroenteritis; fever during the infectious illness is sometimes low grade or absent (with a median duration of 4 days); in about half of the patients, it disappears at the time of first seizure occurrence [20] in contrast to febrile seizures and febrile status epilepticus. The clinical course of this disorder is typically biphasic with an initial acute catastrophic phase followed by a chronic refractory epilepsy phase.

After the onset, seizures rapidly became frequent or exacerbated into SE showing resistant to treatment with a variety of antiepileptic drugs (AEDs). It is not uncommon for children with FIRES to have hundreds of seizures a day during the acute phase. Seizures are focal (simple motor with facial twitching or complex partial seizures with lateral deviation of the head, chewing movements, and some autonomous features, suggesting a mesial temporal lobe involvement) with a strong tendency to become bilateral tonic-clonic. Also,

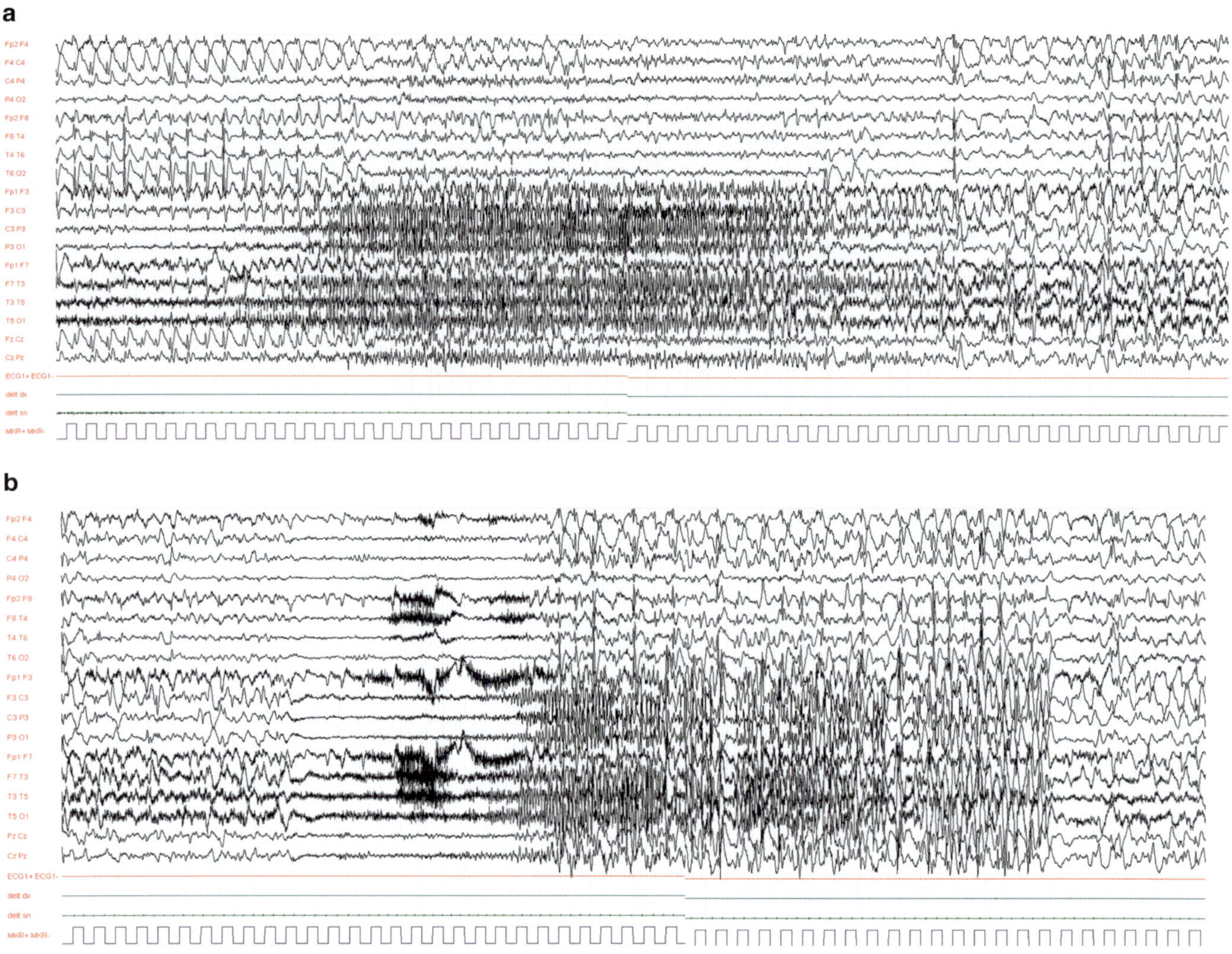

Fig. 30.4 Ictal EEG during a status epilepticus in a 4 years old patient with FIRES. Seizures are brief but subsequent. (**a**) On the right hemisphere there are spikes and spikes and waves discharges as last part of a previous seizure. At the same time a new seizure is staring on the left hemisphere characterized by repetitive spikes over left fronto-temporal region. (**b**) Seizure ends abruptly and after few seconds one more ictal clinical discharge is evident on the same side

myoclonic seizures of facial and oro-buccal muscles have been reported. Consciousness is decreased, including the interictal period. The duration of this acute phase is variable. It can last from a few days to several months. Usually no patient had neurological features other than seizures during the acute phase of illness. Ictal and interictal electroencephalography (EEG) studies revealed focal, generalized, or more frequently bilateral, multifocal pattern, and the location of the epileptic foci was predominantly frontotemporal (Fig. 30.4). Background focal or generalized slowing is common. The EEG between seizures shows slow waves resembling an "encephalitis" pattern.

30.4 Conclusions

Focal slowing is the main electroencephalographic abnormality seen acutely in children with febrile status epilepticus. The findings are quite consistent over time and in different patient populations. If focal slowing is associated with a development of epilepsy later in life is uncertain. Studies to date are not sufficient in order to assess the risk of focal slowing for the development of epilepsy. Future clinical studies, better understanding of animal models, and results from genetic studies might help in this field of knowledge.

References

1. Hauser WA, Kurland LT. The epidemiology of epilepsy in Rochester, Minnesota, 1935 through 1967. Epilepsia. 1975;16:1–66.
2. Nelson KB, Ellenberg JH. Predictors of epilepsy in children who have experienced febrile seizures. N Engl J Med. 1976;295:1029–33.
3. Berg AT, Shinnar S. Complex febrile seizures. Epilepsia. 1996;37:126–33.
4. Hesdorffer DC, Benn EK, Bagiella E, et al. Distribution of febrile seizure duration and associations with development. Ann Neurol. 2011;70:93–100.
5. Shinnar S, Hesdorffer DC, Nordli DR Jr, et al. Phenomenology of prolonged febrile seizures: results of the FEBSTAT study. Neurology. 2008;71:170–6.
6. Shinnar S, Bello JA, Chan S, et al. MRI abnormalities following febrile status epilepticus in children: the FEBSTAT study. Neurology. 2012;79:871–7.
7. Parameter P. The neurodiagnostic evaluation of the child with a first simple febrile seizure. Pediatrics. 1996;97:769–75.
8. Lennox MA. Febrile convulsions in childhood, a clinical and electroencephalographic study. Am J Dis Child. 1949;78:868–82.
9. Frantzen E, Lennox-Buchthal M, Nygaard A. Longitudinal EEG and clinical study of children with febrile convulsions. Electroencephalogr Clin Neurophysiol. 1968;24:197–212.
10. French JA, Williamson PD, Thadani VM, Darcey TM, Mattson RH, Spencer SS, et al. Characteristics of medial temporal lobe epilepsy: I. Results of history and physical examination. Ann Neurol. 1993;34:774–80.
11. Shinnar S, Hesdorffer DC, Nordli DR Jr, Pellock JM, O'Dell C, Lewis DV, et al. Phenomenology of prolonged febrile seizures: results of the FEBSTAT study. Neurology. 2008;71:170–6.
12. Nordli DR, Moshe S, Frank M, Pellock JM, Lewis DV, Marmarou A, et al. Acute EEG findings in children with febrile status epilepticus. Epilepsia. 2005;46(Suppl. 8):266.
13. Aicardi J, Chevrie JJ. The significance of electroencephalographic paroxysms in children less than 3 years of age. Epilepsia. 1973;14:47–55.
14. Yucel O, Aka S, Yazicioglu L, Ceran O. Role of early EEG and neuroimaging in determination of prognosis in children with complex febrile seizure. Pediatr Int. 2004;46:463–7.
15. Kajitani T, Kimura T, Sumita M, Kaneko M. Relationship between benign epilepsy of children with centro-temporal EEG foci and febrile convulsions. Brain and Development. 1992;14:230–4.
16. Baram TZ, Gerth A, Schultz L. Febrile seizures: an appropriate-aged model suitable for long-term studies. Brain Res. 1997;98:265–70.
17. van Baalen A, Häusler M, Boor R, et al. Febrile infection-related epilepsy syndrome (FIRES): a nonencephalitic encephalopathy in childhood. Epilepsia. 2010;51(7):1323–8.
18. van Baalen A, Stephani U, Kluger G, Häusler M, Dulac O. FIRES: febrile infection responsive epileptic (FIRE) encephalopathies of school age. Brain and Development. 2009;31(1):91.
19. van Baalen A, Vezzani A, Häusler M, Kluger G. Febrile infection-related epilepsy syndrome: clinical review and hypotheses of epileptogenesis. Neuropediatrics. 2017;48(1):5–18.
20. Kramer U, Chi CS, Lin KL, et al. Febrile infection-related epilepsy syndrome (FIRES): pathogenesis, treatment, and outcome: a multicenter study on 77 children. Epilepsia. 2011;52(11):1956–65.

31 Paediatric Status Epilepticus

Nicola Specchio and Nicola Pietrafusa

31.1 Introduction

Status epilepticus (SE) is one of the most common paediatric neurologic emergencies, requiring timely identification and emergency treatment to reduce morbidity and mortality [1]. The estimated annual incidence of status epilepticus in children ranges from 10 to 38 per 100,000 and is higher in younger children especially in the first year of life [2].

Short-term mortality rate in 30 days or until discharge ranges from 2.1 to 6% in studies conducted after the 2000s and from 2.7 to 11.5% in studies conducted before 2000. The global reduction during the last years can be explained by more aggressive treatments and best practices in paediatric intensive care units [3]. Mortality is higher in the first 6 months for the higher incidence of symptomatic SE in the youngest children. Long-term mortality ranges from 2.3 to 11% depending on the duration of follow-up [4].

Regarding morbidity, increased risk of developmental deterioration, occurs with longer nonconvulsive status epilepticus (NCSE). Morbidities and mortality of SE may be a direct consequence of the SE itself or might be attributed to the underlying disease responsible for SE [5–7]. Neurological deficits are reported in 6–30% of SE patients; however, varying outcome measures have been used to study the neurocognitive outcome, making comparison difficult [3]. The evaluation and management of SE are similar in adults and children; however, specific conditions and syndromes with convulsive status epilepticus (CSE) and NCSE occur in children [8].

N. Specchio (✉) · N. Pietrafusa
Rare and Complex Epilepsy Unit,
Department of Neuroscience and Neurorehabilitation,
Bambino Gesù Children's Hospital, Rome, Italy
e-mail: nicola.specchio@opbg.net

31.2 Classification of SE

The definition and classification of SE have been updated in the 2015 by the International League Against Epilepsy (ILAE) task force on classification of SE to include four axes where EEG plays a critical role. SE is now defined as "a condition resulting either from the failure of the mechanisms responsible for seizure termination or from the initiation of mechanisms, which lead to abnormally prolonged seizures (after time point t1). It is a condition, which can have long-term consequences (after time point t2), including neuronal death, neuronal injury, and alteration of neuronal networks, depending on the type and duration of seizures" [9].

As it is widely acknowledged, the proposed classification should be adapted to peculiarities of paediatric SE. Particularly aetiologies underlying SE in children often differ from those evident in adults [10], and this have an impact on prognosis in the two populations, even assuming the same seizure type and duration. Therefore, using the 2015 classification, the following discussion on paediatric SE will consider the peculiarity of this population.

Age and aetiology are the most relevant factors rather than seizure duration in order to define the risk of long-term consequences of SE in childhood. More large epidemiologic studies are needed for further redefining the long-term outcome in the paediatric population.

The pivotal point of the classification is the semiology: SE is now divided into status epilepticus with prominent motor symptoms, including all convulsive forms (CSE), and those without prominent motor symptoms representing the nonconvulsive forms of status epilepticus (NCSE); the classification also includes the level of impairment of consciousness (comatose vs. non-comatose).

The Axis 2 considers the aetiology. Paediatric SE has several causes, and identification of these causes is essential to the overall therapeutic approach and the formulation of prognosis. In the paper on paediatric SE by *Aicardi and Chevrie*, including 239 children, 113 cases were symptomatic, and 126 were cryptogenic (unknown). In those with symptomatic

O. Mecarelli (ed.), *Clinical Electroencephalography*, https://doi.org/10.1007/978-3-030-04573-9_31

SE, 63 out of 113 had acute CNS insults (including treatable disorders such as bacterial meningitis, encephalitis, dehydration or electrolyte disorders, toxic ingestions, or subdural hematoma), and 50 out of 113 had remote symptomatic cause, also referred to as a chronic encephalopathy (e.g., anoxia, progressive encephalopathy, nonprogressive encephalopathy, brain malformation, cerebral palsy, and Sturge-Weber syndrome). In those with cryptogenic SE, 67 out of 126 were associated with fever (a prolonged, or complex, febrile seizure) [11]. Aetiology differs by age: in the Richmond study, the most common cause of SE in adults was cerebrovascular disease (25.2%), whereas fever or infection (35.7%) was the most common cause in children [12]. Symptomatic SE has a greatest frequency in the very young and has a higher morbidity and mortality. It occurs less frequently after 1 year of age. Idiopathic SE (in children without an underlying neurologic abnormality) becomes more common after 6 months [13]. It should be considered that SE in childhood often occurs in the context of genetic epilepsy syndromes, but there is always a trigger for the status itself, such as fever, electrolyte disturbance, or other intrinsic factors.

The Axis 3 of the classification includes EEG correlates of SE. In NCSE, a correct diagnosis usually needs an EEG [14]. Clinical suspicion of NCSE arises in patients who have disturbance of consciousness with or without minor motor phenomena (e.g., perioral or periorbital low-amplitude jerking). In some cases, only EEG can reveal the epileptiform or rhythmic discharges that lead to diagnosis. The task force recommends describing the EEG correlate of status in a patient using the following descriptors, name of pattern, morphology, location, time-related features, modulation, and effect of intervention, and use the proposed terminology by the American Clinical Neurophysiology Society [15] and the diagnostic "Salzburg EEG criteria for NCSE" [16]. A recent retrospective study using EEG recordings from patients admitted for neurological symptoms or signs of NCSE confirmed the high clinical utility for the "Salzburg EEG criteria for NCSE" [17]. The sensitivity was 97.7% (95% CI 87.9–99.6), and specificity was 89.6% (95% CI 80.8–94.6); overall accuracy was 92.5% (95% CI 88.3–97.5). The positive predictive value was 84.0% (95% CI 74.1–91.5), and negative predictive value was 98.6% (95% CI 94.4–100).

Starting from Axis 4, we will describe the electro-clinical features of the peculiar forms of CSE/NCSE that might be seen in some paediatric age groups.

31.2.1 Convulsive Status Epilepticus

In convulsive SE, the clinical presentation is most often clear, and artefacts obscure the EEG; thus the EEG is of little value. In the new classification, SE with prominent motor symptoms includes: tonic-clonic SE, myoclonic SE, focal motor SE, tonic SE, and hyperkinetic SE. Epilepsia partialis continua (EPC) appears as a subclass of focal motor status [9]. Symptoms of EPC are often not only motor but, rather, sensorimotor in nature. Therefore, a broader definition of EPC includes these and other sensory variants that are often referred in the ILAE task force report to aura continua (with the latter also including cognitive and emotional variants). EPC is defined as "a condition of continuously repeated fragments of epileptic seizures (motor or sensory), with preserved consciousness, lasting > 1h, and representing locally restricted epileptic activity" [18].

EPC has many possible causes comprising both focal and systemic aetiologies such as Rasmussen's encephalitis and other inflammatory causes, stroke, focal cortical dysplasia and other brain malformations, neoplastic disease, brain trauma, mitochondrial and metabolic disorders, and non-ketotic hyperglycemia [19].

EPC is reported to present irregularly occurring focal discharges of cortical origin [20] that commonly consist of discrete spikes, sharp waves or slow wave activity, and periodic lateralized epileptiform discharges [21]. Long-term video-EEG recordings show that EPC persists during sleep and that there is no major modification of seizure frequency by the sleep and wake cycle. However, a normal EEG (about one-fifth of patients with EPC) does not exclude the diagnosis of epilepsy or a cortical origin of the disorder [22]. In Rasmussen's encephalitis, as early as 4 months after disease onset, EEG shows polymorphic delta waves over the affected hemisphere, mainly in temporal and central regions. This may be accompanied by epileptiform abnormalities which may evolve into (subclinical) ictal EEG patterns [23]. During the disease course, in most cases, contralateral asynchronous slow waves and epileptiform discharges occur. However, ictal patterns are rarely recorded from contralateral electrodes [24–26].

31.2.2 Nonconvulsive Status Epilepticus

EEG appearance of NCSE in paediatric population is fundamentally influenced by age, cerebral maturity, presence of encephalopathy, and underlying epilepsy syndromes, and NCSE does not correspond itself to a set of EEG criteria. Several different epileptic encephalopathies occur in neonates, infants, and children. In other less-specific cases, encephalopathy can be due to numerous aetiologies, including peripartum anoxia, metabolic disorders, infection, or genetic aetiologies, in which NCSE may present less-specific features. Moreover, NCSE in paediatric population is not a single disease entity but a pattern of reactions depending on cortical maturation and on the clinical situation. Published criteria include descriptions of the name of pattern, morphology, location, time-related features, modulation, and effect of intervention [9] and use the recently proposed terminology by the American Clinical Neurophysiology Society [15] and the diagnostic "Salzburg EEG criteria for NCSE" [17] as a practical guide for diagnosis. More studies are needed to assess the clinical utility for the "Salzburg EEG criteria" for paediatrics NCSE. Below we will describe the main NCSE EEG patterns of the most common epileptic syndromes of the paediatric age.

31.2.3 SE Occurring in Neonatal and Infantile-Onset Epilepsy Syndromes

- *Tonic Status* (e.g., *in Ohtahara Syndrome or West Syndrome see Chap. 23).*
- *SE in Severe Myoclonic Encephalopathy of Infancy (Dravet Syndrome)*
  Dravet syndrome (DS) is a severe, intractable epilepsy syndrome that occurs in the first year of life, characterized by fever-sensitive, multiple seizure types, and psychomotor developmental delay after seizure onset. SCN1A mutations, usually de novo, are found in 70 to 80% of patients with DS [27]. Febrile or afebrile SE occurs in DS, both convulsive and nonconvulsive types. The frequency of SE usually decreases with age. NCSE has been previously described as *obtundation status epilepticus* [28]. This is reported in the about 40% of patients [28, 29], and it is characterized by altered awareness, autonomic symptoms, or erratic subtle myoclonus that commonly involves the fingers and orobuccal muscles and isolated massive myoclonic jerks [30]. A CSE can precede or follow this condition. The EEG is usually characterized by a diffuse dysrhythmia of slow waves, intermixed with focal and diffuse spikes, sharp waves of higher voltage in the anterior regions and the vertex, with a certain time correspondence between the spikes and the myoclonic jerks except during intercalated myoclonic fits. A pseudo-rhythmic diffuse high-amplitude, irregular slow waves, gradually slowing down in frequency, and bursts of bilateral, diffuse high-voltage slow waves, occasionally notched with small spikes, have been also described [29–31]. *Wakai* et al. *(1996) and Oguni* et al. *(2001)* described a complex partial status with an irregular unilateral spike-and-waves complex [29, 32]. Rarely an absence status can be observed: The EEG is characterized by a subcontinuous sequence of slow polyspikes and waves diffuse on both hemispheres, with an anterior predominance and clinically by a fluctuating consciousness disturbance without motor manifestations [30]. Myoclonic status is also rare [33]: In many cases the recurrence in clusters of myoclonic jerks can culminate into a convulsive seizure. The massive jerks are frequently mixed with numerous asynchronous and arrhythmic distal jerks, often difficult to differentiate also polygraphically from nonepileptic myoclonus. An acute encephalopathy characterized by non-inflammatory cerebral edema, followed by prolonged consciousness disturbance, with high morbidity and mortality after SE has been described (5.6% of patients with DS); it is more likely to occur in patients with DS who had high fever [34]. It is important to educate caregivers about early symptoms and signs of NCSE: An early rescue management can help to prevent prolonged status epilepticus and its associated complications (Fig. 31.1).
- *Febrile SE* (see Chap. 30).

31.2.4 SE Occurring in Childhood and Adolescence

- *Autonomic SE in early-onset benign childhood occipital epilepsy (Panayiotopoulos syndrome).*
  Prolonged seizures are not a characteristic feature of the self-limited focal epilepsies except for Panayiotopoulos syndrome (PS) [35]. This syndrome also known as early-onset benign childhood occipital epilepsy has a peak incidence at 4 to 5 years old. Autonomic seizures are the main clinical seizure type of this syndrome. Pallor, emesis, and vomiting are seen at the onset, which are often not associated with an alteration in consciousness. After the autonomic changes, motor manifestations may occur and include eye deviation, head turning, or hemi-convulsion. Although CSE is rarely seen, brief hemi-convulsion is reported in 40% of children with PS [35]. The duration of autonomic seizures is usually longer than 10 min, and 50% can last longer than 30 min configuring an autonomic status epilepticus [36]. The electrical ictal discharge consists of rhythmic theta or delta activity, usually intermixed with small spikes. Rhythmical spike-and-wave discharges have been observed. Onset is unilateral, more often posterior but sometimes anterior and not well localized. Data on the electrographic seizure termination pattern in subjects not given acute antiepileptic drugs are based on only a few recorded seizures. Termination is usually abrupt but occasionally may be stuttering [37, 38]. In Specchio et al. (2010) series the electrical ictal discharge is characterized by low-voltage fast activity followed by rhythmic epileptic activity of 1–2.5 Hz predominantly in the occipital regions, increasing in voltage and decreasing in frequency with rapid bilateral frontotemporal spreading that is followed by rhythmic spike-and-wave discharges with occipital predominance. Usually background activity is slow and desynchronized [39] (Fig. 31.2).
- *NCSE in specific childhood epilepsy syndromes and aetiologies.*

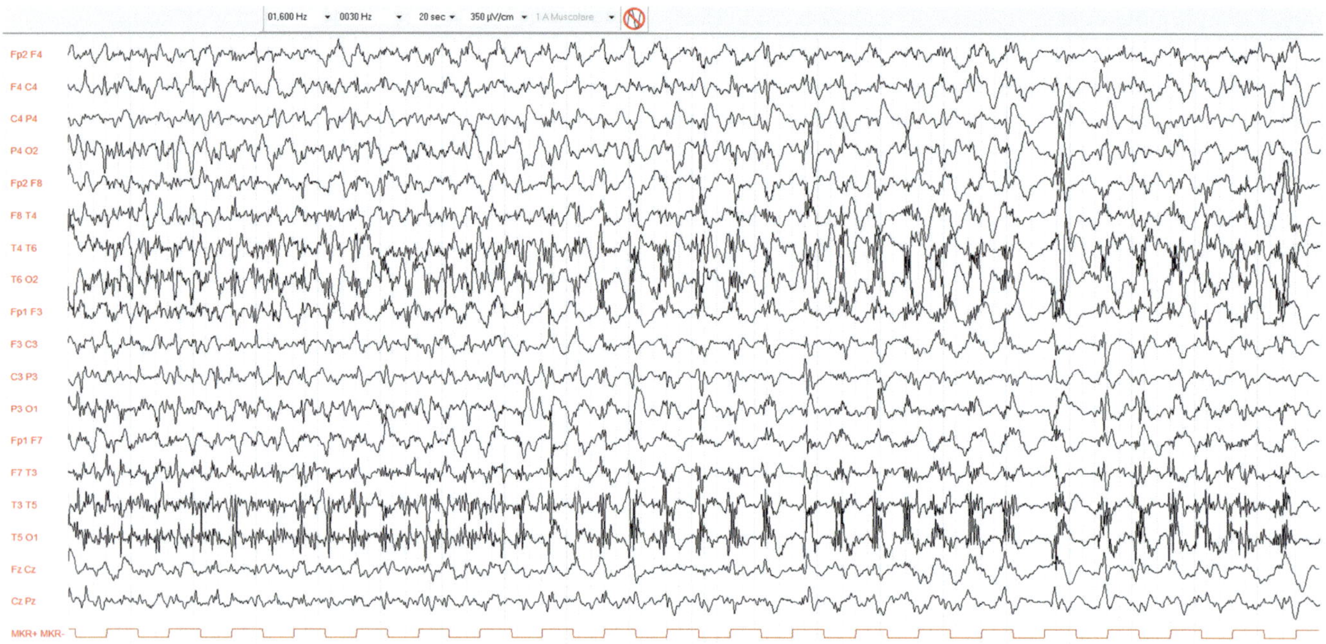

Fig. 31.1 An obtundation status in a 3-year and 4-month-old boy characterized by altered awareness, autonomic symptoms, subtle myoclonus that involves orobuccal muscles. The EEG is usually characterized by a diffuse dysrhythmia of diffuse slow and sharp waves

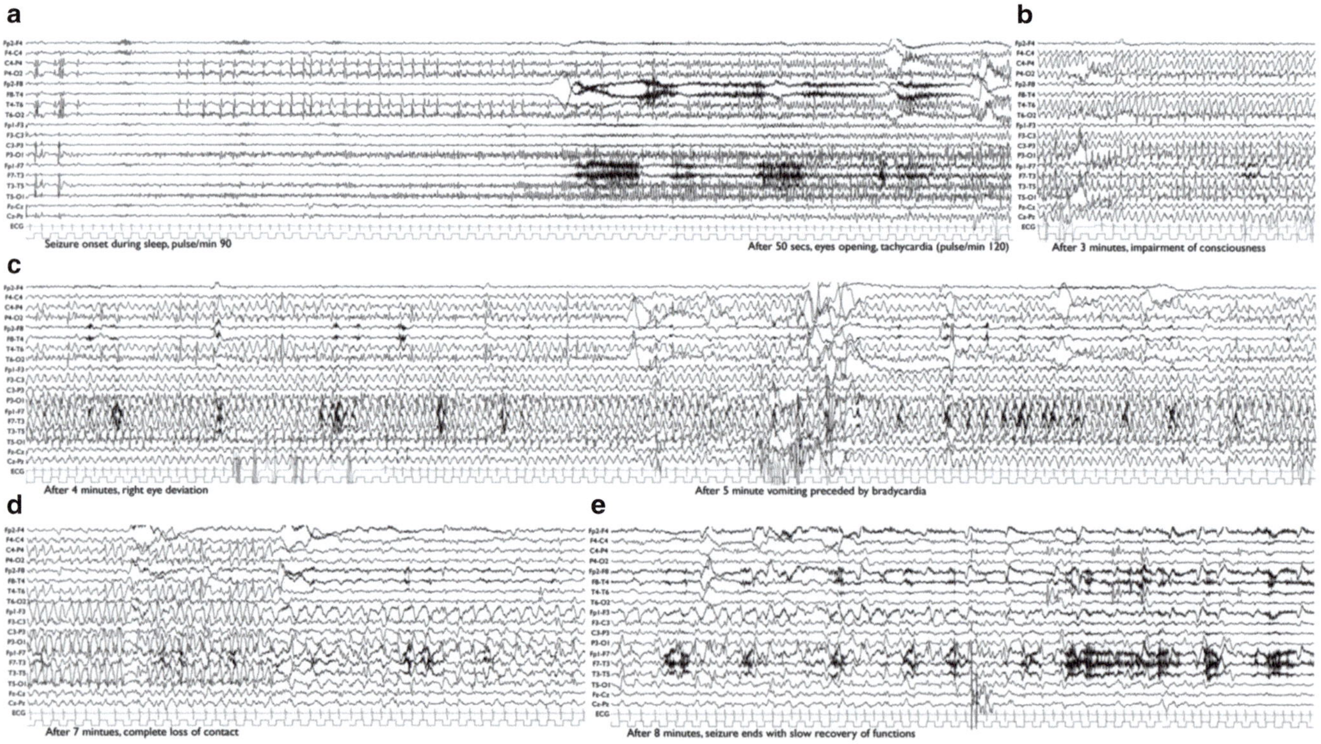

Fig. 31.2 Ictal recording (video/EEG) of a 7-year-old girl. (**a**) The ictal discharge starts during sleep over the left occipital area with low-voltage fast activity, increasing in amplitude and decreasing in frequency and quickly involving the temporal and parietal areas. Persisting over the right occipital area in the first part of the seizure is independent spike-and-wave activity lasting 22 s. After 50 s, the patient opens her eyes and tachycardia is evident. (**b**) After 3 min, the discharge is bilateral with more pronounced spike-and-wave activity over the left posterior area. (**c**) This is followed by eye deviation and then vomiting with an EEG counterpart characterized by 2.5-Hz spikes and waves over the left occipital region and delta waves over the frontal and temporal areas. (**d**, **e**) After 7 min, the patient has complete loss of consciousness (**d**), after which the seizure ends (**e**); slow waves are evident and involve mainly the left hemisphere

31.3 Ring Chromosome 20

Ring chromosome 20 is a rare clinical genetic syndrome often associated with intractable epilepsy. Seizures may occur anytime between birth and adolescence. However, seizures are rarely seen before a year of age. Behavioural and psychiatric problems are common although cognitive impairment may not be present. Multiple seizures can be seen and usually remain refractory to medical treatment. Nearly all children experience NCSE with an ictal EEG characterized by continuous bilateral repetitive irregular spikes with frontal predominance, followed by rhythmic or irregular high-amplitude slow waves at 3–4 Hz with interspersed multifocal, irregular spikes. Usually the frequency of the spike-and-wave discharges increases, and the slow waves can get polymorphic. Usually background activity is slow and/or suppressed [40] (Fig. 31.3).

31.4 Angelman Syndrome

Angelman syndrome is a genetic syndrome with clinical features, including ataxia, cognitive impairment, epilepsy, and typical facial features [41]. Myoclonic and atypical absence seizures are seen most frequently. Baseline EEG always shows high-amplitude generalized spikes and slow waves that are often pronounced in the posterior regions. Children with Angelman syndrome have an increased risk of developing a

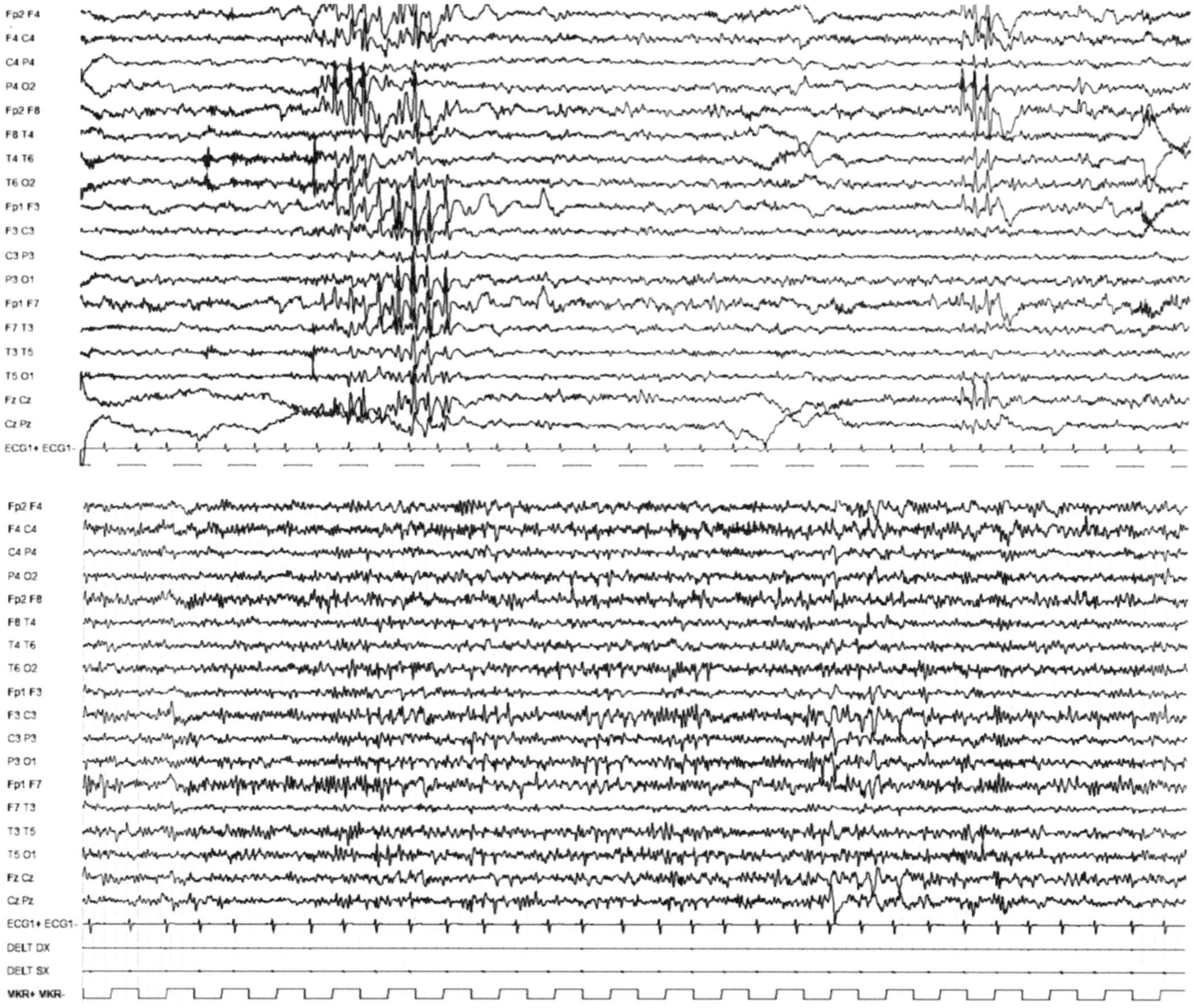

Fig. 31.3 Ictal EEG of NCSE in a 17 years old boy with r(20) syndrome. It is characterized by continuous bilateral spike waves and slow spike waves over the frontal regions. From the clinical point of view, the patient had a partial impairment of consciousness, able to answer simple questions and to perform some tasks

NCSE [42]. NCSE should be suspected in these children when parents report regression of neurodevelopment, decreasing alertness, excessive drooling, or increasing irritability and sleep, even if the other clinical manifestations of habitual seizures are not present. With NCSE, there are continuous or waxing and waning rhythmic sharp wave discharges with frontocentral predominance. Usually background activity is slow and/or suppressed Comparison with a baseline EEG is essential for a timely diagnosis of NCSE in these children [43].

31.5 Rett Syndrome

Rett syndrome (RTT), an X-linked, dominant neurodevelopmental disorder caused by mutations in the MECP2 gene, presents with acquired microcephaly, autistic regression, hand usage loss, and stereotypies [44]. Epilepsy is frequent and has been reported to correlate with mutation type, general disease severity, and BDNF polymorphism [45]. ESES (between the ages of 4 and 7 years) is common among those patients with an early onset of epilepsy with a pattern characterized by continuous or subcontinuous unilateral, multifocal, or generalized spikes usually during 50% of slow-wave sleep. Usually background activity is disorganized and desynchronized. In *Nissenkorn* et al. *(2010)* series, a total of 21.42% of the girls with early epilepsy onset developed ESES [45]. EEG pattern had a disorganized background resembling hypsarrhythmia. From a clinical point of view, all patients deteriorated in communication and motor skills during this period, two patients with preserved speech variant had no seizures at all, two patients evolved into NCSE, and in six patients there was unchanged seizure pattern.

31.6 Epilepsy with Myoclonic-Atonic Seizures

Otherwise traditionally known as myoclonic-astatic epilepsy (Doose syndrome) is relatively common syndrome constituting approximately 1 to 2% of childhood-onset epilepsies. It is more common in males, and onset is usually between 3 and 4 years of age. Doose syndrome is characterized by multiple different seizure types. Myoclonic, astatic or atonic, absence, tonic, clonic, generalized tonic-clonic seizures can occur, with frequent explosive-onset seizures [46]. All seizure types can result in SE, common in this syndrome, including NCSE, previously called "status of minor seizures", as well as myoclonic and absence SE [47]. During SE, rhythms consisting of generalized continuous or waxing and waning slow spike-and-wave activity with interposed slow waves can be seen. Discharges of 2–3 Hz with interspersed multifocal, irregular spikes, polyspikes, and slow wave complexes can be observed. This type of activity can lead to clinically multifocal, erratic myoclonic jerks on a background of mild tonic contraction [48]. The ictal activity then may blend into a burst-suppression pattern, and myoclonus occurs in association with EEG bursts during sleep [49] (Fig. 31.4).

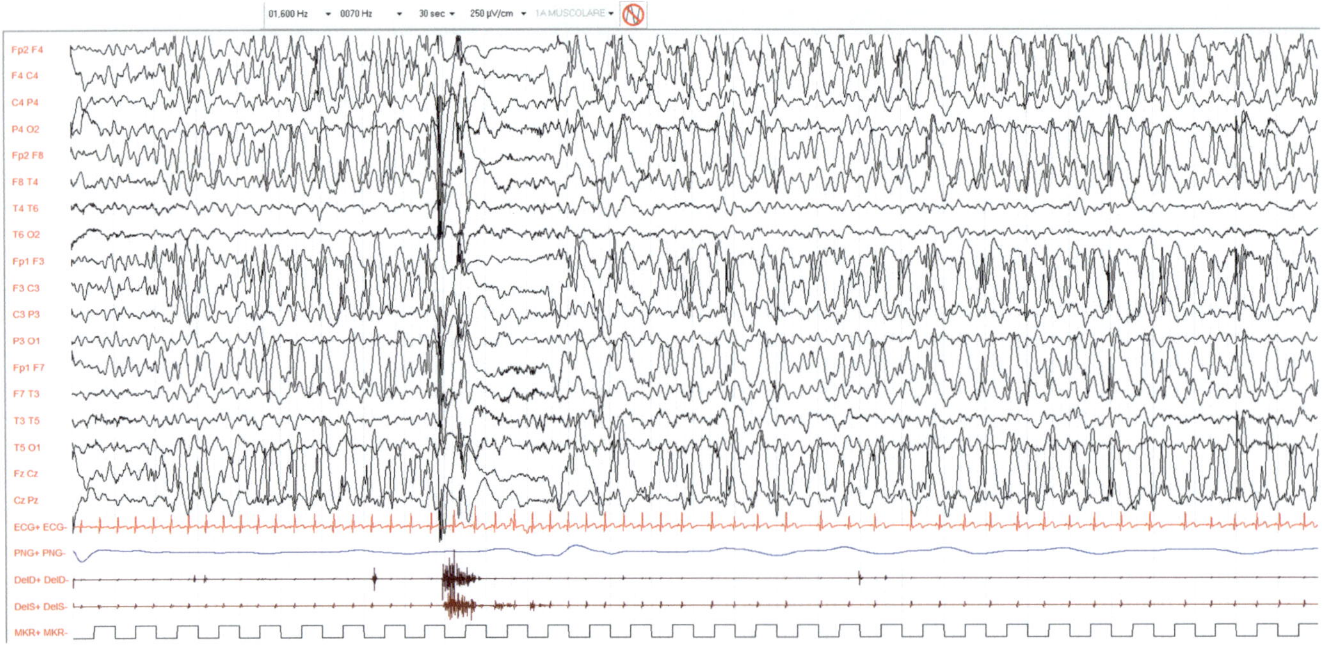

Fig. 31.4 A 3 years and 5 month old boy with Doose Syndrome. NCSE, rhythms consisting of generalized continuous or sub-continuous slow spike–wave activity with interposed slow waves can be seen

31.7 Myoclonic Status in Nonprogressive Encephalopathy (MSNPE)

Myoclonic status in nonprogressive encephalopathies (MSNPE) is characterized by recurrence of long-lasting myoclonic status appearing in infants and young children with nonprogressive encephalopathy [50, 51]. It is characterized by the recurrence of long-lasting atypical status epilepticus associated with attention impairment and continuous polymorphous jerks, mixed with other complex abnormal movements, in infants suffering from a nonprogressive encephalopathy [51, 52].

In the Caraballo series, three main subgroups have been identified:

- Children with genetic aetiology (deletion of the short arm of chromosome 4 [Wolf-Hirschhorn syndrome or 4p-syndrome], Rett syndrome, Prader-Willi syndrome, and others) presented myoclonic absences and rhythmic myoclonias. EEG shows a subcontinuous delta-theta activity involving the central areas and rhythmic delta waves with superimposed spikes mainly involving the parietooccipital regions and often activated by eye closure; the EMG recording shows frequent erratic, sometimes rhythmic myoclonias with related EEG paroxysms.
- Children affected by a cortical malformation (bilateral polymicrogyria) have an EEG pattern characterized by subcontinuous multifocal slow spike-and-waves, predominating in frontocentral regions; negative myoclonus mixed with dyskinetic movements on the EMG recording, associated with irregular and subcontinuous slow spike-and-wave discharges, might be seen.
- Children, with perinatal anoxic injury, presents a SE initially characterized by subcontinuous generalized spike-and-wave-type paroxysms related to rhythmic myoclonia of the face and limbs and after weeks by theta waves with very slow pseudo-rhythmic continuous spikes in the central regions and vertex [51] (Fig. 31.5).

31.8 SE in Other Childhood Myoclonic Encephalopathies (Mitochondrial Diseases Causing SE)

SE is a prominent feature of a number of mitochondrial disorders.

Alpers' or Alpers-Huttenlocher disease is a rare autosomal recessive hepato-cerebral disorder starting in infancy or childhood [53]. Prominent neurologic symptoms are epilepsy (especially EPC), ataxia, developmental regression, and cortical blindness. Liver involvement may be silent and slowly progressive, and patients are at high risk of valproic acid-induced liver failure [54]. Alpers' disease is a heterogeneous disorder [55], and most cases are caused by recessive mutations in the POLG1. Almost all patients present with refractory convulsive SE characterized by focal clonic and complex focal seizures; EEG often shows unilateral occipital rhythmic high-amplitude delta with superimposed (poly) spikes (RHADS). In Wolf series, RHADS persisted for several days, throughout treatment with various antiepileptic drugs [56] (Fig. 31.6).

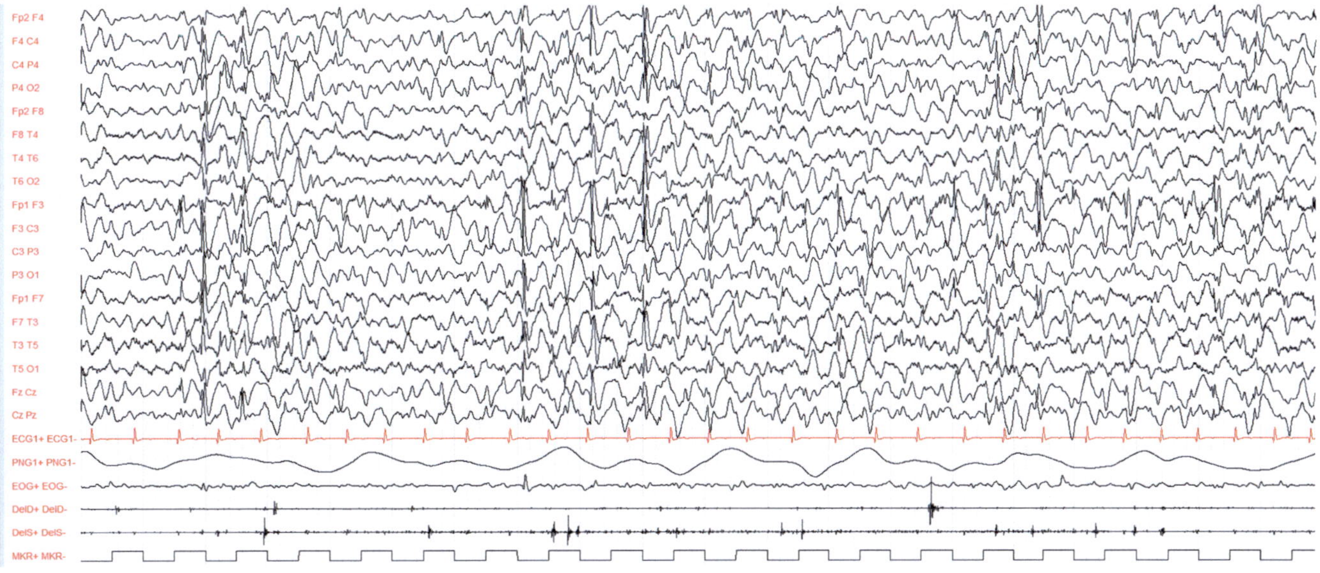

Fig. 31.5 Myoclonic status in non-progressive encephalopathy (MSNPE). Multiple spikes and spikes and waves discharges are evident intermingled with high amplitude slow waves. EMG traces reveal erratic myoclonic jerks of upper limbs

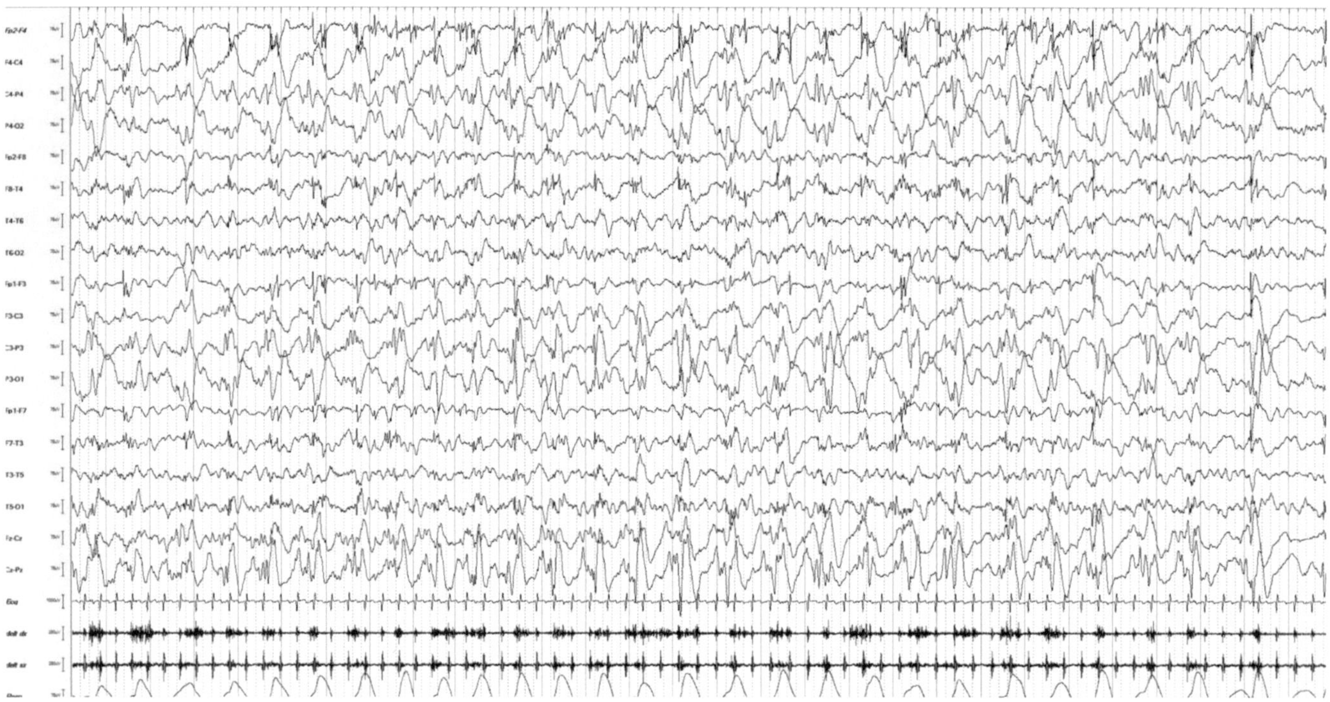

Fig. 31.6 A 9 month old girl with POLG1-related epilepsy with rhythmic high-amplitude delta with superimposed (poly)spikes (RHADS). EEG shows diffuse polymorphic theta-delta activity of medium-high voltage, associated with RHADS over the frontal and central electrodes of both hemispheres

31.9 Atypical Absence SE and Tonic Status in Lennox-Gastaut Syndrome

Lennox-Gastaut syndrome (LGS) is a severe epilepsy syndrome characterized by multiple seizure types including tonic, atonic, atypical absence, and generalized tonic-clonic seizures [57]. Between 50 and 75% of patients with LGS have episodes of NCSE, which usually consist of subcontinuous atypical absences characterized by the alternation of tonic attacks and episodes of confused behaviour, frequently with erratic myoclonic activity of the face and upper limbs, which can last for hours to weeks [58]. Hoffman-Riem et al. (2000) examined the incidence of NCSE in 101 paediatric and adult patients with LGS: NCSE was described in 85% of LGS patients and CSE in 67% [59].

EEG in atypical absence SE is characterized by generalized continuous or subcontinuous diffuse irregular 2–2.5 Hz frontotemporal spike and polyspikes and slow-wave discharges. Clinically a decrease in response to external stimuli with frequent head nodding (electromyogram can show a brief atonic seizure, which was time-locked by a diffuse spike-and-wave burst). Rhythmic and polymorphic diffuse delta activity of 1.5–2 Hz is also described [60–62]. NCSE likely contributes to the severe cognitive impairment in LGS in addition to the underlying aetiology [59].

EEG in tonic SE is characterized by generalized repetitive runs of polyspikes at high frequencies of 16–20 Hz, beginning with low voltage and increasing high voltage and a 10 Hz recruiting rhythm of high voltage from onset. The runs of polyspikes can be intermingled with slow waves. Background activity may be disorganized and desynchronized [63]. Clinically an alternation of tonic attacks and episodes of tonic seizures with sleep/drowsiness or confused behaviour, frequently with erratic myoclonic activity of the face and upper limbs, which can last for hours to weeks might be seen (Fig. 31.7a, b).

31.10 ESESS/CSWSS/Epilepsy-Aphasia Spectrum

Encephalopathy with electrical status epilepticus in sleep (ESES), ESES syndrome, and continuous spikes and waves during sleep (CSWS) has been used interchangeably to define patients with an EEG pattern of near-continuous spike-and-wave discharges during non-REM sleep and acquired neuropsychological deficits.

EEG pattern is characterized by presence of generalized bilateral and symmetric 1.5–3 Hz spike-and-wave frequency [64]. Some authors have suggested the cut-off value of at least 85%. Other contemporary reports have suggested that lower burdens of spikes (up to 50%) may be associated with reversible cognitive impairment and thus warrant treatment [65].

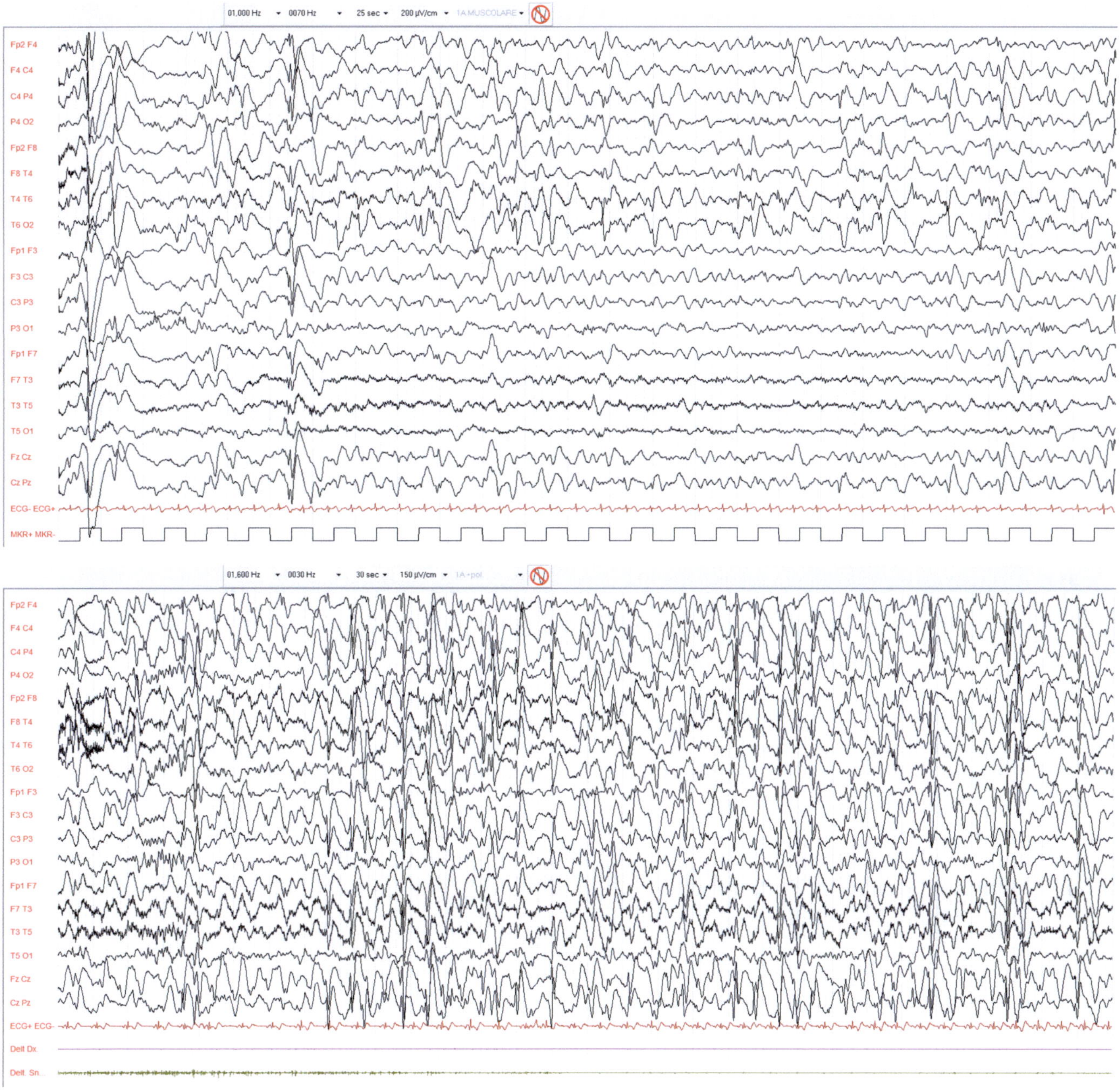

Fig. 31.7 A 15 years old girl with Lennox-Gastaut syndrome. EEG taken 1 days after start of an atypical absence status shows. Continuously occurring generalized 2/s sharp and slow waves, maximal over the anterior regions. The pattern also can be read as triphasic waves. The EEG and the condition remained unchanged with several AEDs

ESES/CSWS/epilepsy-aphasia spectrum is an acquired condition characterized by a triad of epilepsy, cognitive or behavioural impairment, and EEG abnormality of ESES/CSWS.

This epilepsy syndrome is typically age related, presenting at an age between 2 and 14 years, with a peak at 4–8 years. While the ESES EEG pattern resolves during puberty, cognitive deficits often remain [66].

Epilepsy-aphasia spectrum is a spectrum of disorders ranging from severe epileptic encephalopathy with CSWS and Landau-Kleffner syndrome (LKS) to the mild condition of childhood epilepsy with centrotemporal spikes [67, 68]. The common underlying pathway is a ion channel dysfunction (SCN2A, KCNQ2, KCNB1, KCNA2, and GRIN2A) [69]. Despite the fact that the ESES/CSWS pattern can be seen in ESES/CSWS/epilepsy-aphasia spectrum, it can also concur with other syndromes such as Rett syndrome, Rolandic epilepsy, Landau-Kleffner syndrome, 8p deletion syndrome and 9p duplication syndrome, Costeff syndrome,

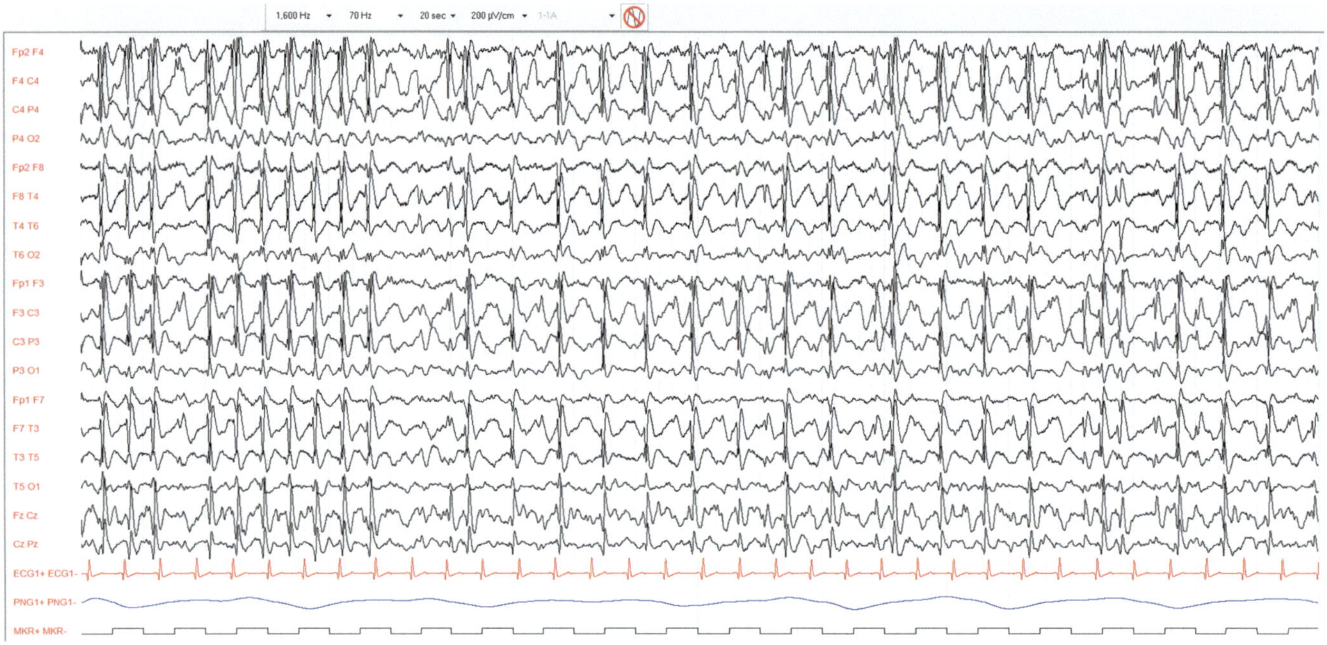

Fig. 31.8 A 14 years old boy with GRIN2A mutation. The EEG shows a near-continuous spike and wave discharges during non-REM sleep

Christianson syndrome, tuberous sclerosis complex, Cohen syndrome and autism spectrum disorders, and brain malformations (include porencephaly, polymicrogyria, pachygyria, cortical atrophy, and hydrocephalus) [45, 66, 70–73]. Immunity disorders with evidence of onco-neuronal antibodies have been also reported [74] (Fig. 31.8).

31.11 Myoclonic Status in Progressive Myoclonus Epilepsies

Progressive myoclonus epilepsy (PME) represents an epilepsy syndrome characterized by myoclonic jerks, generalized seizures, mental retardation, and ataxia. This entity encompasses many hereditary neurodegenerative diseases, including neuronal ceroid lipofuscinosis, dentatorubral-pallidoluysian atrophy, Gaucher disease, mitochondrial encephalopathy with ragged red fibres, Lafora disease, and Unverricht-Lundborg disease [75].

Epilepsy in these disorders results from pathological processes underline the disease and patients gradually become refractory to antiepileptic drugs (AEDs) and develop repeated episodes of SE at advanced stages of the illness.

Myoclonic SE is characterized by the generalized or multifocal myoclonus with a predominant involvement of face, limbs, and trunk during wakefulness. Ictal EEG shows often a temporal correlation between the generalized or focal spikes, polyspikes or spike bursts/sharp waves, and the myoclonus.

Some patients present massive, generalized myoclonus evolved into a condition with persistent increase of muscle tonus, with breathing difficulties, and with repetitive, semi-rhythmic jerking of the limbs resembling a clonic-tonic SE although ictal EEG findings were similar to those of myoclonic SE. In other patients, secondarily generalized clonic or tonic-clonic seizures were clearly identified as the main component of SE [76].

31.11.1 SE Occurring Mainly in Adolescence and Adulthood

– *Myoclonic status in juvenile myoclonic epilepsy (JME).* Myoclonic SE is very rare in JME. It is often triggered by excessive alcohol intake, sleep deprivation, poor patient compliance, and inadequate AEDs. Asynchronous and asymmetric myoclonic jerk with a predominant involvement of the upper limbs and oropharyngeal muscles and confused behaviour are the clinical signs of myoclonic SE in JME, and EEG (with polygraphy) documents a positive and negative myoclonus, correlating with repetitive, continuous, rhythmic generalized polyspike-and-wave discharges [77]. A mixed absence-myoclonic SE is also reported in juvenile myoclonic epilepsy [78].
– *Absence Status Epilepsy (ASE)*
Childhood absence epilepsy is one of the most common epilepsy syndromes in school-age children. The estimated incidence of ASE is 6% of all adult SE and 25% of SE in

children and adults combined [79]. The clinical features of ASE may include confusion, change in alertness, agitation, eye blinks, and myoclonic jerks but almost never involves coma. ASE may occur in primary or symptomatic generalized epilepsy syndromes. Approximately 3% of the individuals diagnosed with absence epilepsy may develop absence SE [79] with characteristic EEG findings of generalized, synchronous 3-Hz spike-and-wave complexes intermixed with slowing of the EEG background [80].

References

1. Brophy GM, Bell R, Claassen J, Alldredge B, Bleck TP, Glauser T, et al. Guidelines for the evaluation and management of status epilepticus. Neurocrit Care. 2012;17:3–23.
2. Nishiyama M, Nagase H, Tanaka T, Fujita K, Maruyama A, Toyoshima D, et al. Demographics and outcomes of patients with pediatric febrile convulsive status epilepticus. Pediatr Neurol. 2015;52:499–503.
3. Jafarpour S, Stredny CM, Piantino J, Chapman KE. Baseline and outcome assessment in pediatric status epilepticus. Seizure. 2018. https://doi.org/10.1016/j.seizure.2018.04.019.
4. Lv RJ, Wang Q, Cui T, Zhu F, Shao XQ. Status epilepticus-related etiology, incidence and mortality: a meta-analysis. Epilepsy Res. 2017;136:12–7.
5. Barnard C, Wirrell E. Does status epilepticus in children cause developmental deterioration and exacerbation of epilepsy? J Child Neurol. 1999;14:787–94.
6. Barry E, Hauser WA. Status epilepticus: the interaction of epilepsy and acute brain disease. Neurology. 1993;43:1473–8.
7. Krumholz A, Sung GY, Fisher RS, Barry E, Bergey GK, Grattan LM. Complex partial status epilepticus accompanied by serious morbidity and mortality. Neurology. 1995;45:1499–504.
8. Riviello JJ. Pediatric status epilepticus: initial management and the special syndromes of status epilepticus in children. In: Drislane FW, Kaplan PW, editors. Status epilepticus: a clinical perspective. Totowa, NJ: Humana Press; 2018. p. 333–52.
9. Trinka E, Cock H, Hesdorffer D, Rossetti AO, Scheffer IE, Shinnar S, et al. A definition and classification of status epilepticus - report of the ILAE task force on classification of status epilepticus. Epilepsia. 2015;56:1515–23.
10. Neligan A, Shorvon SD. Prognostic factors, morbidity and mortality in tonic-clonic status epilepticus: a review. Epilepsy Res. 2011;93:1–10.
11. Aicardi J, Chevrie JJ. Convulsive status epilepticus in infants and children: a study of 239 cases. Epilepsia. 1970;11:187–97.
12. DeLorenzo RJ, Towne AR, Pellock JM, Ko D. Status epilepticus in children, adults, and the elderly. Epilepsia. 1992;33(Suppl 4):S15–25.
13. Morton LD, Garnett L, Towne A, Waterhouse E, Brown A, Byers SF, et al. Mortality of status epilepticus in the first year of life. Epilepsia. 2001;42(Suppl 7):165.
14. Young GB, Jordan KG, Doig GS. An assessment of nonconvulsive seizures in the intensive care unit using continuous EEG monitoring: an investigation of variables associated with mortality. Neurology. 1996;47:83–9.
15. Hirsch LJ, Laroche SM, Gaspard N, Gerard E, Svoronos A, Herman ST, et al. American clinical neurophysiology society's standardized critical care EEG terminology: 2012 version. J Clin Neurophysiol. 2013;30:1–27.
16. Beniczky S, Hirsch LJ, Kaplan PW, Pressler R, Bauer G, Aurlien H, et al. Unified EEG terminology and criteria for nonconvulsive status epilepticus. Epilepsia. 2013;54(Suppl 6):28–9.
17. Leitinger M, Trinka E, Gardella E, Rohracher A, Kalss G, Qerama E, et al. Diagnostic accuracy of the Salzburg EEG criteria for nonconvulsive status epilepticus: a retrospective study. Lancet Neurol. 2016;15:1054–62.
18. Mameniškienė R, Bast T, Bentes C, Canevini MP, Dimova P, Granata T, et al. Clinical course and variability of non-Rasmussen, nonstroke motor and sensory epilepsia partialis continua: a European survey and analysis of 65 cases. Epilepsia. 2011;52:1168–76.
19. Mameniškienė R, Wolf P. Epilepsia partialis continua: a review. Seizure. 2017;44:74–80.
20. Chauvel P, Liegeois-Chauvel C, Marquis P, Bancaud J. Distinction between the myoclonus-related potential and the epileptic spike in epilepsia partialis continua. Electroencephalogr Clin Neurophysiol. 1986;64:304–7.
21. Pandian JD, Thomas SV, Santoshkumar B, Radhakrishnan K, Sarma PS, Joseph S, et al. Epilepsia partialis continua - a clinical and electroencephalography study. Seizure. 2002;11:437–41.
22. Dulac O, Dravet C, Plouin P, Bureau M, Ponsot G, Gerbaut L, et al. Nosological aspects of epilepsia partialis continua in children. Arch Fr Pediatr. 1983;40:689–95.. [article in French]
23. Granata T, Gobbi G, Spreafico R, Vigevano F, Capovilla G, Ragona F, et al. Rasmussen's encephalitis: early characteristics allow diagnosis. Neurology. 2003;60:422–5.
24. So NK, Gloor P. Electroencephalographic and electrocorticographic findings in chronic encephalitis of Rasmussen type. In: Andermann F, editor. Chronic encephalitis and epilepsy: Rasmussen's syndrome. Boston: Butterworth- Heinemann; 1991. p. 37–45.
25. Ian Andrews P, McNamara JO, Lewis DV. Clinical and electroencephalographic correlates in Rasmussen's encephalitis. Epilepsia. 1997;38:189–94.
26. Bien CG, Granata T, Antozzi C, Cross JH, Dulac O, Kurthen M, et al. Pathogenesis, diagnosis and treatment of Rasmussen encephalitis: a European consensus statement. Brain. 2005;128:454–71.
27. Saitoh M, Shinohara M, Hoshino H, Kubota M, Amemiya K, Takanashi JL, et al. Mutations of the SCN1A gene in acute encephalopathy. Epilepsia. 2012;53:558–64.
28. Dalla Bernardina B, Capovilla G, Chiamenti C, Trevisan E, Colamaria V, Fontana E. Myoclonic epilepsies, advances in neurology series. In: Wolf P, Dam MJ, editors. Advances in epileptology, vol. 16. New York: Raven Press; 1987. p. 175–9.
29. Oguni H, Hayashi K, Awaya Y, Fukuyama Y, Osawa M. Severe myoclonic epilepsy in infants – a review based on the Tokyo Women's medical university series of 84 cases. Brain Dev. 2001;23:736–48.
30. Bureau M, Bernardina BD. Electroencephalographic characteristics of Dravet syndrome. Epilepsia. 2011;52(Suppl. 2):13–23.
31. Ohmori I, Ohtsuka Y, Murakami N, Asano T, Hattori J. Analysis of ictal EEG in severe myoclonic epilepsy in infancy. Epilepsia. 2001;42(Suppl 6):54.
32. Wakai S, Ikehata M, Nihira H, Ito N, Sueoka H, Kawamoto Y, et al. "Obtundation status (Dravet)" caused by complex partial status epilepticus in a patient with severe myoclonic epilepsy in infancy. Epilepsia. 1996;37:1020–2.
33. Dravet C, Bureau M, Oguni H, Fukuyama Y, Cokar O. Severe myoclonic epilepsy in infancy (Dravet syndrome). In: Roger J, Bureau M, Dravet C, Genton P, Tassinari CA, Wolf W, editors. Epileptic syndromes in infancy, childhood and adolescence. 4th ed. Montrouge: John Libbey Eurotext; 2005. p. 89–113.
34. Tian X, Ye J, Zeng Q, Zhang J, Yang X, Liu A, et al. The clinical outcome and neuroimaging of acute encephalopathy after status epilepticus in Dravet syndrome. Dev Med Child Neurol. 2018;60:566–73.

35. Panayiotopoulos CP. Vomiting as an ictal manifestation of epileptic seizures and syndromes. J Neurol Neurosurg Psychiatry. 1988;51:1448–51.
36. Ferrie CD, Caraballo R, Covanis A, Demirbilek V, Dervent A, Fejerman N, et al. Autonomic status epilepticus in panayiotopoulos syndrome and other childhood and adult epilepsies: a consensus view. Epilepsia. 2007;48:1165–72.
37. Beaumanoir A. Occipital seizures and epilepsies in children. In: Andermann F, Beaumanoir A, Mira L, Roger J, Tassinari CA, editors. Occipital seizures and epilepsies in children. London: John Libbey and Company Ltd; 1993. p. 71–86.
38. Vigevano F, Lispi ML, Ricci S. Early onset benign occipital susceptibility syndrome: video-EEG documentation of an illustrative case. Clin Neurophysiol. 2000;111(Suppl 2):S81–6.
39. Specchio N, Trivisano M, Claps D, Battaglia D, Fusco L, Vigevano F. Documentation of autonomic seizures and autonomic status epilepticus with ictal EEG in Panayiotopoulos syndrome. Epilepsy Behav. 2010;19:383–93.
40. Inoue Y, Fujiwara T, Matsuda K, Kubota H, Tanaka M, Yagi K, et al. Ring chromosome 20 and nonconvulsive status epilepticus. A new epileptic syndrome. Brain. 1997;120:939–53.
41. Galván-Manso M, Campistol J, Conill J, Sanmartí FX. Analysis of the characteristics of epilepsy in 37 patients with the molecular diagnosis of Angelman syndrome. Epileptic Disord. 2005;7:19–25.
42. Pelc K, Boyd SG, Cheron G, Dan B. Epilepsy in Angelman syndrome. Seizure. 2008;17:211–7.
43. Weber P. Levetiracetam in nonconvulsive status epilepticus in a child with angelman syndrome. J Child Neurol. 2010;25:393–6.
44. Amir RE, Van den Veyver IB, Wan M, Tran CQ, Francke U, Zoghbi HY. Rett syndrome is caused by mutations in X-linked MECP2, encoding methyl-CpG-binding protein 2. Nat Genet. 1999;23:185–8.
45. Nissenkorn A, Gak E, Vecsler M, Reznik H, Menascu S, Ben Zeev B. Epilepsy in Rett syndrome – the experience of a National Rett Center. Epilepsia. 2010;51:1252–8.
46. Trivisano M, Specchio N, Cappelletti S, Di Ciommo V, Claps D, Specchio LM, et al. Myoclonic astatic epilepsy: an age-dependent epileptic syndrome with favorable seizure outcome but variable cognitive evolution. Epilepsy Res. 2011;97:133–41.
47. Kelley SA, Kossoff EH. Doose syndrome (myoclonic-astatic epilepsy): 40 years of progress. Dev Med Child Neurol. 2010;52:988–93.
48. Guerrini R, Aicardi J. Epileptic encephalopathies with myoclonic seizures in infants and children (severe myoclonic epilepsy and myoclonic-astatic epilepsy). J Clin Neurophysiol. 2003;20:449–61.
49. Kobayashi K, Inoue T, Kikumoto K, Endoh F, Miya K, Oka M, et al. Relation of spasms and myoclonus to suppression-burst on EEG in epileptic encephalopathy in early infancy. Neuropediatrics. 2007;38:244–50.
50. Dalla Bernardina B, Fontana E, Darra F. Myoclonic epilepsies, advances in neurology series. In: Delgado-Escueta AV, Guerrini R, Medina MT, Genton P, Bureau MDC, editors. Myoclonic epilepsies, advances in neurology series. Philadelphia: Lippincott Williams & Wilkins; 2004. p. 153–6.
51. Caraballo RH, Cersósimo RO, Espeche A, Arroyo HA, Fejerman N. Myoclonic status in nonprogressive encephalopathies: study of 29 cases. Epilepsia. 2007;48:107–13.
52. Dalla Bernardina B, Fontana E, Darra F. Myoclonic status in non progressive encephalopathies. In: Bureau M, Genton P, Dravet C, Delgado-Escueta A, Tassinari CA, Thomas P, Wolf P, editors. Epileptic syndromes in infancy, childhood and adolescence. 5th ed. Montrouge: John Libbey Eurotext Ltd; 2012. p. 431–9.
53. Wiltshire E, Davidzon G, Dimauro S, Akman HO, Sadleir L, Haas L, et al. Juvenile Alpers disease. Arch Neurol. 2008;65:121–4.
54. Bicknese AR, May W, Hickey WF, Dodson WE. Early childhood hepatocerebral degeneration misdiagnosed as valproate hepatotoxicity. Ann Neurol. 1992;32:767–75.
55. Uusimaa J, Finnilä S, Vainionpää L, Kärppä M, Herva R, Rantala H, et al. A mutation in mitochondrial DNA-encoded cytochrome c oxidase II gene in a child with Alpers-Huttenlocher-like disease. Pediatrics. 2003;111:e262–8.
56. Wolf NI, Rahman S, Schmitt B, Taanman JW, Duncan AJ, Harting I, et al. Status epilepticus in children with Alpers' disease caused by POLG1 mutations: EEG and MRI features. Epilepsia. 2009;50:1596–607.
57. Gastaut H, Roger J, Soulayrol R, Tassinari CA, Régis H, Dravet C, et al. Childhood epileptic encephalopathy with diffuse slow spike-waves (otherwise known as "petit mal variant") or Lennox syndrome. Epilepsia. 1966;7:139–79.
58. Arzimanoglou A, Guerrini R, Aicardi J. Lennox-Gastaut syndrome. In: Aicardi's epilepsy in children. Philadelphia: Lippincott Williams & Wilkins; 2004. p. 38–50.
59. Hoffmann-Riem M, Diener W, Benninger C, Rating D, Unnebrink K, Stephani U, et al. Nonconvulsive status epilepticus--a possible cause of mental retardation in patients with Lennox-Gastaut syndrome. Neuropediatrics. 2000;31:169–74.
60. Livingston JH, Brown JK. Non-convulsive status epilepticus resistant to benzodiazepines. Arch Dis Child. 1987;62:41–4.
61. Ohtsuka Y, Sato M, Oka E. Nonconvulsive status epilepticus in childhood localization-related epilepsy. Epilepsia. 1999;40:1003–10.
62. Bauer G, Trinka E. Nonconvulsive status epilepticus and coma. Epilepsia. 2010;51:177–90.
63. Tassinari CA, Dravet C, Roger J, Cano JP, Gastaut H. Tonic status epilepticus precipitated by intravenous benzodiazepine in five patients with Lennox–Gastaut syndrome. Epilepsia. 1972;13:421–35.
64. Patry G, Lyagoubi S, Tassinari CA. Subclinical "electrical status epilepticus" induced by sleep in children: a clinical and electroencephalographic study of six cases. Arch Neurol. 1971;24:242–52.
65. McVicar KA, Ballaban-Gil K, Rapin I, Moshé SL, Shinnar S. Epileptiform EEG abnormalities in children with language regression. Neurology. 2005;65:129–31.
66. Nickels K, Wirrell E. Electrical status epilepticus in sleep. Semin Pediatr Neurol. 2008;15:50–60.
67. Rudolf G, Valenti MP, Hirsch E, Szepetowski P. From rolandic epilepsy to continuous spike-and-waves during sleep and Landau-Kleffner syndromes: insights into possible genetic factors. Epilepsia. 2009;50(Suppl 7):25–8.
68. Tsai MH, Vears DF, Turner SJ, Smith RL, Berkovic SF, Sadleir LG, et al. Clinical genetic study of the epilepsy-aphasia spectrum. Epilepsia. 2013;54:280–7.
69. Kessi M, Peng J, Yang L, Xiong J, Duan H, Pang N, et al. Genetic etiologies of the electrical status epilepticus during slow wave sleep: systematic review. BMC Genet. 2018;19:40.
70. Zanni G, Barresi S, Cohen R, Specchio N, Basel-Vanagaite L, Valente EM, et al. A novel mutation in the endosomal Na^+/H^+ exchanger NHE6 (SLC9A6) causes Christianson syndrome with electrical status epilepticus during slow-wave sleep (ESES). Epilepsy Res. 2014;108:811–5.
71. Pacheva I, Panov G, Gillberg C, Neville B. A girl with tuberous sclerosis complex presenting with severe epilepsy and electrical status epilepticus during sleep, and with high-functioning autism and mutism. Cogn Behav Neurol. 2014;27:88–95.
72. Carmi N, Lev D, Leshinsky-Silver E, Anikster Y, Blumkin L, Kivity S, et al. Atypical presentation of Costeff syndrome-severe psychomotor involvement and electrical status epilepticus during slow wave sleep. Eur J Paediatr Neurol. 2015;19:733–6.
73. Lesca G, Rudolf G, Labalme A, Hirsch E, Arzimanoglou A, Genton P, et al. Epileptic encephalopathies of the Landau-Kleffner and

continuous spike and waves during slow-wave sleep types: genomic dissection makes the link with autism. Epilepsia. 2012;53:1526–38.
74. Nabbout R. Autoimmune and inflammatory epilepsies. Epilepsia. 2012;53:58–62.
75. Minassian BA, Striano P, Avanzini G. Progressive myoclonus epilepsies: state-of-the-art. Epileptic Disord. 2016;18(Suppl 2):S1–158.
76. Miyahara A, Saito Y, Sugai K, Nakagawa E, Sakuma H, Komaki H, et al. Reassessment of phenytoin for treatment of late stage progressive myoclonus epilepsy complicated with status epilepticus. Epilepsy Res. 2009;84:801–9.
77. Fanella M, Egeo G, Fattouch J, Casciato S, Lapenta L, Morano A, et al. Oxcarbazepine-induced myoclonic status epilepticus in juvenile myoclonic epilepsy. Epileptic Disord. 2013;15:181–7.
78. Gélisse P, Crespel A. Mixed myoclonic-absence status epilepticus in juvenile myoclonic epilepsy. Epileptic Disord. 2015;17:95–6.
79. Knake S, Rosenow F, Vescovi M, Oertel WH, Mueller HH, Wirbatz A, et al. Incidence of status epilepticus in adults in Germany: a prospective, population-based study. Epilepsia. 2001;42:714–8.
80. Cascino GD. Nonconvulsive status epilepticus in adults and children. Epilepsia. 1993;34(Suppl 1):S21–8.

Status Epilepticus in Adults

32

Fabio Minicucci, Matteo Impellizzeri, and Giovanna Fanelli

32.1 Introduction

32.1.1 Epidemiology

The estimate of the annual incidence of Status Epilepticus (SE) varies depending on cases, and the values are between 9,9/100.000 and 41/100.000 inhabitants [1–5]. This wide variability can also be justified by different recruitment parameters. A higher incidence in the population over 60 years (from 54 to 86/100.000) has been observed [6]. Estimations of mortality associated with the SE vary in relation to multiple parameters. Hauser [7] points out that 2% is the maximum mortality value to be attributed only to the SE. It is commonly estimated that morbidity is higher in the generalized convulsive SE, while a different mortality has not been demonstrated according to the symptoms of the seizures. Unfavorable prognostic factors are lasting longer than 1 h, anoxic etiology, and an old age [8, 9]. Rather than the presence or absence of a clinical correlate of the ictal patterns it is the condition of coma decisive in the prognostic evaluation [10].

32.1.2 Etiology

No etiology can be ruled out [11] but more often should be considered: cranial traumas, cerebrovascular diseases, brain tumors, CNS infections, metabolic diseases, intoxication, or electrolyte disorders. The list of possible causes of SE is however almost unlimited, and no etiology can be excluded [12]. In about 15% of patients, no cause triggering the SE is identified; this aspect is more frequent in patients with a previous diagnosis of epilepsy.

Much more useful is the differentiation between symptomatic SE of an acute pathology, where prognosis and therapy have uncertain implications, and symptomatic SE of remote pathologies or appearing in the context of an already known epilepsy. The prognosis of acute symptomatic SE is worse in the acute phase.

32.1.3 Definition and Diagnosis

Gastaut was the real promoter of the nosographic autonomy of the SE defining it as "crises that last for a sufficiently long period of time or that are repeated with a frequency sufficient to produce a stable and lasting epileptic condition." In this way Gastaut provides the description of a pathological condition adaptable to all cases of SE, but it presents some gaps in clinical practice because of times and methods of emergency treatment. If a seizure is defined as "a transient occurrence of signs and/or symptoms due to abnormal excessive or synchronous neuronal activity in the brain," the SE is "a condition resulting from the failure of the mechanism responsible for seizure termination or from the initiation of mechanisms which lead to abnormally prolonged seizures (after time point T1). It is a condition that can have long-term consequences (after time point t2), including neuronal death, neuronal injury, and alteration of neuronal networks, depending on the type and duration of seizures."

How long must a seizure last for an SE to be defined? How many seizures must appear in an hour or 30 min to talk about SE? Dobesberger et al. [13] after an evaluation of a wide range of seizures recorded in video-EEG have come to propose "2 min of convulsive seizure activity, which could serve as a time point to consider treatment to prevent SE." As definition of prolonged seizures, they suggest an upper limit of 7 min in focal seizures with a loss of awareness and 11 min

F. Minicucci (✉)
Department of Neurology, Chief of Epilepsy Center, Ospedale San Raffaele, Milan, Italy
e-mail: minicucci.fabio@hsr.it

M. Impellizzeri · G. Fanelli
Department of Neurology, Ospedale San Raffaele, Milan, Italy

O. Mecarelli (ed.), *Clinical Electroencephalography*, https://doi.org/10.1007/978-3-030-04573-9_32

in focal simple seizures. In their study they also found that a "history of SE, temporal seizure onset, and lesional MRI findings are factors associated with significantly longer epileptic seizures". These time parameters are generally in agreement with the hypothesis in the Epilepsy Foundation of America (EFA) Working Group document [14], which established that treatment should not be unnecessarily delayed. As already reported, contrary to what has been done in the past, not all clinical settings require such rapid intervention. The proposed classification of SE establishes a different time of intervention depending on the characteristics of the SE (generalized convulsive epileptic state or a focal state with impaired consciousness or a state of absence).

The diagnosis of SE is primarily clinical, but without the aid of the EEG, it is not always possible to suspect or confirm it. This is due to the fact that focal SE are easily mistaken with confusing status of other origin or may be hidden by symptoms such as motor deficits or coma. This situation occurs more frequently in patients with SE from acute pathologies or in those patients admitted to the intensive care unit; in these latter the vigilance and consciousness is often difficult to assess because of the underlying pathology and because of pharmacological sedation. For this reason, the EEG is still the cornerstone of the diagnosis of SE, and its use is basic for a complete understanding of the symptoms. The EEG must obviously be correlated with the data emerging from the neuroimaging, which are now essential to indicate the basic etiology and, in some patients, to better understand the data provided by neurophysiological evaluation.

The classification shown in Table 32.1 [15] in the first axis below repeats partially the one proposed by Gastaut [16]; today it is still valid for some patients. The classification starts from the assumption that the SE is, in the majority of cases, the succession of seizures and post-critical phases more or less prolonged and without complete recovery between one episode and another. For example, a focal motor SE is the continuous repetition of focal motor seizures separated by a post-critical phase in which the patient does not completely recover the motor function of the body district affected by the epileptic phenomenon. However this classification introduces the concept according to which it is possible that the SE does not appear as an alternation of seizures but as a substantially continuous epileptic condition; this happens, for example, in the case of "continuous partial epilepsy" or in "absence status." Other classification hypotheses follow this line with not substantial changes from the clinical point of view.

However, there are classifications based on other parameters other than seizures semeiology. The one suggested by Shorvon [17] largely follows the classification of epileptic syndromes made by the International League Against Epilepsy (ILAE) and includes the SE in more complex clinical settings where age, type of epilepsy, and general clinical context help to better identify individual patients and individualize therapeutic treatment.

Table 32.1 Classification of Status Epilepticus (Simplified from Trinka et al. [15])

I. Axis: Semeiology
(A) With prominent motor symptoms
A.1 Convulsive SE (CSE, synonym: tonic-clonic SE)
A.2 Myoclonic SE (prominent epileptic myoclonic jerks)
A.3 Focal motor
A.4 Tonic status
A.5 Hyperkinetic SE
(B) Without prominent motor symptoms (i.e., nonconvulsive SE, NCSE)
B.1 NCSE with coma (including so-called "subtle" SE)
B.2 NCSE without coma
B.2.a. Generalized
B.2.a.a Typical absence status
B.2.a.b Atypical absence status
B.2.a.c Myoclonic absence status
B.2.a.c Myoclonic absence status
B.2.b. Focal
B.2.c Unknown whether focal or generalized
Boundaries
Epileptic encephalopathies
Coma with non evolving epileptiform EEG pattern
Behavioral disturbance (e.g., psychosis) in patients with epilepsy
Acute confusional status, (e.g., delirium) with epileptiform EEG pattern
II. Axis: Etiology
Acute (e.g., stroke, intoxication, malaria, encephalitis)
Remote (e.g., posttraumatic, postencephalitic, poststroke)
Progressive (e.g., brain tumor, Lafora's disease and other PMEs, dementias)
SE in defined electroclinical syndromes
Unknown (i.e., cryptogenic)
III. Axis: EEG
1. Location: generalized (including bilateral synchronous patterns), lateralized, bilateral independent, multifocal
2. Name of the pattern: Periodic discharges, rhythmic delta activity or spike-and-wave/sharp-and-wave plus subtypes
3. Morphology: sharpness, number of phases (e.g., triphasic morphology), absolute and relative amplitude, polarity
4. Time-related features: prevalence, frequency, duration, daily pattern duration and index, onset (sudden vs. gradual), and dynamics (evolving, fluctuating, or static)
5. Modulation: stimulus-induced vs. spontaneous
6. Effect of intervention (medication) on EEG
IV. Axis: Age

32.2 EEG Pattern According to Clinical Manifestation

32.2.1 Generalized SE with Prominent Motor Signs

32.2.1.1 Tonic-Clonic SE

According to its clinical manifestation, SE appears with a sequence of events that are not different from those of the single seizures. The number of seizures for each hour is variable as well as the duration of the single seizures.

Almost all the primary CNS pathologies, but also some systemic diseases, can be the cause of this kind of SE (electrolyte diseases, hypoglycemia, and others) (Figs. 32.1, 32.2, and 32.3); this demonstrates that SE should be considered as a symptom of an underlying disease that must be sought in all patients without a previous history of epilepsy.

Of all the SE, this is the one that most easily changes its clinical characteristics over time (mostly after the pharmacological treatment). Moreover, especially if carried out with drugs able of inducing deep sedation, the therapy can remove clinical manifestations leaving partial seizures that can only be detected with the EEG.

The initial pattern is a classical EEG one with generalized seizures alternated with periods of amplitude attenuation, with progressive recovery until the onset of the subsequent seizure. However, this SE is rarely registered, maybe because clear clinical evidence of the problem induces the treatment of seizures without waiting for EEG confirmation. The typical EEG pattern is often hidden by muscle artifacts and can be described as the appearance of a recruiting fast activity that begins with a rapid discharge, grows in amplitude and decreases in frequency until the appearance of very wide slow waves, clinically related to the clonic phase. Frequently, it is possible to find a "focal" seizure or the appearance of repeated partial seizures on which a secondary generalization is established in an unpredictable way. According to Gastaut [16], even SE with a clear focal onset should be classified as generalized as tonic-clonic (Figs. 32.4 and 32.5).

At the beginning of the 1990s, Treiman et al. [18] suggested and described the progressive clinical-EEG modification of the SE over time. In clinical practice we often find more complex clinical-EEG patterns than those described above. The different approaches adopted in these complex cases (much more frequently in acute symptomatic SE) need theoretical basis that would consider the SE as a dynamic process that slowly overturns the classic rules of alternating appearance of critical and intercritical EEG patterns. This is most likely due to various factors such as the etiology and its evolution over time, the consequences of the seizures on the brain and on the whole organism, the therapy administered,

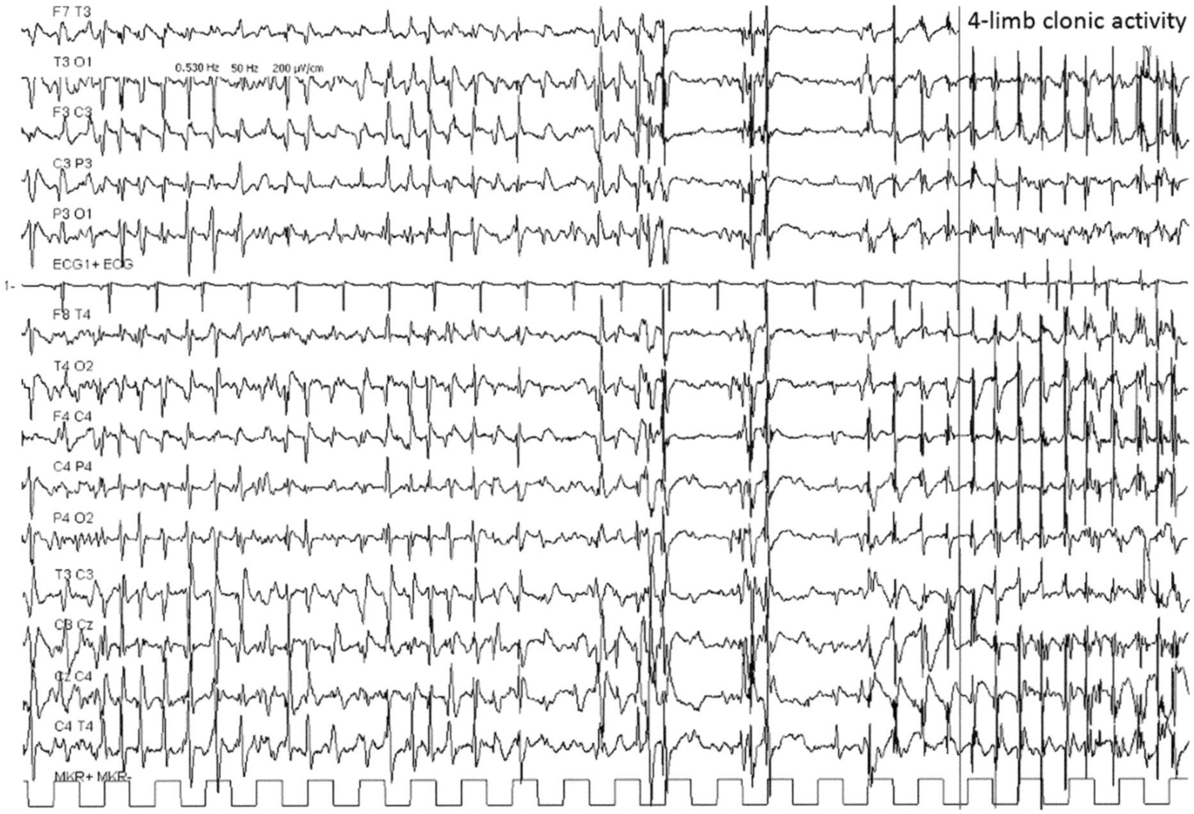

Fig. 32.1 Generalized convulsive epileptic status in a 63-year-old patient affected by a chronic renal failure, since 2 days confused and slowed down. Three hours before the execution of the EEG, appearance of generalized tonic-clonic seizures repeated without recovery of vigilance between one episode and another. Hematologic data not indicative of uremic encephalopathy. CT encephalon with modest, bilateral, and subcortical vascular outcomes. The EEG shows GPEDs (generalized, periodic epileptiform discharges), bilateral and synchronous on which muscular artifacts linked to bilateral and symmetric clones are superimposed. On the onset of the seizure, two short amplitude attenuations almost completely interrupt the underlying pathological activity

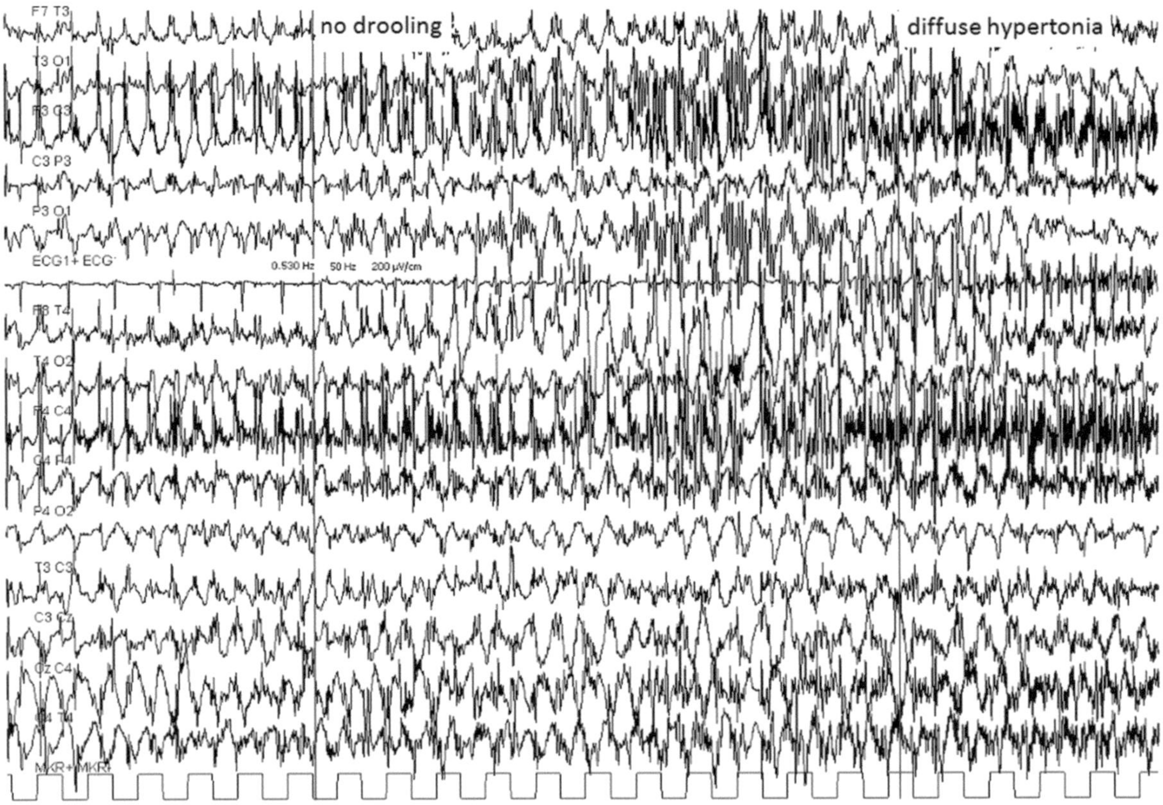

Fig. 32.2 Same patient of Fig. 32.1. The artifacts related to clonic manifestations changes in relation to the appearance of a "tonic" clinical phase. The widespread and progressive increase of rapid components could also be linked to a modification of muscular artifacts, while the slower components do not undergo variations due to clinical modifications

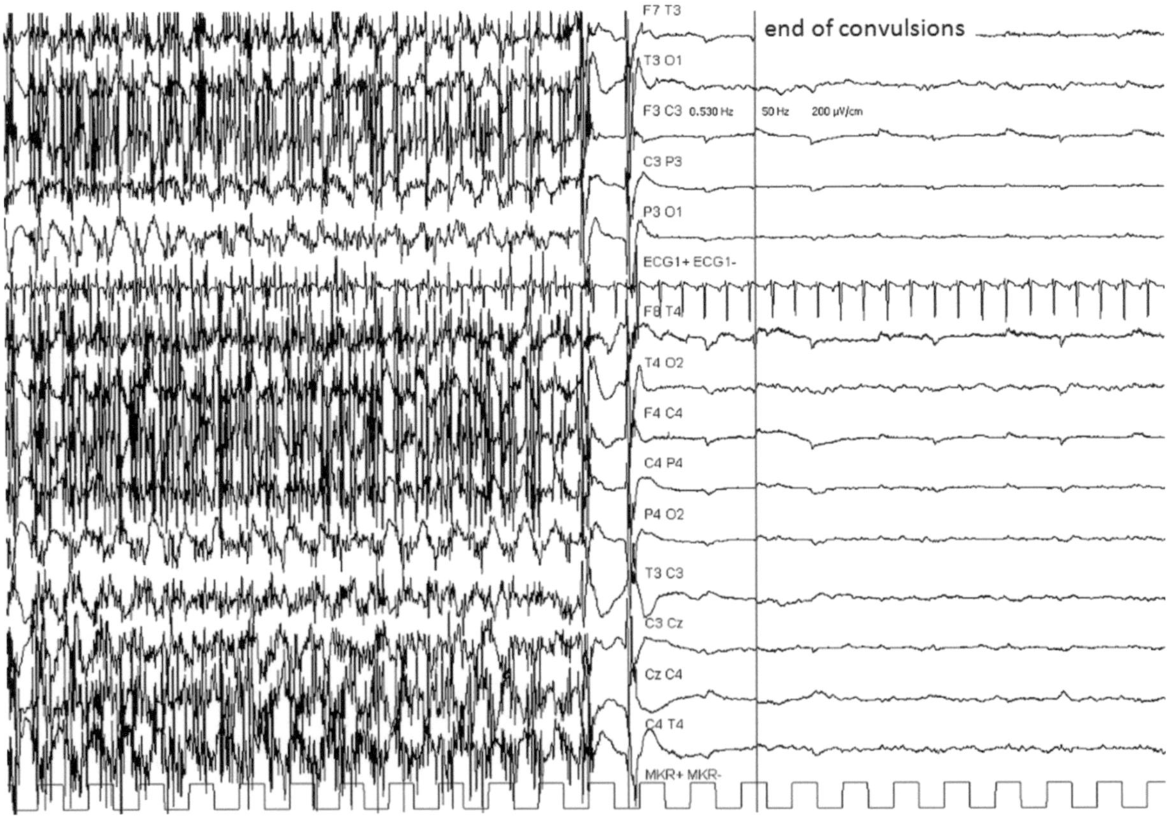

Fig. 32.3 Same patient as in Fig. 32.1. End of the crisis. Abrupt disappearance of both EEG and artifactual activity without significant asymmetries in post-crypt. The amplification of the path used to visualize the crisis, however, makes it difficult to correctly evaluate the underlying activity

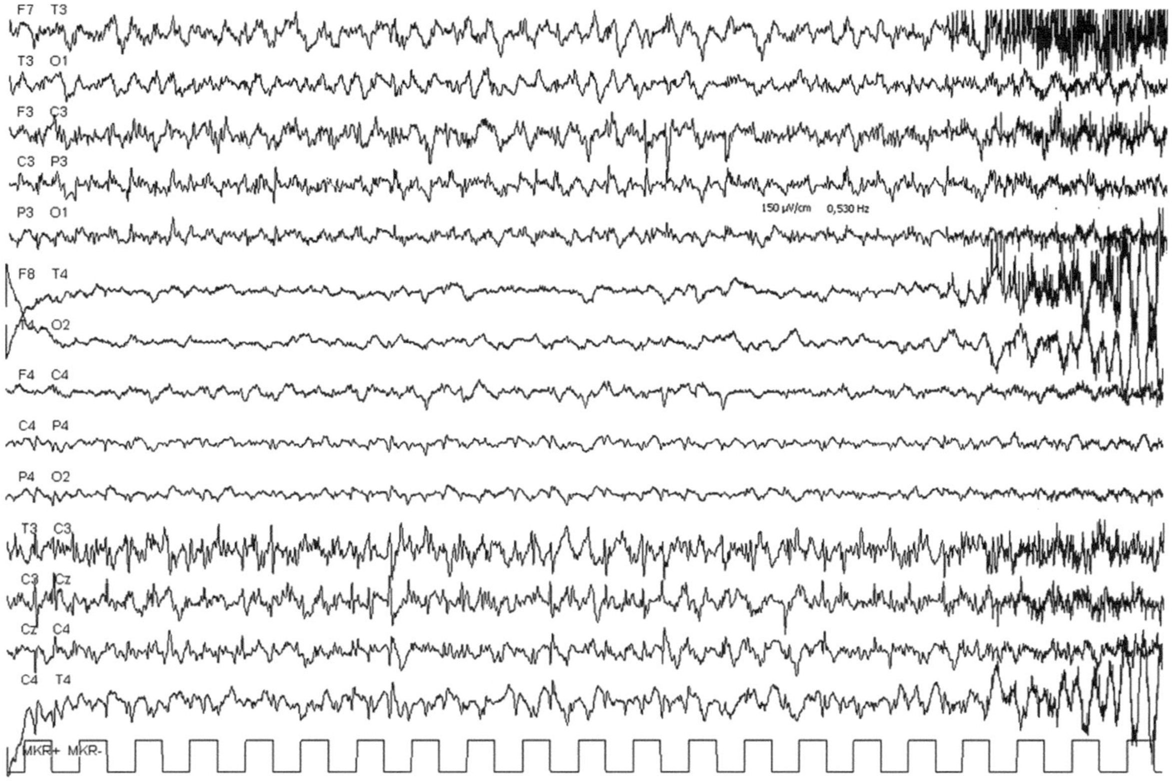

Fig. 32.4 Continuous epileptic activity in a 68-year-old patient with a metastatic lesion in left temporal area. Initially he is clinically with acinetic mutism. The background is asymmetric with rhythmic, irregular delta activity on the left hemisphere with fast frequency and spike waves with partial contralateral diffusion. The appearance of adversary seizure with rapid secondary generalization is characterized by an attenuation of the slow components rather than an increase of the rapid ones

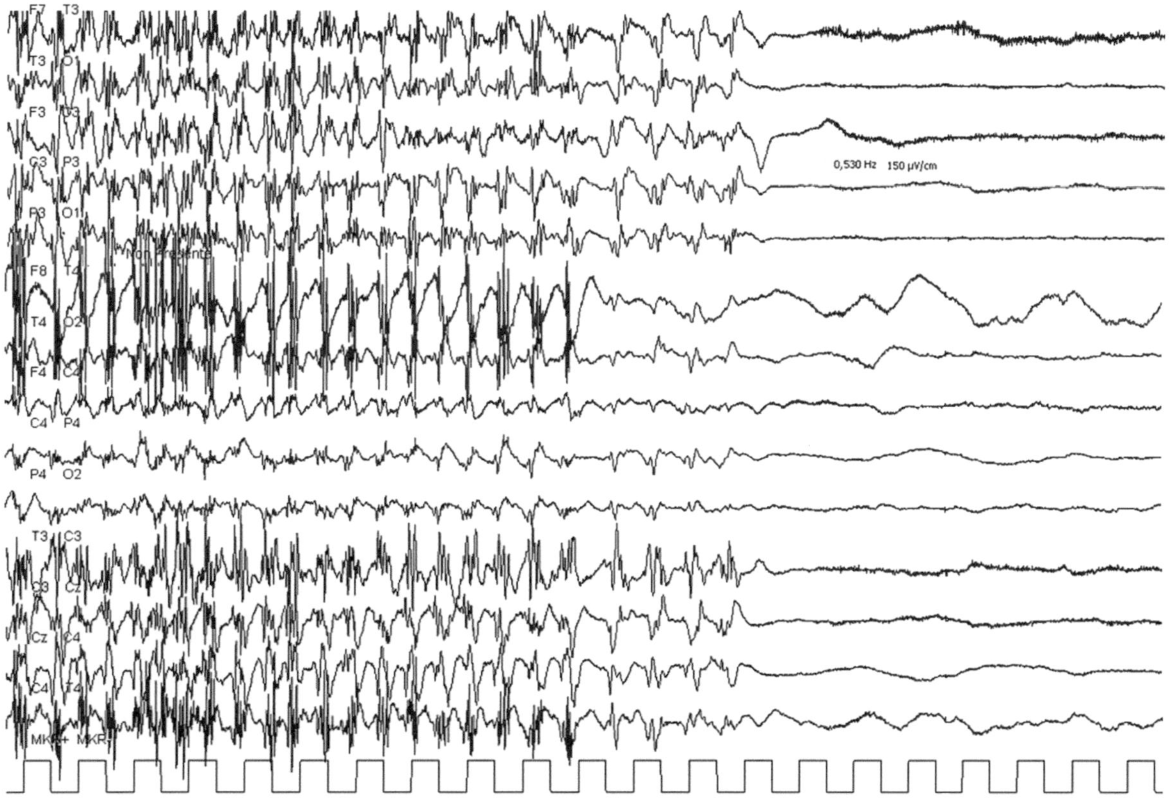

Fig. 32.5 Continuous epileptic activity. Same patient as in Fig. 32.4. End of the secondarily generalized seizure. Sudden disappearance of epileptiform anomalies subjected to muscular artifacts. Disappearance also of the previous continuous activity

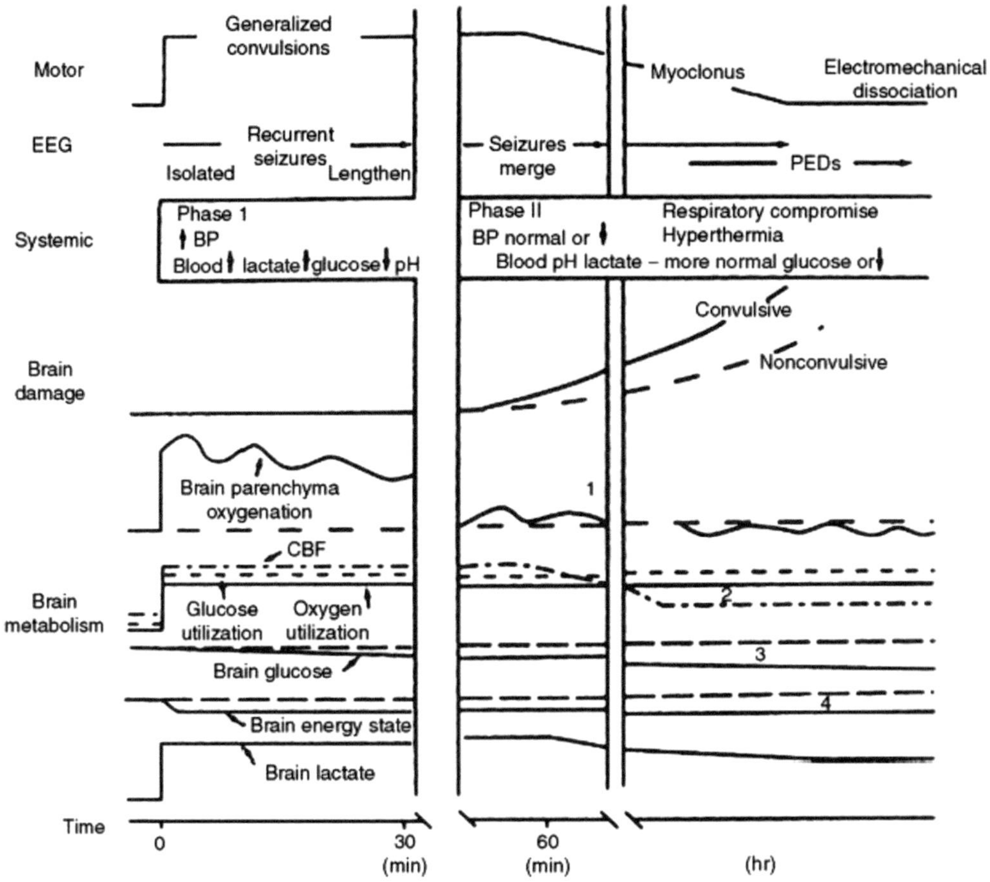

Fig. 32.6 Modified scheme from the original by Lothman on the progressive pathophysiological alterations induced by the epileptic status. (Modified by: Lothman EW Neurology 1990: 40 (Suppl. 2): 13–23, with permission)

or, more frequently, the sum of all these factors. Some studies seem to support this hypothesis. Studies on experimental models [19] (Fig. 32.6) indicated that SE should be considered as a dynamic process that recognizes stereotypical stages. Not only the EEG pattern but also the clinical phenomenology demonstrate a progressive disappearance of evident seizures. The more or less complex ictal manifestations progressively give way to the decline of cortical functions and to clonic contractions in more limited body areas [20]. In summary, from the literature it can be concluded that a complex clinical-EEG pattern would be established. The progressive systemic and local complications of the SE would take precedence over the typical aspects of the seizures up to a sort of "electromechanical" dissociation.

32.2.1.2 Tonic SE

It appears usually in Lennox-Gastaut syndrome, but some cases are described also in idiopathic generalized epilepsies [21]. It is characterized by tonic seizures affecting a more or less large body districts and seizures with few clinical manifestations like winking, deviation of the ocular globes, or only respiratory changes. The single seizures have a variable duration, but generally they last less than 1 min. They appear in both wakefulness and sleep state and may present a frequency of more than 60 episodes per hour. The impairment of consciousness is variable, and the SE, usually resistant to treatment, can last up to 4 months. Usually there are no permanent deficits at the end of the SE. The EEG is fundamental for the diagnosis. This SE can occur with generalized repetitive runs of polyspikes at high frequencies of 16–20 Hz, beginning with low voltage and increasing high voltage (100 microV) and at 10 Hz recruiting rhythm of high voltage from onset. The trait of polyspikes can be interspersed with slow waves (Fig. 32.7).

32.2.1.3 Myoclonic SE

It is characterized by the presence of myoclonic manifestations not localized to a specific body district and without other precise features (including impairment of consciousness). For this reason, it is difficult to consider it as an unique entity, even according to Gastaut. Shorvon classifies this according to the clinical contexts or epileptic syndrome in which it occurs (idiopathic and symptomatic generalized epilepsies, progressive myoclonic, etc.). The myoclonic SE in coma patients is of particular importance. This is usually sign of severe systemic and widespread diseases affecting

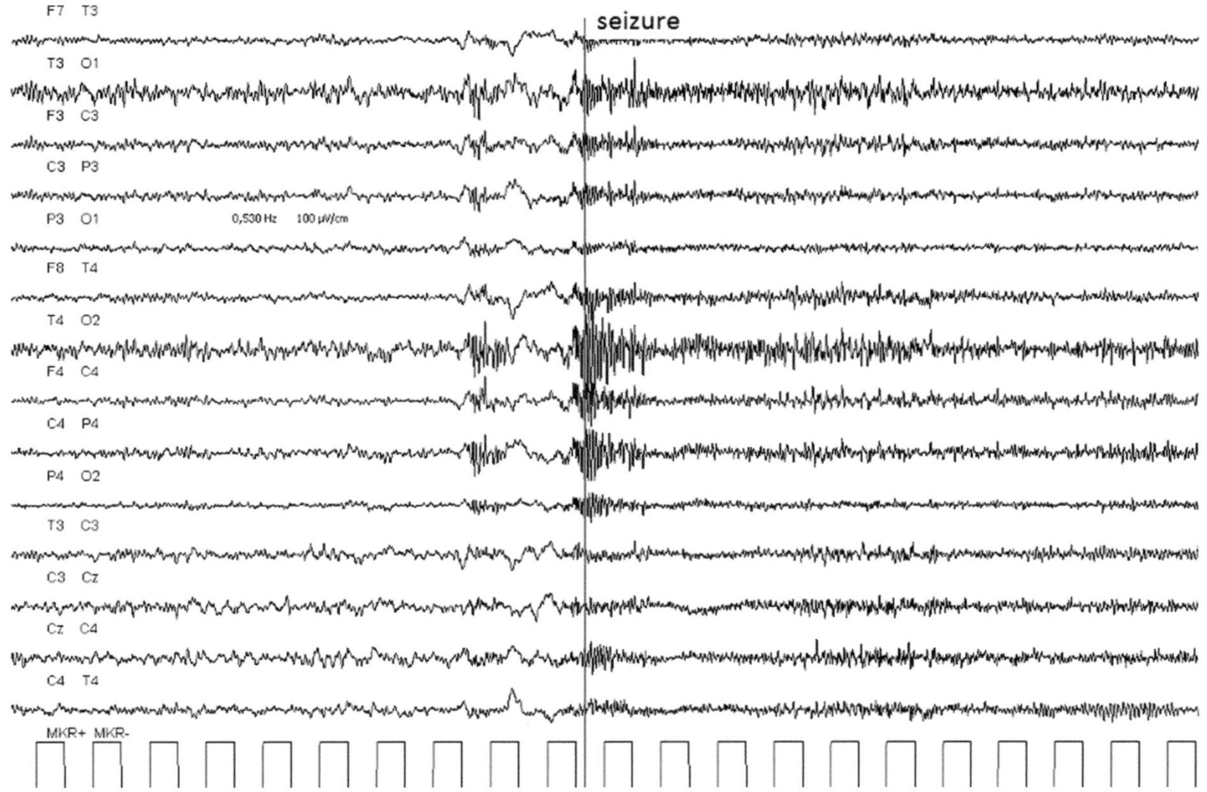

Fig. 32.7 Generalized tonic status epilepticus in a 23-year-old patient with a previous diagnosis of symptomatic generalized epilepsy. Registration after sleep deprivation. The EEG during the falling asleep phase highlights the appearance of bilateral, symmetrical, and peak of rapid activity on the posterior regions and with a progress that is only partly recruited and indicative of a tonic seizure. In the next hour of the recording time, similar frames of variable duration from 7 to 12 s were repeated with an interval less than 10 min. The clinical correlate was a modest tonic flexion movement of the head and trunk

the CNS, cerebral anoxic-ischemic disorders, systemic metabolic disorders and encephalopathies due to physical agents, and inflammatory or degenerative diseases. Within the myoclonic SE, other seizures often occur like tonic-clonic, (only) tonic, or (only) clonic.

It should be noted that in postanoxic encephalopathies, seizures can be triggered by stimuli and that the appearance of epileptic manifestations is in any case described as an unfavorable prognostic factor.

In myoclonic SE, even if the myoclonic manifestations are often very limited and lateralized, the subtle SE with few motor symptoms must be included.

32.2.2 Focal SE

In the past, the focal SE was usually divided into "simple partial status" and "partial complex status." The distinction between the two clinical conditions was made in analogy with the old classification of epileptic seizures, based on the presence or absence of consciousness. Unfortunately, the term consciousness has a non-univocal meaning, and this is the reason why the distinction between the two clinical phenomena has recently been questioned. The historical reason for this subdivision is strictly linked to the old hypothesis of a temporal localization of the conscience disorder.

Theoretically, it is possible that for each kind of partial seizure, there is at least one kind of SE consisting of a recurrence of that seizure over time. In clinical practice some SE types are more easily found: the focal motor, the sensory, the aphasic or dysphasic, the visual, and the vegetative status. Considering patients with severe conscience and vigilance disorders, in clinical practice it is common to encounter focal critical EEG patterns without evident clinical correlation.

32.2.2.1 Focal Motor SE

The seizures are characterized by the recurrence of partial motor seizures with variable clinical characteristics depending on the motor area involved, not necessarily with a Jacksonian march but, in any case, without loss of consciousness or vegetative symptoms both during seizures and in intercritical periods. In some cases, the epileptic manifestations occur with repetitive sequence of single myoclonic contractions limited to a body district. Those manifestations could be either a part of an SE with well-differentiated recurring single seizures or the only evident and continuous element of the epileptic condition. This last type of manifestation is usually known as *continuous partial epilepsy* or *Kojevnikov syndrome*, and it is symptomatic of acute CNS injury or of a progressive encephalopathy [22]. The term "subtle" has been introduced to define those partial motor status (single, repetitive clones, affecting a body district, and ocular globes) that arise in patients in a coma; for this reason the "subtle" SE must not be inserted in the simple partial ones. In some patients, clinical seizures occur with critical EEG patterns with "recruiting" characteristics affecting the motor area. In some other conditions, the EEG pattern may be more masked. If the SE presents with single myoclonic manifestations, the EEG pattern is often represented by periodic discharges that not necessarily involve the motor area (Figs. 32.8 and 32.9).

32.2.2.2 Dysphasic or Aphasic SE

The diagnosis is based on the occurrence of a speech disorder that could be either a paroxysmal disorder with episodes interspersed with a complete recovery of the language or a more stable clinical manifestation that is maintained even in intercritical phases [23–28]. EEG support is essential to distinguish this from other clinical conditions with similar symptoms. EEG seizures do not have any peculiar characteristics, except for the localization on the language (Fig. 32.10) areas (Figs. 32.11, 32.12, 32.13, and 32.14).

32.2.2.3 Focal Sensory Status Epilepticus

The characteristics of the seizures are obviously connected with the involvement of the sensory area, but descriptions of this type of SE in the literature are rare [29]. Gastaut expressed his doubts on the need to identify as SE also those conditions of continuous dysesthesias accompanying seizures with a clear involvement of the somatosensory projection areas.

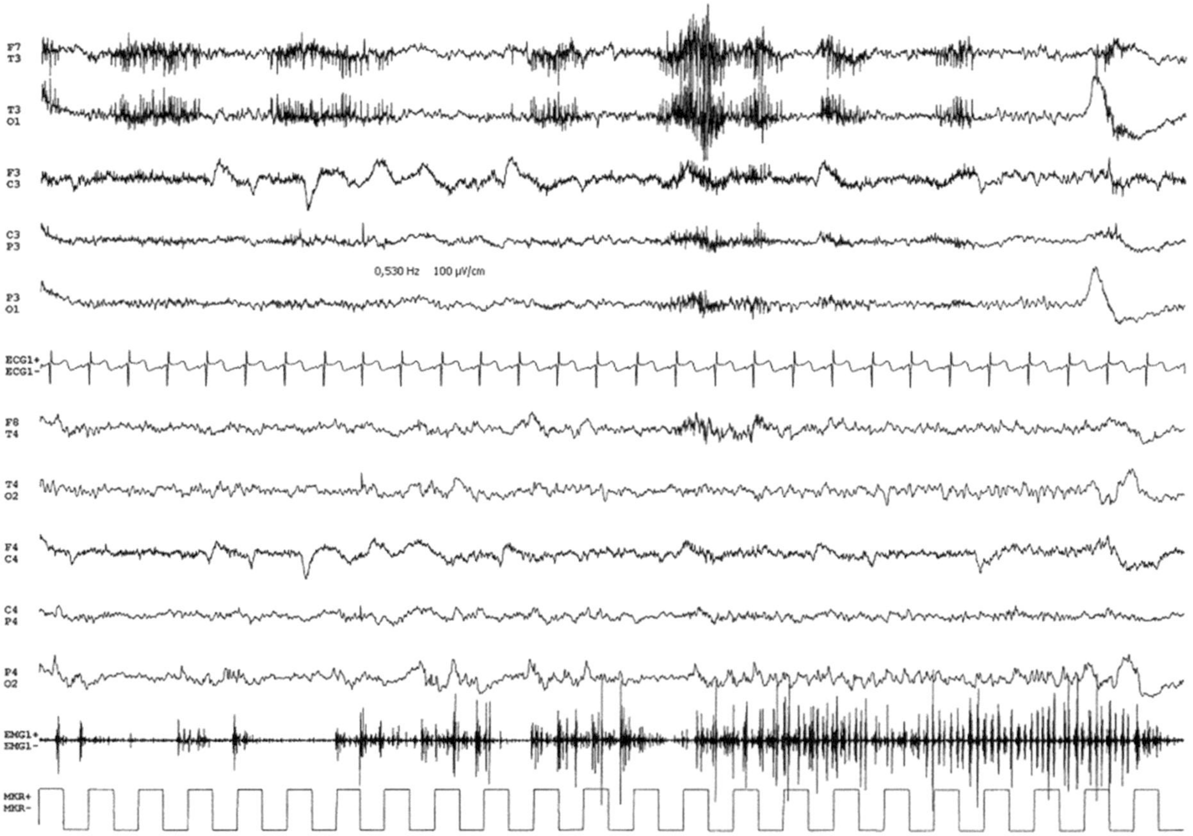

Fig. 32.8 Motor focal epileptic status in a 78-year-old patient with a previous lesion in the right frontoparietal region. Since a few hours, the appearance of myoclonic manifestations in the left upper limb was only at times collected in a shorter sequence forming a focal seizure. EEG (electromyogram [EMG] m. left brachial biceps), normal organization of the left hemisphere, while on the right it is observed an excess of irregular theta components with maximum expression on temporo-occipital. The theta components (probably non-artifactual) accompanied the recording of the EMG activity with a discrete temporal correlation only during the longest sequence

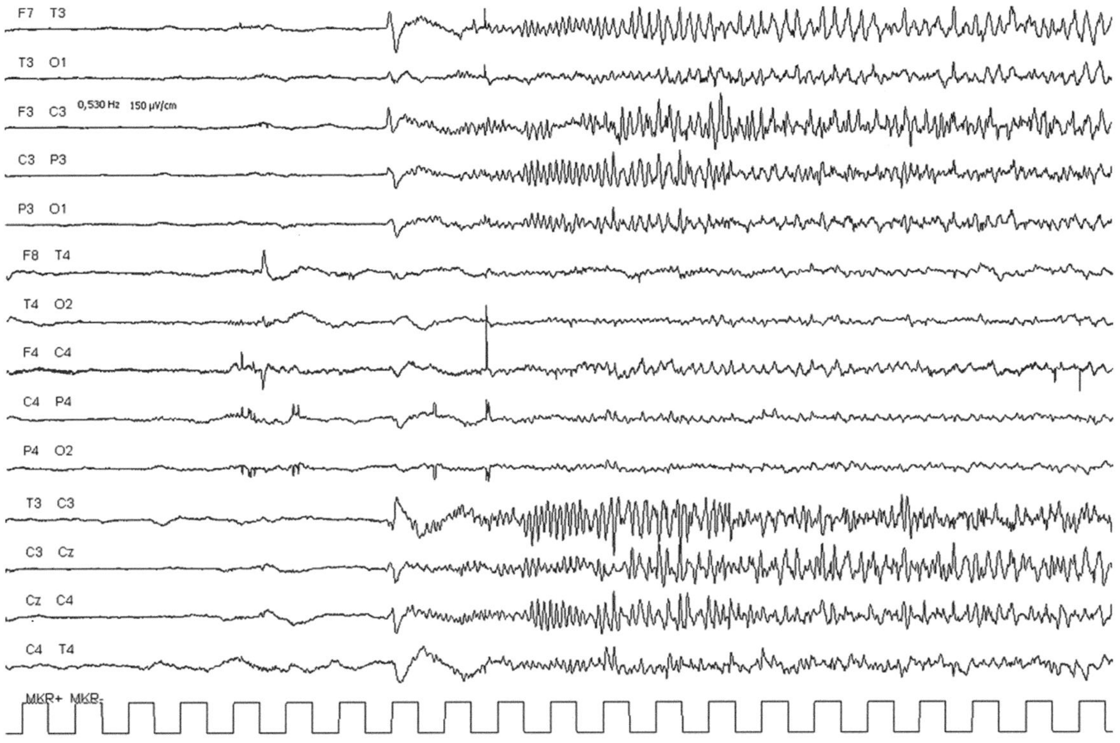

Fig. 32.9 Focal epileptic status in a 59-year-old patient without major pathological early events, with sudden onset of adverse episodes and only the first one with secondary generalization. Subsequent negative assessments for diseases affecting the central nervous system. Examination performed 1 h after the administration of benzodiazepines in the emergency department. Patient in a coma without significant clinical manifestations. The EEG path shows the appearance of a seizure with recruited activity in a frontocentral left onset. Similar episodes have occurred two more times before the modification of therapeutic attitudes

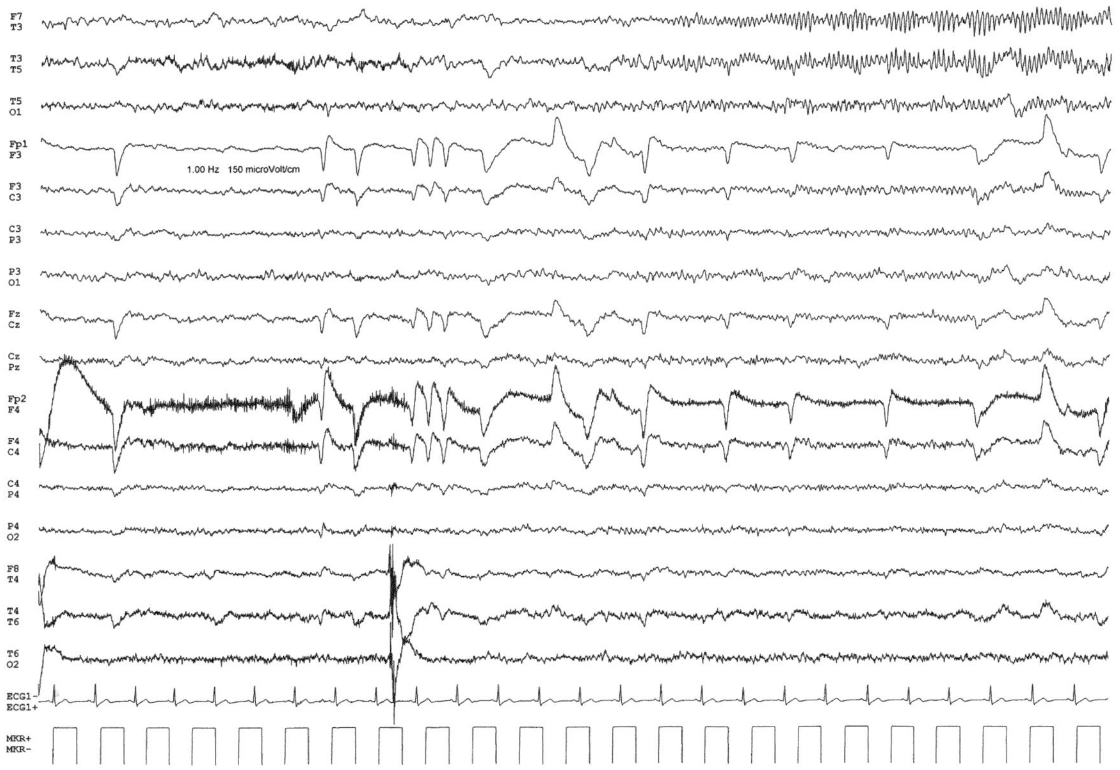

Fig. 32.10 Focal aphasic SE in a 73-year-old patient with a neoplastic lesion in the area of left temporal cortex. Two days after diagnostic biopsy was done. Continuous short episodes of aphasia lasting less than 1 min. The left temporal area shows the presence of a sudden appearance of focal seizures with evolving spatiotemporal features

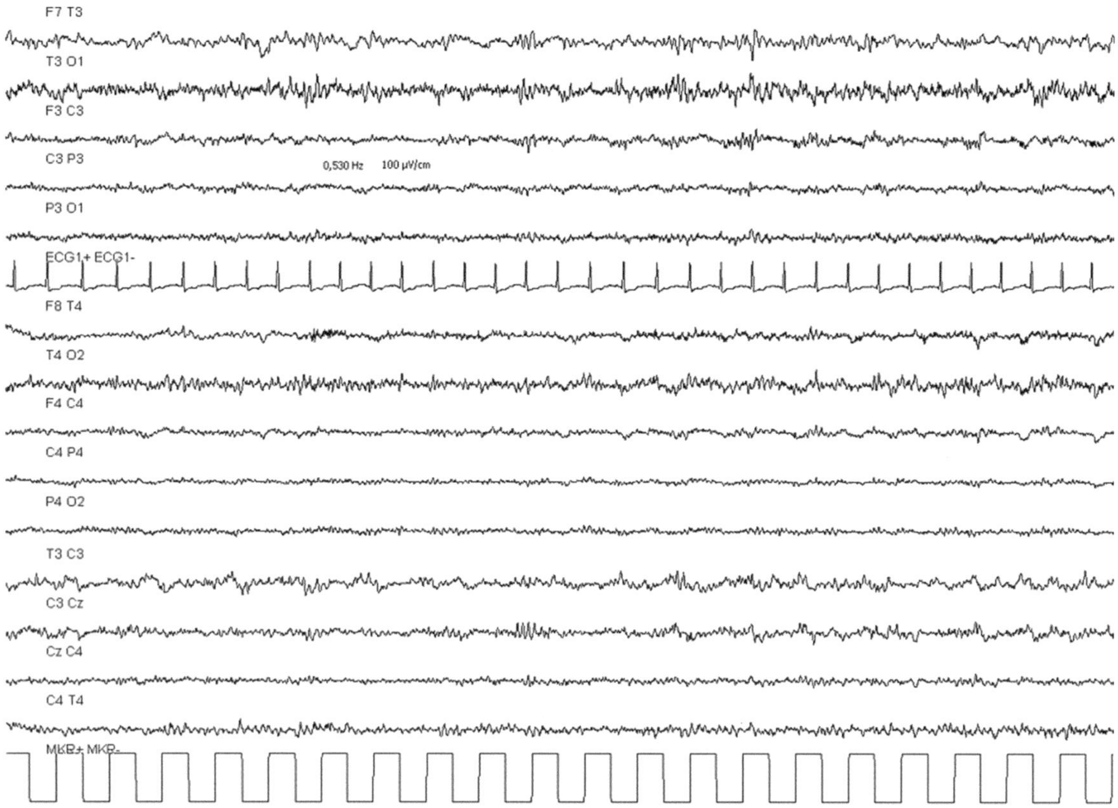

Fig. 32.11 Focal aphasic epileptic status in a 64-year-old patient with appearance from some hours of confusion and short-term transient episodes of expressive aphasia. Previous left-handed temporal infarct lesion. Right-handed. The right hemisphere shows an organization within normal limits. On the left, a minimum progressive increase of the slow temporal arhythmic components

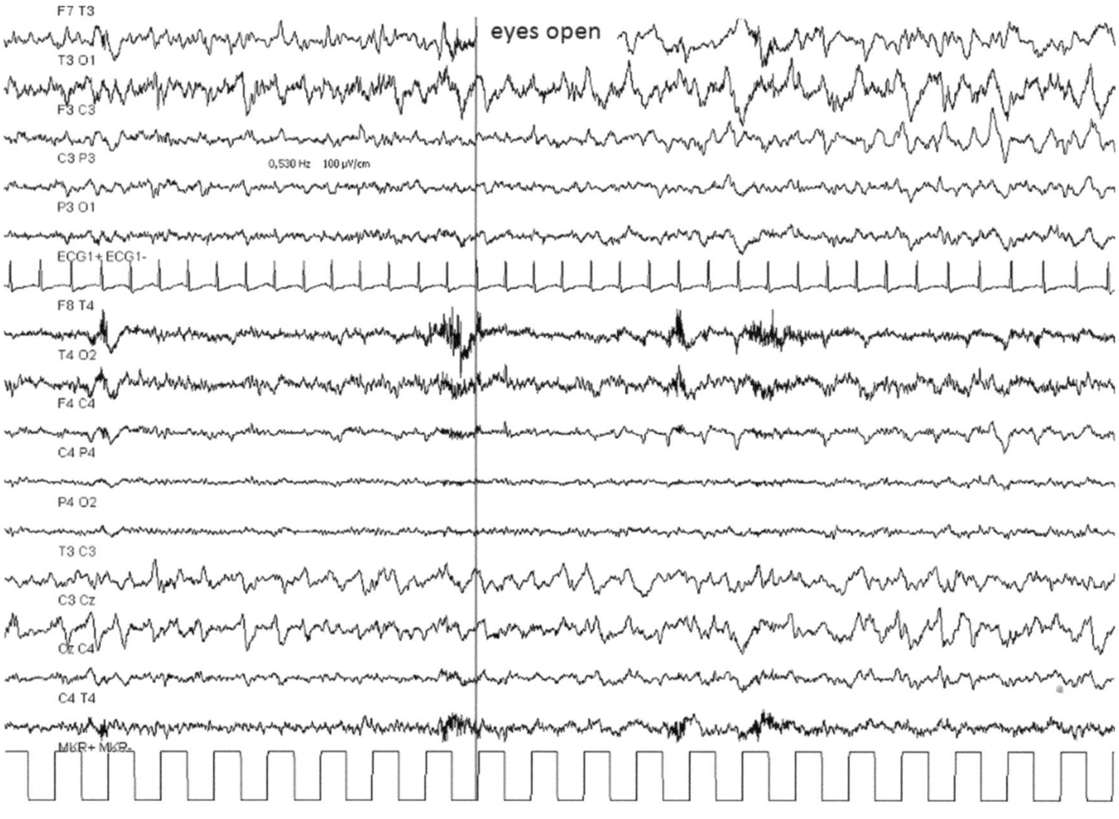

Fig. 32.12 Focal aphasic epileptic status. Same patient as in Fig. 32.11 (sequence in timeline). Development of a left critical temporal EEG without subjective or objective clinical manifestations

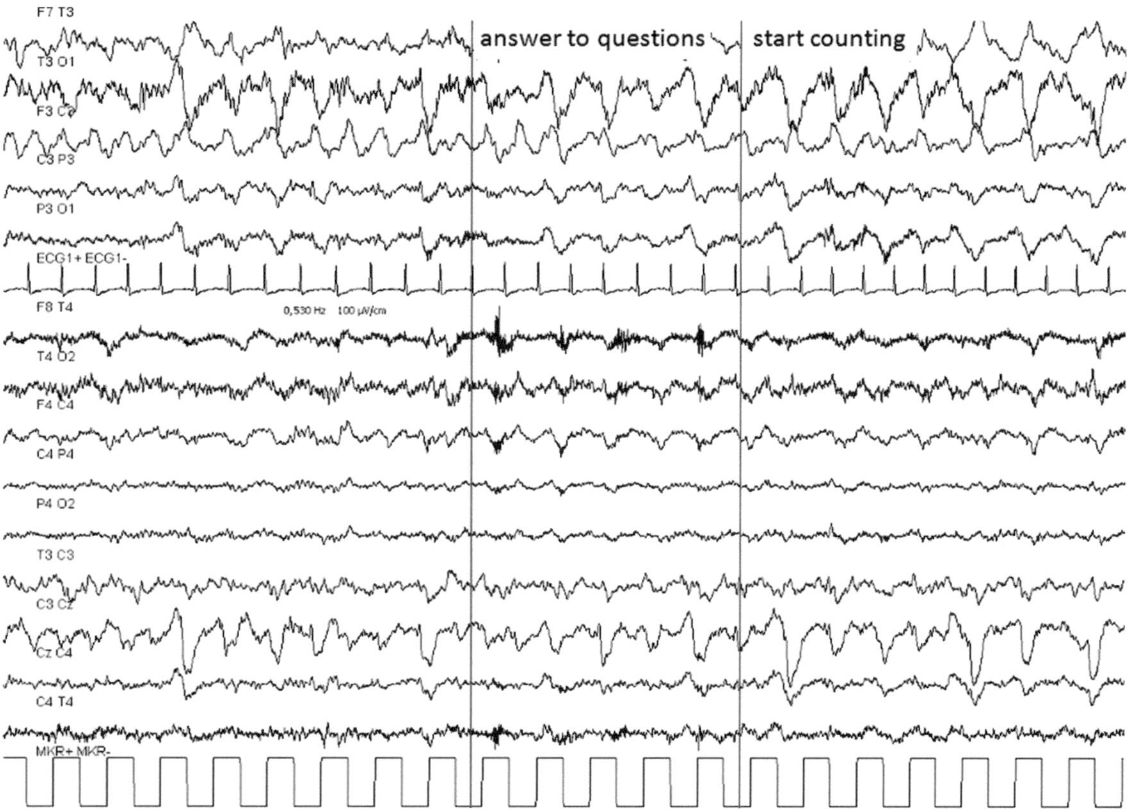

Fig. 32.13 Aphasic focal epileptic status. Same patient as in Fig. 32.11 (sequence in time line). Continuation of the seizure without clear clinical findings even if the patient is asked to count

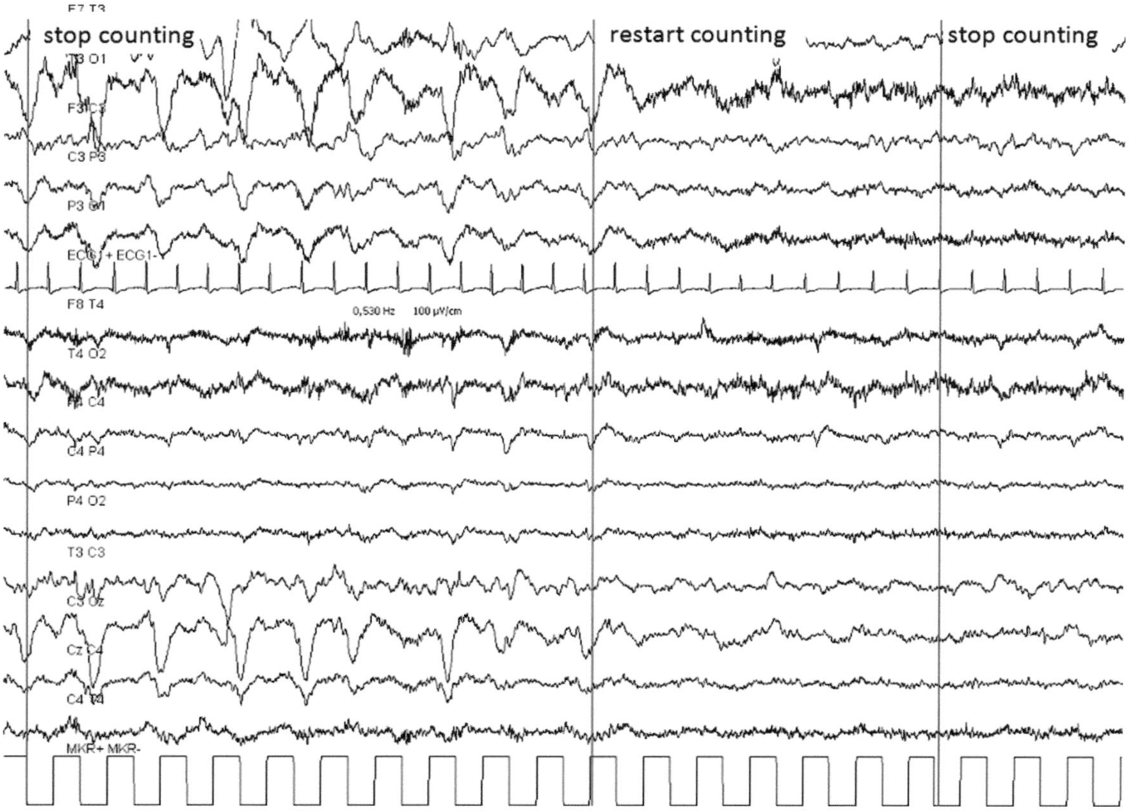

Fig. 32.14 Aphasic focal epileptic status. Same patient as in Fig. 32.11 (sequence in time line). End of seizure concomitant with the end of a temporary inability to count. On the temporal regions, in the post-critic phase, arhythmic delta components are not present before the seizure

32.2.2.4 SE with Visual Seizures

It must refer to very simple visual elements and not to hallucinations or complex visual illusions. If it is defined in this manner, the phenomenon is described as extremely rare.

32.2.2.5 Autonomic SE

Its existence as a phenomenon, which can manifest itself even without more evident signs, is obviously debatable. Vomiting and headache may be accompanied by focal seizures; it is considered possible the abdominal pain as the only symptom of a seizure that may occur as an SE. Gastaut reports the case of a patient in whom, in the context of neurophysiological diagnostics for "abdominal seizures" [30], an SE has been observed for some hours with EEG demonstration of the seizures.

32.2.2.6 Unilateral or Erratic SE

This SE could be seen only in children.

32.3 Diagnostic Criteria of Nonconvulsive Status Epilepticus (NCSE)

The Nonconvulsive Status Epilepticus (NCSE) on the basis of the clinical correlation can be distinguished between generalized and focal (without prominent motor symptoms) [31].

32.3.1 Historical Background

32.3.1.1 Generalized NCSE

Traditionally were distinguished the "absence SE" and the "atonic and acinetic SE". In the "absence SE," the typical absence status and the atypical absence status are differentiated. The clinical manifestations are characterized by a situation of lapses in awareness, sometimes with staring. The contact with the environment is more or less complete, such as it is easily confused with many other epileptic and non-epileptic conditions. Usually this type of SE is related to generalized idiopathic or symptomatic epilepsies.

The typical absence status occurs in children or adolescents with idiopathic generalized epilepsy in which these clinical features appears in the presence of repeated sequences of spike-and-wave complexes with an average frequency of 3 Hz. The atypical one occurs in patients with symptomatic generalized epilepsy in which the EEG pattern is characterized by continuous spike-and-wave complexes at frequencies lower than 3 Hz. Clinical signs might be also different, and variable tonic, atonic, or myoclonic manifestations may be present. In some patients the continuous discharges of sharp wave/slow waves are replaced by a modification of the background with a theta or delta activity, on which an overlapping discharge of activity at 10 Hz or occasional burst of spike-and-wave complexes occurs (Figs. 32.15, 32.16, and 32.17).

This category should also include absence status with prolonged confusional statuses, usually occurring in women after menopause or related to an abrupt withdrawal of benzodiazepine therapy in patients without prior history of epilepsy. In these patients, absence status are often the only epileptic clinical feature. The first EEG characteristic that can be noticed is the gap between the marked alteration of the background activity and the few clinical symptoms. Epileptiform transients have a variable morphology, except for those NCSE in idiopathic epilepsies, and in these cases, the SE expresses itself with regular spike-and-wave complexes at 3 Hz frequency. In the other cases, the transients are irregular complexes of atypical spike-and-wave (not at 3 Hz) or polyspike-wave whose frequency can vary from 1.5 to 4 Hz, without evident clinical manifestations. The sequences of these transients are of variable duration and may be more or less interspersed with normal background activity or pathologic lateralized activity.

32.3.1.2 Focal Status Without Prominent Motor Symptoms (Partial Complex SE)

In 1975, Gastaut and Tassinari [16] suggested that there might be two clinical forms of focal or partial complex SE (i.e., with a modification of consciousness). The first type (cyclic) (Figs. 32.18, 32.19, 32.20, and 32.21) required the presence of repetitive focal "complex" seizures from the clinical point of view clearly related with psychomotor, psychosensory, or psycho-affective symptoms. In the second type (noncyclic), the clinical condition was stable with a period of mental confusion or psychiatric symptoms. In the last, there were frequently behavioral automatisms that, even if not clearly organized in seizures, could recall epileptic symptoms without a clear recovery of a normal mental state.

Later Treiman and Delgado-Escueta [32] described three possible EEG features to make the diagnosis:

1. Recognizable EEG patterns.
2. Evident response to the administration of benzodiazepines e.v.
3. Intercritical EEG with stable focal epileptiform anomalies (usually with frontal or temporal localization) (Fig. 32.22).

32.3.2 Current Diagnostic Criteria

In 1994 Granner and Lee [33] described EEG aspects of a large series of patients with also clinical features suggestive for NCSE described as a state with slowness in behavior and

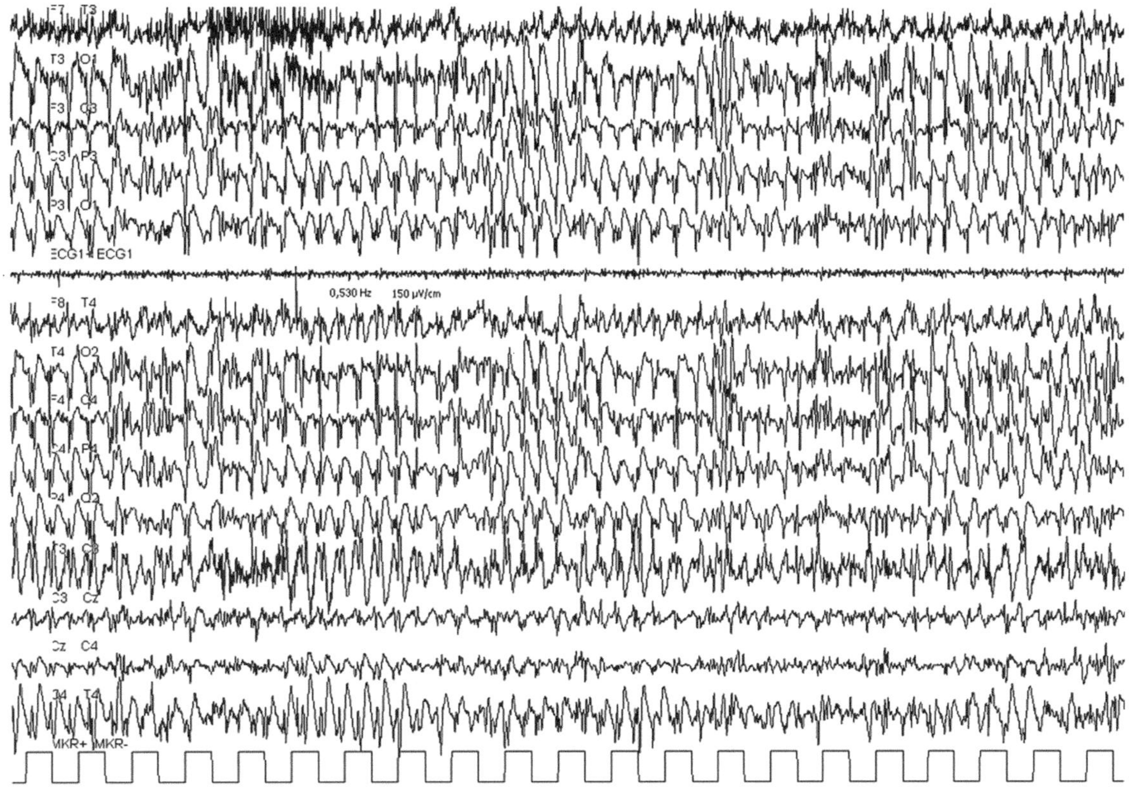

Fig. 32.15 Epileptic status of absence in a 35-year-old patient without clear precedents of epilepsy. Recent, abrupt withdrawal of benzodiazepine therapy. Slow down, confused. EEG: continuous, irregular, symmetric pick and poly-peak wave complex with maximum frontal expression and a prevalent frequency at 3.5 Hz

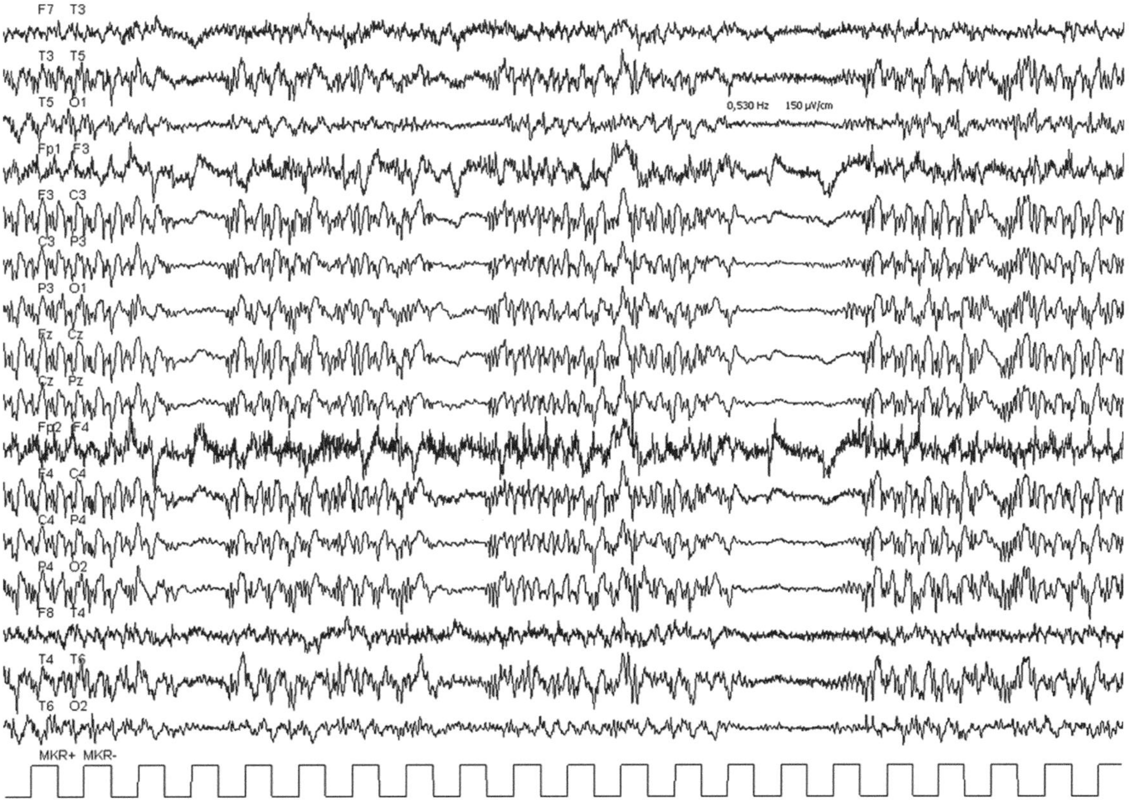

Fig. 32.16 Epileptic status of absence in a 57-year-old patient without previous episodes of epilepsy. Confusion state with sudden onset in full well-being. Brain MR not significant. EEG: poly-peak wave complex, symmetrical, diffuse projection, better expressed on the anterior regions and with a prevalent frequency of 3.5–4.0 Hz. The pathological activity is collected in sequences of a few seconds and separated by intervals of 1–3 s with recovery of a normal background activity

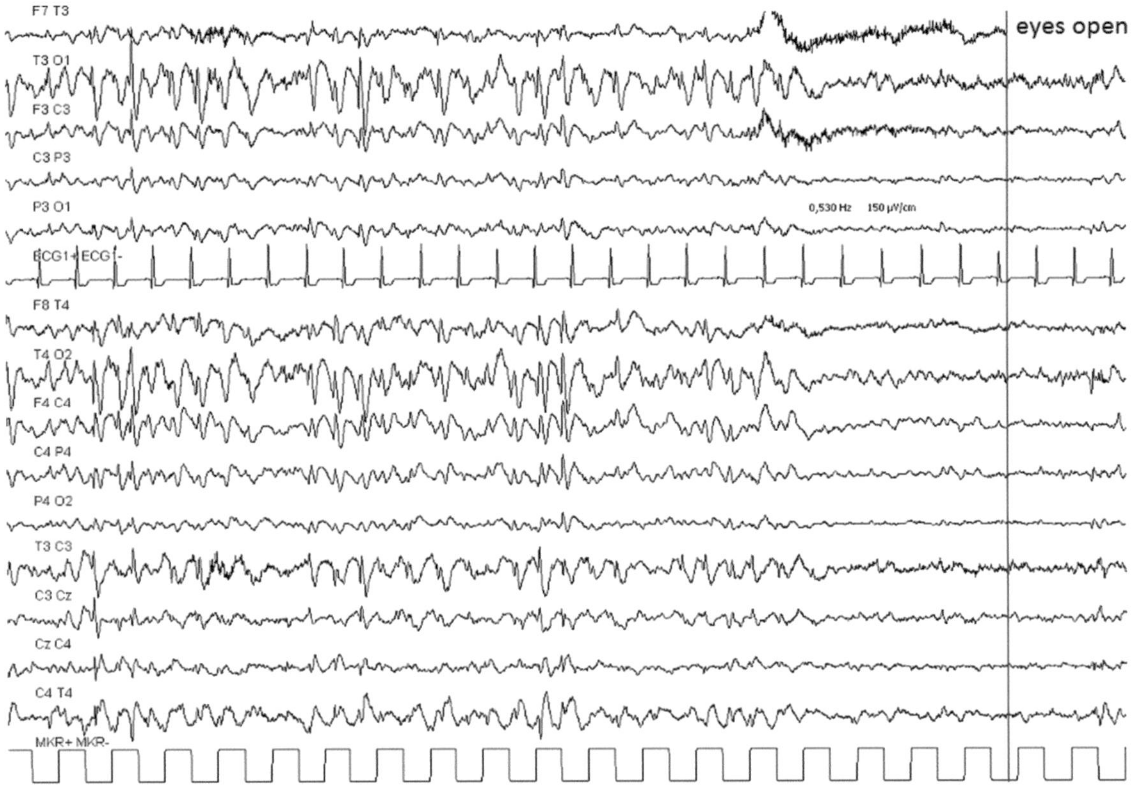

Fig. 32.17 Epileptic status of atypical absence in a 47-year-old patient with a previous diagnosis of symptomatic generalized epilepsy. For a few days, modest increase of psychomotor retardation after reduction of therapy prescribed for ataxia and somnolence. EEG: continuous complex slow wave, bilateral and synchronous more evident on the posterior regions. The pathological activity presents a temporary suspension after the opening of the eyes

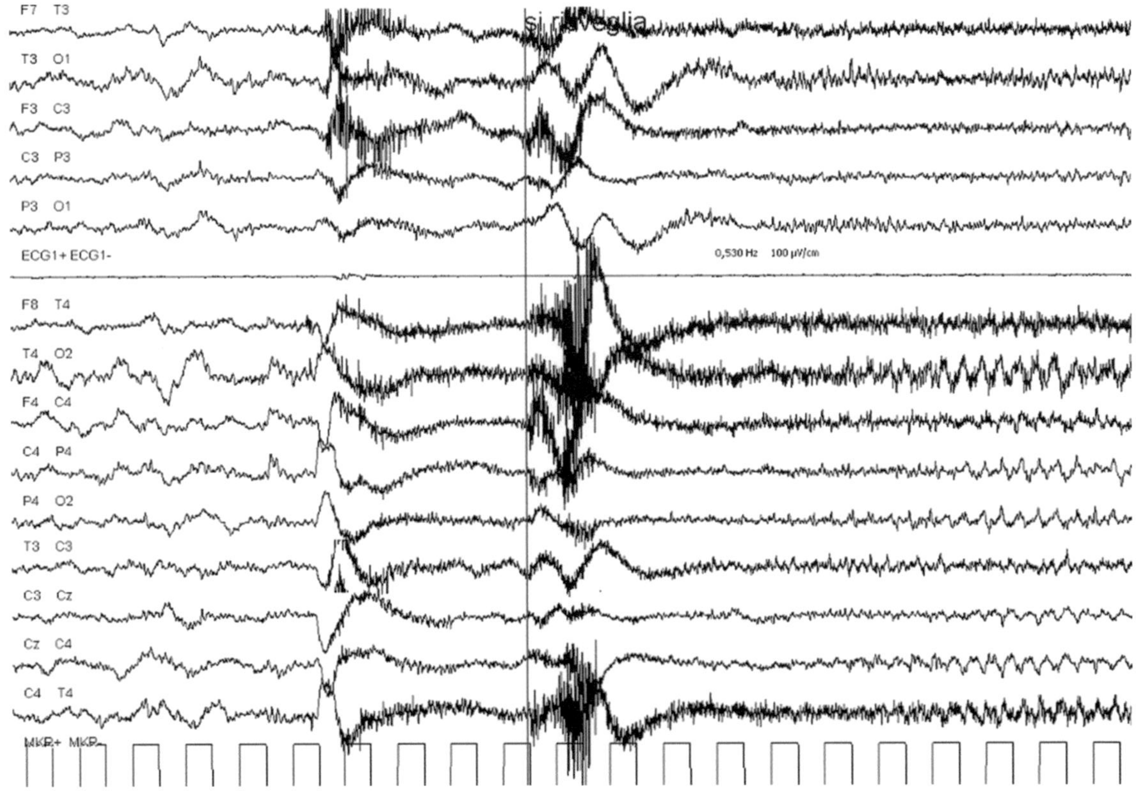

Fig. 32.18 Epileptic status in limbic encephalitis in a 72-year-old patient with a progressive decay of superior cortical functions for about 15 days. Episodes are reported during which the patient seems to present visual hallucinations preceded by abrupt dystonic facial movements. The recording in sleep shows an abrupt electroencephalographic awakening without certain pathological characteristics. After the appearance of artifactual linked to a short, abrupt tonic contraction of the left side of the face, a "recruiting" picture of activity with a right center-temporal onset corresponds to which, from the clinical point of view, corresponds to a motor stop without automatisms

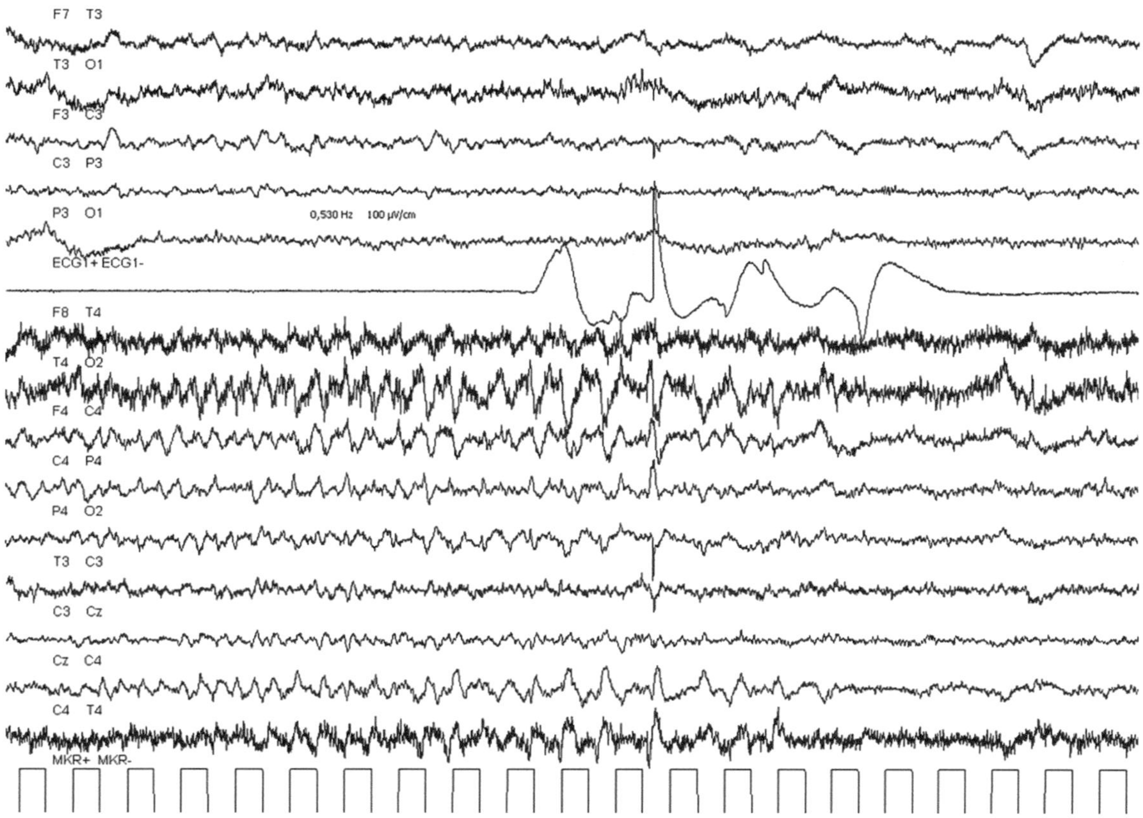

Fig. 32.19 Epileptic status in limbic encephalitis. Same patient as in Fig. 32.18. End of right central-temporal seizure

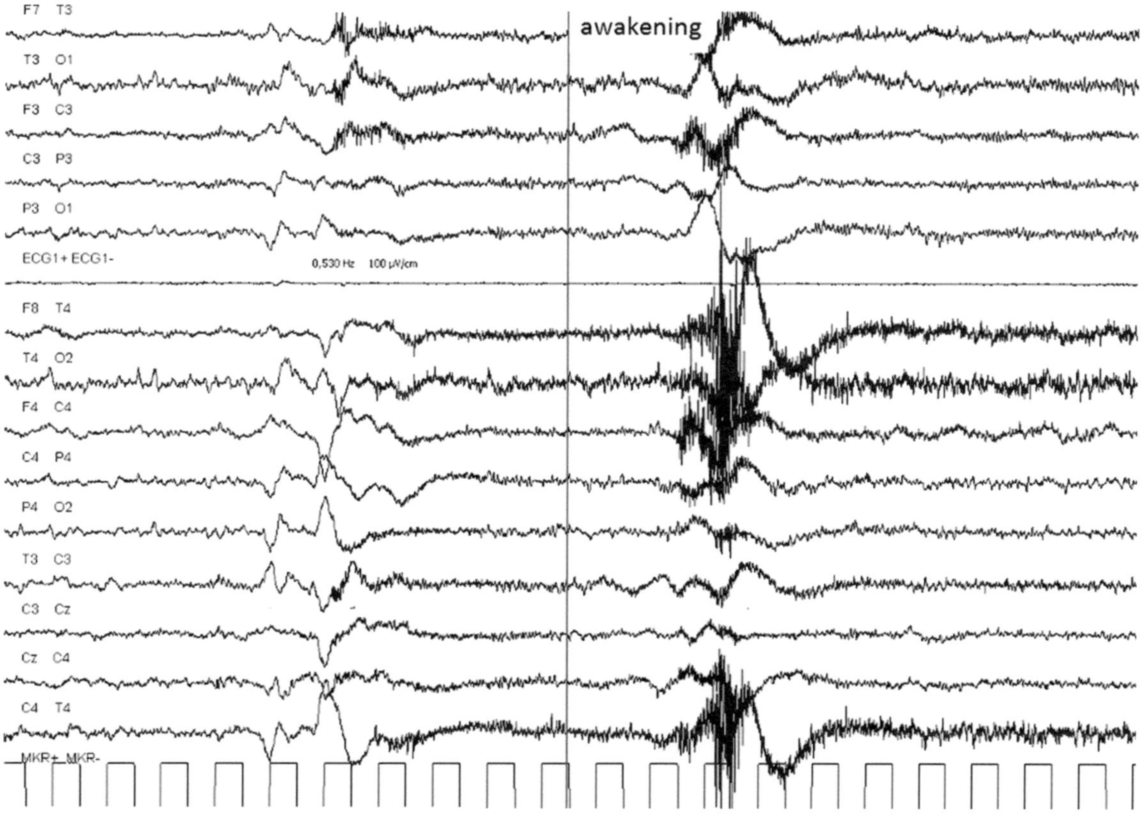

Fig. 32.20 Status epilepticus in limbic encephalitis. Same patient as in Fig. 32.18, 15 min later. The initial sequence of events is substantially analogous to that of the previous seizure, including the tonic contraction of the always right side of the face. The right derivations maintain a prevalence of theta components, while on the left a non-congruous alpha activity is organized on the posterior regions with the usual organization of the patient's path but similar to the one of previous seizure

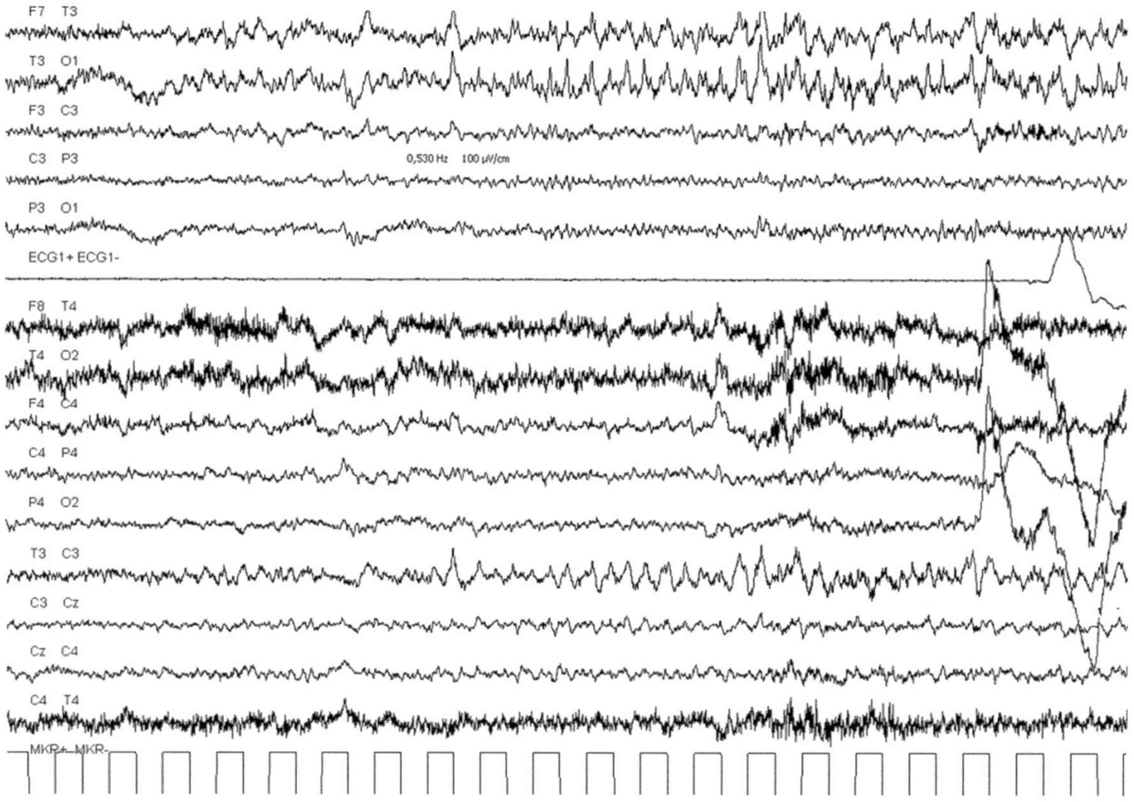

Fig. 32.21 Epileptic status in limbic encephalitis. Same patient as in Fig. 32.18. Development of the seizure on the left temporal regions with substantially overlapping of clinical manifestations

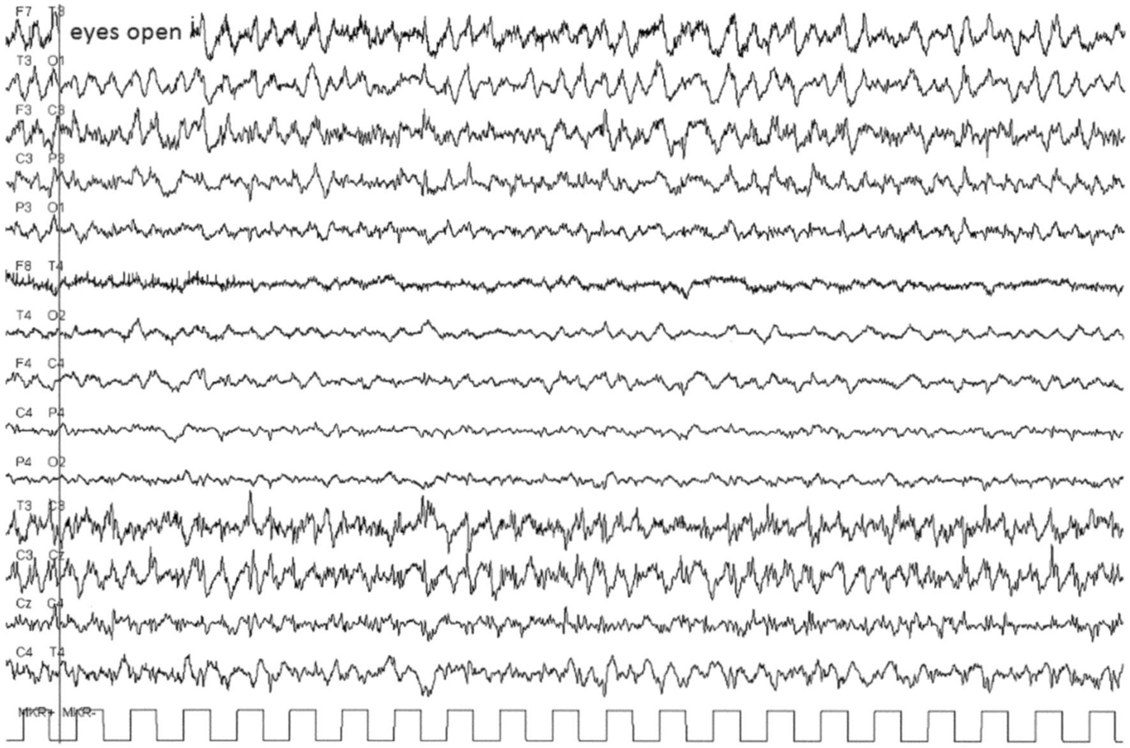

Fig. 32.22 Continuous epileptic activity in a 59-year-old patient with continuous adverse episodes and occasional secondary generalization. Apparently vigilant, not responsive after treatment with benzodiazepines. The left hemisphere has a continuous, rhythmic, 1,5 Hz delta activity over which alpha and continuous beta components overlap

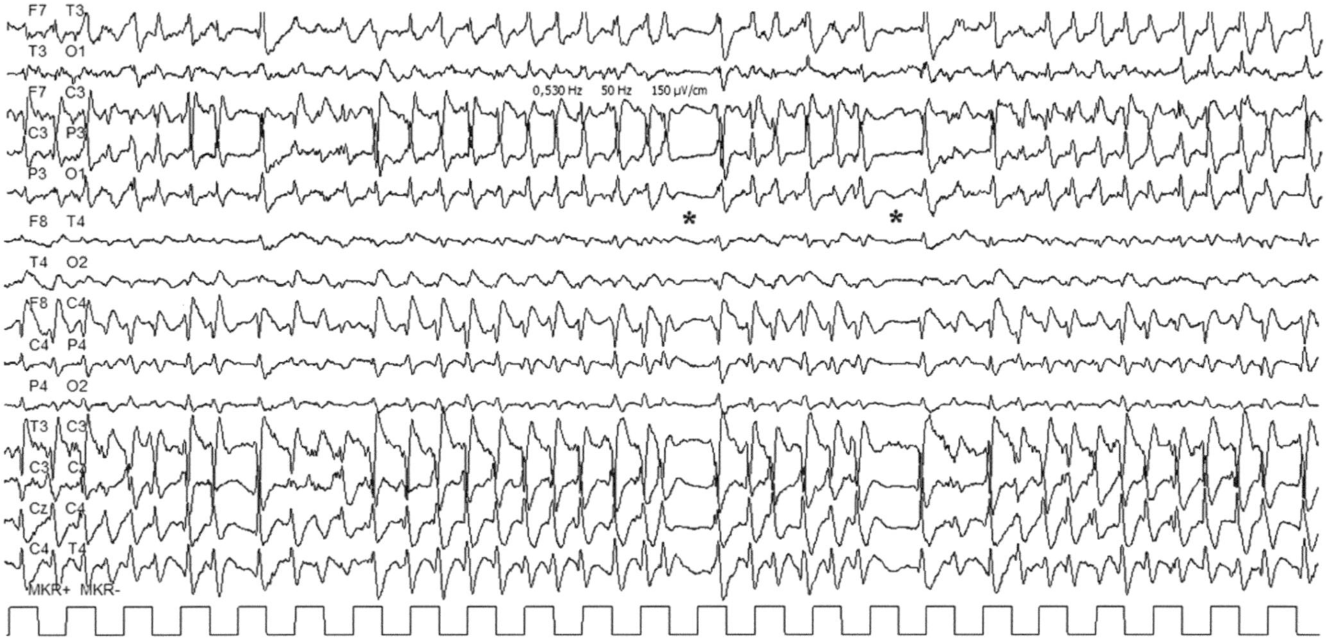

Fig. 32.23 Continuous epileptic activity with attenuations in a 59-year-old patient with SE with left focal seizures and on therapy with phenytoin and benzodiazepine. Of note continuous periodic anomalies relatively regular on which short periods of "attenuation" of the graphoelements are inserted

mentation, confusion, and sometimes stupor and coma. They describe three different distributions of activity (generalized, focal, generalized with some focal aspect) and four EEG patterns (spike-and-wave, atypical spike-and-wave, multiple spike-and-wave, and rhythmic delta with intermittent spikes). The persistence of this activity can vary over the time. The EEG activity was not organized in single seizure but appears like a continuous epileptiform activity or persistent with brief breaks (Fig. 32.23) or intermittent. They also provided some information about the modification of SE after administration of benzodiazepine [34].

In 1996 Young et al. [34] proposed a different method of diagnosis of NCSE based on EEG features. These was partially modified in 2005 by Chong and Hirsch [35]. They claimed some EEG characteristics as essential to indicate the presence of this kind of status. NCSE is present if any pattern satisfying any one of the following three primary criteria:

1. Repetitive generalized or focal spikes, sharp waves, spike-and-wave, or sharp-and-slow wave complexes at ≥3/s.
2. Repetitive generalized or focal spikes, sharp waves, spike-and-wave, or sharp-and-slow wave complexes at <3/s and the secondary criterion.
3. Sequential rhythmic, periodic, or quasiperiodic waves at 1/s and unequivocal evolution in frequency (gradually increasing or decreasing by at least 1/s, e.g., from 2 to 3/s), morphology, or location (gradual spread into or out of a region involving at least two electrodes). Evolution in amplitude alone is not sufficient. Change in sharpness without other change in morphology is not adequate to satisfy evolution in morphology.

The secondary criterion is "significant improvement in clinical status or appearance of previously absent normal EEG patterns (such as a posterior dominant rhythm) temporally coupled to acute administration of a rapidly acting AED. Resolution of the 'epileptiform' discharges leaving diffuse slowing without clinical improvement and without appearance of previously absent normal EEG patterns would not satisfy the secondary criterion."

Subsequently Sutter and Kaplan [36] suggested to consider the diagnosis of a NCSE with six different patterns.

1. Frequent or continuous focal electrographic seizures, with ictal patterns that appear and disappear with change in amplitude, frequency, and/or spatial distribution.
2. Frequent or continuous generalized spike-and-wave discharges in patients without a previous history of epileptic encephalopathy or epilepsy syndrome.
3. Frequent or continuous generalized spike-and-wave discharges, which showed significant changes in intensity or frequency (usually a faster frequency) when compared to baseline EEG, in patients with an epileptic encephalopathy or epilepsy syndrome.

4. PLEDs or BIPEDs that occurred in patients in a coma herein after a generalized tonic-clonic status epilepticus (subtle status epilepticus).
5. EEG patterns that were less easy to interpret including frequent or continuous EEG abnormalities (spikes, sharp waves, rhythmic slow activity, PLEDs, BIPEDs, GPEDs, triphasic waves) in patients whose EEGs showed no previous similar abnormalities, in the context of acute cerebral damage (e.g., anoxic brain damage, infection, trauma).
6. Frequent or continuous generalized EEG abnormalities in patients with epileptic encephalopathies in whom similar interictal EEG patterns were seen but in whom clinical symptoms were suggestive of NCSE.

Kaplan et al. [31] subsequently resume the hypothesis with some clarifications.

In patients without a known epileptic encephalopathy:

1. Repetitive generalized or focal spikes, polyspike, sharp waves, spike-and-wave, or sharp-and-slow wave complexes at >2.5/s.
2. Above, with discharges <2.5/s but with EEG and clinical improvement after rapid onset antiepileptic drugs, typically BZPs. Testing for patient responsiveness and improvement in EEG, increases in EEG reactivity, and appearance of EEG background activity.
3. Above, with discharges <2.5/s with focal ictal phenomena (e.g., facial twitching, gaze deviation, nystagmus, limb myoclonus).
4. Rhythmic waves (theta-delta) at >0.5 Hz with:
   (a) Incrementing onset (increase in voltage with increase or decrease in frequency).
   (b) Evolution in pattern (increase or decrease in frequency (>1 Hz), or location [changes in discharge voltage (amplitude) or morphology are not sufficient].
   (c) Decrementing termination (voltage or frequency).
   (d) Post-PED background slowing or attenuation. A, b, and c may be acutely abolished by IV BZPs.

In patients with known epileptic encephalopathy:

1. Frequent or continuous generalized spike-and-wave discharges, which show an increase in profusion or frequency when compared to baseline EEG with observable changes in the clinical status.
2. Regression (improvement) of clinical or EEG features with IV BZPs.

Finally, Beniczky et al. first [37] and then M. Leitinger et al. [38] added some clarifications concerning the modalities of evolution of the EEG pattern but always starting from the previous considerations made by the other authors. The authors argued that the fundamental differences with the previous criteria suggested by the ACNS are related to define the criteria of evolution. This is to obtain a more detailed and unambiguous operating criterion. They suggest at least three undoubted criteria of change in frequency, morphology, and location.

(a) Evolution in frequency is defined as at least two consecutive changes in the same direction by at least 0.5/s, e.g., from 2 to 2.5 to 3/s or from 3 to 2 to 1.5/s.
(b) Evolution in morphology is defined as at least two consecutive changes to a novel morphology.
(c) Evolution in location is defined as sequentially spreading into or sequentially out of at least two different standard 10–20 electrode locations. In order to qualify as present, a single frequency or location must persist at least three cycles (e.g., 1/s for 3 s or 3/s for 1 s) (Fig. 32.24).

These criteria may vary if the patient has a previous diagnosis of epileptic encephalopathy [39].

A different clinical approach was proposed by Epilepsy Research Foundation workshop [40] with an analysis of NCSE in different clinical conditions. A similar one was subsequently proposed by Sutter and Kaplan [36], and they also note the characteristics of the main forms of NCSE in adults:

(a) Status epilepticus in Lennox-Gastaut syndrome: Spike and polyspike-wave continuous or paroxysmal, irregular at 2–2.5 Hz maximum on the frontotemporal regions.
(b) Typical absence status: Spike and polyspike anterior waves, at 3–4 Hz, continuous or paroxysmal.
(c) Complex partial status:
    Limbic: Continuous or waxing and waning periodic or pseudoperiodic sharp wave discharges interspersed with low-voltage spikes and polyspike-and-waves with uni- or bilateral frontocentral predominance and usually generalized slow and/or suppressed background activity. Waxing and waning rhythmic delta activity, only.
    Nonlimbic: Continuous or waxing and waning periodic or pseudoperiodic sharp waves and spike-and-wave discharges with unilateral, focal onset and frequent seizure progression into generalized sharp wave and slow and/or suppressed wave discharges usually with frontal predominance and generalized slow background activity
(d) Nonconvulsive status after generalized tonic-clonic status epilepticus: PLEDs or GPEDs continuous or

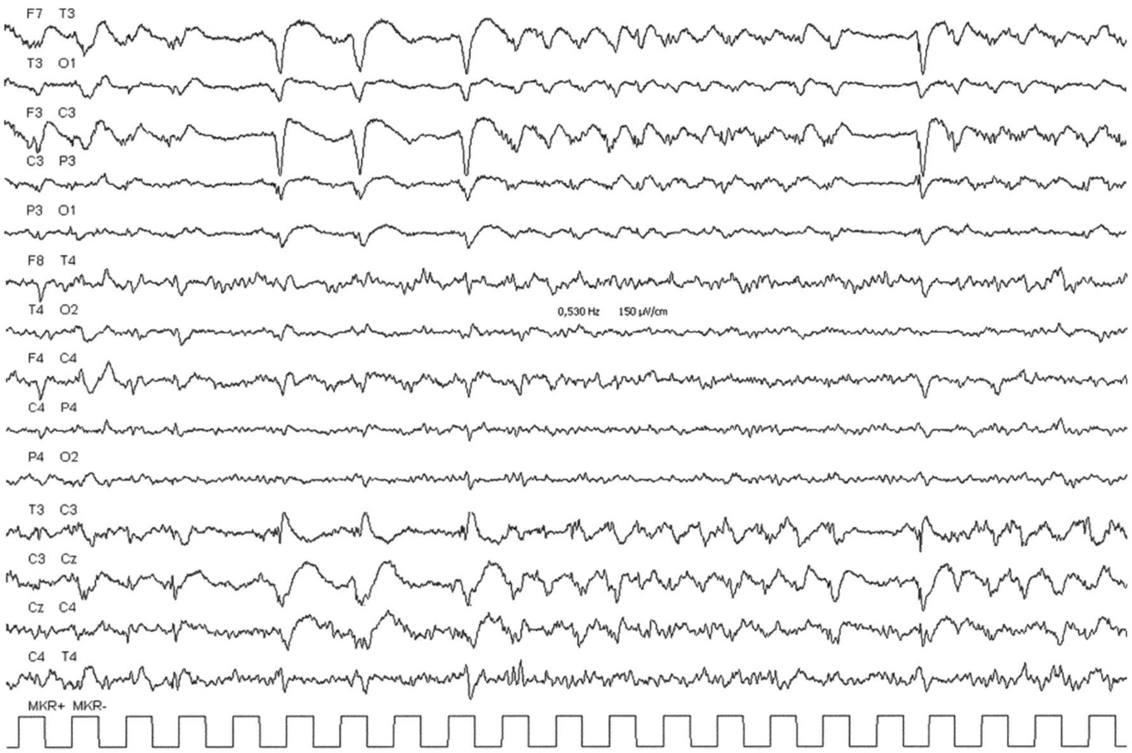

Fig. 32.24 Fluctuating activity in a 53-year-old patient with an acute vascular ischemic lesion on frontotemporal region of the left hemisphere. Continuous modification of LPDs with fluctuating intervals between the discharges and short runs of LRDA is present

paroxysmal often localized in anterior areas with a depression of the background activity.

(e) Subtle status: Continuous or paroxysmal GPEDs on a depressed background activity up to 3–5 s.

(f) Continuous aura: Unilateral presence of continuous or paroxysmal rhythmic spike-and-wave or slow rhythmic activity greater than 200 uV on a slow or depressed background activity.

32.4 Suspected Epileptic Status or the "Ictal-Interictal Continuum"

Some EEG patterns [41] do not meet the above criteria to diagnose a status epilepticus, or, alternatively, their meaning is still under discussion. In everyday clinical practice, this leads to an evident problem in the pharmacological management of patients. These frames have been partially remembered in the previous paragraph concerning the possibility to observe the modifications of the seizures' EEG pattern over time, but it is not the only problem of a diagnosis in these situations.

The term "ictal-interictal continuum" defined by Chong and Hirsch [35] expresses the set of those EEG patterns present in patients with variable impairment of central nervous system functions in which an epileptic mechanism can be supposed as a partial contributing factor. In these cases, it should be defined a "possible status epilepticus" but is still open a debate on the meaning of each single pattern [42].

32.4.1 Intermittent Rhythmic Delta Activity

Intermittent rhythmic delta activity occurring over the frontal regions, occasionally also posteriorly, is usually bilateral and synchronous, but its presence only on one hemisphere must be distinguished from other slow components of the EEG because of the poor localization value. Intermittent rhythmic delta activity on temporal regions has instead a possible relationship with the location of the origin site of epileptic seizures. The sequences occur in a short time but clearly do not relate with the SE [43].

32.4.2 Generalized or Lateralized Rhythmic Activity (RDA or LRDA)

The generalized rhythmic delta activity (RDA) is characterized by a repetition of waves with a relatively stable morphology and duration without a free interval. Obviously, to define the delta activity, it must have a frequency lower than 4 Hz, and the duration of a cycle of the rhythm pattern should vary less than 50% compared to the sequent. The study of Gaspard et al. [44] demonstrates that the LRDA has the same probability of LPDs and GPDs (these ones with an overlap of rapid activity) to associate with evident epileptic seizures. The RDA was ruled out as prognostic factor of SE, as opposed to the LRDA [45] (Figs. 32.25 and 32.26).

32.4.3 Generalized Periodic Discharges (GPDs)

According to literature [46], GPDs may result from severe dysfunction or disruption of the thalamocortical pathways, to the impairment of cortical inhibitory interneurons or both [47].

Trinka et al. [42] describe these elements as a repetition of a waveform with relatively uniform morphology and duration and without an interval between consecutive waveforms. This range varies from 0.5 s to several seconds. They generally do not have more than three phases, and the duration of the single elements is not more than 0.5 s. Sometimes they are so close and steep that they look like spike-and-wave complexes. The correlation between GPD and NCSE is not demonstrated and is commonly denied. However, it is admitted in any case that the presence of these GPDs is a generic sign of "cortical irritation." It is not clear whether antiepileptic drugs are able to facilitate the recovery of the correct function (Fig. 32.27).

32.4.4 Lateralized Periodic Discharges (LPDs or PLEDs)

Lateralized periodic discharges (LPD, previously periodic lateralized epileptiform discharges or PLEDs) [47–50] can occur in a broad range of conditions, in which the patient is fully alert or with impaired consciousness down to the level of coma. As with other EEG patterns, LPDs can be found in a variety of etiologies with cortical or subcortical pathology [51, 52].

There is a long-lasting debate whether they represent an ictal, interictal, or semiictal pattern [53–56]. In some patients, they can appear in the form of PLED-proper or PLED-plus, with superimposed faster activity, the last related to a greater risk of seizure recurrence [57] (Fig. 32.28). PLEDs can appear asynchronously on the two hemispheres (BIPLEDs) [58] (Fig. 32.29) or can be multifocal (multifocal PLEDs). They are single transients or EEG complexes that occur periodically on a generally depressed background activity. These EEG elements can associate with motor manifestations (myoclonic contraction of contralateral body segments). Somatosensory stimuli and modification of level of vigilance might change the possibility to observe GPED and LPD [59]. Synchronous or not on the two hemispheres were considered

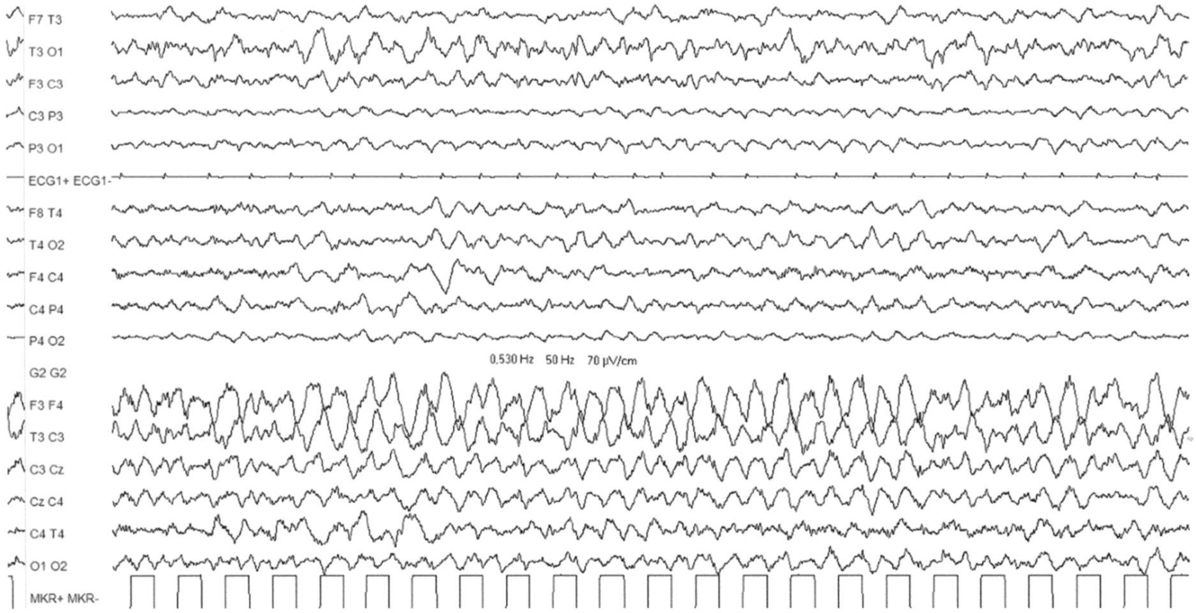

Fig. 32.25 RDA. An 82-year-old patient with subacute confusional state. Prolonged run of RDA with short period without delta waves. Asymmetric alpha components are present with a left prevalence on the frontotemporal regions, but delta activity is not different on the two hemispheres

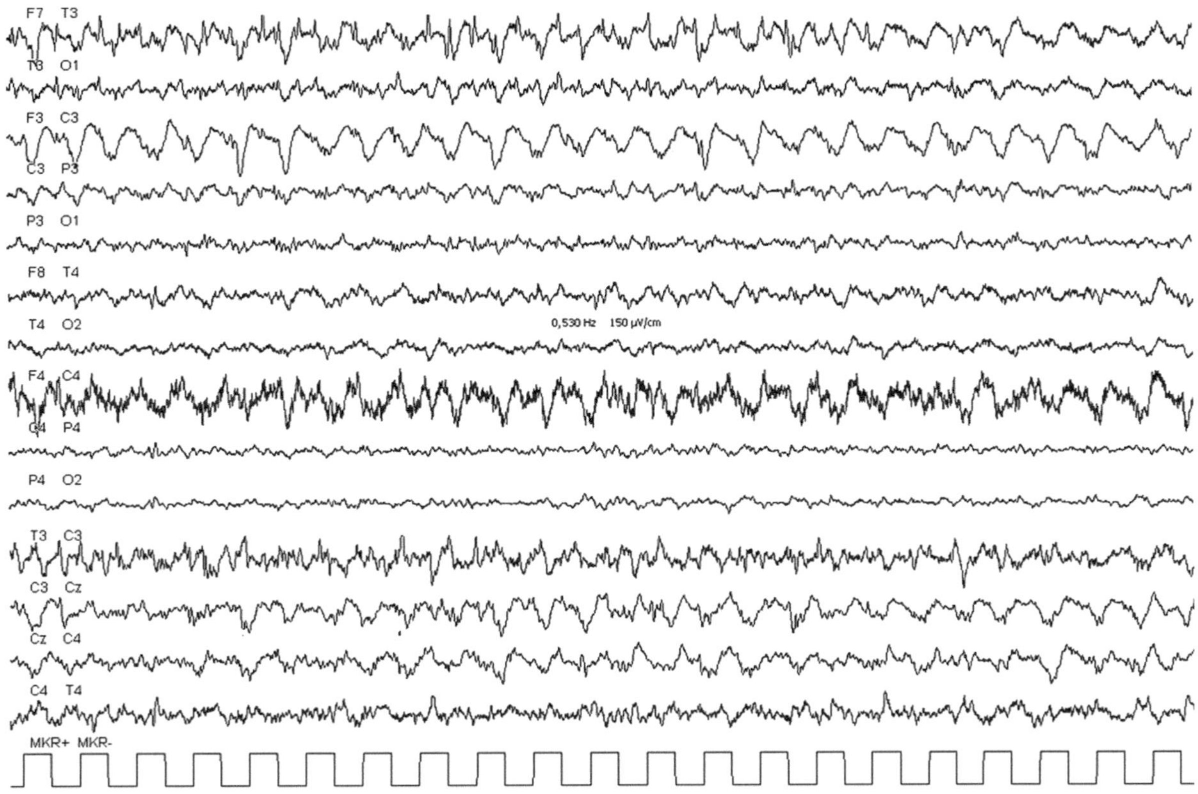

Fig. 32.26 RDA or continuous epileptic activity? A 33-year-old patient with recent head trauma and mild confusional state. Subcontinuous delta activity with more evident on the frontal area without clear asymmetry. More arhythmic and faster EEG also with spike appearance components is superimposed on the left frontotemporal region of the scalp

as a pathognomonic EEG sign of particular pathologies [60, 61]. First of all the herpetic encephalitis but also other infectious diseases or acute and subacute focal pathologies of the CNS and metabolic disorders have been associated with this particular EEG transient. Moreover, it has been associated with a greater risk of seizure recurrence [54] (Figs. 32.30, 32.31, and 32.32). In some patients, the morphological characteristics of the GPEDs are very similar to those of the so-called triphasic waves. Although Kaplan [31] described the characteristics of these two elements, there is still overlap between the two descriptions, and this limits the clinical utility of the differentiation.

32.4.5 Triphasic Waves (TWs)

Triphasic waves (TWs) appear in toxic and metabolic encephalopathies and frequently occur with behavior, cognition, and motor deficit. So it is clinically indistinguishable from NCSE. In the new classification, they are now termed "continuous 2 Hz generalized PDs with triphasic morphology." They are described as rhythmic complexes occurring in clusters, with amplitude 100–300 uV with a blunted, low-amplitude initial negative-phase. TWs may be distinguished pharmacotherapeutically from NCSE, when EEG rhythmic activity resolves after BZPs, but without concomitant clinical improvement. Some authors suggested considering NCSE in any patient who present with altered consciousness or confusional state and "atypical" TWs. Some authors [35, 62, 63] proposed EEG features to distinguish "toxic-metabolic" TWs from NCSE waves, but these criteria need to be confirmed; shorter phase one duration, multispikes and less background slowing, predominant phase two, unusual asymmetry in amplitude, and different increased with stimulation could be the main EEG features for the differential diagnosis.

32.4.6 Stimulus-Induced Rhythmic, Periodic, or Ictal Discharges (SIRPIDs)

In comatose patients, ictal-appearing or periodic discharges may be evoked after any alerting stimulus [64]. They are reproducible and often correlate with the duration of the

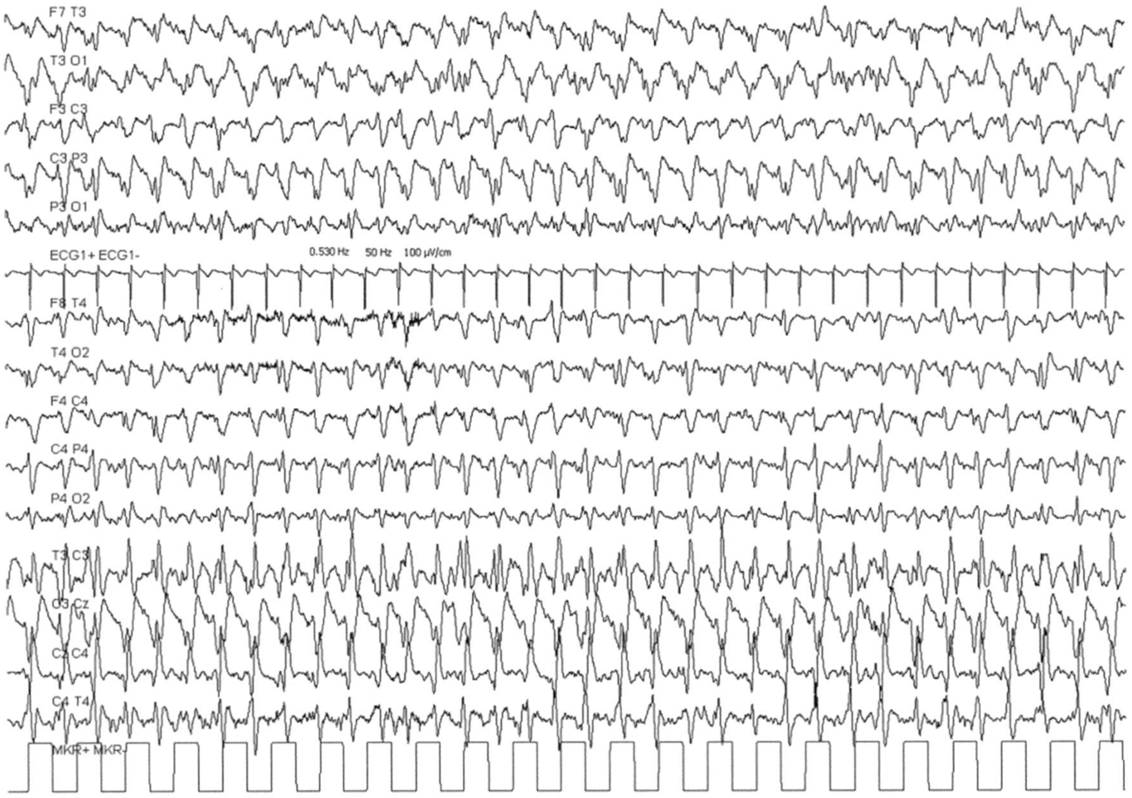

Fig. 32.27 GPEDs in a 42-year-old patient with renal insufficiency. Appearance of somnolence and related asynchronous bilateral myoclonic manifestations. The EEG path shows graphical elements with an almost-periodic course that have a triphasic appearance only on some derivations. The amplitude of the elements and the activity interposed between them are not symmetrical

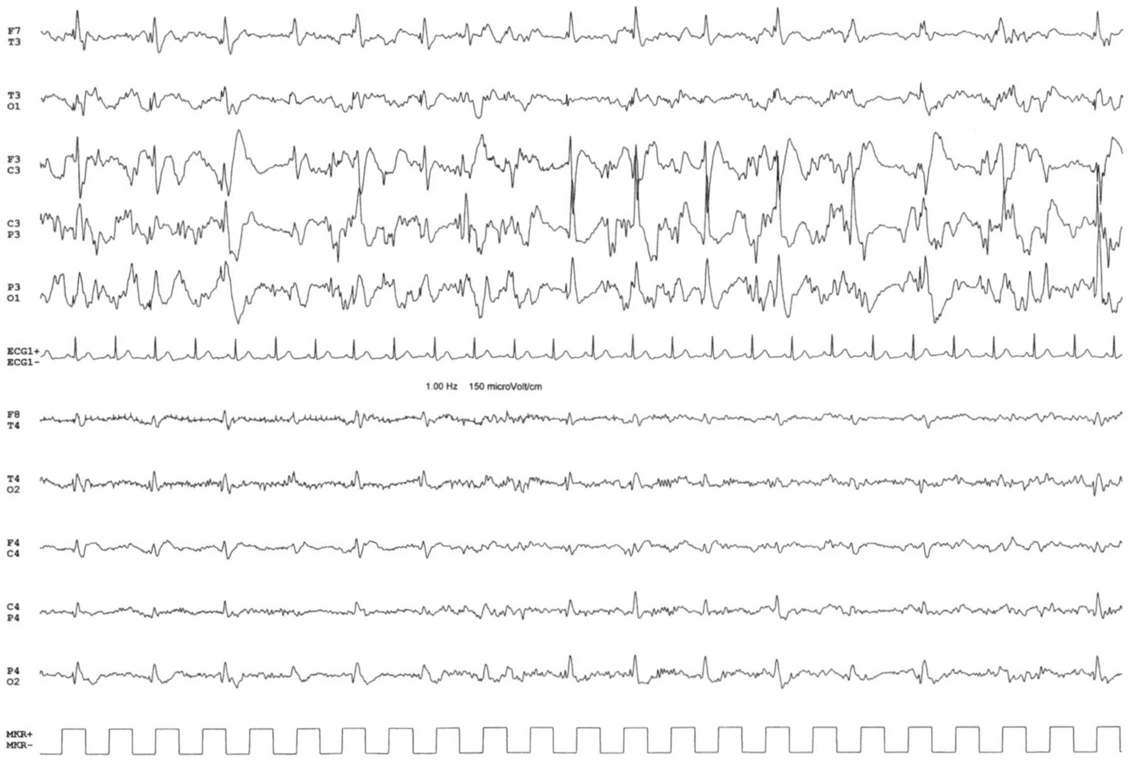

Fig. 32.28 LPDs in a 56-year-old patient with recent subarachnoid hemorrhage from anterior cerebral artery aneurism. Coma without recovery after surgery 2 days before. LPDs are presents bilaterally maximum on the frontoparietal area with minimum variation of intervals between epileptic discharges. In left frontoparietal area, also faster EEG component is more evident. It is difficult to exclude the presence of "PLEDs plus"

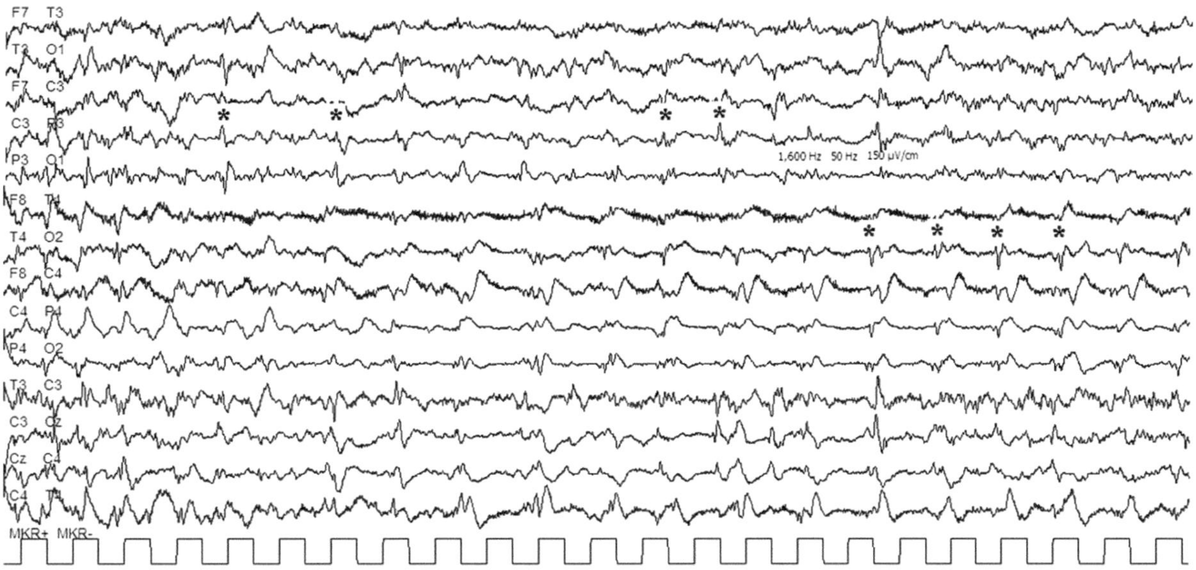

Fig. 32.29 BIPLEDs in a 71-year-old patient with cryptococcal meningoencephalitis. Suspension phase of continuous barbiturate infusion set for generalized convulsive epileptic status. Complex frame with poor interhemispheric synchronization and stability of the background activity. Elements with almost-periodic progression and with different morphology (*) appear asynchronously irregularly and on the right and left central frontocentral temporal regions. On the remaining path, there were independent critical EEG frames on the two hemispheres

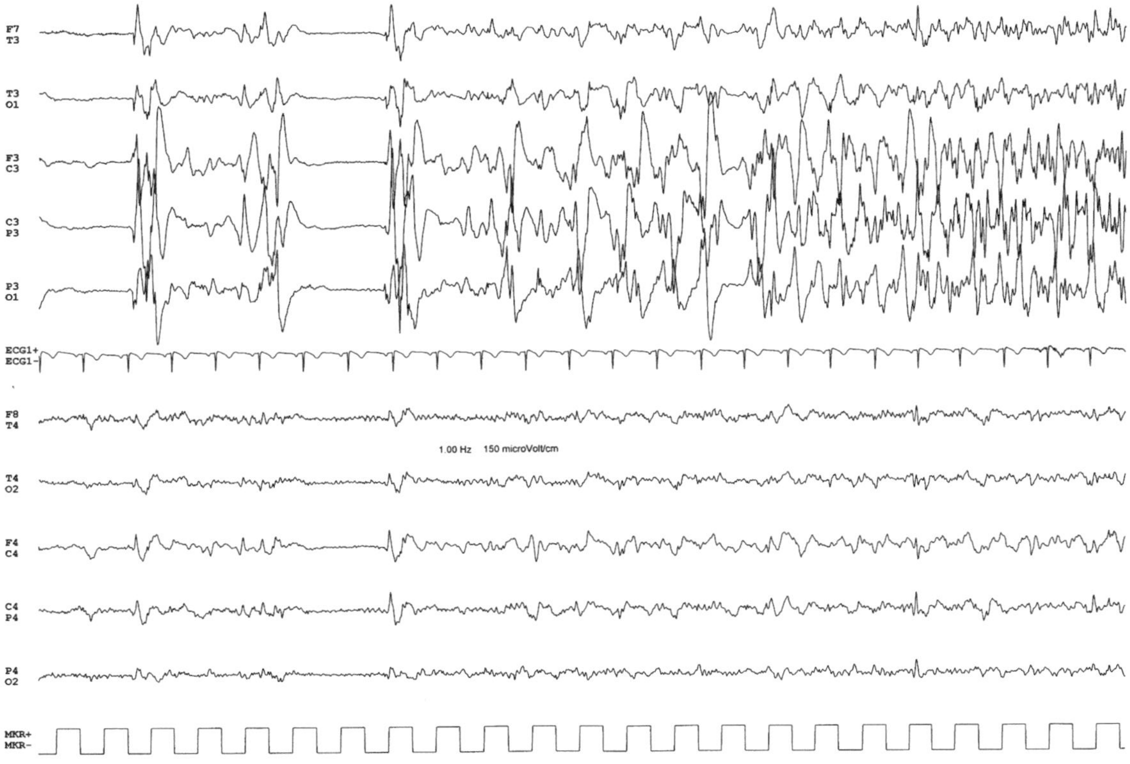

Fig. 32.30 The same patient of Fig. 32.28. A focal left frontocentral seizure breaks the regular sequence of LPDs more evident in the same area of the scalp

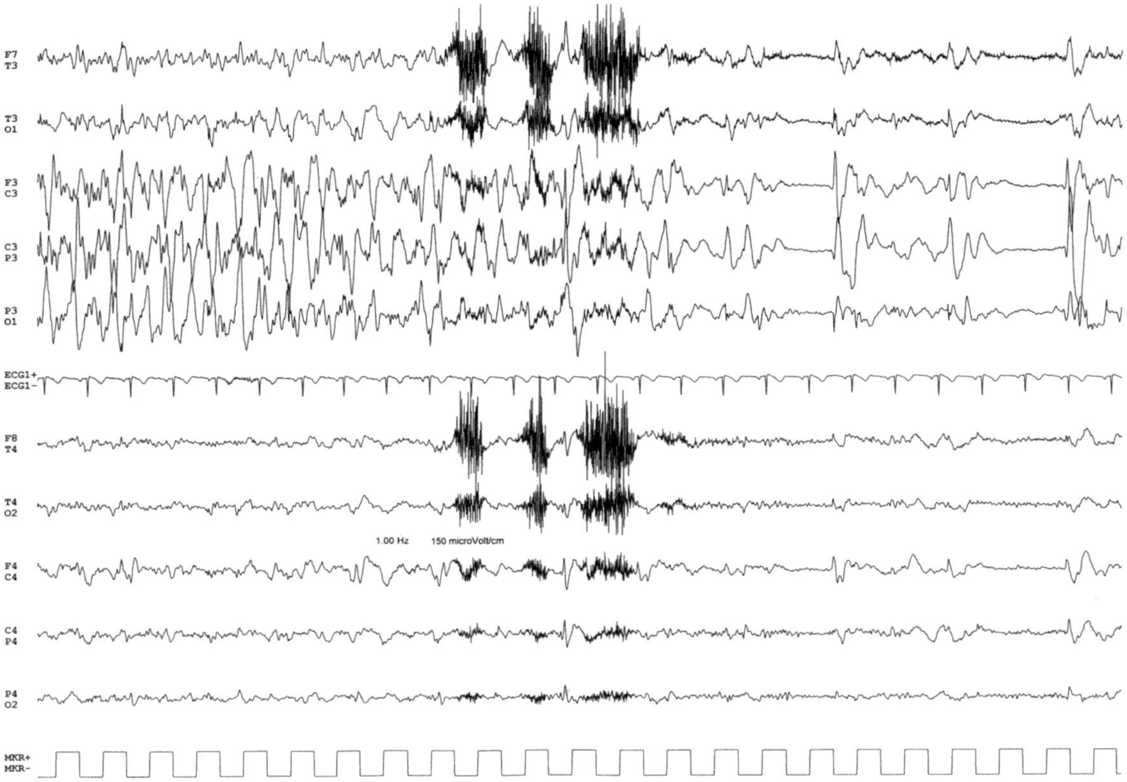

Fig. 32.31 The same patient of Fig. 32.28. Approximatively after 20 s the seizure stop and LPD restart with the same frequency

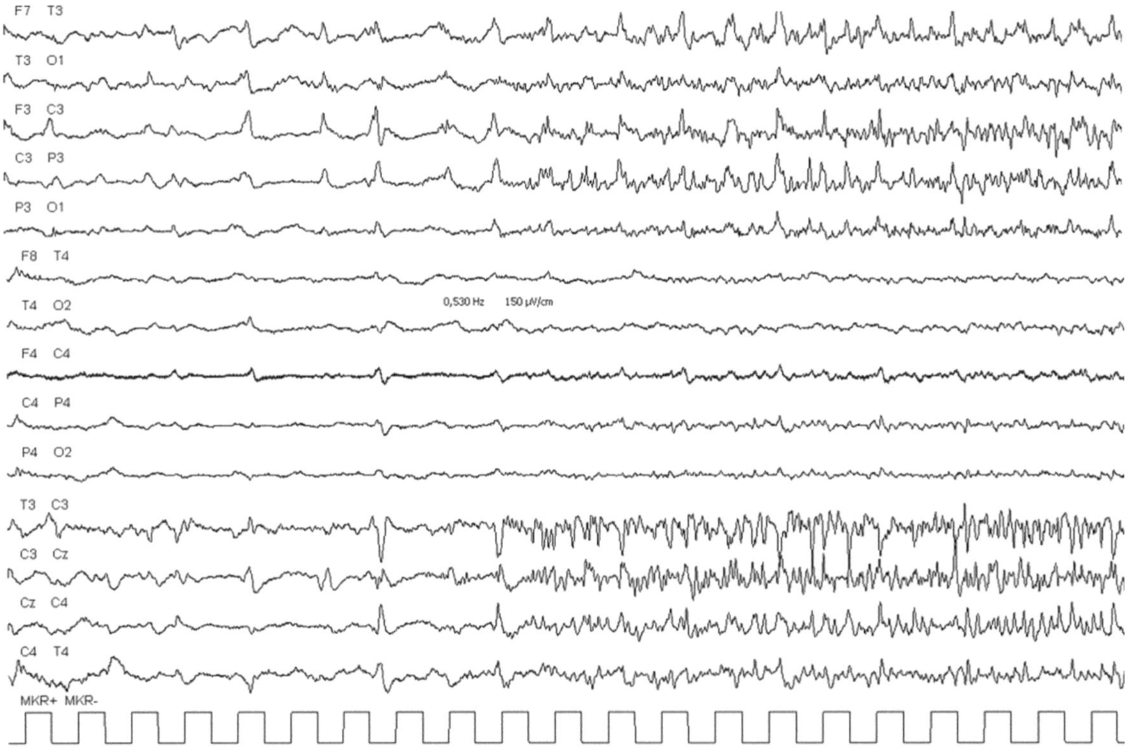

Fig. 32.32 PLEDs and seizure in a 54-year-old patient with left frontal hemorrhagic lesion. Complete control of seizure with continuous infusion of barbiturates. Phase of progressive reduction of the therapy. The track shows PLEDs on the left hemisphere with a maximum frontal expression. Without any clinical manifestation, it is observed a critical EEG that progressively interrupts the sequence of the periodic elements

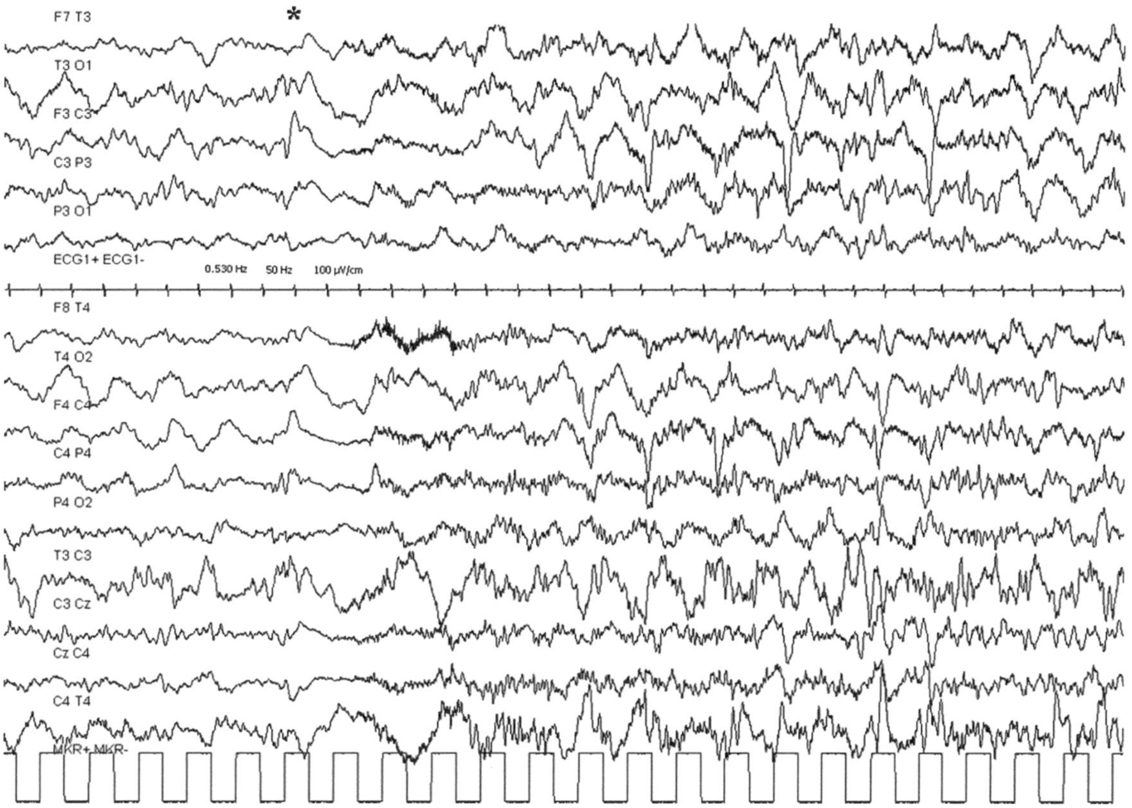

Fig. 32.33 SIRPIDs in a 67-year-old patient with recent right frontal hemorrhage. No clear seizures have been observed. The patient was sedated to promote assisted breathing. Initial frame of bilateral alteration of the general organization with a probable depression of the alpha and theta components on the right derivations. After the painful stimulus (*), an abrupt disappearance of the slow components in a synchronous manner with an evidence of beta activity of a small amplitude maximum on the right frontocentral regions. "Recruiting" aspect with a progressive increase in amplitude and a reduction in frequency. This frame could also occur spontaneously with similar characteristics

stimulation and with the prognosis of the patient. They usually occur in deeply comatose patients with or without clinical seizures [65]. This EEG pattern could be closely related to spontaneous seizures, and it potentially indicates a modification of pharmacological strategies. It must be carefully differentiated from other EEG reactions to alerting stimuli (Fig. 32.33).

32.4.7 Burst-Suppression Patterns

The pattern consists of periodic high-voltage, sharply contoured waveforms, including spikes and polyspikes, at times with a buildup or bursts of spikes alternating with periods of severe suppression or even isoelectricity. The bursts last from less than a second to 10 s or more, and the period of suppression may be a second to 10 s or much longer. The suppression period may have a variable degree of residual activity of low voltage or is completely isoelectric.

Burst-suppression pattern can be found in very different conditions: some rare childhood encephalopathies (e.g., Ohtahara syndrome) but also in severe encephalopathies like in the cerebral hypoxia [66], a condition of a sedative intoxication or a severe hypothermia [67] (Figs. 32.34 and 32.35). These are the reasons why the pattern is reconnected to a possible status epileptic even if paradoxically its obtaining during barbiturate therapy for a status epileptic is considered the therapeutic goal to be achieved (Fig. 32.36).

32.5 EEG and Therapy in Status Epilepticus

The use of the EEG to monitor the effect of therapy in SE is important in management of the SE. In clinical practice, the administration of benzodiazepine e.v. is frequently used to verify the presence of a suspected SE. As reported above, this test has been included in the criteria for the diagnosis of

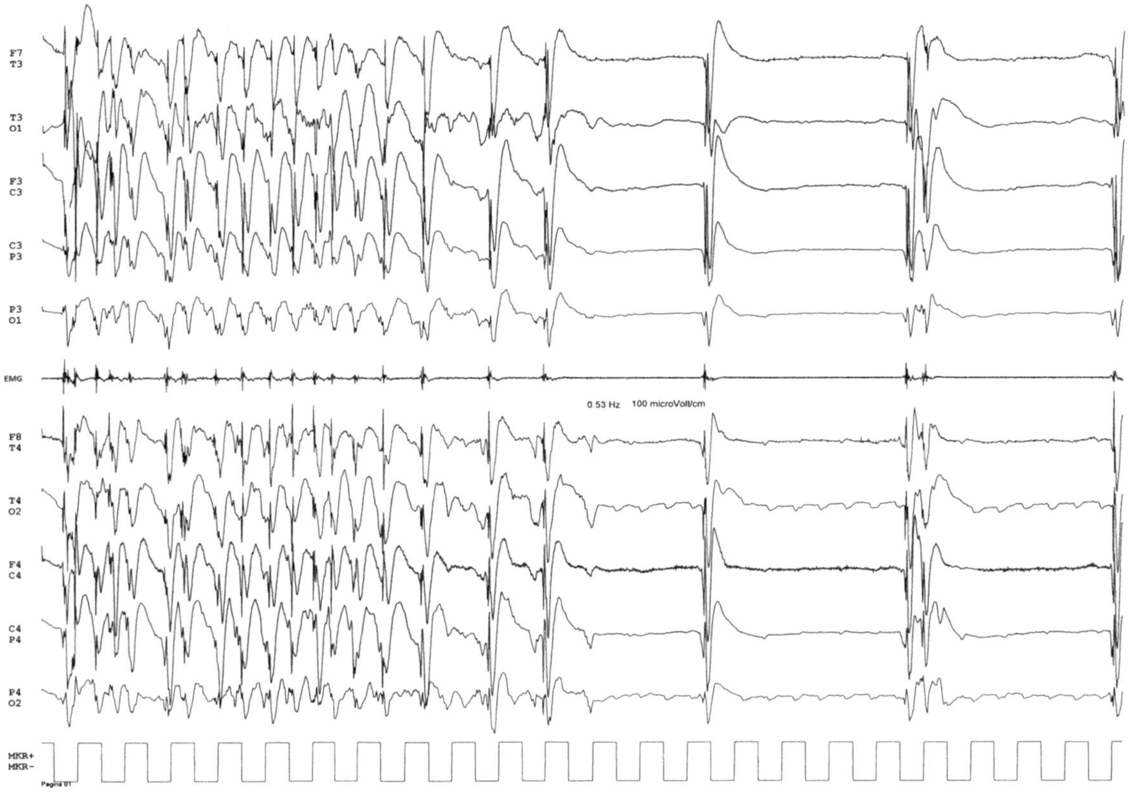

Fig. 32.34 Postanoxic encephalopathy in a 33-year-old patient. Continuous epileptiform discharges with an irregular frequency less than 2.5 Hz and clinically related to myoclonia at the right shoulder (see EMG line). The pages are related to a period of 40 s after start of propofol infusion. Appearance of long interval of flat recordings of EEG activity

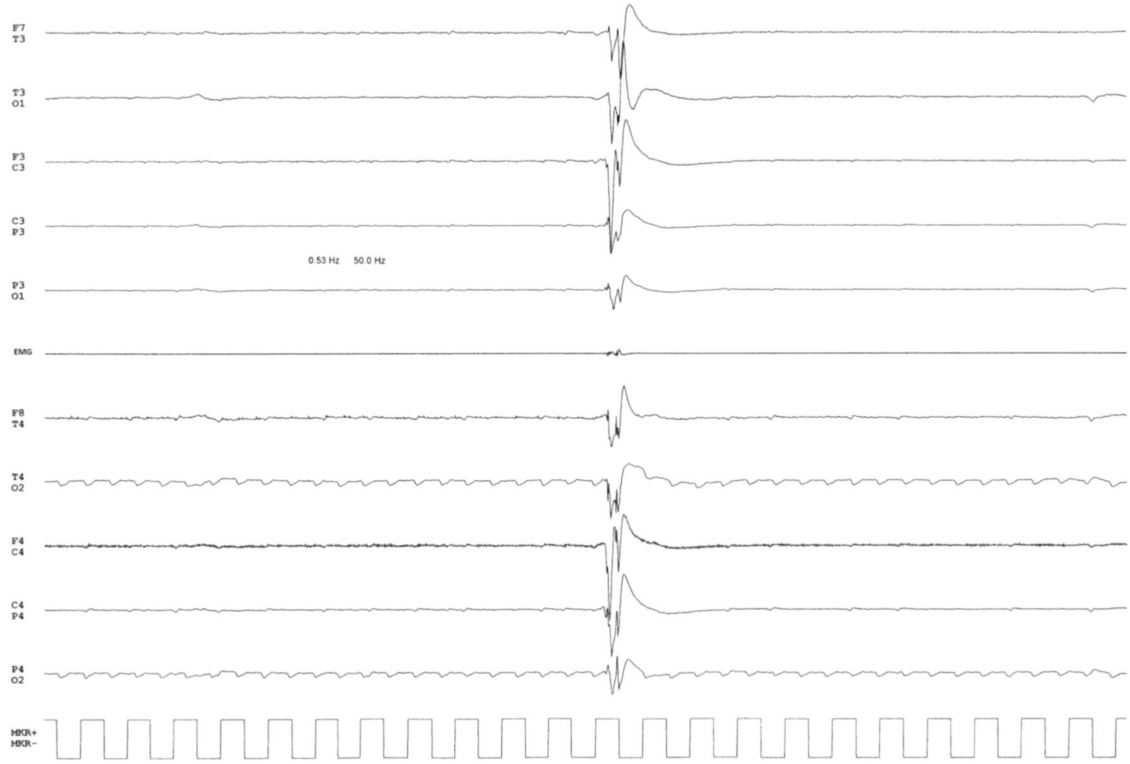

Fig. 32.35 Same patients of Fig. 32.34 (10 min later). EMG line with residual but still presence of muscle activation synchronous with EEG epileptic discharges. The last doesn't show any clear difference in morphology compared with the previous one, but the period of EEG silence is markedly increased

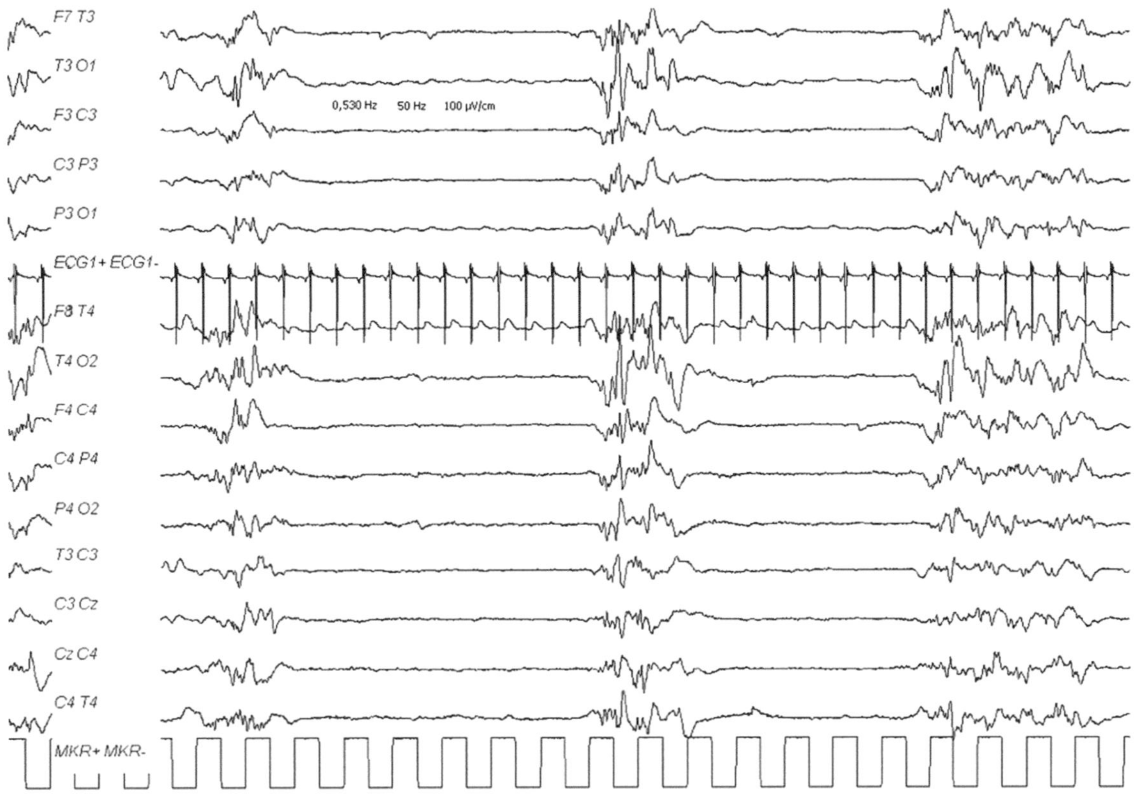

Fig. 32.36 Suppression-burst pattern after prolonged cardiac arrest 24 h before recording

NCSE. Kaplan asserts that the disappearance of EEG abnormalities after diazepam administration is a nonspecific element that is also present in other non-epileptic situations. It must also be taken into account that at least 40% of the SEs do not respond to the first-line therapy and therefore it is evident that the nonresponse to diazepam cannot be considered as demonstrating that that EEG pattern is not a status epilepticus (Figs. 32.37 and 32.38). Remember also that a positive response to the administration of benzodiazepines e.v. could be demonstrated only after disappearance of the seizures for at least 30 min. The EEG is also necessary to determine the correct dose of barbiturates by continuous infusion in patients with refractory status epilepticus. There are no other methods for a correct evaluation of efficacy, because the necessary dosages are extremely different from case to case and because, during deep sedation obtained in this way, clinical manifestations are easily suppressed even in the presence of electrically detectable seizures [68]. Whether it is necessary to reach a pattern of suppression or suppression-burst is a matter of debate in the literature [69]. Although suppression pattern is an electrically more stable pattern, it is burdened by greater toxic side effects (Fig. 32.39).

32.6 Conclusion

The use of EEG remains the fundamental criterion for diagnosis, classification, and therapy of SE. Even in the most evident clinical situations, the EEG is useful both to confirm the clinical diagnosis and to monitor the correct effectiveness of the therapy. Neurological urgency should not miss the EEG in the instrumental diagnostic kit also because the SE is a reversible condition. The current health economy rarely allows its implementation around the clock, but mortality, morbidity, and lengthening of hospital stays should be a valid argument for changing this attitude [70]. Surely, this is a difficult electroencephalography that requires a proven experience, which must however be part of the training not only of the neurophysiologist but also of the neurologist [71].

Acknowledgments A special thanks to the EEG technicians of San Raffaele Hospital of Milan, Alessandra Amato, Sara Bruno, Aldo Elia, Claudia Paleari, and Amelia Tirelli, for the competence in carrying out of the exams. We also mentioned Laura Schieppati e Lucrezia Nava for English translation of the text and Marco Vabanesi and Marco Cursi for the relevant contribution to the activity of our laboratory.

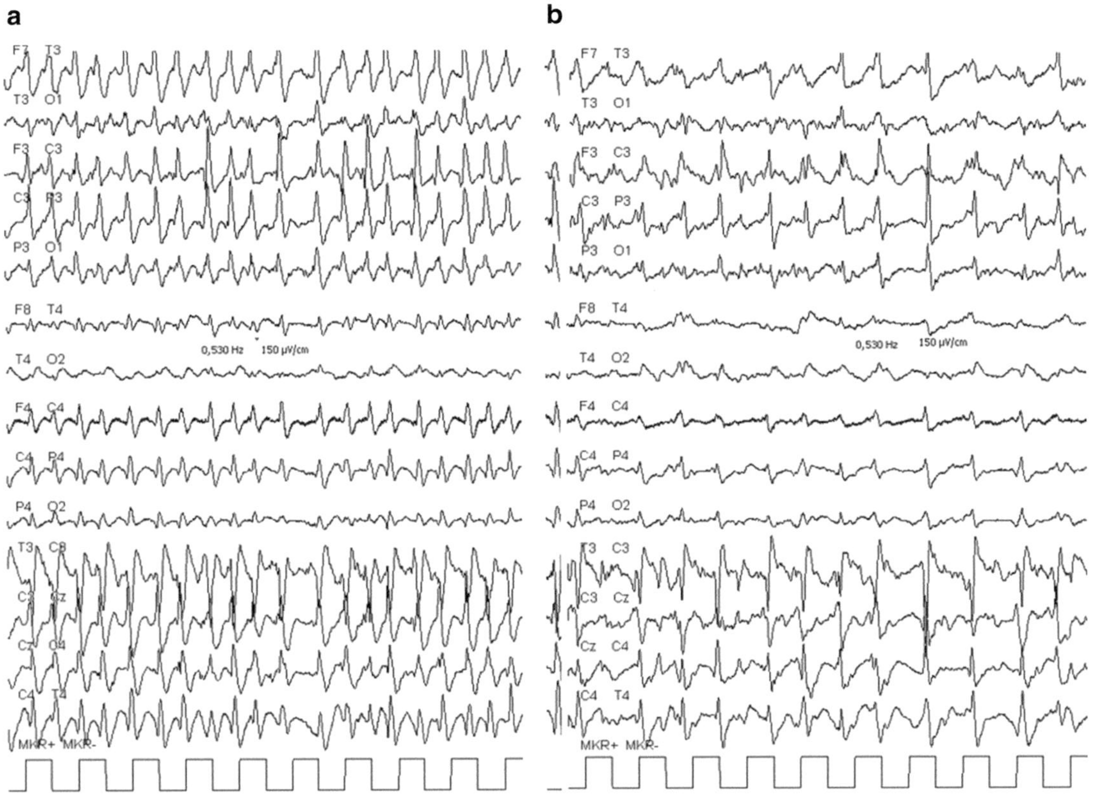

Fig. 32.37 Progressive change of PLEDs during therapy. (**a**) Continuous periodic elements prevailing in amplitude on the left hemisphere. (**b**) After 30 min, reduction of the contralateral diffusion of the elements and increase of the period between them

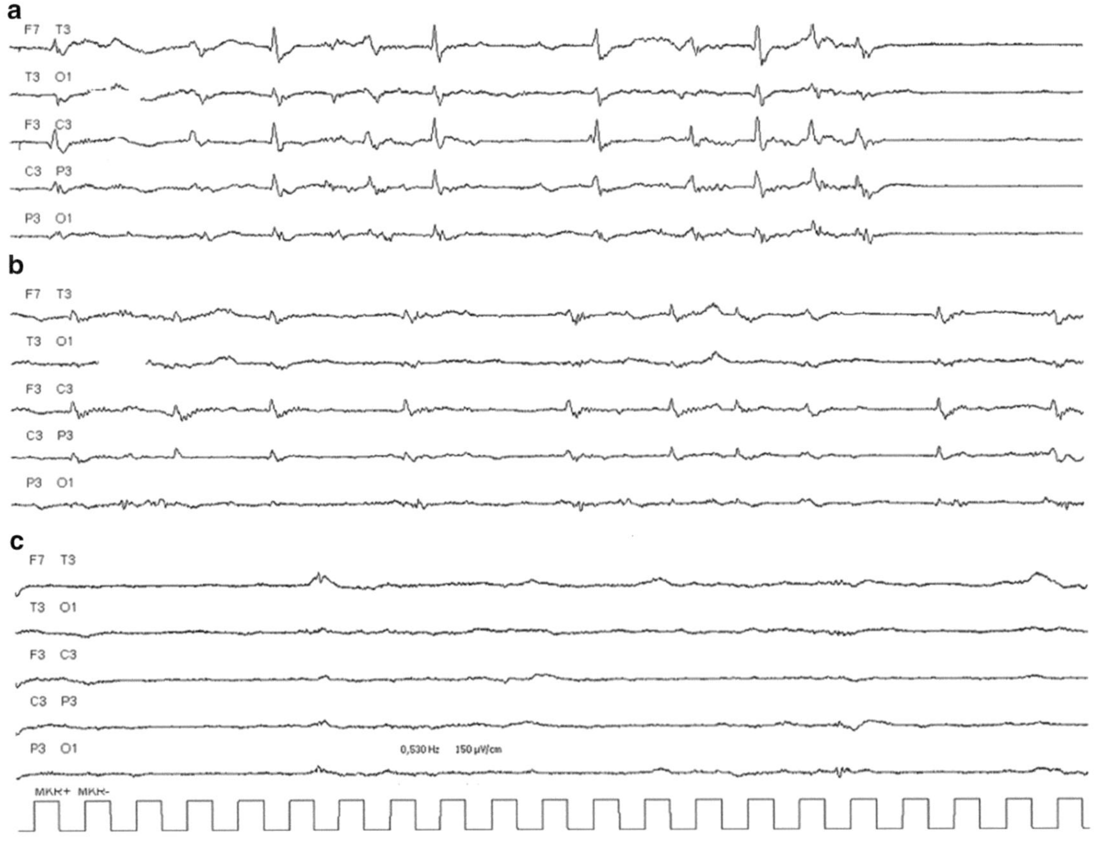

Fig. 32.38 Progressive modification of the PLEDs during therapy. (**a**–**c**) Same patient of Fig. 32.28 at subsequent times. Only left derivations. The periodic elements are progressively reduced in amplitude, and their appearance occurs with less and less frequency

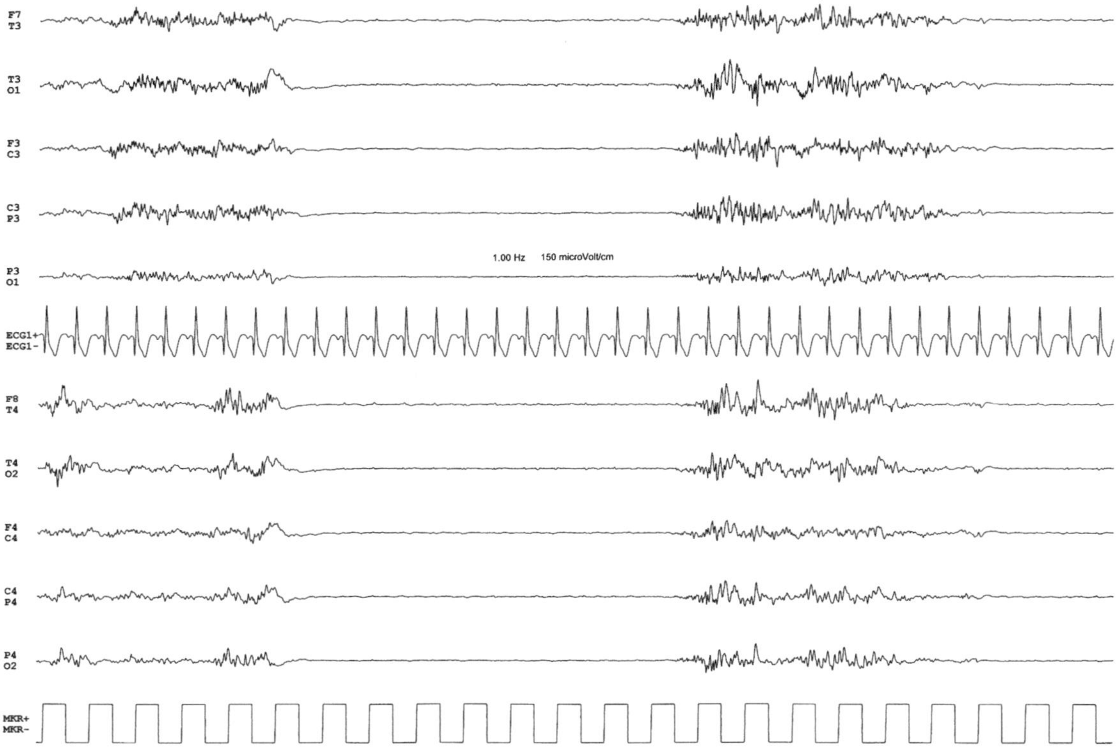

Fig. 32.39 Suppression-burst. Examination performed during a continuous infusion of barbiturates. The track shows the characteristic pattern with an alternation of irregular activity sequences, essentially symmetrical, interrupted by periods of abrupt attenuation in amplitude with disappearance of the background activity. The F8-T4 derivation highlights a synchronous rhythmic artifact with the cardiac activity

References

1. Hesdorffer DC, Logroscino G, Cascino G, et al. Incidence of status epilepticus in Rochester, Minnesota, 1965–1984. Neurology. 1998;50(3):735–41.
2. Coeytaux A, Jallon P, Galobardes B. Incidence of status epilepticus in French-speaking Switzerland: (EPISTAR). Neurology. 2000;55(5):693–7.
3. DeLorenzo RJ, Pellock JM, Towne AR, et al. Epidemiology of status epilepticus. J Clin Neurophysiol. 1996;13(5):458.
4. Knake S, Rosenow F, Vescovi M, et al. Incidence of status epilepticus in adults in Germany: a prospective, population-based study. Status Epilepticus Study Group Hessen (SESGH). Epilepsia. 2001;42(6):714–8.
5. Vignatelli L, Tonon C, D'Alessandro R. Bologna Group for the Study of Status Epilepticus. Incidence and short-term prognosis of status epilepticus in adults in Bologna, Italy. Epilepsia. 2003;44(7):964–8.
6. Waterhouse EJ, DeLorenzo RJ. Status epilepticus in older patients: epidemiology and treatment options. Drugs Aging. 2001;18(2):133–42.
7. Hauser WA. Status epilepticus: epidemiologic considerations. Neurology. 1990;40(5 Suppl 2):9–13.
8. Towne AR, Pellock JM, Ko D, et al. Determinants of mortality in status epilepticus. Epilepsia. 1994;35:27–34.
9. Shneker BF, Fountain NB. Assessment of acute morbidity and mortality in non status epilepticus. Neurology. 2003;61:1066–73.
10. Rossetti AO, Logroscino G, Bromfield EB. A clinical score for prognosis of status epilepticus in adult. Neurology. 2006;66:1736–8.
11. Aminoff MJ, Simon RP. Status epilepticus. Causes, clinical features and consequences in 98 patients. Am J Med. 1980;69(5):657–66.
12. Tan RY, Neligan A, Shorvon SD. The uncommon causes of status epilepticus. Epilepsy Res. 2010;91:111–22.
13. Dobesberger J, Ristić AJ, Walser G, et al. Duration of focal complex, secondarily generalized tonic–clonic, and primarily generalized tonic–clonic seizures: a video-EEG analysis. Epilepsy Behav. 2015;49:111–7.
14. Treatment of convulsive status epilepticus. Recommendations of the epilepsy foundation of America's working group on status epilepticus. JAMA. 1993;270(7):854–9.
15. Trinka E, Cock H, Hesdorffer D, et al. A definition and classification of status epilepticus – report of the ILAE task force on classification of status Epilepticus. Epilepsia. 2015;56(10):1515–23.
16. Gastaut H, Tassinari C. Status epilepticus. In: Redmond A, editor. Handbook of electroencephalography and clinical neurophysiology, vol. 13. Amsterdam: Elsevier; 1975. p. 39–45.
17. Shorvon S. Status epilepticus: its clinical features and treatment in children and adults. Cambridge: Cambridge University Press; 1994.
18. Treiman DM, Walton NY, Kendrick C. A progressive sequence of electroencephalographic changes during generalised convulsive status epilepticus. Epilepsy Res. 1990;5:49–60.
19. Lothman EW. The biochemical basis and pathophysiology of status epilepticus. Neurology. 1990;40(Suppl 2):13–23.
20. Florea B, Beniczky SA, Demény H. Semiology of subtle motor phenomena in critically ill patients. Seizure. 2017;48:33–5.
21. Kobayashi E, Thomas P, Andermann F. Tonic status epilepticus in patients with idiopathic generalized epilepsy. Epileptic Disord. 2005;7(4):327–31.
22. Mameniškienė R, Wolf P. Epilepsia partialis continua: a review. Seizure. 2017;44:74–80.

23. Gastaut H. Aphasia: the sole manifestation of focal status epilepticus. Neurology. 1979;29(12):1638.
24. Wells CR, Labar DR, Solomon GE. Aphasia as the sole manifestation of simple partial status epilepticus. Epilepsia. 1992;33(1):84–7.
25. DeToledo JC, Minagar A, Lowe MR. Persisting aphasia as the sole manifestation of partial status epilepticus. Clin Neurol Neurosurg. 2000;102(3):144–8.
26. Thomas P, Kullmann B, Chatel M. Status epilepticus with aphasic manifestation. Rev Neurol. 1991;147(3):246–50.
27. Grimes DA, Guberman A. De novo aphasic status epilepticus. Epilepsia. 1997;38(8):945–9.
28. Herskovitz M, Schiller Y. Prolonged ictal aphasia: a diagnosis to consider. J Clin Neurosci. 2012;19(11):1605–6.
29. Takaya S, Matsumoto R, Namiki C, et al. Frontal nonconvulsive status epilepticus manifesting somatic hallucinations. J Neurol Sci. 2005;234(1–2):25–9.
30. Tiamkao S, Pratipanawatr T, Jitpimolmard S. Abdominal epilepsy: an uncommon of non-convulsive status epilepticus. J Med Assoc Thai. 2011;94(8):998–1001.
31. Kaplan P. EEG criteria for nonconvulsive status epilepticus. Epilepsia. 2007;48(Suppl 8):39–41.
32. Treiman DM, Delgado-Escueta AV. Complex partial status epilepticus. Adv Neurol. 1983;34:69–81.
33. Granner MA, Lee S. Nonconvulsive status epilepticus: EEG annalysis in a large series. Epilepsia. 1994;35:42–7.
34. Young GB, Jordan KG, Doig GS. An assessment of nonconvulsive seizures in the intensive care unit using continuous EEG monitoring: an investigation of variables associated with mortality. Neurology. 1996;47:83–9.
35. Chong DJ, Hirsch LJ. Which EEG patterns warrant treatment in the critically ill? Reviewing the evidence for treatment of periodic epileptiform discharges and related patterns. Clin Neurophysiol. 2005;22(2):79–91.
36. Sutter R, Kaplan PW. Electroencephalographic criteria for nonconvulsive status epilepticus: synopsis and comprehensive survey. Epilepsia. 2012;53(Suppl 3):1–51.
37. Beniczky S, Hirsch LJ, Kaplan PW, et al. Unified EEG terminology and criteria for nonconvulsive status epilepticus. Epilepsia. 2013;54(Suppl 6):28–9.
38. Leitinger M, Beniczky S, Rohracher A, et al. Salzburg consensus criteria for non-convulsive status epilepticus: approach to clinical application. Epilepsy Behav. 2015;49:158–63.
39. Leitinger M, Trinka E, et al. Diagnostic accuracy of the Salzburg EEG criteria for non-convulsive status epilepticus: a retrospective study. Lancet Neurol. 2016;15:1054–62.
40. Walker M, Cross H, Smith S, et al. Nonconvulsive status epilepticus: Epilepsy Research Foundation workshop reports. Epileptic Disord. 2005;7(3):253–96.
41. Hirsch LJ, Brenner RP, Drislane FW, et al. The ACNS subcommittee on research terminology for continuous EEG monitoring: proposed standardized terminology for rhythmic and periodic EEG patterns encountered in critically ill patients. J Clin Neurophysiol. 2005;22:128–35.
42. Trinka E, Leitinger M. Which EEG patterns in coma are nonconvulsive status epilepticus? Epilepsy Behav. 2015;49:203–22.
43. Brigo F. Intermittent rhythmic delta activity patterns. Epilepsy Behav. 2011;20:254–6.
44. Gaspard N, Manganas L, Rampal N. Similarity of lateralized rhythmic delta activity to periodic lateralized epileptiform discharges in critically ill patients. JAMA Neurol. 2013;70(10):1288–95.
45. Rodriguez Ruiz A, Vlachy J, Lee JW, et al. Association of periodic and rhythmic electroencephalographic patterns with seizures in critically ill patients. JAMA Neurol. 2017;74(2):181–8.
46. Van Putten MJ, Hofmeijer J. Generalized periodic discharges: pathophysiology and clinical considerations. Epilepsy Behav. 2015;49:228–33.
47. Bremer F. Considérations sur l'origine et la nature des ondes cérébrales. Electroencephalogr Clin Neurophysiol. 1949;1(2):177–93.
48. Chatrian GE, Shaw CM, Leffman H. The significance of periodic lateralized epileptiform discharges in EEG: an electrographic, clinical and pathological study. Electroencephalogr Clin Neurophysiol. 1964;17:177–93.
49. Brenner RP, Schaul N. Periodic EEG patterns: classification, clinical correlation, and pathophysiology. J Clin Neurophysiol. 1990;7(2):249–67.
50. Snodgrass SM, Tsuburaya K, Ajmone-Marsan C. Clinical significance of periodic lateralized epileptiform discharges: relationship with status epilepticus. J Clin Neurophysiol. 1989;6(2):159–72.
51. Raroque HG Jr, Purdy P. Lesion localization in periodic lateralized epileptiform discharges: gray or white matter. Epilepsia. 1995;36(1):58–62.
52. Gurer G, Yemisci M, Saygi S, et al. Structural lesions in periodic lateralized epileptiform discharges (PLEDs). Clin EEG Neurosci. 2004;35(2):88–93.
53. Pohlmann-Eden B, Hoch DB, Cochius JI, et al. Periodic lateralized epileptiform discharges a critical review. J Clin Neurophysiol. 1996;13(6):519–30.
54. Baykan B, Kinay D, Gokyigit A, et al. Periodic lateralized epileptiform discharges: association with seizures. Seizure. 2000;9(6):402–6.
55. Assal F, Papazyan JP, Slosman DO, et al. SPECT in periodic lateralized epileptiform discharges (PLEDs): a form of partial status epilepticus? Seizure. 2001;10(4):260–5.
56. Garzon E, Femandes RM, Sakamoto AC. Serial EEG during human status epilepticus: evidence for PLEDs as an ictal pattern. Neurology. 2001;57(7):1175–83.
57. Reiher J, Rivest J, Grand'Maison F, et al. Periodic lateralized epileptiform discharges with transitional rhythmic discharges: association with seizures. Electroencephalogr Clin Neurophysiol. 1991;78(1):12–7.
58. De la Paz D, Brenner RR. Bilateral independent periodic lateralized epileptic discharges. Arch Neurol. 1981;38:713–5.
59. Schwartz MS, Prior PF, Scott DF. The occurrence and evolution in the EEG of a lateralized periodic phenomenon. Brain. 1973;96(3):613–22.
60. Cobb WA, Hill D. Electroencephalogram in subacute progressive encephalitis. Brain. 1950;73(3):392–404.
61. Alajouanine T, Nehlil J. Clinical and electroencephalographic verification of a probable case of subacute sclerosing leukoencephalitis. Rev Neurol. 1955;93(2):435–7.
62. Kaya D, Bingol CA. Significance of atypical triphasic waves for diagnosing nonconvulsive status epilepticus. Epilepsy Behav. 2007;11(4):567–77.
63. Boulanger JM, Deacon C, Lecuyer D, et al. Triphasic waves versus nonconvulsive status epilepticus: EEG distinction. Can J Neurol Sci. 2006;33(2):175–80.
64. Hirsch LJ, Claassen J, Mayer SA, et al. Stimulus-induced rhythmic, periodic, or ictal discharges (SIRPIDs): a common EEG phenomenon in the critically ill. Epilepsia. 2004;45(2):109–23.
65. Hirsch LJ, Pang T, Claassen J, et al. Focal motor seizures induced by alerting stimuli in critically ill patients. Epilepsia. 2008;49(6):968–73.
66. Zaret BS. Prognostic and neurophysiological implications of concurrent burst suppression and alpha patterns in the EEG of post-anoxic coma. Electroencephalogr Clin Neurophysiol. 1985;61(4):199–209.
67. Trinka EHJ. EEG in coma and brain death. Clin Neurophysiol. 2011;42(3):141–8.
68. DeLorenzo RJ, Waterhouse EJ, Towne AR, et al. Persistent nonconvulsive status epilepticus after the control of convulsive status epilepticus. Epilepsia. 1998;39(8):833–40.
69. Krishnamurthy KB, Drislane FW. Depth of EEG suppression and outcome in barbiturate anesthetic treatment for refractory status epilepticus. Epilepsia. 1999;40(6):759–62.
70. Brenner RP. How useful is EEG and EEG monitoring in the acutely ill and how to interpret it? Epilepsia. 2009;50(Suppl 12):34–7.
71. Kaplan PW. Assessing the outcomes in patients with nonconvulsive status epilepticus: nonconvulsive status epilepticus is underdiagnosed, potentially overtreated, and confounded by comorbidity. J Clin Neurophysiol. 1999;16(4):341–52.

33 Chromosomal Abnormalities and Cortical Malformations

Maurizio Elia

33.1 Chromosomal Abnormalities

Chromosome abnormalities are often associated with neurodevelopmental disorders and particularly with intellectual disability (ID). They represent a relatively rare etiology of epilepsy, but seizures are more frequently present in patients with ID than in the general population. Consequently, chromosome abnormalities play an important role especially when there is the co-occurrence of epilepsy and ID.

Different genetic tools such as karyotyping, high-resolution chromosome banding, and fluorescent in situ hybridization (FISH) have contributed to the discovery of a certain number of abnormalities involving rather large chromosome regions. In the last few decades, some new "molecular karyotype" techniques have been implemented, based on DNA hybridization, such as array comparative genomic hybridization (aCGH), multiplex ligation-dependent probe amplification (MLPA), and single nucleotide polymorphisms (SNP) array. In particular, aCGH has allowed to investigate the entire genome for micro-rearrangements, namely, copy number variations (CNVs) in the same experiment.

However, many of the studies published have been carried out on small groups of patients or on single cases with chromosome abnormalities and epilepsy, usually without providing sufficient information on the clinical and EEG phenotype, in order to correctly classify epilepsy.

Discovering chromosome abnormalities in patients with epilepsy may be important in order to verify whether they are correlated with peculiar clinical and EEG phenotypes and to clarify whether epileptogenesis is determined by the abnormal function of a candidate gene localized in the region of the chromosome anomaly. This is the case, for instance, of fragile X syndrome (FraXS) and Angelman syndrome (AS) that will be included in this chapter. The former, originally diagnosed with the evidence of a fragile site at the Xq27.3 region, when lymphocytes are grown in a folic acid-deprived medium, is now recognized as caused by a mutation of FMR1 gene; the latter has been correlated with the maternal copy of the ubiquitin-protein ligase gene (UBE3A), localized on the 15q11–13 region.

I will discuss here only those chromosome abnormalities or gene mutations, discovered by means of older and newer techniques, that have been strongly associated with clinical and EEG patterns so characteristic to suggest to the clinician a specific genetic diagnosis.

33.1.1 1p36 Deletion Syndrome

1p36.3 deletions account approximately for 0.5–1.2% of idiopathic ID. The prevalence, once estimated 1:10.000, is now considered to be 1:5000, making this genetic condition the most common terminal deletion [1, 2]. According to a recent review, more than 300 cases of 1p36 deletion syndrome have been reported in literature [3]. 1p36 deletion may be the result of pure terminal deletions, interstitial deletions of varying sizes, or more complex rearrangements. Deletions of the paternally inherited chromosome are usually larger than those of the maternally inherited chromosome [1].

Haploinsufficiency for KCNAB2 has been proposed as a significant risk factor for epilepsy in subjects with 1p36.3 deletion syndrome [4], but probably this is not the only gene responsible for epileptogenesis in this syndrome. In fact, the human gamma-aminobutyric acid A receptor delta-subunit gene GABRD and the proto-oncogene SKI have also been suggested to contribute to pathogenesis of epilepsy and neurodevelopmental disorders in 1p36 deletion syndrome [3].

1p36.3 deletion syndrome is typically characterized by craniofacial dysmorphic features, brachydactyly/camptodactyly, short feet, and sensorineural hearing impairment. More rare findings are epicanthal folds, highly arched palate, oral-facial clefting, congenital heart malformations, hypothyroidism, and visual inattentiveness. All subjects present developmental delay or ID of moderate to profound degree,

M. Elia (✉)
Unit of Neurology and Clinical Neurophysiopathology, Oasi Research Institute, IRCCS, Troina, Italy
e-mail: melia@oasi.en.it

O. Mecarelli (ed.), *Clinical Electroencephalography*, https://doi.org/10.1007/978-3-030-04573-9_33

and more than 85% of them show early muscle hypotonia. The majority of the patients achieves independent walking, but gait appears broad-based or ataxic. Behavior disturbances have been reported, mostly characterized by aggressiveness, self-injury, and autism spectrum disorder [1].

Brain neuroimaging may show cerebral atrophy, dilation or asymmetry of the lateral ventricles, hydrocephalus, myelination delay, focal dysplasias, polymicrogyria, subependimal heterotopia, and leukodystrophy [1, 3, 5].

Interictal EEG—A multicenter retrospective study of 91 subjects with 1p36.3 deletion syndrome has reported an interictal EEG at the onset characterized by spikes, polyspikes, or spike-and-wave complexes over the rolandic regions (6 cases), the temporo-occipital regions (18 cases), or multifocal/generalized (14 cases). Furthermore, in the majority of the patients, a slow activity was evident over the temporo-parieto-occipital regions. Only three patients (two of whom with seizures) had a normal EEG and five showed a hypsarrhythmic pattern. Interictal EEG remained unchanged in almost all cases, showing high-voltage diffuse or multifocal spikes, intermixed with slow waves in patients with drug-resistant epilepsy, slow background activity, and focal spikes in subjects with partially controlled seizures or seizure-free [5]. A more recent review of the literature confirms these data, reporting 31 cases of focal spikes in the interictal EEG at the onset (7 rolandic, 18 temporo-posterior or temporo-occipital, 1 right centrotemporal, 1 bilateral frontal, and 4 no better specified focal). There were also 20 cases with multifocal or generalized spikes or polyspikes and 10 cases with spike-and-wave discharges. Abnormal delta-theta wave activity mainly on the posterior temporo-parieto-occipital areas and asymmetry of slow activities were present in most patients. Thirty-one patients with seizures had a normal EEG, and 29 showed hypsarrhythmia [3].

Seizures and ictal EEG—Seizures are present in more than 60% of cases, with a predominance for female sex, and they are polymorphous: more commonly spasms, but also focal, generalized tonic-clonic, myoclonic, atonic, and absence seizures. It is arduous to define the age at seizure onset, since most reports fail to specify it. Anyway, seizures usually start in the first year of life (about 80% of cases during the first 6 months of age). Approximately 22% of patients develop an epileptic encephalopathy at a median age of 5 months [1–3, 5].

Two different patterns have been recognized: (1) patients with a few seizures in infancy, transiently treated with antiepileptic drugs, with no recurrence of the seizures during or after the first year of age [6, 7], and (2) patients suffering from enduring convulsions and requiring long-term medication [8]. Taking in count the literature data, 18.8% (36/191) of subjects with seizures develop a drug-resistant epilepsy [3]. The onset of refractory epilepsy in 1p36 deletion syndrome might be associated with the onset of infantile spasms and their degree of response to high-dose steroids [5].

33.1.2 2q24.4 Deletion Syndrome

Patients with a clinical and EEG picture of Dravet syndrome (DS) who are negative for SCN1A mutations may present SCN1A exonic or larger deletions involving SCN1A and contiguous genes [9–12]. These deletions account for 2–3% of all DS cases and for about 12.5% of patients with DS who are negative for mutations on sequencing [13].

Deletions extending beyond SCN1A and including variable numbers of contiguous genes can be associated with additional dysmorphic features, depending on the genes involved [9], or with a more severe epilepsy phenotype when other voltage-gated sodium channels (VGSC) α subunit genes clustered on chromosome 2q such as SCN2A, SCN3A, SCN7A, and SCN9A are involved [12, 14]. Clinical phenotype may be characterized by microcephaly, bitemporal narrowing or frontal bossing, down-slanting or short palpebral fissures, bulbous nose or broad nasal bridge, low-implanted ears, thick helix, bow-shaped mouth, anterior open bite, single palmar creases bilaterally, and partial syndactyly between the second and third toes [9, 14]. In a review of 43 previously published cases with a del(2)(q24.3q31.1), for the 22 seizure-positive cases, 2q24.3 region constituted the smallest commonly deleted region among the majority of the cases. The most common dysmorphic features were ear abnormalities, microcephaly, micrognatia, and brachysyndactyly [12].

MRI is usually normal, although one patient at 14 months of age showed diffuse lesions in the periventricular white matter and basal ganglia. Postmortem brain examination showed abnormalities as seen in Leigh syndrome, with spongiosis and increased gliosis of the internal and external pallidum, and less pronounced lesions in the pons and mesencephalon (central tegmental tract) [11].

Interictal EEG—The interictal EEG picture is that typical of DS [13, 15].

Seizures and ictal EEG—Seizures start always in the first year of life, with severe drug resistance, mild to severe ID, autistic behavior, ataxia, and muscle hypotonia. Ictal EEG picture shows the typical patterns of DS, i.e., absences, generalized tonic-clonic, myoclonic, and focal seizures [13, 15].

33.1.3 4p⁻ Syndrome (Wolf-Hirschhorn Syndrome)

The 4p⁻ syndrome or Wolf-Hirschhorn syndrome (WHS) is a rare malformative condition caused by the distal deletion of the short arm of chromosome 4 (region 4p16), which is sporadic in approximately the 85% of cases or originates from an unbalanced translocation in the remaining 15% of cases. The deleted region can be of paternal or maternal origin. The frequency of WHS is estimated as 1:50,000 births with a female predilection of 2:1. However, this prevalence figure may be underestimated, taking in count missed diagnoses due to lack of recognition or inadequate genetic analysis [16–19].

The shortest area regarded as the WHS critical region (WHSCR) is restricted to a 165-kb interval on 4p16.3. WHSC1 gene may be involved in the pathogenesis of WHS, such as in Pitt-Rogers-Danks syndrome which represents the result of an allelic variation and is usually milder than WHS [20]. Also the HOX7 (MSX1) gene has been found deleted in patients with WHS, and this was the first demonstration of the involvement of a homeobox gene in a human malformative condition Anyway, this gene anomaly has not been reported in all subjects with WHS [21, 22]. A new critical region has been proposed, WHSCR2, distally contiguous with WHSCR. One of the candidate genes included in WHSCR2 is LETM1 which likely plays a role in epileptogenesis. More recently, an additional chromosome region for seizures has been suggested, falling within the terminal 1.5 Mb on 4p, not including LETM1 [23]. On the basis of a genotype-phenotype analysis, WHS should be distinguished in a "classical" form and a "mild" form, the latter correlated with shorter deletions [20].

WHS is clinically characterized by severe prenatal and postnatal growth delay, low birth weight, severe ID, microcephaly, "Greek warrior helmet" profile of the face, cleft of the lip or palate, ocular coloboma, and heart septal defects. In about one third of cases, death occurs in the first year of age for systemic severe malformations, heart failure, and pulmonary infections [16–19].

In WHS, the following neuropathological abnormalities have been observed: microcephaly, anomalous pattern of the cortical gyri, heterotopia, dysplasia of the lateral geniculate bodies and dentate nuclei, and corpus callosum hypoplasia [24].

Interictal EEG—Two types of EEG patterns have been reported. The first type was characterized by frequent, diffuse, atypical slow spike and wave complexes, often occurring in long bursts, elicited by slow wave sleep. The second type included frequent, high-amplitude, fast spike-polyspike and wave complexes over the centro-posterior regions, triggered by eye closure (Fig. 33.1) [19, 25].

Seizure and Ictal EEG—Although the precise frequency of seizures in WHS is unknown, they occur in 50–100% of subjects reported in literature. Seizure onset is usually in the first year of age but definitely before 2 years of age [19, 26].

Clinical and EEG features of epilepsy in WHS have been described in detail only in a few cases. They are clonic or tonic, involving one side with or without secondary generalization, generalized tonic-clonic from the onset, in clusters, often triggered by fever. Unilateral or generalized tonic-clonic status epilepticus may occur. Focal seizures, myoclonic

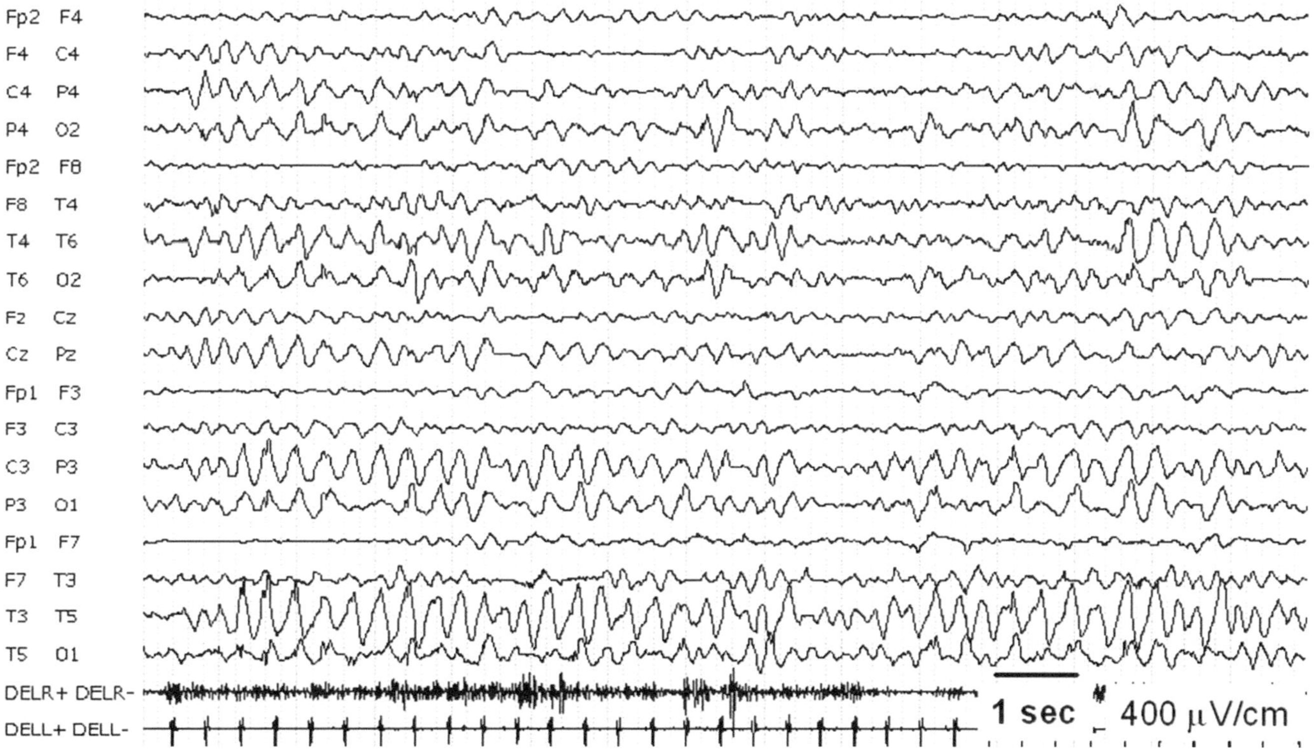

Fig. 33.1 Wakefulness EEG of a 1-year-old female with $4p^-$ syndrome. Long sequences of high-voltage slow waves and spike-and-wave complexes are evident over the parieto-temporo-occipital regions of both hemispheres, prominent on the left one (*R* right, *L* left, *DELT* deltoid muscle)

seizures, tonic spasms, or migrating partial seizures are rarer [19, 26–29].

A peculiar ictal EEG pattern has been observed in some studies. After the onset of unilateral or generalized tonic-clonic seizures in the first year of age, the patients develop frequent atypical absences accompanied by myoclonic jerks mainly involving the eyelids and axorizomelic muscles, induced by eye closure. EEG shows generalized spike-and-wave complexes [19, 30].

The prognosis of epilepsy in WHS is rather favorable. Seizures are controlled by valproic acid alone or in association with ethosuximide. In some cases, benzodiazepines and levetiracetam should be considered as treatment options. Sodium bromide is effective for preventing status epilepticus and for treating migrating partial seizures [19, 26–28, 31, 32].

33.1.4 5q14.3 Deletion Syndrome

Although 5q14.3 deletion has been associated with a Rett-like phenotype, most of the patients do not show acquired microcephaly and developmental regression after a normal interval but show muscle hypotonia, severe ID, early onset seizures, and sometimes autistic behavior, stereotypic hand movements, and episodic hyperventilation [33, 35].

Other characteristic dysmorphic signs include broad and high forehead, relatively large, backward rotated ear lobes, mildly upward-slanting palpebral fissures, and cupid bowed or tented upper lip [36]. Periventricular heterotopias or simplified gyral pattern on brain MRI are other possible features [34, 37].

MEF2C is the candidate gene for this syndrome. It encodes for a transcriptor factor, and its activity relies on the recruitment of many other transcription factors, as well as on translational and posttranscriptional modifications [38]. Patients with MEF2C defects showed diminished MECP2 and CDKL5 expression, and MEF2C mutations in vitro resulted in diminished transactivation of both the MECP2 and CDKL5 promoters [36]. A mutational screening for MEF2C microdeletion can be considered in patients with early onset Rett-like phenotype and negative for MECP2, CDKL5, and FOXG1 mutation or deletion.

Interictal EEG—Generalized spike-wave or polyspike-wave discharges have been reported in four patients [39].

Seizures and ictal EEG—Seizure onset is between 1 and 10 months of age, usually with infantile spasms. Febrile seizures, atypical absences, myoclonic, and focal seizures may also occur [15, 37, 39].

33.1.5 6q Terminal Deletion Syndrome

The 6q terminal deletion syndrome is a rare condition characterized by ID, facial dysmorphic features, genital hypoplasia, and structural CNS abnormalities. We described five patients with 6q terminal deletion (9 to 16 Mb large) and a specific electroclinical pattern [40]. Subsequently, other seven patients with 6q subtelomere deletion and a similar clinical and EEG pattern were reported with a size of the deletion ranging from 3 to 13 Mb [41, 42]. It has been calculated that 6q terminal deletion is present in about 0.05% of patients with ID and/or development delay [43].

Brain MRI is characterized by colpocephaly and dysgenesis of the corpus callosum, thalami, and brainstem [40].

In a more recent review, 28 cases with pure 6q terminal deletion were counted [43]. A comparison of the case with the smallest deletion (~0.4 Mb; 3 known genes) reported to date and the case that has the largest deletion (<11 Mb; >34 known genes) showed no specific phenotype differences. The region of greatest interest resulted the smallest overlapped portion of the most distal part of chromosome 6q. The genes located in the region within 0.4 Mb of the 6q terminus were PSMB1, TBP, and PDCD2. The TBP gene has been proposed as a candidate gene for phenotype in patients with 6q terminal deletion. However, the possibility of other genes playing a role in the phenotype resulting from this deleted region cannot be ruled out. To confirm this, a study on 12 patients with 6q terminal deletion and developmental brain abnormalities, including also periventricular nodular heterotopia, suggested that C6orf70 gene might play a major role in the control of neuronal migration [44].

Interictal EEG—Interictal EEG is characterized by posterior spike-and-wave complexes which become more pronounced during NREM sleep (Fig. 33.2) [40, 41].

Seizures and ictal EEG—There are no ictal EEG pictures of 6q terminal deletion in literature up to now. Epilepsy starts in the first or second decade of life. In almost all cases, seizures had a focal onset, characterized by the ictal signs of vomiting, cyanosis, and head and eye version with or without loss of consciousness. The ictal signs and the EEG patterns in these patients suggest that the seizures originate from the occipital lobes. Given the early onset of seizures, it is conceivable that an age-related low threshold of emetic centers causes the ictal vomiting, as occurs in Panayiotopoulos-type occipital epilepsy. No status epilepticus or prolonged seizures occur. Prognosis of epilepsy is generally good, in terms of both seizure control and evolution [40, 41].

33.1.6 Trisomy 12p Syndrome

This represents a rare condition (estimated prevalence 1:50,000), which can be caused by a de novo occurrence (also in a mosaic fashion) or by an unbalanced translocation, and is characterized by severe ID, absent language, and generalized hypotonia. The main dysmorphic features include round face, short neck, high and prominent forehead, flat

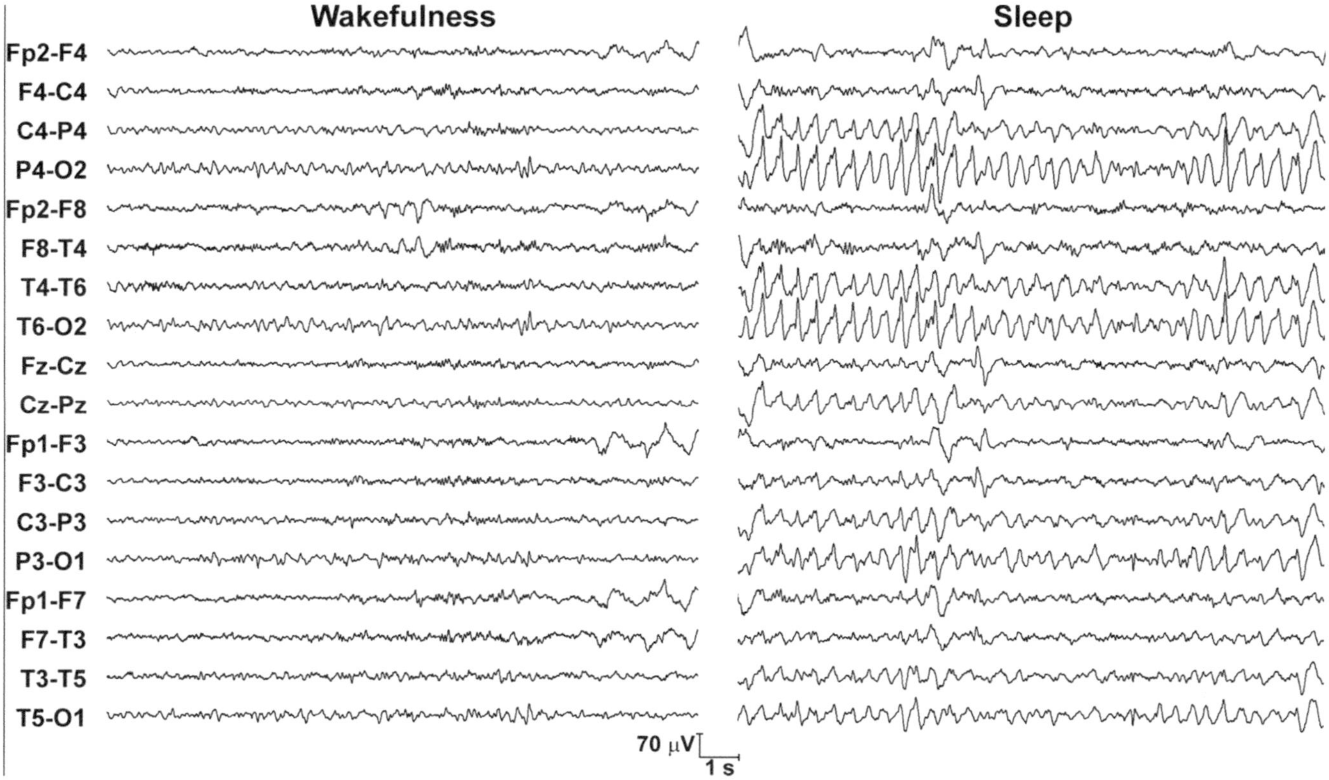

Fig. 33.2 Wakefulness EEG of a 19-year-old male with 6q terminal deletion showing sharp waves over the occipital regions of the right hemisphere (**a**). During non-REM sleep, high-voltage rhythmical delta activity is present over the temporo-parietal regions (**b**)

occiput, hypertelorism, epicanthus, broad nasal bridge, long philtrum, prominent lower lip, low-set ears, and micrognathia [45–47].

Brain neuroimaging discloses calcifications of the basal ganglia, cortical and subcortical atrophy, "mega cisterna magna," and signal alteration of the white matter [45–47].

It is noteworthy that in the 12p13 region, deleted in this chromosome abnormality, there is a cluster of three genes coding for potassium voltage-gated channels which might be relevant for epileptogenesis [45–47].

Interictal EEG, seizures, and ictal EEG—In some cases, a typical electroclinical pattern has been found, characterized by absences with myoclonias, starting after 3 years of age, associated with generalized spike- and polyspike-and-wave complexes at the interictal and ictal EEG (Fig. 33.3) [45–47].

Seizures are present in about 30% of cases, and they present mostly as febrile or afebrile generalized tonic-clonic, or myoclonic fits. They are usually controlled by valproic acid in monotherapy or associated with ethosuximide [45, 46].

33.1.7 Ring Chromosome 14 Syndrome

Ring chromosome 14 is a rare chromosomal anomaly which occurs as a mosaicism. The patients present early onset epilepsy, severe or profound ID, language disturbance, microcephaly, and facial dysmorphisms. Ocular anomalies, such as cortical cataract, retinopathy, and refractive errors, may be present [47].

Neuroimaging shows hypoplasia of the corpus callosum, left temporal hypodensity, cortical atrophy, mild dilatation of the left temporal horn, mild bilateral fronto-temporo-parietal atrophy, cystic hypophysis anomaly, mild external hydrocephaly, sphenoid wing cyst, cerebral and white matter hypoplasia, hippocampal dysmorphisms, and cerebellar structural anomalies [48–51].

Ring chromosome 14 represents the smallest form of 14q monosomy. Two hypotheses could explain the presence of seizures in r(14) syndrome: ring instability, resulting in monosomy 14 in a proportion of cells, or haploinsufficiency of critical genes, with a decreased expression of genes contained on the adjacent 14q arm. FOXG1B gene, included in the 14q11q13 region, with a well-known role in the development of the brain and telencephalon, has been suggested as a candidate gene for epilepsy [51].

Interictal EEG—In a recent retrospective study on 22 patients with ring 14 chromosome syndrome, 15 of them had a slow and poorly organized EEG background activity, with interposed discontinuous rhythmic monomorphous bifrontal or temporo-posterior high-voltage slow waves. Epileptiform abnormalities, such as spike-and-wave complexes, slow

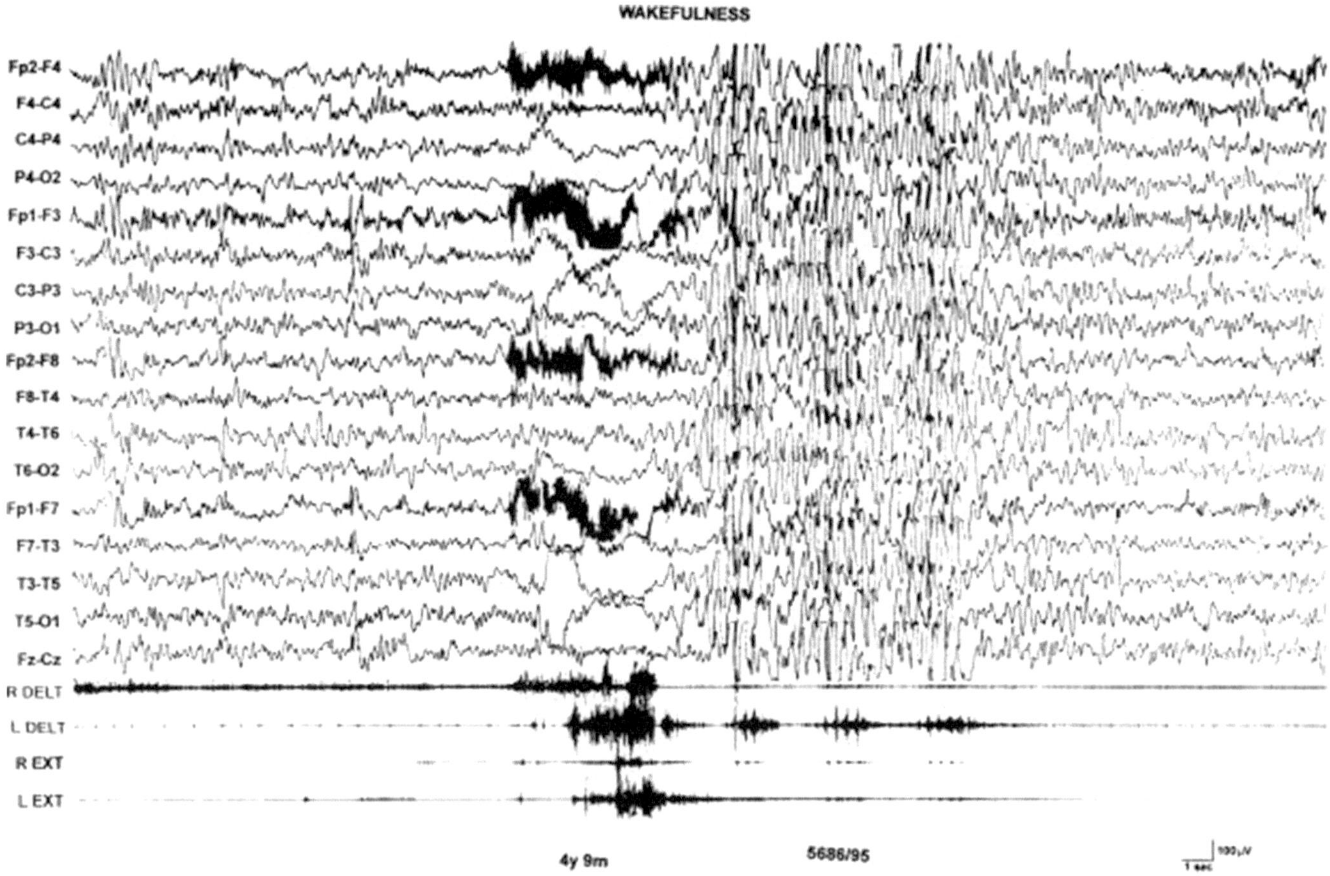

Fig. 33.3 Wakefulness EEG of a 4-year-old female with trisomy 12p syndrome. A myoclonic absence is recorded, characterized by a diffuse spike-and-wave discharge, accompanied by rhythmical myoclonic jerks, prevalent at the left deltoid muscle, superimposed over a tonic contraction (*R* right, *L* left, *DELT* deltoid muscle, *EXT* forearm extensor muscles)

spikes, sharp waves, fast rhythms over the fronto-central or fronto-temporal regions, and more diffuse during sleep, were present in seven subjects. In five patients, paroxysmal generalized abnormalities were preceded by unusual unilateral or bilateral posterior recruiting spikes or fast rhythms. Follow-up EEG evaluation showed the persistence of the bursts of rhythmic high-voltage slow waves over the posterior or fronto-central areas. In sporadic cases with a good seizure outcome, EEG revealed only theta activities over the temporal regions or was normal [51].

Seizures and ictal EEG—Epilepsy has an early onset, mostly in the first year of age. Seizure at onset was reported to be of generalized, tonic-clonic, myoclonic-tonic, and clonic types in 9 out of 22 patients. Focal hemiclonic seizures were present in two subjects and focal seizures with secondary generalization, mainly starting from the mid-temporal and frontal regions, in 11 subjects. Seizures were often prolonged or in clusters, correlated with sleep, and resistant to the different antiepileptic drugs used; convulsive and nonconvulsive status epilepticus have been reported in some cases [51].

At the EEG, in focal seizures, the fast generalization of the ictal discharge can hide its focal origin, or focal discharge can appear during an apparently generalized seizure. Focal seizures originate mainly from fronto-temporal and mid-posterior regions. Generalized tonic seizures are characterized by a generalized desynchronization on EEG. Irregular or asymmetric 2.5–3 Hz spike-and-wave discharges clinically correlated with eyelid myoclonic absences may be rarely present. In patients with nonconvulsive status epilepticus, an EEG pattern with bilateral frontal high-voltage continuous rhythmic or pseudo-rhythmic delta activity is evident [51].

33.1.8 Angelman Syndrome

Angelman syndrome (AS) is a genetic malformative condition characterized by severe ID with absent or very limited verbal language, ataxia, myoclonus, paroxysmal laughter, and seizures [47, 52, 53].

The prevalence of AS has been reported as 1:62,000, but this epidemiological finding could be underestimated, and a higher prevalence, 1:12,000, has been recently suggested [53, 54]. In more than 70% of cases, a deletion of the long arm of the chromosome 15 is recognizable, with a maternal origin (15q11–13 region); in approximately 2–3% of cases, a uniparental paternal disomy is present; about 3–5% of cases are associated with a defect of the *imprinting center*, leading to the absence of the typical maternal DNA methylation pattern. Furthermore, from 1997 up today, several sporadic and familial cases (5–10%) with mutations of the UBE3A (ubiquitin-protein ligase E3A) gene, located in the 15q11–13 region, have been reported. Fifty percent of these mutations involves exons 8 and 9 of UBE3A gene [47, 55].

The abovementioned genotypes determine AS variable phenotypes, more severe in subjects with 15q11–13 deletion, less severe in those with UBE3A mutations, and milder in those with uniparental paternal disomy and with *imprinting center* defect [47, 56].

Among the different known transgenic animal models, the GABRB3 knockout shows clinical and EEG features similar to those found in humans. Up to now, it is unclear how the inactivation of UBE3A gene is able to cause AS. It has been hypothesized that the UBE3A gene might act by means of a defect of activation of Plic-1 protein, which regulates the number of $GABA_A$ receptors containing the β3 subunit on the cell membrane, reducing the strength of the GABAergic synapses [57, 58].

Neuroimaging usually shows nonspecific anomalies. Frequently, cerebral atrophy of variable degree and dilation of lateral ventricles are observed [59].

Interictal EEG—EEG picture in AS is rather peculiar, is similar in the different phenotypes, and is characterized by a slow background activity and paroxysmal abnormalities, mostly spike-and-wave complexes, prominent over the occipital or frontal regions. Diffuse spike-and-wave complexes, accompanied by myoclonias, sometimes rhythmical and bilateral, sometimes quasi-continuous and apparently not correlated with the paroxysmal abnormalities are often recorded (Fig. 33.4).

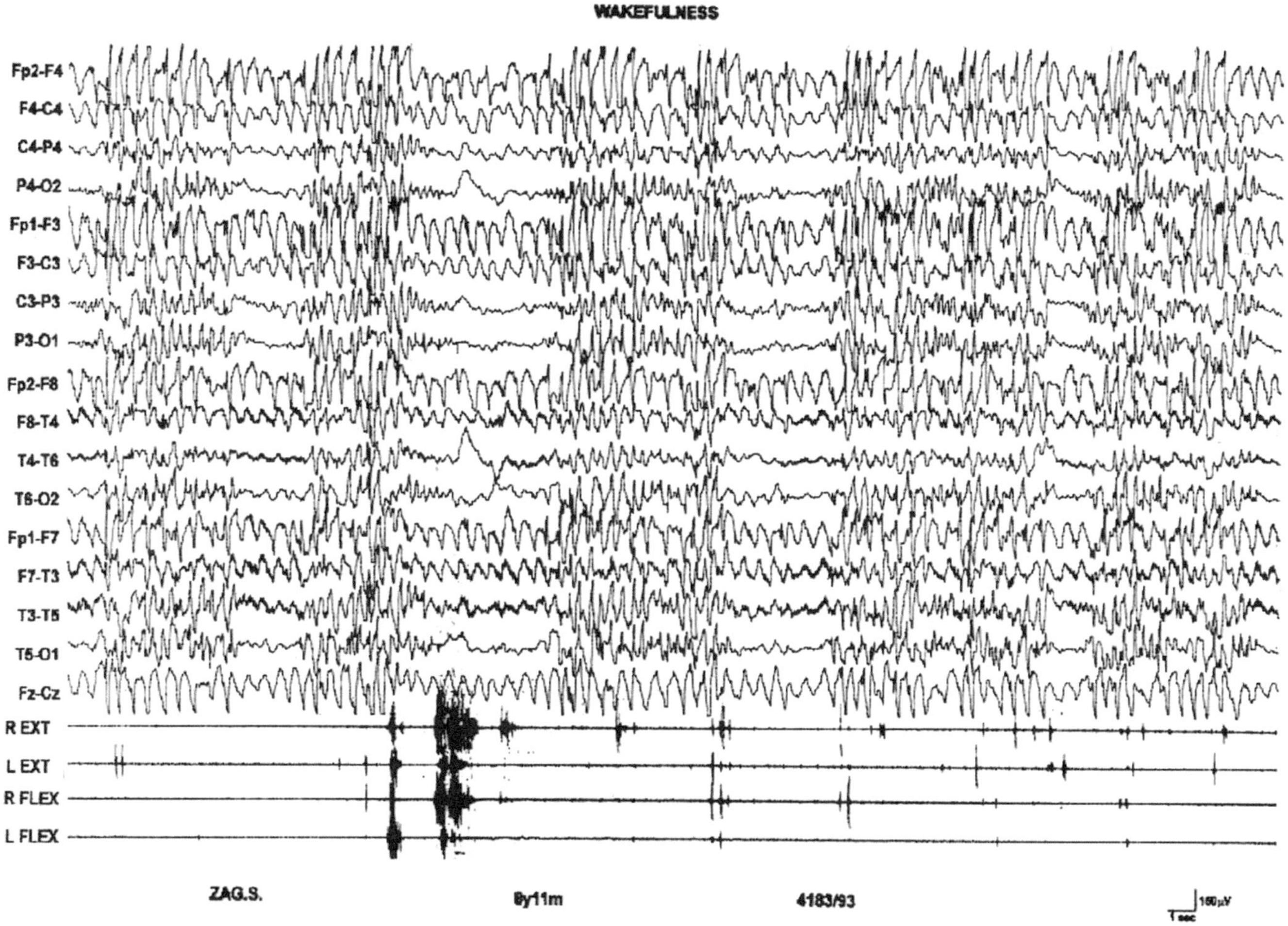

Fig. 33.4 An 8-year-old female with Angelman syndrome. At wakefulness EEG, a slow background activity and quasi-continuous spike-and-wave discharges, better represented over the frontal regions, are present. Surface EMG of forearm extensor and flexor muscles records numerous bilateral, sometimes rhythmical and bilateral, myoclonic jerks which are inconstantly correlated with paroxysmal abnormalities (*R* right, *L* left, *EXT* forearm extensor muscles, *FLEX* forearm flexor muscles)

In the sleep stages 1–2, spike-and-wave complexes become continuous, and spindles are not easily recognizable; in the stages 2–3 of the subsequent sleep cycles, the activation of paroxysmal abnormalities is reduced, and spindles are better represented (Fig. 33.5). In slow sleep, myoclonus disappears, and it reappears at the awakening and during REM sleep, when a theta activity on the vertex and rolandic regions is evident.

Two females have been reported with the typical EEG trait of AS but with mutations of MECP2 gene and a diagnosis of Rett syndrome [60, 61].

Back-averaging study of myoclonus in AS has demonstrated that it has a cortical origin, with a rostro-caudal activation pattern. Furthermore, in some patients, a quasi-continuous focal or multifocal rhythmical cortical myoclonus, at about 11 Hz of frequency, involving hands or face, has been described [62].

Seizures and ictal EEG—Seizures are present in approximately 90% of cases, start in the first year of age, and are polymorphous: spasms, myoclonic, myoclonic-atonic, generalized tonic-clonic, focal seizures, myoclonic absences, and febrile convulsions [47, 63]. The typical ictal EEG pattern of AS is the so-called myoclonic status, which is clinically correlated with an obtundation status, an impairment of the gait, more frequent myoclonic jerks, and hyperactivity. At the EEG, quasi-continuous spike-and-wave complexes diffuse over both hemisphere, correlated or not with myoclonic jerks, are evident (Figs. 33.6 and 33.7) [47, 64, 65].

An earlier onset and a greater severity of seizures are common in patients with 15q11–13 deletion, in comparison with the other genotypes [56].

Epilepsy is rather benign in the evolution, and treatment is based on valproic acid, also in association with ethosuximide, or benzodiazepines [47, 66]. Lamotrigine, topiramate, and levetiracetam have been reported as helpful in a few cases [47, 67]. Cortical myoclonus can be treated with high dosages of piracetam [62]. In adults, drug withdrawal might be considered in the management of epilepsy despite the persistence of epileptiform abnormalities [66].

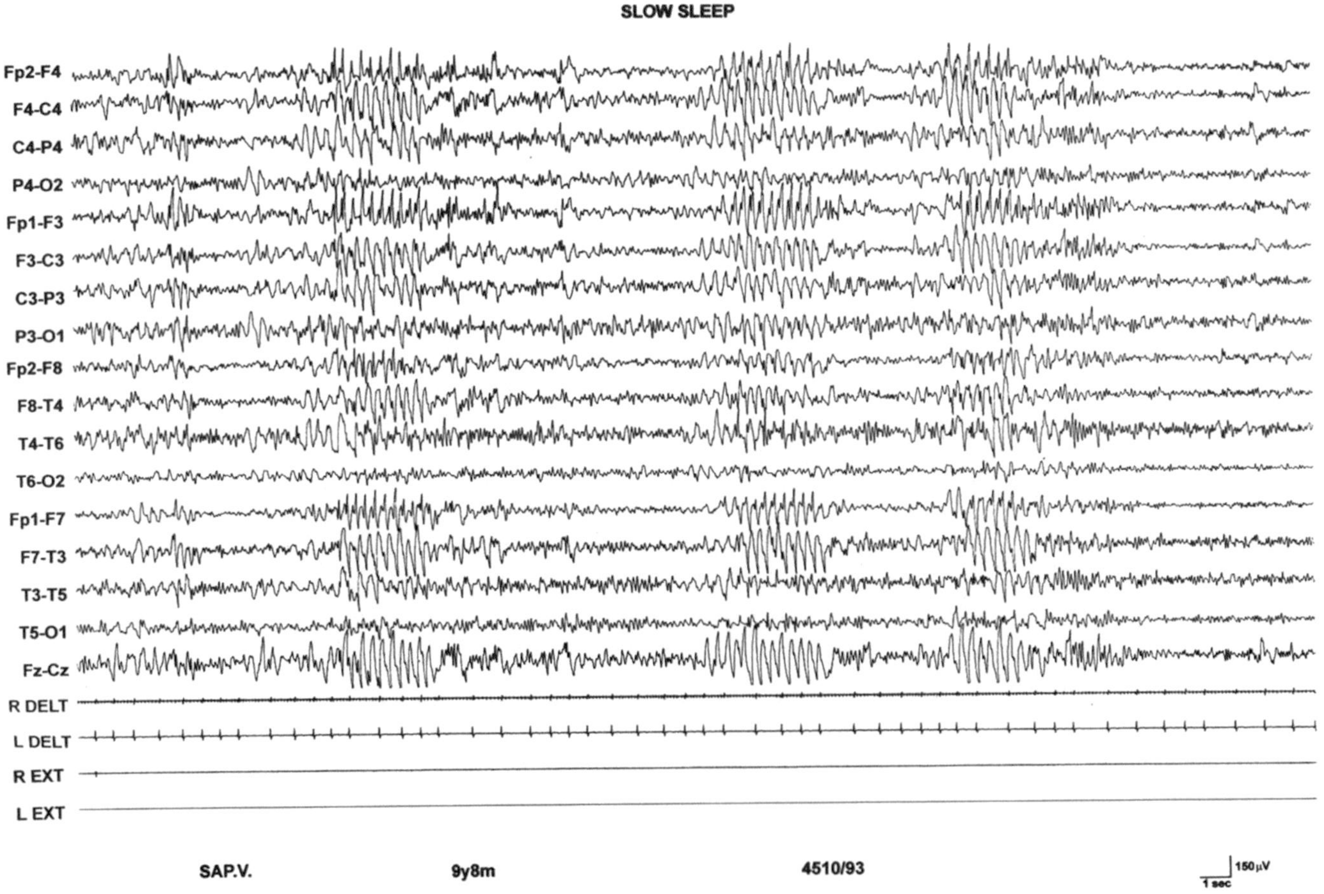

Fig. 33.5 A 9-year-old female with Angelman syndrome. Sleep EEG shows diffuse spike-and-wave discharges, prevalent over the anterior regions of both hemispheres and the vertex. Spindles are bilaterally and symmetrically represented. There are no myoclonic jerks at surface EMG of forearm muscles (*R* right, *L* left, *DELT* deltoid muscle, *EXT* forearm extensor muscles)

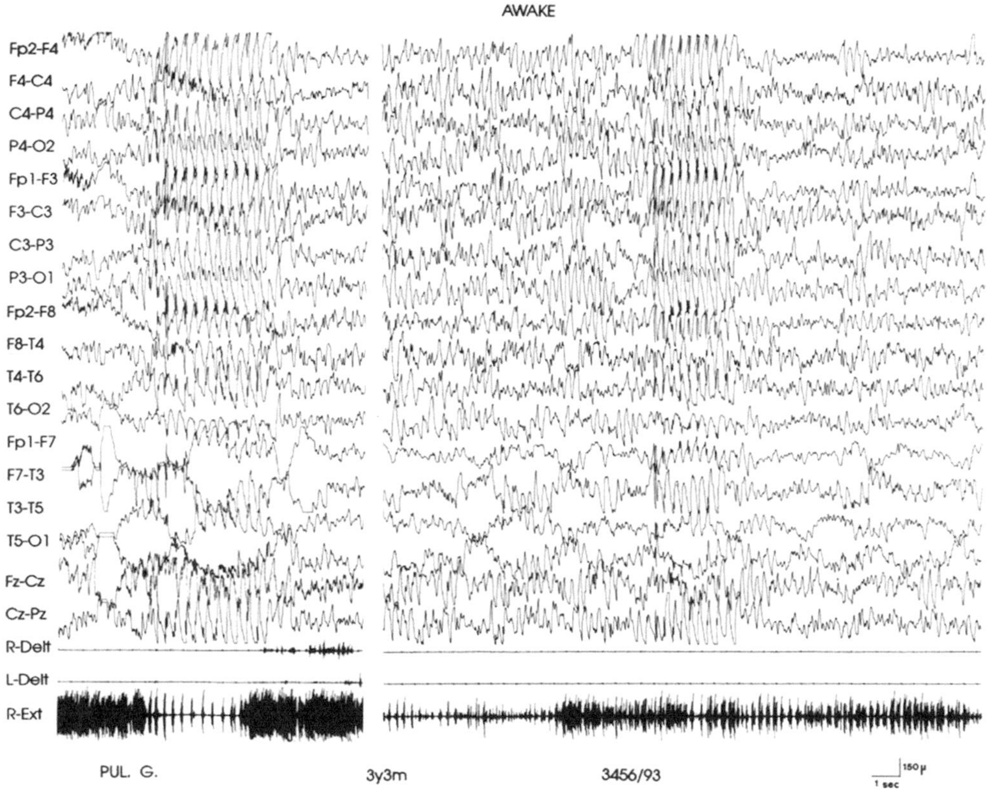

Fig. 33.6 A 3-year-old male with Angelman syndrome. On the left side, a short generalized discharge of spike-and-wave complexes is evident, and it is timely correlated with rhythmical losses of muscle tone, determining an absence with myoclonus. On the right side, EEG shows spike-and-wave complexes over the anterior regions of both hemispheres and another short spike-and-wave discharge. In this case, the correlation with myoclonus is less evident (*R* right, *L* left, *DELT* deltoid muscle, *EXT* forearm extensor muscles)

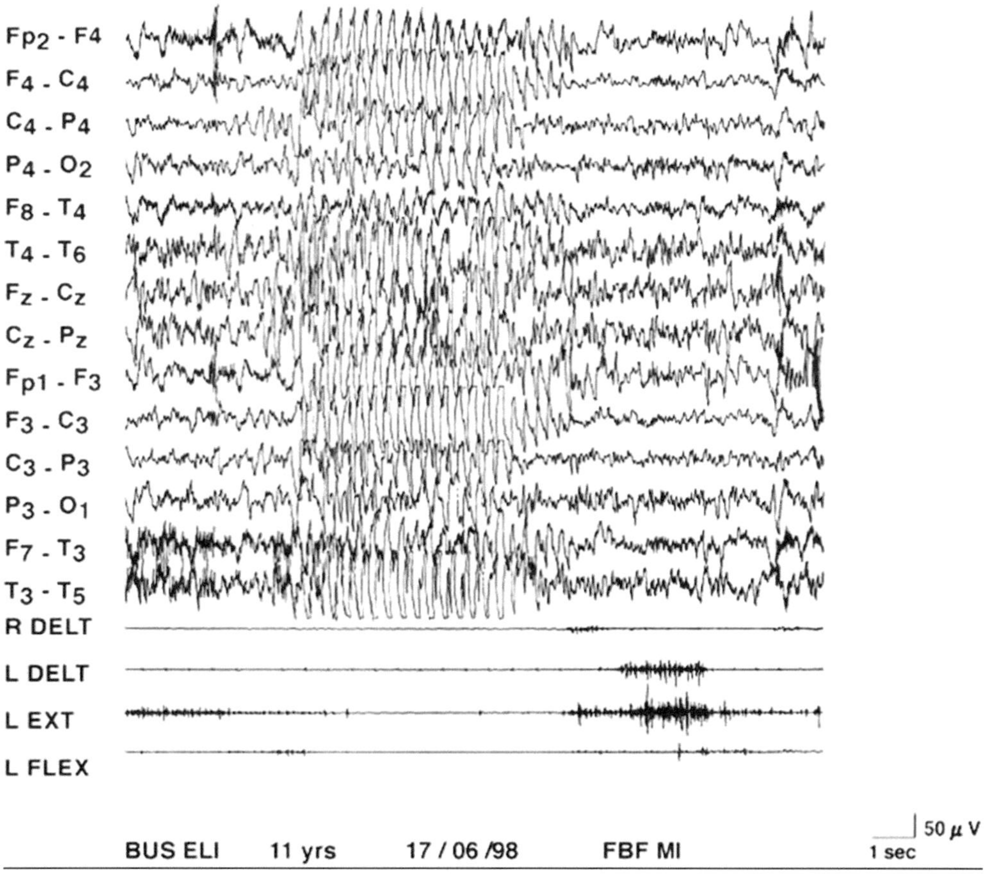

Fig. 33.7 An 11-year-old female with Angelman syndrome. Ictal EEG disclosing an atypical absence, correlated with an interruption of the motor activity at surface EMG of deltoid and forearm extensor muscles (*R* right, *L* left, *DELT* deltoid muscle, *EXT* forearm extensor muscle, *FLEX* forearm flexor muscle)

33.1.9 Inv Dup (15) Syndrome

The inverted duplication of proximal chromosome 15 [inv dup (5)] or isodicentric 15 chromosome [idic (15)] is the most common chromosome marker or extra structural abnormal chromosome (ESAC). Its prevalence is estimated to be 1:30,000 [47].

Phenotype is very variable, with ID, behavioral disturbances, autism spectrum disorder, and epilepsy. In the majority of cases, neuroimaging does not reveal specific alterations; enlarged ventricles, enlarged subarachnoid spaces, thinning of the corpus callosum and increased signal density around the posterior horns of the lateral ventricles, moderate volume increase of the cerebrospinal fluid surrounding the left temporal pole, and mild brain atrophy have been reported [68, 69].

There are many evidences that phenotype is more severe when the inverted and duplicated 15 chromosome segment is larger. Anyway, some other reports seem to contradict this statement [70]. Certainly, phenotype is strictly correlated with the extension of the region and with the gene dosages, when it contains the PWS/AS critical region. Among genes with a sure role in determining phenotype of inv. dup (15) syndrome, there are those coding for the subunits α5 and β3 of GABA receptor and P gene. Tetrasomy of these genes could alter the activity of GABA receptor and then cause some of the main clinical features of this syndrome, such as seizures, hyperactivity, aggressiveness, and autism spectrum disorder.

Other genes, such as SLC12A6, located more distally, coding for cation chloride cotransporter, and expressed in the brain, or CHRNA7, coding for a subunit of nicotinic acethylcholine receptors, located on 15q11.2–q13.3, could be involved in the pathogenesis of seizure [47, 71].

Interictal EEG—In a recent retrospective study of 35 patients with inv. dup (15), the interictal EEG was differentiated: slow or sharp waves, biphasic spikes-polyspikes more prominent over both frontal regions, often quasi-continuous, sometimes diffuse to the entire brain; fast ill-defined spike-and-wave complexes, usually in runs of variable duration, over both fronto-centro-temporal regions; fast activity at 12–20 Hz bilaterally over fronto-centro-temporal areas (Fig. 33.8); and slow background activity. Sleep spindles

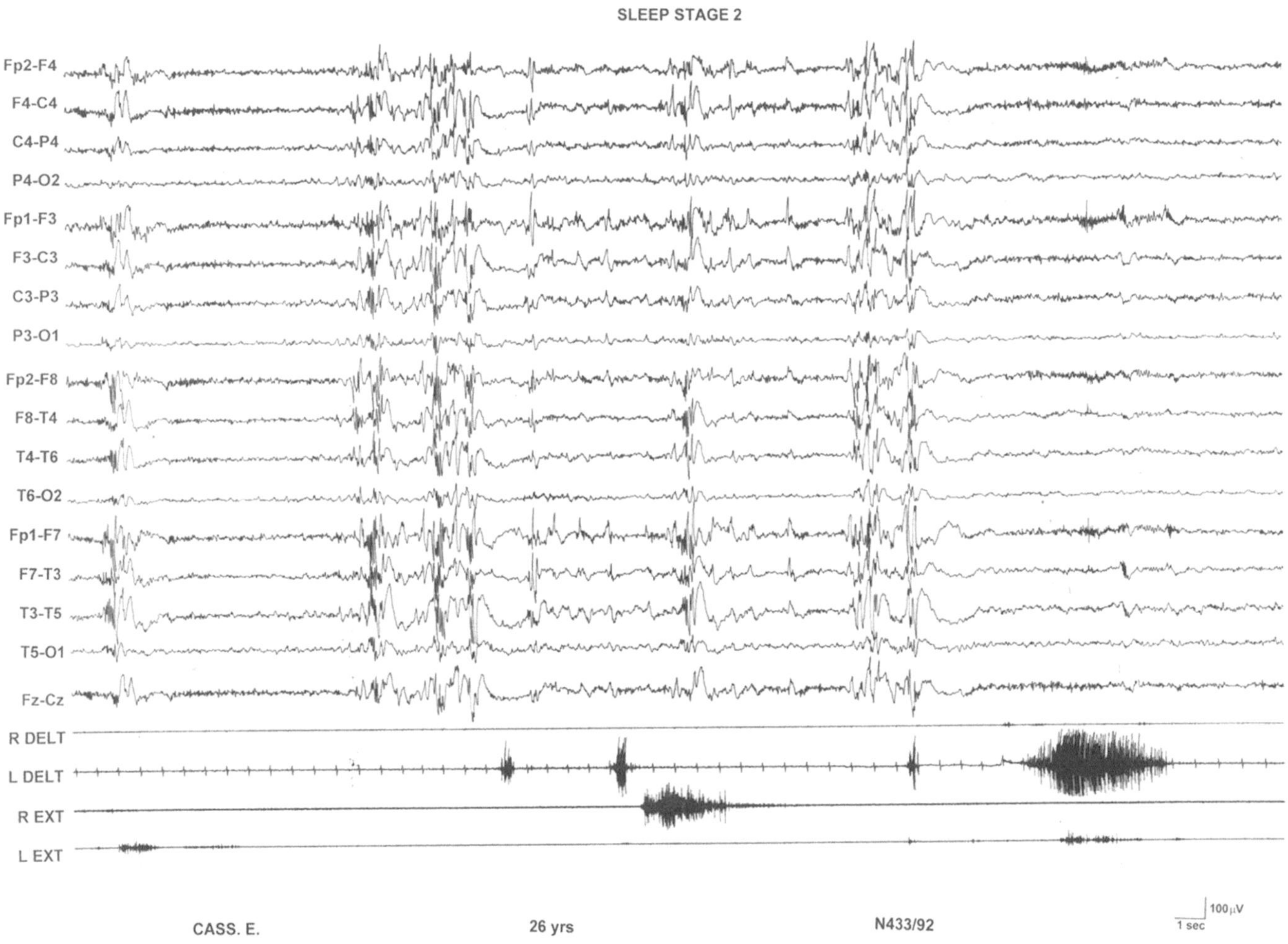

Fig. 33.8 A 26-year-old female with inv. dup (15) syndrome. Sleep EEG shows numerous short fast polyspike discharges, without clinical correlation, as in the typical Lennox-Gastaut syndrome (*R* right, *L* left, *DELT* deltoid muscle, *EXT* forearm extensor muscle)

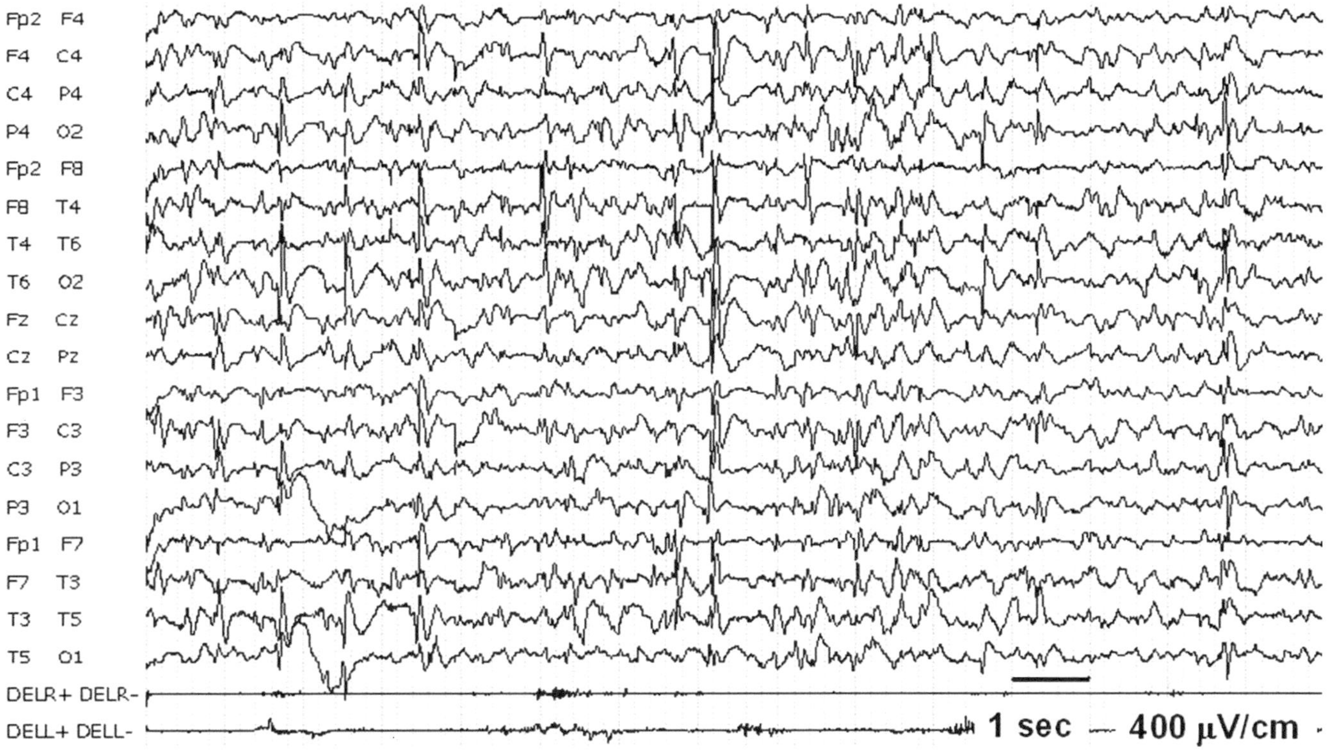

Fig. 33.9 A 2-year-old male with inv. dup (15) syndrome. Wakefulness interictal EEG is characterized by numerous high-voltage, multifocal or diffuse spikes and slow spike-and-wave complexes (*R* right, *L* left, *DELT* deltoid muscle)

were recognizable in most patients [71]. These findings were confirmed in a recent review of the literature [69].

In the first year of life, the EEG picture can be that of an epileptic encephalopathy, with a poorly organized and reactive background activity and numerous multifocal epileptiform abnormalities (Fig. 33.9).

Seizure and ictal EEG—Seizures usually start between 2 months and 9 years of age and affect 65–80% of patients. In about 32% of cases, the first seizures are infantile spasms associated with an hypsarrhythmic EEG [69, 71]. In the first year of age, also episodes with the EEG characteristics of very short tonic seizures, i.e., diffuse fast paroxysmal activity discharges, are typically recorded (Fig. 33.10).

In about 25% of cases, first seizures are tonic, either focal or generalized, triggered by sleep with a later onset (up to 10 years); 30% of patients develop atypical absences, by age 1–7 years. All such patients later developed a Lennox-Gastaut syndrome [71, 72]. Focal, myoclonic, and atonic seizures are present in about 30%, 27%, and 28% of cases, respectively [69]. On the basis of a further very recent retrospective study of 45 patients with inv. dup (15) syndrome, it was possible to define four definite epileptic syndromes: generalized epilepsy, focal epilepsy, epileptic encephalopathy with spasms as the only seizure type, and epileptic encephalopathy with epileptic spasms associated with other seizure types [73].

Ictal EEG has been recorded only sporadically and shows diffuse spikes followed by high-voltage spikes and waves in the right frontal-temporal regions during an episode of head rotation to the right followed by rotation to the left, tonic adduction of the arms, chewing movements, and loss of consciousness (Fig. 33.11a, b); diffuse fast spikes followed by voltage decrease; mild diffuse attenuation of background activity with low-amplitude, rhythmic theta activity; or diffuse delta bursts followed by an electrodecremental response [69].

Epilepsy results well controlled in 35.7% of patients, satisfactorily controlled (seizure reduction >75%) in 7.1%, partially controlled (seizure reduction <50%) in 21.4%, and drug-resistant in 35.7%. Valproate, lamotrigine, and rufinamide seem to be the most effective AEDs [71].

33.1.10 15q13.3 Deletion Syndrome

15q13.2–13.3 deletion has been first described as a recurrent CNV associated with ID and epilepsy [74]. Subsequently, many other papers described this abnormality in association with a broad phenotype including polymorphous dysmorphisms, schizophrenia, severe neurodevelopmental disorders, autism spectrum disorder, and epilepsy [75–78]. The most frequent dysmorphic features are hypertelorism,

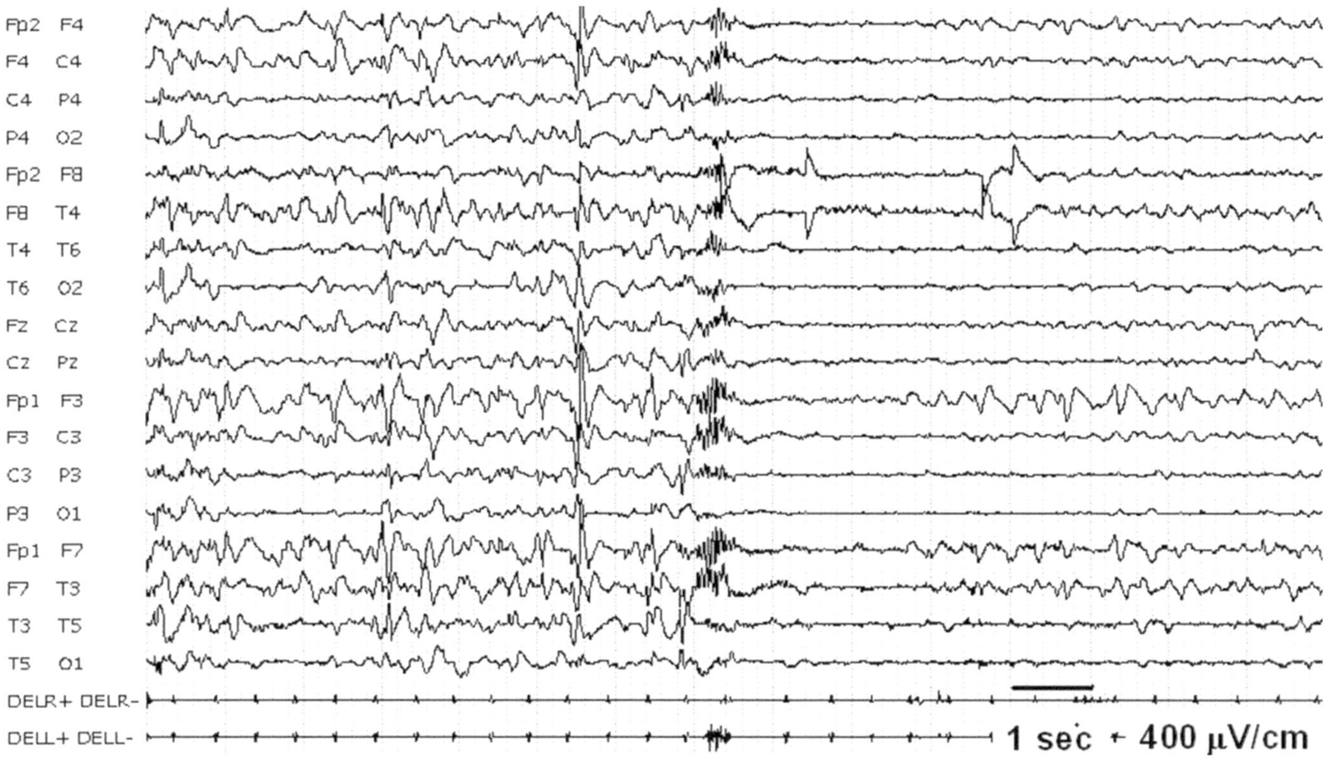

Fig. 33.10 The same patient of Fig. 33.9, at 3 years of age. EEG recording of a short tonic seizure, characterized by a short sequence of diffuse fast activity, followed by diffuse desynchronization. At surface EMG of deltoid muscles, a short tonic contraction, more intense on the left side, is evident (*R* right, *L* left, *DELT* deltoid muscle)

upslanting palpebral fissures, prominent philtrum with full everted lips, and clinodactyly [74].

The breakpoints 4 and 5 (BP4 and BP5) have been associated with the epilepsy phenotype [74]. A more severe phenotype has been found in the homozygous loss state [79, 80].

Recently, 15q13.3 deletion has been proposed as a common risk factor for epilepsy, since it is detected in about 1% of patients with idiopathic generalized epilepsy with or without other neurological manifestations [75, 81].

Haploinsufficiency of CHRNA7, which encodes for the α7 subunit of the acetylcholine receptor, is considered as the most likely responsible factor for the phenotype [75, 82]. No specific brain abnormalities have been reported in association to this CNV [15].

Interictal EEG—Focal (frontal, central, or parietal) spike/slow waves or generalized spike-and-wave complexes are present in some patients [77].

Seizures and ictal EEG—Absences have been recently reported in three patients with 15q13.3 deletion out of 570 children with epilepsy and ID [83]. Two other families with multiple affected individuals, presenting with absences or myoclonic absences associated to mild ID, have been described. The ictal EEG showed generalized polyspike-and-wave or spike-and-wave discharge. Apparently, the seizures persisted in the elderly and were difficult to control, requiring an association of at least two AEDs [84].

33.1.11 Ring Chromosome 20 Syndrome

Ring chromosome 20 is a rare chromosome anomaly. Until now, 170 cases of ring chromosome syndrome have been reported in literature [85]. Reported cases are almost exclusively sporadic and in mosaicism [47]. Phenotype is characterized by ID of variable degree, usually without major dysmorphic features; in approximately 90% of cases, drug-resistant seizures are present [47]. In some cases, MRI structural abnormalities (i.e., cortical dysplasias or hypoplasia of the corpus callosum or cerebellum) or PET neurotransmitter dysfunctions (i.e., reduced uptake of 18F-fluoro-l-DOPA) involving the frontal lobes and basal ganglia have been reported [86–89].

Telomeric regions involved in ring chromosome 20 contain some genes implied in the genesis of autosomal dominant epilepsies, such as benign neonatal familial convulsions or autosomal dominant frontal lobe epilepsies which are very different from ring chromosome 20 epilepsy. The mecha-

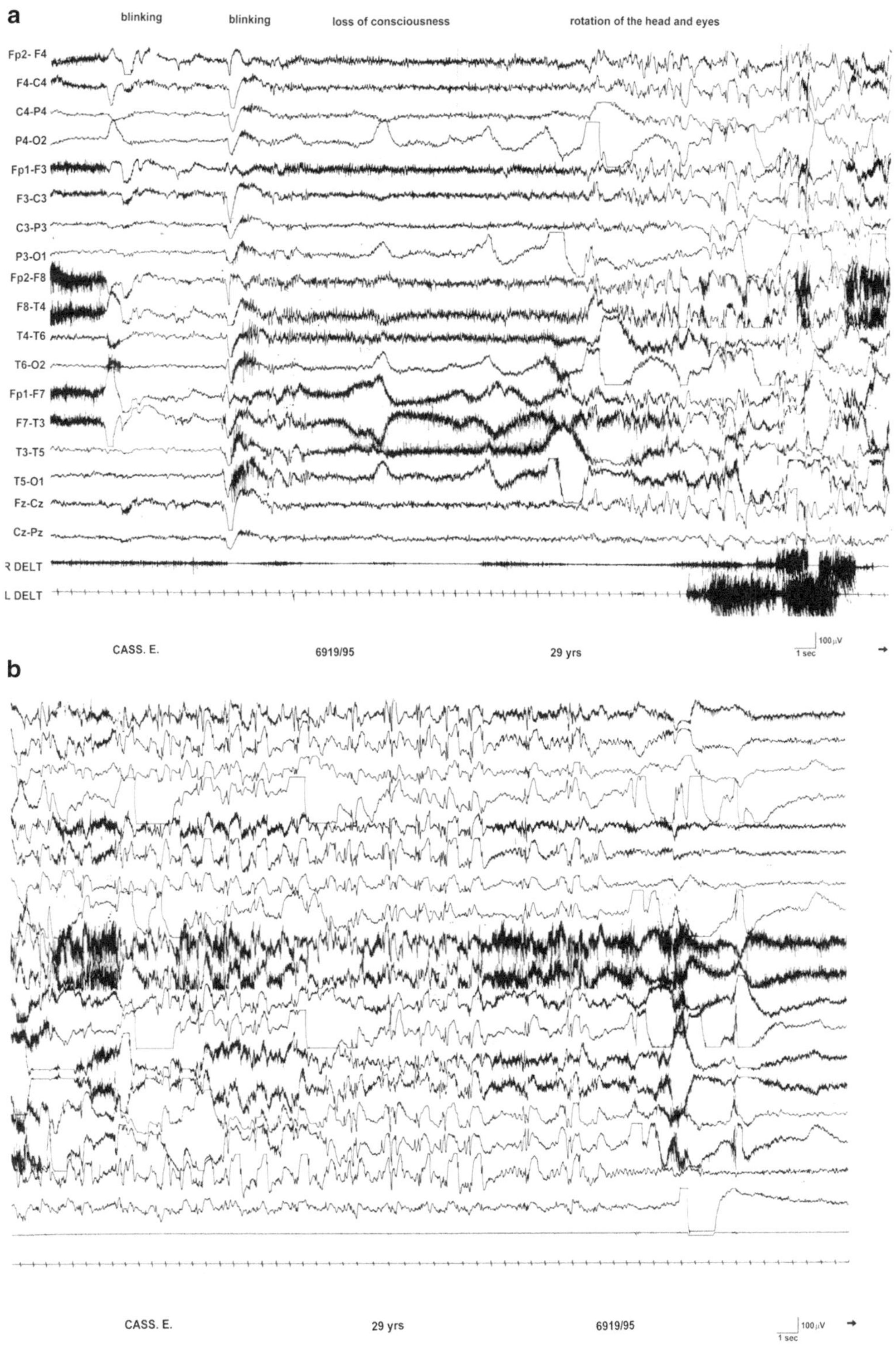

Fig. 33.11 (**a**, **b**) A 29-year-old female with inv. dup (15) syndrome. Ictal EEG is characterized by repetitive artifacts correlated with eye blinking, followed by diffuse desynchronization, and diffuse spikes (**a**) and spike-and-wave complexes (**b**). The patient presents loss of consciousness, generalized hypertonia, and head and eye deviation (*R* right, *L* left, *DELT* deltoid muscle)

nism of epileptogenesis in this syndrome is not well understood, since many of the patients have not deletions, and deleted genes are rather heterogenous. Alteration of gene expression derived from telomere position could be a possible explanation [47].

Interictal EEG—Slow waves, spikes, or spike-and-wave complexes most prominent over the fronto-central regions are often evident (Fig. 33.12). A peculiar EEG pattern, apparently subclinical, characterized by multifocal 5 Hz theta waves, mostly localized over the temporal regions, which persists after administration of diazepam intravenously [90]. More recently, a peculiar 3–7 Hz cortical rhythm has been found in ring chromosome 20 patients arising from the sensory-motor system [91].

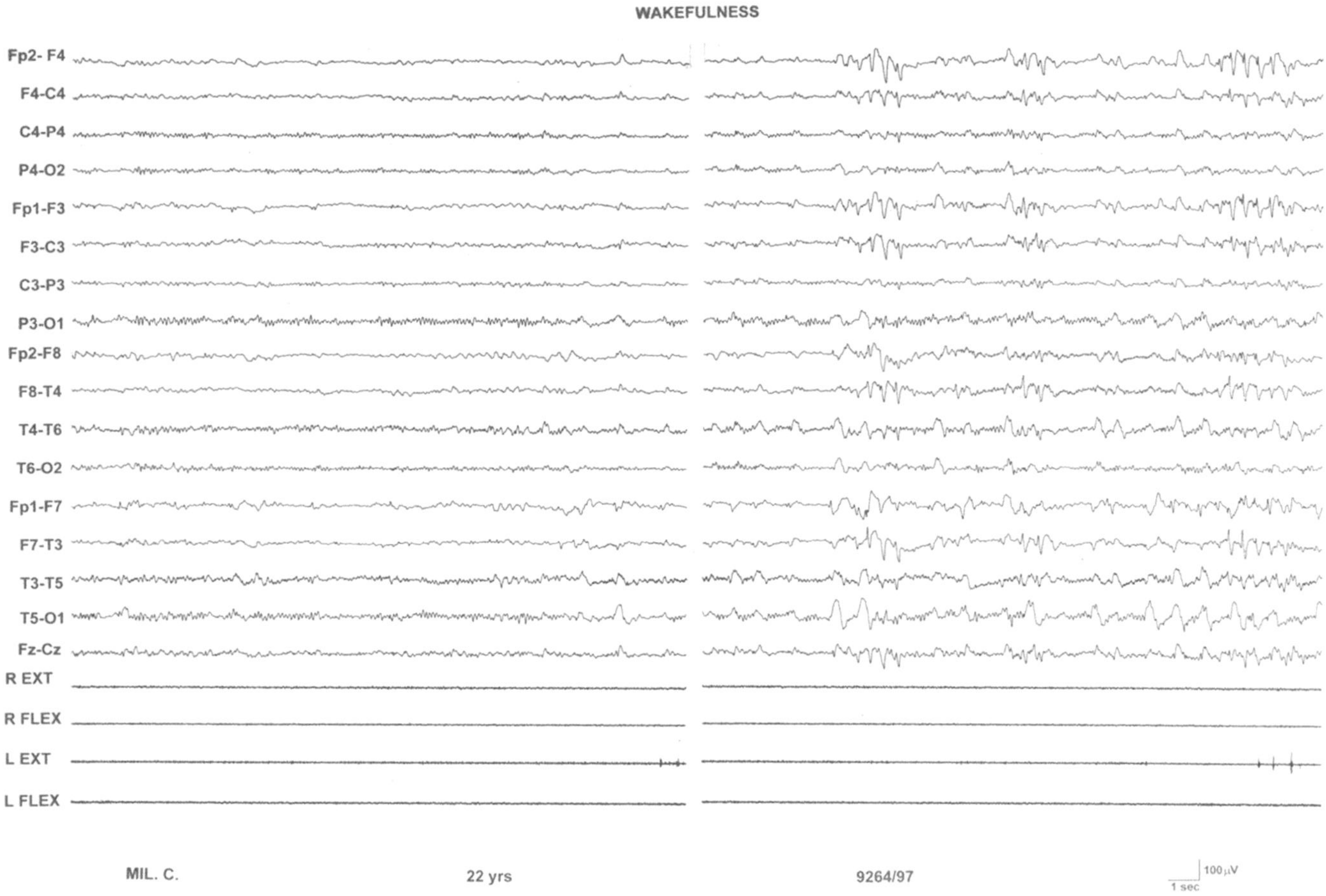

Fig. 33.12 A 22-year-old male with ring chromosome 20 syndrome. On the left side, wakefulness interictal EEG shows theta waves over the left temporal regions; on the right side, diffuse, repetitive sequences of theta waves and spike-and-wave complexes, prominent over the frontal regions of both hemispheres (*R* right, *L* left, *EXT* forearm extensor muscles, *FLEX* forearm flexor muscles)

The total duration of paroxysmal anomalies appeared significantly longer in patients (31–692 min) compared to controls (0–48 min) in a long-term EEG recording study [92].

Seizures and ictal EEG—Epilepsy, invariably drug-resistant, has an age-dependent course, and cognitive outcome is inversely correlated with age at seizure onset. When seizure onset occurs in childhood, terrifying hallucinations associated with focal motor seizures, often sleep-related, or dyscognitive seizures, are often the typical features, with a possible evolution in epileptic encephalopathy and non-convulsive status epilepticus [93, 94]. Subsequently, epilepsy is associated with non-convulsive status epilepticus, focal seizures with motor and autonomic features, and eyelid myoclonia [94]. Reflex seizures evoked by video games or by psychical stimuli have been sporadically reported [86, 95]. During non-convulsive status epilepticus, patients present a consciousness disturbance with bizarre or persevering behaviors, motor or verbal automatisms, fear, and perioral or eye myoclonia. The episodes of status occur daily or weekly and last also for hours [47, 87].

Ictal EEG is characterized by sequences of slow waves mixed with spikes, and spike-and-wave frequency can change during the episode (Fig. 33.13).

Drug-resistant frontal lobe seizures, recurrent non-convulsive status epilepticus, and characteristic EEG features represent a typical electroclinical triad which is specifically observed in all the patients with ring chromosome 20 syndrome [85].

Regarding treatment, there are no effective antiepileptic drugs for this epileptic syndrome, although valproate associated with lamotrigine was helpful in two children with non-convulsive status epilepticus. Vagal nerve stimulation was beneficial in one case [96].

33.1.12 Down Syndrome

Down syndrome (DS) or trisomy 21 is the commonest chromosome abnormality in subjects with ID, with an estimated prevalence of 1:800 live births. The phenotype is typical: ID of variable degree, short stature, muscle hypotonia, microceph-

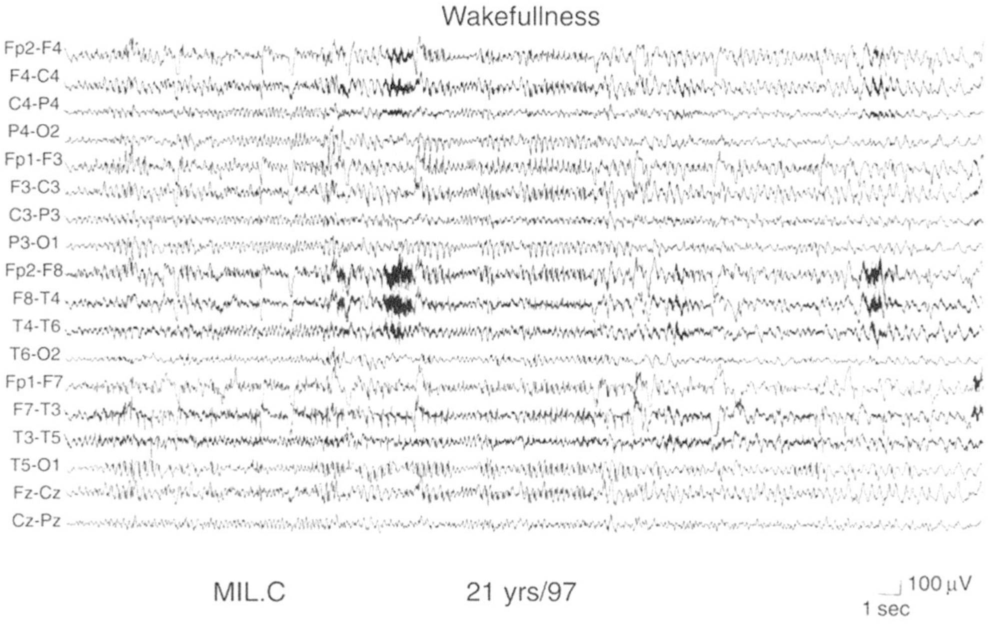

Fig. 33.13 The same patient of Fig. 33.12 at age 21 years. Ictal EEG, during nonconvulsive status epilepticus, characterized by sequences of slow waves intermixed with spikes; the frequency of the spike-and-wave complexes changes during the recording

aly, flat occiput, upslanting palpebral fissures, microtia, short neck, simian crease, and congenital heart malformations [47].

Trisomy 21 is due to a nondisjunction of chromosomes 21 during meiosis in 95% of cases; approximately 4% of patients present an unbalanced translocation and 1% a mosaicism; in a minimal percentage of cases, a duplication of the 21q22.3c critical region is present [59].

Gene imbalance in trisomy 21 determines developmental cell alterations in different tissues, such as the brevi and heart. Cortical gyri show a simplified pattern, and cytoarchitectural anomalies have been described, such as reduction of the GABAergic granular cells, lower neuronal density, delayed myelination, and dysgenesis of the dendritic spines [47].

Interictal EEG—Background activity is frequently slow, and bilateral hypsarrhythmia is evident in children with infantile spasms. Hypsarrhythmia reappears between spasms and clears after intravenous administration of diazepam, determining a pattern which is similar to that observed in idiopathic West syndrome (Fig. 33.14). In patients with Lennox-Gastaut syndrome, wakefulness EEG shows numerous slow waves mixed with spikes, prevalent over the frontal regions; during sleep, spike-and-wave complexes and polyspikes appear over the same regions [47, 59].

In adults, diffuse background slowing is the dominant EEG abnormality (60%). Epileptiform activity is present in 18% of cases, over the frontal, central, or temporal regions [97].

Seizures and ictal EEG—Seizures are present and heterogeneous in 10% of cases with DS [98]. In a large Italian cohort of patients with DS, 49% of subjects had infantile spasms, 33.7% had focal seizures, and 17.3% had generalized seizures. Febrile seizures were recorded in 4.8% subjects [99]. Patients with trisomy 21 may present a peculiar Lennox-Gastaut syndrome, characterized by late onset and high occurrence of reflex seizures, mostly precipitated by sudden unexpected sensory stimulations, usually preceding or accompanying the onset of the Lennox-Gastaut syndrome picture [100] (Fig. 33.15).

Some other cases have been reported with benign myoclonic epilepsy or with reflex seizures but without the features of the Lennox-Gastaut syndrome. The age at onset of spontaneous and reflex seizures tends to coincide in DS (2–24 years). Reflex seizures are evoked by different unexpected stimuli, their frequency is high. The same stimulus can evoke different types of seizures, such as atypical absences or tonic seizures [47, 59].

In adult patients with DS, a late myoclonic epilepsy with photosensitivity may appear, often associated with an Alzheimer-type dementia. At the EEG, myoclonic and generalized tonic-clonic seizures are recorded [47, 101, 102].

Outcome of seizures and response to treatment are strictly related to the type of epilepsy presented by the patients. In the majority of cases, myoclonic seizures are controlled by valproic acid or benzodiazepines; for drug-resistant infantile spasms, a short treatment with corticosteroids can be useful [47].

33.1.13 Fragile X Syndrome

The fragile X syndrome (FraXS) represents the most common familial form of ID known, affecting approximately 1:1500 males. Phenotype of FraXS includes ID, seizures, macroorchidism, large and prominent ears, narrow face, and signs of connective tissue dysplasia. A psychiatric phenotype is also recognizable in FraXS, with hyperactivity, language disorders, and autistic traits (i.e., tactile defensiveness, eye contact avoiding, stereotypies, hand biting, tantrums).

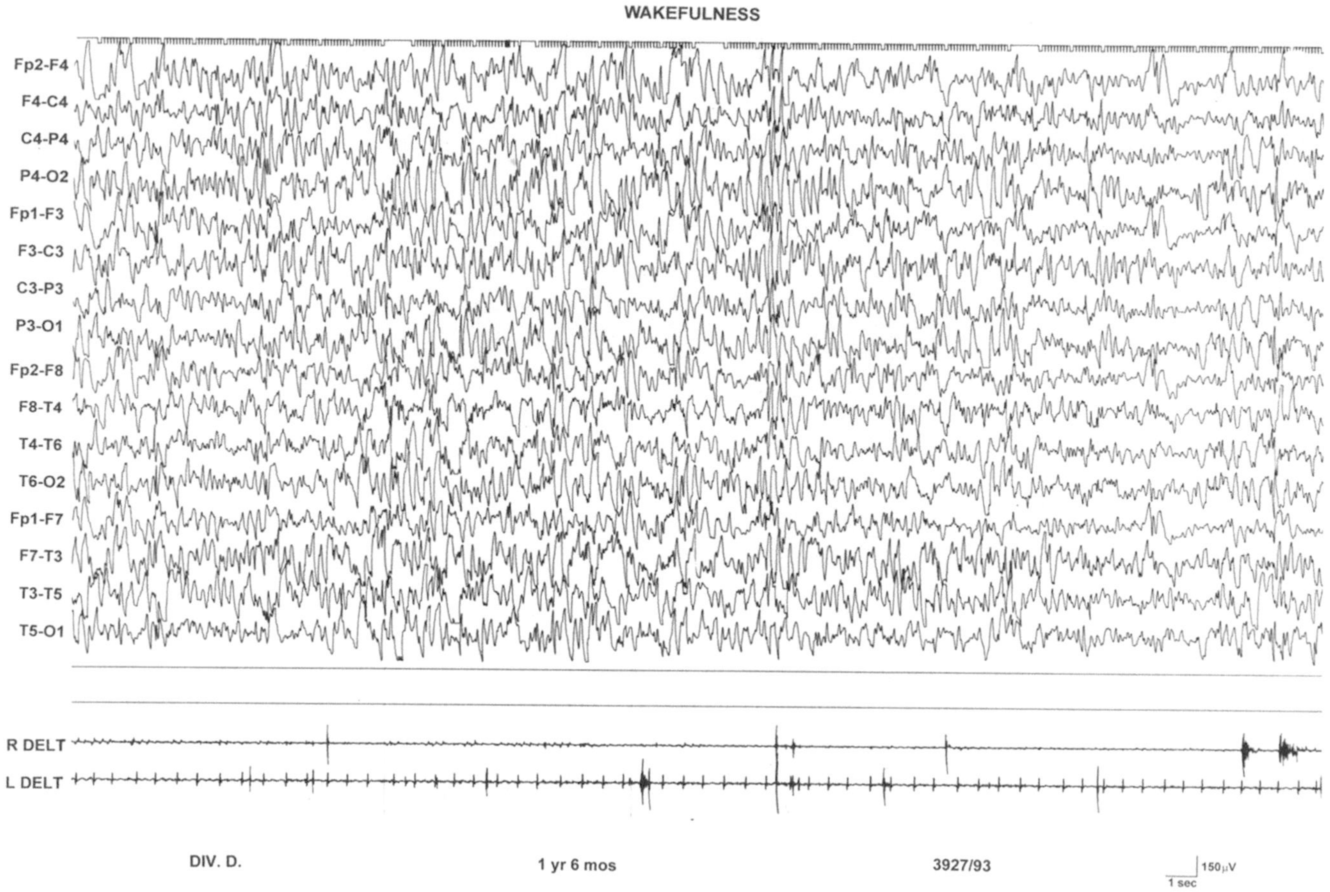

Fig. 33.14 A 1-year-old male with Down syndrome. Interictal EEG shows a hypsarrhythmic pattern (*R* right, *L* left, *DELT* deltoid muscle)

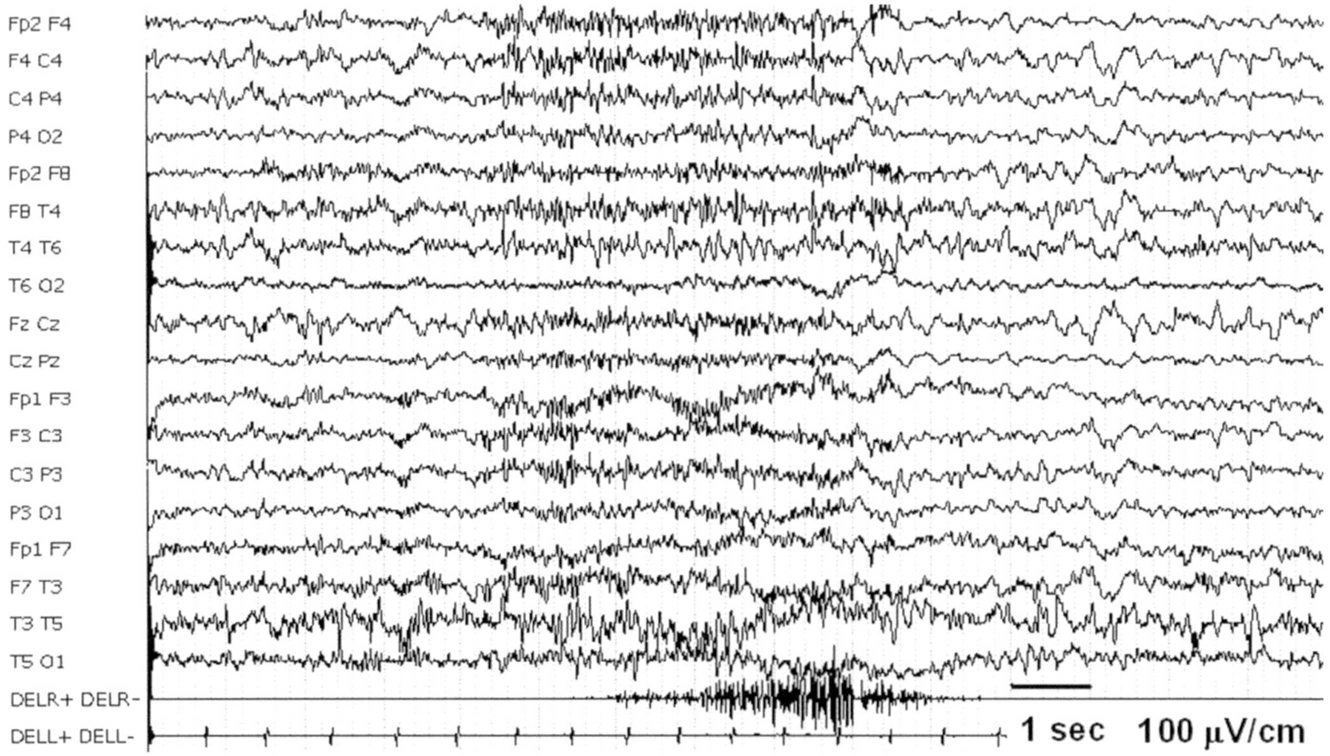

Fig. 33.15 A 43-year-old female with Down syndrome. Ictal EEG during sleep. The seizure is characterized by a diffuse fast activity discharge. At surface EMG of deltoid muscles, an asymmetrical tonic contraction, prevalent on the right side, is present (*R* right, *L* left, *DELT* deltoid muscle)

Originally, the demonstration of the fragile site at Xq27.3 region was dependent on the use of folate-deficient tissue culture media. More recently, molecular genetic studies revealed that FraXS results from a mutation in a (CGG) repeat in the FMR1 gene. In normal subjects, FMR1 allele contains 6–52 copies of the CGG repeat; in patients with FraXS, ≥200 repeats are present, and this determines the transcriptional silencing of the gene and the absence of the FMR protein (full mutation). An intermediate range of CGG repeats (50–200) characterizes the premutation status [47, 103].

The main neuropathologic findings in FraXS are abnormally long and thin cortical dendrites and abnormal dendrite spine morphology [104]. Furthermore, an abnormally enlarged hippocampal volume has been found in FraXS patients at MRI [105].

An increased susceptibility to audiogenic seizures is present in FraX knockout mice at all the ages tested, and these results support the validity of this animal model also for epilepsy and seizures in the human FraXS [106]. In addition, the introduction of the human FMR1 gene in knockout mice is able to revert the epileptic phenotype [107].

This evidence in the animal model and the presence of giant somatosensory evoked potentials (SEPs) in patients with FraXS seem indicate a relationship between FMR protein (FMRP) absence and cortical hyperexcitability [108]. FMRP may have a role in mRNA regulation in dendrites. Dendritic spines are longer and more frequently present an immature morphology in the pyramidal cells of the V stratum of the visual cortex in FMR1 knockout mice, mossy fibers of the hippocampal dentate gyrus have an altered distribution, GluR1 receptor cortical expression is depressed, and long-term potentiation is reduced [109–112]. A reduced number of mGlu5 receptors are tightly linked to the constituents of postsynaptic density and, in particular, to the constitutive forms of Homer proteins, with possible consequent alterations in synaptic plasticity [113].

Interictal EEG—Background activity is normal or slow, and a peculiar EEG pattern characterized by multifocal spikes, prevalently localized over the centro-temporal regions, is evident in approximately 40–50% of cases. These paroxysmal abnormalities appear at 3–4 years of age and persist up to 12–13 years, with a marked activation in NREM sleep (Fig. 33.16). In a retrospective and prospective study on 193 patients with FraXS, this EEG pattern was, respectively, found in 43.5% and 48% of cases at all ages, in 50.3% and 52% of subjects younger than 12 years. Spikes tended to disappear in adulthood, and if present, they were usually nonspecific [114].

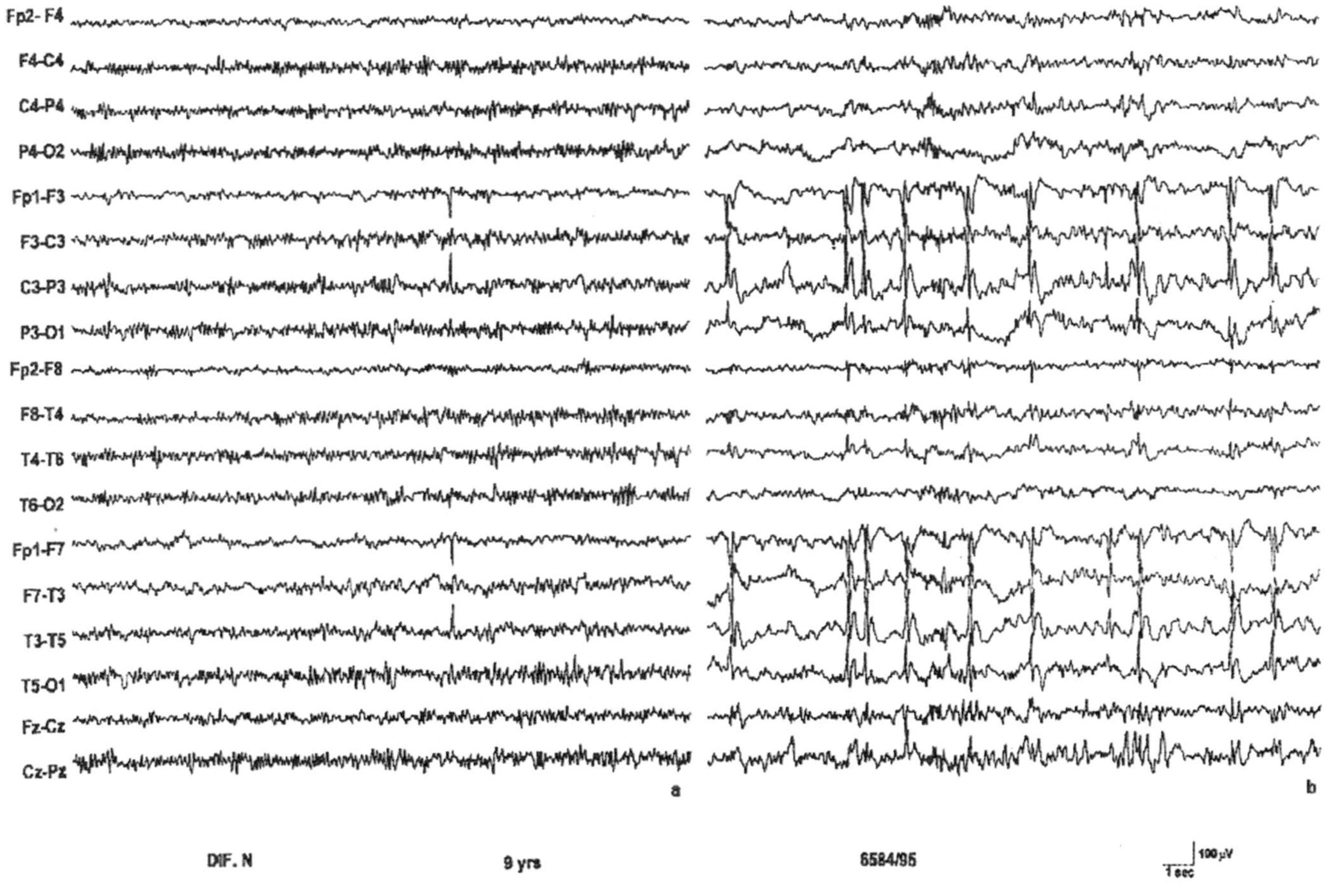

Fig. 33.16 A 9-year-old male with fragile X syndrome. On the left side, wakefulness EEG shows a single high-voltage spike localized over the right centro-temporal regions; on the right side, during sleep, there is a marked activation of paroxysmal abnormalities over the same regions

Seizures and ictal EEG—Ictal EEG figures of FraXS have never been published in literature. The prevalence of seizures ranges between 17 and 30%, respectively, in a retrospective and prospective population. The age at onset is between 2 and 9 years. Focal seizures with unawareness (originating from frontal or temporal lobes) predominate (>85%), in respect to other types of seizures, such as generalized tonic-clonic seizures or focal seizure without loss of consciousness [114]. Nine patients with FraXS and status epilepticus have been reported [115].

The choice of the antiepileptic drug depends from the type of epilepsy or seizures. At least 80% of patients reach a good control of seizures.

33.1.14 Klinefelter Syndrome

Klinefelter syndrome (KS) is a relatively common genetic condition characterized by mild or moderate ID, behavior disturbances, infertility, tall stature, long limbs, hypogonadism, ginecomasty, and reduced hair. The estimated prevalence is around 1.7:1000 males. The abnormality consists of a meiotic nondisjunction of sexual chromosomes, which determines the presence of one or more supplementary X chromosomes. The mosaic forms derive from a post-zygotic nondisjunction of X chromosomes [47, 59].

Neuropathology is not specific, and only one case with polymicrogyria and megalencephaly has been reported [116].

Interictal EEG—Background activity can be slow, and focal or generalized paroxysms are present (Figs. 33.17 and 33.18).

Seizures and ictal EEG—Seizures are present in 2–10% of cases. Generalized seizures are more frequent than focal ones, with atypical absences, generalized tonic-clonic seizures. One case with West syndrome has been described [117]. Seizures are easily controlled by therapy [47, 118, 119].

33.1.15 Xp11.22–11.23 Duplication Syndrome

A group of nine subjects with a microduplication at Xp11.22–11.23 has been identified at a diagnostic genome array screening of 2400 subjects with ID. The duplication was either familial or sporadic. The phenotype is characterized by a cognitive disturbance (from borderline functioning to severe ID), speech delay, poor speech articulation, hoarse and/or nasal voice, early puberty, overweight, nonspecific facial dysmorphic features, and lower-extremity anomalies, including flat or arched feet, fifth-toe hypoplasia, and syndactyly. Neuroimaging does not show specific abnormalities [120].

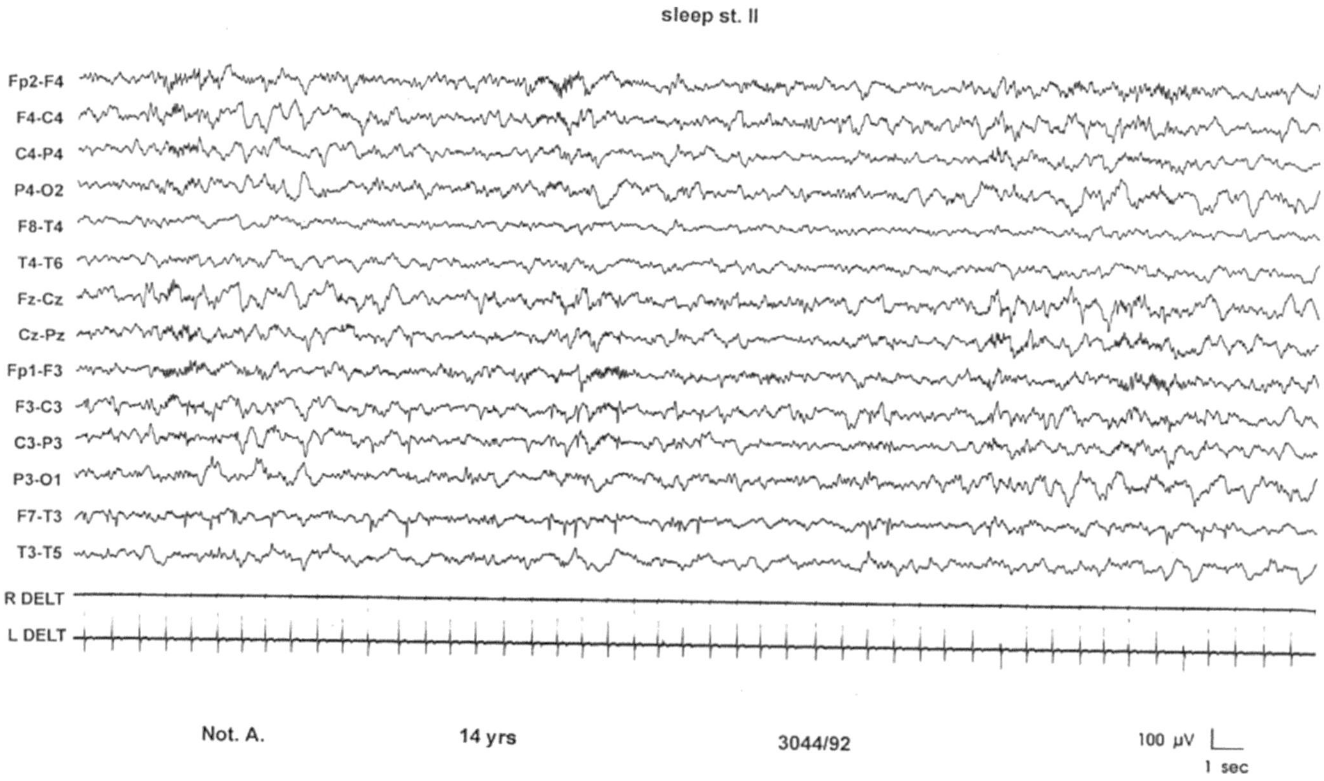

Fig. 33.17 A 14-year-old male with Klinefelter syndrome. During sleep EEG, focal spikes are recorded over the left fronto-centro-temporal regions and vertex (*R* right, *L* left, *DELT* deltoid muscle)

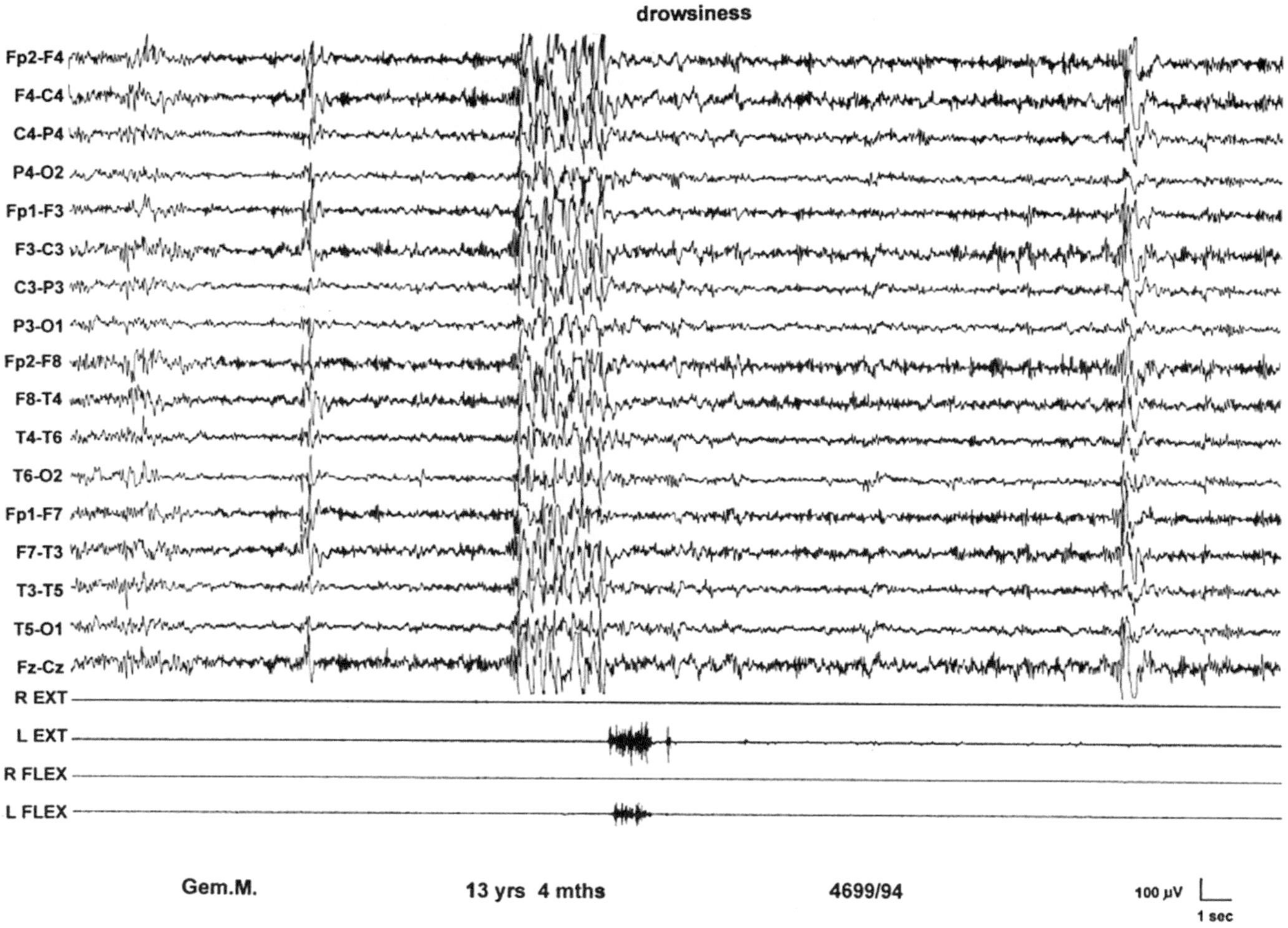

Fig. 33.18 A 13-year-old male with Klinefelter syndrome. EEG during drowsiness presents numerous diffuse spikes and spike-and-waves (*R* right, *L* left, *EXT* forearm extensor muscles, *FLEX* forearm flexor muscles)

Xp11.2 is a gene-rich, rearrangement-prone region within the critical linkage interval for several neurogenetic disorders harboring X-linked mental retardation (MRX) genes which could be responsible for the syndrome phenotype [121].

Interictal EEG—A study contributed to better define the neurological phenotype of this new syndrome [120]. Electrical status epilepticus during sleep (ESES) was present in five of nine patients, particularly in younger ones (from 5 to 13 years), and was associated with speech delay in all cases. ESES was controlled by antiepileptic drugs in three out of five patients; the other two patients remained untreated.

Seizures and ictal EEG—Epilepsy was reported in about one third of cases, with different types of seizures starting in infancy or in childhood, such as clonic jerks of the limbs and staring, generalized tonic-clonic seizures during sleep, and absences. Outcome was favorable [120].

33.1.16 XYY Syndrome

The XYY syndrome is characterized by an extra copy of the Y chromosome, with an incidence of 1:1000 males. Males with 47, XYY syndrome are sometimes taller than average and have a variable risk of cognitive, language, and behavioral deficits. Neuroimaging is generally normal in the cases reported [122].

Interictal EEG—In a series of four patients with XYY, EEG background activity was normal; focal EEG profile showed rolandic-like focal paroxysms localized over the vertex area or over central-temporal regions, markedly activated during sleep; these EEG traits were independent of the presence or not of seizures. However, other cases with slow background activity, with generalized or multifocal paroxysmal abnormalities, and with hypsarrythmia have been described [122].

Seizures and ictal EEG—Seizures, when present, may present features such as age of onset, clinical characteristic evolution, and good response to antiepileptic drugs, which are very similar to those of rolandic epilepsy [122].

33.2 Cortical Malformations

Malformations of cortical development represent another group of etiologies that can determine neurodevelopmental disorders and epilepsy in the first years of life. They are characterized by a wide spectrum of syndromes. There are very severe conditions that present with marked delay of psychomotor development and early and drug-resistant seizures but also milder clinical pictures that are discovered late, often after the occurrence of seizures in subjects without neurological signs.

Recently, the advances in the technology of noninvasive neuroimaging techniques, such as high-field MRI, facilitated diagnosis and structural and topographic classification of these syndromes.

Cortical malformations may occur as sporadic or familial forms. Genetic studies, i.e., Sanger sequencing, next-generation sequencing (NGS), and whole exome or genome sequencing (WES, WGS), allowed to discover a great number of genes regulating the development of the CNS.

Here, I will describe the main cortical malformative syndromes, focusing special attention to the specific interictal and ictal EEG pictures. They are classically distinguished taking into account the different phases of the intrauterine CNS development in which they occur: malformations secondary to abnormal neuronal and glial proliferation or apoptosis (tuberous sclerosis complex, focal cortical dysplasias type II, hemimegalencephaly); malformations due to abnormal neuronal migration (lissencephaly, subcortical band heterotopia, periventricular nodular heterotopia); and malformations secondary to abnormal postmigrational development (schizencephaly, polymicrogyria, focal cortical dysplasias type I and III).

33.2.1 Tuberous Sclerosis Complex

Tuberous sclerosis complex (TSC) is a neurocutaneous syndrome involving the CNS, retina, skin, kidney, heart, and lungs with an estimated prevalence ranging from 1:30,000 to 1:50,000. The characteristic cerebral lesions are represented by the cortical tubers, the subependymal nodules, and the giant cell tumors. Cortical tubers, highly epileptogenic, often multiple, are hamartomas easily recognizable at MRI, as enlarged gyri with an atypical form and with an altered signal intensity (Fig. 33.19) [123–125].

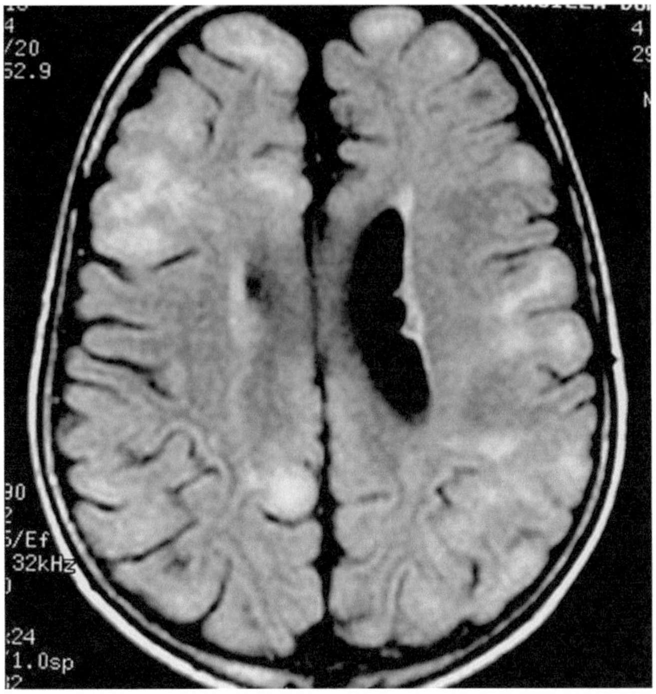

Fig. 33.19 Brain MRI of a 4-year-old male with tuberous sclerosis. Numerous cortical tubers are present over both hemispheres

TSC can occur in a sporadic or familial way, and in this case, it has autosomal dominant inheritance. TSC is caused by mutations of the TSC1 (tuberin) or TSC2 (hamartin) genes, respectively, localized in the 9q34 and 16p13.3 regions. The TSC1-TSC2 protein complex integrates cues from growth factors, the cell cycle, and nutrients to regulate the activity of mammalian target of rapamycin (mTOR), p70S6 kinase (S6K), 4E-BP1, and ribosomal S6 proteins. Mutations leading to loss of function of the TSC1 or TSC2 genes result in enhanced Rheb-GTP signaling and consequent mTOR activation, causing increased cell growth, ribosome biogenesis, and mRNA translation; the result is overgrowth of normal cells and production of abnormal cells in many organs [126].

Approximately 50% of the familial cases are caused by TSC1 mutations; among sporadic cases, TSC2 mutations are present in about 50% of cases, and TSC1 mutations are found in 10% of cases. Somatic mosaicism is present in 8–15% of cases.

Studies on genotype-phenotype correlation suggested that TSC1 mutations are usually correlated with a milder clinical picture: lower frequency of seizures, minor cognitive dysfunction, minor number of tubers and subependymal nodules, and milder impairment of the kidney, retina, and skin [123–125].

Interictal EEG—When EEG is recorded between the neonatal period and the seizure onset, focal or multifocal

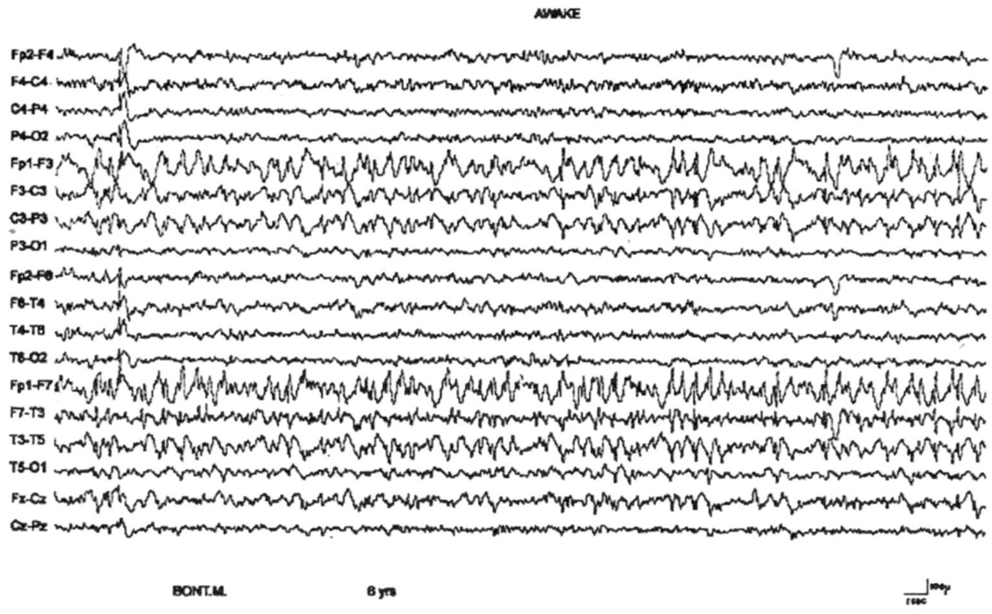

Fig. 33.20 A 6-year-old male with tuberous sclerosis. Wakefulness EEG shows quasi-continuous sharp waves and spikes over the left fronto-central-temporal (correlated with the localization of a large cortical tuber)

paroxysmal abnormalities are evident. Children with infantile spasms show a wakefulness EEG characterized by multifocal paroxysms, with the morphology of high-voltage spikes and irregular slow waves, at 2–3 Hz, sometimes with a typical hypsarrhythmic pattern.

Subsequently, this pattern tends to disappear, and interictal EEG shows only focal or multifocal spikes or slow waves (Fig. 33.20).

These paroxysms are localized over the temporal or occipital regions at first, often correlated with the tubers, but after 2 years of age, they can be observed also over the frontal regions.

NREM sleep is characterized by activation of paroxysmal abnormalities. They become generalized in the evolution and synchronous polyspike-and-wave discharges, sometimes followed by short abrupt flattenings are evident. Spindle can be poorly recognizable (Fig. 33.21). During REM sleep, epileptiform activity is less frequent, and diffuse paroxysms tend to disappear.

In some patients, interictal EEG is seen in Lennox-Gastaut syndrome, but this pattern actually could be the evolution of a frontal epilepsy to a secondary generalization [123, 124].

Seizures and ictal EEG—Seizures are polymorphous: infantile spasms in 50% of cases, but also tonic seizures, focal seizures, atypical absences, and generalized tonic-clonic seizures. They start before 15 months of age. In about one third of cases, prognosis is severe. A correlation between number and size of tubers and severity of epilepsy has been proposed.

Infantile spasms, at EEG, are characterized by a focal discharge of spikes or polyspikes originating from central, temporal, or occipital regions, followed by irregular diffuse slow waves and by a sudden desynchronization of the background activity. Paroxysmal activity disappears during the cluster of spasms and re-emerges at the end (Fig. 33.22).

It is possible to identify three different clinical and EEG phenotypes of epilepsy in TSC.

1. Onset with spasms or focal seizures; spasms may present a focal component (unilateral or bilateral with eye deviation or eye myoclonias) or may be "pseudoperiodic," in clusters lasting also many minutes; they can evolve in tonic seizures with a focal component.
2. An epileptic encephalopathy from the onset; the background activity is slow with quasi-continuous diffuse or multifocal paroxysmal abnormalities during wakefulness and sleep; seizures are polymorphous, frequent, and drug-resistant.
3. A focal epilepsy, with variable frequency of rather stereotyped seizures (Fig. 33.23) [123, 124].

Treatment of seizures in TSC depends from the specific clinical and EEG aspects of epilepsy.

Among the new antiepileptic drugs, vigabatrin demonstrated the higher efficacy in the treatment of infantile spasms associated to TSC. Response to vigabatrin is much quicker than that observed with steroids, benzodiazepines, and valproic acid; however, focal seizures can persist after the disappearance of spasms. However, the high risk of visual field alterations limits the use of this drug. Lamotrigine determines a seizure reduction higher than 50–80% of cases. Its efficacy is prolonged, but responders prevalently belong to the group of patients with focal seizures. Felbamate may be helpful, but it determines a risk of severe aplastic anemia. Also topiramate has been successfully used in patients with focal seizures with or without secondary generalization [123].

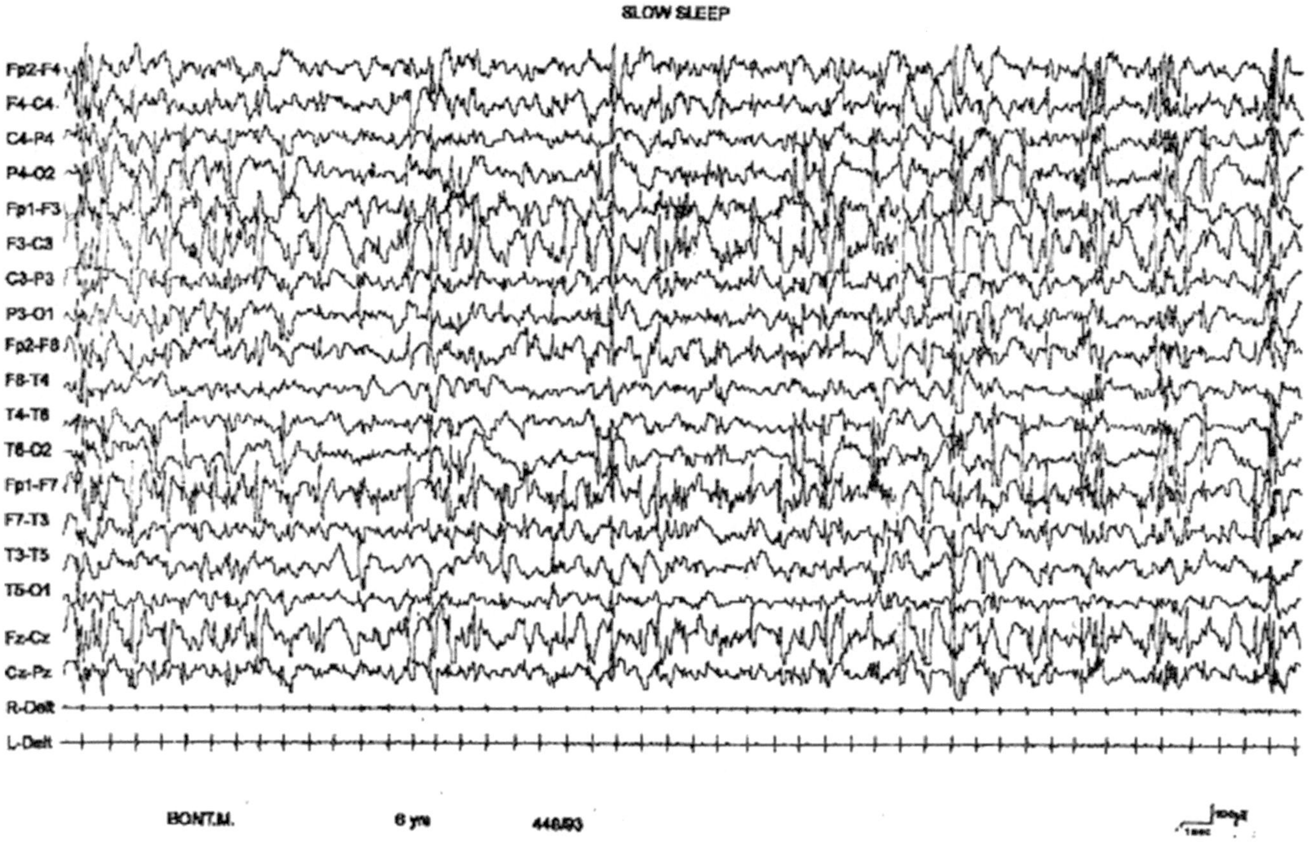

Fig. 33.21 The same subject of Fig. 33.20. During sleep, paroxysmal abnormalities become quasi- continuous over both hemispheres (*R* right, *L* left, *DELT* deltoid muscle)

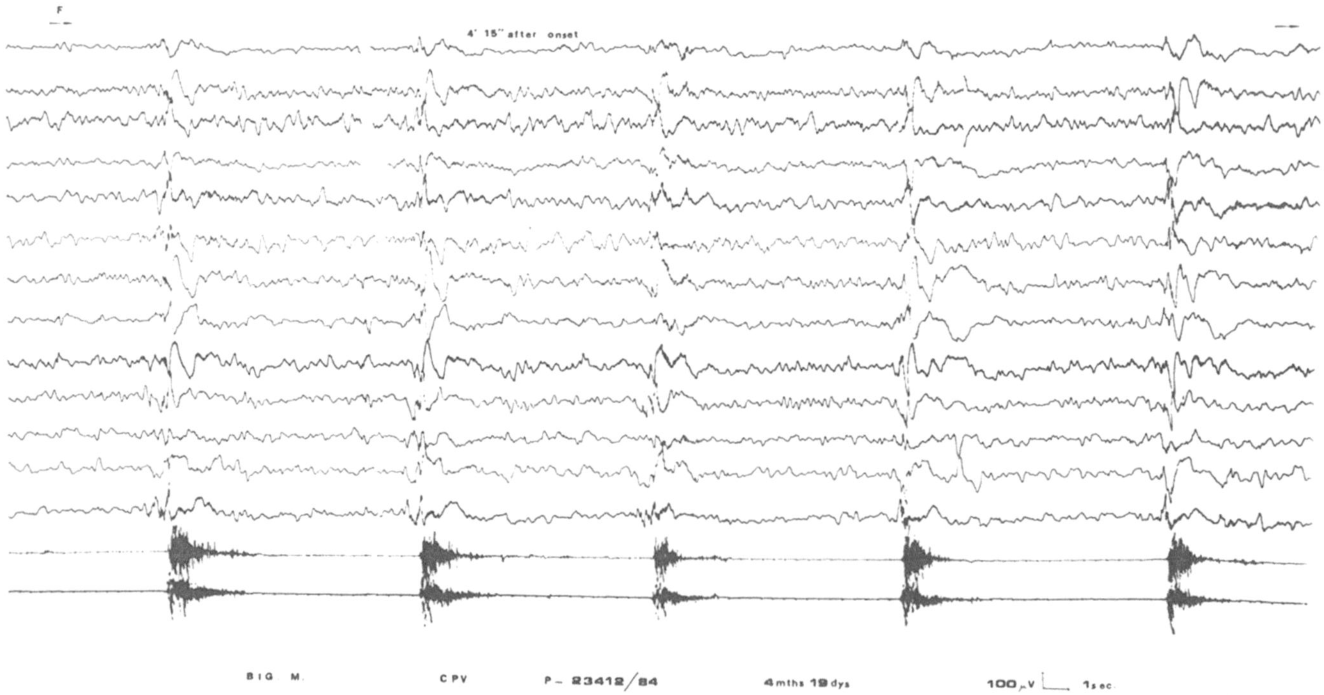

Fig. 33.22 Male at 4 months of age with tuberous sclerosis. Ictal EEG shows a long series of spasms which interrupts hypsarrhythmia. Spasms are characterized by repetitive synchronous and symmetrical muscle contractions, corresponding to high-voltage diffuse slow complexes at the EEG

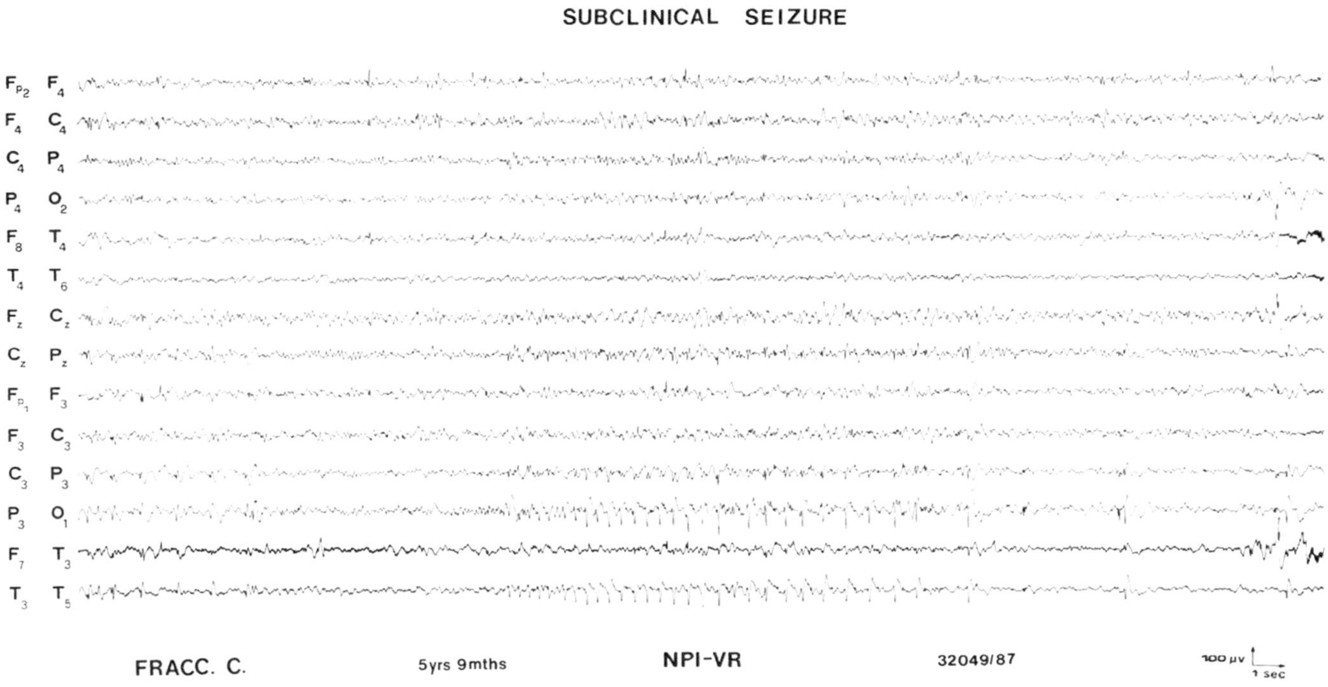

Fig. 33.23 A 5-year-old female with tuberous sclerosis. A subclinical focal seizure, characterized by rhythmical spikes, is recorded over the left temporo-occipital regions

Multimodality imaging, including MRI scans, positron emission tomography, and magnetoencephalography, has been used to localize epileptogenic tubers and peritubular regions. Surgical resection of epileptogenic foci has yielded excellent results: seizures have been stopped in 57% of drug-resistant patients. If antiepileptic drugs fail and no clear epileptogenic tuber is identified, alternative therapies, such as ketogenic diet, and vagus nerve stimulation can be considered [125].

There is now also particular interest in the potential role of mTOR inhibitors in treating seizures, neurodevelopmental disabilities, and other extra-neurological manifestations of TSC. Although no mTOR inhibitors are currently indicated specifically for the treatment of seizures associated with TSC, the results of some studies suggest that sirolimus and everolimus may be effective [127].

33.2.2 Focal Cortical Dysplasias Type II

The new classification supports the classification of focal cortical dysplasias (FCDs) type II as a malformation due to abnormal proliferation. FCDs type II are malformations presenting with disrupted cortical lamination and specific cytologic abnormalities, which differentiate FCDs type IIa (dysmorphic neurons without balloon cells) and FCDs type IIb (dysmorphic neurons and balloon cells).

FCDs type IIa are rarely detected at MRI. FCDs type IIb are often characterized by hypo-, de-, or dysmyelination (blurring) in the subcortical white matter. The white matter signal alterations frequently taper from a gyrus or a sulcus toward the ventricle, reflecting the involvement of radial glial-neuronal units. This is named "transmantle sign" and is almost exclusively found in FCD type IIb [128].

Using WES in blood, saliva and brain biopsy specimens from FCD type II patients, somatic mutations of mTOR, and other five genes involved in mTOR pathways (PIK3CA, PIK3R2, AKT3, TSC1, and TSC2) were identified. In addition to somatic mutations, also germline mutations of DEP domain containing 5 (DEPDC5), nitrogen permease regulator-like 3 (NPRL3), and TSC1 genes have been associated with FCDs type II [129].

Interictal EEG—In FCDs type IIb, stereo-EEG, subdural and epidural, and sometimes surface recordings are characterized by total absence of background activity and a distinctive pattern of repetitive, high amplitude, fast spikes, followed by high amplitude slow waves, interspersed with relatively flat periods. Sometimes, also repetitive bursts of low-amplitude high-frequency oscillations intermixed with flat periods can be recorded. During sleep, fast spikes become more evident, activated in frequency, and spread into contiguous nonlesional areas. During REM sleep, these paroxysms are markedly reduced [128].

Seizures and ictal EEG—Seizure presentation is age and location related. In a recent study, six different ictal patterns were described in FCDs. In FCDs type II, the most prevalent resulted pattern 3 (burst of polyspikes followed by low-voltage fast activity, LVFA), pattern 1 (LVFA), and pattern 2 (preictal spiking followed by LVFA). Better postsurgical outcome is associated with patterns including LVFA [130].

Seizures are often drug-resistant. Pathogenic mutations of mTOR genes open the way to new treatment options with mTOR inhibitors. The ketogenic diet can be effective. Surgery and neurostimulation techniques, such as vagus nerve stimulation, have demonstrated variable clinical outcomes [131].

33.2.3 Hemimegalencephaly

Hemimegalencephaly (HME) is a rare cortical malformation characterized by the enlargement of one cerebral hemisphere, associated with developmental delay, contralateral hemiplegia, and severe epilepsy with onset in the first months of life. It can be isolated or syndromic, in Proteus syndrome, neurofibromatosis, hypomelanosis of Ito, Klippel-Weber-Trenaunay syndrome, TSC, and linear sebaceous nevus syndrome.

An abnormal gyral pattern (pachygyria, polygyria, or polymicrogyria), as well as increased thickness of the cortex of the enlarged hemisphere are present at neuropathology or neuroimaging.

The similarities in neuropathology between HME, FCD type II, and TSC strongly suggest a pathogenic link between these malformations, leading to the introduction of the common term of "mTORopathies."

De novo somatic mutations in PIK3CA, AKT3, and MTOR, encoding regulators of the mTOR signaling pathway, have been reported, and recent studies reported pathogenic germline and mosaic mutations in multiple phosphatidylinositol 3-kinase (PI3K)-AKT3-mTOR signaling genes (i.e., DEPDC5, PIK3CA, mTOR, and TSC2) [132].

Interictal EEG—Three different EEG patterns have been described: (1) triphasic complexes of very large voltage characterized by a small negative wave, followed by a large amplitude, positive slow spike, and a very slow wave, which formed a "plateau," often associated with a monomorphic, sharp theta activity; (2) an asymmetrical suppression-burst pattern, with bursts of "alpha-like" activity interrupted by hypoactive phases on the affected hemisphere and high-voltage bursts of polymorphous polyspikes on the unaffected side; and (3) a large amplitude asymmetrical "alpha-like" activity, at 7–12 Hz, scarcely modified by waking state. "Alpha-like" pattern was associated with a relatively favorable outcome than triphasic complexes; prognostic significance of the suppression-burst was less clear [133].

Seizures and ictal EEG—Seizures have a very early onset, also in neonatal age. Semiology is characterized by repeated tonic seizures in series, usually asymmetric because of a greater involvement of the side contralateral to the brain malformation, associated with homolateral eye deviation; they can be preceded by short, clonic, unilateral jerks. Also atonic seizures, spasms, and myoclonic jerks can be observed. In one case, ictal EEG was characterized by focal theta activity followed by isolated periodic high-voltage diffuse triphasic delta wave complexes. In a neonate, epileptic negative myoclonus has been recorded. In the evolution, epilepsy can assume a picture resembling Ohtahara syndrome before, usually after the third month of life, then can present electroclinical features typical of West and Lennox-Gastaut syndrome, finally a focal epilepsy or epilepsia partialis continua is evident.

Seizures are almost invariably resistant to antiepileptic drugs, and early surgery is needed to remove or functionally disconnect the epileptogenic area within the affected hemisphere, in order to control seizures, protect the healthy hemisphere from damage, and prevent cognitive impairment [132, 134–136].

33.2.4 Lissencephaly

Classical lissencephaly (LIS) represents a very severe neurodevelopmental disorders due to a rare abnormality of neuronal migration occurring between the 12th and 16th week of pregnancy, determining a smooth and thickened cortex constituted by four layers instead of six layers (agyria-pachygyria, Fig. 33.24). Miller-Dieker syndrome (MDS) is a LIS accompanied by profound ID, often by the absence of

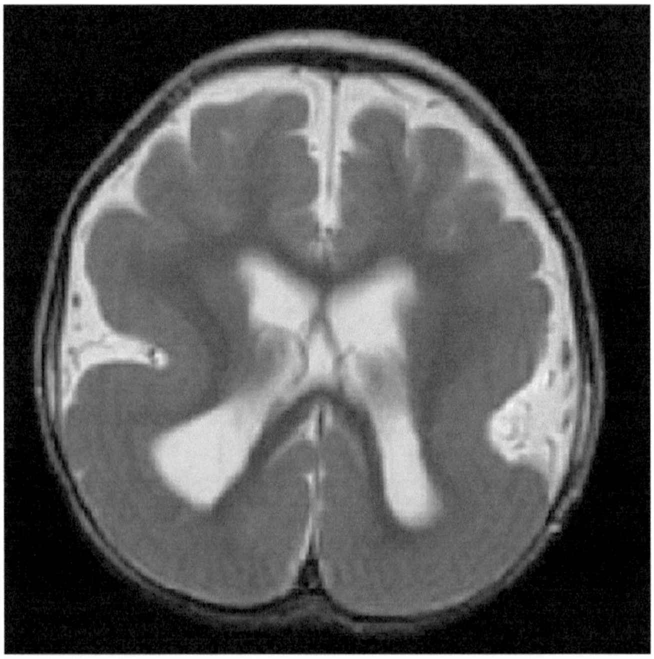

Fig. 33.24 Brain MRI of a 4-year-old male with lissencephaly (TUBA1A mutation). The typical posterior-to-anterior gradient of agyria-pachygyria

psychomotor milestones, and facial dysmorphisms such as bitemporal narrowing, short nose, prominent upper lip, and jaw hypoplasia [137].

In the 17p13.3 region, the LIS1 (PAFAH1B1) gene has been identified, and it codifies for an enzyme regulating the platelet-activating factor (PAF). LIS1 gene plays an important role in stabilizing neuronal microtubules which intervene in the CNS development. Approximately 65% of patients with LIS present a LIS1 mutation (deletion of the entire gene in 40% of cases, intragenic mutation in 25% of cases). Missense mutations are correlated with a milder phenotype than truncating mutations or deletions. Mutations of the doublecortin gene (DCX or XLIS) determine LIS in males and subcortical band heterotopia (SBH) in females. Lissencephaly is prevalently posterior in patients with LIS1 mutations, anterior in those with DCX mutations. MDS is caused by large deletions of LIS1 gene, and sometimes of two other genes, CRK and YWHAE, in approximately 92% of cases [137–139].

Another form of lissencephaly in males is X-linked lissencephaly with corpus callosum agenesis and ambiguous genitalia (XLAG). The anatomoclinical picture is characterized by agyria-pachygyria with posterior-to-anterior gradient, mild thickening of the cerebral cortex (6–7 mm versus 15–20 mm observed in LIS or DCX-associated lissencephaly), the absence of the corpus callosum, poorly delineated and capitate basal ganglia, postnatal microcephaly, early onset epilepsy, hypothalamic dysfunction, chronic diarrhea, and ambiguous genitalia. XLAG has been associated with mutations of the aristaless-related homeobox (ARX) gene [137].

Autosomal recessive lissencephaly with abnormalities of the cerebellum, hippocampus, and brainstem represents a further subtype, due to mutations of reelin (RELN) gene mapping in the 7q22 region and codifying for a protein which controls cell interactions and positioning during CNS development [137].

Finally, mutations of the tubulin α -1A (TUBA1A) gene have been found in patients with lissencephaly (posterior-to-anterior gradient), associated to other abnormalities of hippocampus, corpus callosum, internal capsula, and brainstem [137, 140–142].

Interictal EEG—In LIS, a characteristic EEG pattern, with unusually diffuse high-voltage fast rhythms, has been described from the first year of age. This activity can be alternated with theta e delta rhythms (Fig. 33.25) [143]. The EEG may not show typical hypsarrhythmia [137].

More recently, three distinct EEG patterns have been described in LIS patients: (1) diffuse bi-hemispheric

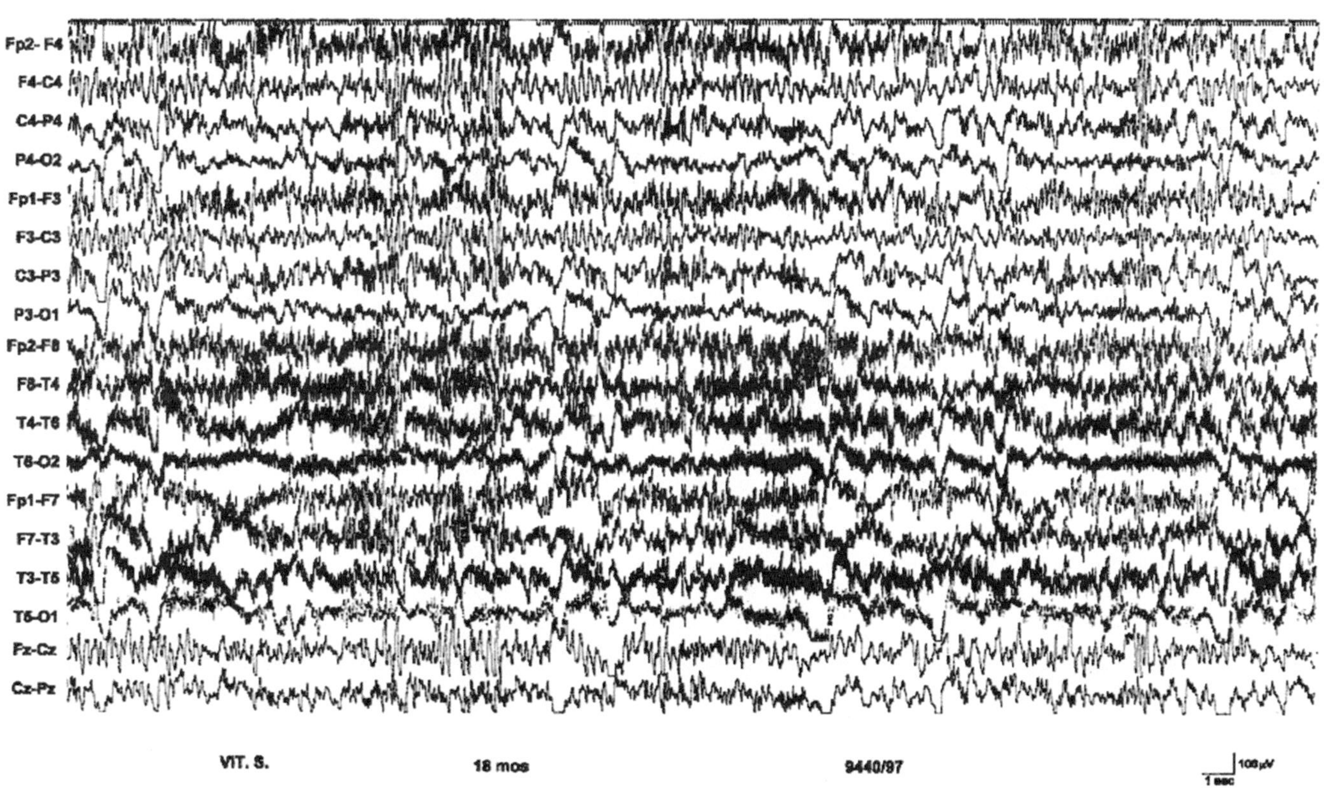

Fig. 33.25 Male at 18 months of age with isolated lissencephaly. Wakefulness EEG reveals a diffuse high-voltage theta activity, prominent over the anterior regions

distribution of high-voltage 8 Hz alpha with intermingled 14–16 Hz beta activity; (2) diffuse bi-hemispheric distribution of high-voltage rather sharp 1.5–2.5 Hz slow waves, with amplitude fluctuations of cortical activity; and (3) very high-voltage generalized 1–1.5 Hz sharp waves [144].

Seizures and ictal EEG—In LIS, seizures, present in more than 90% of cases, usually start before 6 months of age and are polymorphous: more often spasms, but also tonic-clonic, myoclonic, focal, tonic, or atonic seizures and atypical absences (Figs. 33.26, 33.27, and 33.28) [137, 145, 146].

In XLAG tonic, multifocal myoclonic and generalized tonic-clonic seizures have been reported with a very early onset [147].

In patients with TUBA1A mutations, epilepsy presents with infantile spasms or astatic-myoclonic seizures early on, evolving to atypical absences, myoclonic and atonic drop seizures, focal seizures, and tonic and tonic-clonic seizures in later childhood [142].

Outcome is very poor regarding epilepsy which is almost intractable, since reduction of seizures can be obtained with old and new antiepileptic drugs (phenobarbital, valproate, lamotrigine) and with corticosteroids [146]. Death occurs in the majority of cases before adult age.

33.2.5 Subcortical Band Heterotopia (Double Cortex)

Subcortical band heterotopia (SBH) or double cortex is characterized by simplified cortical gyri and, often, by thickening

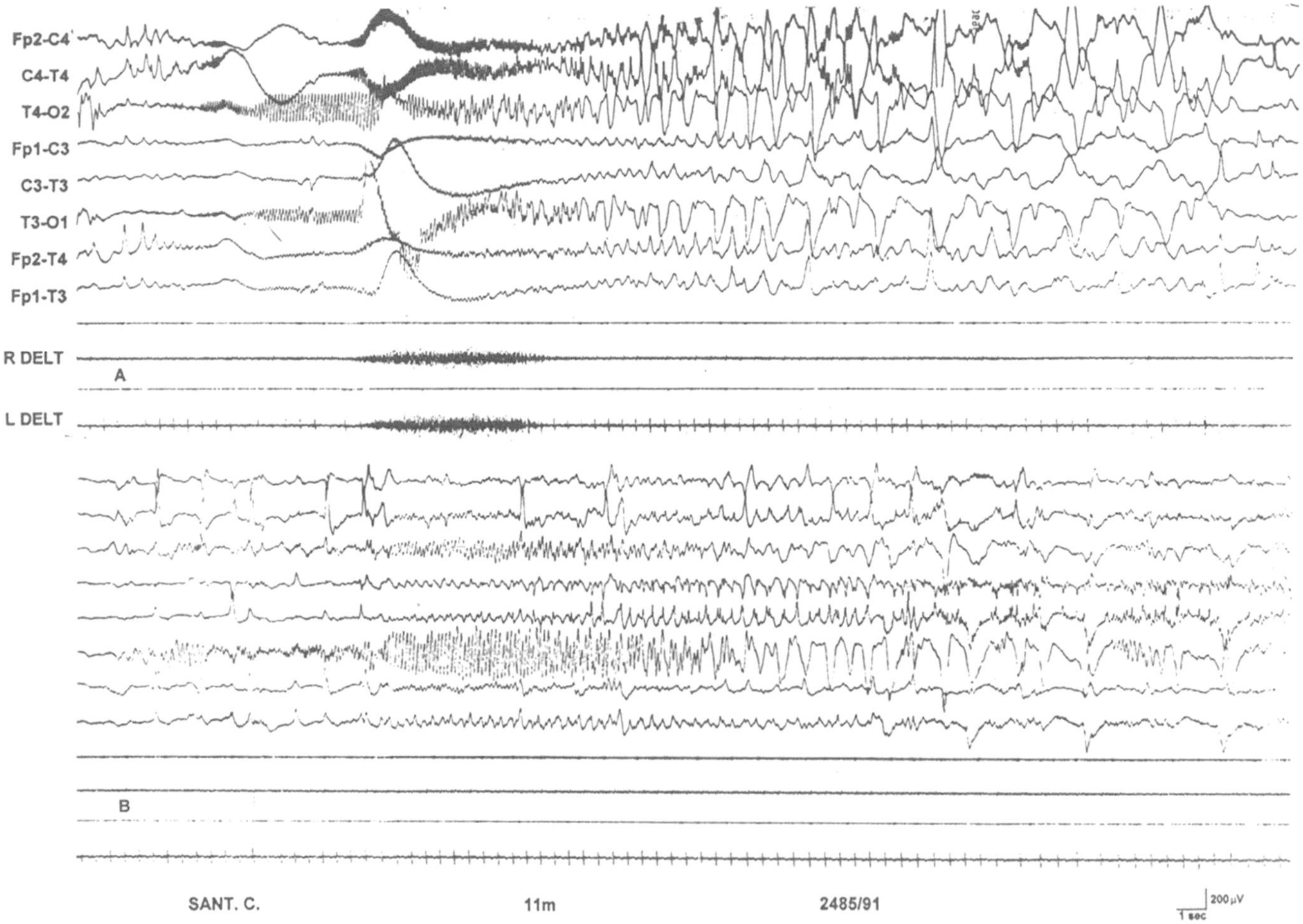

Fig. 33.26 Female at 11 months of age with lissencephaly and cerebellar hypoplasia. On the top, ictal recruiting activity starting from the right posterior regions, rapidly spreading to the contralateral hemisphere, followed by spike and spike-and-wave activity. At surface EMG of deltoid muscles, a short tonic contraction is evident. On the bottom, after the end of the seizure, a second seizure starts from the left hemisphere and promptly diffuses to the contralateral hemisphere, apparently without motor manifestations (*R* right, *L* left, *DELT* deltoid muscle)

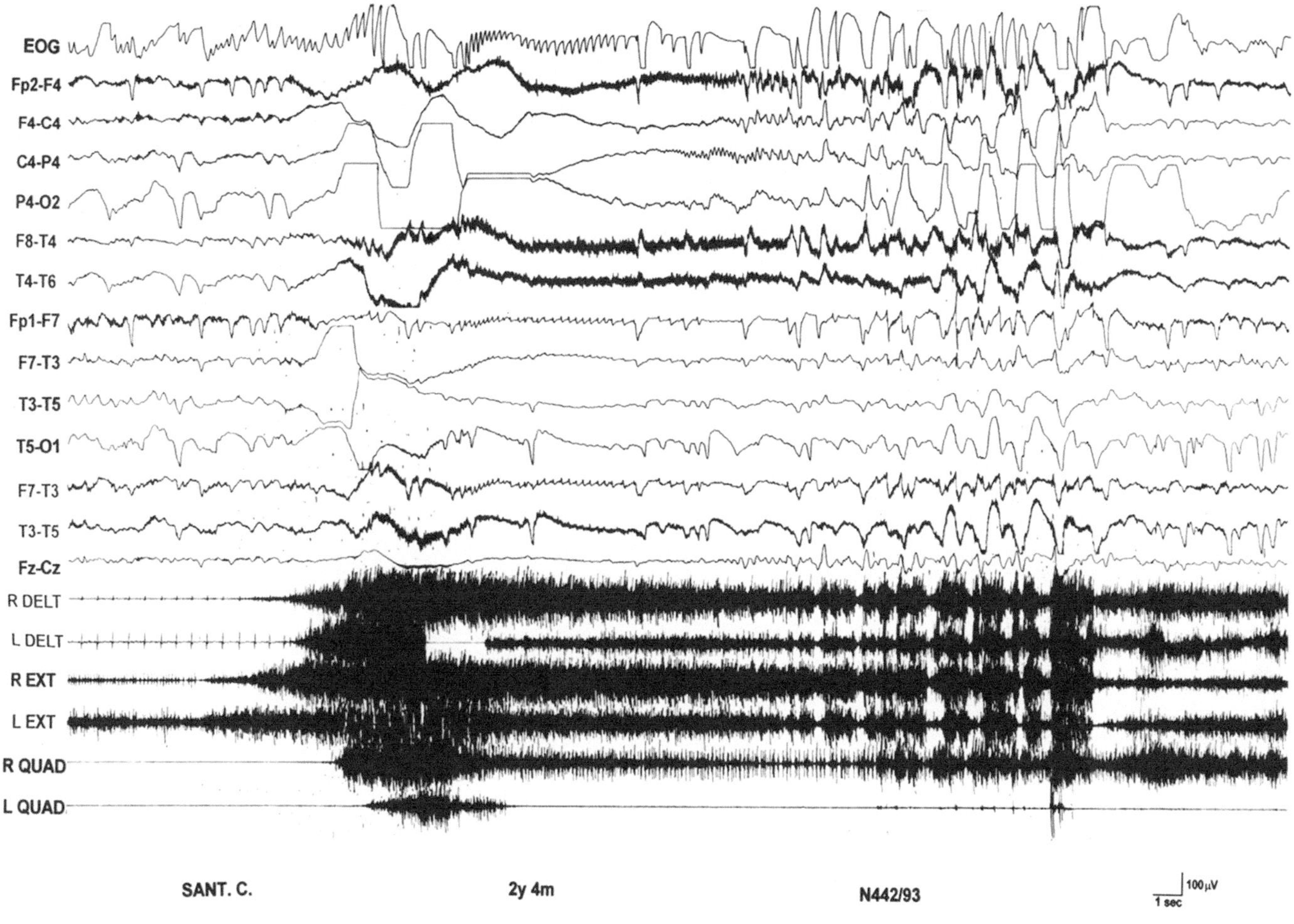

Fig. 33.27 The same patient of Fig. 33.26. EEG shows a tonic seizure with diffuse desynchronization. The appearance of the spike-and-slow wave complexes is correlated with shorter rhythmical tonic contractions (*R* right, *L* left, *DELT* deltoid muscle, *EXT* forearm extensor muscles, *QUAD* quadriceps femoris muscle)

of the cortex. A thin band of white matter divides the cortex from another band of gray matter (heterotopia) of variable thickness and extension (Fig. 33.29).

Mutations of doublecortin (DCX) gene, localized in the Xq22.3–q24 region, are responsible for SBH. These mutations have been reported in all familial cases and in 38–91% of sporadic cases. All the females with DCX gene mutations present a prevalently anterior double cortex; on the other hand, one quarter of those with an anterior pattern of double cortex and all those with a posteriorly predominant or unilateral double cortex do not have DCX mutations. In these cases, an intragenic deletion is found by means of MLPA assay, or the involvement of other genes, or a mosaic condition can be suspected. Rare reports of males with SBH, determined by DCX or LIS1 mutations, have been described.

The main clinical features of females with SBH are ID and epilepsy (in approximately 95% of cases).

ID degree appears correlated with the thickness of the subcortical band and with the coexistence of an overlying cortical pachygyria. The subjects with pachygyria and with larger ventricle dilation present an earlier onset of seizures [137, 145].

Interictal EEG—During wakefulness, frequent multifocal paroxysmal abnormalities are evident; during sleep, spike-and-wave or polyspike-and-wave complexes or sequences of fast paroxysmal activity, prominent over the frontal regions, are recorded (Figs. 33.30 and 33.31).

Seizures and ictal EEG—The typical pattern of Lennox-Gastaut syndrome, with tonic, atonic, generalized tonic-clonic, and atypical absence seizures is present. Using depth electrodes, the epileptiform activity may originate directly from

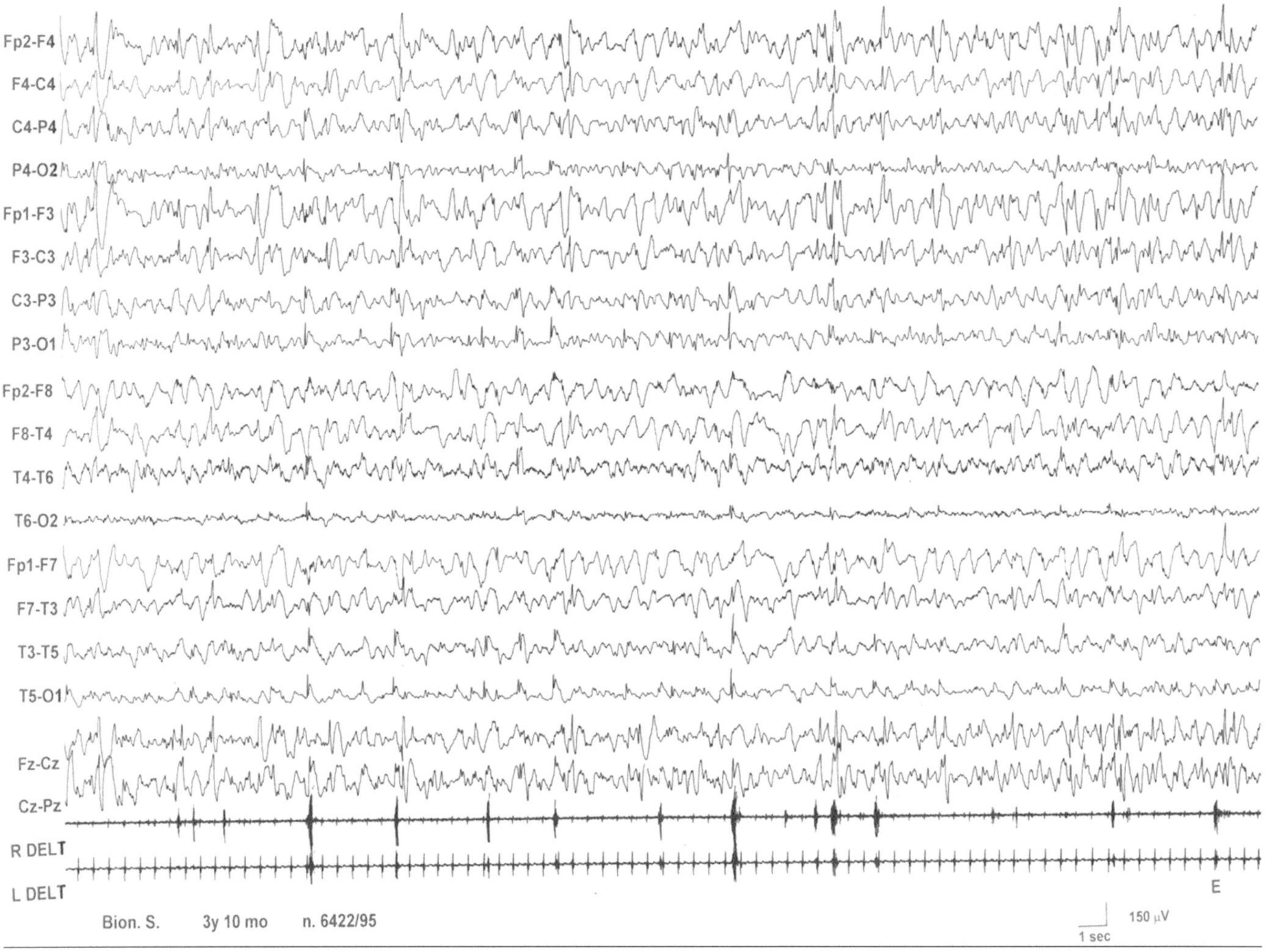

Fig. 33.28 A 3-year-old male with classical lissencephaly. EEG shows numerous diffuse spike-and-wave complexes, prominent over the anterior regions, often correlated with myoclonic jerks at surface EMG of deltoid muscles (*R* right, *L* left, *DELT* deltoid muscle)

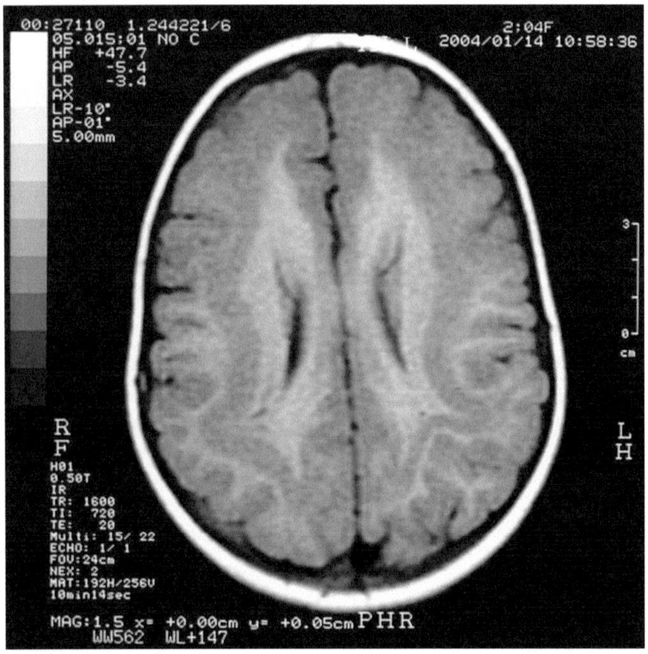

Fig. 33.29 Brain MRI of a 2-year-old female with subcortical band heterotopia (double cortex)

the heterotopic neurons. Approximately 65% of patients with SBH have intractable seizures. Callosotomy has been helpful in controlling atonic seizures in a few cases [137, 145].

33.2.6 Bilateral Periventricular Nodular Heterotopia

Bilateral periventricular nodular heterotopia (PNH) is characterized by subependymal gray matter nodules, confluent and symmetric, along the lateral ventricles (Fig. 33.32). PNH has an X-linked inheritance in females, with a high rate of lethality in males. Almost all familial cases, and 26% of sporadic cases are associated with filamin (FLNA) gene mutations (splicing or nonsense mutations, intragenic deletions), mapping in the Xq28 region. FLNA gene promotes orthogonal ramification of actin filaments and links them to membrane glycoproteins, influencing neuronal migration.

Females with FLNA mutations have a normal or borderline intellectual functioning and an epilepsy of variable severity.

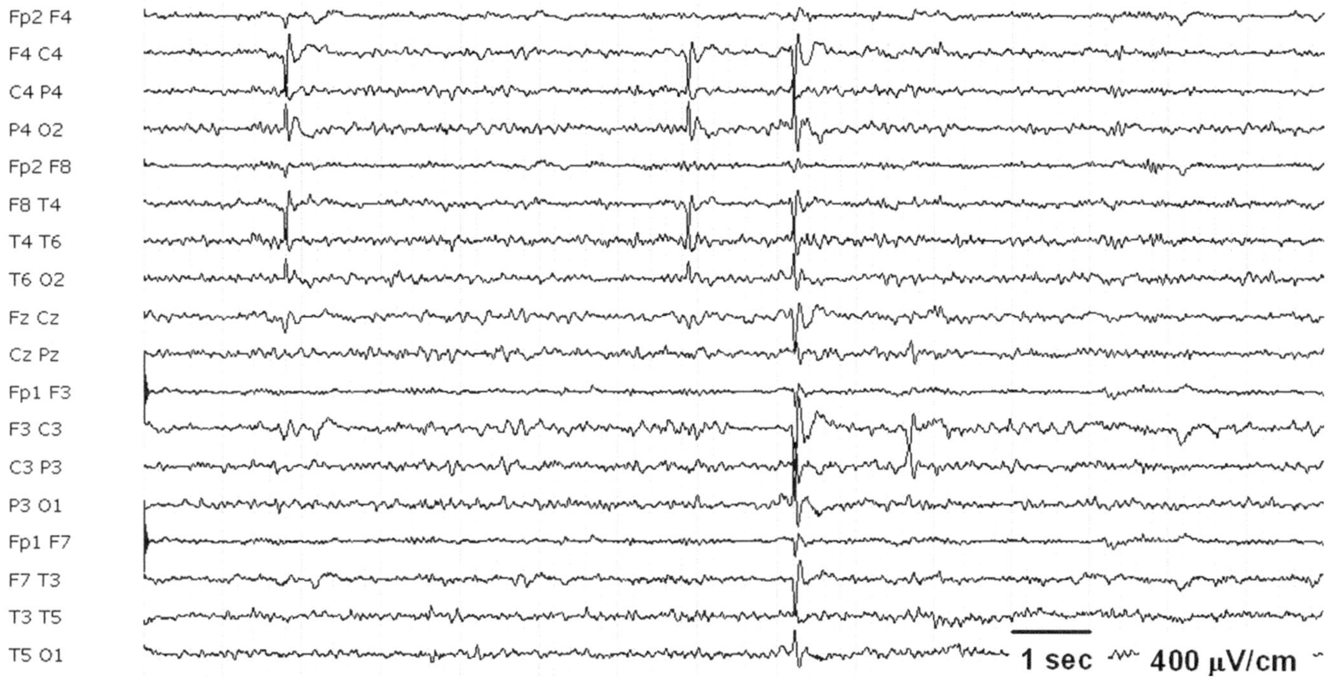

Fig. 33.30 Wakefulness EEG of a 3-year-old female with subcortical band heterotopia. High-voltage spikes are diffuse or asynchronously localized over the centrotemporal regions of both hemispheres, with right prevalence

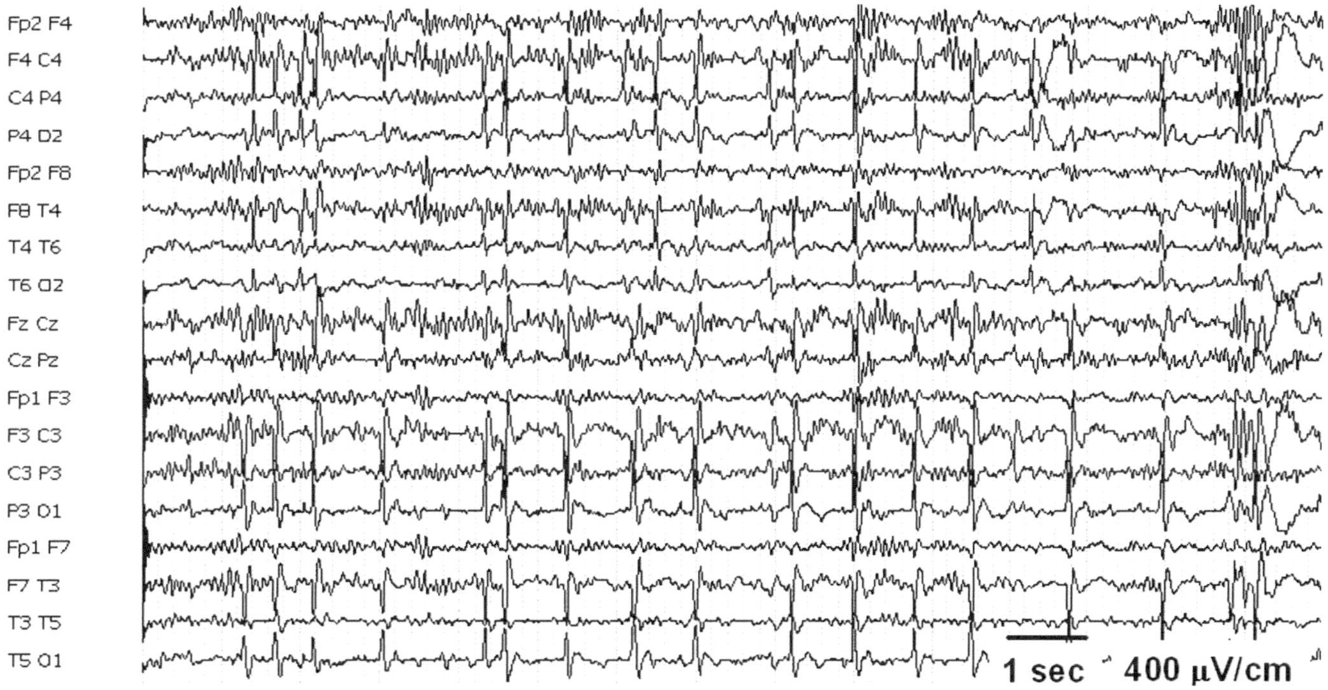

Fig. 33.31 Sleep EEG of the same patient of Fig. 33.30, at 3 years of age. Epileptiform abnormalities are diffuse and quasi-continuous over both hemispheres. Diffuse fast activity, more represented over the fronto-central regions and vertex, is evident

A rare form of autosomal recessive PNH associated with microcephaly and severe ID has been reported in two siblings, and it was due to a mutation of ADP-ribosylation factor guanine nucleotide-exchange factor-2 (ARFGEF2) gene.

Many other sporadic cases of PNH have been reported in association with more complex malformative syndrome, chromosomal abnormalities, or copy number variants [126, 137].

Interictal EEG—Background activity is usually normal, and sleep physiological elements are preserved. Photic

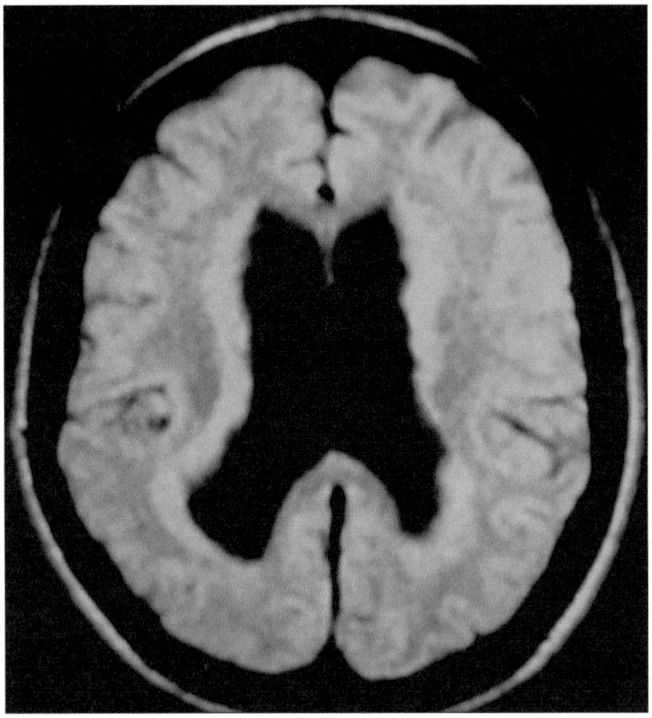

Fig. 33.32 Brain MRI of a 30-year-old female with bilateral periventricular nodular heterotopia

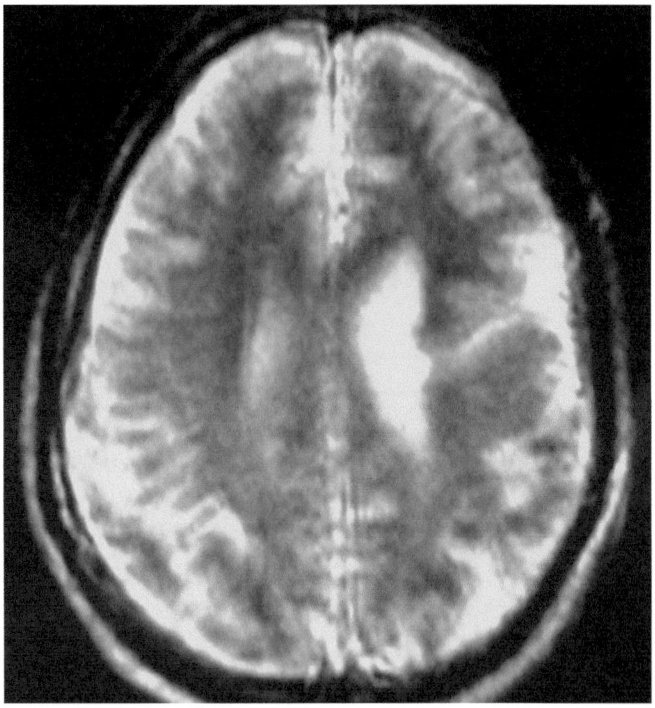

Fig. 33.33 Brain MRI of an 8-year-old male with polymicrogyria and schizencephaly at the left frontal cortex

driving at the intermittent photic stimulation is bilateral and symmetric in patients with bilateral PNH but asymmetrically represented over the affected hemisphere.

In the majority of cases, paroxysmal abnormalities are focal. Bilateral asynchronous abnormalities over the temporal regions are present in patients with symmetrical or asymmetrical PNH. In patients with unilateral PNH, abnormalities can be concordant with neuroimaging, but they are frequently multifocal. During NREM sleep, paroxysms tend to diffuse and to present as polyspike discharges [148].

Seizures and ictal EEG—About 88% of patients with PNH present epilepsy with a variable onset age (from infancy to adult age).

Three different ictal patterns have been proposed: (1) a spike-and-slow wave burst rapidly followed by a discharge of fast spikes which diffuse to the ipsilateral or contralateral hemisphere; (2) a tonic seizure correlated with fast spikes, rapidly involving the entire hemisphere where PNH is located; and(3) recruiting theta rhythms rapidly diffusing to the affected hemisphere.

Different asynchronous seizures can start from both hemispheres in cases of asymmetrical PNH.

Seizures are frequently drug-resistant. Outcome is worse when PNH is asymmetrical or unilateral, with or without extension to the overlying cortex [137, 148].

33.2.7 Schizencephaly

Schizencephaly is characterized by a unilateral or bilateral cerebral cleft, which can result in a communication between ventricle and subarachnoid spaces. The walls of the fissure are separated (open-lip schizencephaly) or appose each other (closed-lip schizencephaly) (Fig. 33.33). Schizencephaly may have different localizations but generally is found at the perisylvian region, and its edges are often covered by polymicrogyric cortex.

Schizencephaly has been correlated with different environmental factors, such as prenatal cytomegalovirus infection, but in some cases, mutations of the homeobox gene EMX2, mapping on 10q26.1 region, have been found.

The clinical phenotype is very heterogeneous. Patients with bilateral schizencephaly may present microcephaly, severe psychomotor delay, and spastic quadriplegia; those with unilateral schizencephaly tend to show milder neurological signs [137, 149].

Interictal EEG—Focal epileptiform abnormalities correlated with the localization of the schizencephaly are present; they increase in frequency and tend to diffuse during drowsiness and sleep (Fig. 33.34) [137, 150]. The frequency of EEG abnormalities is not different in patients with unilateral and bilateral schizencephaly [149].

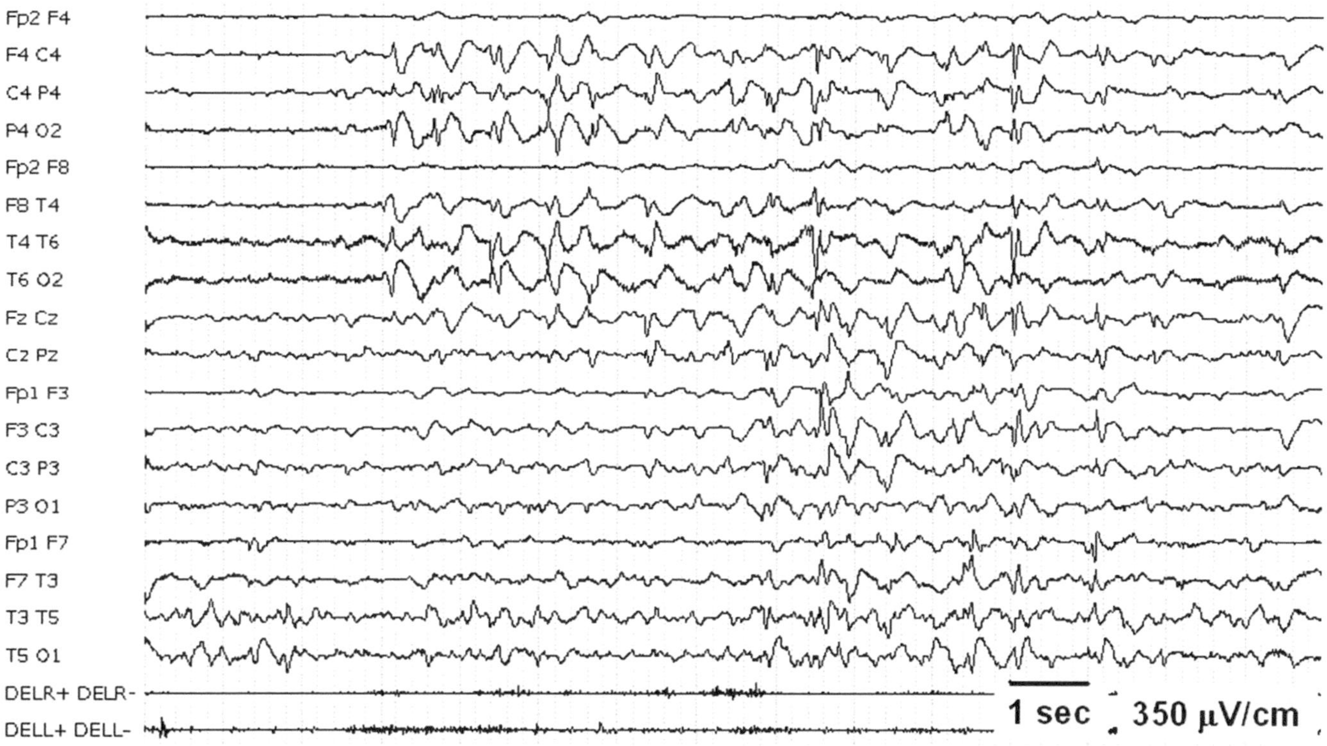

Fig. 33.34 A 1-year-old male with schizencephaly. Wakefulness EEG reveals high-voltage spike-and-slow-wave complexes, mostly localized over the right posterior regions and diffused contralaterally (*R* right, *L* left, *DELT* deltoid muscle)

Seizures and ictal EEG—Epilepsy is present in 36–65% of patients. Seizures start before 3 years of age and are drug-resistant in 9–38% of cases. Seizures are mostly focal, and their semiology strictly depends on the schizencephaly localization. Infantile spasms and myoclonic, tonic, and atonic seizures are rarely observed (Fig. 33.35). A young boy with unilateral schizencephaly and epilepsia partialis continua presented a normal scalp electroencephalogram (EEG) but an abnormal intracranial EEG, with synchronized periodic lateralized epileptiform discharges [151]. The extent of the cortical malformation in patients with schizencephaly does not correlate statistically with the severity of the clinical and EEG features of epilepsy, but in some series, seizures were more frequent in unilateral schizencephaly, with an onset ranging from 21 months to 21 years of age. It has been hypothesized that reorganization of cortical and subcortical circuits, together with the frequent presence of genesi of the corpus callosum, could prevent the occurrence and the diffusion of epileptic discharges. Surgery can be proposed in unilateral forms and callosotomy in bilateral ones complicated by tonic or atonic seizures [137, 149, 150].

33.2.8 Polymicrogyria

This term defines a disorder of the cortical organization with an increased number of small and prominent gyri divided by shallow and large sulci, determining a knobbly aspect of the cortical surface. Two histological types of polymicrogyria (PMG) are recognized: the unlayered form, in which the molecular layer is continuous and does not follow the profile of gyri, and the underlying neurons are radially distributed, without a laminar organization; the four-layered form, with an intracortical laminar necrotic layer, consequent late disorder of migration, and cortical disorganization.

PMG can be focal, unilateral, bilateral, symmetric or asymmetric, and isolated or associated with other cortical malformations, such as schizencephaly.

Clinical spectrum is wide, including normal neurological development, mild and selective cognitive dysfunctions with and without epilepsy, and severe and drug-resistant epileptic encephalopathies.

Specific PMG syndromes have been described: bilateral perisylvian PMG, bilateral parasagittal parieto-occipital

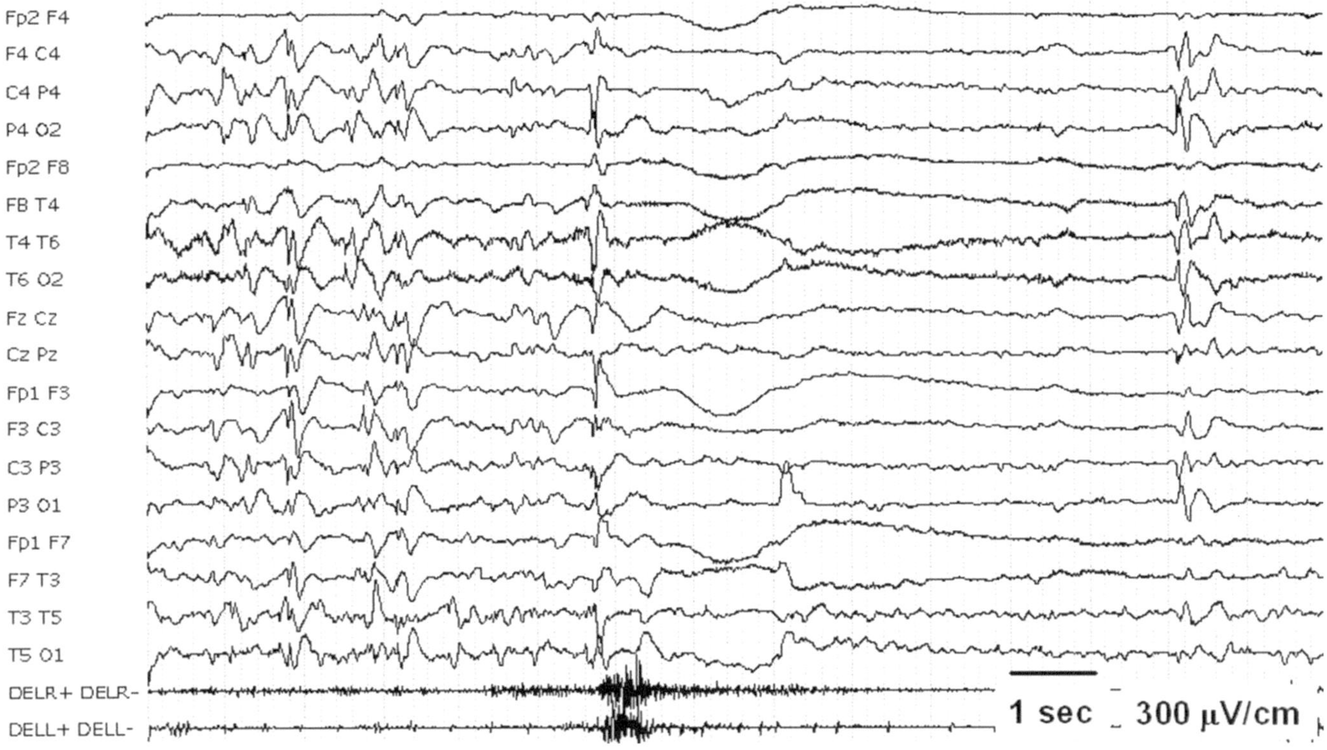

Fig. 33.35 The same child of Fig. 33.34. EEG recording of a seizure characterized by a diffuse slow complex and subsequent desynchronization; at surface EMG of deltoid muscles, a short tonic contraction is present (*R* right, *L* left, *DELT* deltoid muscle)

PMG, frontal and fronto-parietal PMG, unilateral or multilobar PMG, and bilateral generalized PMG.

Bilateral perisylvian PMG has been observed in sporadic and familial cases, associated with a missense mutation of SRPX2 gene (Xq22), with chromosome 22q11.2 deletion, with twin pregnancies complicated by twin-twin transfusion syndrome [137], with severe neonatal encephalopathy and mutation of MECP2 gene [152], with MELAS syndrome due to A3243G mitochondrial mutation [153]. The clinical picture in bilateral perisylvian PMG is characterized by facio-pharyngo-glosso-masticatory diplegia, ID, spastic quadriplegia, and epilepsy [137].

Bilateral parasagittal parieto-occipital PMG involves the mesial regions of the parietal and occipital lobes. Only sporadic cases with normal or mildly impaired cognitive level and mostly drug-resistant focal seizures beginning between 20 months and 15 years of age have been described [137, 154].

Frontal PMG has been reported in children with ID, spastic quadriplegia, and epilepsy. The majority of cases are sporadic, but its presence in probands born from consanguineous parents or in sibs suggests an autosomal recessive inheritance. Frontoparietal PMG (Fig. 33.36) is a recessive disorder described in familial cases and associated with mutations of the G protein-coupled receptor 56 (GPR56) gene, mapping on 16q13 region and involved in the regulation of the cortical pattern. Recently, frontoparietal PMG has been reclassified as a cobblestone malformation, associated with N-glycosylation defect [137, 155].

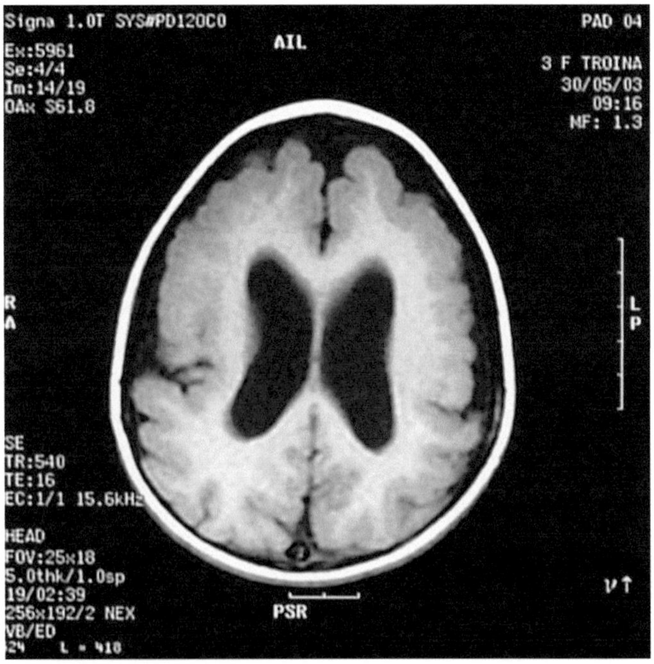

Fig. 33.36 Brain MRI of a 3-year-old female with frontoparietal polymicrogyria

Unilateral PMG has been found in association with mutations of PAX6 (paired-box transcription factor) gene, mapping on 11p13 region. This disorder is very often characterized by hemiparesis, ID, and focal seizures [137, 156, 157].

Multilobar PMG can present with status epilepticus during sleep (ESES), accompanied by focal seizures and, sometimes, atonic seizures [137, 158].

Bilateral generalized PMG entirely affects both hemispheres but is prominent at the perisylvian regions. Patients show cognitive and motor delay and epilepsy with a variable outcome [159].

Recently, TUBB2B mutations have been found in association with PMG, with different localizations (anterior asymmetric and involving perisylvian regions, diffuse and bilateral) and with other malformative features (dysmorphism of basal ganglia, hypoplasia of the internal capsula, corpus callosum agenesis) [137].

PMG, isolated or complicated by other malformations, has been associated with some pathogenic copy number variants, such as 1p36.3, 2p16–p23, 4q21–q22, 6q26–q27, and 21q2 [137].

Interictal EEG—In the bilateral perisylvian PMG, interictal EEG can be normal. In cases with focal seizures, multifocal spikes are recorded; in patients with generalized seizures, frequent slow waves are evident, bilaterally, but prominent over the centro-temporal regions, with intermingled bilateral or unilateral spikes or sharp waves or diffuse spike-and-wave complexes.

In the bilateral parasagittal parieto-occipital PMG, interictal EEG can be also normal. However, in the majority of cases, focal or bilateral paroxysmal abnormalities, localized over the parieto-occipital, parieto-temporal, or centro-parietal regions, are evident. More rarely, diffuse paroxysms are recorded [154].

In the frontal PMG, frontal slow and sharp waves or diffuse paroxysms are observed [160].

Interictal EEG reports regarding the frontoparietal PMG are sporadic. Bilateral, synchronous and asyncronous sharp waves, spikes and polyspikes are present (Figs. 33.37 and 33.38) [155].

In the unilateral PMG, epileptiform abnormalities are localized over the affected hemisphere. Patients without seizures and with normal interictal EEG have been reported [156, 157, 161]. In a series of cases with hemispheric PMG, focal electrical status has been described, presenting with continuous epileptiform abnormalities over a focal area on awakeness, which become bilateral and synchronous during sleep [162]. In another more recent review of cases with unilateral PMG, a typical ESES was constantly recorded [161].

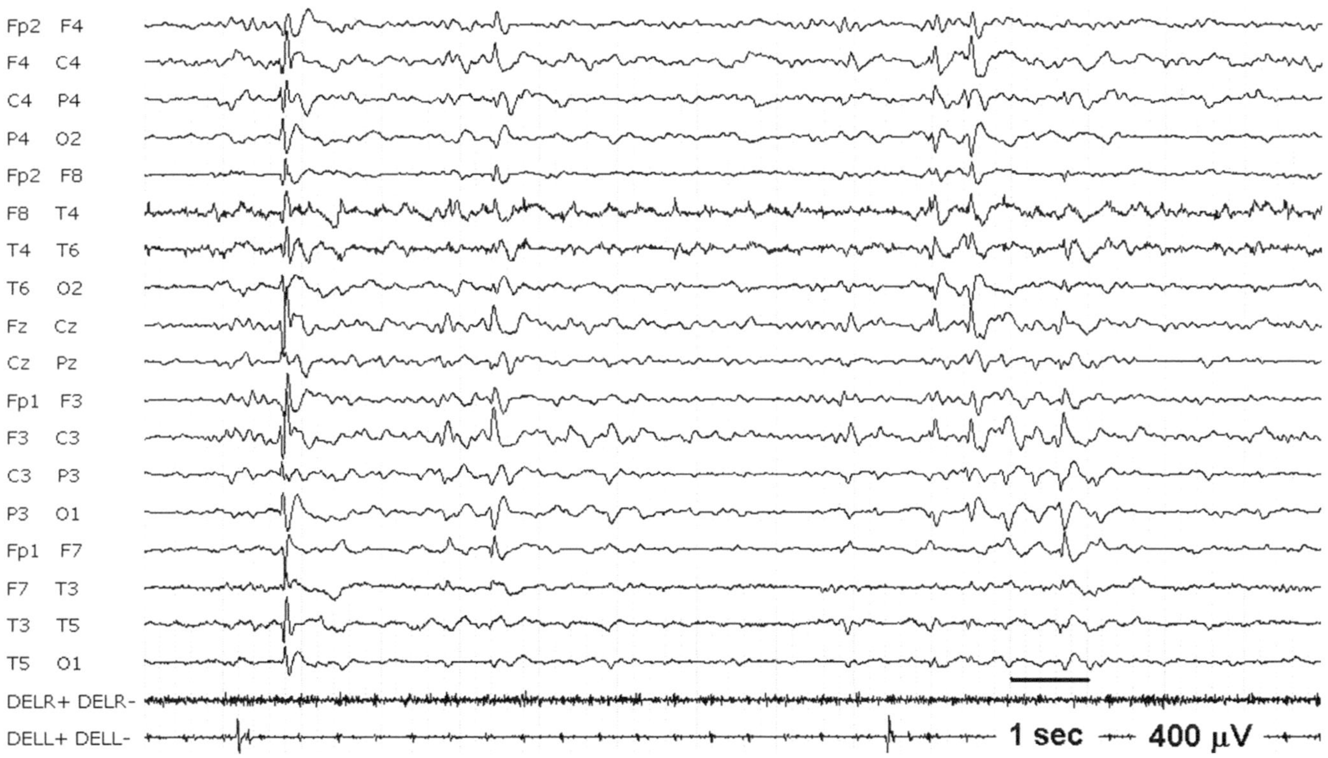

Fig. 33.37 The same child of Fig. 33.36. At age 8, wakefulness EEG in veglia shows high-voltage spikes and spike-and-slow wave complexes, asynchronously localized over the fronto-centro-parietal regions of both hemispheres; a bisynchronous discharge is also evident (*R* right, *L* left, *DELT* deltoid muscle)

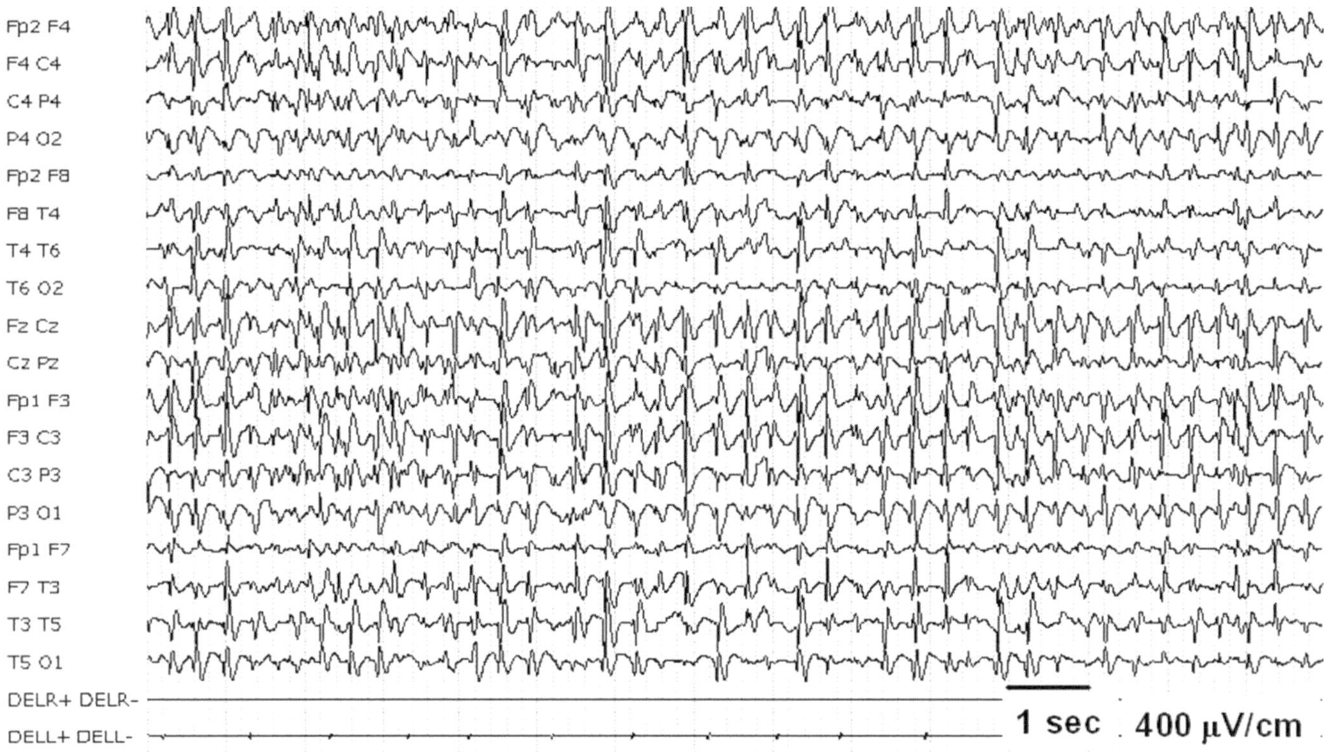

Fig. 33.38 The same child of Fig. 33.37 at age 8. Sleep EEG discloses a diffuse continuous spike-and-wave pattern (*R* right, *L* left, *DELT* deltoid muscle)

In the multilobar PMG, ESES is frequently observed between 2 and 10 years of age. All patients present also focal or multifocal spikes during wakefulness, prominent over the centro-parietal regions of the hemisphere from which start focal seizures [158].

In the bilateral generalized PMG, interictal EEG shows focal, multifocal (ventral, temporal, frontal), or diffuse epileptiform abnormalities [159].

Seizures and ictal EEG—In the bilateral perisylvian PMG, seizures start between 4 and 12 years of age and are drug-resistant in approximately 65% of cases. Atypical absence, tonic, atonic, or tonic-clonic seizures are frequent, also in the framework of a Lennox-Gastaut syndrome. Focal seizures are rare [137].

In the bilateral parasagittal parieto-occipital PMG, focal seizures with a possible apparently generalized or parieto-occipital onset are recorded [137, 154].

In the frontal and frontoparietal PMG, epilepsy is almost always present, polymorphous, with focal (with or without unawareness), generalized tonic-clonic seizures, or atypical absences. Outcome is variable [137, 154, 160].

In the unilateral PMG, focal, generalized tonic-clonic seizures, atypical absences, and negative and positive myoclonus are most commonly reported, between 9 months and 9 years of age [137, 156, 157, 161].

In the multilobar PMG, epilepsy starts between 14 months and 5 years of age, with sporadic focal motor seizures and atypical absences. ESES appears at the same time with atonic seizures. They are of variable intensity and duration and if very fast can determine an abrupt fall. At video EEG, the atonic event is correlated with a diffuse spike-and-wave complex. Focal motor seizures can occur with unilateral clonic jerks of the face. Seizure outcome is good with remission before adolescence, but neuropsychological impairment, typical of ESES, may persist [137, 158, 163].

In the bilateral generalized PMG, generalized, febrile, myoclonic, or atonic seizures occur also from the neonatal period [159].

Recently, a series of 58 cases with different types of PMG was retrospectively studied, and the results suggested that also PMG-related drug-resistant epilepsy warrants a comprehensive presurgical evaluation, including SEEG investigations, given that the epileptic zone may only partially overlap with the PMG or include solely remote cortical areas. Indeed, seizure freedom was reached in 72% of patients with PMG (mostly unilateral) who underwent corticectomy or hemispherotomy. These data support that surgery may play a role in the treatment of PMG whatever it is its extent [164].

33.2.9 Focal Cortical Dysplasia Types I and III

FCD types I and III are classified as secondary to abnormal postmigrational development because evidence suggests that they can result from injury to the cortex during later stages of cortical development.

FCD type I presents with abnormal cortical layering and is subdivided into three subtypes: (1) FCD type Ia, with abnormal radial cortical lamination; (2) FCD type Ib, with abnormal tangential cortical lamination; and (3) FCD type Ic, with abnormal radial and tangential cortical lamination. Prenatal and perinatal insults are frequently associated in children with FCD type I.

FCDs type III are characterized by cortical lamination abnormalities associated with a main lesion, usually close to or affecting the same cortical region. Four subtypes of FCD type III are now recognized: (1) cortical lamination abnormalities in the temporal lobe associated with hippocampal sclerosis (FCD type IIIa); (2) cortical lamination abnormalities adjacent to a glial or glioneuronal tumor (FCD type IIIb); (3) cortical lamination abnormalities adjacent to vascular malformation (FCD type IIIc); and (4) cortical lamination abnormalities adjacent to any other lesion acquired during early life (FCD type IIId) [126, 128].

Interictal EEG—Comparing scalp EEG in patients with FCD types I and II, no statistical differences for asymmetry of alpha rhythm and sleep spindles, intermittent slowing, and type and extent of interictal pattern were found; continuous irregular slowing was more frequently observed in FCD type I [165].

In a young girl with FCD type 1b, who underwent surgery, interictal pattern at electrocorticography disclosed multifocal 2 Hz spike-and-waves asynchronous over the right and left hemispheres, with sporadic spreading to the cortical surface, and especially to frontopolar electrodes [166].

The interictal EEG in FCDs type III involving the temporal regions are similar to those observed in extratemporal areas. Isolated spikes, a repetitive intermittent or almost continuous spike activity, and a paroxysmal fast pattern were frequently recorded during wakefulness and non-REM sleep in patients with FCD and hippocampal sclerosis [167].

Seizures and ictal EEG—In FCD type I, the most prevalent seizure-onset patterns at stereoelectroencephalography were slow wave or baseline shift followed by LVFA and LVFA [130]. In a study carried out on 215 consecutive patients with FCDs type I, two subgroups were distinguished: isolated FCDs, characterized by more frequent seizures, negative MRI, multilobar involvement, and worse postsurgical seizure control, and FCDs associated with hippocampal sclerosis and tumors, with a clinical picture similar to that of patients with HS or with tumors alone [168].

A study correlated ictal onset patterns in temporal lobe epilepsy patients with FCD associated with hippocampal sclerosis (type IIIa), and invasive EEG recordings showed that about 40% of seizures arose from the amygdala/hippocampus complex, 35% from the temporal neocortex with the FCD, 22% were simultaneously recorded from both areas, and 2% from the contralateral hemisphere [167].

Although literature data on surgery outcome of patients with FCD IIIa are controversial, some evidences demonstrate that these patients may have a favorable evolution when both pathologies (FCD and hippocampal sclerosis) are removed [167].

References

1. Battaglia A. Del 1p36 syndrome: a newly emerging clinical entity. Brain Dev. 2005;27:358–61.
2. Battaglia A, Hoyme HE, Dallapiccola B, Zackai E, Hudgins L, McDonald-McGinn D, et al. Further delineation of deletion 1p36 syndrome in 60 patients: a recognizable phenotype and common cause of developmental delay and mental retardation. Pediatrics. 2008;121:404–10.
3. Greco M, Ferrara P, Farello G, Striano P, Verrotti A. Electroclinical features of epilepsy associated with 1p36 deletion syndrome: a review. Epilepsy Res. 2018;139:92–101.
4. Heilstedt HA, Burgess DL, Anderson AE, Chedrawi A, Tharp B, Lee O, et al. Loss of the potassium channel b-subunit gene, KCNAB2, is associated with epilepsy in patients with 1p36 deletion syndrome. Epilepsia. 2001;42:1103–11.
5. Bahi-Buisson N, Guttierrez-Delicado E, Soufflet C, Rio M, Daire VC, Lacombe D, et al. Spectrum of epilepsy in terminal 1p36 deletion syndrome. Epilepsia. 2008;49:509–15.
6. Kurosawa K, Kawame H, Okamoto N, Ochiai Y, Akatsuka A, Kobayashi M, et al. Epilepsy and neurological findings in 11 individuals with 1p36 deletion syndrome. Brain Dev. 2005;27:738–82.
7. Seo GH, Kim JH, Cho JH, Kim GH, Seo EJ, Lee BH, et al. Identification of 1p36 deletion syndrome in patients with facial dysmorphism and developmental delay. Korean J Pediatr. 2016;59:16–23.
8. Shapira SK, McCaskill C, Northrup H, Spikes AS, Elder FF, Sutton VR, et al. Chromosome 1p36 deletions: the clinical phenotype and molecular characterization of a common newly delineated syndrome. Am J Hum Genet. 1997;61:642–50.
9. Madia F, Striano P, Gennaro E, Malacarne M, Paravidino R, Biancheri R, et al. Cryptic chromosome deletions involving SCN1A in severe myoclonic epilepsy of infancy. Neurology. 2006;67:1230–5.
10. Mulley JC, Nelson P, Guerrero S, Dibbens L, Iona X, McMahon JM, et al. A new molecular mechanism for severe myoclonic epilepsy of infancy: exonic deletions in SCN1A. Neurology. 2006;67:1094–5.
11. Suls A, Claeys KG, Goossens D, Harding B, Van Luijk R, Scheers S, et al. Microdeletions involving the SCN1A gene may be common in SCN1A-mutation-negative SMEI patients. Hum Mutat. 2006;27:914–20.
12. Davidsson J, Collin A, Olsson ME, Lundgren J, Soller M. Deletion of the SCN gene cluster on 2q24.4 is associated with severe epilepsy: an array-based genotype-phenotype correlation and a comprehensive review of previously published cases. Epilepsy Res. 2008;81:69–79.
13. Marini C, Scheffer IE, Nabbout R, Mei D, Cox K, Dibbens LM, et al. SCN1A duplications and deletions detected in Dravet syndrome: implications for molecular diagnosis. Epilepsia. 2009;50:1670–8.

14. Pereira S, Vieira JP, Barroca F, Roll P, Carvalhas R, Cau P, et al. Severe epilepsy, retardation, and dysmorphic features with a 2q deletion including SCN1A and SCN2A. Neurology. 2004;63:191–2.
15. Coppola A, Elia M. Copy number variants and epilepsy: new emerging syndromes. In: Striano P, editor. Epilepsy towards the next decade. New trends and hopes in epileptology. London: Springer International Publishing Switzerland; 2015. p. 1–14.
16. Guthrie RD, Aase JM, Asper AC, Smith DW. The 4p⁻ syndrome. A clinically recognizable chromosomal deletion syndrome. Am J Dis Child. 1971;122:421–5.
17. Centerwall WR, Thompson WP, Allen IE, Fobes CD. Translocation 4p⁻ syndrome. Am J Dis Child. 1975;129:366–70.
18. Battaglia A, Carey JC, Wright TJ. Wolf-Hirschhorn (4p⁻) syndrome. Adv Pediatr Infect Dis. 2001;48:75–113.
19. Battaglia A, Carey JC. Seizure and EEG patterns in Wolf-Hirschhorn (4p⁻) syndrome. Brain Dev. 2005;27:362–4.
20. Zollino M, Lecce R, Fischetto R, Murdolo M, Faravelli F, Selicorni A, et al. Mapping the Wolf-Hirschhorn syndrome phenotype outside the currently accepted WHS critical region and defining a new critical region, WHSCR-2. Am J Hum Genet. 2003;72:590–7.
21. Campbell K, Flavin N, Ivens A, Robert B, Buckingham M, Williamson R. The human homeobox gene HOX7 maps to 4p16.1 and is deleted in Wolf-Hirschhorn syndrome patients. Am J Hum Genet. 1989;45(Suppl):A179.
22. Ivens A, Flavin N, Williamson R, Dixon M, Bates G, Buckingham M, et al. The human homeobox gene HOX7 maps to chromosome 4p16.1 and may be implicated in Wolf-Hirschhorn syndrome. Hum Genet. 1990;84:473–6.
23. Zollino M, Orteschi D, Ruiter M, Pfundt R, Steindl K, Cafiero C, et al. Unusual 4p16.3 deletions suggest an additional chromosome region for the Wolf-Hirschhorn syndrome-associated seizures disorder. Epilepsia. 2014;55:849–57.
24. Gottfried M, Lavine L, Roessmann U. Neuropathological findings in Wolf-Hirschhorn (4p⁻) syndrome. Acta Neuropathol. 1981;55:163–5.
25. Battaglia D, Zampino G, Zollino M, Mariotti P, Acquafondata C, Lettori D, et al. Electroclinical patterns and evolution of epilepsy in the 4p⁻ syndrome. Epilepsia. 2003;44:1183–90.
26. Battaglia A, Filippi T, South ST, Carey JC. Spectrum of epilepsy and electroencephalogram patterns in Wolf-Hirschhorn syndrome: experience with 87 patients. Dev Med Child Neurol. 2009;51:373–80.
27. Kagitani-Shimono K, Imai K, Otani K, Kamio N, Okinaga T, Toribe Y, et al. Epilepsy in Wolf-Hirschhorn syndrome (4p⁻). Epilepsia. 2005;46:150–5.
28. Itakura A, Saito Y, Nishimura Y, Okazaki T, Ohno K, Sejima H, et al. Successful treatment of migrating partial seizures in Wolf-Hirschhorn syndrome with bromide. Brain Dev. 2016;38:658–62.
29. Motoi H, Okanishi T, Kanai S, Yokota T, Yamazoe T, Nishimura M, et al. Wolf-Hirschhorn (4p⁻) syndrome with west syndrome. Epilepsy Behav Case Rep. 2016;6:39–41.
30. Sgrò V, Riva E, Canevini MP, Colamaria V, Rottoli A, Minotti L, et al. 4p(−) syndrome: a chromosomal disorder associated with a particular EEG pattern. Epilepsia. 1995;36:1206–14.
31. Worthington JC, Rigby AS, Quarrell OW. Seizure frequency in adults with Wolf-Hirschhorn syndrome. Am J Med Genet A. 2008;146A:2528–31.
32. Karalok ZS, Arhan EP, Erdogan KM, Gurkas E. Excellent response to levetiracetam in epilepsy with Wolf-Hirschhorn syndrome. Childs Nerv Syst. 2016;32:9–11.
33. Le Meur N, Holder-Espinasse M, Jaillard S, Goldenberg A, Joriot S, Amati-Bonneau P, et al. MEF2C haploinsufficiency caused by either microdeletion of the 5q14.3 region or mutation is responsible for severe mental retardation with stereotypic movements, epilepsy and/or cerebral malformations. J Med Genet. 2010;47:22–9.
34. Cardoso C, Boys A, Parrini E, Mignon-Ravix C, McMahon JM, Khantane S, et al. Periventricular heterotopia, mental retardation, and epilepsy associated with 5q14.3–q15 deletion. Neurology. 2009;72:784–92.
35. Engels H, Wohlleber E, Zink A, Hoyer J, Ludwig KU, Brockschmidt FF, et al. A novel microdeletion syndrome involving 5q14.3–q15: clinical and molecular cytogenetic characterization of three patients. Eur J Hum Genet. 2009;17:1592–9.
36. Zweier M, Gregor A, Zweier C, Engels H, Sticht H, Wohlleber E, et al. Mutations in MEF2C from the 5q14.3q15 microdeletion syndrome region are a frequent cause of severe mental retardation and diminish MECP2 and CDKL5 expression. Hum Mutat. 2010;31:722–33.
37. Hotz A, Hellenbroich Y, Sperner J, Linder-Lucht M, Tacke U, Walter C, et al. Microdeletion 5q14.3 and anomalies of brain development. Am J Med Genet. 2013;161A:2124–33.
38. Potthoff MJ, Arnold MA, McAnally J, Richardson JA, Bassel-Duby R, Olson EN. Regulation of skeletal muscle sarcomere integrity and postnatal muscle function by Mef2c. Mol Cell Biol. 2007;27:8143–51.
39. Myers KA, Nasioulas S, Boys A, McMahon JM, Slater H, Lockhart P, et al. ADGRV1 is implicated in myoclonic epilepsy. Epilepsia. 2018;59:381–8.
40. Elia M, Striano P, Fichera M, Gaggero R, Castiglia L, Galesi O, et al. 6q terminal deletion syndrome is associated with a distinctive EEG and clinical pattern. A report of five cases. Epilepsia. 2006;47:830–8.
41. Striano P, Malacarne M, Cavani S, Pierluigi M, Rinaldi R, Cavaliere ML, et al. Clinical phenotype and molecular characterization of 6q terminal deletion syndrome: five new cases. Am J Med Genet A. 2006;140:1944–9.
42. Bertini V, De Vito G, Costa R, Simi P, Valetto A. Isolated 6q terminal deletions: an emerging new syndrome. Am J Med Genet A. 2006;140:74–81.
43. Lee JY, Cho YH, Hallford G. Delineation of subtelomeric deletion of the long arm of chromosome 6. Ann Hum Genet. 2011;75:755–64.
44. Conti V, Carabalona A, Pallesi-Pocachard E, Parrini E, Leventer RJ, Buhler E, et al. Periventricular heterotopia in 6q terminal deletion syndrome: role of the C6orf70 gene. Brain. 2013;136:3378–94.
45. Guerrini R, Bureau M, Mattei MG, Battaglia A, Galland MC, Roger J. Trisomy 12p syndrome: a chromosomal disorder associated with generalized 3-Hz spike-and-wave discharges. Epilepsia. 1990;31:557–66.
46. Elia M, Musumeci SA, Ferri R, Cammarata M. Trisomy 12p and epilepsy with myoclonic absences. Brain Dev. 1998;20:127–30.
47. Genton P, Bahi-Buisson N, Kaminska A, Elia M, Gobbi G. Epilepsies and chromosomal disorders. In: Bureau M, Genton P, Dravet C, Delgado-Escueta A, Tassinari CA, Thomas P, Wolf P, editors. Epilepsy syndromes in infancy, childhood and adolescence. 5th ed. London: John Libbey Eurotext Ltd.; 2012. p. 545–74.
48. Shirasaka Y, Ito M, Okuno T, Fujii T, Nozaki K, Mikawa H. Ring 14 chromosome with complex partial seizures: a case report. Brain Dev. 1992;14:257–60.
49. Ville D, De Bellescize J, Nguyen MA, Testard H, Gautier A, Perrier J, et al. Ring 14 chromosome presenting as early-onset isolated partial epilepsy. Dev Med Child Neurol. 2009;51:917–22.
50. Specchio N, Trivisano M, Serino D, Cappelletti S, Carotenuto A, Claps D, et al. Epilepsy in ring 14 chromosome syndrome. Epilepsy Behav. 2012;25:585–92.
51. Giovannini S, Marangio L, Fusco C, Scarano A, Frattini D, Della Giustina E, et al. Epilepsy in ring 14 syndrome: a clinical and EEG study of 22 patients. Epilepsia. 2013;54:2204–13.
52. Zori RT, Hendrickson J, Woolven S, Whidden EM, Gray B, Williams CA. Angelman syndrome: clinical profile. J Child Neurol. 1992;7:270–80.

53. Clayton-Smith J, Laan L. Angelman syndrome: a review of the clinical and genetic aspects. J Med Genet. 2003;40:87–95.
54. Kyllerman M. On the prevalence of Angelman syndrome. Am J Med Genet. 1995;59:405.
55. Russo S, Cogliati F, Viri M, Cavalleri F, Selicorni A, Turolla L, et al. Novel mutations of ubiquitin protein ligase 3A gene in Italian patients with Angelman syndrome. Hum Mutat. 2000;15:387.
56. Lossie AC, Whitney MM, Amidon D, Dong HJ, Chen P, Theriaque D, et al. Distinct phenotypes distinguish the molecular classes of Angelman syndrome. J Med Genet. 2001;38:834–45.
57. DeLorey TM, Olsen RW. GABA and epileptogenesis: comparing gabrb3 gene-deficient mice with Angelman syndrome in man. Epilepsy Res. 1999;36:123–32.
58. Dan B, Boyd SG. Angelman syndrome reviewed from a neurophysiological perspective. The UBE3A-GABRB3 hypothesis. Neuropediatrics. 2003;34:169–76.
59. Guerrini R, Gobbi G, Genton P, Bonanni P, Carrozzo R. Chromosomal abnormalities. In: Engel Jr J, Pedley TA, editors. Epilepsy: a comprehensive textbook. Philadephia: Lippincott-Raven Publishers; 1997. p. 2533–46.
60. Laan LA, Vein AA. A Rett patient with a typical Angelman EEG. Epilepsia. 2002;43:1590–2.
61. Valente KD. Another Rett patient with a typical Angelman EEG. Epilepsia. 2003;44:873–4.
62. Guerrini R, De Lorey TM, Bonanni P, Moncla A, Dravet C, Suisse G, et al. Cortical myoclonus in Angelman syndrome. Ann Neurol. 1996;40:39–48.
63. Viani F, Romeo A, Viri M, Mastrangelo M, Lalatta F, Selicorni A, et al. Seizure and EEG patterns in Angelman's syndrome. J Child Neurol. 1995;10:467–71.
64. Dalla Bernardina B, Fontana E, Sgrò V, Colamaria V, Elia M. Myoclonic status in non-progressive encephalopathies. In: Roger J, Bureau M, Dravet C, Genton P, Tassinari CA, Wolf P, editors. Epileptic syndromes in infancy, childhood and adolescence. 3nd ed. London: John Libbey & Co. Ltd; 1992. p. 137–44.
65. Elia M. Myoclonic status in nonprogressive encephalopathies: an update. Epilepsia. 2009;50(Suppl 5):41–4.
66. Sueri C, Ferlazzo E, Elia M, Bonanni P, Randazzo G, Gasparini S, et al. Epilepsy and sleep disorders improve in adolescents and adults with Angelman syndrome: a multicenter study on 46 patients. Epilepsy Behav. 2017;75:225–9.
67. Franz DN, Glauser TA, Tudor C, Williams S. Topiramate therapy of epilepsy associated with Angelman's syndrome. Neurology. 2000;54:1185–8.
68. Battaglia A. The inv dup(15) or idic(15) syndrome: a clinically recognisable neurogenetic disorder. Brain Dev. 2005;27:365–9.
69. Verrotti A, Sertorio F, Matricardi S, Ferrara P, Striano P. Electroclinical features of epilepsy in patients with Inv Dup(15). Seizure. 2017;47:87–91.
70. Chifari R, Guerrini R, Pierluigi M, Cavani S, Sgrò V, Elia M, et al. Mild generalized epilepsy and developmental disorder associated with large inv dup(15). Epilepsia. 2002;43:1096–100.
71. Battaglia A, Bernardini L, Torrente I, Novelli A, Scarselli G. Spectrum of epilepsy and electroencephalogram patterns in idic (15) syndrome. Am J Med Genet A. 2016;170:2531–9.
72. Battaglia A, Gurrieri F, Bertini E, Bellacosa A, Pomponi MG, Paravatou-Petsotas M, et al. The inv dup(15) syndrome: a clinically recognizable syndrome with altered behavior, mental retardation, and epilepsy. Neurology. 1997;48:1081–6.
73. Matricardi S, Darra F, Spalice A, Basti C, Fontana E, Dalla Bernardina B, et al. Electroclinical findings and long-term outcomes in epileptic patients with inv dup (15). Acta Neurol Scand. 2018;137(6):575–81.. [Epub ahead of print]
74. Sharp AJ, Mefford HC, Li K, Baker C, Skinner C, Stevenson RE, et al. A recurrent 15q13.3 microdeletion syndrome associated with mental retardation and seizures. Nat Genet. 2008;40:322–8.
75. Dibbens LM, Mullen S, Helbig I, Mefford HC, Bayly MA, Bellows S, et al. Familial and sporadic 15q13.3 microdeletions in idiopathic generalized epilepsy: precedent for disorders with complex inheritance. Hum Mol Genet. 2009;18:3626–31.
76. Ben-Shachar S, Lanpher B, German JR, Qasaymeh M, Potocki L, Nagamani SC, et al. Microdeletion 15q13.3: a locus with incomplete penetrance for autism, mental retardation, and psychiatric disorders. J Med Genet. 2009;46:382–8.
77. van Bon BW, Mefford HC, Menten B, Koolen DA, Sharp AJ, Nillesen WM, et al. Further delineation of the 15q13 microdeletion and duplication syndromes: a clinical spectrum varying from non-pathogenic to a severe outcome. J Med Genet. 2009;46:511–23.
78. Masurel-Paulet A, Andrieux J, Callier P, Cuisset JM, Le Caignec C, Holder M, et al. Delineation of 15q13.3 microdeletions. Clin Genet. 2010;78:149–61.
79. Lepichon JB, Bittel DC, Graf WD, Yu S. A 15q13.3 homozygous microdeletion associated with a severe neurodevelopmental disorder suggests putative functions of the TRPM1, CHRNA7, and other homozygously deleted genes. Am J Med Genet. 2010;152A:1300–4.
80. Endris V, Hackmann K, Neuhann TM, Grasshoff U, Bonin M, Haug U, et al. Homozygous loss of CHRNA7 on chromosome 15q13.3 causes severe encephalopathy with seizures and hypotonia. Am J Med Genet. 2010;152A:2908–11.
81. Helbig I, Mefford HC, Sharp AJ, Guipponi M, Fichera M, Franke A, et al. 15q13.3 microdeletions increase risk of idiopathic generalized epilepsy. Nat Genet. 2009;41:160–2.
82. Mulley JC, Dibbens LM. Chipping away at the common epilepsies with complex genetics: the 15q13.3 microdeletion shows the way. Genome Med. 2009;1:33.
83. Muhle H, Mefford HC, Obermeier T, von Spiczak S, Eichler EE, Stephani U, et al. Absence seizures with intellectual disability as a phenotype of the 15q13.3 microdeletion syndrome. Epilepsia. 2011;52:e194–8.
84. Coppola A, Bagnasco I, Traverso M, Brusco A, Di Gregorio E, Del Gaudio L, et al. Different electroclinical picture of generalized epilepsy in two families with 15q13.3 microdeletion. Epilepsia. 2013;54:e69–73.
85. Gago-Veiga AB, Toledano R, García-Morales I, Pérez-Jiménez MA, Bernar J, Gil-Nagel A. Specificity of electroclinical features in the diagnosis of ring chromosome 20. Epilepsy Behav. 2018;80:215–20.
86. Takahashi Y, Shigematsu H, Kubota H, Inoue Y, Fujiwara T, Yagi K, et al. Nonphotosensitive video game-induced partial seizures. Epilepsia. 1995;36:837–41.
87. Inoue Y, Fujiwara T, Matsuda K, Kubota H, Tanaka M, Yagi K, et al. Ring chromosome 20 and nonconvulsive status epilepticus. A new epileptic syndrome. Brain. 1997;120:939–53.
88. Gomes Mda M, Lucca I, Bezerra SA, Llerena J Jr, Moreira DM. Epilepsy and ring chromosome 20: case report. Arq Neuropsiquiatr. 2002;60:631–5.
89. Biraben A, Semah F, Ribeiro MJ, Douaud G, Remy P, Depaulis A. PET evidence for a role of the basal ganglia in patients with ring chromosome 20 epilepsy. Neurology. 2004;63:73–7.
90. Canevini MP, Sgro V, Zuffardi O, Canger R, Carrozzo R, Rossi E, et al. Chromosome 20 ring: a chromosomal disorder associated with a particular electroclinical pattern. Epilepsia. 1998;39:942–51.
91. Avanzini P, Vaudano AE, Vignoli A, Ruggieri A, Benuzzi F, Darra F, et al. Low frequency mu-like activity characterizes cortical rhythms in epilepsy due to ring chromosome 20. Clin Neurophysiol. 2014;125:239–49.
92. Freire de Moura M, Flores-Guevara R, Gueguen B, Biraben A, Renault F. Long-term EEG in patients with the ring chromosome 20 epilepsy syndrome. Epilepsia. 2016;57:e94–6.
93. Vignoli A, Canevini MP, Darra F, La Selva L, Fiorini E, Piazzini A, et al. Ring chromosome 20 syndrome: a link between epilepsy

onset and neuropsychological impairment in three children. Epilepsia. 2009;50:2420–7.
94. Vignoli A, Bisulli F, Darra F, Mastrangelo M, Barba C, Giordano L, et al. Epilepsy in ring chromosome 20 syndrome. Epilepsy Res. 2016;128:83–93.
95. Roubertie A, Petit J, Genton P. Ring chromosome 20: an identifiable epileptic syndrome. Rev Neurol (Paris). 2000;156:149–53.
96. Chawla J, Sucholeiki R, Jones C, Silver K. Intractable epilepsy with ring chromosome 20 syndrome treated with vagal nerve stimulation: case report and review of the literature. J Child Neurol. 2002;17:778–80.
97. Lefter S, Costello DJ, McNamara B, Sweeney B. Clinical and EEG features of seizures in adults with down syndrome. J Clin Neurophysiol. 2011;28:469–73.
98. Romano C, Tinè A, Fazio G, Rizzo R, Colognola RM, Sorge G, et al. Seizures in patients with trisomy 21. Am J Med Genet. 1990;7:298–300.
99. Verrotti A, Cusmai R, Nicita F, Pizzolorusso A, Elia M, Zamponi N, et al. Electroclinical features and long-term outcome of cryptogenic epilepsy in children with down syndrome. J Pediatr. 2013;163:1754–8.
100. Ferlazzo E, Adjien CK, Guerrini R, Calarese T, Crespel A, Elia M, et al. Lennox-Gastaut syndrome with late-onset and prominent reflex seizures in trisomy 21 patients. Epilepsia. 2009;50:1587–95.
101. De Simone R, Puig XS, Gélisse P, Crespel A, Genton P. Senile myoclonic epilepsy: delineation of a common condition associated with Alzheimer's disease in down syndrome. Seizure. 2010;19:383–9.
102. Aller-Alvarez JS, Menéndez-González M, Ribacoba-Montero R, Salvado M, Vega V, Suárez-Moro R, et al. Myoclonic epilepsy in down syndrome and Alzheimer disease. Neurologia. 2017;32:69–73.
103. Elia M, Musumeci SA, Ferri R, Ayala GF. Chromosome abnormalities and epilepsy. Epilepsia. 2001;42(Suppl 1):24–7.
104. Rudelli RD, Brown WT, Wisniewski K, Jenkins EC, Laure-Kamionowska M, Connell F, et al. Adult fragile X syndrome. Clinico-neuropathologic findings. Acta Neuropathol. 1985;67:289–95.
105. Reiss AL, Lee J, Freund L. Neuroanatomy of fragile X syndrome: the temporal lobe. Neurology. 1994;44:1317–24.
106. Musumeci SA, Bosco P, Calabrese G, Bakker C, De Sarro GB, Elia M, et al. Audiogenic seizures susceptibility in transgenic mice with fragile X syndrome. Epilepsia. 2000;41:19–23.
107. Musumeci SA, Calabrese G, Bonaccorso CM, D'Antoni S, Brouwer JR, Bakker CE, et al. Audiogenic seizure susceptibility is reduced in fragile X knockout mice after introduction of FMR1 transgenes. Exp Neurol. 2007;203:233–40.
108. Ferri R, Musumeci SA, Elia M, Del Gracco S, Scuderi C, Bergonzi P. BIT-mapped somatosensory evoked potentials in the fragile X syndrome. Neurophysiol Clin. 1994;4:413–26.
109. Irwin SA, Idupulapati M, Gilbert ME, Harris JB, Chakravarti AB, Rogers EJ, et al. Dendritic spine and dendritic field characteristics of layer V pyramidal neurons in the visual cortex of fragile-X knockout mice. Am J Med Genet. 2002;111:140–6.
110. Ivanco TL, Greenough WT. Altered mossy fiber distributions in adult Fmr1 (FVB) knockout mice. Hippocampus. 2002;12:47–54.
111. Li J, Pelletier MR, Perez Velazquez JL, Carlen PL. Reduced cortical synaptic plasticity and GluR1 expression associated with fragile X mental retardation protein deficiency. Mol Cell Neurosci. 2002;19:138–51.
112. Huber KM, Gallagher SM, Warren ST, Bear MF. Altered synaptic plasticity in a mouse model of fragile X mental retardation. Proc Natl Acad Sci U S A. 2002;99:7746–50.
113. Giuffrida R, Musumeci S, D'Antoni S, Bonaccorso CM, Giuffrida-Stella AM, Oostra BA, et al. A reduced number of metabotropic glutamate subtype 5 receptors are associated with constitutive homer proteins in a mouse model of fragile X syndrome. J Neurosci. 2005;25:8908–16.
114. Musumeci SA, Hagerman RJ, Ferri R, Bosco P, Dalla Bernardina B, Tassinari CA, et al. Epilepsy and EEG findings in males with fragile X syndrome. Epilepsia. 1999;40:1092–9.
115. Gauthey M, Poloni CB, Ramelli GP, Roulet-Perez E, Korff CM. Status epilepticus in fragile X syndrome. Epilepsia. 2010;51:2470–3.
116. Budka H. Megalencephaly and chromosomal anomaly. Acta Neuropathol (Berl). 1978;43:263–6.
117. Inoue H, Orita T, Matsushige T, Hasegawa S, Ichiyama T. Klinefelter's syndrome complicated with west syndrome in a 4-month-old boy. Brain Dev. 2012;34:148–50.
118. Elia M, Musumeci SA, Ferri R, Scuderi C, Del Gracco S, Stefanini MC. Seizures in Klinefelter's syndrome: a clinical and EEG study of five patients. Ital J Neurol Sci. 1995;16:231–8.
119. Tatum WO 4th, Passaro EA, Elia M, Guerrini R, Gieron M, Genton P. Seizures in Klinefelter's syndrome. Pediatr Neurol. 1998;19:275–8.
120. Broli M, Bisulli F, Mastrangelo M, Fontana E, Fiocchi I, Zucca C, et al. Definition of the neurological phenotype associated with dup (X)(p11.22–p11.23). Epileptic Disord. 2011;13:240–51.
121. Giorda R, Bonaglia MC, Beri S, Fichera M, Novara F, Magini P, et al. Complex segmental duplications mediate a recurrent dup(X) (p11.22–p11.23) associated with mental retardation, speech delay, and EEG anomalies in males and females. Am J Hum Genet. 2009;85:394–400.
122. Torniero C, Bernardina BD, Fontana E, Darra F, Danesino C, Elia M. Electroclinical findings in four patients with karyotype 47, XYY. Brain Dev. 2011;33:384–9.
123. Curatolo P. Tuberous sclerosis complex. From basic science to clinical phenotypes. London: Mac Keith Press; 2003.
124. Elia M. L'epilessia nella sclerosi tuberosa. In: Schepis C, editor. Argomenti in tema di sclerosi tuberosa. Troina: Multigrafica Troinese VCR srl; 2004. p. 55–64.
125. Randle SC. Tuberous sclerosis complex: a review. Pediatr Ann. 2017;46:e166–71.
126. Barkovich AJ, Guerrini R, Kuzniecky RI, Jackson GD, Dobyns WB. A developmental and genetic classification for malformations of cortical development: update 2012. Brain. 2012;135:1348–69.
127. Franz DN, Capal JK. mTOR inhibitors in the pharmacologic management of tuberous sclerosis complex and their potential role in other rare neurodevelopmental disorders. Orphanet J Rare Dis. 2017;12:51.
128. Blümcke I, Thom M, Aronica E, Armstrong DD, Vinters HV, Palmini A, et al. The clinicopathologic spectrum of focal cortical dysplasias: a consensus classification proposed by an ad hoc task force of the ILAE diagnostic methods commission. Epilepsia. 2011;52:158–74.
129. Becker AJ, Beck H. New developments in understanding focal cortical malformations. Curr Opin Neurol. 2018;31:151–5.
130. Lagarde S, Bonini F, McGonigal A, Chauvel P, Gavaret M, Scavarda D, et al. Seizure-onset patterns in focal cortical dysplasia and neurodevelopmental tumors: relationship with surgical prognosis and neuropathologic subtypes. Epilepsia. 2016;57:1426–35.
131. Guerrini R, Duchowny M, Jayakar P, Krsek P, Kahane P, Tassi L, et al. Diagnostic methods and treatment options for focal cortical dysplasia. Epilepsia. 2015;56:1669–86.
132. Aronica E, Mühlebner A. Neuropathology of epilepsy. Handb Clin Neurol. 2017;145:193–216.
133. Paladin F, Chiron C, Dulac O, Plouin P, Ponsot G. Electroencephalographic aspects of hemimegalencephaly. Dev Med Child Neurol. 1989;31:377–83.
134. Vigevano F, Bertini E, Boldrini R, Bosman C, Claps D, di Capua M, et al. Hemimegalencephaly and intractable epilepsy: benefits of hemispherectomy. Epilepsia. 1989;30:833–43.

135. Guzzetta F, Battaglia D, Lettori D, Deodato F, Sani E, Randò T, et al. Epileptic negative myoclonus in a newborn with hemimegalencephaly. Epilepsia. 2002;43:1106–9.
136. Di Rocco C, Battaglia D, Pietrini D, Piastra M, Massimi L. Hemimegalencephaly: clinical implications and surgical treatment. Childs Nerv Syst. 2006;22:852–66.
137. Guerrini R, Parrini E. Epilepsy and malformations of cerebral cortex. In: Bureau M, Genton P, Dravet C, Delgado-Escueta A, Tassinari CA, Thomas P, Wolf P, editors. Epilepsy syndromes in infancy, childhood and adolescence. 5th ed. London: John Libbey Eurotext Ltd; 2012. p. 607–29.
138. Hattori M, Adachi H, Tsujimoto M, Arai H, Inoue K. Miller-Dieker lissencephaly gene encodes a subunit of brain platelet-activating factor acetylhydrolase. Nature. 1994;370:216–8.
139. Pilz DT, Quarrell OWJ. Syndromes with lissencephaly. J Med Genet. 1996;33:319–33.
140. Poirier K, Keays DA, Francis F, Saillour Y, Bahi N, Manouvrier S, et al. Large spectrum of lissencephaly and pachygyria phenotypes resulting from de novo missense mutations in tubulin alpha 1A (TUBA1A). Hum Mutat. 2007;28:1055–64.
141. Sohal AP, Montgomery T, Mitra D, Ramesh V. TUBA1A mutation-associated lissencephaly: case report and review of the literature. Pediatr Neurol. 2012;46:127–31.
142. Mencarelli A, Prontera P, Stangoni G, Mencaroni E, Principi N, Esposito S. Epileptogenic brain malformations and mutations in tubulin genes: a case report and review of the literature. Int J Mol Sci. 2017;18:E2273.
143. Gastaut H, Pinsard N, Raybaud C, Aicardi J, Zifkin B. Lissencephaly (agyria-pachygyria): clinical findings and serial EEG studies. Dev Med Child Neurol. 1987;29:167–80.
144. Menascu S, Weinstock A, Farooq O, Hoffman H, Cortez MA. EEG and neuroimaging correlations in children with lissencephaly. Seizure. 2013;22:189–93.
145. Guerrini R, Sicca F, Parmeggiani L. Epilepsy and malformations of the cerebral cortex. Epileptic Disord. 2003;5(Suppl 2):S9–S26.
146. Herbst SM, Proepper CR, Geis T, Borggraefe I, Hahn A, Debus O, et al. LIS1-associated classic lissencephaly: a retrospective, multicenter survey of the epileptogenic phenotype and response to antiepileptic drugs. Brain Dev. 2016;38:399–406.
147. Gupta B, Ramteke P, Paul VK, Kumar T, DAS P. Ambiguous genitalia associated with an extremely rare syndrome: a case report of XLAG syndrome and review of the literature. Turk Patoloji Derg. 2017. https://doi.org/10.5146/tjpath.2017.01391. [Epub ahead of print].
148. Battaglia G, Chiapparini L, Franceschetti S, Freri E, Tassi L, Bassanini S, et al. Periventricular nodular heterotopia: classification, epileptic history, and genesis of epileptic discharges. Epilepsia. 2006;47:86–97.
149. Lopes CF, Cendes F, Piovesana AM, Torres F, Lopes-Cendes I, Montenegro MA, et al. Epileptic features of patients with unilateral and bilateral schizencephaly. J Child Neurol. 2006;21:757–60.
150. Granata T, Freri E, Caccia C, Setola V, Taroni F, Battaglia G. Schizencephaly: clinical spectrum, epilepsy, and pathogenesis. J Chil Neurol. 2005;20:313–8.
151. Lv Y, Ma D, Meng H, Zan W, Li C. A case of schizencephaly has a normal surface EEG but abnormal intracranial EEG: epilepsia partialis continua or dystonia? Clin EEG Neurosci. 2013;44:319–23.
152. Geerdink N, Rotteveel JJ, Lammens M, Sistermans EA, Heikens GT, Gabreëls FJ, et al. MECP2 mutation in a boy with severe neonatal encephalopathy: clinical, neuropathological and molecular findings. Neuropediatrics. 2002;33:33–6.
153. Keng WT, Pilz DT, Minns B, FitzPatrick DR. A3243G mitochondrial mutation associated with polymicrogyria. Dev Med Child Neurol. 2003;45:704–8.
154. Guerrini R, Dubeau F, Dulac O, Barkovich AJ, Kuzniecky R, Fett C, et al. Bilateral parasagittal parietooccipital polymicrogyria and epilepsy. Ann Neurol. 1997;41:65–73.
155. Chang BS, Piao X, Bodell A, Basel-Vanagaite L, Straussberg R, Dobyns WB, et al. Bilateral frontoparietal polymicrogyria: clinical and radiological features in 10 families with linkage to chromosome 16. Ann Neurol. 2003;53:596–606.
156. Pascual-Castroviejo I, Pascual-Pascual SI, Viaño J, Martinez V, Palencia R. Unilateral polymicrogyria: a common cause of hemiplegia of prenatal origin. Brain Dev. 2001;23:216–22.
157. Mitchell TN, Free SL, Williamson KA, Stevens JM, Churchill AJ, Hanson IM, et al. Polymicrogyria and absence of pineal gland due to PAX6 mutation. Ann Neurol. 2003;53:658–63.
158. Guerrini R, Genton P, Bureau M, Parmeggiani A, Salas-Puig X, Santucci M, et al. Multilobar polymicrogyria, intractable drop attack seizures, and sleep-related electrical status epilepticus. Neurology. 1998;51:504–12.
159. Chang BS, Piao X, Giannini C, Cascino GD, Scheffer I, Woods CG, et al. Bilateral generalized polymicrogyria (BGP): a distinct syndrome of cortical malformation. Neurology. 2004;62:1722–8.
160. Guerrini R, Barkovich AJ, Sztriha L, Dobyns WB. Bilateral frontal polymicrogyria: a newly recognized brain malformation syndrome. Neurology. 2000;54:909–13.
161. Caraballo RH, Cersósimo RO, Fortini PS, Ornella L, Buompadre MC, Vilte C, et al. Congenital hemiparesis, unilateral polymicrogyria and epilepsy with or without status epilepticus during sleep: a study of 66 patients with long-term follow-up. Epileptic Disord. 2013;15:417–27.
162. Teixeira KC, Cendes F, Guerreiro CA, Guerreiro MM. Focal electrical status (FES): a new finding associated with polymicrogyria. J Clin Neurophysiol. 2009;26:155–9.
163. Bartolini E, Falchi M, Zellini F, Parrini E, Grisotto L, Cosottini M, et al. The syndrome of polymicrogyria, thalamic hypoplasia, and epilepsy with CSWS. Neurology. 2016;29(86):1250–9.
164. Maillard LG, Tassi L, Bartolomei F, Catenoix H, Dubeau F, Szurhaj W, et al. Stereoelectroencephalography and surgical outcome in polymicrogyria-related epilepsy: a multicentric study. Ann Neurol. 2017;82:781–94.
165. Krsek P, Pieper T, Karlmeier A, Hildebrandt M, Kolodziejczyk D, Winkler P, et al. Different presurgical characteristics and seizure outcomes in children with focal cortical dysplasia type I or II. Epilepsia. 2009;50:125–37.
166. Buoni S, Zannolli R, Miracco C, Macucci F, Hayek J, Burroni L, et al. Focal cortical dysplasia type 1b as a cause of severe epilepsy with multiple independent spike foci. Brain Dev. 2008;30:53–8.
167. Fauser S, Schulze-Bonhage A. Epileptogenicity of cortical dysplasia in temporal lobe dual pathology: an electrophysiological study with invasive recordings. Brain. 2006;129:82–95.
168. Tassi L, Garbelli R, Colombo N, Bramerio M, Lo Russo G, Deleo F, Milesi G, Spreafico R. Type I focal cortical dysplasia: surgical outcome is related to histopathology. Epileptic Disord. 2010;12:181–91.

34 Paroxysmal Nonepileptic Events

Barbara Mostacci and Lidia Di Vito

Paroxysmal nonepileptic events are, like epileptic seizures, time-limited behavioral, cognitive, motor, sensory, and/or vegetative alterations. Unlike epilepsy, however, they do not depend on excessive cortical activity, but either are the result of neurological or systemic disturbances affecting the cerebral functions or have a psychogenic origin. The diagnostic work-up and the differentiation from epileptic seizures rely on the clinical description or visual analysis of the episodes and on several tests and exams.

This chapter will deal with the two conditions that pose the major issues of differential diagnosis with epilepsy: syncope and psychogenic seizures.

34.1 Syncope

34.1.1 Definition and Classification

Syncope is a transient self-limited episode of loss of consciousness resulting from cerebral hypoperfusion [1]. The classification is mainly based on the underlying mechanisms that lead to the transient global hypoperfusion, including the following.

34.1.1.1 Neurally Mediated Syncope (Reflex Syncope)

This is a group of conditions in which the cardiovascular effector mechanisms controlling circulation become overactive, resulting in vasodilatation and/or bradycardia causing a fall of blood pressure and consequently cerebral perfusion [2].

Vasovagal syncope is the most common type of this category and is also the most common cause of non-traumatic transient loss of consciousness, with an estimated 30–40% of people experiencing at least one episode in their lifetime [3]. It is typically triggered by emotional distress or prolonged orthostatism.

Carotid sinus syndrome results from an extreme reflex response to carotid sinus stimulation and may be elicited by rotation or turning of the head or pressure on the carotid sinus (i.e., shaving, tight collars or neckwear, or tumor compression). It is more common in the elderly and primarily in men [4].

Situational syncope may be triggered by different activities such as micturition, defecation, coughing, or swallowing.

34.1.1.2 Orthostatic Hypotension Syncope

Syncope occurs as a consequence of the body's inability to maintain an adequate blood pressure for cerebral perfusion on assuming the upright position [3, 5]. It may be drug-induced (alcohol, vasodilators, diuretics, beta-adrenergic blockers), due to volume depletion (inadequate fluid intake, diarrhea, vomiting, etc.) or caused by a primary autonomic failure (pure autonomic failure, multiple system atrophy, Parkinson's disease with autonomic failure, Lewy body dementia) or secondary autonomic failure (diabetes, amyloidosis, spinal cord injuries).

34.1.1.3 Cardiac Syncope

This category includes mainly syncope due to cardiac arrhythmias. Bradycardia and asystole are the commonest causes. However, supraventricular and ventricular tachyarrhythmias may also trigger syncope.

Less frequently syncope may be caused by valvular or structural heart disease (e.g., severe aortic stenosis, severe mitral stenosis, large left atrial myxoma, acute myocardial infarction) or pulmonary embolism.

34.1.1.4 Syncope Secondary to Cerebrovascular Causes

A transient ischemic attack in the vertebrobasilar distribution is a rare cause of syncope, often accompanied by posterior circulation symptoms (i.e., dizziness and loss of balance).

B. Mostacci (✉) · L. Di Vito
IRCCS Istituto delle Scienze Neurologiche di Bologna, Bologna, Italy
e-mail: b.mostacci@isnb.it

O. Mecarelli (ed.), *Clinical Electroencephalography*, https://doi.org/10.1007/978-3-030-04573-9_34

Steal syndrome due to subclavian stenosis is a rare condition that may provoke a syncope in case of intense or prolonged use of ipsilateral arm muscles. However, syncope as a solitary manifestation of these conditions is extremely rare [6].

34.1.2 Clinical Features

Syncope semiology includes the rapid onset of loss of consciousness with or without warning symptoms. Symptoms and signs generally fall into two groups [7].

Symptoms of the first group depend on the cause of syncope and include palpitations in arrhythmia or sensation of forthcoming swoon, pallor, and sweating in vasovagal syncope. Carotid sinus syncope generally has no prodromes.

Symptoms of the second group are the consequence of cerebral and retinal hypoperfusion and are therefore less specific, including visual disturbances, loss of consciousness and postural control, stiffness, and myoclonic jerks. When the latter are present, syncope is called "convulsive," and differential diagnosis with epilepsy may be more difficult. As in epileptic seizures, eyes usually remain open in the course of syncope; the most consistent ocular motor sign accompanying syncope is an upward turning of the eyes which can be preceded by a few seconds of downbeat nystagmus [8].

The circumstances in which the episode has occurred together with associated symptoms and signs are important to reach a correct diagnosis.

Several clinical features are useful for differential diagnosis of syncope and epilepsy.

In syncope, stiffness and jerks typically last for a shorter time, and jerks do not present with the typical frequency and amplitude evolution pattern observed in tonic-clonic seizures. Shmuely et al. reported that the number of myoclonic jerks has a strong diagnostic potential in differentiating syncope from convulsive seizures, fewer than 10 jerks indicating syncope and more than 20 seizures.

Loss of tone during transient loss of consciousness strongly favors syncope and argues against a convulsive seizure [9].

Automatisms, such as lip-licking, chewing, fumbling, and reaching for the head as well as growling or moaning vocalizations, are more frequent in epileptic seizures; however they were reported in case series of induced reflex syncope [1, 10].

Recovery from syncope is typically prompt and complete without residual neurologic findings. Enuresis may be observed, while fecal incontinence and tongue biting are very rare [11].

34.1.3 Diagnostic Work-Up

A thorough clinical history taking, together with physical examination, including orthostatic blood pressure measurement, and a basal ECG represent the basic diagnostic work-up, to be performed in all patients presenting with suspected syncope.

Additional exams may be required, depending on the suspected etiology, including cardiac evaluation, echocardiogram, ECG monitoring, and exercise stress testing in the suspicion of a cardiac syncope or provocation tests in reflex syncope [3].

The best-known provocation technique to induce neurally mediated or orthostatic hypotension syncope is tilt-table testing. The most used tilt-table method consists in relatively long duration (20–45 min) passive head-up position on a table with a footboard. A positive test is characterized by the onset of a syncope associated with a documented cardioinhibitory and/or a vasodepressor response causing hypotension. If the passive tilt is nondiagnostic, a pharmacological provocation with nitroglycerine or isoproterenol may be performed [12].

When carotid sinus hyperexcitability is suspected, a carotid sinus massage under ECG monitoring is useful for diagnostic confirmation.

34.1.4 EEG Findings

Although EEG is usually not recommended in the work-up of syncope, several specific features were described and may be of value for shading light on the pathophysiology of the typical clinical signs. The first EEG pattern of syncope to be reported was the "slow-flat-slow" pattern [13, 14], shown in Fig. 34.1. In the first slow phase, the background alpha rhythm is supplanted by a slow activity, decreasing in frequency from theta to delta waves while wave amplitude increases. This slow phase may last for up to 10 s; then the slow activity disappears abruptly, leaving a "flat" EEG whose duration depends on the duration of insufficient flow. The third phase consists of slow activity, in which frequency and amplitude evolve in the reverse order than the first slow phase, and hypersynchronous delta activity may be observed. This pattern is generally thought to denote more severe cerebral hypoperfusion. Accordingly, a second pattern consisting of slow activity only, corresponding to the first "slow" phase of the "slow-flat-slow" pattern, is thought to be associated with shorter or less severe hypoperfusion [7]. Flat EEG is invariably associated with loss of consciousness and postural control; conversely the relation between the level of consciousness and the degree of EEG slowing at the beginning of the episode remains unclear [7]. Motor phenomena occur at various phases and seem to be related to cortical ischemia, with slow EEG resulting from a reduced cortical function and flat EEG periods depending on suppression of cortical activity. Myoclonic jerks are mostly seen during the slow EEG phase, both at the onset of syncope and during its

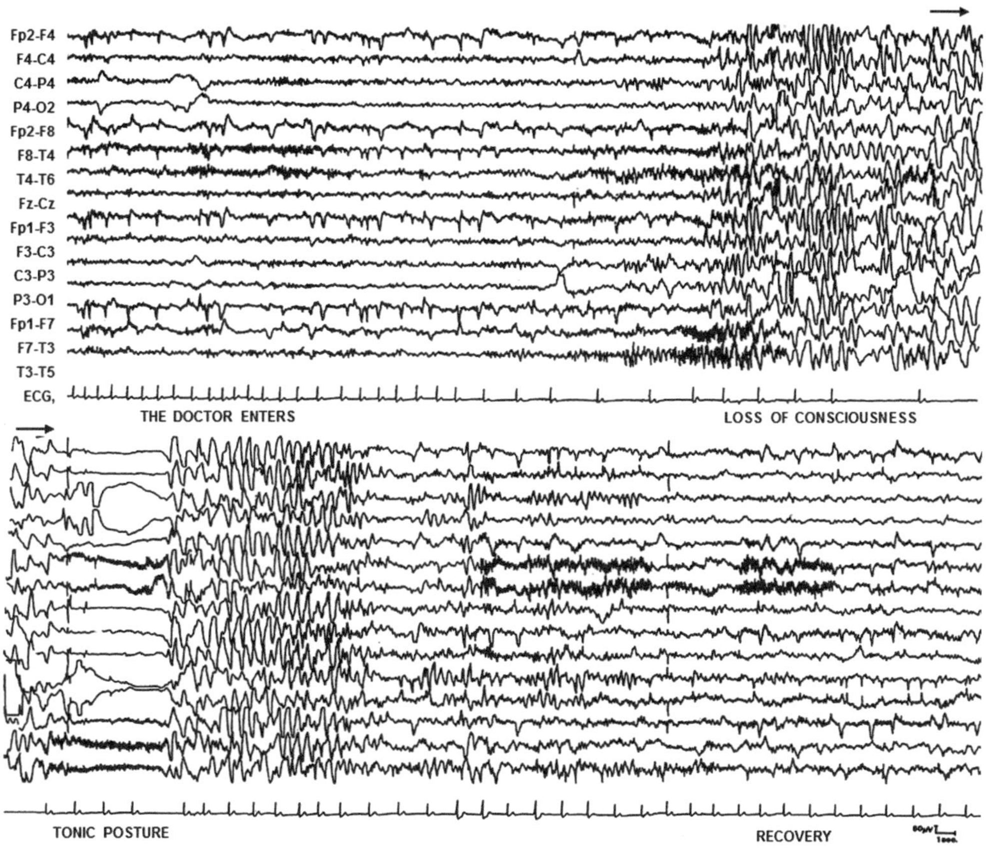

Fig. 34.1 A typical "slow-flat-slow" pattern in an 8-year-old child. After the onset of bradycardia, observable in the ECG trace, the background rhythm is supplanted by a slow, ample, theta-delta activity. During this phase a brief pause on ECG may be noticed and loss of consciousness supervenes. The slow activity then disappears abruptly, leaving a brief flattening on the EEG during which a tonic posture appears. ECG then returns to a normal rhythm, while a second slow phase activity appears on the EEG, evolving from hypersynchronous ample delta waves to theta activity. Subsequently the normal background activity resumes and so does consciousness

conclusion [9, 15]. They are likely of cortical origin and are thought to result from cortical hyperexcitability related to impaired cortical function and cortical disinhibition. Their abolition with electroencephalographic flattening suggests dependence on cortical activity.

Flaccidity invariably occurs during slowing of the EEG, while tonic postures, stertorous breathing, and roving cyc movements mostly occur during the flat EEG as a result of brainstem disinhibition related to loss of cortical function.

Interictal EEG is usually normal, but a specific EEG slowing, either focal or diffuse, can be observed.

Mecarelli et al. compared the EEG performed in basal condition and during hyperventilation (HV) in patients with neurally mediated syncope versus healthy controls. They found that syncope subjects presented more abundant and pronounced delta-theta activities and alpha slowing. In particular, the patients presented more frequently with slow activities and a peculiar intermittent rhythmic delta activity during prolonged HV (Fig. 34.2). These "pseudoparoxysmal" EEG changes are distinct, both from the common slowing observed during HV in adult subjects and from epileptiform activity [16]. Simultaneous transcranial Doppler and EEG recording performed in patients presenting this EEG pattern suggested that changes in the sympathetic modulation of cerebral vasoconstriction may explain both the pathophysiology of vasovagal syncope and the typical EEG findings [17].

34.1.5 Syncope in Epilepsy

As a rare and challenging condition, syncope may be the expression of an epileptic seizure. Epileptic syncope is typically preceded (and sometimes accompanied) by signs suggesting a temporal seizure, such as psychic or visceral aura, behavioral arrest, unresponsiveness, staring, gestural and oral automatisms, unilateral hypertonia, head turning, and more rarely clonic lateralized movements. It is usually secondary to ictal asystole or sudden bradycardia with concomitant severe hypotension [18–20].

In a series of 26 patients with a video-EEG-ECG recording of an ictal asystole, a typical electroclinical sequence was described. Ictal bradycardia and subsequent asystole arise after more than 30 s after the onset of seizures, and, clinically, seizure symptoms either continue or are replaced by syncope symptoms, while EEG discharges either continue or are supplanted by diffuse slowing (and, clinically, atonia supervenes) and/or EEG suppression (with hypertonia). On average normal EEG activity resumes after 10 s from the recovery of cardiac activity, while skin flushing and late

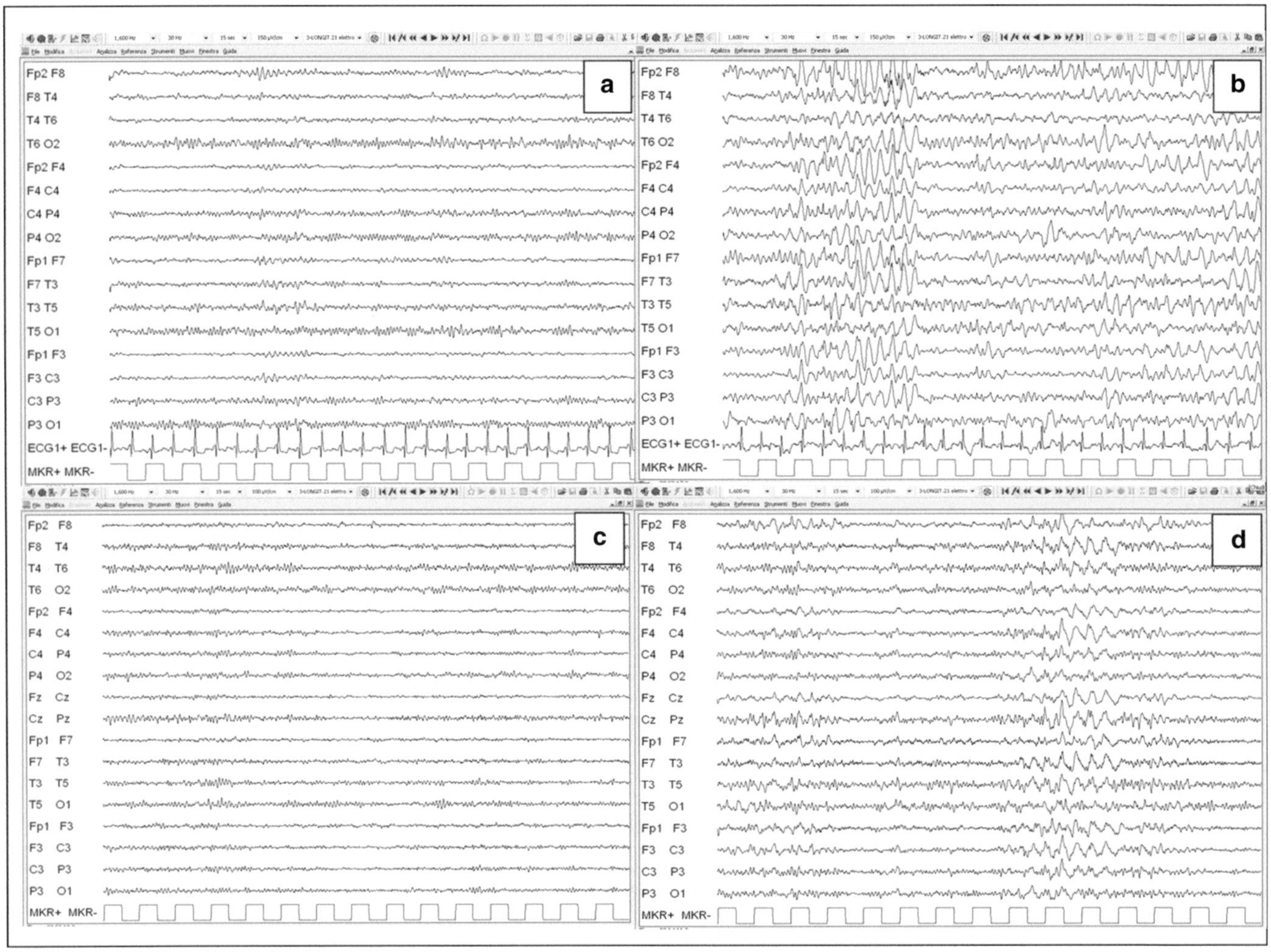

Fig. 34.2 EEG slow "pseudoparoxysmal" patterns after 3 min of hyperpnea in a 16-year-old (**a**, **b**) and in a 21-year-old (**c**, **d**) patients with recurrent vasovagal syncopes (Reproduced from Mecarelli and Zarabla 2009 [21])

myoclonic jerks may appear [20]. Figure 34.3 shows an example of ictal asystole with syncope.

It has also been reported that a syncope can occasionally trigger a seizure in patients with epilepsy [22], probably as a result of the transient cerebral hypoxia.

34.2 Psychogenic Nonepileptic Seizures

34.2.1 Definition and Overview

Psychogenic nonepileptic seizures (PNES) are paroxysmal attacks assumed to be the physical manifestation of a psychic disturbance, the most accredited interpretation being a dissociative response to potentially distressing stimuli. They are not a distinct nosological entity, and most of them are classified as a subtype of conversion disorders in the DSM V [23].

They have been variously named, including functional seizures, hysterical seizures, nonepileptic attack disorder, and pseudoseizures. It is currently advised that the latter should be avoided, as it implies deceit.

PNES are frequently seen in epilepsy centers, where these disturbances represent the final diagnoses for 9 to 50% of patients referred for refractory epilepsy [24–28].

The most common age at presentation is between the third and the fourth decade, and the female to male ratio is 3–4:1 [29, 30].

Patients with intellectual and learning disability and with mild traumatic injury are at greater risk for developing PNES [31, 32]. Although data from different studies are not consistent

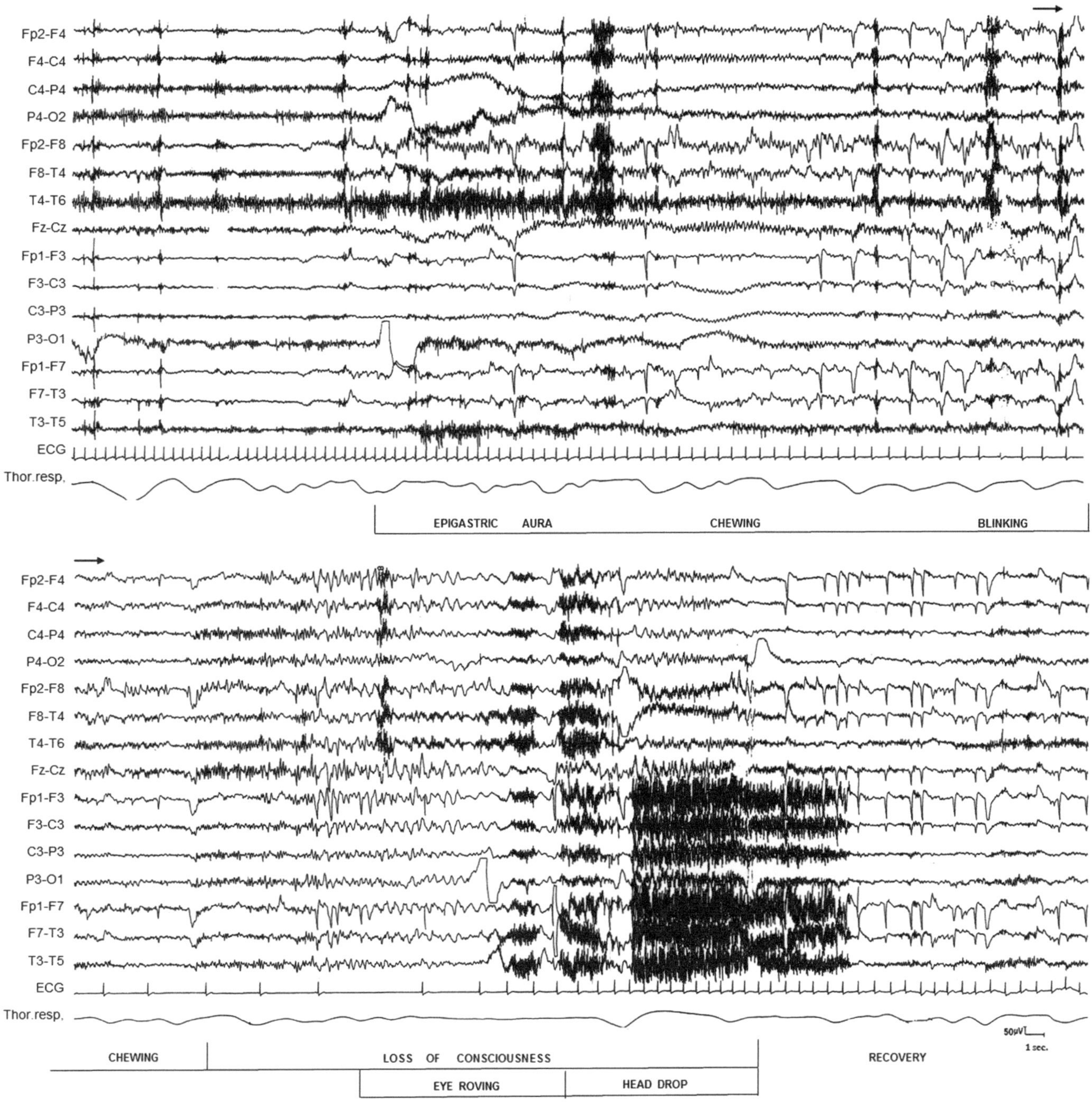

Fig. 34.3 Ictal EEG tracing of a 35-year-old woman with temporal lobe epilepsy. The patient reports an epigastric aura; then she starts chewing, swallowing, and then blinking. She answers correctly to the questions. The automatisms continue for several seconds; then loss of consciousness, accompanied by pallor, eye roving, and head drop, supervenes. During the first part of the seizure, the EEG shows a recruiting discharge over the right temporal lobe, rapidly spreading to the homolateral hemisphere and then contralaterally. Concomitantly to the loss of consciousness, diffuse sharp slow waves appear, followed by a brief EEG flattening and then by a theta activity over the right hemisphere, while the left hemisphere tracing is covered by artifacts. At the beginning of the seizure, the ECG shows tachycardia followed by a progressive decrease of the heart rate, leading to asystole lasting more than 5 s associated with apnea. The bradycardia and subsequent asystole are concomitant to the loss of consciousness, while recovery occurs several seconds after restoring the normal heart rate

concerning specific abnormalities or brain regions, there is evidence of a higher frequency of structural and functional abnormalities in patients with PNES compared to healthy controls [33].

A history of psychological trauma, particularly physical and sexual abuse, and a major life event in the year preceding diagnosis are very common [31, 32, 34–40].

Up to 10% of patients with PNES have comorbid epilepsy [29]. This comorbidity poses peculiar diagnostic difficulties as PNES onset typically follows epilepsy, presenting as a "pseudoresistance" to AEDs, particularly when the new seizures resemble the epileptic ones. Similar diagnostic dilemmas may arise when PNES occur de novo after epilepsy surgery, mimicking a surgical failure [41, 42]. Conversely, preexisting PNES may disappear after epilepsy surgery [42].

Several models were proposed and will not be discussed here, in which biological factors, comorbidities, experiences, and major life events could interact resulting in recurrent PNES [23, 29].

34.2.2 Clinical Ictal Features

Situational features more common in PNES than epileptic seizures (ES) are stressor events as seizure precipitants, habitual presence of "significant" witnesses (including physicians) [27, 30], and gradual onset (contrasting with the abrupt onset of ES) [27, 43]. The occurrence predominantly or exclusively during sleep is very specific of ES. However, PNES may occur during behavioral sleep, with EEG revealing normal waking activity ("pseudosleep") which, on the contrary, is very specific to PNES [26, 44–46].

Prodromal feelings are frequent and may suggest hyperventilation (light headedness, acral paresthesias, and palpitations) [25].

PNES usually last for more than 2 min and may be longer than 30 min, which is very unusual for ES [27, 46].

A motor behavior is frequently reported as part of the attack. The features most often reported in seizures mimicking generalized tonic-clonic seizures (GTCS) are asynchronous out-of-phase limb movements, or absence of in-phase limb movements, side-to-side head/body turning, forward pelvic thrusting, thrashing, and grabbing behavior [27, 46]. The retention of verbal responsiveness during PNES resembling GTCS is pathognomonic for PNES [47].

An important caveat is the resemblance of several motor features with seizures arising from (or propagating to) the frontal mesial structures, during which, to add complexity, awareness is often maintained during bilateral motor attacks, postictal signs are lacking, and ictal EEG may be normal [48–52]. However, movements in PNES generally involve the head and neck, whereas in mesial frontal lobe seizures, they are generalized or mainly involve the lower limbs and trunk. Features strongly pointing toward epilepsy include also turning to a prone position [49], tonic posturing in abduction of upper extremities [48], short-duration, highly stereotyped pattern and frequent or exclusive occurrence during sleep [48, 53].

Tonic posturing and opisthotonus can occur in PNES [26, 47, 48, 54] and the "arc de cercle" described by Charcot and Richer in 1887 is highly specific to these attacks. PNES often exhibit a discontinuous pattern with motor activity alternating with brief periods of rest, in contrast to the epileptic pattern [46, 47, 53, 55]. Motor activity resumes at the same frequency after pauses, and this leads to peculiar artifacts on the ECG and EEG as described later in this chapter [56].

PNES may present also as prolonged limpness without motor symptoms, possibly associated with apparent atonia [26, 35, 47, 54, 55]. Some minimal movements, such as intermittent eye blinking, swallowing, or mouthing movements, may be present [47] and so may be slumping forward [47], staring [26], or avoidance behavior [54]. Eyes are frequently closed, sometimes forcefully. This PNES pattern, which is also sometimes referred to as "pseudosyncope," does not really resemble any seizure type with the exception of very rare conditions like absence status or focal frontal status, in which, however, atonia is rare and the eyes are usually open. As a general rule, episodes with loss of consciousness lasting more than 5 min with immediate and complete recovery are not evocative of organic disturbances [53, 55]. However, caution is needed if the event has not been observed since the beginning, as a long-lasting unresponsiveness can represent the postictal phase following a GTCS [30].

Eye closure is a very important tool for differential diagnosis [27, 43, 46]. Eyes are closed during 55–96% of PNES. Conversely, eyes are open at the beginning or throughout 92–100% of ES, including episodes arising from sleep [27]. A forceful closure with active opposition to opening is very specific to PNES [26, 57].

Although individual ictal features may suggest a specific epileptic seizure type, the temporal sequence of events in PNES is often variable or not congruent with an epileptic discharge spreading [54, 55, 58].

Self-injury is uncommon in PNES. Tongue biting is rare and, when it occurs, is typically on the tip and not in the lateral or anterolateral tongue as in GTCS [27].

Postictal stertorous breathing, agitation, confusion, headache, and fatigue are uncommon after PNES [43, 46, 51, 59]. Ability to recall the seizure, in episodes with apparent impaired awareness, is specific to PNES [46, 53, 58, 60].

Though the absence of stereotypy is specific to PNES, stereotyped events were recorded in 67–90% of video-EEG studies recording multiple PNES in the same patient [27].

A fearsome and frequent complication of PNES (occurring in up to 78% of patients) [61] is psychogenic status, a condition in which the seizure lasts for a long time. It may rarely constitute the onset of a PNES disorder and can lead to intubation, use of anesthetics, and tracheostomy, if misdiagnosed for status epilepticus.

34.2.3 EEG Findings

34.2.3.1 Interictal EEG

Since interictal EEG alone does not allow the physician to make nor exclude the diagnosis of epilepsy, it cannot result in the diagnosis of PNES. Furthermore, some potential confounders should be kept in mind. EEG abnormalities, which can be found in up to 15% of the general population (less than 1% with an epileptiform appearance), are more common in patients with PNES independent of comorbid epilepsy [62, 63], as well as in borderline personality disorder and in relatives of patients with epilepsy, common conditions in PNES [25, 53, 54, 64]. Generalized epileptiform discharges can occur during drug withdrawal even in patients without epilepsy.

Furthermore, up to 37% of patients with PNES had a report of "epileptiform" abnormalities [65, 66] which, when re-evaluated at an epilepsy center, revealed to be normal variants [65], as in the case reported in Fig. 34.4.

Diagnostic levels of certainty of PNES were proposed by an International League Against Epilepsy (ILAE) Task Force, and an interictal EEG with no epileptiform activity is required, together with history or clinician-witnessed attack, to formulate a possible or probable diagnosis [30].

34.2.3.2 Ictal EEG

By definition, EEG has no alteration before, during, and after a psychogenic attack. However, this might be insufficient for a diagnosis because of two reasons. First, ictal scalp EEG may be normal even during seizures with sensory or very subtle behavioral symptoms and retained awareness [26, 57] and in mesial frontal lobe seizures [52], two types of seizures in which even semiology is often uninformative or challenging.

Second, motion artifacts can obscure the EEG or even be mistaken for ictal discharges. Figure 34.5 shows typical rhythmic artifacts in a PNES resembling GTCS.

However, an EEG, not obscured by artifacts, showing no ictal epileptiform activity in an attack in which it should be expectable if it were epileptic, together with a compatible history and an epileptologist-witnessed event, allows a diagnosis of clinically established PNES according to the diagnostic criteria of the ILAE Task Force [30].

A highly specific and sensitive rhythmic artifactual pattern on the EEG in PNES resembling GTCS has been described in a study. It consists of rhythmic movements with a stable frequency contrasting with the typical patterns observed during GTCS, characterized by rhythms in

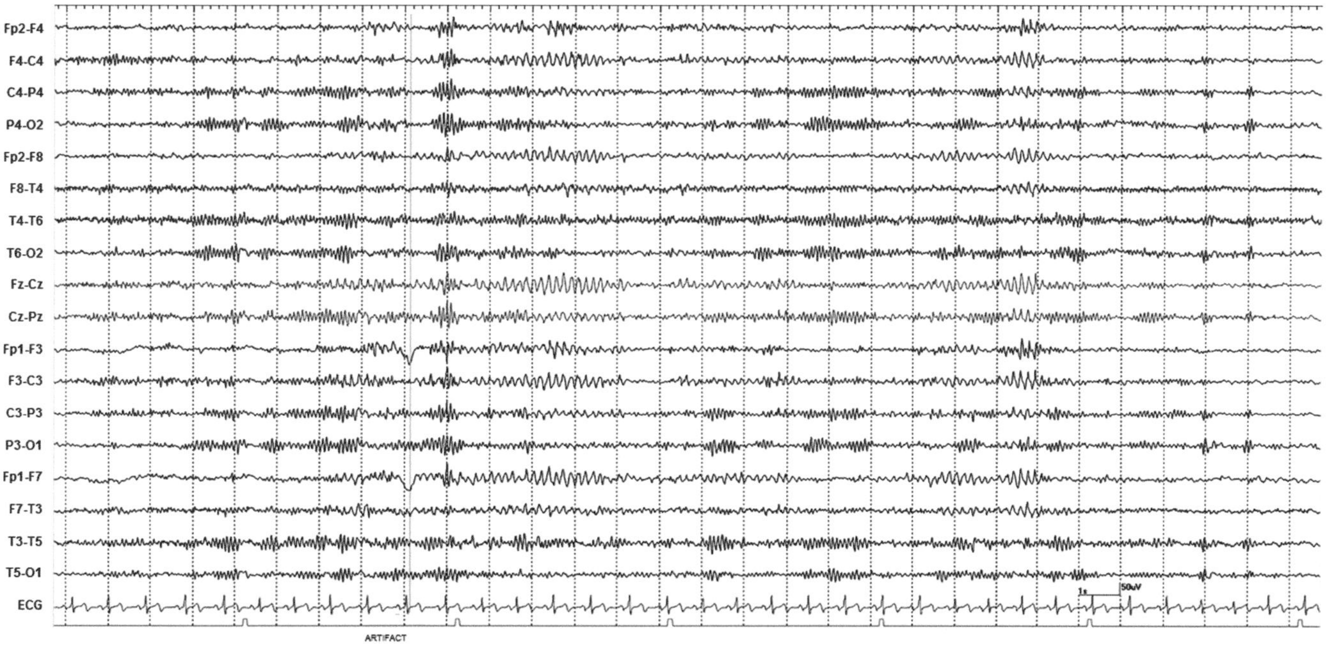

Fig. 34.4 EEG tracing of a 28-year-old woman who experienced three unclear episodes of brief "blackouts" followed by panic, breathing difficulties, and palpitations. A theta activity at 5–6 Hz, most prominent on the central vertex and diffuse over both frontal regions, may be observed, with a sinusoidal and, occasionally, spiky, appearance with a wax and wane pattern, mostly presenting on wakefulness fluctuations. This pattern was previously misinterpreted as "generalized epileptiform discharges" by neurologists who were not epileptologists, and antiepileptic treatment was started. When re-evaluated at our center, it was identified as a "midline theta rhythm," a normal variant

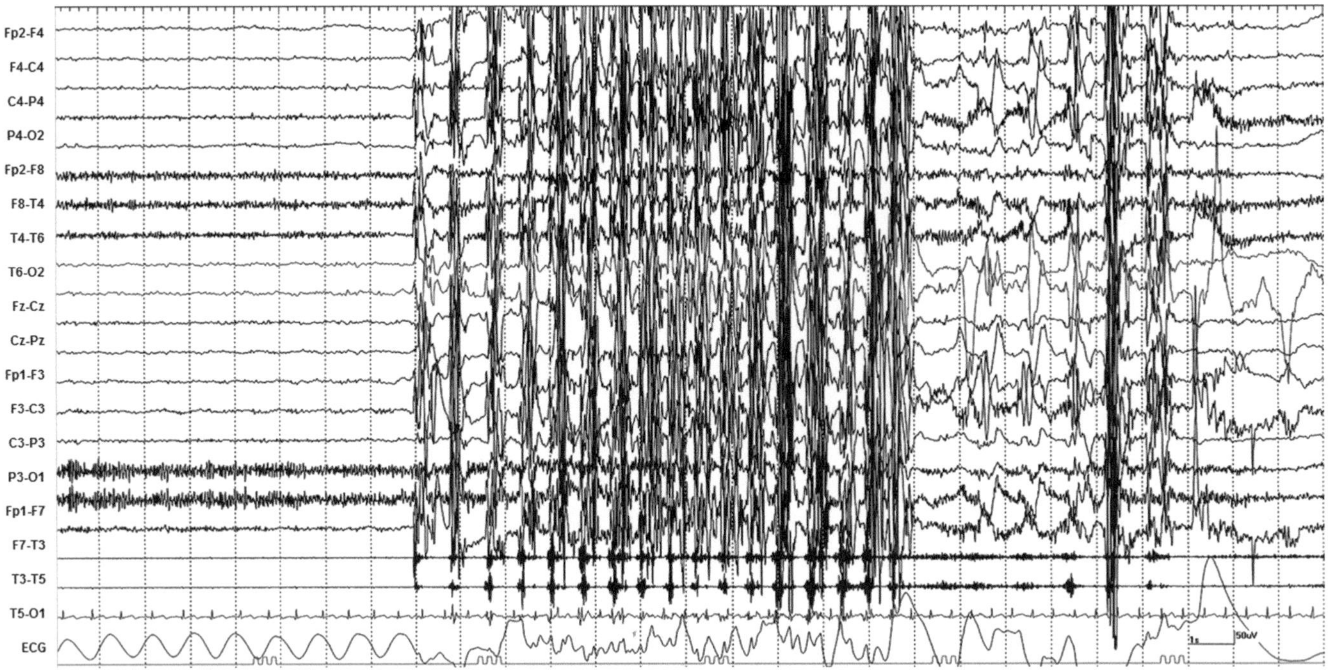

Fig. 34.5 Polygraphic tracing of a 13-year-old girl during an episode of intermittent "generalized" hypertonia with trunk and limb rhythmic jerks, induced by hyperpnea. The EEG shows rhythmic motor artifacts, corresponding to the muscle jerks on the EMG trace, with a rather constant frequency and a discontinuous pattern with a period of rest and subsequent brief resumption in the course of the event

the frequency of delta and beta range evolving from one to the other during the course of the seizure. This was documented with a time-frequency mapping of the EEG artifacts. The PNES pattern reflects a relative stability of limb movement frequency throughout the seizures, which differs from what happens in a GTCS. As a further very specific element, the authors described brief pauses in rhythmic movement, followed by resumption of movement at the same frequency ("on-off-on" pattern), which can be observed clinically and confirmed by analysis of the artifacts [56].

The concomitant recording of an ECG, which should be routinely performed, may offer additional information. Although in PNES an increase in heart rate might be observed, this is generally less significant, rapid, and sustained than the one typically observed during focal seizures with impaired awareness (temporal lobe seizures) and after a GTCS. Relative heart rate during and after a "staring seizure" proved to be a good diagnostic tool in one study: the increase by 30% of baseline rate during the spell had a 97% positive predictive value for epilepsy. Relative heart rate measurement showed a sensitivity of 83% and specificity of 96% [67]. The importance of ictal heart rate was not confirmed by another study in which, however, heart rate increases in the pre-ictal phase and decreases in the postictal phase significantly in PNES compared with ES [68].

34.2.3.3 Video-EEG Telemetry

Video-EEG monitoring is considered the "gold standard" investigation for PNES. Provided the abovementioned limitations on type of seizures and artifacts, in the presence of a suggestive history, the video recording of a typical event and the simultaneous recording of an EEG trace which does not show alteration, but instead keeps being a normal awake EEG before, during, or after the event, allow the diagnosis of documented PNES, according to the ILAE criteria [30]. It is paramount to record the habitual attack, and, when different kinds of seizures are reported, ideally all the types should be recorded, in order not to miss possible comorbid ES [30]. Figures 34.6 and 34.7 show examples of diagnostic tracings.

A typical event occurs within the first hours of video-EEG monitoring in the majority of patients according to several authors [30, 63, 66]. Indeed, according to a large study, more than 90% of the events are recorded in the first 30 min [69]. The presence of additional professional personnel in the EEG lab increases the chance to record an event [69].

Therefore, outpatient monitoring can be cost-effective, especially when provoking techniques are used [69]. Besides verbal suggestion, which should always accompany the others, they include prolonged photic stimulation and hyperventilation, compression of body parts, placing a tuning fork or moistened patches on the skin, intravenous administration of saline or other placebo, and hypnosis [29]. Induction may be used to start or stop the seizure. Although

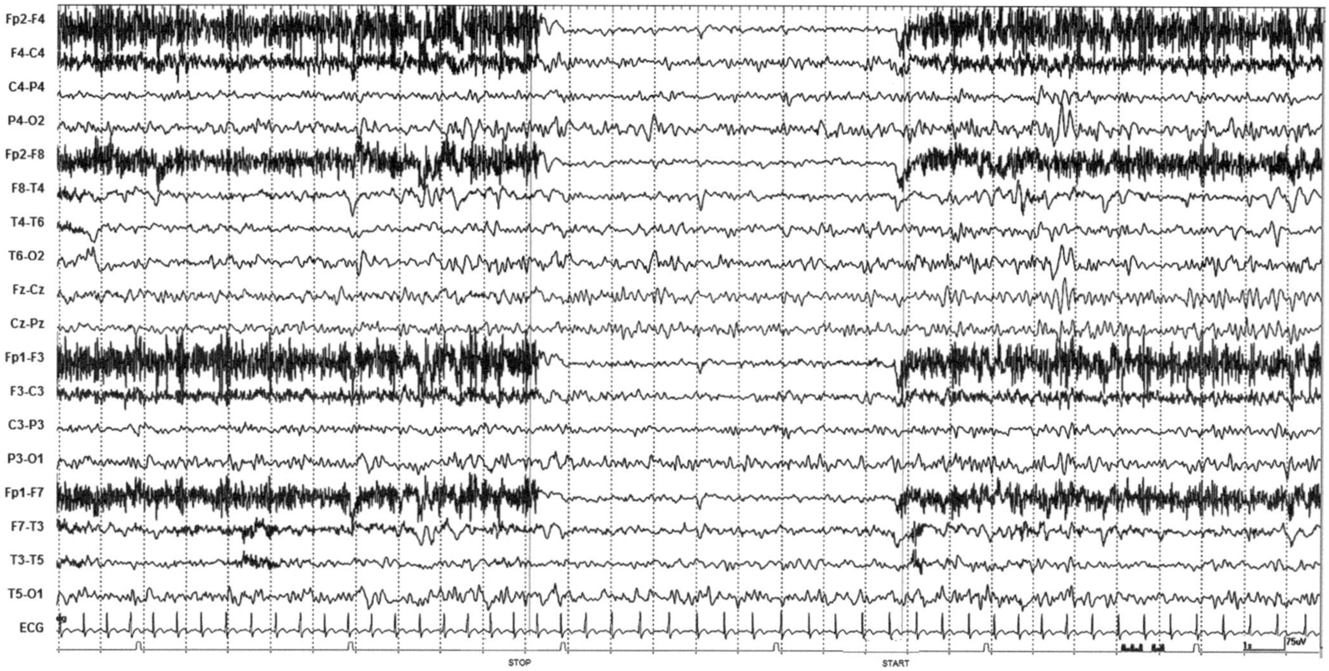

Fig. 34.6 EEG recording of a 6-year-old girl during which numerous episodes of bilateral rapid eyelid movements, with inconstant upward revulsion, were recorded. The EEG shows motor artifacts on the frontal regions during two episodes, while the background activity does not modify during and in between the events persisting as a normal wakefulness activity

Fig. 34.7 EEG tracing of a 38-year-old woman with a history of focal temporal lobe epilepsy and PNES, recorded during a status of apparent persistent impaired consciousness, subcontinuous facial jerks, and upper arms' "tremor," increasing during the medical visit. The EEG tracing shows a normal wakefulness activity with superimposed rhythmic muscular artifacts on the anterior derivations

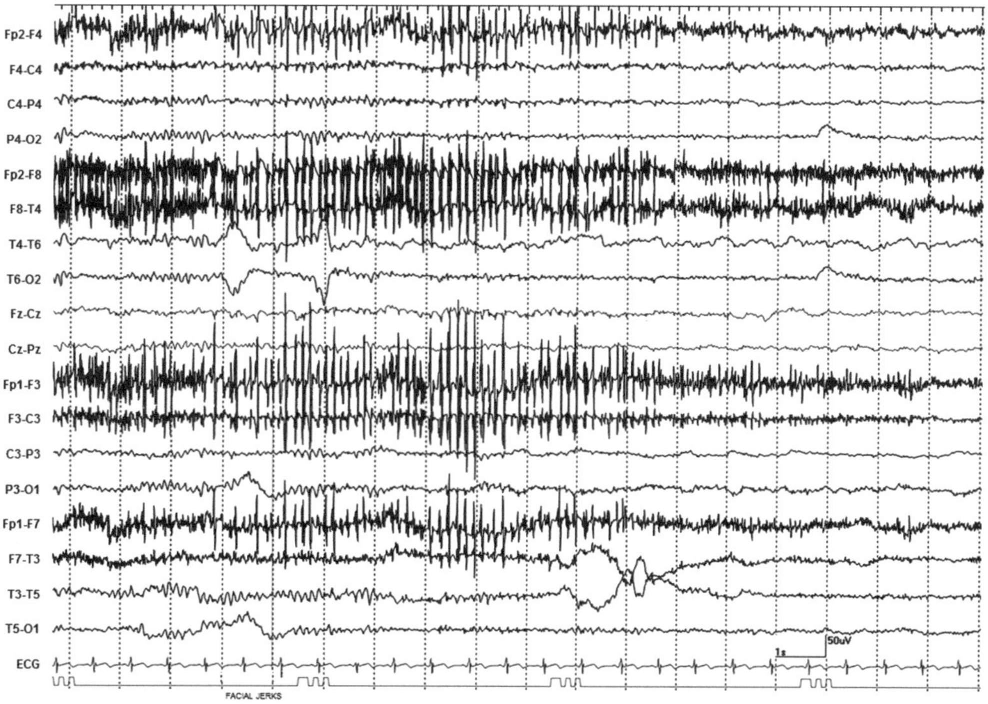

the use of placebo/nocebo poses ethical concerns, and some have questioned their specificity [70, 71], according to the majority of studies, induction maneuvers are highly sensitive and their specificity approaches 100% [29], significantly reducing time to diagnosis. Figure 34.8 shows the usefulness of nocebo/placebo in inducing and stopping a seizure in a challenging case.

Clinicians should review videos of the events with patients and families, in particular in cases of comorbidity with epilepsy, teaching them to differentiate PNES from ES in order

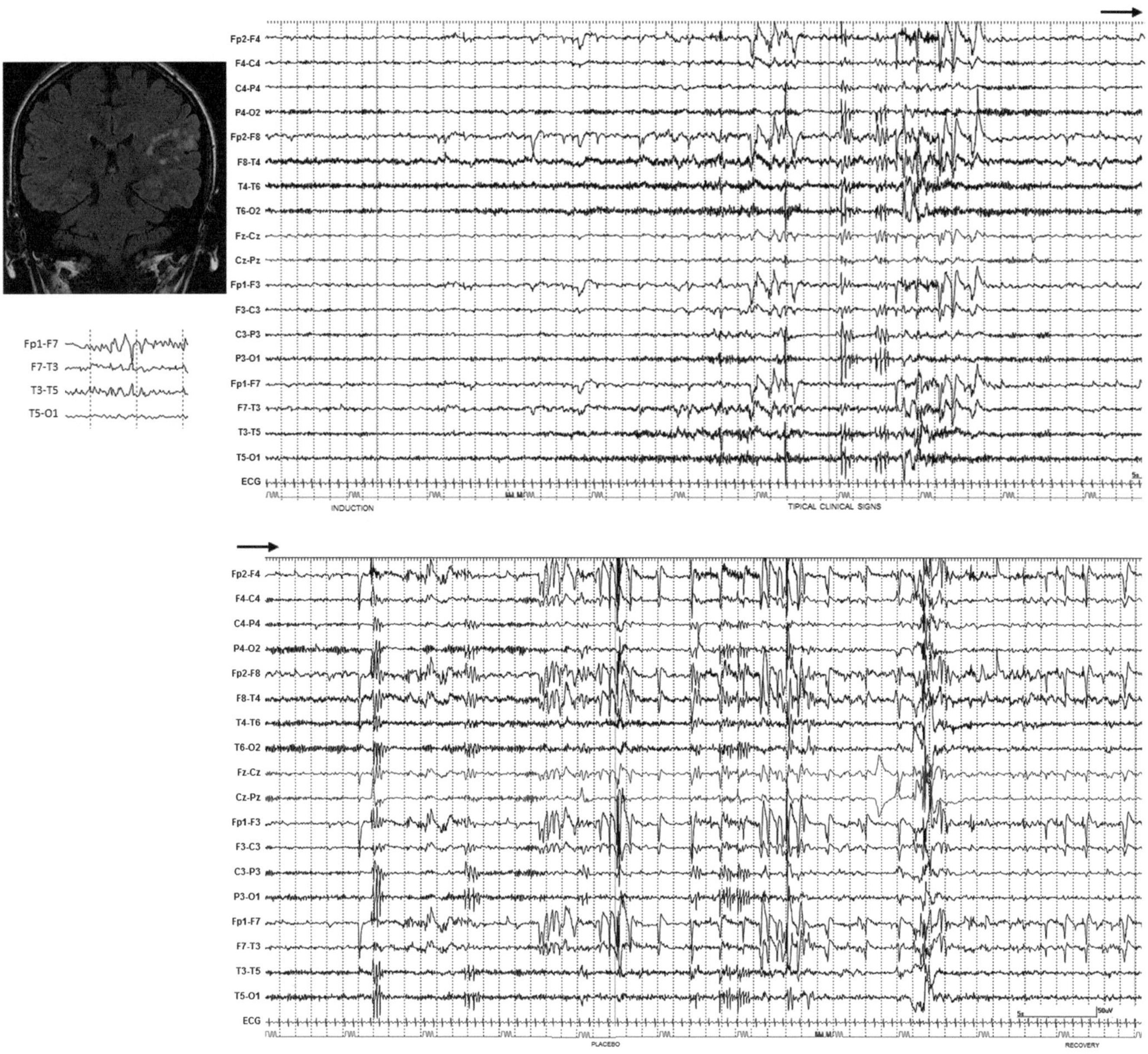

Fig. 34.8 Interictal focal spikes and MRI showing a parietal dysplasia in a 35-year-old woman who had a diagnosis of refractory epilepsy until a typical episode was recorded following intravenous saline nocebo administration. The episode consists of paroxysmal strabismus, aphasia, and lip protrusion and regresses after intravenous placebo

to correctly classify the subsequent events and guide management decisions, avoiding overtreatment [29].

34.2.4 Other Exams

Home video recording alone may have a high accuracy in selected patients when reviewed by experienced observer and in conjunction with a clear clinical history [30, 72]. An important caveat is that the onset of the seizure is frequently missed, and, therefore, the postictal phase of an ES may be mistaken for a PNES. Motor attacks seem more accurately recognized with this technique [30, 72]. In any case home video recording is a good screening tool before video-EEG recording.

Serum prolactin and CPK assays demonstrate with a good level of accuracy the absence of a postictal rise contrasting with the large majority of GTCS and most focal seizures with impaired awareness [30].

A validated linguistic approach proved useful to distinguish PNES from ES on the ground of the communication style patients used to describe their own seizures in German, English, and Italian [73–75].

Acknowledgments We thank Lara Alvisi for her precious technical assistance and Paolo Tinuper for support and advice.

References

1. Van Dijk JG, Thijs RD, van Zwet E, et al. The semiology of tilt-induced reflex syncope in relation to electroencephalographic changes. Brain. 2014;137(Pt 2):576–85.
2. Hainsworth R. Pathophysiology of syncope. 2004;14(Suppl 1):18–24.
3. Moya A, Sutton R, Ammirati F, et al. Task force for the diagnosis and Management of Syncope, European Society of Cardiology (ESC), European Heart Rhythm Association (EHRA), Heart Failure Association (HFA), Heart Rhythm Society (HRS), Guidelines for the diagnosis and management of syncope (version 2009). Eur Heart J. 2009;30:2631–71.
4. Parry SW, Steen N, Bexton RS, et al. Pacing in elderly recurrent fallers with carotid sinus hypersensitivity: a randomized double-blind placebo-controlled crossover trial. Heart. 2009;95:405–9.
5. Freeman R, Wieling W, Axelrod FB, et al. Consensus statement on the definition of orthostatic hypotension, neurally mediated syncope and the postural tachycardia syndrome. Clin Auton Res. 2011;21:69–72.
6. Chan-Tack KM. Subclavian steal syndrome: a rare but important cause of syncope. South Med J. 2001;94:445–7.
7. Wieling W, Thijs RD, van Dijk N, et al. Symptoms and signs of syncope: a review of the link between physiology and clinical clues. Brain. 2009;132.(Pt 10:2630–42.
8. Lempert T, von Brevern M. The eye movements of syncope. Neurology. 1996;46:1086–8.
9. Shmuely S, Bauer PR, van Zwet EW, et al. Differentiating motor phenomena in tilt-induced syncope and convulsive seizures. Neurology. 2018;90:e1339.
10. Lempert T, Bauer M, Schmidt D. Syncope: a videometric analysis of 56 episodes of transient cerebral hypoxia. Ann Neurol. 1994;36:233–7.
11. Puppala VK, Dickinson O, Benditt DG. Syncope: classification and risk stratification. J Cardiol. 2014;63(3):171–7.
12. Brignole M, Alboni P, Benditt DG, et al. Guidelines on management (diagnosis and treatment) of syncope—update 2004. Europace. 2004;6:467–537.
13. Gastaut H, Fischer-Williams EM, Lugaresi B. Electroencephalographic study of syncopes. II. Electro-clinical correlations in 25 subjects recorded during syncope. Rev Neurol. 1956;95:542–7.
14. Gastaut H, Fischer-Williams EM. Electro-encephalographic study of syncope; its differentiation from epilepsy. Lancet. 1957;273:1018–25.
15. Stephenson J. Fits and faints. Oxford: Blackwell Scientific Publications; 1990.
16. Mecarelli O, Pulitano P, Vicenzini E, et al. Observations on EEG patterns in neurally-mediated syncope: an inspective and quantitative study. Neurophysiol Clin. 2004;34(5):203–7.
17. Vicenzini E, Pro S, Strano S, Pulitano P, et al. Combined transcranial Doppler and EEG recording in vasovagal syncope. Eur Neurol. 2008;60(5):258–63.
18. Tinuper P, Bisulli F, Cerullo A, et al. Ictal bradycardia in partial epileptic seizures: autonomic investigation in three cases and literature review. Brain. 2001;124.(Pt 12:2361–71.
19. Rubboli G, Bisulli F, Michelucci R. Sudden falls due to seizure-induced cardiac asystole in drug-resistant focal epilepsy. Neurology. 2008;70(20):1933–5.
20. Nguyen-Michel VH, Adam C, Dinkelacker V, et al. Characterization of seizure-induced syncopes: EEG, ECG, and clinical features. Epilepsia. 2014;55(1):146–55.
21. Mecarelli O, Zarabla A. Manifestazioni parossistiche non epilettiche. In: Mecarelli O, editor. Manuale Teorico pratico di Elettroencefalografia. Italy: Wolters Kluwer Health, Lippincott Williams & Wilkins; 2009. p. 405.
22. Gastaut H, Broughton R, de Leo G. Syncopal attacks compulsively self-induced by the Valsalva manoeuvre in children with mental retardation. Electroencephalogr Clin Neurophysiol Suppl. 1982;35:323–9.
23. Reuber M, Brown RJ. Understanding psychogenic nonepileptic seizures-phenomenology, semiology and the integrative cognitive model. Seizure. 2017;44:199–205.
24. Gates JR, Ramani V, Whalen S, et al. Ictal characteristics of pseudoseizures. Arch Neurol. 1985;42:1183–7.
25. Lesser RP. Psychogenic seizures. Neurology. 1996;46:1499–507.
26. Hovorka J, Nezada T, Herman E, et al. Psychogenic non-epileptic seizures, prospective clinical experience: diagnosis, clinical features, risk factors, psychiatric comorbidity, treatment outcome. Epileptic Disord. 2007;9(Suppl 1):S52–8.
27. Mostacci B, Bisulli F, Alvisi L, et al. Ictal characteristics of psychogenic nonepileptic seizures: what we have learned from video/EEG recordings--a literature review. Epilepsy Behav. 2011;22(2):144–53.
28. Pana R, Labbé A, Dubeau F, et al. Evaluation of the "non-epileptic" patient in a tertiary center epilepsy clinic. Epilepsy Behav. 2018;79:100–5.
29. Widdess-Walsh P, Mostacci B, Tinuper P, et al. Psychogenic non-epileptic seizures. Handb Clin Neurol. 2012;107:277–95.
30. LaFrance WC Jr, Baker GA, Duncan R, et al. Minimum requirements for the diagnosis of psychogenic nonepileptic seizures: a staged approach. A report from the International League Against Epilepsy Nonepileptic Seizures Task Force. Epilepsia. 2013;54(11):2005–18.
31. Duncan R, Oto M. Predictors of antecedent factors in psychogenic nonepileptic attacks: multivariate analysis. Neurology. 2008a;71:1000–5.
32. Kerr WT, Janio EA, Braesch CT, et al. An objective score to identify psychogenic seizures based on age of onset and history. Epilepsy Behav. 2018;80:75–83.
33. Mcsweeney M, Reuber M, Levita L. Neuroimaging studies in patients with psychogenic non-epileptic seizures: a systematic meta-review. Neuroimage Clin. 2017;16:210–21.
34. Alper K, Devinsky O, Perrine K, et al. Nonepileptic seizures and childhood sexual and physical abuse. Neurology. 1993;43:1950–3.
35. Abubakr A, Kablinger A, Caldito G. Psychogenic seizures: clinical features and psychological analysis. Epilepsy Behav. 2003;4:241–515.
36. Binzer M, Stone J, Sharpe M. Recent onset pseudoseizures – clues to aetiology. Seizure. 2004;13:146–55.
37. Fleisher W, Staley D, Krawetz P, et al. Comparative study of trauma-related phenomena in subjects with pseudoseizures and subjects with epilepsy. Am J Psychiatry. 2002;159:660–3.
38. Fiszman A, Vieira Alves-Leon S, Gomes Nunes R, et al. Traumatic events and posttraumatic stress disorder in patients with psychogenic nonepileptic seizures: a critical review. Epilepsy Behav. 2004;5:818–25.
39. Rechlin T, Loew TH, Joraschky P. Pseudoseizure "status". J Psychosom Res. 1997;42:495–8.
40. Reuber M, Enright SM, Goulding PJ. Postoperative pseudostatus: not everything that shakes is epilepsy. Anaesthesia. 2000;55:74–8.
41. Parra J, Iriarte J, Kanner AM, et al. De novo psychogenic nonepileptic seizures after epilepsy surgery. Epilepsia. 1998;39:474–7.
42. González Otárula KA, Tan YL, Dubeau F, et al. Psychogenic non-epileptic seizures in patients with surgically treated temporal lobe epilepsy: Presurgical and de novo postsurgical occurrence. Epilepsy Behav. 2017;75:252–5.
43. Syed TU, LaFrance WC Jr, Kahriman ES, et al. Can semiology predict psychogenic nonepileptic seizures? A prospective study. Ann Neurol. 2011;69(6):997–1004.
44. Thacker K, Devinsky O, Perrine K, et al. Nonepileptic seizures during apparent sleep. Ann Neurol. 1993;33:414–8.
45. Benbadis SR, Lancman ME, King LM, et al. Preictal pseudosleep: a new finding in psychogenic seizures. Neurology. 1996;47:63–7.

46. Avbersek A, Sisodiya S. Does the primary literature provide support for clinical signs used to distinguish psychogenic nonepileptic seizures from epileptic seizures? J Neurol Neurosurg Psychiatry. 2010;81(7):719–25.
47. Gulick TA, Spinks IP, King DW. Pseudoseizures: ictal phenomena. Neurology. 1982;32(1):24–30.
48. Kanner AM, Morris HH, Luders H, et al. Supplementary motor seizures mimicking pseudoseizures: some clinical differences. Neurology. 1990;40(9):1404–7.
49. Saygi S, Katz A, Marks DA, et al. Frontal lobe partial seizures and psychogenic seizures: comparison of clinical and ictal characteristics. Neurology. 1992;42:1274–7.
50. Geyer JD, Payne TA, Drury I. The value of pelvic thrusting in the diagnosis of seizures and pseudoseizures. Neurology. 2000;54:227–9.
51. Azar NJ, Tayah TF, Wang L, et al. Postictal breathing pattern distinguishes epileptic from nonepileptic convulsive seizures. Epilepsia. 2008;49:132–7.
52. Tinuper P, Bisulli F, Cross JH, et al. Definition an diagnostic criteria of sleep-related hypermotor epilepsy. Neurology. 2016;86(19):1834–42.
53. Mellers JDC. The approach to patients with "non-epileptic seizures". Postgrad Med J. 2005;81:498–504.
54. Luther JS, McNamara JO, Carwile S, et al. Pseudoepileptic seizures: methods and video analysis to aid diagnosis. Ann Neurol. 1982;12:458–62.
55. Meierkord H, Will B, Fish D, et al. The clinical features and prognosis of pseudoseizures diagnosed using video-EEG telemetry. Neurology. 1991;41:1643–6.
56. Vinton A, Carino J, Vogrin S, et al. "Convulsive" nonepileptic seizures have a characteristic pattern of rhythmic artifact distinguishing them from convulsive epileptic seizures. Epilepsia. 2004;45:1344–50.
57. DeToledo JC, Ramsay RE. Patterns of involvement of facial muscles during epileptic and nonepileptic events: review of 654 events. Neurology. 1996;47:621–5.
58. Leis AA, Ross MA, Summers AK. Psychogenic seizures: ictal characteristics and diagnostic pitfalls. Neurology. 1992;42:95–9.
59. Ettinger AB, Weisbrot DM, Nolan E, et al. Postictal symptoms help distinguish patients with epileptic seizures from those with nonepileptic seizures. Seizure. 1999;8:149–51.
60. Bell WL, Park YD, Thompson EA, et al. Ictal cognitive assessment of partial seizures and pseudoseizures. Arch Neurol. 1998;55:1456–9.
61. Reuber M, Pukrop R, Mitchell AJ, et al. Clinical significance of recurrent psychogenic nonepileptic seizure status. J Neurol. 2003;250:1355–62.
62. Reuber M, Fernández G, Bauer J, et al. Interictal EEG abnormalities in patients with psychogenic nonepileptic seizures. Epilepsia. 2002;43:1013–20.
63. Woollacott IOC, Scott C, Fish DR, et al. When do psychogenic nonepileptic seizures occur on a video/EEG telemetry unit? Epilepsy Behav. 2010;17:228–35.
64. De la Fuente JM, Tugendhaft P, Mavroudakis N. Electroencephalographic abnormalities in borderline personality disorder. Psychiatry Res. 1998;77:131–8.
65. Benbadis S, Tatum W. Overinterpretation of EEGs and misdiagnosis of epilepsy. J Clin Neurophysiol. 2003;20:42–4.
66. Lobello K, Morgenlander JC, Radtke JA, et al. Video/EEG monitoring in the evaluation of paroxysmal behavioral events: duration, effectiveness and limitations. Epilepsy Behav. 2006;8:261–6.
67. Opherk C, Hirsch LJ. Ictal heart rate differentiates epileptic from non-epileptic seizures. Neurology. 2002;58:636–8.
68. Reinsberger C, Perez DL, Murphy MM, et al. Pre- and postictal, not ictal, heart rate distinguishes complex partial and psychogenic nonepileptic seizures. Epilepsy Behav. 2012;23(1):68–70.
69. Kandler R, Lawrence S, Pang C, et al. Optimising the use of EEG in non-epileptic attack disorder: results of a UK national service evaluation. Seizure. 2018;55:57–65.
70. Devinsky O, Fisher R. Ethical use of placebos and provocative testing in diagnosing nonepileptic seizures. Neurology. 1996;47:866–70.
71. Gates JR. Provocative testing should not be used for nonepileptic seizures. Arch Neurol. 2001;58:2065.
72. Chen DK, Graber KD, Anderson CT, et al. Sensitivity and specificity of video alone versus electroencephalography alone for the diagnosis of partial seizures. Epilepsy Behav. 2008;13:115–8.
73. Reuber M, Monzoni C, Sharrack B, et al. Using interactional and linguistic analysis to distinguish between epileptic and psychogenic nonepileptic seizures: a prospective, blinded multirater study. Epilepsy Behav. 2009;16:139–44.
74. Plug L, Sharrack B, Reuber M. Conversation analysis can help to distinguish between epilepsy and non-epileptic seizure disorders: a case comparison. Seizure. 2009;18:43–50.
75. Papagno C, Montali L, Turner K, et al. Differentiating PNES from epileptic seizures using conversational analysis. Epilepsy Behav. 2017;76:46–50.

Sleep Diseases

35

Liborio Parrino, Andrea Melpignano, and Giulia Milioli

The fountains mingle with the river
And the rivers with the Ocean,
The winds of Heaven mix for ever
With a sweet emotion;
Nothing in the world is single;
All things by a law divine
In one spirit meet and mingle.
—Percy Bysshe Shelley

35.1 Insomnia

Insomnia refers to a set of different clinical pictures in terms of onset, course, etiology, and therapeutic approach. The sleepless individual can complain of having difficulty falling asleep, not being able to maintain a continuous sleep all night, waking up too early in the morning, or simply having a non-restorative sleep. Each of these subjective disorders, also called nocturnal markers of insomnia, has an identifiable neurophysiological correlation within polysomnography, indicating a non-exclusively mental origin of insomnia. Accordingly, the new DSM-5 [1] and the ICDS-3 consider insomnia a disorder and not simply the symptom of an organic or psychiatric disease. However, in clinical practice, the diagnosis of insomnia is almost exclusively anamnestic. According to the European guidelines [2], the diagnostic procedure for insomnia, and its comorbidities, should include a clinical interview consisting of a sleep history (sleep habits, sleep environment, work schedules, circadian factors), the use of sleep questionnaires and sleep diaries, questions about somatic and mental health, a physical examination, and additional measures if indicated (i.e., blood tests, electrocardiogram, electroencephalogram). Wearable actigraph devices record movements that can be used to estimate sleep parameters with specialized algorithms in computer software programs. This technology is being used increasingly in clinical settings as actigraphy has the advantage of providing objective information on sleep habits in the patient's natural sleep environment and/or when extended monitoring is clinically indicated. Although actigraphy has been well validated for the estimation of nighttime sleep parameters across age groups, the accuracy of sleep-onset latency and daytime sleeping is limited [3]. Moreover, when polysomnographic (PSG) recordings are applied, in many cases, conventional sleep patterns of insomniac individuals do not differ significantly from those of good sleepers, and a number of patients with insomnia underestimate the actual objective sleep time. Accordingly, PSG may be useful to rule out other sleep disorders (e.g., sleep-disordered breathing, periodic limb movement disorder) in patients who appear to meet criteria for a chronic insomnia disorder. The discrepancy between subjective and objective data represents a critical issue and raises the question whether alternative metrics of sleep quality (e.g., the analysis of sleep microstructure or related physiological parameters) are more pertinent than the conventional measures of sleep latency, total sleep time, and wake after sleep onset [4].

L. Parrino (✉) · A. Melpignano · G. Milioli
Department of Medicine and Surgery, Sleep Medicine Center, University of Parma, Parma, Italy
e-mail: liborio.parrino@unipr.it

35.1.1 Insomnia and Instrumental Findings

Although questionnaires and sleep logs may supply relevant information regarding sleep habits, self-reports of sleep latency, number of awakenings, and nocturnal wakefulness are often imprecise due to insomniacs' underestimation of total sleep time. In contrast, PSG can offer objective data on the typical features of insomnia. In particular, sleep macrostructure shows altered metrics with a longer sleep latency, more stage 1 sleep and less SWS sleep [5–7]. In a meta-analysis of PSG studies comparing good sleepers (n. 485) and patients with chronic insomnia disorder (n. 582) [8], Baglioni et al. described consistent differences in sleep latency, total sleep time, sleep efficiency, and wake after sleep onset (with a difference of 12 min in subjective data collected from diaries). A reduction in REM sleep and SWS (slow wave sleep) was also detected. Finally, PSG features may be exploited to evaluate and compare different therapies (CBT or drug) applied in the treatment of insomnia [9, 10].

O. Mecarelli (ed.), *Clinical Electroencephalography*, https://doi.org/10.1007/978-3-030-04573-9_35

Besides conventional PSG measures, integrative information can be supplied by sleep microstructure. In several studies, EEG spectral analysis in insomniacs revealed an increase of power in beta and sigma band during NREM sleep compared to healthy sleepers [11, 12]. Increased activity in the beta frequency band also during rapid eye movement (REM) sleep has been reported [13–15]. Increased activities in NREM and REM sleep in faster frequency bands suggest an excessive cortical activation and link insomnia to physiological and emotional hyperactivation as predisposing, precipitating, and maintaining factors [16].

Accordingly, insomnia reflects also an altered hormonal and autonomic condition. Compared to good sleepers, insomniacs usually present a higher metabolic rate as well as a faster cardiac rhythm on a 24 h basis [17], and the presence of chronic insomnia (with TST shorter than 5 h) is associated with an increased risk of arterial hypertension and acute cardiovascular diseases [18]. In other words, the impact of insomnia is not simply confined to the sleep metrics (subjective or objective) but reverberates also on the global balance of the living system with a heavy biological burden on wellness and health.

35.1.2 CAP Role in Insomnia

A microstructural component that is always altered in pathologic sleep is the cyclic alternating pattern (CAP).

CAP is a periodic EEG activity occurring under conditions of reduced vigilance (sleep, coma). It is characterized by sequences of CAP cycles defined by an A phase (transient electrocortical events that are distinct from background EEG activity) and by the following B phase (return to background EEG activity).

CAP translates a neurophysiological condition of unstable sleep, and the amount of CAP correlates significantly with the subjective perception of sleep quality [19].

Good sleep quality is associated with low CAP values that undergo age-related differences across the life span.

The enhancement of CAP time and CAP rate is a regular feature in insomniac patients, independent of cultural or genetic factors. A study on a large sample of Caucasian patients with primary insomnia showed that CAP parameters consistently correlate with sleep quality and it can be useful to quantify the effectiveness of hypnotic treatment [20]. Similar findings were described on insomniac Japanese patients in a randomized crossover comparative study with placebo which demonstrated that zolpidem medication consolidates sleep stability with a reduction of CAP rate and improves sleep perception [21].

The subtle information supplied by CAP parameters is clinically useful in insomniac patients who show a mismatch between subjective reports (poor sleep quality, nocturnal awakenings) and conventional PSG parameters. Compared to normal controls, insomniacs with sleep misperception (also defined paradoxical insomnia) show significantly higher amounts of CAP rate in stage 1 and in stage 2, but not in slow-wave sleep. Misperceptors report lower but longer amounts of subjective awakenings (mean: 4) in contrast to objective findings (mean: 11). The mismatch is related to the high amounts of CAP between successive awakenings which are merged together by the patient in a single experience. In other words, if sleep between two successive awakenings is superficial (expressed by sleep stages 1 and 2), unstable (as reflected by increased amounts of CAP), and fragmented (increased arousal index), the time separating the two events is perceived as continuous wake. Misperceptors interpret as wakefulness their difficulty to maintain consolidated sleep [22].

In conclusion, an increased amount of CAP is a typical PSG finding in insomniac patients, even without a clear-cut sleep macrostructure disruption.

Therefore, PSG microstructural measures can feature an important role in the objective identification of a sleep disorder, even when conventional sleep measures appear unaltered.

The additional value of sleep microstructure is also supported by the tight association between CAP and autonomic arousals, which are often neglected in the evaluation of biological price of chronic insomnia.

Finally, microstructural investigation can shed light on the treatment strategies of insomnia as CAP parameters allow us to discriminate hypnotic drugs from placebo, benzodiazepines from Z-drugs, and zopiclone from zolpidem [23].

35.2 Parasomnias

Parasomnias are defined as undesirable motor events or experiences that occur during sleep onset, inside sleep, or during arousal from sleep. Parasomnias may occur during NREM sleep (NREM parasomnias: disorders of arousal, confusional arousals, sleepwalking, sleep terrors) and REM sleep (REM parasomnias: REM behavior disorder, recurrent sleep paralysis, nightmare disorder).

The main pathophysiological mechanism of parasomnias is a boundary failure between wakefulness and sleep [24].

Parasomnias play a relevant role in clinical practice, although they are common and usually benign during childhood when they are considered as an expression of a non-completed brain maturation. In adulthood they may trigger severe injuries to the patient or to the bed partner and cause social impairment and related medicolegal issues.

35.2.1 NREM Sleep Parasomnias (Disorders of Arousal)

This group includes confusional arousals, sleepwalking, and sleep terrors which are not distinct conditions but rather a continuum of behavioral patterns. They derive from a partial arousal from deep NREM sleep, less frequently from superficial NREM sleep. During the episodes the subject presents a reduced or absent responsiveness and impaired cognition functionality or a dreamlike imagery. Usually patients are amnesiac for the episode. Eating behavior can occur during sleep in a condition of full awareness (nocturnal eating syndrome [25]) or unconsciousness (sleep-related eating syndrome [26]).

Typically the events occur during the first third of sleep, when SWS is predominant. The confusional state can last several minutes or longer [27].

35.2.1.1 Confusional Arousal

The episodes are characterized by mental confusion or confused behavior that occurs while the patient is sleeping. The subjects seem disoriented, nonresponsive to external stimuli, and cognitively impaired but do not show signs of fear. Confusional arousals usually begin with a sitting up in bed and looking around in a dazed deportment without walking outside the bed [28].

During the episodes violent behaviors may appear, especially if the patient is abruptly awakened. Sometimes confusional arousals coexist with sleepwalking. A confusional arousal emerging from REM sleep is rare. Intracerebral recording demonstrated, during an episode of confusional arousal, the occurrence of fast EEG activities in motor, cingulate, insular temporopolar areas and the concomitant presence of slower activity in frontal regions [29].

35.2.1.2 Sleepwalking

With this term we mean a group of behaviors that typically begin from an arousal during deep NREM sleep and proceed to leaving the bed with an impaired state of consciousness [30].

35.2.1.3 Sleep Terror (Pavor Nocturnus)

Episodes of intense fright or terror, usually associated with agitation and screaming, that arise suddenly from NREM sleep. They are common in childhood. The patients during episodes are not completely responsive and are totally inconsolable [31]. Commonly a strong autonomic activity is present (tachycardia, flushing, mydriasis, sweating).

35.2.2 PSG Features of NREM Parasomnias

EEG can show brief periods of delta activity, a stage 1-like pattern, or repetitive microsleeps or a diffuse, poorly reactive, alpha rhythm.

Especially in sleepwalking, diagnostic PSG may detect high-amplitude hypersynchronous delta waves and, sometimes, frequent arousals from slow-wave sleep. However, these findings do not have a high specificity, since they have been described in the normal population and in subjects with sleep-related breathing disorders [32] (Fig. 35.1).

Video-PSG is mandatory for the diagnosis. A disorder of arousal must be distinguished from sleep apnea-related arousals, paroxysmal arousals in sleep-related hypermotor epilepsy (SHE), or RBD (REM Behavior Disorder). PSG allows us to identify possible triggering factors, such as sleep apnea or periodic limb movements. Sleep deprivation [33], acoustic stimulation during sleep [34], hypnotic agents (e.g., Z-drugs [35]), or antidepressant drugs can evoke parasomnias in predisposed individuals [36].

In NREM parasomnia sleep macrostructure is usually well preserved, but sleepwalkers show numerous awakenings from SWS and decreased delta power [37].

Sleep microstructure can exhibit some alterations. In adult with somnambulism, power spectral analyses of slow-wave activity show high quantity of slow-wave sleep disruption (principally during the first sleep cycle) or a significant increase in delta power just prior to an arousal. An increased slow-wave activity across all NREM sleep cycles has been reported [38, 39].

35.2.3 REM Parasomnias

35.2.3.1 REM Behavior Disorder

REM behavior disorder (RBD) is characterized by abnormal behaviors during REM sleep that may cause injury or sleep disruption. The main finding is an EMG abnormality during REM sleep characterized by an excess of muscle tone (REM without atonia or RWA) and/or an excess of phasic EMG twitch activity during REM sleep [40] (Fig. 35.2).

These abnormal behaviors seem to resemble the dream content (i.e., dream-enacting behavior).

Acting out dreams may consist in many different motor manifestations, such as talking, limb twitching, yelling, punching, kicking, and developing dangerous patterns for the patient or for the bed partner.

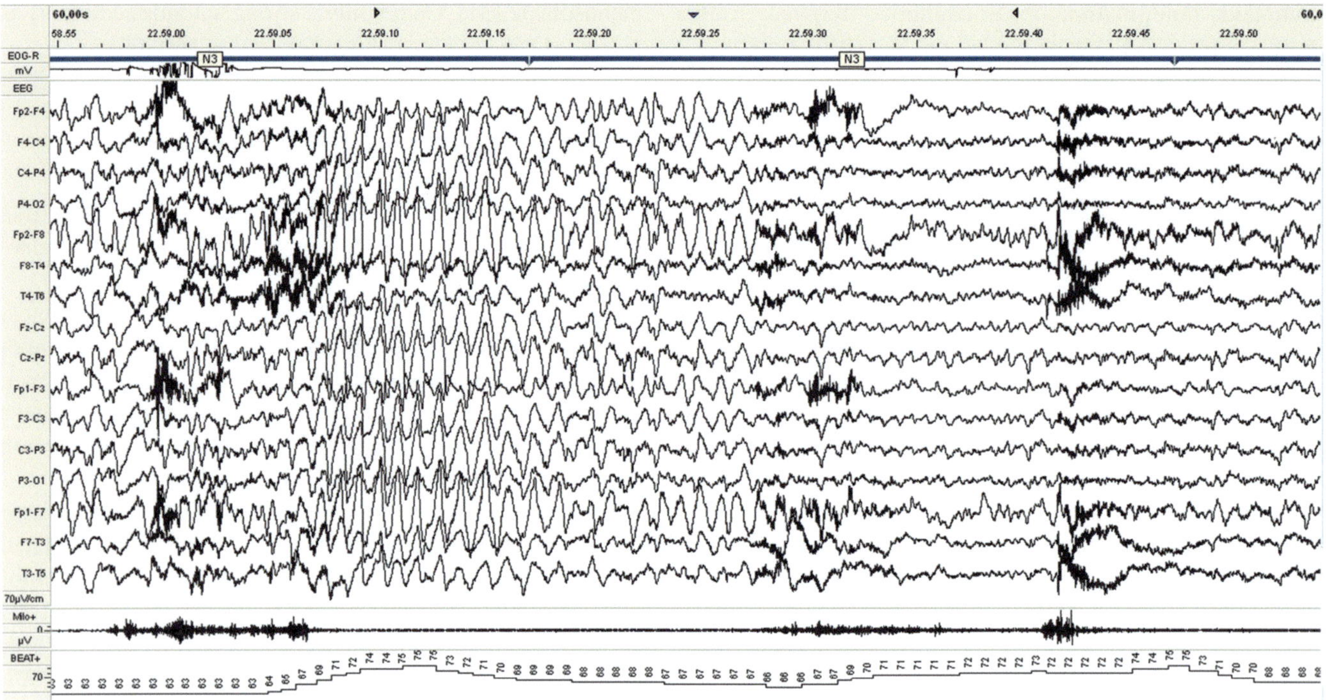

Fig. 35.1 Hypersynchronous delta activity in N3 associated with confusional arousal and sleepwalking in a patient with NREM parasomnia

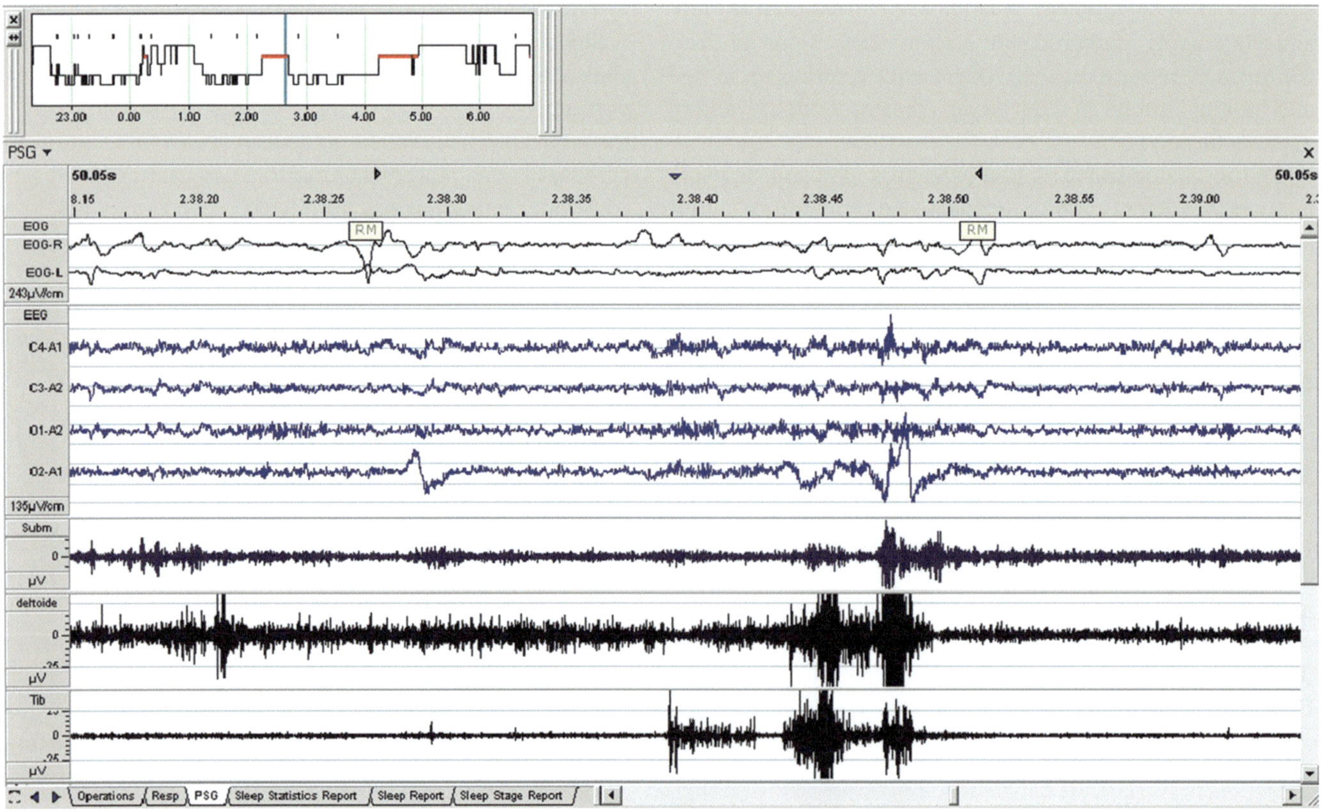

Fig. 35.2 Persistent EMG activity in the chin and phasic EMG activity in tibialis anterior and deltoid muscles in a patient with REM behavior disorder (50 s of recording)

RBD exists both in an acute form and a chronic form. Acute forms are mainly caused by tricyclic antidepressants, serotonin-selective reuptake inhibitors, beta-blockers, or abrupt alcohol withdrawal [41].

The chronic form can be idiopathic (iRBD), when no causes are found, or associated with neurological disorders (secondary form). The main associations are with neurodegenerative disorders, narcolepsy [42], or various kinds of brain stem lesions (ischemic, malignancy, inflammatory, or autoimmune) [43]. The most consistent association of RBD is with Parkinson disease, Lewy body dementia, and multiple system atrophy [44]. Accordingly, RBD can be considered a prodromal stage of synucleinopathies [45].

PSG reveals an excessive amount of continued or intermittent loss of REM atonia and/or excessive phasic muscle twitch activity of the submental and/or limb EMGs during REM sleep.

In the evaluation of RBD, any (tonic/phasic) chin EMG activity combined with bilateral phasic activity of the flexor digitorum superficialis muscles in >27% of REM sleep (scored by 30-s epochs) reliably distinguishes RBD patients from controls.

RDB patients may present a decreased autonomic reactivity, for example, a lack in tachycardia during phasic sleep events. In addition, REM sleep also shows a higher prevalence of PLMs (periodic limb movements), which are less connected to EEG arousals or to sleep disruption compared to patients with a PLM disorder or a restless legs syndrome [46].

The architecture of macrostructure is preserved with a maintenance of a NREM-REM cyclicity. However, a larger representation of SWS can be detected with a higher delta power [47].

PSG recording is fundamental also to rule out some mimicking conditions such as arousal disorders, seizures in sleep, although rare in REM sleep, nightmares, post-traumatic stress disorder, or sleep-related respiratory disorders with RBD-like motor events during the breathing recovery [48].

35.3 Sleep-Related Movement Disorders

Some very common disorders are included in this category such as restless legs syndrome (RLS), periodic limb movement disorder (PLMD), bruxism, and propriospinal myoclonus.

Sleep movements can provoke a severe sleep disruption with serious daytime consequences. Recently, they have been associated to increased vascular risk [49]. Usually these movements are simple, stereotyped, and unintentional. Their classification is founded on the body part involved or on the kind of movement. They are also separated in two different groups: primary and associated to other conditions.

35.3.1 Restless Legs Syndrome and Periodic Limb Movements

RLS is a sensorimotor disorder; its main feature is an unpleasant sensation in lower limbs which generates an uncontainable urge to move them. Limb movement induces a transient relief. This sensation appears in rest condition, especially when the patient is waiting to sleep [50]. In this scenario the patient complains of severe secondary insomnia. RLS is usually associated, when eventually the patient falls asleep, to periodic limb movement (PLM). PLM consist in phasic motor events involving usually lower limbs, which arise in sleep, most frequently in light NREM sleep and more commonly in the first sleep cycles of the night. Sometimes they can emerge while the subject is falling asleep (PLM during wake).

PLM jerks appear as toe extension and ankle dorsiflexion with, sometimes, flexion of the knee and hip. Thus, they resemble the Babinski sign and spinal cord flexor reflex, phenomena connected to the spinal disinhibition caused by a lesion of the pyramidal system [51]. The contraction duration is between 0.5 and 10 s, and the episode must be composed of at least four consecutive movements. Between consecutive episodes the time range is 5–90 s. The majority of PLM events are separated by intervals of 20–40 s. Their detection is achieved by means of surface electromyogram of the tibialis anterior muscle. It is possible to record PLM on other muscles or using actigraphy. In the presence of two isolated movements of tibialis anterior muscles, these limb movements are considered as bilateral and thus as a unique phenomenon if they are separated by an interval shorter than 5 s. Otherwise they are considered as monolateral if the interval is longer than 5 s.

The consequences of PLM on sleep are still a matter of debate. They are often associated with EEG arousals or with a heart-breathing rate activation or blood pressure increase [52].

The EEG arousal may precede, be concomitant, or follow the movement. These observations suggest that limb jerks are endowed into a dynamic physiologically oscillating process of sleep, with a 20–40 s periodism which involves different systems, including cortical, vegetative, and behavioral functions. PLM has a close relationship with the oscillations of CAP, which acts as a permissive window (in particular, phase A).

A certain amount of limb movements are physiological during sleep in healthy individuals. In adults, a PLM index (number of limb jerks/hours of sleep) is pathological if higher than 15 [53].

A high PLM index is a common finding in many different sleep disorders such as narcolepsy, RBD, and OSAS. PLM is frequently associated with RLS (80%) [54] and can be considered a PSG marker of this pathology. PLM has been

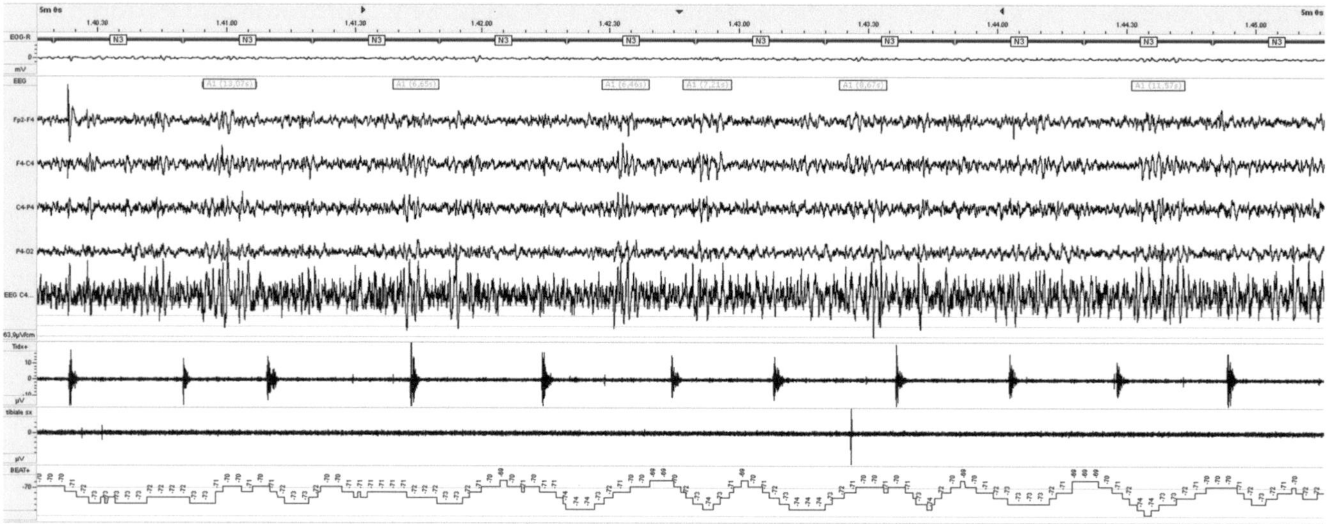

Fig. 35.3 A 5 min sample of PSG of a patient with PLMD. The PSG shows repetitive contractions on the right tibialis muscle associated EEG arousal that may precede, be concomitant, or follow the movement. An increase in the heart rate is synchronous with the movement

reported in other neurological or medical conditions such as heart failure [55] with or without periodic breathing, renal failure, Parkinson disease, Gilles de la Tourette syndrome, spinocerebellar ataxia, iron deficiency and in association with drug administration (SSRI, tricyclic, phenothiazines, lithium). In RBD, PLM events are often present in REM sleep [54].

A PLM > 15 related to poor sleep quality is defined as PLM disorder (PLMD) which is usually described by the patient as difficulty in maintaining sleep, non-restorative sleep, or agitated sleep [53] (Fig. 35.3). Habitually, the patient is not aware about the movements. For this reason it is advisable to perform a PSG with leg EMG or an actigraphic study. It is important to rule out other sleep disorders which can produce sleep movements such as OSAS, insomnia, and epilepsy.

PLM must be distinguished from sleep starts (brief nonperiodic motor events lasting 20–100 ms, typical of sleep-wake transitions), REM twitches (phasic muscle tone increases arising in REM sleep), fragmentary myoclonus (incidental EMG findings of small movements of the corners of the mouth, fingers or toes, or by no visible movement at all), and nocturnal leg cramps (prolonged and painful contraction of the gastrocnemius muscle, rarely the tibialis, with a complete arousal of the patient).

35.3.2 Propriospinal Myoclonus at Sleep Onset

Propriospinal myoclonus (PSM) at sleep onset is a disorder of the transition from wakefulness to sleep, rather than a classically defined sleep disorder. This condition is rare and consists of sudden and brief (less than 500 ms) myoclonic jerks which occur during the falling asleep shift (less frequently, during intrasleep wakefulness and upon the final awakening), involving the abdomen, trunk, neck, and sometimes limbs. Patients often report a transient prodrome anticipating motor manifestations [56].

Myoclonic jerks can be isolated or organized in sequences and induce an arousal and secondary insomnia. PSM is usually spontaneous but sometimes can be triggered by external stimuli. PSM is never associated to loss of consciousness.

EMG findings reveal that jerks origin from a single myelomere and diffuse rostrally and caudally at the same time. The propagation velocity is 2–16 ms (less than the physiologic velocity of the voluntary pyramidal system). PSM can be idiopathic or caused by a medullary lesion of various nature.

PSG shows myoclonic nonperiodic EMG bursts and EEG reveals an alpha activity. In particular, myoclonic jerks are associated to an EEG alpha activity spreading from the posterior to the anterior regions. Epileptiform discharges are totally absent. EEG desynchronization, mental activity, or the onset of sleep spindles and K-complexes interrupts jerk occurrence. EEG back-averaging techniques show absence of a premotor cortical potential. PSG is mandatory to rule out other conditions such as epileptic myoclonus, sleep starts, phasic REM twitches, fragmentary myoclonus, or psychogenic myoclonus.

35.3.3 Sleep-Related Bruxism

Bruxism consists of an excess of repetitive and rhythmic masticatory activity occurring during sleep (or wakefulness), which induce a detrimental effect on sleep structure and/or mandibular pain and/or temporal cephalalgia or tooth injury [53]. These movements are connected to the typical noise caused by tooth scraping. In physiological sleep, non-volitional movements of masticatory muscles are common. These movements can be phasic or tonic. A normal frequency is defined as 1–2 episodes per hour.

Bruxism prevalence is high in children and tends to decrease over age. Primary forms are more frequent but secondary forms are also reported. They can be related to different conditions such as Parkinson disease, drug administration, Down syndrome, cerebral palsy, OSAS, or parasomnia such as RBD.

Etiology is still unknown. Psychosocial components and a genetic predisposition may play a role in the pathogenesis [57]. The role of dental imperfection or of occlusal defects is uncertain. High level of catecholamine in urine has been reported, and this could mean a relationship with stressing situations [58].

Performing a complete video-PSG is not mandatory for the diagnosis. Nevertheless, PSG may be useful to prove the disorder and rule out possible associations with sleep-related respiratory disorders, gastroesophageal reflux, RBD, night terrors, facio-mandibular myoclonus, or epilepsy.

In mild cases, PSG sensitivity is not high due to the night-to-night variability in RMMA (rhythmic masticatory movement activity) and tooth grinding.

PSG must include EMG on masseter muscles (at least one) and video-audio recording to detect the typical noise of grinding. Phasic and tonic muscular activity are scored as movement or artifacts on the EEG channels and as EMG contractions on masseter muscles (Fig. 35.4). Phasic RMMA last from 0.25 to 2 s, with a 1.2 Hz frequency. Tonic activity is more prolonged. It is possible to observe mixed patterns. A single episode of bruxism must be separated from another by an absence of muscle activity of at least 3 s. It is possible to evaluate muscle activity with EMG and observe RMMA with video.

Bruxism can arise in all sleep stages, but it is more frequent in light sleep. Rarely, RMMA can be present in REM sleep. In some patients RMMA occur exclusively in REM sleep.

Bruxism episodes are often associated to EEG arousals and microarousals (up to 80%) and autonomic activation, starting with a raise in sympathetic cardiac activity and with a faster EEG activity in the seconds/minutes preceding a RMMA [59].

Though a clear sleep disruption is rare in bruxism, RMMA induce always microstructure perturbation with an increase of CAP phase A3 subtypes which act as "permissive windows" for the occurrence of RMMA during sleep [60].

35.4 Epilepsy

35.4.1 Impact of NREM and REM Sleep

During NREM sleep, virtually every cell in the brain discharges synchronously [61]. Synchronous synaptic effects, whether excitatory or inhibitory, could augment the magnitude and propagation of postsynaptic responses, including epileptic discharges. Background EEG effects seem to be exacerbated by sudden surges of afferent stimulation associated with transient, synchronous phasic arousal events. Generalized seizures, particularly generalized tonic-clonic or myoclonic convulsions, tend to occur during NREM sleep

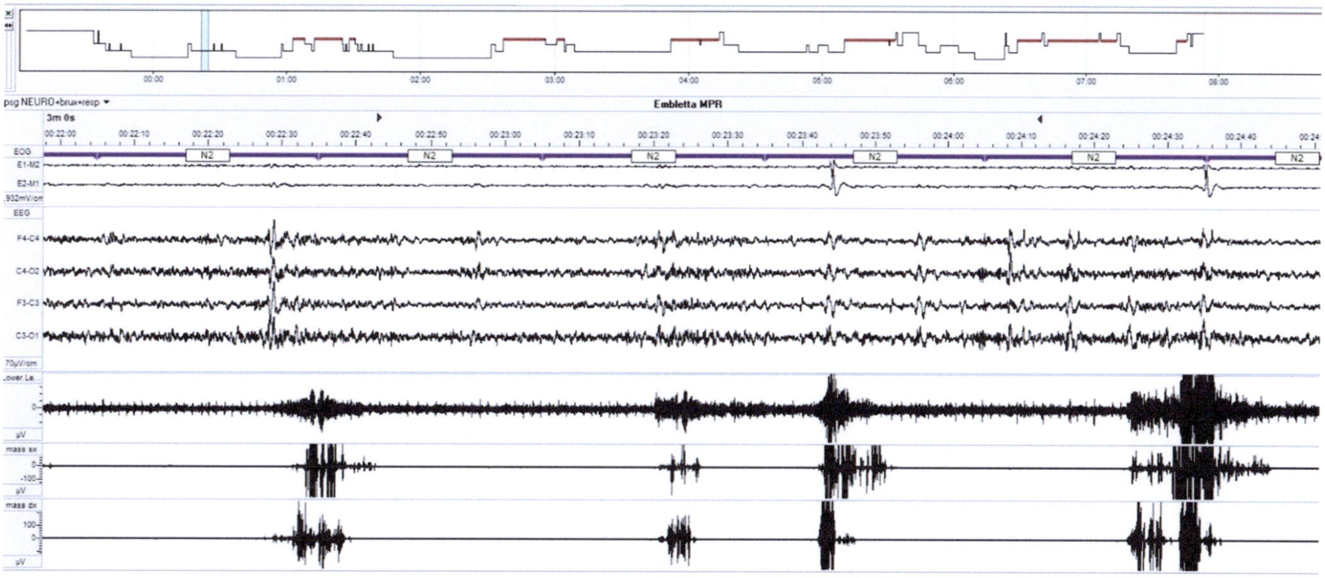

Fig. 35.4 Regular bilater contractions of masseter muscles during N2 in patient with bruxism

or transitional arousal periods characterized by background EEG synchronization, often with phasic events that include sleep EEG transients such as sleep spindles, K-complexes, and ponto-geniculo-occipital waves. In the majority of patients with primary generalized epilepsy, frequent brief bursts of spikes, polyspikes, and spike-wave-like discharges are associated with K-complexes or spindles, which are specific phasic EEG patterns of NREM sleep [62].

Most epileptic syndromes show non-persistence of ictal and interictal discharges during REM sleep. Characterized by asynchronous cellular discharge patterns [63] and skeletal motor paralysis, REM sleep is resistant to propagation of epileptic EEG potentials and to clinical motor accompaniment [64], even though spontaneous phasic activity and focal EEG discharges persist at this time and may be evoked by photic stimulation. Although antigravity muscle tone is preserved in NREM sleep and waking, thus, permitting seizure-associated movement, profound lower motor neuron inhibition occurs in REM, creating virtual paralysis and preventing seizure-related movement.

These findings indicate that substrates of state-specific components rather than integrity of the state per se can be salient determinants of seizure propagation, regardless of the epileptic syndrome.

35.4.2 CAP and Epilepsy

Pioneering contributions in the early 1990s [65–67] focused attention on the dynamic relationship between epileptic paroxysms and EEG phasic events during sleep. These studies highlighted the relevance of arousal instability as an important triggering factor of epileptic paroxysms. In primary generalized epilepsy, in temporal lobe epilepsy, and in patients with focal lesional frontotemporal epilepsy, interictal discharges are commonly activated during unstable sleep, with a number of EEG paroxysms per minute of sleep significantly higher during CAP compared to non-CAP. Phase A has a significant activation influence, whereas phase B exerts a powerful and prolonged inhibitory action. On the contrary, despite the high burst frequency during NREM sleep, interictal epileptiform discharges in benign epilepsy with Rolandic spikes are not modulated by the arousal-related mechanisms of CAP. A sleep condition of highly fluctuating vigilance constitutes a favorable substrate also for the occurrence of focal epileptic seizures. In patients affected by focal epilepsy, the great majority of nocturnal partial motor seizures occur during NREM sleep, more frequently in CAP than in non-CAP sleep and in phase A than in phase B.

35.4.3 Sleep-Related Hypermotor Epilepsy

In 2016, the syndrome previously known as nocturnal frontal lobe epilepsy (NFLE) was defined as sleep-related hypermotor epilepsy or SHE [68]. Clinically, SHE is characterized by short-lasting seizures (<2 min) patterned by repetitive and stereotyped motor events in the same subject. Besides complex hypermotor seizures, paroxysmal arousals and minor motor events are the most common clinical manifestations, occurring most commonly during the night. Most seizures occur periodically during non-REM sleep (Fig. 35.5).

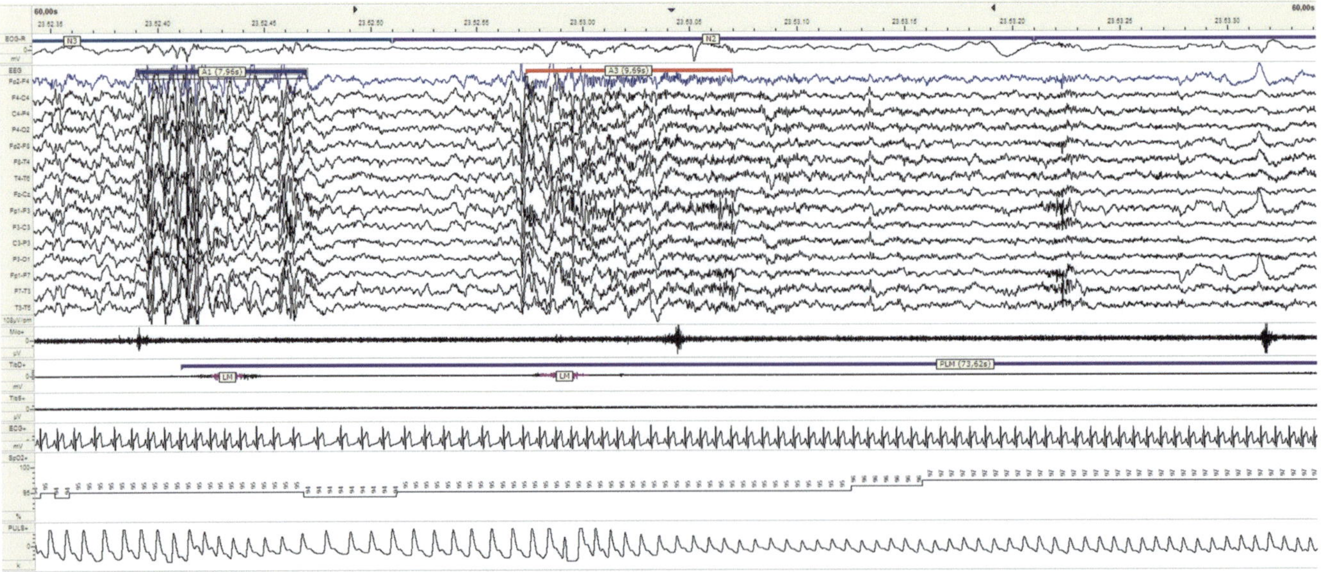

Fig. 35.5 60 s of PSG recording of a patient with a sleep-related hypermotor epilepsy. High-amplitude generalized epileptic discharges, with right frontal prevalence, associated with a minor motor event, trigger the onset of A phases of CAP

Differential diagnosis between SHE and parasomnias can represent a challenging issue. In the large majority of patients, neurologic and neuropsychological assessment is normal [69]. Diagnosis of SHE cannot be excluded even when interictal and ictal features are lacking in the EEG, both during sleep and wakefulness. Clinical history is the starting point for the diagnosis of SHE. According to the new definition, diagnostic criteria of SHE are based on three levels of certainty: witnessed (possible) SHE, video-documented (clinical) SHE, and video-EEG-documented (confirmed) SHE.

New insights into the biology of SHE occurred with the discovery of an autosomal dominant form and identification of the first gene, CHRNA4, encoding a neuronal nicotinic receptor subunit [70].

Further investigation has ascertained that SHE shows similar clinical features both in familial and sporadic cases, although autosomal dominant inheritance is characterized by a marked intrafamilial variation in severity [71, 72]. Three individuals affected by a possible SHE with genetic transmission were described in 1872 by Darwin and Galton [73].

Although SHE may have diverse etiologies, it is defined by clinical manifestations (hypermotor seizures), possibly resulting from shared downstream mechanisms occurring during sleep/wake oscillation changes, suggesting a unique pathogenic network [74, 75].

Because ictal discharges may arise not only from frontal lobe [76, 77] but also from various extrafrontal areas [78], this might suggest the ictal involvement of common cortico-subcortical networks [79] or a release phenomenon of stereotyped inborn fixed motor pattern. Tassinari et al. [80] claim that genetically determined motor behaviors essential for survival (feeding, locomotion, reproduction, etc.) are under the control of central pattern generators (CPGs), neuronal aggregates located in the brain stem and spinal cord. During sleep, transient arousals triggered by epileptic events or brain dysfunction can "activate" or "release" CPGs responsible for involuntary behavioral patterns. In NREM sleep, where muscle tone is still operative, EEG synchrony allows multiple levels of expression (from N1 to N3), and a variety of motor events can take place from seizures to parasomnias. Whether the outcome is a muscle jerk or a major epileptic attack will depend on a number of ongoing factors (sleep stage, delta power, motor chain, body position, etc.), but all events will share the common trait of arousal-activated phenomena. These findings suggest that arousal during sleep is the common condition for the onset of motor patterns which are already written in the brain codes (GPG) but require a certain degree of activation (arousal) to become visibly apparent. In this case, arousal acts as a trigger releasing or facilitating an encoded "kinetic melody" [75, 80, 81]. Stereo-EEG investigation of sleep, nocturnal epilepsy, and parasomnias can shed light upon the specific epileptogenic networks involved during ictal activity and unveil the local electrophysiological dissociated substrate of parasomnias [82, 83].

A common feature is the onset of all episodes during NREM sleep, with different distributions within the sleep stages. Major attacks prevail in N3, leading abruptly to a wake condition. Paroxysmal arousals and minor motor events may recur every night, sometimes several times per night, arising mainly from CAP in stage 2 [84].

Patients affected by SHE frequently report a poor sleep quality, fatigue, and excessive daytime sleepiness ascribed to the presence of recurrent seizures and motor episodes during sleep. In these patients, enhanced sleep fragmentation and higher percentages of wakefulness are common polysomnography findings, as well as increased amounts of CAP rate [85]. The presence of an epileptic focus in the frontal regions likely represents an internal disturbance that interferes subcontinuously with the stability of NREM sleep. Though extremely short-lived, the interictal epileptiform discharges in SHE is an activating event sharing the same pathways of arousal instability.

PSG recordings show that increased arousal instability is very common in SHE, particularly when multiple events occur during sleep (Fig. 35.6). Some studies suggest that macrostructural sleep disturbances and enhanced arousal instability are part of the syndrome. In SHE, stereotyped manifestation not only involve motor behaviors but also polysomnographic (PSG) patterns [74]. Baseline PSG recordings of 40 patients (20 males and 20 females; mean age, 31 ± 10 years) with a diagnosis of SHE were compared with those of 24 age- and gender-balanced healthy subjects without sleep complaints (controls). SHE patients showed a significant increase in wake after sleep onset, slow-wave sleep duration, and REM latency, whereas REM sleep was significantly lower. SHE patients also showed a significant increase of CAP time, CAP rate (72 vs 32% in the control group), CAP cycles, and mean duration of CAP sequences. These findings were associated with a significant enhancement of all subtypes of the A phases of CAP (mainly subtype A1). A total of 139 epileptic motor events supported by video-PSG evidence were counted. NREM sleep included 98% of all seizures, which were especially abundant in the first sleep cycles, decreasing in frequency together with the progressive decline of deep sleep. Ninety percent of total NREM seizures occurred during a CAP sequence, and CAP-related seizures occurred in association with a phase A.

In SHE patients, the robust enhancement of sleep instability was associated with an increased amount of all phase A subtypes of CAP, especially phase A1, without relevant changes of respective percentages. Studies of scalp mapping obtained with electromagnetic tomography during sleep show that slow-wave activity (0.25–2.5 Hz), a main

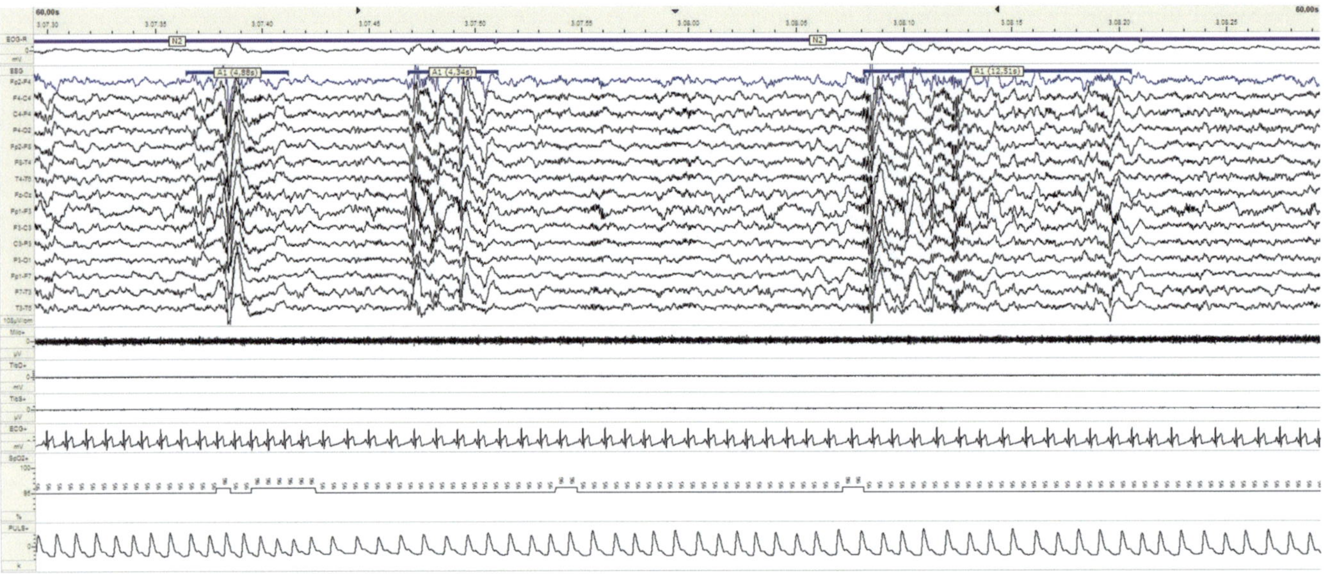

Fig. 35.6 A CAP sequence (unstable sleep) in NREM sleep modulated by epileptic activity in a case of sleep-related hypermotor epilepsy

component of A1 phases of CAP, has a major representation over the frontal and prefrontal regions, whereas fast activities (7–12 Hz), mainly associated with phases A2 and A3, have a parieto-occipital prevalence (Ferri et al. 2005). These findings suggest a primary role of the high-amplitude low-frequency CAP phase A components, that is, EEG delta activity or K-complexes, on the occurrence of ictal episodes [84, 86–90]. In this perspective, subtype A1 of CAP could be considered as frontal lobe arousals, periodically causing an increase of cerebral excitability that triggers the onset of frontal seizures.

According to these premises, diagnosis of SHE based exclusively on video-recorded phenomena, without EEG support, is not satisfactory, especially for paroxysmal arousals and minor motor events [91]. Moreover, a number of sleep parasomnias may occur during NREM sleep, and differentiating these conditions from SHE only through visual patterns can be problematic [79, 92–94]. Therefore, only the integrated evaluation of nocturnal video-EEG features, PSG metrics, and underlying regulatory sleep processes can help to clarify diagnostic uncertainties. These integrative criteria for the diagnosis of SHE can supply precious information on the effects of antiepileptic treatment.

35.5 Hypersomnia of Central Origin

Hypersomnia of central origin is represented by narcolepsy type 1, narcolepsy type 2, idiopathic hypersomnia, and Kleine-Levin syndrome. Hypersomnia can also be due to medical disorders, medication, and psychiatric diseases or be secondary to insufficient sleep [53].

35.5.1 Narcolepsy Types 1 and 2

Narcolepsy type 1 (NT1) is a chronic, non-degenerative, neurological disorder characterized by excessive daytime sleepiness and cataplexy (a generalized or focal sudden, short-lasting, loss of muscle tone during wake provoked by intense emotion, particularly positive, without loss of consciousness). Cataplexy can be considered a pathognomonic manifestation of narcolepsy type 1 [95].

The cause of NT1 is a massive loss of orexin-producing neurons localized in the lateral hypothalamus [96]. An autoimmune origin for the selective cell loss is suspected: almost 90% of NT1 patients exhibit a specific HLA haplotype positivity (DQB1*0602) [97]. This haplotype is found in 20% of healthy individuals (for this reason it is especially useful if negative in doubtful cases). One of the main diagnostic criteria is the low level of orexin in the CSF (below 110 pg/mL) or < 1/3 of the mean values obtained in normal subjects with the same standardized assay. If low CSF level of orexin is found, a diagnosis of NT1 can be done even if cataplexy is not present [53].

Other manifestations consist of phenomena of REM sleep dissociation such as sleep paralysis, hallucination during sleep onset or during awakenings, intense and even lucid dreaming, and sometimes REM without atonia.

Daytime sleepiness is characteristically incoercible and sudden (sleep attacks) and can appear in situations of passive activity but sometimes may occur in more active circumstances. Usually the daytime sleep lasts less than 20 min and it is deeply restoring. One of the hallmarks of narcolepsy is an early appearance, within 15 min after the sleep onset, of REM sleep (sleep-onset REM periods—SOREMPs). In addition to these features, a difficulty in maintenance of nocturnal sleep is often reported.

Narcolepsy type 2 is not a well-defined pathologic entity, and it is also called "narcolepsy without cataplexy." Orexin level is normal (in the 8% of cases, an intermediate level was found) or not measured. Other features of NT1 can be part of the clinical picture. About 45% of narcolepsy type 2 cases have been reported to be HLA DQB1*0602 positive, so HLA haplotype alone cannot determine the narcolepsy type [98].

Both types of narcolepsy can be caused by a central nervous system disorder such as autoimmune or paraneoplastic syndrome, neoplasia, or other hypothalamic lesions.

35.5.2 Objective Findings

If a clear history of cataplexy is present, a nocturnal PSG is not mandatory, but it is useful to rule out other conditions that can worsen sleepiness such as sleep apneas and PLM. During nocturnal PSG, SOREMPs are often detected (Fig. 35.7). For diagnostic purposes, SOREMPs are explored during the multiple sleep latency test which consists of five nap opportunities. This test is performed the day after the video-PSG and allows to measure sleep latency (i.e., the propensity to fall asleep/an objective measurement of sleepiness). Narcoleptic subjects show a mean sleep latency below 8 min (characteristically <3 min) and the presence of at least two SOREMPs (for the diagnosis a single SOREMP is sufficient if one SOREMP occurs during the PSG). The minimal duration of nocturnal PSG is 7 h.

An actigraphic study with a sleep log lasting at least 7 days is endorsed to rule out insufficient sleep syndrome, shift work, or other circadian sleep disorders which can mimic a narcolepsy [53].

Sleep macrostructure in narcolepsy is not dramatically altered (with a possible presence of a SOREMP), but an increase in stage N1 is reported [99]. Shorter REM latency, sleep fragmentation with repetitive awakening, middle-of-the-night insomnia, or a REM without atonia with RDB can be found. As a translation of impaired arousal regulation, a significant decrease in CAP rate is reported [100, 101].

35.6 Sleep-Related Breathing Disorders

Sleep-related breathing disorders are divided into obstructive sleep apnea (OSA) disorders, central sleep apnea (CSA) disorders, sleep-related hypoventilation disorders, and sleep-related hypoxemia disorder, depending upon the pathophysiologic mechanism of respiration abnormalities during sleep.

35.6.1 Obstructive Sleep Apnea

OSA is the most frequent sleep-related breathing disorder characterized by repetitive collapse of the upper airways during sleep, leading to episodes of complete (apnea) or partial (hypopnea) upper airway obstruction. These events, lasting a minimum of 10 s, often result in reduction of blood oxygen saturation and brief arousals from sleep (Figs. 35.8 and 35.9).

The prevalence of OSA (3–7% in men and 2–5% in women) enhances with age, weight increase, and presence of certain medical conditions [102]. The gold standard for the diagnosis of OSA is the overnight PSG involving simultaneous recordings of multiple physiological signals, including the electroencephalogram (EEG), electrooculogram (EOG), electromyogram (EMG), oronasal airflow, thoracic and abdominal effort, and oxyhemoglobin saturation (Fig. 35.8).

PSG allows identification and classification of all types of respiratory events, i.e., apnea, hypopnea, and respiratory effort-related arousal (RERA). An apnea is defined as the complete cessation of airflow for at least 10 s and is further classified as obstructive, central, or mixed, based on whether effort to breathe is present during the event. The obstructive apnea is characterized by continuous or increased inspiratory effort throughout the entire period of absent airflow

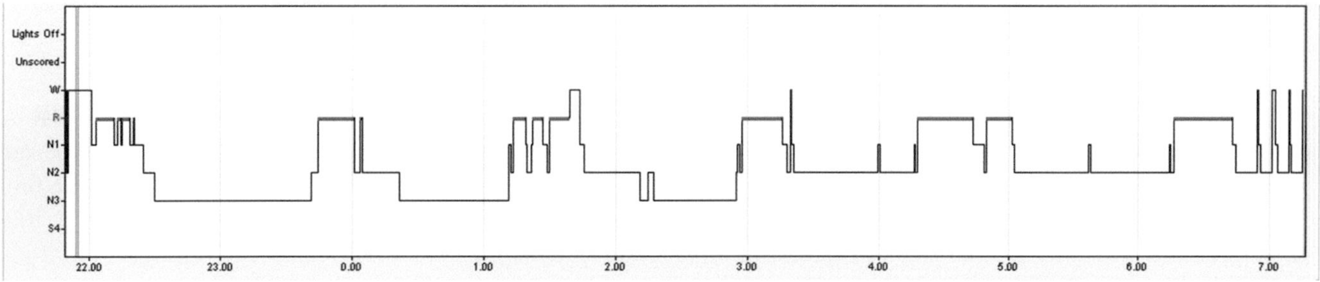

Fig. 35.7 A hypnogram of a 19-year-old patient with narcolepsy type 1. In this case we can observe a sleep-onset REM period (SOREMP) episode

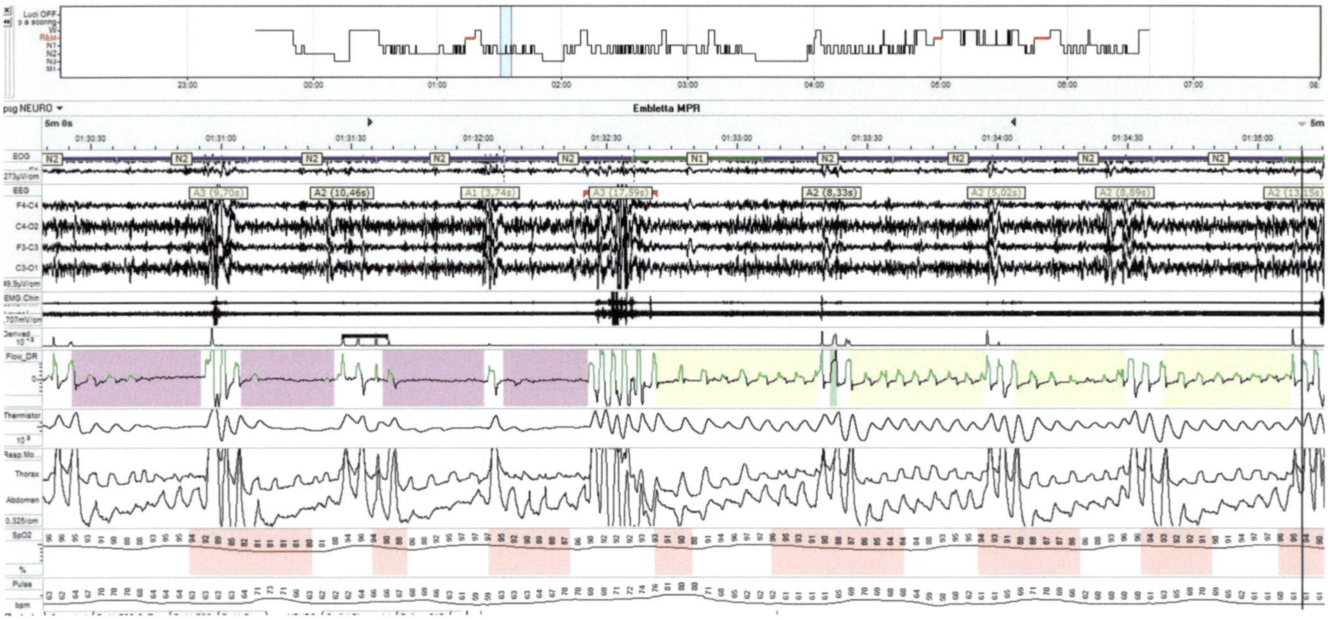

Fig. 35.8 Obstructive apneas and hypopneas in PSG. In the pink purple boxes, the obstructive sleep apnea events; in the yellow boxes, the hypopneas events; in the pink boxes, the desaturation events (5 min window)

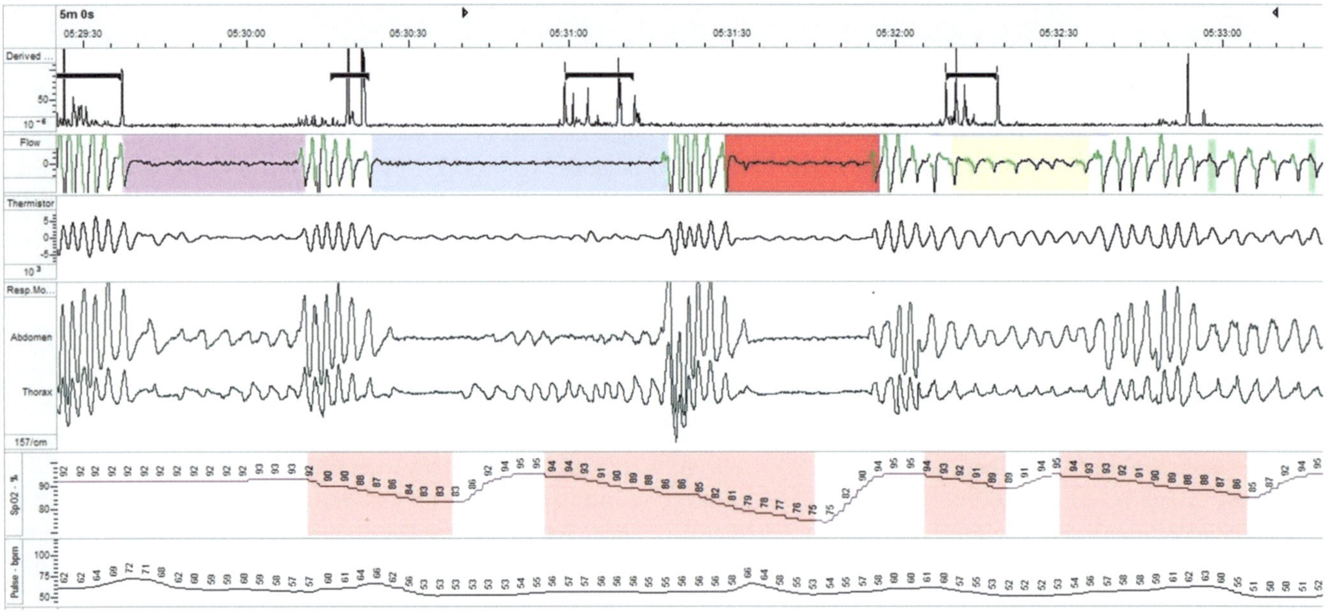

Fig. 35.9 Obstructive, mixed, and central apneas and hypopnea in PM. In the purple box, obstructive sleep apnea event; in the blue box, mixed apnea event; in the red box, the central apnea; in the yellow box, the hypopneas; in the pink boxes, the desaturation events (5 min window)

(Figs. 35.8 and 35.9), whereas central apnea is associated with absent inspiratory effort (Fig. 35.9). An initial period of central apnea followed by a period of obstructive sleep apnea constitutes a mixed apnea (Fig. 35.9) [103].

A hypopnea is defined as a reduction in airflow (30% in nasal airflow) that is followed by an arousal from sleep or a decrease in oxyhemoglobin saturation [103] (Figs. 35.8 and 35.9).

The more subtle respiratory events are RERA defined by obstructive upper airway airflow reductions (which do not meet the criteria of apnea or hypopnea) associated with progressive negative esophageal pressure lasting at least 10 s and culminating in an arousal (Fig. 35.10) [103].

Sleep apnea severity is assessed by the respiratory disturbance index (RDI), which is the number of apneas, hypopneas, and RERA occurring per hour of sleep.

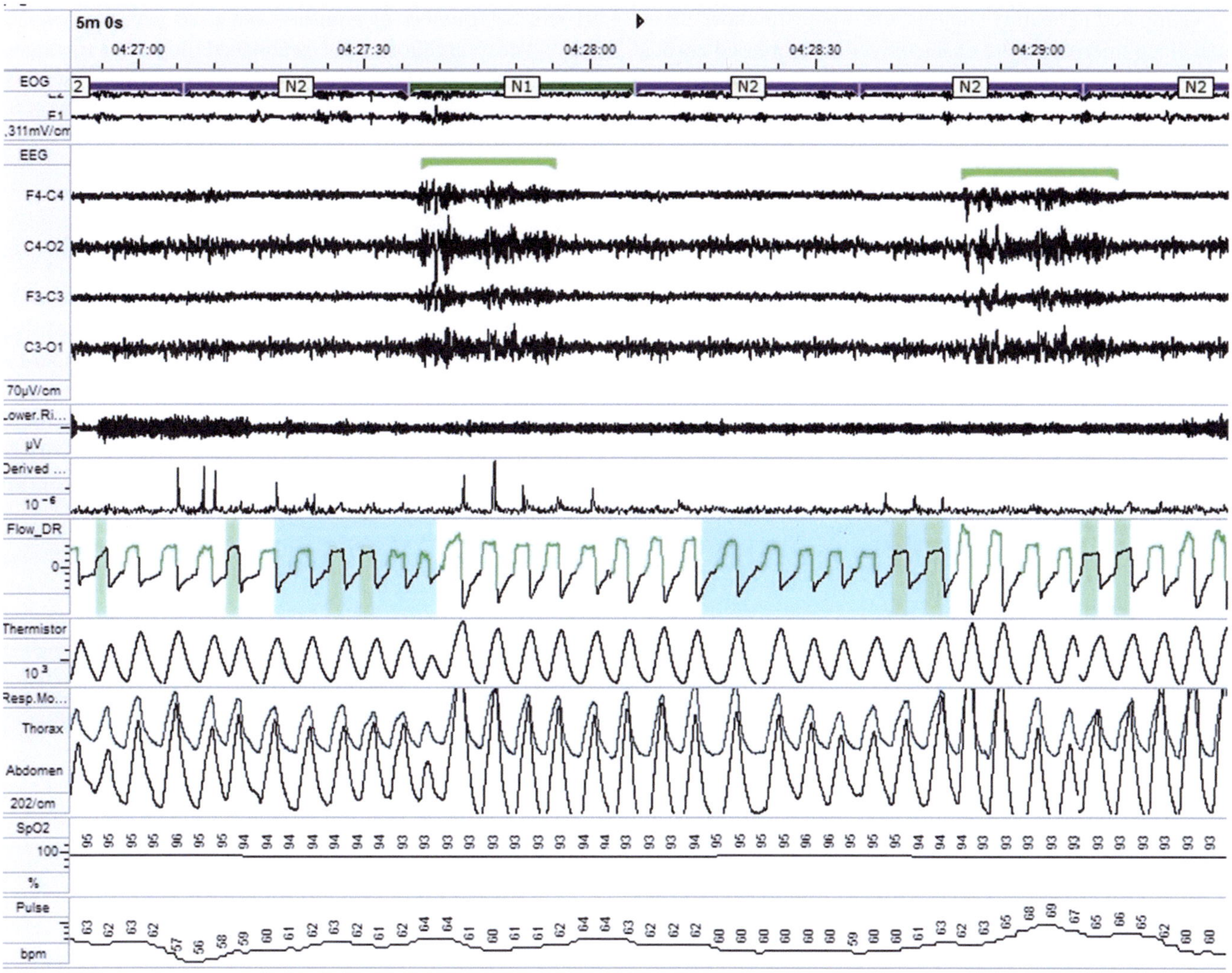

Fig. 35.10 Respiratory effort-related arousals (RERA) in PSG: in the light blue box, the RERA. The EEG arousals are highlighted with the green lines (5 min window)

Although considered as a "gold standard," the PSG is an expensive and technically intense procedure. For these reasons portable monitoring (PM) is becoming an increasingly accepted cost-effective alternative approach [104]. Although PM is less time-consuming, it lacks neurological signals (EEG, EOG, EMG) and therefore precludes the identification of arousals and the use of this criterion in the definition of respiratory events.

The apnea-hypopnea index (AHI), the number of apneas and hypopneas for hours of sleep, is the parameter used for OSA severity classification in PM. Although the AHI is the most commonly used parameter to evaluate OSA, a number of studies show that arousal scoring in OSA patients is important to clarify the impact of this disease on sleep [105, 106].

In terms of sleep architecture, patients with OSA often show reduction of slow-wave sleep and REM sleep with increase in NREM stage 2. Increased time spent awake after sleep onset and shortened sleep latency are other findings.

Immediately preceding the recovery of normal breathing, the EEG may provide evidence of a brief cortical arousal from sleep, the submental electromyogram may demonstrate a burst of activity indicating activation of upper airway dilating muscle, and microphones may record a sudden resumption of loud snoring. At the time of cortical arousals, there is often a surge in both sympathetic nervous system activity and systemic blood pressure. The respiratory events may be also accompanied by bradyarrhythmias, tachyarrhythmias, or both. Some studies have shown that the sleeping brain can even solve respiratory events with involvement of slow EEG activity (subcortical arousal) without involving a cortical arousal. The latter is triggered only when thalamocortical structures fail to modulate breathing or when ascending reticular volleys are required to restore respiration [107].

Compared to healthy subjects, OSA patients show abnormal sleep microstructure characterized by increased cortical arousals index and enhanced amounts of CAP, with longer and more desynchronized EEG patterns. The increase of A3 subtypes permits scoring of CAP also in REM sleep. All CAP-related respiratory events originate in close temporal connection with a phase B, while effective breathing is always recovered during a phase A (especially A2 and A3). These data suggest that phase B of CAP offers a vulnerable background for upper airway collapse and for attenuation of biochemical and neural mechanisms in the control of the ventilatory drive [108].

The best treatment for moderate-to-severe OSAS is the application of continuous positive airway pressure (CPAP) devices. In OSAS patients effectively treated with nasal CPAP, therapy induces an immediate enhancement of sleep N3, a more consolidated REM sleep, a reduction of stages N1 and N2, number of arousals, and CAP rate. However, a normal sleep architecture is established only after sustained CPAP treatment. The improvement is associated with a robust reduction of A3 subtypes and an expansion of A1 percentages [109].

35.6.2 Central Sleep Apnea Syndromes

Central sleep apnea (CSA) is characterized by an unstable ventilatory drive during sleep, resulting in repetitive central sleep apnea or hypopnea events (Fig. 35.11). CSA syndromes include CSA with Cheyne-Stokes breathing (CSB), CSA due to high-altitude periodic breathing, primary CSA, central apnea induced by drugs and medical conditions, and treatment-emergent central sleep apnea.

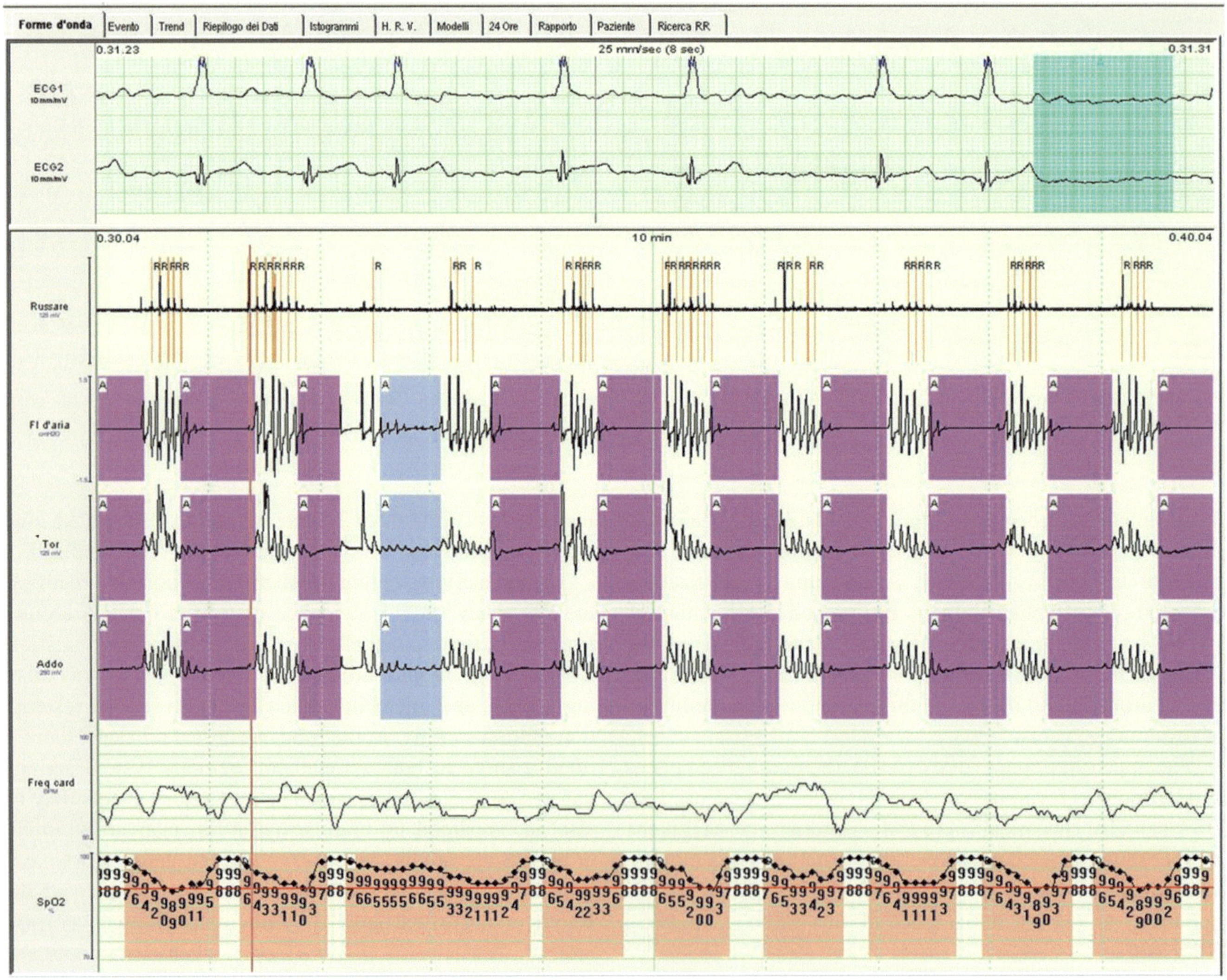

Fig. 35.11 Recurrent central apnea events in patients with atrial fibrillation (10 min window)

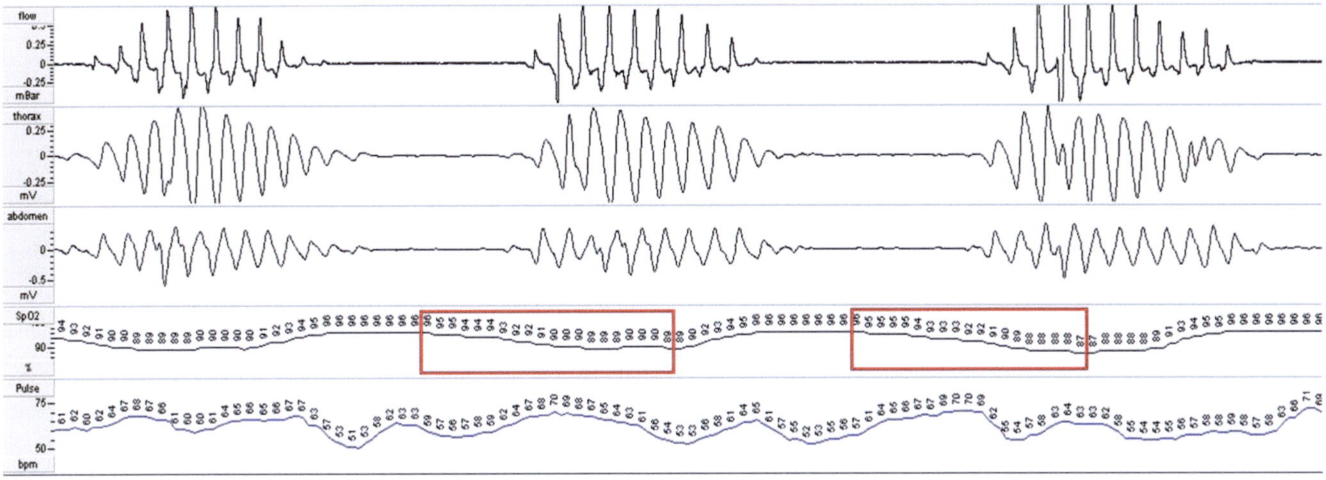

Fig. 35.12 PM in a patient with Cheyne-Stokes breathing (3 min window)

Primary CSA is uncommon and may constitute <5% of patients referred to a sleep lab [110]. Conversely, within certain clinical populations, the presence of CSA may be extremely high (congestive heart failure, neurological disorders, and sometimes renal failure) [111].

Typically, CSA is considered to be the primary diagnosis when ≥50% of apneas and hypopneas are scored as central in PSG or PM. CSA is usually characterized by normal or reduced $PaCO_2$ levels (normocapnic or hypocapnic) and a respiratory cycle length (apnea or hypopnea plus hyperpnea duration) shorter than 45 s.

CSB is a type of periodic breathing with a crescendo-decrescendo cyclic pattern separated by central apneic or hypopneic events. In CSB, the respiratory cycle length is longer than 45 s (Fig. 35.12).

Treatment-emergent CSA is a type of CSA syndrome characterized by the development or persistence of central apneas or hypopneas during application of CPAP (central apnea index ≥5 events) in patients with predominant obstructive events (obstructive or mixed apneas or hypopneas) during the diagnostic sleep study. The percentage of treatment-emergent CSA patients varies from 2 to 20%, depending on the characteristics of the investigated population [112].

During PSG with CPAP, the treatment-emergent CSA patients show adequate treatment during REM sleep and stage N3 sleep but persistent sleep fragmentation and repetitive episodes of central events during stages N1 and N2 [53].

35.7 Conclusions

Sleep or sleeplike states occur throughout the animal kingdom and appear encoded in our genes. Sleep is also essential for survival. The ultimate outcome of prolonged sleep deprivation in animals is death. The amount of recommended sleep is age-dependent, ranging between 7 and 9 h in adults and between 7 and 8 h in elderly [113]. Mortality hazard increases significantly in individuals reporting sleep durations ≤6 and ≥8 h.

Sleep is also a health imperative. The risk of arterial hypertension rises significantly in subjects that chronically sleep <5 h [114] with 7 to <8 h sleep per night as the referent category [115]. After adjustment for age and sex, sleeping length shorter or longer than 7.7 h/night is associated with an increased BMI. Type 2 diabetes and impaired glucose tolerance are more commonly found when usual sleep times last ≤6 or ≥9 h/night [116]. The risk of chronic diseases becomes even greater when health is jeopardized by sleep disorders, in particular OSAS and persistent insomnia [117]. These considerations strongly indicate that sleep is a mandatory and nonnegotiable daily experience and that any factor disrupting or impairing sleep duration and quality represents a severe menace of disability and death.

References

1. American Psychiatric Association. Diagnostic and statistical manual of mental disorders. 5th ed. Arlington, VA: American Psychiatric Association; 2013.
2. Riemann D, Baglioni C, Bassetti C, Bjorvatn B, Dolenc Groselj L, Ellis JG, et al. European guideline for the diagnosis and treatment of insomnia. J Sleep Res. 2017;26:675–700.
3. Martin JL, Hakim AD. Wrist actigraphy. Chest. 2011;139:1514–27.
4. Sateia MJ, Buysse DJ, Krystal AD, Neubauer DN, Heald JL. Clinical practice guideline for the pharmacologic treatment of chronic insomnia in adults: an American Academy of sleep medicine clinical practice guideline. J Clin Sleep Med JCSM. 2017;13:307–49.
5. Merica H, Blois R, Gaillard JM. Spectral characteristics of sleep EEG in chronic insomnia. Eur J Neurosci. 1998;10:1826–34.

6. Gaillard JM. Is insomnia a disease of slow-wave sleep? Eur Neurol. 1976;14:473–84.
7. Frankel BL, Coursey RD, Buchbinder R, Snyder F. Recorded and reported sleep in chronic primary insomnia. Arch Gen Psychiatry. 1976;33:615–23.
8. Baglioni C, Regen W, Teghen A, Spiegelhalder K, Feige B, Nissen C, et al. Sleep changes in the disorder of insomnia: a meta-analysis of polysomnographic studies. Sleep Med Rev. 2014;18:195–213.
9. Miller CB, Espie CA, Bartlett DJ, Marshall NS, Gordon CJ, Grunstein RR. Acceptability, tolerability, and potential efficacy of cognitive behavioural therapy for insomnia disorder subtypes defined by polysomnography: a retrospective cohort study. Sci Rep. 2018;8:6664.
10. Winkler A, Auer C, Doering BK, Rief W. Drug treatment of primary insomnia: a meta-analysis of polysomnographic randomized controlled trials. CNS Drugs. 2014;28:799–816.
11. Perlis ML, Smith MT, Andrews PJ, Orff H, Giles DE. Beta/gamma EEG activity in patients with primary and secondary insomnia and good sleeper controls. Sleep. 2001;24:110–7.
12. Spiegelhalder K, Regen W, Feige B, Holz J, Piosczyk H, Baglioni C, et al. Increased EEG sigma and beta power during NREM sleep in primary insomnia. Biol Psychol. 2012;91:329–33.
13. Freedman RR. EEG power spectra in sleep-onset insomnia. Electroencephalogr Clin Neurophysiol. 1986;63:408–13.
14. Perlis ML, Merica H, Smith MT, Giles DE. Beta EEG activity and insomnia. Sleep Med Rev. 2001;5:363–74.
15. Marzano C, Ferrara M, Sforza E, De Gennaro L. Quantitative electroencephalogram (EEG) in insomnia: a new window on pathophysiological mechanisms. Curr Pharm Des. 2008;14:3446–55.
16. Bonnet MH, Arand DL. Hyperarousal and insomnia: state of the science. Sleep Med Rev. 2010;14:9–15.
17. Bonnet MH, Arand DL. 24-hour metabolic rate in insomniacs and matched normal sleepers. Sleep. 1995;18:581–8.
18. Li Y, Vgontzas AN, Fernandez-Mendoza J, Bixler EO, Sun Y, Zhou J, et al. Insomnia with physiological hyperarousal is associated with hypertension. Hypertension. 2015;65:644–50.
19. Parrino L, Ferri R, Bruni O, Terzano MG. Cyclic alternating pattern (CAP): the marker of sleep instability. Sleep Med Rev. 2012;16:27–45.
20. Terzano MG, Parrino L, Spaggiari MC, Palomba V, Rossi M, Smerieri A. CAP variables and arousals as sleep electroencephalogram markers for primary insomnia. Clin Neurophysiol. 2003;114:1715–23.
21. Ozone M, Yagi T, Itoh H, Tamura Y, Inoue Y, Uchimura N, et al. Effects of zolpidem on cyclic alternating pattern, an objective marker of sleep instability, in Japanese patients with psychophysiological insomnia: a randomized crossover comparative study with placebo. Pharmacopsychiatry. 2008;41:106–14.
22. Parrino L, Milioli G, De Paolis F, Grassi A, Terzano MG. Paradoxical insomnia: the role of CAP and arousals in sleep misperception. Sleep Med. 2009;10:1139–45.
23. Parrino L, Boselli M, Spaggiari MC, Smerieri A, Terzano MG. Multidrug comparison (lorazepam, triazolam, zolpidem, and zopiclone) in situational insomnia: polysomnographic analysis by means of the cyclic alternating pattern. Clin Neuropharmacol. 1997;20:253–63.
24. Terzaghi M, Sartori I, Tassi L, Didato G, Rustioni V, LoRusso G, et al. Evidence of dissociated arousal states during NREM parasomnia from an intracerebral neurophysiological study. Sleep. 2009;32:409–12.
25. Milano W, De Rosa M, Milano L, Capasso A. Night eating syndrome: an overview. J Pharm Pharmacol. 2012;64:2–10.
26. Inoue Y. Sleep-related eating disorder and its associated conditions. Psychiatry Clin Neurosci. 2015;69:309–20.
27. Nobili L, Arnulf I. Parasomnias: pathophysiology and psychopathology. In: Bassetti CL, Dogas Z, Peigneux P, editors. European sleep medicine textbook. Regensburg: European Sleep Research Society; 2014. p. 377–88.
28. Ohayon MM, Priest RG, Zulley J, Smirne S. The place of confusional arousals in sleep and mental disorders: findings in a general population sample of 13,057 subjects. J Nerv Ment Dis. 2000;188:340–8.
29. Terzaghi M, Sartori I, Tassi L, Rustioni V, Proserpio P, Lorusso G, et al. Dissociated local arousal states underlying essential clinical features of non-rapid eye movement arousal parasomnia: an intracerebral stereo-electroencephalographic study. J Sleep Res. 2012;21:502–6.
30. Sleep-related movement disorders and disorders of motor control. In: Walters E, Baumann C, editors. Parkinson Disease and other movement disorders: motor behavioural disorders and behavioural motor disorder. 2014.
31. Ohayon MM, Guilleminault C, Priest RG. Night terrors, sleepwalking, and confusional arousals in the general population: their frequency and relationship to other sleep and mental disorders. J Clin Psychiatry. 1999;60:268–76.. quiz 277
32. Bargiotas P, Arnet I, Frei M, Baumann CR, Schindler K, Bassetti CL. Demographic, clinical and polysomnographic characteristics of childhood- and adult-onset sleepwalking in adults. Eur Neurol. 2017;78:307–11.
33. Pilon M, Zadra A, Joncas S, Montplaisir J. Hypersynchronous delta waves and somnambulism: brain topography and effect of sleep deprivation. Sleep. 2006;29:77–84.
34. Pilon M, Desautels A, Montplaisir J, Zadra A. Auditory arousal responses and thresholds during REM and NREM sleep of sleepwalkers and controls. Sleep Med. 2012;13:490–5.
35. Hwang T-J, Ni H-C, Chen H-C, Lin Y-T, Liao S-C. Risk predictors for hypnosedative-related complex sleep behaviors: a retrospective, cross-sectional pilot study. J Clin Psychiatry. 2010;71:1331–5.
36. Yeh Y-W, Chen C-H, Feng H-M, Wang S-C, Kuo S-C, Chen C-K. New onset somnambulism associated with different dosage of mirtazapine: a case report. Clin Neuropharmacol. 2009;32:232–3.
37. Montplaisir J, Petit D, Pilon M, Mongrain V, Zadra A. Does sleepwalking impair daytime vigilance? J Clin Sleep Med JCSM. 2011;7:219.
38. Guilleminault C, Poyares D, Aftab FA, Palombini L, Abat F. Sleep and wakefulness in somnambulism: a spectral analysis study. J Psychosom Res. 2001;51:411–6.
39. Guilleminault C, Kirisoglu C, da Rosa AC, Lopes C, Chan A. Sleepwalking, a disorder of NREM sleep instability. Sleep Med. 2006;7:163–70.
40. Schenck CH, Mahowald MW. REM sleep behavior disorder: clinical, developmental, and neuroscience perspectives 16 years after its formal identification in SLEEP. Sleep. 2002;25:120–38.
41. Parish JM. Violent dreaming and antidepressant drugs: or how paroxetine made me dream that I was fighting Saddam Hussein. J Clin Sleep Med JCSM. 2007;3:529–31.
42. Bonakis A, Howard RS, Williams A. Narcolepsy presenting as REM sleep behaviour disorder. Clin Neurol Neurosurg. 2008;110:518–20.
43. Iranzo A, Graus F, Clover L, Morera J, Bruna J, Vilar C, et al. Rapid eye movement sleep behavior disorder and potassium channel antibody-associated limbic encephalitis. Ann Neurol. 2006;59:178–81.
44. Boeve BF, Silber MH, Saper CB, Ferman TJ, Dickson DW, Parisi JE, et al. Pathophysiology of REM sleep behaviour disorder and relevance to neurodegenerative disease. Brain J Neurol. 2007;130:2770–88.
45. Iranzo A, Fernández-Arcos A, Tolosa E, Serradell M, Molinuevo JL, Valldeoriola F, et al. Neurodegenerative disorder risk in idiopathic REM sleep behavior disorder: study in 174 patients. PLoS One. 2014;9:e89741.
46. Fantini ML, Michaud M, Gosselin N, Lavigne G, Montplaisir J. Periodic leg movements in REM sleep behavior disor-

der and related autonomic and EEG activation. Neurology. 2002;59:1889–94.
47. Ferini-Strambi L, Zucconi M. REM sleep behavior disorder. Clin Neurophysiol. 2000;111(Suppl 2):S136–40.
48. Iranzo A, Santamaría J. Severe obstructive sleep apnea/hypopnea mimicking REM sleep behavior disorder. Sleep. 2005;28:203–6.
49. Alessandria M, Provini F. Periodic limb movements during sleep: a new sleep-related cardiovascular risk factor? Front Neurol. 2013;4:116.
50. Ekbom KA. Restless legs syndrome. Neurology. 1960;10: 868–73.
51. Bara-Jimenez W, Aksu M, Graham B, Sato S, Hallett M. Periodic limb movements in sleep: state-dependent excitability of the spinal flexor reflex. Neurology. 2000;54:1609–16.
52. Pennestri M-H, Montplaisir J, Fradette L, Lavigne G, Colombo R, Lanfranchi PA. Blood pressure changes associated with periodic leg movements during sleep in healthy subjects. Sleep Med. 2013;14:555–61.
53. American Academy of Sleep Medicine. International classification of sleep disorders. 3rd ed. Darien, IL: American Academy of Sleep Medicine; 2014.
54. Manconi M, Ferri R, Zucconi M, Fantini ML, Plazzi G, Ferini-Strambi L. Time structure analysis of leg movements during sleep in REM sleep behavior disorder. Sleep. 2007;30:1779–85.
55. Hanly PJ, Zuberi-Khokhar N. Periodic limb movements during sleep in patients with congestive heart failure. Chest. 1996;109:1497–502.
56. Vetrugno R, Provini F, Meletti S, Plazzi G, Liguori R, Cortelli P, et al. Propriospinal myoclonus at the sleep-wake transition: a new type of parasomnia. Sleep. 2001;24:835–43.
57. Hermesh H, Schapir L, Marom S, Skopski R, Barnea E, Weizman A, et al. Bruxism and oral parafunctional hyperactivity in social phobia outpatients. J Oral Rehabil. 2015;42:90–7.
58. Lobbezoo F, Lavigne GJ, Tanguay R, Montplaisir JY. The effect of catecholamine precursor L-dopa on sleep bruxism: a controlled clinical trial. Mov Disord. 1997;12:73–8.
59. Carra MC, Huynh N, Lavigne G. Sleep bruxism: a comprehensive overview for the dental clinician interested in sleep medicine. Dent Clin N Am. 2012;56:387–413.
60. Macaluso GM, Guerra P, Di Giovanni G, Boselli M, Parrino L, Terzano MG. Sleep bruxism is a disorder related to periodic arousals during sleep. J Dent Res. 1998;77:565–73.
61. Steriade M, McCormick DA, Sejnowski TJ. Thalamocortical oscillations in the sleeping and aroused brain. Science. 1993;262:679–85.
62. Shouse MN, Scordato JC, Farber PR. Sleep and arousal mechanisms in experimental epilepsy: epileptic components of NREM and antiepileptic components of REM sleep. Ment Retard Dev Disabil Res Rev. 2004;10:117–21.
63. Jones BE. Paradoxical REM sleep promoting and permitting neuronal networks. Arch Ital Biol. 2004;142:379–96.
64. Shouse MN, Siegel JM, Wu MF, Szymusiak R, Morrison AR. Mechanisms of seizure suppression during rapid-eye-movement (REM) sleep in cats. Brain Res. 1989;505:271–82.
65. Terzano MG, Parrino L, Garofalo PG, Durisotti C, Filati-Roso C. Activation of partial seizures with motor signs during cyclic alternating pattern in human sleep. Epilepsy Res. 1991;10:166–73.
66. Terzano MG, Parrino L, Anelli S, Boselli M, Clemens B. Effects of generalized interictal EEG discharges on sleep stability: assessment by means of cyclic alternating pattern. Epilepsia. 1992;33:317–26.
67. Terzano MG, Parrino L, Spaggiari MC, Barusi R, Simeoni S. Discriminatory effect of cyclic alternating pattern in focal lesional and benign rolandic interictal spikes during sleep. Epilepsia. 1991;32:616–28.
68. Tinuper P, Bisulli F, Cross JH, Hesdorffer D, Kahane P, Nobili L, et al. Definition and diagnostic criteria of sleep-related hypermotor epilepsy. Neurology. 2016;86:1834–42.
69. Provini F, Plazzi G, Tinuper P, Vandi S, Lugaresi E, Montagna P. Nocturnal frontal lobe epilepsy. A clinical and polygraphic overview of 100 consecutive cases. Brain J Neurol. 1999;122(Pt 6):1017–31.
70. Phillips HA, Scheffer IE, Berkovic SF, Hollway GE, Sutherland GR, Mulley JC. Localization of a gene for autosomal dominant nocturnal frontal lobe epilepsy to chromosome 20q 13.2. Nat Genet. 1995;10:117–8.
71. Ross SA, Wong JY, Clifford JJ, Kinsella A, Massalas JS, Horne MK, et al. Phenotypic characterization of an alpha 4 neuronal nicotinic acetylcholine receptor subunit knock-out mouse. J Neurosci. 2000;20:6431–41.
72. De Fusco M, Becchetti A, Patrignani A, Annesi G, Gambardella A, Quattrone A, et al. The nicotinic receptor beta 2 subunit is mutant in nocturnal frontal lobe epilepsy. Nat Genet. 2000;26:275–6.
73. Parrino L, Pavesi G. When sleep-related hypermotor epilepsy (SHE) met Charles Darwin and Francis Galton. Neurology. 2017;89:502–5.
74. Parrino L, De Paolis F, Milioli G, Gioi G, Grassi A, Riccardi S, et al. Distinctive polysomnographic traits in nocturnal frontal lobe epilepsy. Epilepsia. 2012;53:1178–84.
75. Tassinari CA, Cantalupo G, Högl B, Cortelli P, Tassi L, Francione S, et al. Neuroethological approach to frontolimbic epileptic seizures and parasomnias: the same central pattern generators for the same behaviours. Rev Neurol (Paris). 2009;165:762–8.
76. Nobili L, Francione S, Mai R, Cardinale F, Castana L, Tassi L, et al. Surgical treatment of drug-resistant nocturnal frontal lobe epilepsy. Brain J Neurol. 2007;130:561–73.
77. Ryvlin P, Minotti L, Demarquay G, Hirsch E, Arzimanoglou A, Hoffman D, et al. Nocturnal hypermotor seizures, suggesting frontal lobe epilepsy, can originate in the insula. Epilepsia. 2006;47:755–65.
78. Nobili L, Cossu M, Mai R, Tassi L, Cardinale F, Castana L, et al. Sleep-related hyperkinetic seizures of temporal lobe origin. Neurology. 2004;62:482–5.
79. Bisulli F, Vignatelli L, Provini F, Leta C, Lugaresi E, Tinuper P. Parasomnias and nocturnal frontal lobe epilepsy (NFLE): lights and shadows--controversial points in the differential diagnosis. Sleep Med. 2011;12(Suppl 2):S27–32.
80. Tassinari CA, Rubboli G, Gardella E, Cantalupo G, Calandra-Buonaura G, Vedovello M, et al. Central pattern generators for a common semiology in fronto-limbic seizures and in parasomnias. A neuroethologic approach. Neurol Sci. 2005;26(Suppl 3): s225–32.
81. Parrino L, Halasz P, Tassinari CA, Terzano MG. CAP, epilepsy and motor events during sleep: the unifying role of arousal. Sleep Med Rev. 2006;10:267–85.
82. Parrino L. Down the rabbit-hole: new perspectives from stereo-EEG in the investigation of sleep, nocturnal epilepsy and parasomnias. Sleep Med Rev. 2016;25:1–3.
83. Gibbs SA, Proserpio P, Terzaghi M, Pigorini A, Sarasso S, Lo Russo G, et al. Sleep-related epileptic behaviors and non-REM-related parasomnias: insights from stereo-EEG. Sleep Med Rev. 2016;25:4–20.
84. Terzaghi M, Sartori I, Mai R, Tassi L, Francione S, Cardinale F, et al. Coupling of minor motor events and epileptiform discharges with arousal fluctuations in NFLE. Epilepsia. 2008;49:670–6.
85. Zucconi M, Oldani A, Smirne S, Ferini-Strambi L. The macrostructure and microstructure of sleep in patients with autosomal dominant nocturnal frontal lobe epilepsy. J Clin Neurophysiol. 2000;17:77–86.
86. Sforza E, Montagna P, Rinaldi R, Tinuper P, Cerullo A, Cirignotta F, et al. Paroxysmal periodic motor attacks during sleep: clinical and polygraphic features. Electroencephalogr Clin Neurophysiol. 1993;86:161–6.

87. Terzano MG, Monge-Strauss MF, Mikol F, Spaggiari MC, Parrino L. Cyclic alternating pattern as a provocative factor in nocturnal paroxysmal dystonia. Epilepsia. 1997;38:1015–25.
88. Provini F, Plazzi G, Montagna P, Lugaresi E. The wide clinical spectrum of nocturnal frontal lobe epilepsy. Sleep Med Rev. 2000;4:375–86.
89. Nobili L, Sartori I, Terzaghi M, Stefano F, Mai R, Tassi L, et al. Relationship of epileptic discharges to arousal instability and periodic leg movements in a case of nocturnal frontal lobe epilepsy: a stereo-EEG study. Sleep. 2006;29:701–4.
90. Terzaghi M, Sartori I, Mai R, Tassi L, Francione S, Cardinale F, et al. Sleep-related minor motor events in nocturnal frontal lobe epilepsy. Epilepsia. 2007;48:335–41.
91. Vignatelli L, Bisulli F, Provini F, Naldi I, Pittau F, Zaniboni A, et al. Interobserver reliability of video recording in the diagnosis of nocturnal frontal lobe seizures. Epilepsia. 2007;48:1506–11.
92. Zucconi M, Ferini-Strambi L. NREM parasomnias: arousal disorders and differentiation from nocturnal frontal lobe epilepsy. Clin Neurophysiol. 2000;111(Suppl 2):S129–35.
93. Derry CP, Davey M, Johns M, Kron K, Glencross D, Marini C, et al. Distinguishing sleep disorders from seizures: diagnosing bumps in the night. Arch Neurol. 2006;63:705–9.
94. Derry CP, Harvey AS, Walker MC, Duncan JS, Berkovic SF. NREM arousal parasomnias and their distinction from nocturnal frontal lobe epilepsy: a video EEG analysis. Sleep. 2009;32:1637–44.
95. Dauvilliers Y, Arnulf I, Mignot E. Narcolepsy with cataplexy. Lancet. 2007;369:499–511.
96. Burgess CR, Scammell TE. Narcolepsy: neural mechanisms of sleepiness and cataplexy. J Neurosci. 2012;32:12305–11.
97. Mignot E, Lin X, Hesla PE, Dement WC, Guilleminault C, Grumet FC. A novel HLA DR17,DQ1 (DQA1–0102/DQB1–0602 positive) haplotype predisposing to narcolepsy in Caucasians. Sleep. 1993;16:764–5.
98. Oka Y, Inoue Y, Kanbayashi T, Kuroda K, Miyamoto M, Miyamoto T, et al. Narcolepsy without cataplexy: 2 subtypes based on CSF hypocretin-1/orexin-a findings. Sleep. 2006;29:1439–43.
99. Pizza F, Vandi S, Iloti M, Franceschini C, Liguori R, Mignot E, et al. Nocturnal sleep dynamics identify narcolepsy type 1. Sleep. 2015;38:1277–84.
100. Ferri R, Miano S, Bruni O, Vankova J, Nevsimalova S, Vandi S, et al. NREM sleep alterations in narcolepsy/cataplexy. Clin Neurophysiol. 2005;116:2675–84.
101. Terzano MG, Smerieri A, Del Felice A, Giglia F, Palomba V, Parrino L. Cyclic alternating pattern (CAP) alterations in narcolepsy. Sleep Med. 2006;7:619–26.
102. Young T, Peppard PE, Gottlieb DJ. Epidemiology of obstructive sleep apnea: a population health perspective. Am J Respir Crit Care Med. 2002;165:1217–39.
103. The AASM Manual for the Scoring of Sleep and Associated Events. Version 2.1. American Academy of Sleep Medicine. 2014.
104. Collop NA, Anderson WM, Boehlecke B, Claman D, Goldberg R, Gottlieb DJ, et al. Clinical guidelines for the use of unattended portable monitors in the diagnosis of obstructive sleep apnea in adult patients. Portable monitoring task force of the American Academy of sleep medicine. J Clin Sleep Med JCSM. 2007;3:737–47.
105. Masa JF, Corral J, Gomez de Terreros J, Duran-Cantolla J, Cabello M, Hernández-Blasco L, et al. Significance of including a surrogate arousal for sleep apnea-hypopnea syndrome diagnosis by respiratory polygraphy. Sleep. 2013;36:249–57.
106. Milioli G, Bosi M, Grassi A, Riccardi S, Terzano MG, Cortelli P, et al. Can sleep microstructure improve diagnosis of OSAS? Integrative information from CAP parameters. Arch Ital Biol. 2015;153:194–203.
107. Poyares D, Guilleminault C, Rosa A, Ohayon M, Koester U. Arousal, EEG spectral power and pulse transit time in UARS and mild OSAS subjects. Clin Neurophysiol. 2002;113:1598–606.
108. Terzano MG, Parrino L, Boselli M, Spaggiari MC, Di Giovanni G. Polysomnographic analysis of arousal responses in obstructive sleep apnea syndrome by means of the cyclic alternating pattern. J Clin Neurophysiol. 1996;13:145–55.
109. Parrino L, Smerieri A, Boselli M, Spaggiari MC, Terzano MG. Sleep reactivity during acute nasal CPAP in obstructive sleep apnea syndrome. Neurology. 2000;54:1633–40.
110. Central sleep apnea. In: Carney PR, Berry RB, Geyer JD, editors. Clinical sleep disorders. Philadelphia, PA: Lippincott Williams and Wilkins; 2004. pp. 331–46.
111. Javaheri S. Sleep disorders in systolic heart failure: a prospective study of 100 male patients. The final report. Int J Cardiol. 2006;106:21–8.
112. Javaheri S, Smith J, Chung E. The prevalence and natural history of complex sleep apnea. J Clin Sleep Med JCSM. 2009;5:205–11.
113. Hirshkowitz M, Whiton K, Albert SM, Alessi C, Bruni O, DonCarlos L, et al. National Sleep Foundation's updated sleep duration recommendations: final report. Sleep Health. 2015;1:233–43.
114. Vgontzas AN, Liao D, Bixler EO. Insomnia and hypertension. Sleep. 2009;32:1547.
115. Gottlieb DJ, Redline S, Nieto FJ, Baldwin CM, Newman AB, Resnick HE, et al. Association of usual sleep duration with hypertension: the sleep heart health study. Sleep. 2006;29:1009–14.
116. Luyster FS, Strollo PJ, Zee PC, Walsh JK. Boards of directors of the American Academy of sleep medicine and the Sleep Research Society. Sleep: a health imperative. Sleep. 2012;35:727–34.
117. McDermott M, Brown DL, Chervin RD. Sleep disorders and the risk of stroke. Expert Rev Neurother. 2018;18(7):523–31.

Traumatic Brain Injury

36

Francesco Brigo and Oriano Mecarelli

36.1 Introduction

Traumatic brain injury (TBI) is a medical-surgical emergency with relevant socioeconomic consequences. Several conditions can cause TBI, including accidents occurring at home or at work, sport-related injuries, or motor vehicle accidents. TBI is a frequent reason for referral to emergency rooms and for hospitalization, particularly among young and elderly patients.

TBI is a clinically heterogeneous condition, comprising mild to severe forms. It is classified by injury severity at presentation according to level of consciousness after TBI assessed with the Glasgow Coma Scale (GCS): a total GCS score of 3–8 indicates severe TBI, a score of 9–12 corresponds to moderate TBI, and a score of 13–15 corresponds to mild TBI [1].

Mild TBI (sometimes termed “concussion,” particularly in the old medical literature) is characterized by confusion and amnesia, sometimes associated with a preceding transient loss of consciousness. In more severe cases—sometimes associated with skull fracture or penetrating open-head injuries from a foreign object (e.g., bullet)—the clinical symptoms include a more severe and longer impairment of consciousness and neurological deficits related to the intracerebral lesions.

Computed tomography (CT) is the preferred neuroimaging investigation in the acute phase of TBI and is used to identify the location, type, and extent of brain injury and the presence of skull fractures. Before the advent of imaging, electroencephalogram (EEG) was commonly used in the first assessment of patients with acute TBI. Currently, CT and other neuroimaging techniques have substituted EEG as first-line investigation for the diagnosis of cerebral lesions following head trauma. However, EEG still has a relevant role in monitoring brain functional activity in patients with TBI and in detecting post-traumatic epileptogenic foci.

F. Brigo (✉)
Department of Neurosciences, Biomedicine and Movement Sciences, University of Verona, Verona, Italy

Department of Neurology, Hospital Franz Tappeiner, Merano, Italy

O. Mecarelli
Department of Human Neurosciences, Sapienza University of Rome, Rome, Italy

36.2 EEG in the Acute Post-traumatic Phase

When the brain injury is severe enough to cause coma, the EEG recording shows features characteristic of this condition (Fig. 36.1). In Chap. 46, the EEG patterns typically encountered in comatose patients are described in detail; these patterns should be carefully considered in the prognostic evaluation of TBI for the close correlation between clinical and EEG findings in acute post-traumatic coma [2].

Depending on the severity, extent, and location of TBI, the EEG may show focal, multifocal, or widespread abnormalities, the degree of which is directly proportional to the severity of the TBI [2]. They are usually much more frequent and evident in children than adults. A TBI with direct trauma and contrecoup may result in bilateral abnormalities, usually more prominent at the site of direct trauma.

In patients with traumatic subdural hematoma, the EEG shows an amplitude reduction compared to the opposite hemisphere. If the extent of subdural hematoma is small, the EEG can be normal or shows only a reduced amplitude or absence of beta activity and posterior dominant alpha rhythm; if the amount of subdural blood is larger, ipsilateral slowing may occur. Focal epileptiform abnormalities are rare and may also appear after surgical evacuation.

Post-traumatic subarachnoid hemorrhage can cause amplitude asymmetry, particularly if associated with local cortical damage or subdural hematoma.

EEG features associated with mild TBI usually show a slight slowing of the overall activity and background alpha rhythm, which may disappear after minutes or hours. Experimental data in animals show that mild TBI initially

O. Mecarelli (ed.), *Clinical Electroencephalography*, https://doi.org/10.1007/978-3-030-04573-9_36

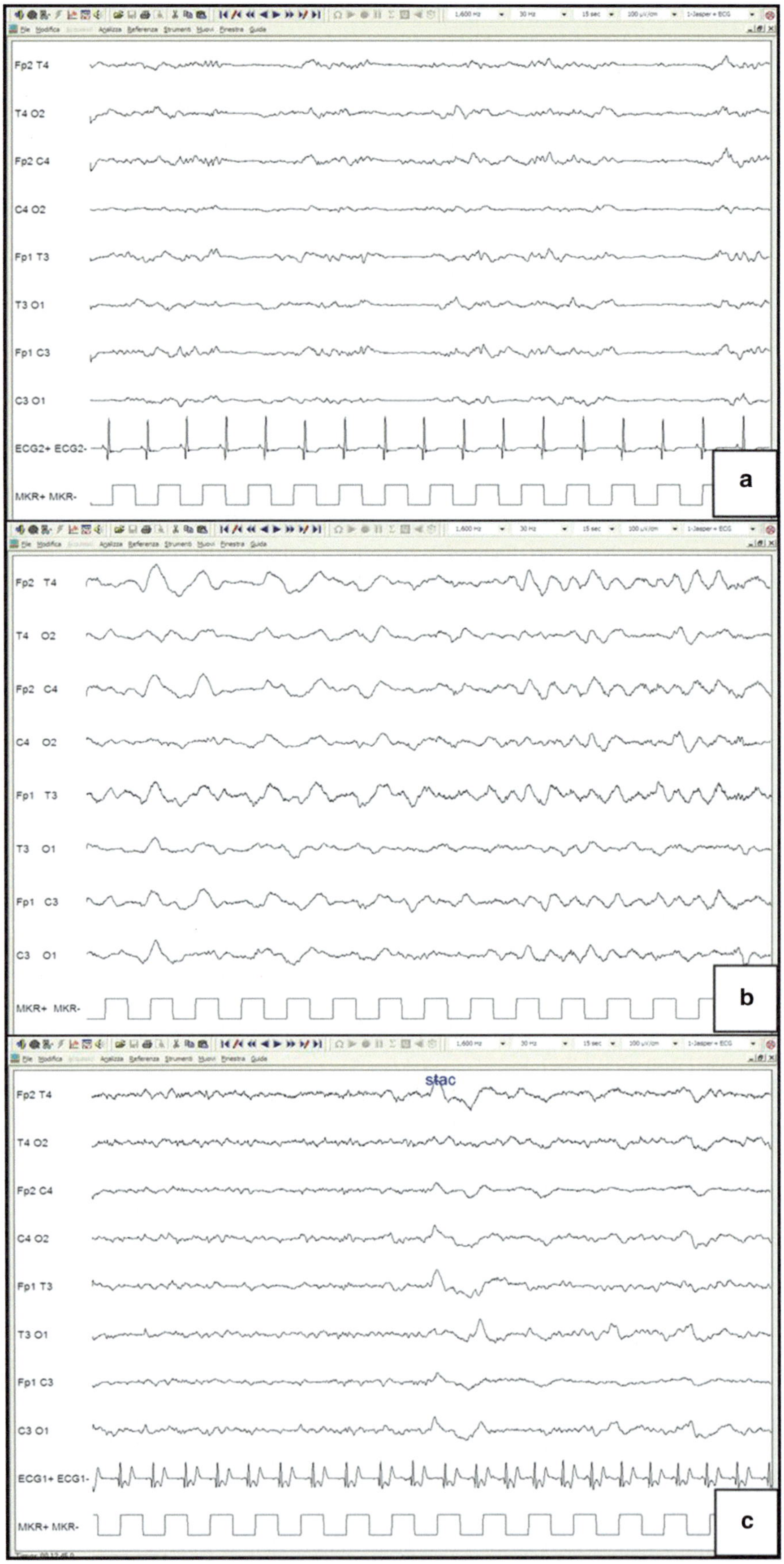

Fig. 36.1 24-year-old comatose patient following polytrauma due to motor vehicle collision. (**a**) The EEG, recorded 2 days after the TBI and under pharmacological sedation, shows amplitude depression. (**b**) Four days after the TBI, the clinical picture has improved; the EEG shows a widespread mono- and polymorphic delta activity, with theta sequences. This EEG pattern corresponds to the clinical picture of fluctuating consciousness. (**c**) Five days after the TBI, the EEG shows reactivity to acoustic stimulation

leads to epileptiform changes, followed by amplitude depression, widespread slowing, and subsequent EEG normalization; this sequence occurs rapidly over time [3]. These EEG abnormalities probably do not reflect a structural brain damage but represent transient changes in cortical excitability, cerebral circulation, or local post-traumatic edema.

36.3 EEG in the Chronic Post-traumatic Phase

A severe TBI may cause different degrees of neurological impairment, usually severe enough to lead to persistent neurological deficits (e.g., hemiplegia, cognitive impairment, behavioral changes, etc.). Mild TBI is often associated with symptoms that are less specific and severe (headache, dizziness, weakness, memory impairment, irritability, anxiety and/or depression, sleep disorders, etc.), may persist for months or even years, and are difficult to assess objectively.

The EEG in severe TBI shows changes correlated with the type of cerebral lesion and the overall clinical picture. They include widespread or focal slowing, generalized or focal decrease of amplitude, and focal epileptiform activities [4]; depending on the severity of TBI, sleep patterns may be disrupted or completely absent. However, none of these changes is specific or pathognomonic of TBI, as they can be found also in other conditions (Fig. 36.2).

The EEG findings of chronic subdural hematoma are focal amplitude reduction or slowing, rarely associated with epileptiform abnormalities. Focal epileptiform abnormalities may also develop after brain surgery, particularly after craniotomy or operations associated with major cortical damage. They may also occur, although more rarely, after minor neurosurgical procedures such as positioning of ventricular shunt.

There is scant literature about EEG findings in patients with mild TBI [5]. They include EEG slowing and amplitude attenuation of posterior dominant alpha rhythm with increased theta activity, particularly over temporal regions. However, these EEG changes are usually transient: they become less visible over time and disappear within hours or days, although may persist for weeks or months even in patients recovering without complications.

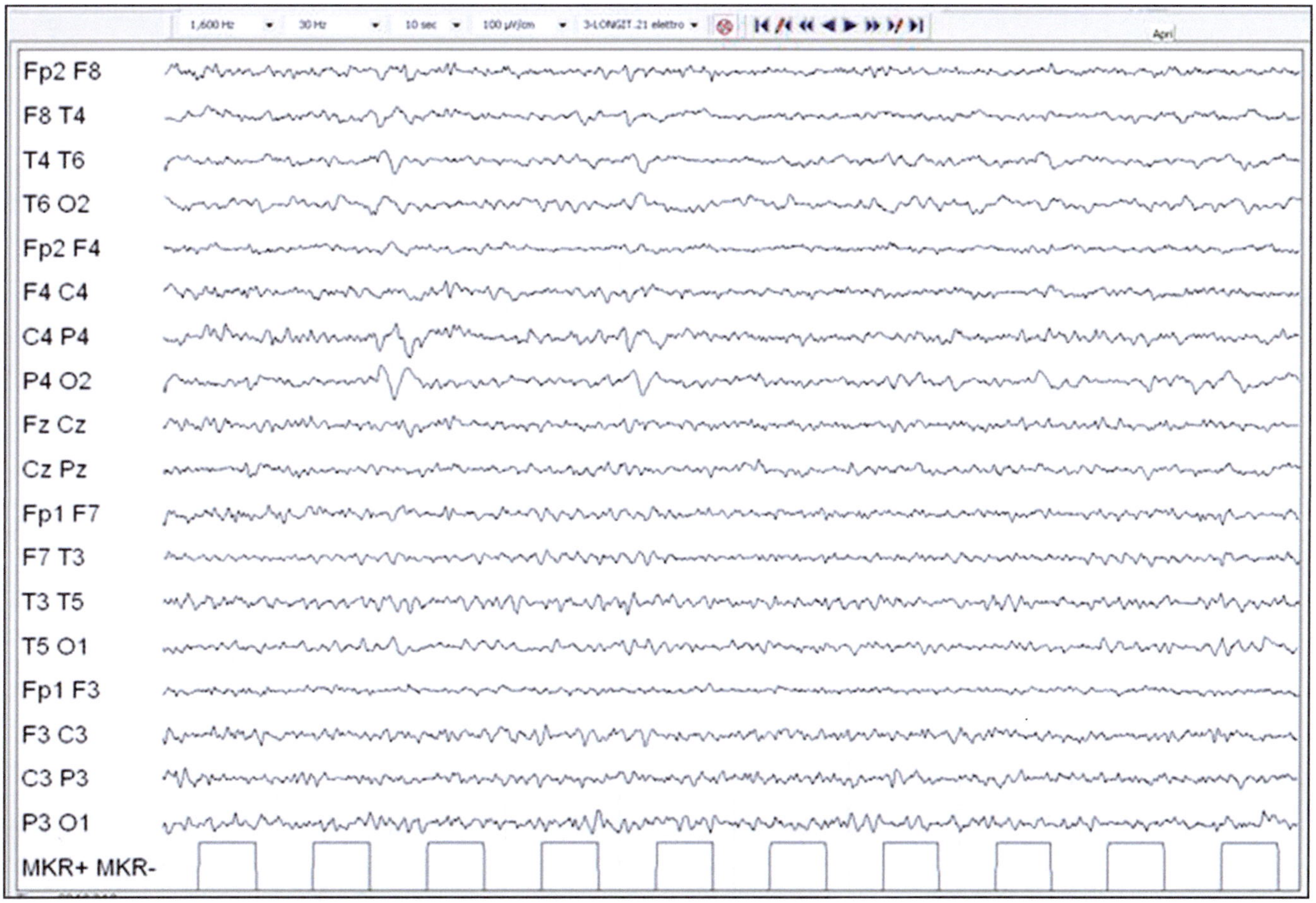

Fig. 36.2 39-year-old patient. The patient had a severe TBI at the age of 12 years, with multiple cerebral lesions and coma. Several EEG recordings performed over the years have shown a slowing of background alpha rhythm and a widespread theta-delta activity, prevalent over right hemispheric regions. Isolated sharp waves can be seen over right temporal-parietal region

EEG recordings obtained in post-traumatic patients are often of low-amplitude and scarcely organized as expression of anxiety (suppression of posterior dominant alpha rhythm).

In late stages after a TBI, the EEG features do not correlate closely with clinical symptoms: a normal EEG does not rule out an underlying brain injury and does not reflect the severity of the initial trauma, whereas mild and nonspecific EEG changes do not support, by themselves, a diagnosis of post-traumatic syndrome [3]. The EEG recording is therefore of little value in follow-up after TBI; quantitative EEG has not provided robust evidence to support its routinary use in clinical practice [3].

36.4 Breach Effect

EEG recordings obtained in patients with open-head injuries may show breach rhythm (more properly termed "breach effect," BE [6]), which by itself is not indicative of brain dysfunction and should be considered as the consequence of a skull defect. The breach effect is defined as a focal increase in the amplitude of EEG activity recorded by electrodes placed over or close to the area of a skull defect, such as after craniotomy or cranial surgery [6].

Differentiating true epileptiform abnormalities from physiological BE may be challenging, particularly because of the sharply contoured appearance and high amplitude of BE.

The following aspects should be considered to differentiate BE from true epileptiform abnormalities [6]:

1. If the EEG shows BE, it is very important to have a high threshold for epileptiform activity. Conversely, it is important not to overlook true epileptiform abnormalities arising from the same region where BE is seen.
2. In pure BE there is no spread of activity to other cerebral regions.
3. BE may attenuate in amplitude or disappear during sleep; conversely, sleep may facilitate the appearance of focal interictal epileptiform abnormalities.
4. BE can be admixed with underlying mu rhythm, which may be misinterpreted as true epileptiform activity. The attenuation of BE when the patient is asked to move the contralateral hand suggests an enhanced underlying mu rhythm; conversely, the lack of reactivity doesn't rule out a normal pattern.
5. Similarly, BE admixed with background alpha rhythm may resemble sharp waves, particularly on temporo-occipital derivations in bipolar montage. The attenuation of BE recorded over posterior regions after eye opening suggests an enhanced underlying posterior dominant alpha rhythm.
6. When a skull defect is over the temporal regions, benign epileptiform patterns such as wicket spikes can become more prominent and hence be misinterpreted as true epileptiform abnormalities.
7. Reducing too much high-frequency filters' values to attenuate the BE may filter out the admixed higher frequencies, resulting in a sharply contoured activity which may be misinterpreted as true epileptiform.
8. Reducing too much high-frequency filters' values to attenuate muscle artifacts carries the same risk. Muscle artifacts can be easily distinguished by BE because of the much higher frequency of their components.
9. Reducing sensitivity is recommended to better analyze the features of BE with excessively high amplitude.
10. Excessive emphasis on "phase reversals" in the context of BE should be avoided. Phase reversals are not always indicative of abnormalities and should therefore be evaluated in a "conservative" way.

36.5 Post-traumatic Epilepsy

Post-traumatic epilepsy is defined as the occurrence of at least two unprovoked epileptic seizures occurring after 1 week following a TBI (late post-traumatic seizures) or the occurrence of one late post-traumatic seizure and a risk of seizure recurrence of at least 60% over the following 10 years [7].

Differentiating between early post-traumatic seizures occurring within 1 week from the TBI and post-traumatic seizures occurring afterward is extremely relevant in clinical practice. Early post-traumatic seizures occur "at the time of a systemic insult or in close temporal association with a documented brain insult" [8] and have a lower risk of seizure recurrence than unprovoked late post-traumatic seizures. One study has systematically assessed the risk of seizure recurrence over the next 10 years following a cerebral injury (stroke, central nervous system infection, or TBI) [9]. The risk of a subsequent seizure after a single early post-traumatic seizure was 13.4% (95% CI: 7.0 to 24.8%); conversely, the risk of seizure recurrence was much higher (46.6%; 95% CI: 30.4 to 66.3%) after the occurrence of a single late post-traumatic seizure (unprovoked seizure) [9]. Hence, not every single late post-traumatic seizure carries a risk of seizure recurrence higher than 60%. The risk of seizure recurrence following a single late (unprovoked) post-traumatic seizure should therefore be assessed in each patient, taking into consideration the presence of the following additional risk factors for post-traumatic epilepsy: cerebral contusion and intracerebral hematoma, skull fracture, bony skull defect or penetrating injuries (e.g., bone or metal fragments, craniectomy or cranial surgery), loss of consciousness or amnesia lasting more than 1 day, post-traumatic seizures within the first week, and age $\geq$ 65 years at the time of injury [10, 11].

The incidence of post-traumatic seizures ranges from 4 to 53% [11]; this rather imprecise estimate is due to the high clinical heterogeneity of studies, which differ for severity of TBI included and duration of follow-up, and often does not distinguish between early and late post-traumatic seizures.

Overall, TBI is one of the most commonly identified causes of acquired epilepsy; it is responsible for approximately 4% of all structural epilepsies. Epileptic seizures may occur even several years after the TBI, and their occurrence depends mainly on the severity of the trauma. An epidemiological study has shown that the cumulative risk of developing post-traumatic seizures within 5 years from the TBI is 0.5% among patients with mild TBI, 1.2% in those with moderate, and 10% in those with severe TBI [10].

The treatment with antiepileptic drugs (e.g., carbamazepine or phenytoin) reduces the risk of early post-traumatic seizures [12] but does not prevent the occurrence of post-traumatic epilepsy or reduce mortality [13]. A long-term prophylactic treatment with antiepileptic drugs seems therefore not justified [14].

In patients with post-traumatic epilepsy, baseline EEG may show theta/delta slowing, usually focal, associated with well-defined epileptiform abnormalities (spikes, sharp waves, spike and wave complexes, etc.) (Figs. 36.3 and 36.4). Most seizures have focal onset, with or without evolution to bilateral tonic-clonic seizures; the EEG pattern is that typically encountered in these seizure types.

Although the prognostic role of EEG in predicting post-traumatic epilepsy still needs to be fully elucidated [15], the presence of abnormal findings in the EEG recorded at the time of discharge from the hospital seems to increase the subsequent risk of late post-traumatic seizures in patients with moderate TBI [16].

Finally, it is worth considering that in patients with a previous diagnosis of epilepsy, the TBI can accentuate the pre-existing epileptiform abnormalities.

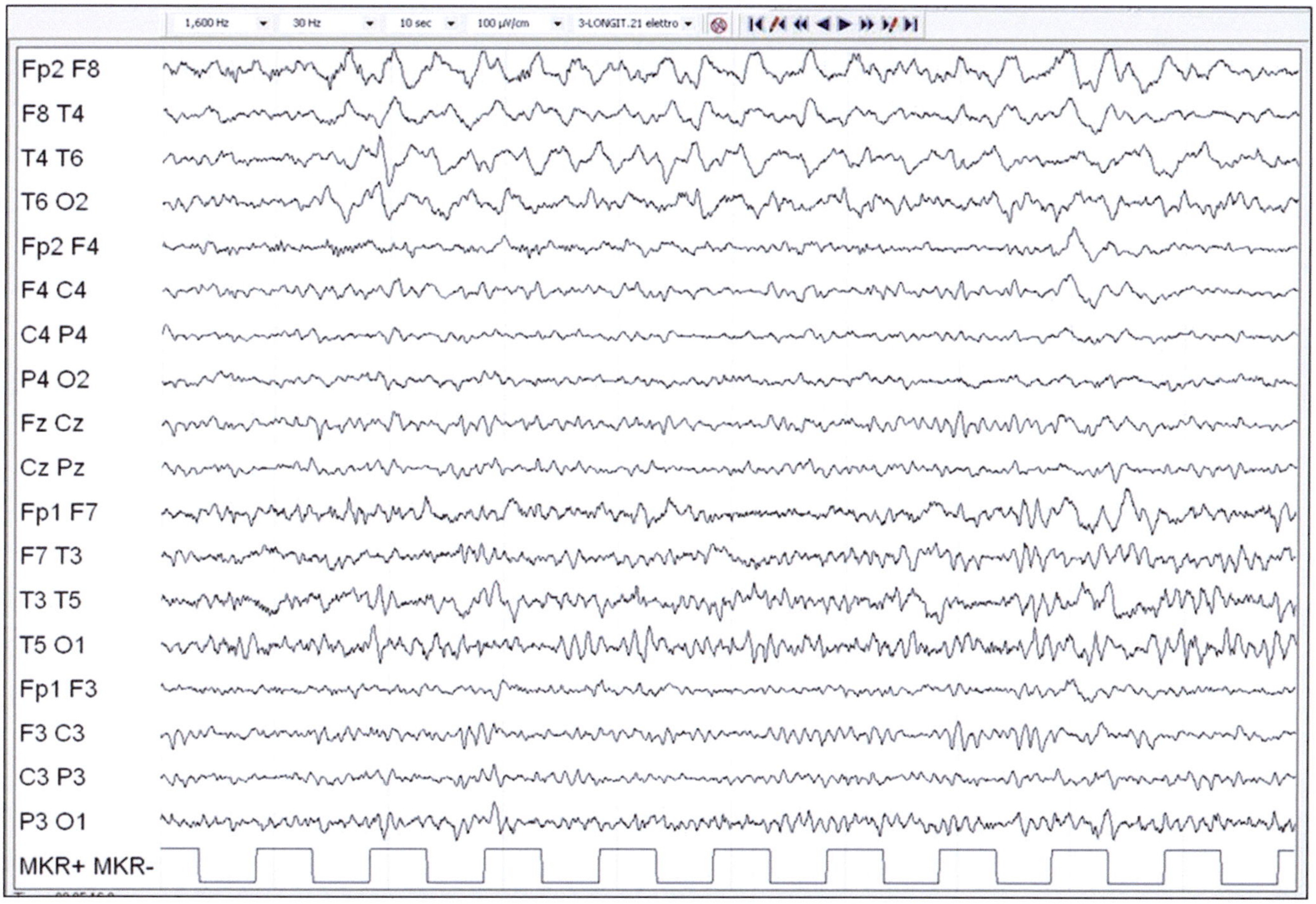

Fig. 36.3 46-year-old patient. The patient had a severe TBI with brain contusions in right hemisphere and remained comatose for approximately 3 months. Subsequently, the status improved, albeit with neurological deficits. Two epileptic seizures occurred 2 years after the trauma, without seizure recurrence under antiepileptic therapy. The baseline EEG recording shows a background alpha rhythm which is scarcely visible on the right with intermittent sequences of rhythmic delta potentials at 2–2.5 Hz over the right temporal region, intermixed with sporadic sharp waves

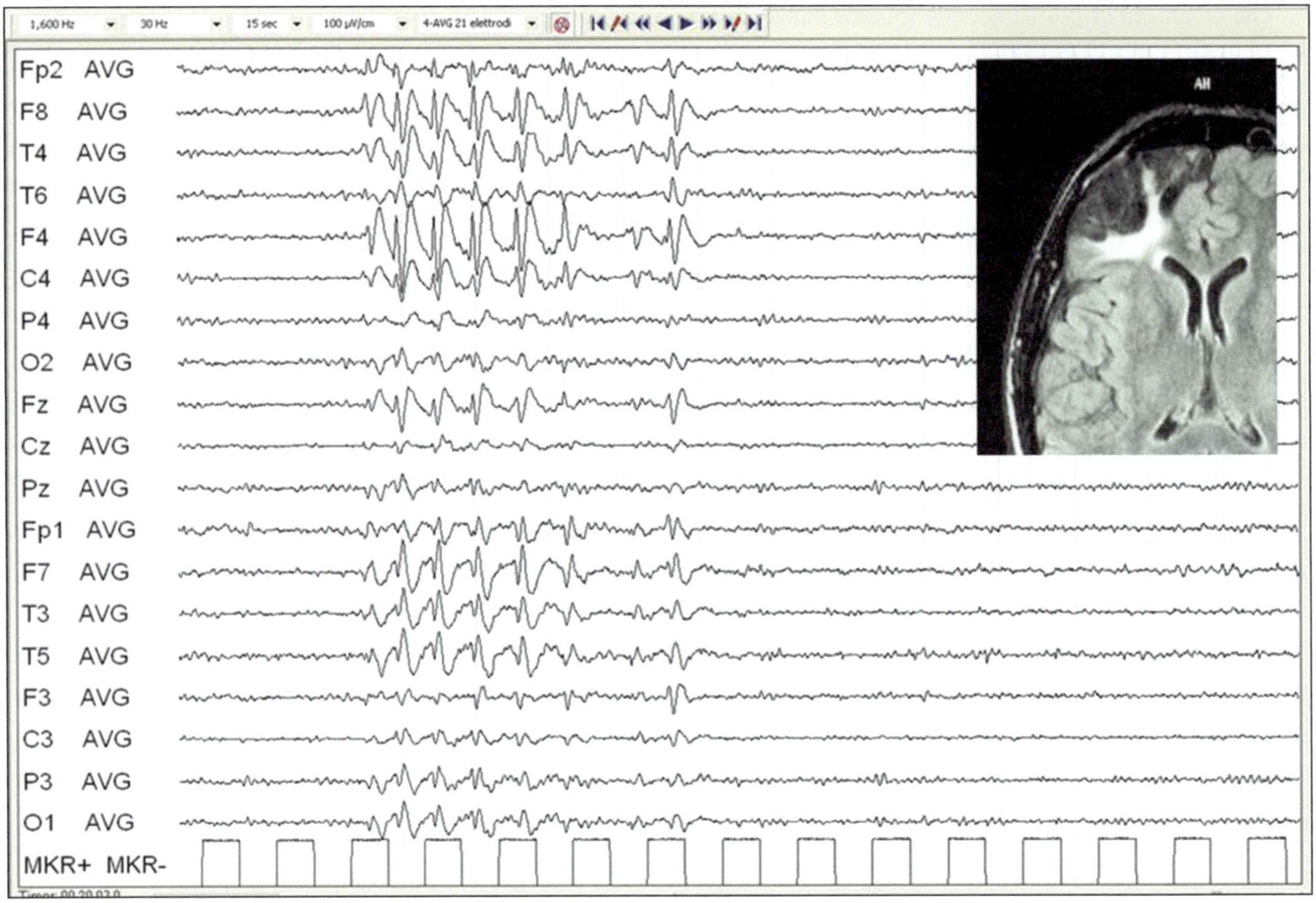

Fig. 36.4 32-year-old patient. TBI with right frontal brain contusion. A focal to bilateral tonic-clonic seizure occurred 30 months after the TBI. The magnetic resonance imaging shows the post-traumatic cerebral lesion. The baseline EEG (recorded more than 4 years after the trauma) shows an epileptogenic focus in right frontal-temporal regions, with tendency to spread contralaterally

References

1. Hawryluk GW, Manley GT. Classification of traumatic brain injury: past, present, and future. Handb Clin Neurol. 2015;127:15–21.
2. Galovic M, Schmitz B, Tettenborn B. EEG in inflammatory disorders, cerebrovascular diseases, trauma, and migraine. In: Schomer DL, Lopes da Silva F, editors. Niedermeyer's electroencephalography: basic principles, clinical applications, and related fields. 7th ed. Oxford: Oxford University Press; 2018. p. 371–412.
3. Nuwer MR, Hovda DA, Schrader LM, Vespa PM. Routine and quantitative EEG in mild traumatic brain injury. Clin Neurophysiol. 2005;116:2001–25.
4. Ronne-Engstrom E, Winkler T. Continuous EEG monitoring in patients with traumatic brain injury reveals a high incidence of epileptiform activity. Acta Neurol Scand. 2006;114:47–53.
5. Williams CS, Spitz MC, Foley JF, Weaver LK, Lindblad AS, Wierzbicki MR. Baseline EEG abnormalities in mild traumatic brain injury from the BIMA study. Undersea Hyperb Med. 2016;43:521–30.
6. Brigo F, Cicero R, Fiaschi A, Bongiovanni LG. The breach rhythm. Clin Neurophysiol. 2011;122:2116–20.
7. Fisher RS, Acevedo C, Arzimanoglou A, Bogacz A, Cross JH, Elger CE, Engel J Jr, Forsgren L, French JA, Glynn M, Hesdorffer DC, Lee BI, Mathern GW, Moshé SL, Perucca E, Scheffer IE, Tomson T, Watanabe M, Wiebe S. ILAE official report: a practical clinical definition of epilepsy. Epilepsia. 2014;55:475–82.
8. Beghi E, Carpio A, Forsgren L, Hesdorffer DC, Malmgren K, Sander JW, Tomson T, Hauser WA. Recommendation for a definition of acute symptomatic seizure. Epilepsia. 2010;51:671–5.
9. Hesdorffer DC, Benn EK, Cascino GD, Hauser WA. Is a first acute symptomatic seizure epilepsy? Mortality and risk for recurrent seizure. Epilepsia. 2009;50:1102–8.
10. Annegers JF, Hauser WA, Coan SP, et al. A population-based study of seizures after traumatic brain injuries. N Engl J Med. 1998;30:20–4.
11. Frey LC. Epidemiology of posttraumatic epilepsy: a critical review. Epilepsia. 2003;44(Suppl 10):11–7.
12. Temkin NR. Preventing and treating posttraumatic seizures: the human experience. Epilepsia. 2009;50(Suppl 2):10–3.
13. Thompson K, Pohlmann-Eden B, Campbell LA, Abel H. Pharmacological treatments for preventing epilepsy following traumatic head injury. Cochrane Database Syst Rev. 2015;8:CD009900.
14. D'Ambrosio R, Perucca E. Epilepsy after head injury. Curr Opin Neurol. 2004;17:731–5.
15. Young GB, Wang JT, Connolly JF. Prognostic determination in anoxic-ischemic and traumatic encephalopathies. J Clin Neurophysiol. 2004;21:379–90.
16. De Reuck J. Risk factors for late-onset seizures related to cerebral contusions in adults with a moderate traumatic brain injury. Clin Neurol Neurosurg. 2011;113:469–71.

37 Cerebral Tumors

Marianna Brienza, Patrizia Pulitano, and Oriano Mecarelli

37.1 The Role of EEG in Brain Tumors

Neuroimaging, histology and immunohistochemistry represent the cornerstones in the diagnosis and characterization of cerebral tumors. Seizures can also occur in patients with brain tumors at any stage of the disease: they can be an early symptom, at onset, or appear later or even never. Furthermore, patients can have a single provoked seizure, before or after surgery; in these cases, one single ictal episode is sufficient for epilepsy diagnosis [1]. EEG is an important diagnostic tool in brain tumors, with or without related epilepsy, for many and for different reasons. It can confirm the clinical diagnosis of seizure, especially in case of first provoked seizure, with a high localization value for the epileptogenic focus. EEG can also be used to identify epileptic activity in the absence of clinically manifest seizures. It can show interictal epileptiform discharges or aspecific alterations in the tumor and peritumoral areas, suggesting damage of specific neural networks allowing the identification of the epileptogenic area: this is of fundamental importance to address surgery, especially in case of dual pathology. EEG can also be useful during follow-up, to monitor antiepileptic therapy and for monitoring brain functions during awake surgery.

M. Brienza · O. Mecarelli (✉)
Department of Human Neurosciences, Sapienza University of Rome, Rome, Italy
e-mail: marianna.brienza@uniroma1.it; oriano.mecarelli@uniroma1.it

P. Pulitano
Azienda Ospedaliero-Universitaria Policlinico Umberto I, Rome, Italy
e-mail: patrizia.pulitano@uniroma1.it

37.2 EEG Patterns: Correlation with Site and Type of Brain Tumors

Although up-to-date there are no unequivocally and pathognomonic EEG patterns of specific brain tumors and considering that not all tumors are associated to EEG alterations, some EEG abnormalities may be considered highly suggestive.

Cortical tumors can cause EEG slowings, as sequences of slow-wave activities, theta and delta. These abnormalities consist of polymorphic and irregular waves, with poor or absent reactivity to different stimuli and without changes during sleep (Fig. 37.1). They can be focal, with or without contralateral transmission and/or diffuse. Anterior temporal lobe tumors, especially fibrillary astrocytomas and oligodendrogliomas, usually show more localized focal slowings on EEG than tumors in the posterior temporal area; spikes, spike-wave and sharp-wave patterns have also been described. Focal abnormalities may also be observed in parietal lobe tumors.

A characteristic type of a focal slow pattern is represented by the Broad Sharp Waves (BSWs), also known as Z waves, because of a zed-like shape of the complex. BSWs have been defined as focal or lateralized paroxysmal, high voltage, sharply contoured delta waves, distinguished from the background activity; they were first described in 1936 and numerous efforts have been made during years for their final definition. According to literature, Zeta waves consist of a first slowly negative phase followed by a relatively more prolonged positive phase - crossing the baseline - lastly followed by another slowly negative phase returning to baseline. [2, 3] Therefore, they are a type of delta waves with a distinctive, sharply diphasic waveform [4]. When zeta waves occur in runs of two or three graphoelements, they have a total duration between 1 and 3 s and an amplitude between 100 and 400 μV. To highlight them, it is then necessary to use very low high-pass filters and a compact time base. They may be more frequently observed in the frontal or temporal regions, but they may also occur in any region of the scalp. Z

O. Mecarelli (ed.), *Clinical Electroencephalography*, https://doi.org/10.1007/978-3-030-04573-9_37

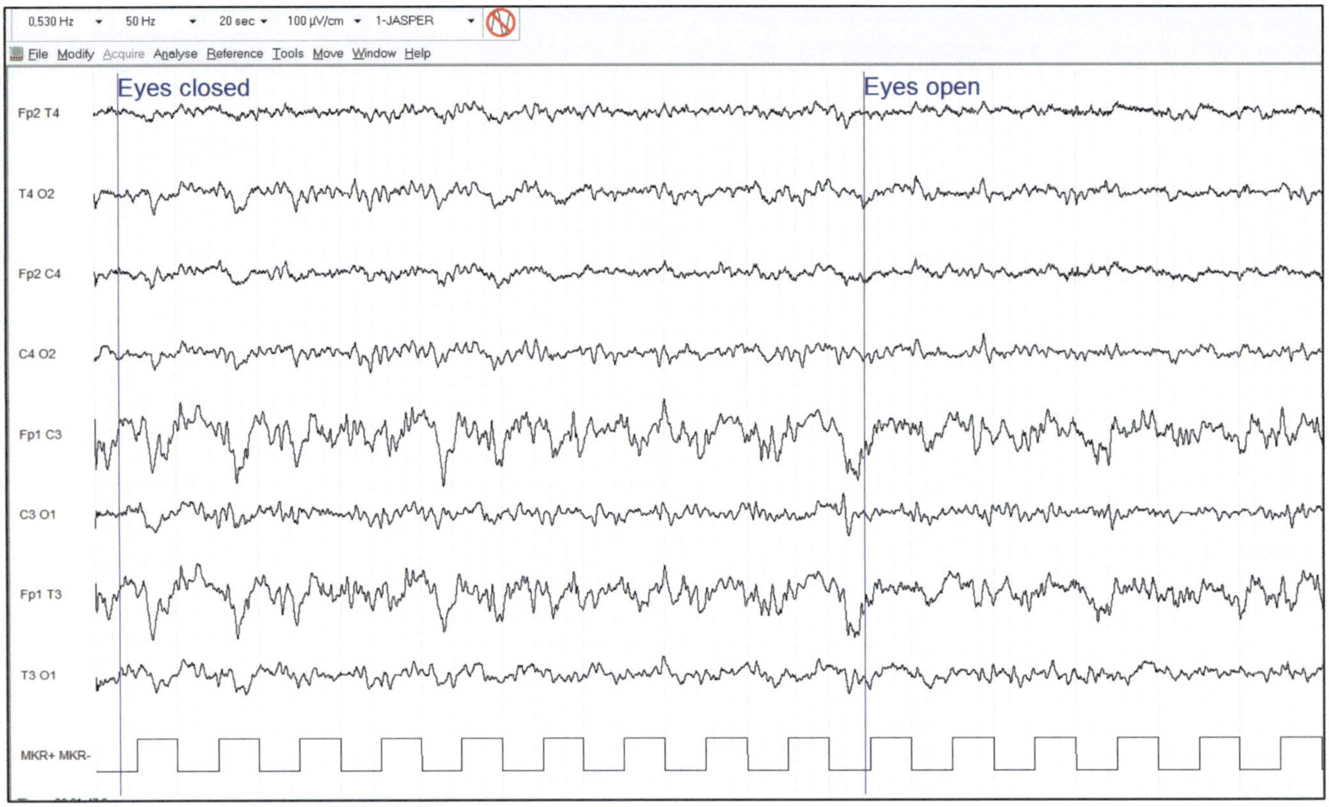

Fig. 37.1 Left frontal slow-wave activity, with superimposed fast rhythms, in a 54-year-old male patient with left frontal low-grade astrocytoma: this subcontinuous activity remains unchanged with eyes open

waves are rarely bilateral, but they can be bisynchronous—especially in frontal areas—and they are unreactive to opening/closing of the eyes and to other stimuli. Zeta waves are typical—but not exclusive—of brain tumors, as they can also be observed in severe brain lesions, usually with an acute or subacute onset and a space occupying character (i.e., contusion, hemorrhage, infarction, etc.) (Fig. 37.2).

In addition to focal slow waves, diffuse slowings can occur as sequences of bilateral theta and, more frequently, delta waves (Intermittent Rhythmic Delta Activity, IRDA): they may be prevalent in any region of the scalp, but they are more typical in the anterior and posterior regions and defined as FIRDA (Frontal Intermittent Rhythmic Delta Activity), when frontal (Fig. 37.3) and OIRDA (Occipital Intermittent Rhythmic Delta Activity), when occipital. They may be associated with slowing and/or depression of background activity, especially when the tumor is located in the posterior areas. Differently from focal anomalies, bilateral slow activity may be reactive to the various stimuli; it is also increased during the phase of falling asleep, it generally disappears in NREM sleep and it reappears in the REM phase. The etiology and significance of this slow activity are still unclear. FIRDA was initially considered a projected rhythm originating from subcortical, deep midline structures and its appearance has been associated with ventricular dilatation and intracranial hypertension. Subsequently, it has been suggested that this pattern may reflect a pathological hyperactivity occurring in diffuse gray matter disease, in both cortical and subcortical areas, whereas polymorphic irregular localized delta activity occurs in focal white matter lesions or in thalamic lesions. These slow patterns should be considered non-specific of brain tumors, as they can be observed in various encephalopathies (e.g., metabolic encephalopathy, cerebral edema, Creutzfeldt-Jakob disease, dementia with Lewy bodies, cortico-basal degeneration, progressive supranuclear palsy, subcortical lesions, etc.) [5].

Focal epileptiform abnormalities as spikes, spike-wave and sharp-wave complexes may be recorded also in the peritumoral areas. These are not necessarily correlated with clinical epileptic seizures and their appearance may not have a strong relevance for the tumor localization, as these elements can be generated in the areas adjacent to the tumor or also in the contralateral ones. Nevertheless, a careful identification of these EEG abnormalities is important to detect potential epileptogenic lesions associated with the tumor (dual pathology). Ictal epileptiform discharges may also represent an early sign of brain neoplasms and they can precede the appearance of focal slow waves by months or even years. These abnormalities are more frequently observed in the frontal and temporal regions. Lateralized Periodic Discharges (LPDs) may be recorded in

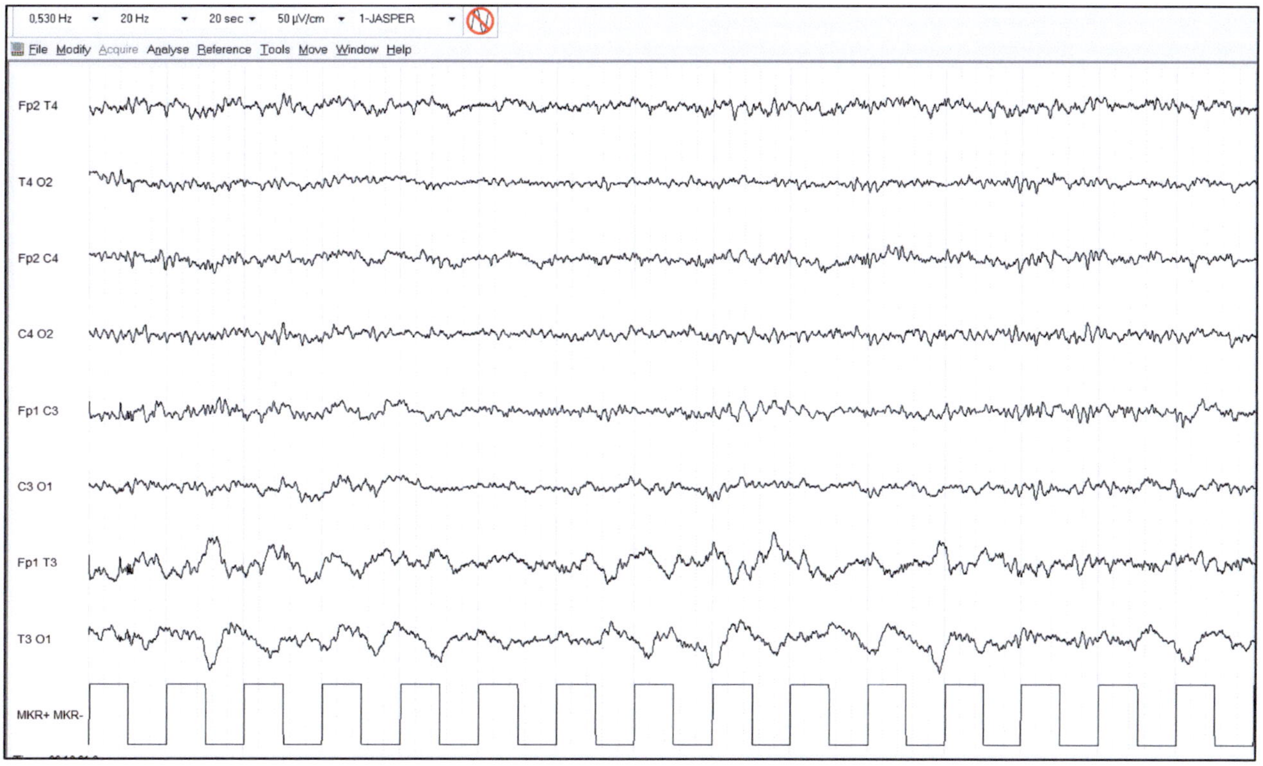

Fig. 37.2 Slow Z-like waves in a 59-year-old male patient with left temporal cerebral metastasis

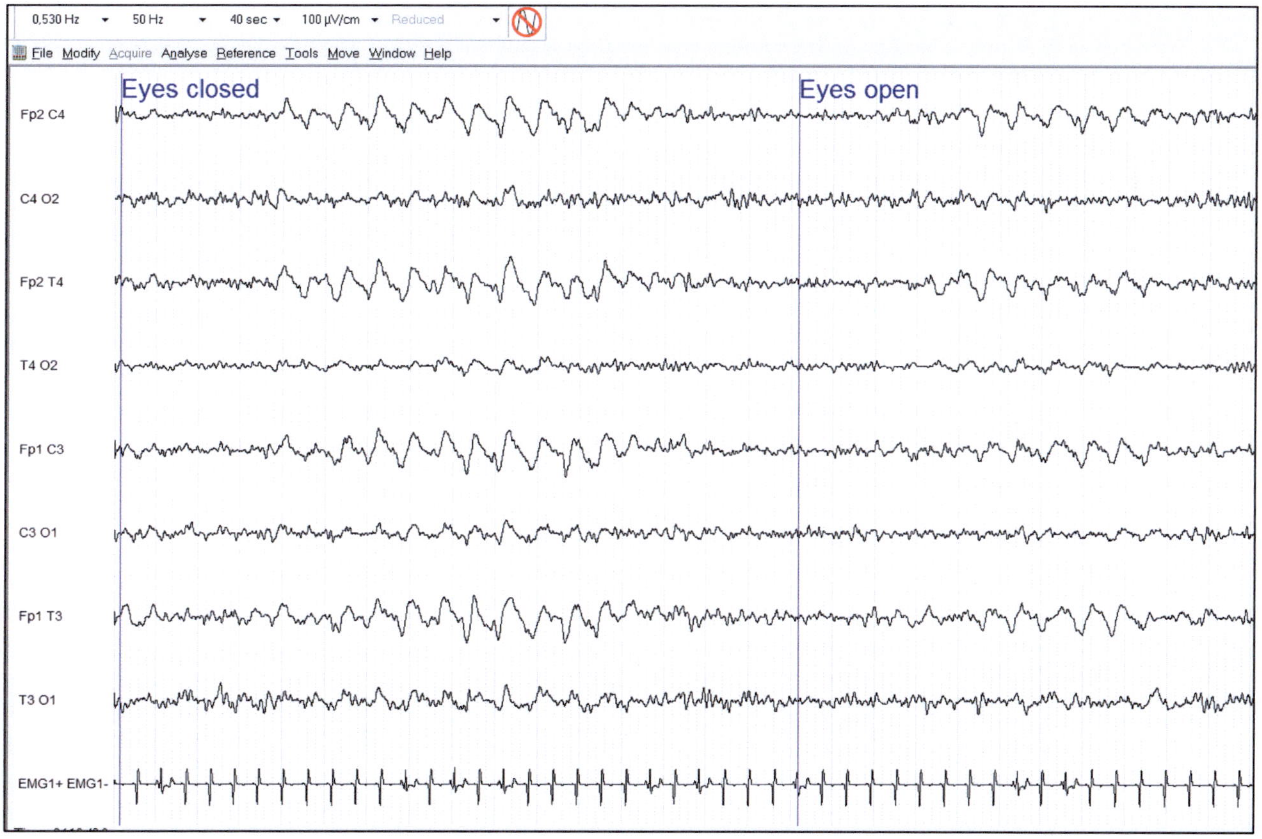

Fig. 37.3 Bilateral Frontal Intermittent Rhythmic Delta Activity (FIRDA) in a 60-year-old male patient with cerebral transcallosal glioblastoma. In this patient, FIRDA is evident both with closed and open eyes

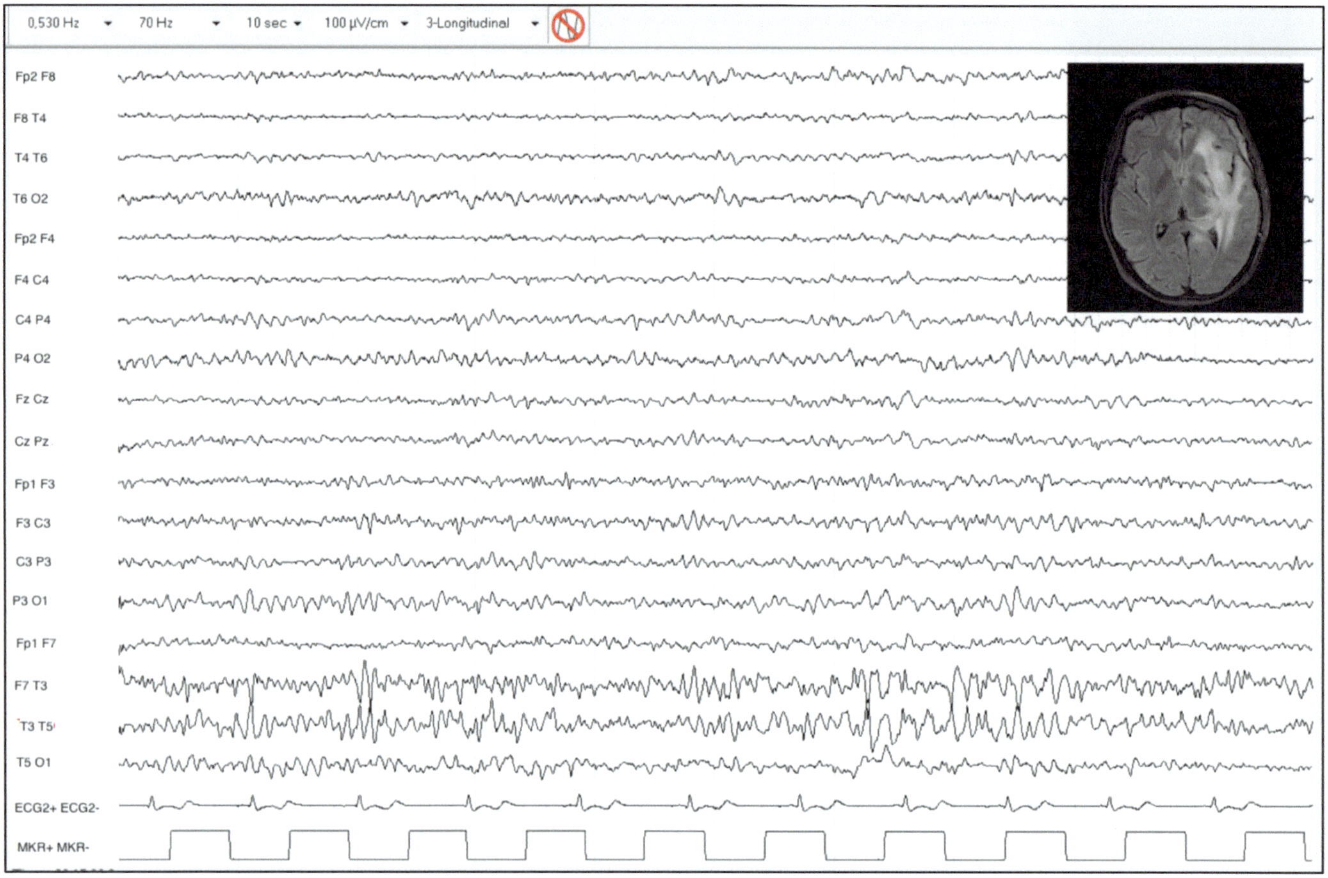

Fig. 37.4 Focal epileptiform activity localized in left temporal area in a 22-year-old female patient with fronto-temporo-parietal glioblastoma. Note that the epileptiform activity is well localized despite the large extent of the tumor

over 10% of patients with brain tumors, but they are not characteristics, as they may also be found in cerebrovascular diseases, infectious inflammatory diseases of CNS, traumatic brain injuries, etc. (Figs. 37.4, 37.5 and 37.6). Status epilepticus, with focal onset, appears in 7% of brain tumors, usually due to high-grade destructive lesions [6].

In basal ganglia tumors, EEG can be normal, or Intermittent Rhythmic Delta Activity (IRDA) can be observed. Subtentorial, periventricular, thalamic, hypothalamic and midbrain tumors generally induce the appearance of a focal or—more frequently—widespread slow rhythmic activity (delta and/or theta) with a concomitant reduction of amplitude and frequency of the background activity. The diffuse or focal background slowing may be related to the involvement of the reticulo-thalamocortical pathways. Slow patterns are often increased by hyperventilation and decreased by eye-opening. EEG patterns similar to those observed in dysmetabolic encephalopathies, characterized by bilateral triphasic frontal waves, have also been described in some thalamic and diencephalic tumors. There have also been reports of 12–14 Hz "spindles" during awake EEG, whereas spindling in healthy brains is only observed during sleep: however, this is a rare phenomenon [7, 8]. Furthermore, there has been a report of dissociation between cerebral hemispheres during sleep, one hemisphere later than the other in cycling through the normal sleep stages. High-voltage and epileptiform EEG activities may be observed in case of a tumor-induced local over-excitation of the thalamus, which propagates to the cortex. The abnormal activity at theta and spindle frequencies appears when a small portion of the brain is forced into an over-inhibited state due to the tumor, in which there is an increase in the firing of the inhibitory thalamic reticular neurons. The effect is highlighted when there is a concurrent decrease in the firing of excitatory thalamic relay neurons which are, in any case, inhibited by the reticular ones. This is likely due to a decrease in the responsiveness of the peritumoral region to cholinergic inputs from the brainstem and a corresponding depolarization of thalamic reticular neurons and hyperpolarization of thalamic relay neurons, similar to the mechanism active during slow-wave sleep. Thus, there is a wide range of reported abnormal EEG phenomena associated with subcortical and especially thalamic tumors. However, it is important to consider that subcortical brain tumors may not give any EEG alterations: it has been reported that around 10–30% of subjects exhibit indeed normal EEGs in the presence of thalamic tumors [9].

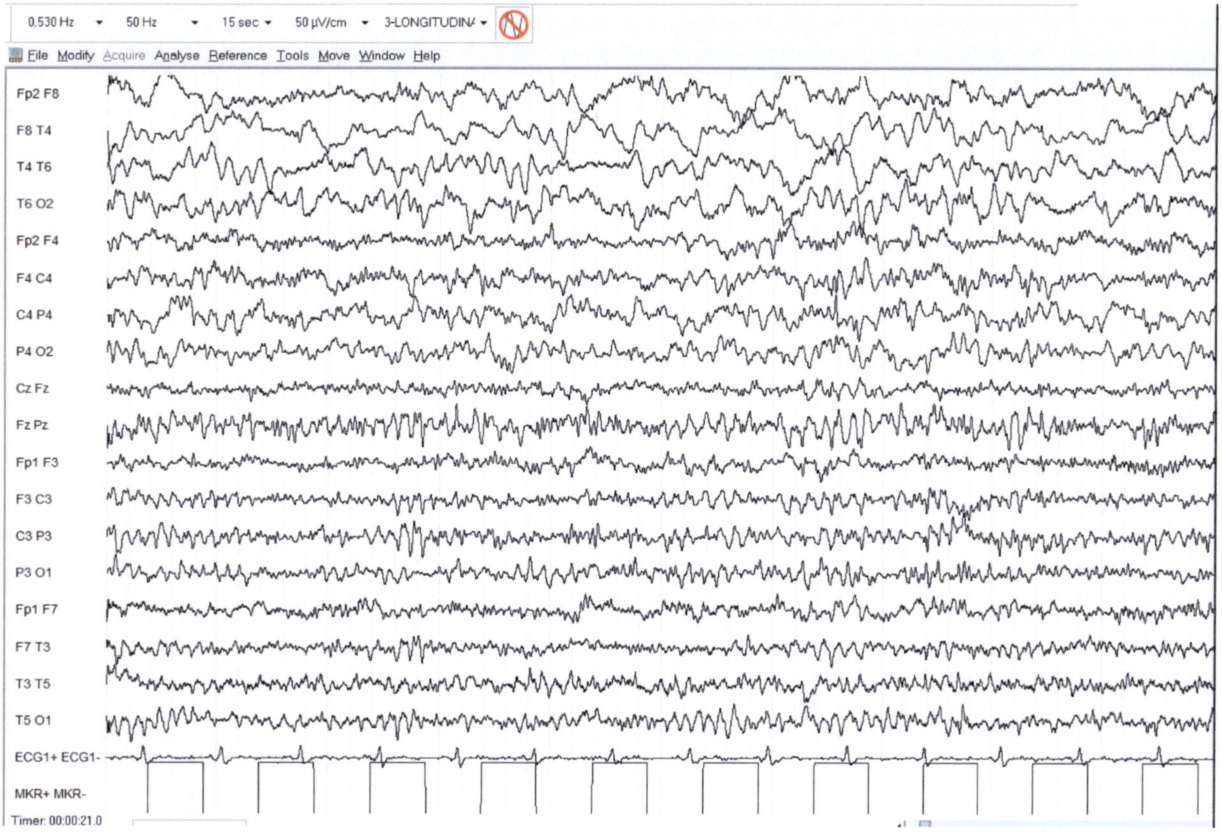

Fig. 37.5 Focal polymorphic slow activity in right fronto-centro-temporal areas in a 56-year-old female patient with temporal astrocytoma. Note the EEG asymmetry, with background activity better represented in left hemisphere

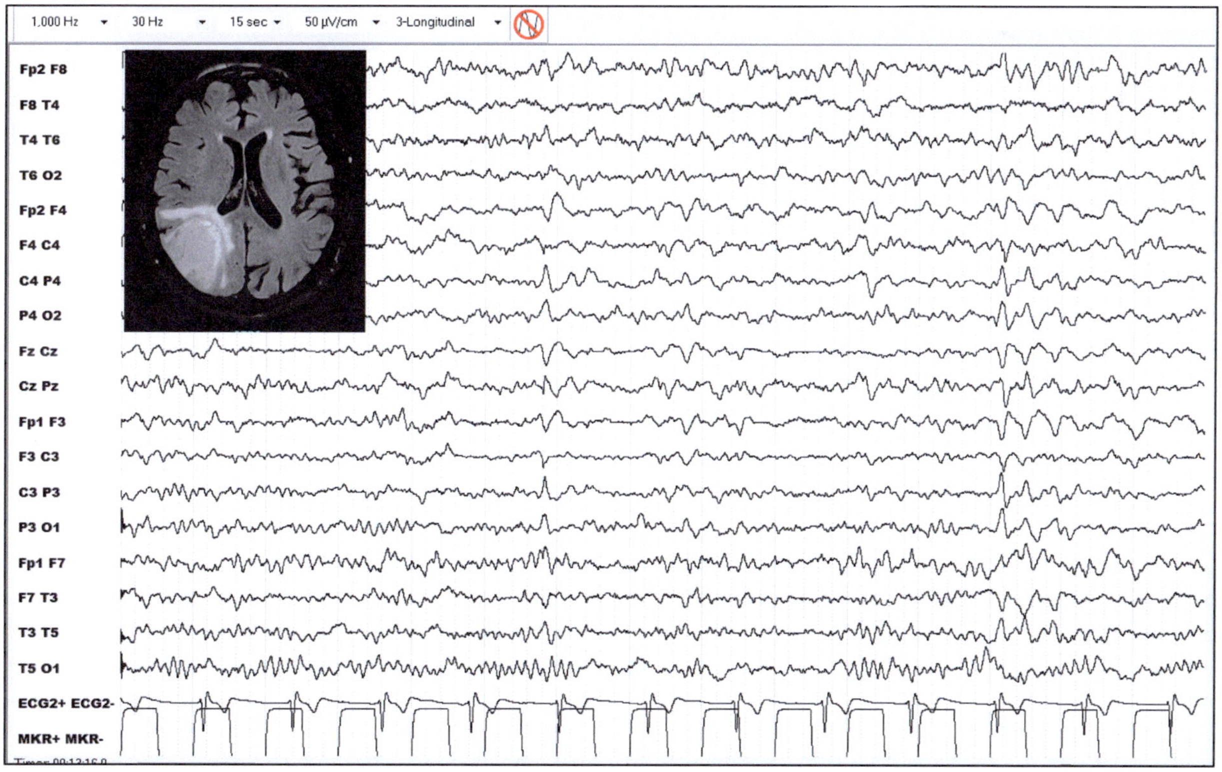

Fig. 37.6 A 77-year-old patient with right temporo-occipital glioblastoma. Asymmetric EEG with alpha activity, evident only in posterior regions of the left hemisphere. Slow-wave activity is recorded on the right hemisphere, with tendency to contralateral anterior transmission. In left temporal areas, sporadic sharp waves are also observed, possibly due to the involvement of contralateral networks

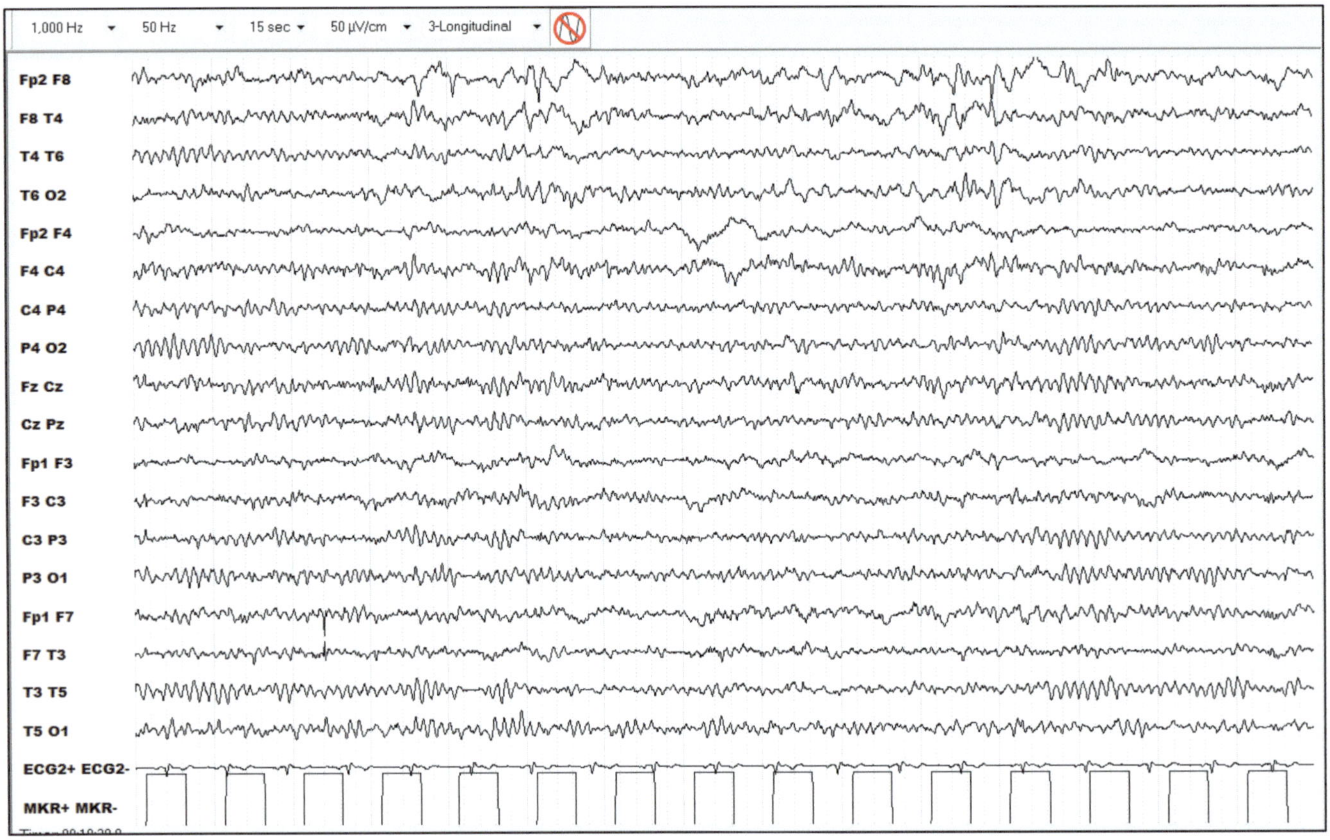

Fig. 37.7 Dysembrioplastic neuroectodermal tumor in a 53-year-old male patient: brief sequences of slowings and sporadic spikes in anterior temporal region

In case of sellar tumors, EEG might show slow waves in the temporal areas or widespread slowings due to intracranial hypertension. Focal EEG abnormalities, although infrequent, can be found in tumors of corpus callosum, possibly related to interhemispheric disconnection or infiltration of the cingulate gyri [10] or associated cortical dysplasia [11]. In 10–15% of pontocerebellar tumors, slowings can be observed in temporal and temporo-occipital areas, both in correspondence of the tumor site, as well as in the contralateral areas, or even bilaterally.

37.2.1 Cortical Tumors: Focus on Dysembryoplastic Neuro Ectodermal Tumors

Dysembryoplastic Neuro Ectodermal Tumors (DNETs) are rare neoplasms. They are World Health Organization (WHO) grade 1 neoplasms, typically present as isolated cortical lesions and with no associated edema [12]. DNETs are an important cause of refractory focal epilepsy and they represent almost 10% of all the tumors resected in patients with pharmaco-resistant focal epilepsy. Their most frequent location is in the temporal lobe, where they are sometimes associated to cortical abnormalities (e.g., focal cortical dysplasia) in the context of dual pathology. For this reason, EEG abnormalities may be due to the tumor, to the intrinsic epileptogenic properties of dysplasic cortex, or to both. Ictal EEG abnormalities are represented by focal discharges while interictal EEG patterns are characterized by slowings, with or without spikes (Fig. 37.7). These patterns may be located in the region of the scalp corresponding to the tumor or even in other areas, suggesting the presence of global structural changes or alterations of different cortical networks: this latter case is associated with a poor seizure's prognosis. [13, 14]

37.2.2 Subcortical Tumors: Focus on Hypothalamic Hamartoma

Among subcortical tumors, Hypothalamic Hamartoma (HH) deserves a particular mention. HHs are well-recognized congenital malformations of the brain, defined as benign, tumor-like nodules of disorganized but mature cells, mostly composed of a combination of neuronal or ganglion cells, glial cells and blood vessels [15]. These tumors induce a broad neuroendocrine syndromic spectrum which includes central precocious puberty, psychiatric and behavioral disorders and epilepsy. A symptomatic epilepsy, often drug-resistant, is the main symptom and it is related to the sessile type of HH [16]. Seizure semiology is mainly characterized by brief paroxysms of sudden, unmotivated, unnatural laughter (gelastic seizures) or, less frequently, crying (dacristic seizures); consciousness may be preserved and occasional cases of status epilepticus have been reported. Associated manifestation includes facial contraction, mimicking a grimace or smile and clonic buccal, palpebral and ocular movements. Autonomic features including facial flushing, pupillary dilatation, lacrimation, blood pressure and heart rate changes have been reported. In patients with HH, stereotactic depth EEG studies have shown that gelastic seizures are associated with an ictal discharge within the hamartoma itself, and in vitro studies have demonstrated intrinsic pacemaker-like properties of GABAergic neurons in the hamartoma. Although the intrinsic epileptogenicity of the hamartoma is well known and also confirmed by the reduction of seizure after tumor removal, the involvement of other cortical networks is plausible, as demonstrated by EEG recordings [17, 18]. Thus, although scalp EEG recordings do not show any abnormalities in many cases, these are present and sometimes even peculiar in others. Interictal non-epileptiform EEG changes were reported as an intermittent slow activity or as a background slow activity. Interictal epileptiform activity is characterized by sharp waves and spikes or epileptiform discharges, initially only during sleep and typically localized in the frontal or temporal regions [19]. Ictal patterns may be regional, lateralized to one hemisphere, or non-localizable. When focal, EEG alterations involve the anterior cingulate cortex, premotor frontal cortex, opercular areas and temporal cortex [20]: it is generally believed that the behavioral and motor manifestations constituting nongelastic partial seizures represent spread of seizure activity from the HH to specific frontal and temporal cortical regions [21]. The development of generalized seizures is usually accompanied by more widespread EEG abnormalities and neurobehavioral disturbances. Typically, EEG shows an increase in the amount of interictal spike-wave activity, an increase in the degree of bilateral synchrony and the eventual appearance of abundant generalized spike-and-wave patterns, particularly prominent in sleep, without any lateralization/focality [22]. In case of seizures with only gelastic semiology, video-EEG recordings can be useful to confirm the diagnosis in many cases.

37.2.3 Extra-axial Tumors: Focus on Meningioma

Meningiomas are usually benign (except for atypical and anaplastic variants), slow-growing tumors account for approximately 30% of all primary brain tumors, constituting the largest subset of all intracranial tumors [23]. They can occur at any age, but most commonly in the middle age. Women are more likely to develop intracranial meningiomas, with a female/male ratio of nearly 2:1. Meningiomas are more often spontaneous, but they can occur in association with other diseases in a minority of cases (e.g., neurofibromatosis 2) also as "meningiomatosis" which is approximately 1–5% in surgical series [24]. Rare meningiomas are accompanied by other estrogen-dependent tumors, such as carcinomas of the breast or endometrium [25]. The majority of meningiomas are intradural and arise at intracranial, intraspinal, or orbital locations. Intracranial meningiomas favor sites of arachnoidal granulations and produce increased intracranial pressure, including symptoms of mass effect and focal neurologic deficits. In contrast to intraparenchymal tumors, such as gliomas and metastases, seizures are relatively less common in meningiomas [26]. The frequency and the type of seizures depend on its location. Seizure frequency in supratentorial meningioma is estimated from 29 to 67% [27]. Lesions in the temporal lobe frequently cause focal seizures with impairment of awareness and gustatory and olfactory auras. Focal motor or sensory seizures are common with perirolandic lesions. Focal seizures are also frequent with tumors in the supplementary motor cortical area and the associative somatic sensory area. Generalized tonic-clonic seizures may occur as a bilateral diffusion of focal epileptic activity [28]. Few studies focus on seizure outcomes after resections of meningiomas. Chozick and colleagues [29] assessed the incidence of postoperative seizures in 158 patients with meningiomas. They identified six clinical variables predictive of the occurrence of postoperative seizures: preoperative seizure history, preoperative language disturbance, parietal location of the tumor, extent of tumor removal, postoperative medication status, postoperative hydrocephalus. In contrast, it has been reported that there was no statistically significant association between extent of surgical resection and the development of delayed seizures [29, 30]. Wirsching and colleagues, [31] in their study about the risk factors for postoperative epilepsy, observed that on postoperative EEG recordings, focal slowing, but not slowing of the background rhythm, was associated with persistence of preoperative epilepsy, while focal or background slowings occurred equally in patients with and without postoperative new-onset epilepsy. Epileptiform potentials on postoperative EEG recordings are generally associated with a poor postsurgical seizure's outcome [31]. Therefore, EEG is a widely available technique, and epileptiform discharges on EEG recordings predict seizure recurrence upon withdrawal of antiepileptic drugs (Fig. 37.8) [32].

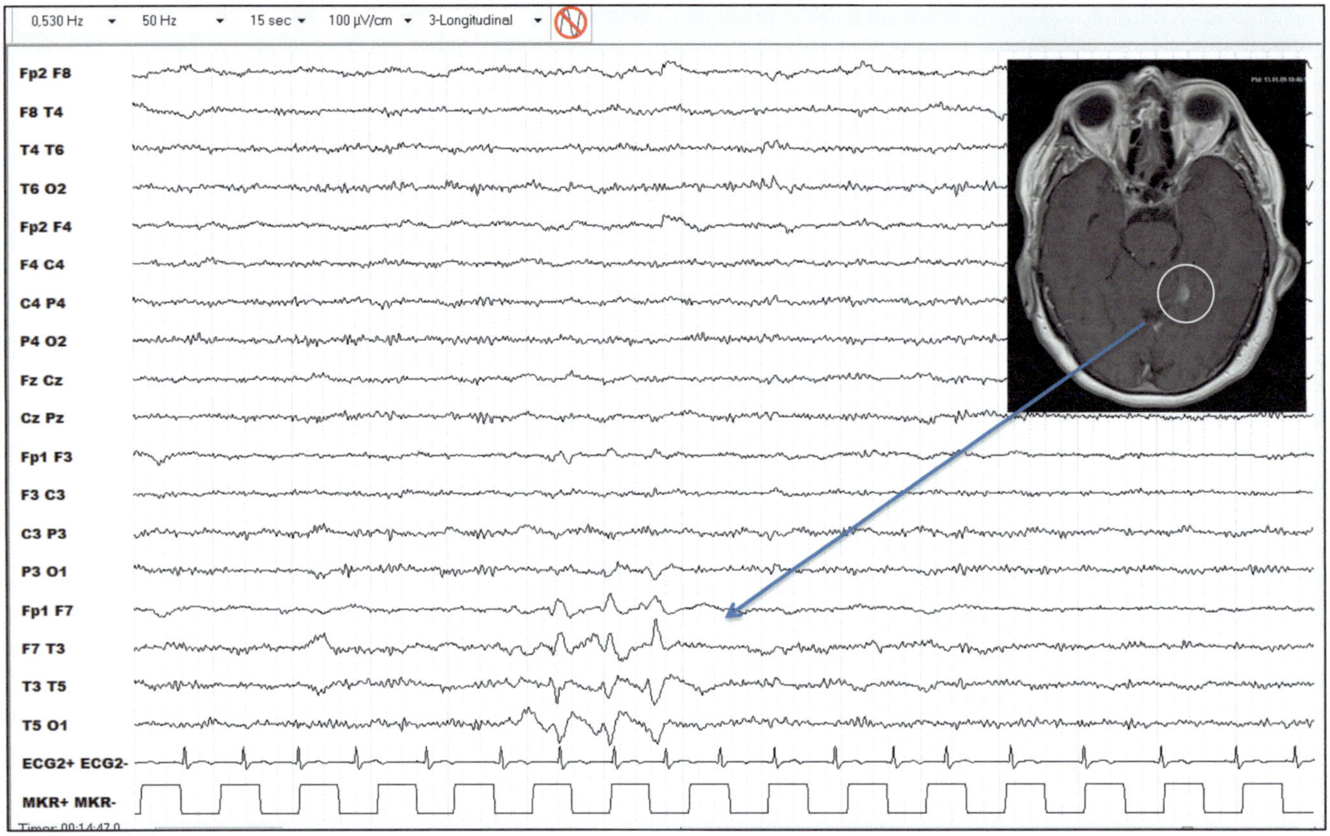

Fig. 37.8 EEG focal epileptiform abnormalities correlated with left temporo-mesial meningioma in a 78-year-old female patient

37.3 Tumor-Related Epilepsy: Neurophysiological Basis and Considerations

Tumor-related epilepsy is a complex field of neurosciences: it represents a common bridge between two pathologies—epilepsy and brain tumors—whose pathophysiological relationships are undoubted, but not yet fully clarified. Literature suggests that seizures occur in approximately one quarter to one half of patients with intracerebral tumors [33], although prevalence rates over 70% have been observed [34]. Seizures that occur consequently to brain tumors account for approximately 5% of new-onset seizures and more than 10% of lesional focal epilepsy [35]. All brain tumors, primary and metastatic, can potentially cause seizures: the probability of seizure developing depends however strongly upon the histological type and grade of tumor, its location, and any other cerebral pathologies associated. The 2016 WHO classification formulates tumor entities based on both histological and molecular information [36]. Among primary tumors, low grade ones seems more associated with epilepsy; epilespy identification in high-grade tumors is conditioned by the shorter observation period, due to the short survival. Neurogliomas (DNETs and gangliogliomas) have a seizure incidence of 80–100%, low-grade gliomas of 60–85%, and glioblastoma of 30–60% [37]. The acronym LEATs (Long-term Epilepsy-Associated Tumors) is often used to identify highly differentiated glial and glioneuronal low-grade tumors (WHO I–II), with a benign biologic behavior and clinical course, often characterized only by epilepsy; however, some of these show recurrence or even malignant transformation [38, 39]. The common and peculiar aspect of these tumors, differing from each other by immunohistochemical and histopathologic characteristics, is the high epileptogenicity: they are responsible for 10% of structural symptomatic epilepsies and they represent the focal most frequent brain pathology in adult epilepsy surgery after hippocampal sclerosis. LEATs usually have cortical localization, especially in the temporal and frontal lobes; they are well circumscribed and not infiltrating and they cause symptomatic epilepsy with recurring seizures, often resistant to pharmacological treatments. Seizures are more common in cortical tumors than in those of subcortical areas, with a seizure frequency of 56% compared with 15%, respectively; frontal, temporal, insular and centroparietal regions are the most common cortical regions associated with symptomatic seizures and incidence rates are higher for tumors located in eloquent areas, as opposed to functionally subtle or "clinically silent" areas [40].

The pathophysiology of tumor epileptogenesis is multifactorial, and it is not fully clarified. LEATs of glioneuronal origin are highly epileptogenic, most likely because of the intrinsic hyperexcitability of dysplastic neurons inside the tumor itself. Moreover, they can be associated with other adjacent brain lesions, such as focal cortical dysplasia, characterized by architectural alterations of cortical lamination with or without cytoarchitectural anomalies (hypertrophy of pyramidal neurons). This association, classified by the International League Against Epilepsy as FCD III B, contributes to the high epileptogenic potential of these neoplasms and influences their surgical prognosis [41, 42]. The coexistence of two adjacent brain lesions, both potentially epileptogenic, is also defined "dual pathology" [43]. Gliomas have no intrinsic neural component and their epileptogenic potential can be due to functional and/or structural factors. An imbalance between excitatory and inhibitory neurotransmitters (a reduction in GABAergic transmission, an increase in glutamatergic inputs) or other local factors increasing local excitability (pH shifts, increased gap junction-mediated connectivity, blood-brain barrier alterations) leads to an alteration of peritumoral networks, with increased predisposition to seizures development; this "epileptocentric" hypothesis is more plausible for slow-growing tumors, with gliosis and chronic inflammation in the peritumoral cortex. More traditionally, the alternative "tumor-ocentric" hypothesis considers epileptogenicity directly following the structural alterations induced by the tumor itself (mass effect, edema) that lead to local hypoperfusion, deafferentation processes, neoangiogenesis, vascular alterations and infiltration of peritumoral tissue [44, 45].

37.4 EEG After Brain Surgery

After complete resection of the tumor, EEG could still show some abnormalities. They are represented, in a first phase, by focal and/or widespread slowings with or without epileptiform abnormalities: these patterns can regress spontaneously, persist or evolve into an epileptic focus (Fig. 37.9). Furthermore, in the postoperative EEGs, it is possible to observe specific alterations due to the injury of the cranial bones and meninges occurred during surgery. These are defined as "breach rhythm," more evident in the rolandic area and often misinterpreted as an epileptic activity. "Breach rhythm" consists of sequences of mixed frequency activity (theta, alpha and beta) and sporadic spikes: it is basically due to variations of cranial impedance, it is not reactive to stimuli, and it is clearly evident both in wakefulness and in sleep.

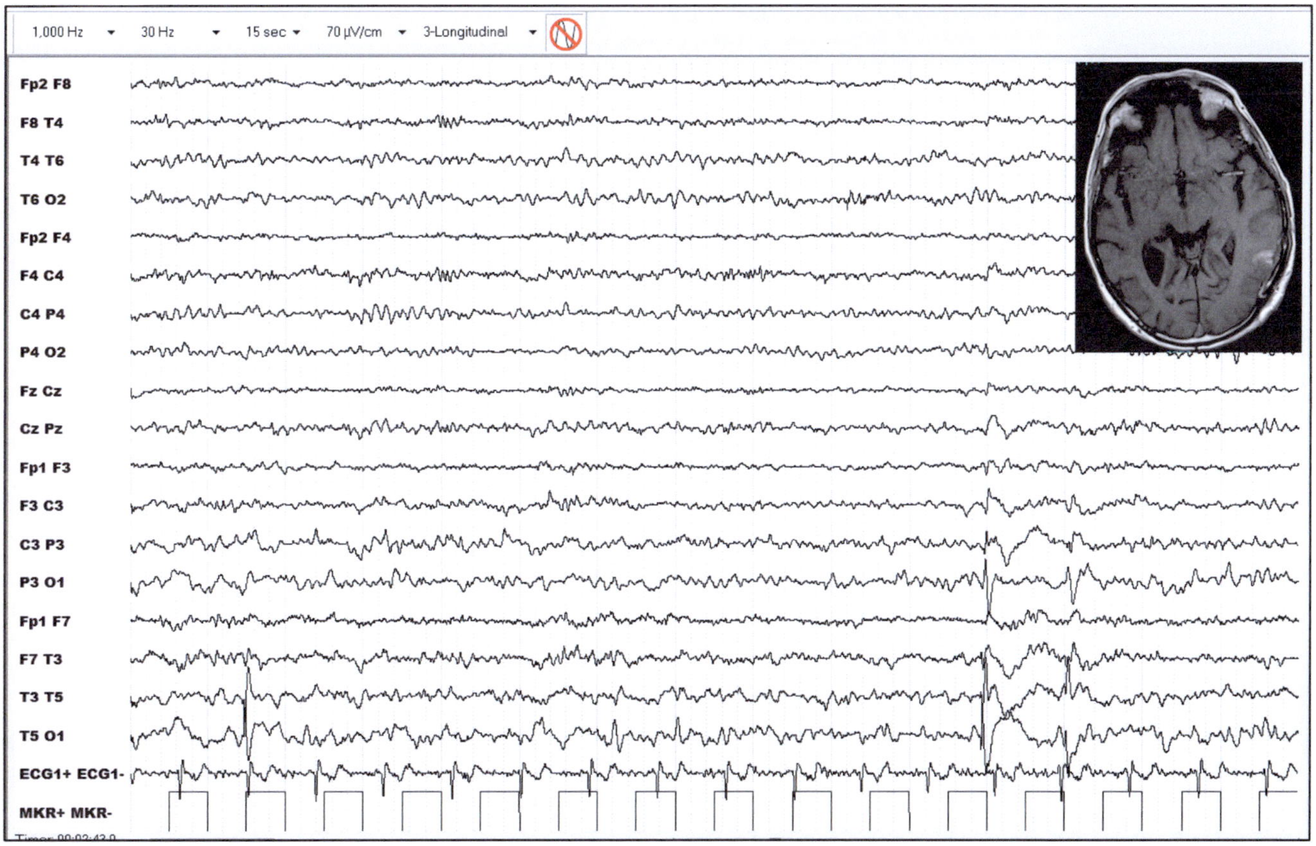

Fig. 37.9 An example of left hemispheric slow activity with concomitant sporadic spikes and spike-and-wave complexes in homolateral temporal region in an 84-year-old male patient after surgical resection of glioblastoma

References

1. Fisher RS, Cross JH, French JA, et al. Operational classification of seizure types by the International League Against Epilepsy: Position Paper of the ILAE Commission for Classification and Terminology. Epilepsia. 2017;58:522–30.
2. Magnus O, Van der Holst M. Zeta waves: a special type of slow delta waves. EEG Clin Neurophysiol. 1987;67:140–6.
3. Dunne JW, Silbert PL. Zeta waves: a distinctive type of intermittent delta wave studied prospectively. Clin Exp Neurol. 1991;28: 238–43.
4. Stern JM. Atlas of EEG patterns. 2nd ed. Philadelphia: Lippincott Williams & Wilkins; 2013.
5. Brigo F. Intermittent rhythmic delta activity patterns. Epilepsy Behav. 2011;20:254–6.
6. Knudsen-Baas KM, Power KN, Engelsen BA, Hegrestad SE, Gilhus NE, Storstein AM. Status epilepticus secondary to glioma. Seizure. 2016;40:76–80.
7. Janati A, Hester RL. Spindle activity in the waking electroencephalogram: report of a case with hemispheric glioblastoma. Clin Electroencephal. 1986;17:1–5.
8. Steriade M. Corticothalamic resonance, states of vigilance, and mentation. Neuroscience. 2000;101:243–76.
9. O'Connor SC, Robinson PA. Analysis of the electroencephalographic activity associated with thalamic tumors. J Theor Biol. 2005;233:271–86.
10. Gastaut H, Regis H, Gastaut JL, Yermenos E, Low MD. Lipomas of the corpus callosum and epilepsy. Neurology. 1980;30:132–8.
11. Fuga M, Tanaka T, Yamamoto Y, Hasegawa Y, Murayama Y, Takahashi-Fujigasaki J. Lipoma in the corpus callosum presenting with epileptic seizures associated with expanding perifocal edema: a case report and literature review. Case Rep Neurol Med. 2015;2015:520208.
12. Stark J, Friedman E, Thompson S, Von Allmen G, Bhattacharjee M, Tandon N. Atypical presentations of dysembryoplastic neuroepithelial tumors. Epilepsia. 2018;59:e14–7
13. Labate A, Briellmann RS, Harvey AS, et al. Temporal lobe dysembryoplastic neuroepithelial tumor: significance of discordant interictal spikes. Epileptic Disord. 2004;6:107–14.
14. Radhakrishnan A, Abraham M, Vilanilam G, et al. Surgery for "long-term epilepsy associated tumors (LEATs)": seizure outcome and its predictors. Clin Neurol and Neurosurg. 2016;141:98–105.
15. Coons SW, Rekate HL, Prenger EC, et al. The histopathology of hypothalamic hamartomas: study of 57 cases. J Neuropathol Exp Neurol. 2007; 66: 131–41.
16. Striano S, Striano P. Clinical features and evolution of the gelastic seizures–hypothalamic hamartoma syndrome. Epilepsia. 2017;58(Suppl. 2): 12–5.
17. Specchio N, Rizzi M, Trivisano M, et al. Acute intralesional recording in hypothalamic hamartoma: description of 4 cases. Acta Neurol Belg. 2015;115:233–9.
18. Scholly J, Staack AM, Kahane P, et al. Hypothalamic hamartoma: epileptogenesis beyond the lesion? Epilepsia. 2017;58(Suppl. 2): 32–40.
19. Harvey AS, Freeman JL. Epilepsy in hypothalamic hamartoma: clinical and EEG features. Semin Pediatr Neurol. 2007;14:60–4.
20. Kovac S, Diehl B, Wehner T, et al. Gelastic seizures: incidence, clinical and EEG features in adult patients undergoing video-EEG telemetry. Epilepsia. 2014;56::e1–5.
21. Leal AJ, Moreira A, Robalo C, et al. Different electroclinical manifestations of the epilepsy associated with hamartomas connecting to the middle or posterior hypothalamus. Epilepsia. 2003;44:1191–5.
22. Freeman JL, Harvey AS, Rosenfeld JV, et al. Generalized epilepsy in hypothalamic hamartoma: evolution and postoperative resolution. Neurology. 2003;60:762–7.
23. Claus EB, Bondy ML, Schildkraut JM, Wiemels JL, Wrensch M, Black PM. Epidemiology of intracranial meningioma. Neurosurgery. 2005;57:1088–95.
24. Antinheimo J, Sankila R, Carpen O, Pukkala E, Sainio M, Jaaskelainen J. Population-based analysis of sporadic and type 2 neurofibromatosis-associated meningiomas and schwannomas. Neurology. 2000;54:71–6.
25. Black PM. Meningiomas. Neurosurgery. 1993; 32: 643–57.
26. Burger PC, Scheithauer BW. Meningiomas. In: Burger PC, Scheithauer BW, editors. AFIP atlas of tumor pathology: tumors of the central nervous system. Washington, DC: American Registry of Pathology; 2007.
27. Chan RC, Thompson GB. Morbidity, mortality, and quality of life following surgery for intracranial meningiomas. A retrospective study in 257 cases. J Neurosurg. 1984;60:52–60
28. Regis J, Sanson M, Kalamarides M. Recurrent multiple meningioma and generalized seizure. Neurochirurgie. 2005;51:129–35.
29. Chozick BS, Reinert SE, Greenblatt SH. Incidence of seizures after surgery for supratentorial meningiomas: a modern analysis. J Neurosurg. 1996;84:382–6.
30. Rothoerl RD, Bernreuther D, Woertgen C, Brawanski A. The value of routine electroencephalographic recordings in predicting postoperative seizures associated with meningioma surgery. Neurosurg Rev. 2003;26:108–12.
31. Wirsching HG, Morel C, Gmür C, et al. Predicting outcome of epilepsy after meningioma resection. Neuro-Oncology. 2016;18: 1002–10.
32. Callaghan N, Garrett A, Goggin T. Withdrawal of anticonvulsant drugs in patients free of seizures for two years. A prospective study. N Engl J Med. 1988;318:942–6.
33. Lynam L, Lyons M, Drzkowski J, et al. Frequency of seizures in patients with newly diagnosed brain tumors: a retrospective review. Clin Neurol Neurosurg. 2007;109:634–8.
34. Lebrun C, Fontaine D, Ramaioli A, et al. Nice Brain Tumor Study Group. Long-term outcome of oligodendrogliomas. Neurology. 2004;62:1783–7.
35. Benerjee P, Filippi D, Hauser W. The descriptive epidemiology of epilepsy – a review. Epilepsy Res. 2009;85:31–45.
36. Louis DN, Perry A, Reifenberger G, et al. World Health Organization histological classification of tumours of the central nervous system. Acta Neuropathol. 2016;131:803–20.
37. Kerkhof M, Vecht CJ. Seizure characteristics and prognostic factors of gliomas. Epilepsia. 2013;54(Suppl 9):12–7.
38. Majores M, von Lehe M, Fassunke J, Schramm J, Becker AJ, Simon M. Tumor recurrence and malignant progression of gangliogliomas. Cancer. 2008;113:3355–563.
39. Luyken C, Blumcke I, Fimmers R, et al. The spectrum of long-term epilepsy-associated tumors: long term seizure and tumor outcome and neurosurgical aspects. Epilepsia. 2003;44:822–30.
40. Politsky J. Brain tumor-related epilepsy: a current review of the etiologic basis and diagnostic and treatment approaches. Curr Neurol Neurosci Rep. 2017;17:70.
41. Blümcke I, Thom M, Aronica E, et al. The clinicopathologic spectrum of focal cortical dysplasias: a consensus classification proposed by an ad hoc task force of the ILAE diagnostic methods commission. Epilepsia. 2011;52:158–74.
42. Cossu M, Fuschillo D, Bramerio M, et al. Epilepsy surgery of focal cortical dysplasia-associated tumors. Epilepsia. 2013;54(Suppl 9): 115–22.
43. Palmini A, Paglioli E, Duval Silva V. Developmental tumors and adjacent cortical dysplasia: single or dual pathology? Epilepsia. 2013;54(Suppl 9):18–24.
44. Nowell M, Miserocchi A, McEvoy AW. Tumors in epilepsy. Semin Neurol. 2015;35:209–17.
45. Pallud J, Capelle L, Huberfeld G. Tumoral epileptogenicity: how does it happen? Epilepsia. 2013;54 Suppl 9):30–4.

Cerebrovascular Diseases

38

Oriano Mecarelli and Edoardo Vicenzini

CerebroVascular Disease (CVD) clinical course may be extremely various after acute onset, from clinical stability to recovery or also worsening of the neurological status. Stroke recurrence may be fatal in the first hours after the ictal event and general systemic and iatrogenic complications may also occur in subacute phases, worsening the neurological conditions. A small percentage of CVD patients may also present epileptic seizures in the acute phase (convulsive or nonconvulsive), as well as they may later develop poststroke epilepsy. Considering the extreme variability in the CVD clinical course, continuous EEG monitoring or seriated recordings in stroke acute phase may be helpful for describing in real-time the dynamic status of cerebral functions. Later, in the post-acute and chronic phases, EEG may reveal early signs of diffuse cerebral damage, in cases of deterioration, as well as the possible development of an epileptogenic focus.

38.1 Cerebral Blood Flow (CBF) and Electric Cortical Activity During Cerebral Ischemia

EEG changes appear soon as CBF is reduced from the normal values of 70–50 mL/100 g/min to 35–25 mL/100 g/min: at this perfusion level, slowing of alpha rhythm and beta activity reduction is observed, consequent to synaptic transmission failure. A more consistent CBF reduction, up to 25–18 mL/100 g/min, induces more evident EEG slowings, with the appearance of a prevalent theta activity. At perfusion levels below 18 mL/100 g/min, EEG slowings of the delta band appear. At last, below the critical threshold of 12–10 mL/100 g/min, global suppression of the cortical electrical activity is observed, evolving in the clinical and EEG condition of brain death if blood flow is not rapidly restored. Summarizing, EEG is a very sensible tool to evaluate cerebral functional activity related to cerebral perfusion levels, revealing that slowings appear already when CBF is reduced at a level of 35 mL/100 g/min and that, between CBF levels of 35 to 10 mL/100 g/min, these alterations may still be reversible (Table 38.1) [1–3]. It must be also emphasized that EEG changes occur as early as 10 s after a significant decrease in CBF, while abnormalities in diffusion-weighted MRI appear later, after at least 12 min of ischemia [4].

During a focal cerebral ischemia a more global brain involvement can be also present, due to the synaptic and axonal transmission failure and spontaneous neurotransmitters release changes (including glutamate increase). In addition, important metabolic changes occur, including decline in protein synthesis, anaerobic metabolism, energetic failure, ionic disturbances and cytotoxic edema. All these changes may result in global EEG slowings, even in the contralateral hemisphere, during an acute focal cerebral ischemia [3, 5]. Thus, in the acute stroke phase, EEG recordings may reveal more extensive dysfunctional patterns, even when neuroimaging - especially CT - is still unremarkable. Almost 40% of acute stroke patients have indeed normal CT scans, while, on the other hand, almost half of these patients show already focal and/or lateralized EEG alterations.

Table 38.1 EEG changes associated with different Cerebral Blood Flow (CBF) levels

CBF (mL/100 g/min)	EEG changes
70–50	Normal
50–35	No significant changes
35–25	Mild slowing alpha rhythm, Reduction of beta activity
25–18	Increased slow activity (>theta)
18–12	Delta activity, progressively of lower amplitude
<12–10	Suppression of activity (development of irreversible neuronal injury)

O. Mecarelli (✉)
Department of Human Neurosciences,
Sapienza University of Rome, Rome, Italy
e-mail: oriano.mecarelli@uniroma1.it

E. Vicenzini
Azienda Ospedaliero-Universitaria Policlinico Umberto I,
Rome, Italy

O. Mecarelli (ed.), *Clinical Electroencephalography*, https://doi.org/10.1007/978-3-030-04573-9_38

Continuous EEG (cEEG) monitoring is the most valid method for prolonged cerebral ischemia detection and before infarction occurs, possibly identifying a window of therapeutic intervention to prevent irreversible injury. Visual examination and interpretation of cEEG is the gold standard, but it may be scarcely achievable for various reasons (long and expensive evaluation, need for expert neurophysiologists, etc.). For this purpose, qualitative evaluation of cEEG can be assisted by quantitative EEG (qEEG) analysis. During prolonged EEG monitoring, commercial software can calculate the power spectrum of the cerebral signals and reveal how these cange over time. qEEG spectrograms are usually presented in a colored graphs and they define "spectral trends," allowing to easily highlight changes, such as an increase in activity in a specific frequency band, even by less experts.

EEG may also be an important diagnostic tool when patients do not present with a clear neurological status—such as motor or sensitive deficits—and when they are admitted at the hospital with, for example, only isolated superior cognitive function deficits and language disturbances. Following an acute stroke, patients may indeed present a confusional state, aphasia or dysarthria that may be misinterpreted as the final clinical neurological diagnosis; in these cases, an emergency EEG may reveal focal slowings with sporadic epileptiform abnormalities or quasiperiodic EEG patterns or even typical non convulsve status epilepticus patterns. All these findings may be highly suggestive of an acute ischemic damage, notwithstanding acute CT scans may still be normal. On the other hand, a normal EEG in a patient with clear focal neurological signs may rule out a more extensive, severe ischemic damage and it may also suggest the diagnosis of other stroke-mimicking conditions, like migraine with aura. However, it is necessary to underline that a normal EEG is not reliable to allow the exclusion of an ischemic damage, since small cerebral cortical infarctions, smaller than 3 cm of diameter, may not show any EEG changes at all and since small subcortical lacunar infarction also shows a normal EEG in most of the cases.

38.2 Acute Ischemic Stroke

EEG changes in hemispheric acute ischemic stroke consist substantially in: ipsilateral slowing and desynchronization of background alpha activity with partial or absent reactivity; widespread arhythmic delta-theta activity in the involved hemisphere, more evident in frontotemporal regions; focal or generalized epileptiform discharges. These features are of variable intensity, according to the stroke severity and metabolic disturbances. In extensive infarctions, electrocerebral activity may be markedly decreased in the affected hemisphere during the first few days. In severe cases, a slow activity of variable degree appears also in the hemisphere contralateral to the ischemic damage, more frequently in the form of bilateral Frontal Intermittent Rhythmic Delta Activity (FIRDA) and intermittent diffuse bursts of delta activity; these changes are related to cerebral edema and to the displacement of midline structures (Fig. 38.1). In children, this rhythmic delta activity may be more evident in the posterior areas (Occipital Intermittent Rhytmic Delta Activity, OIRDA).

Ictal and interictal epileptiform abnormalities are detected rarely in the first days after stroke, usually originating in the affected hemisphere and, sometimes, with contralateral diffusion. In reality, the scarce evidence of these abnormalities may be mainly due to the fact that EEG recordings are not always performed routinely in the acute stroke phase and the chances to record an epileptic activity can instead be improved with the more extensive up-to-date use of cEEG in stroke units.

Epileptic abnormalities in stroke patients consist of spikes, sharp waves, spike-and-wave, or sharp-wave-and-slow-wave complexes, sometimes configuring a periodic pattern (Lateralized Periodic Discharges, LPDs or Bilateral Independent Lateralized Periodic Discharges, BI-LPDs). These discharges may be recorded both in patients without clear manifest epileptic seizures, as well as preceding - or following - a seizure. LPDs usually occur early, in the first 24 h and during the first days after stroke, they are generally transitory and disappear within 4 weeks. As time lapses, these periodic discharges tend to be smaller in voltage and lower in frequency, to be replaced by monomorphic slow waves of high voltage or sporadic spikes or sharp waves, until their total disappearance. These lateralized periodic activities persist also during NREM and REM sleep, with scarce reactivity to stimuli.

The EEG characteristics of LPDs are describe extensively in details in Chap. 13; they are expression of an "irritative" cortical pattern and usually represents an "ictal-interictal continuum". strictly associated with the convulsive or non-convulsive seizures [6]. Recently, we have prospectively studied 232 patients with ischemic and hemorrhagic strokes, in which EEG monitoring was performed within 24 h from symptoms onset. In this cohort we observed focal or diffuse slowing of background activity in 84% of the cases and epileptiform abnormalities in 16%, LPDs accounting for approximately 40% (6% of the whole cohort of patients). In patients with LPDs, this pattern preceded and/or followed the epileptic seizures (identifying a convulsive SE in the majority of patients) in 71.4% (Fig. 38.2). These findings suggest that LPDs in the acute phase of stroke are not frequent but, when present, they are closely related to early epileptic seizures [7].

In regard to LPDs pathogenesis in acute ischemic stroke, the increased release of excitatory amino acids - such as glutamate and aspartate- in the ischemic penumbra and the localized cortical hyperexcitability are responsible of both the EEG abnormalities and of the epileptic seizures. In some cases, this excitotoxicity continues for a long time after

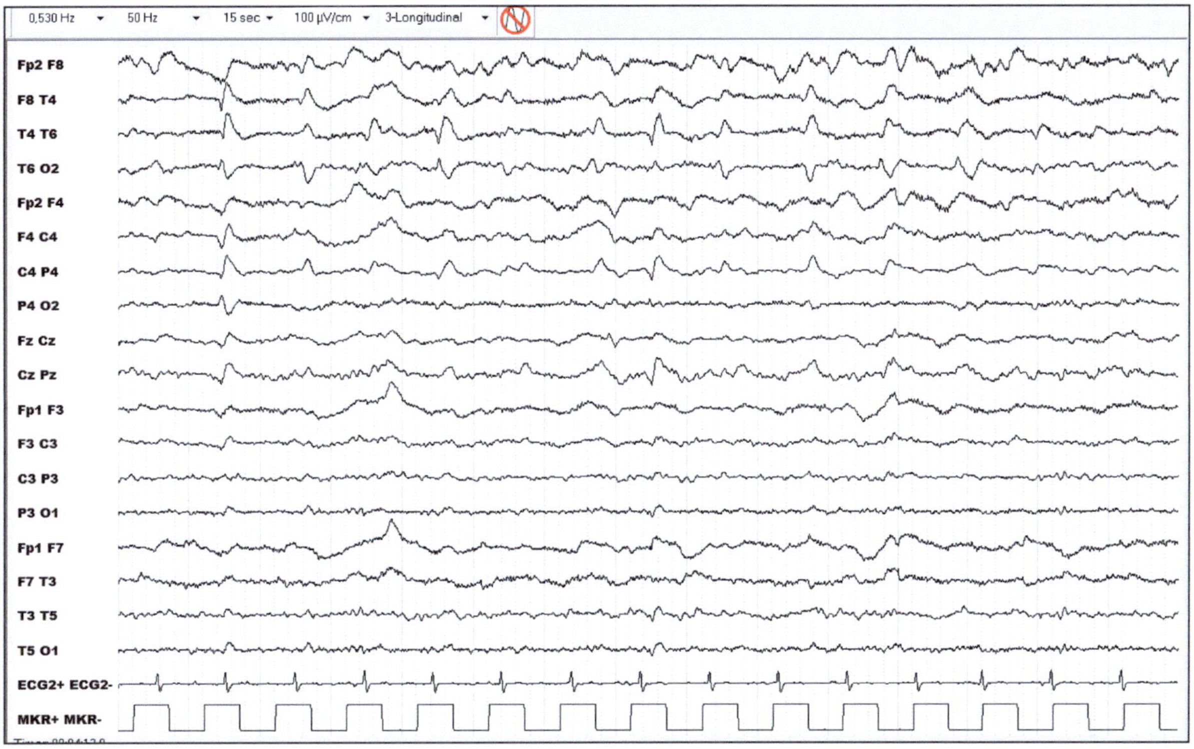

Fig. 38.1 A 67-year-old patient with acute massive left hemisphere ischemic stroke occurred the day before this EEG recording. A marked right frontotemporal polymorphic delta activity, spreading contralaterally is clearly evident. In the right temporal regions, a periodic lateralized discharge-like pattern is also noted, without a clinical correlate. Background alpha activity is suppressed bilaterally

stroke onset, as the result of the anatomical damage induced by ischemia. Also metabolic transitory changes during acute stroke phase, such as fever or hyperglycemia, may also be involved in the LPDs genesis [8–10]. Hartings et al. [11] have demonstrated that, in a rat model model of focal ischemia, LPDs appeared over penumbral regions in the injured hemisphere, while Intermittent Rhythmic Delta Activity (IRDA) recurred in the contralateral hemisphere, dominant in the frontoparietal areas. This phenomenon occurs also in humans after stroke and it suggests that the periodic and rhythmic contralateral patterns appear as a consequence of the disrupted cortico-subcortical connections and/or disconnected fiber tracts innervating the cortex.

LPDs appear more frequently in embolic strokes rather than in atherosclerotic strokes and LPD patients seem to have a worse prognosis and outcome [12]. The decision whether to treat or not to treat these EEG changes is controversial, except for patients with clear clinical seizures: moreover they are in general, even refractory to the antiepileptic treatment (Fig. 38.3) [13].

Rarely, a nonperiodic epileptiform activity may be observed only in the healthy contralateral unaffected hemisphere. This activity is defined Contralateral Epileptiform Transients in Stroke (CETS) and consists of nonperiodic spikes, sharp waves, or spike-and-wave complexes, occurring isolated or in bursts during awake, controlaterally to the stroke. These discharges are not associated with clinical seizures and they seem to last longer than LPDs [14].

The cEEG in acute stroke phase allows also evaluating the changes in sleep EEG patterns, which consist in a lower sleep efficacy and a reduced sleep spindle activity in the side of the lesion. When sleep efficiency and spindle activity are preserved, outcome is more favorable.

Other rare EEG alterations in stroke may be represented by the wicket spikes, at 6–11 Hz of frequency and 60–200 µV of amplitude. Wicket spikes are dominant in the left temporal regions, but sometimes they are bilateral and asynchronous; they are observed mainly during drowsiness and they disappear in slow sleep. Very rarely, it is possible to record (during awake or drowsiness) Subclinical Rhythmic Electrographic Discharges of Adults (SREDA), consisting in discharges of theta activity (5–7 Hz), with sinusoidal or arciform morphology, dominant in temporoparietal areas, lasting from seconds to minutes.

Ischemic damage could also involve the subcortical areas or the brainstem. In bulbar and pontine lesions, EEG may be completely normal or show minimal diffuse monomorphic slow abnormalities, with a background activity partially reactive to nociceptive stimuli. The EEG partial reactivity has been in the past considered, along with REM disappearance during sleep, pathognomonic of lesions occurring in the pons. In locked-in syndrome, however, due to damage in the

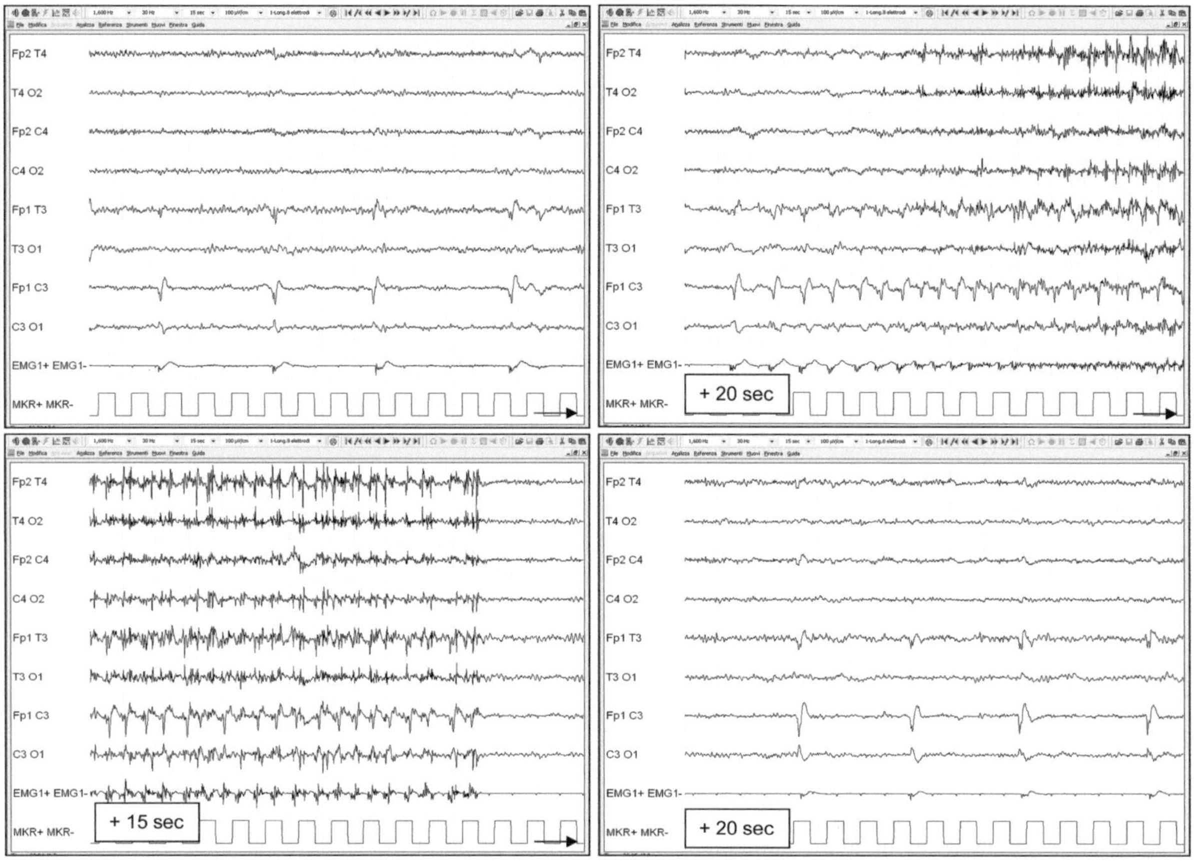

Fig. 38.2 An 89-year-old patient with left frontotemporal cortical ischemic stroke. EEG recorded within 12 h from symptoms onset shows LPDs in the left hemisphere, with myoclonic contralateral facial and upper limb jerks. LPDs increase over time and evolve into a diffuse epileptic discharge, with a tonic-clonic seizure. About 20 s after the epileptic discharge stops, LPDs and ictal pattern reappear, configuring a pattern of convulsive status epilepticus

medial and ventral pons, alpha rhythm could show only minimal slowing, generally preserving the reactivity to stimuli. More rostral cerebral damage—in the mesencephalon or in the diencephalon—will induce a rhythmic slow activity, synchronous and symmetric on both hemispheres, generally more evident in the anterior frontal regions. If the lesion is located more caudally in the mesencephalon, a diffuse background activity of low voltage could be observed, sometimes associated with slow lateralized abnormalities. In these cases, a thalamic damage could be hypothesized, with a secondary involvement of the posterior hypothalamus. The different effects of rostral and caudal subcortical lesions on EEG patterns could be explained by the different specialization of the superior and inferior reticular activating system. The damage of rostral part of reticular formation—normally inducing the desynchronization of EEG activity—would then lead to a slow hypersynchronization or, in the early phases, to an alpha hypersynchronization; conversely, lesions in the caudal part - normally having a synchronizing effect- would then lead to desynchronized, low-voltage EEG activity. In patients with thalamic or midbrain lesions, hypersomnia may be observed, particularly in patients with bilateral paramedian thalamic stroke, with an increase of slow-wave sleep and REM sleep [15].

cEEG monitoring in acute ischemic stroke provides real-time and dynamic data on cerebral dysfunction, adding useful information to clinical and imaging-based outcome prediction [1]. During the first 24 h, focal or diffuse slowings—as well as epileptic specific patterns—could be indeed observed, eventually correlated with clinical seizures. The reduction of the EEG slowings in the following days, with the reappearance of a more stable background activity, is constantly associated with a good clinical recovery, whereas the increase of the slow EEG bands could be associated to a worsening of the clinical status. In general, the delta-theta activities tend to be less diffuse after 1 week from stroke onset and dominant in the temporal areas. EEG normalization, in cases without clinical worsening or complications, is usually achieved after about 6 months. EEG evolution has also been correlated with neuroradiological imaging and it has been shown to be even more strictly correlated with the clinical outcome rather than with the Rankin score at admission [16]. The presence of a continuous slow and polymorphic activity in the ischemic

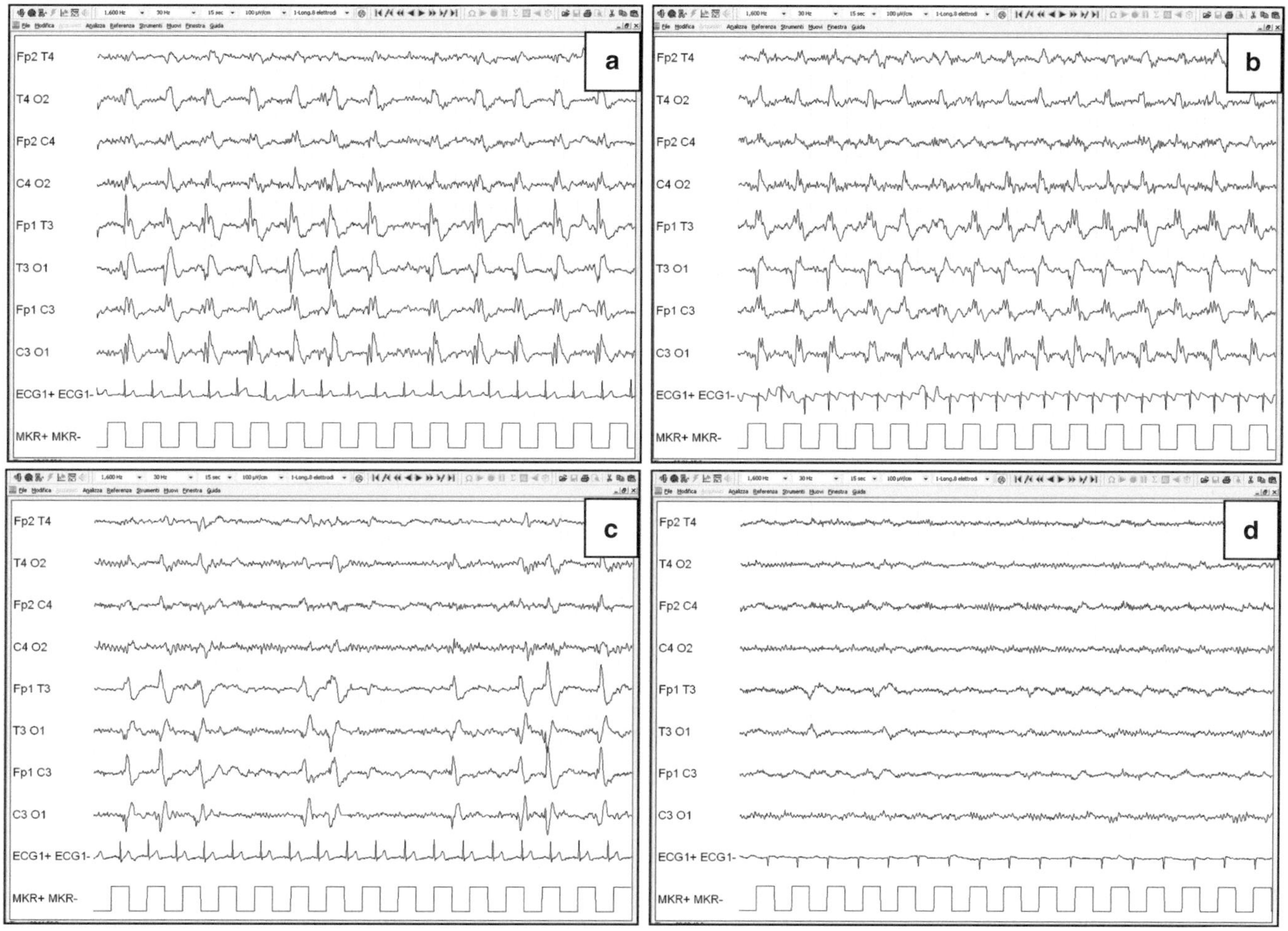

Fig. 38.3 A 72-year-old patient with acute confusional state and aphasia. CT scan showed a left temporoparietal ischemic stroke. EEG recorded 18 h after admission shows a severe LPDs pattern, more evident in the left hemisphere, but with tendency to contralateral diffusion (**a**). 48 h later, even after benzodiazepine i.v. administration, LPDs persist (**b**). 4 days later, despite ongoing antiepileptic treatment, LPDs still persist, even if less evident and less organized, with the reappearance of background irregular alpha activity (**c**). 10 days later (**d**), EEG shows a more regular and stable alpha rhythm (more in the right side) and sequences of rhythmic anterior delta waves (more in the left side), with superimposed isolated sharp waves in T3. Patient showed a good recovery and outcome

hemisphere, concomitant with depression of alpha or beta frequencies, has been described as poor prognostic factors. On the other hand, absence of slowings with minimal changes in the background alpha rhythm and sporadic appearance of theta/delta activities with minimal asymmetries are related to a better prognosis [1]. Finnigan et al. [17] reported that quantitative EEG (qEEG) measures from acute cortical stroke patients can help monitoring brain pathophysiology and predict stroke evolution. These authors calculated an "acute Delta Change Index" (aDCI), evaluating the changes of the delta power in the ischemic region, across the acute and poststroke periods. The correlation between the initial qEEG and the 30-day NIHSS (National Institutes of Health Stroke Scale) scores was strongly evident, and even better than the initial lesion volumedetected with diffusion weighted images at MRI. Successively, the same authors demonstrated that also the Delta/Alpha power Ratio (DAR) and the evaluation of relative alpha power have a potential prognostic value of stroke evolution [17]. Other authors have used, as a prognostic index for disability or death at 6 months after stroke, the pairwise-derived Brain Symmetry Index (pdBSI) and the (Delta+Theta)/(Alpha+Beta) ratio (DTABR) [18]. The pdBSI is a slight modification of the spatial BSI; it estimates the normalized difference between the spectral densities of each bipolar signal from each hemisphere and it is more sensitive for focal EEG asymmetries. EEG pdBSI and DTABR were significantly correlated with NIHSS at admission and with the modified Rankin scale score at month 6th, even if these correlations are moderate [3]. It is also relevant to underline the importance of EEG changes in the unaffected hemisphere. For instance, an increase in the contralateral delta power was correlated with a poor outcome [19].

cEEG monitoring can support to evaluate the effects of specific treatments. Hypervolemic hypertensive therapy, with the increase of cerebral blood flow above the ischemic threshold, induces a normalization of detected pre-hypervolemic treatment EEG focal slow activity [20]. Already in 1998, Jordan [21] described a distinctive early EEG pattern in spontaneous acute ischemic stroke and defined RAWOD (Regional Attenuation WithOut Delta), characterized by regional or hemispheric attenuation of all frequencies, without appearance of delta activity. This pattern would be an early expression of massive global hemisphere damage; patients with RAWOD are unlikely to benefit from thrombolysis, but they may be candidates for early surveillance and intervention for cerebral edema. De Vos et al. [22] performed cEEG monitoring during thrombolysis in acute hemispheric stroke patients using BSI, which has been shown to have a positive correlation with NIHSS. The results of the study demonstrate that cEEG monitoring, using BSI, is technically feasible and provides real-time information about the effect of thrombolysis in acute hemispheric stroke patients. All these data underline again that EEG monitoring could be not only a valid support to clinical monitoring, but it also may be useful to monitor the efficacy of therapeutic strategies.

Finally, the measurement of ultraslow activity (<0.5 Hz), including phenomena associated with Spreading Depolarization and Depression (SD), should be of high clinical significance. There is, indeed, unequivocal neurophysiologic evidence that SD occurs in acute stroke and that it contributes to lesion progression [23]. However, at present, in patients with structural brain lesions, the SD has been recorded only during electrocortigraphy, with subdural or intraparenchymal electrodes [24].

Transient Ischemic Attacks (TIAs) are brief episodes of focal neurological deficits resulting from focal transient cerebral ischemia, not associated with a permanent cerebral infarction [25]. In the past, TIAs were operationally define as any focal cerebral ischemic event with symptoms lasting <24 h. Recently, however, it was demonstrated that this arbitrary time threshold was too broad and a new definition has been proposed by several groups. TIAs have been now defined as brief episodes of neurological dysfunction caused by focal brain or retinal ischemia, with clinical symptoms typically lasting less than 1 h, always without evidence of acute cerebral infarction. Considering their usual short presentation, EEG recordings during TIA are extremely rare. However, focal mild theta slowing in the affected hemisphere has been described, sometimes with sharp morphology of waves, even in the presence of a normal background alpha rhythm, sometimes asymmetric. When a more important delta slowing in the temporal region is observed, it may be argued that ischemia is more severe and that recovery may be slower, even if the background alpha rhythm is preserved.

38.3 Intraparenchymal Hemorrhage

Hemorrhagic stroke accounts for approximately 10-20% of all strokes, provoked by a weakened atherosclerotic small vessel that ruptures and bleeds into the surrounding brain. Blood accumulates and compresses, destroying, the surrounding brain tissue. When the bleeding occurs in brain cortical areas, a delta-theta slow activity may be observed in the affected hemisphere in the early phases, more evident in the frontotemporal regions, sometimes rhythmic and intermittent. The background alpha rhythm is preserved or sometimes disregulated in the affected hemisphere; the contralateral hemisphere is scarcely involved by the above-mentioned EEG changes (Fig. 38.4).

qEEG analysis demonstrated an asymmetry of the mu rhythm, depressed in the affected hemisphere. The entity of EEG abnormalities has been related to the size of the vessel involved and to the bleeding cortical localization. When the bleeding occurs in deeper brain areas, originating from the striate arteries and causing small subcortical bleedings, EEG could show minimal alterations or be normal. If the clinical neurological status worsens and consciousness deficits appears, coma EEG characteristic patterns will appear, starting with more diffuse and marked slowings until global cortical activity attenuation/suppression; this last condition may be typical when the bleeding extends to the lateral ventricles and a severe cerebral edema occurs.

Similar to ischemic stroke, cEEG monitoring in IntraCerebral Hemorrhage (ICH) has proven useful for the prognosis. Claassen et al. [26] have studied 102 consecutive patients with ICH who underwent cEEG monitoring. In these patients, epileptic seizures occurred in one third and half of these were purely electrographic, associated with hemorrhages expanding in volume. More than half of electrographic seizures were detected within the first hour of cEEG; however, cEEG showed the maximal yield for capturing potentially epileptogenic abnormalities within the first 48 h of recording. Though seizures were found to be associated with hematoma volume increase, they were not significantly associated with increasing midline shift. Among the EEG abnormalities, periodic discharges were recorded in 17% of patients (LPDs: 13%, GPDs: 6%, BI-LPDs: 1%) and they were more frequently observed in patients with hemorrhage sizes greater than 60 mL on CT scans. Periodic discharges were more frequently observed in hemorrhages located closer to the cortex, and they were independently associated with a poor outcome.

EEG recordings in ICH patients show, in addition to epileptiform discharges and focal or diffuse slowings, the occurrence of sleep pattern alterations, with K complexes and spindle's disappearance. During clinical recovery after an hemorrhagic event, the EEG activity generally

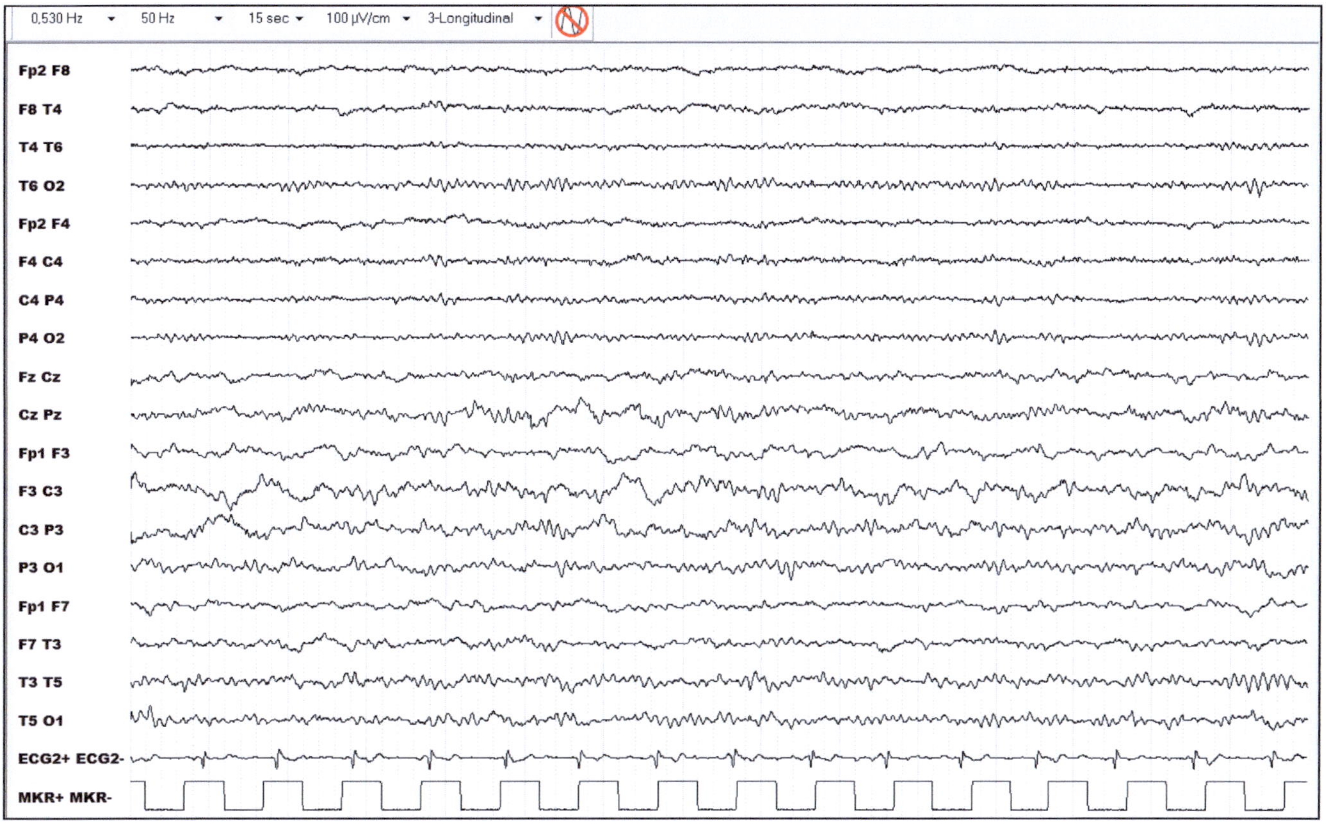

Fig. 38.4 A 51-year-old patient, 18 h after intraparenchymal left frontotemporal hemorrhage. EEG shows polymorphic delta activity in the site of hemorrhage; background alpha activity persists in both posterior regions, more regularly represented in the right side

improves, even though epileptiform and focal slow abnormalities could persist even up to 1 month after the acute event.

Subcortical hemorrhages involving the thalamus, the brainstem and the cerebellum have different effects on the EEG, according to the extent and severity of the hemorrhage [15]. When damage is localized in the thalamus, a delta homolateral activity may be observed. Lesions in the anteroventral thalamus will induce an alpha rhythm reduction, while lesions in the posterior thalamus areas will cause an alpha activity increase. During sleep, a thalamic damage will also induce the spindle's disappearance. Mesencephalic lesions could induce a monomorphic diffuse slow activity at 6–7 Hz, while bulbo-pontine lesions may be associated with a more diffuse electrocortical depression. Bulbo-pontine hemorrhages may also appear with an alpha background activity, reactive - or only partially reactive - to stimuli. Hemorrhagic lesions in the cerebellum are considered at higher risk of herniation, rostro-caudal deterioration and dramatical increase of the intracranial pressure; generally, EEG is not performe routinely in these patients, for logistic reasons. However, a diffuse delta activity has been described in rare monitored cases, prevailing in the contralateral cerebral hemisphere.

38.4 Subarachnoid Hemorrhage

Spontaneous SubArachnoid Hemorrhage (SAH) from aneurysmal rupture has an overall estimated annual incidence rate of 9 per 100,000, and it is the main cause of sudden death after stroke [27]. The presence of blood in the subarachnoid space lowers the seizure threshold and induces frequently clinical epileptic seizures, focal or generalized, convulsive or nonconvulsive. For these reasons, cEEG monitoring may be particularly helpful in these often critically ill patients. Claassen et al. [28] studied a cohort of patients with poor-grade SAH, using an invasive multimodality monitoring including minidepth EEG. In these patients, intracortical seizures were observed in 38%, whereas only 8% of patients had a surface seizure correlate. In literature, NonConvulsive Status Epilepticus (NCSE) was identified with prolonged monitoring in up to 14% after SAH, with onset between 2 and 20 days from initial hemorrhage; prolonged monitoring—beyond 24 h— could then further increase the yield of capturing nonconvulsive seizures and status epilepticus [27, 29].

Blood presence in the subarachnoid spaces causes various EEG changes, related with the extension of the hemorrhage and with the severity of the clinical picture. EEG abnormalities are therefore variable: slowing of the background rhythm; appearance of focal or diffuse theta-delta activity, sometimes with anterior rhythmicity; patterns of diffuse suppression, with or without persistence of activity bursts. Sometimes, the most dominant slowings or attenuation can be observed on the side of the initial hemorrhage. In addition, periodic epileptiform patterns, most frequently LPD, but also GPDs or BI-LPDs, can be observed in SAH patients. Claassen et al., [28] in their study on nonconvulsive seizures after SAH, classified EEG by visual inspection in three categories: (1) *ictal pattern*, defined as any epileptic discharge lasting for 10 s or more, with clear evolution in frequency, morphology and location; (2) *ictal-interictal continuum*, defined as repetitive generalized or focal epileptiform abnormalities (as LPDs or GPDs), without clear evolution to ictal pattern; (3) *non-ictal pattern*, defined as conditions different from 1) and 2). The periodic patterns can be as frequent as 23–48% [30, 31] and they seem to be more common in older patients and in those with nonconvulsive seizures and NCSE.

Vasospasm is the most frequent complication after SAH, and it is the most common cause of SAH survivor's late ischemic complications. EEG monitoring shows slowings in the areas where the vasospasm is more evident and a seriated monitoring could be helpful in intensive care units, to soon detect this condition. In patients with high-grade SAH, in whom delayed cerebral ischemia due to vasospasm is undetectable by clinical examinations, qEEG measures can be really helpful. A decrease in alpha/delta ratio may be a sensitive method of detecting delayed cerebral ischemia, with reasonable specificity [32]. Furthermore, compressed spectral arrays remain a reliable screening method for seizure identification and they can also display long periods of activity suppression, as consequence of seizures or sedation [33] (Fig. 38.5).

38.5 Subdural Hematoma

Acute SubDural Hematoma (SDH) is usually provoked by head trauma, with death in more than half of patients. Prognostic factors include severity of trauma, old age, neurologic condition at admission and the increase of intracranial pressure. EEG is useful in evaluating patients with SDH because it provides diagnostic and prognostic information.

The reported EEG features in patients with SDH include focal or hemispheric slowings, asymmetries of background activity, FIRDA and epileptiform activity, including LPDs. Rudzinski et al. [34] revised the EEGs of patients who underwent evacuation for acute or subacute SDH and described, in this series of patients, a combination of various EEG patterns. Epileptiform discharges - predominantly bilateral - are present in 87% of patients and 43% of these had LPDs, focal or multifocal. A typical finding is the presence of midline

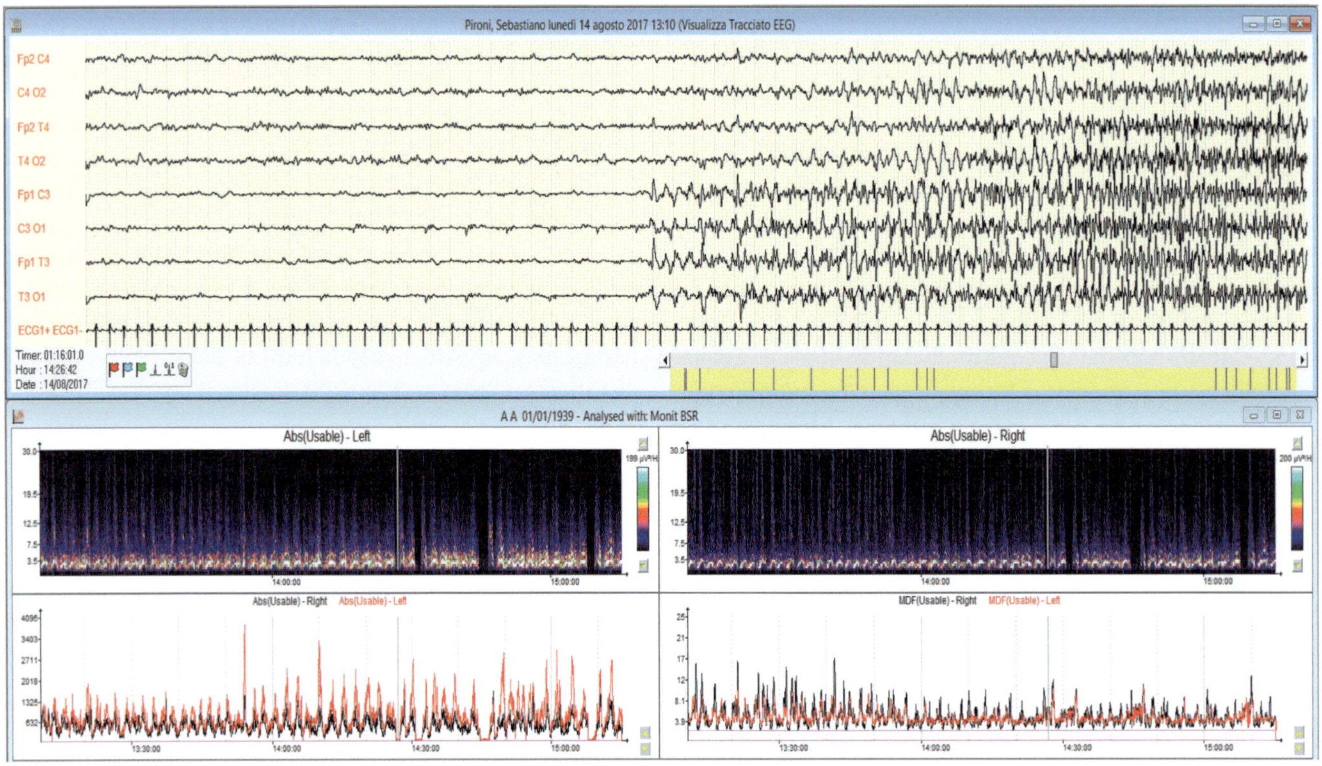

Fig. 38.5 Continuous EEG monitoring (cEEG) in a stroke patient with convulsive status epilepticus. Raw EEG (top) demonstrates a prolonged and intermittent ictal pattern, originating from the left hemisphere. Quantitative absolute power and frequency trends (bottom) show the recurrence of seizures in about 150 min of recording

epileptiform discharges, which occurred in 62% of the patients with epileptiform discharges, and these are significantly associated with the degree of midline shift on brain imaging. The 92% of patients had bilateral slowings that, in about half of the cases, is predominant in one hemisphere. Focal slowings, ipsilateral to the side of SDH, are observed in 62% of patients, predominantly in the temporal and frontal regions. FIRDA is demonstrated in 29%. Asymmetry of the EEG tracing is present in all the patients, consisting in a cerebral activity amplitude increase (42%) or decrease (33%) in the side of SDH while, in the remaining patients, asymmetries varied over time. In regard to prognosis, the midline epileptiform discharges and LPDs were strongly associated with the midline shift on neuroimaging and with poor functional outcome at hospital discharge. Improvement in follow-up EEGs over time may be predictive of good long-term functional outcome. Very recently, Pollandt et al. [35] reviewed the cEEG of a large series of adult patients with SDH. Almost all the patients received antiseizure prophylaxis but - despite the antiepileptic treatment - 41, 1% had epileptic seizures (16% with status epilepticus) and 32% had epileptiform abnormalities on the EEG. Surprisingly, seizures and epileptiform abnormalities were not associated with poor long-term outcome, even if they are associated with longer intensive care unit and hospital length of stay (Figs. 38.6 and 38.7).

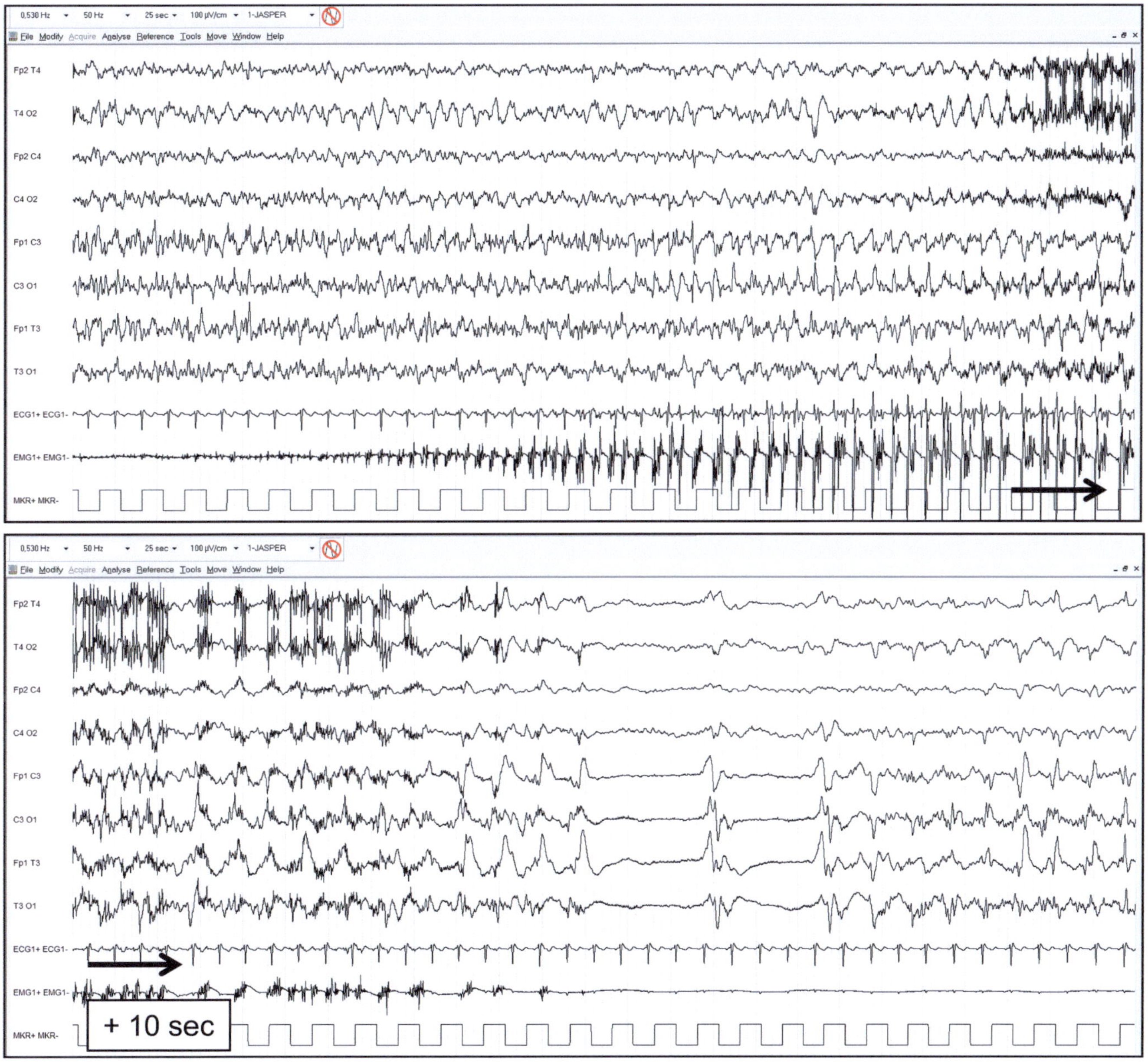

Fig. 38.6 A 78-year-old patient with extensive left posttraumatic subdural hematoma. Four days later after onset, focal convulsive status epilepticus with right hand and face myoclonic jerks and secondary generalization, refractory to antiepileptic treatment. EMG recorded in the deltoid

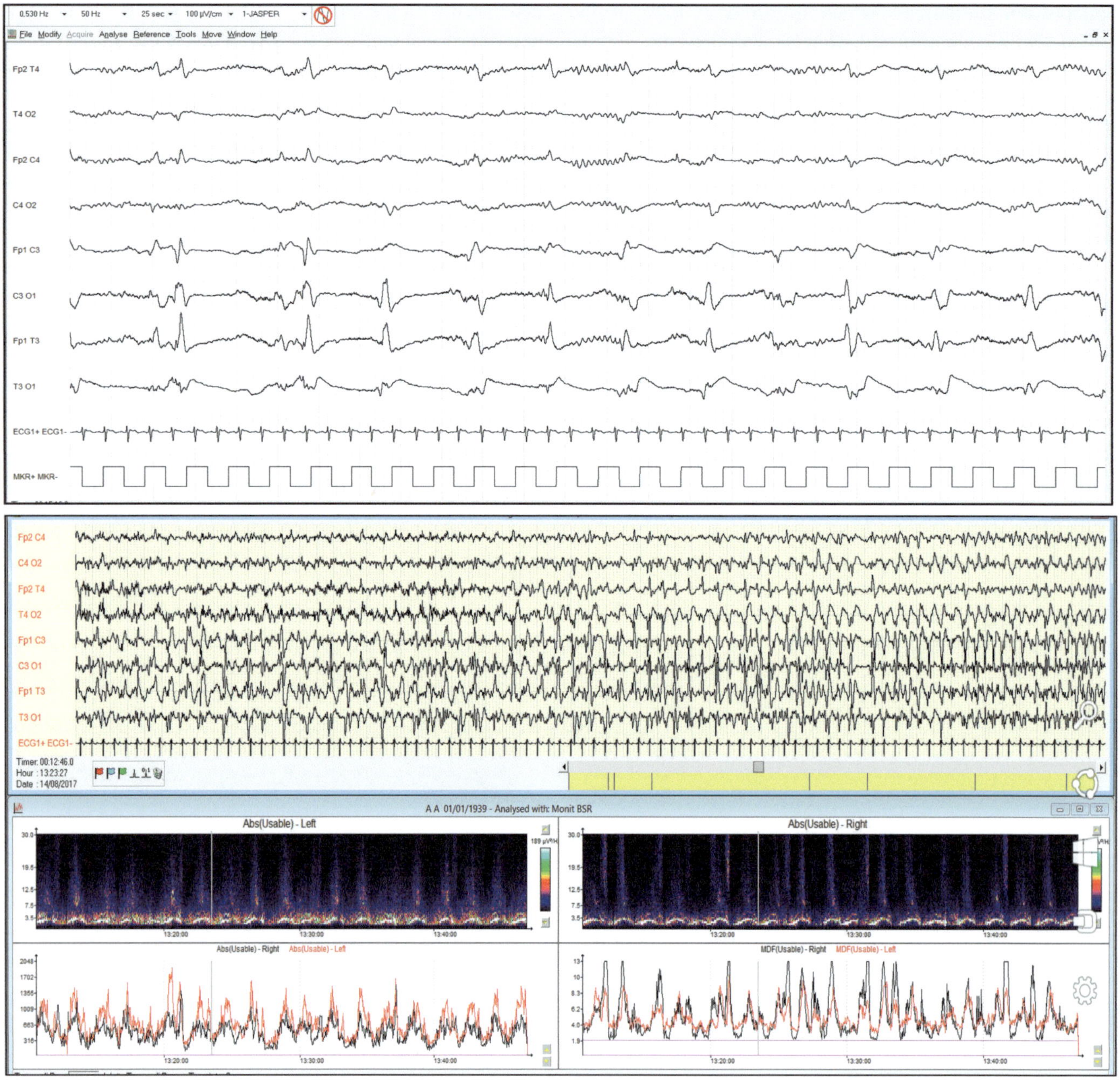

Fig. 38.7 The same case described in Fig. 38.6. Between-seizure EEG shows left LPDs. After 7 days of refractory status epilepticus, the patient died. Raw EEG (top); quantitative absloute power and frequency trends (bottom)

38.6 Other Cerebrovascular Diseases

In cases of chronic or minimal blood flow reduction in the posterior circulation, EEG findings may be completely unremarkable or with minimal, non-specific abnormalities (such as diffuse background activity of low amplitude, with superimposed fast frequencies). However, in most cases, alpha activity is clearly detectable and more evident during intermittent photic stimulation (IPS). Sometimes, during IPS, a symmetrical photic driving of high amplitude in the occipital regions may be observed, associated with a more intense blinking reflex. Sequences of theta-sharpened rhythms may be observed in the temporal areas, generally predominant in the left side. Hyperventilation, to be executed with caution in these patients, does not generally affects background rhythms, especially when in basal conditions they show a low EEG voltage. Typical sleep patterns also remain unchanged, with low amplitude.

These non-specific EEG changes due to *vertebrobasilar hypoperfusion* may be originated by the chronic-reduced vascularization—with consequent hyperexcitability—in the occipital cortex (higher photic driving), in the temporal regions (sharp theta temporal waves) and in the brain stem (background activity of low amplitude and scarcely synchronized). Basilar artery occlusion may produce an infarct in the ventral pons, with or without the tegmentum involvement. If the the tegmentum is spared, the pons lesion causes the "locked-in" syndrome; the patient in this case is mute and tetraplegic but the EEG is normal, with a reactive alpha rhythm. In comatose patients with infarct involving the ventral pons and tegmentum bilaterally, EEG may show a diffuse alpha activity, with absent or scarce reactivity (alpha coma pattern) [15].

During *drop attacks,* EEG changes are ininfluent. In very rare cases recorded, an ictal monolateral discharge in occipital region, spreading to the whole posterior areas of both hemispheres and lasting 30–90 s has been described. This ictal activity may persist even for the following days and has been compared with SREDA.

Subclavian steal syndrome is a peculiar hemodynamic condition that occurs when, in relation to a subclavian artery stenosis or occlusion blood flow is maintained to the arm through the ipsilateral vertebral artery, showing blood flow direction inversion—i.e., away from the brain—especially during flow increase in the ipsilateral arm, as it may occur during arm physical excercise. EEG may show non-specific EEG slowing in the affected hemisphere, related to the severity of blood flow reduction and prevalent in the posterior areas.

Thrombosis of the cerebral venous system is an uncommon cause of cerebral infarction in respect to arterial disease but its prompt diagnosis is important to reduce the risk of poor outcome and disability. Most of the patients may experience various clinical symptoms, mimicking many neurological conditions such as meningitis, encephalopathy, benign intracranial hypertension and stroke. Neuroimaging study could be not indicative for diagnosis if the venous system is not investigated, but EEG recording might be in these cases helpful. The most common EEG finding is a diffuse delta slowing of electrical activity, coexisting with focal abnormalities and clinical focal symptoms. In one third of the patients, diffuse slowings and epileptiform abnormalities [15] may also be observed. The epileptiform abnormalities are represented by LPDs that precede and/or follow an epileptic seizure or SE (Fig. 38.8).

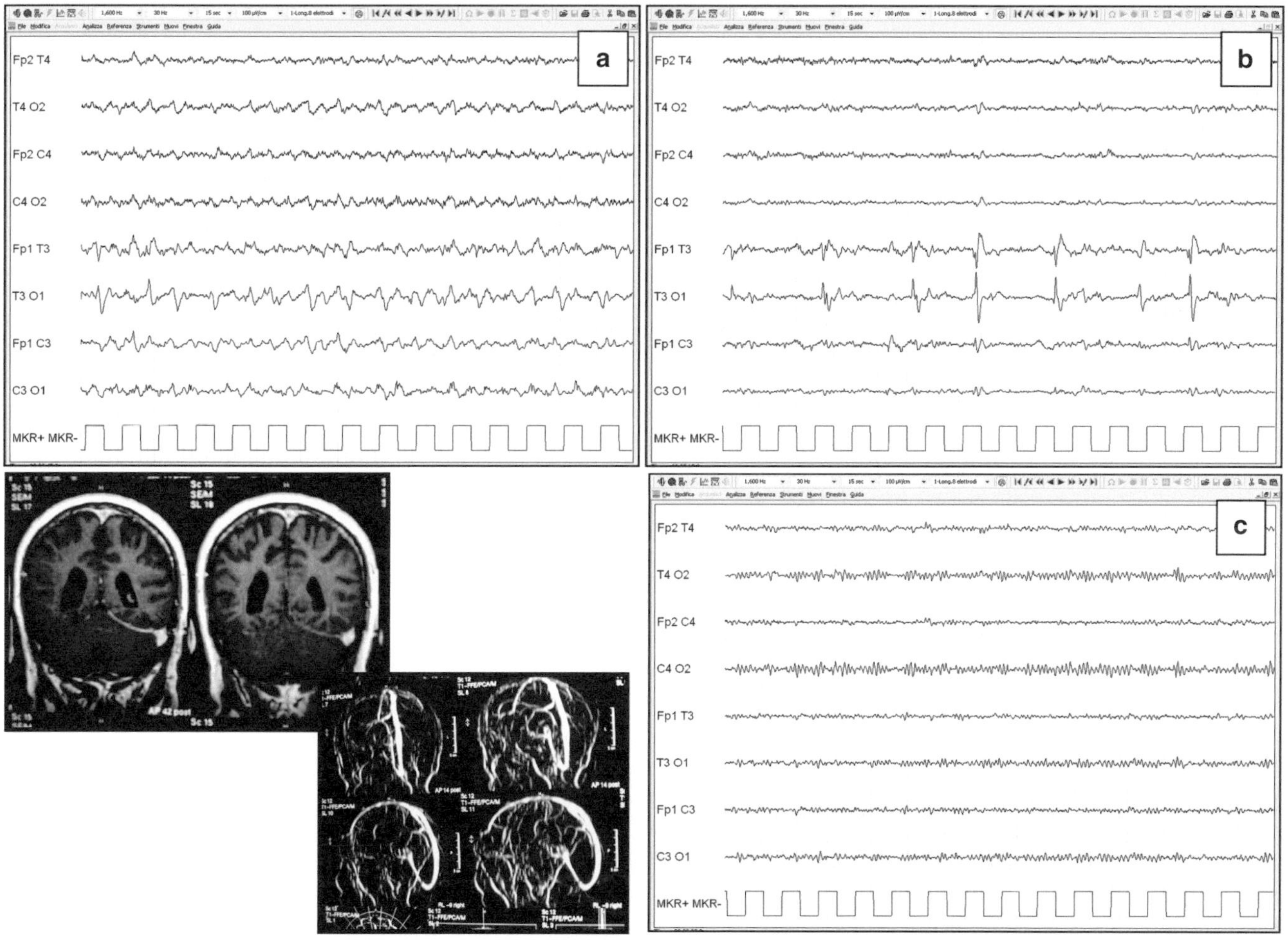

Fig. 38.8 A 56-year-old patient admitted for headache and confusional state. Cerebral CT scan was normal at admission. Emergency EEG shows diffuse delta-theta slowings, prevalent in the left posterior temporal regions (**a**). 24 h later (**b**), EEG appears with attenuated background activity and LPDs in the left temporal area. Cerebral MRI reveals left transverse sinus thrombosis. 10 days later EEG is normalized, except but persistance of mild alpha asymmetry (right > left) (**c**)

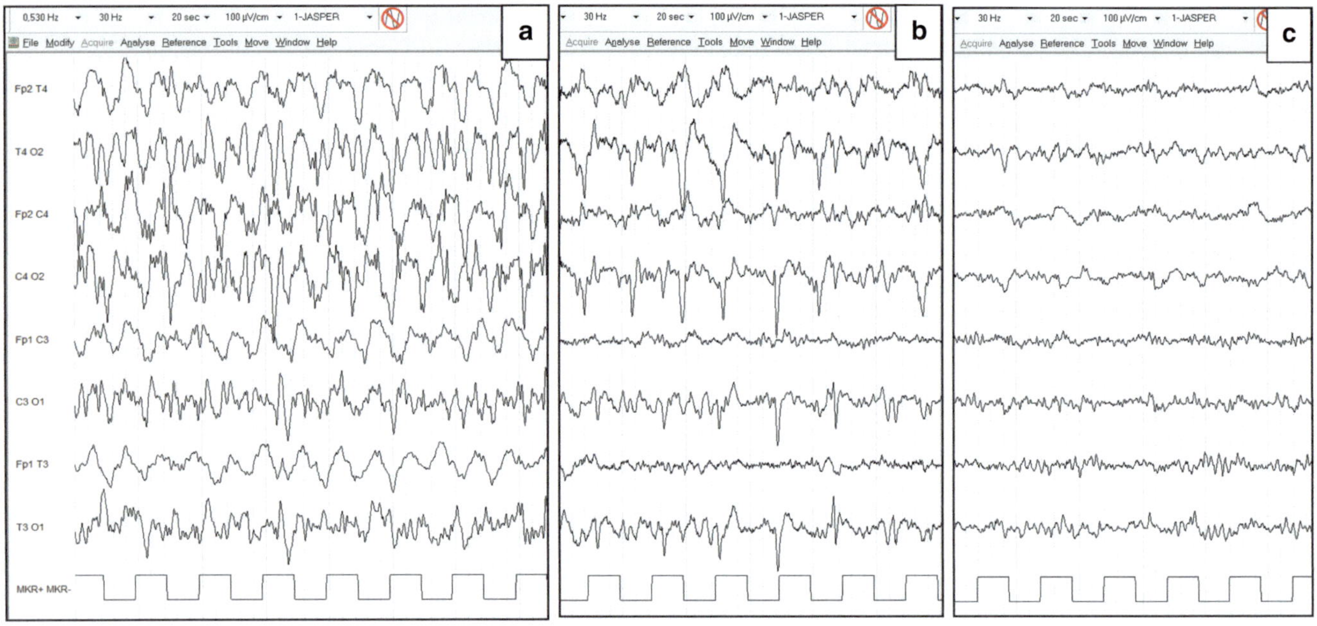

Fig. 38.9 A 52-year-old patient with posterior reversible encephalopathy syndrome. First EEG recorded 3 days after symptom onset (**a**) shows rhythmic bilateral anterior delta activity with continuous epileptiform abnormalities in the posterior areas, dominant in the right hemisphere. This EEG pattern is still present 5 days later, even though less relevant and more localized in the right posterior region (**b**). 4 days later, EEG shows only central occipital slowing with alpha rhythm reappearance (**c**)

Transient Global Amnesia (TGA) is a clinical syndrome characterized by the sudden onset of anterograde amnesia, accompanied by repetitive questioning, sometimes with a retrograde component, lasting up to 24 h, without compromise of other neurologic functions [36].

Attacks usually last for 1–8 h, but they should be less than 24 h. Pathogenesis of TGA has been disputed over years to be the result from different mechanisms, such as venous congestion with Valsalva-like activities before symptom onset, arterial thromboembolic ischemia and vasoconstriction due to hyperventilation. The differential diagnoses that need to be considered are acute confusional state, focal epileptic manifestations, psychogenic amnesia and transient ischemic attack. Clinical history and course of the attack are crucial for the diagnosis and, in the very acute phases, EEG is always normal, helping in the differentiation between TGA and temporal epilepsy. In particular, Transient Epileptic Amnesia (TEA) [37] is a rare ictal manifestation of temporal epilepsy, usually occurring in middle- or old-age patients, often during waking phase. Epileptic seizures with memory impairment are more numerous and shorter than the attacks typical of TGA, and the ictal EEG recording obviously allows a correct and definitive differential diagnosis.

Posterior Reversible Encephalopathy Syndrome (PRES) is a neurotoxic state associated with reversible vasogenic edema and that presents with various neurological symptoms, including seizures and SE, convulsive or nonconvulsive. Epileptic seizures were mostly of occipital origin, but generalized seizures are also described. The majority of patients with PRES has abnormal EEG findings, characterized by diffuse theta/delta slowings, associated or not with focal epileptiform discharges (Fig. 38.9) [38].

Acknowledgments We are grateful to Dr. Patrizia Pulitano for her help in selecting and editing the EEG figures.

References

1. Jordan KG. Emergency EEG and continuous EEG monitoring in acute ischemic stroke. J Clin Neurophysiol. 2004; 21: 341–52.
2. Gaspard N. Current clinical evidence supporting the use of continuous EEG monitoring for delayed cerebral ischemia detection. J Clin Neurphysiol. 2016; 33: 211–6.
3. van Putten MJAM, Hofmeijer J. EEG monitoring in cerebral ischemia: basic concepts and clinical applications. J Clin Neurophysiol. 2016; 33: 203–10.
4. Kohno K, Back T, Hoehn-Berlage M, Hossmann KA. A modified rat model of middle cerebral artery thread occlusion under electrophysiological control for magnetic resonance investigations. Magn Reson Imaging. 1995; 13: 65–71.
5. Melamed E, Lavy S, Portnoy Z, Sadan S, Carmon A. Correlation between regional cerebral blood flow and EEG frequency in the contralateral hemisphere in acute cerebral infarction. J Neurol Sci. 1975; 26: 21–7.
6. Kaplan PW. EEG criteria for non convulsive status epilepticus. Epilepsia. 2007; 48.(Suppl. 8): 39–41.
7. Mecarelli O, Pro S, Randi F, et al. EEG patterns and epileptic seizures in acute phase stroke. Cerebrovasc Dis. 2011; 31: 191–8.
8. Pohlmann-Eden B, Hoch DB, Cochius JI, Chiappa KH. Periodic lateralized epileptiform discharges–a critical review. J Clin Neurophysiol. 1996; 13: 519–30.

9. Neufeld M, Vishnevskaya S, Treves T, et al. Periodic lateralized epileptiform discharges (PLEDs) following stroke are associated with metabolic abnormalities. Electroencephalogr Clin Neurophysiol. 1997; 102: 295–8.
10. Kalamangalam GP, Diehl B, Burgess RC. Neuroimaging and neurophysiology of periodic lateralized epileptiform discharges: observations and hypotheses. Epilepsia. 2007; 48: 1396–405.
11. Hartings JA, Williams AJ, Tortella FC. Occurrence of nonconvulsive seizures, periodic epileptiform discharges, and intermittent rhythmic delta activity in rat focal ischemia. Exp Neurol. 2003; 179: 139–49.
12. Cillesen JPM, van Huffelen AC, Kappelle LJ, et al. Electroencephalography improves the prediction of functional outcome in the acute stage of cerebral ischemia. Stroke. 1994; 25: 1968–72.
13. Chong DJ, Hirsch LJ. Which EEG patterns warrant treatment in the critically ill? Reviewing the evidence for treatment of periodic epileptiform discharges and related patterns. J Clin Neurophysiol. 2005; 22: 79–91.
14. Verma NP, Kooi KA. Contralateral epileptiform transients in stroke (CETS). Epilepsia. 1986; 27: 437–40.
15. Galovic M, Schmitz B, Tettenborn B. EEG in inflammatory disorders, cerebrovascular diseases, trauma, and migraine. In: Schomer DL, Lopes daSilva FH, editors. Niedermeyer's electroencephalography. Basic principles, clinical applications, and related fields. 7th ed. Oxford: Oxford University Press; 2018. p. 371–412.
16. Finnigan SP, Rose SE, Walsh M, et al. Correlation of quantitative EEG in acute ischemic stroke with 30-day NIHSS score. Stroke. 2004; 35: 899–903.
17. Finnigan SP, Walsh M, Rose SE, Chalk JB. Quantitative EEG indices of sub-acute ischaemic stroke correlate with clinical outcomes. Clin Neurophysiol. 2007; 118: 2525–32.
18. Sheorajpanday RVA, Nagels G, Weeren AJTM, et al. Quantitative EEG in ischemic stroke: correlation with functional status after 6 months. Clin Neurophysiol. 2011; 122: 874–83.
19. Assenza G, Zappasodi F, Pasqualetti P, et al. A contralesional EEG power increase mediated by interhemispheric disconnection provides negative prognosis in acute stroke. Restor Neurol Neurosci. 2013; 31: 177–88.
20. Jordan KG, Stringer WA. Correlative xenon enhanced CT cerebral blood flow (XeCTCBF) and EEG to functionally stratify acute cerebral infarction. Neurology. 1991; 4(Suppl 1): 336.
21. Jordan KG. Regional attenuation without delta (RAWOD): a distinctive EEG pattern that can aid in the diagnosis and management of in acute cerebral infarctions (SACI). Neurology. 1998; 50(Suppl 1): A43.
22. De Vos CC, van Maarseveen SM, Brouwers PJAM, van Putten MJAM. Continuous EEG monitoring during thrombolysis in acute hemispheric stroke patients using the brain symmetry index. J Clin Neurophysiol. 2008; 25: 77–82.
23. Dreier JP. The role of spreading depression, spreading depolarization and spreading ischemia in neurological disease. Nat Med. 2011; 17: 439–47.
24. Jeffcote T, Hinzman JM, Jewell SL, et al. Detection of spreading depolarization with intraparenchimal electrodes in the injured human brain. Neurocrit Care. 2014; 20: 21–31.
25. Easton DJ, Saver JL, Albers GW, et al. Definition and evaluation of transient ischemic attack. Stroke. 2009; 40: 2276–93.
26. Claassen J, Jetté N, Chum F, et al. Electrographic seizures and periodic discharges after intracerebral hemorrhage. Neurology. 2007; 69: 1356–65.
27. Maciel CB, Gilmore EJ. Seizures and epileptiform patterns in SAH and their relation to outcomes. J Clin Neurophysiol. 2016; 33: 183–95.
28. Claassen J, Perotte A, Albers D, et al. Nonconvulsive seizures after subarachnoid hemorrhage: multimodal detection and outcomes. Ann Neurol. 2013; 74: 53–64.
29. Claassen J, Mayer SA, Hirsch LJ. Continuous EEG monitoring in patients with subarachnoid hemorrhage. J Clin Neurophysiol. 2005; 22: 92–8.
30. Claassen J, Hirsch LJ, Frontera JA, et al. Prognostic significance of continuous EEG monitoring in patients with poor-grade subarachnoid hemorrhage. Neurocrit Care. 2006; 4: 103–12.
31. Crepeau AZ, Kerrigan JF, Gerber P, et al. Rhythmical and periodic EEG patterns do not predict short-term outcome in critically ill patients with subarachnoid hemorrhage. J Clin Neurophysiol. 2013; 30: 247–54.
32. Claassen J, Hirsch LJ, Kreiter KT, et al. Quantitative continuous EEG for detecting delayed cerebral ischemia in patients with poor-grade subarachnoid hemorrhage. Clin Neurophysiol. 2004; 115: 2699–710.
33. Carlson C. Can we screen EEGs more efficiently? Spectrographic review of EEG data. Epilepsy Curr. 2015; 15: 24–5.
34. Rudzinski LA, Rabinstein AA, Chung SY, et al. Electroencephalographic findings in acute subdural hematoma. J Clin Neurophysiol. 2011; 28: 633–41.
35. Pollandt S, Ouyang B, Bleck TP, Busl KM. Seizures and epileptiform discharges in patients with acute subdural hematoma. J Clin Neurophysiol. 2017; 34: 55–60.
36. Arena JE, Rabinstein AA. Transient global amnesia. Mayo Clin Proc. 2015; 90: 264–72.
37. Zeman A, Butler C. Transient epileptic amnesia. Curr Opin Neurol. 2010; 23: 610–6.
38. Kamiya-Matsuoka C, Tummala S. Electrographic patterns in patients with posterior reversible encephalopathy syndrome and seizures. J Neurol Sci. 2017; 375: 294–8.

39 Cerebral Infectious Diseases

Chiara Davassi, Patrizia Pulitano, and Oriano Mecarelli

39.1 Infectious Meningitis

EEG studies on meningitis reveal that EEG abnormalities are absent or only mild in viral (aseptic) meningitis, while they are more pronounced in bacterial meningitis [1].

39.1.1 Bacterial Meningitis

Bacterial infections of the meninges (dura mater, arachnoid and pia mater) are distinguished in acute meningitis, also defined purulent, and subacute/chronic meningitis that often affect the basal portion of the brain. These latter may be caused also by non-bacterial organisms, such as fungi and parasites.

Acute bacterial meningitis is a life-threatening infection that requires prompt diagnosis and treatment. Ninety-five percentage of patients present with two of the following four symptoms: fever, nuchal rigidity, altered mental status and headache [2]. Its incidence is about 5 per 100,000 adults per year in developed countries. The principal causative pathogens in adults are *Streptococcus pneumoniae* (pneumococcus) and *Neisseria meningitidis* (meningococcus), responsible for about 80% of all cases [3]. The organisms causing meningitis in hospitalized patients (nosocomial meningitis) differ from those of community-acquired meningitis and they include Gram-negative rods (e.g., *Escherichia coli*, *Klebsiella* spp., *Pseudomonas aeruginosa*, *Acinetobacter* spp., E*nterobacter* spp.), staphylococci and streptococci other than *S. pneumoniae*.

C. Davassi · O. Mecarelli (✉)
Department of Human Neurosciences, Sapienza University of Rome, Rome, Italy
e-mail: chiara.davassi@uniroma1.it; oriano.mecarelli@uniroma1.it

P. Pulitano
Azienda Ospedaliero-Universitaria Policlinico Umberto I, Rome, Italy
e-mail: patrizia.pulitano@uniroma1.it

Although EEG may be heterogeneous, the most common finding in purulent meningitis consists of diffuse slow-wave abnormalities of variable severity. A single EEG may not be pivotal for the specific diagnosis, but seriated recordings are useful to follow the course of the disease, for the early detection of complications or relapses, and for indication of the presence of additional brain damage in the case when the meningitis evolves into a meningoencephalitis. Fuvrthermore, EEG allows recognizing epileptiform discharges even before the development of clinical epileptic seizures, correlating with a poor prognosis and a higher mortality. Thus, EEG provides clinicians an instrument to eventually establish a preventive antiepileptic therapy.

Other EEG abnormal patterns observed in bacterial meningitis include triphasic waves and occasional frontal delta wave activity (Frontal Intermittent Rhythmic Delta Activity, FIRDA), although these are more typical of other etiologies [4]. It is reasonable to consider slowings in the delta range as the only abnormality that may suggest clinicians to a likely etiological diagnosis, more often observed in bacterial than in viral meningitis (Fig. 39.1) [1]. Lateralized Periodic Discharges (LPDs) have been described in pneumococcal infections, especially when a brain lesion occurs [5]. Another possibility is the formation of bacterial brain abscesses that may represent either the cause or the consequence of bacterial meningitis. In such cases, EEG shows focal unilateral delta slowings [6], although other EEG changes are possible, including epileptiform focal abnormalities, focal suppression of the background activity, and LPDs [4].

Subacute and chronic infectious meningitides are commonly defined as inflammations of the meninges evolving during weeks to months, without resolution of Cerebro Spinal Fluid (CSF) abnormalities.

Also called "basal meningitis", due to their tendency to involve the basal regions of the brain and the brainstem, several pathogens are recognized. Bacterial causes of subacute

O. Mecarelli (ed.), *Clinical Electroencephalography*, https://doi.org/10.1007/978-3-030-04573-9_39

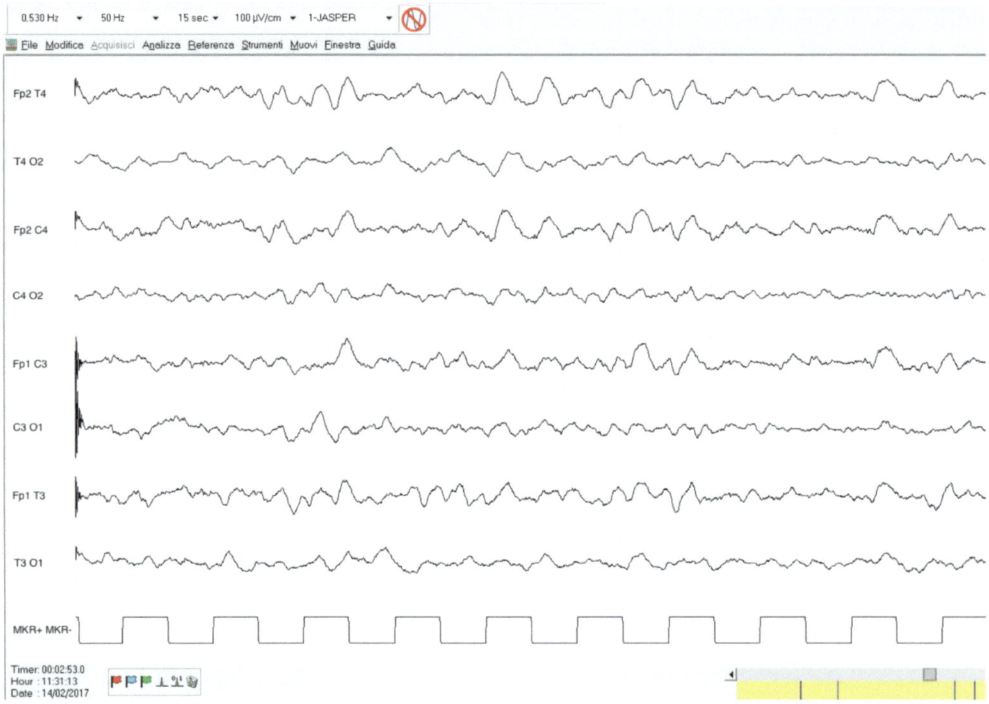

Fig. 39.1 Example of bilateral Frontal Intermittent Rhythmic Delta Activity (FIRDA) in a 70-year-old male patient affected by streptococcal meningitis

and chronic meningitis include *Mycobacterium tuberculosis* and syphilis. *Mycobacterium tuberculosis* represents the most common bacterial agent.

Tuberculous Meningitis (TBM) is an aggressive form of extrapulmonary disease, more common in patients coinfected with HIV. *Mycobacterium tuberculosis* may reach the meninges and the CNS through the blood, 4–8 weeks after primary infection, giving rise to an inflammation that involves the cranial nerves and that may generate a blockage of CSF flow with obstructive hydrocephalus. However, although it may follow a primary infection, TBM is more frequently due to reactivation of an old subclinical tuberculoid focus that had previously been inactive, sometimes even for many years [7].

TBM in immunocompetent adults is typically preceded by non-specific symptoms like anorexia, fatigue, weight loss, fever, myalgia and headache. Characteristic clinical features are vomiting, meningeal signs, focal deficits, vision loss, cranial nerve palsies and increased intracranial pressure [8].

The EEG findings in TBM vary according to the site of the inflammatory process and to the presence of other conditions, such as hydrocephalus and increased intracranial pressure.

In basal meningitis, EEG may be normal or may show only mild, non-specific changes. The involvement of the cerebral cortex and of the meninges results in moderate to severe slowing of EEG activity. The degree of the slowings depends on several factors, which include the magnitude of cortical involvement, the rate of progression of the process, the level of consciousness and the medications administered.

Some authors report heterogeneous EEG patterns and their presence in the early phase appear to be associated with a poor outcome. Among them, the most frequent are the diffuse slowing of background activity and the Intermittent Rhythmic Delta Activity (IRDA); on the other hand, lateralized epileptiform discharges (consisting in spike or multiple spike and wave complexes) appear to be rare (Fig. 39.2). IRDA is a non-specific finding and may occur in increased intracranial pressure, being attributed to a diffuse gray matter disease, involving both cortical and subcortical areas. Significant right to left asymmetry in voltage and frequency has also been observed [7, 9, 10].

39.1.2 Viral Meningitis

Viral meningitis, also known as aseptic meningitis, is a nonbacterial form of meninges infection. The most commonly involved viruses are enterovirus, Herpes Simplex Virus (HSV), and Varicella-Zoster Virus (VZV) [11].

Clinically, viral meningitis is characterized by fever, headache and signs of meningeal irritation, although a mild degree of drowsiness is not uncommon [12]. As the clinical picture of bacterial and viral meningitis are similar, CSF analysis is essential for their distinction, to identify the virus, and to decide whether or not to initiate antiviral therapy [11].

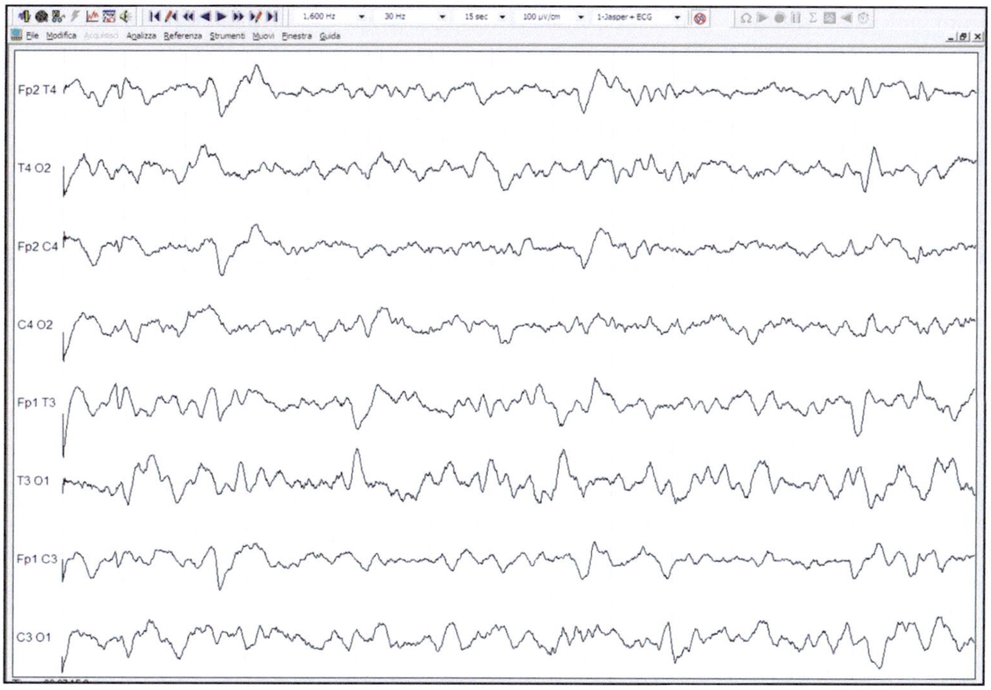

Fig. 39.2 3-year-old child with tubercular meningitis complicated by hydrocephalus, after derivation. EEG shows focal epileptiform abnormalities in left temporo-occipital regions and a widespread slowing of the background activity

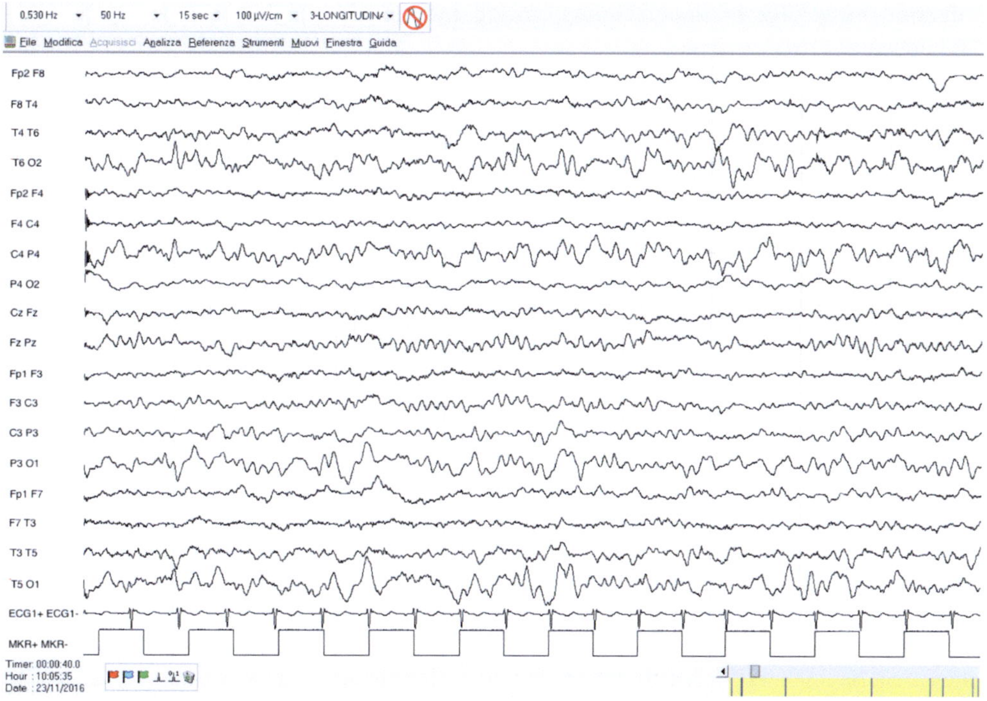

Fig. 39.3 High-voltage slowings in posterior regions in a 6-year-old child with viral meningitis

EEG is usually normal. However, non-specific EEG changes occur in 33–50% of patients especially in young children, consisting essentially in generalized, sometimes prevalent in posterior regions, continuous or intermittent slowings (Fig. 39.3). Epileptiform abnormalities are infrequent, and their occurrence suggests a diagnosis of encephalitis [12].

39.2 Infectious Encephalitis

Encephalopathies due to infections may result from the direct invasion of brain parenchyma by various agents (bacteria, viruses, parasites, fungi), from the effects of a systemic infection during sepsis ("Sepsis-Associated Encephalopathies," SAE) or, indirectly, from the aberrant immunologic reaction to the infectious pathogen ("post-infectious encephalitis"). The latter may occur either as a consequence of an otherwise benign infectious disease or after a vaccination. Most infectious encephalitides have non-specific EEG patterns. Among those with characteristic EEG abnormalities, Herpes Virus Encephalitis (HVE), Subacute Sclerosing Pan Encephalitis (SSPE) and prion diseases are described.

Herpes virus encephalitis is an acute encephalitis characterized by fever, altered mental status, focal neurological symptoms and generalized or focal epileptic seizures. Symptoms usually appear in hours to days. Differently from the other acute encephalitides (VZV and arboviruses, including West Nile, Toscana, tick-borne, Japanese and others) that cause widespread infection in the brain and tend to determine only diffuse delta to theta slowing [9, 13], HVE induces characteristics focal or multifocal EEG abnormalities likewise epileptic discharges. Besides providing a diagnostic support, EEG in HVE appears to have a prognostic role, as an early normal EEG seems to be predictive of good outcome [14, 15]. HVE is caused in 90% of all cases by HSV-1, whereas HSV-2 leads to disseminated infection especially in immunocompromised individuals and neonates [15].

EEG findings in HVE may consist in focal or diffuse slow waves, focal epileptiform abnormalities, electrical seizures, attenuation/disorganization of background activity, or periodic lateralized discharges [16]. The EEG activity in HVE reflects the virus tendency to affect temporal and orbital frontal lobes and the cingulate gyrus, although it may also cause a more widespread cerebral involvement.

EEG shows initially delta slowings in the temporal lobe. Later, isolated sharp waves appear on this slow activity and, as the disease progresses - between the 2nd and 14th day of progression -, LPDs appear. The periodic complexes consist of sharply shaped slow waves or polyphasic spikes with a duration of complexes of 200–600 ms and an amplitude of 100 to about 500 μV, recurring at a rather constant interval of 1.5–2.5 s, but sometimes ranging from 1 to 5 s. These lateralised alterations may become bilateral as the disease involves the contralateral hemisphere [16]. When bilateral, they can be bilateral independent (BIPDs) or multifocal (MfPDs) or generalised (GPDs) [13].

PLDs localised in the affected temporal lobe are then considered the most characteristic abnormalities for the diagnosis of HVE.

Seizure discharges are common in the affected brain areas, consisting of epileptiform fast rhythmic activity, with or without clinical correlate [4].

Attenuation of background activity is another EEG finding in HVE, coexisting or not with periodic patterns. Although periodic sharp waves and the other EEG findings are not pathognomonic of this condition, the localization of these abnormalities in the temporal lobe is considered very characteristic and helpful in the early diagnosis, enabling the prompt start of antiviral therapies [16].

In refractory or fatal cases, a burst suppression pattern may be observed, with generalized EEG attenuation following a burst of LPDs or polyspikes, indicating a poor prognosis. In nonfatal HVE, with the resolution of the infection, the EEG periodic abnormalities become infrequent and intermittent and they are replaced by a slow activity that may persist even for few months. However EEG recovers usually slowly to almost normal activity on seriated examinations during a period of 20–30 days, with the clinical improvement often preceding the electrographic normalization. Figs. 39.4 and 39.5 show the progression of EEG pattern in HVE in two cases.

Subacute sclerosing panencephalitis is a progressive and usually fatal encephalitis, secondary to measles virus infection, that causes a widespread CNS demyelination with a higher risk in subjects who had the infection earlier, before the age of 2 years. It is a late complication, occurring with a latency of about 6 years after the first infection. Its pathogenesis seems to be related to an abnormal immune response that may favor the permanence and replication of the mutant virus in the CNS [17].

The main clinical symptoms are represented by poor school performance and progressive intellectual deterioration, personality changes and behavior abnormalities, followed by stereotyped myoclonic jerks and other neurological symptoms such as pyramidal, extrapyramidal, visual, cerebellar and autonomic symptoms, seizures, and coma.

EEG recording is essential for the diagnosis. Typical Periodic Complexes (PCs) are found in 65–83% of individuals with SSPE and they are described as stereotyped, bilaterally synchronous and symmetrical 100–800 μV, 1–3 Hz slow-wave complexes, sometimes with sumperimposed spikes or sharp waves (Fig. 39.6). Their duration ranges from 0.5 to 3 s, and the interval between complexes varies from 3 to 20 s, although in the early phases, they can recur as long as every 5 min [17]. Due to the variable but long interval between them, periodic complexes in SSPE are suggested to be named as Periodic, Long-Interval Diffuse Discharges (PLIDDs), in contraposition with those observed in Creutzfeldt–Jakob disease presenting shorter (0.5–3 s) intervals (Periodic Short-Interval Diffuse Discharges, PSIDDs) [18]. PCs are usually

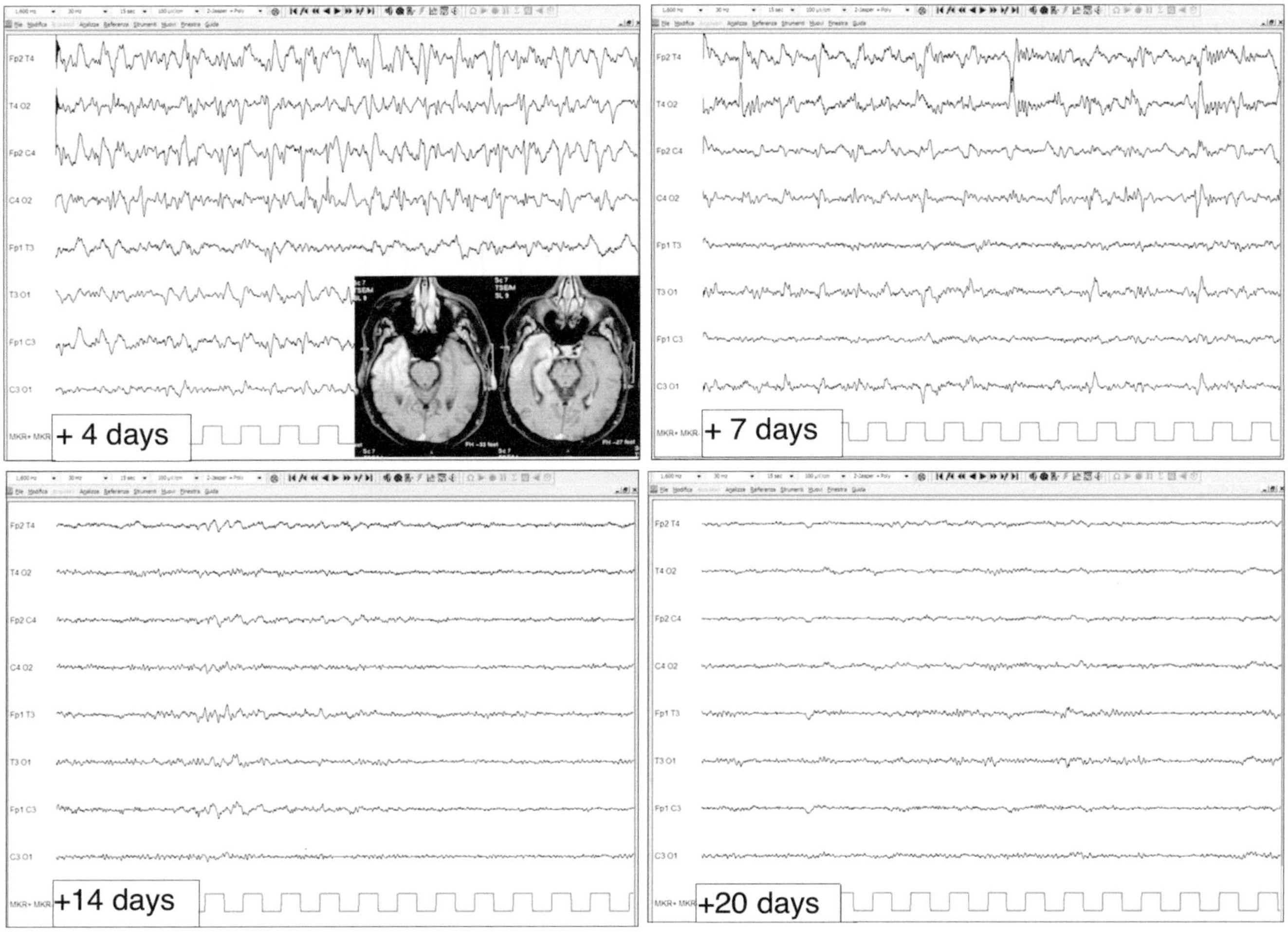

Fig. 39.4 EEG evolution of a 64-year-old male patient with right temporal herpetic encephalitis. Four days after symptoms onset (fever, confusion and focal seizures), EEG showed right quasi-periodic spikes and sharp waves, with a tendency to contralateral transmission. After 7 days, the abnormalities were less represented, maintaining a quasi-periodic recurrence. After 14 days, sporadic slow sequences were only evident, especially in the contralateral hemisphere. After 20 days, EEG normalization was observed. MRI showed in the small boxes.

present during awake and sleep; during sleep, however, there could be differences in their morphology and frequency and they may also disappear; in the early sleep phases, PCs could be elicited by external stimuli [17, 19]. PCs are recognizable throughout SSPE early stages and they are often related to the myoclonias, which may precede or succeed the PCs in the EEG. Less commonly, periodic complexes can disappear with high body temperatures, lose their rhythmicity with variable intervals between them, or be preceded by bisynchronous occipital spikes. Other atypical findings include, focal spikes, slow wave and random spikes in the frontal regions, and multifocal paroxysmal, high-amplitude slow waves alternating with fast waves [18].

Even if the PLIDDs are typically observed in SSPE, they are also reported in some toxic encephalopathies (like baclofen or ketamine intoxication) and in anoxic brain injury.

Periods of short-lasting (1–4 s) bioelectrical suppression may follow PCs. FIRDA are also recognized in more than half of the patients with SSPE during waking and light sleep. Although classically considered prominent in later stages of the disease, in the study conducted by Demir in 2013, [20] they appear especially in the early stages, so that they may be considered as a transitory phenomenon that could evolve into other types of EEG abnormalities. Independent from the PCs, epileptogenic discharges as focal or multifocal spikes and/or unilateral or bilateral generalized paroxysmal abnormalities have been reported in the EEGs of patients with SSPE [20].

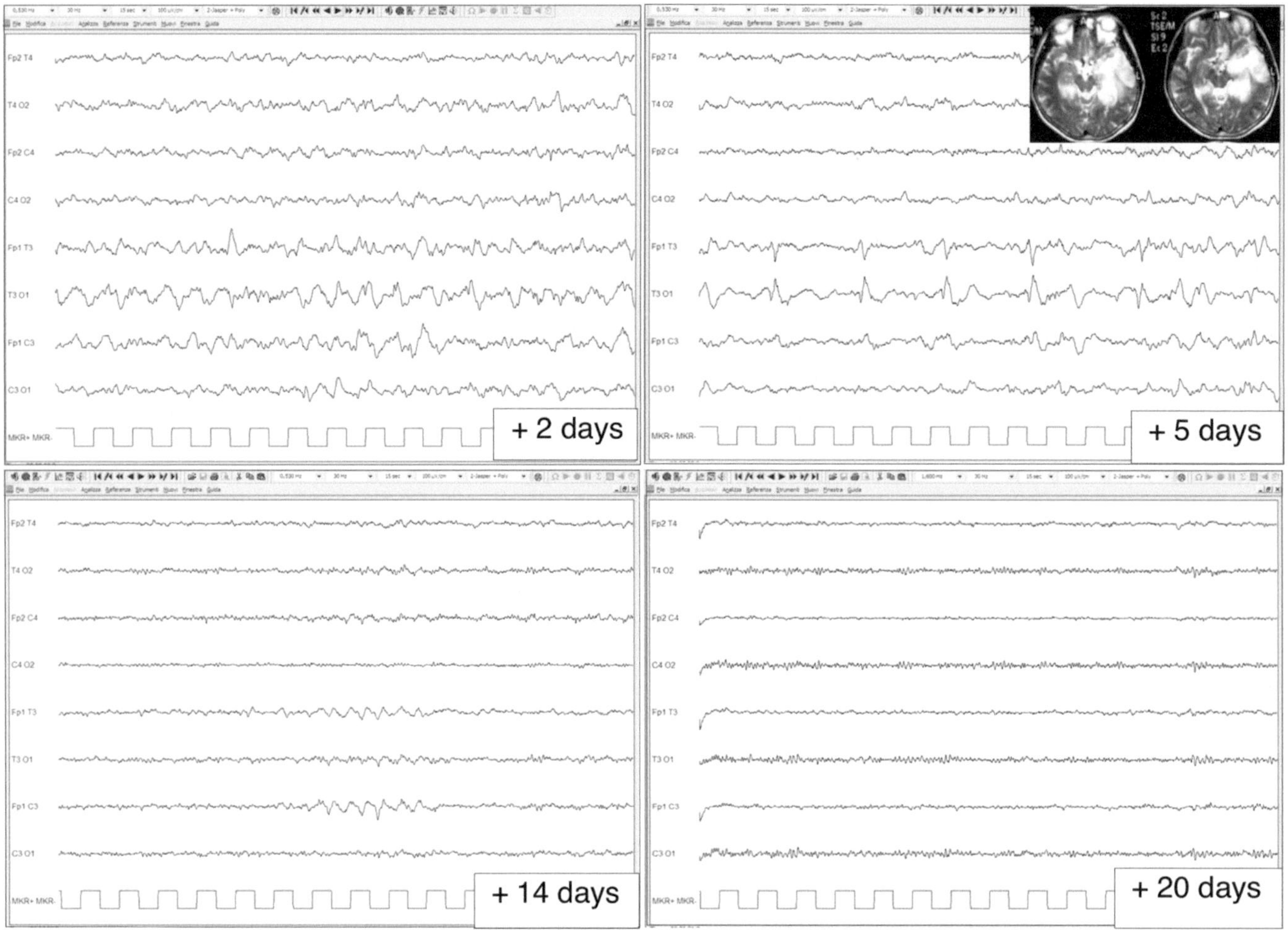

Fig. 39.5 Herpes virus encephalitis EEG progression in a 56-year-old female patient. Two days after symptoms onset, EEG showed left temporal monomorphic slow activity with sporadic spikes. After 5 days, lateralized periodic discharges appeared in the same. Rare monomorphic delta activity in anterior regions was observed after 14 days. After 20 days, EEG normalization was observed. MRI showed in the small boxes.

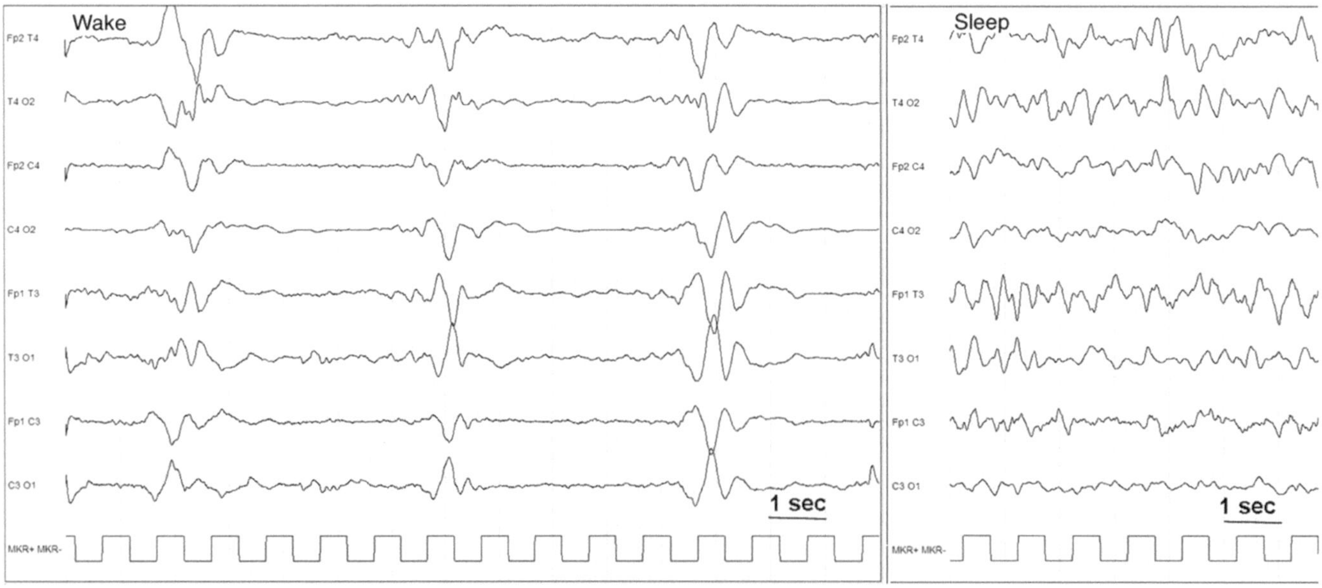

Fig. 39.6 10-year-old child affected by subacute sclerosing panencephalitis. Characteristic periodic, long-interval diffuse discharges are observed during awake state; these abnormalities tend to disappear during sleep

39.3 Prion Diseases

Prion Diseases (PrDs) are a group of neurodegenerative disorders caused by an abnormally proteinaceous infectious particles, called prions. Prion diseases result from the conversion of a normal, cell-surface glycoprotein (PrP^{C}) into a conformationally altered protein isoform (PrP^{Sc}) that, in the absence of the nucleid acids, becomes infectious. For the characteristic neuropathological changes that include spongiform vacuolation, neuronal loss, PrP^{Sc} deposition, amyloid plaque formation, and gliosis, prionic diseases are also called spongiform encephalitis. PrDs are classified into three groups: sporadic, genetic and acquired. The sporadic form is called sporadic Creutzfeldt-Jakob Disease (sCJD). The genetic forms are subdivided into genetic CJD (gCJD), Gerstmann-Sträussler-Scheinker Disease (GSSD), and Familial Fatal Insomnia (FFI). The acquired forms include *kuru*, iatrogenic CJD (iCJD), and variant CJD (vCJD).

39.3.1 Sporadic Creutzfeldt–Jakob Disease (sCJD)

sCJD is the most common subtype, accounting for 85% of the spongiform encephalitis, with an incidence of 1 to 1.5 per million per year [21].

Clinical symptoms rapidly include progressive dementia, cerebellar dysfunction and visual, speech and gait abnormalities. Dementia is the major symptom, followed by spontaneous or induced myoclonia. Pyramidal and extrapyramidal dysfunction, as well as behavioral changes with agitation, confusion and depression may also be observed. At the late stage of the disease, patients become unresponsive to external stimuli [22]. In almost 40% of patients, the initial symptom at presentation is represented by cognitive deterioration while cerebellar symptoms - as well as behavioral symptoms and visual dysfunction - are the initial manifestation in approximately only 15–20% of cases. Extrapyramidal and pyramidal symptoms are usually observed during the disease progression. Although myoclonus is infrequent as a presenting symptom, it is observed during the clinical course in almost the totality of cases. Epileptic seizures, either focal or generalized, usually occur later in the progression of the disease, in the 8–9% of cases. Symptoms appear in a rapidly progressive course and death occurs often within 1 year.

EEG is an essential part of the diagnostic process and it is included, together with clinical and CSF features (presence of abnormal protein 14-3-3), both in the WHO and in the MRI-CJD diagnostic criteria of sCJD [21, 23].

EEG activity changes over the sCJD course with different features. In the early stage (first 8–9 weeks), characterized clinically by cognitive and behavioral disturbances, nonspecific EEG abnormalities are usually observed; these are represented by diffuse slowing and disorganization of background activity and occasional predominantly frontal Generalized Rhythmic Delta Activity (GRDA).

In the middle stage, after a time average of 10 weeks and clinically dominated by abundant myoclonic jerks and sensorimotor and cerebellar dysfunction, an almost pathognomonic EEG pattern appears: continuous generalized bisynchronous Periodic Sharp Wave Complexes (PSWCs) (Fig. 39.7).

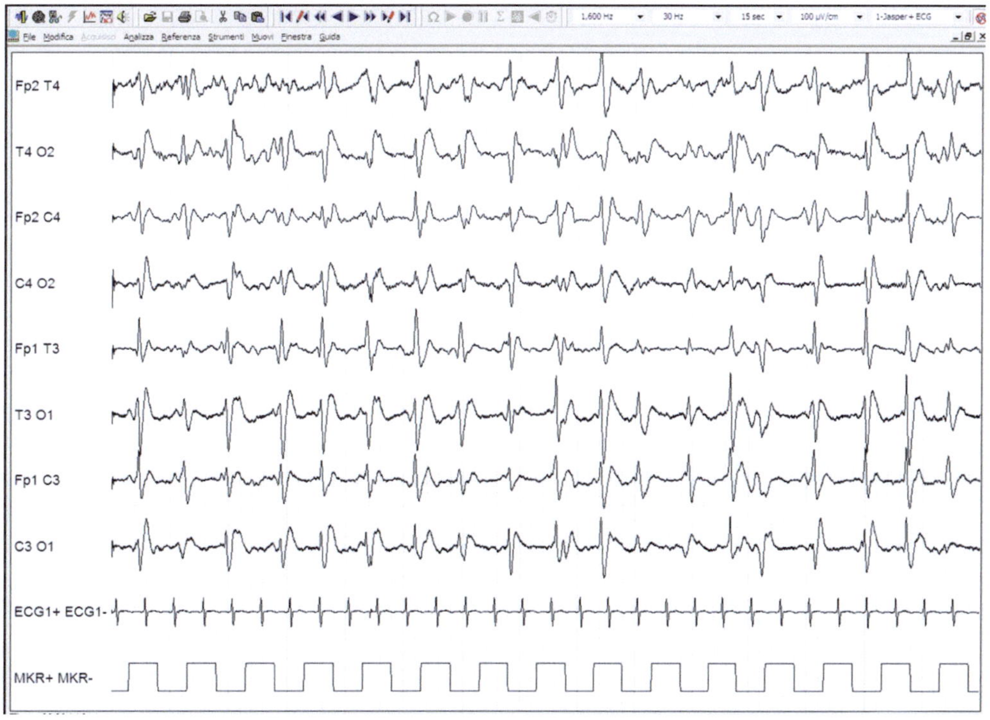

Fig. 39.7 Periodic short-interval diffuse discharges, predominant in the left hemisphere, in a 64-year-old female patient with sporadic Creutzfeldt-Jakob disease

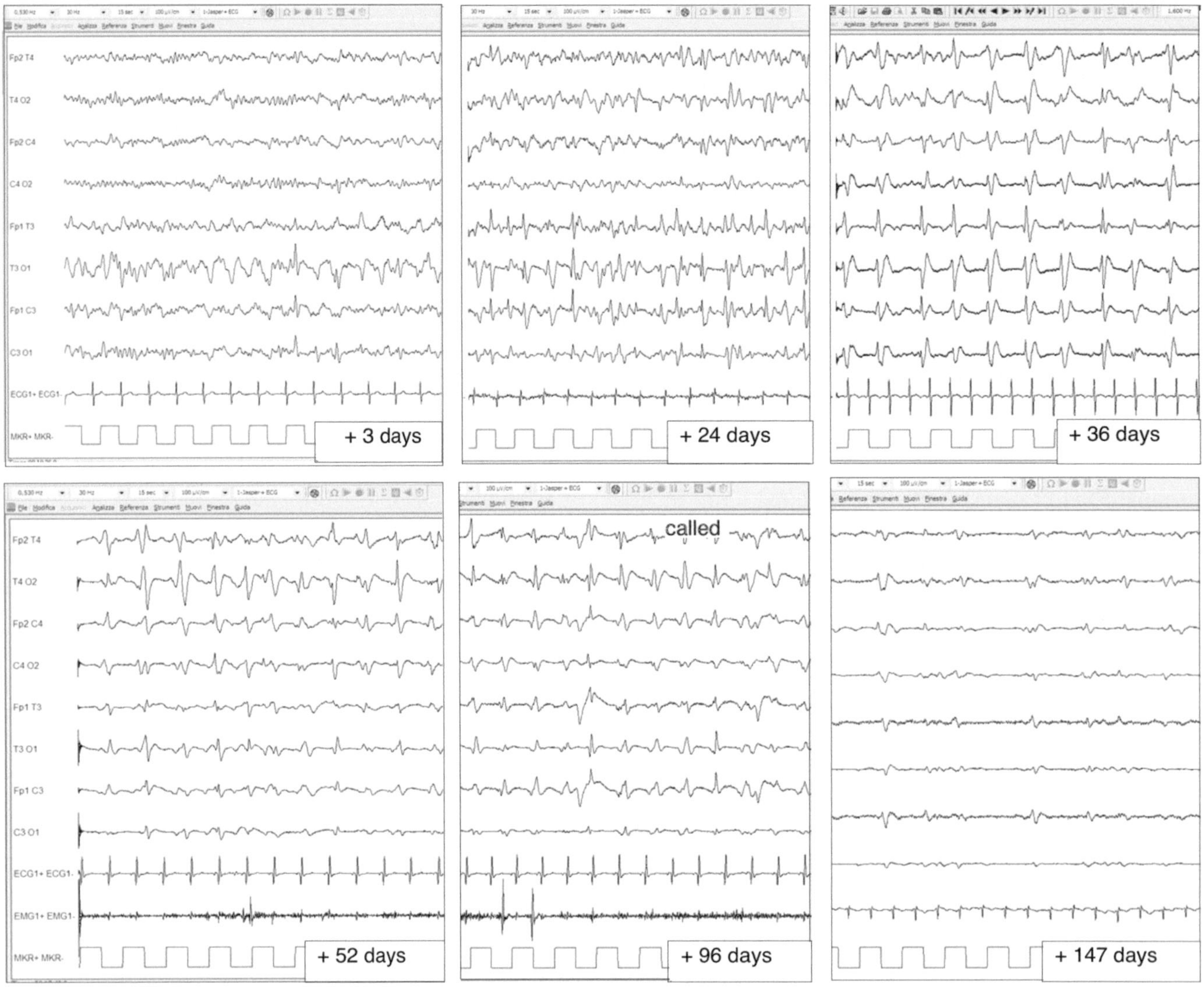

Fig. 39.8 EEG evolution in a 71-year-old female patient with sporadic Creutzfeldt-Jacob disease. EEG performed 3 days after hospital admission showed left temporal slow activity with rare sharp waves. At that phase, she appeared disoriented and manifested behavioral alterations, headache and visual disturbances. EEG performed after 24 days demonstrated left quasi-periodic epileptiform abnormalities. After 36 days, EEG showed a diffuse periodic activity predominant in the left hemisphere. From days 52 and 96, periodic complexes were more evident in the right hemisphere and the EEG activity was poorly reactive to acoustic and nociceptive stimuli; the patient also did not show reactions to external stimuli and had myoclonic jerks, not always correlated to periodic EEG abnormalities. Three days before exitus (day 147), electrocortical diffuse attenuation with low-amplitude periodic abnormalities was recorded

In the last stage, usually lasting 3 to 4 months and clinically characterized by a severe dementia evolving to akinetic mutism or even coma, unreactive EEG tracings with predominantly slow waves, low-voltage activity, or—rarely—an alpha-coma pattern may be observed. In more advanced stages, burst suppression and then diffuse suppression patterns are likely evident (Fig. 39.8) [4].

Atypical EEG patterns may also be observed, with bifrontal sharp waves that are quasi-periodic or even with multifocal spike-and-wave discharges [4].

However, PSWCs are the hallmark EEG finding in patients with sCJD and may be missed if the EEG is performed too early or, less commonly, too late in the course of the disease [24]. For this reason, it is essential to perform seriated EEG recordings overall the disease course.

Typical PSWCs may consist of both simple sharp waves, biphasic or triphasic, and complexes with mixed spikes, polyspikes and slow waves of 150–300 μV amplitude, with a typical 100–600 ms duration, recurring every 0.5–2 s. PSWCs occur, in average, 12 weeks after the first symptoms, typically together with the appearance of myoclonic jerks [24, 25]. Topographically, PSWCs commonly reveal a bilateral voltage distribution with a fronto-precentral midline maximum.

PSWCs may or may not be related to the myoclonic jerks. Myoclonus in CJD can be classified according to its time course as periodic, rhythmic, or irregular and, in relation to the EMG pattern, as positive or negative. Polygraphic study reveals that positive EMG bursts of periodic myoclonus are always time-locked with PSWCs [26, 27].

PSWCs may also occur lateralized, especially at early disease stage, but with usual development into the typical sCJD bilateral PSWCs during the course of the disease [23].

However, differently from the LPDs, sCJD-associated lateralized PSWCs are not consistent with the transitory EEG discharges occurring during an acute brain lesion and they are influenced by external stimulation and sleep, being prominent during wakefulness and usually decreasing-until disappearing-during sleep.

With regard to EEG reactivity, it is important to underline that in the early stages, when PSWCs may still be absent, they may appear after external stimuli. As the disease progresses, photic, acoustic and somatosensory stimulations may also induce modifications in PSWCs frequency or even determine their appearance. Particularly, low-frequency intermittent photic stimulation may induce the appearance of rhythmic periodic complexes with frequency identical to that of the stimulation.

Moreover, seizures have been reported during the late phases of disease, and seizure-like EEG activity, in particular nonconvulsive status epilepticus must be carefully distinguished from PSWCs. Most problems concern the responsiveness of both PSWCs and epileptic activity to antiepileptic drugs, such as benzodiazepines. Therefore, EEG response to AEDs alone is not sufficient to conclude that the periodic discharges represent the EEG correlates of seizures [28, 29].

The following table (Table 39.1) summarises the clinical-electrophysiological correlations during the progression of sCJD.

With regard to PolySomnoGraphic (PSG) analysis, sleep abnormalities in patients with CJD, with or without sleep complaints are frequently observed. The most commonly observed PSG abnormalities are loss of normal sleep EEG architecture and the presence of sleep-disordered breathing. The lack of sleep spindles, K-complexes and vertex waves seems to be the main finding. Furthermore, REM sleep is less represented, as well as slow-wave sleep [30]. Terzano and colleagues (1995) [31] published a case report of serial PSGs in a single patient with CJD, which suggested that loss of physiologic sleep patterns might be associated with disease progression and follow this order: Sequences of sporadic sharp waves; pseudo-periodic discharges cyclically alternating with slow pseudo-rhythmic theta-delta activity; slow activity at 0.5–4 Hz poorly rhythmic.

Table 39.1 Clinical-electrophysiological correlations during the progression of sCJD

sCJD stages	Clinical features	EEG features
Stage I	Mild cognitive impairment Cerebellar dysfunction Behavioral disorders Visual alterations	Diffuse slowing and disorganization of background activity Predominantly frontal Generalized Rhytmic Delta Activity-GRDA
Stage II	Myoclonic jerks Extrapyramidal and pyramidal dysfunction Cerebellar dysfunction	Continuous generalized or even lateralized (initially) Periodic Sharp Wave Complexes (PSWCs)
Stage III	Severe dementia Severe myoclonic jerks Akinetic mutism Stupor/coma till death	PSWCs tend to disappear Slow waves Low-voltage activity Alpha coma (rare) Burst suppression Diffuse suppression

39.3.2 Genetic CJD (gCJD)

gCJD cases are associated with point mutations or insertions within the open reading frame of the PRioN Protein (PRNP) gene. Up to date, more than 20 mutations have been described. The clinical presentation of gCJD overlaps between mutations and may resemble patients with sCJD, although it seems to be associated with a younger age at onset and a longer clinical course [21, 24]. On the contrary, EEG abnormalities may be different . Although a typical CJD-EEG is more frequent in gCJD than in the other forms of genetic spongiform encephalopathies (Familial Fatal Insomnia and Gerstmann-Sträussler-Scheinker syndrome), overall PSWCs are uncommon in patients with gCJD, occurring in only about 10% of them [24].

39.3.2.1 Variant Creutzfeldt-Jakob Disease (vCJD)

vCJD, also known as “mad cow disease,” is strictly associated with Bovine Spongiform Encephalopathy (BSE), currently believed to be the only non-human PrD to be directly transmissible to humans. Transmission from affected cattle occurs through meat consumption. Compared to patients with sCJD, those affected by vCJD are usually younger, with a median age of onset at around 27 years (range 12–74 years). The mean disease duration is longer, ≈14.5 months compared with sCJD. Even if psychiatric symptoms may characterize the early stages of sCJD, prominent psychiatric symptoms are regularly the presenting symptoms in vCJD and they may be the only clinical feature for more than 6 months before clear neurologic symptoms arise [21].

PSWCs do not occur in patients with vCJD and this absence is considered characteristic, so that their absence is one of the diagnostic criteria for vCJD [32]. Normal EEG or non-specific slow-wave activity may be found.

39.3.2.2 Iatrogenic CJD (iCJD)

iCJD cases are very rare and may result from the use of cadaveric-derived human pituitary hormones, dura mater grafts, corneal transplants, reuse of EEG implanted depth electrodes, or other neurosurgical equipment.

EEG shows an evolutive pattern similar to that of the sCJD. Both PSWCs, lateralized or generalized, and slow-wave activity, focal or diffuse, have been described. Obviously, since this form is the result from the direct inoculation of the pathogen, the presence of prevailing EEG abnormalities in a specific cerebral site is more frequent, especially in the initial phases. In two patients contaminated with bifrontal deep electrodes, Wieser et al. (2004) [33] described the evolutionary phases of the EEG pattern during the course of the disease, from incubation to death, consisting of:

- Regional progressive unspecific slowing of background activity at the site of the infected electrode.
- Regional sharper slow theta-activity.
- Occasional frontal delta activity.
- PSWCs, first intermittent and with regional accentuation, then more stereotyped and finally symmetrical and generalized with prefrontal-midline maximum.
- Progressive disappearance of periodic complexes with attenuation/suppression of EEG activity.

The best solution to eradicating cross-contamination risk should be to remove and incinerate all materials coming in contact with any tissue other than the skin. However, due to the elevated costs of some invasive instruments, hospitals are generally reluctant to discard and replace them. On the other hand, some expensive instruments cannot endure the hard treatment that has been shown to ensure complete inactivation of prions (e.g., 1-h immersion in bleach or lye followed by 1-h autoclaving at 132 °C). Finally, the accuracy of more recently studied "gentle" methods to inactivate the proteins (e.g., immersion in detergents and proteinases in an alkaline solution or exposure to gaseous H_2O_2) still lacks verification in multiple independent laboratories.

In this situation, the best solution could be the institution of regional centers with a set of instruments dedicated for use on patients with proven or highly probable CJD. Hospitals should be able to access to these instruments, sharing the cost of their purchase, storage and handling. After their use, the instruments would be returned to the centers and decontaminated using "harsh" methods for durable instruments and one or more "gentle" methods for fragile instruments. Therefore, in order to avoid disease transmission through invasive instruments, patients with proven or highly probable CJD should undergo invasive procedures conducted with appropriate isolation protocols and dedicated instruments. Patients with possible CJD, even if unlikely, should be operated using the same isolation protocols, but with non-dedicated instruments. The instruments should be labeled and quarantined until a correct diagnosis had been established and then either sent to the regional center for dedicated instruments or returned to hospital service, depending on the diagnosis [34].

39.4 Neurosyphilis

Syphilitic involvement of the CNS can occur early or late in the course of the disease. According to the clinical pictures, Neuro Syphilis (NS) can present under the following forms: asymptomatic NS, syphilitic meningitis, meningovascular NS and parenchymal NS (including General Paresis (GP) and tabes dorsalis). GP has a peak incidence in 10–20 years after syphilitic infection. The clinical spectrum of GP is very wide and may include cognitive impairment, a delusional or apathetic state, dysarthria, myoclonus, intention tremor, seizures, hyperreflexia, and Argyll Robertson pupils [35].

EEG abnormalities depend on the brain structures involved, the rate of progression of the disease and the age of the patient. Epileptic discharges have been described, as seizures are known to occur in GP and meningovascular NS with a frequency from 14 to 60% [36]. Background EEG activity is slowed with bursts of diffuse or predominant anterior slow waves, which increase in relation to the progression of the disease. In some patients, LPDs have also been described, mostly on the fronto-temporal areas, in the absence of lesions detectable with neuroimaging. After pharmacological therapy, the improvement of the clinical conditions is generally observed, not necessarily related to the normalization of EEG abnormalities.

39.5 HIV-Related CNS Diseases

Human Immunodeficiency Virus (HIV), the viral pathogen responsible for Acquired Immuno Deficiency Syndrome (AIDS), is a neuroinvasive, neurotrophic and neurovirulent virus. Thus, it is able to determine meningoencephalitis independently from the occurrence of secondary opportunistic CNS infection, during the entire progression of the disease. The early CNS infection is usually asymptomatic, but CSF and imaging studies can detect abnormalities even during the "asymptomatic" period that presage later neurological events.

The most common CNS manifestation of HIV is the so-called HIV-Associated Neurocognitive Disorder (HAND), a chronic neurodegenerative condition characterized by cognitive, central motor, and behavioral abnormalities [37].

EEG in the asymptomatic phase of the disease is mostly normal, although a focal or diffuse slowing of background activity may be appreciated. As the disease progresses, slow activity increases, and rarely epileptic discharges may be found.

Furthermore, through opportunistic infections of the CNS, HIV increases the risk of other neurological manifestations. Toxoplasmosis, CNS lymphoma, cryptococcal or tuberculous meningitis and Progressive Multifocal Leukoencephalopathy (PML) are strongly associated with the occurrence of acute or chronic repeated seizures.

Although new-onset seizures are reported in a variable percentage of patients with HIV infection, ranging from 3 to 17% according to different studies, most of patients have unspecific EEG abnormalities, while epileptiform discharges are seen infrequently. This means that EEG is relatively insensitive in the setting of seizures associated with HIV infection. However, patients with more advanced HIV disease and those with neuroimaging abnormalities seem to be more likely to have abnormal EEG [38].

39.6 Brain Abscess and Subdural Empyema

Brain abscess and subdural empyema are severe life-threatening infectious diseases caused by bacteria, fungi or parasites. Both can result from contiguous site infections (such as skull osteomyelitis, chronic otitis, mastoiditis, sinusitis and dental infections), from the direct access of microorganisms after head trauma or neurosurgical procedures or from metastatic inoculation of the brain from distant extracranial sources (pulmonary, infection, endocarditis). The microbial dissemination tends to provoke multiple cerebral abscesses, while specific localizations are related to the area of primary infection or altered tissue integrity.

Neurological function can be impaired in different ways: direct destruction of nervous tissue, infarction after inflammatory occlusion of veins and arteries, or compression caused by a mass effect. EEG abnormalities vary according to several factors, such as the localization of the abscess, which may be supratentorial or subtentorial, and its severity. Supratentorial abscesses may be characterized by slow-wave focal activity, sometimes intermixed with epileptiform abnormalities (spikes or sharp waves) and associated with a diffuse slowing or attenuation/suppression of background activity on the interested hemisphere (Fig. 39.9). Clinical and/or electrographic seizures are not uncommon [4]. EEG in subtentorial abscesses is often normal, although non-specific slowing of background activity, sometimes with sequences of bilateral, monomorphic delta-theta waves, predominant in the anterior regions can be observed . In subdural empyema, EEG can show a depression of background activity in the infectious site in the late stages, with slow and epileptiform focal abnormalities, indicating a cortical involvement.

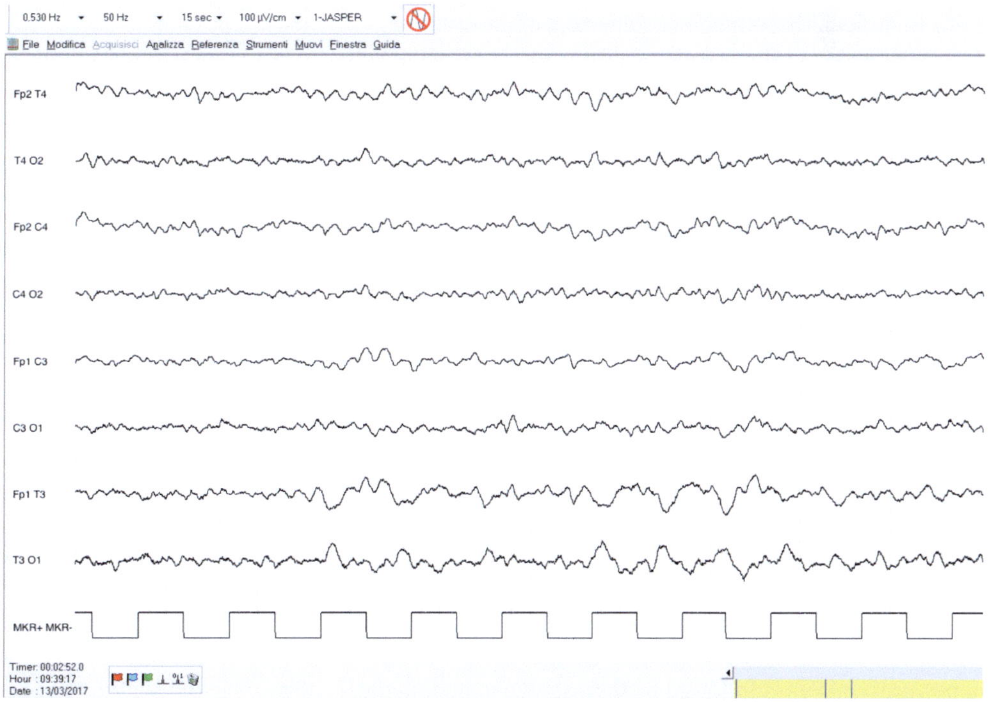

Fig. 39.9 45-year-old male patient with left temporal cerebral abscess. EEG shows focal monomorphic delta activity in the site of the abscess

39.7 Parasitic Brain Infections

Parasites that are able to affect the CNS include cestodes [(*Taenia solium*: neurocysticercosis), *Echinococcus granulosus* (cerebral cystic echinococcosis), *E. multilocularis* (cerebral alveolar echinococcosis)], nematodes (*Toxocara canis* and *T. cati* neurotoxocariasis), and protozoa [(*Toxoplasma gondii*: neurotoxoplasmosis), *Plasmodium falciparum* (cerebral malaria), and *Trypanosoma brucei* gambiense/rhodesiense (sleeping sickness) or *Trypanosoma cruzi* (cerebral Chagas disease)]. Adults or larvae of helminths or protozoa enter the CNS and cause meningitis, encephalitis, ventriculitis, myelitis, ischemic stroke, bleeding, venous thrombosis, or cerebral abscess, clinically manifesting as headache, epilepsy, weakness, cognitive decline, impaired consciousness, confusion, coma, or focal neurological deficits [39].

39.7.1 Neurotoxoplasmosis

Neurotoxoplasmosis is caused by the obligate intracellular protozoal parasite *Toxoplasma gondii*; the primary hosts are the cats and humans may represent an intermediate host, infected through the oral or the transplacental route.

Common sources of human infection are the consumption of undercooked meat from lamb or pork that contains viable tissue cysts or direct ingestion of oocytes from contaminated soil, water, goat's milk, or unwashed vegetables. In adults, most *T. gondii* infections are subclinical, but severe clinical manifestations occur in immune-compromised patients, especially in HIV-infected patients, in whom toxoplasmic encephalitis is particularly common. Involvement of the cerebral gray or white matter in these patients results in encephalitis with cerebral tissue destruction or abscess formation. Furthermore, it can result in a CNS mass lesion, presenting with headache, epilepsy, hemiparesis, psychosis and cognitive dysfunction. The basal ganglia, the thalami and the cortico-medullary junction are the most frequently affected structures [39].

EEG in infants with congenital infections may show several abnormalities: slowing of background activity; sequences of delta slow activity, both focal and diffuse; epileptiform patterns (even hypsarrhythmia). In adults, especially when toxoplasmosis gives rise to a mass lesion, EEG is demonstrative of focal slow abnormalities, sometimes intermixed with sharp waves.

39.7.2 Neurocysticercosis

Neurocysticercosis is caused by encysted larval stages of the tapeworm *Taenia solium*. Ingestion of eggs from the feces of tapeworm carriers is followed by their spread to neural, muscular or ocular tissue. Neurocysticercosis is the most common helminthic disease of the CNS, particularly in endemic areas where the parasite exchange between humans and pigs is maintained. Cerebral manifestations of neurocysticercosis include epilepsy (50–70%); headache (40%); hydrocephalus (33%); meningitis; aneurysm formation; stroke. Ischemic stroke occurs in 4–12% of the neurocysticercosis patients. Seizures, predominantly focal, are caused by the perilesional inflammation, stroke, vasculitis, or calcified granulomas [39].

EEG slow and epileptiform abnormalities may be focal or diffuse and their entity depends on the type, site and severity of the cerebral lesion.

39.7.3 Neurotoxocariasis

The genus *Toxocara* includes *Toxocara canis* and *Toxocara cati*, for which the definitive host is, respectively, the upper digestive tract of dogs and foxes. Human infection is the result of accidental ingestion of embryonated eggs from soils or ingestion of infected raw fruits and vegetables. These embryonated eggs then hatch in the small intestine and release immature larvae, which migrate to the liver via the portal circulation, then lungs and left heart, from where they further disseminate through the systemic circulation, especially to the muscles, optic nerves and, in rare cases, to the central nervous system [38]. Asymptomatic CNS infection is probably common. Clinically evident neurotoxocariasis consists of a wide spectrum of neurological manifestations such as eosinophilic meningitis, encephalitis, meningoencephalitis, ependymitis, arachnoiditis, vasculitis, meningomyelitis, meningoradiculitis, epilepsy, dementia or optic neuritis [39–41].

Encephalic/meningeal toxocariasis involvement was associated with a broad range of clinical manifestations including headache, seizures, focal deficits, confusional state and cognitive impairment, with or without fever [41].

EEG abnormalities, slow and epileptiform, depend on the lesion characteristics, especially on their location, that may be multiple, cortical, or subcortical.

39.7.4 Cerebral Cystic Echinococcosis (Cystic Hydatidosis)

Cerebral cystic echinococcosis is caused by infection with larvae of *Echinococcus granulosus*, a tapeworm which requires canines as definitive hosts and herbivores or humans as intermediate hosts.

Cystic echinococcosis is a self-limiting but potentially fatal disease, with CNS involvement in only 1–3% of cases

[39]. Generally, cysts are located within the parenchyma, the subarachnoid space, or the ventricles. Patients may present with headache, vomiting, hemiparesis and other focal neurological deficits, or seizures. EEG generally shows polymorphic focal slow-wave delta activity or sequences of monomorphic slow rhythms. Rarely, epileptiform discharges can be appreciated.

39.7.5 Trypanosomiasis

African trypanosomiasis (sleeping sickness) is caused by *Trypanosoma brucei*, which is transmitted via the bite of the tsetse fly. African trypanosomiasis follows two stages. In stage one the parasite proliferates within the hemolymphatic system, followed by stage two, in which the parasite invades the CNS, resulting in meningoencephalitis with progressive neurological dysfunction and a disrupted sleep–wake pattern. Patients are sleepy by day, but awake and restless by night. Encephalopathy may progress to an apallic syndrome/vegetative state/unresponsive wakefulness [39].

Wake EEG shows a diffuse slowing of background activity with bursts of bisynchronous slow waves recurring every 5–10 s. In more advanced stages of the disease, EEG activity becomes slower, background activity tends to disappear, and epileptic discharges are often observed, associated or not with clinical seizures. Sleep EEG doesn't show the typical NREM sleep graphoelements and a disorganization of sleep architecture is observed. Sleep is fragmented with frequent arousals, associated with muscle tone, respiratory and cardiac alterations, especially in the deepest sleep stages.

American trypanosomiasis (Chagas disease) is caused by *Trypanosoma cruzi*. In the acute stages, Chagas disease presents mainly with myocarditis and with megaesophagus and megacolon in the chronic stages. CNS involvement manifests as acute meningitis, which is a hallmark of the disease, or as multifocal, nodular encephalitis due to reactivation, occasionally complicated by a brain abscess. Also, patients with cardio-embolic stroke have been described. Isolated cases with CNS involvement may also present with dementia, confusion, or sensory or motor deficits. Cerebral Chagas disease is frequently associated with HIV [39]. As in other parasitoses, EEG slow and epileptiform abnormalities may be focal or diffuse, and their entity depends on the type, site, and severity of the cerebral lesion.

39.7.6 Cerebral Malaria

Cerebral malaria is the most severe complication of malignant tertian malaria. It is caused by *Plasmodium falciparum*, developing within the red blood cells.

It is clinically defined as unarousable coma in the absence of other potential causes but the presence of malaria-infected erythrocytes. Impaired consciousness with coma may occur spontaneously or may develop at least 1 h after termination of a seizure, following 1–3 days of fever, or after correction of hypoglycemia. Some patients develop headache, delirium or coma, following progressive weakness or prostration due to cerebral edema manifesting as brainstem signs or retinal changes, often associated with systemic complications. Some patients develop cortical infarcts or cerebral sinus venous thrombosis. Survivors have an increased risk of long-term complications such as cognitive impairment, speech and language problems, behavioral difficulties, or epilepsy [39].

Even in patients with minimal neurological manifestations, EEG may show mild alterations. When CNS involvement is wide, EEG abnormalities are significant and consist in bilateral theta-delta waves and, rarely, spikes and sharp waves. Electrical and clinical seizures are frequently observed.

References

1. Bartel P, Schutte CM, Becker P, van der Meyden C. Discrimination between viral and nonviral meningitis by visually analyzed and quantitative electroencephalography. Clin Electroencephalogr. 1999;30:35–8.
2. VanDemark M. Acute bacterial meningitis: current review and treatment update. Crit Care Nurs Clin North Am. 2013; 25: 351–61.
3. Heckenberg SG, Brouwer MC, van de Beek D. Bacterial meningitis. Handb Clin Neurol. 2014;121:1361–75.
4. Galovic M, Schmitz B, Tettenborn B. EEG in inflammatory disorders, cerebrovascular diseases, trauma and migraine. In: Shomer DL, Lopes da Silva FH, editors. Niedermeyer's electroencephalography: basic principles, clinical applications, and related fields. 7th ed. New York: Oxford University Press; 2018. p. 371–412.
5. Pardal-Fernández JM, Bengoa M, Carrascosa-Romero MC. Periodic Lateralized Epileptiform Discharges (PLEDs) and pneumococcal meningoencephalitis. Eur J Paediatr Neurol. 2012;16:749–52.
6. Sáez-Llorens X, Nieto-Guevara J. Brain abscess. Handb Clin Neurol. 2013;112:1127–34.
7. Konno S, Sugimoto H, Nemoto H, et al. Triphasic waves in a patient with tuberculous meningitis. J Neurol Sci. 2010;291:114–7.
8. Zunt JR, Baldwin KJ. Chronic and subacute meningitis. Continuum (Minneap Minn). 2012;18:1290–318.
9. Kalita J, Misra UK. EEG changes in tuberculous meningitis: a clinicoradiological correlation. Electroencephalogr Clin Neurophysiol. 1998;107:39–43.
10. Patwari AK, Aneja S, Ravi RN, Singhal PK, Arora SK. Convulsions in tuberculous meningitis. J Trop Pediatr. 1996;42:91–7.
11. Jarrin I, Sellier P, Lopes A, et al. Etiologies and management of aseptic meningitis in patients admitted to an internal medicine department. Medicine (Baltimore). 2016;95(2):e2372.
12. Pollak L, Klein C, Schiffer J, Flechter S, Rabey J. Electroencephalographic abnormalities in aseptic meningitis and noninfectious headache. A comparative study. Headache. 2001;41:79–83.
13. Young GB. Encephalopathy of infection and systemic inflammation. J Clin Neurophysiol. 2013;30:454–61.

14. Sutter R, Kaplan PW, Cervenka MC, et al. Electroencephalography for diagnosis and prognosis of acute encephalitis. Clin Neurophysiol. 2015;126:1524–31.
15. Jordan B, Kösling S, Emmer A, Koch A, Müller T, Kornhuber M. A study on viral CNS inflammation beyond herpes encephalitis. J Neurovirol. 2016;22:763–73.
16. Lai CW, Gragasin ME. Electroencephalography in herpes simplex encephalitis. J Neurophysiol. 1988;5:87–103.
17. Gutierrez J, Issacson RS, Koppel BS. Subacute sclerosing panencephalitis: an update. Dev Med Child Neurol. 2010;52:901–7.
18. Yemisci M, Gurer G, Saygi S, Ciger A. Generalised periodic epileptiform discharges: clinical features, neuroradiological evaluation and prognosis in 37 adult patients. Seizure. 2003;12:465–72.
19. Ekmekci O, Karasoy H, Gokcay A, Ulku A. Atypical EEG findings in subacute sclerosing panencephalitis. Clin Neuro- physiol. 2005;116: 1762–7.
20. Demir N, Cokar O, Bolukbasi F, et al. A close look at EEG in subacute sclerosing panencephalitis. J Clin Neurophysiol. 2013;30: 348–56.
21. Takada LT, Geschwind MD. Prion diseases. Semin Neurol. 2013; 33:348–56.
22. Imran M, Mahmood S. An overview of human prion diseases. Virol J. 2011;8:559.
23. Zerr I, Kallenberg K, Summers DM, et al. Updated clinical diagnostic criteria for sporadic Creutzfeldt-Jakob disease. Brain. 2009;132: 2659–8.
24. Wieser HG, Schindler K, Zumsteg D. EEG in Creutzfeldt–Jakob disease. Clin Neurophysiol. 2006;117:935–51.
25. Marquetand J, Knake S, Strzelczyk A, et al. Periodic EEG patterns in sporadic Creutzfeldt-Jakob-disease can be benzodiazepine-responsive and be difficult to distinguish from non-convulsive status epilepticus. Seizure. 2017;53:47–50.
26. Hashimoto T, Iwahashi T, Ishii W, Yamamoto K, Ikeda S. EEG–EMG polygraphic study of dystonia and myoclonus in a case of Creutzfeldt–Jakob disease. Epilepsy Behav Case Rep. 2015:4: 30–2.
27. Binelli S, Agazzi P, Canafoglia L, et al. Myoclonus in Creutzfeldt-Jakob disease: polygraphic and video-electroencephalography assessment of 109 patients. Mov Disord. 2010;25:2818–27.
28. Lapergue B, Dermeret S, Denys V, et al. Sporadic Creutzfeldt-Jacob disease mimicking nonconvulsive status epilepticus. Neurology. 2010;74:1995–9.
29. Fernandez-Torre JL, Solar DM, Astudillo A, Cereceda R, Acebes A, Calatayud MT. Creutzfeldt-Jakob disease and nonconvulsive status epilepticus: a clinical and electroencephalographic follow-up study. Clin Neurphysiol. 2004;115:316–9.
30. Kang P, de Bruin GS, Wang LH, et al. Sleep pathology in Creutzfeldt-Jakob disease. J Clin Sleep Med. 2016;12:1033–9.
31. Terzano MG, Parrino L, Pietrini V, et al. Precocious loss of physiologic sleep in a case of Creutzfeldt Jakob disease: a serial polygraphic study. Sleep. 1995;18:849–58.
32. World Health Organisation. The revision of the surveillance case definition for variant Creutzfeldt–Jakob Disease (vCJD). Report of a WHO consultation Edinburgh, United Kingdom. 2001. http://whqlibdoc.who.int/hq/2002/WHO_CDS_CSR_EPH_2001.5.pdf.
33. Wieser HG, Schwarz U, Blättler T, et al. Serial EEG findings in sporadic and iatrogenic CreutzfeldtJakob disease. Clin Neurophysiol. 2004;115:2467–78.
34. Brown P, Farrell M. A practical approach to avoiding iatrogenic Creutzfeldt-Jakob disease (CJD) from invasive instruments. Infect Control Hosp Epidemiol. 2015;36:844–8.
35. Chen YY, Zhang YF, Qiu XH, et al. Clinical and laboratory characteristics in patients suffering from general paresis in the modern era. J Neurol Sci. 2015;15:79–83.
36. Noone ML, Sinha S, Taly AB, Chandrika S. Periodic lateralized epileptiform discharges in neurosyphilis. Epilepsia. 2007;48: 390–3.
37. Singer EJ, Valdes-Sueiras M, Commins D, Levine A. Neurologic presentations of AIDS. Neurol Clin. 2010;28:253–75.
38. Siddiqi OK, Elafros MA, Sikazwe I, et al. Acute EEG findings in HIV-infected Zambian adults with new-onset seizure. Neurology. 2015;84:1317–22.
39. Finsterer J, Auer H. Parasitoses of the human central nervous system. J Helminthol. 2013;87:257–70.
40. Deshayes S, Bonhomme J, de La Blanchardière A. Neurotoxocariasis: a systematic literature review. Infection. 2016;44:565–74.
41. Sánchez SS, García HH, Nicoletti A. Clinical and magnetic resonance imaging findings of Neurotoxocariasis. Front Neurol. 2018;9:53.

40 Autoimmune and Inflammatory Encephalopathies

Andrea Stabile and Flavio Villani

40.1 Autoimmune Encephalitides

Autoimmune encephalitides represent a group of neurological disorders characterized by various symptoms suggestive of limbic or diffuse cortical dysfunction occurring in association with antibodies directed to intracellular or cell-surface neuronal antigens. In the past 10 years, an increasing number of antibodies have been identified, but only in 2016 criteria for autoimmune encephalitis, based on conventional neurological evaluation and standard diagnostic tests, such as cerebrospinal fluid (CSF) analysis, magnetic resonance imaging (MRI), and electroencephalography (EEG), have been proposed (Table 40.1).

Antibody testing still remains essential to confirm diagnosis and refine therapy, but initiation of an immunomodulatory treatment should not be delayed [1]. Compared to previous guidelines for encephalitis diagnosis [2, 3], these criteria underline the most common clinical and paraclinical features of autoimmune encephalitis [4]. EEG findings are rarely specific. However, EEG may play an important role in the diagnosis of definite form of encephalitis (e.g., extreme delta brush [5]), in the differential diagnosis of other disorders or to reveal subclinical seizures and nonconvulsive status epilepticus (SE) [1].

Annual incidence of encephalitides of any etiology reaches 2–3 cases/100,000 in Northern Europe. Among them, 40% are infectious, 40% are due to unknown causes, and at least 20% have a supposed immune-mediated etiology [6]. Autoimmune encephalitides can be classified according to the autoantibody specificity in two major groups: encephalitides associated with antibodies against neuronal intracellular antigens and encephalitides associated with antibodies against neuronal surface antigens (Table 40.2).

Table 40.1 Diagnostic criteria for possible autoimmune encephalitis, adapted from ref. [1]

Diagnosis can be made when all three of the following criteria have been met:
1. Subacute onset (rapid progression of less than 3 months) of working memory deficits (short-term memory loss), altered mental status[a], or psychiatric symptoms
2. At least one of the following:
• New focal CNS findings
• Seizures not explained by a previously known seizure disorder
• CSF pleocytosis (white blood cell count of more than 5 cells per mm^3)
• MRI features suggestive of encephalitis[b]
3. Reasonable exclusion of alternative causes[c]

CNS central nervous system

[a]Altered mental status defined as decreased or altered level of consciousness, lethargy, or personal change

[b]Brain MRI hyperintense signal on T2-weighted fluid-attenuated inversion recovery (FLAIR) sequences highly restricted to one or both medial temporal lobes or in multifocal areas involving gray matter, white matter, or both, compatible with demyelination or inflammation

[c]CNS infections, especially herpes simplex virus encephalitis; septic encephalopathy; metabolic encephalopathy; drug toxicity; cerebrovascular disease; neoplastic disorders; Creutzfeldt-Jakob disease; epileptic disorders; rheumatologic disorders (e.g., lupus, sarcoidosis, other); Kleine-Levin; Reye syndrome (children); mitochondrial diseases; inborn errors of metabolism (children)

Antibodies directed to neuronal intracellular antigens target both intranuclear (Hu, Ri, Ma1, Ma2/Ta) and cytoplasmic (CRMP5/CV2, GAD) neuronal proteins and are not directly pathogenic but indicate a cytotoxic T-cell-mediated immune response against neurons. At this category belong the "well-characterized" onconeural antibodies (anti-Hu, Yo, CRMP5/CV2, Ri, Ma2, amphiphysin antibodies), directed against neural antigens expressed by tumors, which, even in the absence of a detected neoplasm, can be used to classify encephalitis as a "definite paraneoplastic syndrome" [9]. By contrast, *antibodies directed to neuronal surface antigens*

A. Stabile
Division of Clinical and Experimental Epileptology, Foundation IRCCS Neurological Institute "Carlo Besta", Milan, Italy

Department of Neurology, San Gerardo Hospital ASST Monza, University of Milano Bicocca, Monza, Italy

F. Villani (✉)
Epilepsy Monitoring Unit "Paolo Zorzi", Division of Clinical and Experimental Epileptology, Foundation IRCCS Neurological Institute "Carlo Besta", Milan, Italy
e-mail: flavio.villani@istituto-besta.it

O. Mecarelli (ed.), *Clinical Electroencephalography*, https://doi.org/10.1007/978-3-030-04573-9_40

Table 40.2 Antibodies in the diagnosis of autoimmune encephalitis, adapted from ref. [1]

	Syndrome	Frequency of cancer	Main type of cancer
Antibodies against neuronal intracellular antigens			
Hu	LE	>95%	SCLC
Ri [7][a]	Encephalitis [7]	...	Breast cancer [7]
Ma1 [7]	LE [7]	>90% [8]	Diverse (lung, skin, gastrointestinal, and renal) [7]
Ma2/Ta	LE[b]	>95%	Testicular seminoma
CRMP5/CV2 [7]	LE [7]	>90% [8]	Thymoma, SCLC [7]
GAD	LE[c]	25%[d]	Thymoma, SCLC
Antibodies against neuronal surface antigens			
NMDAR	Anti-NMDAR encephalitis	Varies with age and gender	Ovarian teratoma[e]
AMPAR	LE	65%	Thymoma, SCLC
$GABA_B$ receptors	LE	50%	SCLC
$GABA_A$ receptors	Encephalitis	<5%	Thymoma
mGluR5	Encephalitis	70%	Hodgkin's lymphoma
Dopamine2 receptors	Basal ganglia encephalitis	0%	...
LGI1	LE	5–10%	Thymoma
CASPR2	Morvan's syndrome[f] or LE	20–50%	Thymoma[g]
DPPX6	Encephalitis[h]	<10%	Lymphoma

LE limbic encephalitis, *SCLC* small-cell lung carcinoma, *CRMP5/CV2* collapsin response-mediator protein 5, *GAD* glutamic acid decarboxylase, *NMDAR* N-methyl-D-aspartate receptor, *AMPAR* α-amino-3-hydroxy-5-methylisoxazole-4-propionic acid receptor, *GABA* γ-aminobutyric acid, *mGluR5* metabotropic glutamate receptor 5, *LGI1* leucine-rich glioma inactivated 1, *CASPR2* contactin-associated protein-like 2, *DPPX6* dipeptidyl-peptidase-like protein 6

[a]More associated with opsoclonus myoclonus syndrome

[b]LE frequently associated with hypothalamic and mesencephalic involvement

[c]GAD autoantibodies occur more frequently in patient with stiff person syndrome and cerebellar ataxia. The association with cancer preferentially occurs in patients with LE

[d]Tumor found more frequently in men older than 50 years

[e]Ovarian teratoma usually found in young women aged 12–45 years

[f]Morvan's syndrome usually has a more chronic clinical course but might present with predominant cognitive and behavioral symptoms fulfilling criteria of possible autoimmune encephalitis

[g]Thymoma associated with Morvan's syndrome rather than LE

[h]Encephalitis associated with diarrhea and hyperekplexia

target synaptic receptors (NMDAR, AMPAR, GABA receptor, mGluR5, dopamine-2 receptors) as well as ion channels, such as voltage-gated potassium channel (VGKC) and associated proteins (LGI1, CASPR2, DPPX6) and exert a direct pathogenic effect on neuronal cells. These encephalitides differ from the first group in several important aspects, among them are (1) association with malignancy is much less consistent and (2) symptoms can more commonly be reversed by treatment, since they are due to functional disruption of the target antigens [1, 7, 8].

Table 40.3 Diagnostic criteria for definite autoimmune LE, adapted from ref. [1]

Diagnosis can be made when all four[a] of the following criteria have been met:
1. Subacute onset (rapid progression of less than 3 months) of working memory deficits, seizures, or psychiatric symptoms suggesting involvement of the limbic system
2. Bilateral brain abnormalities on T2-weighted FLAIR MRI highly restricted to medial temporal lobes[b]
3. At least one of the following:
• CSF pleocytosis (white blood cell count of more than 5 cells per mm^3)
• EEG with epileptic or slow-wave activity involving the temporal lobes
4. Reasonable exclusion of alternative causes (see Table 40.1, point 3)

[a]If one of the first three criteria is not met, a diagnosis of definite LE can be made only with the detection of antibodies against cell-surface or onconeural proteins

[b]Fluorodeoxyglucose (FDG) positron emission tomography (PET) can be used to fulfill this criterion

40.1.1 Anti-intracellular Neuronal Antigen Encephalitides

A substantial number of patients affected by encephalitides associated with antibodies directed to intracellular neuronal antigens present with a well-defined syndrome, represented by LE. Recently, new diagnostic criteria have been proposed for autoimmune LE (Table 40.3).

Although antibodies status is not considered, it is still a fundamental piece of information for the diagnosis. In patients not satisfying the other indicated criteria, it may confirm the diagnosis of autoimmune LE. Furthermore, since LE can recognize a paraneoplastic origin, mostly when associated with onconeural antibodies, the presence of a particular antibody type clarifies the immunological subgroup with comorbidities, tumor association, and prognosis [1]. Clinically, LE displays seizures with a focal onset. Focal seizures originating from the temporal lobe represent the most common type, even if generalized and focal motor or sensory seizures, suggesting an extratemporal involvement, may occur. Seizures may be the presenting symptom and rapidly become drug-resistant [10, 11]. EEG has a fundamental role in identifying interictal and ictal epileptiform activities [12], to monitor patients with subclinical or clinically overt SE [13], and, finally, to monitor the response to immunological and antiepileptic drug treatment [12]. Among the EEG findings of LE, nonspecific irregular theta-delta abnormalities are considered the most common. They are variable in severity and sometimes intermixed with a relatively well-retained background activity. Generalized slowing correlates with clinical and MRI evidence of a more widespread CNS engagement; instead, focal slowing classically involves the temporal regions [11], less frequently the frontal regions [12], and rarely the entire hemisphere. Focal epileptiform activity is observed in 50% of patients, particularly in those with clinical seizures and mesial temporal regions MRI abnormalities [11]. They are most prominent at the anterior temporal electrodes, consistent with an origin from the mesial temporal region [14]. Most patients have unilateral temporal epileptiform activity, but bilateral or multifocal independent temporal spikes and sharp waves have also been registered. Epileptiform abnormalities may be associated with focal slowing in the same region. Rarely, a limited number of patients, all of whom with clinical and electrographic seizures, showed periodic lateralized epileptiform discharges (PLEDs) predominantly involving the temporal region and representing in this setting either a peri-ictal phenomenon or an acute or subacute irritative focus [11]. Interestingly, the neuropsychiatric symptoms of LE with a prolonged waxing and waning course remarkably overlap the clinical features of a possible mesial temporal or limbic SE. In prolonged cases of LE, scalp EEG usually does not show any ictal patterns but reveals a nonspecific diffuse or focal rhythmic delta activity (RDA). Attenuation of this activity after benzodiazepines administration accompanied by subsequent clinical improvement could be taken as evidence of seizures or even a nonconvulsive limbic SE [15].

40.1.2 Anti-cell-Surface Neuronal Antigen Encephalitides

There are currently 16 known disorders with autoantibodies against cell-surface neuronal antigens, more than 10 manifesting as autoimmune encephalitides [16]. Since 2007, when the first target of autoimmune encephalitis was characterized molecularly (NMDAR) [17], the rate of discovery has been almost one new autoantigen per year, the most recent being at this moment IgLON5 [18] and neurexin-3α [19].

40.1.2.1 Anti-NMDAR Encephalitis

Anti-NMDAR encephalitis is a multistage diffuse cortico-subcortical encephalopathy, which presents with a severe syndrome characterized by a precise sequence of symptoms [20]. Young individuals are predominantly affected with a female predominance (F:M 4:1). Underlying tumor is present in 0–5% of children younger than 12 years and in 58% of women older than 18 years (usually an ovarian teratoma) [21]. In teenagers and adults, the clinical presentation can recognize the following stages: (1) a *prodromal phase*, in which fever, respiratory tract infections, gastrointestinal symptoms, and headache can occur [22]; (2) an *early stage*, with abnormal behavior (psychosis, delusion, hallucinations, agitation, irritability, aggression, or catatonia) and insomnia, memory deficit, and speech dysfunction; and (3) a *later stage*, within 1–2 weeks, characterized by movement disorders (orofacial dyskinesia, choreoathetoid involuntary movements, alternating with mutism and catatonia), autonomic instability, hypoventilation, and often reduced consciousness, requiring admission to intensive care unit (ICU) [1, 23]. Seizures can take place at any stage but tend to occur earlier in males. Indeed, adult male patients more often have focal seizures at onset and psychiatric or cognitive symptoms occurring few days later (median 12 days) [24]. In addition, young children more frequently present with abnormal movements or seizures. MRI abnormalities have been described either at cortical level (usually in the limbic mediotemporal cortex) or subcortically in the brainstem, the basal ganglia, or the cerebellum. Rarely, FLAIR hyperintensities or contrast enhancement in cortical meninges or basal ganglia is detected. In some patients, mesial temporal or frontotemporal atrophy can develop [17, 20, 25–28]. Treatment can improve dramatically this condition, if started promptly. Two independent predictors of good outcome are the lower severity of symptoms, with no need for ICU admission, and the early initiation of immunotherapy and tumor removal, when appropriate. Relapse risk is esteemed around 12% within 2 years [21]. On the basis of these data, criteria for anti-NMDAR encephalitis have been proposed (Table 40.4).

Although no EEG abnormalities may be present at disease onset, widespread interictal epileptiform activity can be seen in some patients during the *early stage* of the disease. Seizures have been reported in 76% of adults and 77% of children, and only a small percentage of patients have an EEG correlate [5]. At *later stages* this activity is more commonly replaced by high-amplitude diffuse or predominantly frontotemporal slowing [20]. In a series of 23 patients under continuous EEG (cEEG), monitoring diffuse slowing of the background activity was present in the 91% of patients whereas focal slowing only in 34%. Generalized RDA was observed in the 47.8% of patients, and 61% of patients had electrographic seizures [5] (Fig. 40.1). Other authors confirmed these data: at the disease peak stage, nearly all (98.4%) patients had an abnormal EEG with diffuse slowing being the most common correlate [22, 29, 30]. At the same stage of disease, abnormal brain MRI rate was 46.8%, suggesting that EEG was more sensitive than MRI for diagnosis [30]. Ikeda et al. were the first to suggest that anti-NMDAR encephalitis could have a specific EEG pattern that they termed "burst and slow complexes" [31]. A novel, unique, electrographic pattern has been confirmed in subsequent studies and has been named *extreme delta brush* (*EDB*). EDB consists in a continuous rhythmic delta (1–3 Hz) activity with superimposed bursts of rhythmic beta (20–30 Hz) activity "riding" on each delta wave. It is most often sym-

Table 40.4 Diagnostic criteria for anti-NMDAR encephalitis, adapted from ref. [1]

Probable anti-NMDAR encephalitis[a]
Diagnosis can be made when all three of the following criteria have been met:
1. Rapid onset (less than 3 months) of at least four of the six following major groups of symptoms:
• Abnormal (psychiatric) behavior or cognitive dysfunction
• Speech dysfunction (logorrhea, verbal reduction, mutism)
• Seizures
• Movement disorders, dyskinesias, or rigidity/abnormal postures
• Decreased level of consciousness
• Autonomic dysfunction or cerebral hypoventilation
2. At least one of the following laboratory study results:
• Abnormal EEG (focal or diffuse slow or disorganized activity, epileptic activity, or extreme delta brush)
• CSF pleocytosis or oligoclonal bands
3. Reasonable exclusion of other disorders (see Table 40.1, point 3)
Diagnosis can also be made in the presence of three of the above groups of symptoms accompanied by a teratoma
Definite anti-NMDAR encephalitis
Diagnosis can be made in the presence of one or more of the six major groups of symptoms and IgG anti-glutamate receptor N1 subunit antibodies[b], after a reasonable exclusion of other disorders (see Table 40.1, point 3)

IgG Immunoglobulin G

[a]Patients with a history of herpes simplex virus encephalitis in the previous weeks might have relapsing immune-mediated neurological symptoms (post-herpes simplex encephalitis)

[b]Antibody testing should include testing of CSF. If only serum is available, confirmatory tests should be included (e.g., live neurons or tissue immunohistochemistry in addition to cell-based assay)

metric and synchronous, spreads over all head regions, and does not vary with sleep-wake cycles, stimulation, or level of arousal (Fig. 40.2). It has been reported in 30% of the cases [5]. EDB may emerge early in the disease course, mainly at the peak stage, and gradually disappear at the recovery stage [30]. The ictal versus interictal nature of this novel pattern is still unclear. Since neither benzodiazepines nor antiepileptic drugs were able to determine a clinical or electrographical improvement of patients with EDB, it has been considered lying on the ictal-interictal continuum [32]. Currently, the prognosis of patients with EDB is still controversial [30]. Previous studies have shown that EDB patients had a worse outcome: they were hospitalized and monitored with cEEG longer and were unexpectedly more likely to have a normal brain MRI and, generally, demonstrated a higher Rankin Scale score at discharge (4.0 ± 0.8 vs 3.1 ± 1.1 seen in patients without EDB), suggesting that this pattern could be predictive of a more aggressive phenotype [5, 33, 34]. Early detection of EDB pattern in a coherent clinical context, as well as in atypical cases [30], should raise a strong suspicion of anti-NMDAR encephalitis, prompting early treatment. Hence, cEEG monitoring is highly recommended in a patient affected by an encephalitis of unknown cause [5]. Abbas et al. reported in a case of NMDAR encephalitis besides EDB the abrupt onset of short (5 s) paroxysmal rhythmic activity evolving in frequency and amplitude. Such a pattern is termed as *brief ictal rhythmic discharge* (*BIRD*). From a practical perspective, patients with these abnormalities,

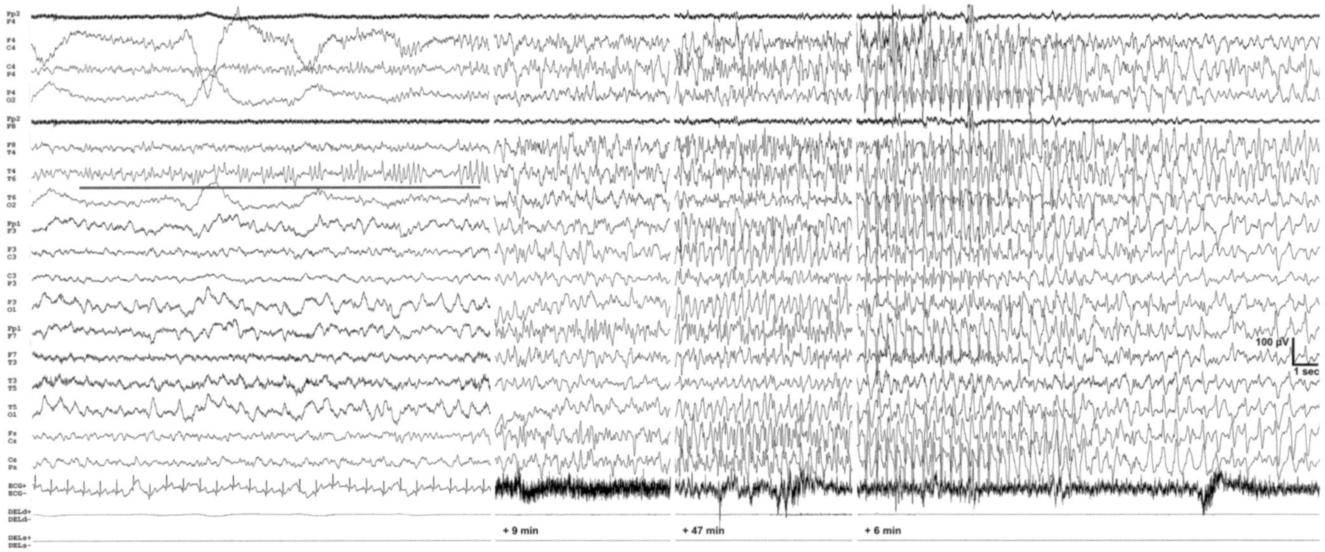

Fig. 40.1 Electrographic seizure in a 21-year-old female patient with anti-NMDAR encephalitis under cEEG monitoring. Marked asymmetry of the background activity still represented on the right hemisphere; on the left hemisphere, background activity is substituted by high-amplitude irregular theta-delta waves. The ictal rhythmic discharge starts on the right posterior temporal regions (*underlined*) and spreads diffusely over homo- and contralateral cerebral areas

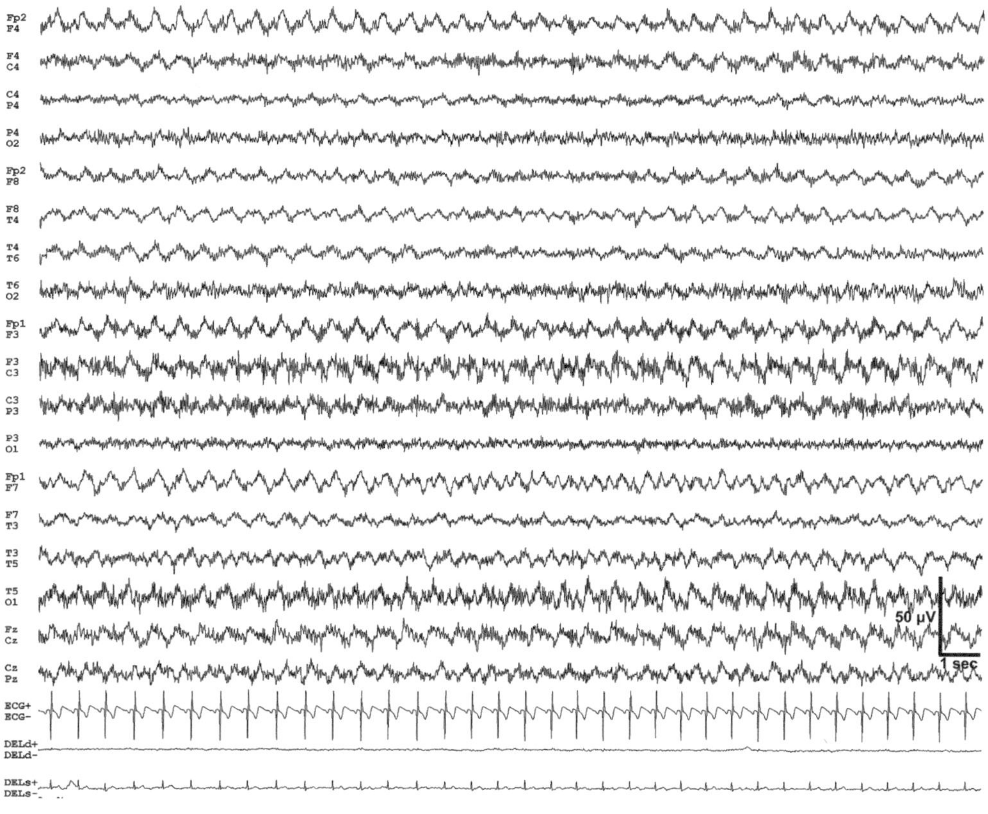

Fig. 40.2 Extreme delta brush: the pattern is observed in the same patient with anti-NMDAR encephalitis under cEEG monitoring. The EEG tracing shows rhythmic delta activity, at 1.5–2 Hz, with superimposed fast activity in the beta range, bilaterally diffuse, but predominant on the anterior and temporal regions of the left hemisphere

similarly to PLEDs, have a significantly higher risk of developing full-length electrographic seizures [35, 36]. Focusing on a small case series of nine children aged 1.5–15 years with anti-NMDAR encephalitis, Gitiaux et al. found two main electro-clinical presentations correlating with cognitive outcome: one group presented mostly unilateral, focal, or hemispheric, continuous slow (0.5–3 Hz) waves with persistence of normal background activity and physiological figures on at least one hemisphere on waking and sleep EEG. These abnormalities were associated with abnormal movements (myoclonic jerks or dystonic postures) contralateral to the focal or unihemispheric slow-wave activity. These movements either had no EEG changes or were accompanied by an increase in frequency of slow activity, sometimes generating rhythmic discharges, and disappearing in sleep. These features predict a better outcome. In the second group, high-amplitude diffuse slow waves with lack of physiological background activity during waking and sleep states were associated with severe neurological impairment, generalized dystonia with choreoathetosis, and orofacial dyskinesia, with no EEG correlate. This group showed a poor outcome [37]. In another small series of three patients with anti-NMDAR encephalitis under cEEG monitoring, Da Silva-Júnior et al. indicated that generalized RDA is a common finding. This pattern usually persists for minutes-hours and is replaced by periods of nonspecific irregular theta or delta activity. It is synchronous; occurs in a monotonous manner not clearly evolving in frequency, voltage, or field; is not related to body or facial movements; and does not disappear with intravenous benzodiazepine administration. Like EDB, it could be absent on routine EEG recordings and may remain unchanged for months after disease onset. Hence, serial or cEEG may be necessary to discover its presence. The significance of generalized RDA and EDB is still incompletely understood. Although generalized RDA was recognized as a form of nonconvulsive SE in previous cases [38], it should not be interpreted as indicative of ictal activity or nonconvulsive SE, unless clear frequency, voltage, or field evolution and both electrographic and clinical response to a benzodiazepine have been observed [33].

40.1.2.2 Anti-VGKC-Complex Encephalitides: Anti-LGI1 and Anti-CASPR2 Encephalitis

From 2000 LE associated with VGKC autoantibodies has been described in the literature [39, 40]. In 2010, direct immunoprecipitation using patients' serum or CSF with high titer of VGKC antibodies clearly demonstrated that the target antigen was not the VGKC but, in some patients, two related proteins part of the VGKC-complex, LGI1 and CASPR2 [41, 42]. LGI1 antibodies were detected in patients with LE [41], whereas CASPR2 antibodies were associated with Morvan's syndrome or, less frequently, neuromyotonia [42]. At present, no other relevant antigens have been identified, and in up to 74% of the patients with positive VGKC antibodies (more frequently with low titers), the antigens are unknown [43].

Anti-LGI1 Encephalitis

Anti-LGI1 encephalitis has been traditionally described as a LE characterized by some peculiar aspects. Males are affected more frequently (M:F 2:1). Annual incidence has been estimated around 0.83 per million people in the Netherlands. In van Sonderen's series tumor analysis comprised neuroendocrine pancreas tumor, thymoma, abdominal mesothelioma, in situ rectal carcinoma, and breast cancer, with an overall cancer incidence estimated around 11% [44].

The most common initial symptoms are seizures and cognitive disorder, with memory disturbance in nearly all patients and spatial disorientation in a half of the cases. Behavioral changes are also highly frequent and include apathy, disinhibition, egocentrism, and compulsive behavior. Other frequent symptoms are insomnia, autonomic dysfunction, and sexual dysfunction. Focal seizures may be of different types: dyscognitive, autonomic, motor, or gelastic seizures, mostly with a temporal lobe origin, and a tonic-clonic evolution. Tonic-clonic seizures usually occur simultaneously with or after cognitive decline onset [44, 45]. A highly specific seizure type is represented by *faciobrachial dystonic seizures* (*FBDS*) [46], also reported in recent literature as tonic-dystonic seizures [45] or motor spasms [47]. FBDS usually start several weeks before cognitive symptoms and are frequently unrecognized. They consist in sudden, short, involuntary contractions, involving the arm and the face (or leg) [44]. In some patients a groaning or a brief anarthria may also occur. When lower limbs are involved, falls with trauma are possible. Initially FBDS are often unilateral, but with time can evolve into bilateral, asynchronous seizures, occurring either independently or with a short delay ("à bascule"). These seizures can be registered during wakefulness and sleep. In some patients they are provoked by motor triggers, such as change of position or orthostatism, by surprise, such as an unexpected noise, or by emotion and stress. A sensory aura has been reported preceding FBDS in some cases. Its frequency can increase with time from more than weekly to a median value of 35 per day. Consciousness can be retained during isolated episodes, whereas it can be lost in those patients with FBDS rapidly turned into temporal or frontal lobe seizures [45]. Although a non-epileptic pathophysiology was hypothesized in the past, several findings support the fact that FBDS originate in the motor cortex [45]. In general, the recognition of these seizures is a clue for early diagnosis of anti-LGI1 encephalitis. In a series reported by van Sonderen et al., a total of 47% of patients had FBDS, while another 66% of patients had focal seizures with mainly dyscognitive or autonomic features, early in the disease course [44]. A few cases presenting with pilomotor seizures have also been reported [48]. Tonic-clonic seizures are more easily recognized but usually occur later in the disease course [44]. Early identification of FBDS and initiation of immunotherapy have shown to accelerate recovery and prevent secondary limbic engagement [46, 49]. According to van Sonderen et al., interictal EEG has been found positive for focal slowing in about 25% of cases. Focal dyscognitive, autonomic, gelastic, or motor seizures are usually associated with epileptic discharges, whereas FBDS have remained with no clear EEG correlate for long time, making their recognition difficult [44]. In another series, EEG abnormalities were detected in 75% of patients: focal, diffuse slowing in 62% of patients and ictal activity in 53% of cases [45]. FBDS electrographic features have progressively been delineated over time. An *electrodecremental event* (*EDE*), characterized by a brief (~500 ms) generalized attenuation, was the first EEG correlate reported by Andrade et al. as a case to support the cortical, epileptic origin for these unusual phenomena [50, 51] (Fig. 40.3). The second element was added in 2016 by Navarro et al. who described in seven patients with isolated FBDS a *frontal region slow wave* (mean duration 577 ± 320 ms; mean amplitude 71 ± 34 mV). It preceded seizure muscle activation and was recorded from two or more adjacent fronto-polar, frontal, or central electrodes, contralaterally to FBDS-related muscle contractions [45]. This transient likely represented the *direct current* (*DC*) *shift* preceding the EDE, already visible in a previous report [51]. In 2018 Wennberg et al. have referred to this DC shift with a more accurate descriptor, termed *infraslow activity* (*ISA*). In artifact-free recordings, obtained using clinical amplifiers equipped with a low-frequency analog filter of 0.07 Hz, they found that ISA reliably preceded clinical onset of the motor spasms (FBDS) by ~1.2 s and preceded the EDE by ~700 ms, thus recognizing the EDE and the associated ISA as the EEG correlate of FBDS. Pre-spasm ISA was invariably recorded contralaterally to FBDS, with a voltage topographic maximum over the mid-frontal region. Bilaterally synchronous motor spasms are less easily clinically recognizable as FBDS and can appear more intense, with more obvious leg involvement. Occasionally brief series of FBDS can occur as two or three ipsilateral spasms spaced over 3–5 s. The initial spasm was invariably preceded by clearly identifiable ISA, while no ISA could be detected before the second or third event in these series. Furthermore, this premovement transient was different from the *Bereitschaftspotential* in timing and topography and was an order of magnitude higher in amplitude [47]. Classical EEG epileptic activities during LE were found in patients with temporal seizures and cognitive

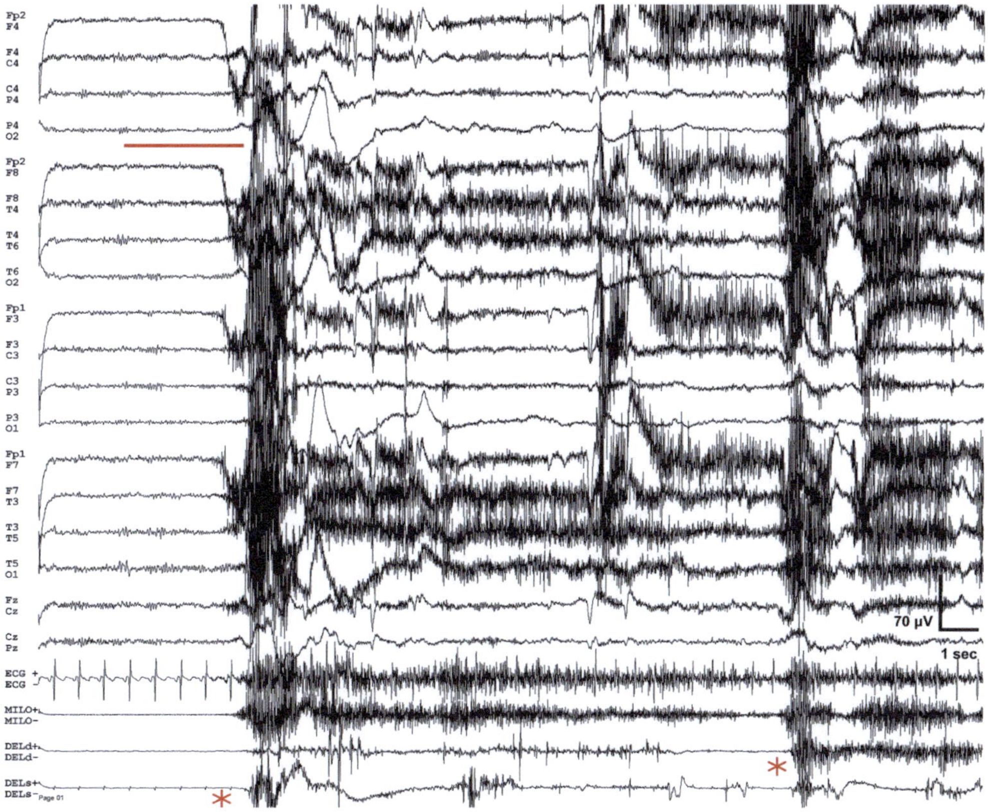

Fig. 40.3 Video-polygraphic recording of a FBDS in a 77-year-old male with anti-LGI1 encephalitis. *Asterisks* mark the muscular activity of two FBDS, the first engaging the left arm and the second the right one. Note the activation of the mylohyoid muscle (*MILO* electrode) preceding the motor spasm of the upper limbs in both cases. An EDE has been recognized (*underline*) short before the first FBDS

impairment. In this context, a slowing of background activity was frequently observed. Interictal epileptic spikes and sharp waves were preferentially generated by the temporal or frontal lobes during sleep or drowsiness. Seizures can begin either with a unilateral or bilateral flattening of the background over several seconds or with a similar focal slow wave as those associated with FBDS. Sometimes, FBDS can be observed 10–30 s before the temporal seizure. After muscular activation, a rhythmic activity, generally irregular, distributed bilaterally over frontal and temporal lobes was detected [45]. Not all temporal seizures had a clinical correlate. Electrographically, unusually frequent (up to dozens of times per day) subclinical temporal lobe seizures in absence of interictal spikes have been identified as an independent diagnostic marker of anti-LGI1 encephalitis [50–52].

Anti-CASPR2 Encephalitis

Recently, the clinical spectrum of CASPR2 autoimmunity has been investigated. After studying a series of 38 patients having CASPR2 antibodies, van Sonderen et al. defined a set of core symptoms and signs observed in most patients: cerebral symptoms (altered cognition and epilepsy), cerebellar symptoms, peripheral nerve hyperexcitability, autonomic dysfunction, insomnia, neuropathic pain, and weight loss. 77% of patients had ≥3 core symptoms and 61% had ≥4. The course of disease is often less rapid; the disorder predominates in males, and approximately 25% of patients have relapses. 42% of patients developed a LE. 26% of them had symptoms beyond the limbic system, such as cerebellar dysfunction or pain (LE plus). EEG was positive for epileptic activity in 40% of patients; 33% of patients showed a slow background and was normal in the remainders [53].

40.1.2.3 Anti-AMPAR Encephalitis

Antibodies directed to subunits 1/2 of the AMPAR were associated with a type of encephalitis presenting with prominent limbic features. Often patients hid a lung, breast, or thymus cancer and partially responded to treatment. EEG changes included diffuse theta activity with temporal epileptic activity, frontotemporal delta and slow alpha activity, posterior temporal theta, and bilateral temporal sharp activity [54]. In 2015 Höftberger et al. recognized four distinct syndromes in patient with anti-AMPAR antibodies: LE (55%), limbic dysfunction along with multifocal/diffuse encephalopathy (36%), LE preceded by motor deficits (in one patient), and psychosis with bipolar features (in another single patient). In their series anti-AMPAR encephalitis was prevalent in female patients (F:M 14:8) and was paraneoplastic in 64% of cases. When available, EEG showed a general slowing in 29% of cases, unihemispheric focal slowing, lateralized periodic focal slowing, and focal spike waves with frontotemporal polymorphic delta. Epileptiform activity was detected in 23% of patients (often without clinical seizures). In another 23% of cases, EEG was normal [55].

40.1.2.4 Anti-$GABA_B$ Receptor Encephalitis

$GABA_B$ receptor encephalitis was described by Lancaster et al. in 15 patients with LE associated with SCLC in a third of cases and/or with concurrent GAD antibodies. All patients experienced seizures. EEG showed diffuse slowing and bilateral PLEDs [56]. In 2013 Höftberger et al. reported a series of 20 patients with anti-$GABA_B$ receptor antibodies. The M:F ratio was 12:8. Nearly all (95%) of these patients developed a LE, 85% of them in association with prominent seizures. In this context, EEG detected temporal lobe epileptic activity with or without general slowing in 58% of patients [57].

40.1.2.5 Anti-$GABA_A$ Receptor Encephalitis

Petit-Pedrol et al. found in the serum and the CSF of six patients affected by a severe form of encephalitis with refractory seizures and SE a high titer of antibodies directed against α1/β3 subunits of $GABA_A$ receptor. This new kind of encephalitis affected five male patients and one female in a wide range of age (3–63 years, median 22 years). All patients developed a rapidly progressive encephalopathy with extensive cortical-subcortical MRI abnormalities that eventually resulted in refractory seizures, with evolution to SE in 83% of the cases. One of them also had epilepsia partialis continua (EPC). In all patients, epileptic symptoms were preceded or associated with behavioral or cognitive changes. EEG showed seizures in all patients, with ictal activity originating from the temporal lobe, frontotemporal cortex, or occipital cortex. Two patients had generalized periodic discharges; three patients showed a generalized slowing [58].

40.1.3 Hashimoto Encephalopathy or Steroid-Responsive Encephalopathy Associated with Autoimmune Thyroiditis

Hashimoto encephalopathy (HE) is a disorder predominantly affecting women with overt or subclinical thyroid disease, usually hypothyroidism. Most patients improve after steroid administration with or without levothyroxine [59]. Hence, in 2006 the disorder was renamed as steroid-responsive encephalopathy with autoimmune thyroiditis (SREAT) [60]. Criteria have been proposed for diagnosis of HE (Table 40.5). Since the underlying pathogenic mechanism is unclear, it should be classified as probable autoimmune encephalitis [1].

The hallmark presenting feature is a nonspecific encephalopathy characterized by mental status alteration ranging from confusion to coma [62]. Seizures are reported in 52–66% of cases and SE in 12% [63]. At EEG, mild to severe generalized slowing is the most common finding in both children and adults and is found in 85–98% of cases [59, 64–66]. Schäuble et al. studied the EEG of 17 patients with HE: all of them showed a generalized slowing, which corresponded to the clinical severity of the underlying encephalopathy. In this study, they also reported lateralized slowing independent from focal abnormalities detected by neurologic examination or neuroimaging studies; the cause of these findings remains unexplained [67]. Rodriguez et al. documented the improvement of the EEG abnormalities over a few hours after steroid administration and fluctuating side-to-side EEG changes, consisting in decreased amplitude of the background activity over one alternating hemisphere, in addition to generalized slowing, in HE. The authors hypothesized that a vascular alteration may be, at least partially, responsible for the focal cerebral dysfunction seen in HE [68]. Other EEG abnormalities include typical and atypical triphasic waves, frontal intermittent rhythmic delta activity (FIRDA), and epileptiform discharges [69]. Less frequently, photomyogenic and photoparoxysmal response has been described [67].

Table 40.5 Diagnostic criteria for HE, adapted from ref. [1]

Diagnosis can be made when all six of the following criteria have been met:
1. Encephalopathy with seizures, myoclonus, hallucinations, or stroke-like episodes
2. Subclinical or mild overt thyroid disease (usually hypothyroidism)
3. Brain MRI normal or with nonspecific abnormalities
4. Presence of serum thyroid TPO, TG antibodies[a]
5. Absence of well-characterized neuronal antibodies in serum and CSF
6. Reasonable exclusion of alternative causes

TPO thyroid peroxidase, *TG* thyroglobulin
[a]There is no disease-specific cutoff value for these antibodies (detectable in 13% of healthy individuals) [61]

40.2 Inflammatory Encephalopathies

40.2.1 Rasmussen Encephalitis

Rasmussen encephalitis (RE) is a rare inflammatory neurologic disorder characterized by intractable focal seizures, EPC, unilateral cortical deficits, and progressive unihemispheric brain atrophy. Children and young adults are prevalently affected (median age 6 years), even if adult cases have been described [70]. Estimated incidence is 2.4 cases per ten million people aged 18 years or younger per year in Germany [71]. The clinical course of the disease includes three stages:

1. A *prodromal stage*, with a relatively low seizure frequency and rarely mild hemiparesis, which may last years (median duration 7.1 months).
2. The *acute stage*, characterized by frequent seizures arising from one cerebral hemisphere, EPC, in about 50% of patients [72–74] and neurological deterioration with progressive hemiparesis, hemianopia, cognitive decline, and

aphasia when dominant hemisphere is involved [75]. The median duration of this stage is 8 months.

3. A *residual stage* with permanent stable neurological deficits and persisting difficult-to-treat seizures, despite less frequent than before.

Diagnosis of RE is performed according to the 2005 European consensus statement criteria (Table 40.6).

RE initial manifestations are seizures and SE in up to 20% of cases at onset, with focal motor seizures the most frequent (Fig. 40.4). Despite considered the hallmark of RE, EPC occurs in 56–92% of the patients [78–80]. EPC consists in a spontaneous regular or irregular myoclonic muscle twitching of cortical origin (Fig. 40.5). It is confined to one part of the body (mostly distal muscles or face), can be enhanced by action or sensory stimuli, and continues for a period of hours, days, or weeks (Fig. 40.6) [73]. EPC has three peculiarities: (1) it is refractory to antiepileptic drugs; (2) it does not have the general tendency to Jacksonian spread; and (3) it does not stop after the usual short time of focal motor seizures [72, 81–84]. The scalp EEG may not detect ictal epileptic activity related to this phenomenon because of the restrict cortical area or the unfavorable orientation of the dipole of the discharge with respect to the recording electrodes [85]. At RE onset EEG findings are confined to the affected hemisphere and consist in the slowing of background activity and sleep disorganization, focal slow and epileptic abnormalities, early ictal and interictal hemispheric abnormalities (Fig. 40.7), and subclinical ictal discharges. Over time the epileptic activity increases and tends to spread, involving the unaffected hemisphere. Seizure onset, though multifocal, remains clearly unilateral, so that the early recording of seizures from the unaffected hemisphere should lead to questioning RE diagnosis [80, 86]. So and Gloor studied extensively EEG changes in RE patients. In their series the abnormalities varied widely and were partly dependent on the stage of the disease, with early traces tending to show unilateral abnormalities and later EEGs bilateral changes with more widespread epileptiform transients. All patients showed slow-wave activity, usually polymorphic theta-delta activity. Interictal epileptiform discharges were evident in 89% of patients. 30% had multiple

Table 40.6 Diagnostic criteria for RE, adapted from ref. [76]

RE can be diagnosed if either 3/3 criteria of part A or 2/3 criteria of part B are present. Check first for the features of part A. then, if they are not fulfilled, of part B. in addition, if no biopsy is performed, MRI with administration of gadolinium and cranial CT need to be performed to document the absence of gadolinium enhancement and calcifications and to exclude the differential diagnosis of a unihemispheric vasculitis [77]
Part A:
1. Clinical: Focal seizures (with or without EPC) and unilateral cortical deficits
2. EEG: Unihemispheric slowing with or without epileptiform activity and unilateral seizures onset
3. Unihemispheric focal cortical atrophy and at least one of the following:
• Gray or white matter T2/FLAIR hyperintense signal
• Hyperintense signal or atrophy of the ipsilateral caudate head
Part B:
1. Clinical: EPC or progressive[a] unilateral cortical deficits
2. MRI: Progressive unihemispheric focal cortical atrophy
3. Histopathology: T-cell dominated encephalitis with activated microglial cells (typically, but not necessarily forming nodules) and reactive astrogliosis. Numerous parenchymal macrophages, B cells, or plasma cells or viral inclusion bodies exclude the diagnosis of RE

CT computed tomography

[a]Progressive means that at least two sequential clinical examinations or MRI studies are required to meet the respective criteria. To indicate clinical progression, each of these examinations must document a neurological deficit, and this must increase over time. To indicate progressive hemiatrophy, each of these MRIs must show hemiatrophy, and this must increase over time.

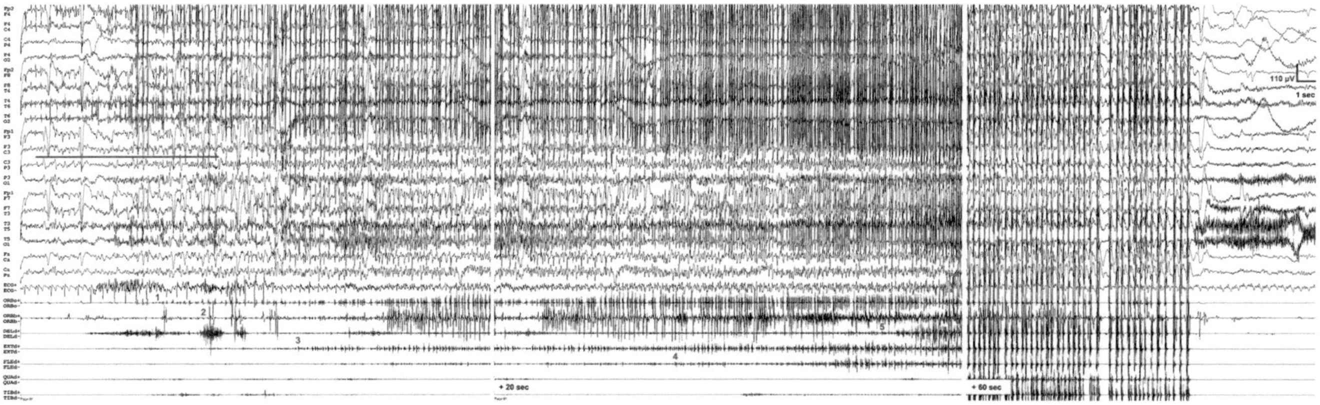

Fig. 40.4 Video-polygraphic recording of right focal motor seizure in a 23-year-old female patient with RE affecting the left hemisphere. EPC involves the right facial muscles; arrhythmic repetitive short bursts of muscle activity were recorded on the orbicularis oculi and orbicularis oris electrodes, coinciding with muscular artifacts on the EEG. The ictal discharge of the right faciobrachial-crural motor seizure starts on the left frontocentral region. Muscles progressively involved by the ictal spreading have been numbered: *1*, orbicularis oculi muscle; *2*, orbicularis oris muscle; *3*, extensor carpi muscle; *4*, flexor carpi muscles; and *5*, deltoid muscle. Ipsilateral lower limb muscles have been later engaged

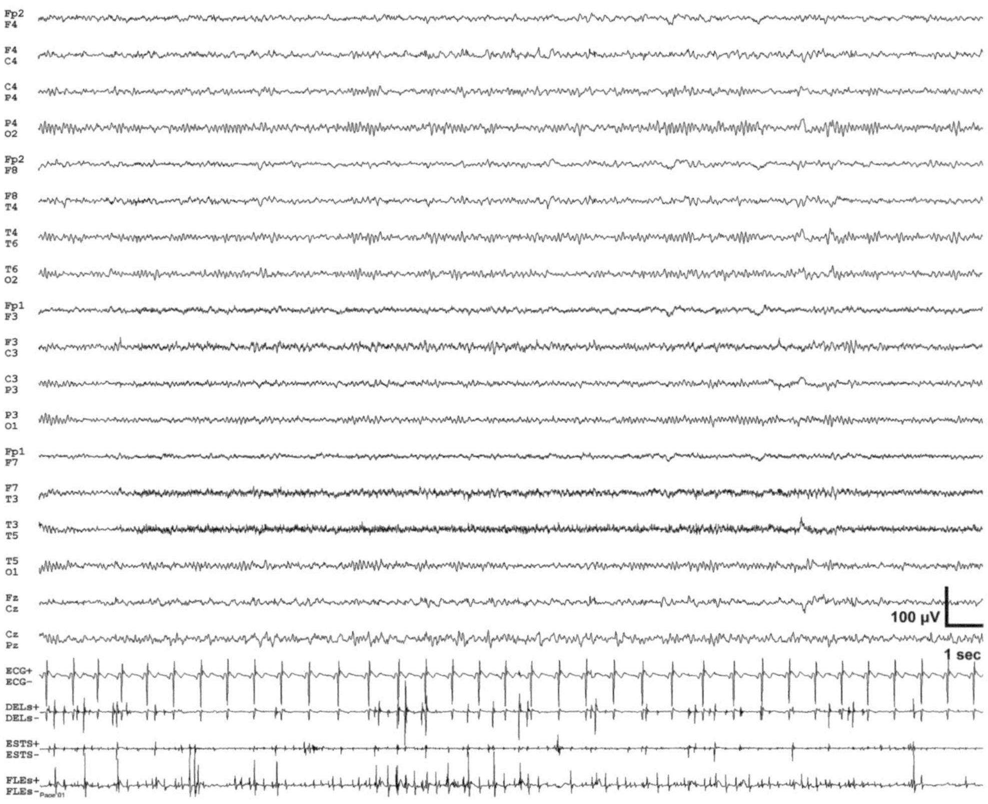

Fig. 40.5 EPC involving the left upper limb of a 24-year-old male patient with RE at rest. Muscular traces show brief asynchronous potentials repeating with an erratic unpredictable pattern over time (without a Jacksonian march, typical of a motor seizure)

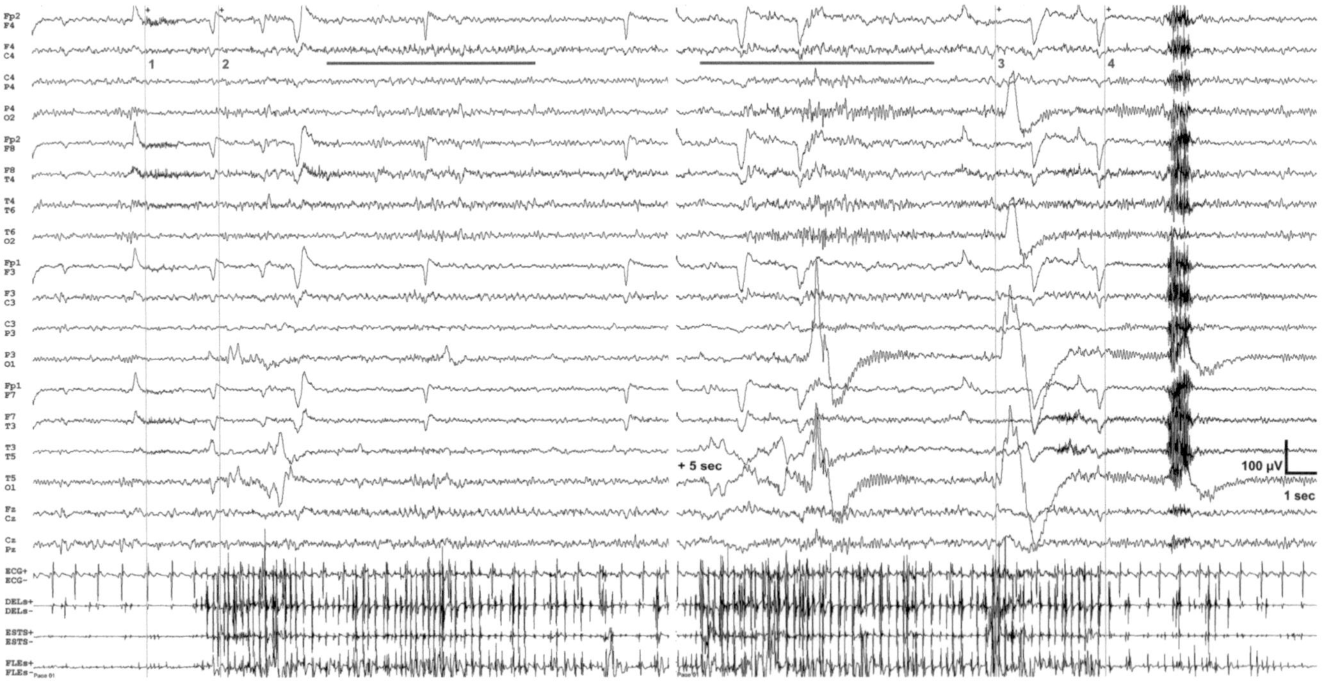

Fig. 40.6 EPC affecting the left upper limb of a 24-year-old male patient with RE increased by voluntary action. At point *1*, patient opened his eyes; at point *2*, he was requested to close his left hand; at point *3*, he was requested to stop the voluntary contraction of the hand; at point *4*, patient closed his eyes. During the voluntary activation of his left-hand muscles, a significant increase in frequency and amplitude of the irregular muscle potentials has been recorded. Over the contralateral frontocentral region (*F4-C4*), a rhythmic activity in the alpha range (8.5–9.5 Hz) has been *underlined* and recognized as a possible correlate of the EPC

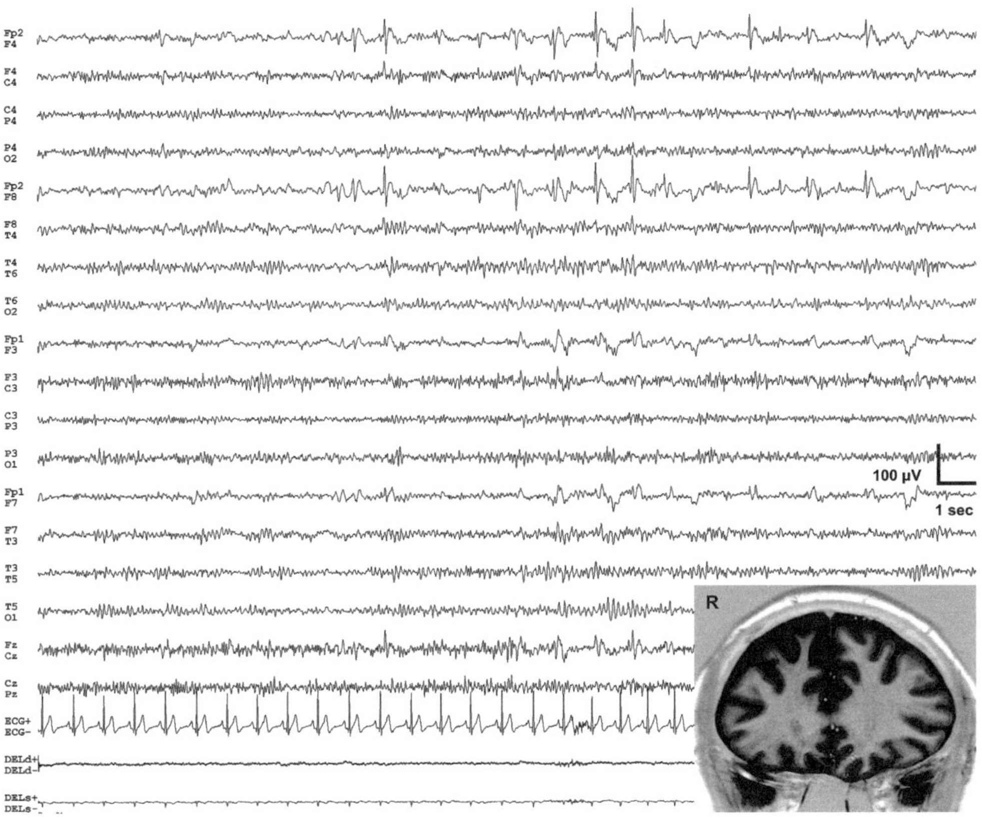

Fig. 40.7 An example of unihemispheric interictal abnormalities in a 47-year-old male patient with RE. High-amplitude spikes and slow waves stand out over the right anterior frontal region, which represents the area of the right hemisphere severely affected by the encephalitis. In the right corner at the bottom of the figure, an Inversion Recovery section of patient's brain MRI documenting the relevant right frontal cerebral atrophy produced by the chronic inflammatory process

independent foci lateralized to one hemisphere, and a further 13% had a similar condition but generating bilaterally synchronous discharges. Bilateral multiple independent foci occurred in 13% of patients. Among patients with recorded seizures, only 16% of cases had a localized onset. By the time that hemiparesis and neuroradiological alterations had occurred, bilateral disturbance of background activity was present in 76%, bilateral slow-wave abnormalities in 81%, and bilateral multiple independent interictal epileptiform discharges in 34%, while 6% had seizures arising independently from the two hemispheres. Often EPC was not clearly detected at scalp EEG, which may just record uncharacteristic, polyphasic slow waves [86].

Magnetoencephalography (MEG) can detect epileptiform abnormalities not revealed by EEG [87]. In 2017 Rossi Sebastiano et al. used MEG to evaluate five RE children in two distinct time-points, separated by a 6-month period. They showed epileptic foci located in different areas of the affected hemisphere in all RE patients, supporting the hypothesis of a "migratory" behavior of the spike generators in RE, which probably reflects the patchy progression of the inflammatory/degenerative process [88].

40.2.2 Multiple Sclerosis

The prevalence of epilepsy is increased threefold in multiple sclerosis (MS) and is even higher in patients with severe forms [89–92]. Nowadays it is well recognized that gray-matter lesions in multiple sclerosis are common at disease onset, particularly in patients with epilepsy [93]. Furthermore, the higher cumulative incidence of epilepsy in patients with progressive disease and advanced disability appears to be in line with the increase of the gray-matter lesions burden [92]. Nonetheless, seizures are still rare events in MS, and in some patients the coexistence of seizures and MS may be due to chance [94]. Focal seizures, with or without tonic-clonic evolution, are the most frequent type, whereas ab initio generalized tonic-clonic seizures are quite rare [95–98]. Furthermore, SE is frequently reported in epileptic MS patients, and sometimes EPC has been described [99–104]. EEG abnormalities can be found in 20–60% of MS patients, related to the location of the lesions and disease course [97, 105]. There are no specific EEG patterns in MS patients with seizures, nor EEG predicts the outcome and response to antiepileptic therapy [98]. Common interictal findings are a diffuse asynchronous theta activity or synchronous rhythmic slow waves and sometimes, especially during a chronic progressive course, a generalized voltage reduction, likely related to a variable degree of cortical atrophy. Occasionally, focal slow waves or localized flattened EEG activity may be found. Interictal paroxysmal activity seems to be quite rare, and an EEG improvement or deterioration usually does not correlate with clinical state. Furthermore, hyperventilation may worsen background activity and also precipitate non-epileptic ictal symptoms (focal paraesthesias or tonic spasms at the extremities) [106]. Sometimes, unusual EEG abnormalities can be also found, such as PLEDs [103, 104].

40.2.3 Primary CNS Vasculitis

Primary CNS vasculitis (PCNSV) is a rare neurological condition diagnosed when all three of the following criteria are met: (1) history or clinical findings of an acquired neurological deficit of unknown origin, (2) cerebral angiogram with classic features of vasculitis or a CNS biopsy sample showing vasculitis, and (3) no evidence of systemic vasculitis or any other disorder to which the angiographic or pathological features could be secondary [107, 108]. In a retrospective study of 101 patients with PCNSV, Salvarani et al. reported that 16% of patients experienced seizures among other various neurological symptoms. EEGs, obtained from 38 patients, showed abnormal findings in 74% of cases. Although electroencephalographic findings were abnormal in most patients, they generally were minor and nonspecific [109].

40.2.4 Systemic Inflammatory Diseases: Neuropsychiatric Systemic Lupus Erythematosus, Neuro-Behçet's Disease, and Neurosarcoidosis

40.2.4.1 Neuropsychiatric Systemic Lupus Erythematosus

Neuropsychiatric symptoms are considered one of the major manifestations of systemic lupus erythematosus (SLE) [110–112]. Most seizures in SLE represent single isolated events; recurrent seizures are less common (12–22%). Generalized tonic-clonic seizures are the most common (67–88%), but focal seizures have also been described. EEG abnormalities are frequent (60–70%) in SLE patients with seizure disorder, but typical epileptiform patterns are only present in 24–50% and are predictive of seizure recurrence (positive predictive value 73%, negative predictive value 79%) [113, 114].

40.2.4.2 Neuro-Behçet's Disease

Behçet's disease (BD) is a rare multisystem disease of unknown cause characterized by an inflammatory perivasculitis which can arise in almost any tissue [115, 116]. Neurological involvement, known as neuro-Behçet's disease (NBD), is one of the most serious causes of long-term morbidity and mortality [117], and it is reported in ~5% of the patient with BD [118]. Epileptic seizures were reported in 2.2–5% of cases [119–121]. Focal seizures were reported at onset in one case series [122]; EPC was reported in another [123]. Generalized seizures are the predominant type [121]. EEG recordings show nonspecific abnormalities [124].

40.2.4.3 Neurosarcoidosis

Sarcoidosis is an inflammatory multisystem disorder of unknown cause that can affect any part of the nervous system. The prevalence of neurological involvement is estimated to be about 5–15% [125, 126]. The diagnosis of neurosarcoidosis requires a compatible clinical or radiological picture of sarcoidosis and histological confirmation of noncaseating granulomas [127, 128]. Seizures may be the first symptom of neurosarcoidosis [129–131]. Most reports indicate a poor prognosis with severe progressing or relapsing course when seizures are associated with sarcoidosis [132–134]. Any type of seizures may appear. EEG may be characterized by generalized or focal slowing with spikes or sharp waves, especially in the presence of a mass lesion or localized encephalopathy [129].

40.3 Status Epilepticus in Autoimmune/Inflammatory Encephalopathies

40.3.1 New-Onset Refractory Status Epilepticus and Febrile Illness-Related Epilepsy Syndrome

The cause of SE is often easily identified with a standardized approach, based on medical history, neurological examination, and basic laboratory tests [135]. Nevertheless, in up to 20% of cases, this initial workup may be unrevealing, and one of the uncommon causes of SE has to be considered [136, 137]. In a small but non-negligible group of patients, mostly previously healthy young adults and children, an extensive diagnostic workup fails to reveal the cause of SE. This group may represent up to 60% of cases of de novo refractory SE [138, 139]. This entity has received various names and acronyms in the past, such as new-onset refractory status epilepticus (NORSE) in adults [140–142] and idiopathic catastrophic epileptic encephalopathy [143], febrile infection or febrile illness-related epilepsy syndrome (FIRES) [144, 145], acute encephalitis with refractory repetitive partial seizures (AERRPS) [146], or devastating epilepsy in school-age children (DESC) [147] in children. In 2017 an expert panel set out to standardize definitions of NORSE and FIRES. According to the consensus definitions, NORSE is a clinical presentation, not a specific diagnosis, in a patient without active epilepsy or other preexisting relevant neurological disorder, with new onset of refractory SE without a clear acute or active structural, toxic, or metabolic cause. This includes patients with viral or autoimmune causes [148]. In a recent study of patients with NORSE, Gaspard et al. found that an etiology could ultimately be identified in 48% of cases, and the most frequent etiologies were non-paraneoplastic autoimmune encephalitides (19%) and paraneoplastic encephalitides (18%) [142]. If no cause is found after extensive evaluation, this is considered a "cryptogenic NORSE" or "NORSE of unknown etiology" [148]. It is possible that some cryptogenic cases correspond to autoimmune encephalitis associated with antibodies yet to be identified [142].

FIRES has to be considered a subcategory of NORSE that requires a prior febrile illness, with fever starting between 2 weeks and 24 h prior to the onset of refractory SE. This applies to all ages [148]. Although the pathophysiology remains elusive, nascent evidence suggests a role for a post-infectious cytokine-mediated mechanism [149]. The diagnosis of FIRES and NORSE is typically given late, if at all, in a patient's clinical course. The development of a specific diagnostic test for their early identification is needed. A CSF or serological marker is currently not available. Although brain MRI may disclose suggestive findings [150], they are usually absent in the early phase. EEG can be performed early and continuously throughout the course of SE. In a retrospective analysis of children with FIRES, three common features were noted: (1) seizures were initially brief and relatively infrequent, with a gradual evolution to SE; (2) beta-delta complexes resembling extreme delta brush were observed; and (3) seizures had a characteristic electrographic pattern, typically beginning with prolonged focal fast activity, followed by the gradual appearance of well-formed rhythmic spike or spike-and-wave complexes. Shifting ictal activity was frequently observed [151]. Whether or not these findings show any specificity to NORSE and FIRES is still unclear, and further investigations are needed [149].

References

1. Graus F, Titulaer MJ, Balu R, Benseler S, Bien CG, Cellucci T, et al. A clinical approach to diagnosis of autoimmune encephalitis. Lancet Neurol. 2016;15:391–404.
2. Venkatesan A, Tunkel AR, Bloch KC, Lauring AS, Sejvar J, Bitnun A, et al. Case definitions, diagnostic algorithms, and priorities in encephalitis: consensus statement of the international encephalitis consortium. Clin Infect Dis. 2013;57:1114–28.
3. Britton PN, Eastwood K, Paterson B, Durrheim DN, Dale RC, Cheng AC, et al. Consensus guidelines for the investigation and management of encephalitis in adults and children in Australia and New Zealand. Intern Med J. 2015;45:563–76.
4. Leypoldt F, Armangue T, Dalmau J. Autoimmune encephalopathies. Ann N Y Acad Sci. 2015;1338:94–114.
5. Schmitt SE, Pargeon K, Frechette ES, Hirsch LJ, Dalmau J, Friedman D. Extreme delta brush: a unique EEG pattern in adults with anti-NMDA receptor encephalitis. Neurology. 2012;79:1094–100.
6. Granerod J, Ambrose HE, Davies NW, Clewley JP, Walsh AL, Morgan D, et al. Causes of encephalitis and differences in their clinical presentations in England: a multicentre, population-based prospective study. Lancet Infect Dis. 2010;10:835–44.
7. Lancaster E, Dalmau J. Neuronal autoantigens-pathogenesis, associated disorders and antibody testing. Nat Rev Neurol. 2012;8:380–90.
8. Toledano M, Pittock SJ. Autoimmune Epilepsy. Semin Neurol. 2015;35:245–58.
9. Graus F, Delattre JY, Antoine JC, Dalmau J, Giometto B, Grisold W, et al. Recommended diagnostic criteria for paraneoplastic neurological syndromes. J Neurol Neurosurg Psychiatry. 2004;75:1135–40.
10. Gultekin SH, Rosenfeld MR, Voltz R, Eichen J, Posner JB, Dalmau J. Paraneoplastic limbic encephalitis: neurological symptoms, immunological findings and tumour association in 50 patients. Brain. 2000;123:1481–94.
11. Lawn ND, Westmoreland BF, Kiely MJ, Lennon VA, Vernino S. Clinical, magnetic resonance imaging, and electroencephalographic findings in paraneoplastic limbic encephalitis. Mayo Clin Proc. 2003;78:1363–8.
12. Kaplan PW, Sutter R. Electroencephalography of autoimmune limbic encephalopathy. J Clin Neurophysiol. 2013;30:490–504.
13. Sutter R, Fuhr P, Grize L, Marsch S, Rüegg S. Continuous video-EEG monitoring increases detection rate of nonconvulsive status epilepticus in the ICU. Epilepsia. 2011;52:453–7.
14. Hamer HM, Najm I, Mohamed A, Wyllie E. Interictal epileptiform discharges in temporal lobe epilepsy due to hippocampal sclerosis versus medial temporal lobe tumors. Epilepsia. 1999;40:1261–8.
15. Kaplan PW, Rossetti AO, Kaplan EH, Wieser HG. Proposition: limbic encephalitis may represent limbic status epilepticus. A review of clinical and EEG characteristics. Epilepsy Behav. 2012;24:1–6.
16. Dalmau J. NMDA receptor encephalitis and other antibody-mediated disorders of the synapse: the 2016 Cotzias lecture. Neurology. 2016;87:2471–82.
17. Dalmau J, Tüzün E, Wu HY, Masjuan J, Rossi JE, Voloschin A, et al. Paraneoplastic anti-N-methyl-D-aspartate receptor encephalitis associated with ovarian teratoma. Ann Neurol. 2007;61:25–36.
18. Sabater L, Gaig C, Gelpi E, Bataller L, Lewerenz J, Torres-Vega E, et al. A novel non-rapid-eye movement and rapid-eye-movement parasomnia with sleep breathing disorder associated with antibodies to IgLON5: a case series, characterisation of the antigen, and post-mortem study. Lancet Neurol. 2014;13:575–86.
19. Gresa-Arribas N, Planagumà J, Petit-Pedrol M, Kawachi I, Katada S, Glaser CA, et al. Human neurexin-3α antibodies associate with encephalitis and alter synapse development. Neurology. 2016;86:2235–42.
20. Irani SR, Bera K, Waters P, Zuliani L, Maxwell S, Zandi MS, et al. N-methyl-D-aspartate antibody encephalitis: temporal progression of clinical and paraclinical observations in a predominantly non-paraneoplastic disorder of both sexes. Brain. 2010;133:1655–67.
21. Titulaer MJ, McCracken L, Gabilondo I, Armangué T, Glaser C, Iizuka T, et al. Treatment and prognostic factors for long-term outcome in patients with anti-NMDA receptor encephalitis: an observational cohort study. Lancet Neurol. 2013;12:157–65.
22. Dalmau J, Lancaster E, Martinez-Hernandez E, Rosenfeld MR, Balice-Gordon R. Clinical experience and laboratory investigations in patients with anti-NMDAR encephalitis. Lancet Neurol. 2011;10:63–74.
23. Vincent A, Bien CG, Irani SR, Waters P. Autoantibodies associated with diseases of the CNS: new developments and future challenges. Lancet Neurol. 2011;10:759–72.
24. Viaccoz A, Desestret V, Ducray F, Picard G, Cavillon G, Rogemond V, et al. Clinical specificities of adult male patients with NMDA receptor antibodies encephalitis. Neurology. 2014;82:556–63.
25. Dalmau J, Gleichman AJ, Hughes EG, Rossi JE, Peng X, Lai M, et al. Anti-NMDA-receptor encephalitis: case series and analysis of the effects of antibodies. Lancet Neurol. 2008;7:1091–8.
26. Iizuka T, Sakai F, Mochizuki H. Update on anti-NMDA receptor encephalitis. Brain Nerve. 2010;62:331–8.

27. Shimazaki H, Ando Y, Nakano I, Dalmau J. Reversible limbic encephalitis with antibodies against the membranes of neurones of the hippocampus. BMJ Case Rep. 2009;2009:bcr07.2008.0509.
28. Sansing LH, Tüzün E, Ko MW, Baccon J, Lynch DR, Dalmau J. A patient with encephalitis associated with NMDA receptor antibodies. Nat Clin Pract Neurol. 2007;3:291–6.
29. Veciana M, Becerra JL, Fossas P, Muriana D, Sansa G, Santamarina E, et al. EEG extreme delta brush: an ictal pattern in patients with anti-NMDA receptor encephalitis. Epilepsy Behav. 2015;49:280–5.
30. Zhang Y, Liu G, Di Jiang M, Li LP, Su YY. Analysis of electroencephalogram characteristics of anti-NMDA receptor encephalitis patients in China. Clin Neurophysiol. 2017;128:1227–33.
31. Ikeda A, Matsui M, Hase Y, Hitomi T, Takahashi Y, Shibasaki H, et al. "Burst and slow complexes" in nonconvulsive epileptic status. Epileptic Disord. 2006;8:61–4.
32. Chong DJ, Hirsch LJ. Which EEG patterns warrant treatment in the critically ill? Reviewing the evidence for treatment of periodic epileptiform discharges and related patterns. J Clin Neurophysiol. 2005;22:79–91.
33. da Silva-Júnior FP, Castro LH, Andrade JQ, Bastos CG, Moreira CH, Valério RM, et al. Serial and prolonged EEG monitoring in anti-N-methyl-d-aspartate receptor encephalitis. Clin Neurophysiol. 2014;125:1541–4.
34. VanHaerents S, Stillman A, Inoa V, Searls DE, Herman ST. Early and persistent "extreme delta brush" in a patient with anti-NMDA receptor encephalitis. Epilepsy Behav Case Rep. 2014;2:67–70.
35. Yoo JY, Rampal N, Petroff OA, Hirsch LJ, Gaspard N. Brief potentially ictal rhythmic discharges in critically ill adults. JAMA Neurol. 2014;71:454–62.
36. Abbas A, Garg A, Jain R, Mazibrada G, Jacob S. Extreme delta brushes and BIRDs in the EEG of anti-NMDA-receptor encephalitis. Pract Neurol. 2016;16:326–7.
37. Gitiaux C, Simonnet H, Eisermann M, Leunen D, Dulac O, Nabbout R, et al. Early electro-clinical features may contribute to diagnosis of the anti-NMDA receptor encephalitis in children. Clin Neurophysiol. 2013;124:2354–61.
38. Kirkpatrick MP, Clarke CD, Sonmezturk HH, Abou-Khalil B. Rhythmic delta activity represents a form of nonconvulsive status epilepticus in anti-NMDA receptor antibody encephalitis. Epilepsy Behav. 2011;20:392–4.
39. Buckley C, Oger J, Clover L, Tüzün E, Carpenter K, Jackson M, et al. Potassium channel antibodies in two patients with reversible limbic encephalitis. Ann Neurol. 2001;50:73–8.
40. Thieben MJ, Lennon VA, Boeve BF, Aksamit AJ, Keegan M, Vernino S. Potentially reversible autoimmune limbic encephalitis with neuronal potassium channel antibody. Neurology. 2004;62:1177–82.
41. Lai M, Huijbers MG, Lancaster E, Graus F, Bataller L, Balice-Gordon R, et al. Investigation of LGI1 as the antigen in limbic encephalitis previously attributed to potassium channels: a case series. Lancet Neurol. 2010;9:776–85.
42. Irani SR, Alexander S, Waters P, Kleopa KA, Pettingill P, Zuliani L, et al. Antibodies to Kv1 potassium channel-complex proteins leucine-rich, glioma inactivated 1 protein and contactin-associated protein-2 in limbic encephalitis, Morvan's syndrome and acquired neuromyotonia. Brain. 2010;133:2734–48.
43. Klein CJ, Lennon VA, Aston PA, McKeon A, O'Toole O, Quek A, et al. Insights from LGI1 and CASPR2 potassium channel complex autoantibody subtyping. JAMA Neurol. 2013;70:229–34.
44. van Sonderen A, Thijs RD, Coenders EC, Jiskoot LC, Sanchez E, de Bruijn MA, et al. Anti-LGI1 encephalitis: clinical syndrome and long-term follow-up. Neurology. 2016;87:1449–56.
45. Navarro V, Kas A, Apartis E, Chami L, Rogemond V, Levy P, et al. Motor cortex and hippocampus are the two main cortical targets in LGI1-antibody encephalitis. Brain. 2016;139:1079–93.
46. Irani SR, Michell AW, Lang B, Pettingill P, Waters P, Johnson MR, et al. Faciobrachial dystonic seizures precede Lgi1 antibody limbic encephalitis. Ann Neurol. 2011;69:892–900.
47. Wennberg R, Steriade C, Chen R, Andrade D. Frontal infraslow activity marks the motor spasms of anti-LGI1 encephalitis. Clin Neurophysiol. 2018;129:59–68.
48. Rocamora R, Becerra JL, Fossas P, Gomez M, Vivanco-Hidalgo RM, Mauri JA, et al. Pilomotor seizures: an autonomic semiology of limbic encephalitis? Seizure. 2014;23:670–3.
49. Irani SR, Stagg CJ, Schott JM, Rosenthal CR, Schneider SA, Pettingill P, et al. Faciobrachial dystonic seizures: the influence of immunotherapy on seizure control and prevention of cognitive impairment in a broadening phenotype. Brain. 2013;136:3151–62.
50. Andrade DM, Tai P, Dalmau J, Wennberg R. Tonic seizures: a diagnostic clue of anti-LGI1 encephalitis? Neurology. 2011;76:1355–7.
51. Irani SR, Schott JM, Vincent A, Smith SJ. Tonic Seizures: a diagnostic clue of anti-LGI1 encephalitis? Neurology. 2011;77:2140–1.. author reply 2141–3
52. Steriade C, Mirsattari SM, Murray BJ, Wennberg R. Subclinical temporal EEG seizure pattern in LGI1-antibody–mediated encephalitis. Epilepsia. 2016;57:e155–60.
53. van Sonderen A, Ariño H, Petit-Pedrol M, Leypoldt F, Körtvélyessy P, Lancaster E, et al. The clinical spectrum of Caspr2 antibody-associated disease. Neurology. 2016;87:521–8.
54. Lai M, Hughes EG, Peng X, Zhou L, Gleichman AJ, Shu H, et al. AMPA receptor antibodies in limbic encephalitis alter synaptic receptor location. Ann Neurol. 2009;65:424–34.
55. Höftberger R, van Sonderen A, Leypoldt F, Houghton D, Geschwind M, Gelfand J, et al. Encephalitis and AMPA receptor antibodies: novel findings in a case series of 22 patients. Neurology. 2015;84:2403–12.
56. Lancaster E, Lai M, Peng X, Hughes E, Constantinescu R, Raizer J, et al. Antibodies to the GABA(B) receptor in limbic encephalitis with seizures: case series and characterisation of the antigen. Lancet Neurol. 2010;9:67–76.
57. Höftberger R, Titulaer MJ, Sabater L, Dome B, Rózsás A, Hegedus B, et al. Encephalitis and GABAB receptor antibodies: novel findings in a new case series of 20 patients. Neurology. 2013;81:1500–6.
58. Petit-Pedrol M, Armangue T, Peng X, Bataller L, Cellucci T, Davis R, et al. Encephalitis with refractory seizures, status epilepticus, and antibodies to the GABAA receptor: a case series, characterisation of the antigen, and analysis of the effects of antibodies. Lancet Neurol. 2014;13:276–86.
59. Chong JY, Rowland LP, Utiger RD. Hashimoto encephalopathy: syndrome or myth? Arch Neurol. 2003;60:164–71.
60. Castillo P, Woodruff B, Caselli R, Vernino S, Lucchinetti C, Swanson J, et al. Steroid-responsive encephalopathy associated with autoimmune thyroiditis. Arch Neurol. 2006;63:197–202.
61. Hollowell JG, Staehling NW, Flanders WD, Hannon WH, Gunter EW, Spencer CA, et al. Serum TSH, T(4), and thyroid antibodies in the United States population (1988 to 1994): National Health and nutrition examination survey (NHANES III). J Clin Endocrinol Metab. 2002;87:489–99.
62. Hilberath JM, Schmidt H, Wolf GK. Steroid-responsive encephalopathy associated with autoimmune thyroiditis (SREAT): case report of reversible coma and status epilepticus in an adolescent patient and review of the literature. Eur J Pediatr. 2014;173:1263–73.
63. Montagna G, Imperiali M, Agazzi P, D'Aurizio F, Tozzoli R, Feldt-Rasmussen U, et al. Hashimoto's encephalopathy: a rare proteiform disorder. Autoimmun Rev. 2016;15:466–76.
64. Fatourechi V. Hashimoto's encephalopathy: myth or reality? An endocrinologist's perspective. Best Pract Res Clin Endocrinol Metab. 2005;19:53–66.

65. Forchetti CM, Katsamakis G, Garron DC. Autoimmune thyroiditis and a rapidly progressive dementia: global hypoperfusion on SPECT scanning suggests a possible mechanism. Neurology. 1997;49:623–6.
66. Lee SW, Donlon S, Caplan JP. Steroid responsive encephalopathy associated with autoimmune thyroiditis (SREAT) or Hashimoto's encephalopathy: a case and review. Psychosomatics. 2011;52:99–108.
67. Schäuble B, Castillo PR, Boeve BF, Westmoreland BF. EEG findings in steroid-responsive encephalopathy associated with autoimmune thyroiditis. Clin Neurophysiol. 2003;114:32–7.
68. Rodriguez AJ, Jicha GA, Steeves TD, Benarroch EE, Westmoreland BF. EEG changes in a patient with steroid-responsive encephalopathy associated with antibodies to thyroperoxidase (SREAT, Hashimoto's encephalopathy). J Clin Neurophysiol. 2006;23:371–3.
69. Pedroso JL, Knobel M, Barsottini OG, Caboclo LO, Knobel E. The relevance of electroencephalogram as a follow-up test in Hashimoto encephalopathy course after corticosteroids therapy. Acta Neurol Belg. 2012;112:409–11.
70. Varadkar S, Bien CG, Kruse CA, Jensen FE, Bauer J, Pardo CA, et al. Rasmussen's encephalitis: clinical features, pathobiology, and treatment advances. Lancet Neurol. 2014;13:195–205.
71. Bien CG, Tiemeier H, Sassen R, Kuczaty S, Urbach H, von Lehe M, et al. Rasmussen encephalitis: incidence and course under randomized therapy with tacrolimus or intravenous immunoglobulins. Epilepsia. 2013;54:543–50.
72. Thomas JE, Reagan TJ, Klass DW. Epilepsia partialis continua. A review of 32 cases. Arch Neurol. 1977;34:266–75.
73. Obeso JA, Rothwell JC, Marsden CD. The spectrum of cortical myoclonus. From focal reflex jerks to spontaneous motor epilepsy. Brain. 1985;108:193–224.
74. Longaretti F, Dunkley C, Varadkar S, Vargha-Khadem F, Boyd SG, Cross JH. Evolution of the EEG in children with Rasmussen's syndrome. Epilepsia. 2012;53:1539–45.
75. Oguni H, Andermann F, Rasmussen TB. The natural history of the syndrome of chronic encephalitis and epilepsy: a study of the MNI series of forty-eight cases. In: Andermann F, editor. Chronic encephalitis and epilepsy. Rasmussen's syndrome. Boston: Butterworth-Heinemann; 1991. p. 7–35.
76. Bien CG, Granata T, Antozzi C, Cross JH, Dulac O, Kurthen M, et al. Pathogenesis, diagnosis and treatment of Rasmussen encephalitis: a European consensus statement. Brain. 2005;128:454–71.
77. Derry C, Dale RC, Thom M, Miller DH, Giovannoni G. Unihemispheric cerebral vasculitis mimicking Rasmussen's encephalitis. Neurology. 2002;58:327–8.
78. Oguni H, Andermann F, Rasmussen TB. The syndrome of chronic encephalitis and epilepsy. A study based on the MNI series of 48 cases. Adv Neurol. 1992;57:419–33.
79. Bien CG, Widman G, Urbach H, Sassen R, Kuczaty S, Wiestler OD, et al. The natural history of Rasmussen's encephalitis. Brain. 2002;125:1751–9.
80. Granata T, Gobbi G, Spreafico R, Vigevano F, Capovilla G, Ragona F, et al. Rasmussen's encephalitis: early characteristics allow diagnosis. Neurology. 2003;60:422–5.
81. Juul-Jensen P, Denny-Brown D. Epilepsia Partialis continua. Arch Neurol. 1966;15:563–78.
82. Bancaud J, Bonis A, Talairach J, Bordas-Ferrer M, Buser P. Kojewnikow syndrome and somato-motor attacks (clinical, E.E.G., E.M.G. and S.E.E.G. study). Encéphale. 1970;59:391–438.
83. Wieser HG, Graf HP, Bernoulli C, Siegfried J. Quantitative analysis of intracerebral recordings in epilepsia partialis continua. Electroencephalogr Clin Neurophysiol. 1978;44:14–22.
84. Cockerell OC, Rothwell J, Thompson PD, Marsden CD, Shorvon SD. Clinical and physiological features of epilepsia partialis continua. Cases ascertained in the UK. Brain. 1996;119:393–407.
85. Mameniškienė R, Wolf P. Epilepsia partialis continua: a review. Seizure. 2017;44:74–80.
86. So NK, Gloor P. Electroencephalographic and electrocorticographic findings in chronic encephalitis of the Rasmussen type. In: Andermann F, editor. Chronic encephalitis and epilepsy. Rasmussen's syndrome. Boston: Butterworth-Heinemann; 1991. p. 37–45.
87. Barkley GL, Baumgartner C. MEG and EEG in epilepsy. J Clin Neurophysiol. 2003;20:163–78.
88. Rossi Sebastiano D, Visani E, Duran D, Freri E, Panzica F, Chiapparini L, et al. Epileptic spikes in Rasmussen's encephalitis: migratory pattern and short-term evolution. A MEG study. Clin Neurophysiol. 2017;128:1898–905.
89. Marrie RA, Reider N, Cohen J, Trojano M, Sorensen PS, Cutter G, et al. A systematic review of the incidence and prevalence of sleep disorders and seizure disorders in multiple sclerosis. Mult Scler. 2015;21:342–9.
90. Martínez-Juárez IE, López-Meza E, González-Aragón Mdel CF, Ramírez-Bermúdez J, Corona T. Epilepsy and multiple sclerosis: increased risk among progressive forms. Epilepsy Res. 2009;84:250–3.
91. Catenoix H, Marignier R, Ritleng C, Dufour M, Mauguière F, Confavreux C, et al. Multiple sclerosis and epileptic seizures. Mult Scler. 2011;17:96–102.
92. Burman J, Zelano J. Epilepsy in multiple sclerosis: a nationwide population-based register study. Neurology. 2017;89:2462–8.
93. Gasparini S, Ferlazzo E, Ascoli M, Sueri C, Cianci V, Russo C, et al. Risk factors for unprovoked epileptic seizures in multiple sclerosis: a systematic review and meta-analysis. Neurol Sci. 2017;38:399–406.
94. Koch M, Uyttenboogaart M, Polman S, De Keyser J. Seizures in multiple sclerosis. Epilepsia. 2008;49:948–53.
95. Spatt J, Chaix R, Mamoli B. Epileptic and non-epileptic seizures in multiple sclerosis. J Neurol. 2001;248:2–9.
96. Kinnunen E, Wikström J. Prevalence and prognosis of epilepsy in patients with multiple sclerosis. Epilepsia. 1986;27:729–33.
97. Poser CM, Brinar VV. Epilepsy and multiple sclerosis. Epilepsy Behav. 2003;4:6–12.
98. Thompson AJ, Kermode AG, Moseley IF, MacManus DG, McDonald WI. Seizures due to multiple sclerosis: seven patients with MRI correlations. J Neurol Neurosurg Psychiatry. 1993;56:1317–20.
99. Hess DC, Sethi KD. Epilepsia partialis continua in multiple sclerosis. Int J Neurosci. 1990;50:109–11.
100. Spatt J, Goldenberg G, Mamoli B. Epilepsia partialis continua in multiple sclerosis. Lancet. 1995;345:658–9.
101. Nyquist PA, Cascino GD, Rodriguez M. Seizures in patients with multiple sclerosis seen at Mayo Clinic, Rochester, Minn, 1990–1998. Mayo Clin Proc. 2001;76:983–6.
102. Striano P, Striano S, Carrieri PB, Boccella P. Epilepsia partialis continua as a first symptom of multiple sclerosis: electrophysiological study of one case. Mult Scler. 2003;9:199–203.
103. Maingueneau F, Honnorat J, Isnard J, Tommasi-Davenas C, Derex L, Nighoghossian N, et al. Partial non-convulsive status epilepsy in multiple sclerosis. Neurophysiol Clin. 1999;29:463–72.
104. Chabolla DR, Moore JL, Westmoreland BF. Periodic lateralized epileptiform discharges in multiple sclerosis. Electroencephalogr Clin Neurophysiol. 1996;98:5–8.
105. Iragui-Madoz V. Electrophysiology of multiple sclerosis. In: Daly DD, Pedley TA, editors. Current practice of clinical electroencephalography. 2nd ed. New York: Raven Press; 1990. p. 708–38.
106. Grabow JD. Optimal recordings techniques and activation procedures: children and adults. In: Wada JA, Ellingson RJ, editors. Clinical neurophysiology of epilepsy. Amsterdam: Elsevier Science; 1990. p. 39–77.
107. Calabrese LH, Mallek JA. Primary angiitis of the central nervous system. Report of 8 new cases, review of the literature,

and proposal for diagnostic criteria. Medicine (Baltimore). 1988;67:20–39.
108. Salvarani C, Brown RD Jr, Hunder GG. Adult primary central nervous system vasculitis. Lancet. 2012;380:767–77.
109. Salvarani C, Brown RD Jr, Calamia KT, Christianson TJ, Weigand SD, Miller DV, et al. Primary central nervous system vasculitis: analysis of 101 patients. Ann Neurol. 2007;62:442–51.
110. Jennekens FG, Kater L. The central nervous system in systemic lupus erythematosus. Part 1. Clinical syndromes: a literature investigation. Rheumatology (Oxford). 2002;41:605–18.
111. Herranz MT, Rivier G, Khamashta MA, Blaser KU, Hughes GR. Association between antiphospholipid antibodies and epilepsy in patients with systemic lupus erythematosus. Arthritis Rheum. 1994;37:568–71.
112. Mackworth-Young CG, Hughes GR. Epilepsy: an early symptom of systemic lupus erythematosus. J Neurol Neurosurg Psychiatry. 1985;48:185.
113. Appenzeller S, Cendes F, Costallat LT. Epileptic seizures in systemic lupus erythematosus. Neurology. 2004;63:1808–12.
114. González-Duarte A, Cantú-Brito CG, Ruano-Calderón L, García-Ramos G. Clinical description of seizures in patients with systemic lupus erythematosus. Eur Neurol. 2008;59:320–3.
115. Sakane T, Takeno M, Suzuki N, Inaba G. Behçet's disease. N Engl J Med. 1999;341:1284–91.
116. Verity DH, Wallace GR, Vaughan RW, Stanford MR. Behçet's disease: from Hippocrates to the third millennium. Br J Ophthalmol. 2003;87:1175–83.
117. Kural-Seyahi E, Fresko I, Seyahi N, Ozyazgan Y, Mat C, Hamuryudan V, et al. The long-term mortality and morbidity of Behçet syndrome: a 2-decade outcome survey of 387 patients followed at a dedicated center. Medicine (Baltimore). 2003;82:60–76.
118. Akman-Demir G, Serdaroglu P, Tasçi B. Clinical patterns of neurological involvement in Behçet's disease: evaluation of 200 patients. The Neuro-Behçet Study Group. Brain. 1999;122:2171–82.
119. Al-Fahad SA, Al-Araji AH. Neuro-Behcet's disease in Iraq: a study of 40 patients. J Neurol Sci. 1999;170:105–11.
120. Siva A, Kantarci OH, Saip S, Altintas A, Hamuryudan V, Islak C, et al. Behçet's disease: diagnostic and prognostic aspects of neurological involvement. J Neurol. 2001;248:95–103.
121. Aykutlu E, Baykan B, Serdaroglu P, Gökyigit A, Akman-Demir G. Epileptic seizures in Behçet disease. Epilepsia. 2002;43:832–5.
122. Mead S, Kidd D, Good C, Plant G. Behcet's syndrome may present with partial seizures. J Neurol Neurosurg Psychiatry. 2000;68:392–3.
123. Aktekin B, Doğan EA, Oğuz Y, Karaali K. Epilepsia partialis continua in a patient with Behçet's disease. Clin Neurol Neurosurg. 2006;108:392–5.
124. Al-Araji A, Kidd DP. Neuro-Behçet's disease: epidemiology, clinical characteristics, and management. Lancet Neurol. 2009;8:192–204.
125. Stern BJ, Krumholz A, Johns C, Scott P, Nissim J. Sarcoidosis and its neurological manifestations. Arch Neurol. 1985;42:909–17.
126. James DG, Sharma OP. Neurosarcoidosis. Proc R Soc Med. 1967;60:1169–70.
127. Lynch JP 3rd. Neurosarcoidosis: how good are the diagnostic tests? J Neuroophthalmol. 2003;23:187–9.
128. Moore FG, Andermann F, Richardson J, Tampieri D, Giaccone R. The role of MRI and nerve root biopsy in the diagnosis of neurosarcoidosis. Can J Neurol Sci. 2001;28:349–53.
129. Krumholz A, Stern BJ, Stern EG. Clinical implications of seizures in neurosarcoidosis. Arch Neurol. 1991;48:842–4.
130. Sponsler JL, Werz MA, Maciunas R, Cohen M. Neurosarcoidosis presenting with simple partial seizures and solitary enhancing mass: case reports and review of the literature. Epilepsy Behav. 2005;6:623–30.
131. Besur S, Bishnoi R, Talluri SK. Neurosarcoidosis: rare initial presentation with seizures and delirium. QJM. 2011;104:801–3.
132. Gullapalli D, Phillips LH 2nd. Neurologic manifestations of sarcoidosis. Neurol Clin. 2002;20:59–83.
133. Delaney P. Seizures in sarcoidosis: a poor prognosis. Ann Neurol. 1980;7:494.
134. Delaney P. Neurologic manifestations in sarcoidosis: review of the literature, with a report of 23 cases. Ann Intern Med. 1977;87:336–45.
135. Brophy GM, Bell R, Claassen J, Alldredge B, Bleck TP, Glauser T, et al. Guidelines for the evaluation and management of status epilepticus. Neurocrit Care. 2012;17:3–23.
136. Tan RY, Neligan A, Shorvon SD. The uncommon causes of status epilepticus: a systematic review. Epilepsy Res. 2010;91:111–22.
137. Watemberg N, Segal G. A suggested approach to the etiologic evaluation of status epilepticus in children: what to seek after the usual causes have been ruled out. J Child Neurol. 2010;25:203–11.
138. Hirsch LJ, Gaspard N. Status Epilepticus. Continuum (Minneap Minn). 2013;19:767–94.
139. Jayalakshmi S, Vooturi S, Sahu S, Yada PK, Mohandas S. Causes and outcomes of new onset status epilepticus and predictors of refractoriness to therapy. J Clin Neurosci. 2016;26:89–94.
140. Wilder-Smith EP, Lim EC, Teoh HL, Sharma VK, Tan JJ, Chan BP, et al. The NORSE (new-onset refractory status epilepticus) syndrome: defining a disease entity. Ann Acad Med Singap. 2005;34:417–20.
141. Costello DJ, Kilbride RD, Cole AJ. Cryptogenic new onset refractory status epilepticus (NORSE) in adults-infectious or not? J Neurol Sci. 2009;277:26–31.
142. Gaspard N, Foreman BP, Alvarez V, Cabrera Kang C, Probasco JC, Jongeling AC, et al. New-onset refractory status epilepticus: etiology, clinical features, and outcome. Neurology. 2015;85:1604–13.
143. Baxter P, Clarke A, Cross H, Harding B, Hicks E, Livingston J, et al. Idiopathic catastrophic epileptic encephalopathy presenting with acute onset intractable status. Seizure. 2003;12:379–87.
144. Kramer U, Chi CS, Lin KL, Specchio N, Sahin M, Olson H, et al. Febrile infection-related epilepsy syndrome (FIRES): pathogenesis, treatment, and outcome: a multicenter study on 77 children. Epilepsia. 2011;52:1956–65.
145. van Baalen A, Häusler M, Boor R, Rohr A, Sperner J, Kurlemann G, et al. Febrile infection-related epilepsy syndrome (FIRES): a nonencephalitic encephalopathy in childhood. Epilepsia. 2010;51:1323–8.
146. Sakuma H. Acute encephalitis with refractory, repetitive partial seizures. Brain and Development. 2009;31:510–4.
147. Mikaeloff Y, Jambaqué I, Hertz-Pannier L, Zamfirescu A, Adamsbaum C, Plouin P, et al. Devastating epileptic encephalopathy in school-aged children (DESC): a pseudo encephalitis. Epilepsy Res. 2006;69:67–79.
148. Hirsch LJ, Gaspard N, van Baalen A, Nabbout R, Demeret S, Loddenkemper T, et al. Proposed consensus definitions for new-onset refractory status epilepticus (NORSE), febrile infection-related epilepsy syndrome (FIRES), and related conditions. Epilepsia. 2018;59:739–44.
149. Gaspard N, Hirsch LJ, Sculier C, Loddenkemper T, van Baalen A, Lancrenon J, et al. New-onset refractory status epilepticus (NORSE) and febrile infection-related epilepsy syndrome (FIRES): state of the art and perspectives. Epilepsia. 2018;59:745–52.
150. Meletti S, Slonkova J, Mareckova I, Monti G, Specchio N, Hon P, et al. Claustrum damage and refractory status epilepticus following febrile illness. Neurology. 2015;85:1224–32.
151. Farias-Moeller R, Bartolini L, Staso K, Schreiber JM, Carpenter JL. Early ictal and interictal patterns in FIRES: the sparks before the blaze. Epilepsia. 2017;58:1340–8.

41 Aging and Degenerative Disorders

Francesco Brigo and Oriano Mecarelli

41.1 EEG Changes in the Elderly

Cerebral aging is associated with characteristic changes of main EEG patterns recorded during wakefulness and sleep [1]. In wakefulness the amplitude of background alpha rhythm is lower in adults and elderly people compared to the adolescent, particularly in the occipital region, and sometimes an instability of alpha can be seen due to a scarce tendency to synchronization. However, these changes are sometimes the mere expression of anxiety and are therefore less evident during and after hyperventilation. When the alpha rhythm is well synchronized, such as during quite wakefulness with closed eyes, the EEG recorded in the elderly may show a tendency toward an anterior diffusion of the background activity; the typical posterior dominance is therefore less evident (Fig. 41.1). Over the years, a progressive slowing of alpha rhythm of approximately 0.08 Hz/year occurs after the age of 60. In our experience, patients in their 80s have a mean alpha rhythm of 8.5–9 Hz. Individuals who are over 100 years old have a physiological reduction of alpha frequency to 7.5–8 Hz [2]. Figures 41.2 and 41.3 show examples of changes in background activities at different ages, assessed both visually and quantitatively. After the age of 50, subharmonics of background activity at 4–5 Hz (slow alpha variant) and an asynchronous and asymmetrical background rhythm can be seen. The mu rhythm is less visible in elderly compared to younger subjects, and the photic drive during intermittent photic stimulation is less evident.

With increasing age, the beta activity is less represented and has lower amplitude, particularly over precentral regions, especially for 25–30 Hz frequencies. Compared to males with the same age, females have greater amount of beta activity [3, 4].

After the age of 60, slow focal activities (theta and/or delta) are more represented and prevalent over left anterior temporal region. Very small amount of theta and delta sequences are nevertheless considered normal for the age. Hyperventilation can lead to a slow widespread theta-delta activity and an increase in a focal temporal slowing already present in baseline EEG recording.

During the first phases of NREM sleep, a reduction in amplitude and frequency of sleep spindles and K complexes can be seen, with a reduced voltage of vertex waves and positive occipital sharp transients of sleep (POSTS). A shorter duration of phases 3 and 4 of NREM sleep with a lower density of delta waves can occur, together with a reduction in REM (rapid eye movements) latency, duration, and density. Overall, there is a reduction in the total number of hours spent to sleep, which is more superficial and characterized by frequent interruptions due to nocturnal awakenings.

In conclusion, different criteria should be used when assessing the EEG of elderly subjects: if the same criteria valid for young and adult individuals were adopted, more than 50% of EEG recordings in subjects older than 60 years would be classified abnormal. The most relevant changes include the alpha rhythm (of lower amplitude and lower frequency and with tendency to anteriorization), theta-delta activities (more evident, particularly over left and temporal regions), and beta activity (less evident and of lower voltage, particularly among men) [1].

41.2 Use and Advantages of the EEG Recording in the Elderly

EEG recordings are usually required in the elderly for syncopal episodes, confusional states, epileptic seizures with motor phenomena, and episodes of transient loss of consciousness [5]. Based on the available literature (mostly unselected and homogeneous case series), approximately

F. Brigo (✉)
Department of Neurosciences, Biomedicine and Movement Sciences, University of Verona, Verona, Italy

Department of Neurology, Hospital Franz Tappeiner, Merano, Italy

O. Mecarelli
Department of Human Neurosciences, Sapienza University of Rome, Rome, Italy

O. Mecarelli (ed.), *Clinical Electroencephalography*, https://doi.org/10.1007/978-3-030-04573-9_41

Fig. 41.1 EEG recorded in a 75-year-old subject. The background 9–10 Hz alpha rhythm shows anteriorization

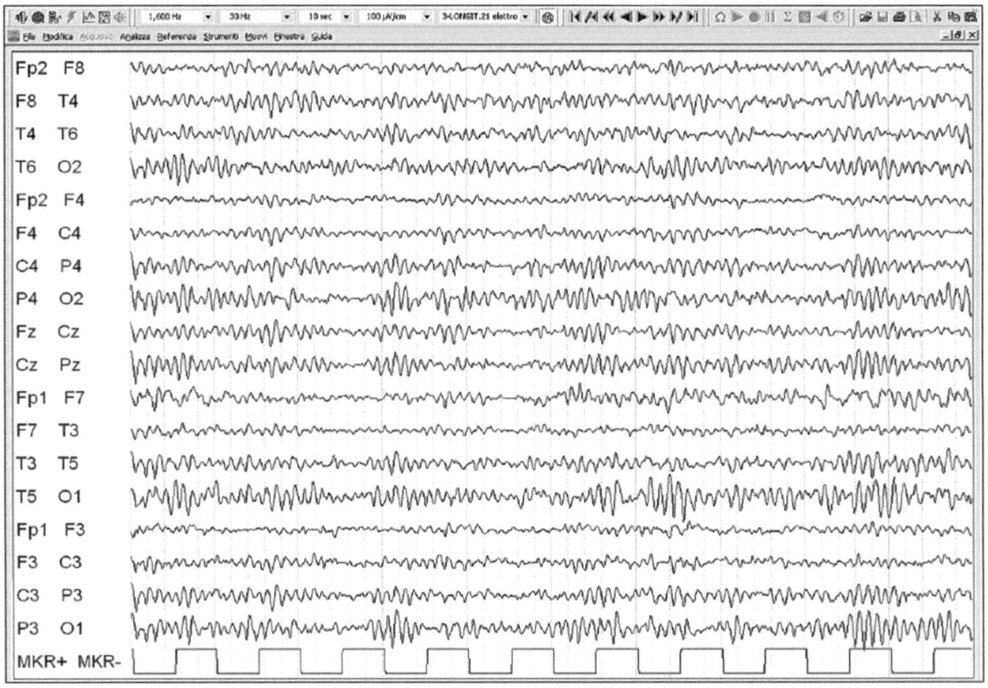

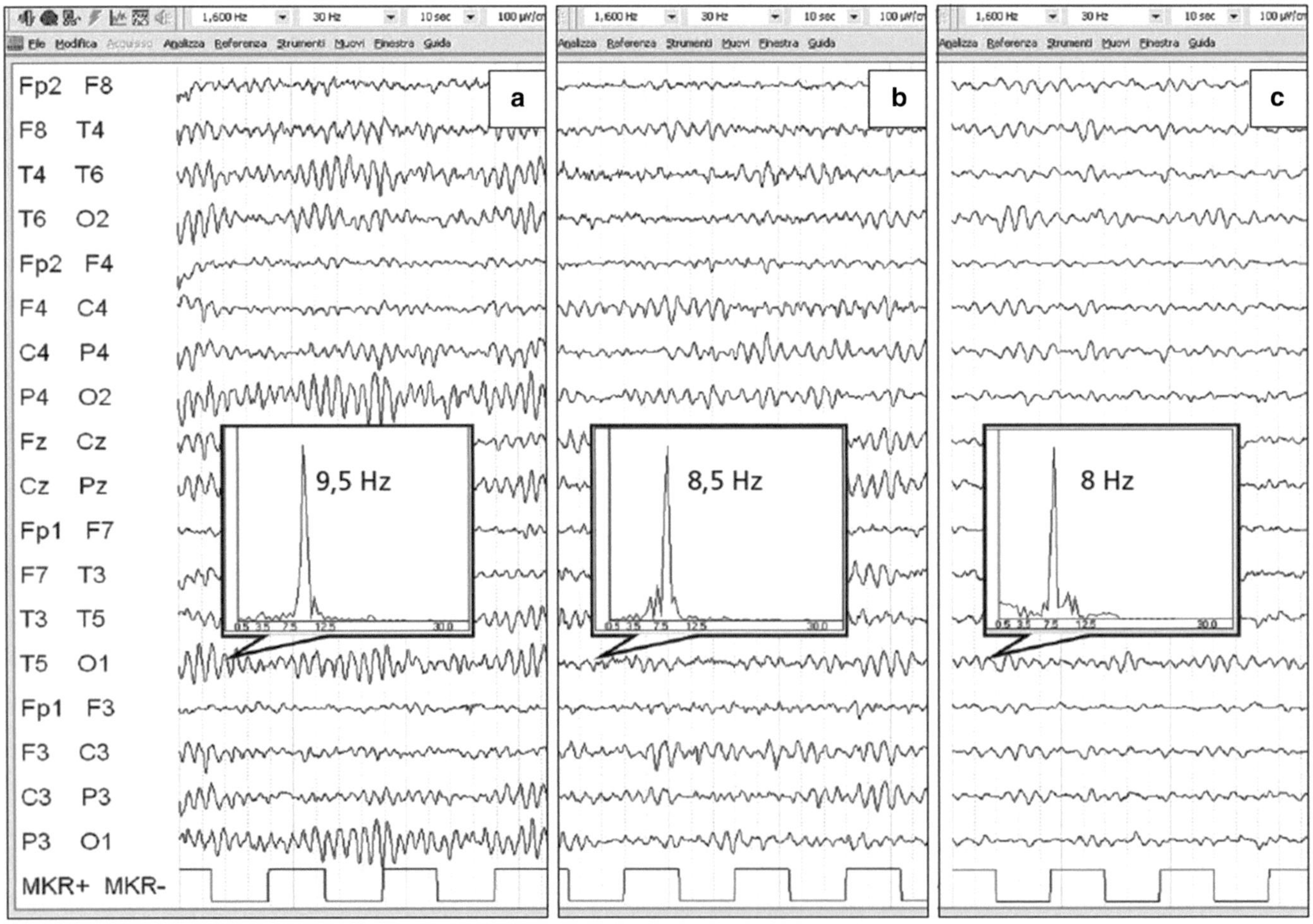

Fig. 41.2 EEG recorded in subjects of 75 (**a**), 83 (**b**), and 91 years (**c**). The peak of alpha power corresponds to 9.5, 8.5, and 8 Hz, respectively

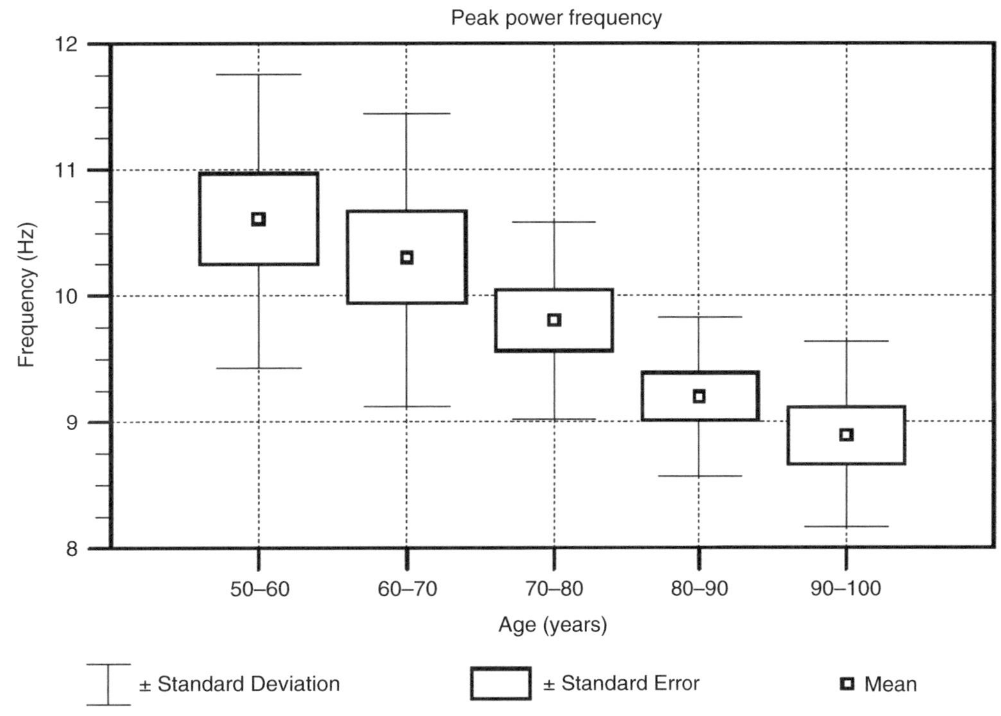

Fig. 41.3 Results of a quantitative EEG study conducted in subjects aged between 50 and 100 years without neuropsychiatric and systemic diseases, grouped according to age (10 individuals each); the peak of alpha power decreases progressively as the age increases [personal data]

50% of the EEGs are abnormal, particularly for the presence of focal and/or widespread slowing, which are encountered more frequently in patients older than 80 years. Epileptiform abnormalities are rarely seen.

In the elderly subjects, it is important that the recordings include an ECG monitoring and last long enough to detect fluctuations in vigilance. Whenever possible a video-EEG recording should also be obtained for differential diagnosis [6], since approximately 50% of the paroxysmal episodes requiring EEG are nonepileptic events. In the elderly, the EEG should be recorded not for detecting focal and/or widespread slowing but to correlate the cognitive deficit or the consciousness impairment with nonconvulsive status epilepticus/seizures and toxic-dismetabolic or infective encephalopathies. In these conditions, the EEG can be more sensitive than neuroimaging, particularly in the initial stages [7]. For instance, in elderly individuals taking several drugs, the EEG can reveal signs compatible with drug toxicity, such as a slowing of the background activity incongruous with the age of the subjects.

41.3 Dementia Syndromes

Dementia is a brain disorder characterized by a progressive deficit of cognitive functions with subsequent impairment of social and working activities. Primary degenerative dementias (Alzheimer's disease, frontotemporal dementia, dementia with Lewy bodies) represent approximately 60–70% of cases, the vascular dementias the 20–30%, and other etiologies (e.g., dementia associated with Parkinson's disease, Huntington chorea, progressive supranuclear palsy) the remaining 10–20%.

The electroencephalogram (EEG) is noninvasive, inexpensive, highly available, and sensitive to changes in the functional state of the human brain. These features explain why EES has been used for many years in dementia research, with the aim of differentiating subjects with various types and severity of cognitive impairment from healthy individuals. Visual EEG analysis is routinely used in clinical practice. A more accurate differential diagnosis between the various subtypes of dementia relies on quantitative EEG (qEEG), which requires extensive technical knowledge in the field of digital signal processing.

The EEG may prove useful in the diagnosis of dementia, because there is usually a good correlation between the degree of cognitive impairment and the EEG changes [1]. In dementia syndromes EEG changes include a progressive slowing of posterior dominant alpha rhythm, a progressive increase in theta-delta activity, and a reduction in beta activity. A highest amount of slowing is related with a more rapid course of disease.

The EEG may also indicate whether the dementia is associated with a focal or a diffuse process or if the cognitive impairment is due to a continuous epileptic activity (i.e., nonconvulsive status epilepticus [7]). Finally, a normal or near-normal EEG in a patient with cognitive deficits suggests the presence of depressive pseudodementia or frontotemporal dementia [1].

41.3.1 Alzheimer's Disease

Usually, in the initial stages of the disease, the EEG shows a nonspecific slowing of alpha rhythm, later evolving into a widespread theta-delta activity and a decrease in beta activity (Fig. 41.4a). In patients with mild cognitive impairment, the EEG can be normal. In some patients the dominant posterior rhythm can still be within the alpha frequency; however, if previous EEGs are available, a slowing of the frequency can be observed. With disease progression bursts of bilateral slow potentials appear, prevalently over anterior regions (Fig. 41.4b). Epileptiform abnormalities are rare and may have a triphasic morphology. Sometimes these graphoelements are periodic and more evident over middle posterior head regions.

In Alzheimer's disease the slowing of the EEG tracing is directly correlated with the degree of cognitive impairment. In mild cognitive impairment, the EEG is normal or may show only a modest increase of theta activity associated with reduced beta activity. Patients with Alzheimer's disease typically show a reduced reactivity of alpha rhythm to eye opening (partial alpha blockade) (Fig. 41.5) and during memory testing, perhaps related to a reduced dopaminergic tone.

The polysomnography shows a progressive reduction in total sleep time, affecting both NREM and REM. Compared to nondemented subjects with the same age, patients with Alzheimer's disease have a higher sleep fragmentation and a reduction of sleep spindles and K complexes.

Studies with quantitative EEG have provided promising results to identify EEG biomarkers of the progressive cognitive impairment, such as increased power of theta-delta frequency bands, a corresponding reduced power of fast alpha-beta frequencies [8], and the reduced reactivity of alpha rhythm to eye opening and during memory testing [9, 10]. EEG coherence is reduced in Alzheimer's disease, suggesting a reduced interaction between different cerebral areas [11].

EEG network analysis methods are emerging as potential biomarkers for the diagnosis of AD and promising tools for studying disease progression and for early recognition of mild cognitive impairment, particularly if combined with spectral methods [12]; their place in clinical practice still needs to be further assessed.

Results of studies assessing the role of EEG in the diagnosis of dementia should however be interpreted with caution, paying attention to the presence of age-matched controls, which is necessary to avoid overestimation of EEG slowing, and to the sample size [13].

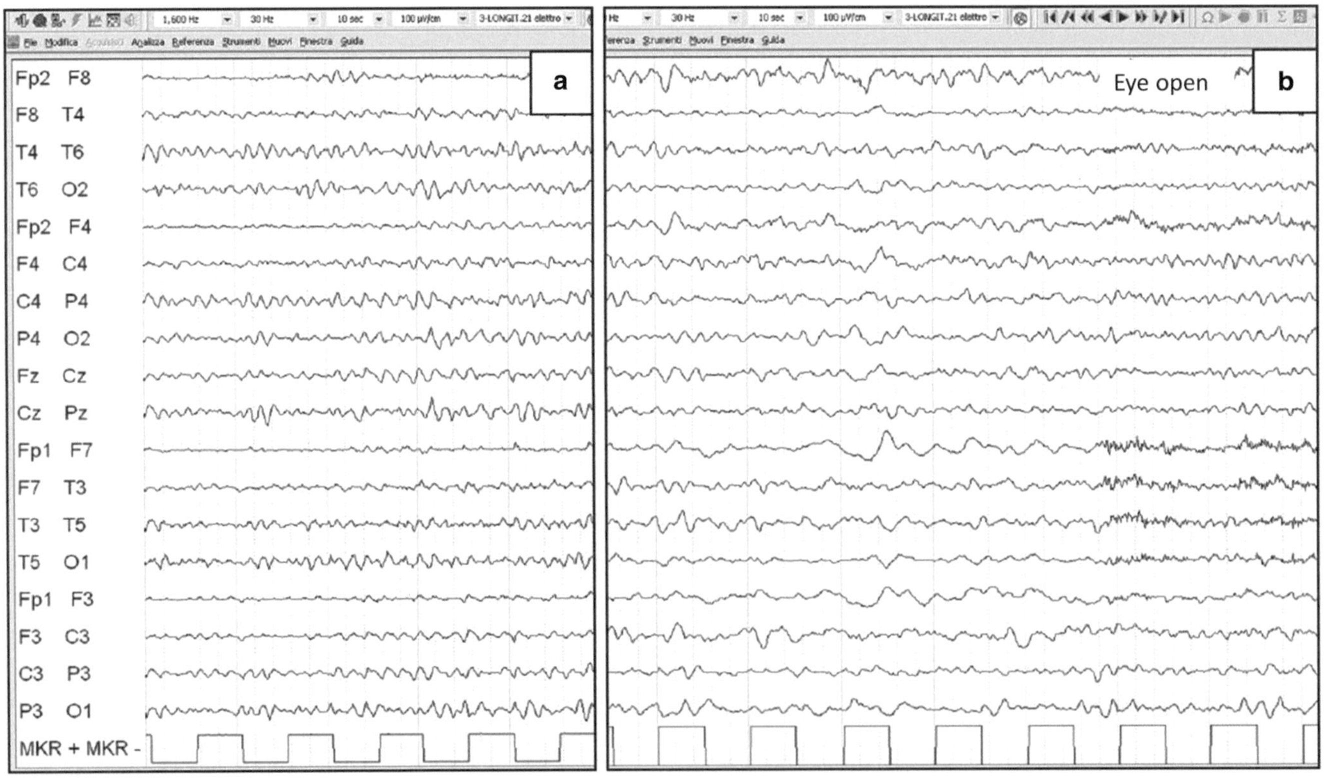

Fig. 41.4 EEG recordings obtained in the same patient with Alzheimer's disease. (**a**) In the initial stage, the EEG recording shows a modest slowing of background activity. (**b**) In a later stage, the tracing is diffusely slowed, particularly over middle anterior regions. The eye opening leads to a background activity which is better synchronized and more rapid (paradoxical alpha)

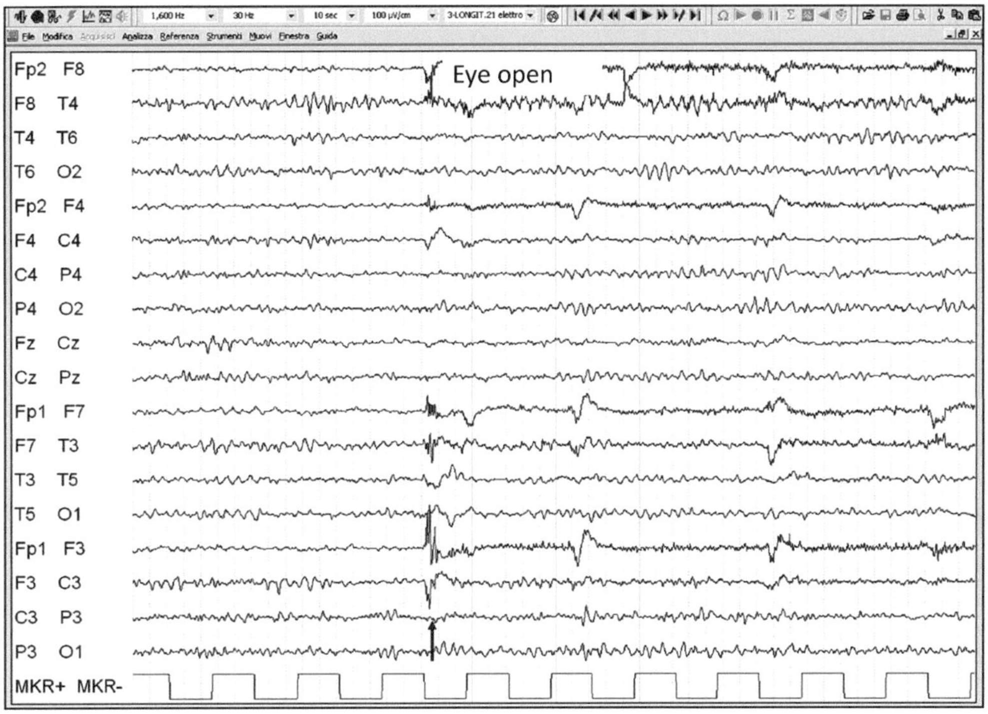

Fig. 41.5 A 65-year-old patient with initial Alzheimer's disease. The EEG shows a partial alpha blockade

41.3.2 Dementia with Lewy Bodies

Dementia with Lewy bodies is the second most common neurodegenerative cause of dementia after Alzheimer's disease. In this dementia syndrome, EEG changes in the initial phases include slowing of background activity and bursts of theta-delta activity, prevalent over frontal regions. Overall, EEG changes in dementia with Lewy bodies are usually more severe than those detected in Alzheimer's disease, particularly for the prominent and precocious theta slowing over temporal regions [14]. Bilateral frontal intermittent rhythmic delta activity (FIRDA) seems to occur more frequently than in patients clinically diagnosed with Alzheimer's disease and has therefore been proposed as a supportive diagnostic feature for this condition [15].

41.3.3 Frontotemporal Dementia

The visual inspection of EEG recordings in patients with frontotemporal dementia does not usually show relevant differences with those of healthy subjects [16]. However, a quantitative analysis may inconstantly reveal theta activity over frontoparietal regions or a reduction of beta activity [17].

41.4 Multi-infarct Dementia

In this type of dementia, the EEG shows focal or multifocal slowing, even in the presence of a preserved background rhythm (Fig. 41.6). The presence of an alpha rhythm, even in later stages of the disease, suggests a multi-infarct dementia, whereas in primary dementia a global slowing of background activity is usually seen in early stages. The EEG changes (slowing of background activity) correlate with cortical atrophy and leukoencephalopathy seen on neuroimaging [18]. In multi-infarct dementia, epileptiform abnormalities may also occur and are more common than in Alzheimer's disease; they are usually sharp waves, sometimes with a quasiperiodic pattern of recurrence, and are frequently associated with large and superficial infarcts.

41.4.1 Subcortical Dementia

In Parkinson's disease without dementia, the EEG shows no relevant changes, apart from those related to aging and concomitant diseases. Theta rhythmic artifactual activities due to tremor are frequently seen, particularly over posterior regions (Fig. 41.7). Parkinson's dementia (i.e., dementia associated with Parkinson's disease) is a clinical

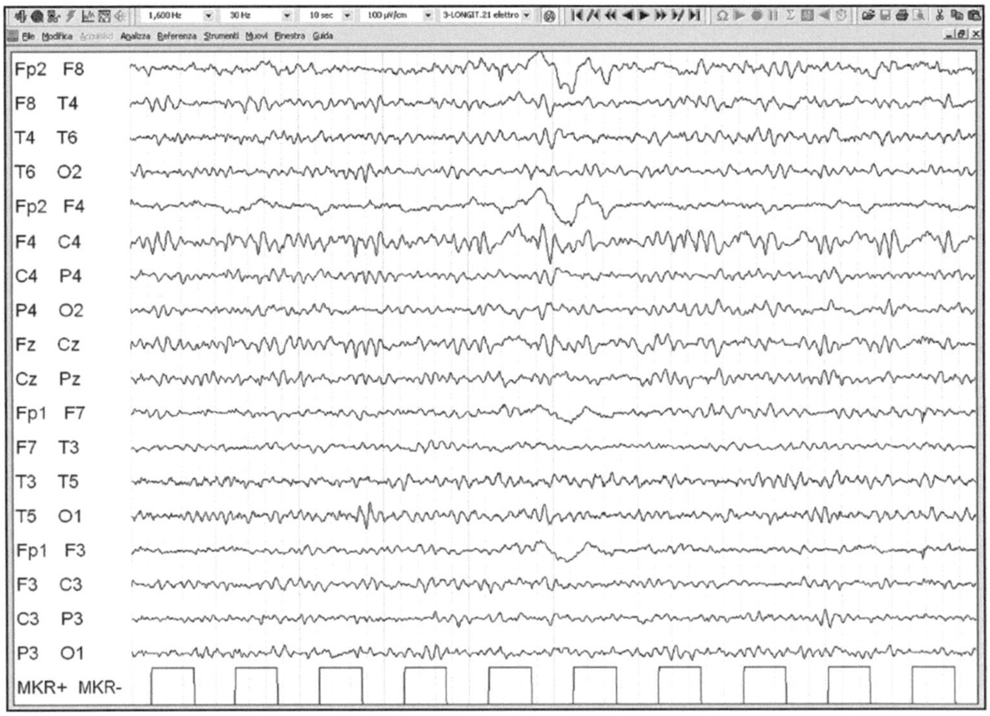

Fig. 41.6 A 73-year-old patient with multi-infarct dementia. The EEG shows a preserved background activity with middle anterior delta slowing, prevalent on the right side, and sporadic sharp waves in frontocentral regions

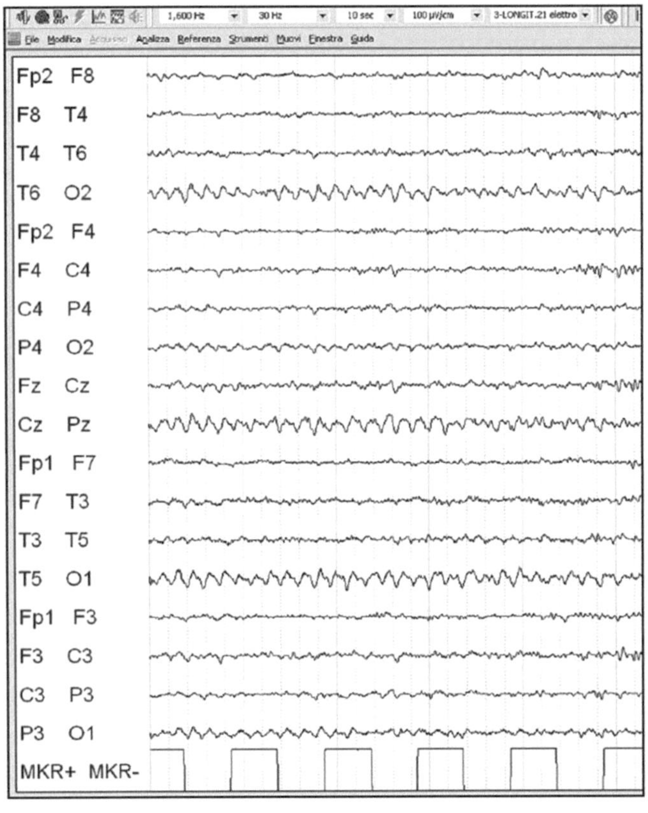

Fig. 41.7 Artifactual activity due to tremor in a patient with Parkinson's disease. The EEG artifacts are characterized by 6 Hz monomorphic theta middle posterior sequences, which might be misinterpreted as cerebral abnormalities

syndrome characterized by slowness of mental processing, impaired cognition, apathy, and depression. It is often associated with an early nonspecific slowing of background activity. During the course of the disease, there is a progressive slowing of the background activity, with a widespread monomorphic theta activity, sometimes admixed with slower (delta) sequences over frontotemporal regions, mostly on the left side (Fig. 41.8). The polysomnography is characterized by an increased sleep latency and a reduced total sleep time, with increased amount of first NREM stages and reduced slow sleep stages and REM. There are also frequent nocturnal awakenings. Quantitative EEG studies have shown that spectral analysis (increase of spectral powers in delta and theta frequency bands, with decrease in alpha and beta bands) can discriminate between dementia associated with Parkinson's disease and Parkinson's disease without dementia and differentiate mild cognitive impairment from normal cognition in patients with Parkinson's disease [19].

In dementia associated with Huntington's disease, the EEG recorded in most advanced stages shows a slowing and destructuration of background activity, with increased slowing predominant anteriorly. In initial stages there is often a low-voltage activity. In patients with myoclonic seizures, the EEG shows polyspike and polyspike-wave complexes.

In dementia associated with progressive supranuclear palsy, the EEG shows a progressive slowing of the alpha rhythm and the progressive appearance of slowing, also

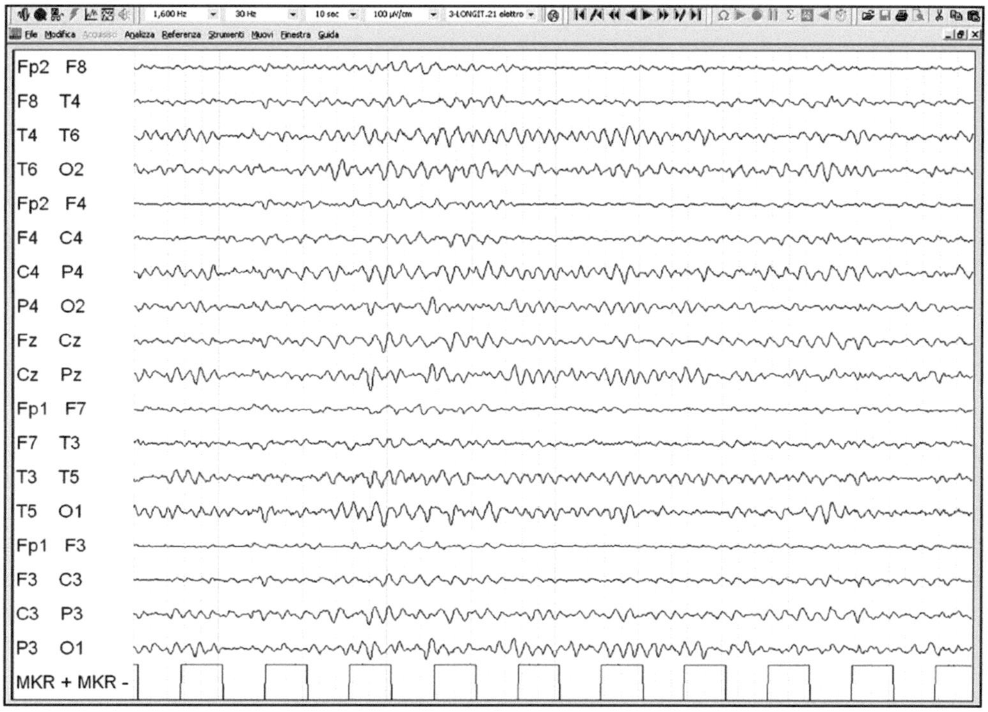

Fig. 41.8 A 75-year-old patient with Parkinson's disease. The EEG shows a 7.5 Hz background activity with widespread theta activity prevalent over left central and temporal posterior regions

manifesting as frontal intermittent rhythmic delta activity or bitemporal (temporal intermittent rhythmic delta activity). In initial stages of disease, the EEG is mostly normal.

References

1. Babiloni C, Del Percio C, Buján A. EEG in dementing disorders. In: Schomer DL, Lopes da Silva F, editors. Niedermeyer's electroencephalography: basic principles, clinical applications, and related fields. 7th ed. New York, NY: Oxford University Press; 2018. p. 413–32.
2. Hubbard O, Sunde D, Goldensohn ES. The EEG in centenarians. Electroencephalogr Clin Neurophysiol. 1976;40:407–17.
3. Giaquinto S, Nolfe G. The EEG in the normal elderly: a contribution to the interpretation of aging and dementia. Electroencephalogr Clin Neurophysiol. 1986;63:540–6.
4. Brenner RP, Ulrich RF, Reinolds CF. EEG spectral analysis in healthy, elderly men and women: sex differences. Electroencephalogr Clin Neurophysiol. 1995;94:1–5.
5. Widdess-Walsh P, Sweeney BJ, Galvin R, McNamara B. Utilization and yield of EEG in the elderly population. J Clin Neurophysiol. 2005;22:253–5.
6. Kipervasser S, Neufeld MY. Video-EEG monitoring of paroxysmal events in the elderly. Acta Neurol Scand. 2007;116:221–5.
7. Bottaro FJ, Martinez OA, Fernandez Pardal MM, et al. Nonconvulsive status epilepticus in the elderly: a case-control study. Epilepsia. 2007;48:966–72.
8. Huang C, Wahlund L, Dierks T, Julin P, Winblad B, Jelic V. Discrimination of Alzheimer's disease and mild cognitive impairment by equivalent EEG sources: a cross-sectional and longitudinal study. Clin Neurophysiol. 2000;111:1961–7.
9. Van der Hiele K, Vein AA, van der Welle A, et al. EEG and MRI correlates of mild cognitive impairment and Alzheimer's disease. Neurobiol Aging. 2007;28:1322–9.
10. Van der Hiele K, Vein AA, Reijntjes RHAM, et al. EEG correlates in the spectrum of cognitive decline. Clin Neurophysiol. 2007;118:1931–9.
11. Jelles B, Scheltens PH, van der Flier WM, et al. Global dynamical analysis of the EEG in Alzheimer's disease: frequency-specific changes of functional interactions. Clin Neurophysiol. 2008;119:837–41.
12. Horvath A, Szucs A, Csukly G, Sakovics A, Stefanics G, Kamondi A. EEG and ERP biomarkers of Alzheimer's disease: a critical review. Front Biosci (Landmark Ed). 2018;23:183–220.
13. Van der Hiele K, Bollen ELEM, Vein AA, et al. EEG markers of future cognitive performance in the elderly. J Clin Neurophysiol. 2008;25:83–9.
14. Cromarty RA, Elder GJ, Graziadio S, et al. Neurophysiological biomarkers for Lewy body dementias. Clin Neurophysiol. 2016;127:349–59.
15. Calzetti S, Bortone E, Negrotti A, Zinno L, Mancia D. Frontal intermittent rhythmic delta activity (FIRDA) in patients with dementia with Lewy bodies: a diagnostic tool? Neurol Sci. 2002;23(Suppl 2):S65–6.
16. Yener GG, Leuchter AF, Jenden D, Read SL, Cummings JL, Miller BL. Quantitative EEG in frontotemporal dementia. Clin Electroencephalogr. 1996;27:61–8.
17. Malek N, Baker MR, Mann C, Greene J. Electroencephalographic markers in dementia. Acta Neurol Scand. 2017;135:388–93.
18. Erkinjuntti T, Larsen T, Sulkava R, Ketonen L, Laaksonen R, Palo J. EEG in the differential diagnosis between Alzheimer's disease and vascular dementia. Acta Neurol Scand. 1988;77:36–43.
19. Cozac VV, Gschwandtner U, Hatz F, Hardmeier M, Rüegg S, Fuhr P. Quantitative EEG and cognitive decline in Parkinson's disease. Parkinsons Dis. 2016;2016:9060649.

42 Systemic and Dismetabolic Disorders

Francesco Brigo and Oriano Mecarelli

42.1 Introduction

Several systemic and metabolic disorders may cause an impairment of cerebral functions with different pathophysiological mechanisms. The function of neurons and glial cells is affected by disturbances of blood sugar levels, electrolytes, impaired liver or renal function, alkalosis or acidosis, and hypoxia.

Neuroimaging investigations are often not sensitive enough to appropriately evaluate these clinical conditions. The EEG represents therefore a useful method for assessing brain functional activity, to support clinical diagnosis and to monitor follow-up (neuromonitoring).

In systemic and metabolic disorders, the EEG changes reflect the diffuse cerebral impairment. Widespread EEG slowing sometimes associated with epileptiform activity is a typical pattern encountered in these conditions; however, it is not pathognomonic of systemic and metabolic disorders and is not specific of a certain etiology [1, 2].

EEG can also demonstrate the improvement of cerebral function following therapy of the underlying systemic or metabolic disorder. These conditions—which may be acute, subacute, or chronic—are usually characterized by various degree of impairment of vigilance and cognitive functions and are sometimes associated with motor or non-motor epileptic seizures. If cerebral impairment is severe and prolonged enough to produce an irreversible condition, without return to the previous cerebral function, the EEG and the neurophysiological monitoring are of utmost importance both to detect negative prognostic factors and to diagnose brain death [2].

F. Brigo (✉)
Department of Neurosciences, Biomedicine and Movement Sciences, University of Verona, Verona, Italy

Department of Neurology, Hospital Franz Tappeiner, Merano, Italy

O. Mecarelli
Department of Human Neurosciences, Sapienza University of Rome, Rome, Italy

42.2 Liver Disease

Liver disease may cause a cerebral impairment of various degrees, termed hepatic encephalopathy (HE). It is a reversible impairment of neuropsychiatric function associated with acute or chronic liver failure, due to toxic catabolites which accumulate and interfere with cerebral functions. The biochemical mechanisms leading to HE are different, including hyperammonia, impaired metabolism of glutamine, and changes in neurotransmitters [2].

In terms of physiopathology, it is important to distinguish HE due to acute liver failure following necrosis of liver cells (for instance, as a consequence of fulminant hepatitis) from chronic HE due to portosystemic shunt. Portosystemic shunt, which may occur in patients without structural liver damage or in patients with cirrhosis of different degree of severity, is a bypass of the liver by the extrahepatic circulatory system. Both in acute and chronic hepatic disease, the filtering function of the liver is impaired.

Usually the increased blood levels of toxins, accumulating as a consequence of the impaired liver catabolism, are associated with a progressive impairment of cortical functions. This leads to confusion, behavioral changes, motor deficit, and—if the condition persists over time—motor and non-motor epileptic seizures and even status epilepticus.

In the initial stages, HE is characterized by irritability, apathy or euphoria, and impairment of cognitive functions. In milder cases, patients have no clinically overt neuropsychiatric symptoms, but neurophysiological and psychometric evaluations may nonetheless reveal subclinical deficits. In this stage, constructional apraxia can occur, due to altered spatial perception. A typical symptom of patients with initial HE is asterixis, a tremor of the hand observed when the wrist is extended, which resembles a bird flapping its wings ("flapping tremor"); it is due to a recurrent and transient loss of muscular tone involving hands and arms. In more advanced stages, the impairment of vigilance and the behavioral changes become more severe, leading to stupor or coma.

O. Mecarelli (ed.), *Clinical Electroencephalography*, https://doi.org/10.1007/978-3-030-04573-9_42

According to the West Haven criteria, the severity of HE is classified and graded based on the clinical manifestations, the degree of impairment of vigilance, cognitive functions, and behavior [3, 4]:

- Grade I: Changes in behavior, mild confusion, slurred speech, and disordered sleep.
- Grade II: Lethargy and moderate confusion.
- Grade III: Marked confusion (stupor), incoherent speech, and patient sleeping but arousable.
- Grade IV: Coma and unresponsiveness to pain.

The EEG is a useful method to monitor the impaired cerebral functions in acute or chronic liver disease [2]. The mildest cases are characterized by nonspecific changes, such as widespread theta activity, sometimes prominent over frontal-temporal regions and associated with a normal posterior dominant alpha rhythm. In subsequent phases a widespread theta-delta activity is seen, sometimes manifesting as frontal intermittent delta activity (FIRDA) or occipital intermittent delta activity (OIRDA) [5]. The posterior dominant alpha rhythm is further slowed and only partly responsive to eye opening. Sharply contoured elements, sometimes with bi- or triphasic morphology, can coexist. The impairment of cognitive functions is clinically evident and worsens over time in parallel with the slowing of EEG activity and the appearance of bi- and triphasic sharp waves. The triphasic waves, although not pathognomonic of liver impairment, are typically observed and are frequently seen in most advanced phases of hepatic disease; the morbidity and mortality associated with this EEG pattern depend on the underlying etiology [6]. Triphasic waves are high-amplitude graphoelements (100–300 μV) repeating periodically at 1.5–3 Hz, usually predominant over frontal regions. They are bisynchronous, although the amplitude may be asymmetric. As their name suggests, triphasic waves consist of three phases: a surface-positive high-amplitude (greater than 70 μV) wave is preceded and followed by negative waves with smaller amplitude [6]. The high-amplitude positive wave steeply declines, whereas the final negative wave has a gradually ascending "asymptotic" morphology. Sometimes biphasic or polyphasic waves can coexist. Although initially described in patients affected by liver failure, triphasic waves have been described in a large number of conditions, including renal failure and postanoxic encephalopathy.

The most severe stages of HE are characterized by coma with arrhythmic delta activity progressively reducing in frequency and amplitude and eventually leading to isoelectric tracing. Figures 42.1, 42.2, and 42.3 show EEG patterns recorded in various stages of HE and examples of triphasic waves [6].

Apart from triphasic waves, epileptiform abnormalities are not frequently seen in HE. However epileptiform activities (spikes, focal sharp waves, spike-wave complexes) can sometimes appear, usually associated with isolated or recurrent epileptic seizures and even status epilepticus. If nonconvulsive, status epilepticus requires EEG for the diagnosis. The occurrence of epileptic seizures is a negative prognostic factor (Fig. 42.4).

Over time, different classifications of EEG changes in HE have been proposed with the aim of correlating EEG patterns with the degree of liver impairment. In 1957 Parsons-Smith et al. proposed a first classification, based exclusively on qualitative criteria [7], which was revised and updated in 1999 by Amodio et al. [8] (Table 42.1). This classification was deemed to be too operator-dependent and not suitable for comparing large case series. Thus, in 1977 Conn et al. proposed a semiquantitative classification based on mean frequency of background activity assessed over posterior regions (Table 42.2) [3]. In 1984 Van der Rijt et al. proposed a classification in four grades based on quantitative features and spectral analysis [9]; this classification was further modified in 1999 by Amodio and coworkers [8]. This classification considers both the mean dominant frequency and the relative power of theta and delta band (Table 42.3).

The use of quantitative EEG in patients with HE should be validated in a large number of patients. However, it shows changes in brain activity occurring before clinical symptoms, eliminates the intra-rater variability, and provides quantitative data which can be compared with those obtained with other techniques. In our experience, patients with liver disease and cirrhosis but without HE have a higher relative power of theta-delta bands and a slowing of alpha, compared to control subjects. The quantitative EEG, together with other neurophysiological investigations (e.g., evoked potentials), may provide data suggesting an initial impairment of cerebral function in patients without clinically overt HE.

Besides qualitative and quantitative EEG analyses [10], automatized procedures based on artificial neural network-expert systems have been used to detect the different EEG patterns encountered in various stages of the disease. Amodio et al. have analyzed these procedures, concluding that although further improvements are needed, they are already able to differentiate normal and clearly altered EEG patterns [11].

The visual analysis of EEG remains therefore essential for providing a global qualitative assessment of the cerebral function in HE, even if EEG changes are nonspecific and may be influenced by accompanying metabolic disturbances (e.g., hyponatremia) or drugs. A quantitative analysis, which should include the background frequency with mean dominant frequency or spectral band analysis [12], could increase

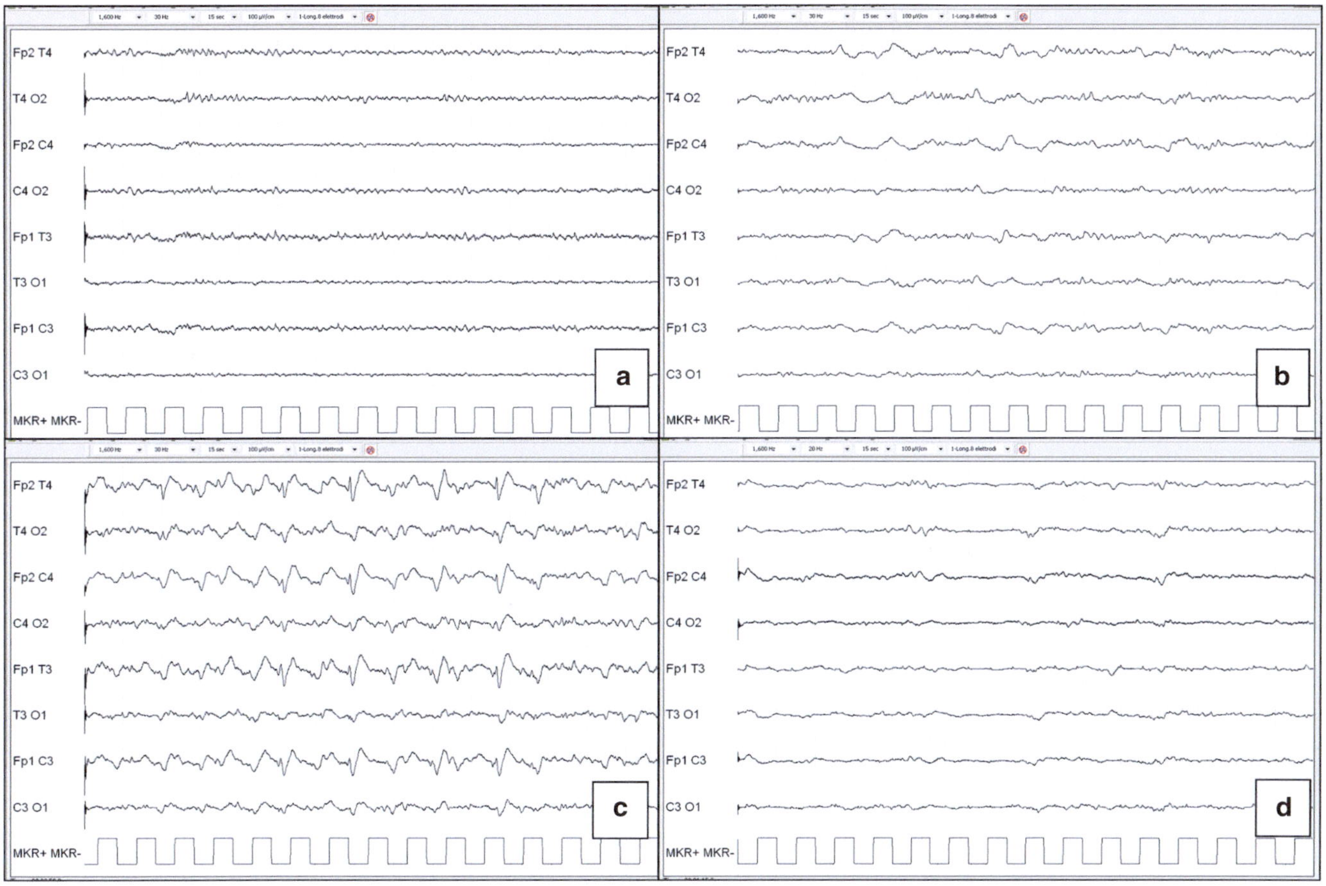

Fig. 42.1 Hepatic encephalopathy in a 57-year-old patient with cirrhosis. (**a**) Normal EEG recording. (**b**) Slowing of alpha rhythm and appearance of delta waves predominant over anterior regions. (**c**) Typical pattern with sharply contoured bi-triphasic waves. (**d**) Low-amplitude pattern with widespread theta-delta activity

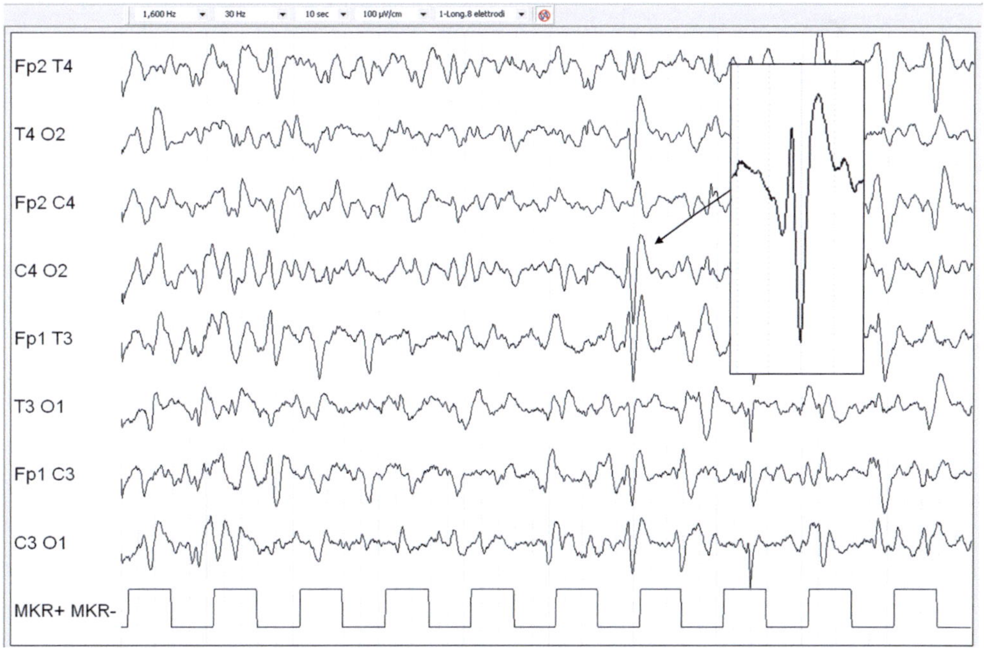

Fig. 42.2 Advanced stage of hepatic encephalopathy with widespread slowing and sharply contoured bi-triphasic waves

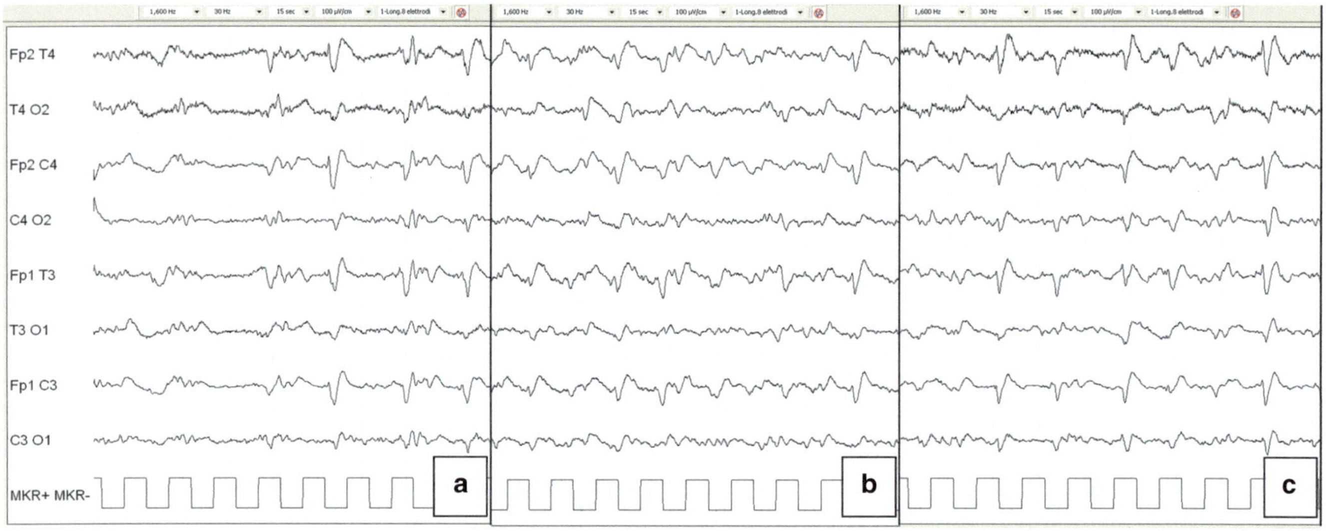

Fig. 42.3 EEG recordings showing triphasic waves in three different patients (**a**, **b**, and **c**) with hepatic encephalopathy

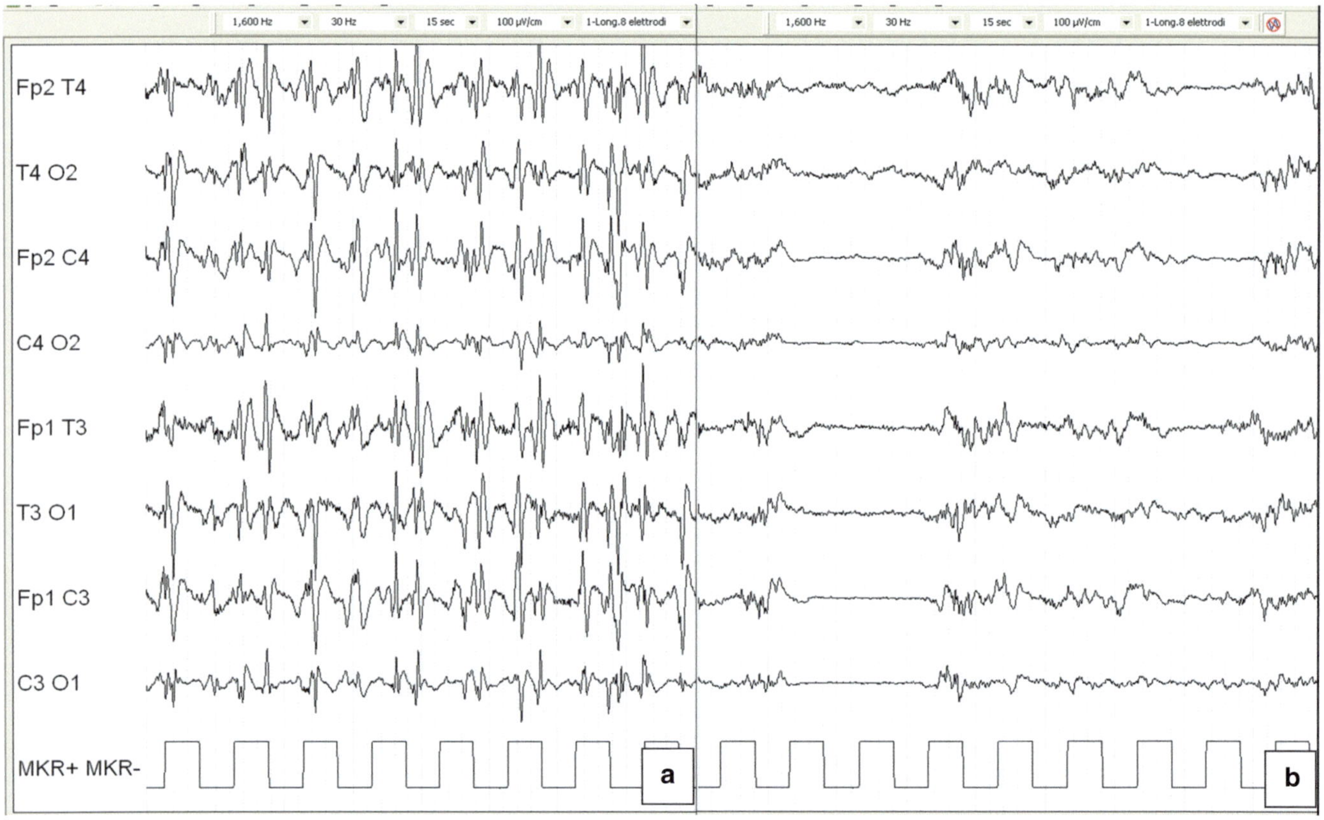

Fig. 42.4 A 45-year-old patient with severe liver failure and coma, followed by death. (**a**) Widespread epileptiform activity, without apparent clinical correlate. (**b**) After intravenous administration of sodium thiopental, the activity temporarily disappears but reappears after approximately 10 min

the reliability of the EEG. As emphasized by the joint Practice Guideline by the American Association for the Study of Liver Diseases and the European Association for the Study of the Liver, "in most situations, EEG requires an institutional setup and neurological expertise in evaluation, and the cost varies among hospitals" [4].

The EEG is also extremely useful to monitor the efficacy of pharmacological treatment, as the improvement in clinical and biochemical parameters goes in parallel with a progressive reduction of slowing, the disappearance of sharp graphoelements, and the reappearance of a normal background activity.

Table 42.1 Qualitative classification of EEG alterations according to Amodio et al. [8] (reproduced with permission)

Score	Description
0: Normal EEG	Well-structured EEG with stable and symmetrical posterior basic rhythm >8 and <13 Hz dominant in the posterior regions. Such activity has medium amplitude (30 ± 50 mV) and is reactive to eye opening. No slow activities or irritative signs are present
1: Normal-limit EEG	Unstable or suppressed alpha rhythm frequently replaced by high prevalence of diffuse beta rhythm (corresponding to grade A of Parsons-Smith's classification)
2: Mild signs of encephalopathy	Low-frequency alpha rhythm (8 Hz) disturbed by random waves in the theta range over both hemispheres (corresponding to grade B of Parsons-Smith's classification)
3: Distinctive features of encephalopathy	Background activity in the theta range, diffused over both hemispheres. Random appearance of high waves in the delta range (roughly corresponding to grade C of Parsons-Smith's classification)
4: Signs of severe encephalopathy	Severe disorganization of EEG activity without any normal element. Diffuse asynchronous theta and delta waves over both hemispheres with or without triphasic waves (roughly corresponding to grades D–E of Parsons-Smith's classification)

Table 42.2 Semiquantitative visual assessment, according to Conn's classification based on the main frequency of background activity [3]

Grade 0	Normal alpha frequency: 8.5–12 Hz
Grade 1	Main frequency of background activity: 7–8 Hz
Grade 2	Main frequency of background activity: 3–4 Hz
Grade 3	Main frequency of background activity: 1–2 Hz

Table 42.3 Spectral analysis-based classification, according to Amodio et al. [8]

Grade 0	Mean dominant frequency > 7.3 Hz and theta relative power < 35%
Grade 1	Mean dominant frequency > 7.3 Hz and theta relative power ≥ 35%
Grade 2	Mean dominant frequency ≤ 7.3 Hz and delta relative power < 45%
Grade 3	Mean dominant frequency ≤ 7.3 Hz and delta relative power ≥ 45%

Most liver diseases show the same evolution of the EEG pattern described above.

Approximately 30% of patients with acute viral hepatitis have EEG changes, even in patients without neurological deficits. These EEG changes are nonspecific and include slowing of posterior dominant alpha rhythm and the appearance of a 5–6 Hz theta activity predominant over anterior regions. In severe cases of infective and toxic acute hepatitis, the EEG pattern is that typically encountered in advanced HE.

In patients undergoing liver transplantation, EEG changes reflect impaired cerebral function during surgical operation or in postsurgical phases, due to hypoxia, sepsis, anesthesia, or lack of normalization of liver functions. In this scenario, epileptic seizures are frequent and may also manifest as convulsive and nonconvulsive status epilepticus. A continuous EEG monitoring or seriate EEG recordings are essential to assess the efficacy of therapy and to differentiate between epileptic and nonepileptic events. After liver transplantation, seriate EEG recordings show a progressive normalization of background activity in patients whose EEG prior to transplantation was severely impaired (Figs. 42.5 and 42.6); this can be observed also with spectral electroencephalogram analysis [13]. In our experience, the EEG is often required, particularly in patients with acute liver failure, to assess the cerebral function before transplantation. In these cases, the EEG may allow the neurophysiologist to provide a prognostic judgment on the reversibility of the cerebral impairment and the need for acute transplantation.

Liver failure may also occur as a consequence of rare conditions.

Reye syndrome is a rapidly progressive infantile encephalopathy associated with fat degeneration of the liver. It often begins several days after apparent recovery from a viral illness, especially varicella or influenza, sometimes treated with aspirin. In this condition, the EEG changes are widespread and similar to those previously reported in HE and correlate with impairment of vigilance and consciousness. In Reye syndrome 14- and 6-Hz positive spikes have also been reported [14].

The Wilson syndrome (hepatolenticular degeneration) is a severe autosomal recessive disease characterized by impairment of cellular copper transport leading to copper accumulation in the liver, brain, and cornea. The clinical picture includes psychic and motor symptoms (usually extrapyramidal: dystonia, tremor, parkinsonism); the EEG shows nonspecific widespread theta-delta activity, which can be prevalent over anterior regions (Fig. 42.7). Epileptiform abnormalities associated with epileptic seizures are rare. In this syndrome the EEG is not particularly useful, also because the clinical picture is dominated by symptoms reflecting copper accumulation in the basal ganglia.

42.3 Renal Disease

EEG changes can occur both in acute and chronic renal failure and correlate with urea blood levels.

Acute renal failure manifests usually with agitation and confusion (sometimes associated with myoclonus and tremor) and may be severe enough to evolve into coma. In these patients the EEG shows a slowing of the background alpha rhythm and widespread theta sequences, and in later stages a diffuse slowing admixed with sharply contoured graphoelements sometimes with triphasic morphology [2, 15]. These patients often have myoclonic or generalized

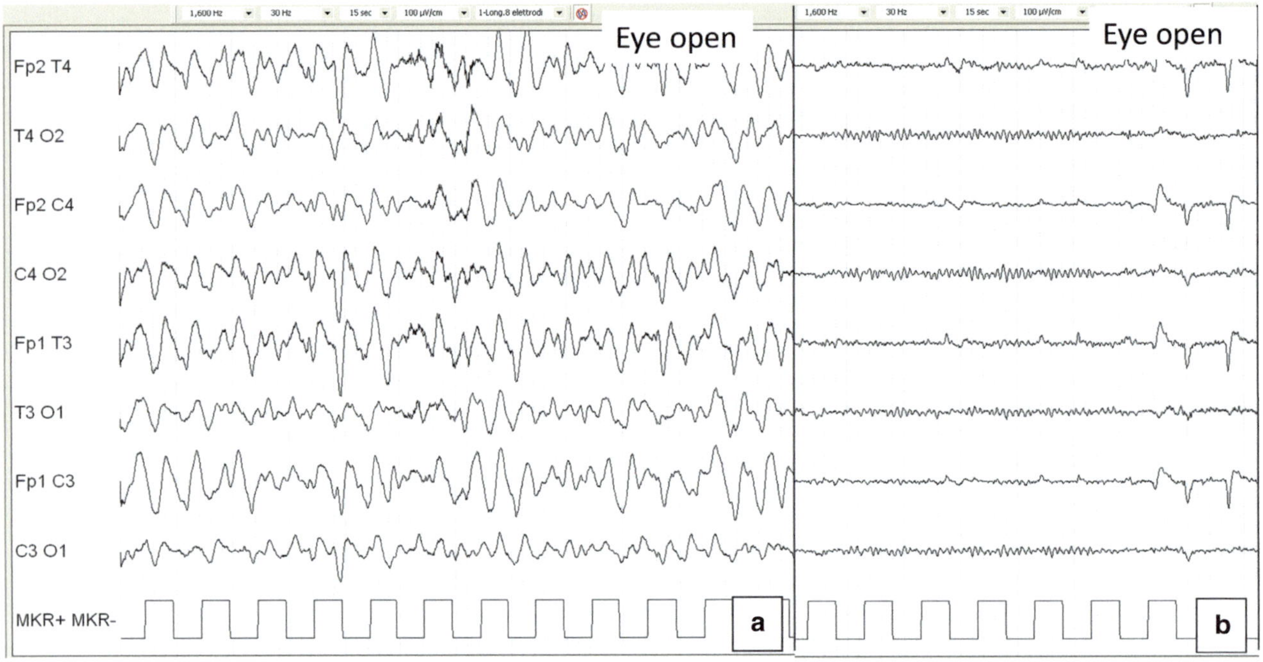

Fig. 42.5 A 37-year-old patient with liver transplantation for fulminant hepatitis. (**a**) Baseline EEG recording showing widespread delta slowing and sharply contoured bi-triphasic waves. (**b**) Three days after the transplantation, the EEG is normal

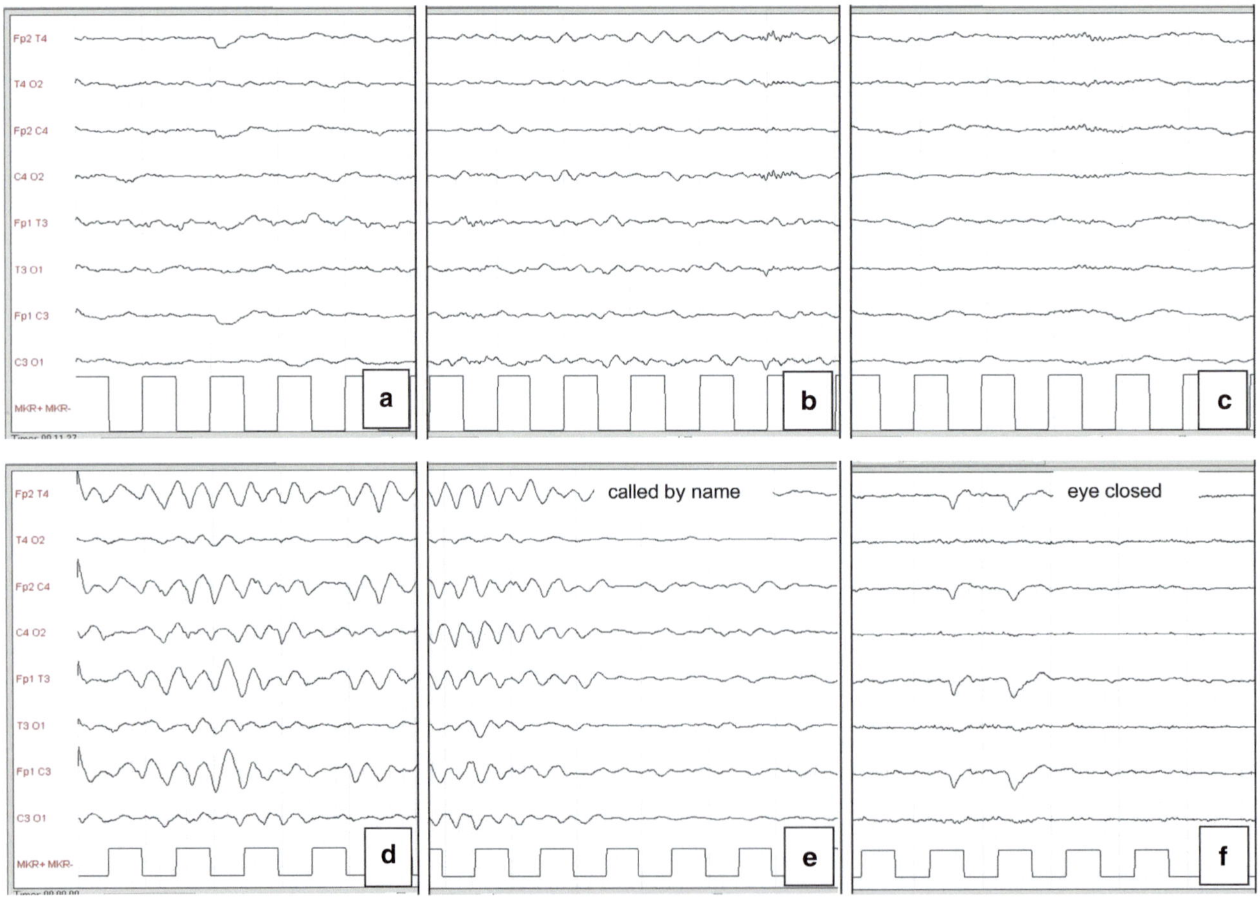

Fig. 42.6 A 14-year-old patient with fulminant hepatitis due to drug intoxication admitted for severe comatose state. EEG recordings performed at days 1 (**a**), 2 (**b**), and 3 (**c**) following admission show low-amplitude slow activity admixed with fast activities. (**d**) EEG recording performed 24 h after the liver transplantation shows widespread slow monomorphic activities, prevalent over anterior regions. (**e**) Four days after the liver transplantation, the EEG corresponds to wakeful state. Filters: 1.6–30 Hz; amplification: 50 μV/cm (**a**, **b**, **c**); 100 μV/cm (**d**, **e**, **f**)

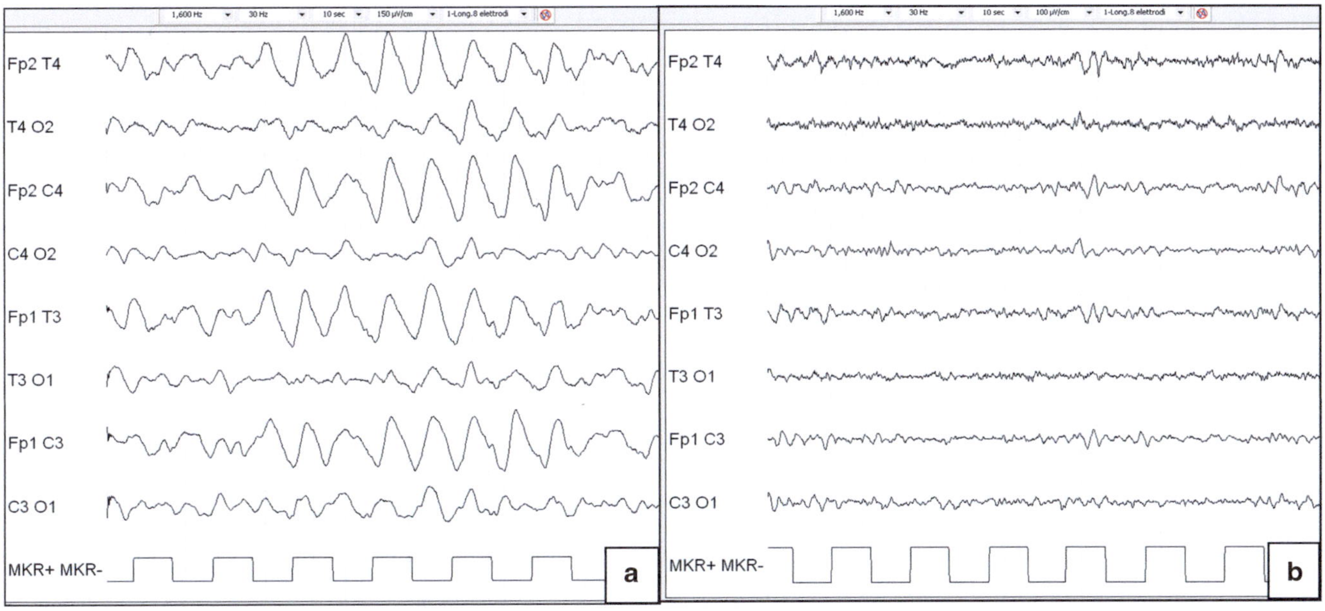

Fig. 42.7 A 15-year-old patient with Wilson's disease admitted for severe liver failure. (**a**) Widespread monomorphic slowing, prevalent over anterior regions. (**b**) Three days after the liver transplantation, the EEG has markedly improved

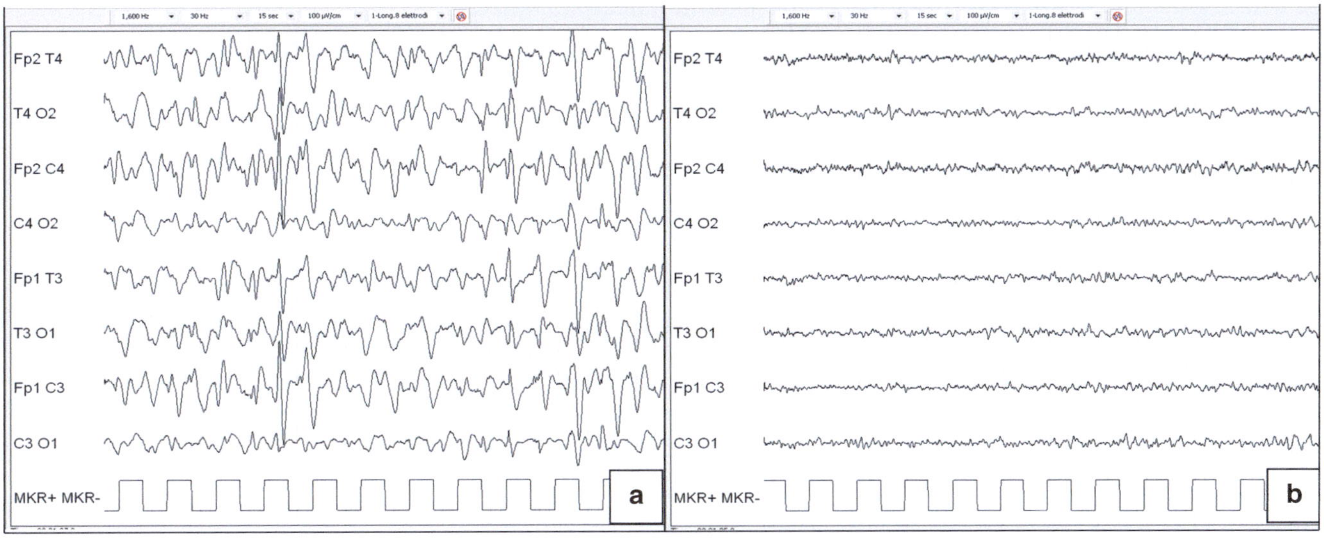

Fig. 42.8 A 53-year-old patient with chronic renal failure for over 30 years. (**a**) The baseline EEG recording shows widespread slowing and bi-triphasic high-amplitude graphoelements. (**b**) Two hours after the end of dialysis, the previous pattern has disappeared

tonic-clonic seizures, and even status epilepticus, with the typical EEG patterns. The epileptiform abnormalities usually reduce or disappear after pharmacological treatment and dialysis (Fig. 42.8).

Chronic renal failure is associated with cognitive deficits and mild EEG changes, even after years of disease. Sometimes fluctuations of cognitive functions may occur, associated with widespread theta and/or delta activity correlated with urea levels. Spikes or generalized spike-wave complexes can be rarely seen in intercritical recordings, and there is an increased tendency to photosensitivity. In these patients sleep abnormalities are also frequently encountered.

42.4 Cardiorespiratory Disease

A severe heart or respiratory failure may cause cerebral anoxia. Severe anoxia leads to a severe impairment of consciousness, associated with reduced amplitude and slowing of background alpha rhythm, and the subsequent appearance of widespread theta and delta activity. In case of severe and prolonged anoxia, the EEG initially shows a burst-suppression pattern which may subsequently evolve into isoelectric tracing, corresponding to cerebral death.

If normal ventilation and cerebral oxygenation are restored before an irreversible brain damage has occurred, the EEG pattern may show an inverse evolution from isoelectric tracing to burst-suppression and slowed background activity [16].

Epileptic seizures occur frequently both in acute and in post-acute phases following anoxia (massive myoclonic seizures, tonic-clonic seizures, convulsive and nonconvulsive status epilepticus), with the corresponding EEG patterns. A prolonged EEG monitoring is required to identify subclinical seizures and to monitor cortical postanoxic myoclonic seizures, which may be particularly refractory to pharmacological treatment.

Chronic respiratory failure can cause an encephalopathy characterized by headache, papilledema, increased intracranial pressure, and tremor. The EEG shows widespread theta-delta activity, sometimes associated with triphasic waves prevalent over anterior regions. Also in this case, the EEG changes can be reversible following a prompt and effective therapeutic management.

The EEG pattern associated with congenital heart defect is a widespread slowing of various degrees, reflecting the cerebral hypoxia. Focal slowing and epileptiform abnormalities, focal or generalized, sometimes associated with epileptic seizures can also be seen. The frequency of epileptiform abnormalities increases with the age, probably because of the higher susceptibility to epileptogenic lesions following cerebral hypoxia.

During open-heart surgery procedures, cerebral hypoxia may occur as a consequence of extracorporeal circulation, hypothermia, and anesthesia. In these cases the EEG shows a generalized reduction of amplitude with widespread slowing admixed with burst-suppression pattern.

42.5 Disorders of Glucose Metabolism

42.5.1 Hypoglycemia

The brain functions depend on blood glucose levels. Glucose is the main metabolic substrate of neurons, and some neuroimaging techniques assess glucose consumption in different cerebral areas as an indirect way of measuring corresponding degrees of cerebral activity.

EEG changes correlate with the severity of hypoglycemia and particularly with the rapidity of onset. Diabetic patients with long disease duration may have no EEG changes even during episodes of severe hypoglycemia. Conversely, a sudden drop in glucose levels can cause a severe impairment of cerebral function and consciousness severe enough to cause coma.

In initial phases the EEG typically shows a slowing of background alpha rhythm and subsequently, if hypoglycemia persists, the appearance of theta activity and then delta activity, initially predominant anteriorly and then becoming widespread. Epileptiform abnormalities, not necessarily associated with seizures, are not frequent.

After intravenous administration of glucose, the EEG recording normalizes rapidly, although focal abnormalities (slowing or sharply contoured elements) may persist over time, particularly if hypoglycemia has lasted for a long time or a preexisting cerebrovascular disease is present.

42.5.2 Hyperglycemia

The EEG changes in hyperglycemia are usually less marked than those observed in hypoglycemia. Slowing or fast activities, sometimes associated with sharp elements, can be seen particularly in patients with high glucose levels.

The patients with diabetes are more prone to cerebrovascular lesions, and consequently the EEG can show focal, slow, or sharply contoured graphoelements.

Neurological complications, including epileptic seizures, are more likely to occur when hyperglycemia is associated with ketoacidosis: focal motor seizures associated with rolandic epileptogenic foci and occipital seizures are quite frequent, whereas status epilepticus occurs rarely (Fig. 42.9).

Severe hyperglycemia can lead to diabetic coma, with EEG features typically encountered in dysmetabolic coma.

42.6 Electrolyte Disturbances

42.6.1 Hypocalcemia

Hypoparathyroidism, usually as a complication of thyroidectomy, is a common cause of hypocalcemia. Hypocalcemia usually manifests with increased neuromuscular excitability and tetany and with generalized or focal epileptic seizures [17]. The symptoms, which depend on the degree of hypocalcemia and the speed of the decrease in the serum calcium concentration, can be controlled by supplementation with calcium and vitamin D.

Muscular tetany is not associated with changes of cerebral activity, since it has a peripheral genesis. However, severe hypocalcemia is a highly epileptogenic condition. Serum calcium concentration does not seem to correlate with the severity of seizures or with the frequency of epileptiform abnormalities.

Baseline EEG usually shows a slowing of background rhythm with evolution from alpha to theta and diffuse increase in slow wave activity in the theta and delta range, admixed with spikes and sharp waves. These abnormalities are often worsened by hyperventilation. In most severe cases, generalized spikes or sharp-wave burst of delta activity with sharp components can occur.

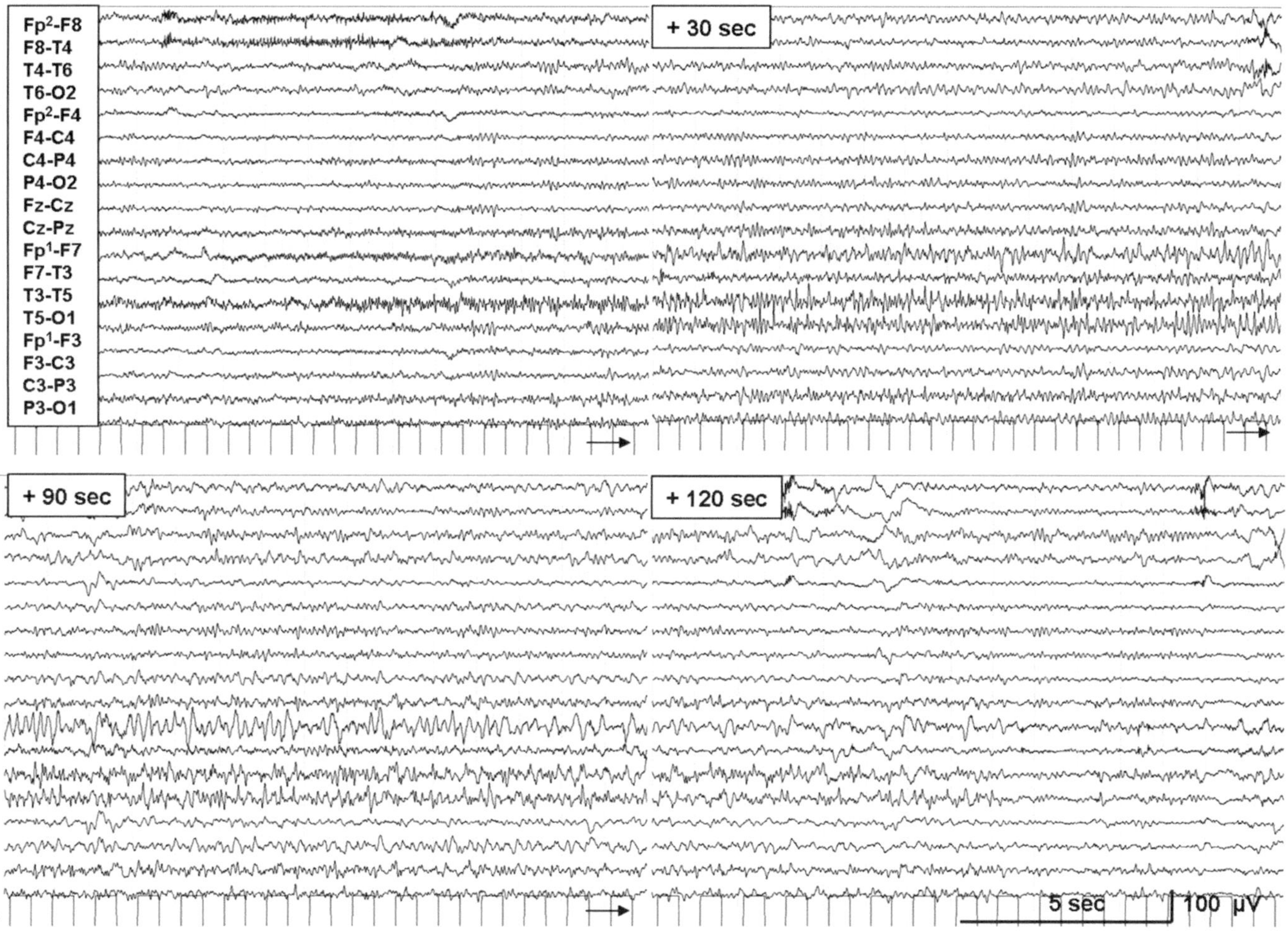

Fig. 42.9 A 52-year-old patient, admitted for behavioral changes and confusion. The only abnormal bioumoral parameter is glucose (350 mg/dL). During the following days, the patient had epileptic seizures with stared gaze and aphasia. EEG recorded during the seizures show prolonged (>120 s) epileptiform activity over left temporal region, with tendency to spread over contralateral regions

Of note, hypocalcemia is a frequent cause of acute neonatal seizures.

42.6.2 Hypercalcemia

Hypercalcemia can have different causes (hyperplasia or neoplasia of parathyroids, hyperfunction of parathyroids secondary to renal failure, vitamin D intoxication, paraneoplastic syndrome with/without bone metastases) [17]. Its main neurologic manifestations are drowsiness, lethargy, weakness, and confusion. The clinical symptoms are associated with slowing of background activity, due to theta 4–6 Hz components associated with bursts of 1–2 Hz delta waves, which may have a spiky appearance similar to triphasic waves. Periodic bioccipital epileptiform discharges can also occur, probably due to a reversible cerebral vasoconstriction. Usually EEG changes appear when serum calcium levels are higher than 13 mg/100 mL.

42.6.3 Hyponatremia

Severe hyponatremia (below 116 mg/dL) and water intoxication cause slowing of background alpha rhythm and a widespread delta activity, sometimes with rhythmic bursts prevalent over the anterior regions. Triphasic waves and periodic lateralized discharges have also been reported. Epileptic seizures and status epilepticus occur frequently. EEG changes do not disappear immediately after correction of hyponatremia.

42.7 Thyroid Disorders

42.7.1 Hyperthyroidism

Hyperthyroidism is usually associated with increased frequency of the background alpha rhythm, sometimes with fast activity at 15–30 Hz; often spikes or sharp waves, widespread or focal, can coexist. Widespread slowing in theta-delta range, increased by hyperventilation, may be seen. An increased mu rhythm over rolandic regions has also been reported. Epileptic seizures may occur.

The sleep is also altered, with reduction of deeper phases and frequent episodes of awakening; sleep spindles have a frequency higher than 14 Hz. The duration of REM phases is approximately the same during the whole night.

In patients with hyperthyroidism occurring acutely, the impairment of cerebral functions is usually severe, and the EEG shows delta monomorphic slowing, predominant over posterior regions, sometimes associated with fast activities. Marked and widespread slowing has been described in Hashimoto thyroiditis associated with hyperthyroidism.

42.7.2 Hypothyroidism

Hypothyroidism can be congenital or acquired. In this condition the EEG shows a slowed background alpha rhythm, of low voltage, scarcely reactive to eye opening, and fast activities at 15–20 Hz or more rarely a widespread theta-delta activity.

The EEG in children with congenital myxedema has a slow widespread activity of high amplitude, with reduced reactivity to stimulations and delayed appearance of physiological graphoelements (e.g., sleep spindles).

The EEG changes are usually reversible after treatment, provided that hypothyroidism did not lead to a dismetabolic encephalopathy with periodic epileptiform discharges similar to those encountered in Creutzfeldt-Jakob disease. Hypothyroidism can also cause a nonconvulsive status epilepticus.

42.7.3 Hashimoto Encephalopathy

The Hashimoto encephalopathy (steroid-responsive encephalopathy associated with autoimmune thyroiditis, SREAT) is a rare form of autoimmune encephalopathy characterized by high titer of antithyroid peroxidase antibodies, even in absence of alterations in thyroid function [18]. The encephalopathy might be due to an autoimmune cerebral vasculitis or the consequence of an autoimmune reaction directed against an antigen shared by thyroid and brain tissue. It is more common among women and may affect patients of any age, including children and elderly subjects. It manifests with psychiatric symptoms, cognitive deficits, myoclonus, and epileptic seizures (both focal and generalized). Brain magnetic resonance imaging can yield normal result or reveal leukoencephalopathy, whereas the CSF examination can be normal or show increased protein levels with oligoclonal bands (in this case other etiologies, such as toxic, dismetabolic, or infectious disorders, need to be excluded). This entity should be differentiated by Creutzfeldt-Jakob disease, other rapidly progressive dementias, and limbic encephalitis.

The EEG shows widespread slowing, sometimes prevalent over posterior or frontal-central regions; in this case their appearance may resemble frontal intermittent rhythmic delta activity. In most severe cases, widespread high-amplitude delta waves can be seen, sometimes with bi- or triphasic morphology (Fig. 42.10). Some authors have reported periodic lateralized discharges, particularly over temporal-parietal regions, and cases of epilepsia partialis continua and nonconvulsive status epilepticus [19].

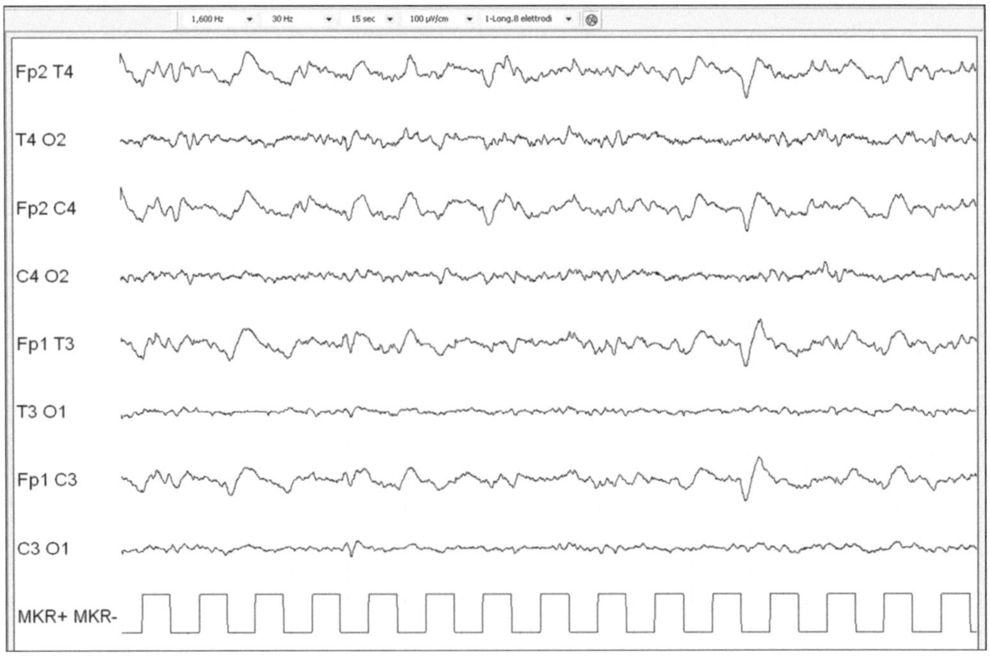

Fig. 42.10 A 46-year-old patient with Hashimoto encephalopathy. The EEG shows a widespread slowing, prevalent anteriorly and associated with isolated sharp waves

The treatment with steroids typically leads to a marked improvement of psychiatric and cognitive deficits and to the normalization of the EEG.

42.8 Other Hormonal Disorders

42.8.1 Hypercortisolism and Cushing's Syndrome

In hypercortisolism and Cushing's syndrome, the EEG is often normal or sometimes shows widespread beta activity or a small amount of theta 4–7 Hz activity.

The treatment with steroids can lead to a slowing of alpha rhythm and to the appearance of theta activity and periodic 1–3 Hz delta components, predominant over anterior regions.

42.8.2 Hypocortisolism

Hypocortisolism causes slowing of alpha rhythm and a theta-delta activity, sometimes manifesting with periodic bursts that disappear after hormonal replacement and correction of electrolyte imbalance.

42.8.3 Hypopituitarism and Hyperpituitarism

In hypopituitarism the EEG changes correlate with the severity of the metabolic-hormonal disorder (hypocortisolism, hypothyroidism). In case of tumor of the pituitary gland, they are also directly related to the damage to the surrounding cerebral tissue. The EEG shows theta-delta slowing, bilateral, synchronous, and often predominant posteriorly, which can be increased by hyperventilation.

Hyperpituitarism is associated with theta-delta slowing of various degrees and sometimes with fast activity of approximately 20 Hz not modified by eye closure.

42.9 Eclampsia

Eclampsia is a toxic-metabolic syndrome characterized by the onset of hypertension, proteinuria, multiorgan dysfunction, and seizures after 20 weeks of gestation. In the acute phase, the EEG shows a slowing and desynchronization of the posterior dominant alpha rhythm associated with widespread theta-delta activity of various degrees [20]. Epileptic seizures can occur and are associated with the typical EEG patterns. The EEG monitoring during treatment of eclampsia shows a rapid normalization parallel to the improvement of the clinical picture [2].

42.10 Acute Porphyria

Porphyrias are rare metabolic disorders caused by altered activities of enzymes within the heme biosynthetic pathway. Patients with acute intermittent acute porphyria may have confusion and psychiatric symptoms, associated with theta-delta activities prevalent over anterior regions, and sometimes admixed with sharply contoured elements [21]. In stable phases, usually manifesting with abdominal pain and polyneuropathy, the EEG is usually normal. Epileptic seizures are relatively frequent and are associated with the typical corresponding EEG patterns.

References

1. Kaplan PW. The EEG in metabolic encephalopathy and coma. J Clin Neurophysiol. 2004;21:307–18.
2. Sutter R, Pang T, Kaplan PW. EEG in metabolic disorders, intoxications, and epileptic encephalopathies. In: Schomer DL, Lopes da Silva F, editors. Niedermeyer's electroencephalography: basic principles, clinical applications, and related fields. 7th ed. New York, NY: Oxford University Press; 2018. p. 433–66.
3. Conn HO, Leevy CM, Vlahcevic ZR, Rodgers JB, Maddrey WC, Seeff L, Levy LL. Comparison of lactulose and neomycin in the treatment of chronic portal-systemic encephalopathy. A double-blind controlled trial. Gastroenterology. 1977;72:573–83.
4. Vilstrup H, Amodio P, Bajaj J, Cordoba J, Ferenci P, Mullen KD, Weissenborn K, Wong P. Hepatic encephalopathy in chronic liver disease: 2014 practice guideline by the American Association for the Study of Liver Diseases and the European Association for the Study of the Liver. Hepatology. 2014;60:715–35.
5. Brigo F. Intermittent rhythmic delta activity patterns. Epilepsy Behav. 2011;20:254–6.
6. Brigo F, Storti M. Triphasic waves. Am J Electroneurodiagnostic Technol. 2011;51:16–25.
7. Parsons-Smith BG, Summerrsskill WHJ, Dawson AM, Sherlock S. The electroencephalogram in liver disease. Lancet. 1957;2:867–71.
8. Amodio P, Marchetti P, Del Piccolo F, de Tourtchaninoff M, Varghese P, Zuliani C, Campo G, Gatta A, Guerit JM. Spectral versus visual EEG analysis in mild hepatic encephalopathy. Clin Neurophysiol. 1999;110:1334–44.
9. Van der Rijt CD, Schalm SW, De Groot GH, De Vlieger M. Objective measurement of hepatic encephalopathy by means of automated EEG analysis. Electroencephalogr Clin Neurophysiol. 1984;57:423–6.
10. Amodio P, Gatta A. Neurophysiological investigation of hepatic encephalopathy. Metab Brain Dis. 2005;20:369–79.
11. Amodio P, Pellegrini A, Ubiali E, Mathy I, Del Piccolo F, Orsato R, Gatta A, Guerit JM. The EEG assessment of low-grade hepatic encephalopathy: comparison of an artificial neural network-expert system (ANNES) based evaluation with visual EEG readings and EEG spectral analysis. Clin Neurophysiol. 2006;117:2243–51.
12. Guerit JM, Amantini A, Fischer C, Kaplan PW, Mecarelli O, Schnitzler A, Ubiali E, Amodio P, members of the ISHEN commission on Neurophysiological Investigations. Neurophysiological investigations of hepatic encephalopathy: ISHEN practice guidelines. Liver Int. 2009;29:789–96.
13. Ciancio A, Marchet A, Saracco G, Carucci P, Lavezzo B, Leotta D, Capellero B, Nobili M, Smedile A, Rizzetto M. Spectral electroencephalogram analysis in hepatic encephalopathy and liver transplantation. Liver Transpl. 2002;8:630–5.

14. Yamada T, Young S, Kimura J. Significance of positive spike bursts in Reye's syndrome. Arch Neurol. 1977;34:376–80.
15. Hughes JR. EEG in uremia. Am J EEG Technol. 1984;24:1–10.
16. Scollo-Lavizzari G, Bassetti C. Prognostic value of EEG in post-anoxic coma after cardiac arrest. Eur Neurol. 1987;26:161–70.
17. Nardone R, Brigo F, Trinka E. Acute symptomatic seizures caused by electrolyte disturbances. J Clin Neurol. 2016;12:21–33.
18. Mocellin R, Walterfang M, Velakoulis D. Hashimoto's encephalopathy: epidemiology, pathogenesis and management. CNS Drugs. 2007;21:799–811.
19. Arain A, Abou-Khalil B, Moses H. Hashimoto's encephalopathy: documentation of mesial temporal seizure origin by ictal EEG. Seizure. 2001;10:438–41.
20. Thomas SV, Somanathan N, Radhakumari R. Interictal EEG changes in eclampsia. Electroencephalogr Clin Neurophysiol. 1995;94:271–5.
21. Reichenmiller HE. EEG findings in acute porphyria. Electroencephalogr Clin Neurophysiol. 1970;29:214–5.

43 Migraine

Chiara Davassi, Patrizia Pulitano, and Oriano Mecarelli

43.1 Migraine and the Role of EEG

The last International Classification of Headache Disorders (ICHD-3 beta) [1] distinguishes primary headaches, not ascribable to other medical causes, and secondary headaches. Among the former, migraine - affecting 11% of the adult population [2] - is the headache that most creates diagnostic problems with epilepsy, not only because it can resemble a seizure - especially when preceded by aura - but also because pain may represent itself as an epileptic manifestation, either ictal or postictal. The term "aura" denotes recurrent attacks of focal neurologic symptoms that can include visual, sensory, speech, motor, or other central nervous symptoms which duration is >5 and <60 min for each symptom, usually followed by the headache. In hemiplegic migraine, unilateral weakness is supposed to last for a period <72 h.

Migraine is characterized by functional disturbances of the central nervous system at several levels, with a dynamic pattern over time (ictal/interictal). It may be preceded by typical or atypical aura and sometimes it may present only with symptoms of aura, not followed by pain (aura sine emicrania). This last scenario is the one that may be the most confused with an epileptic seizure. Furthermore, among its complications, there is a special entity, the migraine aura-triggered seizure, formerly known as "migralepsy", whose nature is still controversial. Lastly, epilepsy and headache may coexist, and the postictal headache can show the same characteristics as migraine headache. In patients presenting with headache and in whom atypical associated symptomatology makes a seizure disorder reasonably probable, epileptiform activity on EEG would significantly raise the probability of epilepsy. EEG in such cases, represents indeed a useful tool to differentiate a migraine attack from an epileptic attack.

EEG usefulness in the study of migraine has been matter of discussion for a long time, either as a diagnostic tool or as a follow-up examination. Its execution was considered and encouraged especially before the advent of neuroimaging, in order to figure out whether migraine could be secundary to a brain lesion [3].

American Academy of Neurology (AAN) guidelines reaffirmed in 2014 [4] the impropriety of requesting EEG as a routine examination in patients with headache, an opinion already expressed in 1995 [5]. Nowadays EEG, in addition to other neurophysiological studies, though plays a role in the investigation of the still not completely known pathophysiology of migraine.

However, it is important for clinicians to know which abnormalities may be found in migraineurs, to not misinterpret them.

43.1.1 Interictal EEG Abnormalities

There is little evidence of EEG changes during migraine attacks, while there is extensive literature concerning the interictal phases. Studies designed to determine whether headache patients have an increased prevalence of EEG abnormalities report conflicting results, varying from total normal findings to alterations such as "hypersynchronous bursts" of focal slowing.

43.1.1.1 Background Activity Abnormalities

Diffuse or localized slowings has been reported by some authors in a variable percentage of headache patients, with a slight predominance in migraineurs [6, 7]. EEG abnormalities in migraine patients in-between attacks were more often reported in the posterior regions [8] (Fig. 43.1). Neufeld et al. [9] did not find significant differences in background interictal activity between patients and healthy controls.

C. Davassi · O. Mecarelli (✉)
Department of Human Neurosciences, Sapienza University of Rome, Rome, Italy
e-mail: chiara.davassi@uniroma1.it; oriano.mecarelli@uniroma1.it

P. Pulitano
Azienda Ospedaliero-Universitaria Policlinico Umberto I, Rome, Italy
e-mail: patrizia.pulitano@uniroma1.it

O. Mecarelli (ed.), *Clinical Electroencephalography*, https://doi.org/10.1007/978-3-030-04573-9_43

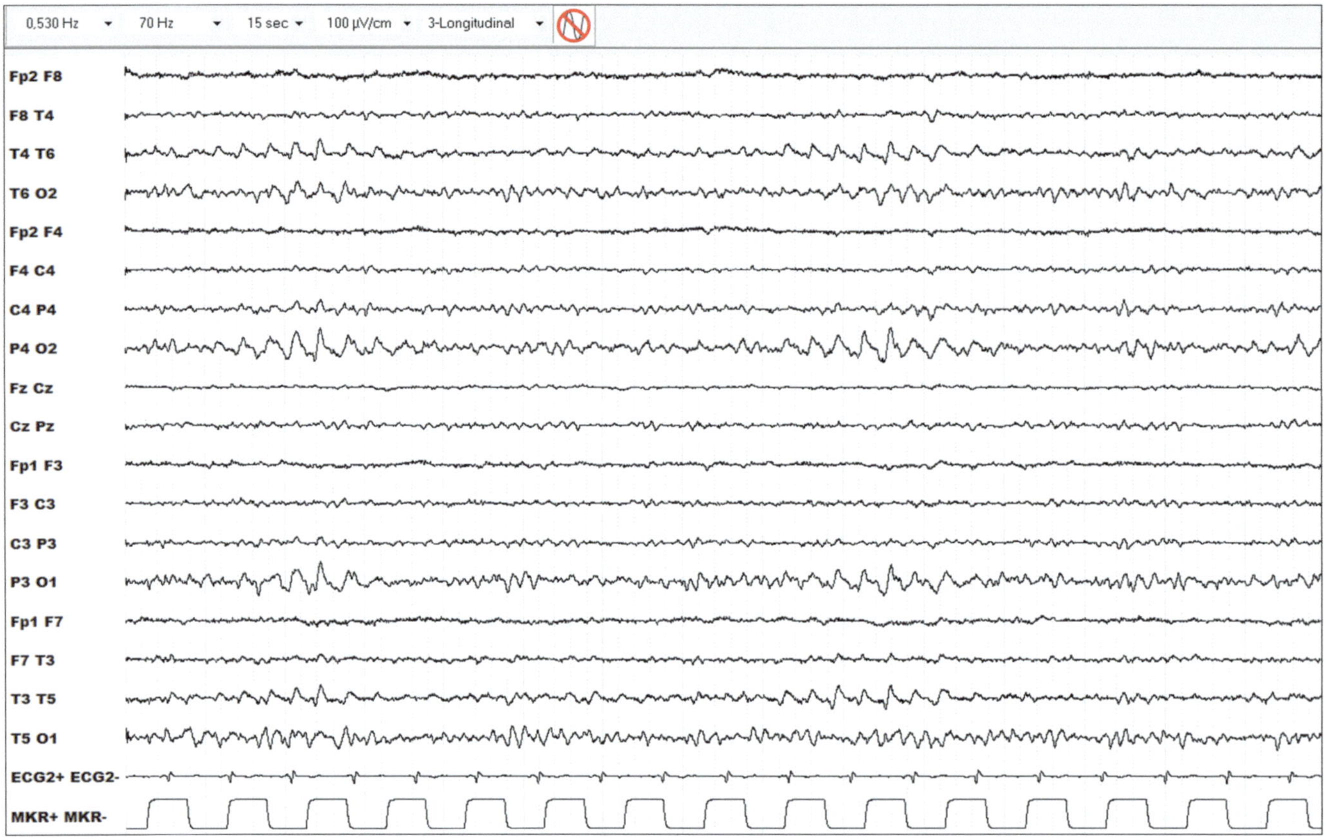

Fig. 43.1 Example of interictal abnormalities in a patient with migraine without aura. A pattern of monomorphic rhythmic delta activity is detectable over the posterior areas

Their major findings were a higher alpha power and a higher peak alpha reactivity in controls as compared to migraineours. These findings may suggest some differences in the electrophysiologic background in the two groups [9]. An increase in theta activity was also observed in a recent blinded, controlled study using quantitative EEG in adult patients with migraine [10].

43.1.1.2 Intermittent Photic Stimulation-Induced Abnormalities

An enhanced Photic Driving Response (PDR), especially at 20 Hz frequency flashes during Intermittent Photic Stimulation (IPS), defined as "H response", is considered almost specific for migraine by some authors (11) (Fig. 43.2). Nevertheless, a recent case-control study demonstrated that visual EEG inspection overestimates this phenomenon; spectral EEG analysis, on the contrary, revealed that this finding was true only in 60% of migraineurs that were considered instead positive at visual EEG analysis (38% of the whole sample). Furthermore, PDR power appeared to be significantly superior in episodic migraine as compared with chronic migraine [11].

43.1.1.3 HV-Induced Abnormalities

Some abnormalities are reported to occur during Hyper Ventilation (HV). Considering the last 10 years' literature on the topic, a case-controlled study showed, as the only significant difference between the two groups, the presence of Anterior Theta Activity and Frontal Intermittent Rhythmic Delta Activity (FIRDA) during hyperventilation in the migraine group (Fig. 43.3).

However, changes in EEG activity seemed not necessarily to be correlated with the occurrence of headache during HV, neither when preceded by aura [12].

43.1.1.4 Epileptiform Abnormalities

Epileptiform abnormalities are uncommon and the association between migraine and epilepsy is debatable, although some epileptic syndromes - such as childhood epilepsy with centro-temporal spikes, childhood occipital epilepsies and perhaps even childhood absence epilepsy - seem to be associated with a higher prevalence of migraine [9].

43.1.2 Ictal EEG Abnormalities

In migraine without aura there are no EEG abnormalities, according to some authors [13]. On the contrary, different types of EEG abnormalities have been reported during migraine with aura, both in children and in adults.

During visual aura, either slow waves, depression of background activity amplitude, or normal EEGs have been

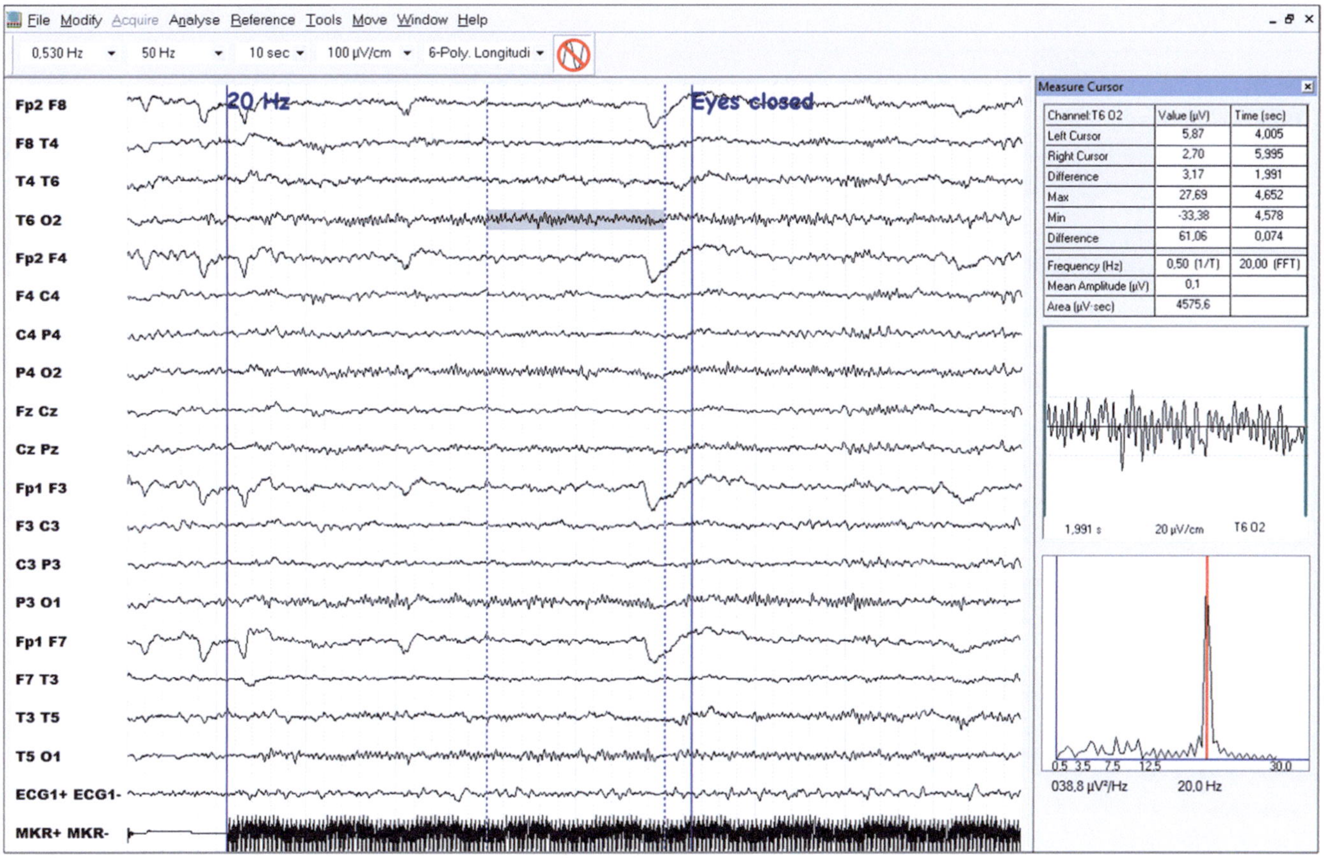

Fig. 43.2 Photic Driving Response (PDR) at Intermittent Photic Stimulation (IPS) at 20 Hz in a migraineur male patient during interictal period

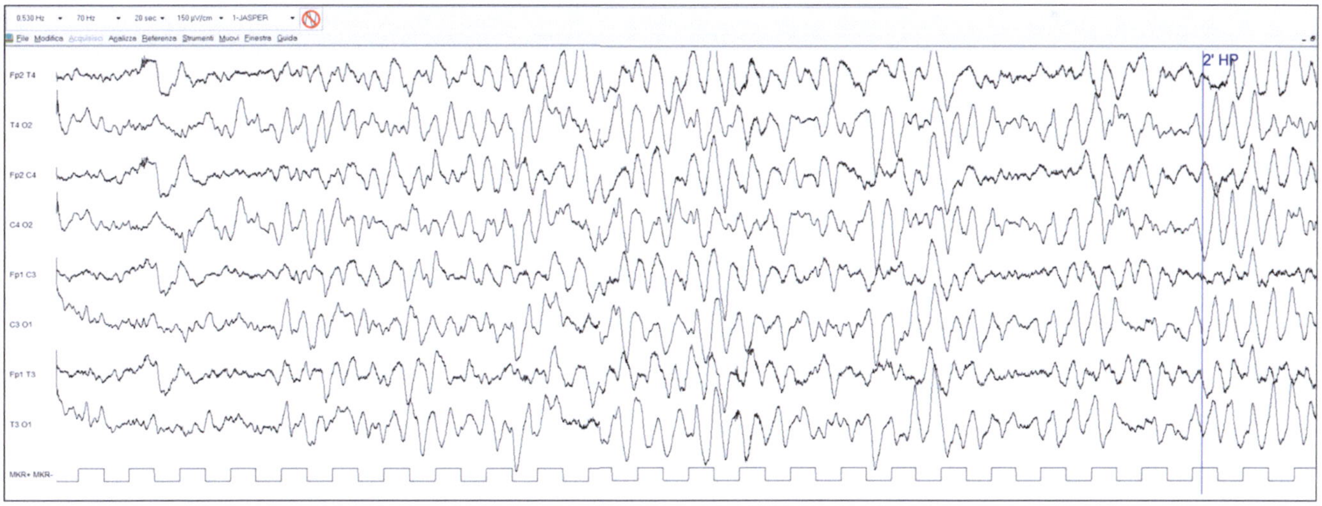

Fig. 43.3 Hyperventilation in an 18-year-old male migraine patient during interictal period: high-voltage diffuse delta activity (3–4 Hz), predominant in the anterior regions. During the activation procedure, the patient developed a strong bifrontal migraine

reported. The most definitely abnormal EEGs with unilateral or bilateral delta activity have been recorded during attacks of hemiplegic migraine and during attacks of migraine with disorders of consciousness [13]. Patients with short-lasting auras usually show no EEG changes [14]. In patients in whom aura is >1 h but <24 h, unilateral slow-wave abnormalities in the migraneous hemisphere and either temporo-occipital or diffuse abnormalities were observed (Fig 43.4 and 43.5), associated with slight hypoperfusion. In the following day, occipital rhythmic slow-wave abnormalities on the migraneous hemisphere, with a good reactivity at eyes opening was recorded [15].

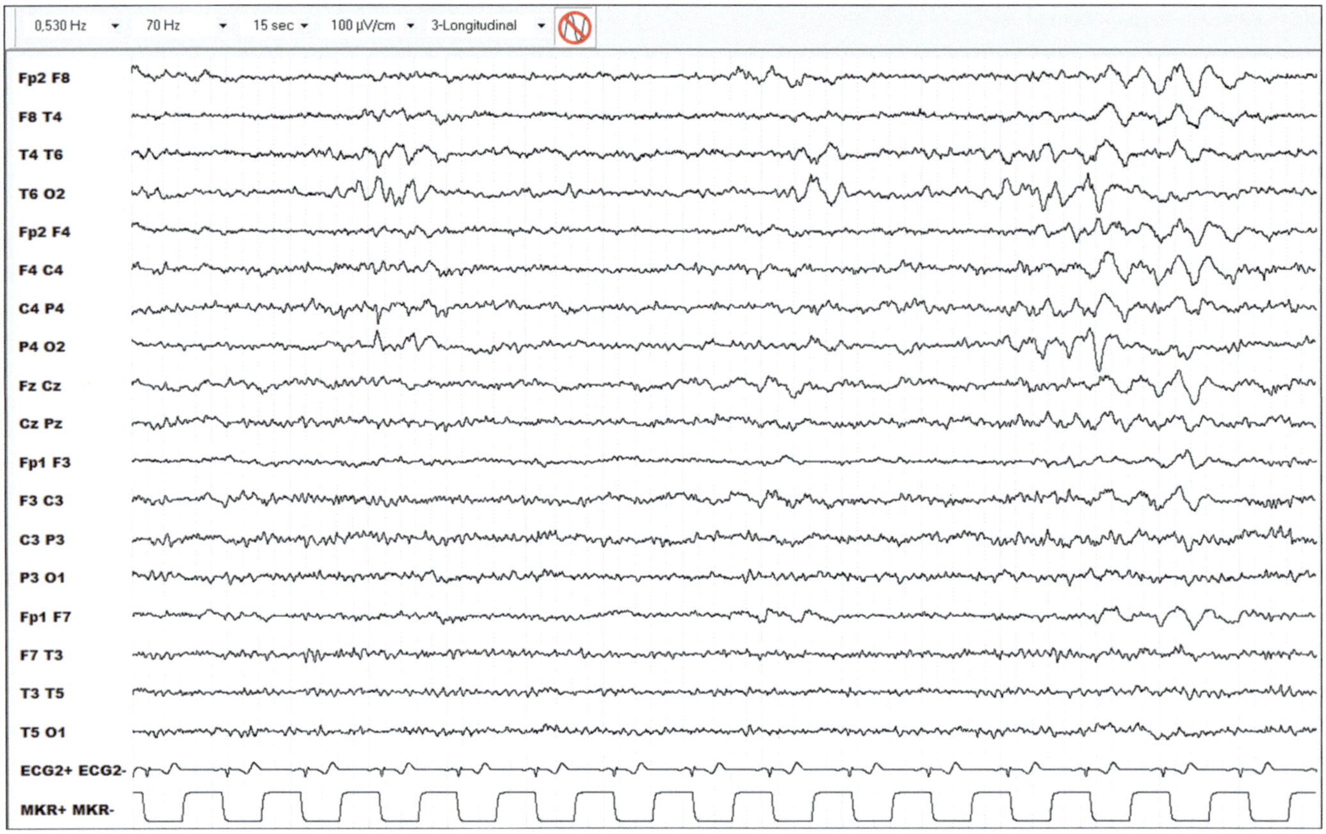

Fig. 43.4 EEG recorded during long-lasting visual aura in a 37-year-old female patient: sharpened slow wave abnormalities in the migrainous hemisphere, predominant on the posterior regions

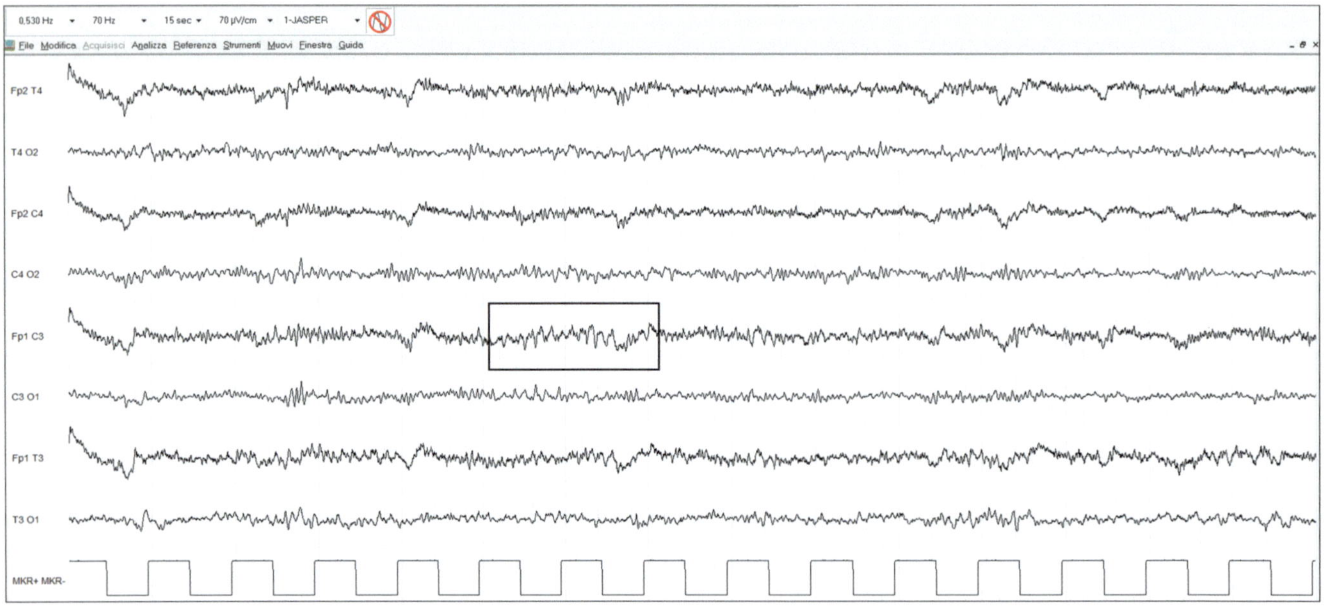

Fig. 43.5 Focal theta activity in left central areas in a 40-year-old male patient during sensory aura

Ozkan et al. (2012) in a prospective study demonstrated the predominance of abnormalities in children with migraine, either with or without aura, in respect to those affected by tension-type headache. EEG abnormalities, prevalent during the attack, are variable, consisting of: intermittent generalized slow waves; focal fronto-temporal or occipital sharp and/or slow waves; bilateral fronto-centro-temporal or temporo-occipital slow waves [16].

Basilar migraine with a reduced state of consciousness a type of aura that is associated with signs of bilateral brainstem dysfunction is often associated with bilateral frontocentral paroxysmal slow activity [17].

In 2016, Chastan et al. [18] described a full sporadic hemiplegic migraine attack with right hyposthenia during a 72-hour video—EEG recording and made clinical—neurophysiological correlations during the episode (Fig 43.6). EEG was normal at the beginning of visual aura while, after 15 minutes, posterior slow waves appeared in the migraneous hemisfere, spreading progressively to the anterior regions of both hemispheres.

43.1.3 Quantitative EEG (qEEG)

qEEG has been used in several studies on migraine with controversial results. However, only a few researchers have studied qEEG during spontaneous attacks. Brain mapping using quantitative topographical EEG [19] showed unilateral reduction of alpha activity during and within 3 days of a migraine attack with visual aura [20, 21], as well as in migraine without aura on the side of the headache, and in patients with menstrual migraine, up to 24 h before the attack (Fig. 43.7) [20].

A study by Bjørk and Sand [17] on qEEG before, during and after migraine attack showed that frontocentral delta power increased, whereas frontocentral theta and alpha power tended to increase within 36 h before the next attack, compared with the interictal period. Occipitoparietal alpha and theta and temporal alpha power were more asymmetric before the attack in comparison with the interictal period. During attacks, posterior alpha power increased slightly. Post-ictal power and power asymmetry of EEG bands were not significantly different from baseline. According to these observations, EEG activity seems then to change shortly before the attack. This suggests that migraineurs are most susceptible to attack when anterior qEEG delta power and posterior alpha and theta asymmetry values increase. Cholinergic brainstem and/or basal forebrain nuclei and thalamo-cortical connections remodulation before migraine attack are probably responsible of these changes. Posterior alpha power was increased during attack, whereas frontocentral beta power also was slightly increased. Temporal beta power asymmetry tended to be higher during the attack. Ictal EEG showed a moderately increased occipitoparietal alpha activity [17, 22]. This is in contrast to the results of Schoenen et al., [20] who reported unilateral alpha and theta reduction in common migraine attacks.

43.2 Migraine and Epilepsy

The relationship between migraine and epilepsy is a relevant topic, still a matter of debate among physicians, also regarding the most appropriate terminology to be used. While in the most recent ILAE classification of seizures and epilepsies (2017) [23] this aspect has not been considered, in the ICHD-3 beta classification [1], "Headache attributed to epileptic seizure" is reported, including two entities: "hemicrania epileptica" and "postictal headache". Furthermore, "migraine aura-triggered seizure", as a complication of migraine, is also described in the 1st chapter of the same classification.

According to their temporal occurrence, four types of association between headache and epileptic seizure are recognized: (1) pre-ictal headache, (2) headache as the expression of an epileptic manifestation, (3) postictal headache and (4) interictal headache [24].

With regard to headache as the expression of an epileptic manifestation, it is known that although headache often represents only the beginning of a seizure, rarely head pain is the only manifestation of an epileptic seizure.

This condition represents the so-called pure epileptic headache, in contrast with the "headache followed without discontinuity by other epileptic manifestations", thus actually being an epileptic seizure beginning with headache.

The term "hemicrania epileptica", accepted by the ICHD-2 and still present in the ICHD-3 beta [1] refers to a unilateral migraine attack coinciding with EEG (scalp and/or deep) epileptic activity, localized homolateral to migraine pain. Some authors consider this term just a useless terminological complication, suggesting that it should be classified as a type of ictal epileptic headache (IEH) [24, 25]. IEH is considered a secondary headache disorder, as the condition is primarily an epileptic condition with headache presenting as a manifestation of the seizure.

Although the accurate pathophysiology of hemicrania epileptica is uncertain, it has been suggested that the increased cerebral blood flow observed during the pre-ictal or ictal period may trigger trigeminovascular activation, resulting in headache [25].

The neocortical dysexcitability is thought to be the main pathological mechanism underlying the onset of both

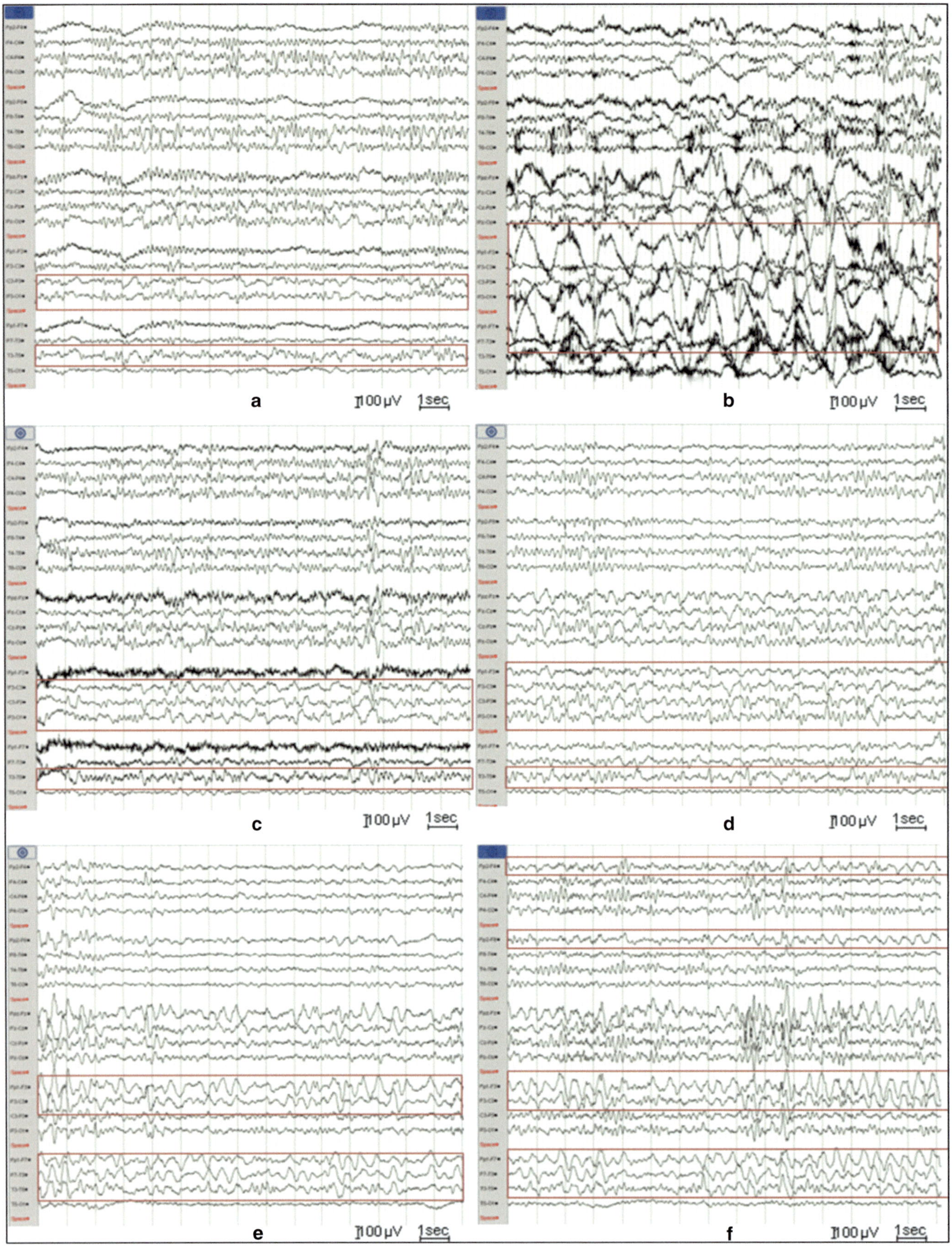
a
100 µV
1 sec
b
100 µV
1 sec
c
100 µV
1 sec
d
100 µV
1 sec
e
100 µV
1 sec
f
100 µV
1 sec

Fig. 43.6 EEG abnormalities during the full duration of a hemiplegic migraine attack. (**a**) Slow waves in the left temporo-parietal region. (**b**) Superimposition of left rhythmic frontal slow waves of very large amplitude. (**c**) Left temporoparietal slow waves spreading forward towards the left central region. (**d**) Left temporo-parieto-central slow waves spreading forward towards the left frontal region. (**e**) Disappearance of slow waves from the left parietal region. Persistence of temporo-frontal slow waves becoming rhythmic. (**f**) Left temporo-frontal slow waves spreading toward the right frontal region with bifrontal rhythmic delta activity. EEG abnormalities are framed in red colour. (From Chastan N, Lebas A, Legoff F, Parain D, Guyant-Marechal L. Clinical and electroencephalographic abnormalities during the full duration of a sporadic hemiplegic migraine attack. Neurophysiol Clin. 2016;46:307–311, with permission)

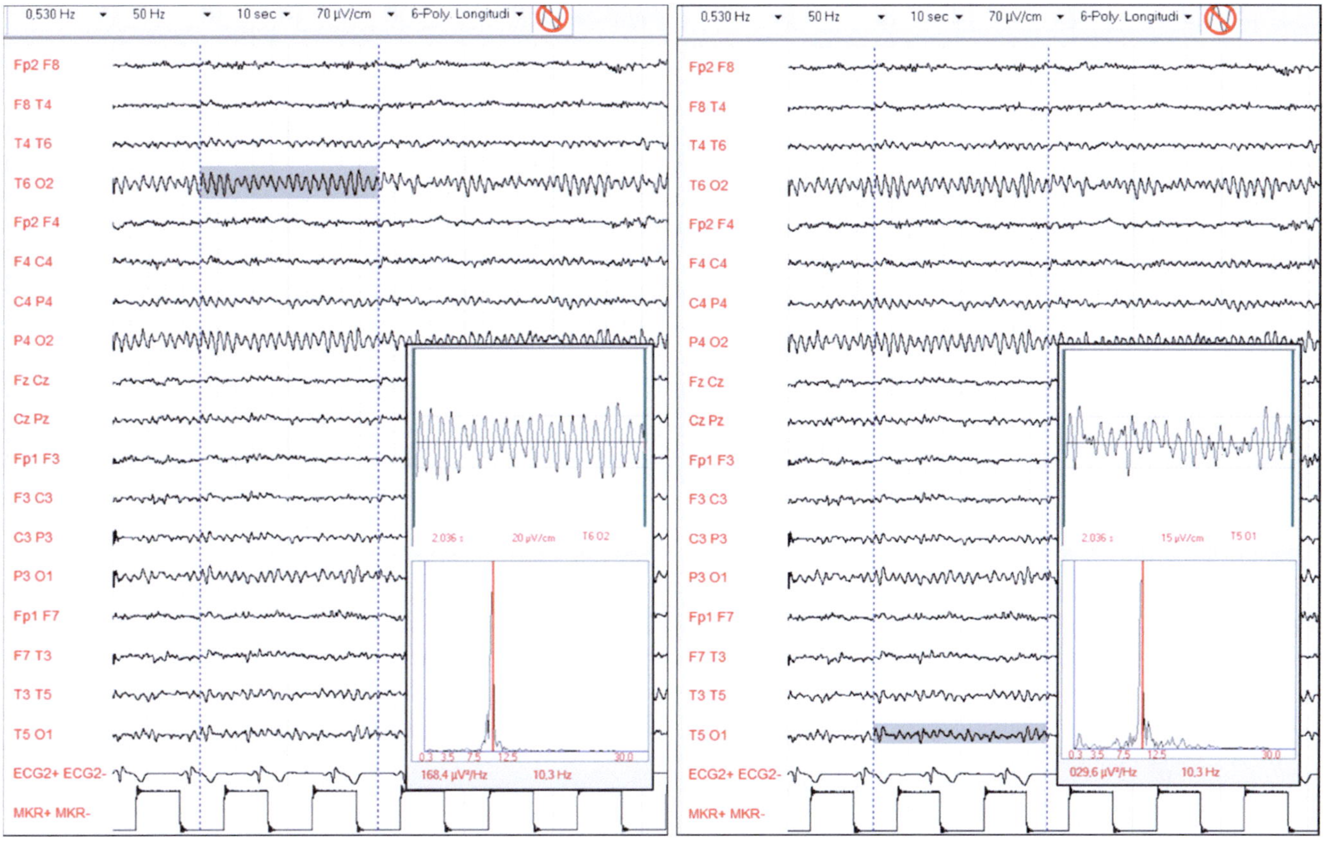

Fig. 43.7 EEG recorded after 24 h from the cessation of migraine with visual aura in a 25-year-old woman: note the difference in amplitude of the alpha rhythm, evidenced by the spectral analysis, between the affected (left) and the contralateral hemisphere

migraine and epilepsy with Cortical Spreading Depression (CSD), being the connecting point between them. CSD is characterized by a slowly propagating wave (2–6 mm/min) of sustained strong neuronal depolarization that generates transitory intense spike activity as progressing into brain tissue, followed by a neural suppression which may last for minutes. As CSD begins, an excitatory phase during which neurons depolarize is observed, releasing potassium and start firing. This is followed by a depressed neuronal activity, usually recorded as an EEG flattening, during which cells repolarize and extracellular potassium levels are restored. In certain areas of the cortex, after multiple episodes of CSD, epileptiform abnormalities may occur [26, 27].

CSD can also lead to increased ongoing activity in central trigeminovascular neurons in the spinal trigeminal nucleus and exerts a similar effect on the activity of meningeal nociceptors, causing migraine and aura symptoms [28].

In both CSD and epileptic seizures, the onset and propagation of depolarization are triggered when a certain threshold of membrane potential is reached, which is lower for CSD than for seizures. Moreover, the onset of CSD and that of the epileptic seizure may facilitate each other. These two phenomena lead to the same effect: neuronal depolarization and hypersynchronization. Consequently, it is possible that a paroxysmal activity may induce headache without any associated ictal symptoms when the epileptic discharge predominantly activates CSD and trigeminovascular system [27].

As the detection of CSD with standard methods is probably impossible [29], currently clinical monitoring of spreading depolarizations is limited to patients who require neurosurgical interventions (such as surgical aneurysm ligation after subarachnoid haemorrhage, placement of extraventricular drainage, decompressive hemicraniectomy or evacuation of a haematoma) that allow the placement of a subdural electrode strip [30].

Just a few cases of ictal epileptic headaches confirmed by ictal epileptiform EEG discharges have been reported, and these cases vary considerably with respect to their patterns of headache and EEG abnormalities. Different EEG patterns were described, mainly consisting in rhythmic focal spikes in the posterior cortex. Nevertheless, many other patterns have been observed, such as generalized spike-or-polyspike-and-wave discharges, rhythmic theta-delta activity and spike-and-waves in the left temporal regions. Finally, even rhythmic theta activity and spikes in the left parietal regions or bilateral continuous spike-and-wave discharges have been described [25, 27].

In regard to treatment, ictal headache patients may respond to intravenous injection of benzodiazepines. However, benzodiazepines have also been proven to be ineffective in several instances; thus, response to intravenous medication treatment does not necessarily match with a diagnosis of IEH [31].

It could be very difficult to demonstrate the ictal EEG changes and the potential response to intravenous AED administration in patients with short-lasting headache. This means that epileptic activity in reported cases with ictal epileptic headache was sufficiently prolonged and sustained to be considered as a non-convulsive status epilepticus. One interesting finding in patients with ictal epileptic headache is that many of them show photosensitivity [25].

On the other hand, in the absence of EEG epileptic features during aura and migraine, we should consider the manifestation as an epileptic seizure preceded ("pre-ictal migraine") and possibly triggered by migraine ("migraine-triggered seizure") [24]. With regard to the latter, the term "migraine aura-triggered seizure" should be used in the rare conditions, in which the triggering mechanism can be really demonstrated; otherwise, the term "pre-ictal migraine-like headache" is more appropriate.

A key role in the recognition of a headache as part of the seizure is played by the time interval between pain and the seizure occurrence. If the interval exceeds 1 h, conventionally the definition is "interictal headache". If there is no interval, the differentiating criterion between an epileptic headache and a pre-ictal headache should be the presence or absence of epilepsy-compatible EEG discharges, beginning at onset of headache and continuing during the following seizure. Anyway, since not always epileptiform discharges are detectable at the scalp EEG during an epileptic aura, its absence is not an absolute exclusive criterion. Most problems arise in the differentiation between a migraine attack with visual aura preceding an epileptic seizure and an epileptic seizure of occipital origin beginning with visual symptoms and migraine-like headache, as it occurs in childhood benign epileptic forms. Besides the presence of a time interval between the migrainous attack and the seizure, as already stated before, another discriminating element could be the duration and characteristics of the visual aura, usually shorter and consisting in coloured circular elements when of epileptic nature [32].

Until now, we have focused on the migrainous headache, but we know that other pre-ictal forms of headache ("pre-ictal non-migraine-like headache"), such as tension-type headache, occur with a frequency lower than 10% [32].

Finally, PostIctal Headache (PIH) is the most common association between headache and seizures, occurring between 12 and 52% of persons with epilepsy [32].

Most studies have defined PIH as a headache that begins after - or immediately after - a seizure. However, postictal headache have been reported to occur up to 3 h after the seizure. Longer durations between seizure end and headache onset are more likely considered as interictal headaches [33].

Incidence varies according to the type of epilepsy and the region of focus [34]. It is more frequent after generalized tonic-clonic seizures, particularly when prolonged and repetitive. Moreover, it's not rare in focal epilepsy syndromes. Among these, very commonly associated with headache are the occipital childhood forms, both Panayiotopoulos syndrome and Gastaut type of benign occipital epilepsy [31].

Prolonged EEG recordings of postictal headache in patients with occipital lobe epilepsy show absence of any ictal discharge, but the presence of postictal delta activities in the posterior head regions [35, 36].

References

1. Headache Classification Committee of the International Headache Society (IHS). The International Classification of Headache Disorders, 3rd edition (beta version). Cephalalgia. 2013; 33:629–808.
2. Steiner TJ. Headache in the world: public health and research priorities. Expert Rev Pharmacoecon Outcomes Res. 2013;13:51–7.
3. Kramer U, Nevo Y, Harel S. Electroencephalography in the evaluation of headache patients: a review. Isr J Med Sci. 1997;33:816–20.
4. American Academy of Neurology. Electroencephalogram in the evaluation of headache https://www.aan.com/Guidelines/Home/GuidelineDetail/47
5. Anon. Practice parameter: the electroencephalogram in the evaluation of headache (summary statement). Report of the Quality Standards Subcommittee of the American Academy of Neurology. Neurology. 1995;45:1411–3.
6. Prensky AL, Sommer D. Diagnosis and treatment of migraine in children. Neurology. 1979;29:506–10.
7. Mariani E, Moschini V, Pastorino G, Rizzi F, Severgnini A, Tiengo M. Patter-reversal visual-evoked potentials and EEG correlations in common migraine patients. Headache. 1988;28:269–71.
8. Slatter KH. Some clinical and EEG findings in patients with migraine. Brain. 1968;91:85–98.

9. Neufeld MY, Treves TA, Korczyn AD. EEG and topographic frequency analysis in common and classic migraine. Headache. 1991;31:232–6.
10. Bjørk MH, Stovner LJ, Engstrøm M, Stjern M, Hagen K, Sand T. Interictal quantitative EEG in migraine: a blinded controlled study. J Headache Pain. 2009;10:331–9.
11. Fogang Y, Gérard P, De Pasqua V, et al. Analysis and clinical correlates of 20 Hz photic driving on routine EEG in migraine. Acta Neurol Belg. 2015;115:39–45.
12. Tan HJ, Suganthi C, Dhachayani S, Rizal AM, Raymond AA. The electroencephalogram changes in migraineurs. Med J Malaysia. 2007;62:56–8.
13. Sand T. EEG in migraine: a review of the literature. Funct Neurol. 1991;6:7–22.
14. Lauritzen M, Trojaborg W, Olesen J. EEG during attacks of common and classical migraine. Cephalalgia. 1981;1:63–6.
15. Parain D, Hitzel A, Guegan-Massardier E, et al. Migraine aura lasting 1–24 h in children: a sequence of EEG slow-wave abnormalities vs. vascular events. Cephalalgia. 2007;27:1043–9.
16. Ozkan M, Teber ST, Deda G. Electroencephalogram variations in pediatric migraines and tension-type headaches. Pediatr Neurol. 2012;46:154–7.
17. Bjørk M, Sand T. Quantitative EEG power and asymmetry increase 36 h before a migraine attack. Cephalalgia. 2008;28:960–8.
18. Chastan N, Lebas A, Legoff F, Parain D, Guyant-Marechal L. Clinical and electroencephalographic abnormalities during the full duration of a sporadic hemiplegic migraine attack. Neurophysiol Clin. 2016;46:307–11.
19. Sauer S, Schellenberg R, Hofmann HC. Functional imaging of headache—first steps in an objective quantitative classification of migraine. Eur J Med Res. 1997;2:367–76.
20. Schoenen J, Jamart B, Delwaide PJ. Topographic EEG mapping in common and classic migraine during and between attacks. In: Clifford Rose F, editor. Advances in headache research. London: Smith Gordon; 1987. p. 25–33.
21. Cerquiglini A, Guidetti V, Seri S. Computerized EEG topography in childhood migraine between and during attacks. Cephalalgia. 1993;13:53–6.
22. Bjørk MH, Stovner LJ, Nilsen BM, Stjern M, Hagen K, Sand T. The occipital alpha rhythm related to the "migraine cycle" and headache burden: a blinded, controlled longitudinal study. Clin Neurophysiol. 2009;120:464–71.
23. Scheffer IE, Berkovic S, Capovilla G, et al. ILAE classification of the epilepsies position paper of the ILAE Commission for Classification and Terminology. Epilepsia. 2017;58:512–21.
24. Cianchetti C, Pruna D, Ledda MG. Epileptic seizures and headache/migraine: a review of types of association and terminology. Seizure. 2013;22:679–85.
25. Kim DW, Lee SK. Headache and epilepsy. J Epilepsy Res. 2017;7:7–15.
26. Broberg M, Pope KJ, Olsson T, Shuttleworth WC, Willoughby JO. Spreading depression: evidence of five electroencephalogram phases. J Neurosci Res. 2014;92:1384–94.
27. Zhang X, Levy D, Kainz V, Noseda R, Jakubowski M, Burstein R. Activation of central trigeminovascular neurons by cortical spreading depression. Ann Neurol. 2011;69:855–65.
28. Fanella M, Morano A, Fattouch J, et al. Ictal epileptic headache in adult life: electroclinical patterns and spectrum of related syndromes. Epilepsy Behav. 2015;53:161–5.
29. Bastany ZJ, Askari S, Dumont GA, Speckmann EJ, Gorji A. Non-invasive monitoring of spreading depression. Neuroscience. 2016;1:1–12.
30. Drenckhahn C, Winkler MK, Major S, et al. Correlates of spreading depolarization in human scalp electroencephalography. Brain. 2012;135:853–68.
31. Saitowitz Z, Flamini R, Berenson F. Ictal epileptic headache: a review of current literature and differentiation from migralepsy and other epilepsies. Headache. 2014;54:1534–40.
32. Cianchetti C, Avanzini G, Dainese F, Guidetti V. The complex interrelations between two paroxysmal disorders: headache and epilepsy. Neurol Sci. 2017;38:941–8.
33. Ekstein D, Schachter SC. Postictal headache. Epilepsy Behav. 2010;19:151–5.
34. Ito M, Nakamura F, Honma H, et al. Clinical factors associated with post-ictal headache in patients with epilepsy. Acta Neurol Scand. 2000;102:129–31.
35. Andermann F, Zifkin B. The benign occipital epilepsies of childhood: an overview of the idiopathic syndromes and of the relationship to migraine. Epilepsia. 1998;39(Suppl 4):9–23.
36. Ogunyemi A, Adams D. Migraine-like symptoms triggered by occipital lobe seizures: response to Sumatriptan. Can J Neurol Sci. 1998;25:151–3.

Psychiatric Disorders

44

Chiara Davassi, Patrizia Pulitano, and Oriano Mecarelli

44.1 Depressive Disorders

According to DSM-5 [1], depressive disorders are classified in Major Depressive Disorder (MDD), persistent depressive disorder (formerly called dysthymia), premenstrual dysphoric disorder, depressive disorder due to another medical condition, other specified depressive disorder, and unspecified depressive disorder.

Common symptoms are the presence of sad, empty or irritable mood, accompanied by somatic and cognitive changes that significantly affect the individual's daily life. Differences are represented by duration, timing or presumed etiology.

Most evidences about EEG abnormalities relate to MDD, which represents the classic condition in this group. It is characterized by discrete episodes of at least 2-week duration involving definite changes in affect, cognition, neurovegetative functions, and inter-episode remissions.

Few studies have reported background EEG abnormalities in MDD patients and there are no established EEG features considered characteristic of MDD. Temporal slow waves were found to be significantly more common in depressed patients than in age-matched controls, and those depressed patients with temporal slow-wave activity had a lower probability of having a family history of mood disorders [2]. Abnormal mid-frontal theta activity has also been described: it is thought to reflect Anterior Cingulate Cortex (ACC) activity and it has been linked with focused and sustained attention or concentration as well as with mental efforts.

C. Davassi · O. Mecarelli (✉)
Department of Human Neurosciences, Sapienza University of Rome, Rome, Italy
e-mail: chiara.davassi@uniroma1.it; oriano.mecarelli@uniroma1.it

P. Pulitano
Azienda Ospedaliero-Universitaria Policlinico Umberto I, Rome, Italy
e-mail: patrizia.pulitano@uniroma1.it

The ACC is involved in several cognitive and emotive functions. It is subdivided into ventral and dorsal aspects. The subgenual (sgACC; BA25) and rostral aspects (BA24ab and BA32) constitute the ventral ACC, considered the "affective" region, as it is connected with limbic and subcortical structures as well as with the orbital Pre-Frontal Cortex (PFC). The sgACC, specifically, has been implicated in visceral responses to emotive processing, in emotive memory formation and in regulating reward contingencies. The dorsal aspect of ACC (composed of BA24 and BA32) constitutes the "cognitive" ACC as it is strictly connected with the Dorso Lateral Pre Frontal Cortex (DLPFC). Few studies have examined baseline ACC theta activity in depressed non-medicated individuals versus controls, with controversial results, as theta power/amplitude reductions and increases have been both observed in MDD. Theta activity, examined using standardized low-resolution electromagnetic tomography (sLORETA) in the ACC, showed the MDD population displaying increased sgACC theta activity. Altered theta activity in the sgACC may reflect emotion regulation abnormalities in MDD. Furthermore, elevated baseline sgACC theta activity and rostral ACC theta activity have been shown to predict a positive antidepressant response [3].

Moreover, data arising from studies of spectral analysis of background EEG activity suggested asymmetry in brain activity, especially Frontal Brain Asymmetry (FBA), as a potential marker for depression [4]. Henriques and Davidson, in 1991, found that subjects with depression have less activation in the left frontal cortex compared with the right frontal cortex [4, 5]. Previously depressed subjects also exhibit diminished left-sided anterior and right-sided posterior activation compared with never-depressed subjects [6]. Thus, a pattern of relatively less left than right frontal activity may represent a risk marker for MDD. In support of this, it seems that increased relative right fronto-cortical activity tends to emerge during the processing of negative information and emotions, while greater relative

O. Mecarelli (ed.), *Clinical Electroencephalography*, https://doi.org/10.1007/978-3-030-04573-9_44

left fronto-cortical activity is associated with positive information/affective processing [3, 7].

Furthermore, right parietal hypoactivity - associated with emotional under-arousal - has been noted in MDD. Right parietotemporal activity is thought to be involved in modulating emotion-related autonomic arousal; thus, decreased right parietotemporal activity may reflect diminished emotional arousal in the disorder. Notably, depressed patients with comorbid anxiety, characterized by a hyperaroused state, display right parietotemporal hyperactivity while those without anxiety exhibit decreased activity in this region [3].

Finally, polysomnographic studies found that MDD is associated with abnormal sleep architecture. Some authors suggested that major depression may be related to a combination of diminished Slow-Wave Sleep (SWS) duration and increased Rapid Eye Movement (REM) sleep density. REM density was proposed as a possible biological marker for the disorder [8]. Patients may have prolonged sleep-onset latency and frequent nocturnal awakenings resulting in sleep fragmentation and poor sleep efficiency. Depressed patients often have decreased REM sleep latency and prolonged REM sleep periods early in the night, leading to an overall increase in the proportion of REM sleep. In addition, REM sleep in depressed patients is characterized by more frequent rapid eye movements than in controls. The relative excess of REM sleep corresponds to a decrease of stage SWS. Not only is time spent in SWS decreased in depressed patients compared with controls, but also the distribution of Slow-Wave Activity (SWA), a marker of SWS intensity, is also abnormal. In fact, contrary to healthy subjects who have maximal SWA during the first sleep cycle, depressed patients have peak SWA during subsequent cycles [9].

44.2 Bipolar and Related Disorders

Bipolar Disorders (BDs) are severe, chronic mental disorders affecting 1–4% of the population worldwide [10]. BDs, also known as manic-depressive illness, are characterized by unusual shifts in mood, energy and activity levels that interfere with the ability to achieve daily life activities. These moods range from manic episodes, consisting in periods of extremely euphoric and energized behavior, to depressive episodes, resulting in very sad, or hopeless periods. Less severe manic periods are known as hypomanic episodes [11].

In the DSM-5 [1], bipolar and related disorders are separated from the depressive disorders and placed between “schizophrenia spectrum and other psychotic disorders” and “depressive disorders”, as they are considered a bridge between the two diagnostic classes in terms of symptomatology, family history and genetics. The conditions included in this group are bipolar I disorder, bipolar II disorder, cyclothymic disorder, substance/medication-induced bipolar and related disorder, bipolar and related disorder due to another medical condition, other specified bipolar and related disorder, unspecified bipolar and related disorder.

With regard to EEG abnormalities in BDs they are less defined than in other psychiatric disorders, such as schizophrenia or MDD. Most studies on BDs patients have described normal EEG [2]. However, a background of fast (beta) activity and temporal lobe dysrhythmias, consisting of paroxysmal runs of theta activity, which may become generalized and interposed with slow waves and occasional sharp wave and spike activity, have been also reported [12].

Spectral EEG analysis reports are heterogeneous and do not always consider the potential effects of drugs on oscillatory dynamics (see Chap. 45) [13]. Some authors reported indeed in BDs a generalized increased power in all frequencies, mostly in the beta bands, despite clinical euthymia [12, 14], whereas others reported reduced alpha power in euthymic BD patients [12, 14].

Finally, sleep studies in BDs patients evidenced variations in sleep architecture, disruption of the 24-hour sleep-wake cycle and increased sleep fragmentation. Polysonnographic findings in both manic and depressed bipolar subjects include a disruption in sleep continuity, increased time spent in stage 1 sleep, shortened REM latency and an increase in the density of REM sleep [15].

44.3 Anxiety Disorders

Anxiety disorders are the most prevalent psychiatric disorders with lifetime prevalence rates of nearly 30% [16, 17].

They include symptoms of excessive fear and anxiety and related behavioral disturbances that can interfere with daily activities such as job performance, school work and relationships. According to the types of objects or situations that induce fear, anxiety, or avoidance behavior and to the age of onset, in DSM-5 [1], they are organized in separation anxiety disorder, selective mutism, specific phobia, social anxiety disorder, panic disorder, agoraphobia, generalized anxiety disorder, anxiety disorder due to another medical condition, other specified anxiety disorder, and unspecified anxiety disorder.

Differently from the previous edition of the manual, Obsessive-Compulsive Disorder (OCD) and Post-Traumatic Stress Disorder (PTSD) are no longer in this chapter, representing the former distinct section and being the latter now listed among the trauma- and stressor-related disorders.

Anxiety disorders are not correlated to specific EEG patterns, but a trend for a decrease in amplitude of alpha rhythm - which appears less confined to the posterior regions - has been described. A desynchronization of the background activity and the presence of fast activity, predominantly in the anterior regions (Fig. 44.1) is often appreciated in healthy people experiencing anxiety feelings. In subjects

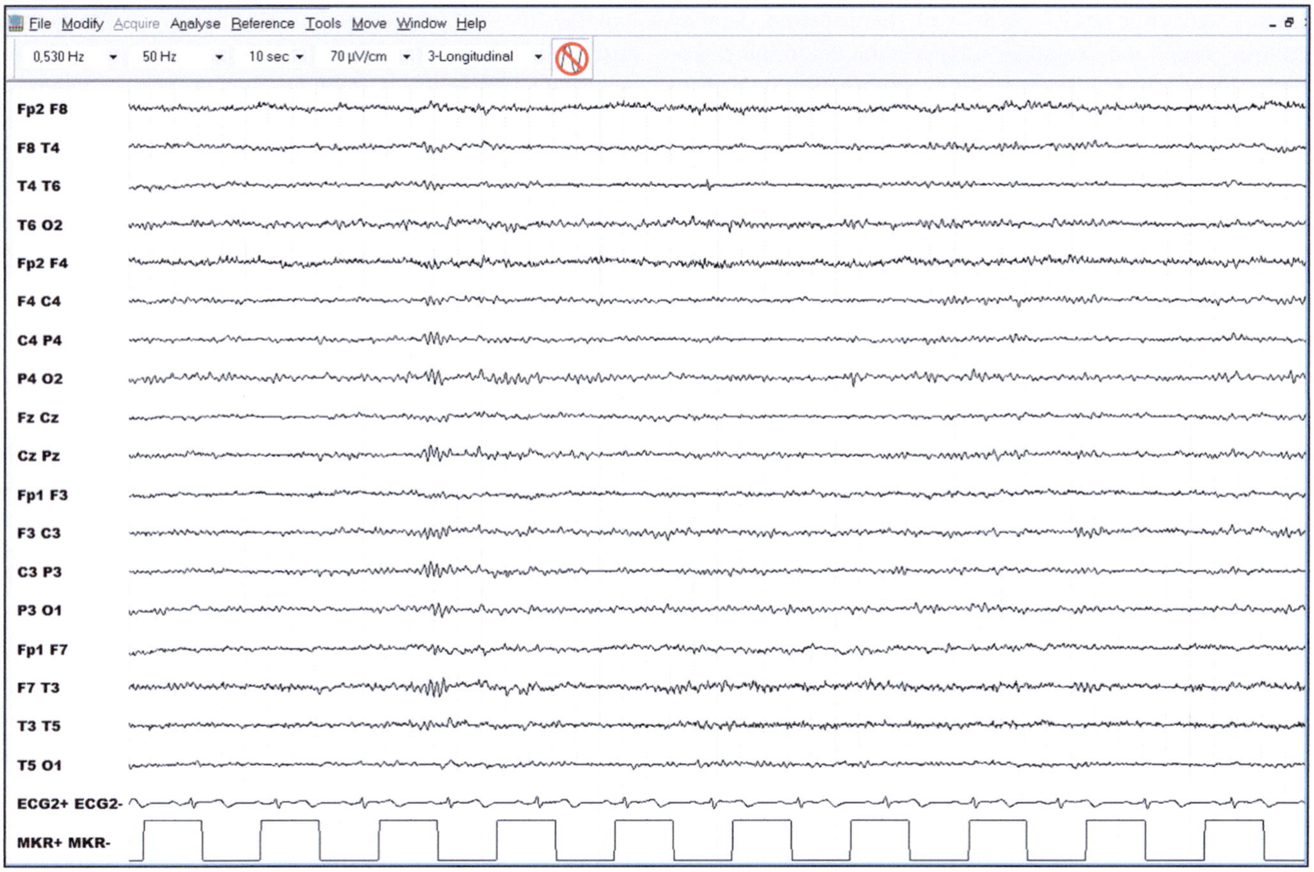

Fig. 44.1 Desynchronization of background activity in a male patient with generalized anxiety disorder. Note the diffuse low-amplitude fast activity, predominant in the anterior regions

with anxiety disorders, this pattern may become, on the other hand, persistent. Moreover, they can show theta sequences in temporal regions that, sometimes, can be emphasized by hyperventilation, although this activation procedure usually promotes the reappearance of alpha rhythm as a consequence of psychophysical relaxation.

EEG studies are very few and if we exclude those on OCD and PTSD, it is hard to draw strong conclusions from them. Most of them are on panic disorder, generalized anxiety disorder, and social anxiety disorder and show in the first two a basal cortical hypoactivity, reflected by abnormal elevations in slow spectral frequencies; in the last one, a tonic hyperarousal of the cortex, with increased high-frequency spectral EEG is observed. Overall, basal instability of the cortical arousal system was reported in quantitative EEG (qEEG) studies as a common, non-specific, feature of most patients with anxiety disorders [18]. This is represented by changed spectral power of theta and alpha bands in most of the brain areas and of beta range, especially in frontal and central brain regions [19].

With regard to sleep EEG findings, patients with anxiety disorders typically have prolonged sleep latency, reduced sleep efficiency and shortened total sleep time. However, in contrast to patients with major depression, REM sleep latency is usually not shortened. Furthermore, a reduction of slow-wave sleep is not as common as in other mental disorders, such as in schizophrenia [18, 19].

44.4 Schizophrenia Spectrum and Other Psychotic Disorders

Schizophrenia spectrum and other psychotic disorders, according to DSM-5 [1], include schizophrenia, other psychotic disorders and schizotypal disorder.

They are defined by the presence of "positive symptoms," - consisting in abnormalities in one or more of the following five domains: delusions, hallucinations, disorganized thinking, grossly disorganized, or abnormal motor behavior, including catatonia - and "negative symptoms" associated with disruptions to normal emotions and behaviors, such as "flat affect", reduced feelings of pleasure in everyday life, difficulty in beginning and sustaining activities and reduced speaking [1, 20].

Although early studies found prevalence rates for EEG abnormalities in schizophrenia of 20–60%, a recent paper by

Endres and colleagues - with well-characterized, healthy control groups and excluding subjects with comorbidities or under medications - revealed EEG abnormalities in about 7% of people with schizophrenia or related disorders, indicating how these are under the influence of other several factors, such as medication and comorbidities [21].

Intermittent Rhythmic Theta Activity (IRTA) and Intermittent Rhythmic Delta Activity (IRDA), mostly with frontal distribution, were the main EEG abnormalities observed in this population (Fig. 44.2) [21].

With regard to qEEG, the most frequently reported abnormalities include increased absolute slow activity power and decreased absolute alpha activity power, which is normalized after antipsychotic medical treatment [22].

Clinically, EEG may be useful in diagnosing conditions other than schizophrenia that may present with psychosis and other psychiatric abnormalities likely ascribable to schizophrenia. Among these, the most important is temporal lobe focal epilepsy. A possible link between epilepsy and schizophreniform disorder has been a matter of discussion for a long time. The observation of different psychotic syndromes in patients with temporal lobe epilepsy led to the "temporal lobe hypothesis" for schizophrenia. Psychotic symptoms are described in 7% of patients with pharmacoresistant focal epilepsy, predominantly as interictal and postictal psychoses, rarely as ictal psychosis [21]. When ictal psychoses occur, they represent typically focal phenomena arising from the temporal lobe, that elicit the activation of limbic system and neocortical temporal areas. Transient ictal psychoses may be secondary to continuous epileptic discharges that cause no other epileptic symptoms [23]. Interictal psychosis typically begins years after the onset of pharmacoresistant epilepsy and it is independent from seizures. Clinically, the first manifestations are auditory hallucinations, combined with strong affective components. Postictal psychosis manifests 10–20 years after the onset of pharmacoresistant epilepsy. It occurs after clusters of seizures and can last from a few days to several weeks. Clinically, the most frequent symptoms are paranoia, visual and auditory hallucinations. Therefore, increased EEG epileptiform abnormalities in schizophreniform patients might be a sign of increased risk for developing epilepsy or an indicator of a specific pathomechanism in a subgroup of psychotic patients potentially treatable with antiepileptic drugs, such as valproate [21].

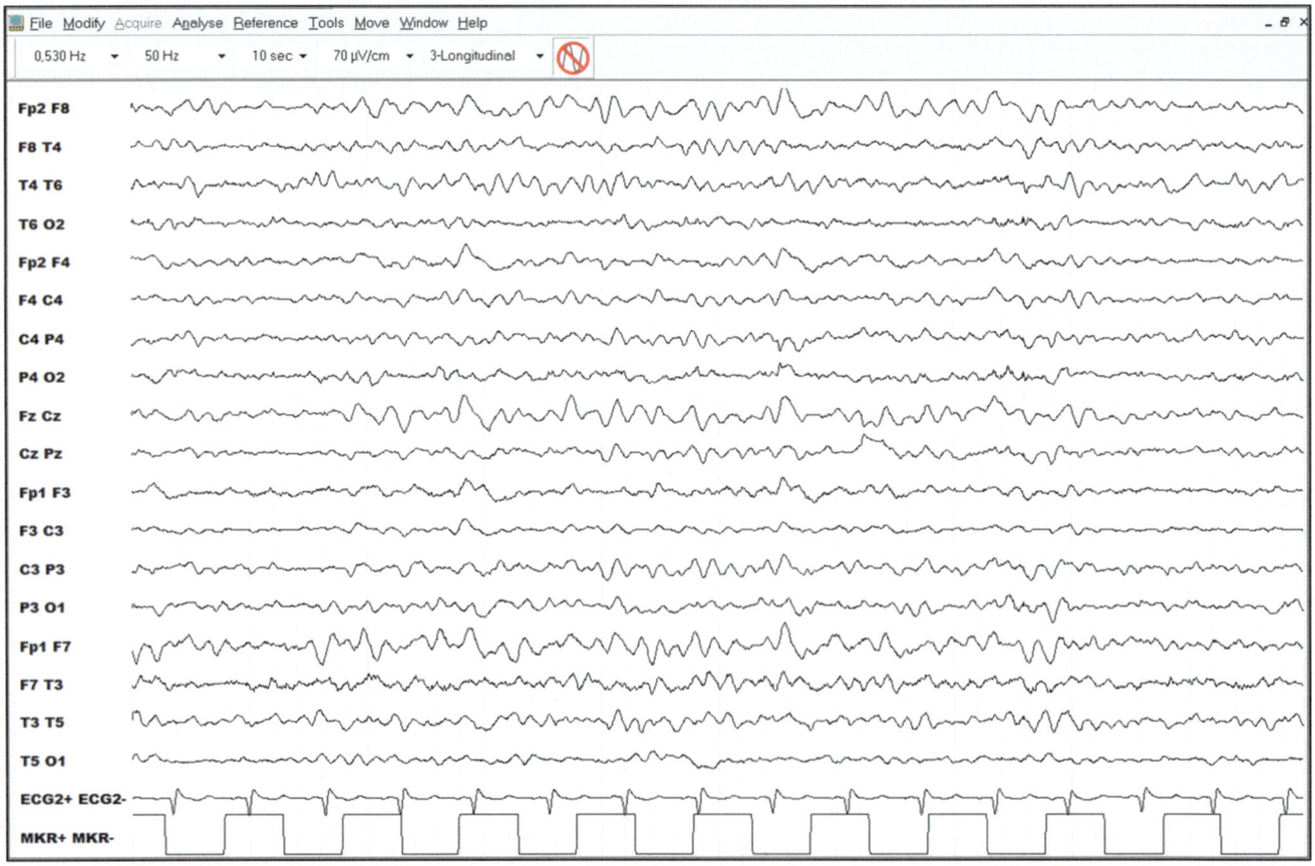

Fig. 44.2 Generalized slowing of background activity at 4–6 Hz, more evident in the frontal areas, in a 40-year-old female schizophrenic patient

Finally, sleep architecture is also altered in subjects with schizophrenia, showing difficulties in initiating sleep, reduced duration of SWS and a shorter REM sleep latency [24].

44.5 Attention-Deficit/Hyperactivity Disorder (ADHD)

Included in the chapter of neurodevelopmental disorders in DSM 5 [1], ADHD is a common neurodevelopmental disorder, whose worldwide prevalence is estimated at approximately 5% [25].

It is characterized by inattention, disorganization, and/or hyperactivity-impulsivity. Inattention and disorganization determine inability to focus on tasks, seeming not to listen and losing materials, at levels inconsistent with age or development. Hyperactivity-impulsivity entails overactivity, fidgeting, inability to stay seated, intruding into other people's activities, and inability to wait, all symptoms that are excessive for age or developmental level. DSM-5 distinguishes between three subtypes of the disorder: predominantly hyperactive-impulsive type, predominantly inattentive type, and combined type [1].

Qualitative EEG observations reported in early studies on children with ADHD consisted in abnormalities such as excessive slow-wave and/or abnormal spike-and-wave activity. Epileptiform abnormalities have been observed in children with ADHD with a wide range of prevalence (5–15%) reported in different studies and without a specific relation with the risk of developing epileptic seizures [26]. In sleep-deprived EEG, epileptiform abnormalities have been described in about 25% of patients with ADHD with central, frontal and temporal localization in more than half (Fig. 44.3) [27].

Rolandic spikes have been found in 5.6% of children with ADHD without epilepsy in a study by Holtman and colleagues and these abnormalities seem to be present predominantly in children who exhibit more hyperactive–impulsive symptoms [26, 28].

With regard to qEEG evaluation, the most consistent EEG finding in ADHD is elevated fronto-central theta absolute power, together with a lower beta1 absolute power, in comparison with non-ADHD controls. The combination of these two EEG markers is called the "THeta to Beta Ratio" (THBR) [29]. Furthermore, powers of all frequency bands, and in particular the beta power in the frontal region, are

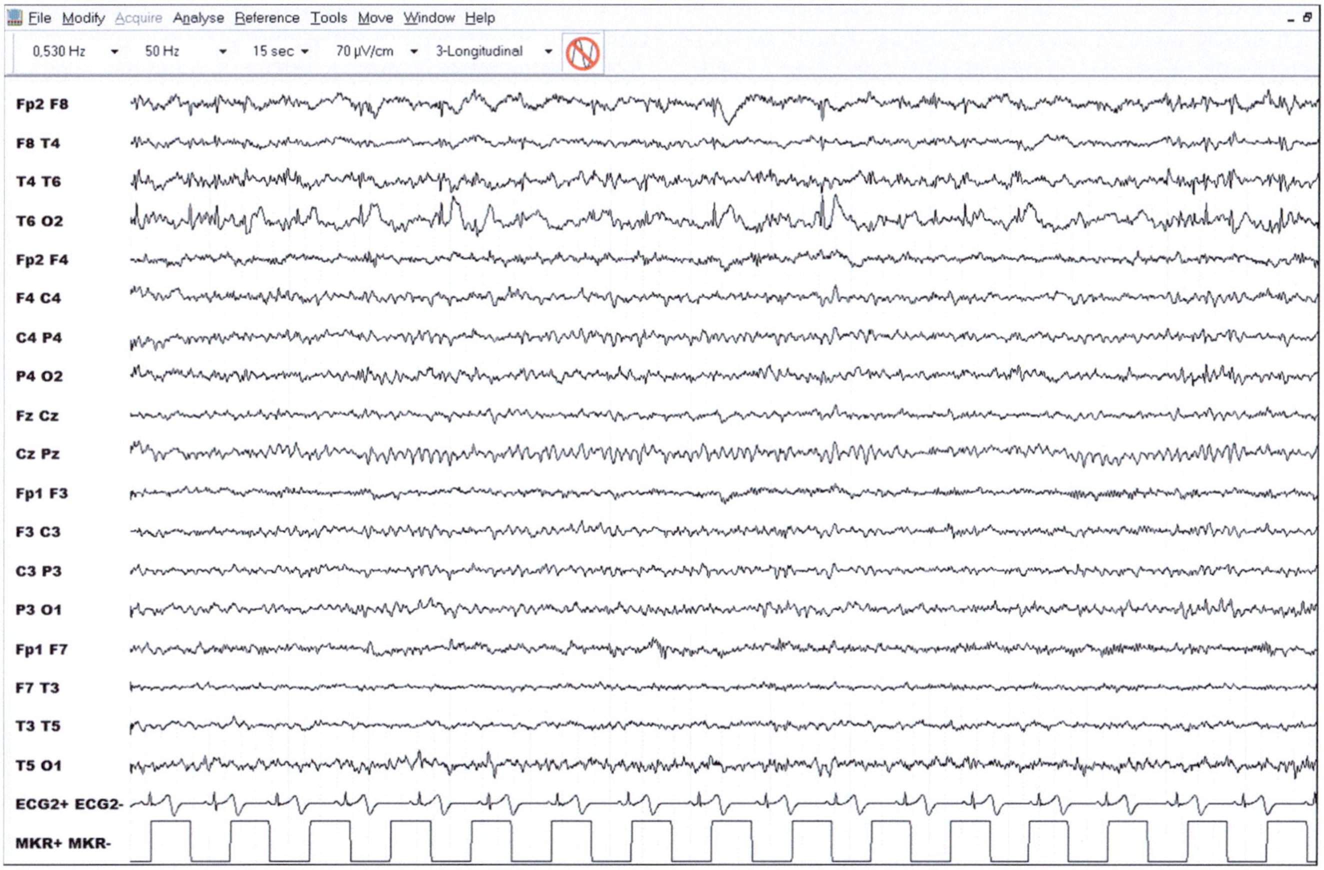

Fig. 44.3 A 20-year-old male patient affected by ADHD since childhood. Delta slowings with epileptiform abnormalities (spikes and spike-wave complexes) are evident in the right temporal regions

reported to be significantly higher in children with ADHD compared with control children [30].

In 2013, the US Food and Drug Administration (FDA) recognized, through the approvation of the Neuropsychiatric EEG-Based ADHD Assessment Aid (NEBA), the value of THBR measured at electrode CZ combined with a clinical evaluation as a confirmatory support in the diagnosis of ADHD. Nevertheless, this test is still not suggested by the American Academy of Neurology (AAN) and should not replace a standard clinical evaluation, because of the high false-positive diagnostic rate of EEG theta/beta power ratio and frontal beta power [31].

Sleep disorders are reported with prevalence ranging from 25% to 43%, without specific alterations of sleep architecture. More specifically, people with ADHD have a significantly higher number of movements during both non-REM and REM sleep and a significantly higher level of arousals from sleep as compared with the healthy population [32].

44.6 Autism Spectrum Disorder (ASD)

Listed among the neurodevelopmental disorders in DSM-5, Autism Spectrum Disorder (ASD) is characterized by persistent deficits in social communication and social interaction across multiple contexts, including deficits in social reciprocity, nonverbal communicative behaviors used for social interaction, and skills in developing, maintaining and understanding relationships. In addition to the social communication deficits, the diagnosis of ASD requires the presence of restricted, repetitive patterns of behavior, interests, or activities [1].

The worldwide population prevalence of ASD is about 1% [33] and the prevalence of epilepsy in children with ASD is significantly higher than in the healthy pediatric population. Considering the frequent co-occurrence of autism and epilepsy, ranging from 13% to 40%, it is comprehensible that the results from studies using EEG to detect epileptic paroxysmal discharges is highly variable, ranging from 22.0 to 60.8% [34].

Epileptiform EEG abnormalities are predominantly focal and they are observed in several brain regions, but more preferentially in the frontal and the temporal lobes [34].

The incidence of EEG abnormalities in non-epileptic patients with ASD varies in the different studies, ranging from 8 to 20%. A large study using prolonged EEG recordings found epileptiform activity in 60.7% of ASD patients without clinical evidence of epilepsy only during sleep, remarking the importance of performing ambulatory 24 h EEG in these patients. Many different localizations of the EEG epileptiform abnormalities were observed in this study, with the right temporal site as the most common locus suggesting that the right hemisphere - potentially involved in social deficits - is a site of dysfunction in ASD. Moreover, bitemporal and left temporal epileptiform abnormalities are also consistent with sites of potential language dysfunction in these patients. Less frequently, generalized spike-wave activity has been recorded and it presumabily indentifies a different subgroups of ASD patients [35].

EEG is often performed in ASD children, due to occurrence of clinical episodes that could be interpreted as possible absence or focal dyscognitive epileptic seizures. For this reason, EEG plays a fundamental role in the differential diagnosis with epilepsy. Nevertheless, it is difficult to correlate interictal epileptiform abnormalities with clinical episodes - such as staring - if they are not observed during the EEG recording. A large retrospective study on ASD children with episodes of staring or inattention demonstrated the absence of EEG correlation in almost the entire sample, showing in only 3% the presence of potentially significant EEG abnormalities. Therefore, given the improbability of staring or reduced responsiveness in children with ASD to be of epileptic origin and considering the low yield of potentially significant interictal EEG abnormalities, it should be carefully considered whether to carry out routine EEG in children with ASD [36]. However, since the frequent occurrence of epileptic abnormalities during sleep and the scarce collaboration of children with ASD during routine examinations, when the clinical suspect of epileptic seizures is very strong, it may be decisive to perform a prolonged EEG recording, including sleep (Fig. 44.4). Furthermore, it would be advisable to eventually use video EEG recording, to correlate the suspected episodes to the EEG activity. When the poor cooperation of the patient hampers the video-EEG recording in a laboratory, this should be performed at home, through ambulatory EEG and with the aid of the family, that should predispose a home video recording set.

qEEG studies show increased slow and fast frequency bands power (determining a so-called U-shaped pattern of electrophysiological power alterations), abnormal functional connectivity (overall local over-connectivity and long-range under-connectivity), and enhanced power in the left hemisphere of the brain, compared with the right hemisphere, across all frequency bands [37].

With regard to sleep characteristics, polysomnography studies show most of the abnormalities related to REM sleep. The main sleep architecture abnormalities include increased proportion of stage N1 sleep, reduced REM sleep latency, and immature organization of eye movements into discrete bursts. Other alterations reported are increased undifferentiated sleep, decreased time in bed and decreased total sleep time [38].

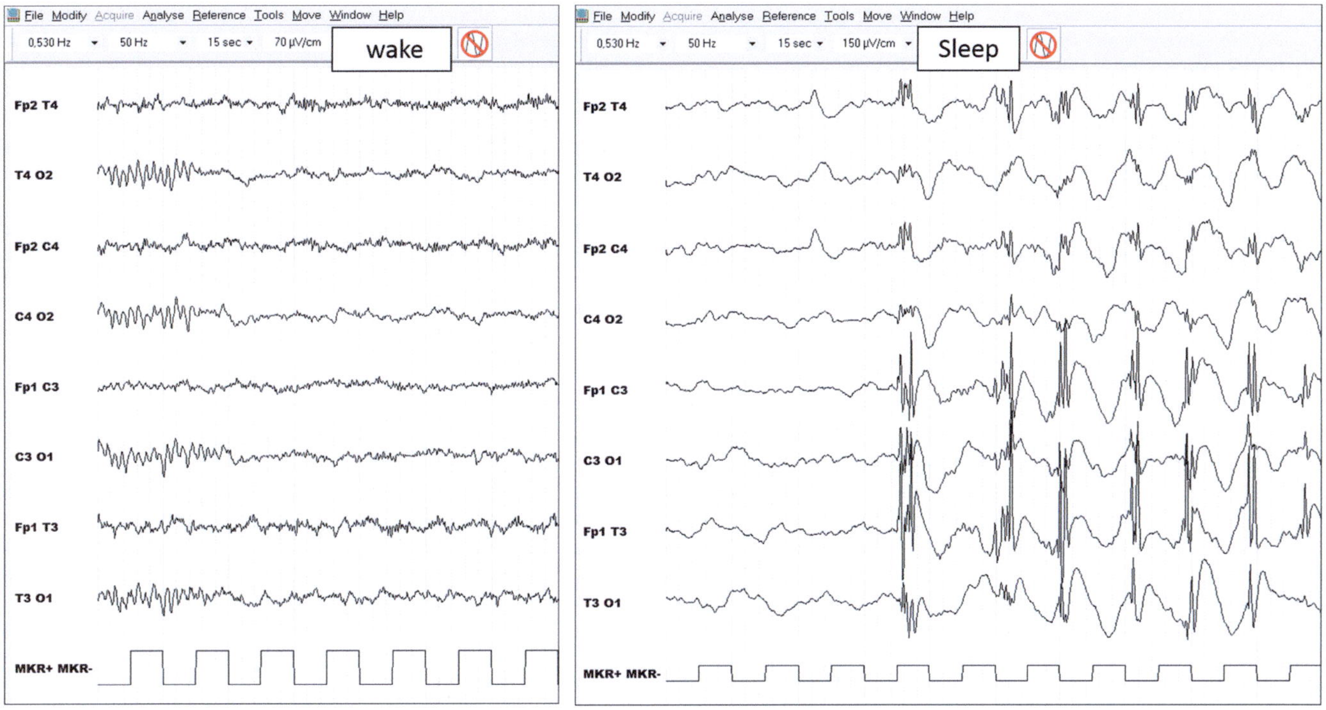

Fig. 44.4 Example of an ambulatory EEG performed at home in a 17-year-old male patient with autism. During awake, alpha rhythm in the posterior regions is detectable. As the patient falls asleep, a sub-continuous epileptic activity (spike- and polyspike-wave complexes) become markedly evident in the left hemisphere, with tendency to the contralateral diffusion

References

1. American Psychiatric Association. Diagnostic and statistical manual of mental disorders. 5th ed. Arlington: American Psychiatric Association; 2013.
2. Krystal AD. Psychiatric disorders and EEG. In: Shomer DL, da Silva FHL, editors. Niedermeyer's electroencephalography: basic principles, clinical applications, and related fields. 6th ed. Philadelphia: Lippincott Williams & Wilkins; 2011.
3. Jaworska N, Blier P, Fusee W, Knott V. α power, α asymmetry and anterior cingulate cortex activity in depressed males and females. J Psychiatr Res. 2012;46:1483–91.
4. Niemiec A, Lithgow B. Alpha-band characteristics in EEG spectrum indicate reliability of frontal brain asymmetry measures in diagnosis of depression. Conf Proc IEEE Eng Med Biol Soc. 2005;7:7517–20.
5. Henriques JB, Davidson RJ. Left frontal hypoactivation in depression. J Abnorm Psychol. 1991;100:535–45.
6. Henriques JB, Davidson RJ. Regional brain electrical asymmetries discriminate between previously depressed and healthy control subjects. J Abnorm Psychol. 1990;99:22–31.
7. Davidson RJ. Anterior electrophysiological asymmetries, emotion, and depression: conceptual and methodological conundrums. Psychophysiology. 1998;35:607–14.
8. Baglioni C, Nanovska S, Regen W, et al. Sleep and mental disorders: a meta-analysis of polysomnographic research. Psychol Bull. 2016;142:969–90.
9. Murphy MJ, Peterson MJ. Sleep disturbances in depression. Sleep Med Clin. 2015;10:17–23.
10. Merikangas KR, Akiskal HS, Angst J, et al. Lifetime and 12-month prevalence of bipolar spectrum disorder in the National Comorbidity Survey replication. Arch Gen Psychiatry. 2007;64:543–52.
11. National Institute of Mental Health. Bipolar Disorders. 2016. https://www.nimh.nih.gov/health/topics/bipolar-disorder/index.shtml. Accessed 26 Jan 2018.
12. El-Badri SM, Ashton CH, Moore PB, Marsh VR, Ferrier IN. Electrophysiological and cognitive function in young euthymic patients with bipolar affective disorder. Bipolar Disord. 2001;3:79–87.
13. Başar E, Güntekin B, Atagün I, Turp Gölbaşı B, Tülay E, Ozerdem A. Brain's alpha activity is highly reduced in euthymic bipolar disorder patients. Cogn Neurodyn. 2012;6:11–20.
14. Kam JW, Bolbecker AR, O'Donnell BF, Hetrick WP, Brenner CA. Resting state EEG power and coherence abnormalities in bipolar disorder and schizophrenia. J Psychiatr Res. 2013;47:1893–901.
15. Gonzalez R, Tamminga C, Tohen M, Suppes T. Comparison of objective and subjective assessments of sleep time in subjects with bipolar disorder. J Affect Disord. 2013;149:363–6.
16. Bandelow B, Michaelis S. Epidemiology of anxiety disorders in the 21st century. Dialogues Clin Neurosci. 2015;17:327–35.
17. Kessler RC, Berglund P, Demler O, Jin R, Merikangas KR, Walters EE. Lifetime prevalence and age-of-onset distributions of DSM-IV disorders in the National Comorbidity Survey Replication. Arch Gen Psychiatry. 2005;62:593–602.
18. Clark CR, Galletly CA, Ash DJ, Moores KA, Penrose RA, McFarlane AC. Evidence-based medicine evaluation of electrophysiological studies of the anxiety disorders. Clin EEG Neurosci. 2009;40:84–112.
19. Bandelow B, Baldwin D, Abelli M, et al. Biological markers for anxiety disorders, OCD and PTSD—a consensus statement. Part I: neuroimaging and genetics. World J Biol Psychiatry. 2016;17:321–65.
20. National Institute of Mental Health. Schizophrenia. 2016. https://www.nimh.nih.gov/health/topics/schizophrenia/index.shtml. Accessed 26 Jan 2018.

21. Endres D, Perlov E, Feige B, et al. Electroencephalographic findings in schizophreniform and affective disorders. Int J Psychiatry Clin Pract. 2016;20:157–64.
22. Begić D, Popović-Knapić V, Grubišin J, et al. Quantitative electroencephalography in schizophrenia and depression. Psychiatr Danub. 2011;23:355–62.
23. González MC, Gil Villar MP, Calvo Medel D, et al. Epileptic peri-ictal psychosis, a reversible cause of psychosis. Neurologia. 2013;28:81–7.
24. Poulin J, Daoust AM, Forest G, Stip E, Godbout R. Sleep architecture and its clinical correlates in first episode and neuroleptic-naive patients with schizophrenia. Schizophr Res. 2003;62:147–53.
25. Polanczyk G, De Lima M, Horta B, Biederman J, Rohde L. The worldwide prevalence of ADHD: a systematic review and metaregression analysis. Am J Psychiatry. 2007;164:942–8.
26. Socanski D, Herigstad A, Thomsen PH, Dag A, Larsen TK. Epileptiform abnormalities in children diagnosed with attention deficit/hyperactivity disorder. Epilepsy Behav. 2010;19:483–6.
27. Millichap JJ, Stack CV, Millichap JG. Frequency of epileptiform discharges in the sleep-deprived electroencephalogram in children evaluated for attention-deficit disorders. J Child Neurol. 2011;26:6–11.
28. Holtmann M, Becker K, Kentner-Figura B, Schmidt MH. Increased frequency of rolandic spikes in ADHD children. Epilepsia. 2003;44:1241–4.
29. Loo SK, Cho A, Hale TS, McGough J, McCracken J, Smalley SL. Characterization of the theta to beta ratio in ADHD: identifying potential sources of heterogeneity. J Atten Disord. 2013;17:384–92.
30. Kamida A, Shimabayashi K, Oguri M, et al. EEG power spectrum analysis in children with ADHD. Yonago Acta Med. 2016;59:169–73.
31. Gloss D, Varma JK, Pringsheim T, Nuwer MR. Practice advisory: the utility of EEG theta/beta power ratio in ADHD diagnosis: report of the guideline development, dissemination, and implementation Subcommittee of the American Academy of Neurology. Neurology. 2016;87:2375–9.
32. Stephens RJ, Chung SA, Jovanovic D, et al. Relationship between polysomnographic sleep architecture and behavior in medication-free children with TS, ADHD, TS and ADHD, and controls. J Dev Behav Pediatr. 2013;34:688–96.
33. Lai MC, Lombardo MV, Baron-Cohen S. Autism. Lancet. 2014;383:896–910.
34. Yasuhara A. Correlation between EEG abnormalities and symptoms of autism spectrum disorder (ASD). Brain Dev. 2010;32:791–8.
35. Chez MG, Chang M, Krasne V, Coughlan C, Kominsky M, Schwartz A. Frequency of epileptiform EEG abnormalities in a sequential screening of autistic patients with no known clinical epilepsy from 1996 to 2005. Epilepsy Behav. 2006;8:267–71.
36. Hughes R, Poon WY, Harvey AS. Limited role for routine EEG in the assessment of staring in children with autism spectrum disorder. Arch Dis Child. 2015;100:30–3.
37. Wang J, Barstein J, Ethridge LE, Mosconi MW, Takarae Y, Sweeney JA. Resting state EEG abnormalities in autism spectrum disorders. J Neurodev Disord. 2013;5:24.
38. Devnani PA, Hegde AU. Autism and sleep disorders. J Pediatr Neurosci. 2015;10:304–7.

45 Effects on EEG of Drugs and Toxic Substances

Marianna Brienza, Patrizia Pulitano, and Oriano Mecarelli

45.1 Pharmaco-Electroencephalography: History, Methodology, and Basic Principles

Pharmaco-electroencephalography (P-EEG) is a noninvasive tool used to assess the effects of drugs on the central nervous system by processing the EEG signals, directly revealing the spontaneous synchronized postsynaptic neuronal activity of the cortex with high temporal resolution [1].

The basis of the P-EEG can be dated back to 1931, when Hans Berger first experienced the effects of subcutaneous cocaine on the alpha rhythm that he had just discovered. Over the last few years, in line with the technological evolution and the introduction of the quantitative analysis of EEG, P-EEG has become increasingly important, especially for its various applications in clinical and experimental fields.

Although it is well known that EEG activity is affected by many substances acting on the central nervous system, the interest in increasing this knowledge and the best methodology by which to assess it are relatively recent.

EEG can be considered a sensitive and reproducible biomarker in different conditions, such as in the early detection of cognitive impairment [2], localization of epileptogenic foci, physiopathologic characterization of sleep and sleep disorders, evaluation of the depth of anesthesia, etc. Similarly, EEG could be used as a biomarker of the effects of specific drugs on the CNS to classify psychotropic drugs, evaluate drug-to-drug interactions, and monitor the side effects and toxicity. Moreover, the use of quantitative methods for data processing and statistical data analysis provides a description of the direct and indirect effects of active compounds on brain functions, thus generating pharmacodynamics outcome measures which, together with pharmacokinetic data, may be used to study the pharmacodynamic-pharmacokinetic relationships [3]. Thus, EEG can be useful for all phases of clinical research on drug effects.

The study of P-EEG is complex, as it is affected by a high inter- and intraindividual variability and it should be adapted to the clinical and experimental needs for which it is required (comparison studies, case-control studies, evaluations on healthy patients, large-scale experimental studies vs. single patient evaluations, etc.).

In all cases, before the evaluation, a meticulous medical history is essential to detect all the possible variables that may affect the EEG activity. Physiological anamnesis is important to obtain information about developmental milestones, irregularities of the menstrual cycle, type of work, sleep-wake cycle, and usual behaviors during the day: for example, to evaluate the effect of a drug on arousal, it is important to know if the patient has slept sufficiently the night before the registration and, in general, how is his sleep-wake cycle. It's necessary to ask the patient if he smokes cigarettes, drinks coffee, and/or makes use of ethanol or other psychotropic substances for therapeutic or recreational use, because of the well-known effects of these substances on the CNS.

With regard to the recording methods, many guidelines have been drafted over the years, trying to standardize data acquisition and processing techniques among EEG laboratories: the final purpose should be the identification of a shared and comparable analytical algorithm beyond interindividual and interlaboratory differences and, if possible, the individuation of peculiar EEG features of specific drugs.

The latest guidelines from the International Pharmaco-EEG Society (IPEG) summarise the requirements for the recording and computerized evaluation of P-EEG data in humans.

A detailed description of the methods and techniques of acquisition, processing, and statistical analysis of the EEG signal is beyond the scope of this chapter and, therefore, we refer to the full text of the guidelines [3].

M. Brienza · O. Mecarelli (✉)
Department of Human Neurosciences, Sapienza University of Rome, Rome, Italy
e-mail: marianna.brienza@uniroma1.it; oriano.mecarelli@uniroma1.it

P. Pulitano
Azienda Ospedaliero-Universitaria Policlinico Umberto I, Rome, Italy
e-mail: patrizia.pulitano@uniroma1.it

O. Mecarelli (ed.), *Clinical Electroencephalography*, https://doi.org/10.1007/978-3-030-04573-9_45

The recording should be performed in a quiet environment and the patient should be relaxed. A configuration of 21 electrodes according to the international 10–20 system is usually enough: however, it is possible to add further electrodes to study the activity of specific cortical areas and, eventually, to make a P-EEG brain map. Electrooculography is necessary, to identify and exclude ocular artifacts, while electrocardiogram monitors cardiac activity and indirectly highlights the patient's state during the recording.

The recording must be performed with open and closed eyes for a sufficient time: guidelines recommend a vigilance-controlled EEG for 5 min followed by a resting EEG recording with closed eyes for 5–15 min. The variable duration of the latter depends on the purpose of the registration: sessions of 5 min (with a minimum of 2-min artifact-free signal) are sufficient to quantify EEG activity and to demonstrate pharmacological effects on spectral parameters, while longer recordings are necessary to evaluate the effects of drugs on vigilance and wakefulness (or sleepiness) [3–5].

Data processing provides the representation in time and frequency domain, the latter indispensable for spectral analysis, to evaluate EEG band power (absolute and relative), Peak Power Frequency (PPF), Main Dominant Frequency (MDF), Spectral Edge Frequency (SEF), and Median Frequency (MF). Time domain EEG parameters are useful to evaluate the effect of specific anesthetic drugs on brain activity: among them, Burst Suppression Ratio (BSR) is used as an indirect index of the level of anesthesia.

A reliable assessment of the EEG effects of a drug cannot forget considering the status of the basal EEG, necessary to make comparisons between basal and drug-induced activity. Thus, more recordings at specific time points should be performed.

Although different substances may be responsible for the same EEG pattern and despite the large interindividual variability, some EEG features may be considered characteristic and sometimes peculiar of specific drugs.

45.2 Effects of Drugs on EEG

45.2.1 Antiepileptic Drugs (AEDs)

AEDs can induce EEG changes, sometimes not detectable by the simple qualitative analysis and whose evaluation is often far from easy. This is due to several reasons: the principal is that epilepsy is a chronic disease which involves the rearrangement of brain networks in addition to the epileptic focus, and this influences the EEG activity. Moreover, epilepsy is a dynamic pathology and it may involve changes in EEG over time, regardless of the patient's treatment. Persons with epilepsy often take more than one antiepileptic drug, and their EEG tracings may be modified by several substances. To avoid these confounding factors, many studies on antiepileptic drugs EEG changes has been conducted in healthy volunteers. However, even in this case, there are some limitations, above all the time-limited therapy and the low dosages. Therefore, it is clear that EEG modifications induced by AEDs are still not totally defined and sometimes controversial [6, 7].

On the basis of literature data, the modifications induced by AED will be briefly described, subdividing them into two topics: the effects on the background activity and the effects on the ictal and interictal epileptiform activity.

45.2.1.1 Effects of AEDs on Background Activity

The main old-generation AEDs are barbiturates (PB), diphenylhydantoin (DPH), carbamazepine (CBZ), valproic acid (VPA), and benzodiazepines (BDZs).

PB was the first AED on the market, since 1912. It is still a widely used drug, both in mono- and in polytherapy, for the treatment of focal and/or generalized epilepsies. At low dosages, PB typically induces an increase in rapid EEG rhythms (15–35 Hz), more evident in the anterior regions than in lesional areas. At higher dosages, a progressive slowing of the alpha rhythm and a corresponding increase in theta-delta activity can be observed. Acute administration of high dosages of barbiturates can induce a pattern of burst suppression, which may result in a pattern of cortical suppression (Fig. 45.1).

Among the older-generation AEDs, DPH induces mainly a slowing of alpha rhythm and an increase in slow theta-delta activity, even at therapeutic dosages and in the absence of clinical signs of toxicity. In case of overdose, a paroxysmal, hypersynchronous delta activity may occur.

It was reported that CBZ may cause slowing of background EEG. The correlation between the entity of slowing and the serum concentration of CBZ is controversial: some studies found significant correlations between the percentage of delta, theta and alpha 2 power bands and serum levels of CBZ [8]. In particular, with the increase of serum concentration of CBZ, the percentage of power progressively increased in the theta band, while it decreased in the alpha 2 band (Fig. 45.2). The percentage of theta and alpha 2 power was found to reach maximum and minimum levels, respectively, when the peak values of serum concentration of CBZ were attained [9]. Therefore, it can be affirmed that CBZ induces a slowing of the background activity through a mechanism not fully clarified, but similar to that of some tricyclic antidepressants (TCA) with which CBZ shares the biochemical structure (Fig. 45.3).

At therapeutic dosages, VPA does not determine qualitative EEG modifications. However, the quantitative EEG analysis also showed a slight slowing of the alpha

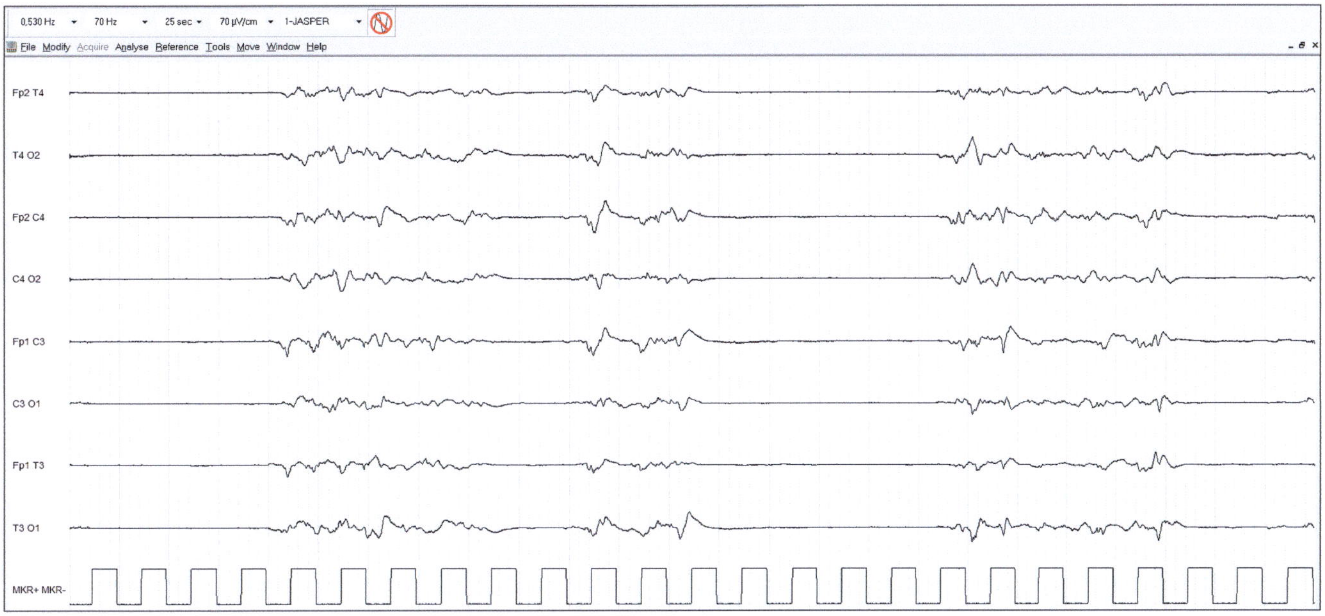

Fig. 45.1 A 35-year-old male patient admitted to the emergency department of our hospital due to acute ingestion of unspecified amount of barbiturate (sodium phenobarbital). EEG documents a burst suppression pattern with plasma barbiturate concentrations corresponding to 82 μg/mL

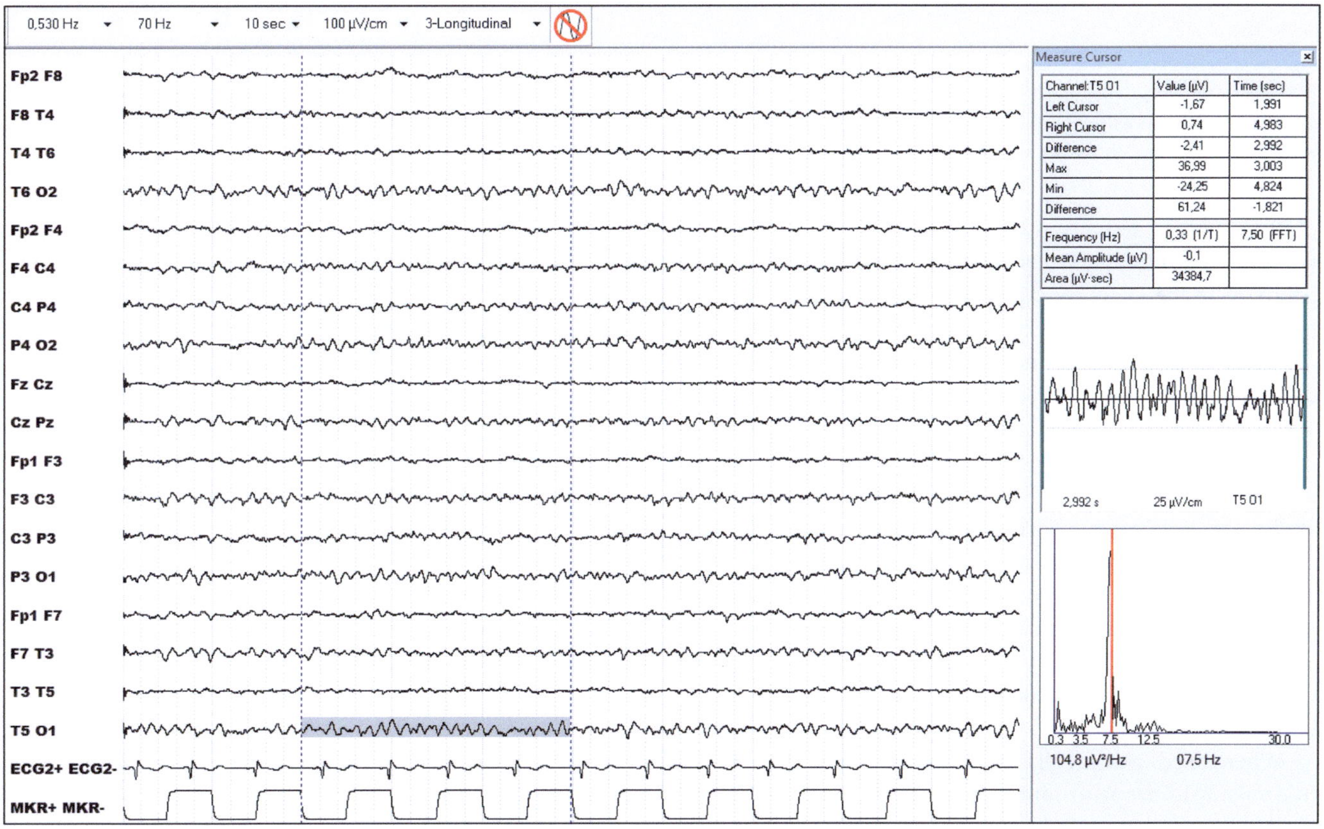

Fig. 45.2 A 65-year-old female patient under chronic treatment with carbamazepine. EEG shows an alpha background rhythm at 7.5–8 Hz, without clinical signs of toxicity

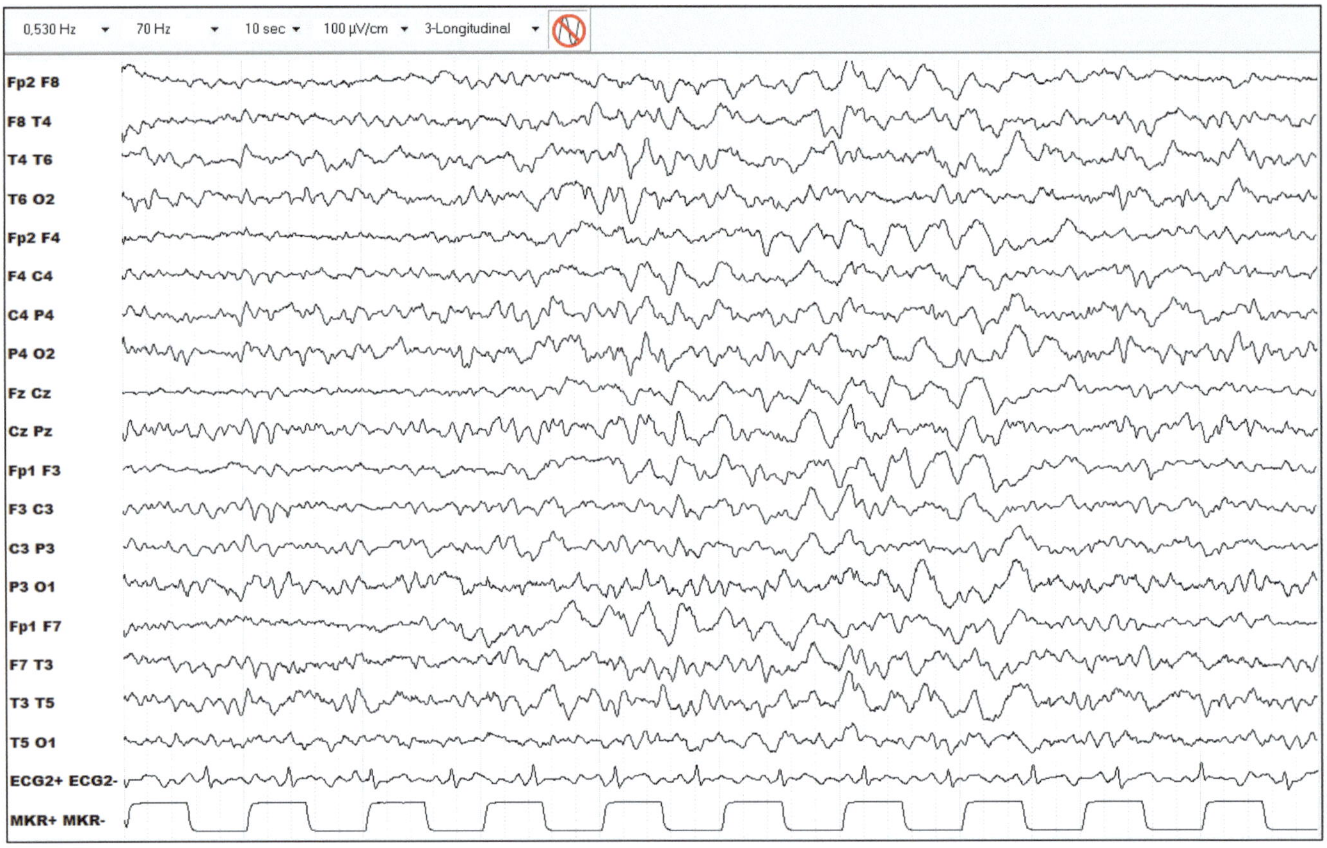

Fig. 45.3 EEG recorded in a 42-year-old female patient after a single dose of 2400 mg of carbamazepine. The patient was poorly reactive to external stimuli and the EEG showed a global slowing of the background activity with sequences of monomorphic and rhythmic delta potentials, prevalent in the medium-anterior areas

rhythm and an equally slight increase in both theta and beta bands. It has also been demonstrated that VPA causes a decrease in the synchronization of delta and theta bands in patients with generalized epilepsy. Toxic dosages of VPA produce diffuse delta activity, which in the case of VPA encephalopathy become hypersynchronous and paroxysmal, with superimposed spikes and bi-triphasic waves. Burst suppression pattern, secondary to VPA-induced hyperammonemic encephalopathy, is also described [10]. Furthermore, studies of topographic analysis in the frequency domain, conducted in patients with normal EEG treated in monotherapy with VPA, demonstrated that VPA (wich has multiple actions on sodium and calcium channel as well as on GABA turnover) decreased the low gamma range (30-40 Hz), while CBZ, a sodium-channel modulator, altered brain topography in the 50–60 Hz [11].

When used chronically at therapeutic dosages, BDZs (diazepam, lorazepam, nitrazepam, clonazepam, clobazam, etc.) induce the appearance of a characteristic fast activity of medium/low amplitude, generally bilateral and symmetric and more prominent in the anterior areas. Also in this case, the overdose of BDZ induces, in addition to the fast activity, a slow diffuse abnormalities (Fig. 45.4).

The newAEDs generation seems to have a better safety profile than the older ones, but an overlapping therapeutic efficacy. Those currently available are vigabatrin (VGB), felbamate (FBM), gabapentin (GBP), lamotrigine (LTG), tiagabine (TGB), topiramate (TPM), oxcarbazepine (OXC), levetiracetam (LEV), pregabalin (PGB), zonisamide (ZNS), lacosamide (LCM), eslicarbazepine acetate (ESL), and perampanel (PER). Nevertheless, of the aforementioned drugs, some are currently underused for relevant adverse events (VGB, FBM), or for low antiepileptic efficacy (PGB, GBP, TGB).

Among the new AEDs, OXC (a member of dibenzazepine family as CBZ) induces a slowing of alpha rhythm and an increase in the power of the slow bands, but less than CBZ; an increase of delta and theta activities and a slight slowdown of alpha rhythm is also caused by TPM and GBP [12].

LTG is a phenyltriazine derivative which acts through inhibition of voltage-activated sodium channels and possibly calcium channels, preventing the release of glutamate [13]. It seems to have an EEG activating effect: in persons with epilepsy, it increases the fast frequencies (alpha and beta), decreases the slow frequencies (theta-delta), and also increases the reactivity of the alpha rhythm and the power of

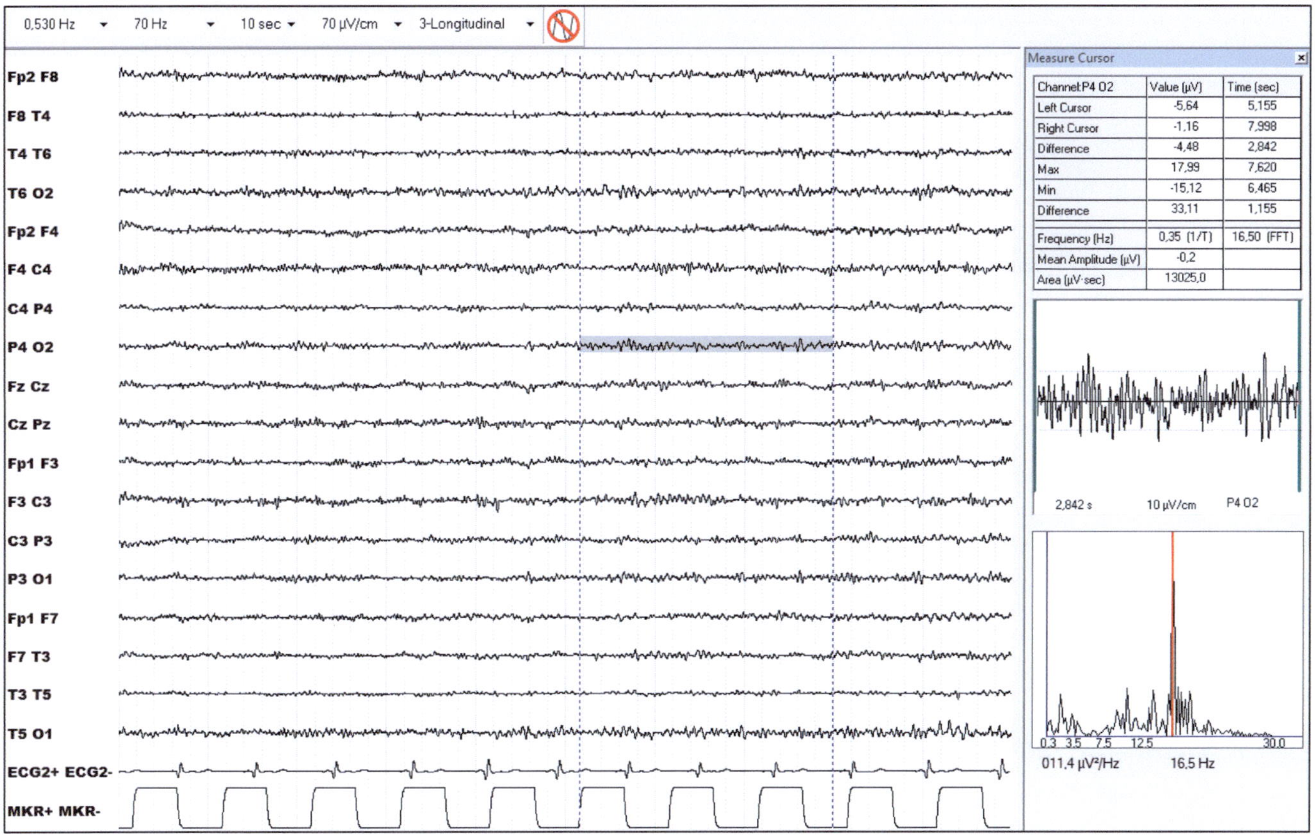

Fig. 45.4 EEG recorded in a 40-year-old male patient under chronic treatment with clonazepam (6 mg/day): diffuse, but prevalent in anterior areas, fast activity at 16–21 Hz

the beta band during the performance of attention tests. It has also recently been shown that LTG induces a reduction in thalamocortical synchronization functions in patients with generalized epilepsy, thus reducing the absolute power of the slow bands [14, 15]. However, topographic analysis in the frequency domain has demonstrated that LTG, as CBZ, induces significant power decrease in gamma band at 50-60 Hz (11).

LEV binds synaptic vesicle protein 2A, inhibits calcium release from intraneuronal stores and, thus, excessive synchronized neuronal activity [16]. It does not seem to induce any modification of the background EEG activity; however, the appearance of a burst suppression pattern, in a patient with a postanoxic coma, has been described in a case of LEV overdose [17].

ESL and LCM bind voltage-dependent sodium channels at an inactive state and prolong it reducing the channel firing, while PER is a selective noncompetitive AMPA receptor antagonist. Currently, there are no available literature data about their effect on the background EEG activity: according to our clinical experience, ESL does not seem to induce any changes.

In conclusion, the low or absent impact on background activity of new AEDs could reflect their better tolerability than old AEDs, with scarce repercussions on cognitive profile.

45.2.1.2 Effects of AEDs on Ictal and Interictal Epileptiform Activity

BDZs usually have a drastic and positive effect on ictal epileptic activity, especially if it is generalized, and for this reason they represent the first-line treatment of the status epilepticus. Their action on interictal activity is less relevant, especially if it is focal (Fig. 45.5a–c).

Chronic treatment with barbiturates (PB) has a good effect on both ictal and interictal activity, and acute treatment is used for the management of status epilepticus (second-line therapy).

DPH generally has a positive effect on epileptic activity, both in acute (it is considered a second-line drug for the treatment of status epilepticus) and in chronic administration, while the effects on interictal activity are more controversial. However, rare cases in which high-dose DPH has increased ictal activity, also evolving to status epilepticus, have been described.

VPA, at therapeutic dosages, has an excellent effect on the generalized ictal and interictal activity and it is currently also used for acute administration in the status epilepticus as

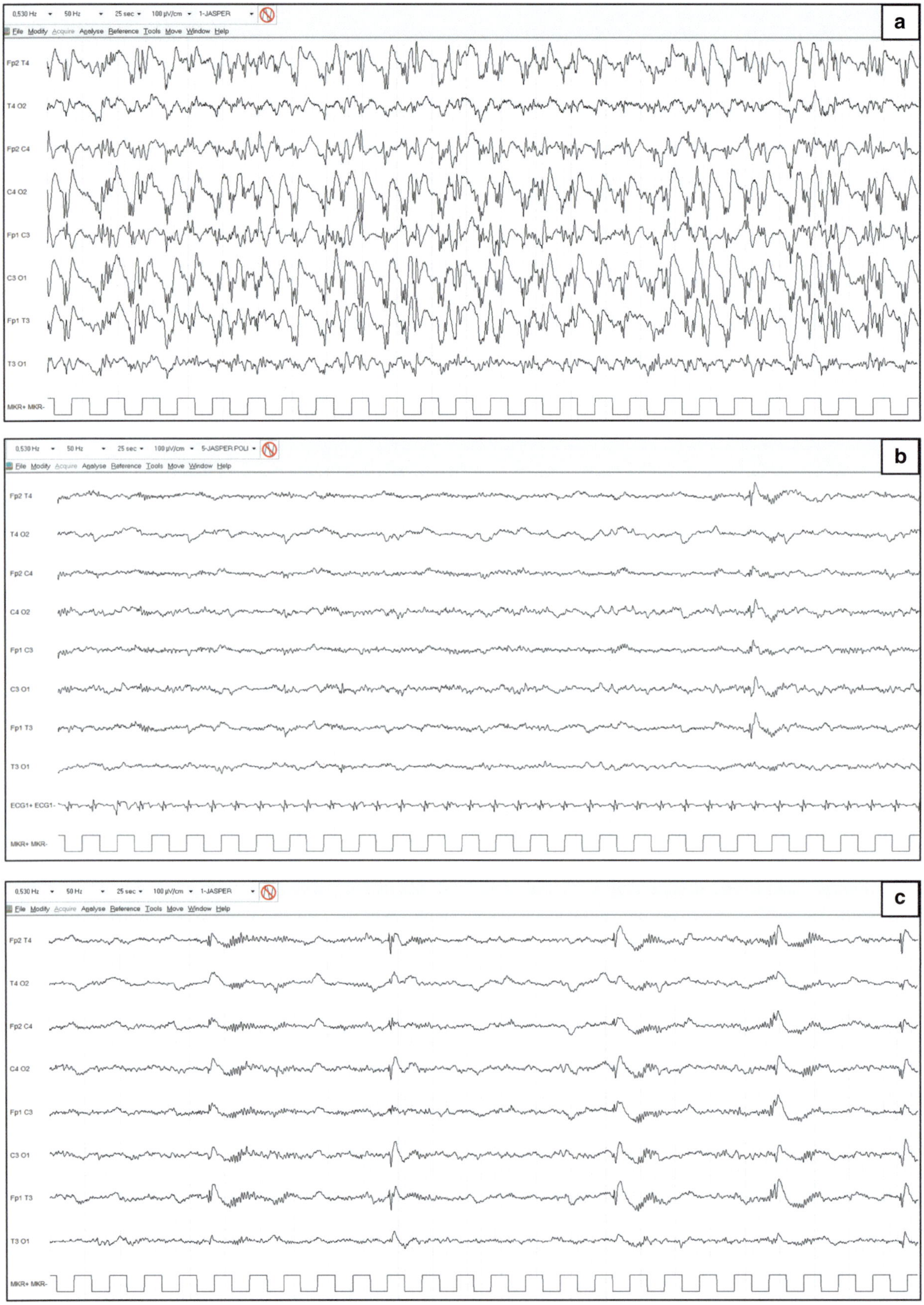

Fig. 45.5 (**a**) Generalized nonconvulsive status epilepticus recorded in a 64-year-old male patient; (**b, c**) 5 and 10 min after i.v. bolus of lorazepam 4 mg administration, the epileptiform activity was almost completely replaced by a diffuse, low-amplitude, fast activity although isolated sharp waves complexes persist followed by bursts of sleep spindles at 14 Hz

second-line therapy. The SANAD (Standard and New Antiepileptic Drugs) study reported that valproate was the most effective and best-tolerated first-line AED for patients with Idiopatic Generalized Epilepsy (IGE), including juvenile myoclonic epilepsy (JME), when it was compared to LTG and TPM [18].

The efficacy of LEV in both focal and generalized ictal discharges has been demonstrated. In particular, it has been reported that LEV reduces the photoparoxysmal response and controls the generalized discharges in juvenile myoclonic epilepsy, so that it may be considered a first choice drug in this rare type of epilepsy [19]. Moreover, our experience with LEV, conducted on a series of patients with generalized epilepsy and with very frequent epileptic discharges, showed a less homogeneous response, more evident when LEV is administered as an add-on therapy. LEV was often able to reduce the average duration of generalized discharges, but not to suppress them or significantly reduce their frequency: in some cases, paradoxically, the discharges have appeared even less prolonged, but more numerous in 24 h [20].

LTG is a generally well-tolerated drug with a broad spectrum of actions, and it is often preferred to VPA, especially in young women, for the treatment of IGE with generalized tonic-clonic and absence seizures. Nevertheless, some studies have reported aggravation of JME with LTG [21], while others have documented an amelioration of seizures in this type of epilepsy [22, 23]. A reduction of photoparoxysmal response was described for both focal and generalized ictal and interictal epileptic activity. In particular, LTG seems to allow a better localization of the epileptic focus by limiting its diffusion.

TPM is a widely used drug, especially for the treatment of IGE. Based on the current limited available data, TPM seems to be better tolerated than VPA, but there were no more benefits in terms of efficacy in TPM compared with VPA [24]. Mecarelli and colleagues performed a study on the clinical and EEG effects of TPM in patients with epilepsy and healthy volunteers. They observed that, in patients with epilepsy, the TPM induced EEG changes consisted of increased delta and theta activities and decreased activity in the fast bands. This recognizable TPM-induced EEG pattern was again evident in the healthy volunteers, in whom they also detected a significant reduction in the alpha rhythm. Their results confirm that TPM needs to be introduced gradually, while patients undergo close neuropsychological and neurophysiological monitoring to detect adverse sedative and cognitive effects. The EEG correlate of these events seems to be an increased activity in the slower frequency bands [25].

LCM is used for the treatment of focal onset seizures (both in mono as add-on therapy) and as second-line therapy for the treatment of status epilepticus [26–28]. Moreover, LCM treatment has shown effective anti-epileptogenic properties in the pilocarpine model of mesial temporal lobe epilepsy in rats: these effects were accompanied by decreases in interictal spike rates in the hippocampus [29].

ESL and PER are two new, well-tolerated, third-generation AEDs: their clinical efficacy on focal onset and generalized seizures are demonstrated, also for drug-resistant epilepsies, and this is reflected in a reduction of epileptic EEG discharges.

45.2.2 Anxiolytic Drugs

Anxiolytic drugs are essentially represented by BDZs (diazepam, clobazam, clonazepam, nitrazepam, lorazepam, etc.), whose effects on EEG have already been described in the section dedicated to the AEDs (some of these molecules are indeed used also in the treatment of epilepsy, especially in emergency). Typically, the chronic use of BDZs induces a more or less marked increase in the EEG fast frequencies, predominant in the anterior areas, associated with a slight decrease in the alpha activity and a mild increase in theta frequencies (higher in the case of BDZs with a more important hypnotic effect). Chronic assumption of BDZs for insomnia induce sleep changes consisting in an increase of total sleep duration and a decrease of sleep latency and night awakenings. However, from a macrostructural point of view, a reduction in the duration of the REM sleep and of the NREM stages 3 and 4 occurs. An increase in K complexes and spindles in NREM stage 2 has also been reported [30].

45.2.3 Antidepressants

Tricyclic antidepressants (TCAs) typically induce an increase of the beta frequencies, a slowing of the alpha activity and a dose-dependent increase in the diffuse theta-delta activities.

Furthermore, numerous studies have been carried out to validate the role of EEG as a biomarker for the response to antidepressant drugs in different psychiatric diseases: in bipolar disorder, for example, some studies suggest that the alpha wavelet power in occipital areas and the alpha asymmetry between anterior and posterior areas could be considered a reliable marker of treatment response [31, 32]. In major depression, other evidences reported no differences in occipital alpha power and in frontal alpha asymmetry. even though a gender and drug class interaction effect was found in frontal alpha asymmetry; right dominant frontal alpha asymmetry in women only was associated with a favorable response to escitalopram and sertraline [33]. Finally, EEG-derived biomarkers as changes in the activity of frequency bands and hemispheric alpha asymmetry, have all been shown to predict response to a various antidepressants [34].

Bupropion is an antidepressant well-known for its effects to lower seizure threshold, as demonstrated by several studies: it would cause the appearance of specific epileptiform graphoelements on EEG (sharp waves, spikes or focal slowings), more frequently in women [35]. Additionally, in contrast with other antidepressants that suppress the REM sleep, bupropion lengthens the REM latency and increases the total REM density [36].

With few exceptions, Selective Serotonin Reuptake Inhibitors (SSRIs) and Serotonin-Norepinephrine Reuptake Inhibitors (SNRIs) decrease REM sleep and suppressed cortical spectral power in experimental models and in healthy and depressed patients. Studies on animal models have shown that duloxetine, as well as vortioxetine, increases vigilance (measured as time awake), yet their effects on brain rhythms were markedly different. Vortioxetine (at a dosage corresponding to 80% serotonin transporter occupancy) significantly increases theta, alpha and gamma power, whereas duloxetine (at the same level of serotonin transporter occupancy), has no effects on theta and gamma power, but decreass alpha power. Besides, the fact that vortioxetine elicited increase of hippocampal and pyramidal neuron firing and frontal cortical gamma oscillatory power in rats [37] indicates that the cellular framework for activating cortical neurons and eliciting gamma is engaged [38–40]. Duloxetine also seems to cause changes in left-frontal qEEG cordance after 1 week of treatment in a pilot sudy on fibromyalgia [41]. The stability of alpha power and asymmetry differences between responders and non-responders to SSRI, suggests that they represent a reasonable positive predictive factors to response to treatment [42].

The use of SSRIs or SNRIs seems generically to be associated with a low risk of epileptic seizure, however twofold in respect to nonusers. Current use of low-dosage TCAs seems not to be associated with seizures; moreover the risk of seizure would be higher at the beginning of the treatment than in longer-term treatment and among patients with major depression [43, 44].

45.2.4 Antipsychotics

Chronic administration of first-generation antipsychotic drugs (chlorpromazine, haloperidol, etc.) at therapeutic dosages induces typical EEG changes: slowdown of the alpha rhythm, increase of theta-delta activity, decrease of beta1 and increase of beta2 bands. Acute intoxication may induce a paroxysmal, widespread delta activity, up to EEG coma patterns.

These drugs could also lower the seizure threshold and, therefore, induce epileptic seizures (especially in already epileptic patients) and, in the most severe cases, also status epilepticus.

Haloperidol determines extremely unpredictable EEG activity, as reported by controversial literature data: while some studies have indicated an increase of alpha and beta power [45], others reported a decrease of alpha power [46].

Among atypical antipsychotics, clozapine was one of the most investigated: it has been demonstrated that chronic treatment with clozapine decreases relative alpha power and mean beta/total spectrum frequency and increases absolute delta/theta power [47]. Moreover, among antipsychotic drugs, clozapine seems to be the most responsible for seizures occurrence: Centorrino et al. further confirmed clozapine's impact on brain electrical activity by conducting a large study on the EEG findings among 323 hospitalized psychiatric patients who were given various antipsychotic medications. The results showed EEG abnormalities, majorly consisting in theta and delta slowings, in 47.1% of clozapine-treated patients, in 38.5% of those treated with olanzapine, in 28% of the risperidone group, and in none of those under quetiapine treatment [48].

As regard to EEG changes induced by lithium carbonate, an increase of beta, theta and delta absolute power was reported [49, 50]. However, it is very interesting to note that in a study of 27 patients affected by bipolar disorder and treated with lithium carbonate, only those who didn't respond to therapy had EEG abnormalities, thus suggesting that the presence of EEG abnormalities may be a biomarker of the lack of therapeutic response [42, 51].

45.2.5 Anesthetics

The Bispectral Index System (BIS) is one of the most widely used EEG parameters during anesthesia, providing information about its level. BIS monitoring uses a single sensor applied in the frontotemporal region, and the EEG signal is converted into a numerical value ranging from 0 (deeply unconscious patient with isoelectric wave) to 100 (awake patient). Originally, BIS monitoring was validated to monitor the depth of anesthesia in patients undergoing surgery (avoiding intraoperative awareness). Clinical studies are currently focusing on the use of BIS in the assessment of the state of consciousness during sedation schemes in patients admitted to ICU, to avoid oversedation [52, 53]. Nevertheless, qualitative EEG is however often required to assess the depth of anesthesia in intensive care units. Regardless of the indications for the EEG execution, the basic principle is the same: anesthetics induce oscillations that alter or disrupt the oscillations produced by the brain during normal information processing; these aesthesia-induced oscillations are readily visible in the electroencephalogram [54].

The effects of anesthetics on EEG depend on several factors: pharmacodynamic characteristics of the drug;

molecular and neural circuit mechanisms of the anesthetic drug; dose administered and plasmatic concentration and metabolism.

The characteristic EEG patterns of some of the most commonly used anesthetics, in relation to their action on CNS, are described in this section.

45.2.5.1 Propofol

Propofol hyperpolarizes and inhibits postsynaptic neurons through its binding to postsynaptic $GABA_A$ receptors. Since the drug is highly liposoluble and the GABAergic inhibitory interneurons are widely distributed in the CNS (cortex, thalamus, brainstem and spinal cord), the action of propofol is carried out at multiple levels. In particular, propofol reduces excitatory inputs from the thalamus to the cerebral cortex by enhancing GABAergic inhibition on the reticular nuclei; it induces GABAergic inhibition of cortical pyramidal neurons; it inhibits arousal by acting on the reticular nuclei and on the inputs from brainstem to hypothalamic nuclei. These actions correspond to specific EEG patterns that, according to the depth of sedation and to the rate of drug administration (bolus vs. continuous infusion), are distinguished by: diffuse low-amplitude fast-activity, anteriorization of the background alpha rhythm, appearance of a widespread slow activity that progressively reduces in frequency and increases in amplitude (theta and delta), "burst suppression" pattern, and electrocortical inactivity (Fig 45.6). When propofol is administered as an induction bolus, patients, in particularly elderly patients, can show the burst suppression pattern immediatly [55].

In addition to its action on the brainstem circuits, propofol also induces unconsciousness through its effects on the thalamocortical and cortico-cortical circuits, which is likely to be expressed through topographic modifications of the alpha rhythm (anteriorization) and appearance of incoherent theta-delta activity.

The appearance of these two simultaneous patterns would suggest the lack of cortical reception of the inputs from the

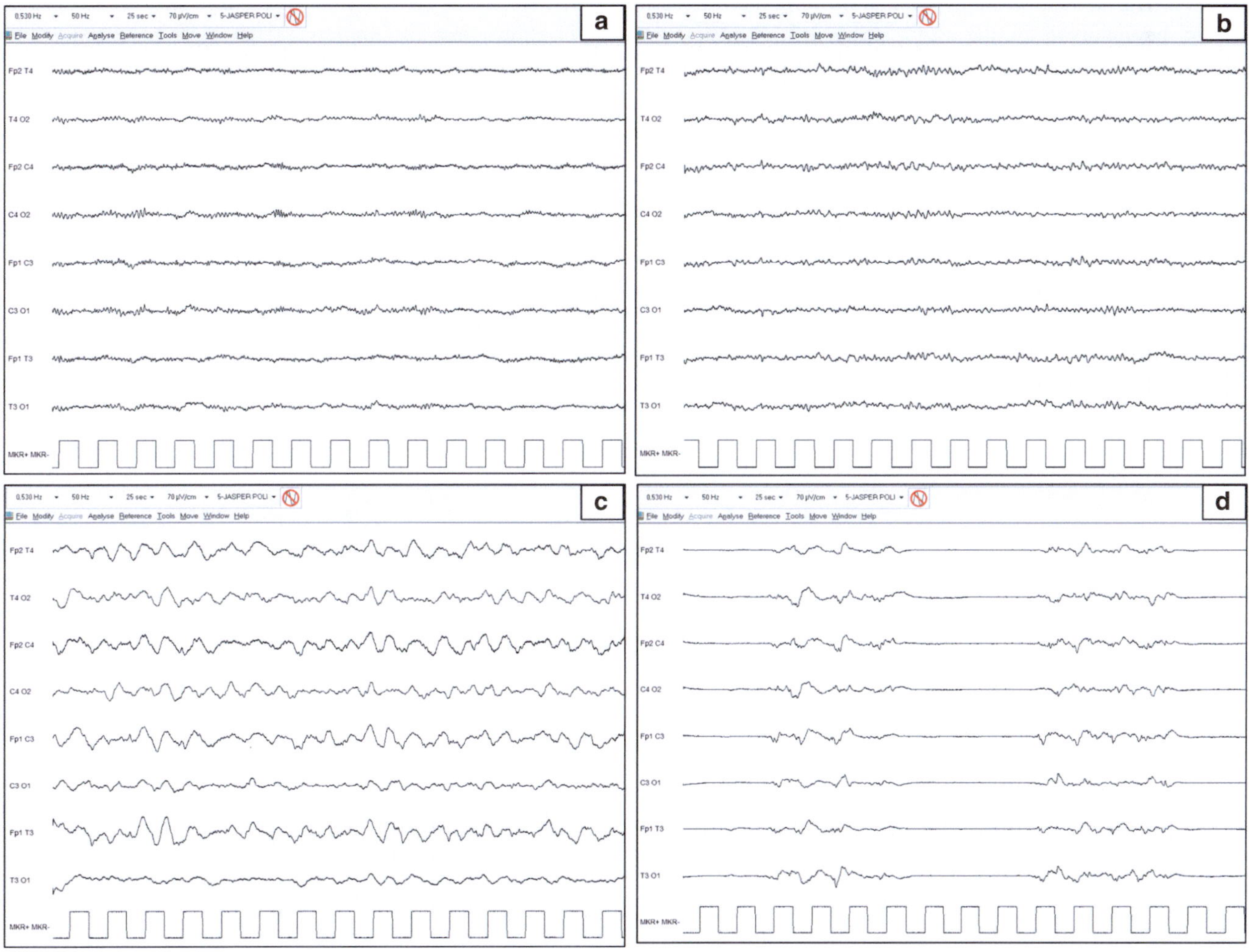

Fig. 45.6 EEG changes during propofol administration: (**a**) low-amplitude fast activity; (**b**) anteriorization of alpha rhythm; (**c**) high-amplitude delta oscillations; (**d**) burst suppression pattern

thalamic relay nuclei. As the effects of the propofol bolus recede, EEG evolves into slow-delta oscillation and alpha oscillation patterns. The transition time from slow oscillations or burst suppression into a combined slow oscillation and alpha oscillation patterns depends on how strong the effect of the propofol bolus had been. Even if no additional propofol is administered after the first bolus, it can take several minutes for the transition to occur [48, 56].

45.2.5.2 Dexmedetomidine

Dexmedetomidine alters the arousal mainly hyperpolarizing the α2-adrenergic presynaptic receptors (α2:α1 selectivity of 1600:1) of the locus coeruleus, thus reducing the release of norepinephrine. Hyperpolarization of the locus coeruleus results in the loss of inhibition on the hypothalamic preoptic area, leading to activation of the GABAergic inputs to the brainstem structures (ventral periaqueductal gray, dorsal raphe nuclei, locus coeruleus, lateral dorsal tegmental nucleus and the pedunculopontine tegmental nucleus). These actions lead to decreased arousal by inhibition of the arousal centers. The activation of hypothalamic inhibitory circuits would be involved in the early stages of NREM sleep. Sedation induced by dexmedetomidine is also enhanced by the reduction of presynaptic norepinephrine release that contributes to the loss of excitatory inputs from the locus coeruleus to the basal forebrain, the thalamus intralaminar nuclei, the cortex and then the thalamocortical connections. The EEG during sedation shows a delta pattern mixed with potentials similar to the spindles of NREM sleep (oscillations at 9–15 Hz that appear at intervals of 1–2 s). The progressive increase in sedation corresponds to the transition to a slower EEG (slow-delta) pattern, similar to that of the deeper phases of NREM sleep [57, 58] (Fig. 45.7).

Both propofol and dexmedetomidine act by inhibiting thalamocortical connections; however, propofol action, even at the same sedation levels, is more effective than dexmedetomidine on these circuits (Fig. 45.8).

45.2.5.3 Ketamine

Ketamine binds N-Metil-D-Aspartate (NMDA) receptors in the brain and in the spinal cord. At low-to-moderate dosages, ketamine blocks inputs to inhibitory interneurons and it allows downstream excitatory neurons to become disinhibited or more active: this clinically results in hallucinations. As the dosage of ketamine is increased, the NMDA receptors on the excitatory glutamatergic neurons are also blocked, with loss of consciousness.

Given the preference of ketamine for NMDA receptors on inhibitory interneurons, whose inhibition results in increased cerebral metabolic rate, cerebral blood flow and hallucinations, ketamine is associated with an active EEG pattern. When ketamine is administered alone in a low dosage, EEG shows fast oscillations in the high beta and a low gamma range, at between 25 and 32 Hz. Compared with propofol and dexmedetomidine, ketamine slow oscillations are less regular [54].

Summarizing, in the earlier stages of continuous anesthesia, we can observe a typical widespread - or prevalent in anterior areas - beta 1 or alpha EEG activity, defined as WAR (Widespread Anteriorly maximum Rhythmic pattern). The frequency of this anesthetic pattern tends to decrease in correlation with the depth of the anesthesia. In association with

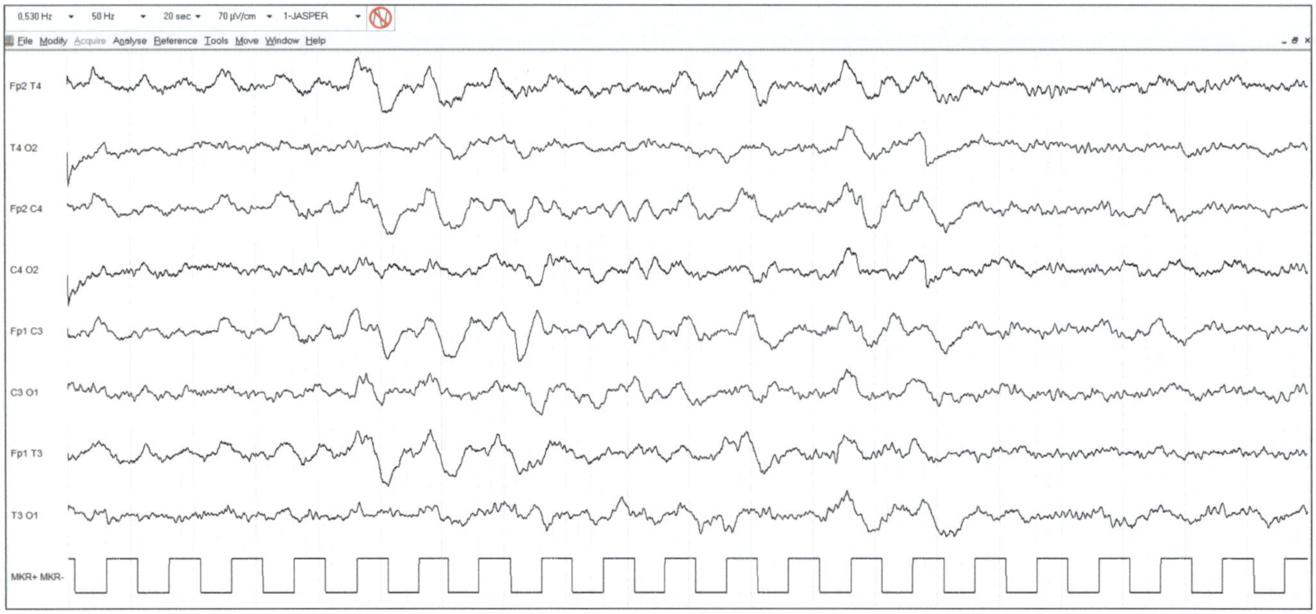

Fig. 45.7 EEG during "light sedation" with dexmedetomidine: high-amplitude slow-delta oscillations with a frequency of 1.5–2 Hz in anterior areas

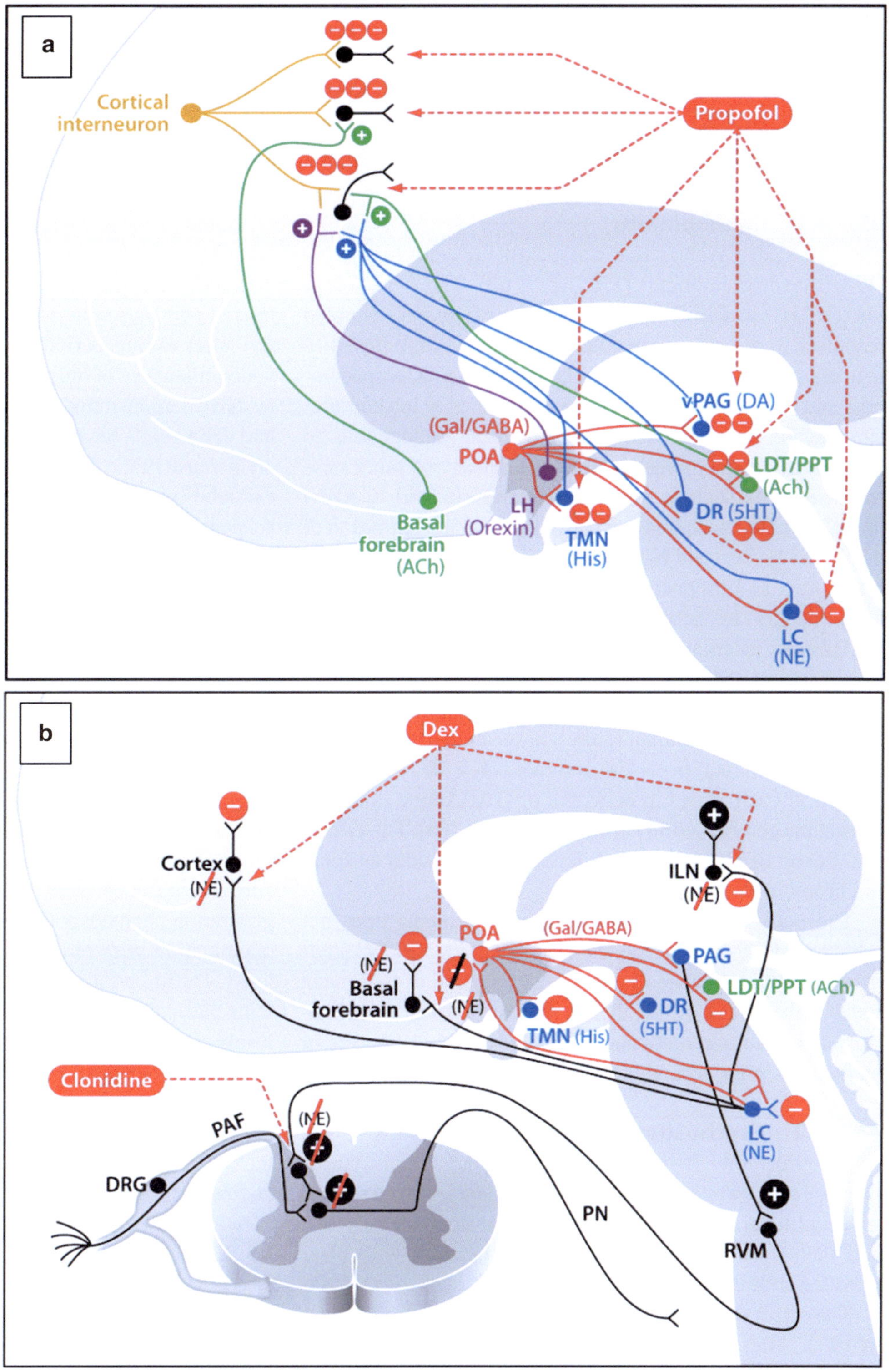

Fig. 45.8 Neurophysiological mechanisms of propofol (**a**) and dexmedetomidine and clonidine (**b**) actions in the brain. (**a**) Propofol enhances GABAergic transmission in the cortex and at the inhibitory projections from the POA to the arousal centers. (**b**) Dexmedetomidine-induced loss of consciousness through NE-mediated inhibition of the POA and decreased noradrenergic signaling in the thalamus and cortex. Clonidine-induced analgesia through enhanced inhibitory activity in the descending pain pathway. Abbreviations: *5HT* serotonin, *ACh* acetylcholine, *DA* dopamine, *DR* dorsal raphe, *DRG* dorsal root ganglia, *GABA* gamma-aminobutyric acid, $GABA_A$ GABA receptor subtype A, $_A$*Gal* galanin, *His* histamine, *ILN* intralaminar nucleus of the thalamus, *LC* locus coeruleus, *LDT* laterodorsal tegmental area, *LH* lateral hypothalamus, *NE* norepinephrine, *PAF* peripheral afferent fiber, *PN* projection neuron, *POA* preoptic area, *PPT* pedunculopontine tegmental area, *RVM* rostral ventral medulla, *TMN* tuberomammillary nucleus, *vPAG* ventral periaqueductal gray. (Modified from Brown EN, Purdon PL, Van Dort CJ. General Anesthesia and Altered States of Arousal: A Systems Neuroscience Analysis. Annual Review of Neuroscience. 2011; 34:601–628, with permission)

this pattern, we can often observe anterior - usually diphasic - slow waves, lasting about 1 s, isolated or in short sequences (Anteriorly maximum Intermittent Slow, AIS). Then, a slower activity, predominant in posterior and temporal areas and characterized by widespread delta potentials (Widespread Persistent Slow, WPS), can occur completely, replacing the WAR. When the rate of anesthetics is too high, the slow activity decreases in amplitude and it is progressively replaced by burst suppression pattern and, then, by electrocerebral inactivity.

45.2.6 Recreational Drugs and Toxic Substances

45.2.6.1 Cannabinoids

The principal psychoactive constituent in cannabinoids is D9-tetrahydrocannabinol (THC) [59, 60]. The CB1 receptor (CB1R) is one of the most abundant G-protein-coupled receptors in the central nervous system, with high densities in areas such as the cerebral cortex, basal ganglia, hippocampus, and cerebellum [61]. CB1Rs are primarily located presynaptically and their activation (by either endogenous or exogenous cannabinoids) inhibits the release of other neurotransmitters, such as gamma-aminobutyric acid (GABA) and glutamate, by decreasing Ca^{2+} influx via the inhibition of adenylate cyclase and N-type Ca^{2+} channels [62]. In the cerebral cortex and hippocampus, this neuromodulation principally occurs in networks of cholecystokinin-containing GABAergic interneurons [63]; thus, it appears that CB1Rs may function as a molecular "brake," regulating the timing and release of GABA and other neurotransmitters [64]. In vitro and in vivo animal studies have shown that CB1Rs modulate gamma (30–80 Hz) and theta (4–7 Hz) bands synchronized oscillations in networks of GABAergic interneurons in the cerebral cortex and hippocampus [65]. The effects of CBD on EEG activity are different if we consider an acute or chronic use.

The occasional use of hashish and marijuana does not seem to induce visible EEG changes. Quantitative EEG studies have rather evidenced that the chronic use of marijuana reduces the power of the alpha and beta bands in the posterior areas. During abstinence, an increase of the power of alpha band in the frontal areas have been observed.

45.2.6.2 Psychostimulant Substances

In general, low dosages of psychostimulant substances increase the power of alpha and beta frequencies and decrease the amplitude and magnitude of the slow frequencies (delta and theta), causing an EEG desynchronization with clear prevalence of the fast components.

The effect of cocaine on EEG was first studied by Berger in 1931. After acute administration, cocaine determines an increase of the power of the beta band with decrease and desynchronization of alpha band. Quantitative EEG studies demonstrate that cocaine-addicted male subjects show substantially significat deficits of low-frequency activity and significant excess of alpha activity. Furthermore, cocaine can induce epileptiform abnormalities and epileptic seizures up to status epilepticus [66].

Morphine and heroin generally induce a dose-dependent slowing of the alpha rhythm and an increase both in the theta and the beta bands. Acute intoxication may lead to a coma state with the related EEG patterns [66].

45.2.6.3 Ethanol

EEGs of ethanol abusers are poorly synchronized, with reduction of the alpha and increase of fast frequencies. With regard to EEG modifications induced by ethanol abuse, it is extremely difficult to distinguish between those alcohol-related and those due to concomitant factors (cortical atrophy after a long period of intoxication, systemic diseases, concomitant use of other drugs, etc.). Quantitative EEG studies have demonstrated a decrease in the power of alpha, theta and delta bands (characteristic of chronic brain damage) and an increase in the power of beta band (due to cortical hyperexcitability state) (Fig. 45.9). During the abuse, but also after suspension (abstinence), interictal epileptic abnormalities can be observed, even with epileptic seizures and/or status epilepticus [66].

45.2.7 Antibiotics

Although the association between seizures and antibiotics has been known since long time, recent literature reviews suggest that this association can be actually considered low or very low (evidence Class III–IV). However, numerous reports underline an increased risk of provoked epileptic seizures, especially with unsubstituted penicillins, fourth-generation cephalosporins, imipenem, and ciprofloxacin, in combination with renal dysfunction, brain lesions and epilepsy. During administration of these antibiotics in patients with particular predispositions, close monitoring of serum levels is suggested [67].

The risk of seizures is mainly related to the concomitance of other medical conditions that may alter the clearance and/or the bioavailability of the drug. The drug's ability to cross the blood-brain barrier (BBB) and/or damage to the BBB is another important risk factor for seizures.

45.2.7.1 Penicillins

The prevalence of seizures in patients receiving penicillin G or oxacillin is estimated to be 3.2 per 1000 patients [68]. Studies on animal models suggest that symptomatic seizures may derive from the interaction of penicillin with GABA, leading to a reduction of GABAergic inhibition allowing excitatory cortical afferents to trigger epileptiform bursts [69, 70].

However, the risk of epileptic seizures varies among the different molecules. As a matter of fact, the association between amoxicillin and clavulanic acid is not related to the

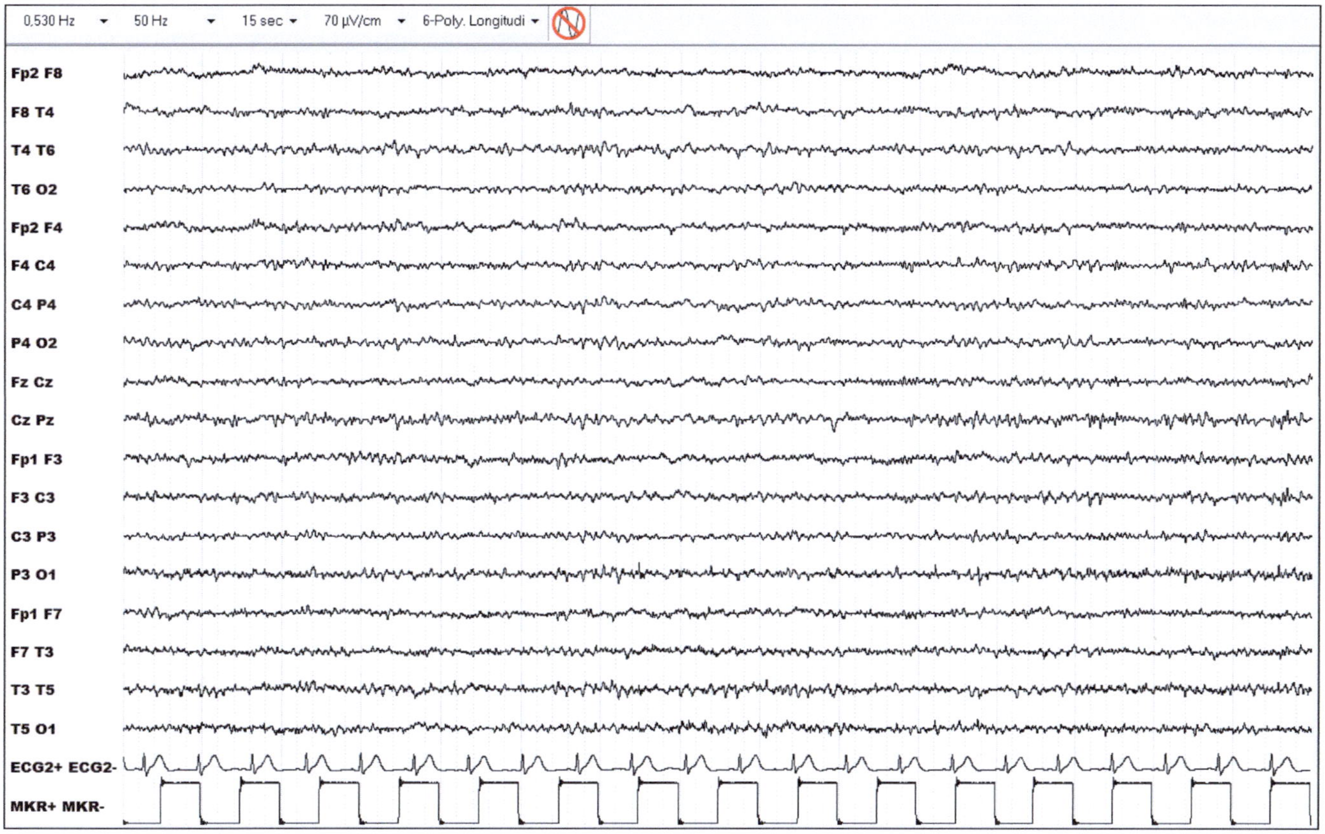

Fig. 45.9 Low-amplitude, diffuse, fast activity in a 49-year-old male chronic ethilist

risk of seizures, probably because of the inability to cross the blood-brain barrier and the poor ability to bind the $GABA_A$ receptor. Nevertheless, some case reports have described specific EEG abnormalities associated with amoxicillin (intermittent generalized short bursts of beta-frequency polyspikes alternated to frontal intermittent rhythmic delta activity (FIRDA) bursts during wakefulness) [71].

On the other hand, cases of nonconvulsive status epilepticus after piperacillin/tazobactam treatment have been reported [72].

45.2.7.2 Cephalosporins

The risk of seizures has been also reported for cephalosporins. All generations may cause seizures but cefepime and cefazoline are the most involved. Cephalosporins may induce encephalopathy with different EEG patterns characterized by several kinds of diffuse abnormalities—especially in fronto-central areas—from diffuse triphasic waves [73, 74] to continuous or intermittent bursts of generalized, high-voltage, 1 to 2 Hz sharp-wave or sharp and slow-wave activity [75]. The mechanism proposed of the cephaloporins-induced seizures is the dose-dependent inhibition of the $GABA_A$ receptors function [76].

45.2.7.3 Carbapenems

Carbapenems are able to penetrate the BBB, with effective treatment of CNS infections. This property, however, may promote seizure induction. Seizure induction could be caused by the structural similarity of the b-lactam ring with the GABA neurotransmitter, enabling carbapenems to interact at the $GABA_A$ receptor and act as a GABA antagonist [77]. Anecdotal cases of encephalopathy caused by imipenem are reported. EEG abnormalities described are diffuse slowing of background activity and intermittent multifocal or generalized epileptiform discharges (rhythmic spikes, polyspikes, sharp waves, spike wave, and sharp-and-slow wave complexes), accompanied by a diffuse low-voltage 10–25 Hz activity. In addition, a generalized photoparoxysmal response induced by intermittent photic stimulation at 20–25 Hz was observed [78].

45.2.7.4 Fluoroquinolones

Animal models suggest that fluoroquinolones inhibit GABAergic transmission by blocking the intracerebral $GABA_A$ receptors at a specific binding site [79]. Fluoroquinolone-associated neurotoxicity may manifest as seizures, delirium, or encephalopathy, and some cases of encephalopathy related to these drugs are reported. In a case report of a nonconvulsive status epilepticus due to levofloxacin, EEG revealed a continuous slow electrical activity with frequent generalized atypical spike-and-wave discharges prevalent in the anterior regions [80].

References

1. Jobert M, Wilson FJ. Advanced analysis of Pharmaco-EEG data in humans. Neuropsychobiology. 2015;72:165–77.
2. Babiloni C, Vecchio F, Lizio R, et al. Resting state cortical rhythms in mild cognitive impairment and Alzheimer's disease: electroencephalographic evidence. J Alzheimers Dis. 2011;26(Suppl 3):201–14.
3. Jobert M, Wilson FJ, Ruigt GSF, et al. Guidelines for the recording and evaluation of Pharmaco-EEG data in man: the international Pharmaco-EEG society (IPEG). Neuropsychobiology. 2012;66:201–20.
4. Jobert M, Schulz H, Jahnig P. On the choice of recording duration in pharmaco-EEG studies. Neuropsychobiology. 1995;32:106–14.
5. Olbrich S, Mulert C, Karch S, et al. EEG vigilance and BOLD effect during simultaneous EEG/fMRI measurement. Neuroimage. 2009;45:319–32.
6. Salinsky MC, Oken BS, Morehead L. Intraindividual analysis of antiepileptic drug effects on EEG background rhythms. Electroencephalogr Clin Neurophysiol. 1994;90:186–93.
7. Salinsky MC, Oken BS, Storzbach D, Dodrill CB. Assessment of CNS effects of antiepileptic drugs by using quantitative EEG measures. Epilepsia. 2003;44:1042–50.
8. Marciani MG, Gigli GL, Stefanini F, et al. Effect of carbamazepine on EEG background activity and on interictal epileptiform abnormalities in focal epilepsy. Int J Neurosci. 1993;70:107–16.
9. Wu X, Xiao CH. Quantitative pharmaco-EEG of carbamazepine in volunteers and epileptics. Clin Electroencephalogr. 1996;27:40–5.
10. Cherian KA, Legatt AD. Burst suppression pattern on electroencephalogram secondary to Valproic acid-induced Hyperammonemic encephalopathy. Pediatr Neurol. 2017;73:88–91.
11. Arzy S, Allali G, Brunet D. Antiepileptic drugs modify power of high EEG frequencies and their neural generators. Eur J Neurol. 2010;17:1308–12.
12. Mecarelli O, Vicenzini E, Pulitano P, et al. Clinical, cognitive, and neurophysiologic correlates of short-term treatment with carbamazepine, oxcarbazepine, and levetiracetam in healthy volunteers. Ann Pharmacother. 2004;38:1816–22.
13. Nicholson A, Appleton RE, Chadwick DW, Smith DF. The relationship between treatment with valproate, lamotrigine, and topiramate and the prognosis of then idiopathic generalized epilepsies. J Neurol Neurosurg Psychiatry. 2004;75:75–9.
14. Clemens B, Ménes A, Piros P, et al. Quantitative EEG effects of carbamazepine, oxcarbazepine, valproate, lamotrigine, and possible clinical relevance of the findings. Epilepsy Res. 2006;70:190–9.
15. Clemens B, Piros P, Bessenyei M, Hollody K. Lamotrigine decreases EEG synchronization in a use-dependent manner in patients with idiopathic generalized epilepsy. Clin Neurophysiol. 2007;118:910–7.
16. Lyseng-Williamson KA. Levetiracetam: a review of its use in epilepsy. Drugs. 2011;71:489–514.
17. Bouchier B, Demarquay G, Guérin C, André-Obadia N, Gobert F. Marked EEG worsening following Levetiracetam overdose: how a pharmacological issue can confound coma prognosis. Clin Neurol Neurosurg. 2017;152:1–4.
18. Schomer DL. In: Lopes da Silva FH, editor. Niedermeyer's electroencephalography: basic principles, clinical applications and related fields. New York: Oxford University Press; 2018.
19. Marson AG, Al-Kharusi AM, Alwaidh M, et al. The SANAD study of effectiveness of valproate, lamotrigine, or topiramate for generalized and unclassifiable epilepsy: an unblinded randomized controlled trial. Lancet. 2007;369:1016–26.
20. Specchio N, Boero G, Michelucci R, et al. Effects of levetiracetam on EEG abnormalities in juvenile myoclonic epilepsy. Epilepsia. 2008;49:663–9.
21. Pro S, Vicenzini E, Pulitano P, et al. Effects of levetiracetam on generalized discharges monitored with ambulatory EEG in epileptic patients. Seizure. 2009;18:133–8.
22. Biraben A, Allain H, Scarabin J, Schück S, Edan G. Exacerbation of juvenile myoclonic epilepsy with lamotrigine. Neurology. 2000;55:1758.
23. Morris G, Hammer A, Kustra R, Messenheimer J. Lamotrigine for patients with juvenile myoclonic epilepsy following prior treatment with valproate: results of an open-label study. Epilepsy Behav. 2004;5:509–21.
24. Machado RA, García VF, Astencio AG, Cuartas VB. Efficacy and tolerability of lamotrigine in juvenile myoclonic epilepsy in adults: a prospective, unblinded randomized controlled trial. Seizure. 2013;22:846–55.
25. Liu J, Wang LN, Wang YP. Topiramate monotherapy for juvenile myoclonic epilepsy. Cochrane Database Syst Rev. 2017;4:CD010008.
26. Mecarelli O, Piacenti A, Pulitano P, et al. Clinical and electroencephalographic effects of topiramate in patients with epilepsy and healthy volunteers. Clin Neuropharmacol. 2001;24:284–9.
27. Misra UK, Dubey D, Kalita J. Comparison of lacosamide versus sodium valproate in status epilepticus: a pilot study. Epilepsy Behav. 2017;76:110–3.
28. Zhu LN, Chen D, Xu D, Tan G, Wang HJ, Liu L. Newer antiepileptic drugs compared to levetiracetam as adjunctive treatments for uncontrolled focal epilepsy: an indirect comparison. Seizure. 2017;51:121–32.
29. d'Orsi G, Pascarella MG, Martino T, et al. Intravenous lacosamide in seizure emergencies: observations from a hospitalized in-patient adult population. Seizure. 2016;42:20–8.
30. Behr C, Lévesque M, Ragsdale D, Avoli M. Lacosamide modulates interictal spiking and high-frequency oscillations in a model of mesial temporal lobe epilepsy. Epilepsy Res. 2015;115:8–16.
31. Manconi M, Ferri R, Miano S, et al. Sleep architecture in insomniacs with severe benzodiazepine abuse. Clin Neurophysiol. 2017;128:875–81.
32. Jernajczyk W, Gosek P, Latka M, Kozlowska K, Święcicki Ł, West BJ. Alpha wavelet power as a biomarker of antidepressant treatment response in bipolar depression. Adv Exp Med Biol. 2017;968:79–94.
33. Bruder GE, Sedoruk JP, Stewart JW, McGrath PJ, Quitkin FM, Tenke CE. Electroencephalographic alpha measures predict therapeutic response to a selective serotonin reuptake inhibitor antidepressant: pre-and post-treatment findings. Biol Psychiatry. 2008;63:1171–7.
34. Arns M, Bruder G, Hegerl U, et al. EEG alpha asymmetry as a gender-specific predictor of outcome to acute treatment with different antidepressant medications in the randomized iSPOT-D study. Clin Neurophysiol. 2016;127:509–19.
35. Baskaran A, Milev R, McIntyre RS. The neurobiology of the EEG biomarker as a predictor of treatment response in depression. Neuropharmacology. 2012;63:507–13.
36. Macaluso M, Zackula R, D'Empaire I, Baker B, Liow K, Preskorn SH. Twenty percent of a representative sample of patients taking bupropion have abnormal, asymptomatic electroencephalographic findings. J Clin Psychopharmacol. 2010;30:312–7.
37. Ott GE, Rao U, Lin KM, Gertsik L, Poland RE. Effect of treatment with bupropion on EEG sleep: relationship to antidepressant response. Int J Neuropsychopharmacol. 2004;7:275–81.
38. Leiser SC, Pehrson AL, Robichaud PJ, Sanchez C. Multimodal antidepressant vortioxetine increases frontal cortical oscillations

unlike escitalopram and duloxetine–a quantitative EEG study in rats. Br J Pharmacol. 2014;171:4255–72.
39. Pehrson AL, Leiser SC, Gulinello M. Treatment of cognitive dysfunction in major depressive disorder—a review of the preclinical evidence for efficacy of selective serotonin reuptake inhibitors, serotonin-norepinephrine reuptake inhibitors and the multimodal-acting antidepressant vortioxetine. Eur J Pharmacol. 2015;753:19–31.
40. Dale E, Zhang H, Leiser SC, et al. Vortioxetine (Lu AA21004) disinhibits pyramidal cell output and enhances theta rhythms and long-term plasticity in the hippocampus. Eur Neuropsychopharmacol. 2013;23:S394.
41. Riga MS, Celada P, Sanchez C, Artigas F. Role of 5-HT3 receptors in the mechanism of action of the investigational antidepressant vortioxetine. Eur Neuropsychopharmacol. 2013;23:S393–4.
42. Hunter AM, Leuchter AF, Cook IA, et al. Brain functional changes and duloxetine treatment response in fibromyalgia: a pilot study. Pain Med. 2009;10:730–8.
43. Bruder GE, Sedoruk JP, Steward JW. EEG alpha measures predict therapeutic response to an SSRI antidepressant: pre and post treatment findings. Biol Psychiatry. 2008;63:1171–7.
44. Bloechliger M, Ceschi A, Rüegg S, et al. Risk of seizures associated with antidepressant use in patients with depressive disorder: follow-up study with a nested case–control analysis using the clinical practice research datalink. Drug Saf. 2016;39:307.
45. Wu C, Liu HY, Tsai HJ, Liu SK. Seizure risk associated with antidepressant treatment among patients with depressive disorders: a population-based case-crossover study. J Clin Psychiatry. 2017;78:e1226–32.
46. Liem-Moolenaar M, Gray FA, de Visser SJ, et al. Psychomotor and cognitive effects of a single oral dose of talnetant (SB223412) in healthy volunteers compared with placebo or haloperidol. J Psychopharmacol. 2010;24:73–82.
47. Yoshimura M, Koenig T, Irisawa S, et al. A pharmaco-EEG study on antipsychotic drugs in healthy volunteers. Psychopharmacology (Berl). 2007;191:995–1004.
48. Knott V, Labelle A, Jones B, Mahoney C. Quantitative EEG in schizophrenia and in response to acute and chronic clozapine treatment. Schizophr Res. 2001;50:41–53.
49. Centorrino F, Price BH, Tuttle M, et al. EEG abnormalities during treatment with typical and atypical antipsychotics. Am J Psychiatry. 2002;159:109–15.
50. Henninger GR. Lithium carbonate and brain function. Cerebral-evoked potentials, EEG and symptom changes during lithium carbonate treatment. Arch Gen Psychiatry. 1978;35:228–33.
51. Thau K, Rappelsberger P, Lovrek A, Petsche H, Simhandl C, Topitz A. Effect of lithium on the EEG of healthy males and females. A probability mapping study. Neuropsychobiology. 1989;20: 158–63.
52. Aiyer R, Novakovic V, Barkin RL. A systematic review on the impact of psychotropic drugs on electroencephalogram waveforms in psychiatry. Postgrad Med. 2016;128:656–64.
53. Avidan MS, Zhang L, Burnside BA, et al. Anesthesia awareness and the bispectral index. N Engl J Med. 2008;358:1097–108.
54. Kelley SD. Monitoring consciousness: using the bispectral index. 2nd ed. Boulder: Covidien; 2010. p. 6.
55. Purdon PL, Sampson A, Pavone KJ, Brown EN. Clinical electroencephalography for anesthesiologists part I: background and basic signatures. Anesthesiology. 2015;123:937–60.
56. Besch G, Liu N, Samain E, et al. Occurrence of and risk factors for electroencephalogram burst suppression during propofol-remifentanil anaesthesia. Br J Anaesth. 2011;107:749–56.
57. Purdon PL, Pierce ET, Mukamel EA, et al. Electroencephalogram signatures of loss and recovery of consciousness from propofol. Proc Natl Acad Sci U S A. 2013;110:E1142–51.
58. Akeju O, Kim SE, Vazquez R, et al. Spatiotemporal dynamics of dexmedetomidine-induced electroencephalogram oscillations. PLoS One. 2016;11:e0163431.
59. Akeju O, Pavone KJ, Westover MB, et al. A comparison of propofol- and dexmedetomidine-induced electroencephalogram dynamics using spectral and coherence analysis. Anesthesiology. 2014;121:978–89.
60. Devane WA, Dysarz FA, Johnson MR, Melvin LS, Howlett AC. Determination and characterization of a cannabinoid receptor in rat brain. Mol Pharmacol. 1988;34:605–13.
61. Pertwee RG, Howlett AC, Abood ME, et al. International union of basic and clinical pharmacology. LXXIX. Cannabinoid receptors and their ligands: beyond CB and CB. Pharmacol Rev. 2010;62:588–631.
62. Glass M, Dragunow M, Faull RL. Cannabinoid receptors in the human brain: a detailed anatomical and quantitative autoradiographic study in the fetal, neonatal and adult human brain. Neuroscience. 1997;77:299–318.
63. Freund TF, Katona I, Piomelli D. Role of endogenous cannabinoids in synaptic signaling. Physiol Rev. 2003;83:1017–66.
64. Eggan SM, Melchitzky DS, Sesack SR, Fish KN, Lewis DA. Relationship of cannabinoid CB1 receptor and cholecystokinin immunoreactivity in monkey dorsolateral prefrontal cortex. Neuroscience. 2010;169:1651–61.
65. Farkas I, Kallo I, Deli L, et al. Retrograde endocannabinoid signaling reduces GABAergic synaptic transmission to gonadotropin-releasing hormone neurons. Endocrinology. 2010;151:5818–29.
66. Katona I, Sperlagh B, Magloczky Z, et al. GABAergic interneurons are the targets of cannabinoid actions in the human hippocampus. Neuroscience. 2000;100:797–804.
67. Ceballos NA, Bauer LO, Houston RJ. Recent EEG and ERP findings in substance abusers. Clin EEG Neurosci. 2009;40:122–8.
68. Sutter R, Ruegg S, Sutter ST. Seizures as adverse events of antibiotic drugs: a systematic review. Neurology. 2015;85:1332–41.
69. Boston Collaborative Drug Surveillance Program. Drug induced convulsions: report from the Boston Collaborative Drug Surveillance Program. Lancet. 1972;2:677–9.
70. Van Duijn H, Schwartzkroin PA, Prince DA. Action of penicillin on inhibitory processes in the cat's cortex. Brain Res. 1973;53:470–6.
71. Wong RK, Prince DA. Dendritic mechanisms underlying penicillin-induced epileptiform activity. Science. 1979;204:1228–31.
72. Raposo J, Teotónio R, Bento C, Sales F. Amoxicillin, a potential epileptogenic drug. Epileptic Disord. 2016;18:454–7.
73. Fernández-Torre JL, Santos-Sánchez C, Pelayo AL. De novo generalised non-convulsive status epilepticus triggered by piperacillin/tazobactam. Seizure. 2010;19:529–30.
74. Pro S, Randi F, Pulitano P, Vicenzini E, Mecarelli O. Reversible encephalopathy induced by cefoperazone: a case report monitored with EEG. Neurol Sci. 2011;32:465–7.
75. De Silva DA, Pan AB, Lim SH. Cefepime-induced encephalopathy with triphasic waves in three Asian patients. Ann Acad Med Singapore. 2007;36:450–1.
76. Martínez-Rodríguez JE, Barriga FJ, Santamaria J, et al. Nonconvulsive status epilepticus associated with cephalosporins in patients with renal failure. Am J Med. 2001;111:115–9.
77. Sugimoto M, Uchida I, Mashimo T, et al. Evidence for the involvement of GABA(A) receptor blockade in convulsions induced by cephalosporins. Neuropharmacology. 2003;45:304–14.
78. Miller AD, Ball AM, Bookstaver PB, Dornblaser EK, Bennett CL. Epileptogenic potential of carbapenem agents: mechanism of action, seizure rates, and clinical considerations. Pharmacotherapy. 2011;31:408–23.
79. Fernández-Torre JL, Velasco M, Gutiérrez R, Fernández-Sampedro M. Encephalopathy secondary to imipenem therapy. Clin EEG Neurosci. 2004;35:100–3.
80. Green MA, Halliwell RF. Selective antagonism of the GABA(A) receptor by ciprofloxacin and biphenylacetic acid. Br J Pharmacol. 1997;122:584–90.
81. Mazzei D, Accardo J, Ferrari A, Primavera A. Levofloxacin neurotoxicity and non-convulsive status epilepticus (NCSE): a case report. Clin Neurol Neurosurg. 2012;114:1371–3.

Disorders of Consciousness

46

Oriano Mecarelli, Marianna Brienza, Antonello Grippo, and Aldo Amantini

46.1 Anatomo-Pathophysiology of Disorders of Consciousness

Disorders Of Consciousness (DOC) result from failure of the arousal system. The current knowledge regarding the anatomo-physiology of vigilance dates back to the 1930s and 1940s, owing to the elegant experiments performed by Bremer [1] and Moruzzi and Magoun [2]. Observing cats with their brainstem sectioned between the pons and midbrain and in the lower part of the bulb, Bremer discovered that rostral section caused a clinical state and an EEG similar to that of sleep (with characteristic synchronised EEG sleep rhythms), while animals with caudal section remained awake but with desynchronised EEG rhythms. Many years later, Dempsey and Morrison [3] demonstrated the presence of a system of non-specific projections (independent from specific sensory nuclei) from the thalami to all the cortical regions. This concept was further demonstrated by Moruzzi and Magoun [2], who observed that the electrical stimulation of the medial mesencephalic tegmentum and of the adjacent areas caused the awakening of slightly anesthetised animals, with corresponding EEG desynchronisation as in normal awakening, in response to sensory stimuli. The sites that induced awakening upon stimulation consisted of a series of neuronal stations extending from the non-specific nuclei of the medial thalamus to the caudal midbrain. These areas corresponded to the complex system of the ascending reticular formation, a system that is widely innervated by axon collaterals of the ascending sensory systems and is, therefore, in a state of tonic activation. Moreover, since this region, in particular the medial thalamus, projected widely to the cerebral hemispheres, the concept of a Reticular Activating System (RAS) that maintained the waking state originated, which inactivation led to a state of unconsciousness. Despite several experimental disagreements [4], the paramedian upper mesencephalic tegmentum and the lower diencephalon began to be considered as the brain system responsible for arousal. The anatomical boundaries of RAS in the upper midbrain are indistinct, since it is scattered throughout the paramedian regions of the rostral part of the pons and of the mesencephalic tegmentum. In the thalamus, RAS includes the posterior, paramedian, parafascicular and medial portions of the centromedian and intralaminar nuclei. In the brainstem, RAS includes the nuclei of the reticular formation, which receive collaterals from the spinal and trigeminal-thalamic pathways and project widely to the entire cortex, and other key structures for arousal, including the raphe nuclei, locus coeruleus, substantia nigra pars compacta, ventral tegmental area and the mesopontine tegmentum, the latter including the pedunculopontine and laterodorsal tegmental nuclei. These nuclei extend throughout the brainstem, sending ascending and descending signals to influence arousal. Furthermore, their dendrites are positioned in the brainstem such as to detect signals that pass to and from the periphery. The dendrites of these neurons form web-like “reticula” around the passing axons and they can detect a wide variety of external sensory or internal thalamic stimuli passing through the surrounding structures. Therefore, these reticular neurons are positioned strategically to respond to both external and internal signals in the control of arousal [5, 6] (Table 46.1).

The sensory stimulation has therefore a double effect; conveying information from somatic structures to the cortex and activating the regions of the central nervous system on which consciousness depends. Moreover, the cortex does not

O. Mecarelli (✉)
Department of Human Neurosciences,
Sapienza University of Rome, Rome, Italy
e-mail: oriano.mecarelli@uniroma1.it

M. Brienza
Department of Human Neurosciences,
Sapienza University of Rome, Rome, Italy
e-mail: marianna.brienza@uniroma1.it

A. Grippo · A. Amantini
SODc Neurofisiopatologia, Dipartimento Neuromuscolo-Scheletrico e degli Organi di Senso, AOU Careggi, Florence, Italy

Unità di Riabilitazione Neurologica,
Fondazione Don Carlo Gnocchi, IRCCS, Florence, Italy
e-mail: antonello.grippo@unifi.it; aldo.amantini@unifi.it

O. Mecarelli (ed.), *Clinical Electroencephalography*, https://doi.org/10.1007/978-3-030-04573-9_46

Table 46.1 Neuroanatomical structures for the regulation of arousal and REM sleep

Function	Neuroanatomical structure	Target	Neurotransmitter
Promotion of arousal	Reticular formation of brainstem	Nucleus pontis oralis	GABA
	Caudal raphe nuclei (medulla and caudal pons)	Spinal cord	Serotonin
	Rostral raphe nuclei (median and dorsal)	Cortex, basal forebrain, locus coeruleus, thalamus, hypothalamus, reticular formation, parabrachial and precoeruleus nuclei	Serotonin
	Locus Coeruleus (rostral pons)	Prefrontal cortex, ventral tegmental area	Norepinephrine
	Parabrachial and precoeruleus nuclei (dorsolateral pons)	Lateral hypothalamus, substantia innominata	Glutamate
	Pedunculopontine nucleus/laterodorsal tegmental nucleus (midbrain and pons)	– Motor cortex – Nucleus pontis oralis – Basal forebrain	Acetylcholine GABA Glutamate
	Ventral tegmental area (midbrain)	Septal area; nucleus accumbens; amygdala; piriform, prefrontal, cingulate, entorhinal cortices	Dopamine
	Posterior hypothalamic nucleus	Locus coeruleus, nucleus pontis oralis	Orexin
	Lateral hypothalamic nucleus	Tuberomammillary nucleus, dorsal raphe nuclei, laterodorsal tegmental nucleus, thalamus, basal forebrain	Orexin
	Tuberomammillary nucleus (hypothalamus)	Diagonal band of Broca, ventral tegmental area, pars compacta of substantia nigra, parabrachial nucleus, cortex	Histamine
Modulation of arousal	Specific and non-specific thalamic nuclei	Diffuse cortical and subcortical connections	Glutamate
	Diagonal band of Broca	– Ventral tegmental area – Cortex	Histamine Acetylcholine
Promotion of REM sleep	Reticular formation of brainstem	Nucleus pontis oralis	Acetylcholine
	Pedunculopontine nucleus/laterodorsal tegmental nucleus (midbrain and pons)	Nucleus pontis oralis	Acetylcholine
	Pars compacta substantia nigra (midbrain)	Dorsal striatum	Dopamine
	Tuberomammillary nucleus	Tuberomammillary nucleus	Glutamate
Promotion of arousal and REM sleep	Diagonal band of Broca	Cortex	Acetylcholine
	Magnocellular preoptic area/substantia innominata	– Cortex – Lateral hypothalamus	Acetylcholine Glutamate
	Nucleus basalis of Meynert/median septum/globus pallidus	Cortex	Acetylcholine
Inhibition of REM sleep	Rostral raphe nuclei (median and dorsal)	Cortex, basal forebrain, Locus coeruleus, thalamus, hypothalamus, reticular formation, Parabrachial nucleus	Serotonin
	Thalamic reticula nucleus	Nucleus pontis oralis	GABA
	Hypothalamic dorsocaudal nucleus	Ventral oral pontine reticular nucleus	GABA

limit to receiving stimuli from the RAS, but also modulates these input information through corticofugal projections towards the reticular formation.

Other anatomical structures more recently considered as fundamental in maintaining the state of consciousness, especially in the transition across the DOC continuum, are the basal forebrain and the hypothalamic systems, that participate in the constitution of the "mesocircuit model".

The mesocircuit model postulates that the anterior forebrain function is markedly downregulated in all severe brain injuries, as a result of widespread disconnection or neuronal death. A crucial role is proposed for neurons within the central thalamus that are known to show progressive deafferentation in proportion to the severity of structural brain injuries [7]. At the mesocircuit level, a broad reduction in corticostriatal, thalamo-cortical and thalamostriatal outflow is expected to produce sufficient loss of afferent inputs to the Medium Spiny Neurons (MSNs) of the striatum, to prevent these neurons from reaching their firing threshold [8]. The direct deafferentation of central thalamic neurons and the active inhibition of some of these cells by the internal globus pallidus, due to loss of their active inhibition by the MSNs in the striatum, cause a large reduction in the synaptic activity of the entire brain, as reflected by the very low cerebral metabolic rates typical in patients with DOC [9]. As evidence of the important role of the anterior forebrain mesocircuit, the expressed behaviour and level of conscious content increase with restoration of its normal patterns of activity [10]. This model can also explain some of the effects of different activating drugs used in DOC [11] and novel strategies, such as Deep Brain Stimulation (DBS), all of which have the effect of restoring activity of cortical frontal, striatal and central thalamic neurons [12]. It also draws a direct connection across similar shifts in frontal cortical and striatal activation during the sleep–wake cycle and the paradoxical behavioural activation observed during the early stages of anaesthesia [13].

Large reductions of arousal level in normal individuals involve broad hyperpolarisation of these neurons via withdrawal of excitatory neuromodulatory influences from orexinergic, cholinergic, noradrenergic, and other brainstem, basal forebrain and hypothalamic systems [14, 15]. Such hyperpolarisation of cortical and thalamic neurons, as progressively occurs across the deeper stages of sleep or with the broad inhibitory effects of anaesthesia, markedly changes the firing patterns of these neuronal populations, influencing the overall pattern of cortico-thalamic dynamics towards more synchronous and dynamically stereotyped waves of activity as compared with the more spatio-temporally differentiated patterns associated with wakeful conscious state [11].

EEG is important for the assessment of waking state, since the electrical activity of cerebral cortex depends on the characteristics of the thalamo-cortical discharge system, an indispensable component for the maintenance of wakefulness. As already described in Chap. 2, the electrical activity recorded at the surface of the skull depends on the summation of the synaptic potentials arising in the dendrites of cortical neurons; therefore, EEG rhythms depend on the synchronisation of the waves derived from the summation of the synaptic potentials generated by the activity of thalamo-cortical neurons. In turn, the rhythms of thalamic activity depend on the important properties of thalamic retransmission neurons, which can be found in two different physiological states: the transmission mode and the burst mode. In the former case, the membrane potential of a retransmission neuron is close to the discharge threshold and the excitatory synaptic potentials generated by the afferent signals produce a discharge, the characteristics of which are related to those of the sensory stimulus. In the latter case, thalamic neurons are hyperpolarised by inhibitory afferent signals. Thalamic retransmission neurons possess a special voltage-dependent calcium channel that is inactive when the membrane potential is close to the threshold. Conversely, when the retransmission neuron is hyperpolarised, the excitatory synaptic potentials generated by the afferent signals determine the transient opening of these calcium channels and the appearance of a calcium current that carries the neuron membrane potential beyond the threshold necessary for the genesis of the action potential. As a consequence, the neuron generates a burst of action potentials causing a further opening of the calcium channels, until the amount of calcium entering the cell is no longer sufficient to trigger a potassium current that hyperpolarises the cell, returning its potential to the initial level at which a new burst-mode cycle is generated. The thalamic retransmission neurons are initially hyperpolarised, due to their mutual interactions with GABAergic inhibitory interneurons of the reticular nucleus of the thalamus, whose dendrites receive collaterals from the axons of the thalamocortical and cortico-thalamic neurons that pass through the nucleus. Neurons of the reticular nucleus hyperpolarise the thalamic retransmission neurons; thus, their ability to reach the threshold of discharge in response to afferent sensory signals depends on the activity of the neurons of the reticular nucleus; when they are hyperpolarised, both retransmission and reticular neurons enter the burst mode.

In retransmission neurons, afferents from the reticular nucleus generate inhibitory synaptic potentials that remove the inactivation of calcium channels; subsequently, modification of the membrane potential generates a burst of action potentials. In turn, thalamic retransmission neurons send excitatory signals to the reticular neurons, which trigger another burst of activity in the reticular neurons. The consequent rhythmic and synchronous discharge of the thalamic retransmission neurons produces waves of excitatory synaptic potentials at the level of the dendrites of the cortical neurons. Depolarisation cycles are recorded as slow and rhythmic EEG waves, and this pattern indicates that the thalamus is unable to retransmit sensory information to the cortex. This type of EEG pattern is observed during deep sleep, but also in pathological conditions characterised by the blockage of the thalamo-cortical transmission, as in coma state. On the contrary, when the thalamus is in transmission mode, as during wakefulness, the desynchronised EEG trace indicates that information regarding sensory stimuli is being relayed. During the normal waking state, the thalamus is maintained in the transmission mode by cholinergic afferents from the rostral pons and from the basal forebrain. The main cholinergic afferents to the thalamic retransmission nuclei originate from the peduncle-pontine nucleus and from the laterodorsal tegmental nuclei of the brainstem. These nuclei, together with the cholinergic neurons of the basal forebrain, innervate the reticular nucleus of the thalamus, reducing its activity, and thus preventing the hyperpolarisation of the thalamic retransmission neurons during the waking state [16].

Knowledge of these anatomo-physiological mechanisms is of fundamental importance in understanding the neuropathological bases of the different types of brain lesions that can cause coma and in making a correct diagnosis of the lesion site. It is known that structural abornalities in different brain regions may have different clinical and electrophysiological aspects. Brainstem sections under the rostral pons have no influence on the state of consciousness; however, acute sections above the inferior colliculus, as well as those of the paramedian reticular formation of the midbrain, always cause coma, even if circumscribed. Posterolateral hypothalamic lesions interrupt the branch passing through the hypothalamus and cause a marked EEG slowing and the induction of coma, even if the branch passing through the thalamus remains intact. In contrast, injuries to the thalamus or its afferents from the reticular nucleus prevent the brain from maintaining a desynchronised or waking state. If the lesions are sufficiently extensive, the EEG rhythm may completely disappear.

46.2 Coma, Vegetative State, and Minimally Conscious State

Coma is defined as a state of deep, unarousable unconsciousness; the patient lies with eyes closed and, as coma deepens, responsiveness to acoustic and/or painful stimuli diminishes or completely disappears [17]. Coma should be considered a self-limiting or transitory condition that usually resolves within 2–4 weeks, evolving into: partial or complete recovery; Vegetative State (VS) or Minimally Conscious State (MCS); death [13].

The causes of coma can be classified in two principal groups: structural brain diseases and diffuse neuronal dysfunction [18]. Structural brain lesions include Space-Occupying Lesions (SOL) and all conditions of increased intracranial pressure (tumours, abscesses, cerebral oedema, hydrocephalus), anoxic-hypoxic brain disease, epidural or subdural haematoma, cerebral haemorrhages, and acute ischaemic stroke. SOL are also characterised by their location above or below the cerebellar tentorium and are classified as supratentorial or infratentorial brain lesions. Structural brain diseases can also be induced by sepsis, CNS infections, or status epilepticus. A condition of diffuse neuronal dysfunction responsible for coma can be caused by different metabolic syndromes (hypo- or hyperglycaemia, hyponatraemia, hypercalcemia, hepatic and renal failure, thyroid diseases) or toxic agents (sedatives, opioids, toxic alcohols, carbon monoxide).

Vegetative state is a condition characterised by the absence of responsiveness and awareness due to a massive dysfunction of the cerebral cortex of both hemispheres, with sufficient integrity of the diencephalon and brainstem to preserve autonomic and motor reflexes and sleep–wake cycles. VS patients have spontaneous eye-opening movements (because the reticular activating system is intact) and completely or partially preserved hypothalamic and brainstem functions. The eyes are open during wake and closed during sleep, and ocular movements, such as blinking, roving and nystagmus, are present; breathing is spontaneous.

However, these patients show no evidence of sustained, reproducible, purposeful, or voluntary behavioural response to various stimuli, and there is no evidence of language comprehension or expression. Cranial nerve functions and spinal reflexes are variably preserved, as is the sleep-wave cycle, but there is no control of the sphincters, leading to bowel and bladder incontinence. It is recommended not to use the term "persistent" for VS; aetiology of the brain injury (traumatic or non-traumatic) and the duration of the VS should instead be specified. The clinical course and outcome of VS depend on its cause: acute traumatic and non-traumatic brain injuries, degenerative and metabolic brain disorders, or severe congenital malformations of the CNS. Recovery from a post-traumatic VS is unlikely after 12 months (and more unlikely in adults than in children), while recovery from a non-traumatic VS after 3 months is rare in both adults and children. Finally, patients with metabolic diseases or congenital malformations who remain in a VS for several months are unlikely to recover consciousness [13, 19, 20].

Minimally conscious state must be distinguished from VS. It is a chronic condition consequent to a severe diffuse brain damage, characterised by an altered state of consciousness and a diminished - but demonstrated - self and environmental awareness. This condition may represent a transitional state reflecting clinical improvement following coma or a VS or, conversely, a progressive deterioration of consciousness as in neurodegenerative disease [13, 21].

In comparison with VS, thalamic lesions are less prevalent in MCS, and the relative sparing of cortico-thalamic connections could explain the minimal preservation of cognitive processes. Behavioural features of MCS patients are: response to simple commands and questions (gestural or "yes-no" responses); intelligible verbalisation in response to the linguistic content of questions; reaching for and grabbing objects, recognising their position; recognising the shape and size of objects; pursuit eye movement or fixation on moving objects; appropriate smiling or crying. However, the behavioural responses to stimuli are inconsistent and sometimes even ambiguous.

MCS was recently subcategorised according to the complexity of patients' behaviour: MCS *plus* describes high-level behavioural responses (i.e. command execution, intelligible verbalisation, or non-functional communication); MCS *minus* describes low-level behavioural responses (i.e. visual pursuit, localisation of nociceptive stimulation, or contingent behaviour such as appropriate smiling or crying in response to emotional stimuli) [22].

46.3 Differential Diagnosis Among Consciousness Disorders

VS and MCS should be placed in differential diagnosis with Akinetic Mutism (AM) and Locked-In Syndrome (LIS).

AM was first described in 1941 by Cairns and colleagues [23] as a mental state in which patients lose the ability to move or to speak. This condition could be explained by dam-

Table 46.2 Clinical and EEG characteristics of disorders of consciousness

Clinical condition	Consciousness	Awareness	Vegetative functions	Motor response	EEG features
MCS	Partially compromised	Preserved	Preserved	Variable/finalistic movements	Aspecific alterations; reactivity +
VS	Absent	Preserved	Preserved	Present but afinalistic	Aspecific alterations; reactivity ±
Coma	Absent	Absent	Partially compromised	Reflex/postural responses	Aspecific and/or peculiar patterns; reactivity ±
BD	Absent	Absent	Absent	Absent (only spinal reflexes)	Electrocerebral inactivity
LIS	Preserved	Preserved/partially compromised	Preserved/partially compromised	Tetraplegia, pseudobulbar palsy	Normal EEG

MCS Minimally Conscious State, *VS* Vegetative State, *BD* Brain Death, *LIS* Locked-In Syndrome

age to the frontal lobe or by the interruption of the complex frontal-subcortical circuits by stroke or degenerative disease [24]. In AM, differently from MCS, speech and movements may be facilitated by exposure to high-intensity sensory or personally salient stimuli.

LIS is a rare and severe condition caused by damage to cortico-spinal and cortico-bulbar pathways due to brainstem lesions. Patients are conscious but cannot respond or move; all voluntary muscles are paralysed, except those used for vertical eye movements and blinking. LIS can be misdiagnosed if the loss of speech and movements is attributed to consciousness impairment. Furthermore, in some cases, LIS may appear to be a VS or MCS at the acute stage, and may only subsequently evolve into the classic LIS features [12]. Most patients in a LIS show an EEG wake pattern similar to that of normal individuals, with preserved consciousness. Thus, the EEG pattern observed in LIS must not be interpreted as an alpha coma pattern and EEG findings may be helpful in differentiating LIS from coma (Table 46.2).

46.4 Clinical Examination of Comatose Patients

Although the clinical definition of coma is universally accepted, the set of causes that underlie this complex condition and the lesion sites are wide, which justifies the great corollary of possible clinical manifestations. Moreover, a careful clinical examination can often be very useful in individuating, with sufficient precision, the level of the lesion.

It is easy to understand that the first clinical approach to a comatose patient depends strictly on the most probable cause of coma (traumatic, metabolic, anoxic, etc.) and the length of time since the condition has been established, which should not be deduced from only a general physical examination. Alterations in body temperature (fever or hypothermia), cardiac activity and blood pressure, skin appearance, and the breath odor are important to the physician when addressing the possible causes of coma. For instance, the presence of multiple contusions and cerebrospinal fluid otorhinorrhaea are suggestive of traumatic injury; cyanosis indicates hypoxia; petechiae are characteristic of systemic infections or haematological diseases; blood pressure and heart rate may be altered in the case of endocranial hypertension; certain breath odors may be suggestive of renal or hepatic dysfunction or alcohol intoxication. Furthermore, the presence of rigor nucalis should always be investigated, in addition to all other signs of meningeal irritation. Neurological examination should, therefore, test the functionality of the main systems involved in the maintenance of consciousness and, at the same time, identify any other localising signs. In comatose patients, the hemispheres can only be examined by assessment of responses to sound, touch and nociceptive stimuli [25]. The state of consciousness is assessed by the responsiveness to environmental stimuli. Two important aspects of the state of consciousness must be evaluated: the level of consciousness, depending on the patient's ability to awake and the content of consciousness, depending on the relevance of the patient's responses. In assessing the level of consciousness, it is necessary to determine the intensity of the stimulation required to arouse the patient: the grading system, from verbal responsiveness to localising responses, non-localising responses and no response, is all needed for the initial assessment of the depth of unresponsiveness, used also to monitor the progress of the clinical status. In case of no response to voice or vigorous shaking, a painful stimulus should be applied to obtain information regarding the laterality of the motor response. It should begin with a modest, lateralised stimulus (compression of the nail beds, the supraorbital ridge, the temporomandibular joint) performed bilaterally and, in the case of no response, a more vigorous midline stimulus may be given in the form of a sternal rub [17]. Patient responses are noted and graded in the specific sections of the Glasgow Coma Scale (GCS). An essential part of neurological examination, especially for its high value in localising brainstem lesions, is the evaluation of cranial nerves and breathing patterns. The most important aspects are: pupillary shape, reaction, and diameter; ocular movements; oculovestibular reflexes. Pupil dilation is mediated by the orthosympathetic innervation of the iris from the superior cervical ganglion. The preganglionic neurons are located in the cervical part of the spinal cord and are under the control of tonic excitatory signals from the hypothalamus. In case of diffuse alterations of the forebrain, the pupils are myotic but reactive to light. Pons lesions can result in a marked myosis with preserved pupillary reactions, due to interruption of the pathways that mediate their dilation; opioids can cause myosis with reactive pupils. The loss of pupillary responses to light is almost always caused by structural changes. Pupils are intermediate (diameter slightly larger than normal) and fixed (unreactive to light) in lesions of the pretectal area of the midbrain, while lesions of the third cranial nerve in the midbrain cause the complete loss of pupillary responses, due to interference with both the descending orthosympathetic system - crossing the midbrain laterally to the nuclei of the third nerve - as well as the parasympathetic system. Unilateral mydriasis can occur from oculomotor nerve injury in the midbrain, since the pupil that loses parasympathetic with preserved orthosympathetic control has a larger diameter than the contralateral. The most common causes of unilateral compression of the oculomotor nerve in comatose patients are attributable to aneurysms of the posterior communicating artery or to the compression of the third cranial nerve by temporal lobe herniation through the tentorium (uncal herniation) [16]. Finally, diencephalic injuries typically result in small and reactive pupils; since this shape is also seen in most types of metabolic encephalopathy, it has limited value in identifying structural causes of coma [15]. The pathways that mediate eye movements run parallel to the RAS at the level of the paramedian tegmentum of the upper part of the brainstem. In comatose patients, the study of oculomotor responses has great value for localisation. Spontaneous and evoked eye movements should be observed. Slow roving eye movements are typical of metabolic encephalopathy and, if conjugate, are expression of an intact ocular motor system. Conjugate lateral deviation of the eyes is typically observed with destructive or irritative lesions: in the former case, the lesion generally involves the frontal eye fields and causes an homolateral deviation of the eyes; in the latter case, the same cortical injury may cause deviation of the eyes away from the side with the lesion, as the result of epileptic activity [15]. The interruption of descending cortico-bulbar pathways for gaze control, passing through the thalamic internal medullary lamina, rather than the internal capsule, may produce "wrong-way eyes", which deviate away from the side with the lesion [26]. Conjugate vertical deviation of the eyes may be due to lesions of the tectal nuclei. Nonconjugate eye deviation, generally with concomitant strabismus, can be a result of monolateral lesions of oculomotor cranial nerves of the medial longitudinal fasciculus (near the midline tegmentum) on that side, between the abducens and oculomotor nuclei. Bilateral lesions of the medial longitudinal fasciculus impair adduction of both eyes, as well as vertical oculocephalic and vestibulo-ocular eye movements, a condition different from bilateral oculomotor nucleus or nerve injuries, with the preservedpupillary light responses [15]. In light of the above considerations, eye movements in a comatose patient can be summarised as follows: spontaneous roving eye movements, indicating the integrity of the brainstem; skewed deviation, suggesting a brainstem lesion; forced deviation of the eyes to one side, generally indicating an ipsilateral hemispheric or contralateral pons lesion; eye deviation away from the side of the lesion, due to seizures [18].

The oculocephalic reflex is tested in comatose - or severely lethargic - patients by keeping their eyes open and briskly rotating the head side-to-side and up–down. The nerves involved in this reflex, known as the "doll's eyes reflex", are the oculomotor nerves and the eighth pair of cranial nerves. If the brainstem is intact, such as in comatose patients due to metabolic encefalopathy, the eyes rotate conjugately in the opposite direction to the head movement. If brainstem gaze centres are damaged, this reflex is reduced or absent [17, 27]. Therefore, "doll's eye reflex" observation in comatose patients indicates brainstem integrity.

Oculovestibular testing with cold/warm (than body temperature) water infusion is a simple test to check integration of ocular and vestibular pathways. After trauma to the external ear canal and tympanum have been excluded, the patient's head should be placed at 30° up from horizontal, and cold/warm water infused into the external auditory canal. In a comatose patient with an intact lower midbrain and pons, eyes will tonically and conjugately deviate towards the side of the cold irrigation and away from the side of the warm irrigation [18, 28]. Normally, evoked conjugate eye movements while testing the reflex indicate that the centres of horizontal gaze and median longitudinal fasciculi are intact. A brainstem lesion interrupting the medial longitudinal fasciculus will instead result in the disconjugated abduction of the eye ipsilateral to the cold irrigated ear, but in failure to the adduction of the opposite eye. Conplete absence of oculovestibular responses, not related to drugs intoxication, is a sign of poor prognosis in coma [14, 29, 30].

Breathing patterns should be carefully evaluated, to identify the coma depth. Gradual deterioration from the periodic breathing (cluster or Cheyne-Stokes) to tachypnea and to irregular breathing and gasping with long, irregular apneic periods [14] may occur in the case of widespread supratentorial lesions, deep bilateral brain lesions and metabolic diseases. The Cheyne-Stokes periodic pattern has been attributed to the isolation of the breathing centres of the brainstem, which renders them more sensitive to CO_2. As the result of hyperventilation, blood CO_2 levels fall below the concentration required to stimulate the regular breathing centres, and breathing gradually stops; CO_2 is then increased during the apnea exceeding the respiratory threshold, and the cycle starts over again. When this pattern is present, it is usually not considered a sign of poor outcome, unless other types of pathological breathing, indicating the presence of structural damage to the brainstem, appear. Lesions of the inferior part of the midbrain or of the pontine tegmentum can cause a central neurogenic hyperventilation, characterised by an increase in the respiratory frequency (>40 acts per minute) and in the depth of the breathing, resulting in alkalosis. This pattern suggests the release of the reflex mechanisms responsible for respiratory control in the lower part of the midbrain. Lower pontine lesions may cause an apneustic breath (a pause of 2–3 s following a full inspiration). In the case of injuries to the dorso-medial part of the bulb, the respiratory rhythm becomes chaotic, irregularly interrupted and each breath varies according to frequency and depth (Biot's breathing pattern) [26], considered a sign of poor prognosis.

Motor responses to pain stimulation is a fundamental indicator of the anatomical site of the brain lesion. An asymmetrical motor response may be suggestive of damage to one cerebral hemisphere. This reflects the importance of performing a bilateral stimulation, since the paralysed limb, often lying extrarotated on the bed, may not respond to the nociceptive stimulus (e.g. in hemiplegia); in this case, stimulation of the sole of the foot can evoke the Babinski sign.

Lesions of the upper part of the midbrain are often clinically characterised by a decorticated posture, both at rest as well as after nocicpetive stimulus, with the upper limbs flexed and the lower limbs extended with toes flexed downwards.

On the other hand, lesions in the lower part of the midbrain or in the upper part of the pons are characterized by a decerebrated posture, with extension of both the upper and lower limbs. The anatomical dividing line between these two postures, decorticated and decerebrated, is the red nucleus in the ventromedial part of the midbrain, responsible for the control of muscle tone in flexor muscle groups of the upper limbs: in a patient with a decorticated posture the red nucleus is intact. Clinical evolution from a decorticated to a decerebrated posture is generally associated with a poor prognosis, since it suggests a rostro-caudal degeneration of the brainstem [16].

Despite the several types of brain injuries that can be responsible for coma, the mechanisms causing consciousness alteration are essentally two: a) the direct damage extension to the diencephalon and midbrain and b) more frequent, the lateral and downward displacement of the subthalamic structures and upper part of the brainstem, with or without herniation of the medial part of the temporal lobe through the tentorium. The term *herniation* refers to the dislocation of a part of the cerebral or of the cerebellar hemispheres from their normal position to an adjacent compartment, at transfalcial or transtentorial level. Transtentorial herniations are classified in: a) central herniation, with downward dislocation and bilateral compression of the upper portion of the brainstem; b) unilateral dislocation of the medial temporal lobe, including the uncal gyrus, through the tentorial opening. The unilateral herniation causes the "uncal syndrome", characterised in the early stages by somnolence with unilateral pupillary dilation, usually homolateral to the mass provoking the dislocation of other structures and consequent to the compression of the oculomotor nerve by the uncal gyrus or by its stretching or deviation over the clivus or against the posterior cerebral artery. The time of dislocation development has important clinical and prognostic value; in case of acutely developed masses (tumours with important cerebral oedema, intraparenchymal haematomas), a 3–5 mm horizontal dislocation is associated with a soporous state, a 5–8 mm displacement with stupor, and a displacement greater than 8–9 mm with a coma state [15, 16]. Other types of herniations are represented by: dislocation of cerebellar hemispheres (tonsillar herniation) through the foramen magnum, with the typical clinical manifestations of diseases of the posterior cranial fossa (neck pain, rigor nucalis, head inclination, dysphagia, alterations in heart rhythm and breathing); subfalcial herniation characterised by displacement of the brain (typically the cingulate gyrus) below the free edge of the falx cerebri, due to raised intracranial pressure; ascending transtentorial herniation, in which SOLs in the posterior cranial fossa cause an upper displacement of the superior parts of the cerebellum through the tentorial notch [31].

Acute Intracranial Hypertension Syndrome (AIHS) deserves a separate mention for its clinical and prognostic relevance, being a medical emergency that requires prompt diagnosis and management. AIHS is defined as the persistent increase of Intra Cranial Pressure (ICP) above 20 mm/Hg, for longer than 5 min and in a patient who is not being stimulated. AIHS commonly occurs in acute brain injury related to trauma, ischaemia or haemorrhage and it is associated with a poor outcome, regardless its etiology [32, 33]. Intra Crania Hypertension (ICH) has been sistematically categorised in four categories, according to the aetiology and pathogenic mechanisms: parenchymatous ICH with an intrinsic cerebral cause; vascular ICH caused by altered cerebral blood circulation; ICH caused by altered cerebrospinal fluid dynamics; and idiopathic [34]. A coma preceded by headache, recurrent vomiting, marked hypertension, papillary oedema, and retinal haemorrhages is expression of ICH, often due to cerebral haemorrhage or to rapidly evolving SOLs, such as glioblastoma and cerebral lymphoma. The early diagnosis of these presenting signs and symptoms is important to allow a sudden medical and/or surgical intervention and to avoid the evolution of a deep coma.

46.5 Neurobehavioural Rating Scales

The *Glasgow Coma Scale (GCS),* created by Teasdale and Jennett in 1974 [35] in an attempt to bring uniformity to the clinical evaluation of disorders of consciousness, is the most widely used scale to assess the three aspects of a patient's responsiveness (eye, verbal, and motor) to external stimuli. The global numerical score obtained from this scale ranges from a maximum of 15 points (full consciousness) to a minimum of 3 points (deep coma). GCS is a very important tool for assessing coma severity, even though it loses its discriminative value in intubated and sedated patients. Furthermore, a criticism to GCS is the poor scoring of the brainstem functionality. Recently, to provide more information regarding the coma severity and prognosis in patients with traumatic brain injury, the arithmetic combination of *GCS scores with pupillary response* to light has been proposed (GCS-P) [36]. The Pupil Reactive Score (PRS) has a value of 2 points if both pupils are unreactive, 1 if only 1 pupil is unreactive and 0 if both pupils normally react to light. Since the total GCS score can range from 3 to 15, after PRS score subtraction from the GCS, the GCS-P has a possible range of values from 1 to 15. Another coma scale for the assessment of patients with consciousness disorders is the *Full Outline of Unresponsiveness (FOUR) score.* This coma scale has four testable components (eye response, motor response, brainstem reflexes and respiration) that can be rated even when in intubated patients. The resulting FOUR score is a good predictor of a poor outcome in a critically ill patient and can detect the occurrence of brain death [25, 37].

The *Glasgow Outcome Scale (GOS)* is the most widely used and accepted measure of outcome following head injury. In the first version of the GOS, patients with a brain injury can be divided into five categories on the basis of the objective degree of recovery: 1, death; 2, vegetative state; 3, severe disability; 4, moderate disability; 5, good recovery [38].

An *extended version of the GOS (GOS-E)* has been proposed, consisting of eight categories: 1, death; 2, vegetative state; 3, lower severe disability; 4, upper severe disability; 5, lower moderate disability; 6, upper moderate disability; 7, lower good recovery; and 8, upper good recovery [39]. The clinical scales for the evaluation of consciousness disorders are shown in Table 46.3.

46.6 EEG Patterns in Coma

To accurately describe the EEG of a comatose patient, several critical points, such as the characteristics of background activity (frequency, continuity and reactivity) and the presence of peculiar EEG patterns need to be taken into account, some of which have a specific prognostic value. With the purpose of uniforming and standardising the EEG description in critically ill patients, the American Clinical Neurophysiology Society recently published a reference paper for the EEG terminology in critical care [40].

46.6.1 Background Activity

Background EEG activity in comatose patients shows a diffuse or localised slowing, which progressively increases in relation to the degree of the encephalopathy responsible for consciousness impairment (Fig. 46.1). As coma state deteriorates, the background activity progressively decreases in amplitude until attenuation (period of activity >10 μV but <50% of the background voltage) or suppression (background activity <10 μV) of the cortical bioelectrical activity occurs (Fig. 46.2). These background changes in EEG are similar to those recorded when the depth of anaesthesia or sedation is increased; thus, the first characteristic to describe background activity is its *predominant frequency* (delta, theta, alpha, or beta) and distribution, with particular regards to its symmetry/asymmetry. A coma EEG tracing can be symmetrical or asymmetrical; *asymmetry* is defined as *mild* (<50% amplitude or 0.5–1 Hz frequency asymmetry) or *marked* (>50% amplitude or >1 Hz frequency asymmetry), and it must be present for most of the recording time (Fig. 46.3). Other important characteristics of the background activity are the *voltage* - classifiable as normal (>20 μV), low (10–20 μV), or suppressed (<10 μV) - and the *continuity.* The background continuity has a significant favourable prognostic value and, accordingly, a prolonged EEG recorded in ICU can be classified into five main categories (Fig. 46.4):

- Continuous—background activity uninterrupted by periods of attenuation or suppression.
- Near continuous—periods of attenuation/suppression <10% of the recording.
- Discontinuous—periods of attenuation/suppression from 11 to 49% of the recording.
- Burst-attenuation/burst-suppression—>50% of the recording is attenuated/suppressed.
- Suppression—the entire recording period contains suppression of background activity.

46.6.2 EEG Reactivity

EEG reactivity to visual, auditory and nociceptive stimuli should always be tested; it consists of changes in amplitude

Table 46.3 Clinical scales for the evaluation of consciousness disorders

Glasgow Coma Scale (GCS)	Score (min 3–max 15)	FOUR Scale	Score (min 0–max 16)	Glasgow Outcome Scale (GOS)	Glasgow Outcome Scale Extended (GOS-E)
Eye Response	4—Eyes open spontaneously 3—Eyes opening to verbal command 2—Eyes opening to pain 1—No eyes opening	Eye Response	4—Eyelids open or opened, tracking or blinking to command 3—Eyelids open but not tracking 2—Eyelids closed but open to loud voice 1—Eyelids closed but opens to pain 0—Eyelids remain closed with pain stimuli	Category number: 5—Good Recovery 4—Moderate Disability 3—Severe Disability 2—Vegetative State 1—Death	Category number: 8—Good recovery *Upper* 7—Good Recovery *Lower* 6—Moderate Disability *Upper* 5—Moderate Disability *Lower* 4—Severe Disability *Upper* 3—Severe Disability *Lower* 2—Vegetative State 1—Death
Verbal Response	5—oriented 4—confused 3—inappropriate words 2—incomprehensible sounds 1—No verbal response	Motor Response	4—Thumbs up, fist, or peace sign 3—localizing to pain 2—Flexion response to pain 1—Extension posture 0—No response to pain or generalized myoclonus status		
Motor Response	6—Obeys commands 5—Localizing pain 4—Withdrawal from pain 3—Flexion response to pain 2—Extension response to pain 1—No motor response	Brain Stem Reflexes	4—Pupil and corneal reflexes present 3—One pupil wide and flexed 2—Pupil or corneal reflexes absent 1—Pupil and corneal reflexes absent 0—Absent pupil, corneal, or cough reflex		
GCS—Pupils score (min 1—max 15)	GCS score: 2: both pupils unreactive 1: one pupil unreactive 0: pupils reactive	Respiration	4—regular breathing pattern 3—Cheyne-Stokes breathing pattern 2—Irregular breathing 1—Trigger ventilator or breathes above ventilator rate 0—Apnea or breathes at ventilator rate		

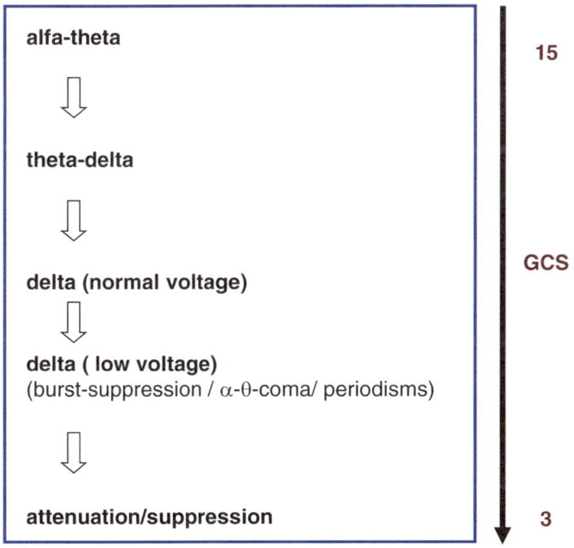

Fig. 46.1 Correlation between the progressive worsening of disorder of consciousness, as documented by Glasgow Coma Scale (GCS) score, and EEG changes

or frequency of the background activity, or in its attenuation. The EEG response to stimuli can be *present*, *absent*, or *unclear* (Figs. 46.5 and 46.6). The appearance of a muscle response or blinking after stimuli should not be considered a form of EEG reactivity. The absence of any reactivity is a sign of a poor prognosis, with the exception of toxic and iatrogenic coma; conversely, EEG reactivity preservation is considered a neurophysiological marker of a more favourable outcome.

The evaluation of EEG reactivity in critically ill patients is not always easy. Technicians should note and transmit all the information regarding the applied stimuli (e.g. modalities, time intervals) to the reporting physicians and monitor any reaction, such as muscle contractions, automatic eye movements, changes in cardiac and respiratory rhythm, and any other reflex and/or autonomic response directly or indirectly related to cortical activity. Pain stimuli are routinely included in the neurological examination of comatose patients (nasal tickling, trapezius squeeze, skin pinches, pressure to fingernail, nipple pinching), with nociceptive

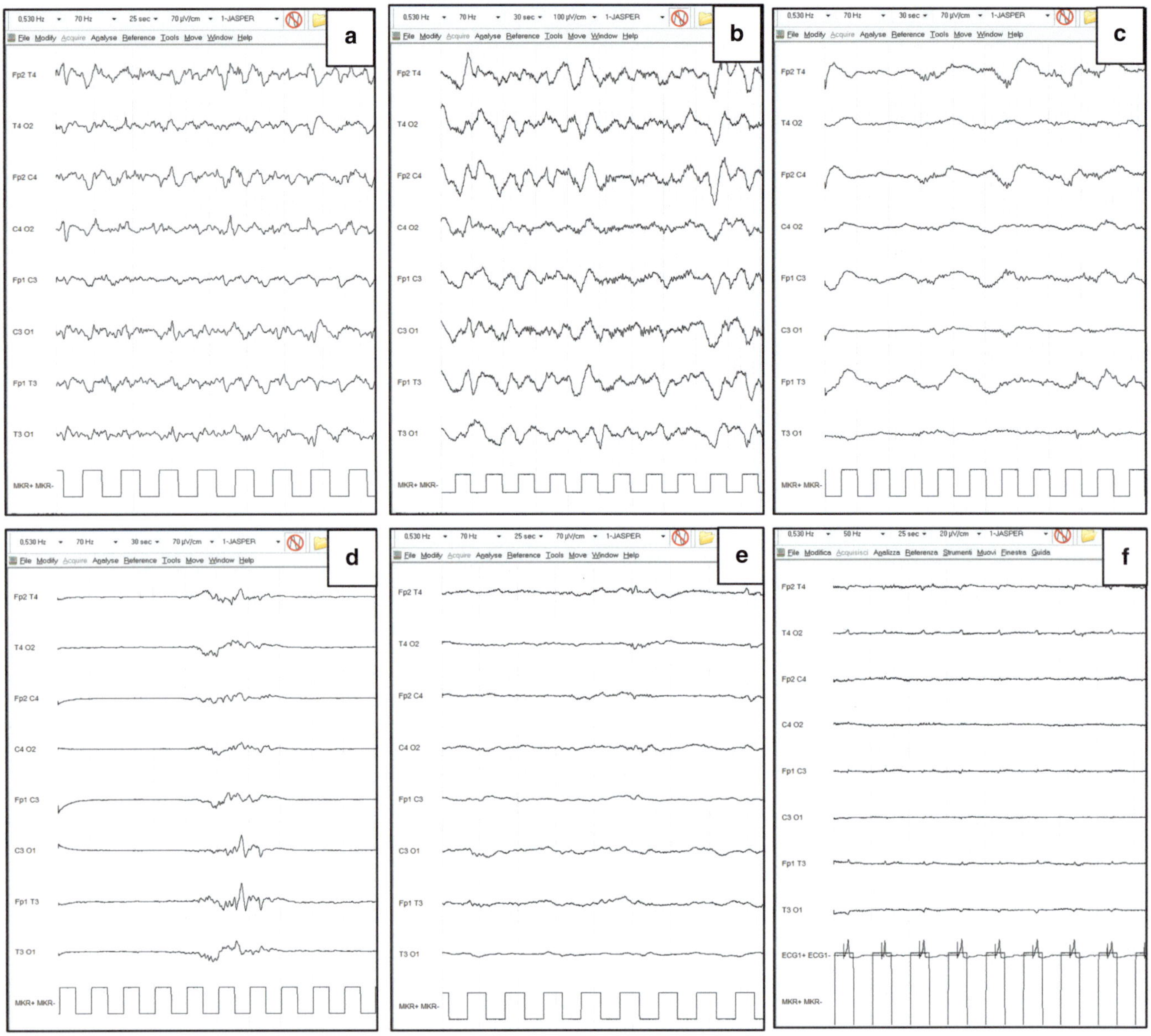

Fig. 46.2 Changes of background activity during various levels of coma. (**a**–**c**) continuous theta-delta diffuse activity progressively decreases in frequency, synchronisation and amplitude. As coma deepens, burst-suppression pattern appears (**d**) and then the background activity is attenuated (**e**) or completely suppressed (**f**)

stimuli appearing to best highlight EEG reactivity. Tsetsou et al. investigated the effects of standardised nociceptive stimuli in comatose patients unreactive to auditory stimuli, using three different painful stimuli: bilateral nipple pinching, nasal pinprick and bilateral fingernail compression. In this prospective study, it was demonstrated that bilateral synchronous nipple pinching appears to be the most nociceptive method to test EEG reactivity [41]. Admiraal et al. recently performed a systematic review aimed at identifying definitions of EEG reactivity and testing methods and found that many different protocols exist; however, the definition of EEG reactivity is neither uniform nor replicable. Therefore, standardisation of the stimulation protocol (stimuli used, duration and intensity of each stimulus) and a more precise definition of EEG reactivity are required [42]. Automated quantitative EEG approaches based on probabilistic description of spectral temporal symmetry potentially improve the objective evaluation of the EEG reactivity and thus assisting in the prediction of the clinical outcome [43].

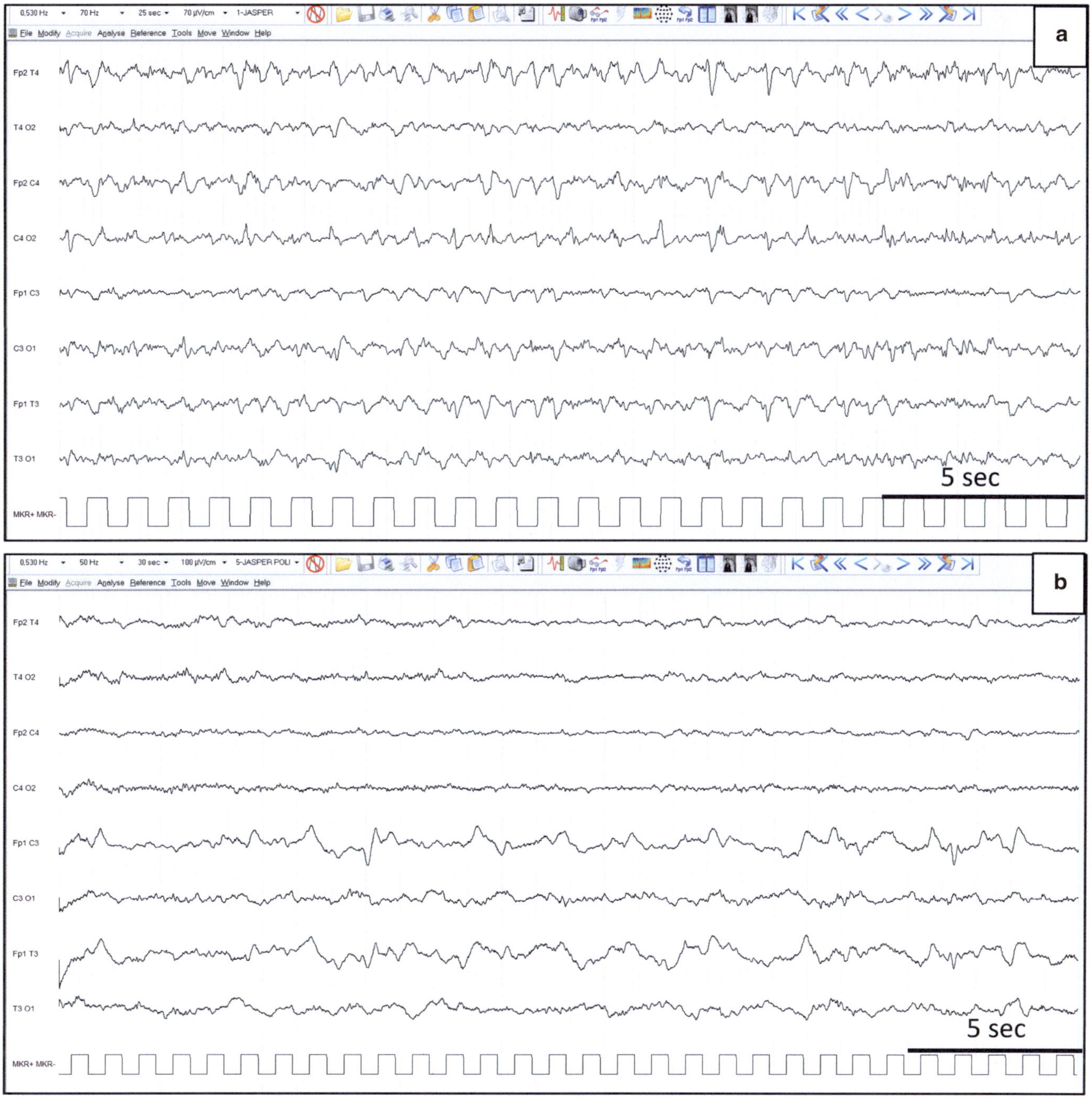

Fig. 46.3 EEG samples demonstrating a symmetric (**a**) or markedly asymmetric background activity (**b**). In (**a**) LFF = 0.53 Hz, HFF = 70 Hz, 70 μV/cm; in (**b**) LFF = 0.53 Hz, HFF = 50 Hz, 100 μV/cm)

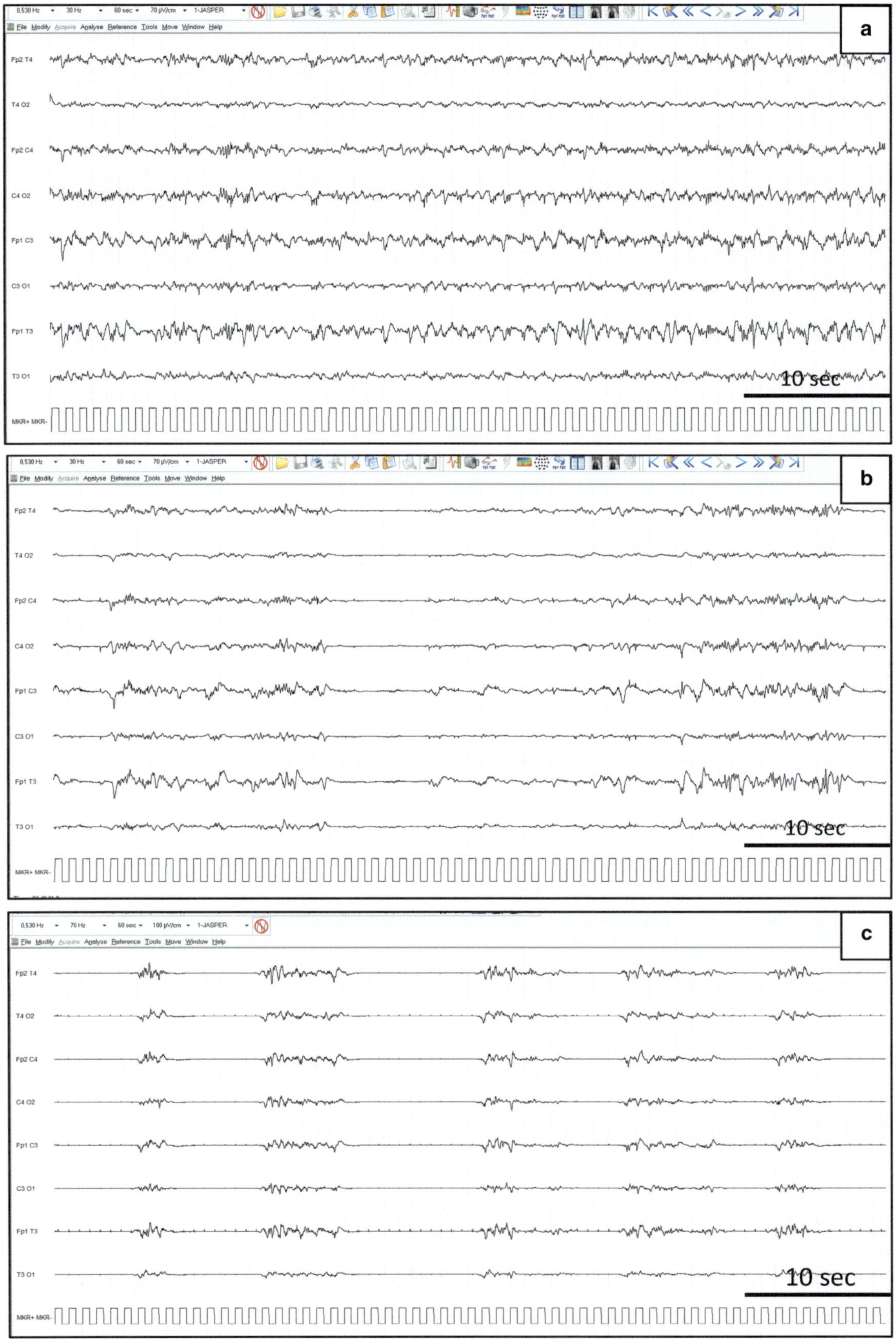

Fig. 46.4 Different types of background activity according to continuity: (**a**) continuous; (**b**) discontinuous; (**c**) burst-suppression. (**a** and **b**) LFF = 0.53 Hz, HFF = 30 Hz, 70 µV/cm. (**c**) LFF = 0.53 Hz, HFF = 70 Hz, 100 µV/cm

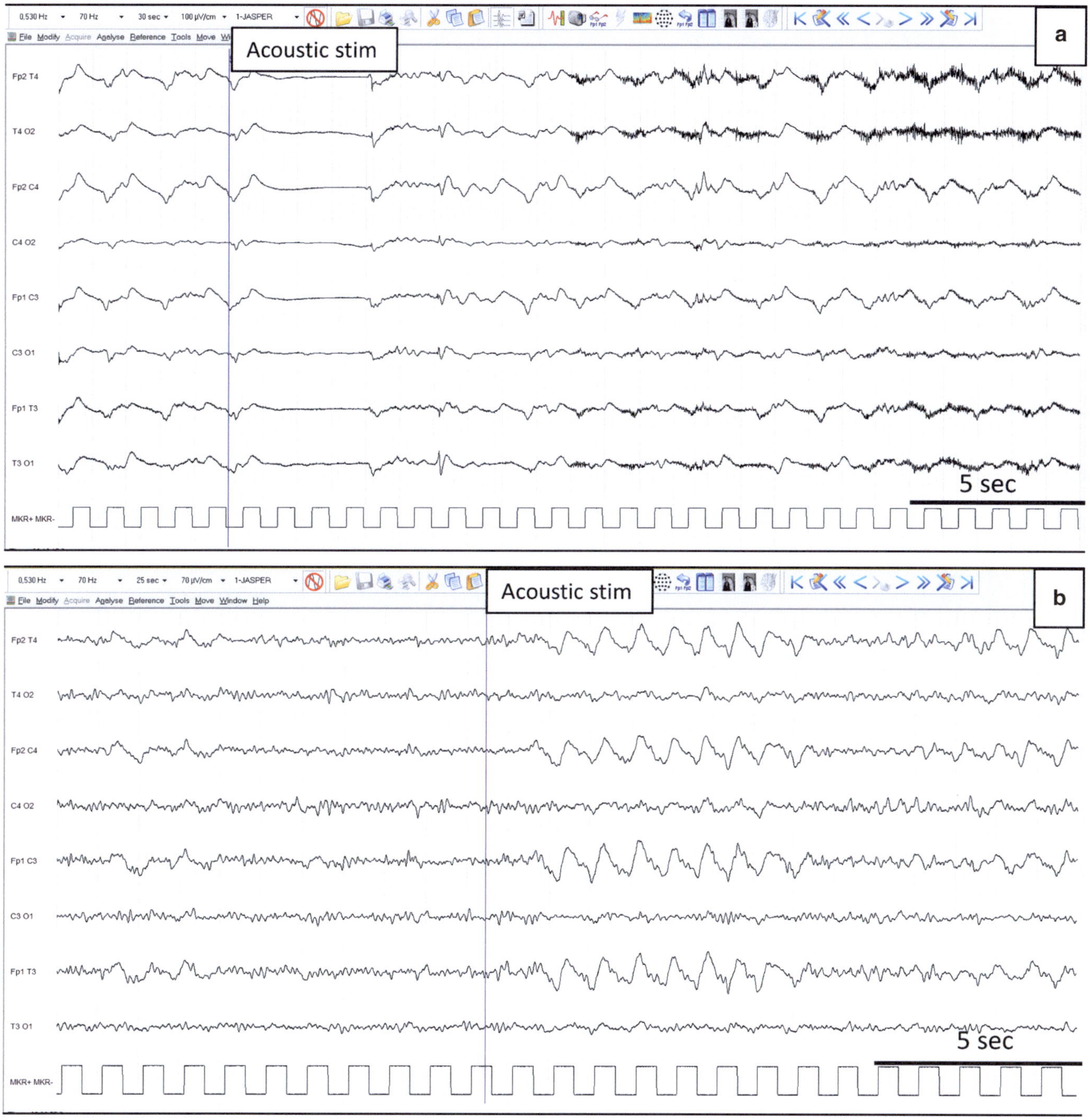

Fig. 46.5 EEG reactivity in comatose patients. In (**a**) the acoustic stimulus induces a short period of diffuse attenuation of tracing (LFF = 0.53 Hz, HFF 70 Hz, 100 μV/cm). In (**b**) the same stimulus induces a frontal intermittent rhythmic delta activity (LFF = 0.53 Hz, HFF = 70 Hz, 70 μV/cm)

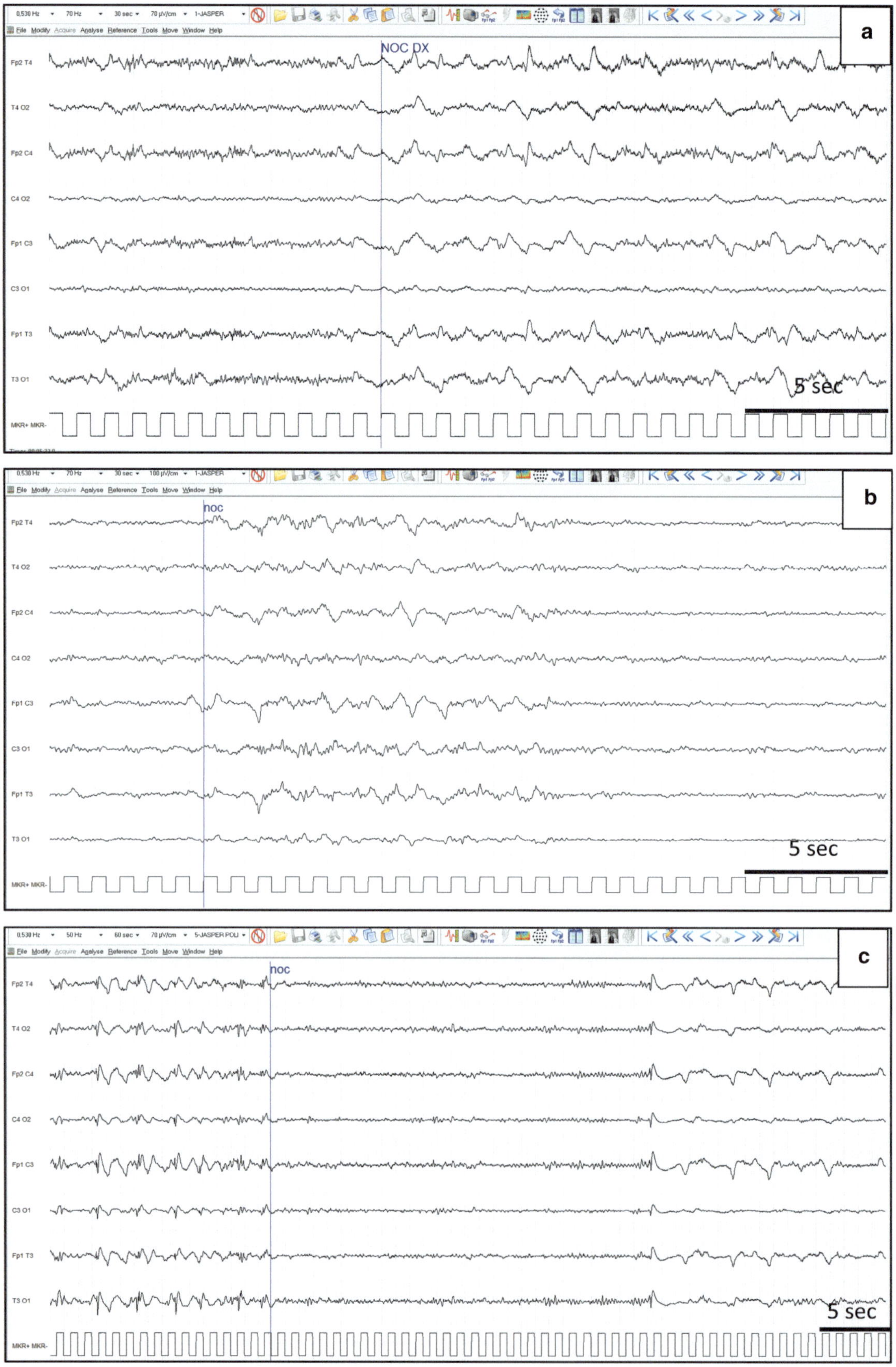

Fig. 46.6 Samples of EEG reactivity to nociceptive stimuli. In (**a** and **b**), the nociceptive stimulus induces the appearance of delta slowings predominant anteriorly, while in (**c**) pain induces a marked diffuse attenuation of tracing (**a**, LFF = 0.53 Hz, HFF = 70 Hz, 70 μV/cm; **b**, LFF = 0.53 Hz, HFF = 70 Hz, 100 μV/cm; **c**, LFF = 0.53 Hz, HFF = 50 Hz, 70 μV/cm)

46.6.3 Peculiar Coma EEG Patterns

46.6.3.1 Periodic and Rhythmic Patterns: Epileptiform Activity

The difference between periodic and rhythmic patterns is based on the presence or absence of an interval between two consecutive waveforms. Periodic activity is generally characterised by discharges, which are defined as waves with no more than three phases or any wave lasting 0.5 s or less (discharges are the opposite of bursts, which are defined as waveforms with at least four phases that last more than 0.5 s). Periodic discharges are therefore characterised by the repetition of a relatively uniform waveform at near regular intervals. Rhythmic EEG patterns are represented by the repetition of delta waves with relatively uniform morphology and duration, without an interval between the consecutive waveforms (Fig. 46.7).

It should be noted that, according to ACNS-standardised critical care EEG terminology [40], an EEG pattern can be qualified as periodic or rhythmic as long as the pattern continues for at least six cycles (1/s for 6 s or 3/s for 2 s).

Based on their localisation, periodic or rhythmic EEG patterns can be:

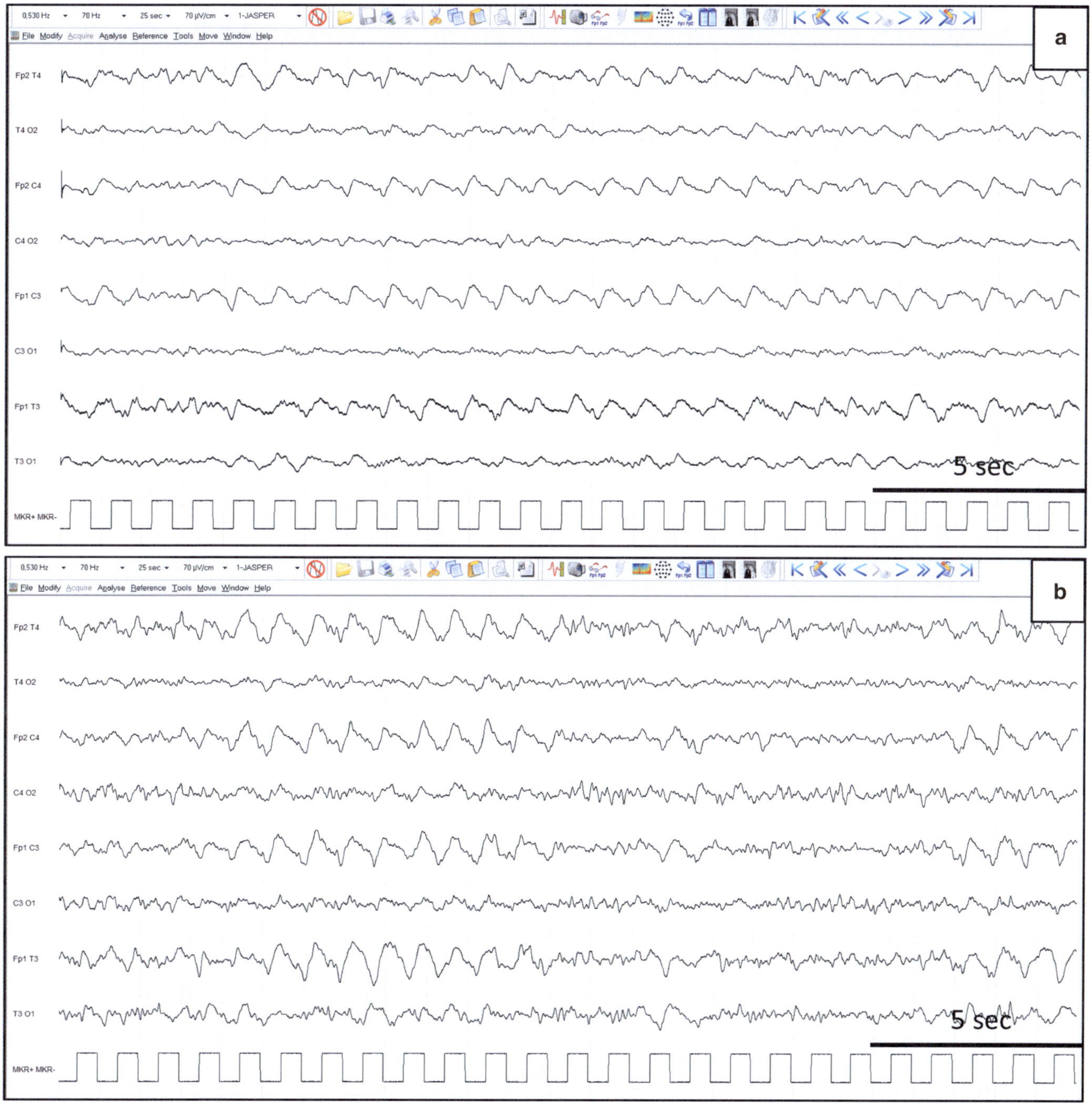

Fig. 46.7 Two samples of generalised rhythmic delta activity, predominant anteriorly. (**a** and **b**) LFF = 0.53 Hz, HFF = 70 Hz; 70 µV/cm

– Generalised (G: Bilateral, bisynchronous and symmetrical).
– Lateralised (L: Unilateral and bisynchronous, but asymmetrical, focal, regional, or hemispheric patterns).
– Bilateral Independent (BI: two asynchronous lateralised patterns, one in each hemisphere).
– Multifocal (Mf: at least three independent lateralised patterns in both hemispheres).

For generalised patterns, it is also necessary to include additional information regarding the predominant site of appearance (frontal, central, or occipital) while, for lateralised patterns, it is important to specify the symmetry vs. asymmetry and the most involved lobes (Figs. 46.8 and 46.9).

Epileptic activity in the EEG of comatose patients may also be recorded as polyspikes, spikes, or sharp waves followed by a slow wave in a regularly repeating and alternating pattern,

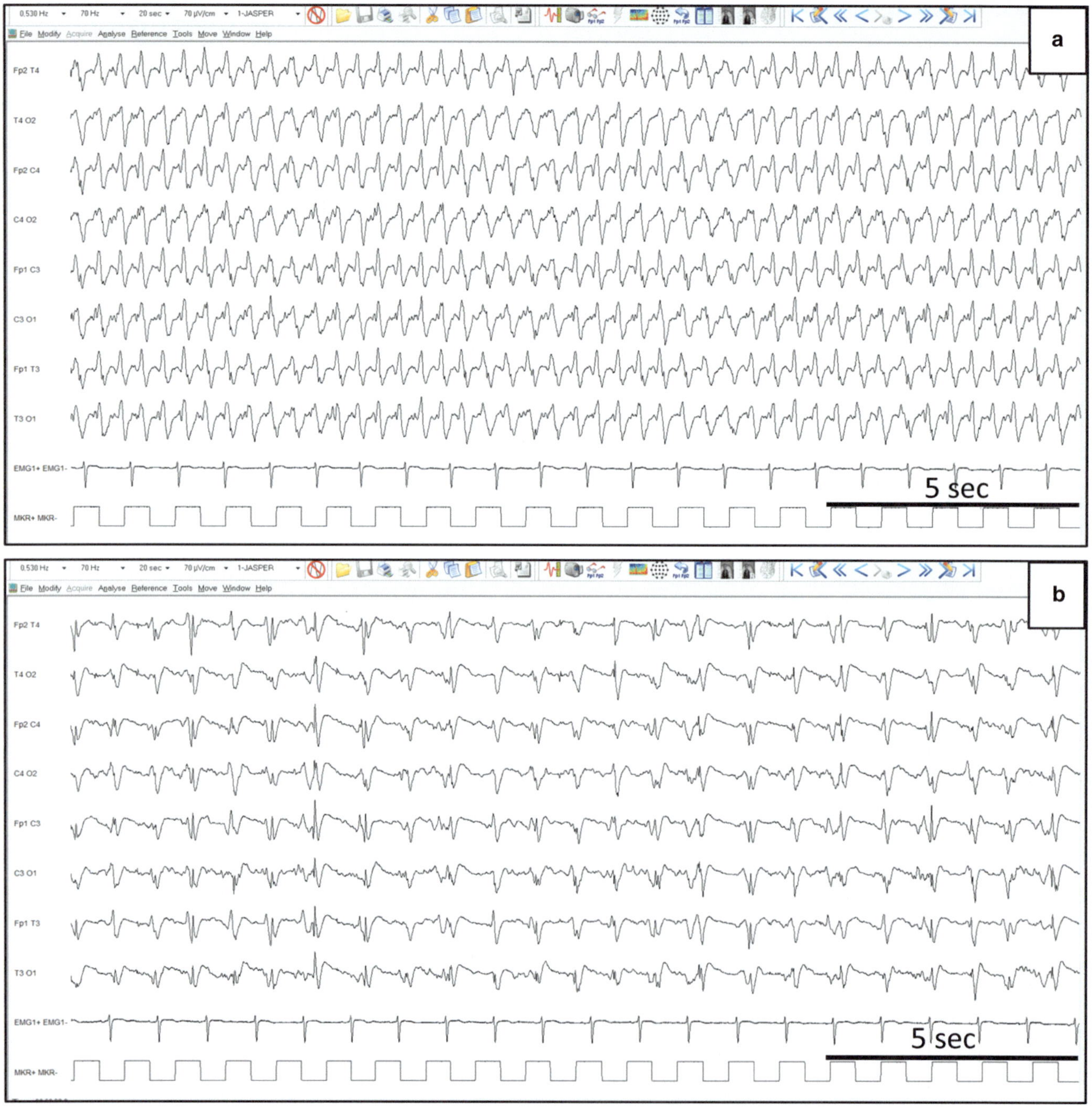

Fig. 46.8 Samples of Generalised Periodic Discharges (GPDs). In (**a**) the spiky GPDs are <0.5 per second, in (**b**) 1 per second (LFF = 0.53 Hz, HFF = 70 Hz, 70 µV/cm)

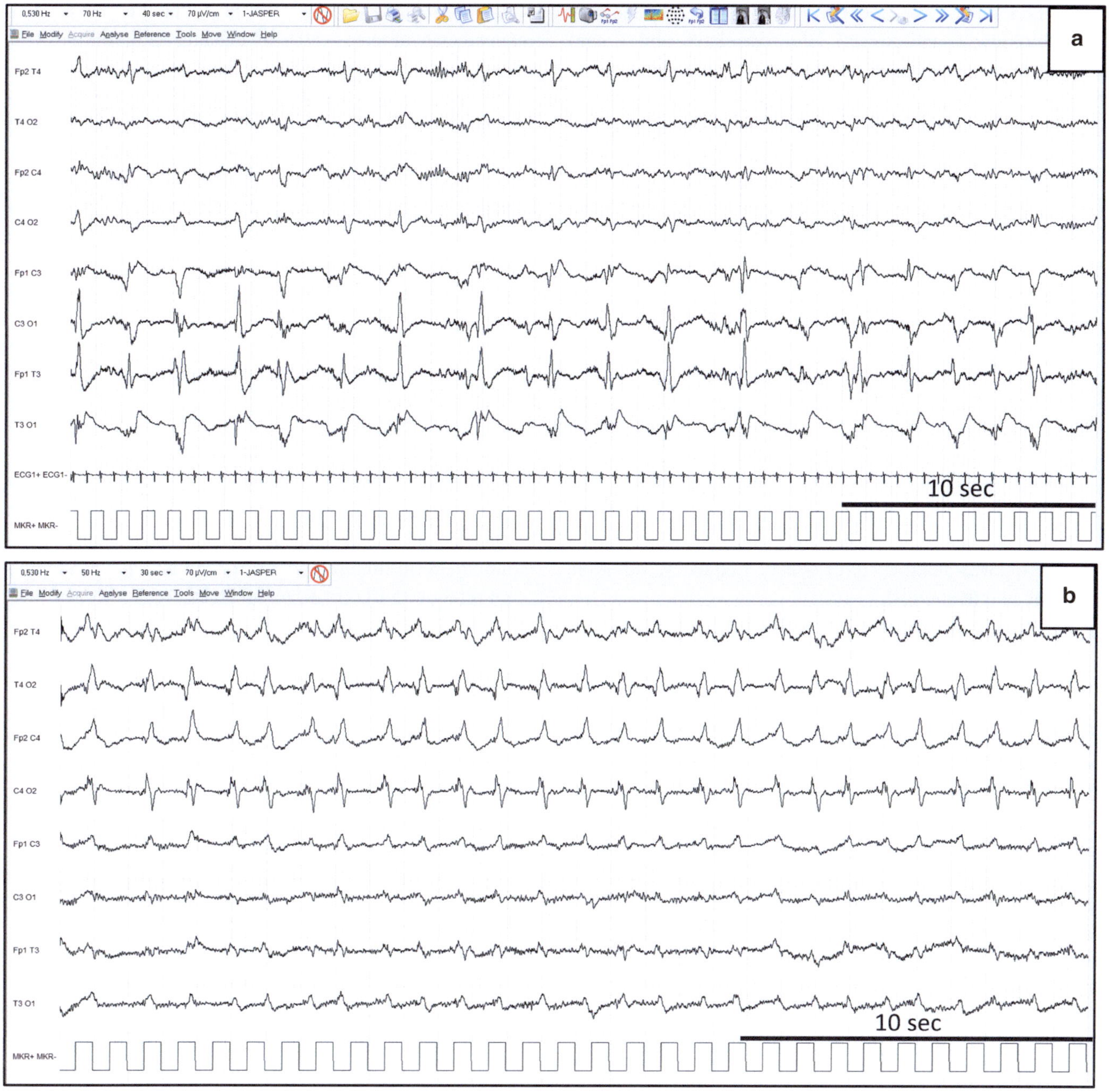

Fig. 46.9 Samples of left (**a**) and right (**b**) 0.5 to 1 per second spiky Lateralised Periodic Discharges (LPDs). LPDs are bilateral, synchronous but clearly asymmetric. (**a**, LFF = 0.53 Hz, HFF = 70 Hz, 70 μV/cm; **b**, LFF = 0.53 Hz, HFF = 50 Hz, 70 μV/cm)

without any interval between one complex and the next. Periodic and rhythmic EEG patterns and epileptic abnormalities have already been described in detail in Chap. 13.

A detailed EEG interpretation using standardised terminology is extremely important, especially in comatose patients. A large, multicentre study evaluating the effects of periodic and rhythmic patterns on seizure risk in critically ill patients highlighted that Lateralised Periodic Discharges (LPDs), Lateralised Rhythmic Delta Activity (LRDA), and Generalised Periodic Discharges (GPDs) are associated with seizures, unlike Generalised Rhythmic Delta Activity (GRDA) [44]. Punia et al. demonstrated that patients with LPDs on continuous EEG during coma are at least seven times more likely to develop epilepsy following an acute brain insult [45].

The definition and classification of Status Epilepticus (SE) by the International League Against Epilepsy (ILAE)

Task Force considers "EEG correlates" as one of four axes (1, semiology; 2, aetiology; 3, EEG correlates; and 4, age) and emphasises that EEG should be performed as early as possible [46].

The ILAE recommends using EEG in an emergency setting with repeated recordings, to highlight the eventual evolution of SE from one form to another. Currently, no evidence-based EEG criteria for SE exist, and none of the ictal EEG patterns of any type of SE are specific; however, EEG is considered indispensable in the diagnosis of Non-Convulsive SE (NCSE).

For the description of EEG patterns in SE, the ILAE Task Force [46] has proposed the following main parameters:

- Location (generalised, lateralised, bilateral independent, or multifocal).
- Type (periodic discharges, rhythmic delta activity, or epileptic activity).
- Morphology (sharpness, number of phases, amplitude, and polarity).
- Time-related features (prevalence, frequency, duration, onset, and dynamics).
- Modulation (spontaneous or stimulus-induced).
- Effects of drugs on the EEG.

Various EEG criteria have been used to identify comatose patients with NCSE, the true incidence of which still remains unknown. The original "Salzburg Consensus Criteria" were modified in accordance with the standardised critical care terminology of the ACNS [40, 47–49].

First, the EEG changes that fulfil the modified Salzburg criteria for NCSE should be continuously present for >10 s; these changes can be represented by Epileptiform Discharges (EDs: spikes, polyspikes, sharp waves, sharp-and-slow wave complexes; the frequency of EDs may be >2.5 or <2.5 Hz) or by Rhythmic Delta Activity (RDA: rhythmic activity <4 Hz; the duration of one cycle should vary by <50% from the duration of the subsequent cycle for the majority of cycle pairs to qualify as rhythmic) [40].

Other parameters defining EEG patterns of NCSE are:

Evolution: at least two unequivocal, sequential changes in frequency (at least two consecutive changes of at least 0.5/s, e.g. from 2 to 2.5/s or from 3 to 2/s), morphology (at least two consecutive changes to a novel morphology), or location (sequentially spreading into or out of at least two different IS 10–20 electrode locations). The criteria for evolution must be reached without the pattern remaining unchanged in frequency, morphology, or location for 5 min or longer [40].

Typical ictal spatio-temporal evolution, which consists of incrementing onset (increase in voltage and change in frequency), evolution of the pattern (change in frequency and location), or decrementing termination (voltage and frequency).

Fluctuation: >3 changes, not more than 1 min apart, in frequency (by at least 0.5/s); >3 changes in morphology; or >3 changes in location, which do not qualify as evolving.

Response to intravenous antiepileptic drugs (IV AEDs): the response to IV AEDs should be tested clinically and by EEG (Figs. 46.10 and 46.11). Clinical improvement is defined as the best performance in one of the following three domains: "say your surname", "repeat 1, 2, 3", and "raise your arms"; if the patient does not respond, the procedure must be repeated following strong tactile stimuli. EEG improvement is defined as a reduction in the pathological pattern to occasional, i.e. 1-9% of epochs.

In comatose patients without any known epileptic encephalopathy, at least one of the following criteria should be fulfilled for the diagnosis of NCSE:

1. EDs >2.5 Hz (i.e. >25 EDs in a 10-s epoch).
2. Typical ictal spatio-temporal evolution of EDs or RDA (>0.5 Hz).
3. Subtle ictal clinical symptoms (minor twitching of the mouth, periorbital region, or extremities) in close temporal relation to EDs or RDA >0.5 Hz.

If the EDs have a frequency <2.5 Hz or there is only RDA with or without fluctuations, the clinical situation should be carefully evaluated and the clinical and EEG response to IV AEDs should be documented. There are four possible responses: no clinical or EEG improvement, only EEG improvement, only clinical improvement, or EEG and clinical improvement. According to the modified Salzburg Consensus Criteria, for clinical practice, all four constellations qualify for NCSE, while for research projects, patients qualify for NCSE only if EEG and/or clinical improvement is documented (Fig. 46.12) [47, 48].

46.6.3.2 Spindle Coma and Beta Coma

The presence of normal sleep transients (i.e. vertex sharp waves, K-complexes, and spindles) in the slow EEGs of comatose patients with acute encephalopathy may be considered a prognostic biomarker for both survival and functional recovery. Chatrian et al. (1963) [50] first described an EEG pattern in patients with acute traumatic encephalopathy characterised by vertex wave, K-complex, and sleep spindle sequences (11–14 Hz), which was named "*spindle coma*". In patients with head injury, it has been hypothesised that the spindle coma may occur due to a pontomesencephalic junction lesion, with functional preservation of the cortex. This pattern was also later described in patients with non-traumatic coma [51] and it is recognised as having a good prognostic value. If the spindle coma pattern is reactive to external stimuli, the outcome is obviously better, although in most cases it remains uncertain; nevertheless, the prognostic value of this pattern is sometimes often uncertain, since the prognosis depends above all

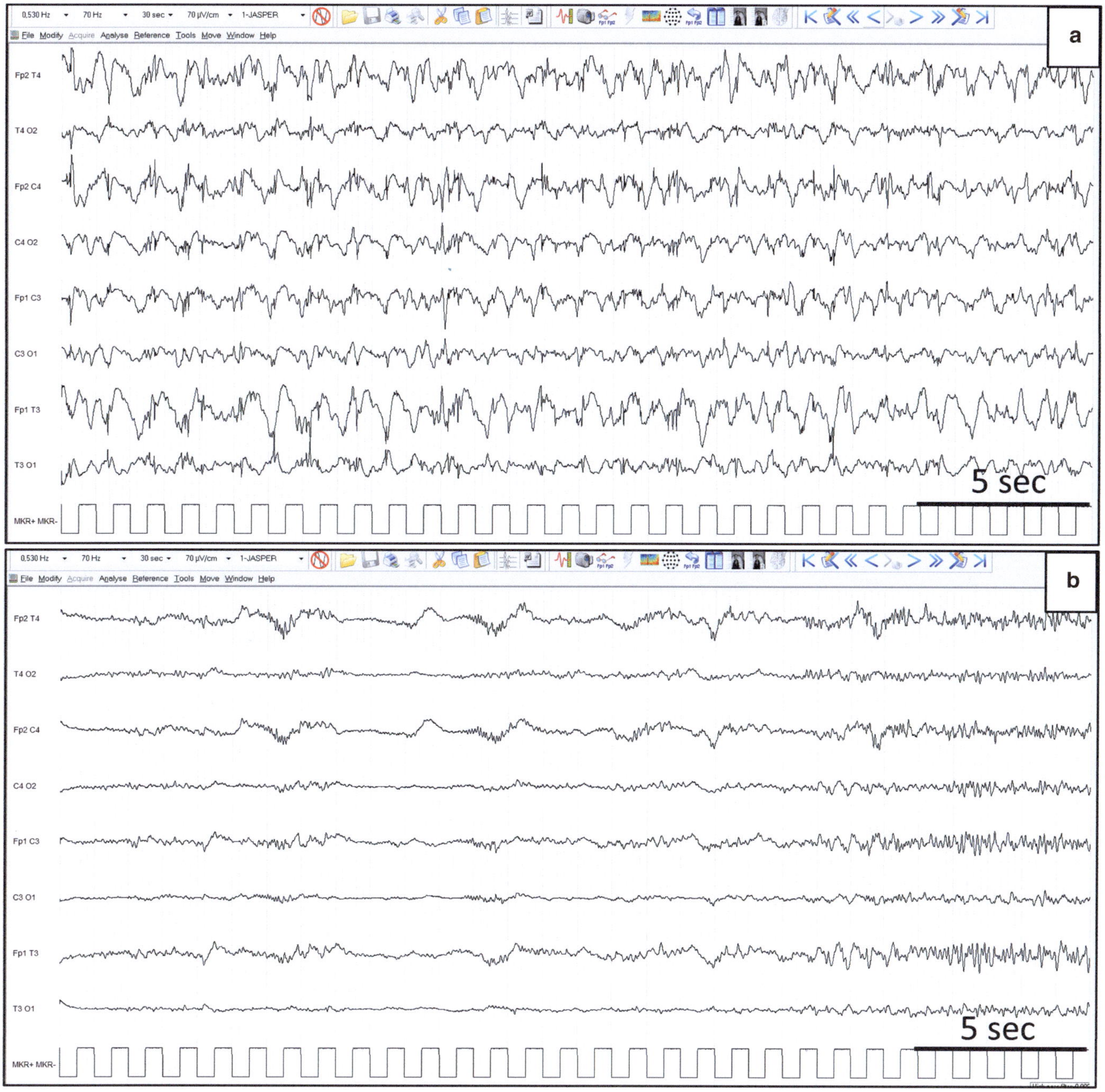

Fig. 46.10 (**a**) EEG pattern of Non-Convulsive Status Epilepticus (NCSE) in a 51-year-old patient with anoxic encephalopathy. In (**b**) EEG improved after a i.v. bolus of midazolam. LFF = 0.53 Hz, HFF = 70 Hz, 70 μV/cm

on the underlying aetiology of the coma [52]. A recent retrospective study investigating the early presence of sleep spindles in the cEEGs of 34 children in the first 24 h after resuscitation from cardiac arrest reported that spindles were recorded in approximately 30% of children and were associated with a favourable neurological outcome at 6 months [53].

The "*beta coma*" pattern is characterised by the presence of diffuse, frontally dominant, beta activity ranging from 12 to 16 Hz. This pattern is most commonly induced by intoxication or withdrawal from benzodiazepines or barbiturates [54], but it may also be the consequence of an acute brainstem lesion (Fig. 46.13).

46.6.3.3 Alpha, Alpha-Theta, and Theta Coma Patterns

The term Alpha Coma (AC) refers to an EEG coma pattern characterised by the presence of diffuse alpha frequency activity; when alpha activity is mixed with theta frequencies,

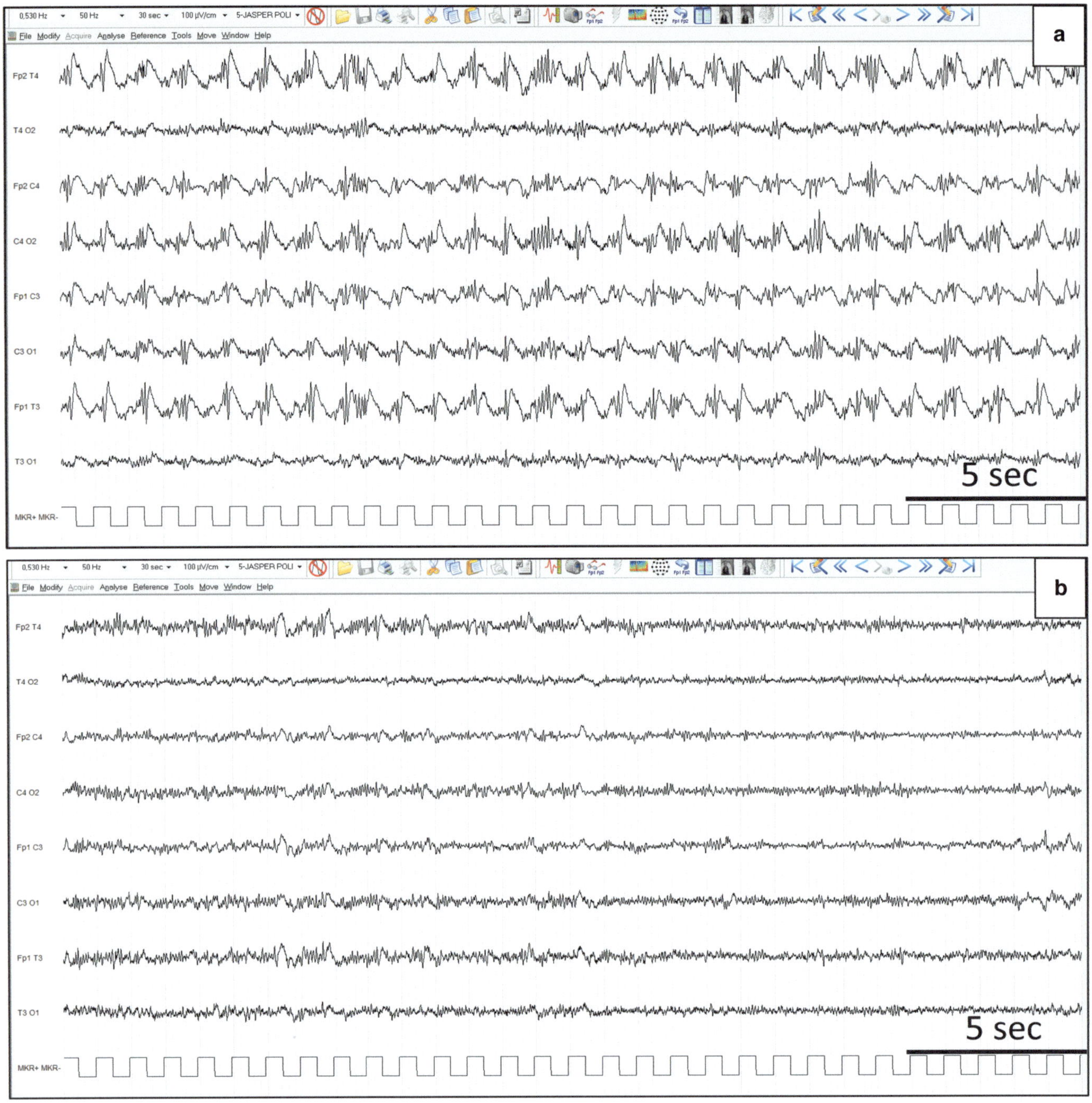

Fig. 46.11 Non-Convulsive Status Epilepticus (NCSE)in a 60-year-old epileptic patient (**a**). After a bolus of lorazepam (4 mg i.v.), epileptic activity disappeared (**b**). LFF = 0.53 Hz, HFF = 50 Hz, 100 μV/cm

the pattern is named Alpha-Theta Coma (ATC), whereas when the rhythmic diffuse activity falls within the theta band range, the pattern is named Theta Coma (TC) (Fig. 46.14).

The most well-known and studied pattern is AC, which was first described in 1953 by Loeb and Poggio in patients with pontomesencephalic haemorrhage [55] and, subsequently, in patients with other acute encephalopathies (anoxic, traumatic, toxic, and dysmetabolic) [56, 57]. An AC pattern following cardiac arrest or traumatic brain injury is characterised by a monomorphic and unreactive alpha activity with a frequency of 8–13 Hz and an amplitude of 10–50 μV, diffuse but predominantly in the frontal regions. If the activity is slower (4–7 Hz), the pattern is defined as ATC or TC. When the AC is due to toxic encephalopathies (overdoses of barbiturates, benzodiazepines, anaesthetics, or antidepressant drugs), beta frequencies may be superimposed on the alpha activity, which may sometimes be predominant in the posterior regions. Given the variety of causes, the AC pat-

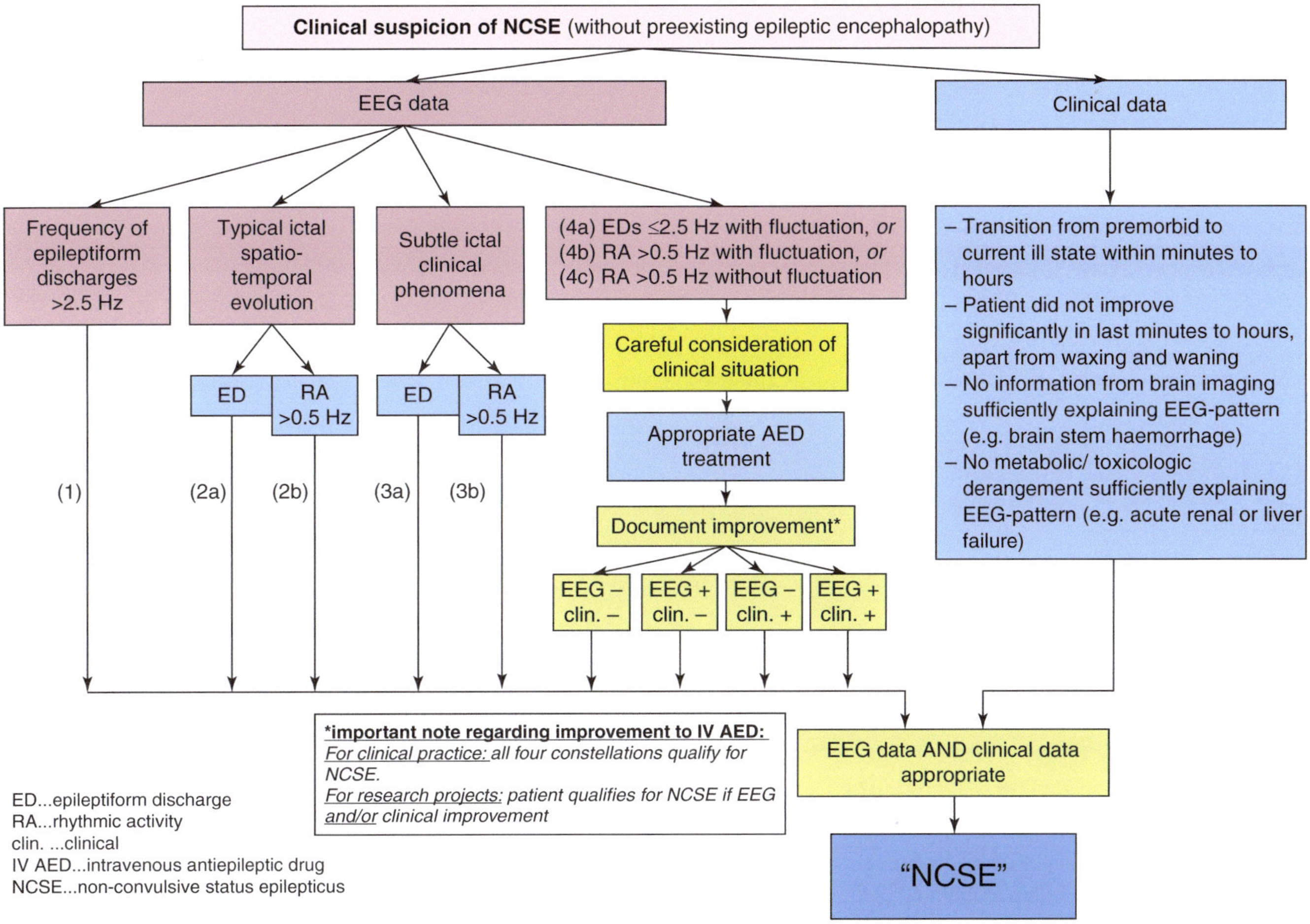

Fig. 46.12 Modified Salzburg criteria for the diagnosis of Non-Convulsive Status Epilepticus (NCSE). From: Trinka E, Leitinger M. Epil & Behav. 2015; 49: 203–222, with permission from Elsevier

tern likely arises from different pathophysiological interactions. In the case of brainstem lesions, there is a deafferentation of thalamo-cortical pathways releasing autonomous cortical alpha rhythm generated from the ascending RAS. A study comparing the alpha pattern between healthy subjects and comatose patients showed a lack of interhemispheric coherence in AC, supporting the hypothesis that when a significant thalamo-cortical disruption is determined, the cortical pacemakers operate independently in each hemisphere [58]. It has also been shown that alpha frequencies can be produced by different generators and networks in normal subjects and patients with AC [59]. Following diffuse cerebral hypoxia or diffuse post-traumatic brain lesions, the cortex is destroyed with preservation of thalamic and brainstem structures; in this case, the alpha activity recorded on the scalp originates from subcortical structures. Finally, drugs or sedatives at toxic doses may produce an AC pattern by a direct effect on cortical alpha generators, with or without impairment of ascending modulating inputs [56].

AC is generally considered a biomarker for poor prognosis; however, outcome also depends on the underlying aetiology of the coma (i.e. a poor prognosis for anoxia or trauma, but a better one for toxic or metabolic encephalopathies). Berkhoff et al. [57] performed a prospective study regarding clinical, EEG, and Somato Sensory-Evoked Potential (SSEP) findings in a series of patients with postanoxic ATC and also reviewed 283 cases of postanoxic ATC reported in the literature. These authors described two types of ATC: incomplete and complete. The *incomplete ATC* is characterised by occipital or diffuse, non-monotonous, hypo-reactive alpha activity; SSEP are usually normal and coma with usually normal brainstem reflexes. Conversely, the *complete ATC* is characterised by diffuse, frontally predominant, monotonous, reactive alpha activity; SSEP usually altered or absent and deep coma, with usually absent brainstem reflexes.

According to Berkhoff et al. [57], the combination of EEG, SSEP, and clinical findings improves the prognostic evaluation of postanoxic ATC; a full recovery is possible in patients with incomplete ATC, whereas complete ATC is invariably associated with a poor outcome. The prognostic significance of complete and incomplete variants of ATC has

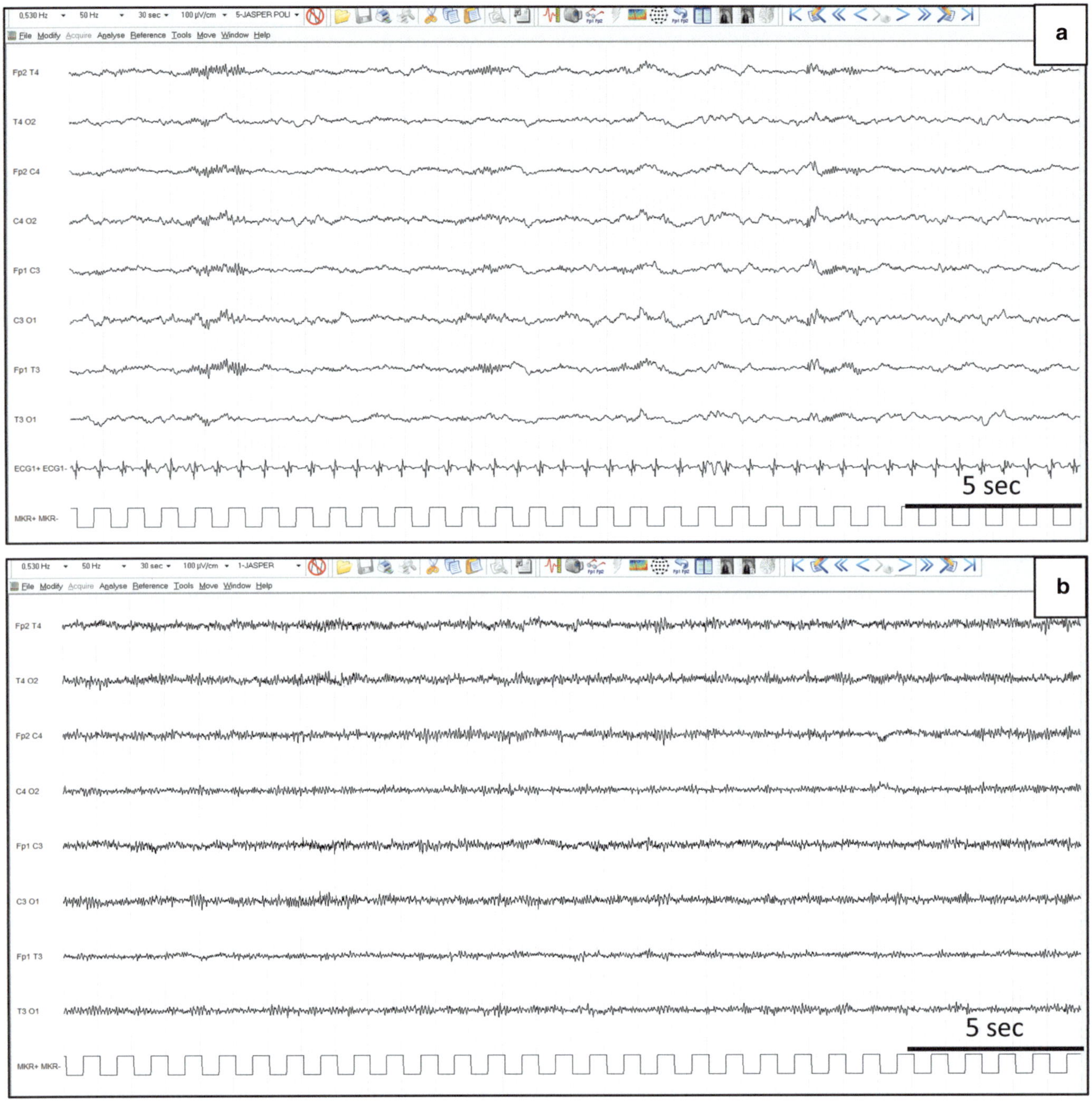

Fig. 46.13 Samples EEG demonstrating the spindle coma pattern (**a**) and the beta coma (**b**: BDZ intoxication). LFF = 0.53 Hz, HFF = 50 Hz; 100 μV/cm

been shown in many recent studies, almost always conducted in patients with postanoxic coma [60, 61].

46.6.3.4 Burst-Attenuation and Burst-Suppression Patterns

The classic definition of a burst-suppression pattern is: "an EEG pattern in which there are generalised and synchronous bursts of high-voltage and mixed-frequency activity alternating with periods of suppression of this activity" [54].

This pattern is observed in comatose patients with diffuse cerebral anoxia (following cardiac arrest), during hypothermia, or as a result of excessive dosage of anaesthetic agents or sedative drugs.

The standardised terminology for EEG in critical care proposed by ACNS [40] specifies the characteristics of the pattern: *bursts* must average more than 0.5 s, have at least four phases, which can last up to 30 s; *the interval between two bursts* may be with *attenuation* (periods of lower voltage

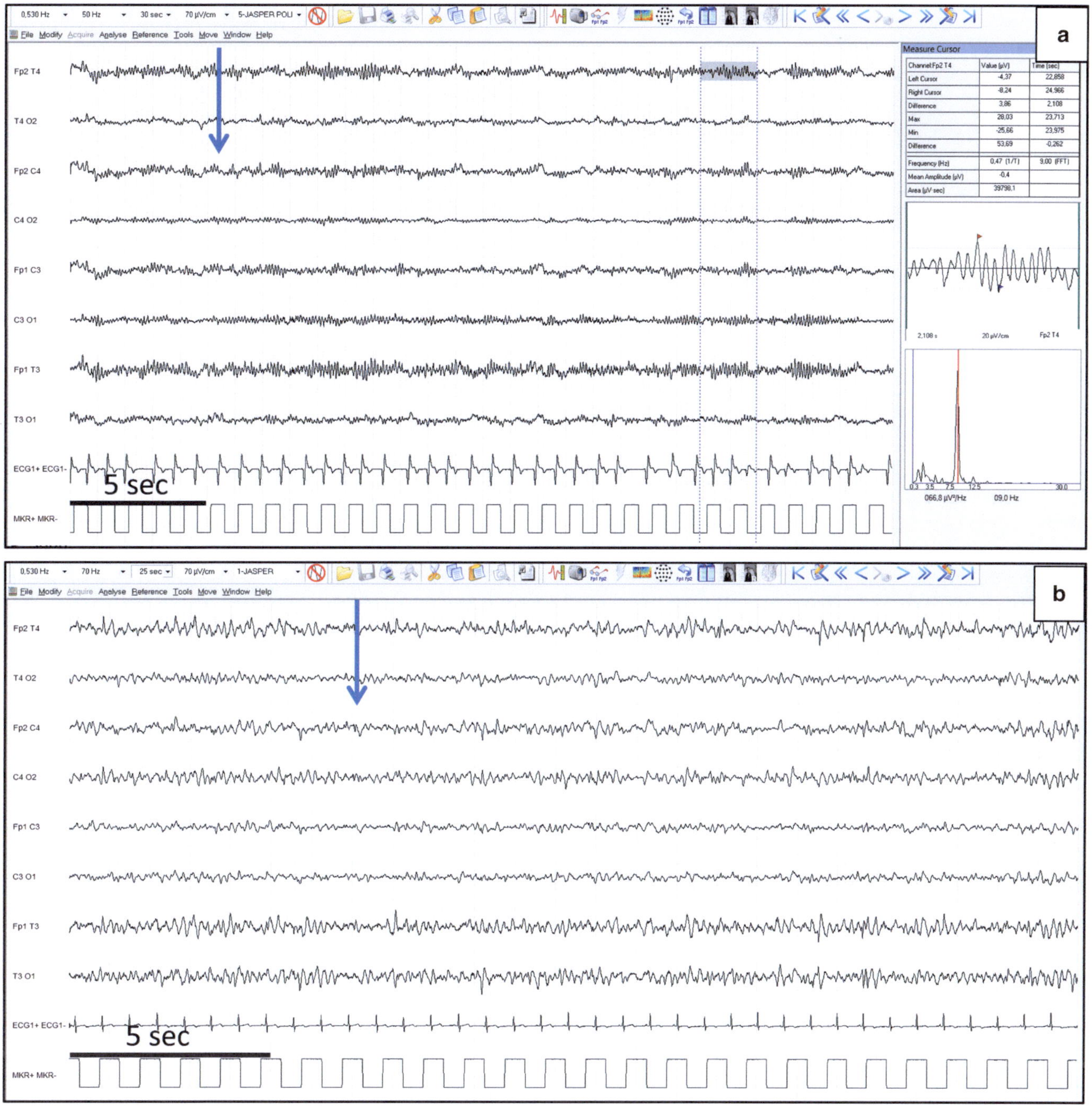

Fig. 46.14 (**a**) Frontally predominant unreactive (at arrow pain stimulus) alpha-coma in a 45-year-old patient with postanoxic encephalopathy. (**b**) unreactive theta coma in 67-year-old patient with post-traumatic encephalopathy. (**a**) LFF = 0.53 Hz, HFF = 50 Hz, 70 μV/cm; (**b**) LFF = 0.53 Hz, HFF = 70 Hz, 70 μV/cm

>10 μV but <50% of the background voltage) or with *suppression* (periods of lower voltage are <10 μV); to define a pattern of *burst-attenuation* or *burst-suppression*, it is necessary that more than 50% of the recording consists of attenuation or suppression, with alternating bursts. Furthermore, it is necessary to report the typical duration of the bursts and interburst intervals, morphology (sharpness) of a typical burst, and the presence or absence of highly epileptiform bursts.

Highly epileptiform bursts are considered present if multiple epileptiform discharges or rhythmic patterns (potentially ictal) occur within the majority (>50%) of bursts, at an average of 1/s or faster (Fig. 46.15).

In addition to ACNS classification, the EEG patterns with bursts may be subdivided into those with *identical bursts* and those without. Bursts are "identical" if they have the same amplitude, duration and shape in defined EEG epochs; inter-

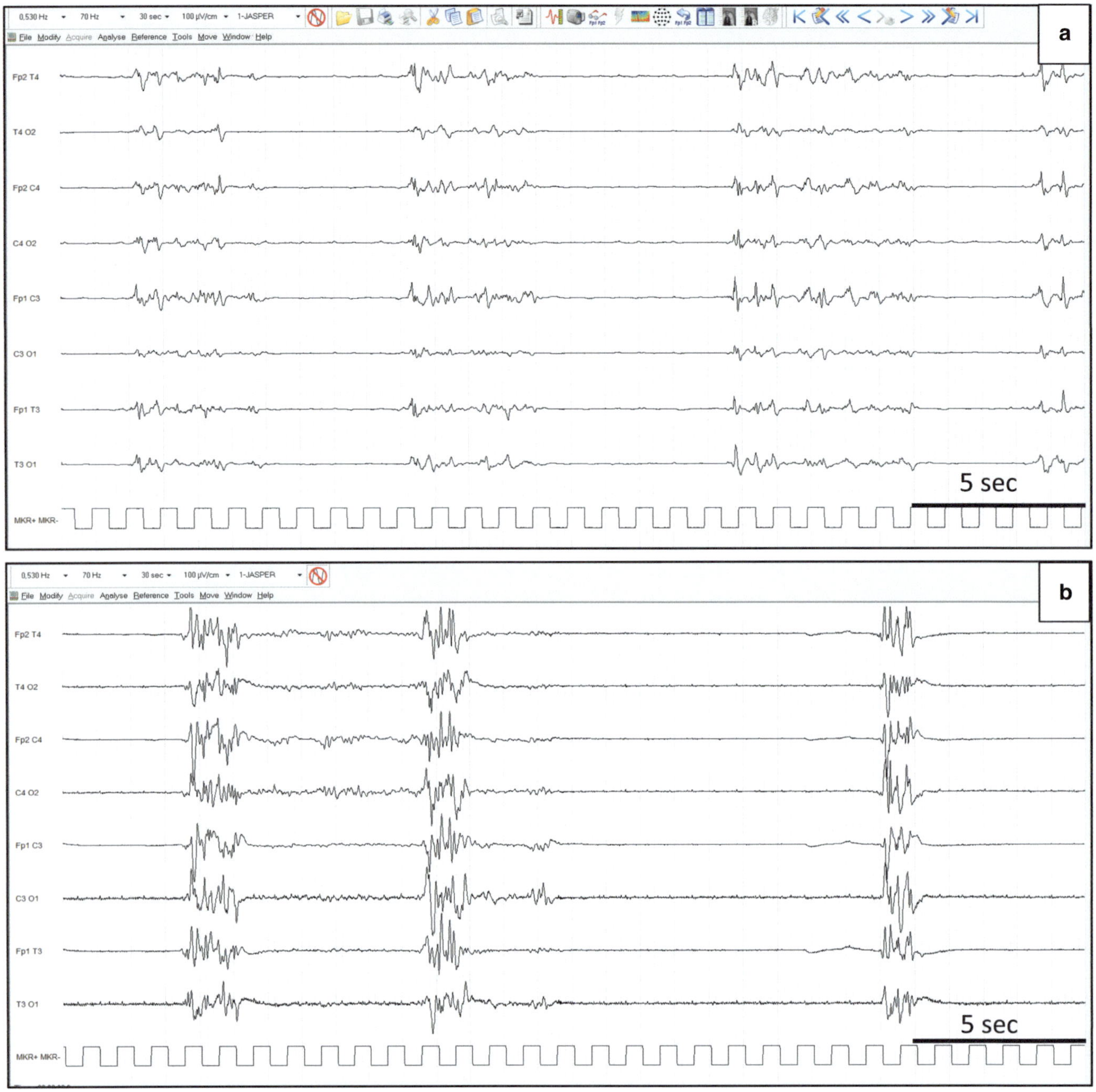

Fig. 46.15 Burst-suppression patterns. (**a**) bursts of generalised activity (>500 ms and >3 phases) interposed with periods of suppressed background activity. (**b**) Burst-suppression pattern with Highly Epileptiform Bursts (HEBs). LFF = 0.53 Hz, HFF = 70 Hz, 100 μV/cm

burst intervals must also be identical. Burst-suppression with identical bursts is a distinct pathological EEG pattern; it is exclusively observed in comatose patients following cardiac arrest and is invariably associated with a poor outcome (Fig. 46.16) [62, 63].

46.6.3.5 Electrocerebral Inactivity

The patterns with attenuation and suppression defined above must be distinguished from *Electro Cerebral Inactivity* (ECI) (the use of terms such as "electrocerebral silence, flat, or isoelectric EEG" to define this condition is discouraged). ECI is characterised by the absence an identifiable electrical activity of cerebral origin over 2 μV (peak to peak), spontaneous or stimulated, in all regions. The ECI is observed in brain death and, for its correct identification, the sensitivity must be increased to a maximum of 2 μV/mm (Fig. 46.17) [64].

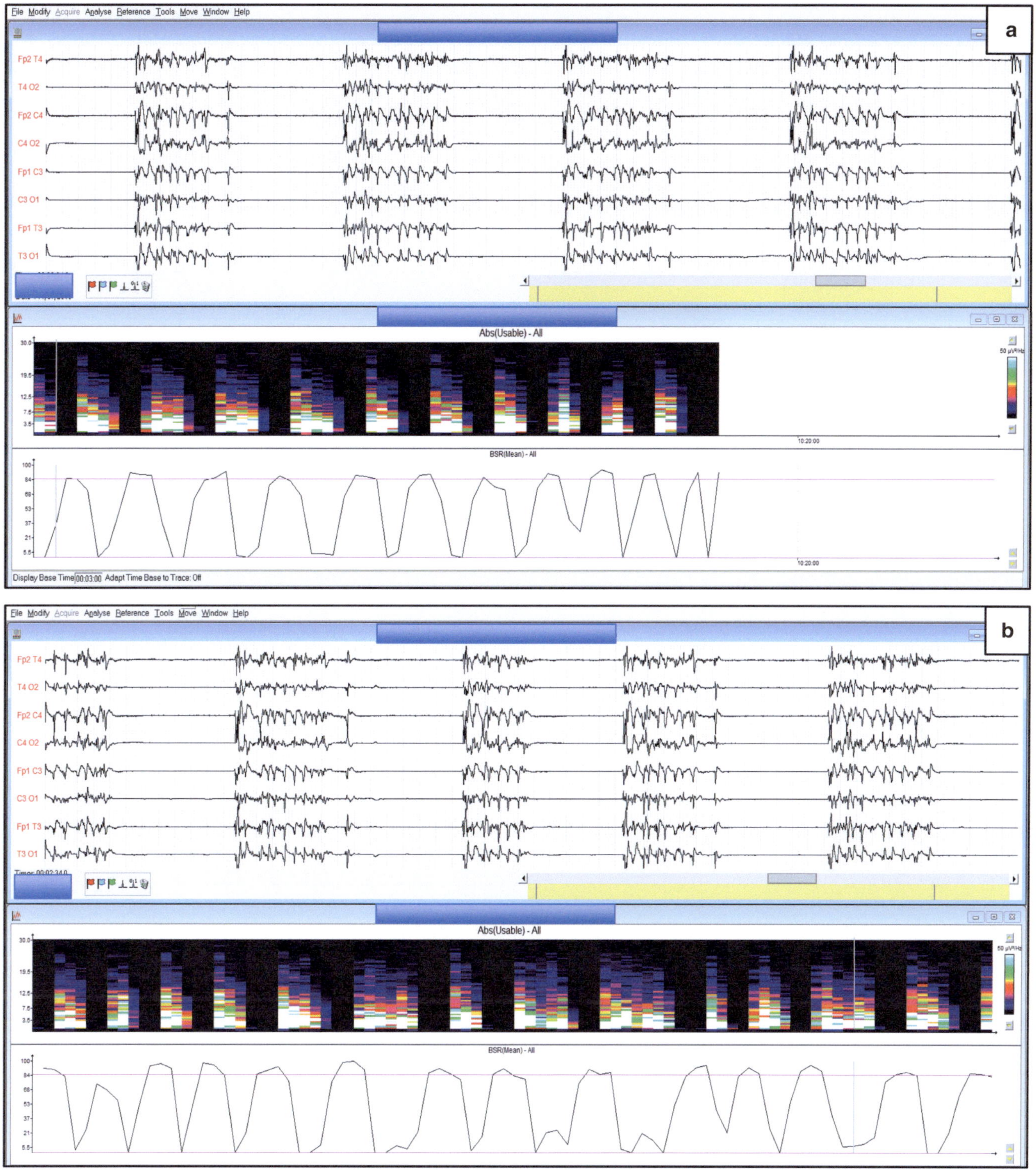

Fig. 46.16 Samples of burst-suppression pattern with identical (**a**) and non-identical (**b**) bursts in two patients with postanoxic encephalopathy. Above, 60 s raw EEG during monitoring; below, Density Spectral Array (DSA) and Burst-Suppression Ratio (BSR). LFF = 0.53, HFF = 70 Hz, 150 μV/cm

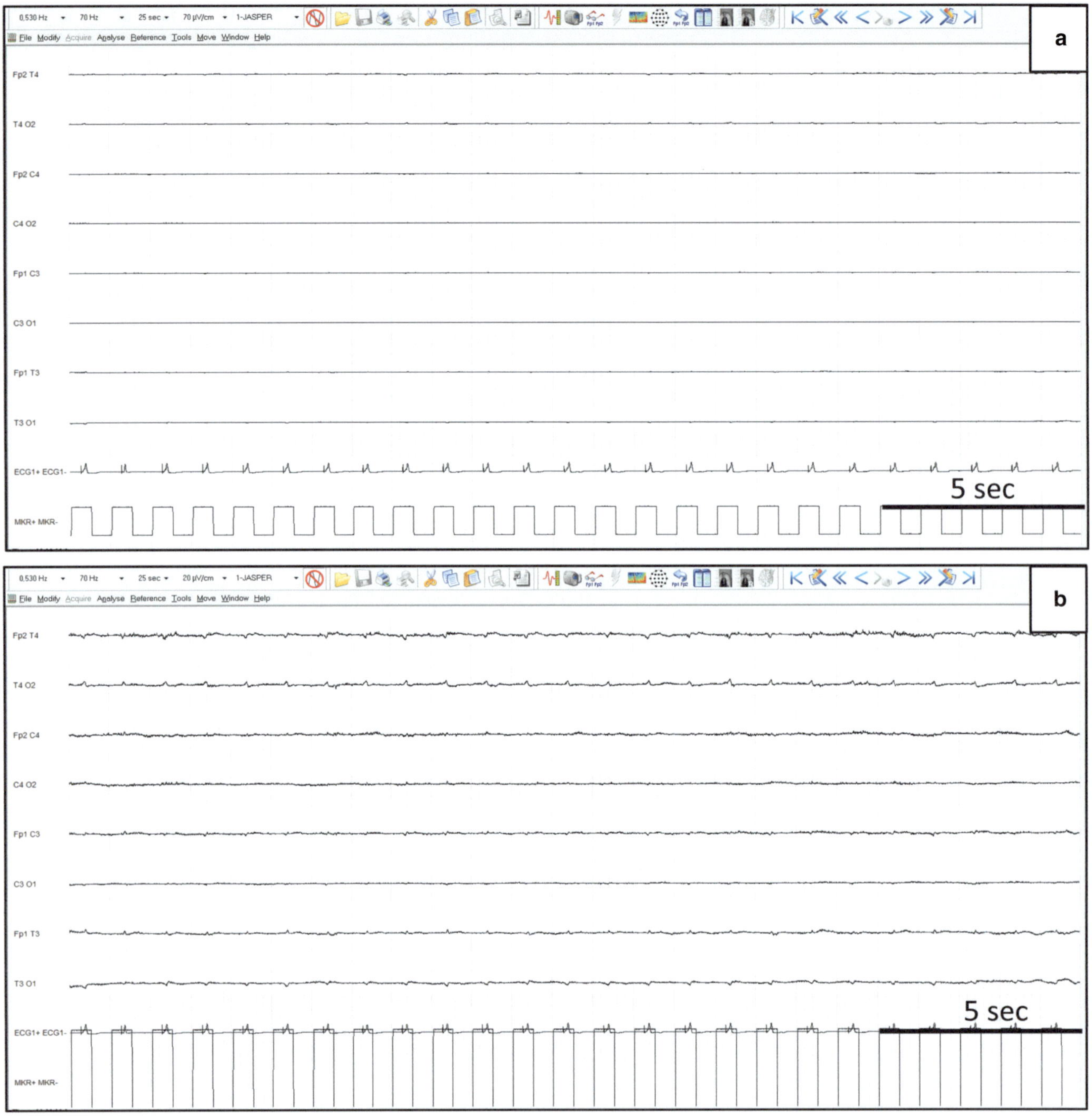

Fig. 46.17 Sample of EEG with electrocerebral inactivity. LFF = 0.53 Hz, HFF = 70 Hz. In (**a**) 70 μV/cm, in (**b**) 20 μV/cm

46.7 EEG Patterns in Vegetative State and Minimally Conscious State

The EEGs in many patients with VS may show a continuous generalised polymorphic theta-delta activity, occasionally reactive (with attenuation) only to nociceptive stimuli. In some patients, the background activity is of very low voltage or suppressed. In <10% of patients with VS, a background rhythm of alpha-theta frequency has been described, without demonstration of reactivity at eyes closing. The recording of ictal or interictal epileptiform abnormalities is unusual. In rare cases, patterns with GPDs, LPDs, triphasic waves, and alpha coma have been described [65].

In patients with MCS, the background activity is more frequently preserved and reactive and the sleep architecture is more recognisable (Fig. 46.18).

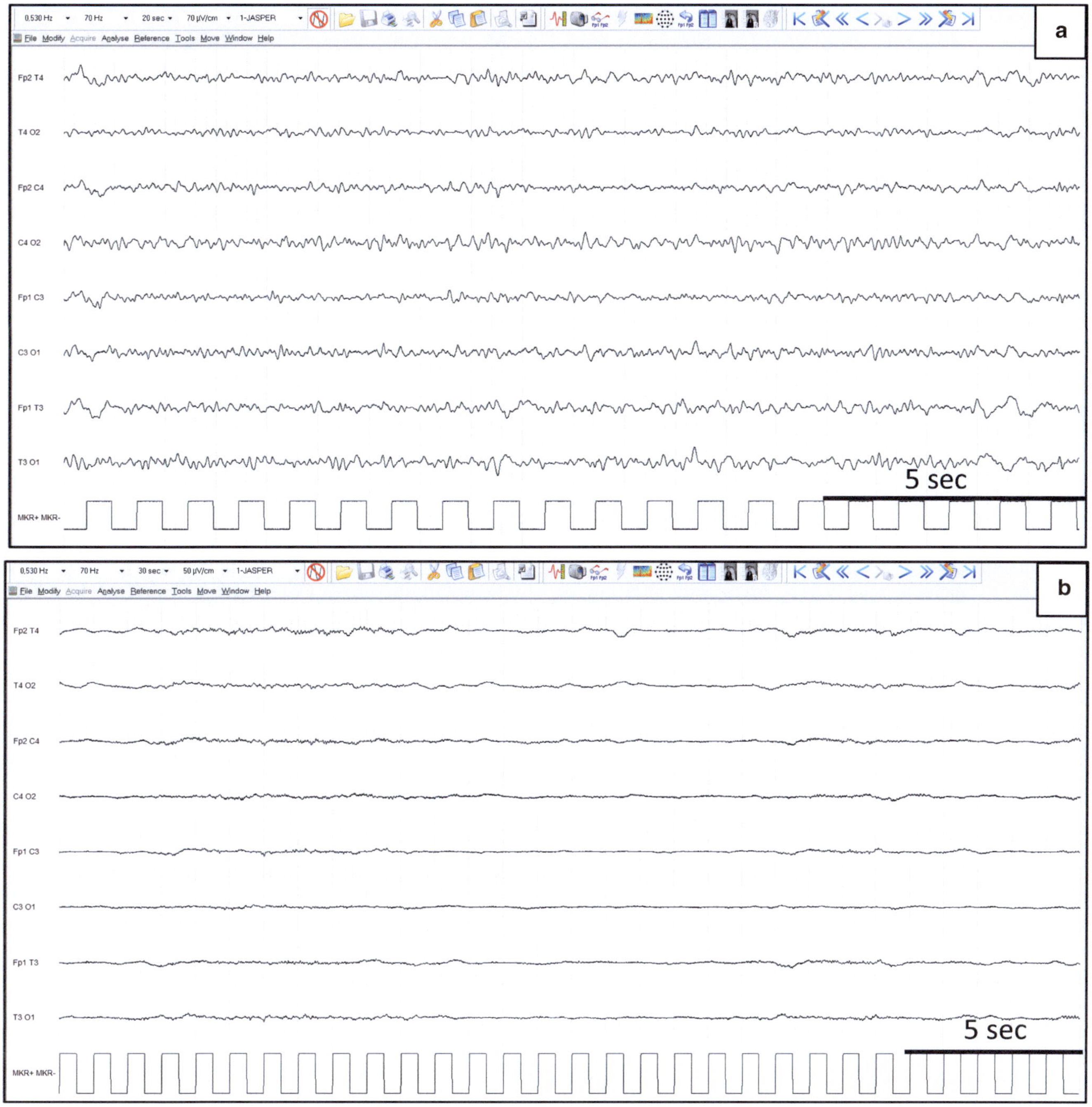

Fig. 46.18 Two samples of EEG in patients with Vegetative State (VS). In (**a**) background activity with theta-alpha frequencies is preserved, but without reactivity (LFF = 0.53 Hz, HFF = 70 Hz, 70 μV/cm). In (**b**) background activity is markedly attenuated (LFF = 0.53 Hz, HFF = 70 Hz, 50 μV/cm)

Forgacs et al. [66] studied the preservation of the EEG organisation during wake and sleep in a large series of patients with VS or MCS (*plus* and *minus*). The EEGs were recorded using a video-EEG system and visually reviewed by clinical neurophysiologists. Wake EEG background was classified into four categories based on the degree of abnormalities observed:

Normal (posterior dominant alpha rhythm at 8–12 Hz, amplitude asymmetry not higher than 50% between hemispheres, normal anteroposterior gradient, no focal or hemispheric slowing).

Mildly abnormal (posterior dominant rhythm asymmetrical or mildly slowed, anteropeterior gradient not well organised, mild focal or hemispheric theta slowing).

Moderately abnormal (posterior rhythms of theta frequency at 4–7 and/or presence of focal or hemispheric theta-delta slowing).

Severely abnormal (diffuse background activity <4 Hz).

During sleep, the presence or absence of characteristic elements of sleep architecture was assessed (vertex waves, spindles, patterns of slow waves, and REM sleep). The results were heterogeneous and related to each individual clinical condition and aetiology of DOC; however, overall, the percentage of moderately or severely abnormal wake EEG decreased from the VS to the MCS *minus* and MCS *plus*. Sleep architecture abnormalities were present in all subjects; vertex waves and spindles were the most preserved sleep pattern, while REM appeared in only 39% of subjects. This study also attempted to elucidate a correlation between the EEG pattern and the results of an fMRI examination during a cognitive task. All patients with fMRI evidence of following covert commands consistently demonstrated well-organised EEG background during wakefulness and spindling activity during sleep [66].

Using high-density EEG, Landsness et al. [67] studied the sleep of 11 patients with VS or MCS with the aim of correlating the EEG changes during sleep to the behavioural changes in vigilance. All patients with MCS showed clear EEG changes associated with behavioural sleep periods. In contrast, patients with VS preserved behavioural sleep (eyes closed) but the EEG patterns remained unchanged during periods with closed eyes, as compared with periods of behavioural wakefulness.

A recent study by Estraneo et al. [68] proposed a modified classification of the EEG patterns of VS and MCS patients into five categories: normal, mildly abnormal, moderately abnormal, diffuse slowing, and low voltage (defined as a predominant slow EEG activity <20 μV over most brain regions). The authors also analysed EEG reactivity following eye opening and closing and following tactile, acoustic, and nociceptive stimulation. The results of this study demonstrated that EEG abnormalities were more severe in VS than in MCS *plus* or MCS *minus* and are prevalent in anoxic aetiology. Reactivity to visual and acoustic stimulation was significantly more frequent in MCS *plus* and MCS *minus* than in VS patients. The patients with normal or mildly abnormal background activity showed higher scores in the Coma Recovery Scale-Revised.

In conclusion, EEG - a time-resolved, low-cost, widespread, and easily reproducible diagnostic technique - may be a valid tool for the classification of patients with persistent DOC and may support neuroimaging in defining the prognosis. However, in addition to the inspective analysis of conventional EEG, high-density EEG recordings should be implemented, as well as the correlation between EEG and other neurophysiological techniques and the quantitative analysis of recorded signals. Spectral power analysis revealed that alpha and theta power are significantly lower in VS than in MCS patients, whereas delta power shows the opposite behaviour. Sitt et al. [69] identified a series of measures that, when combined, allow the classification of the state of consciousness. The authors showed that low-frequency power, EEG complexity, and information exchange constitute the most reliable signatures of consciousness, concluding that a reduced set of EEG measures could ultimately serve as a reliable bedside tool to probe consciousness in patients with DOC.

46.8 EEG in Coma Prognosis

In patients with Acquired Brain Injury (ABI), it is relevant to focus on the prediction of early neurological improvement; however, when patients are still sedated, clinical examination is obviously unreliable, and only instrumental tests are available. Among these, neurophysiological tests (EEG and SSEPs) are important, since they are an extension of clinical examination and integrate with neuroimaging. With respect to the prognostic use of EEG, at least two factors should be considered: the grading system and potential confounding factors (Table 46.4).

It is well-known that the interpretation of EEGs requires more training than the evaluation of other prognostic indicators such as clinical examination and SSEPs, and non-expert interpretation of EEGs introduces the risk of lowering its overall prognostic value. Most grading systems developed decades ago [70–72] evaluated a limited number of EEG features, and standardised terminology had not been adopted; therefore, it is reasonable to assume that the EEG reporters could have been biased by these factors. In particular, grading systems and definitions of malignant and benign EEG patterns varied among studies. Together, these factors hinder accurate recommendations and meta-analysis. For instance, in the first guidelines concerning prognosis of comatose survivors following Cardiac Arrest (CA) [73], EEG was not included among the prognostic indicators, since its prognostic accuracy was considered insufficient based on evidence; thus, standardised terminology evaluating all important features would be preferable to assess which individual features of the EEG are the most predictive. A classification scheme based on clear, strict and standardised definitions of patterns should be used to facilitate comparison among different studies. The variability in classification and rating of the EEG findings has been partly addressed by the introduction of standardised critical care EEG terminology by the ACNS, which has shown high inter-rater agreement, especially for periodic or rhythmic activity [40]. According to this classification, we can identify, for prognostic purposes, the following main EEG patterns: continuous, near continuous, discontinuous, epileptiform discharges, burst-attenuation/

Table 46.4 Classification of coma EEG patterns

EEG grading of anoxic and traumatic encephalopathies in adults (Synek 1988)	EEG classification of coma (Young et al. 1997)
Grade I. Regular alpha, some theta, reactive	Category I. Delta/theta >50% (no theta coma) (a) Reactive (b) Unreactive
Grade II. Predominant theta (a) Normal voltage, reactive (b) Low voltage, unreactive	Category II. Triphasic waves
Grade III. Predominant delta (a) Diffuse delta activity, rhythmic, frontally predominant, reactive (b) Delta activity and spindles (spindle coma) (c) Delta activity of low voltage, discontinuous, irregular, unreactive (d) Predominant delta of medium voltage, either rhythmic or irregular, usually unreactive	Category III. Burst-suppression (a) With epileptiform activity (b) Without epileptiform activity
Grade IV. Burst-suppression and other malignant patterns (a) Burst-suppression, with (i) or without (ii) epileptiform activity (b) Alpha coma, with some reactivity (i) or unreactive (ii) (c) Theta coma (d) Delta of low voltage (<20 μV)	Category IV. Alpha coma/theta coma/spindle coma (unreactive)
Grade V. Suppression (subgrade: Electrocerebral silence—<2 μV)	Category V. Epileptiform activity not in burst-suppression pattern (a) Generalised (b) Focal or multifocal
	Category VI. Suppression (a) <20 μV–>10 μV (b) ≤10 μV

Adapted from: Synek VM. Prognostically important EEG coma patterns in diffuse anoxic and traumatic encephalopathies in adults. J Clin Neurophysiol. 1988; 5: 161–174; and Young GB, McLachlan RS, Kreeft JH, and Demel JD. An Electroencephalographic Classification of Coma. Can J Neurol Sci. 1997; 24: 320–325

burst-suppression, attenuation/suppression, and electrocerebral inactivity. Concerning potential confounding factors, temperature and sedation must be taken into account. Over the last decade, Therapeutic Hypothermia (TH) with a target temperature of 32–34 °C has become the standard of care in the management of patients following CA and has also been proposed in Traumatic Brain Injury (TBI). Moderate TH to the level of 32 °C does not significantly affect the continuity or voltage of EEGs. Only under a temperature of 29 °C do we observe the progressive appearance of periodic complexes, burst-suppression (around 24 °C), and E3 (around 22 °C) [74]. Artifacts from muscle shivering, mechanical ventilation, or electrical equipment that frequently accompany TH may affect the reliability of EEG interpretation; nonetheless, it is apparent that many EEG patterns seen during moderate TH have similar prognostic implications as when seen during normothermia [75]. More relevant than the effect of body temperature per se are its metabolic effects. A decreased body temperature decreases the activity of hepatic enzymes by 7–22% per degree below 37 °C, which can result in significantly higher levels of anaesthetic and a prolonged effect of neuromuscular blockade, and it may be difficult to know whether residual sedation affects the clinical and EEG reactivity, even when recordings are performed 24 h after normothermia is restored.

Concerning sedation, based on their pharmacological effects, we expected propofol and midazolam to decrease the continuity of the EEG, leading to a false prediction of a poor outcome. Firstly, a distinction should be made between patients surviving CA and the other acquired brain injuries. Comatose patients affected by TBI) are treated at an early stage with high doses of propofol or midazolam to control the intracranial pressure, and this treatment induces burst-suppression patterns on EEG. Instead, the typical dosages of propofol (1–2 mg/kg/h) or midazolam (0.03–0.1 mg/kg/h) used in CA patients did not affect the continuity of the EEG; in these patients, the severity of postanoxic injury influenced the EEG much more than sedative drugs [76]. During rewarming, even if we consider the prolonged duration of sedative drugs, the dose will be even lower. In any case, in this condition, the absence of reactivity and the Episodic Low-Amplitude Events (ELAEs) [77] should not be considered as reliable for the prognosis of a poor outcome.

The main role of the EEG in TBI is the detection of acute seizures immediately following brain injury. The EEG can also be helpful in determining the prognosis but with the limitation of timing, since all these comatose patients are treated at an early stage with high doses of propofol or midazolam to control the intracranial pressure, creating unreliable EEG findings. As a consequence, the presence of malignant patterns (e.g. burst-suppression) should be interpreted with caution, since it may be related to ongoing sedation rather than cerebral injury; however, knowing the effects of sedation on EEG activity, a comparison between the dosage of the sedatives and the expected EEG pattern should be considered. Approximately 1 week after the onset of the post-traumatic coma, the EEG has predictive value for a good outcome in the case of the presence of reactivity [78]. Logi et al. [79], using the Synek classification in the post-acute phase, showed that in the presence of a benign EEG pattern (which included dominant theta and alpha activity, delta activity with sleep spindles, and high-amplitude frontally predominant rhythmic delta activity in a background of alpha and theta activity), patients regained consciousness. The absence of EEG reactivity marks a poor prognosis in TBI patients when associated with severe SSEP alterations [80].

Another important indication to perform EEG with a prognostic aim is the case of a coma state following CA. Recent European guidelines [81, 82] have recognised

EEG as a prognostic indicator in Hypoxic–Ischaemic Encephalopathy (HIE) but with caveats owing to the lack of strong statistical evidence from the pooled data of available studies and the newly emerging influence of confounding factors such as sedation, paralysis, and TH. In light of the data published in recent years, the EEG can be useful for both a poor and a good outcome and neurological prognosis. To this end, the classification of different EEG patterns into three categories has been proposed. *Highly malignant EEG patterns* include suppressed background without discharges, suppressed background with continuous periodic discharges, and burst-suppression background with or without discharges. *Malignant EEG patterns* include malignant periodic or rhythmic patterns (abundant periodic discharges, abundant rhythmic polyspike–/spike–/sharp-and-waves, unequivocal electrographic seizure), malignant background (discontinuous background, low-voltage background, reversed anterior-posterior gradient), and unreactive EEG (absence of background reactivity or only stimulus-induced discharges). *Benign EEG* is characterised by the absence of all the malignant features stated above. For proper prognostic use of the EEG, the natural evolution and pathophysiological basis of EEG changes following CA and return to spontaneous circulation should be carefully taken into account. The electrophysiological changes following CA have been studied in several animal models, showing the clear evolution of changes over time including an initial period of complete EEG suppression, a subsequent burst-suppression pattern, and later transition into continuous cortical activity. The duration of EEG suppression and the latency of emergence of a continuous background correlate with neurological outcome and neuropathological injury [83]. Changes in humans may follow a similar pattern, for instance, studies describe similar natural evolution of the EEG signal along with neurological recovery following cardiac and/or respiratory arrest [84].

Thus, different from SSEPs, EEG is a time-dependent indicator because the prognostic value of a single pattern changes over time, at least until 72 h following CA. This factor strongly influences the "optimal" timing of EEG recording and the distinct EEG patterns, assisting with prognostication in post-CA patients. In each time frame, if standardised definitions of EEG patterns are applied, there is at least one EEG pattern that is specific to good and poor outcomes. From a practical point of view, we can distinguish three temporal frames: 12, 24, and 72 h. During the early phase following CA (12 h, Fig. 46.19), continuous and near continuous EEG indicate a good prognosis (false-positive rate, FPR = 0) [75, 85–87]. The value of these EEG patterns for a good prognosis at a very early stage following CA is strengthened when the EEG is used in combination with SSEPs. In fact, both EEG (continuous and quasi-continuous) and SSEP (bilaterally absent) patterns have an FPR = 0, but with opposite prognostic significance (indeed each of these findings is mutually exclusive of the other). The EEG and SSEPs recordings in the same patient increase the number of correctly classified cases (65.2%) in comparison with the number of patients classified by each test individually (EEG predicted a good prognosis in 30.5%; SSEPs predicted a poor prognosis in 34.7%). Moreover, continuous and near continuous EEG are always associated with the presence of cortical SSEPs, whereas bilaterally absent cortical SSEPs are always associated with malignant EEG patterns. This consistency of findings increases the reliability of prediction in a single patient. In literature, there have been reports, albeit rarely, of patients with bilaterally absent

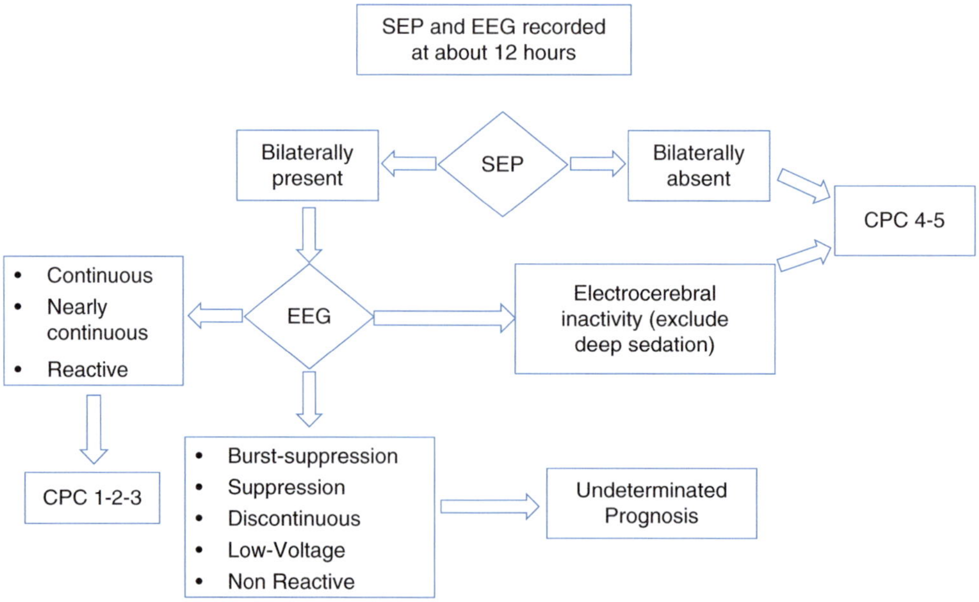

Fig. 46.19 Prognostic significance of Sensory Evoked Potentials (SEP) and EEG at about 12 h after cardiac arrest. CPC (Cerebral Performance Category) is a clinical score of outcome: 1, no or minor neurological deficits; 2, moderate disability; 3, severe disability; 4, unresponsive wakefulness state; 5. death

cortical SSEPs who have recovered consciousness [88], but no indication of the EEG pattern in these patients was reported. The finding of a continuous or near continuous EEG within 12 h following CA in patients with bilaterally absent cortical SEPs requires caution in the interpretation and a repeat SSEPs recording to avoid a false pessimistic prediction. From a pathophysiological point of view, at least during the early stage following CA, the lack of correlation between SSEPs and EEG could be explained by a selective resistance to hypoxia/ischaemia of their generator systems: somatosensory neurons have both "receiving" and "sending" properties, and then the preservation of N20 reflects an intact "receiving mode"; instead, EEG generation mainly reflects multiple cortical synaptic functions, with greater involvement of "sending mode" [89]. Within the first 12 h, continuous and nearly continuous EEG was always associated with the presence of cortical SSEPs, indicating a low degree of severity of hypoxic–ischaemic encephalopathy. At the same time, the bilaterally absent cortical SSEPs were always associated with malignant EEG as an expression of severe hypoxic–ischaemic encephalopathy. Moreover, when malignant EEG was associated with preserved cortical SSEPs, this indicates an intermediate degree of hypoxic–ischaemic encephalopathy and may explain why some of these patients did not have an unfavourable outcome.

At approximately 24 h (Fig. 46.20), the EEG shows less prognostic utility. Continuous quasi-continuous patterns begin to lose the specificity of 100% for good prognosis. Suppression/burst-suppression patterns show a specificity of 100% for poor prediction at 24 h; however, since these EEG patterns occur in a small percentage (4%) of patients with preserved cortical SSEPs [90], the EEG can slightly increase the prediction of a poor outcome as compared with SSEPs. Moreover, at this time point, the suppressed pattern has not yet reached 100% specificity for a poor outcome.

At 72 h, both malignant EEG patterns and bilaterally absent cortical SSEPs indicate a poor prognosis, with an FPR = 0 (Fig. 46.21). This finding suggests two possible scenarios. On one hand, if unfavourable EEG and SSEP patterns are both present, this confirms and strengthens their prognostic value. On the other hand, since malignant EEG occurs in some patients with present SSEPs, this allows the prediction of an unfavourable prognosis in a greater number of patients. Continuous or near continuous patterns in the later time frames usually predict good outcomes; nevertheless, some patients showing continuous and near continuous EEGs in these time frames can have a poor outcome. These errors in prediction can be explained by the occurrence of alpha-theta coma patterns; the pathogenesis of ATC is thought to involve alternative generators and subcortical pathways including the caudate nucleus, amygdala, hypothalamus, brainstem, and basal forebrain [91]. It is conceivable that the organisation of these subcortical circuits, which are responsible for the appearance of a de novo alpha rhythm, does not occur immediately following CA but takes more time to establish, so that a continuous pattern invariably predicts a good outcome only if observed within the first 12 h following CA. There are two possible ways to avoid a false optimistic prediction. Firstly, the SSEP pattern should be taken into account; if cortical responses are absent in both hemispheres, then the prognosis will be poor. If cortical SSEP responses are present, it would be useful to repeat the EEG after a few

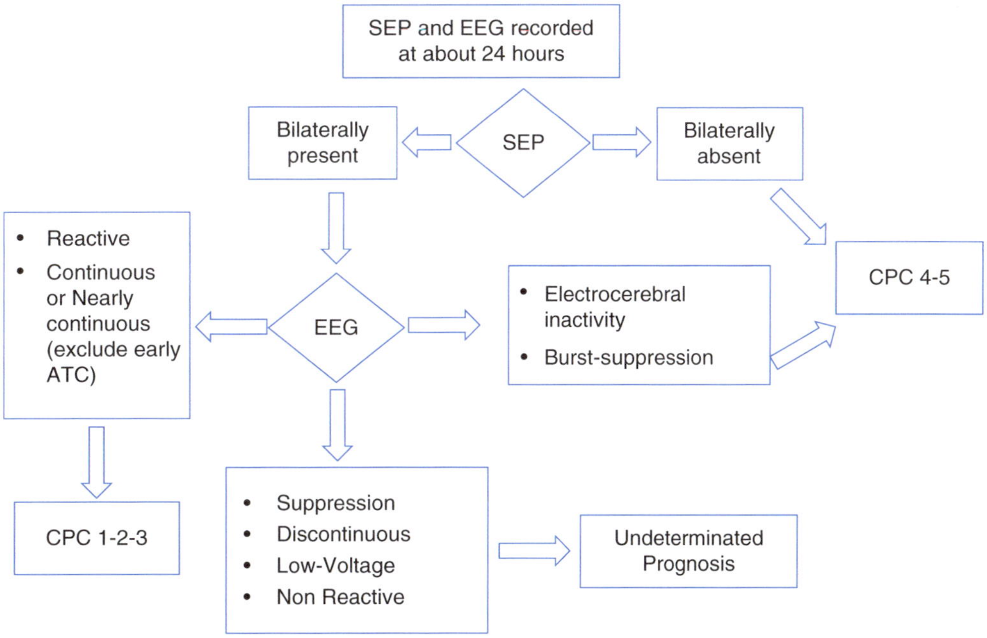

Fig. 46.20 Prognostic significance of Sensory Evoked Potentials (SEP) and EEG at about 24 h after cardiac arrest. CPC (Cerebral Performance Category) is a clinical score of outcome: 1, no or minor neurological deficits; 2, moderate disability; 3, severe disability; 4, unresponsive wakefulness state; 5, death

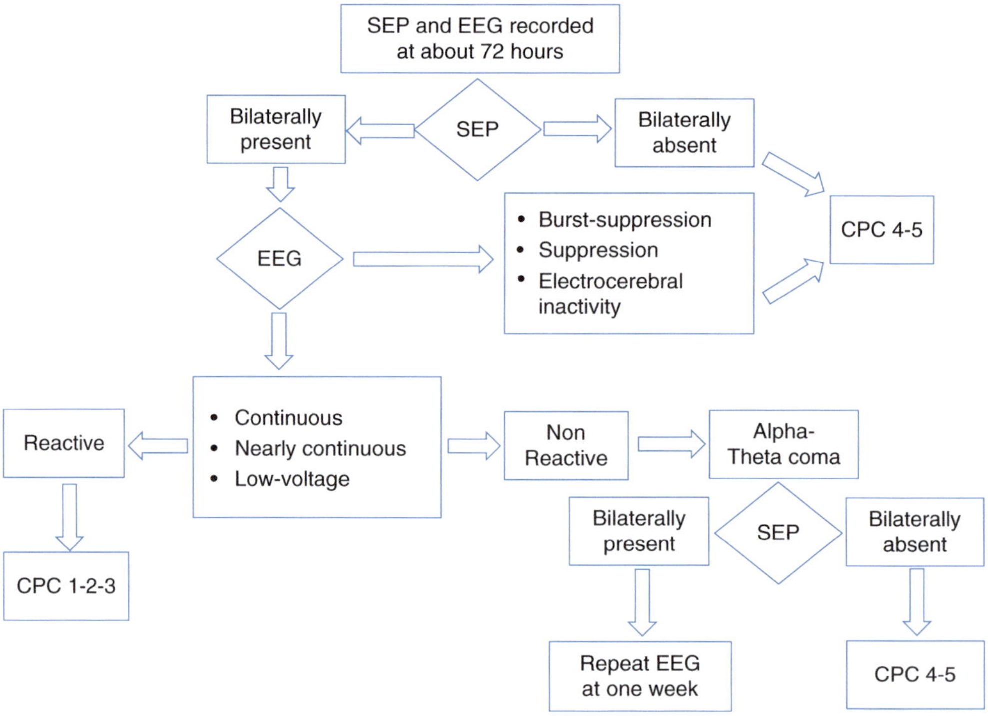

Fig. 46.21 Prognostic significance of Sensory Evoked Potentials (SEP) and EEG at about 72 h after cardiac arrest. CPC (Cerebral Performance Category) is a clinical score of outcome: 1, no or minor neurological deficits; 2, moderate disability; 3, severe disability; 4, unresponsive wakefulness state; 5, death

days. In the case of a true ATC pattern, an evolution towards the malignant patterns (suppressed or low voltage) is to be expected.

Two more features of EEG, reactivity and epileptiform discharges, are time-dependent.

The presence of reactive EEG has a high positive predictive value for a good outcome, with a false positive rate = 0 during early TH (within 12 h of CA), when it is evident despite sedation; however, only a small subgroup of patients with continuous or near continuous EEG shows a reactive EEG in this time frame, likely due to sedation. The absence of reactivity was reported to be indicative of a poor outcome in a prospective study by Oddo and Rossetti (2014) [92], in which all patients with an unreactive EEG during TH went on to have a poor outcome, except for one; however, different findings have also been reported. [63, 87] The absence of reactivity as a negative prognostic indicator should be applied with great caution in the early post-CA period due to the presence of sedation and/or TH. After 48–72 h, when there is less interference from sedation effects, the absence of reactivity becomes more predictive of a poor outcome. One limitation is that all studies exploring the value of EEG reactivity for prognostication evaluated this feature as an “isolated characteristic”. No study included additional analysis of the background EEG patterns. Indeed, a reactive EEG may be associated with a continuous background pattern with physiological rhythms, whereas a nonreactive EEG may represent a low-voltage background pattern. Thus, since the EEG pattern may already contain sufficient information for reliable prognostication, the additional predictive value of reactivity per se is unclear.

Epileptiform activity is usually observed after 24 h [63, 87], but the presence of epileptiform discharges is not invariably predictive of a poor outcome, for instance, in TH-treated patients in any time frame [93–95]. This is why many studies do not include epileptiform activity in the prognostic categories of EEG patterns in HIE coma. Evidence that this pattern is less severe than other malignant patterns is demonstrated by the different percentages of absence of cortical SSEPs in epileptiform (around 20%) and noncontinuous patterns (>65% for burst-suppression, suppression, and isoelectric) [87]; thus, it is conceivable that the former reflects a different grade of encephalopathy severity.

It remains an open issue whether continuous EEG (cEEG) should be preferred to standard EEG (30 min) for prognostication in postanoxic coma. cEEG studies [75, 94, 95] have been useful in identifying the times at which various EEG patterns acquire significant prognostic value and in demonstrating that it is possible to predict good as well as poor outcomes at a very early stage. However, cEEG is not as widely available as standard EEG, and it is also more expensive. Crepeau et al. [75] failed to demonstrate that cEEG was a more effective prognostic tool than standard EEG in clinical practice. Standard EEG can be as informative as cEEG as a predictor of outcome, provided that the timing of the recording is considered.

Background amplitude and continuity are the most relevant features in the postanoxic EEG; however, they remain hard to quantitate by a human observer, with far from perfect inter-rater agreement. Quantitative measures for EEG (qEEG) background continuity and amplitude can improve the prediction of outcome in postanoxic coma. EEG background continuity and the amplitude ratio between bursts and suppressions reliably predict the good and poor outcomes of postanoxic coma [76].

In conclusion, in HIE, the EEG has a high prognostic value for both poor and good outcomes. In fact, when specific EEG patterns are found at a certain time from coma onset, it is possible to predict a neurological outcome with 100% specificity. The continuous and near continuous EEG patterns found within the first 12 h following CA are always associated with a good outcome (recovery of consciousness), whereas an isoelectric pattern (amplitude <2 μV) after 12 h, a burst-suppression pattern after 24 h, and a suppression pattern after 48 h from CA are always associated with a poor outcome. Considering the recent recommendation regarding a multimodal approach [81], an association with SSEP recording is suggested for two reasons: to confirm a poor prognosis (increase certainty) and to increase the number of patients correctly classified (increase sensitivity).

Acknowledgements We are very grateful to Dr. Patrizia Pulitano for her help in selecting and editing the EEG figures.

References

1. Bremer F. L'activitè cerebralè au cours du sommeil et de la narcose. Bull Acad R Soc Belg. 1937;IV:68–86.
2. Moruzzi G, Magoun H. Brainstem reticular formation and activation of EEG. Electroencephalogr Clin Neurophysiol. 1949;1:455–73.
3. Dempsey EW, Morison RS. The production of rhythmically recurrent cortical potentials after localized thalamic stimulation. Am J Physiol. 1942;135:293–300.
4. Steriade M. Arousal: revisiting the reticular activating system. Science. 1996;12:225–6.
5. Jones BE. Arousal systems. Front Biosci. 2003;8:s438–51.
6. McClenathan BM, Thakor NV, Hoesch RE. Pathophysiology of acute coma and disorders of consciousness: considerations for diagnosis and management. Semin Neurol. 2013;33:91–109.
7. Maxwell WL, MacKinnon MA, Smith DH, McIntosh TK, Graham DI. Thalamic nuclei after human blunt head injury. J Neuropathol Exp Neurol. 2006;65:478–88.
8. Grillner S, Hellgren J, Ménard A, et al. Mechanisms for selection of basic motor programs—roles for the striatum and pallidum. Trends Neurosci. 2005;28:364–70.
9. Laureys S, Schiff ND. Coma and consciousness: paradigms (re) framed by neuroimaging. Neuroimage. 2012;61:478–91.
10. Schiff ND. Recovery of consciousness after brain injury: a mesocircuit hypothesis. Trends Neurosci. 2010;33:1–9.
11. Williams ST, Conte MM, Goldfine AM, et al. Common resting brain dynamics indicate a possible mechanism underlying zolpidem response in severe brain injury. Elife. 2013;19:e01157.
12. Schiff ND, Giacino JT, Kalmar K, et al. Behavioural improvements with thalamic stimulation after severe traumatic brain injury. Nature. 2007;448:600–3.
13. Giacino JT, Fins JJ, Laureys S, Schiff ND. Disorders of consciousness after acquired brain injury: the state of the science. Nat Rev Neurol. 2014;10:99–114.
14. Saper CB, Scammell TE, Lu J. Hypothalamic regulation of sleep and circadian rhythms. Nature. 2005;437:1257–63.
15. Llinas RR, Steriade M. Bursting of thalamic neurons and states of vigilance. J Neurophysiol. 2006;95:3297–308.
16. Saper CB, Lumsden AGS. The sensory, motor, and reflex functions of the brainstem. In: Kandel E, Schwartz J, Jessell TM, Siegelbaum SA, Hudspeth AJ, editors. Principles of neural science. 5th ed. New York: McGraw-Hill; 2012. p. 1019–37.
17. Posner JB, Saper CB, Schiff ND, Plum F. Plum and Posner's diagnosis of stupor and coma, vol. 401. 4th ed. New York: Oxford University Press; 2007.
18. Edlow JA, Rabinstein A, Traub SJ, Wijdicks EFM. Diagnosis of reversible causes of coma. Lancet. 2014;384:2064–76.
19. The Multi-Society Task Force on PVS. Medical aspects of the persistent vegetative state (1). N Engl J Med. 1994;330:1499–508.
20. The Multi-Society Task Force on PVS. Medical aspects of the persistent vegetative state (2). N Engl J Med. 1994;330:1572–9.
21. Giacino JT, Kalmar K. Diagnostic and prognostic guidelines for the vegetative and minimally conscious states. Neuropsychol Rehabil. 2005;15:166–74.
22. Bruno MA, Vanhaudenhuyse A, Thibaut A, Moonen G, Laureys S. From unresponsive wakefulness to minimally conscious PLUS and functional locked-in syndrome: recent advances in our understanding of disorders of consciousness. J Neurol. 2011;258:1373–84.
23. Cairns H, Olfield HC, Pennybaker JB, Whineridge D. Akinetic mutism with an epidermoid cyst of the third ventricle. Brain. 1941;34:273–90.
24. Nagaratnam N, Nagaratnam K, Ng K, Diu P. Akinetic mutism following stroke. J Clin Neurosci. 2004;11:25–30.
25. Wijdicks EF. Neurologic examination of the comatose patient and localization principles. In: Wijdicks EFM, editor. The comatose patient. 2nd ed. New York: Oxford University Press; 2008. p. 64–83.
26. Chung CS, Caplan LR, Yamamoto Y, et al. Striatocapsular haemorrhage. Brain. 2000;123:1850–62.
27. Ropper AH, Brown RH. Adams and Victor's principles of neurology. 8th ed. New York: McGraw-Hill; 2005. p. 1333.
28. Huff JS, Stevens RD, Weingart SD, Smith WS. Emergency neurological life support: approach to the patient with coma. Neurocrit Care. 2012;17:S54–9.
29. Jennett B, Adams JH, Murray LS, Grahm DI. Neuropathology in vegetative and severely disabled patients after head injury. Neurology. 2001;56:486–90.
30. Zheng W, Lui G, Wu R. Prediction of recovery from a post-traumatic coma state by diffusion-weighted imaging (DWI) in patients with diffuse axonal injury. Neuroradiology. 2007;49:271–9.
31. Young GB. Impaired consciousness and herniation syndromes. Neurol Clin. 2011;29:765–72.
32. Cremer OL, van Dijk GW, van Wensen E, et al. Effect of intracranial pressure monitoring and targeted intensive care on functional outcome after severe head injury. Crit Care Med. 2005;33:2207–13.
33. Latorre JG, Greer DM. Management of acute intracranial hypertension: a review. Neurologist. 2009;15:193–207.
34. Iencean SM, Ciurea AV. Intracranial hypertension: classification and patterns of evolution. J Med Life. 2008;1:101–7.
35. Teasdale G, Jennett B. Assessment of coma and impaired consciousness: a practical scale. Lancet. 1974;2:81–4.
36. Brennan PM, Murray GD, Teasdale GM. Simplifying the use of prognostic information in traumatic brain injury. Part 1: the GCS-pupils score: an extended index of clinical severity. J Neurosurg. 2018;128:1612–20.

37. Wijdicks EFM, Bamlet WR, Maramattom BV, Manno EM, McClelland RL. Validation of a new coma scale: the FOUR score. Ann Neurol. 2005;58:585–93.
38. Jennett B, Bond M. Assessment of outcome after severe brain damage. Lancet. 1975;1:480–4.
39. Jennett B, Snoek J, Bond M, Brooks N. Disability after severe head injury: observation on the use of the Glasgow outcome scale. J Neurol Neurosurg Psychiatry. 1981;44:285–93.
40. Hirsch LJ, LaRoche SM, Gaspard N, et al. American clinical neurophysiology Society's standardized critical care EEG terminology: 2012 version. J Clin Neurophysiol. 2013;30:1–27.
41. Tsetsou S, Novy J, Oddo M, Rossetti AO. EEG reactivity to pain in comatose patients: importance of the stimulus type. Resuscitation. 2015;97:34–7.
42. Admiraal MM, van Rootselaar AF, Horn J. Electroencephalographic reactivity testing in unconscious patients: a systematic review of methods and definitions. Eur J Neurol. 2017;24:245–54.
43. Hermans MC, Westover MB, van Putten MJAM, Hirsch LJ. Quantification of EEG reactivity in comatose patients. Clin Neurophysiol. 2016;127:571–80.
44. Rodriguez Ruiz A, Vlachy J, Lee JW, et al. Association of periodic and rhythmic electroencephalographic patterns with seizures in critically ill patients. JAMA Neurol. 2017;74:181–8.
45. Punia V, Bena J, Krishnan B, Newey C, Hantus S. New onset epilepsy among patients with periodic discharges on continuous electroencephalographic monitoring. Epilepsia. 2018;59:1612.
46. Trinka E, Cock H, Hesdorffer D, et al. A definition and classification of status epilepticus—report of the ILAE task force on classification of status epilepticus. Epilepsia. 2015;56:1515–23.
47. Leitinger M, Beniczky S, Rohracher A, et al. Salzburg consensus criteria for non-convulsive status epilepticus—approach to clinical application. Epilepsy Behav. 2015;49:158–63.
48. Trinka E, Leitinger M. Which EEG patterns in coma are non-convulsive status epilepticus? Epilepsy Behav. 2015;49:203–22.
49. Leitinger M, Trinka E, Gardella E, et al. Diagnostic accuracy of the Salzburg EEG criteria for non-convulsive status epilepticus: a retrospective study. Lancet Neurol. 2016;15:1054–62.
50. Chatrian GE, White LE Jr, Daly D. Electroencephalographic patterns resembling those of sleep in certain comatose states after injuries to the head. Electroencephalogr Clin Neurophysiol. 1963;15:272–80.
51. Britt CW Jr. Nontraumatic "spindle coma": clinical, EEG, and prognostic features. Neurology. 1981;31:393–7.
52. Kaplan PW, Genoud D, Ho TW, Jallon P. Clinical correlates and prognosis in early spindle coma. Clin Neurophysiol. 2000;111:584–90.
53. Ducharme-Crevier L, Press CA, Kurz JE, et al. Early presence of sleep spindles on electroencephalography is associated with good outcome after pediatric cardiac arrest. Pediatr Crit Care Med. 2017;18:452–60.
54. Husain AM. Electroencephalographic assessment of coma. J Clin Neurophysiol. 2006;23:208–20.
55. Loeb C, Poggio GF. Electroencephalograms in a case with ponto-mesencephalic haemorrhage. Electroencephalogr Clin Neurophysiol. 1953;5:295–6.
56. Kaplan PW, Genoud D, Ho TW, Jaollon P. Etiology, neurologic correlations, and prognosis in alpha coma. Clin Neurophysiol. 1999;110:205–13.
57. Berkhoff M, Donati F, Bassetti C. Postanoxic alpha(theta) coma: a reappraisal of its prognostic significance. Clin Neurophysiol. 2000;111:297–304.
58. McKeown MJ, Young GB. Comparison between the alpha pattern in normal subjects and in alpha pattern coma. J Clin Neurophysiol. 1997;14:414–8.
59. Abusleme IE, Chen JWY. Alternative cerebral generators and circuitry pathways in alpha coma revealed by independent component analysis. Clin Neurophysiol. 2009;120:686–94.
60. Fossi S, Amantini A, Grippo A, Cossu C, Boni N, Pinto F. Anoxic-ischemic alpha coma: prognostic significance of the incomplete variant. Neurol Sci. 2003;24:397–400.
61. Fernandez-Torre JL, Lopez-Delgado A, Hernandez-Hernandez MA, et al. Postanoxic alpha, theta or alpha-theta coma: clinical setting and neurological outcome. Resuscitation. 2018;124:118–25.
62. Hofmeijer J, Tjepkema-Cloostermans MC, van Putten MJ. Burst-suppression with identical bursts: a distinct EEG pattern with poor outcome in post-anoxic coma. Clin Neurophysiol. 2014;125:947–54.
63. Spalletti M, Carrai R, Scarpino M, et al. Single electroencephalographic patterns as specific and time-dependent indicators of good and poor outcome after cardiac arrest. Clin Neurophysiol. 2016;127:2610–7.
64. Kane N, Acharya J, Benickzy S, et al. A revised glossary of terms most commonly used by clinical electroencephalographers and updated proposal for the report format of the EEG findings. Revision 2017. Clin Neurophysiol Pract. 2017;2:170–85.
65. Kulkarni VP, Lin K, Benbadis SR. EEG findings in the persistent vegetative state. J Clin Neurophysiol. 2007;24:433–7.
66. Forgacs PB, Conte MM, Fridman EA, et al. Preservation of EEG organization in patients with impaired consciousness and imaging-based evidence of command-following. Ann Neurol. 2014;76:869–79.
67. Landsness E, Bruno MA, Noirhomme Q, et al. Electrophysiological correlates of behavioural changes in vigilance in vegetative state and minimally conscious state. Brain. 2011;134:2222–32.
68. Estraneo A, Loreto V, Guarino I, et al. Standard EEG in diagnostic process of prolonged disorders of consciousness. Clin Neurophysiol. 2016;127:2379–85.
69. Sitt JD, King J-R, El Karoui I, et al. Large scale screening of neural signatures of consciousness in patients in a vegetative or minimally conscious state. Brain. 2014;137:2258–70.
70. Prior PF, Scott DF. Outcome after severe brain damage. Lancet. 1973;1:770.
71. Synek VM. Prognostically important EEG coma patterns in diffuse anoxic and traumatic encephalopathies in adults. J Clin Neurophysiol. 1988;5:161–74.
72. Young GB, McLachlan RS, Kreeft JH, Demelo JD. An electroencephalographic classification for coma. Can J Neurol Sci. 1997;24:320–5.
73. Wijdicks EF, Hijdra A, Young GB, Bassetti CL, Wiebe S. Practice parameter: prediction of outcome in comatose survivors after cardiopulmonary resuscitation (an evidence-based review): report of the quality standards Subcommittee of the American Academy of Neurology. Neurology. 2006;67:203–10.
74. Stecker MM, Cheung AT, Pochettino A, et al. Deep hypothermic circulatory arrest: II. Changes in electroencephalogram and evoked potentials during rewarming. Ann Thorac Surg. 2001;71:22–8.
75. Crepeau AZ, Fugate JE, Mandrekar J, et al. Value analysis of continuous EEG in patients during therapeutic hypothermia after cardiac arrest. Resuscitation. 2014;85:785–9.
76. Ruijter BJ, Hofmeijer J, Tjepkema-Cloostermans MC, van Putten MJAM. The prognostic value of discontinuous EEG patterns in postanoxic coma. J Clin Neurophysiol. 2018;129:1534–43.
77. Rae-Grant AD, Strapple C, Barbour PJ. Episodic low-amplitude events: an under-recognized phenomenon in clinical electroencephalography. J Clin Neurophysiol. 1991;8:203–11.
78. Fischer C, Mutschler V. Traumatic brain injuries in adults: from coma to wakefulness. Neurophysiological data. Ann Readapt Med Phys. 2002;45:448–55.

79. Logi F, Pasqualetti P, Tomaiuolo F. Predict recovery of consciousness in post-acute severe brain injury: the role of EEG reactivity. Brain Inj. 2011;25:972–9.
80. Amantini A, Grippo A, Fossi S, et al. Prediction of "awakening" and outcome in prolonged acute coma from severe traumatic brain injury: evidence for validity of short latency SEPs. Clin Neurophysiol. 2005;116:229–35.
81. Taccone FS, Baar I, De Deyne C, et al. Neuroprognostication after adult cardiac arrest treated with targeted temperature management: task force for Belgian recommendations. Acta Neurol Belg. 2017;117:3–15.
82. Sandroni C, Cariou A, Cavallaro F, et al. Prognostication in comatose survivors of cardiac arrest: an advisory statement from the European resuscitation council and the European Society of Intensive Care Medicine. Resuscitation. 2014;85:1779–89.
83. Koenig MA, Kaplan PW, Thakor NV. Clinical neurophysiologic monitoring and brain injury from cardiac arrest. Neurol Clin. 2006;24:89–106.
84. Jørgensen EO, Malchow-Møller A. Natural history of global and critical brain ischaemia. Part II: EEG and neurological signs in patients remaining unconscious after cardiopulmonary resuscitation. Resuscitation. 1981;9:155–74.
85. Tjepkema-Cloostermans MC, Hofmeijer J, Trof RJ, et al. Electroencephalogram predicts outcome in patients with postanoxic coma during mild therapeutic hypothermia. Crit Care Med. 2015;43:159–67.
86. Carrai R, Grippo A, Scarpino M, et al. Time-dependent and independent neurophysiological indicators of prognosis in post-anoxic coma subjects treated by therapeutic hypothermia. Minerva Anestesiol. 2016;82:940–9.
87. Grippo A, Carrai R, Scarpino M, et al. Neurophysiological prediction of neurological good and poor outcome in post-anoxic coma. Acta Neurol Scand. 2017;135:641–8.
88. Pfeiffer G, Pfeiffer R, Isenmann S. Cerebral hypoxia, missing cortical somatosensory evoked potentials and recovery of consciousness. BMC Neurol. 2014;14:82–7.
89. van Putten MJ. The N20 in post-anoxic coma: are you listening? Clin Neurophysiol. 2012;123:1460–4.
90. Scarpino M, Lanzo G, Lolli F, et al. Neurophysiological and neuroradiological multimodal approach for early poor outcome prediction after cardiac arrest. Resuscitation. 2018;129:114–20.
91. Fossi S, Amantini A, Grippo A, et al. Anoxic-ischemic alpha coma: prognostic significance of the incomplete variant. Neurol Sci. 2004;24:397–400.
92. Oddo M, Rossetti AO. Early multimodal outcome prediction after cardiac arrest in patients treated with hypothermia. Crit Care Med. 2014;42:1340–7.
93. Amorim E, Rittenberger JC, Baldwin ME, et al. Malignant EEG patterns in cardiac arrest patients treated with targeted temperature management who survive to hospital discharge. Resuscitation. 2015;90:127–32.
94. Hofmeijer J, Tjepkema-Cloostermans MC, van Putten MJ. Burst-suppression with identical bursts: a distinct EEG pattern with poor outcome in postanoxic coma. Clin Neurophysiol. 2014;125:947–54.
95. Sivaraju A, Gilmore EJ, Wira CR, et al. Prognostication of post-cardiac arrest coma: early clinical and electroencephalographic predictors of outcome. Intensive Care Med. 2015;41:1264–72.

47 Brain Death

Oriano Mecarelli and Edoardo Vicenzini

47.1 History of Brain Death Determination

This year recurs the 50th anniversary of publication of the criteria of Harvard Medical School that established brain death as an accepted medical phenomenon [1].

"Brain Death" (BD) is the term for defining death due to the irreversible cessation of all cerebral functions. This term may be actually misleading, since it wrongly implies that there is more than one kind of death, whereas death is instead an unitary phenomenon: in subjects without artificial ventilation, physicians confirm death only with the finding of permanent cessation of respiratory and cardiocirculatory functions; in patients who are receiving mechanical ventilation, it is instead mandatory to determine the irreversible loss of all brain functions, as respiratory and cardiac functions are artificially maintained.

In the 1950s critical care medicine showed rapid development, mainly for the diffusion of artificial ventilation devices and of cardiopulmonary resuscitation procedures; consequently, critical care physicians had firstly involved in the diagnosis and management of the condition of irreversible coma, later defined brain death. Mollaret and Goulon [2] described for the first time in 1959 23 patients with *coma depassé* ("a state beyond coma"), without any brainstem activity and maintained alive only by mechanical ventilation. Subsequently, medical communities and scientific societies worked to create specific definitions of this new entity and to define the guidelines for its determination, especially after the first human-to-human heart transplant in 1967 performed by Christiaan Barnard (1922–2001). At that time, it was indeed already felt the need to define precise criteria for brain death diagnosis, in order to be able to proceed with organ harvest.

It was in 1968 that the "Ad Hoc Committee of Harvard Medical School" defined brain death and described the criteria for its determination. The criteria included unreceptivity and unresponsivity, no movements or breathing, no reflexes, and flat electroencephalogram (confirmatory test that should be utilized when available). The persistence of these conditions had to be revaluated at least 24 h later and hypothermia treatment or administration of CNS depressant drugs was to be excluded [1].

In 1981, the President's Commission for the study of Ethical Problems in Medicine and Behavioral Research in the United States redefined the criteria for the diagnosis of brain death in adults and proposed a legal uniform definition of death (Uniform Determination of Death Act—UDDA). This act reports the following: "An individual who has sustained either (1) irreversible cessation of circulatory and respiratory functions, or (2) irreversible cessation of all functions of the entire brain, including the brain stem, is dead. A determination of death must be made with accepted medical standards" [3]. The UDDA did not define the acceptable diagnostic tests and medical procedures and then the Quality Standards Subcommittee of the American Academy of Neurology (AAN) in 1995 published evidence-based practice parameters for determining brain death in adults [4, 5]. The Guidelines of AAN were then updated in 2010, providing an algorithmic, unified approach to brain death determination in adults [6].

Clinical guidelines for the determination of brain death in children were first published in 1987 and later revised in 2011 [7–9].

O. Mecarelli (✉)
Department of Human Neurosciences, Sapienza University of Rome, Rome, Italy
e-mail: oriano.mecarelli@uniroma1.it

E. Vicenzini
Azienda Ospedaliero-Universitaria Policlinico Umberto I, Rome, Italy
e-mail: edoardo.vicenzini@uniroma1.it

O. Mecarelli (ed.), *Clinical Electroencephalography*, https://doi.org/10.1007/978-3-030-04573-9_47

47.2 Clinical Diagnosis of Brain Death

The prerequisites for BD diagnosis include:

- Knowledge of the proximate cause of coma and confirmation of its irreversibility (history, examination, neuroimaging and laboratory tests).
- Exclusion of confounding variables as severe electrolyte, acid-base and endocrine disturbances.
- Body temperature must be normal or near-normal (>36 °C).
- Systolic blood pressure must be ≥100 mg Hg.
- Exclusion of drug intoxication or poisoning (for the CNS depressant drugs, if available, evaluation of drug plasma levels below therapeutic range).

Neurologic assessment. The three cardinal findings in brain death are:

(a) Coma or unresponsiveness.
(b) Absence of brainstem reflexes.
(c) Absence of spontaneous breathing.

(a) *Coma*. The neurologist must first ascertain that the patient does not present any kind of responsiveness, as documented by the absence of eye opening or eye movements and absence of motor responses (other than spinally mediated reflexes) to noxious stimuli. Some studies reported spontaneous and reflex complex movements after brain death, of spinal or peripheral origin (facial myokymia; transient bilateral finger tremor; repetitive leg movements; cyclical constriction and dilation in light-fixed pupils; cremasteric, plantar, and abdominal reflexes; triple flexion of the lower extremities; deep tendon reflexes; "Lazarus sign"; undulating toe reflex) [10, 11]. Additionally, small changes in tubing pressure of ventilator and ventilator autocycling may falsely suggest a patient-initiated breaths that can be excluded by disconnecting the ventilator [12, 13]. The conclusion of the AAN guidelines is that "for some patients diagnosed as brain dead, complex, non-brain-mediated spontaneous movements can falsely suggest retained brain function" [6].

(b) *Absence of brainstem reflexes*. The neurologist must verify the absence of:
  - *Pupillary reflex* (usually, pupils are fixed in a midsize or dilated position, 4–9 mm diameter, not responding to light; the presence of dilated pupils is compatible with brain death because sympathetic cervical pathways may, however, remain intact; miosis suggests the possibility of drug intoxication; many drugs can influence pupils diameter, but the light response remains preserved [4]).
  - *Oculocephalic and oculovestibular reflexes* (the oculocephalic reflex may be elicited by turning the head to 90° on both sides and by brisk neck flexion: horizontal contralateral or vertical eye movements are absent in brain death; the oculovestibular reflex is tested with the head elevated to 30° by irrigating each ear with 50 mL of cold water, and the normal tonic deviation of the eyes toward the irrigated ear must be absent; the observation of eye movements must be protracted for 1 min after irrigation, and the time between stimulations on each side should be at least 5 min).
  - *Corneal reflex* (the absence of corneal reflex is demonstrated by touching the cornea with a piece of tissue paper or a cotton swab: no eyelids movement should be evoked).
  - *Facial movements* induced by noxious stimuli (deep pressure at temporomandibular joints and at the supraorbital ridge does not determine grimacing or facial muscle movements).
  - *Pharyngeal and tracheal reflexes* (the pharyngeal or gag reflex is elicited by stimulation of the posterior pharynx with a tongue blade or suction device; the tracheal or cough reflex is evoked by the insertion of a catheter into the trachea up to the level of the *carina*, followed by one or two suctioning passes).

(c) *Absence of spontaneous breathing*. The absence of a breathing drive is tested with an apnea test, that induce a CO_2 challenge. For the documentation of $PaCO_2$ increase to above normal levels (*apnea test*) the following prerequisites are necessary: normotension, normothermia, euvolemia, eucapnia ($PaCO_2$ 35–45 mm Hg), absence of hypoxia and no prior evidence of CO_2 retention due to chronic obstructive pulmonary disease or severe obesity. Then, the procedure for the *execution of apnea test* is as follows:
  - Adjust vasopressors to a systolic blood pressure ≥ 100 mm Hg.
  - Pre-oxygenate for at least 10 min with 100% oxygen to a PaO_2 > 200 mm Hg.
  - Reduce ventilation frequency to 10 breaths/min.
  - Reduce Positive End-Expiratory Pressure (PEEP) to 5 cm H_2O.
  - If pulse oximetry oxygen saturation remains >95%, obtain a baseline blood gas analysis.
  - Successively, the patient should be disconnected from the ventilator, delivering 100% O_2 at 6 L/min by an insufflation catheter through the endotracheal tube up to the *carina*.
  - After the disconnection from the ventilator, the patient must be closely observed for respiratory movements for 8–10 min (respiration can manifest itself with abdominal or chest excursions and may include brief gasps).
  - The patient must be reconnected to ventilator if systolic blood pressure decreases to <90 mm Hg and if oxygen saturation is <85%.

– After approximately 8 min from the ventilator disconnection, if no respiratory drive is observed, blood gas analysis (PaO_2, $PaCO_2$, pH, bicarbonate, base excess) can be performed.

The apnea test is considered positive and supportive the clinical diagnosis of brain death if respiratory movements are absent and $PaCO_2$ is ≥60 mm Hg (or $PaCO_2$ increase is >20 mm Hg compared to basal values). If the test is inconclusive ($PaCO_2$ is less than 60 mm Hg), but the patient is hemodynamically stable, the procedure may be repeated with a longer period of time of ventilator disconnection (10–15 min) [4–6].

Apnea testing is considered an indispensable element for brain death diagnosis, but there is insufficient scientific evidence to determine the comparative safety of techniques used [6, 14].

Wijdicks et al. [15] reviewed retrospectively a large series of patients who were declared brain dead and concluded that apnea testing with an oxygen-diffusion technique is safe. Nevertheless, apnea test could not be performed in 7% of the patients because of hemodynamic instability or poor oxygenation at baseline. In 3% of patients, the test was aborted because of hypotension or hypoxemia.

Therefore, once the above clinical conditions are ascertained, there should be no need for an observation period to declare BD diagnosis. Using the criteria universally recognized, recovery of neurologic functions has indeed never been reported, and there is insufficient evidence to determine which would be the minimally acceptable observation period to ensure its irreversibility. In these regards, the length of the observation period is very variable throughout the world and also among the hospitals of the United States. Waiting period between the initial neurologic deterioration until death declaration ranged from <5 to >25 h [16–18]. Lustbader et al. [19] reported that, in the NY State, the time to perform a second neurological evaluation was approximately 3 times longer than that recommended in the guidelines (mean 19.2 vs. 6 h) and that it was associated with markedly higher intensive care unit costs and increased loss of viable organs. Moreover, the time lapse between the two observations may increase the likelihood of premature cardiac arrest, which accounts for up to 12% in literature [19].

47.3 Ancillary Tests

Ancillary tests are optional/confirmatory in the United States and in other parts of the world, but mandatory in many countries [16, 18].

Indications for ancillary tests execution are represented substantially by: difficulties for clinical examination due to anatomic limitations or injuries; apnea test that cannot be completed for hemodynamic instability or hypoxia; limitations to interpreting a positive apnea test (high levels of sedative drugs, severe neuromuscular disease, preexisting CO_2 retention) or apnea test inconclusive in clinically unstable patient; high levels of CNS depressants; less than 24 h since cardiac arrest or recovery from hypothermia therapy; physician or family discomfort with brain death diagnosis (especially when the residual movements and spinal reflexes are disturbing).

The ancillary tests used in the confirmation of brain death are represented by:

(a) Neurophysiological methods to highlight the loss of bioelectrical brain activity (EEG, Evoked Potentials (EPs)).
(b) Methods for the demonstration of cerebral circulatory arrest (Trans Cranial Doppler (TCD); Single-Photon Emission Computed Tomography (Tc99 HMPAO SPECT); conventional and digital subtraction angiography; CT angiography; MRI angiography).

47.3.1 EEG

The characteristic EEG finding in BD is the *Electro Cerebral Inactivity (ECI)*, which is defined as "the absence over all regions of the head of identifiable electrical activity of cerebral origin, whether spontaneous or induced by physiological stimuli (synonyms are electrocerebral silence, flat or isoelectric EEG, but the use of these terms is discouraged)" [20]. Tracings with ECI should be clearly distinguished from the EEG patterns with low-voltage background activity. EEG is a very sensible tool to evaluate cerebral functional activity related to cerebral perfusion: reversible EEG changes appear when the CBF decreases below 35 mL/100 g/min and cortical activity is totally suppressed when CBF reduces below 12/mL/100 g/min. After a few seconds from blood flow arrest, electrical cortical activity is suppressed, and—if the circulation is not readily reestablished—this will cause cells death and irreversible loss of all brain functions (Fig. 47.1).

An EEG with ECI cannot, however, exclude that some subcortical or brainstem functions remain preserved [21, 22], and ECI have been described also in patients with vegetative state. On the other hand, older studies assessing EEG accuracy in BD diagnosis are difficult to be interpreted, since they were performed before the development of explicit guidelines for the clinical BD declaration [23].

More recent studies conducted in countries with precise guidelines have highlighted uncommon discrepancies between clinical and electroencephalographic findings. In 71 consecutive patients declared brain dead using the German guidelines, ECI is present in 94%. In the remaining four patients, EEG tracings could not be interpreted

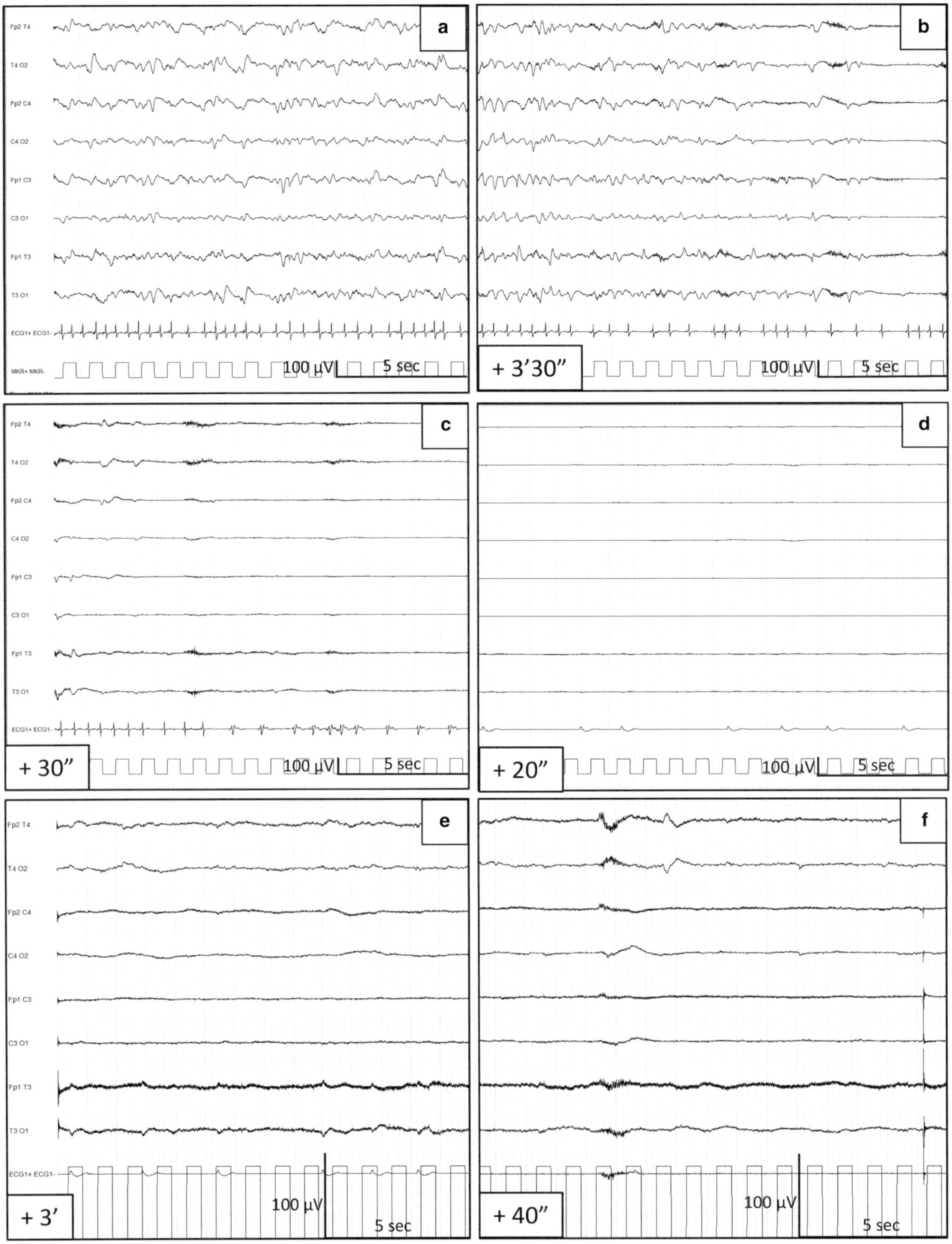

Fig. 47.1 An example of progressive attenuation/suppression of the background activity (**a–c**) up to electrocerebral inactivity (**d–f**), in a 77-year-old patient with cardiorespiratory failure, in absence of artificial ventilation. Note in (**f**) the complete absence of heartbeat. LFF 0.53 Hz, HFF 70 Hz. Sensitivity: **a**, **b**, **c**, **d** = 10 µV/mm; **e**, **f** = 2 µV/mm

because the presence of artifacts [24]. A retrospective study performed using Spanish guidelines showed that EEG tracings confirmed ECI in 96.5% of patients. The remaining patients (3.5%) had most frequently underlying severe brainstem damage with malignant EEG patterns, but no ECI [25]. None of these patients survived. In Italy, EEG is mandatory for brain death diagnosis, and in our series of 66 consecutive patients, we have not found discrepancies between clinical criteria for brain death according to Italian guidelines and ECI [26]. No patients meeting criteria for brain death with ECI in EEG regained neurological functions [25, 26].

In summary, EEG has a long history as a confirmatory test in BD, and it can be easily performed bedside without risks; when clinical BD assessment is performed according to the accepted guidelines, EEG features are rarely discrepant or always concurrent. False positives can occur, mainly due to the depressant effects on electrocerebral activity of sedative drugs or hypothermia. False negatives can be due to electrical interferences in ICU environment and artifacts of various origins. Sometimes, administration of muscle relaxants is necessary to achieve an EEG tracing uncontaminated by EMG activity. Rarely, EEG tracing is uninterpretable or not recordable for the poor condition of the patient's scalp (Fig. 47.2). After all, additional limitations of the EEG as confirmatory test in brain death are represented by its nonavailability 24 h per day at many centers. Despite these limitations, EEG remains the second most common ancillary test to be used [27, 28].

47.3.1.1 Technical Standards for EEG Recording in Brain Death

Various national and international guidelines and laws define the minimum technical standards for EEG recording in suspected cerebral death. The contents of guidelines [6] of the American Clinical Neurophysiology Society, that is an update of the precedent guidelines [3], are summarized [29, 30]:

(a) Electrocerebral inactivity is defined as the absence of nonartifactual electrical activity over 2 μV (peak to peak), at a sensitivity of 2 μV/mm (Fig. 47.3). A calibration signal of 2 or 5 μV is appropriate, and the recording should last 30 min at least.

All major brain areas should be explored with scalp electrodes placed according to 10–20 international system. The montage should include electrode pairs at least

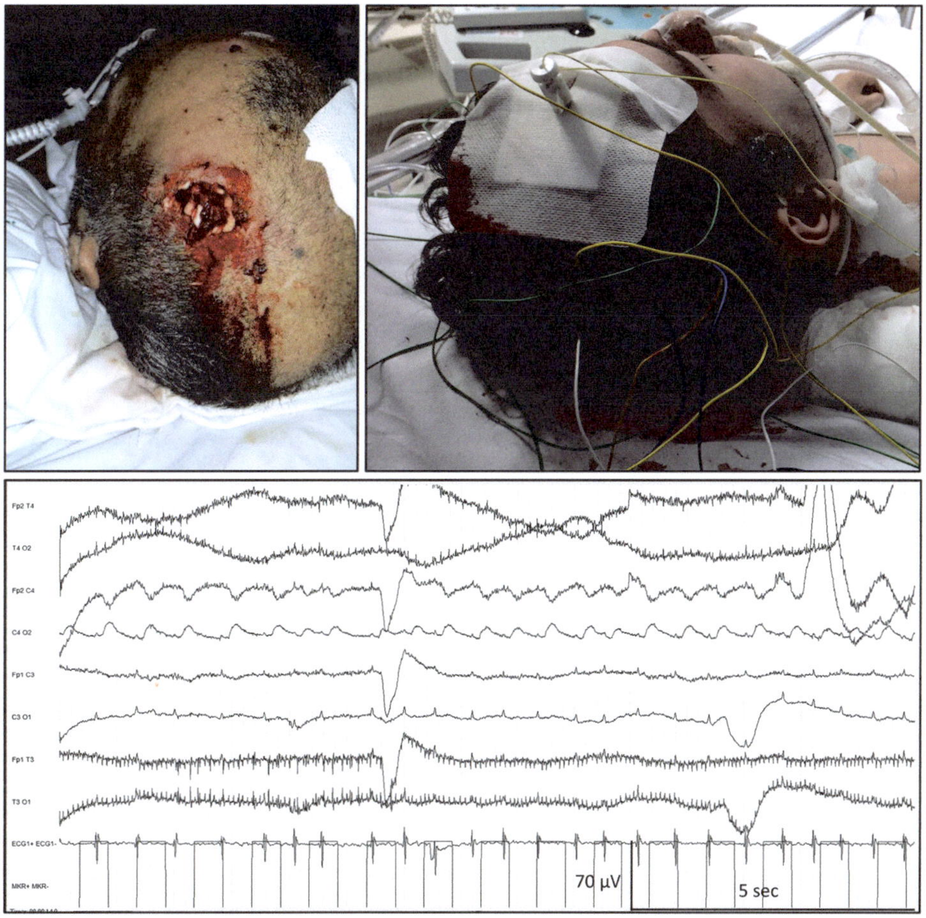

Fig. 47.2 Examples of severe lesions of the scalp, with unvaluable EEG recording (see below)

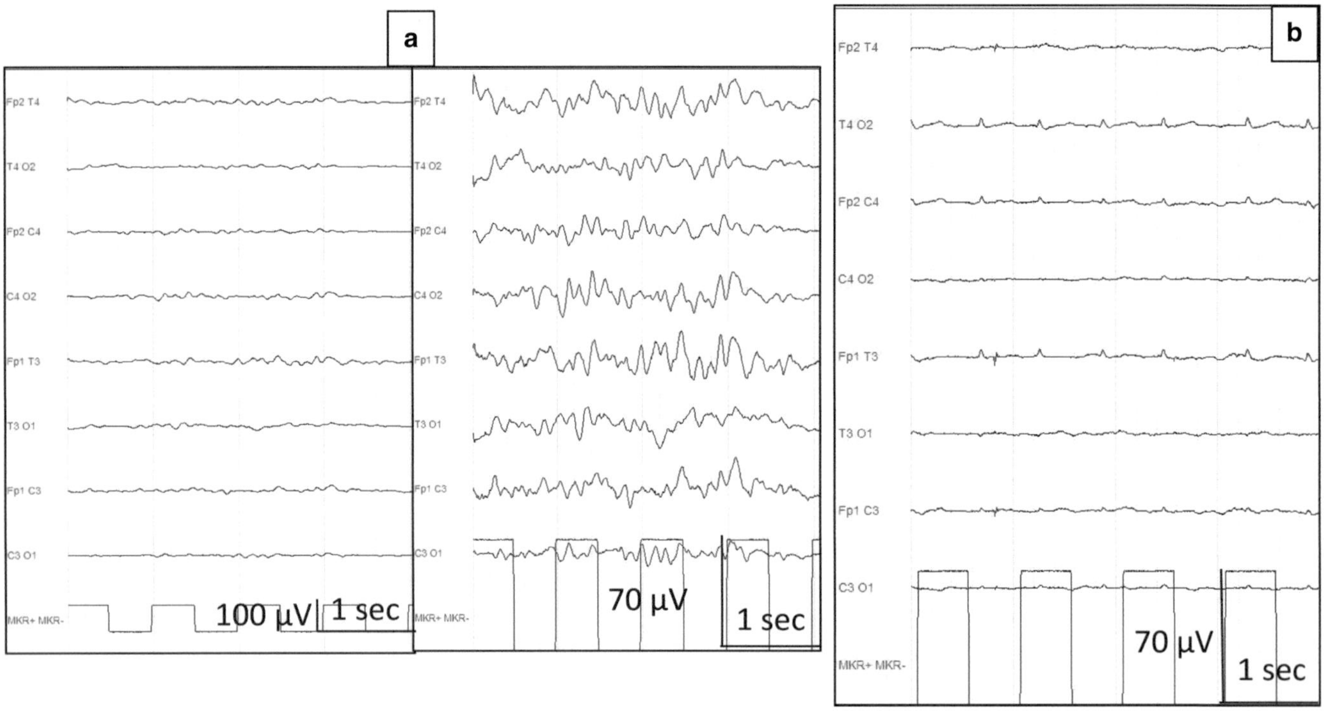

Fig. 47.3 A 56-year-old patient, 2 days after a severe anoxic insult. EEG recording with cerebral activity of low voltage at a sensitivity of 10 µV/mm (**a**, on the left), which is more evident at 2 µV/mm (**a**, on the right). After about 4 h (**b**), the tracing appears with electrocerebral inactivity at sensitivity of 2 µV/mm. LFF 0.53 Hz, HFF 70 Hz

10 cm apart, and an acceptable montage is Fp2-C4, C4-O2, Fp1-C3, C3-O1, T4-Cz (T8-Cz in the modified 10–10 terminology), and Cz-T3 (Cz-T7 in the modified 10–10 terminology).

A montage that includes F8-T6 (F8-P8 in the modified 10–10 terminology), F4-P4, Fz-Pz, F3-P3, and F7-T5 (F7-P7 in the modified 10–10 terminology) should be recommended. The montage must include one channel for ECG (to identify the ECG artifact) and one channel for a noncephalic recording (e.g., on the hand, to document movement-induced artifacts).

In addition, all the preselected laboratory montages should be used.

(b) Electrode impedances should be less than 10.000 ohms, but more than 100 ohms. The integrity of the entire recording system should be tested by touching each electrode of the montage, for verifying the correct connection of all electrodes with the recording machine. The filters should be set between 1 and 30 Hz, and the notch filter (at 60 or 50 Hz) can be used with care and comparing the EEG segments with the notch filter to those without.

(c) To clarify the recording and to accurately assess and identify the various artifacts (physiological, mechanical, electromagnetic or electrostatic, etc.) (Fig. 47.4), it is sometimes necessary to monitor the respiration and the EMG contamination (if EMG activity obscures the EEG tracing, it may be necessary to eliminate it administrating short-term neuromuscular blocking agent) (Fig. 47.5). Furthermore, continuous video-recording is strongly encouraged to help identify any kind of artifacts.

(d) During the recording there should be no reactivity to intense somatosensory, auditory, or visual stimuli. The technician must apply the various standardized stimuli and note on the tracing the time at which they were applied.

(e) The EEG recordings for ECI should be performed by a qualified technologist, under supervision of a qualified electroencephalographer. Sometimes, the interpretation of an EEG performed for BD diagnosis is difficult for technical or physiological variables and, in these cases, the entire procedure should be repeated after a 6-h interval in adults and after at least 24 h in newborns and children. To limit errors in interpretation, it is important that the technologist note all pathophysiologic variables (temperature, blood pressure, oxygen saturation) and all the medications administrated.

47.3.2 Evoked Potentials

Short latency Evoked Potentials (EPs) have the advantage to be a test widely available and noninvasive, able to explore

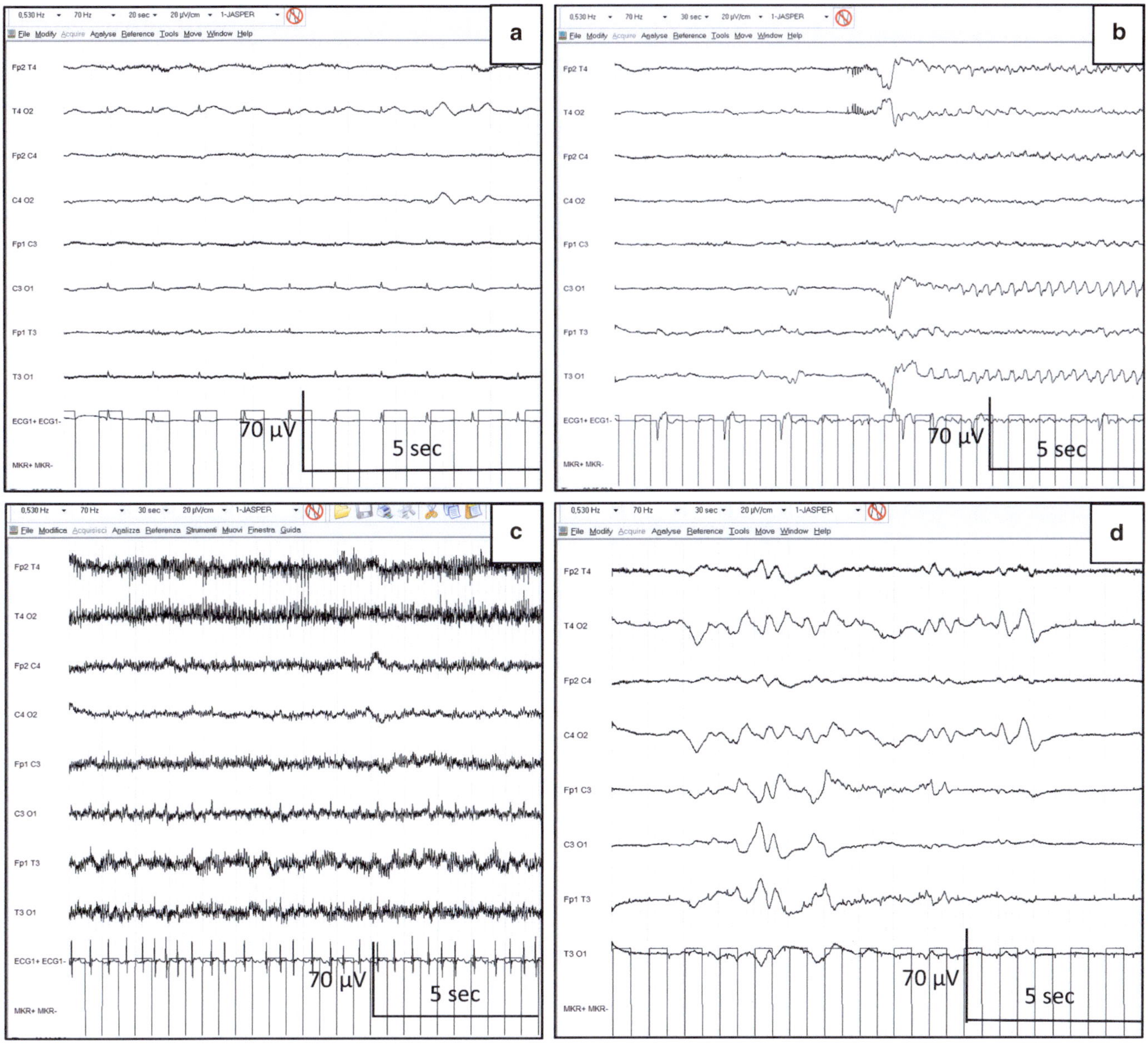

Fig. 47.4 Examples of artifacts during EEG recording for brain death evaluation. (**a**) pulse and ECG artifacts. (**b**) artifact due to atrial fibrillation. (**c**) EMG activity. (**d**) artifacts induced by movements of the nursing staff around the bed

the brainstem structures and less affected by sedation and hypothermia than EEG (Fig. 47.6). The major disadvantages for this technique are represented by the necessity of the expertise in their performance and interpretation, by the possibility of false-negative results, and by the absence of potentials in patients with lesions of cervicomedullary junction.

Somato Sensory Evoked Potentials (SSEPs) assess the functional integrity of posterior columns, medial lemniscus, thalamus, and the sensorimotor cortex, and they are indicative of BD if bilateral absence of N20-P22 response to median nerve stimulation is demonstrated [5]. Generally, the absence of N20 is an indicator of poor prognosis in comatose patients, and it is predictive of BD. However, in BD early phase, the cortical components of SSEPs can be sometimes present, disappearing only over time. Wagner [31] studied the component P14 of SSEPs (presumably generated in the medial lemniscus and cuneate nucleus) and demonstrated that in all 108 patients diagnosed brain dead, the P14 potential on nasopharyngeal electrodes was absent (specificity 100%). However, the P14 potential has two generators: the greater rostral part of the P14 generator dipole is inactivated in BD, whereas the very caudal segments may be still intact for some time; furthermore, the absence of P14 can be due to lesions of the upper cervical cord and medulla. To avoid false-negative or false-positive results, recording with naso-

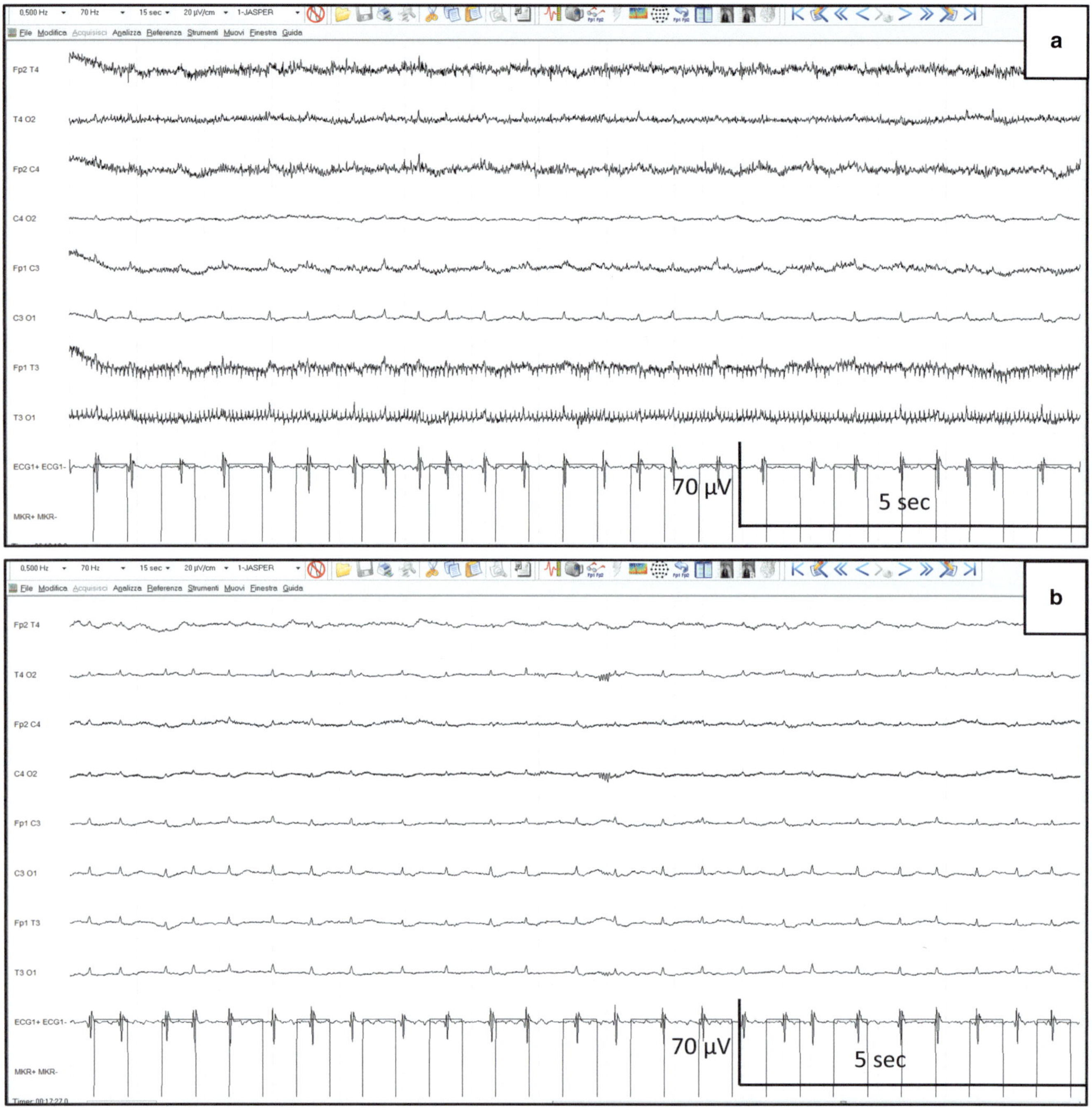

Fig. 47.5 (**a**) EMG activity obscuring the EEG tracing. (**b**) after short-term neuromuscular blocking agent, EMG activity rapidly and transitory disappears (note the persistence of ECG artifact)

pharyngeal electrodes is advisable, but this technique is still not widespread and not sufficiently validated [32].

Brainstem Auditory Evoked Potentials (BAEPs) were found to be 100% sensitive, but only 73.7% specific, and BAEPs may be transiently absent after an anoxic insult [33]. Facco et al., in a series of 130 brain dead patients, demonstrated that BAEPs were absent in 70.8%, while SSEPs confirmed the absence of brainstem activity in 93.7% of cases [34]. These authors concluded that the combined use of SSEPs and BAEPs was able to confirm BD in almost all patients, excluding this diagnosis in a few cases (about 5% in their series) that show residual brainstem activity; they also emphasize the utility of a more complete (not only EEG-based) neurophysiological investigation in BD to improve patients' management and the certainty of diagnosis. Obviously, none of these patients survived, but they were not declared dead until the disappearance of all evoked potentials [34].

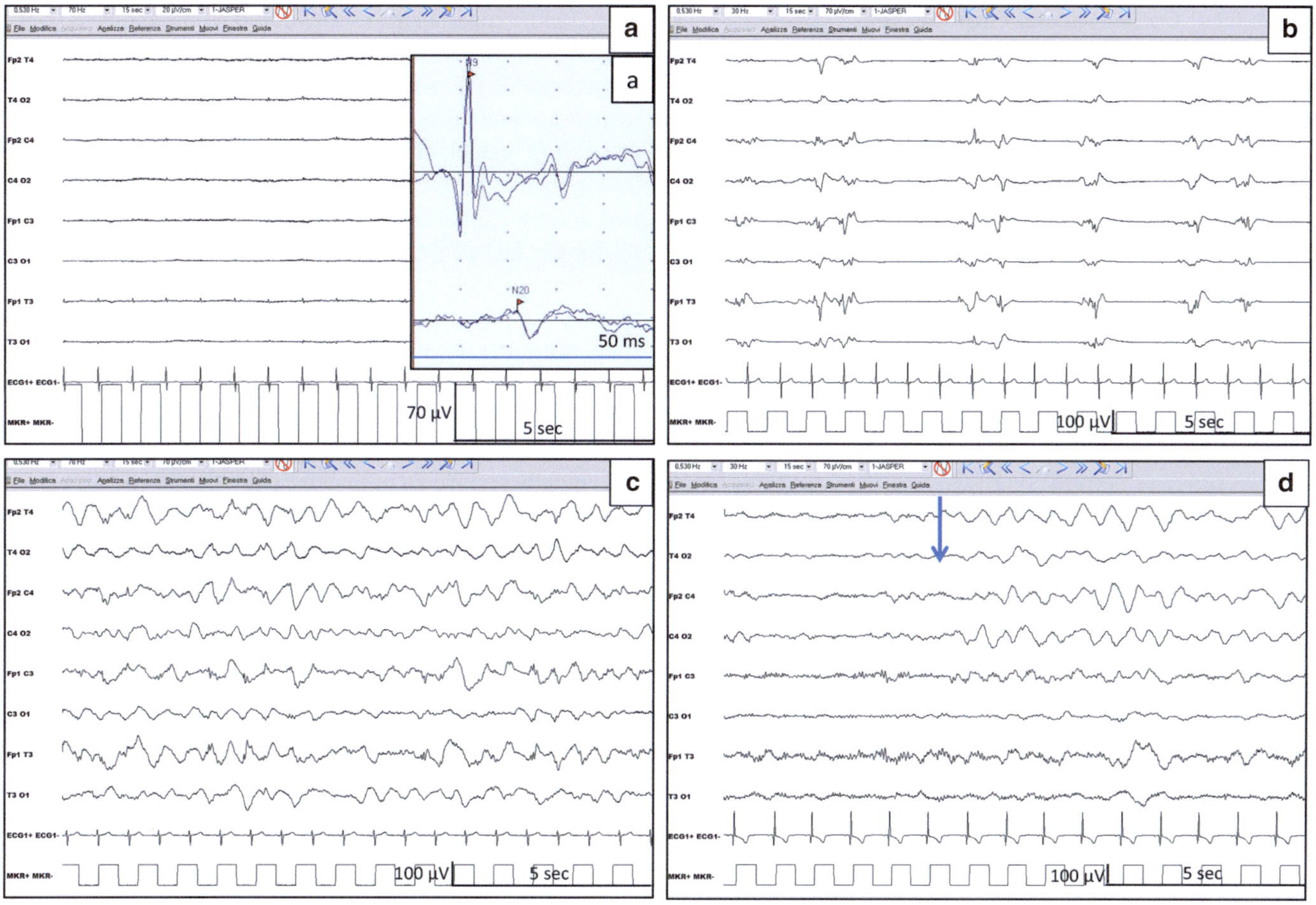

Fig. 47.6 Seriated EEG recordings in a 21-year-old patient with post-traumatic coma, sedated with Sodium Thio Pental (STP). In (**a**) EEG with electrocerebral inactivity; Somato Sensory Evoked Potentials (SSEPs) (**a**) show a persistence of low-voltage, reproducible N20 component (the plasmatic level of STP is 11 µg/mL, and the brainstem reflexes are absent). After 48 h (**b**) EEG with burst-suppression pattern (STP has been suspended, and plasmatic level is 8 µg/mL; the brainstem reflexes had reappeared). After 72 h (**c**) the background EEG activity is continuous and of high amplitude (STP: 5 µg/mL), but unreactive. After 96 h (**d**), EEG is again reactive to acoustic stimulus—at arrow (STP, 2.8 µg/mL)

47.3.3 Assessment of Cerebral Blood Flow

Increase of intracranial hypertension is the condition at the basis of absence of Cerebral Blood Flow (CBF). When the intracranial pressure overrides the mean arterial blood pressure, a mechanical hindrance to blood stream entrance in intracranial arteries, in the intact skull, occurs. This condition is typically referred to as "Cerebral Circulatory Arrest" (CCA), since most techniques aimed at this evaluation actually investigate cerebral circulation and not cerebral perfusion.

Several conventional radiological techniques may be applied to identify CCA: conventional angiography represents the "gold standard," while less invasive techniques, such as CT and MR angiographies, both with perfusion studies, are nowadays also being used. Single-photon emission computed tomography (SPECT) and xenon-CT are dedicated to the investigation of cerebral perfusion, but these investigations may be less commonly available. All these radiological techniques, though expensive, are time-consuming and require the patient to be delivered to the radiological unit to perform the exam, further dilating the time to the final death declaration, a crucial point for eventual organ harvest. Moreover, contrast agent administration may induce further organ damage, eventually reducing the possibility of organ donation. For these reasons, Trans Cranial Doppler (TCD) ultrasound is commonly used for detecting CCA easily and at the bed of the patient, with high sensibility and specificity, when performed with strict protocols. Recently, even the optic nerve sheath diameter evaluation has been correlated with marked intracranial hypertension and, thus, correlated with development of malignant intracranial hypertension and brain death in critically care patients.

47.3.3.1 Conventional Four-Vessel Angiography

Conventional angiography is classically considered to be the gold standard method for CCA diagnosis. This technique is relatively easy to perform and to interpret and may be executed in 30–60 min. Examinations for BD are usually performed with contrast medium injections in the aortic arch with a "pig tail" catheter, but the separate contrast injections performed in either the common or the internal carotid arteries, as well as in both the vertebral arteries, have also been used. Angiographic CCA findings consist in the lack of contrast diffusion in the internal carotid arteries beyond the carotid siphon and beyond the dural penetration of vertebral arteries, with normal visualization of the external carotid arteries (positive control) (Fig. 47.7).

Some opacification in the proximal middle or anterior cerebral arteries are described in 30% of patients [35], and this may be due to the selective injection of individual vessels and to high injection flow rates that force contrast medium into the intracranial vessels [36]. The vein system should not be visualized, though occasional visualization of the superior longitudinal sinus may be possible through meningeal veins. In literature, no false-positive cases have been reported, whereas some false-negative cases are described, where patients have been clinically declared brain dead, but they continue to have some intracranial blood flow [22].

Despite considered the "gold standard," conventional angiography has numerous disadvantages: it is an invasive and expensive procedure, it cannot be performed bedside, and it is not readily available in many hospitals; it requires the insertion of a catheter in the arterial circulation, with potential risk for vessel damage and dissections along the catheter course; the contrast medium may produce organ toxicity, especially for the kidneys, that is unfavorable in case of their harvest [22, 32].

47.3.3.2 Computed Tomography Angiography (CTA) and CT Perfusion

Being nowadays CTA routinely performed in vessel assessment for cerebrovascular diseases, it is the natural evolution of the technique to be used to assess CCA, and it is also well accepted in European countries as an ancillary test for BD determination. As in conventional angiography, CCA is diagnosed when the lack of visualization of intracranial arteries beyond the siphon and beyond the dural penetration of vertebral arteries is observed. CTA is a rapid and widely available method for assessing brain blood flow, far less invasive than conventional angiography; however, as iodinated contrast is to be used, the potential risk of contrast-mediated tissue injury is still present. Systematic reviews have assessed the accuracy of CTA as confirmatory test for BD declaration and reported a pooled sensitivity of 84% [37], and false-positive uncommon cases have been described [38].

In regard to CT perfusion, this technique has been adopted to quantify brain perfusion in stroke, and its subsequent post-processing calculations to generate perfusion parameters (mean transit time, cerebral blood flow, and volume) would also add functional information that could increase sensitivity for the BD diagnosis. However, it requires brain parenchyma appropriate assessment and specific trained personnel to correctly interpret its findings. Further studies will help to standardize the technique [39].

47.3.3.3 Magnetic Resonance Angiography (MRA) and MR Perfusion

In clinically confirmed brain dead patients, MR imaging may demonstrate in BD the lack of the normal intracranial arterial flow voids, due to the intracranial hypertension and to the slowing of blood flow within cerebral arteries. MRA imaging without contrast agents uses the "time-of-flight" sequences that are related to the "moving blood," and, similarly to the other techniques, this will lead to the lack of visualization of the intracranial circulation in CCA. However, MR imaging takes longer time, it is more prone to develop artifacts, and it requires compatibility of the devices that usually these critical patients have attached. MR perfusion with contrast agents may also be considered a promising technique, with data similar to those of the perfusion CT, with no available data in the brain death setting [40–42].

47.3.3.4 Single-Photon Emission Computed Tomography (SPECT)

Brain perfusion scintigraphy with specific brain radionuclide 99mTc-HMPAO (Hexa Methyl Propylene Amine Oxime) represents a well-studied method for BD diagnosis [43]. The radionuclide overrides the blood-brain barrier, with uptake from cerebral neurons after the initial blood flow passage, indicating not only the presence of flow, but also the presence of cerebral activity. Nuclear medicine divisions are necessary to perform this examination, and CCA finding consists in the lack of intracranial tracing uptake, the so-called "hollow skull" [44]. Planar anterior and both lateral images are recommended to be acquired immediately, after between 30 and 60 min and at 2 h after radionuclide injection (740 MBq [20 mCi] -Tc-99 m with a HMPAO and saline 5 mL). Multiprojection static planar imaging can also be used to evaluate the cerebral hemispheres, basal ganglia, thalami, and cerebellum, with progressive 5° rotation of the scanner, 20 s/step, for 360° and for a total exam duration of 25 min. The current use of SPECT is primarily supplemental, to help differentiate overlying scalp from intracerebral activity. The reliability of SPECT to exclude flow and metabolism in the brainstem remains to be scientifically validated. SPECT imaging can be technically difficult in the context of BD con-

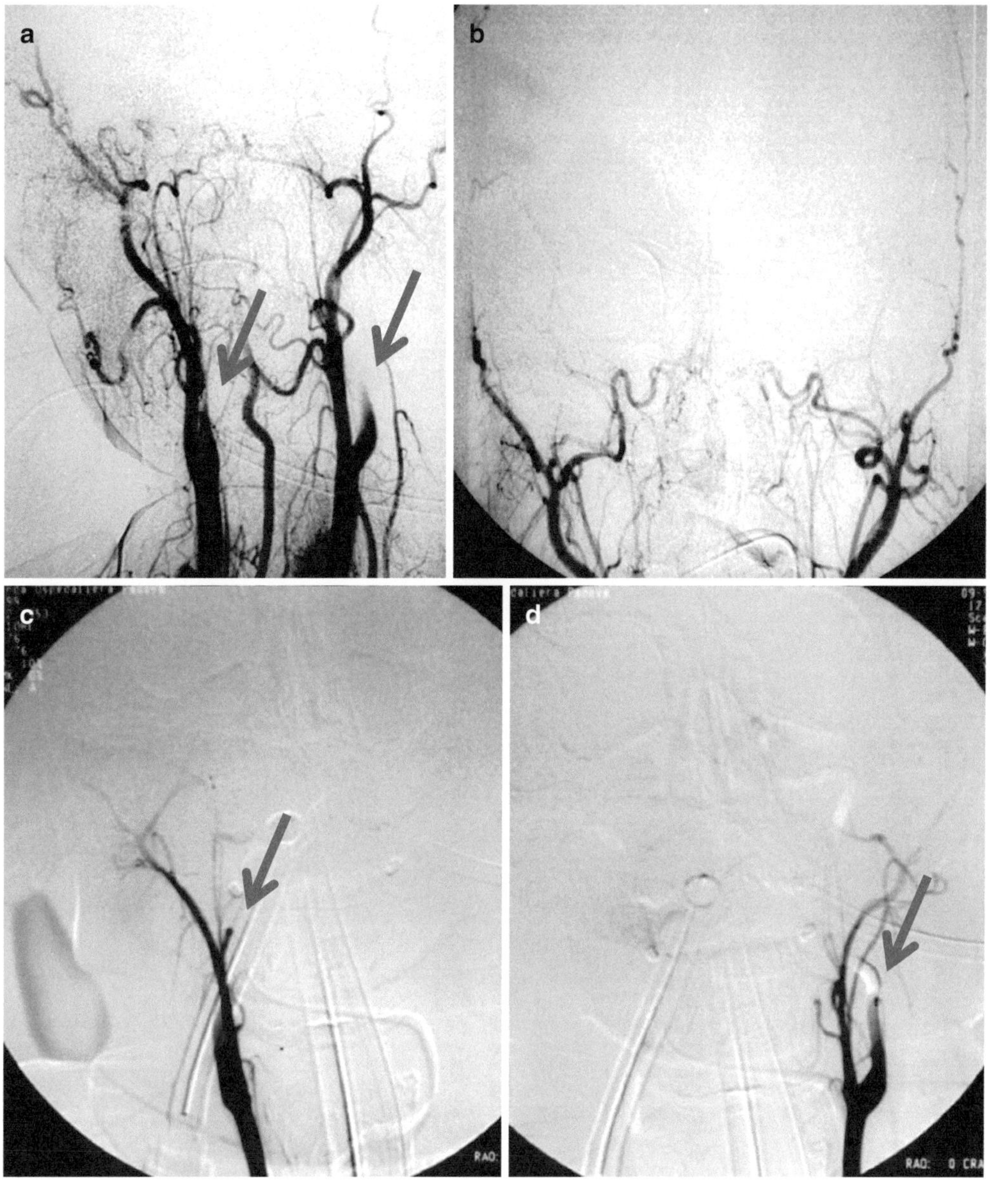

Fig. 47.7 Conventional angiography in brain death during contrast arch injection (**a**, **b**) and during selective common carotid artery injection (**c**, **d**). Arrows show the point of contrast arrest at the level of the internal carotid arteries. Note the normal opacification of the external carotid arteries

firmation. Typical issues encountered for SPECT imaging include indeed the difficulty of bringing the gamma camera detectors sufficiently close to the patient, presence of tubes and lines in the detector orbit acting as impediments to detector rotation, and the requirement of moving the patient to the imaging table. The specificity of SPECT was estimated to be of 100% and sensitivity of 88% [45–47].

47.3.3.5 Transcranial Doppler

In the presence of adequate temporal and occipital bone windows, i.e., in 95% of cases, TCD ultrasound equipments with a 2 MHz probe can easily insonate the intracranial basal cerebral arteries [26, 48, 49]. Characteristic changes of blood flow velocity waveforms are proportional to the increase of intracerebral pressure, up to CCA development. Four pathognomonic stages are identified (Fig. 47.8):

1. Increased resistive indices: the increase of the intracranial pressure induces gradual reduction of diastolic blood flow velocities over systolic flow velocities. This stage, indicative of increased intracranial pressure, is not yet representative of CCA (Fig. 47.8b).
2. Oscillating/reverberating flow: the flow direction in the diastolic phase becomes inverted, i.e., during systole blood flow is directed toward the brain and during diastole is directed away from the brain. When both the phases are equal, this corresponds to the CCA (Fig. 47.8c, d).
3. Systolic spikes: short (<200 ms) and slow velocity (<50 cm/s) ortodromic systolic spikes are expression of further reduction of blood flow movements. High pass filters of ultrasound equipments may participate to cut off slow velocity signals and, thus, should they be set as low as possible (50 Hz) (Fig. 47.8e).

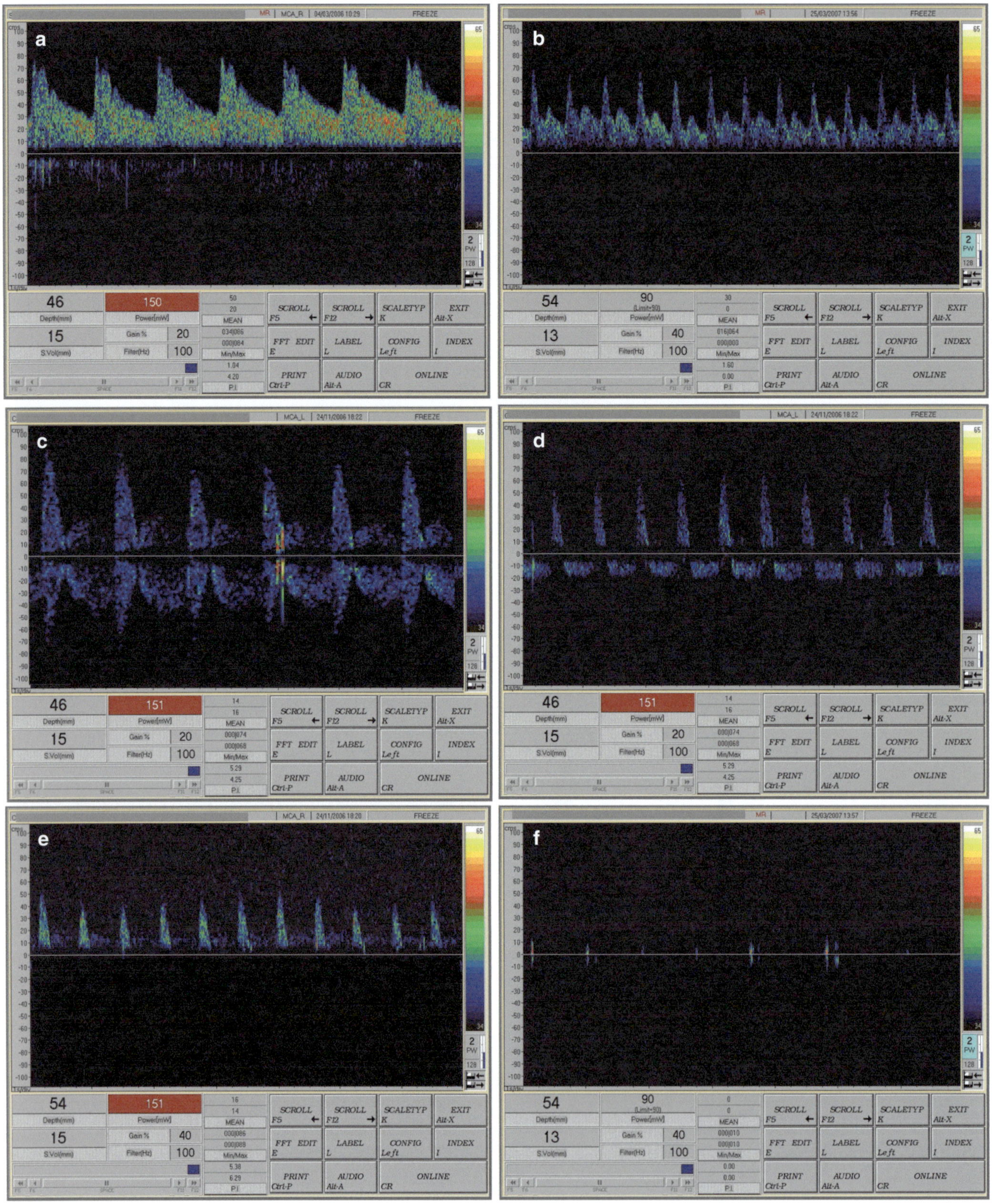

Fig. 47.8 Trans Cranial Doppler (TCD) middle cerebral artery spectrum evolution during intracranial hypertension. (**a**) Normal spectrum; (**b**) increased resistive indices, flow is still present; (**c**, **d**) Oscillating/reverberating flow with various degree of reversal flow reduction, cerebral circulatory arrest (CCA); (**e**) systolic spikes; (**f**) absence of flow

4. Absence of signal: when flow stop becomes more proximal, no signal could be detected in the intracranial arteries (Fig. 47.8f) These findings alone, however, performed in a single examination could also be related to transmission problems through thick and inadequate temporal bone windows and may not be conclusive. Thus, absence of signal is probative of CCA only when the same operator had already performed the examination before, demonstrating the adequacy of the temporal bone windows. In such cases, findings in the vertebral arteries—as well as in the extracranial cervical arteries—represent an important criterion to be added for the diagnosis.

For CCA diagnosis, a single operator should carry out two examinations at a 20–30 min interval, in hemodynamic stable conditions (Systolic Blood Pressure, SBP >100 mm Hg, Mean Arterial Blood Pressure MABP >70 mm Hg), identifying the typical CCA patterns in any of the intracerebral arteries, through temporal and occipital insonation. These findings should also be confirmed in the extracranial circulation. Recently, the use of color-coded transcranial Doppler has also been proposed for the CCA diagnosis, considering that the direct visualization of the brain structures could be of help in discriminating the adequacy of the bone windows and for the detection of the above-described typical Doppler patterns. Though TCD is easily and quickly performed bedside, the main criticism regards the expertise of the operator requiring dedicated, expert and well-formed physicians to obtain a reliable diagnosis. In our experience, CCA diagnosis performed with TCD, when CBF evaluation is requested, is useful to significantly reduce the time to final BD declaration in respect to angiography [26]. Transcranial Doppler—and in general techniques aimed at flow investigation—usually has a very high (up to 100%) specificity, i.e., the identification of CCA consistent with BD diagnosis, but lower sensitivity (90–95%), since the persistence of cerebral blood flow may be observed even after BD, in cases of skull fenestration (decompressive craniectomy, infants with non-ossified fontanelles, ventricular derivation) [50].

An important concept, at the bases of these "false-negative" results, has to be discussed when considering cerebral blood flow for the diagnosis of BD, regardless the technique used. BD is—by definition—the irreversible loss of any cerebral neuronal activity, and it implies that neurons are not functional and they have no metabolism at all. As regards the false-negative persistence, to various degrees, of "blood flow" when BD has already occurred, it has to be underlined that only scintigraphy and PET scans are actually able to really display brain metabolism. All the other techniques, investigating blood flow as "circulation," are based on the assumption that if there is metabolism, there is "flow", but this might not be true backward. As a matter of fact, the condition necessary to induce CCA inside the skull is the increase of the intracranial pressure, overriding the mean arterial blood pressure and, thus, inducing the mechanical forces to interrupt circulation. However, if cerebral damage had already occurred or neuronal degeneration had already developed over time—as it may occur in ICUs during a long follow-up of these neurocritical patients—decompressive craniectomy (or other treatments aimed at reducing ICP, such as ventricular derivation) only reduces the mechanical forces induced by the swollen dead brain, with consequent lowering of intracranial pressure and restoring a "cerebral circulation" (i.e., blood that enters the arterial bed drained out from the vein system), but in absence of cerebral function. To make a simple analogy, in the case of a compartment syndrome for muscular damage, fasciotomy restores blood flow, but if the necrosis had already occurred in the muscle, flow restoration doesn't restore muscular cell activity. Then, to summarize, detection of CCA—regardless of the technique used—in cases of an intact skull has 100% specificity for BD diagnosis. In cases of non-intact skull, when however the brain is swollen and fenestration is not able to compensate for the malignant intracranial pressure, CCA may however occur, and its detection is supportive of BD; usually, in these cases, craniectomies are swollen and hard, and flow spectra may be asymmetric due to the higher "blood movement" in the open skull side and that could be misinterpreted as flow persistence with other techniques (Fig. 47.9). Last, in cases of skull fenestration and clinical and/or instrumental BD suspicion, "persistence" of cerebral blood flow detected with TCD—or with other CBF investigating techniques—only indicates that the assessment of cerebral blood blow cannot be used to support in these cases BD diagnosis and that this false-negative - though "expected" - result only represents that we are evaluating circulation and not metabolism (Fig. 47.10) [51, 52].

Another sonographic exam that can be performed in the follow up neurocritical patients, for the early identification of critical malignant intracranial hypertension, is the Optic Nerve Sheath Diameter (ONSD) measurement [53]. Several clinical studies have indeed correlated the increase of ONSD as a reliable, noninvasive method to detect intracranial hypertension in neurosurgery and ICUs. ONSD is indeed directly connected with the subarachnoid space, and—differently from the inextensible—the intraorbital subarachnoid meningeal prolongation around the optic nerve is free of swelling with the pressure increase in the cerebrospinal fluid. Historically, the sign of the papilledema is a typical expression of this phenomenon. Even though the detection of ONSD enlargement of up to 0.6–0.7 cm could not alone be indicative for BD diagnosis, this very simple measurement performed through the eye during follow-up in ICU could help to identify those patients who—sedated—are developing signs of malignant intracranial hypertension and that could be then at risk of BD development [54].

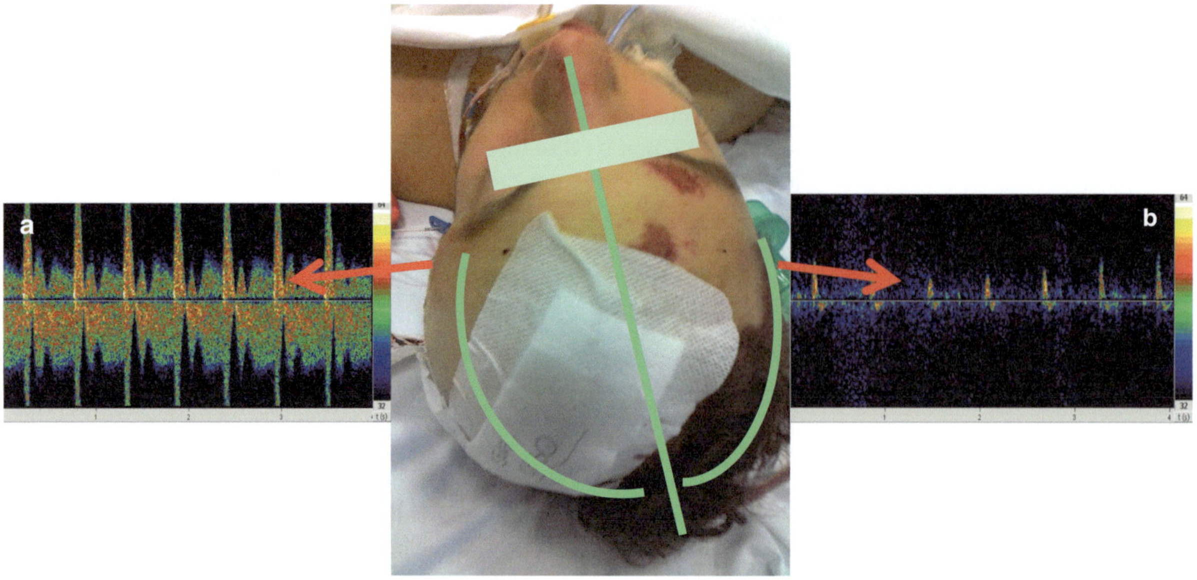

Fig. 47.9 Trans Cranial Doppler (TCD) showing Cerebral Circulatory Arrest (CCA) despite left decompressive craniectomy. TCD spectra are asymmetric, with reverberating flow and high velocities in the open side (**a**) and with only systolic spikes in the intact skull side (**b**). This finding is consistent with higher intracranial pressure in the intact skull side, that induces the disappearance of retrograde flow. In the open side, minimal compensation due to the absence of the bone still preserves higher blood movements with persistance of reverberant flow, though with higher velocities than expected. Decompressive craniectomy is, however, tense and swollen

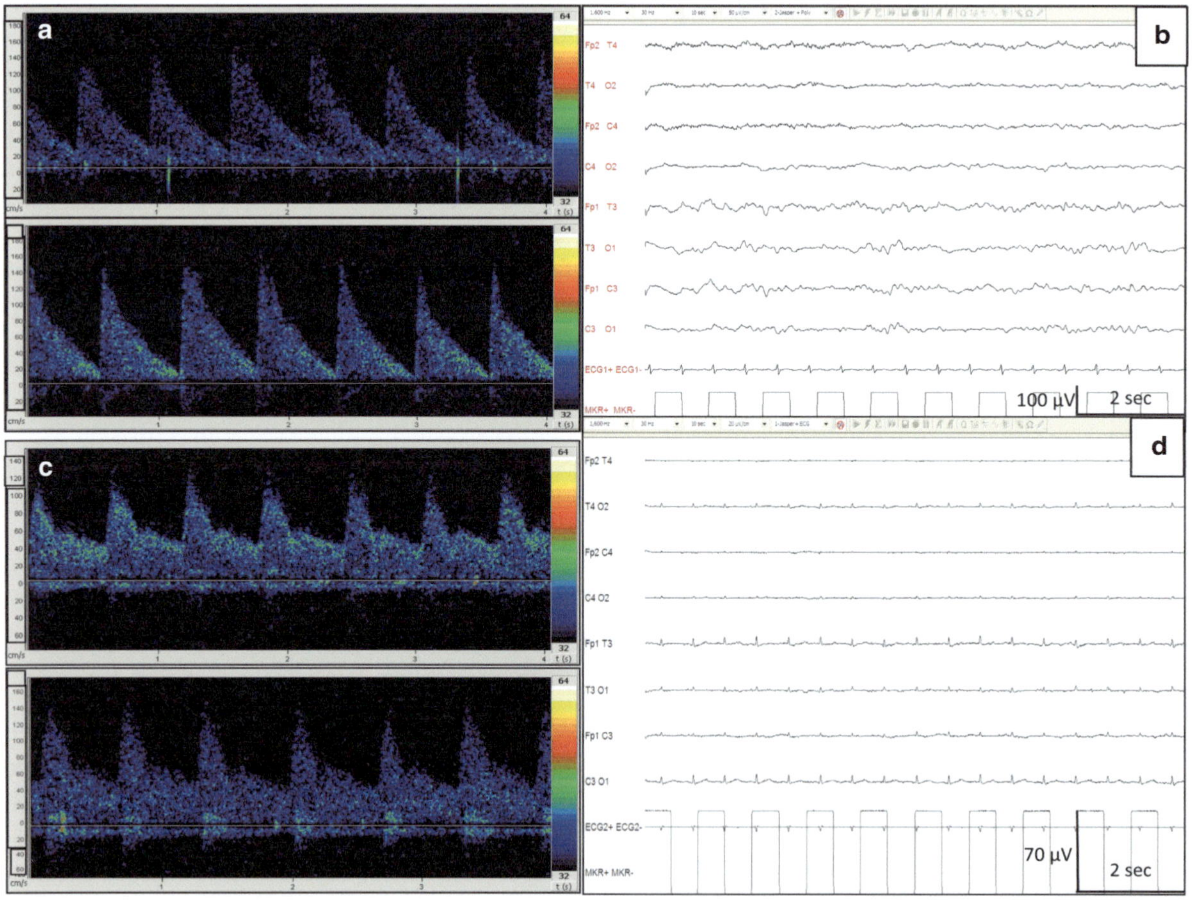

Fig. 47.10 Example of "flow persistence" after decompressive craniectomy; Trans Cranial Doppler (TCD) and EEG coregistration in a patient with right hemisphere hemorrhage due to right siphon aneurism rupture. At the first stage, when the patient clinically worsened, TCD showed only increased resistive indices (**a**), with persistence of asymmetric cerebral activity at EEG (**b**). After decompressive craniectomy, TCD shows normalization of intracranial resistive indices (**c**), but EEG (**d**) shows electro cortical inactivity.

Table 47.1 Principal advantages and disadvantages of ancillary tests

Ancillary test	Advantages	Disadvantages
Neurophysiological tests		
Electro Encephalo Gram (EEG)	– Method used for a long time, well known, widely available – Performed at bedside – Noninvasive, without risks	– Sensitive to confounding factors (i.e., CNS depressant drugs, hypothermia) – Measures predominantly cortical activity – Subject to artifacts and limited by skull injuries
Somato Sensory Evoked Potentials (SSEPs)	– Noninvasive, no risks – Less sensitive than the EEG to confounding factors – Performed at bedside	– Questionable specificity – False-negative early after cardiac arrest – Not widely available
Neuroradiological, neuroimaging, and metabolic techniques for evaluation of cerebral blood flow		
Conventional angiography	– Gold standard for assessment of intracranial blood flow; long history of use – Available at most hospitals – Relatively easy to perform and interpret	– Invasive and with risks for the organs, due to use of contrast medium – Not performed bedside
Computed Tomography Angiography (CTA)	– Widely available	– Requires use of contrast – Not performed bedside – Variable criteria for intracranial circulatory arrest
Magnetic Resonance Angiography (MRA)	– Not requiring the use of iodinated contrast – No risks	– Impractical in critically ill patients and not performed bedside – Variable criteria for intracranial circulatory arrest – Relatively few validating studies
Single-Photon Emission Computed Tomography (SPECT)	– Long history of use – Not requiring the use of iodinated contrast – No risks	– Not available at all hospitals – Not performed bedside
Transcranial Doppler (TCD)	– Performed bedside – Noninvasive; no risks – High specificity and sensitivity	– Acoustic window not present in all patients – Not available at all hospitals – Requires an expert and dedicated physician

In conclusion, ancillary tests, even though they are not mandatory in many countries, will continue to be used when there are factors that interfere with complete clinical assessment or the apnea test cannot be performed. Furthermore, ancillary tests are sometimes used to shorten the duration of the observation period. However, it must be emphasized that the Report of the Quality Standards Subcommittee of the American Academy of Neurology stresses that there is insufficient evidence to determine whether ancillary tests, even those using newer technologies, are able to confirm the complete cessation of all brain functions [6]. Consequently, according to AAN report, ancillary tests are not needed for the clinical BD diagnosis in adults, and they must never replace the neurological clinical examination. Wijdicks, an expert of BD determination, considers ancillary tests "not accurate, not conclusive, not pertinent and not warranted" and considers them to be mandatory by law - or performed as confirmatory - mainly as "a safeguard" [55]. Table 47.1 summarizes the principal advantages and disadvantages of the ancillary tests above described.

47.4 Pediatric Brain Death Determination

The first guidelines for adult BD determination were applied only to children older than 5 years. In the UDDA it is written indeed that "the brains of infants and young children have increased resistance to damage and may recover substantial functions even after exhibiting unresponsiveness for longer periods compared with adults" [3].

A special Task Force of American Academy of Pediatrics developed first clinical guidelines for BD determination in children in 1987 [7] and these guidelines were revised in 2011 [8]. Successively, an international expert panel published a unifying guideline describing death as "the permanent loss of capacity for consciousness and all brainstem functions" [56].

The prerequisites and the clinical neurologic examination for BD diagnosis in children basically follow the same criteria already described for adults: the cause for irreversible acute brain insult must be identified, confounding factors must be excluded, and the brainstem reflexes must be absent. The differences are represented by [57]:

- The first examination must be carried out at least 24 h from ICU admission.
- Two examinations are recommended (in adults: single examination), with an inter-examination observation period of 24 h for term newborns (37-week gestational age) to 30 days of age and 12 h for infants and children (over 30 days to 18 years).
- Body temperature should be maintained over 35 °C.
- $PaCO_2$ at apnea test should be both 20 mm Hg above the baseline and ≥ 60 mm hg.
- The examinations should be performed by different attending physicians "qualified and competent to perform BD examination": pediatric intensivists, neonatologists, pediatric neurologists and neurosurgeons (adult guidelines allow that "it seems reasonable to require that all physicians making a determination of BD are intimately familiar with BD criteria and have demonstrated competence in this complex examination," but they not specify how the physician should be or how the competence should be determined).
- The time of the second neurologic examination is the time of death.

Ancillary tests (EEG and cerebral blow flow study) are not required to establish BD and they are not a substitute for the neurologic examination; they can be performed to reduce the observation period between examinations, but a second clinical evaluation and apnea test should still be performed.

47.5 Brain Death Worldwide

Despite a general consensus on the concept of "brain death," the criteria and the laws for its determination vary among countries (Table 47.2). Wijdicks in 2002 published the results of the first comprehensive survey on BD criteria throughout the world [16]. Legal standards on organ transplantation were present in 69% of 80 countries surveyed and practice guidelines for brain death for adults in 88%. These guidelines specified the exclusion of confounding factors and required irreversible coma and absence of brainstem reflexes for the diagnosis. Apnea test using a $PaCO_2$ measure was recommended only in 59% of the surveyed countries. Differences were also found in the time of observation and required expertise of physicians. Confirmatory ancillary tests were mandatory only in 40% of practice guidelines. Wijdicks concluded that "this survey shows that major differences are not so much in the acceptance of the concept of BD, but in the procedures physicians use to make the final diagnosis".

Table 47.2 Principal characteristics of brain death determination procedures in some European countries

Country	Law	Protocol	No. of physicians	No. of clinical observations	Min time (h) (adults)	Pediatric criteria	Apnea test	EEG	Transplant network
Austria	Yes	Yes	2	2	2	Different	Request	Not req	Present
Belgium	Yes	Yes	1	1	1	Different	Not defined	Mandatory	Present
Croatia	No	Yes	2	2	3	Same	Request	Mandatory	Present
Denmark	Yes	Yes	2	2	1	Different	Request	Optional	Present
Finland	Yes	Yes	2	1	–	Same	Request	Optional	Present
France	Yes	Yes	2	2	2	Same	Request	Mandatory	Present
Germany	Yes	Yes	2	2	2	Different	Request	Mandatory	Present
Greece	Yes	Yes	3	2	12	Different	Request	Not req	Present
Israel	Yes	Yes	2	–	6–10	Different	Request	Optional	Present
Italy	Yes	Yes	3	2	6	± same	Request	Mandatory	Present
Netherlands	Yes	Yes	1	1	–	Different	Request	Mandatory	Present
Norway	Yes	Yes	2	1	–	Same	Request	Mandatory	Present
Portugal	Yes	Yes	2	2	2	Same	Request	Optional	Present
Romania	Yes	Yes	3	2	3	Different	Request	Mandatory	Present
Russian fed	Yes	Yes	3	2	6	Same	Request	Not req	Absent
Spain	Yes	Yes	3	2	6	Different	Request	Optional	Present
Sweden	Yes	Yes	1	2	2	Same	Request	Not req	Present
Switzerland	Yes	Yes	2	1	–	Different	Request	Not req	Present
Turkey	Yes	Yes	2	2	2	Different	Request	Mandatory	Present
United Kingdom	Yes	Yes	2	1	0	Same	Request	Not req	Present

The informations, very often discordant and inaccurate, are taken from the more recent surveys published by Citerio et al. (2014) [58] and by Wahlster et al. (2015) [18]
Not req not required

Successively, the differences and the adherence to the AAN guidelines [6] in BD guidelines among the various hospitals in the United States have been evaluated [17]. The results demonstrated a wide variability in the guidelines' requirements for evaluation of the prerequisites, neurological examination, apnea testing and ancillary test performing. Surprisingly, many institutions do not require a specific level of expertise of physicians and do not consider necessary the availability of neurologists or neurosurgeons on a 24 h basis [17]. Citerio et al. in 2014 [58] published the results of a survey conducted through a web-based questionnaire in 33 European countries. The study demonstrates that, although laws or guidelines for brain death diagnosis are available in all European countries, there are still disparities, in particular regarding the use of ancillary tests as confirmation of the clinical examination. More recently, the practices and perceptions of BD determination worldwide has been assessed by an electronic survey conducted in 91 countries [18]. Overall, legal provisions for brain death are present in 70% of surveyed countries and institutional protocols in 77% of them, but in practice only 22% of low-income vs 97% of high-income countries had an institutional protocol. Among institutions with a formalized brain death protocol, there are marked variabilities in requisite examination findings; apnea testing; necessity and type of ancillary testing (EEG is the most common required test); time to declaration; number and qualifications of physicians present; and distinct pediatric criteria [18].

The high variability in BD determination worldwide is due also to ethical and religious principles. Most Christians accept BD without serious exception. Pope John Paul II in 2000, before an International Transplant Society meeting, affirmed BD to be compatible with catholic principles [59]. The Jewish religion accept BD, with the exception of the most traditionalist part of Judaism. Several Islamic countries, including Saudi Arabia and Iran, permit BD determination and organ transplantation [60]. The BD concept is accepted also in Hindu culture in India and by Shinto-Confucian religious authorities in Japan [61].

47.6 Legal Aspects of Brain Death Determination in Italy

In Italy, BD determination is currently defined by a decree of the Ministry of Health of 12 June 2008, which is valid throughout the entire national territory [62]. The law of 2008 represents a revision of the previous laws, the n. 644 of 2 December 1975 and n. 578 of 29 December 1994. The current decree redefines all the conditions, in patients with severe brain lesions undergoing resuscitation therapies that must lead physicians to immediately alert healthcare management of the presence of a case of irreversible loss of all brain functions. These conditions are literally defined in the law as follows:

- Absence of vigilance and consciousness.
- Absence of brainstem reflexes (pupillary, corneal, oculocephalic and oculovestibular, facial movements induced by noxious stimuli, pharyngeal and tracheal reflexes).
- Absence of spontaneous breathing (apnea test performed according to the methods described above and demonstrating a $PaCO_2 \geq 60$ mm Hg and a pH ≤ 7.40).
- Absence of cerebral electrical activity (EEG mandatory).

The procedure for BD determination can only be started in patients with clear etiopathology of brain injury and exclusion of confounding factors (alterations of thermal and cardiocirculatory homeostasis, major endocrine disorders).

The characteristics of these confounding factors and the procedures to be implemented in the event of their presence have been defined in the Guidelines of the National Transplant Center [63]:

- Body temperature must be maintained above 35 °C.
- Severe hypoglycemia and arterial hypotension must be corrected before BD validation procedures.
- In case of antiepileptic drug administration (including benzodiazepines), the drug level within therapeutic range excludes any possibility of significant interference with BD validation; the administration of other CNS depressant drugs needs to be evaluated singularly, considering pharmacokinetics of specific drug and posology; administration of specific antidotes may be considered when available.

In newborns, BD can be determined only if birth happened after a 38-week gestational period and anyway only after 7 days of extrauterine life.

In patients with postanoxic coma, the observation period can start only 24 h after the anoxic insult, but this latency period can however be drastically reduced if CCA is demonstrated.

The observation period must last 6 h at least, without differences between children and adult patients.

The simultaneous presence of all conditions must be detected twice (at the beginning and at the end of observation period) by three physicians jointly: a neurophysiologist or neurologist or neurosurgeon expert in EEG, a coroner and an anesthesiologist. The time of the first examination is the time of death.

47.6.1 Modalities for the Execution of EEG

The Italian law of 2008 [62] establishes that the mandatory EEG recording of more than 30 min (two continuous recording, at the beginning and at the end of observation period of 6 h) must be performed by a qualified EEG technician, under a supervision of a qualified physician (neurophysiologist or neurologist or neurosurgeon expert of EEG). The EEG must demonstrate the absence of cerebral electrical activity ≥2 μV, spontaneous and/or stimulus-induced (acoustic and nociceptive stimuli). The montage of scalp electrodes and other technical parameters of recording are substantially the same as previously described (see Table 47.3).

The short latency EPs (SSEPs, BAEPs) are considered by the Italian law optional and additional to EEG recording, especially when there are confounding factors.

The demonstration of CCA is mandatory in Italy in:

- Children <1 year of age.
- Treatment with high doses of CNS depressant drugs.

Table 47.3 Technical parameters for EEG as requested by Italian law (DM 11-4-2008, GU n.136 del 12-6-2008) [62]

• *Electrodes and montages*
– At least the following electrodes placed on the scalp according to SI 10–20, with interelectrode distance of 10 cm or more: Fp2, C4, T4, O2, Fp1, C3, T3, O1
– Analog recording: bipolar or monopolar (with ear reference) montage
– Digital recording: monopolar, with display visualization in bipolar montage or monopolar (using ear or FCz as reference electrode)
• *Additional monitoring*
– One channel for ECG (LFF 0.1 Hz, HFF 10–20; max signal input 3200 μV)
– One channel for monitoring movements (e.g., a pair of electrodes placed on the dorsum of the hand; LFF 0.5 Hz, HFF 70 Hz, max signal input 400 μV)
• *Interelectrode impedances* less than 10.000 ohms but more than 100 ohms
• *Sensitivity and filters*
– Analog recording: sensitivity, 2 μV/mm; calibration, 10 μV/5 mm; time constant, 0.1 and 0.3/s
– Digital recording: sensitivity, 2 μV/mm; calibration, 10 μV/5 mm; LFF 0.5 Hz, HFF 70 Hz; sampling rate, ≥128 Hz; digitization depth, 12 bit; max signal input, 200 μV
• Visualization of EEG recording (at least 30 min, with acoustic and nociceptive stimuli)
– Analog recording: paper in continuous scroll
– Digital recording: displays monitor with screen resolution at least 1024 × 768 pixels
• *Storage of digital EEG recording* on unalterable optic or magnetic support (the EEG files must be able to be reviewed on any digital EEG system or PC); the EEG recordings could also be printed—on request—on paper, even in single sheets, with a resolution of at least 300 points/inch
• Recording must be performed only by a qualified EEG technologist, under a direct supervision of a qualified physician (neurophysiologist or neurologist or neurosurgeon EEG expert

- Situations in which the etiopathogenesis of brain injury is uncertain and/or the clinical examination, apnea test, and EEG cannot be performed.
- After an anoxic insult, when physicians decide to start the observation before 24 h from the insult itself. The absence of CBF testing must not be repeated.

The guidelines of the National Transplant Center recommend for the assessment of CCA conventional angiography; single-photon emission computed tomography; transcranial Doppler; and computed tomography angiography [63].

47.6.2 Donation of Organs in Italy

The procedures for the detection of BD are regulated in Italy by the law, and each large hospital is equipped with a commission for the assessment of death, composed of three physicians and with the availability of an EEG technician 24 h/day, to be able to perform the mandatory EEG as soon as possible. BD detection is performed even when his family does not give consent for organ harvesting for transplantation purposes. Once the evaluation procedure for BD has been completed, if the consensus is expressed, the beating heart patient is taken to the operating room for organ harvesting; otherwise, artificial ventilation is suspended and the corpse returned to the family members for the funeral (Fig. 47.11). Despite the law and the correct information that the resuscitators give to the relatives of the critically ill patients, the percentage of opposition to organ donation is about 40%, higher in the regions of Southern Italy than in the North.

In our series of 66 consecutive patients [26], observed over a 1-year period (2010) at Azienda Ospedaliero-Universitaria Policlinico Umberto I (Sapienza University of Rome) and who fulfilled the clinical criteria for BD diagnosis, EEG always demonstrated the electrocortical inactivity, and during the 6 h observation period, no clinical vital signs neither EEG activity did reappear in any of patients. In the time lapse between the two observations requested by law, the premature cardiac arrest occurs only in 4.5% of cases, against 12% reported by Lustbader et al. in hospitals of New York State [19].

While only one observation may be considered medically and scientifically correct, a 6 h delay before BD declaration may be an advantage in those countries such as Italy where, for cultural reasons, additional time is needed to reassure relatives that death has occurred and to explain the reasons and possibly obtain consent to donation. As a matter of fact, in our population time to BD declaration was longer when cerebral blood flow was evaluated: the time to complete the brain death evaluation procedure was 400 ± 17 min with EEG only vs. 443 ± 32 min with TCD up to 525 ± 20 with

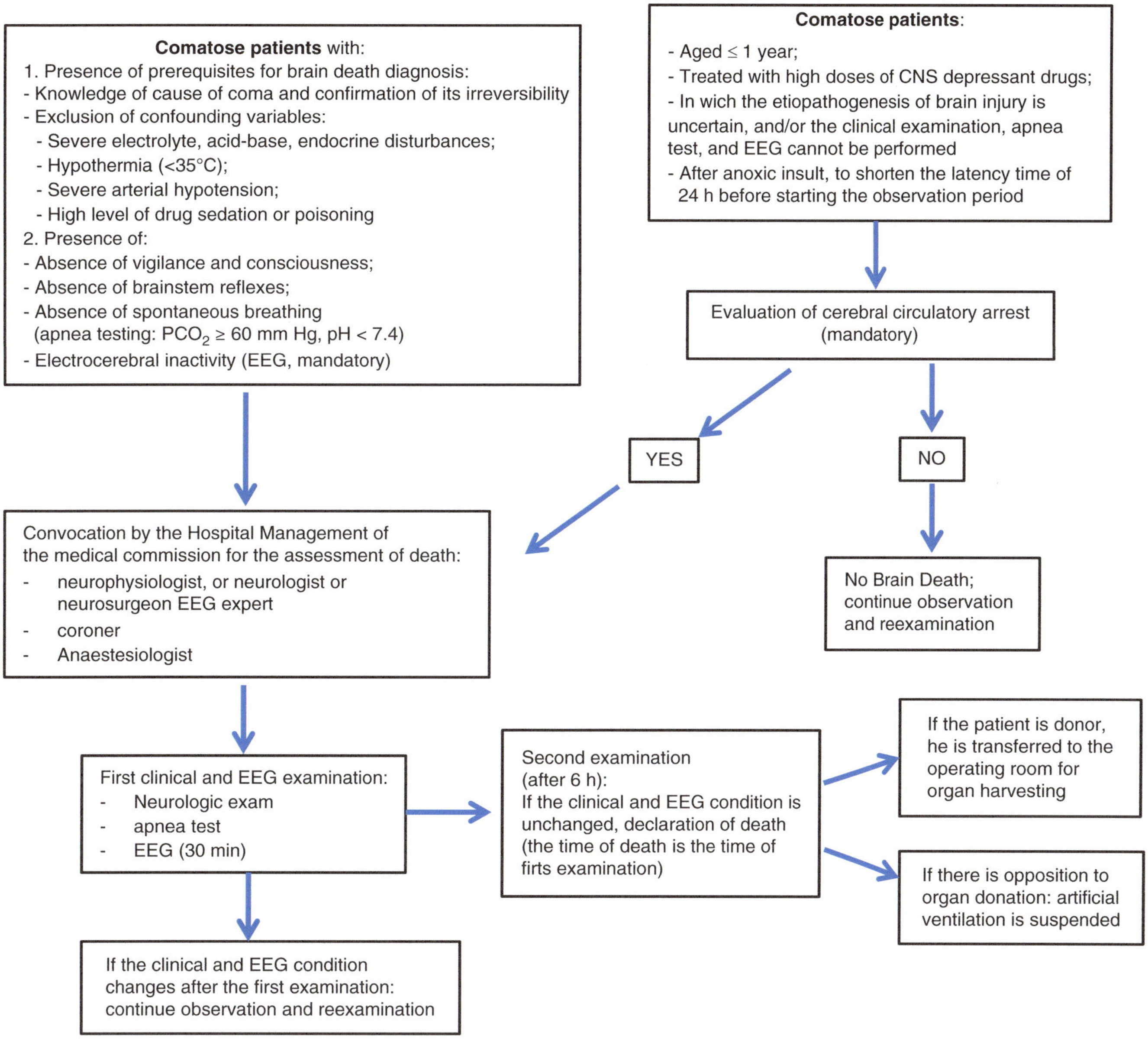

Fig. 47.11 Algorithm for brain death diagnosis according to the Italian law

conventional angiography [26]. In our experience, a multimodal neurophysiological continuous monitoring of comatose patients after severe brain injury may also help to promptly identify cortical electrical inactivity and rapidly diagnose BD.

In Italy, the National Transplant Center performs the following functions:

- Keeps the lists of people awaiting transplantation, with particular reference to the type and urgency of the transplant requested, in order to allow the identification of the recipients.
- Defines the guidelines for regional or interregional centers for transplantation in order to standardize the sampling and transplantation activities in Italy.
- Promotes and coordinates relations with foreign sector institutions in order to facilitate the exchange of organs.

In 2017, the waiting list of patients for organ transplants was 8958 people. BD assessment carried out were 2738 and the donors 1718 (63%), therefore, with a percentage of opposition to donation of 37%. Among the 1718 donors, organs were used only in 1437 (in other cases the organs were not eligible for donation) (Fig. 47.12).

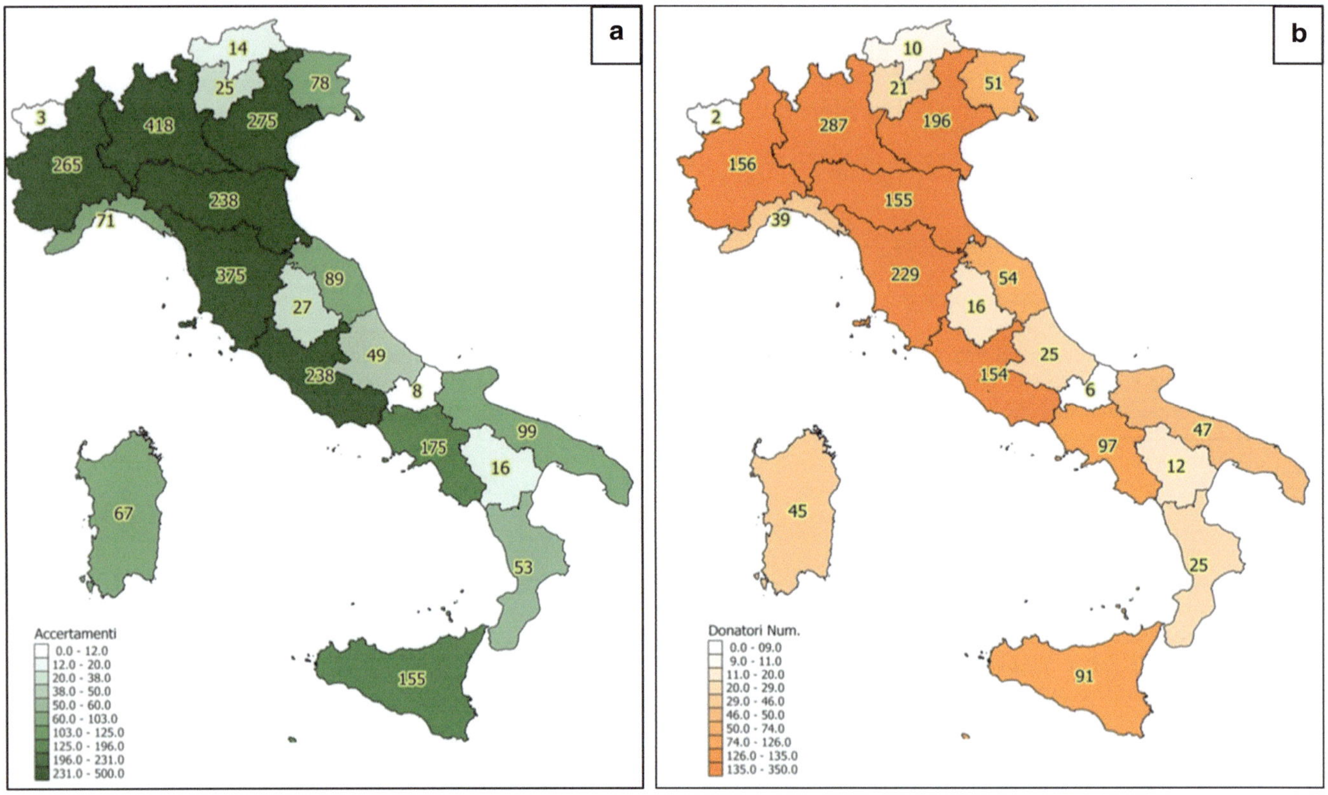

Fig. 47.12 Number of cases of brain death declaration in 2017 (**a**) in the various Italian regions and comparison with the number of organ donors (**b**). Data available on http://www.trapianti.salute.gov.it/cnt

Acknowledgments We are very grateful to Dr. Patrizia Pulitano for her help in selecting and editing the EEG figures.

References

1. Beecher H. A definition of irreversible coma. Report of the ad hoc committee. A definition of irreversible coma. Report of the ad hoc Committee of the Harvard Medical School to examine the definition of brain death. JAMA. 1968;205:337–40.
2. Mollaret P, Goulon M. Le coma dépassé. Rev Neurol. 1959;101:3–15.
3. Guidelines for the determination of death: report of the medical consultants on the diagnosis of death to the President's commission for the study of ethical problems in medicine and biochemical and behavioral research. JAMA. 1981;246:2184–6.
4. Wijdicks EFM. Determining brain death in adults. Neurology. 1995;45:1003–11.
5. Practice parameters for determining brain death in adults (summary statement). Report of the Quality Standards Subcommittee of the American Academy of Neurology. Neurology. 1995;45:1012–4.
6. Wijdicks EFM, Varelas PN, Gronseth GS, Greer DM. Evidence-based guideline update: determining brain death in adults. Report of the Quality Standards Subcommittee of the American Academy of Neurology. Neurology. 2010;74:1911–8.
7. Report of Special Task Force. Guidelines for the determination of brain death in children. American Academy of Pediatrics Task Force on Brain Death in Children. Pediatrics. 1987;80:298–300.
8. Nakagawa TA, Ashwal S, Mathur M, Mysore M, Society of Critical Care Medicine, Section on Critical Care and Section on Neurology of American Academy of Pediatrics, Child Neurology Society. Clinical Report—Guidelines for the determination of Brain Death in Infants and Children: An update of the 1987 Task Force Recommendations. Pediatrics. 2011;128:e720–40.
9. Mathur M, Ashwal S. Pediatric death determination. Semin Neurol. 2015;35:116–24.
10. Saposnik G, Bueri J, Maurino J, et al. Spontaneous and reflex movements in brain death. Neurology. 2008;71:1240–4.
11. Scripko PD, Greer DM. An update on Brain Death Criteria. A simple algorithm with complex questions. Neurologist. 2011;17:237–40.
12. Willatts SM, Drummond G. Brain death and ventilator trigger settings. Anaesthesia. 2000;55:676–84.
13. Wijdicks EFM, Manno EM, Holets SR. Ventilator self-cycling may falsely suggest patient effort during brain death determination. Neurology. 2005;65:774.
14. Lang CJG, Heckmann JG. Apnea testing for the diagnosis of brain death. Acta Neurol Scand. 2005;112:358–69.
15. Wijdicks EFM, Rabinstein AA, Manno EM, Atkinson JD. Pronouncing brain death. Contemporary practice and safety of the apnea test. Neurology. 2008;71:1240–4.
16. Wijdicks EFM. Brain death worldwide. Accepted fact but no global consensus in diagnostic criteria. Neurology. 2002;58:20–5.
17. Greer DM, Varelas PN, Haque S, Wijdicks EFM. Variability of brain death determination guidelines in leading US neurologic institutions. Neurology. 2008;70:284–9.
18. Wahlster S, Wijdicks EFM, Patel V, et al. Brain death declaration. Practices and perceptions worldwide. Neurology. 2015;84:1870–9.
19. Lustbader D, O'Hara D, Wijdicks EFM, et al. Second brain death examination may negatively affect organ donation. Neurology. 2011;76:119–24.
20. Kane N, Acharya J, Benickzy S, et al. A revised glossary of terms most commonly used by clinical electroencephalographers

and updated proposal for the report format of the EEG findings. Revision 2017. Clin Neurophysiol Pract. 2017;2:170–85.
21. Young GB, Lee D. A critique of ancillary tests for brain death. Neurocrit Care. 2004;1:499–508.
22. Kramer AH. Ancillary testing in brain death. Semin Neurol. 2015;35:125–38.
23. Grigg MM, Kelly MA, Celesia GG, Ghobrial MW, Ross ER. Electroencephalographic activity after brain death. Arch Neurol. 1987;44:948–54.
24. Welschehold S, Boor S, Reuland K, et al. Technical aids in the diagnosis of brain death: a comparison of SEP, AEP, EEG, TCD and CT angiography. Dtsch Arztebl Int. 2012;109:624–30.
25. Fernandez-Torre JL, Hernandez-Hernandez MA, Munoz-Esteban C. Non confirmatory electroencephalography in patients meeting clinical criteria for brain death: scenario and impact on organ donation. Clin Neurophysiol. 2013;124:2362–7.
26. Vicenzini E, Pro S, Pulitano P, et al. Current practice of brain death determination and use of confirmatory tests in an Italian university hospital: a report of 66 cases. Minerva Anestesiol. 2013;79:485–91.
27. Shappell CN, Frank JI, Husari K, et al. Practice variability in brain death determination: a call to action. Neurology. 2013;81:2009–14.
28. Orban J-C, Ferret E, Jambou P, Ichai C, AzuRéa Group. Confirmation of brain death diagnosis: a study of French practice. Anaesth Crit Care Pain Med. 2015;34:145–50.
29. American Clinical Neurophysiology Society. Guideline 3: minimum technical standards for EEG recording in suspected cerebral death. J Clin Neurophysiol. 2006;23:97–104.
30. Stecker MM, Sabau D, Sullivan L, et al. American Clinical Neurophysiology Society Guideline 6: minimum technical standards for EEG recording in suspected cerebral death. J Clin Neurophysiol. 2016;33:324–7.
31. Wagner W. Scalp, earlobe and nasopharyngeal recordings of median nerve somatosensory evoked P14 potential in coma and brain death. Brain. 1996;119:1507–21.
32. Busl KM, Greer DM. Pitfalls in the diagnosis of brain death. Neurocrit Care. 2009;11:276–87.
33. Bhattarai BK. An analysis of brain stem evoked potentials (BAEP) in brain death and its usefulness in the diagnosis of brain death. J Anaesth Clin Pharmacol. 2002;18:397–404.
34. Facco E, Munari M, Gallo F, et al. Role of short latency evoked potentials in the diagnosis of brain death. Clin Neurophysiol. 2002;113:1855–66.
35. Savard M, Turgeon AF, Gariépy JL, Trottier F, Langevin S. Selective 4 vessel angiography in brain death: a retrospective study. Can J Neurol Sci. 2010;37:492–7.
36. Braum M, Ducrocq X, Huot JC, et al. Intravenous angiography in brain death: report of 140 patients. Neuroradiology. 1997;39: 400–5.
37. Kramer AH, Roberts DJ. Computed tomography angiography in the diagnosis of brain death: a systematic review and meta-analysis. Neurocrit Care. 2014;21:539–50.
38. Greer DM, Strozyk D, Schwamm LH. False positive CT angiography in brain death. Neurocrit Care. 2009;11:272–5.
39. Shankar JJ, Vandorpe R. CT perfusion for confirmation of brain death. Am J Neuroradiol. 2013;34:1175–9.
40. Heran MK, Heran NS, Shemie SD. A review of ancillary tests in evaluating brain death. Can J Neurol Sci. 2008;35:409–19.
41. Selkuk H, Albayram S, Tureci E, et al. Diffusion-weighted imaging findings in brain death. Neuroradiology. 2012;54:547–54.
42. Luchtmann M, Bernarding J, Beuing O, et al. Controversies of diffusion weighted imaging in the diagnosis of brain death. J Neuroimaging. 2013;23:463–8.
43. Wieler H, Marohl K, Kaiser KP, Klawki P, Frössler H. Tc-99m HMPAO cerebral scintigraphy. A reliable, noninvasive method for determination of brain death. Clin Nucl Med. 1993;18:104–9.
44. Abdel-Dayem HM, Bahar RH, Sigurdsson GH, et al. The hollow skull: a sign of brain death in Tc-99m HM-PAO brain scintigraphy. Clin Nucl Med. 1989;14:912–6.
45. Bertagna F, Barozzi O, Puta E, et al. Residual brain viability, evaluated by (99m)TC-ECD SPECT, in patients with suspected brain death and with confounding clinical factors. Nucl Med Commun. 2009;30:815–21.
46. Berenguer CM, Davis FE, Howington JU. Brain death confirmation: comparison of computed tomographic angiography with nuclear medicine perfusion scan. J Trauma. 2010;68:553–9.
47. Joffe AR, Lequier L, Cave D. Specificity of radionuclide brain blood flow testing in brain death: case report and review. J Intensive Care Med. 2010;25:53–64.
48. Ducrocq X, Hassler W, Moritake K, et al. Consensus opinion on diagnosis of cerebral circulatory arrest using Doppler-sonography: Task Force Group on cerebral death of the Neurosonology Research Group of the World Federation of Neurology. J Neurol Sci. 1998;159:145–50.
49. Monteiro LM, Bollen CW, van Huffelen AC, et al. Transcranial doppler ultrasonography to confirm brain death: a meta-analysis. Intensive Care Med. 2006;32:1937–44.
50. de Freitas GR, André C. Sensitivity of transcranial Doppler for confirming brain death: a prospective study of 270 cases. Acta Neurol Scand. 2006;113:426–32.
51. Vicenzini E, Pro S, Randi F, et al. Transcranial Doppler for brain death after decompressive craniectomy: persistence of cerebral blood flow with flat EEG. Intensive Care Med. 2010;36:2163–4.
52. Vicenzini E, Pulitano P, Cicchetti R, et al. Transcranial Doppler for brain death in infants: the role of the fontanelles. Eur Neurol. 2010;63:164–9.
53. Topcluogu MA, Arsava EM, Bas DF, Kozak HH. Transorbital ultrasonographic measurement of optic nerve sheath diameter in brain death. J Neuroimaging. 2017;25:906–9.
54. Toscano M, Spadetta G, Pulitano P, et al. Optic nerve sheath diameter ultrasound evaluation in intensive care unit: possible role and clinical aspects in neurological critical patients' daily monitoring. Biomed Res Int. 2017;2017:1621428.
55. Wijdicks EFM. The case against confirmatory tests for determining brain death in adults. Neurology. 2010;75:77–83.
56. Shemie SD, Hornby L, Baker A, et al. The international guidelines for determination of death phase 1 participants, in collaboration with the World Health Organization. International Guideline Development for the Determination of Death. Intensive Care Med. 2014;40:788–97.
57. Mathur M, Ashwal S. Pediatric brain death determination. Semin Neurol. 2015;35:116–24.
58. Citerio G, Crippa IA, Bronco A, Vargiolu A, Smith M. Variability in brain death determination in Europe: looking for a solution. Neurocrit Care. 2014;21:376–82.
59. Furton EJ. Brain death, the soul, and organic life. Natl Cathl Bioeth Q. 2002;2:455–70.
60. Akrami SM, Osati Z, Zahedi F, Raza M. Brain death: recent ethical and religious considerations in Iran. Transplant Proc. 2004;36:2883–7.
61. Lock M. Contesting the natural in Japan: moral dilemmas and technologies of dying. Cult Med Psychiatry. 1995;19:1–38.
62. Decreto Ministero della Salute dell' 11 aprile 2008. Aggiornamento del Decreto del 22 agosto 1994, n. 582 relativo al Regolamento recante le modalità per l'accertamento e la certificazione di morte. Gazzetta Ufficiale n. 136 del 12 giugno 2008. http://www.gazzettaufficiale.it/gazzetta/serie_generale/caricaDettaglio?dataPubblicazioneGazzetta=2008-06-12&numeroGazzetta=136
63. Centro Nazionale Trapianti. Linee Guida. Applicazione delle indagini strumentali di flusso ematico cerebrale. Versione aggiornata al 20 febbraio 2009. http://www.trapianti.salute.gov.it

48 Neuromonitoring and Emergency EEG

Marianna Brienza, Chiara Davassi, Patrizia Pulitano, and Oriano Mecarelli

48.1 Intraoperative EEG monitoring

IntraoOperative Neurophysiological Monitoring (IONM) is important for the evaluation of the CNS function during surgical procedures, where injury is possible. IONM can be helpful for the detection of an iatrogenic injury and for mapping of brain structures during the procedure, to avoid their damaging. EEG is one of the oldest and most commonly used modality for intraoperative neuromonitoring. Historically, it has been used at first for the identification of EEG patterns associated with anesthesia to determine the depth of anesthesia and adjusting the drug levels to achieve a predefined neural effect, such as burst suppression. Later, the evolution of intraoperative EEG use was also expanded to include monitoring for assessing cortical perfusion and oxygenation, as well as the identification of epileptiform activities, during a variety of vascular, cardiac and neurosurgical procedures [1, 2]. One of the most relevant application of intraoperative EEG monitoring is Carotid End Arterectomy (CEA). Neuromonitoring can also be useful during cardiovascular surgery and intracranial vessels embolization or during open-heart surgery and cardiopulmonary bypass, where there is risk for ischemic events that could produce both temporary and permanent EEG abnormalities. Among neurophysiologic techniques, EEG provides the fastest feedback with regard to fluctuations in the neurophysiologic dysfunction related to cerebral hypoperfusion. In physiological conditions, Cerebral Blood Flow (CBF) is about 70–50 mL/100 g/min. A reduction of flow to 35–25 mL/100 g/min is not generally able to provoke neuronal damage or to induce EEG modifications. However, a further CBF decrease (<25 mL/100 g/min) causes immediatly cerebral functional changes reflected by reversible EEG modifications and consisting firstly in the decrease in amplitude of the tracing, then in a progressive decrease of the rapid frequencies (alpha-beta) and, finally, in an overall slowdown of cerebral activity with appearance of delta waves. When CBF drops below 12 mL/100 g/min, EEG background activity progressively decreases until it is totally suppressed [3, 4].

Other than ischemic events, there is a wide spectrum of causes for EEG changes during surgery, such as hypotension, hypothermia, emodiluition, embolism and changes in anesthetic drug blood levels. With regard to hypothermia, this may be responsible of specific and evolutive EEG changes. If body temperature remains above 30 °C, hypothermia does not significantly impact electrophysiological findings. At temperatures below 29.6 °C, EEG tracings show a progressive diffuse slowings and periodic and rhythmic abnormalities and when temperature goes under 24.4 °C, a burst suppression or other malignant patterns (i.e., alpha/theta coma) appear. Finally, under 17.8 °C, a pattern of electrocerebral inactivity is reached [5]. During rewarming, the suppressed tracing returns to a burst suppression pattern and, progressively, to a continuous EEG.

48.1.1 EEG Monitoring During Carotid Endarterectomy

CEA is a surgical gold standard procedure for moderate-to-severe symptomatic and selected severe asymptomatic carotid stenosis patients. One of the most serious perioperative complications associated with CEA surgery is stroke, with a 30-day periprocedural stroke rate ranging between 2 and 6% [6]. Several factors contribute to this risk, but the most relevant remains the clamping of the carotid artery, which can induce cerebral ischemia, with consequent irreversible neurologic damage. A meta-analysis of existing literature demonstrated the diagnostic accuracy of EEG in predicting perioperative strokes. As a matter of fact, patients

M. Brienza · C. Davassi · O. Mecarelli (✉)
Department of Human Neurosciences, Sapienza University of Rome, Rome, Italy
e-mail: oriano.mecarelli@uniroma1.it

P. Pulitano
Azienda Ospedaliero-Universitaria Policlinico Umberto I, Rome, Italy

O. Mecarelli (ed.), *Clinical Electroencephalography*, https://doi.org/10.1007/978-3-030-04573-9_48

with strokes after carotid surgery have six times greater chance of experiencing an intraoperative change in EEG during CEA [6].

During CEA, the common carotid artery is temporarily clamped to allow the plaque removal from the internal carotid artery; in this phase, blood flow to the homolateral cerebral hemisphere is provided by collaterals, if the contralateral carotid is also not significantly stenotic and the circle of Willis communicating arteries are functional. If compensatory flow is not sufficient, the clamping performed without shunting (a temporary bypass connecting the sections below and above the blockage) may lead to cerebral ischemia. However, shunts are associated with iatrogenic problems and shunting itself may induce embolic events leading to perioperative stroke, so that they should only be used when necessary.

Based on this premise EEG monitoring is the most sensitive technique for giving indications to shunt positioning [7, 8]. The correlation between severity of EEG changes and degrees of reduction of the regional cerebral blood flow can help the surgeon decide whether there is absolute need for shunting, because mild EEG changes usually reverse with just an increase of systemic blood pressure, while more severe EEG changes require insertion of a temporary intra-arterial shunt.

In order to properly evaluate EEG tracings during CEA, we must consider that general anesthesia provokes itself changes in the EEG activity. This depends mostly on the drugs used, doses and individual responses. Changes in EEG tracings can also happen due to a sudden hypotension. Severe electrocortical depression is observed when arterial blood pressure decreases of about 20–30 mmHg below the mean levels. Surgical stimulation of the vagus nerve or of the carotid glomus can also cause bradycardia or hypotension with consequent EEG modifications and then the cooperation between the surgical equipe, the anesthesiologists and the neurophysiologists is crucial for the proper management of patients undergoing CEA.

Before CEA, it is advisable that patients are submitted to standard EEG recording; this allows neurophysiologists to identify any pre-existing abnormalities, as the presence of both ipsilateral and/or contralateral focal EEG changes may increase the incidence of concomitant EEG abnormalities during clamping. Furthermore, predictors of EEG changes during CEA are represented by preoperative neurologic symptoms, $\geq$ 70% contralateral carotid and bilateral vertebral stenosis: these factors increase the possibility of clamping-induced ischemia, as detected by intraoperative EEG [8].

Chiappa et al. in 1979 classified the EEG changes within 20 sec of ICA clamping in five groups: (1) ipsilateral attenuation, (2) bilateral attenuation, (3) ipsilateral slowing without attenuation, (4) ipsilateral slowing with attenuation and (5) bilateral slowing and attenuation. These authors observed that the most common pattern (47%) was rapid unilateral or bilateral attenuation of background anesthetic-induced fast EEG activity [9].

The ACNS's intraoperative EEG guidelines (2000) defined three degrees of EEG changes caused by ischemia during clamping for CEA, in comparison with the preclamp post-induction baseline: (1) a decrease in background fast activity amplitude >50%, most apparent when using anesthetic agents that generate such fast activity, (2) an increase in delta-theta activity $\geq$50% (decrease in fast activity and increase in slow frequencies may be simultaneous) and (3) all raw EEG activity that progressively diminishes in amplitude and approaches electrocerebral inactivity [2, 10].

These various features of abnormalities, ipsilateral or bilateral, occur promptly after clamping (within 20–40 sec), while ischemic brain lesions need a few minutes to consolidate. Knowing these time intervals can really help surgeons regarding the decision to perform a shunt. For this reason, it may be useful to perform a clamping test for at least 1–2 min, to verify the times of the patient's tolerance after carotid clamping, evaluating the efficiency of collateral circulation.

It is also important to observe the reversal of EEG changes, either after inserting a temporary shunt and/or increasing the systemic blood pressure, because this resulted in a favorable neurologic outcome (Figs. 48.1 and 48.2).

Direct visual analysis of EEG monitoring during CEA offers an increased sensitivity and allows a prompt interaction between the neurophysiologist and the surgeon: the neurophysiologist suggests shunting, if any changes in EEG occurs. However, the methods of quantitative evaluation of EEG are also very useful, which can objectively assess the changes occurring during clamping, making the evaluation less operator-dependent. The most widely used quantitative EEG (qEEG) procedures employ Fast Fourier Transform (FFT) algorithms and the spectral array displays available are the Compressed Spectral Array (CSA), which displays EEG data as a pseudo-three-dimensional plot, and the Density Spectral Array (DSA) that depicts also the same values on a color-coded data. These trends, in addition to a visual inspection of the EEG, are particularly useful during monitoring, because they objectively highlight modifications due to frequency and power variations of EEG signals (Figs. 48.3 and 48.4).

When CBF decreases, alpha and beta relative power decrease, while delta and theta relative power tend to increase. Cursi et al. [11] have studied, for example, the usefulness of the desynchronization index (indicating the reduction of 8–15 Hz band power) for the detection of cerebral hypoperfusion during CEA. The values of desynchronization index exceeding 65% seem to correctly detect patients with cerebral hypoxic risk.

Another quantitative parameter, often used during EEG monitoring in CEA, is the Brain Symmetry Index (BSI). BSI quantifies the mean spectral asymmetry between the hemispheres, calculating the absolute value of the average

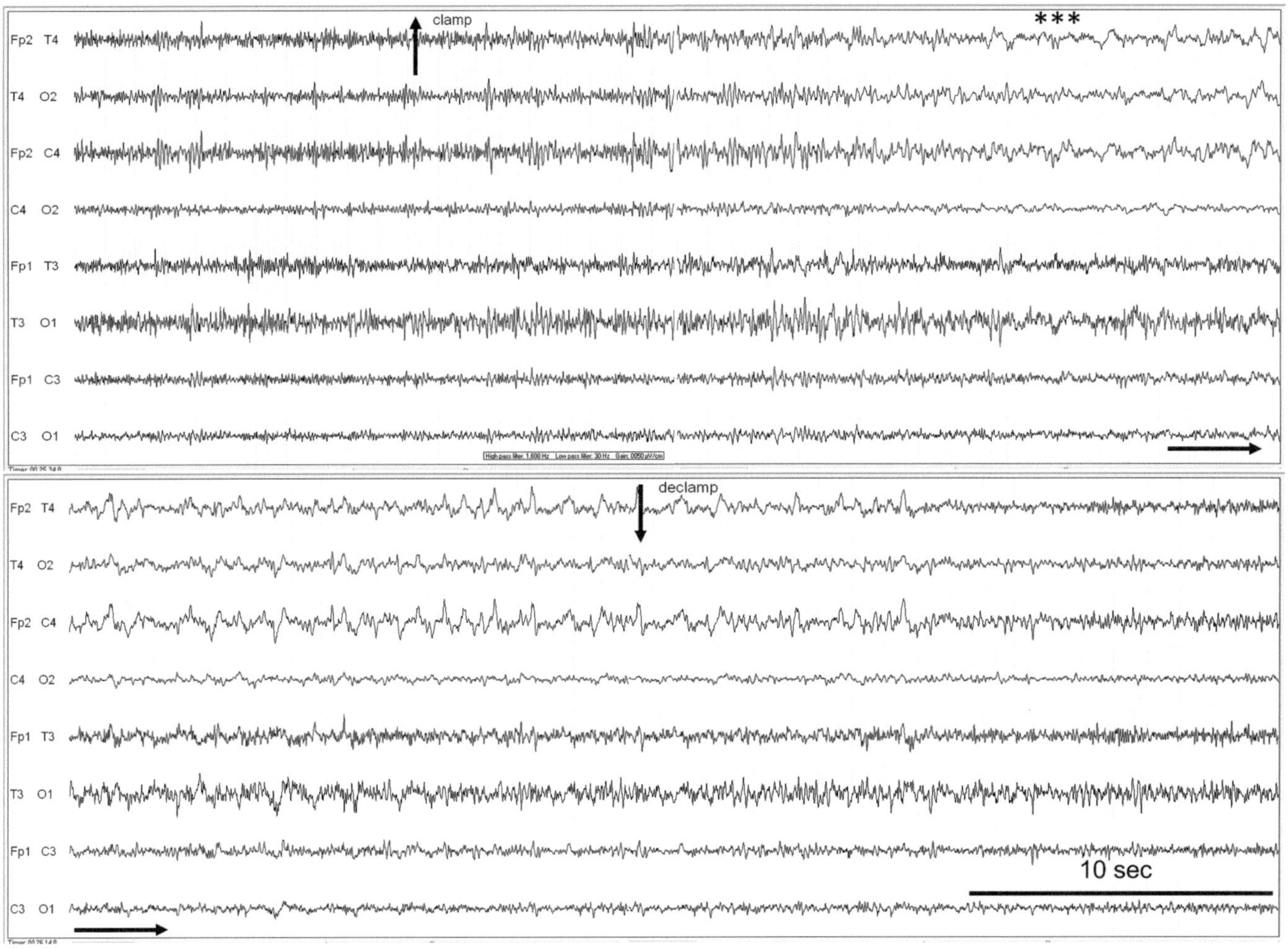

Fig. 48.1 EEG monitoring of 76-year-old patient during carotid endarterectomy. 20 s after clamping (***), EEG showed right delta slowings with tendency to diffusion which disappeared after declamping: this has represented an indication for shunt positioning

spectral density of the right and left hemisphere in the frequency range from 1 to 25 Hz. The BSI is normalized in the range between 0 (perfect symmetry for all channels) and 1 (complete asymmetry), with physiologic values of 0.05 to 0.08. The BSI may assist in the visual EEG analysis during CEA and provides a quantitative measure for EEG asymmetry due to cerebral hypoperfusion. Changes in the BSI of at least 0.06 during clamping test has an excellent correlation with visual EEG assessment and required shunting [3, 12].

Technical notes. In order to perform an intraoperative EEG, technicians need to be experienced and the full cooperation of staff is required. Neurophysiologists should be informed of all clinical and anesthesiological changes, to better interpret EEG patterns. Whereas this happens, bias can be overcome and EEG can be considered as one of the most efficient tools during this kind of surgery. EEG monitoring must be extended from the operative awake to the postoperative awake states. Cup or subdermal needle electrodes can be used: cup electrodes are fixed to the scalp by collodium or EC2, making the best contact and avoiding artifacts due to passive head movements during surgery; needle electrodes can be easily placed, but are also more unstable and have a higher impedance. A bipolar, anterior-posterior, 16 channel montage with placement of 21 electrodes is recommended. According to the intraoperative ACNS's guidelines [1, 10] a number of channels less than 8–12 is insufficient. The high-pass filter should be set at 0.53 Hz, the low-pass filter at 70 Hz, the sensitivity at 5 μV/mm. The aim of the montage is to identify general modifications of the pattern more than to analyze the wave shape of the single elements; for this reason, it is preferable to use a time sweep between 5 and 15 mm/s.

48.1.2 EEG Monitoring in Cardiothoracic Surgery

The indications for EEG monitoring during cardiothoracic surgery include the prompt identification of ischemic damages, both due to cardioembolic events and to hypoperfusion. Particularly important is the role of the EEG during some types of cardiothoracic surgery in which extracorporeal perfusion or hypothermic cardioplegia are used. Ascending

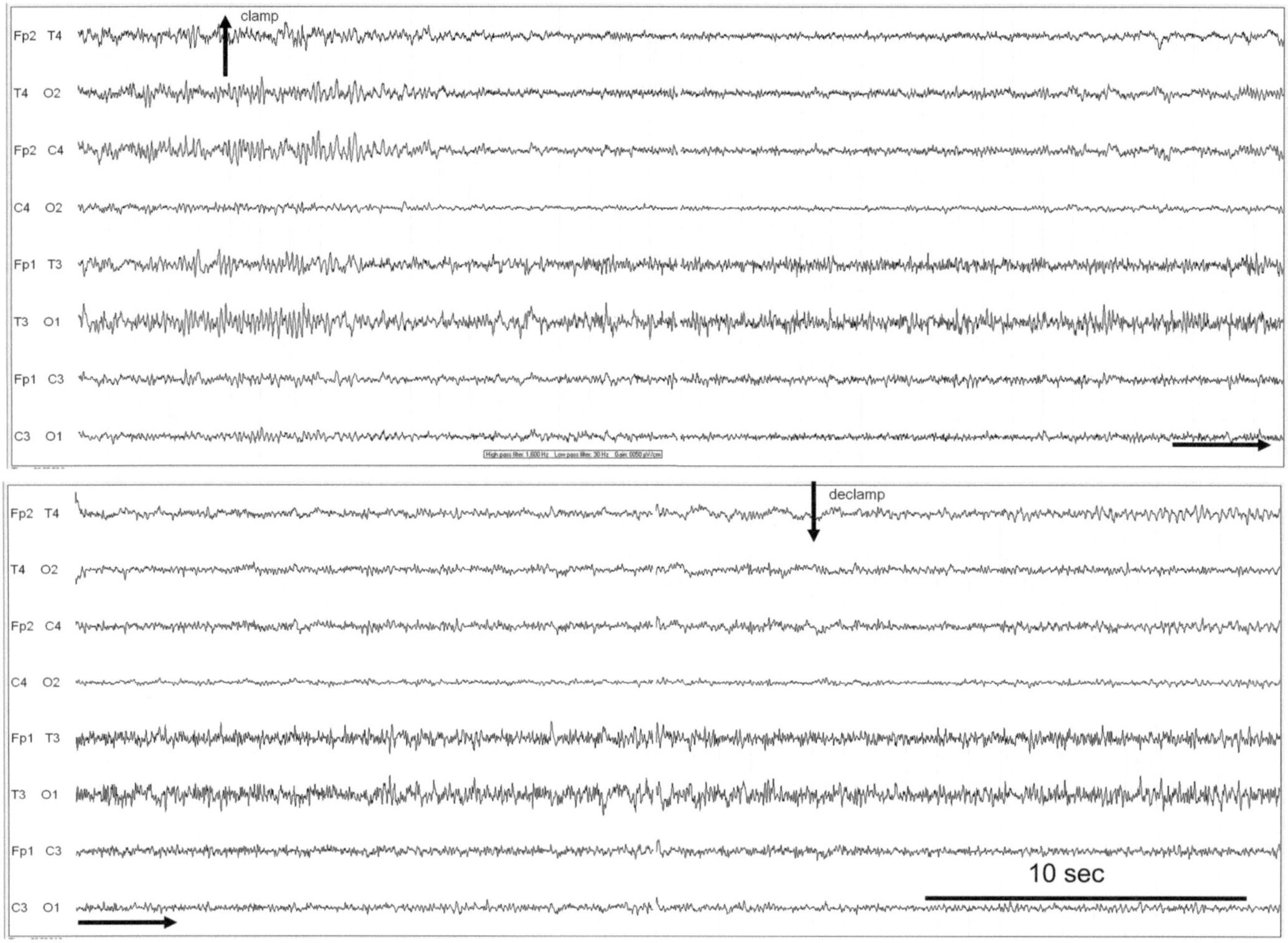

Fig. 48.2 Same patient of Fig. 48.1. After clamping, performed to remove the shunt, a right electrocortical suppression was observed: the suppression promptly disappeared after declamping

aortic and/or aortic arch surgery is a complex procedure that usually requires a Circulatory Arrest (CA) to achieve a surgical field that is free of cannulas and clamps. During this period, there is a high risk of ischemia of all organs, especially of the central nervous system. The safe duration of CA is controversial and will depend on the hypothermia achieved and the concomitant use of cerebral perfusion. The main pathophysiological aspects involved in cerebral ischemia-reperfusion are the consumption of Adenosine Tri Phosphate (ATP), the excitotoxicity of glutamate, the alterations of ionic homeostasis and the formation of oxygen free radicals. Measures that disrupt this cascade of events will theoretically have neuroprotective potential. However, a second pathway of neuronal death by apoptosis has been found, where mitochondria plays a major role and a third pathway due to necroptosis or programmed necrosis that does not depend on caspases. All of this would indicate that some measures that seem effective may have no long-term impact, because what they actually do is delay neuronal death [13]. Hypothermia acts by decreasing intracellular enzyme activity and Cerebral Metabolism Rate for O_2 ($CMRO_2$), thereby improving the balance between the supply and demand for oxygen. For each degree of temperature decrease, the $CMRO_2$ decreases an average of 6–7%, so at 25 °C the $CMRO_2$ decreases to 37% and at 15 °C to 15% of the basal. Cerebral blood flow is also reduced in a linear fashion as opposed to the decrease in the $CMRO_2$ that accelerates below 20 °C [14, 15].

The maximal suppression of $CMRO_2$ occurs at Electro Ccerebral Inactivity (ECI), and cooling to deep hypothermia (≤18 °C) has evolved as the preferred technique for cerebral and systemic organ protection during deep hypothermic CA. However, the cooling time and temperature required to achieve ECI are highly variable among patients [16]. Therefore, EEG monitoring can identify when sufficient hypothermia is reached and permits the verification that it is maintained [17].

48.2 EEG Monitoring in ICU

Multimodal monitoring in ICU using a variety of techniques including clinical and laboratory evaluation, bedside neurophysiological monitoring with continuous or noncontinuous techniques and imaging, is fundamental for patients who

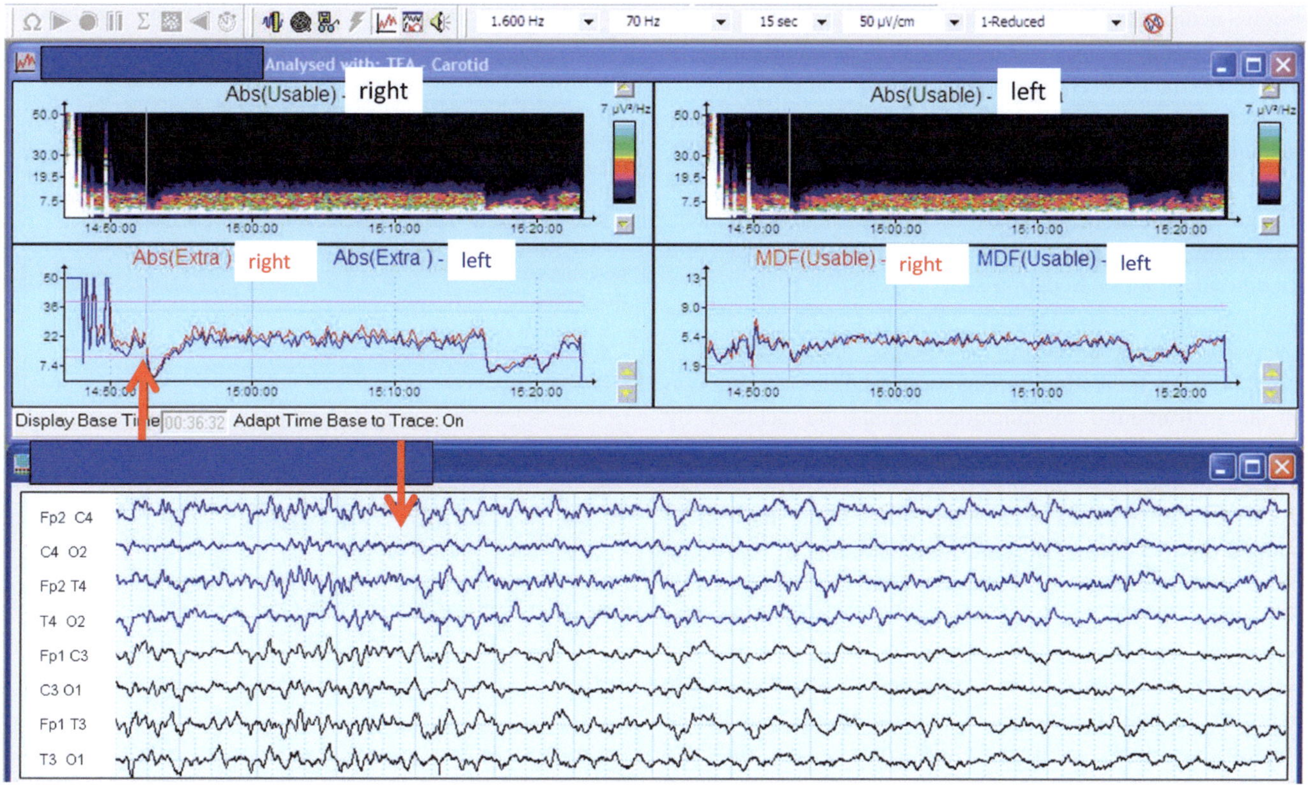

Fig. 48.3 EEG monitoring during left endarterectomy. Raw EEG after clamping (at arrow) showed a diffuse slowing. In the upper part of the figure, the density spectral array of absolute power and the Mean Dominant Frequency (MDF) is showed

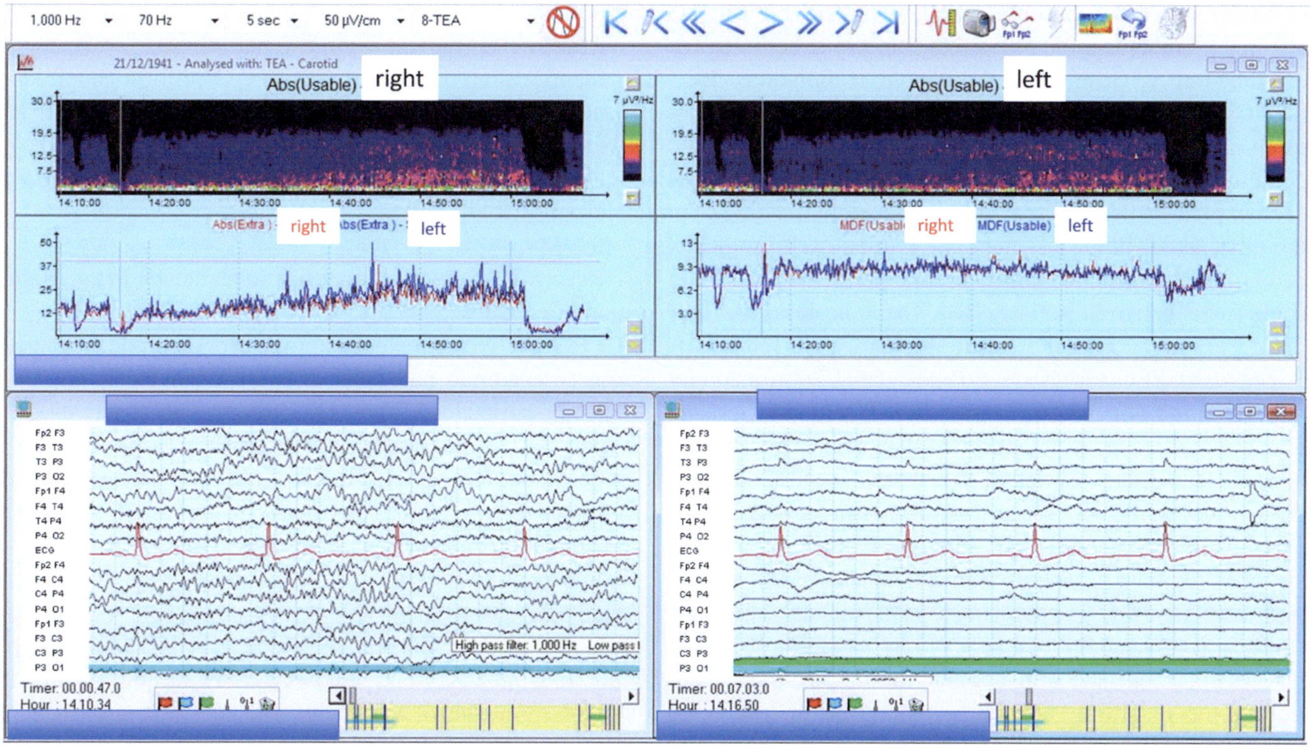

Fig. 48.4 EEG monitoring during right endarterectomy. Clamping caused a marked, sudden suppression of the background activity. In the upper part of the figure, the trends of absolute power of the EEG frequencies and Mean Dominant Frequency (MDF) are shown. In the lower part, raw basal EEG is showed on the left and EEG during clamping on the right side

require neurocritical care. Clinical evaluation, essential precondition to any subsequent investigation, should include, in addition to the general neurological and clinical examination, the use of specific scales that make the contents intelligible through standardized scores: Glasgow Coma Scale (GCS), Full Outline of Un-Responsiveness (FOUR Score) and Glasgow Outcome Scale (GOS) for evaluation of coma state; Confusion Assessment Method for the ICU (CAM ICU) and Richmond Agitation Sedation Scale (RASS) for evaluation of delirium. Moreover, patient's clinical conditions should always be considered during the interpretation of all instrumental exams. Indication, timing and modalities of execution of all instrumental examinations should be decided by the neurophysiologist and the anesthesiologist together.

Among the neurophysiological tools, EEG is recommended in all patients with acute brain injury and unexplained and persistent consciousness disorders. It should be performed in emergency in patients with Convulsive Status Epilepticus (CSE) that do not return to functional baseline within 60 min after seizure medication and in patients with Refractory SE (RSE). EEG is required during therapeutic hypothermia and within 24 h of rewarming to exclude Non Convulsive Status Epilepticus (NCSE) in all comatose patients after cardiac arrest. EEG is suggested in comatose ICU patients, without an acute primary brain condition and with unexplained impairment of mental status or unexplained neurological deficits to exclude NCSE, particularly in those with severe sepsis or renal/hepatic failure. EEG can be useful to detect delayed cerebral ischemia in comatose patients affected by subarachnoid hemorrhage, in whom neurological examination is difficult or unreliable. Continuous EEG (cEEG) monitoring can also be an important diagnostic tool in comatose ICU patients without an acute primary brain condition and with unexplained impairment of mental status or unexplained neurological deficits, to exclude NCSE. On the other hand, EEG does not appear to be useful to detect cerebral ischemia and to target cerebral perfusion pressure in acute ischemic stroke patients [18]. The indications and utility of EEG monitoring in ICU are summarized in Table 48.1.

Table 48.1 Indications and utility of cEEG monitoring in Intensive Care Unit (ICU)

Detection of Non Convulsive Status Epilepticus (NCSE)
Diagnosis, follow-up, and therapy monitoring of seizures and status epilepticus (CSE, NCSE)
Characterization of paroxystic clinical manifestations – Repetitive motor manifestations. – Sudden spasms, nystagmus, ocular deviation, and chewings. – Autonomic paroxystic manifestations (brady-tachycardia, flushing, etc.).
Evaluation of consciousness during particular clinical conditions – Locked-in syndrome. – Serious neuromuscular diseases. – Frontal syndromes. – Akinetic mutism.
Monitoring of the effects of pharmacological therapies – Level of sedation. – Treatment of intracranial hypertension.
Prevention and monitoring of vasospasm – After subaracnoid hemorrhage. – During and after vascular neurosurgical procedures.
Evaluation of altered mental states
Prognosis of coma (>postanoxic and post-traumatic)
Diagnosis of brain death

Standard EEG represents a fundamental instrument for the evaluation of cerebral function in ICU patients. Seriated EEGs provide extremely important data about neurological conditions, helping physicians to elaborate a correct diagnosis and also to decide which treatment is more suitable for every patient. It also provides a helpful tool for the prognosis. New digital equipments offer a noninvasive and easy to perform exams that do not interfere with patients' daily care.

Technicians should take note of any variation of awareness or consciousness of the patient during the whole duration of the recording, as well as of any factor that could influence tracing interpretation. If there is any obstacle to electrodes placement that can generate artifacts, it must be annotated so that the physician can take it into account when reporting the results. It is also very important to collect a detailed medical history and medical therapies. Previous exams, especially neuroradiological, may be useful to better individuate the main clinical aspects.

The most useful information that can be obtained from ICU EEG monitoring are:

- Reactivity of the tracing to external stimuli.
- Identification of focal or diffuse epileptiform abnormalities and evaluation of AntiEpileptic Drugs (AEDs) efficacy.
- Detection of peculiar EEG patterns of coma useful for a prognostic evaluation.

Reactivity to external stimuli is fundamental in the evaluation of comatose patients.

EEG reactivity to external stimuli depends upon the intactness of anatomic pathways different from the lemniscus-thalamus-parietal axis known to carry somatosensory evoked responses [19] and consisting of interconnected stations. This complexand non completely clarified pathway is composed of projections from reticular nuclei of brainstem to diffuse thalamic projection system that relays to the cortex.

In Chap. 46, we have already explained various types of reactivity and testing modalities in comatose patients, through visual (eye opening under light), auditory (clapping, loud name calling) and nociceptive stimuli; while it is assumed that the first stimulus will be more informative, pain is generally viewed as the most effective. Furthermore, pain stimuli are routinely included in the physical examination of coma patients; even if they do not show a behavioral response to external stimuli, a cortical reaction to noxious stimuli can be reflected by a change in EEG background activity [20]. In addition, tactile stimuli should be tested bilaterally on both extremities and the face, in order to avoid any area that may be affected by other kinds of lesions (e.g., spinal lesions).

Focal EEG abnormalities are often suggestive of specific pathologies; for example, Lateralized Periodic Discharges (LPDs) may be indicative of specific conditions such as herpetic encephalitis or intracerebral hemorrhage. Therefore, widespread slow activity is more frequently associated with bilateral, toxic, or dysmetabolic cortical damage, while bilateral and synchronous EEG patterns, often intermittent and monomorphic, are suggestive of deep subcortical lesions. Specific EEG patterns during coma are described in detail in Chap. 46.

The duration of EEG recordings depends on clinical request and it should be at least 30 min.

Other polygraphic data (EKG, EMG, oxygen saturation, PNG) are helpful to obtain more accurate interpretation of the EEG. When available, back-averaging analysis technique may be useful to correlate motor features to cortical epileptiform activity in comatose patients (subtle status epilepticus). This offline analysis method allows an association to be made between cortical epileptiform discharges and correspondent EMG patterns in patients with motor symptoms.

Video-EEG recording results are very useful, especially in patients with epileptic seizures (both convulsive or non-convulsive) or in patients with other motor symptoms, to avoid inadequate pharmacological therapies.

48.2.1 Continuous EEG (cEEG)

As ICU patients often present changes of their electroclinical condition (due to modifications of therapy, sleep-wake rhythm, seizures, etc.), seriated EEG recording results may be often inadequate.

Technological advances have improved the chances to easily collect, analyze and transmit the great deal of information deriving from a long-lasting recording.

Technical improvement converted cEEG from a research tool to a valid diagnostic instrument in the management of ICU patients, integrating the informations with other ICU monitoring systems (blood pressure, intracranial pressure, SaO_2, temperature) (Figs. 48.5 and 48.6).

Among all neuromonitoring tools, EEG has some advantages. It has a good spatial resolution (it can record at the same time the electrical activity of different cortical regions) and an excellent temporal resolution; it can be used to investigate both structural and functional disorders (seizures, post anoxic damages, toxic or dysmetabolic encephalopathies) (Table 48.2).

However, neuromonitoring lasting for days may have management problems. One of the most relevant con-

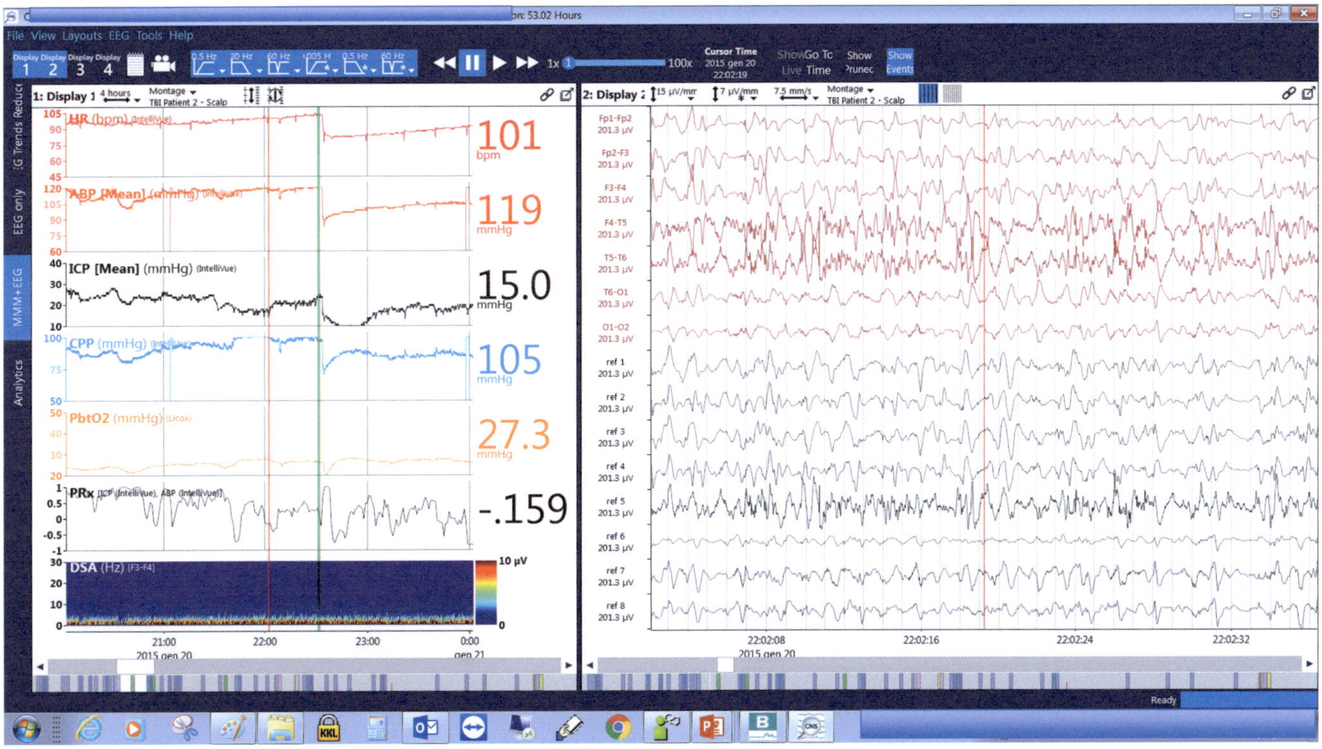

Fig. 48.5 Example of multimodal neuromonitoring in ICU. On the left: *HR* Heart Tate, *ABP* Arterial Blood Pressure, *ICP* Intra Cranial Pressure, *CPP* Cerebral Perfusion Pressure, *PbtO2* Pressure - brain tissue oxygen, *PRx* Pressure Reactivity index, *DSA* Density Spectral Array

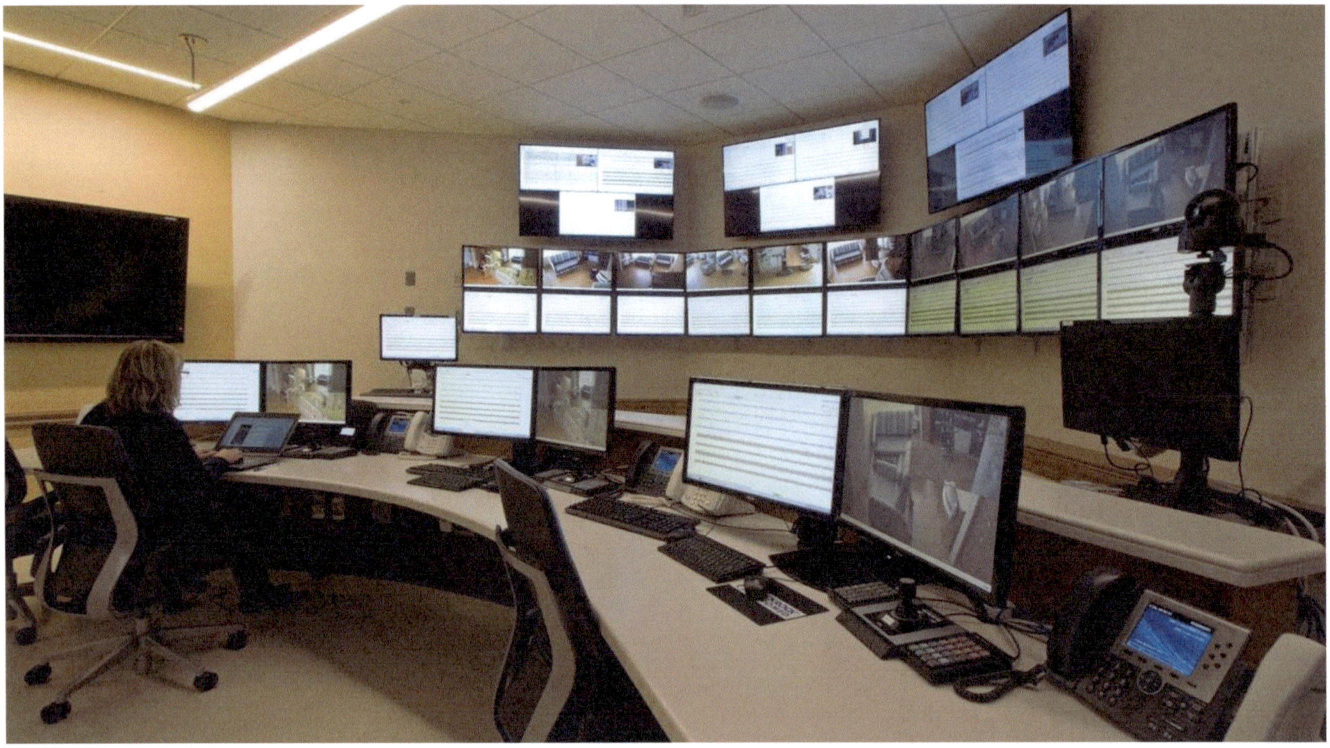

Fig. 48.6 An example of control room in an Intensive Care Unit ICU

Table 48.2 Characteristics of various instrumental techniques for the evaluation of cerebral functions in comatose patients

	Practicality	Spatial resolution	Temporal resolution	Specificity	Interpretation
cEEG	++++	+++	++++	++++	+
Evoked potentials	+++	++	++	++	+
Transcranial Doppler	+++	++	++	++	+
Neuroimaging (CT-MR)	+	++++	+	+++	++
IBP monitoring	++++	+	+++	++	+++

cEEG continuous EEG, *CT* computed tomography, *MR* magnetic resonance, *IBP* intracranial blood pressure

sists in the need to maintaining correct electrodes placement and to assure a valid connection between the patient and the recording equipment. In ICUs, many factors can trigger artifacts: ventilators can cause either mechanical or electric artifacts; caring procedures can produce EEG patterns similar to physiological or pathological conditions. Even an electrode disconnection can produce signals not immediately recognizable as artifacts.

Hirsch et al. [21], in their sample of ICU patients undergoing cEEG monitoring, demonstrated a common periodic pattern as a reaction to various stimuli (Stimulus-Induced Rhythmic, Periodic, or Ictal Discharges, SIRPIDs). SIRPIDs are a relatively common phenomenon in the critically ill patients and their prevalence is reported in 10–34% of EEG neuromonitorings [22]. In order to differentiate SIRPIDs from critical spontaneous activity, a video-EEG recording can be helpful; technical personnel always need to register any stimulus that patients receive. Given the complexity of cEEG recording, a highly trained team is required; it should include neurologists, technicians, nurses and neuro-anesthesiologists.

As a matter of fact, if some patterns could be easily recognized by relatively "nonexpert" personnel, many others may only be detected by experienced neurophysiologists that can give the right interpretation of the trace and can distinguish and exclude eventual artifacts.

Literature shows how cEEG monitoring is extremely helpful in identifying subclinical epileptiform discharges (single nonconvulsive seizures or nonconvulsive status epilepticus) [21, 23]. cEEG monitoring is thus useful in the diagnosis of nonconvulsive epileptic seizures or purely electrical discharges and in the monitoring of status epilepticus when consciousness disorders persist after initial treatment [24]. Symptoms of nonconvulsive seizures can be quite misleading, often wrongly reported as postictal states, psychiatric disorders, strokes, or metabolic encephalopathy. This might explain why nonconvulsive seizures are often underestimated (27–34% of cases) in the ICU [24–27].

A prospective study, conducted by Towne et al., showed that NCSE could be diagnosed via cEEG in 8% of unexplained comas in children or adult patients with no prior history of convulsive seizures [28].

cEEG has demonstrated to be very useful in early diagnosis of ischemic events in patients with any situation leading to a significant decrease in cerebral blood flow. In the case of subarachnoid hemorrhage complicated with vasospasm, ischemic complications are witnessed by a decrease in the alpha/delta ratio during cEEG. This enables an early diagnosis of ischemia at a stage where it is still reversible, helping physicians to quickly adapt therapeutic measures [29]. Other indications are monitoring of all cerebral hemorrhages, severe traumatic brain injuries and encephalitis; in all of these clinical indications, the European Recommendations recently published by the European Society for Intensive Care Medicine (ESICM) reported that continuous EEG was highly beneficial for patients [30].

The diagnosis of nonconvulsive seizures, which can evolve in NCSE, is essential in the ICU, especially in unexplained disorders of consciousness, since their presence has been correlated to a poorer prognosis and a delay in diagnosis appears to increase patient mortality [31]. The persistence of electrical SE has been associated with a higher mortality rate vs. generalized clinical SE, requiring an increase in AE treatment. The possible progression of clinical SE toward subtle SE also validates using EEG monitoring in the care management of generalized SE when disorders of consciousness persist after the initial treatment [27, 32].

Another relevant indication for cEEG is the differential diagnosis between postanoxic encephalopathy and SE, after cardiac arrest. As a matter of fact, after such event, EEG can reveal different types of abnormalities (burst suppression pattern, spike, spike and wave, polyspikes and wave, diffuse polyspikes or triphasic wave activities, often periodic or quasiperiodic). The simultaneous presence of myoclonus and the epileptiform EEG abnormalities should not always be considered, nor treated, as SE, because of the probable subcortical origin of the myoclonus (Fig. 48.7).

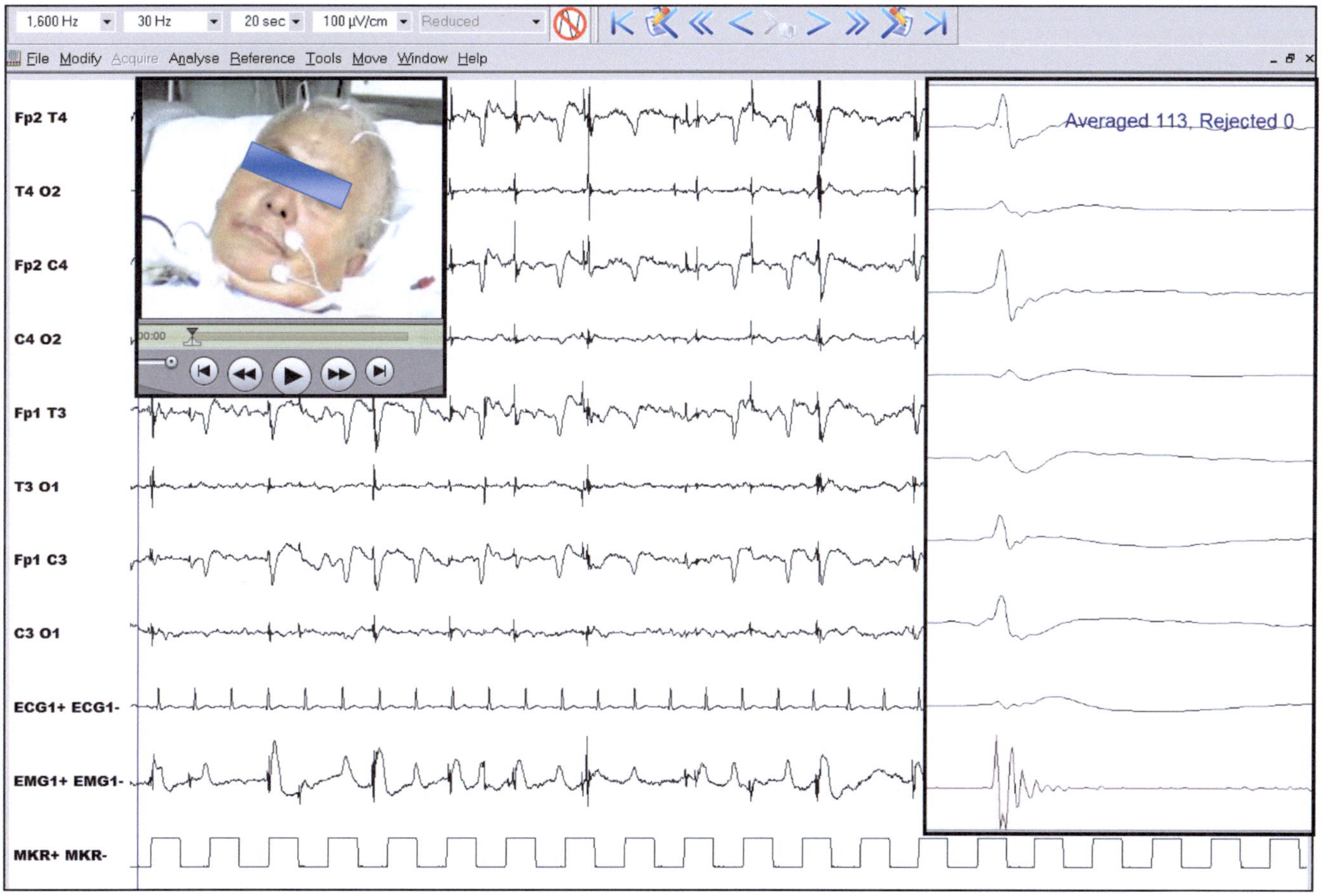

Fig. 48.7 A 71-year-old patient affected by postanoxic encephalopathy due to cardiac arrest. After 15 days diffuse facial myoclonic movements appeared, refractory to antiepileptic treatments. Simultaneous EEG and EMG monitoring didn't show any correlation between cortical and muscular activity (recorded by orbicularis oris muscle), as confirmed by back-averaging analysis

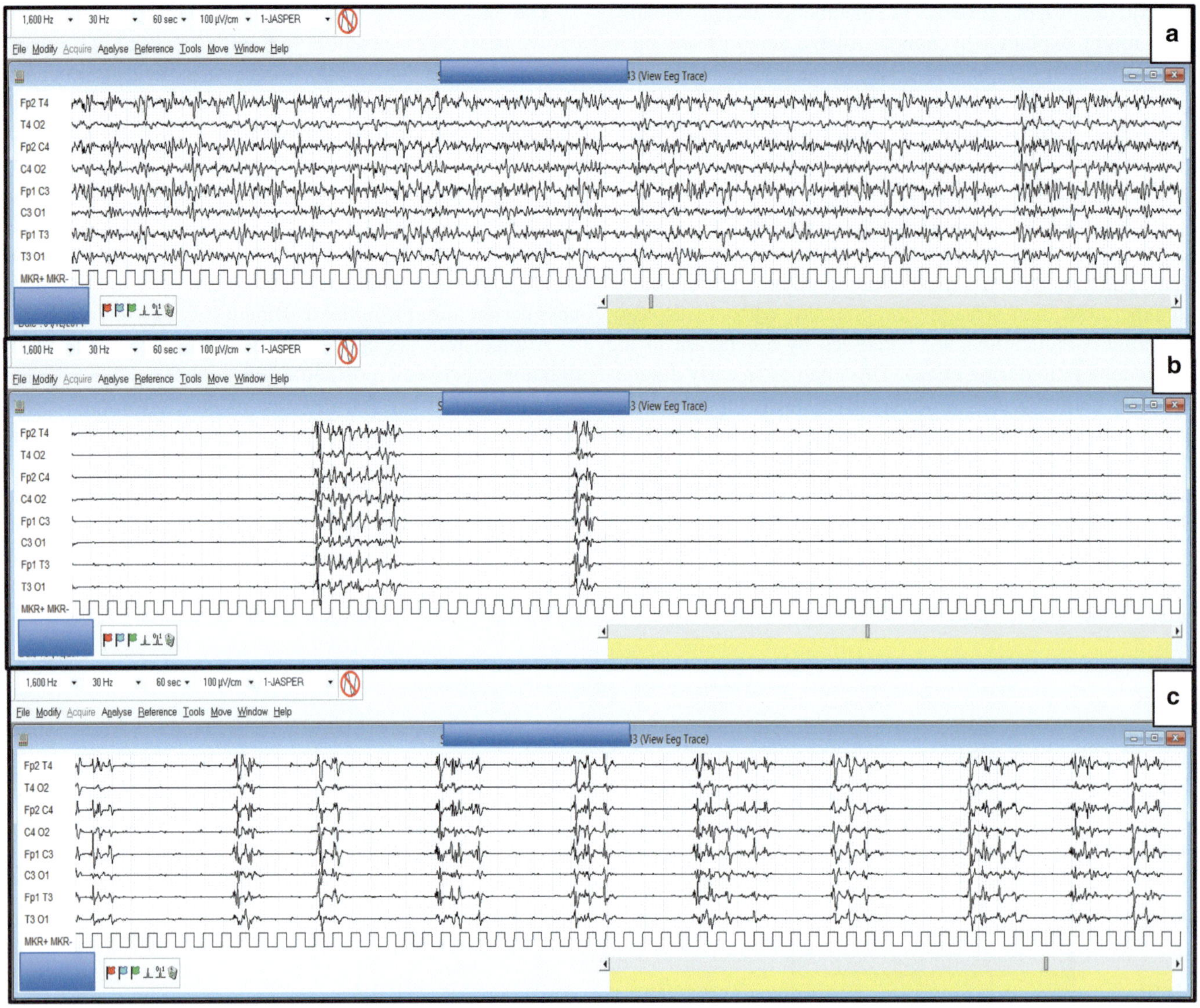

Fig. 48.8 Continuous EEG (cEEG) monitoring in a 76-year-old patient with traumatic brain injury. (**a**) Continuous diffuse epileptiform activity. (**b**) After a bolus of propofol (1 mg/kg) followed by an infusion of 20 mg/kg/h for 35 min, the cEEG showed a pattern of burst suppression with suppression periods >70% of the trace. (**c**) Few minutes after the interruption of propofol infusion, the periods of suppression became progressively shorter

EEG interpretation is always difficult in this context and long-term recording could help prompt detection of these abnormalities and redefine their significance and prognostic value [27, 33, 34].

Finally, cEEG can be used to determine the effects of different kinds of sedation and their optimal level to protect the brain, after severe traumatic brain injury (Fig. 48.8). However, the relevance of cEEG is under discussion in this situation, as most ICUs have the possibility of monitoring the depth of sedation (limiting the oversedation) by the Bi Spectral Index (BIS) [35]. It is based on an algorithm producing a dimensional scale going from 0 (suppressed EEG) to 100 (wake). This scale derives from a combination between direct signal recording from two frontal electrodes (Fp1 and Fp2 electrodes) and data representative of each level of sedation (from a database of EEG recordings). BIS cannot replace cEEG, but it can give an immediate quantitative result restrictively on the depth of anesthesia. For a complete description about the effects of anesthetic drugs on CNS and BIS, consult Chap. 45.

However, inspective analysis of non-processed tracings still represents the main method for revision and evaluation of EEG. Nevertheless, traditional inspective analysis requires a consistent amount of time and it is not very sensitive toward slow-onset abnormalities, such as the progressive decreasing of high waves or relative changes in a specific frequency band. In addition, as previously stated, this method requires a team of experts to be always available. For these reasons,

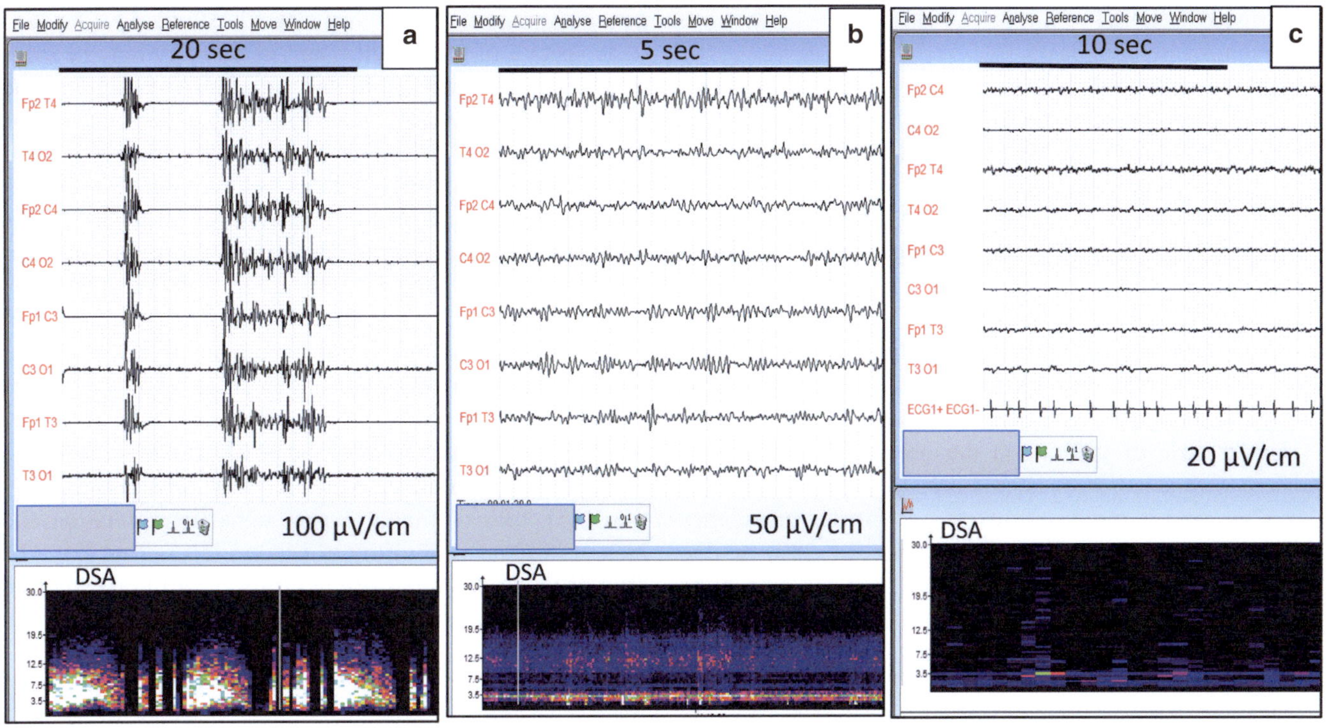

Fig. 48.9 Continuous EEG monitoring in a 56-year-old patient after cardiac arrest: raw EEG and Density Spectral Array (DSA). (**a**) day 1: burst-suppression pattern. (**b**) day 2: areactive alpha-coma of low amplitude. (**c**) day 3: attenuation/suppression of electrocerebral activity. LFF = 1 Hz, HFF = 30 Hz

alternative visualization methods were developed, allowing a simpler display through a quantification of EEG signals. They can be analyzed as number or visualized as graphics. Spectral analysis of cEEG can also be represented in the form of Compressed Spectral Array (CSA), Density Spectral Array (DSA), and amplitude-integrated EEG (aEEG) (Fig. 48.9).

Anyway original, raw tracings must always be available to verify the meaning of some abnormalities or trends. This is because some apparently significant patterns might be artifactual, especially in complex environments such as ICUs. Several programs were developed to automatically identify critical patterns but, up to now, they trigger many false positives.

48.3 Emergency EEG (eEEG)

EEG is a reliable and useful diagnostic tool in a number of clearly defined emergency situations. However, emergency EEG (eEEG) ordering policies at one hospital may not be applicable to others because of differences in staffing, payment difficulties, or local issues. These factors usually limit performing an EEG in emergency departments (EDs) [36].

The term "emergency" for a test means that the results will affect the patient management and outcome; consequently, an emergency test should be performed regardless the time and day. In an ideal situation, the EEG should be available anytime of the day 24/7, and it should only be requested by neurologists. However, the definition of eEEG has not yet been standardized. Varelas et al. defined eEEG an EEG requested from the attending physician—not necessarily a neurologist—for emergency indications on nonelective bases, performed within 1 h from the request [37]. Benbadis in 2008 named "stat" EEG (from the Latin word "statim," meaning immediately) an examination that should be available anytime any day (24 h/7 days), ordered only by neurologists or neurosurgeons, performed stat and interpreted stat (2–4 h from the request) [38]. The risk of this scenario is the abuse of the technique, and it could be ordered inappropriately [36]; an average response time of 3 h from request to initial reading is acceptable for eEEG [38, 39].

In a clinical policy statement, the American College of Emergency Physicians (ACEP) recommended that EEG should be considered in patients suspected of being in a nonconvulsive status epilepticus or in subtle convulsive status epilepticus and concluded that no clear recommendation for ordering eEEG in other clinical situations may be made on the basis of available data [40].

However, based on the clinical experience of many emergency department in the world, the main situations in which eEEG is required are:

- Suspected SENC.
- Diagnosis of brain death.
- Altered mental states.
- Focal neurological deficits especially if there is discordance between clinical and neuroradiological data.
- Coma of uncertain origin.
- Suspected encephalitis, especially of infectious nature.
- Differential diagnosis with Psychogenic Non-Epileptic Seizures (PNES).

Apart from the other indications that have been abundantly discussed above and in the specific chapters, altered mental states deserve a particular mention.

Up to 10% of patients in the emergency department present with seizures or altered mental status (AMS) [40, 41]. The most common causes of AMS in the emergency departments are neurologic, accounting for 28% of discharge diagnoses in one study of 317 patients presenting with AMS [41]. AMS is a significant challenge to the emergency physician, because it is often the clinical feature of a wide spectra of pathologies, and its etiology may be difficult to individuate [42]. Moreover, clinical evaluation can be difficult, especially if a detailed history cannot be obtained and the collaboration of the patient is not complete. Not surprisingly, rates of emergency departments resources use, hospital admission and death for this diagnosis are disproportionately high relative to the percentage of thepopulation this group represents [43]. In these cases, EEG is a very useful diagnostic tool, because it is the only method that could provide an objective picture of the clinical situation. Nevertheless, it is still underused or often even not available in emergency [44]. Proposed reasons for this underuse include lack of availability of a technologist, difficulty and time required for signal acquisition [45], lack of timely expert signal interpretation and lack of awareness of utility of EEG in this setting [39, 41]. Two different examples of the utility of eEEG are showed in Figs. 48.10 and 48.11.

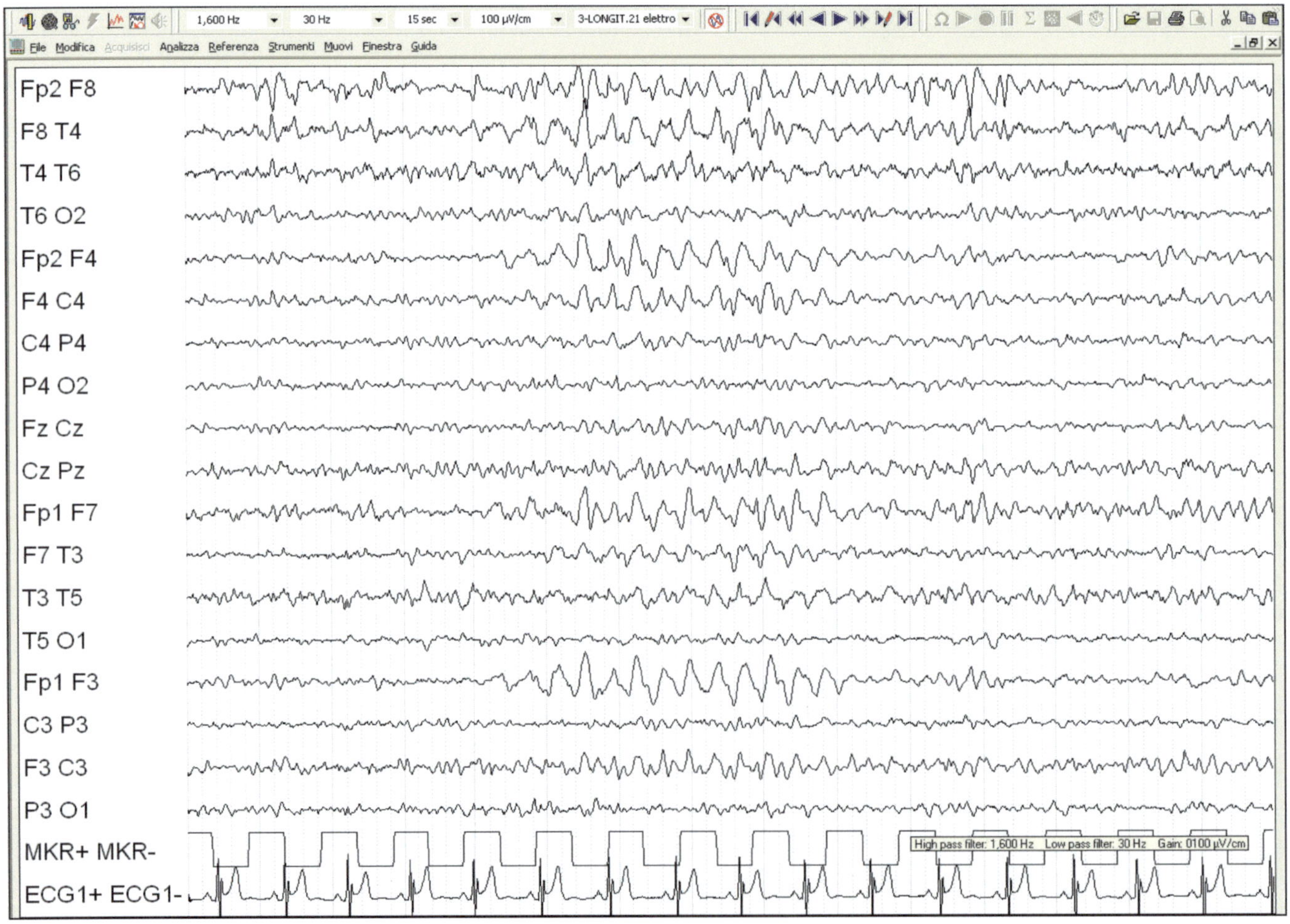

Fig. 48.10 A 27-year-old male patient, admitted to the emergency department for sudden onset of headache, dizziness, and confusion. EEG showed sequences of monomorphic slow waves (3 Hz) in right frontotemporal regions with a tendency to the contralateral transmission and associated with some spikes in phase opposition on F8 electrode. Magnetic resonance angiography showed a cavernous angioma in the same site

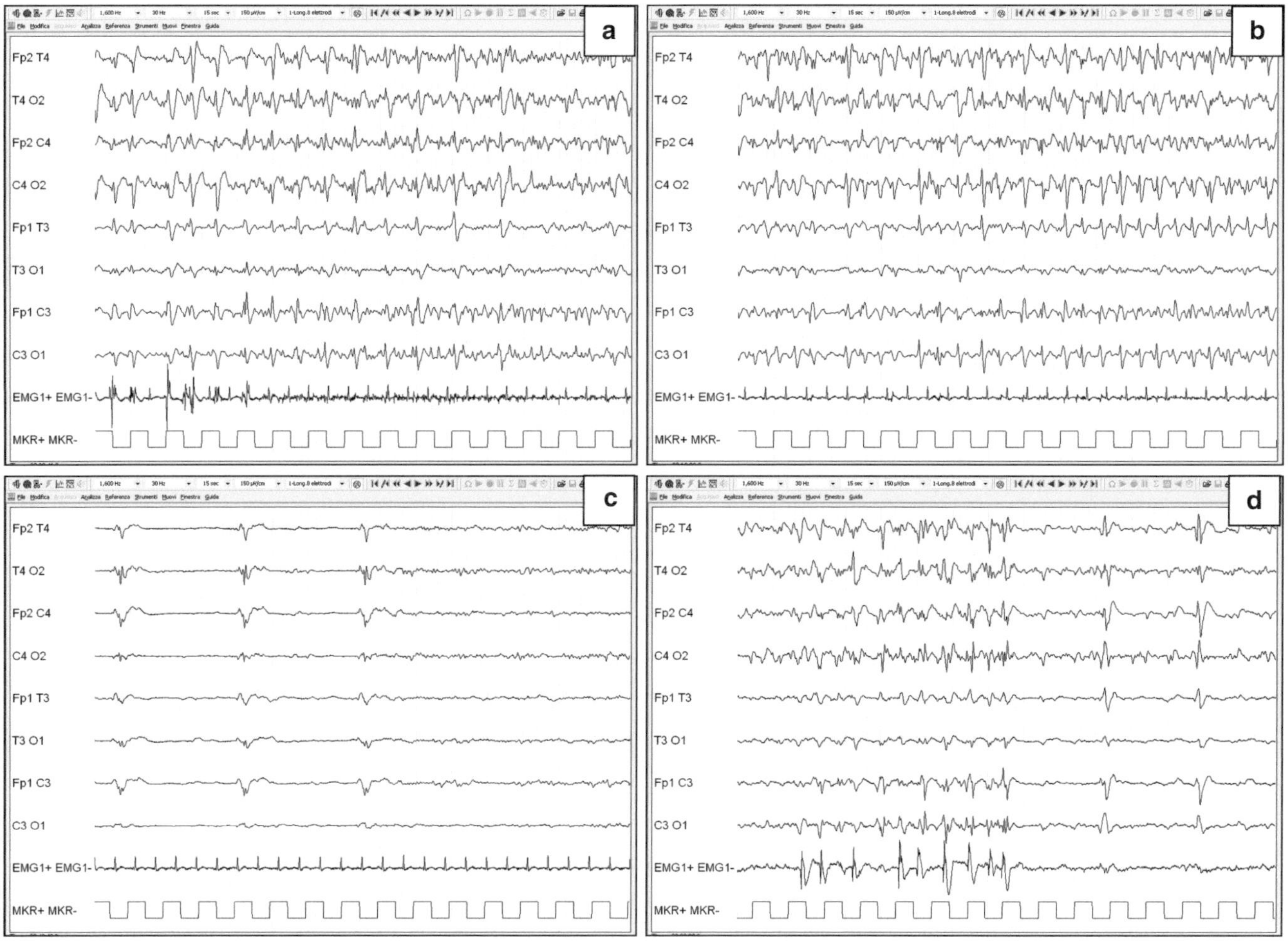

Fig. 48.11 A 55-year-old male patient after liver transplantation. Two days after surgical procedure, sudden onset of altered mental status worsening until coma and left hemisoma clonic movements. MR showed intracerebral right temporal hemorrhage. (**a**) EEG evidenced subcontinuous sequences of epileptiform graphoelements, more evident in the right hemisphere, sometimes related to muscular activity recorded by simultaneous EMG of left deltoid. (**b**) EEG monitoring, during and after administration of levetiracetam (1500 mg, i.v. bolus) showed, despite the disappearance of myoclonic jerks, the persistence of the epileptiform activity. (**c**) EEG abnormalities improved after the administration of Lorazepam (4 mg, i.v. bolus) and they were replaced by sporadic epileptiform abnormalities alternated with periods of electrocortical attenuation. (**d**) the day after, EEG showed more active right epileptiform activity, related to contralateral myoclonic jerks

eEEG is not indicated after a tonic-clonic seizure as it could evidence only minimal, specific, postictal slowings of background activity. However, sometimes, after a tonic-clonic seizure, symptoms as prolonged confusion, behavior disorders, and amnesia can be accompanied by interictal and/or ictal epileptiform abnormalities [46] (Fig. 48.12).

In their prospective study, Praline and colleagues confirm the value of an eEEG in the management of CSE and in the diagnosis of NCSE [47]. Even if a recording of at least 20 min is preferred, also a briefer (5 min) but promptly performed recording could have an adequate reliability [41].

Ziai et al. tested the availability and utility of EEG performed within 30 min in emergency departments in patients with AMS. For this purpose, a standard full-montage EEG lasting 20 min was performed within 30 min of referral by an emergency physician. The entire recording was also compared with abbreviated 5 min EEG. The study demonstrated that the rapid availability of standard full-montage EEG in emergency is feasible and useful to establish a diagnosis in about half of AMS patients; moreover, abbreviated 5-min EEG showed an adequate reliability [41].

Despite the undeniable clinical indications and sensitivity of the eEEG, this is yet poorly utilized in emergency departments. An Italian nationwide epidemiological survey showed that 24 h/ 7 d EEG was available only in 27% of neurology units in the emergency setting [48]. The scenario is the same now as it was 10 years ago.

A more recent survey conducted in the United Kingdom on CSE management demonstrated that only 33% of ICUs have an access to early EEG monitoring, which is stated as essential by NICE guidelines in the management protocol of CSE [49].

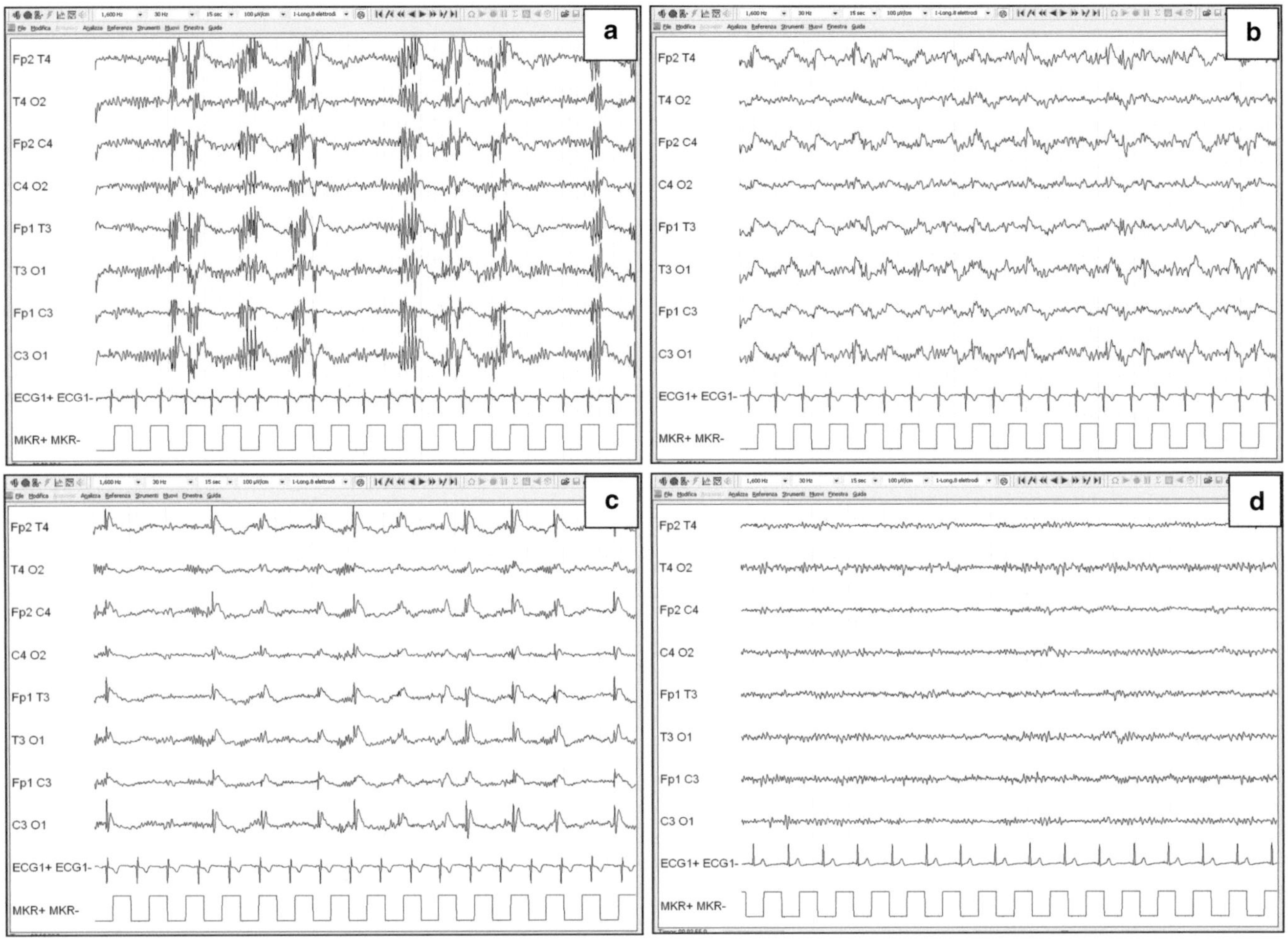

Fig. 48.12 A 66-year-old patient with generalized epilepsy syndrome, admitted to the emergency department because of confusion after two generalized tonic-clonic seizures. eEEG showed a critical pattern of nonconvulsive status epilepticus with diffuse, brief bursts of spikes at 10 Hz followed by a slow wave and alternated with alpha rhythm (**a**). 3 min after the administration of diazepam (10 mg i.v. bolus), EEG showed a diffuse delta activity with interposed spikes and spike-wave complexes (**b**). 20 min later, the alpha rhythm returned to be visible on the posterior regions, while periodic spike-wave complexes are detectable anteriorly (**c**). After 30 min, a second bolus of diazepam was administrated; the epileptiform abnormalities disappeared for the next 24 h (**d**)

References

1. Isley MR, Edmonds HL Jr, Stecker M. Guidelines for intraoperative neuromonitoring using raw (analog or digital waveforms) and quantitative electroencephalography: a position statement by the American Society of Neurophysiological Monitoring. J Clin Monit Comput. 2009;23:369–90.
2. Shils JL, Sloan TB. Intraoperative neuromonitoring. Int Anesthesiol Clin. 2015;53:53–73.
3. Van Putten MJAM, Hofmeijer J. EEG monitoring in cerebral ischemia: basic concepts and clinical applications. J Clin Neurophysiol. 2016;33:203–10.
4. Osman GM, Riviello JJ. Hirsch LJ. EEG in the intensive care unit: anoxia, coma, brain death, and related disorders. In: Schomer DL, Lopes da Silva FH, editors. Niedermeyer's electroencephalography: basic principles, clinical applications and related fields. 7th ed. New York: Oxford University Press; 2018. p. 610–58.
5. Stecker MM, Cheung AT, Pochettino A, et al. Deep hypothermic circulatory arrest: I. Effects of cooling on electroencephalogram and evoked potentials. Ann Thorac Surg. 2001;71:14–21.
6. Thirumala PD, Thiagarajan K, Gedela S, Crammond DJ, Balzer JR. Diagnostic accuracy of EEG changes during carotid endarterectomy in predicting perioperative strokes. J Clin Neurosci. 2016;25:1–9.
7. Ballotta E, Saladini M, Gruppo M, et al. Predictors of electroencephalographic changes needing shunting during carotid endarterectomy. Ann Vasc Surg. 2010;24:1045–52.
8. Simon MV, Chiappa KH, Kilbride RD, et al. Predictors of clamp-induced electroencephalographic changes during carotid endarterectomies. J Clin Neurophysiol. 2012;29:462–7.
9. Chiappa KH, Burke SR, Young RR. Results of electroencephalographic monitoring during 367 carotid endarterectomies. Stroke. 1979;4:381–8.
10. Mizrahi EM, Chatrain G-E, Byrum W, et al. American clinical guidelines on intraoperative electroencephalography. Am Clin Neurophysiol Soc Council. 2000;2000:1–21.
11. Cursi M, Meraviglia MV, Fanelli GF, et al. Electroencephalographic background desynchronization during cerebral blood flow reduction. Clin Neurophysiol. 2005;116:2577–85.
12. Van Putten MJ, Peters JM, Mulder SM, et al. A brain symmetry index (BSI) for online EEG monitoring in carotid endarterectomy. Clin Neurophysiol. 2004;115:1189–94.

13. Fernández Suárez FE, Fernández Del Valle D, González Alvarez A, Pérez-Lozano B. Intraoperative care for aortic surgery using circulatory arrest. J Thorac Dis. 2017;9(Suppl 6):S508–20.
14. Hogue CW, Palin CA, Arrowsmith JE. Cardiopulmonary bypass management and neurologic outcomes: an evidence-based appraisal of current practices. Anesth Analg. 2006;103:21–37.
15. Kimura T, Muraoka R, Chiba Y, et al. Effect of intermittent deep hypothermic circulatory arrest on brain metabolism. J Thorac Cardiovasc Surg. 1994;108:658–63.
16. James ML, Andersen ND, Swaminathan M, et al. Predictors of electrocerebral inactivity with deep hypothermia. J Thorac Cardiovasc Surg. 2014;147:1002–7.
17. Legatt AD, Nuwer MR, Emerson RG. Intraoperative monitoring of central neurophysiology. In: Schomer DL, Lopes da Silva FH, editors. Niedermeyer's Electroencephalopgraphy: basic principles, clinical applications and related fields. 7th ed. New York: Oxford University Press; 2018. p. 833–66.
18. Le Roux P, Menon D, Citerio G, et al. Consensus summary of the international multidisciplinary consensus conference on multimodality monitoring in Neurocritical care. Neurocrit Care. 2014;21:S282–96.
19. Gütling E, Gonser A, Imhof HG, Landis T. EEG reactivity in the prognosis of severe head injury. Neurology. 1995;45:915–8.
20. Tsetsou S, Novy J, Oddo M, Rossetti AO. EEG reactivity to pain in comatose patients: importance of the stimulus type. Resuscitation. 2015;97:34–7.
21. Hirsch LJ, Claassen J, Mayer SA, Emerson RG. Stimulus-induced rhythmic, periodic, or ictal discharges (SIRPIDs): a common EEG phenomenon in the critically ill. Epilepsia. 2004;45:109–23.
22. Johnson EL, Kaplan PW, Ritzl EK. Stimulus-induced rhythmic, periodic, or ictal discharges (SIRPIDs). J Clin Neurophysiol. 2018;35:229–33.
23. Hirsch LJ. Continuous EEG monitoring in intensive care unit: an overview. J Clin Neurophysiol. 2004;21:332–40.
24. Halford J. Electrographic seizures in adults: recognition and examples. In: Husain AM, Sinha SR, editors. Continuous EEG Monitoring. Principle and practice. Switzerland: Springer International Publishing; 2017. p. 87–113.
25. Jordan KG. Continuous EEG and evoked potential monitoring in the neuroscience intensive care unit. J Clin Neurophysiol. 1993;10:445–75.
26. Privitera M, Hoffman M, Moore JL, Jester D. EEG detection of nontonic-clonic status epilepticus in patients with altered consciousness. Epilepsy Res. 1994;18:155–66.
27. André-Obadia N, Parain D, Szurhaj W. Continuous EEG monitoring in adults in the intensive care unit (ICU). Neurophysiol Clin. 2015;45:39–46.
28. Towne AR, Waterhouse EJ, Boggs JG, Garnett LK, Brown AJ, Smith JR Jr, et al. Prevalence of nonconvulsive status epilepticus in comatose patients. Neurology. 2000;54:340–5.
29. Vespa PM, Nuwer MR, Juhasz C, Alexander M, Nenov V, Martin N, et al. Early detection of vasospasm after acute subarachnoid hemorrhage using continuous EEG ICU monitoring. Clin Neurophysiol. 1997;103:607–15.
30. Claassen J, Taccone FS, Horn P, Holtkamp M, Stocchetti N, Oddo M. Recommendations on the use of EEG monitoring in critically ill patients: consensus statement from the neurointensive care section of the ESICM. Intensive Care Med. 2013;39:1337–51.
31. Young GB, Jordan KG, Doig GS. An assessment of nonconvulsive seizures in the intensive care unit using continuous EEG monitoring: an investigation of variables associated with mortality. Neurology. 1996;47:83–9.
32. Rossetti AO, Logroscino G, Bromfield EB. Refractory status epilepticus: effect of treatment aggressiveness on prognosis. Arch Neurol. 2005;62:1698–702.
33. Mani R, Schmitt SE, Mazer M, Putt ME, Gaieski DF. The frequency and timing of epileptiform activity on continuous electroencephalogram in comatose post-cardiac arrest syndrome patients treated with therapeutic hypothermia. Resuscitation. 2012;83:840–7.
34. Navarro V, Engrand N, Gélisse P. The electroencephalogram in status epilepticus. Rev Neurol. 2009;165:329–37.
35. Kamenik M, Möller Petrun A. Bispectral index-guided induction of general anaesthesia. Br J Anaesth. 2014;112:169.
36. Yigit O, Eray O, Mihci E, et al. The utility of EEG in the emergency department. Emerg Med J. 2012;29:301–5.
37. Varelas PN, Spanaki MV, Hacein-Bey L, Hether T, Terranova B. Emergent EEG: indications and diagnostic yield. Neurology. 2003;61:702–4.
38. Benbadis SR. Use and abuse of stat EEG. Expert Rev Neurother. 2008;8:865–8.
39. Quigg M, Shneker B, Domer P. Current practice in administration and clinical criteria of emergent EEG. J Clin Neurophysiol. 2001;18:162–5.
40. ACEP Clinical Policies Committee and the Clinical Policies Subcommittee on Seizures. Clinical policy: critical issues in the evaluation and management of adult patients presenting to the emergency department with seizures. Ann Emerg Med. 2004;43:605–25.
41. Ziai WC, Schlattman D, Llinas R, et al. Emergent EEG in the emergency department in patients with altered mental states. Clin Neurophysiol. 2012;123:910–7.
42. Kanich W, Brady WJ, Huff JS, et al. Altered mental status: evaluation and etiology in the ED. Am J Emerg Med. 2002;20:613–7.
43. American College of Emergency Physicians. Clinical policy for the initial approach to patients presenting with altered mental status. Ann Emerg Med. 1999;33:251–80.
44. Kaplan PW. Assessing the outcomes in patients with nonconvulsive status epilepticus: nonconvulsive status epilepticus is underdiagnosed, potentially overtreated and confounded by comorbidity. J Clin Neurophysiol. 1999;16:341–52.
45. American Clinical Neurophysiology Society. Minimum technical requirements for performing clinical electroencephalography. J Clin Neurophysiol. 2006;23:86–91.
46. Shorvon S, Trinka E. Nonconvulsive status epilepticus and the postictal state. Epilepsy Behav. 2010;19:172–5.
47. Praline J, Grujic J, Corcia P, et al. Emergent EEG in clinical practice. Clin Neurophysiol. 2007;118:2149–55.
48. de Falco FA, Sterzi R, Toso V, et al. The neurologist in the emergency department. An Italian nationwide epidemiological survey. Neurol Sci. 2008;29:67–75.
49. Patel M, Bagary M, McCorry D. The management of convulsive refractory status Epilepticus in adults in the UK: no consistency in practice and little access to continuous EEG monitoring. Seizure. 2015;24:33–7.

EEG Glossary

The first attempt to systematically propose a syllabus for electroencephalographers was made by O'Leary and Knott who in 1955 published in the EEG Journal "Some Minimal Essentials for Clinical Electroencephalographers" [1]. In the following decades, with the EEG being increasingly used in the experimental and clinical field, need to adopt a language as common as possible between various laboratories worldwide became even more pressing. In fact, the multiplicity of terms generated (and sometimes still generates) confusion and misinterpretations, promoting misdiagnosis and making it difficult to compare data between different laboratories.

To overcome this risk, in 1974 "A Glossary of Terms," most commonly used by "Clinical Electroencephalographers," was published in the EEG Journal; this glossary was the result of the work of a group of experts from the International Federation of Clinical Neurophysiology (IFCN) led by Chatrian [2]. Thanks to this document, it was for the first time officially established which term had to be used to correctly describe a specific EEG element, avoiding the proliferation of different terms to indicate the same pattern. Furthermore, the use of terms deemed inappropriate was strongly discouraged.

Similarly, the American Electroencephalographic Society (later to become the American Clinical Neurophysiology Society) wrote its own glossary, published as first edition in 1979, subsequently revised in 1984, 1994 [3], 2006 [4], and 2016 [5].

The IFCN International Glossary was also revised and republished in 1999 by Noachtar et al. [6], basing entirely on the proposal made by Chatrian et al. [2], but updating the terminology according to changes due to technological evolution. The last, updated and revised version of the IFCN glossary has been published in 2017, including a proposal for the report format of the EEG findings [7]. The most relevant entries of the "revised glossary of terms most commonly used by clinical electroencephalographers" by the IFCN, so far the single most authoritative, comprehensive, and updated EEG glossary available in the literature, are reported in the next pages (portions of the text reproduced with permission from [7]).

Activation procedure Any procedure designed to modulate EEG activity, for instance to enhance physiological waveforms or elicit abnormal paroxysmal activity. Examples include eye closing, hyperventilation, photic stimulation, natural or drug-induced sleep, sensory stimulation (acoustic, somatosensory, or pain).

Activity, EEG An EEG wave or sequence of waves of cerebral origin.

Alpha band Frequency band of 8–13 Hz inclusive. Greek letter: α.

Alpha rhythm Rhythm at 8–13 Hz inclusive occurring during wakefulness over the posterior regions of the head, generally with maximum amplitudes over the occipital areas. Amplitude varies but is mostly below 50 μV in the adult, but often much higher in children. Best seen with the eyes closed, during physical relaxation and relative mental inactivity. Blocked or attenuated by attention, especially visual, and mental effort.

Alpha variant rhythms An EEG rhythm recorded most prominently over the posterior regions of the head that differs in frequency, but resembles in reactivity, the alpha rhythm.

Alpha wave Wave with duration of 1/8–1/13 s (77–125 ms).

Amplitude, EEG Is a measure of the change of EEG signals with respect to the mean value, usually measured in microvolts (μV), and often expressed as the difference between the maximum and minimum deviation (i.e., peak-to-peak), or in rectified EEG from baseline to peak. For a variable EEG activity or modulating sinusoidal rhythm a range can be provided.

Amplitude-integrated EEG (aEEG) Involves customized display of EEG activity following signal processing which includes an asymmetric band-pass filter (2–15 Hz), logarithmic amplitude display, rectification, smoothing, and time compression (such that several hours can be viewed on a screen). Widely used in neonatal intensive care unit monitoring, for example, of infants suffering a hypoxic ischemic encephalopathy.

O. Mecarelli (ed.), *Clinical Electroencephalography*, https://doi.org/10.1007/978-3-030-04573-9

Analog-to-digital conversion (AD conversion) Transformation of a continuous, analog signal EEG into its digital representation (a discontinuous series of discrete amplitudes)

Anterior (slow) dysrhythmia A normal EEG activity seen in term and near term infants at 32–44 weeks of post menstrual age; characterized by bilateral frontal delta waves (50–100 μV), seen in isolation or brief runs, typically synchronously and symmetrically.

Application, electrode The process of establishing fixation and electrical connection between an electrode and the subject's scalp or brain.

Arrhythmic activity A sequence of EEG waves with an inconstant periodicity.

Arousal Change from a lower to a higher level of alertness as manifest in EEG activity.

Array, electrode A regular arrangement of electrodes over the scalp or brain, or within the brain substance.

Artifact (1) A physiological potential difference due to an extracerebral source present in EEG recordings, such as eye blinks and movements, electrocardiogram (ECG) or muscle contractions (EMG). (2) A modification of the EEG caused by extracerebral factors, such as instrumental distortion or malfunction, movement of the patient, or ambient electrical noise.

Asymmetry Unequal amplitude, frequency or morphology of EEG activity in channels over homologous areas of the two hemispheres. To be considered abnormal in practice if the amplitude difference exceeds 50% or frequency difference is equal to or greater than 1 Hz in the posterior dominant rhythm, although it should be recognized that these are essentially arbitrary values. It can be quantified by quantitative EEG (qEEG) measures, such as the Brain Symmetry Index (BSI).

Asynchrony The noncoherent occurrence of EEG activities over regions on the same or opposite sides (hemispheres) of the head. For example, two similar waveforms occurring at separate electrodes or channels, but not simultaneously due to a time lag between the channels.

Attenuation Reduction in amplitude of EEG activity (for example, the alpha rhythm is usually attenuated or blocked on eye opening). May occur transiently in response to a physiological or other stimulus, such as electrical stimulation of the brain, or more permanently as a result of pathological conditions, such as cerebral atrophy or ischemia.

Augmentation Increase in amplitude of EEG activity (for example, the alpha rhythm is characteristically augmented upon closing the eyes).

Background activity Any underlying EEG activity representing the setting in which focal or transient activity, either normal or abnormal, appears and from which such underlying pattern is distinguished.

Background slowing The frequency of the background rhythm which is below the normal value for age and state.

Band Range of EEG frequency in a spectrum for a given recording or epoch, i.e., delta, theta, alpha, beta, gamma bands and high frequency oscillations.

Basal electrode Any electrode located in proximity to the base of the skull.

Benign epileptiform transient of sleep (BETS) Use of term discouraged. A normal variant. Small sharp spikes of very short duration (<50 ms) and low amplitude (<50 μV), often followed by a small theta wave, occurring in the temporal regions during drowsiness and light sleep.

Beta band Frequency band of 14–30 Hz inclusive. Greek letter: β.

Beta rhythm or activity Any EEG rhythm between 14 and 30 Hz (wave duration 33–72 ms). Most characteristically recorded over the fronto-central regions of the head during wakefulness. Amplitude of fronto-central beta rhythm varies but is mostly below 30 μV. Blocking or attenuation of the beta rhythm by contralateral movement or tactile stimulation is especially obvious in electrocorticograms. Other beta rhythms are most prominent in other locations or are diffuse, and may be drug-induced (for example, alcohol, barbiturates, benzodiazepines, and intravenous anesthetic agents).

Bilateral Involving both sides of the head (or body).

Bilateral independent periodic discharges (BIPDs) BIPDs are two bilateral independent (i.e., asynchronous) surface-negative bi- or di-, tri- or polyphasic complexes consisting of spike, sharp, or polyspike components, with variably following slow waves, lasting 60–600 ms (typically 200 ms) that occupy at least 50% of a standard 20 min EEG. Amplitude ranges from 50 to 150 μV (occasionally up to 300 μV), which may be asymmetric, usually recurring at 0.5–2 c/s (but very occasionally with intervals of up to 10 s). BIPDs are broadly distributed and waveform morphology stays fairly constant for a given patient and EEG, with intervening background activity usually attenuated and slow. Most BIPDs are ephemeral phenomena that usually resolve within weeks. They occur with acute marked focal destructive lesions (for example, cerebral infarcts, tumors, or herpes simplex encephalitis) or more subacute/chronic pathologies (for example, epilepsy and vascular compromise).

Biphasic wave Complex consisting of two wave components developed on alternate sides of the baseline.

Bipolar derivation (1) Recording from a pair of exploring electrodes. (2) Method of organizing the linkages of electrodes to recording channels.

Bipolar montage Multiple bipolar channels, with no electrode being common to all channels. In most instances, bipolar channels are linked, i.e., adjacent channels from electrodes along the same line of electrodes, or chain, have one electrode in common; so the reference electrode (input terminal 2) in one channel becomes the exploring electrode (input terminal 1) in the next channel of the chain.

Blocking (1) Apparent, temporary obliteration or attenuation of EEG rhythms in response to physiological or other stimuli, such as eye opening on alpha rhythm, or a change in state. (2) A condition of temporary EEG amplifier saturation, caused when the output voltages of the amplifier exceed its operating range sensitivity.

Breach rhythm EEG activity recorded over or nearby a defect in the skull vault (for example, after a fracture, burr hole, or craniotomy), of increased amplitude when compared to homologous areas on the opposite side of the head (usually by a factor of less than 3). The rhythm is composed of fast activity with a spiky appearance along with alpha and/or mu rhythms, due to lack of attenuation and distortion by the skull.

Burst A group of waves with a minimum of four phases and duration longer than 500 ms which appear and disappear abruptly and are distinguished from background activity by differences in frequency, form, and/or amplitude.

Burst suppression Pattern characterized by paroxysmal bursts of theta and/or delta waves, at times intermixed with sharp and faster waves, alternating with intervening periods of attenuation or suppression (below 10 μV) lasting more than 50% of the record.

Channel Complete system for the detection, amplification and display of potential differences between a pair of electrodes, or a computed reference (for example, common average reference). Digital EEG machines simulate a multichannel display by tracing several voltage time plots on a visual display.

Circumferential bipolar montage A montage consisting of linked bipolar derivations encircling the head. Commonly bilateral longitudinal temporal electrode chains are linked together.

Common average reference Computational average potential of all or most electrode signals used as a reference electrode.

Common mode signal Common component of the two signals applied to the two input terminals of a differential EEG amplifier.

Common reference electrode A reference electrode that is common to all channels.

Common reference montage A montage in which each of the channels have the same reference electrode.

Complex A sequence of two or more waveforms having a characteristic composite morphology; and when recurring are seen with a fairly consistent form, distinguished from background activity.

Continuous EEG (cEEG) Prolonged EEG recording and often analysis for monitoring of electrical brain activity.

Continuous slow activity Uninterrupted ongoing slow activity (theta and delta bands) which may be rhythmic, arrhythmic, or polymorphic, which may wax and wane but not regress, and is of variable amplitude and morphology. Typically it is nonresponsive to external stimuli and clearly exceeds the amount considered physiologically normal for the patient's age.

Cycle The complete sequence of recurrent almost sinusoidal oscillatory potential changes undergone by individual waveform components of regularly repeated EEG waves or complexes.

Cycles per second (c/s) Unit of frequency defined as the number of complete cycles in one second. Synonym hertz (Hz).

Delta band Frequency band of 0.1–<4 Hz. Greek letter: δ.

Delta brush Normal neonatal graphoelement, seen at 26–40 weeks of post menstrual age (PMA), maximal around 32–34 weeks, and rare at term; combination of delta wave (0.3–1.5 c/s; 50–300 μV) with superimposed fast activity (>8 Hz; 10–60 μV). Localization changes with PMA.

Delta wave Wave with duration of ¼–2 s (250–2000 ms).

Diffuse Colloquialism: an EEG activity spread over large areas of both sides of the head. This does not imply abnormality as a normal rhythm may be diffusely distributed (for example, alpha activity in some individuals, or slow waves in deep sleep).

Differential amplifier An amplifier whose output is proportional to the voltage difference between its two input terminals.

Differential signal Difference between two signals applied to the respective two input terminals of a differential EEG amplifier.

Diphasic wave Complex consisting of two wave components developed on alternate sides of the baseline.

Dipole An EEG signal vector produced by a separation of negative (sink) and positive (source) potential poles (or current). A dipole is characterized by its strength, location, and orientation. Depending on their orientation, dipoles can be radial (perpendicular to the surface), tangential (parallel to the surface), or a combination of these (oblique).

Disorganization Gross alteration in frequency, form, topography, and/or quantity of physiologic EEG rhythms in: (1) an individual record, relative to previous records in the same subject or the rhythms of homologous regions on the opposite side of the head, or (2) relative to findings in normal subjects of similar age and similar state of vigilance.

Duration (1) The interval from beginning to end of an individual wave or complex. (2) The time that a sequence of waves or complexes or any other distinguishable feature lasts in an EEG record.

Electrocerebral inactivity Absence over all regions of the head of identifiable electrical activity of cerebral origin, whether spontaneous or induced by physiological stimuli or pharmacological agents.

Electrocorticography (ECoG) Technique of recording electrical activity of the brain by means of electrodes applied over or implanted into the cerebral cortex.

Electrode, EEG A conducting device applied over or inserted in a region of the scalp or brain.

Electrodecrement A period of amplitude attenuation usually with superimposed fast activity.

Electrode impedance Total effective resistance to alternating current (AC), arising from ohmic resistance and reactance. Measured between pairs of electrodes or, in some electroencephalographs, between each individual electrode and all the other electrodes connected in parallel. Expressed in ohms (generally kilo-ohms, kΩ).

Electrode resistance Total effective resistance to direct current (DC), through the interface between an EEG electrode and the scalp or brain. Measured between pairs of electrodes or, in some electroencephalographs, between each individual electrode and all the other electrodes connected in parallel. Expressed in ohms (generally kilo-ohms, kΩ).

Encoche frontale Normal neonatal graphoelement in term and near term infants, between 34 and 44 weeks post menstrual age. Frontal broad diphasic sharp waves (50–100 μV); typically bilateral, but may be unilateral. Usually seen in transition from active to quiet sleep.

Epileptiform pattern Describes transients distinguishable from background activity with a characteristic morphology typically, but neither exclusively nor invariably, found in interictal EEGs of people with epilepsy. Epileptiform patterns have to fulfill at least four of the following six criteria:

1. Di- or triphasic waves with sharp or spiky morphology (i.e., pointed peak).
2. Different wave-duration than the ongoing background activity, either shorter or longer.
3. Asymmetry of the waveform: a sharply rising ascending phase and a more slowly decaying descending phase, or vice versa.
4. The transient is followed by an associated slow afterwave.
5. The background activity surrounding epileptiform discharges is disrupted by the presence of the epileptiform discharges.
6. Distribution of the negative and positive potentials on the scalp suggests a source of the signal in the brain, corresponding to a radial, oblique, or tangential orientation of the source. This is best assessed by inspecting voltage maps constructed using common average reference.

Epoch EEG segment with a defined duration. Duration of epochs is determined arbitrarily but should be specified.

Equipotential Applies to regions of the head or electrodes that are at the same potential at a given instant in time.

Event-related potential (ERP) Refer to long latency responses (>70 ms) associated with an event, such as a deviant stimulus (as in mismatch negativity, P3 or P300), anticipation of a response (as in Bereitschaftspotential), or anticipation of a stimulus demanding a response (as in contingent negative variation). Applied mainly to slow (on account of their lower frequency content) "endogenous" evoked potentials elicited by controlled manipulation of the psychological context. Thought to reflect some aspect of higher sensory processing, and therefore sometimes referred to as "cognitive potentials," such as attention, expectancy, novelty detection, stimulus salience, target recognition, task relevance, information delivery, decision-making, stimulus evaluation time, template matching, memory, and closure of cognitive epoch.

Evoked magnetic field Magnetic counterpart of EEG evoked potential.

Evoked potential (EP) Wave or complex elicited by and time-locked to a physiological or nonphysiological stimulus or event, the timing of which can be reliably assessed.

Exploring electrode An electrode that registers electrical potentials from excitable tissue of the nervous system, historically connected to the input terminal 1 of an EEG amplifier, against a reference electrode, connected to the input terminal 2.

Extracerebral potential Any potential that does not originate in the brain, generally referred to as an artifact in EEG. May arise from electrical interference external to the subject and recording system, the subject, the electrodes and their connections to the subject and the electroencephalograph, and the electroencephalograph itself.

Far-field potential A potential generated in a deep neural structure and recorded by electrodes on the head at a distance from the generator, as a result of volume conduction and not mediated by neuronal activity.

Fast activity Activity of frequency higher than the alpha band, i.e., beta and gamma activity, and high frequency oscillations.

Fast alpha variant rhythm A normal variant. Characteristic rhythm at 14–20 Hz, detected most prominently over the posterior regions of the head. May alternate or be intermixed with alpha rhythm, of which it is usually a harmonic frequency. Blocked or attenuated by attention, especially visual, and mental effort.

Fast ripples Part of the high frequency oscillation (HFO) bandwidth, usually defined as being in the range 250–1000 Hz.

Fast wave Wave with duration shorter than alpha waves, i.e., under 1/13 s.

Focal Limited to a small area of the brain in one hemisphere. Focal epileptic seizures are conceptualized as originating within networks limited to one hemisphere, and usually associated with an initially localized epileptiform EEG pattern.

Focus A limited region of the scalp, cerebral cortex, or depth of the brain displaying a given EEG activity, either normal or abnormal.

Foramen ovale electrode A multicontact electrode bundle inserted through the foramen ovale to lie in proximity to the mesial temporal cortex.

Fourteen and 6-Hz positive burst or spikes A normal variant. Burst of arch-shaped waves or spikes at 13–17 c/s and/or 5–7 c/s, but most commonly at 14 and/or 6 c/s, usually seen bilaterally over the posterior temporal and adjacent areas, typically during drowsiness and light sleep, with incidence peaking in adolescence. The sharp peaks of its component waves are positive with respect to other regions. Amplitude varies but is generally below 75 μV.

Frequency Number of complete cycles of repetitive waves or complexes in 1 s. Measured in cycles per second (c/s) or Hertz (Hz).

Frontal intermittent rhythmic delta activity (FIRDA) Fairly regular, approximately sinusoidal or sawtooth waves, mostly occurring in bursts at 1.5–2.5 Hz synchronously over the frontal areas of both sides of the head (occasionally unilateral).

Fronto-central theta A normal variant. Theta rhythm located in the midline, just anterior to the vertex, that occurs during psychological stress and cognitive tasks, particularly problem solving. It appears predominantly in young healthy adults (<30 years of age). The pattern is considered to be a normal response to cognitive tasks.

Gain, voltage The ratio of output signal voltage, V_o, to input signal voltage, V_i, of an EEG channel.

Gamma band Frequency band from >30 to 80 Hz. Greek letter: γ.

Gamma rhythm or activity An EEG rhythm above >30–80 Hz (wave duration 12.5–33 ms).

Generalization Bilateral propagation of EEG activity from limited areas to all regions of the head.

Generalized Loosely: an EEG activity spread over all regions of the head, usually with a frontal, but rarely with an occipital, maximum. Strictly: bilateral EEG discharges appearing reasonably symmetrically and synchronously over homologous regions of the head. For example, generalized epileptic seizures are conceptualized as originating at some point within, and rapidly engaging (i.e., synchronizing), bilaterally distributed networks.

Generalized paroxysmal fast activity (GPFA) Bilateral synchronous bursts of spikes of 2–10 s duration, with frequency between 10 and 25 Hz (typically around 10 Hz) and maximum in the frontal regions that only occurs during sleep. GPFA is considered a feature of Lennox-Gastaut syndrome.

Generalized periodic discharges (GPDs) GPDs are generalized, synchronous, periodic or quasiperiodic complexes that occupy at least 50% of the record. They are high amplitude (typically >100 μV) and have duration of about 0.5 s, with an intervening background activity amplitude usually not more than 35 μV. The morphology of GPDs is variable and consists of sharp or spike and slow wave complexes, triphasic-like waves, and slow wave complexes. Repetition rate usually lies between 0.5 and 2.0 c/s.

Hertz (Hz) Unit of frequency. Synonym: cycles per second (c/s).

High frequency filter (or low pass filter) A circuit that reduces the sensitivity of the EEG signals to relatively high frequencies (for example, above 70 Hz). For each setting of the high frequency filter, this attenuation is expressed as percent reduction in signal amplitude at a given frequency, relative to frequencies unaffected by the filter, i.e., in the mid-frequency band of the signal. Synonym: low pass filter.

High frequency oscillations (HFOs) Transient bursts of EEG activity, spontaneous or evoked, with frequencies beyond 80 Hz. Divided into ripples (80–250 Hz) and fast ripples (250–500 Hz).

High pass filter Synonym: low frequency filter.

Hypersynchrony When describing EEG patterns that are attributed to increased synchronization of neuronal activity (for example, hypnagogic hypersynchrony).

Hyperventilation Deep and regular respiration performed for a period of several minutes. Used as an activation procedure.

Hypnagogic hypersynchrony A normal variant. Paroxysmal bursts of 3–5 c/s, high amplitude (75–350 μV) diffuse, but maximal fronto-central, sinusoidal activity occurring at the onset of sleep in normal infants and children, aged 3 months to 13 years (but typically 4–9 years).

Hypsarrhythmia Characteristic interictal EEG pattern typically, but not invariably, seen in infants with Infantile Spasms (West syndrome). Consists of diffuse very high amplitude (>300 μV) irregular slow waves interspersed with multiregional spikes and sharp waves over both hemispheres, usually with a highly disorganized and asynchronous appearance. It is most frequent during Non-REM sleep, followed by waking and arousal, and is absent or minimal during REM sleep.

Incidence Descriptor used to characterize how often a transient or isolated discharge is seen throughout the recording. Suggested ranges for describing this: ≥1/10 s are abundant, ≥1/min but less than 1/10 s are frequent, ≥1/h but less than 1/minute are occasional, and <1/h are rare.

Index Percent of time an EEG activity is present in an EEG sample. For example: alpha index, spike wave index, daily pattern index.

Infraslow activity EEG activity with frequencies in the EEG below 0.1 Hz.

In-phase signals Waves with no phase difference between them.

Input The signal fed into an EEG amplifier.

Input circuit System consisting of the EEG electrodes and intervening tissues, the electrode leads, jack box, input cable, and electrode selectors.

Input impedance Impedance that exists between the two inputs of an EEG amplifier. Measured in ohms (generally mega-ohms, MΩ) with or without the additional specification of input shunt capacitance (measured in picofarads, pF).

Input voltage Potential difference between the two input terminals of a differential EEG amplifier.

Inter-electrode distance Spacing between pairs of electrodes.

Interhemispheric derivation Recording between a pair of electrodes located on opposite sides of the head (for example, F3-F4).

Intermittent photic stimulation Delivery of intermittent flashes of light to the eyes of a subject. Used as EEG activation procedure.

Intermittent slow activity Slow EEG activity that occurs intermittently and is not caused by drowsiness (usually >100 μV). Intermittent slow activity varies by more than 50% or regresses completely between times of its appearance, and can be polymorphic, arrhythmic, or rhythmical.

Intracerebral electrode Various conducting devices for recording EEG from the surface or within the substance of the brain. Examples include epicortical/subdural, epidural, foramen ovale, and stereotactic [stereotaxic] implanted depth electrodes.

Irregular Applies to EEG waves and complexes of inconstant period and/or uneven contour or morphology.

Isoelectric (1) The record obtained from a pair of equipotential electrodes. (2) Use of term discouraged when describing record of electrocerebral inactivity.

Isolated Occurring singly.

K complex A normal graphoelement. A well delineated negative sharp wave followed by a positive component standing out from the background EEG, with total duration ≥0.5 s, usually maximal in amplitude when recorded from fronto-central derivations and often associated with a sleep spindle.

Lambda wave A normal graphoelement. Diphasic sharp transient occurring over the occipital regions of the head of awake subjects during visual exploration. The main component is positive relative to other areas. Time-locked to saccadic eye movements. Amplitude varies but is generally below 50 μV. Greek letter: λ (note morphology resembling the Greek capital letter lambda).

Laplacian montage Montage that consists of a mathematical transformation involving the second spatial derivative; the Laplacian source of the potential may be approximated by using the weighted average of all the neighboring electrodes as a reference for each site or electrode. This montage may be used for localization of focal abnormalities on digital EEG.

Lateralized Independently involving the right and/or left side of the head (or body).

Lateralized periodic discharges (LPDs) LPDs are unilateral surface negative discharges of spike, sharp or sharp slow-wave polyphasic morphology, usually lasting from 100 to 300 ms that typically recur at quasiperiodic intervals of up to 3/s. The incidence of clinical or electrographic seizures associated with LPDs is high, ranging from 50 to 100%, but there is debate as to whether they represent seizures proper. When contralateral motor movements are time-locked to LPDs they are considered to represent seizure patterns.

Longitudinal bipolar montage A montage consisting of contiguous channels of electrode pairs along longitudinal, mainly antero-posterior, arrays (for example, Fp1-F3, F3-C3, C3-P3, P3-O1).

Low frequency filter (high pass filter) A circuit that reduces the sensitivity of the EEG signal to relatively low frequencies (for example, below 0.5 Hz). For each position of the low frequency filter control, this attenuation is expressed as percent reduction of the signal at a given stated frequency, relative to frequencies unaffected by the filter, i.e., in the mid-frequency band of the channel.

Low voltage EEG A normal variant. Waking record characterized by activity of amplitude not greater than 20 μV over all head regions. With appropriate instrumental sensitivities this activity can be shown to be composed primarily of beta, theta, and, to a lesser degree, delta waves, with or without alpha activity over the posterior areas.

Low voltage fast activity Refers to fast activity (beta rhythm and above), often recruiting, which can be recorded at the onset of an ictal discharge, particularly in intra-cranial depth EEG recording of a seizure.

Magnetoencephalography (MEG) Recording of magnetic fields generated from the cortical neurons.

Monorhythmic delta activity A normal graphoelement in preterm infants (24–34 weeks of post menstrual age). Characterized by relatively stereotyped delta activity (up to 200 μV) predominantly over the posterior regions (occipital, temporal and central).

Montage The arrangement or array of channels on the EEG machine display, defined by the exploring and reference electrodes.

Morphology Refers to the form of EEG waves (i.e., their shape and physical characteristics).

Mu rhythm Rhythm at 7–11 Hz, composed of arch-shaped waves occurring over the central or centro-parietal regions of the scalp during wakefulness. Amplitude varies but is mostly below 50 μV. Blocked or attenuated most clearly by contralateral movement, thought of movement, readiness to move or tactile stimulation. Greek letter: μ.

Multifocal Three or more spatially separated independent foci.

Multiple spike-and-slow-wave complex Use of term discouraged. An epileptiform graphoelement consisting of two or more spikes associated with one or more slow waves.

Multiregional Three or more lobar foci.

Nasopharyngeal electrode Rod electrode introduced through the nose and placed against the nasopharyngeal wall with its tip lying near the body of the sphenoid bone.

Needle electrode Small needle inserted into the subdermal layer of the scalp.

Noise, EEG channel Small fluctuating output of an EEG channel recorded when high sensitivities are used, even if there is no input signal. Measured in microvolts (μV), referenced to the input.

Non-cephalic reference Reference electrode that is placed on body parts other than the head (for example, sternospinal reference).

Notch filter A filter that selectively attenuates a very narrow frequency band, thus producing a sharp notch in the frequency response of an EEG signal. Commonly applied to attenuate electrical noise from mains interference (the frequency of which differs between countries, 50 or 60 Hz), which may occur under unfavorable technical conditions.

Nyquist theorem Accurate digital representation of an EEG signal requires that the sampling rate is at least twice the highest frequency of the signal, i.e., a frequency component of 30 Hz requires at least a sampling rate of 60 Hz.

Occipital intermittent rhythmic delta activity (OIRDA) Fairly regular or approximately sinusoidal waves, mostly occurring in bursts at 2–3 Hz over the occipital areas of one or both sides of the head. Frequently blocked or attenuated by eye opening. An abnormal pattern seen in children's EEGs more frequently than adults, often but not exclusively in association with genetic generalized epilepsies.

Organization Degree to which the posterior dominant rhythm (PDR) conforms to certain characteristics displayed by a majority of subjects in the same age group, without personal or family history of neurologic and psychiatric diseases, or other illnesses that might be associated with dysfunction of the brain.

Out-of-phase signals Two waves of opposite phases.

Output voltage The voltage across the trace display of an EEG channel.

Paper speed Velocity of movement of paper through an analog EEG machine. Expressed in centimeters per second (cm/s) or millimeters per second (mm/s).

Paroxysm Graphoelement phenomenon with sudden onset, rapid attainment of a maximum, and abrupt termination; distinguished from background activity.

Paroxysmal fast Fast frequencies in the beta range or above occurring in trains.

Pattern Any characteristic regular or repetitive EEG activity of approximately constant period.

Peak Point of maximum amplitude of a wave.

Period Duration of complete cycle of individual graphoelement in a sequence of regularly repeated EEG waves or complexes.

Periodic Applies to: (1) EEG waves or complexes occurring in a sequence at an approximately regular rate, (2) EEG waves or complexes occurring intermittently at approximately regular intervals, generally of one to several seconds.

Periodic discharges (PDs) Repetition of a waveform with relatively uniform morphology and duration, with a quantifiable inter-discharge interval between consecutive waveforms, and recurrence of the waveform at nearly regular intervals. Comments: PDs may be generalized (GPDs), lateralized (LPDs), bilateral independent (BIPDs). Old nomenclature for these new terms are GPEDs (=GPDs), PLEDs (=LPDs) and BIPLEDs (=BIPDs). The use of "epileptiform" as an interpretative term is now avoided, since these periodic patterns may or may not be associated with clinical seizures [8].

Phase (1) Time or polarity relationships between a point on a wave displayed in a derivation and the identical point on the same wave recorded simultaneously in another derivation. (2) Time or angular relationships between a point on a wave and the onset of the cycle of the same wave. Usually expressed in degrees or radians.

Phase reversal Simultaneous trace deflections in opposite directions from two or more channels in a bipolar recording montage. Assuming a single generator, phase reversal is due to the same signal being applied to the input terminal 2 of one differential amplifier and to the input terminal 1 of the other amplifier.

Photic driving Physiologic response consisting of periodic activity elicited over the posterior regions of the head, usually induced by repetitive photic stimulation at frequencies of about 1–30 Hz.

Photic stimulation Delivery of intermittent flashes of light to the eyes of a subject, usually from 1 to 60 Hz. Used as EEG activation procedure.

Photomyogenic response A non-cerebral response to intermittent photic stimulation characterized by the appearance in the record of brief repetitive muscle spikes (electromyography artifact) over the anterior regions of the head. These often increase gradually in amplitude as stimuli are continued and cease promptly when the stimulus is withdrawn.

Photoparoxysmal response (PPR) Abnormal response to intermittent photic stimulation characterized by spike-and-slow-wave or polyspike-and-slow-wave complexes. Responses are subclassified into 4 phenotypically different types, from focal occipital spikes (type 1 PPR) time-locked to the flashes to generalized (type 4 PPR) epileptiform discharges, which may outlast the stimulus by a few seconds.

Polarity convention International agreement whereby differential EEG amplifiers are constructed so that negativity at input terminal 1 relative to input terminal 2 of the same amplifier results in an upward trace deflection.

Polarity, EEG wave Sign of potential difference, either positive or negative, existing at a given time between one electrode and another electrode; which may be an exploring and reference electrode in a referential derivation, or two exploring electrodes in a bipolar derivation.

Polygraphic recording Simultaneous monitoring of multiple physiological parameters such as the EEG, respiration, electrocardiogram, electromyogram, eye movements (electrooculogram), oxygen saturation, and leg movements.

Polymorphic activity Irregular EEG waves having multiple forms, which may also vary in frequency and amplitude.

Polyphasic wave Wave consisting of more than two phases developed on alternating sides of the baseline.

Polysomnography (PSG) Polygraphic recording of sleep including EEG, electrooculogram, electromyogram (chin and leg), airflow parameters, and oxygen saturation, along with video. A test used to diagnose sleep disorders.

Polyspike-and-slow-wave complex An epileptiform pattern consisting of two or more spikes associated with one or more slow waves.

Polyspike complex A sequence of two or more spikes.

Positive occipital sharp transient of sleep (POSTS) A normal graphoelement. Sharp transient maximal over the occipital regions, positive relative to other areas, apparently occurring spontaneously during sleep. May be single or repetitive. Amplitude varies but is generally below 50 μV.

Positive rolandic sharp waves (PRSW) Abnormal transients in neonatal period, surface positive, broad-based sharp waves with duration of <0.5 s, localized to central regions (C3/C4/Cz). Associated with white matter injury in preterm infants.

Posterior dominant rhythm (PDR) Rhythmic activity seen at the occipital or parietal regions predominantly during wakefulness while the eyes are kept closed.

Posterior slow waves of youth A normal graphoelement. Isolated slow waves intermixed with the posterior dominant rhythm in young people (typically 4–25 years of age).

Potential (1) Strictly: voltage. (2) Loosely: synonym of electrical activity (waveforms) generated by the nervous system.

Potential field Amplitude distribution of the negative and positive potentials of an EEG signal at the surface of the head, or cerebral cortex or in the depth of the brain, measured at a given instant in time. Represented in diagrams by color codes for negativity and positivity, and by equipotential lines.

Power Spectrum Display of the distribution of frequency-specific power (i.e., amplitude squared), with the waveform frequency plotted on the abscissa and the power plotted on the ordinate of a spectrogram display.

Premature temporal theta Normal graphoelement of preterm infants (24–34 weeks post menstrual age, highest incidence 29–31 weeks). Temporal sharp transients occurring in bursts of rhythmic sharp waves at 4–7 c/s (25–125 μV). Typically bilateral but often asynchronous

Prevalence Proportion of the record or a specified epoch that includes a particular EEG pattern. For example: ≥90% is continuous, 50–89% is abundant, 10–49% is frequent, 1–9% is occasional, and <1% is rare.

Propagation The active neural process whereby electric activity spreads from one area of the brain to another

Quantitative EEG (qEEG) Processing and analysis of portions of digitized EEG data, such as frequency-specific power typically derived by Fourier transform, displayed in various formats. Statistical variables can be compared, such as wave phase and coherence.

Quantity Amount of EEG activity with respect to number of transients or waves. For example, interictal epileptiform discharges: ≥1/10 s are abundant, ≥1/min but less than 1/10 s are frequent, ≥1/h but less than 1/min are occasional, and <1/h are rare.

Quasiperiodic Loosely: applies to EEG waves or complexes that occur at random intervals, which only approach regularity and that are not an exact repeating frequency. Strictly: determined by quantitative computer analysis and defined as having a cycle length (i.e., period) varying by 25–50% from one cycle to the next in the majority (>50%) of cycle pairs.

Reactivity A phenomena in which the EEG pattern clearly and reproducibly changes with sensory (visual, auditory, or noxious) stimulation. Changes may occur in frequency, morphology, and/or amplitude, including attenuation of activity after the stimulus.

Reference electrode (1) In general: any electrode against which the potential variations of another electrode are measured. (2) Specifically: a suitable reference electrode is historically connected to the input terminal 2 of an EEG amplifier and placed so as to minimize the likelihood of recording the same EEG activity as detected by an exploring electrode (connected to the input terminal 1 of the same amplifier), or of other activities.

Referential derivation Recording from a pair of electrodes consisting of an exploring electrode historically connected to the input terminal 1 and a reference electrode usually connected to the input terminal 2 of an EEG amplifier.

Referential montage A montage consisting of referential derivations.

Regional EEG activity that is limited to a region of the scalp overlying a lobe (i.e., frontal, temporal, parietal, occipital).

Regular Applies to waves or complexes of approximately constant period and relatively uniform appearance.

Rhythm EEG activity consisting of waves of approximately constant period.

Rhythmic Applied to regular waves occurring at a constant period and of relatively uniform morphology.

Rhythmic temporal theta A normal graphoelement in preterm infants (GA 24–34 weeks of post menstrual age, maximal 29–32 weeks). Consisting of brief theta bursts (4.5–6 c/s) over the temporal regions, typically symmetrical but not necessarily synchronous.

Rhythmic temporal theta burst of drowsiness A normal variant. Characteristic burst of 4–7 c/s waves whose morphology is frequently notched by faster waves, occurring over the temporal regions of the head during drowsiness, bilaterally or independently.

Rhythm of alpha frequency (1) In general: any rhythm in the alpha band. (2) Specifically: term should be used to designate those activities in the alpha band which differ from the alpha rhythm as regards their topography and/or reactivity and do not have specific appellations (such as mu rhythm and alpha coma).

Rolandic spikes Uni- or bilateral triphasic sharp waves in the centro-temporal area seen in childhood epilepsy with centro-temporal spikes. They often have a tangential (horizontal) dipole oriented with negativity in centro-temporal/parietal areas and positivity in the frontal region, and increase during sleep with a tendency to appear in series.

Sampling rate Frequency in Hz used for sampling the digital EEG. Sampling rates in the 250–500 Hz range are common. Higher sampling rates may be appropriate for specific applications, for example, 1000–2000 Hz in intra-cranial depth EEG.

Sawtooth (saw-tooth) waves Brief runs of rhythmic sharp waves of 4–7 c/s, often of quite high amplitude (up to 125 μV).

Secondary bilateral synchrony Spreading by propagation of an initially focal or regional epileptiform discharge to become generalized.

Seizure pattern, EEG Phenomenon consisting of repetitive epileptiform EEG discharges at >2 c/s and/or characteristic pattern with quasi-rhythmic spatio-temporal evolution (i.e., gradual change in frequency, amplitude, morphology, and location), lasting at least several seconds (usually >10 s). Two other short duration (<10 s) EEG seizure patterns are: electrodecrement and low voltage fast activity seen during clinically apparent epileptic seizures. Frequent interictal epileptiform discharges are usually not associated with clinical seizures and thus should be differentiated from EEG seizure patterns.

Sensitivity Ratio of input voltage to output trace deflection in an EEG channel. Sensitivity is measured in microvolts per millimeter (μV/mm). Example: Sensitivity = input voltage/output trace deflection = 50 μV/10 mm = 5 μV/mm

Sharp wave An epileptiform transient clearly distinguished from the background activity, although amplitude varies. A pointed peak at a conventional time scale and duration of 70–200 ms, usually with a steeper ascending phase when compared to the descending phase. Main component is generally negative relative to other areas, and may be followed by slow wave of the same polarity.

Sharp-and-slow-wave complex An epileptiform pattern consisting of a sharp wave and an associated following slow wave, clearly distinguished from background activity. May be single or multiple.

Sinusoidal Term applies to EEG waves resembling sine waves.

Six Hz spike-and-slow-wave Spike-and-slow-wave complexes at 4–7 c/s, but mostly at 6 c/s occurring generally in brief bursts bilaterally and synchronously, symmetrically or asymmetrically, and either confined to or of larger amplitude over the posterior or anterior regions of the head. Amplitude varies but is generally smaller than that of spike-and-slow-wave complexes repeating at slower rates.

Sleep spindle A normal graphoelement. Train of distinct waves with frequency at 11–16 Hz (most commonly at 12–14 Hz) with a duration ≥0.5 s. Generally higher amplitude over the central regions of the head, occurring during sleep. Amplitude varies but is maximal using central derivations.

Sleep stages Distinctive phases of sleep best demonstrated by polygraphic recordings of the EEG and other variables, including at least eye movements and activity of certain voluntary muscles.

Slow activity Any activity of frequency less than alpha rhythm, i.e., theta and delta bands.

Slow alpha variant rhythms A normal variant. Rhythms mostly at 4–5 Hz, recorded over the posterior regions of the head, that behave like the posterior dominant rhythm in response to activation (i.e., are blocked or attenuated by attention, especially eye opening and mental effort). Generally alternate, or are intermixed, with the alpha rhythm to which they often are harmonically related. They may have a notched morphology but are not generally considered abnormal. Amplitude varies but is frequently close to 50 μV.

Slow wave Wave with duration longer than alpha waves, i.e., over 1/8 s (>125 ms).

Small sharp spikes (SSS) A normal variant. Small sharp spikes of very short duration (<50 ms) and low amplitude (<50 μV), often followed by a small theta wave, occurring in the temporal regions during drowsiness and light sleep.

Somatosensory evoked potential (SEP) Evoked potential in response to somatosensory stimulus, usually electrical stimulation of a sensory or mixed nerve.

Sphenoidal electrode Strictly needle or wire electrode inserted through the soft tissues of the face below the zygomatic arch so that its tip lies near the base of the skull in the region of the foramen ovale, designed to record from the medial temporal lobe structures.

Spike A transient, clearly distinguished from background activity, with pointed peak at a conventional time scale and duration from 20 to less than 70 ms. Amplitude varies but typically >50 μV. Main component is generally negative relative to other areas.

Spike-and-slow-wave complex An epileptiform pattern consisting of a spike and an associated following slow wave, clearly distinguished from background activity. May be single or multiple.

Spindle Group of rhythmic waves characterized by a progressively increasing, then gradually decreasing, amplitude.

Stereotactic (stereotaxic) electroencephalogram (SEEG) Intracerebral EEG recordings using electrodes implanted stereotactically, thus permitting the calculation of electrode coordinates that can be projected on a stereotactic brain atlas or magnetic resonance images to create three-dimensional pictures.

Stimulus-induced rhythmic, periodic, or ictal discharges (SIRPIDs) Sharp transients that are rhythmic, periodic, or ictal appearing discharges in comatose patients that are consistently induced by alerting stimuli including: auditory and other sensory stimulation, such as noxious (airway suctioning) and other patient-care activities. SIRPIDs may be regional or lateralized, bilateral or generalized, and of variable duration. Their pathophysiology and clinical significance is uncertain, but on occasions may be associated with clinical seizures.

Subclinical rhythmic discharges of adults (SREDA) This paroxysmal pattern is usually seen in the adult age group (typically over 50 years) and consists of a mixture of frequencies, often predominantly in the theta range, lasting 40–80 s. It may resemble a seizure discharge but is not accompanied by any clinical signs or symptoms. The significance of this pattern is uncertain, but it should be distinguished from an epileptiform seizure pattern.

Suppression Entirety of an EEG record showing activity below 10 μV (reference derivation).

Symmetry Approximately equal amplitude, frequency and form of EEG activities over homologous areas on opposite sides of the head.

Synchrony The simultaneous occurrence of EEG waves over distinct regions on the same or opposite sides of the head with the same speed and phase.

Temporal intermittent rhythmic delta activity (TIRDA) An EEG pattern characterized by short trains of intermittent and rhythmic delta activity (1–3.5 Hz), often with sawtooth morphology, recorded predominantly over the anterior temporal regions. TIRDA usually occurs during drowsiness and light sleep and may either be unilateral or bilateral, occurring independently. It is associated with temporal lobe epilepsy, and when unilateral is virtually indicative of ipsilateral pathology.

Temporal slow activity of the elderly Pattern of uncertain significance but usually not considered abnormal. Unilateral (most often on the left side) or bilateral, short runs of theta or delta activity intermixed with the background activity over the temporal region(s), in subjects >50 years of age, without clinical abnormalities. Often accentuates during drowsiness and hyperventilation.

Ten-ten (10–10) system System of standardized scalp electrode placement. According to this system, additional scalp electrodes are placed at half distance between the standard electrodes of the ten-twenty system, i.e., 10 percentile increments of the reference curve.

Ten-twenty (10–20) system System of standardized scalp electrode placement recommended by the International Federation of Clinical Neurophysiology. According to this system, the placement of electrodes is determined by measuring the head from 4 external landmarks and taking 10 or 20 percentiles of these measurements.

Theta band Frequency band from 4 to <8 Hz. Greek letter: θ.

Theta rhythm Rhythm with a frequency of 4–<8 Hz.

Theta wave Wave with duration of 1/4 to over 1/8 s (125–250 ms).

Three Hz or three per second spike-and-slow-wave complex Characteristic ictal paroxysmal pattern consisting of a regular sequence of spike-and-slow-wave complexes which: (1) repeat at around 3–3.5 c/s (measured during the first few seconds of the paroxysm), (2) are bilaterally synchronous in their onset and termination (i.e., "generalized"), and usually of maximal amplitude over the frontal areas, and (3) remain approximately synchronous and symmetrical on the two sides of the head throughout the paroxysmal burst. Amplitude varies but can reach values of 1000 μV (1 mV). Characteristic seizure pattern associated with Childhood Absence Epilepsy.

Time constant (TC) Historically the product of the values of the resistance (in mega-ohms, MΩ) and the capacitance (in microfarads, μF) which make up the time constant control of an EEG channel. This product represents the time required for the trace to fall to 37% of the deflection initially produced when a DC voltage difference is applied to the input terminals of the amplifier. Expressed in seconds (s).

Tracé alternant Neonatal EEG pattern of quiet (non-REM) sleep seen in term and near term infants from 34 to 36 weeks post menstrual age onwards, which may persist up to 4 weeks after birth. It is characterized by high amplitude bursts of predominantly slow waves (50–150 μV) alternating with periods of relatively low amplitude activity mixed activities (25–50 μV).

Tracé continu Continuous background activity, consisting of theta and/or delta frequencies (>25 μV), replacing a previously markedly intermittent record during evolution of EEG in preterm infants. Present in active sleep.

Tracé discontinu Normal discontinuous pattern in preterm infants which is characterized by bursts of high amplitude (up to 300 μV) mixed frequency activity regularly interrupted by low amplitude interburst activity (<25 μV). The pattern can still be called discontinuous if there is a modest amount of EEG activity in a single channel or a single transient in multiple channels. The interburst interval depends on the post menstrual age (PMA). It is seen in wakefulness, active and quiet sleep until 30 weeks PMA, then only in quiet sleep, and is rarely seen in infants of 38 weeks PMA.

Transient, EEG Any isolated wave or complex, distinguished from background activity.

Transverse bipolar montage A montage consisting of contiguous channels of electrode pairs along transverse/coronal (i.e., side-to-side) arrays (for example, F7-F3, F3-Fz, Fz-F4, F4-F8).

Triphasic wave (TW) High amplitude (over 70 μV) positive sharp transients (with respect to common average), which are preceded and followed by relatively low amplitude negative waves. The first negative wave generally has lower amplitude than the negative afterwave, and has a steeper slope, which on occasions may be sharp. Usually bilateral with an antero-posterior or a postero-anterior lag, and repetition rate of about 1–<2 c/s. TWs occur typically in runs, and can either regress or increase with arousal or noxious stimuli. Often there is little ongoing or low amplitude (<40 μV) slow background activity between TWs.

Unilateral Confined to one side of the head (or body).

Vertex sharp transient or vertex sharp wave (V wave) A normal graphoelement. Sharply contoured wave with duration <0.5 s, maximal at the vertex, negative relative to other areas, apparently occurring spontaneously during light sleep or in response to a sensory stimulus (usually auditory). Vertex sharp waves may be single or repetitive. Amplitude varies but rarely exceeds 250 μV.

Voltage The difference in electric potential between two points (units: volts).

Volume conduction The passive process by which electrical activity, originating from a generator, spreads through a conductive medium to be detected quite widely by distant (i.e., far-field) recording electrodes, without being mediated by neural activity.

Wave Any change of the potential difference between pairs of electrodes in EEG recording, which may arise in the brain (an EEG wave) or outside of it (i.e., extracerebral potential).

Waveform (wave form) The shape or morphology of an EEG wave.

Wicket spikes or wicket waves Spike-like monophasic surface negative single waves or trains of waves occurring over the temporal regions, typically unilateral, during drowsiness that have an arcuate or mu-like appearance. These are mainly seen in older individuals and represent a benign physiological variant, but may also be seen in patients with a clinical diagnosis of epilepsy.

EEG Reporting

The EEG report should include three main sections: (1) introduction, (2) EEG description, and (3) interpretation, the latter including (a) a judgement on the normality of EEG findings or the degree of abnormality (impression), and (b) correlations with the clinical picture (clinical correlation).

Introduction

This section of the report should include:

History

- Reasons for referral
- Relevant medical and neurological history
- Acute or chronic intake of CNS drugs
- Neuroimaging results
- Note of any previous cranial operations

Technical description

- EEG type (e.g., standard EEG, sleep EEG)
- Technical features (electrode array, EEG duration)
- Patient's level of vigilance and consciousness

EEG Description

The description section should include all the EEG findings, both normal and abnormal, reported in the most objective way possible, avoiding any judgement on their meaning.

The aim is to produce a complete and objective report, to allow other electroencephalographers to draw conclusions on the normality or the degree of abnormality of the EEG on the basis of the written report, ideally without even the need to look at the EEG tracing.

The EEG report should start by describing the background activity should be described, starting from the posterior dominant rhythm. Following features should be reported:

- Frequency (Hz)
- Quantity (persistent or intermittent)
- Localization
- Amplitude (μV)
- Symmetry/asymmetry
- Rhythmicity
- Irregularity

Other nondominant rhythms should be described according to the features reported above.

The reactivity of the EEG upon eye opening-closing or other types of stimulation should be reported, and limb movements or other sources of artifacts should be noticed. When the tracing shows a marked interhemispheric asymmetry, the EEG characteristics of each hemisphere should be described separately.

Any abnormality should be described specifying:

- Morphology (spike, sharp wave, slow wave, etc.)
- Distribution (diffuse or focal)
- Localization
- Symmetry
- Synchrony (Intra and interhemispheric)
- Amplitude
- Timing (Continuous, intermittent, episodic, paroxysmal, etc.)
- Quantity.

The report of the EEG recorded under basal conditions should be followed by the description of EEG during routine activation tests (photostimulation, hyperventilation), specifying the degree of patient's cooperation. The effects of photostimulation and hyperventilation should be described by reporting both normal and abnormal responses. If hyperventilation and/or photostimulation are not performed, the reasons should be mentioned (for example, tests not required for medical reasons or not performed due to lack of collaboration).

The lack of physiological patterns characteristic of wakefulness and/or sleep should be specified, avoiding phrases such as "absence of focal abnormalities" or "absence of epileptic abnormalities" (which should be included in the interpretation section).

The artifacts should be mentioned only when they are debatable (i.e., when there is the doubt that they represent an

O. Mecarelli (ed.), *Clinical Electroencephalography*, https://doi.org/10.1007/978-3-030-04573-9

underlying brain activity), when they are unusual or interfere with the interpretation of the tracing, or when they provide clues to the diagnosis (e.g., myokymia, nystagmus).

Interpretation

The interpretation section should appear at the end of the report and should include the overall impression and the clinical correlation.

Impression

The electroencephalographer should provide a judgement (impression) on the normality or abnormality of the tracing.

While the EEG description is mainly written for the electroencephalographer (who will use it for subsequent comparisons) or for other experts (and therefore should be detailed and objective), the impression (or interpretation) is written primarily for the referring physician, and should therefore be as succinct and readily understandable as possible. Many clinicians are aware that they would not get much additional information by reading the detailed description of the report. If the conclusion it is too long and without explicit correlation to the clinical picture, the whole report in its entirety may appear scarcely useful for the referring physician.

If the EEG is considered abnormal, the degree of abnormality should be scored to facilitate comparison with subsequent tracings. Since this part of the report is largely subjective, the grading will vary from one laboratory to another, but the different degrees should be defined appropriately and the definitions should be used consistently.

After commenting on the normality or degree of abnormality of the EEG tracing, the reasons that led to the conclusion should be briefly reported. When different types of abnormalities have been found, only the most salient should be listed (preferably no more than three or four, otherwise the risk is that the most relevant ones are not adequately emphasized). Confusing and technical terminology should be avoided, and only terms understandable to clinicians of any level of expertise or specialty should be used. If previous EEG tracings are available, a comparison with previous reports should always be included.

Clinical Correlation

The clinical correlation represents the attempt to explain how the EEG tracing relates to the clinical picture and to the reason for referral. The referring physician may not be familiar enough with EEG; hence, a detailed, clear, and accurate terminology readily understandable to clinicians of any level of expertise or specialty should be used.

An abnormal EEG is indicative of cerebral dysfunction. However, the term "cerebral dysfunction" should be used only when abnormalities are relevant and when there is sufficient clinical information to draw conclusions based on the clinical context. Alternatively, a conclusion such as "tracing shows minimal irregularities in brain function" might be more appropriate.

Some types of EEG patterns may be more or less suggestive of specific clinical conditions (e.g., focal delta waves could indicate a structural injury; some types of spikes or sharp waves could suggest a potential epileptogenic focus).

On the other hand, EEG anomalies can be consistent with the clinical information, pointing to the presence of a particular clinical condition: in these cases it can be concluded that the EEG is consistent with or supports the clinical diagnosis.

In the EEG report, the term "compatible with" is used very frequently. However, strictly speaking, each EEG is compatible with virtually any type of clinical condition, so the term is not helpful and should not be used.

In cases where the EEG is strongly suggestive of a given clinical condition, which was not mentioned in the patient's clinical history, it is more prudent to state that the abnormalities detected in the EEG are frequently found in association with some clinical conditions, but they don't necessarily indicate their presence.

An EEG can be defined as diagnostic of a given clinical condition only in the rare cases when clinical episodes occur during the recording and the EEG itself shows electrical abnormalities typically associated with those specific clinical manifestations (for example: a child with abrupt onset of altered awareness concomitant with a generalized discharge of 3 Hz, bilateral and synchronous spike-wave complexes).

In situations where the diagnostic suspicion is inconsistent with the EEG findings, the report should cautiously provide some of the possible reasons for the apparent discrepancy, avoiding any overt criticism of the clinical diagnosis.

If the EEG abnormalities could be partly or entirely attributed to drug therapy or other treatments, this should be clearly stated.

The electroencephalographer should not suggest any changes to the pharmacological treatment or to the clinical approach, but may recommend performing further EEG tracings with additional procedures (for instance: "Depending on the clinical picture, a sleep EEG recording may be useful," or "Since the recording was made immediately after a seizure, a subsequent EEG might be useful to determine if the focal slow waves shown in the tracing is permanent or transitory").

No further explanations are usually required for a normal EEG. However, when the clinical information pose serious doubts between two conditions (for example: psychogenic non-epileptic seizures versus epileptic seizures), it might be appropriate to add a sentence to avoid a misdiagnosis (e.g., "a normal EEG pattern does not exclude the presence of epilepsy. If possible, an EEG recording with provocation methods should be obtained.").

The digitization of EEG recording, reporting, and report transmission often makes it possible to incorporate small samples of the tracing: in this case it is advisable to include selected pages that clearly illustrate the abnormalities described.

The Standardized Computer-Based Organized Reporting of EEG (SCORE)

The best way of reporting an EEG has always been a matter of discussion and a difficult issue. Obviously, adopting a universally accepted glossary represents the first fundamental requirement.

Over the years, several guidelines and recommendations on EEG reporting have been proposed by different scientific societies.

Recently, a standardized computer-based organized reporting of EEG (SCORE) has been developed under the auspices of the International Federation of Clinical Neurophysiology (IFCN) and the International League Against Epilepsy (ILAE) [9, 10].

The SCORE-EEG software can be downloaded for free at following link: http://holbergeeg.com.

The SCORE reporting system, which represents the results of a broad international consensus, is gaining popularity and is increasingly used in several centers worldwide. The IFCN itself has recently proposed an updated report format of the EEG findings, which follows the overall outline and content of SCORE system. Furthermore, the main sections of SCORE (Patient information; Patient referral; Recording conditions; Findings; Diagnostic Significance; and Clinical Comments) correspond to the standard EEG report format of the American Clinical Neurophysiology Society (History; Technical Description; EEG description; Impression; Clinical correlation) [5]. Hence, thanks to its structure and terminology, SCORE represents the single most comprehensive, updated, systematic, and widely accepted EEG report format. Although its inter-rater agreement still needs to be studied, SCORE is a useful tool for EEG reporting and epilepsy monitoring, facilitating communication among different laboratories worldwide.

Details of this computer-based EEG reporting system [7, 9, 10] are summarized and reported below (excerpts have been reproduced with permission from: [7, 9, 10]). Ideally, the electroencephalographer should initially analyze the EEG blinded to clinical data to prevent bias. After EEG description has been completed, it should be evaluated taking into account the whole clinical context to provide a conclusion on the diagnostic significance of the recording.

1. Patient's personal data:
   (a) ***Personal identity number (ID), first and last name, gender, and date of birth*** [obligatory]
   (b) ***Patient's address, handedness, and other personal details*** [optional]
   (c) ***Gestational age*** (for newborns and patients <1 year) [optional]
2. Referral information:
   (a) ***Referring unit/physician*** (name and address)
   (b) ***Clinical question/reason(s) for referral***:
      - Epilepsy-related indications
      - Other differential diagnostic questions
      - Specific pediatric indications
      - Follow-up EEG
      - Assessment of prognosis
      - Research project
      - Other indication (specify)
   (c) ***Diagnosis at referral*** (reported according to the International Classification of Diseases, 10th Edition [ICD-10] list and rare diseases orphaned codes [11]), including neurological condition
   (d) ***Seizure frequency***
   (e) ***Time elapsed since the last seizure***
   (f) ***Current medication*** (particularly CNS drugs)
   (g) ***Neuroimaging*** (Computed Tomography and/or Magnetic Resonance Imaging) ***and functional neuroimaging results*** (normal/abnormal/not performed/results not known)
   (h) ***Additional details on patient history*** (e.g., cognitive impairment due to mental retardation or dementia)
   (i) ***Previous EEG results*** (if available)
3. Recording conditions:
   (a) Administrative data:
      - ***Study identification number***
      - ***Date and time of EEG recording***
      - ***Duration of the EEG recording***
      - ***Names of technologist and physician***
   (b) Technical data:
      - ***EEG Electrode array***, reporting according to Seeck et al. [12] (specify also polygraphic channels, if used)
      - ***EEG type:***
        - Standard
        - Sleep EEG
        - Short-term video-EEG monitoring
        - Long-term video-EEG monitoring

  - Ambulatory recording
  - Long-term video-EEG monitoring
  - Recording in the Intensive Care Unit
  - Intraoperative monitoring
- ***Level of patient's consciousness and vigilance*** (including cooperation):
  - Awake
  - Oriented
  - Good cooperation
  - Poor cooperation
  - Disoriented
  - Drowsy
  - Asleep
  - Unresponsive
  - Comatose
- ***Skull defect or previous brain surgery*** (specify location)
- ***Provocation methods/modulators*** (possibility of specifying how and whether EEG abnormalities are influenced by modulators and procedures):
  - Manual eye closure/opening
  - Hyperventilation (scored as: excellent effort, good effort, poor effort, refused the procedure, unable to do the procedure)
  - Intermittent photic stimulation
  - External sensory stimulation (e.g., auditory or nociceptive)
  - Cognitive tasks
  - Physical effort
  - Sleep deprivation
  - Sleep (natural/induced/after sleep deprivation)
  - Awakening
  - Medication given/withdrawn/reduced during the EEG recording

4. EEG description (Findings)
   - ***Background activity*** (posterior dominant rhythm, mu rhythm, other organized rhythms, each reported according to frequency, amplitude, location, effect of modulators, and clinical significance)
   - ***Background activity of critically ill patients*** (continuous/nearly continuous/discontinuous background activity; burst suppression; burst attenuation; EEG suppression and electrocerebral inactivity)
   - ***Neonatal ongoing activity*** (Table 1)
   - ***Sleep*** (with indications of achieved stages: drowsiness; N1-3; REM). Type and location normal sleep graphoelements can be reported. Clinical significance of any abnormally asymmetrical or absent sleep graphoelement. Presence and name of other sleep patterns such as sleep-onset REM period
   - ***Interictal findings*** They include epileptiform interictal activity, abnormal interictal rhythmic activity, and special patterns (e.g., periodic discharges, burst suppression, burst attenuation)

     For each type of observed interictal pattern, describe the following features:
     - *Morphology:* specify the type of epileptiform activity using the nomenclature from the glossary; for rhythmic or periodic patterns in critically ill patients refer to [8]
     - *Location*: laterality (left, right, midline, bilateral, diffuse) and region (frontal, central, temporal, parietal, occipital)
     - *Propagation* (if any): specify the location of the onset region and the location of the propagation)
     - *Time-related features*: mode of appearance (random/periodic/variable); discharge pattern (e.g., single discharges or in trains/burst); incidence (for single discharges); prevalence (for trains/bursts)
     - *Influence of modulators* (unmodified, increased, decreased, stopped by, triggered by/only during the modulator; changes during sleep; influence of intermittent photic stimulation)
   - ***Clinical episodes*** (for both the ictal and postictal phase):
     - *Name:* epileptic seizure (semiology described according to Blume et al. [13] and named using the current ILAE seizure classification Fisher et al. [14]; psychogenic non-epileptic seizure; electroencephalographic seizure; sleep-related episodes; pediatric episodes; paroxysmal motor events; syncope; other (specify)
     - *Semiology* (reported according to Blume et al. [13])
     - *Ictal EEG activity*: name of ictal pattern; location; source analysis (if done); frequency and amplitude of ictal patterns
     - *Postictal patterns*
     - *Timing and context:* level of consciousness; awareness of the episode; clinical-EEG temporal relationship (clinical start followed by EEG or reverse); number of stereotypical episodes during the EEG recording; state at the start of the episode (from awake or from sleep); duration of the episode; duration of the postictal phase; presence/absence of prodrome; presence/absence of tongue biting
     - *Effect of modulators and procedures* (e.g., clinical and EEG effect of a given medication)
   - ***Transient patterns and rhythmic activity*** (only for neonatal EEG report): name; location; time-related features; clinical significance
   - ***Physiologic patterns and patterns of uncertain significance:*** names and localization
   - ***Artifacts:*** name and type (biological/nonbiological); localization; consequence on diagnostic value of recording

Table 1 Properties scored for the neonatal ongoing activity

Continuity	Normal continuity Normal discontinuity (insert values for burst duration and suppression duration) Tracé alternant (only for "asleep" and >30 weeks) (insert values for burst duration and suppression duration) Excessive background discontinuity (insert values for burst duration and suppression duration) Burst-suppression (only for >30 weeks) (insert values for burst duration and suppression duration) Electrocerebral inactivity
Synchrony	Mostly synchronous Mostly asynchronous
Variability (lability)	No Yes Unclear
Reactivity	No Yes Unclear
Amplitude	Normal Borderline low Borderline high Abnormal low Abnormal high
Significance	Considered normal for age No definite abnormality Considered not normal for age

Reproduced from [9], with permission

- ***Polygraphic channels***: type of channel (e.g., EOG, ECG, EMG, respiration, others) and clinical significance of observed changes
- ***Trend analysis***: results of amplitude-integrated EEG analysis (if done)

5. Diagnostic significance
   EEG findings interpreted in the clinical context.
   They may be categorized as follows:
   - ***Normal EEG recording***
   - ***Abnormal recording***
   - EEG findings in keeping with:
     - Epilepsy (specify which type, according to Scheffer et al. [15])
     - Status epilepticus (classified according to Trinka et al. [16])
     - Psychogenic non-epileptic seizures
     - Other non-epileptic clinical episode
     - Focal CNS dysfunction
     - Diffuse CNS dysfunction
     - Continuous spikes and waves during slow sleep or electrical status epilepticus in sleep
     - Coma
     - Brain death
     - EEG abnormality of uncertain clinical significance
   - ***No definite abnormality***
     - EEG changes since the last (previous) EEG (no change/improved/worsened)
6. Clinical comments
   - Answers to specific questions posed in referral
   - Suggestion of additional investigations

References

1. O'Leary JL, Knott JR. Some minimum essentials for clinical electroencephalographers. Electroencephalogr Clin Neurophysiol. 1955;7(2):293–8.
2. Chatrian GE, Bergamini L, Dondey M, Klass DW, Lennox-Buchthal M, Petersen I. A glossary of terms most commonly used by clinical electroencephalographers. Electroenceph clin Neurophysiol. 1974;37:538–48.
3. American Electroencephalographic Society. Syllabus for clinical electroencphalographers. J Clin Neurophysiol. 1994;11:133–42.
4. Epstein CM, Bej MD, Foldvary-Schaefer N, Lagerlund TD, Helmers SL, Husain AM, American Clinical Neurophysiology Society. Guideline 7: Guidelines for writing EEG reports. J Clin Neurophysiol. 2006;23:118–21.
5. Tatum WO, Selioutski O, Ochoa JG, Munger Clary H, Cheek J, Drislane F, et al. American clinical neurophysiology society guideline 7: guidelines for EEG reporting. J Clin Neurophysiol. 2016;33:328–32.
6. Noachtar S, Binnie C, Ebersole J, Mauguière F, Sakamoto A, Westmoreland B. A glossary of terms most commonly used by clinical electroencephalographers and proposal for the report form for the EEG findings. Guidelines of the International Federation of Clinical Neurophysiology. Clin Neurophysiol. 1999;52:21–41.
7. Kane N, Acharya J, Benickzy S, Caboclo L, Finnigan S, Kaplan PW, Shibasaki H, Pressler R, van Putten MJAM. A revised glossary of terms most commonly used by clinical electroencephalographers and updated proposal for the report format of the EEG findings: Revision 2017. Clin Neurophysiol Pract. 2017;2:170–85.
8. Hirsch LJ, LaRoche SM, Gaspard N, Gerard E, Svoronos A, Herman ST, et al. American clinical neurophysiology society's standardized critical care EEG terminology: 2012 version. J Clin Neurophysiol. 2013;30:1–27.
9. Beniczky S, Aurlien H, Brøgger JC, Hirsch LJ, Schomer DL, Trinka E, Pressler RM, Wennberg R, Visser GH, Eisermann M, Diehl B, Lesser RP, Kaplan PW, Nguyen The Tich S, Lee JW,

Martins-da-Silva A, Stefan H, Neufeld M, Rubboli G, Fabricius M, Gardella E, Terney D, Meritam P, Eichele T, Asano E, Cox F, van Emde Boas W, Mameniskiene R, Marusic P, Zárubová J, Schmitt FC, Rosén I, Fuglsang-Frederiksen A, Ikeda A, MacDonald DB, Terada K, Ugawa Y, Zhou D, Herman ST. Standardized computer-based organized reporting of EEG: SCORE—second version. Clin Neurophysiol. 2017;128(11):2334–46.

10. Beniczky S, Aurlien H, Brøgger JC, Fuglsang-Frederiksen A, Martins-da-Silva A, Trinka E, Visser G, Rubboli G, Hjalgrim H, Stefan H, Rosén I, Zarubova J, Dobesberger J, Alving J, Andersen KV, Fabricius M, Atkins MD, Neufeld M, Plouin P, Marusic P, Pressler R, Mameniskiene R, Hopfengärtner R, van Emde Boas W, Wolf P. Standardized computer-based organized reporting of EEG: SCORE. Epilepsia. 2013;54(6):1112–24.
11. Orphanet: an online rare disease and orphan drug data base. © INSERM. 1997. http://www.orpha.net
12. Seeck M, Koessler L, Bast T, Leijten F, Michel C, He B, et al. The standardized EEG electrode array of the IFCN. Clin Neurophysiol. 2017;128:2070–7.
13. Blume WT, Lüders HO, Mizrahi E, Tassinari C, van Emde Boas W, Jerome E. Glossary of descriptive terminology for ictal semiology: report of the ILAE task force on classification and terminology. Epilepsia. 2001;42:1212–8.
14. Fisher RS, Cross JH, French JA, Higurashi N, Hirsch E, Jansen FE, Lagae L, Moshé SL, Peltola J, Roulet Perez E, Scheffer IE, Zuberi SM. Operational classification of seizure types by the International League Against Epilepsy: Position Paper of the ILAE Commission for Classification and Terminology. Epilepsia. 2017 Apr;58(4):522–30.
15. Scheffer IE, Berkovic S, Capovilla G, Connolly MB, French J, Guilhoto L, et al. ILAE classification of the epilepsies: position paper of the ILAE commission for classification and terminology. Epilepsia. 2017;58:512–21.
16. Trinka E, Cock H, Hesdorffer D, Rossetti AO, Scheffer IE, Shinnar S, et al. A definition and classification of status epilepticus–report of the ILAE task force on classification of status epilepticus. Epilepsia. 2015;56:1515–23.

MIX
Papier aus verantwortungsvollen Quellen
Paper from responsible sources
FSC® C105338

FSC
www.fsc.org

If you have any concerns about our products,
you can contact us on
ProductSafety@springernature.com

In case Publisher is established outside the EU,
the EU authorized representative is:
Springer Nature Customer Service Center GmbH
Europaplatz 3, 69115 Heidelberg, Germany

Printed by Libri Plureos GmbH
in Hamburg, Germany